Scleroderma

Yannick Allanore • John Varga
Christopher P. Denton • Masataka Kuwana
Lorinda Chung • Ami A. Shah
Editors

Scleroderma

From Pathogenesis to Comprehensive Management

Third Edition

Springer

Editors

Yannick Allanore
INSERMU1016, Université Paris Cité,
Service de Rhumatologie, Hôpital Cochin,
Paris, France

John Varga
Department of Internal Medicine
University of Michigan–Ann Arbor
Ann Arbor, MI, USA

Christopher P. Denton
Centre for Rheumatology
University College London, Royal Free Campus
London, UK

Masataka Kuwana
Department of Allergy and Rheumatology
Nippon Medical School
Tokyo, Tokyo, Japan

Lorinda Chung
Department of Medicine and Dermatology
Division of Rheumatology
Stanford University School of Medicine
Palo Alto, CA, USA

Ami A. Shah
Division of Rheumatology
Johns Hopkins University School of Medicine
Baltimore, MD, USA

ISBN 978-3-031-40657-7 ISBN 978-3-031-40658-4 (eBook)
https://doi.org/10.1007/978-3-031-40658-4

This Springer imprint is published by the registered company Springer Nature Switzerland AG
The registered company address is: Gewerbestrasse 11, 6330 Cham, Switzerland

Paper in this product is recyclable.

I am very grateful to my mentors and senior colleagues for their support and guidance in the right path. I express my special thanks to all EUSTAR network members for commitment and stimulating interactions. I thank the patients who gave me their confidence and also inspired my work.

—Yannick Allanore

I gratefully acknowledge Julie, Peter, and Andrew Varga for their unfailing support, patience, and love; my parents who serve as my role models; and the patients I have been privileged to care for, learn from, and be inspired by.

—John Varga

I am indebted to my family and friends for their unwavering support, and gratefully acknowledge the many senior colleagues and mentors that have inspired and guided me, personally and professionally, including Carol Black, Benoit de Crombrugghe, and Jeremy Pearson.

—Christopher P. Denton

I am grateful to the many senior colleagues and mentors who have guided me in science and medicine, and to the patients who have given me motivation and great ideas.

—Masataka Kuwana

I am incredibly grateful to my oldest sister, Delphine, who has suffered from systemic sclerosis for many years, and has served as my inspiration and driving force to search for a cure for this disease. I would also like to acknowledge my parents (Danny and Jenny), my two other sisters (Karine and Alice), my precious children (Reese and Tatum), and my husband (Mike) for their unconditional love and support. Finally I would like to thank my patients who teach me and partner with me to better understand this disease.

—Lorinda Chung

I am deeply grateful to Aalok, Aadarsh, and Aanavi Shah and my parents, Shreenivas and Kokila Vasanawala, for their unwavering love and support; my brother, Shreyas, for being my first scientific teacher; Antony Rosen and Fredrick Wigley for years of selfless mentorship; and my patients who inspire me and teach me every day.

—Ami A. Shah

Foreword

Scleroderma research, funded by the NIH and other agencies, has led to important advances in understanding the disease. Researchers continue to discover new insights about the vascular defects, inflammation, and fibrosis that are hallmarks of scleroderma. Investigations have revealed molecules that may help to identify, and improve screening and guide treatment for, scleroderma patients who may be at increased risk for serious disease manifestations, such as lung disease, pulmonary hypertension or cancer. Recent technological advances in genetics, genomics, and epigenetics have greatly enhanced fundamental knowledge of scleroderma. These advances hold promise for using molecular characteristics to stratify participants in clinical studies, develop innovative targeted therapies, and facilitate precision medicine to improve outcomes for this complex disease.

Despite considerable research progress, there remains an unmet need for effective, targeted therapies for scleroderma. In this book, international scientific and clinical experts studying various aspects of scleroderma present the latest breakthroughs in disease prevention, classification treatment, and management to improve the lives of individuals with scleroderma.

National Institute of Arthritis and Musculoskeletal and Skin Diseases, NIH
Bethesda, MD, USA

Lindsey A. Criswell,

Preface to the Third Edition

Scleroderma (systemic sclerosis) still remains one of the most challenging of all rheumatic diseases to understand and manage. However, scleroderma no longer needs to be viewed with bewilderment and a sense of helplessness. Indeed, in the years since the publication of the first edition of *Scleroderma: From Pathogenesis to Comprehensive Management*, much of our understanding about scleroderma has changed. Progress in biomedical research has been rapid, and new information about scleroderma is now accruing at a phenomenal pace. The number, diversity, and global span of investigators and research consortia focusing on scleroderma; the size of clinical trial cohorts and evolution in trial design and biomarkers; the variety of preclinical disease models; and the power and depth of high-dimensional technologies for data acquisition and analysis are all growing exponentially. Very importantly, the range of treatment strategies is also expanding, and medical innovation is boundless, with new frontiers in cellular, gene, and immunotherapies, including vaccines and CAR-T. Moreover, new targets and druggable pathways can be discovered with the help of machine learning, and timelines for drug development are narrowing. This explosion of new information is truly good news for people living with scleroderma, as well as for students of the disease, while also posing formidable new challenges for anyone seeking to stay abreast of new developments in the field and achieve deeper understanding.

The third edition of *Scleroderma: From Pathogenesis to Comprehensive Management* rises to these challenges. Our goal is to communicate the progress in an up-to-date, authoritative, comprehensive, and accessible manner. Building on the approach established in previous editions, we present a comprehensive and critical survey of current knowledge about the epidemiology, genetics, pathogenesis, classification, clinical manifestations, evaluation, and management of all aspects of scleroderma. We integrate contemporary concepts of pathophysiology and physiology with clinical aspects for each major feature of scleroderma. The book is edited with a broad and global readership in mind to present a uniquely valuable reference for anyone interested in scleroderma, be they clinicians, investigators, students, or other healthcare professionals. Each chapter is written by distinguished international experts in the field, to assure a balanced and global perspective. Up-to-date overview of genetics and functional genomics, a very rapidly evolving area with tremendous implications for both understanding scleroderma and delivering personalized management, is presented in the context of pathophysiology, disease classification and patient stratification, and discovering novel targets and innovative therapeutic approaches. Additional chapters discuss current and evolving biomarker discovery efforts and how these might lead to biomarkers that will have real-life utility in the clinic. The rationale for novel treatments is presented, along with data regarding their efficacy, safety, and appropriate role in patient management. Throughout, each chapter highlights growing awareness of disease heterogeneity and its impact on the practice of individualized "precision" medicine in scleroderma. Finally, we present a series of clinically oriented chapters that highlight current approaches to common and important disease manifestations, and expert opinion for therapeutic conundrums. In this way, both clinicians and non-clinician readers of the book can gain a better understanding of the complex challenges of scleroderma. It is our hope that this third edition of *Scleroderma: From Pathogenesis to Comprehensive Management* will serve not only as a go-to source for authoritative and up-to-date information, but also inspire and catalyze new ideas, collaborations, and discoveries that bring us ever closer to the prevention and cure of scleroderma.

We wish to recognize our esteemed colleague and friend Fredrick Wigley, MD, Professor of Medicine and pioneering founder of the Johns Hopkins Scleroderma Program. Fred, a tireless researcher, inspiring mentor and legendary clinician, was instrumental in creating, and served on prior editions of, *Scleroderma: From Pathogenesis to Comprehensive Management.* We express our gratitude for the superb editorial assistance provided by Margaret Moore (New York). Without her dedication, insights, and unfailing patience, this book would not have come to fruition.

Baltimore, MD, USA	Ami A. Shah
London, UK	Christopher P. Denton
Tokyo, Japan	Masataka Kuwana
Paris, France	Yannick Allanore
Palo Alto, CA, USA	Lorinda Chung
Ann Arbor, MI, USA	John Varga

Contents

Contributors

David J. Abraham Division of Medicine, Department of Inflammation, UCL Centre for Rheumatology, London, UK

Nitin K. Ahuja Division of Gastroenterology & Hepatology, University of Pennsylvania School of Medicine, Philadelphia, PA, USA

Yannick Allanore Service de Rhumatologie A, Université Paris Descartes, Paris, France

Unité INSERM U1016, Université Paris Descartes, Institut Cochin, Paris, France

Cochin Hospital, AP-HP, INSERM U1016, Paris University, Paris, France

Rheumatology Department, Cochin Hospital, APHP, Université Paris Cité, Paris, France

Service de Rhumatologie, Hôpital Cochin, Université de Paris, Paris, France

Yoshihide Asano Department of Dermatology, Faculty of Medicine, University of Tokyo, Tokyo, Japan

Frederic B. Askin Department of Pathology, Johns Hopkins University School of Medicine, Baltimore, MD, USA

Shervin Assassi University of Texas Health Science Centre at Houston, Houston, TX, USA

Elisabeth Bendstrup Department of Respiratory Diseases and Allergy, Aarhus University, Aarhus, Denmark

Elana J. Bernstein Columbia University/New York-Presbyterian Scleroderma Program, Division of Rheumatology, Department of Medicine, Columbia University Vagelos College of Physicians and Surgeons, New York, NY, USA

Francesco Boin Division of Rheumatology, Department of Medicine, Cedars-Sinai Medical Center, Los Angeles, CA, USA

Cosimo Bruni Department of Clinical and Experimental Medicine, Section of Rheumatology, University of Florence, Florence, Italy

Maya H. Buch Department of Rheumatology, Centre for Musculoskeletal Research, School of Biological Sciences, Faculty of Biology, Medicine & Health, University of Manchester, Manchester, UK

NIHR Manchester Biomedical Research Centre, Manchester Academic Health Science Centre, Manchester University Foundation Trust, Manchester, UK

Livia Casciola-Rosen Division of Rheumatology, Johns Hopkins University, Baltimore, MD, USA

Flavia V. Castelino Division of Rheumatology, Massachusetts General Hospital/Harvard Medical School, Boston, MA, USA

Carlo Chizzolini Department of Pathology and Immunology, Centre Médical Universitaire, Geneva University, Geneva, Switzerland

Lorinda Chung Division of Immunology & Rheumatology, Stanford University School of Medicine and Palo Alto VA Health Care System, Palo Alto, CA, USA

Melody Chung Division of Rheumatology, Mid-Atlantic Permanente Group, Gaithersburg, MD, USA

John O. Clarke Division of Gastroenterology & Hepatology, Stanford University School of Medicine, Palo Alto, CA, USA

Bruno Crestani APHP, Service de Pneumologie A, Constitutive Reference Center for Rare Pulmonary Diseases—OrphaLung, FHU APOLLO, Hôpital Bichat, Paris, France

Christopher P. Denton Centre for Rheumatology, Royal Free Hospital, London, UK

Division of Medicine, University College London, London, UK

Centre for Rheumatology and Connective Tissue Diseases, UCL Division of Medicine, Royal Free Hospital, London, UK

UCL Division of Medicine, University College London, London, UK

Centre for Rheumatology, University College London, Royal Free Hospital, London, UK

Jörg H. W. Distler Department of Internal Medicine 3, University of Erlangen-Nuremberg, Erlangen, Germany

Oliver Distler Department of Rheumatology, University Hospital Zurich, Zurich, Switzerland

Robyn T. Domsic University of Pittsburgh, Pittsburgh, PA, USA

Muriel Elhai Department of Rheumatology, University Hospital Zurich, University of Zurich, Zurich, Switzerland

Harrison W. Farber Pulmonary Hypertension Center, Tufts Medical Center, Boston, MA, USA

Carol Feghali-Bostwick Division of Rheumatology and Immunology, Department of Medicine, Medical University of South Carolina, Charleston, SC, USA

Ivan Foeldvari Hamburg Centre for Pediatric Rheumatology, Head of the Juvenile Scleroderma Working Group (JSScWG), Hamburger Zentrum Für Kinder- und Jugendrheumatologie, Hamburg, Germany

Rina S. Fox Department of Medical Social Sciences, Northwestern University Feinberg School of Medicine, Chicago, IL, USA

Tracy M. Frech Vanderbilt University Medical Center and Tennessee Valley Healthcare System Veterans Affairs, Nashville, TN, USA

Daniel E. Furst University of California, Los Angeles, Los Angeles, CA, USA

Armando Gabrielli Fondazione di Medicina Molecolare e Terapia Cellulare, Università Politecnica delle Marche, Ancona, Italy

Francesco Del Galdo Scleroderma Programme, NIHR Biomedical Research Centre and Leeds Institute of Rheumatic and Musculoskeletal Medicine, University of Leeds, Leeds, UK

Luna Gargani Department of Surgical, Medical and Molecular Pathology and Critical Care Medicine, University of Pisa, Pisa, Italy

Shadi Gholizadeh Clinical PsyD Program, California School of Professional Psychology/ Alliant International University-Los Angeles, Alhambra, CA, USA

Jonathan G. Goldin Radiology, Medicine and Biomedical Physics, David Geffen School of Medicine at UCLA, Los Angeles, CA, USA

Computer Vision and Imaging Biomarkers Program, David Geffen School of Medicine at UCLA, Los Angeles, CA USA

Departemt of Radiology, David Geffen School of Medcine, Los Angeles, CA, USA

Pravitt Gourh Scleroderma Genomics and Health Disparities Unit, National Institute of Arthritis and Musculoskeletal and Skin Diseases, National Institutes of Health, Bethesda, MD, USA

Lauren V. Graham Department of Dermatology, Northwestern University, McGraw Medical Center, Chicago, IL, USA

Jean-Marc Guettier Precision Medicine, Sanofi, Boston, MA, USA

Eric Hachulla Univ. Lille, Inserm, CHU Lille, Service de Médecine Interne et Immunologie Clinique, Centre de référence des maladies autoimmunes systémiques rares du Nord et Nord-Ouest de France (CeRAINO), U1286—INFINITE—Institute for Translational Research in Inflammation, Lille, France

Faye N. Hant Division of Rheumatology and Immunology, Medical University of South Carolina, Charleston, SC, USA

Ariane L. Herrick Division of Musculoskeletal and Dermatological Sciences, The University of Manchester, Salford Royal NHS Foundation Trust, Manchester Academic Health Science Centre, Manchester, UK

Kristin B. Highland Department of Pulmonary Medicine, Cleveland Clinic, Cleveland, OH, USA

Monique Hinchcliff Department of Internal Medicine, Section of Rheumatology, Allergy & Immunology, The Anlyan Center, Yale School of Medicine, New Haven, CT, USA

Anna-Maria Hoffmann-Vold Department of Rheumatology, Oslo University Hospital, Oslo, Norway

Alan M. Holmes Centre for Rheumatology, Division of Medicine, University College London, Royal Free Hospital, London, UK

Stephanie M. Hon Pulmonary Hypertension Center, Tufts Medical Center, Boston, MA, USA

Frank H. J. Van den Hoogen Departments of Rheumatology, Radboud University, Nijmegen Medical Center and Sint Maartenskliniek, Nijmegen, The Netherlands

Marie Hudson Division of Rheumatology, Lady Davis Institute for Medical Research, Jewish General Hospital, QC, Canada

Faculty of Medicine, McGill University, QC, Canada

Michael Hughes Department of Rheumatology, Salford Care Organisation, Northern Care Alliance NHS Group, Salford, UK

Division of Musculoskeletal and Dermatological Sciences, Faculty of Biology, Medicine and Health, The University of Manchester and Salford Royal NHS Foundation Trust, Manchester, UK

Marc Humbert Department of Respiratory Medicine, Hôpital Bicêtre, Paris, France

Laura K. Hummers Department of Medicine and Rheumatology, Johns Hopkins University, Baltimore, MD, USA

Nicolas Hunzelmann Department of Dermatology, University of Cologne, Cologne, Germany

Heidi T. Jacobe Department of Dermatology, University of Texas Southwestern Medical Center, Dallas, TX, USA

Bochra Jandali Internal Medicine, Division of Rheumatology and Immunogenetics, University of Texas Health Science Center—Houston, Houston, TX, USA

Lisa R. Jewett Department of Psychiatry, Institute of Community and Family Psychiatry, Jewish General Hospital, QC, Canada

Sindhu R. Johnson Toronto Scleroderma Program, University of Toronto, Toronto, ON, Canada

Bashar Kahaleh Division of Rheumatology, Allergy and Immunology, University of Toledo Medical Center, Toledo, OH, USA

Dinesh Khanna Division of Rheumatology, Department of Internal Medicine, University of Michigan, Ann Arbor, MI, USA

University of Michigan, Ann Arbor, MI, USA

Masataka Kuwana Department of Allergy and Rheumatology, Nippon Medical School Graduate School of Medicine, Tokyo, Japan

Nippon Medical School Graduate School of Medicine, Tokyo, Japan

Linda Kwakkenbos Department of Clinical Psychology, Radboud University, Nijmegen, The Netherlands

Department of IQ Health Care, Radboud University Medical Center, Nijmegen, The Netherlands

Department of Psychiatry, Radboud University Medical Center, Nijmegen, The Netherlands

Jacob M. van Laar Department of Rheumatology and Clinical Immunology, UMC Utrecht, Utrecht, The Netherlands

Robert Lafyatis Division of Rheumatology and Clinical Immunology, Department of Medicine, Scleroderma Center, University of Pittsburgh Medical Center, Pittsburgh, PA, USA

David Lagares Division of Pulmonary and Critical Care Medicine, Massachusetts General Hospital, Harvard Medical School, Boston, MA, USA

Benoit Lechartier Department of Respiratory Medicine, Hôpital Bicêtre, Paris, France

Department of Respiratory Medicine, Lausanne University Hospital, Lausanne, Switzerland

Michael H. Lee Division of Pulmonary and Critical Care Medicine, Department of Medicine, University of California San Francisco, San Francisco, CA, USA

Alain Lescoat Department of Internal Medicine & Clinical Immunology, CHU Rennes, South Hospital, Rennes, France

Vanessa L. Malcarne SDSU/UC San Diego Joint Doctoral Program in Clinical Psychology, San Diego, CA, USA

Department of Psychology, San Diego State University, San Diego, CA, USA

Mirko Manetti Section of Anatomy and Histology, Department of Experimental and Clinical Medicine, University of Florence, Florence, Italy

Javier Martin Institute of Parasitology and Biomedicine López-Neyra, CSIC, Granada, Spain

Stephen C. Mathai Division of Pulmonary and Critical Care Medicine, Department of Medicine, Johns Hopkins University School of Medicine, Baltimore, MD, USA

Marco Matucci-Cerinic Department of Experimental and Clinical Medicine, Careggi Hospital (AOUC), University of Florence, Florence, Italy

Division of Rheumatology, AOUC, Florence, Italy

Unit of Immunology, Rheumatology, Allergy and Rare Diseases (UniRAR), IRCCS San Raffaele Hospital, Milan, Italy

Britta Maurer Department of Rheumatology and Immunology, University Hospital Bern, University of Bern, Bern, Switzerland

Kimberly Doering Maurer Department of Radiology, Duke University Health System, Durham, NC, USA

Maureen D. Mayes Internal Medicine, Division of Rheumatology and Immunogenetics, University of Texas Health Science Center—Houston, Houston, TX, USA

Matteo Mazzola Department of Surgical, Medical and Molecular Pathology and Critical Care Medicine, University of Pisa, Pisa, Italy

Zsuzsanna McMahan Division of Rheumatology, Department of Medicine, McGovern Medical School, Houston, TX, USA

Christopher A. Mecoli Division of Rheumatology, Johns Hopkins University, Baltimore, MD, USA

Sarah D. Mills Department of Health Behavior, University of North Carolina at Chapel Hill, Chapel Hill, NC, USA

Lineberger Comprehensive Cancer Center, University of North Carolina at Chapel Hill, Chapel Hill, NC, USA

Pia Moinzadeh Department of Dermatology and Venerology, University of Cologne, Cologne, Germany

Luc Mouthon Internal Medicine, National Referral Center for Rare Autoimmune and Systemic Diseases, Universite Paris Descartes, Paris, France

Department of Internal Medicine, Centre de Référence Maladies Systémiques Autoimmunes et Autoinflammatoires Rares d'Ile de France de l'Est et de l'Ouest, Assistance Publique Hôpitaux de Paris, France (APHP-CUP), Hôpital Cochin, Paris, France

Université Paris Cité, Paris, France

Ulf Muller-Ladner Justus-Liebig Universität Giessen, Kerckhoff-Klinik GmbH, Bad Nauheim, Germany

Christopher J. Mullin Division of Pulmonary, Critical Care, and Sleep Medicine, Alpert Medical School of Brown University, Providence, RI, USA

Maria-Sinziana Muraru-Carbrune Department of Rheumatology, University Hospital Zurich, University of Zurich, Zurich, Switzerland

Christelle Nguyen Department of Physical and Rehabilitation Medicine, Hôpital Cochin, Paris, France

Nuala O'Donoghue Salford Royal NHS Foundation Trust, Salford, UK

Voon H. Ong University College London, London, UK

Julie J. Paik Division of Rheumatology, Johns Hopkins University School of Medicine, Baltimore, MD, USA

Amy S. Paller Department of Dermatology, Northwestern University Feinberg School of Medicine, Chicago, IL, USA

John D. Pauling Department of Rheumatology, North Bristol NHS Trust, Bristol, UK

Musculoskeletal Research Unit, Bristol Medical School Translational Health Sciences, University of Bristol, Bristol, UK

Markella Ponticos Centre for Rheumatology, Division of Medicine, University College London, Royal Free Hospital, London, UK

Janet L. Poole Occupational Therapy Graduate Program, School of Medicine, University of New Mexico, Albuquerque, NM, USA

Thomas Reifsnyder Department of Surgery/Vascular Surgery and Endovascular Therapy, The Johns Hopkins University School of Medicine, Baltimore, MD, USA

Lisa M. Rooper Department of Pathology, Johns Hopkins Hospital, Baltimore, MD, USA

Antony Rosen Division of Rheumatology, Johns Hopkins University, Baltimore, MD, USA

Muditha Samaranayaka Salford Royal NHS Foundation Trust, Salford, UK

Ami A. Shah Division of Rheumatology, Department of Medicine, Johns Hopkins University School of Medicine, Baltimore, MD, USA

Johns Hopkins University School of Medicine, Baltimore, MD, USA

Sanjiv J. Shah Northwestern University Feinberg School of Medicine, Chicago, IL, USA

Katherine C. Silver Department of Medicine, Medical University of South Carolina, Charleston, SC, USA

Richard M. Silver Division of Rheumatology and Immunology, Medical University of South Carolina, Charleston, SC, USA

Department of Medicine, Medical University of South Carolina, Charleston, SC, USA

Olivier Sitbon School of Medicine, Université Paris-Saclay, Le Kremlin-Bicêtre, France

Department of Respiratory and Intensive Care Medicine, AP-HP, Hôpital Bicêtre, Le Kremlin-Bicêtre, France

INSERM UMR_S 999, Hôpital Marie Lannelongue, Le Plessis-Robinson, France

Vincent Sobanski Univ. Lille, Inserm, CHU Lille, U1286 - INFINITE - Institute for Translational Research in Inflammation, Lille, France

Institut Universitaire de France (IUF), Lille, France

Julia Spierings Department of Rheumatology and Clinical Immunology, UMC Utrecht, Utrecht, The Netherlands

Edward P. Stern Centre for Rheumatology, UCL Royal Free Campus, London, UK

Noelle M. Teske Department of Dermatology, Oregon Health & Science University, OR, USA

Brett D. Thombs Lady Davis Institute for Medical Research, Jewish General Hospital, Montreal, QC, Canada

Department of Psychiatry, McGill University, Montreal, QC, Canada

Department of Epidemiology, Biostatistics, and Occupational Health, McGill University, Montreal, QC, Canada

Department of Medicine, McGill University, Montreal, QC, Canada

Department of Psychology, McGill University, Montreal, QC, Canada

Maria Trojanowska Arthritis and Autoimmune Diseases Center, Boston University School of Medicine, Boston, MA, USA

Rubin M. Tuder Division of Pulmonary Sciences and Critical Care Medicine, Department of Medicine, University of Colorado, Aurora, CO, USA

Alan Tyndall Department of Rheumatology, University Hospital Basel, Basel, Switzerland

Antonia Valenzuela Department of Clinical Immunology and Rheumatology, Pontificia Universidad Católica de Chile, Santiago, Chile

John Varga Division of Rheumatology, Department of Internal Medicine, University of Michigan, Ann Arbor, MI, USA

Elizabeth R. Volkmann Division of Rheumatology, Department of Medicine, University of California, Los Angeles, CA, USA

Jeska de Vries-Bouwstra Department of Rheumatology, Leiden University Medical Center, Leiden, The Netherlands

Athol U. Wells Royal Brompton Hospital, London, UK

Fredrick M. Wigley Division of Rheumatology, Department of Medicine, The Johns Hopkins University School of Medicine, Baltimore, MD, USA

Peter K. Wung Immunology Clinical Development, AbbVie, North Chicago, IL, USA

Elisabetta Zanatta Rheumatology Unit, Department of Medicine (DIMED), University Hospital of Padova, Padova, Italy

Part I

Introduction

John Varga

Historical Perspective of Scleroderma

1

Christopher P. Denton and Marco Matucci-Cerinic

The history of scleroderma reflects the temporal context as well as a growth in knowledge and understanding about multisystem and autoimmune diseases. There are key historic events that are relevant but it was not until the twentieth century that scleroderma emerged as a concept for multisystem diseases. This chapter reviews key aspects of early history that relate to scleroderma and then focuses on the modern era that really reflects advances in biomedical science, genetics and clinical progress in treating connective tissue disease.

In addition to considering how long a distinct medical entity that we would recognize as scleroderma has been recognized, it is useful to place the diagnosis and classification of scleroderma in a historical context. It is clear that there was initially some reluctance to group together all forms of the disease that we would recognize today, and this is perhaps reflective of the advances that have occurred in imaging and laboratory investigation and a greater appreciation of the link between different organ-based manifestations. The milestones in the history of scleroderma bear testimony to the gradual realization of the heterogeneity of the disorder. For a more detailed discussion of the fascinating history of this disease, the reader is referred to the excellent historical review by Rodnan, the "father" of modern-day clinical scleroderma [1].

Early History

It is often considered that the first description of the systemic disease that we recognize as scleroderma was in 1753 by Cario Curzio (Naples Italy) (Fig. 1.1). However, a careful review of the reported case suggests the diagnosis may, in reality, have been *scleroedema* because of the distribution of the skin changes and due to an apparent improvement in the 17-year-old female patient after a combination of therapeutic endeavours that included bloodletting, warm milk and small doses of elemental mercury. In 1836, Fantonetti (1791–1877), a Milanese physician, became the first to use the term *scleroderma* to designate a disease in an adult. However, it is likely that his patient also had scleroedema. The first convincing case of scleroderma was reported in 1842 and then several other cases were published prior to 1847, a year when interest in the disease greatly increased. By 1860 numerous cases had been reported and the first articles that attempted to review the disease were published. Maurice Raynaud (1834–1881) described a patient with *sclerodermie* and cold-induced "asphyxie locale"—this was the first description of the Raynaud phenomenon in scleroderma. Just as for scleroderma it has been speculated that the first cases of the Raynaud phenomenon may have included individuals with an alternative diagnosis underlying their acrocyanosis and vascular insufficiency. Sir William Osler made the diagnosis of scleroderma while at the Johns Hopkins Hospital between 1891 and 1897. Osler appears to have clearly appreciated the systemic nature of the disease, and to recognize the enormous clinical burden that patients with scleroderma endured when he wrote: *In its more aggravated forms diffuse scleroderma is one of the most terrible of all human ills. Like Tithonous, to "whither slowly," and like him to be "beaten down and marred and wasted" until one is literally a mummy, encased in an ever-shrinking, slowly contracting skin of steel, is a fate not pictured in any tragedy, ancient or modern.* Matsui (Japan, 1924) further highlighted the importance of visceral involvement based on several autopsies that he had performed on individuals who had succumbed to the disease. Goetz (Capetown, 1945) further confirmed the multisystem involvement and suggested the disease be named *progressive systemic sclerosis* (SSc). The qualifying term "progressive" was later considered to be inaccurate in some cases that either remained stable or improved or has generally been dropped. It does however serve to highlight the

C. P. Denton (✉)
Centre for Rheumatology, UCL Division of Medicine, London, UK
e-mail: c.denton@ucl.ac.uk

M. Matucci-Cerinic
Department of Experimental and Clinical Medicine, Careggi Hospital (AOUC), University of Florence, Florence, Italy
e-mail: marco.matuccicerinic@unifi.it

Y. Allanore et al. (eds.), *Scleroderma*, https://doi.org/10.1007/978-3-031-40658-4_1

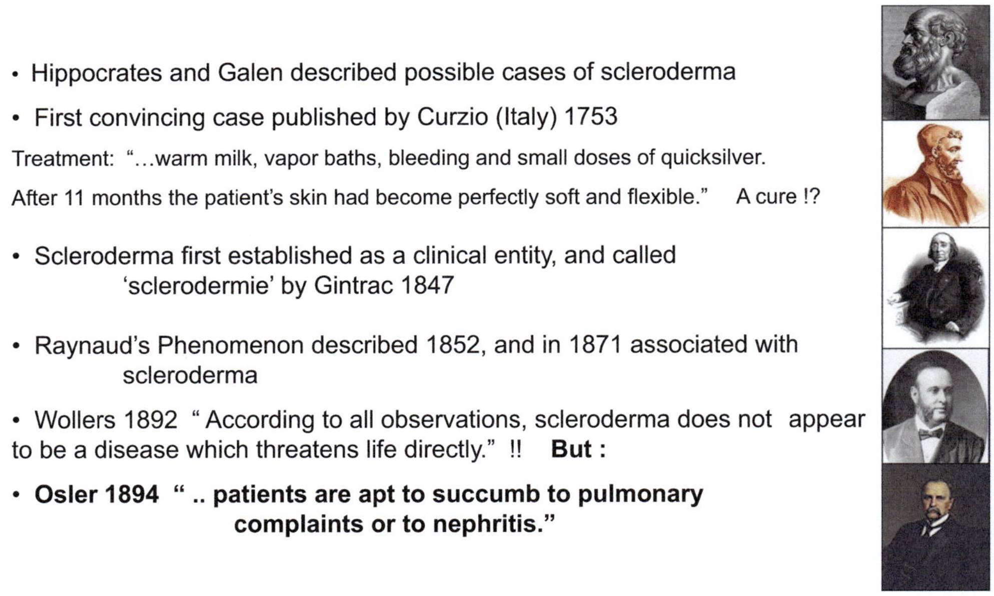

Fig. 1.1 Key figures in the early history of scleroderma. Some of the key historic figures who contributed to the field of scleroderma are listed. Appreciation of the severity of the disease was confounded by clinical variability and the absence of unifying diagnostic criteria or investigational modalities

potential severity of the worst forms of the disease. The potential importance of subtypes of scleroderma began in 1964, when Winterbauer reported cases with the CRST (calcinosis, Raynaud's phenomenon, sclerodactyly and telangiectasias) syndrome. A similar group of patients was reported in 1920, named after the authors, the Thibirge–Weissenbach syndrome. Velayos and colleagues recognized that oesophageal dysmotility was common in these patients; so now it is called the CREST syndrome. In 1969, 58 autopsy cases of scleroderma were compared with matched controls. The organs found to be frequently and significantly involved by this disease were the skin, gastrointestinal tract, lungs, kidneys, skeletal muscle and pericardium. This report first described the systemic nature of vascular pathology in scleroderma with findings of both kidney and lung arterial changes. Rodnan introduced a clinical method to evaluate the extent of skin disease, and correlated this with skin biopsy weight and later with collagen content in the skin. From the same centre in Pittsburgh, Steen and Medsger and others did extensive surveys of large populations of scleroderma patients, defining the clinical course and specific subtypes of the disease. In the 1980s, a subcommittee of world experts established diagnostic criteria [2] and Leroy and colleagues suggested the classification of two major subsets of disease defined by skin involvement: *limited* and *diffuse* [3]. Recent work by several investigators has recognized that scleroderma-specific auto-antibodies occur associated with subtypes of the disease and can be used to predict disease course. Work in the modern era has revealed details of the pathogenesis of the disease and the recognition that scleroderma is a complex polygenetic autoimmune disease associated with a unique disease process involving tissue fibrosis. Although no drug is yet discovered that can be called a successful disease-modifying agent that controls the underlying disease process, major progress has been made in managing specific organ diseases. The discovery of that an angiotensin-converting enzyme inhibitor could reverse the scleroderma renal crisis in the 1970s changed the course of kidney disease and improved the survival of patients. Current therapies for gastrointestinal, cardiac, pulmonary vascular and interstitial lung disease have improved the quality of life and survival. There has been a growing interest in scleroderma around the world, and the emergence of specialist centres that now provide effective patient care and scientific interactions with each other and private industry to discover the causes and new treatment for scleroderma. Although uncommon and without effective disease-modifying therapies, the relevance of scleroderma to a broad range of other medical conditions is now fully appreciated and this has benefited management though translation of treatments into the organ-based complications of scleroderma. In addition, scleroderma provides a potential platform for the development of anti-fibrotic or vascular therapies that could be beneficial in other commoner diseases that are characterized by vascular insufficiency or extracellular matrix overproduction.

Emergence of Systemic Sclerosis as a Clinical Entity

The appreciation of the spectrum of scleroderma and related disorders over the past 40 years has been a gradual process underpinned by growing expertise in the assessment and evaluation of cases and stronger collaboration across medical specialities. This allowed the relationship between systemic sclerosis, localized scleroderma and other autoimmune rheumatic diseases to become established. Additional recognition of conditions such as eosinophilic fasciitis [4] and environmentally triggered diseases fuelled clinical research. Finally, the appreciation of the relationship between isolated Raynaud's phenomenon and evolution into connective tissue disease permitted a broadening of the spectrum to encompass what is currently considered the scleroderma spectrum that is covered in this volume.

Recent History

The late twentieth century was a period of tremendous advance in biomedicine and this is reflected by the growth in understanding of systemic sclerosis. This has occurred in both appreciation of the underlying pathobiology and also the relationship between clinical manifestations of SSc and other organ-based forms of fibrosis and vascular disease. In this way, SSc provides a paradigm for other commoner medical conditions and this has fuelled clinical and translational research and helped to support further research.

Advances in Scleroderma Biology

Underpinned by the work of LeRoy and others, the next generation of researchers have used advances in cell and molecular biology to develop better concepts of pathobiology of SSc that more completely explain the disease. This has most recently included the incorporation of genetic and developmental biology and it is reasonable to assert that models of pathogenesis can now be developed that provide a framework for understanding the disease in its different and diverse forms. Improved outcomes for scleroderma renal crisis emerged in the 1980s and this provided an important demonstration that SSc was indeed treatable and that outcomes even of the most lethal aspects of the disease could be improved. In a similar time frame treatments for gastro-oesophageal disease advanced, with PPIs providing a critical advance in the management of upper GI disease. The International Scleroderma Research Workshop was established by Drs Black and Korn and has provided real stimulus to advance the science of SSc and evolve into the area of translational research. This meeting remains pre-eminent in the field and aims to bring the very best relevant and new science into the arena of scleroderma research. The workshop continues to showcase international efforts and bring the latest advances in basic science into the scleroderma landscape. The workshop together with the Systemic Sclerosis World Congress ensures that the interface between clinical, translational and basic laboratory research is revisited and that progress in understanding disease biology can move to clinical benefit for patients as rapidly as possible.

Progress in Classification Natural History and Clinical Trials Methodology

The past two decades have been a period of clinical progress that has included the development of clinical trials methodology. Important studies have been undertaken, although initially mostly negative, these efforts did confirm the feasibility of clinical trials in SSc and led to a better understanding of the natural history of the disease. Pooled analysis of these early studies has been essential to better understand trial methods and this has provided the foundation for current clinical studies. Early templates for trial design were developed and have been updated, and this is exemplified by the recent publication of a series of points to consider in scleroderma trials [5]. As in other branches of medicine, the availability of valid trial templates is critical as potential therapeutic approaches emerge. The appreciation of the need for cohort enrichment and a clear definition of end-points has emerged from expert discussion over the past three decades and represents an important achievement in recent scleroderma history.

Classification of SSc was first attempted in 1980 and subset criteria were later developed. The new classification criteria were developed by rigorous methodology and with strong international collaboration and were published in 2013 [6]. These reflected expert practice and a growing understaanding of disease h+eterogeneity, although attempts to define robust criteria for early diagnosis of classification of milder disease proved challenging and no real agreement was reached until much more recently when evidence-based approaches such as the prospective VEDOSS project was developed [7].

Important international collaborative groups have emerged including the Scleroderma Clinical Trials Consortium that was established in the 1990s and now have more than 75 member institutions all with a high degree of expertise in clinical research and trials in SSc. This has underpinned recent trials and progress. The first organized group to emerge internationally was the Scleroderma Clinical Trials Consortium. This group links expert centres and was set up in the USA, but has now become a strong international organization. More recently the key international events have been the establishment of EUSTAR, which has developed into an impressive network of scleroderma centres and anchored by a clinical database that is being used for observational clinical research. There are active educational and research programmers and they are now providing very powerful research for study and improved understanding of SSc.

Driven by growing interest from clinicians and supported by patients, scientists and pharmaceutical partners, the World Congress in SSc became established in 2010 and the success of this larger format of international conference for SSc is a testament to the growing interest in the disease and opportunities for better management and strong engagement with patient organizations. FESCA, an umbrella organization for patient groups, was developed in parallel with EUSTAR and the world congress, and offers a real hope for the future with opportunities for a broader political engagement and support. The World Scleroderma Foundation represents the most recent chapter in the history of international collaboration and enterprise (www.worldsclerodermafoundation.net). It provides potential avenues for larger and more inclusive approaches to education and care for SSc underpinned by highest quality research and investigation. It is now formally aligned to EUSTAR and is underpinned by the successful World SSc Congresses. Thus, the recent history of scleroderma is international, collaborative and forward looking and represents the start of the next stage in the journey towards understanding the disease and offering better outcomes for patients.

Over the past few years there has been a much better understanding of the complex needs of systemic sclerosis patients and engagement with patients. This is facilitated by flourishing patient-led organizations and from the links between patients and clinician organizations such as WSF and EUSTAR. There are emerging guidelines and recommendations that aim to give a better standardization of treatment and a secure framework of evidence-based management [8]. This includes taking much greater account of patient needs and the importance of communication. On line resources and social media have generally been a positive force in this endeavour. In addition, there is now a much better understanding of pathogenic processes that allows logical decisions to be made in selecting new potential candidate pathways and mediators for targeting therapeutically. The results of this are a number of positive clinical trials and other studies that provide powerful insight into the disease process. Finally, stem cell transplantation is a proven therapy based upon high-quality clinical trials and although more research is needed, it is encouraging to see hope replacing nihilism in the arena of systemic sclerosis therapy. The approval of drugs for SSc digital ulcer disease and SSc associated lung fibrosis is a testament to the progress that has been made and the feasibility of conducting trials that led to regulatory approval from health authorities.

Some of the key events in the history of scleroderma are listed in Fig. 1.2. This provides an approximate time line that

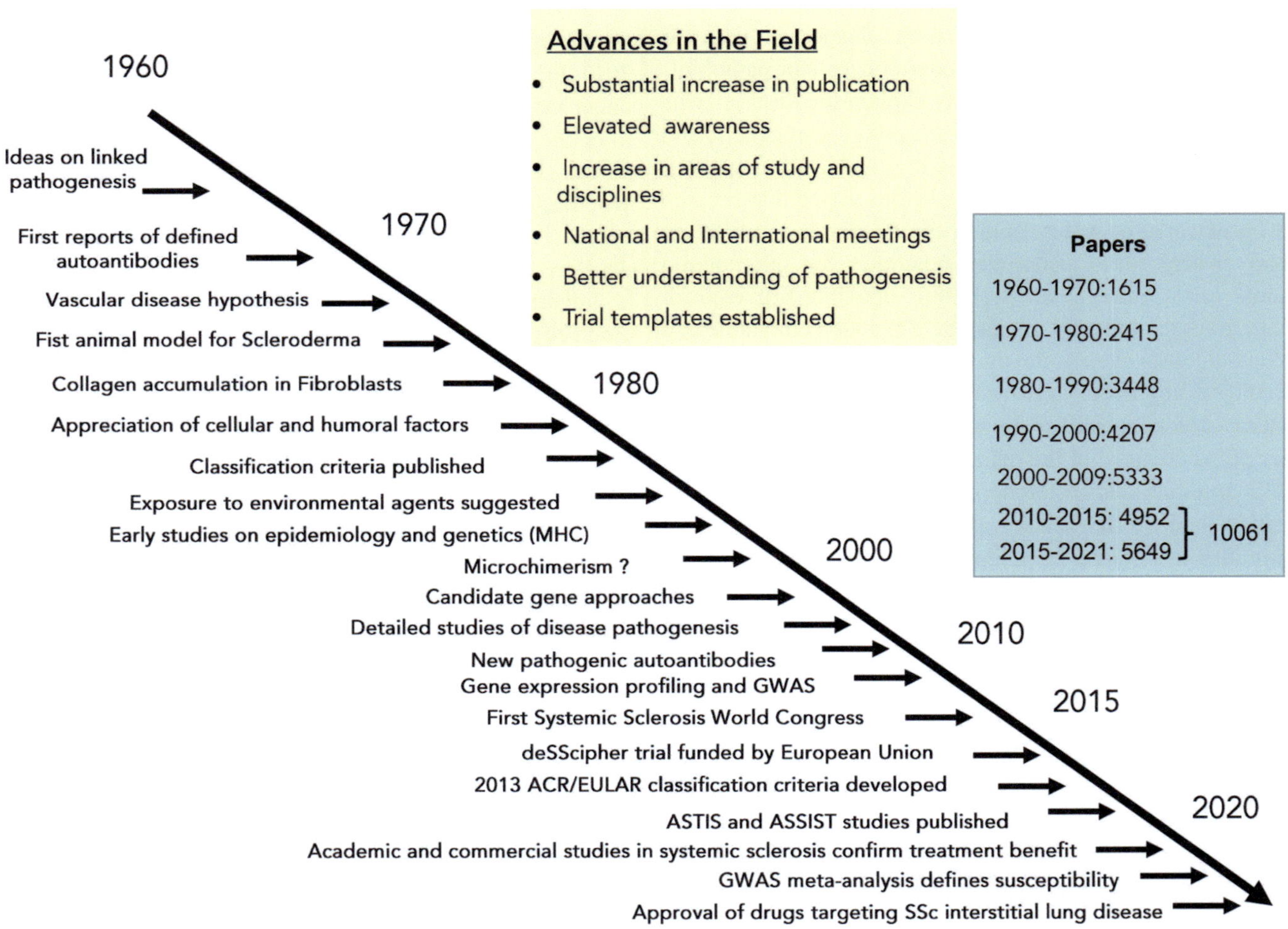

Fig. 1.2 Milestones for translational research in scleroderma. The timeline of translational research into scleroderma illustrates the growing interest in the disease together with better appreciation of its complexity and more candidates for pathogenesis

demonstrates the recent progress in understanding the disease, but it is important to observe that the outcome of the disease in terms of mortality has substantially improved over the past 20 years and that this has come at a time when there is a much better and more complete appreciation of disease burden from non-lethal manifestations. Thus, many more SSc patients are now living with the disease than are dying from it and this raises its own important challenges that are considered in detail in the various sections and subsequent chapters of this textbook.

References

1. Rodnan GP, Benedek TG. An historical account of the study of progressive systemic sclerosis (diffuse scleroderma). Ann Intern Med. 1962;57:305–19.
2. Preliminary Criteria for the Classification of Systemic Sclerosis (scleroderma). Subcommittee for scleroderma criteria of the American Rheumatism Association Diagnostic and Therapeutic Criteria Committee. Arthritis Rheum. 1980;23(5):581–90.
3. LeRoy EC, Medsger TA. Criteria for the classification of early systemic sclerosis. J Rheumatol. 2001;28(7):1573–6.
4. Shulman LE. Diffuse fasciite with hypergammaglobulinemia and eosinophilia: a new syndrome? J Rheumatol. 1974;1(suppl 1):46–9.
5. Khanna D, Furst DE, Allanore Y, Bae S, Bodukam V, Clements PJ, Cutolo M, Czirjak L, Denton CP, Distler O, Walker UA, Matucci-Cerinic M, Müller-Ladner U, Seibold JR, Singh M, Tyndall A. Twenty-two points to consider for clinical trials in systemic sclerosis, based on EULAR standards. Rheumatology. 2015;54:144–51.
6. van den Hoogen F, Khanna D, Fransen J, Johnson SR, Baron M, Tyndall A, Matucci-Cerinic M, Naden RP, Medsger TA Jr, Carreira PE, Riemekasten G, Clements PJ, Denton CP, Distler O, Allanore Y, Furst DE, Gabrielli A, Mayes MD, van Laar JM, Seibold JR, Czirjak L, Steen VD, Inanc M, Kowal-Bielecka O, Müller-Ladner U, Valentini G, Veale DJ, Vonk MC, Walker UA, Chung L, Collier DH, Csuka ME, Fessler BJ, Guiducci S, Herrick A, Hsu VM, Jimenez S, Kahaleh B, Merkel PA, Sierakowski S, Silver RM, Simms RW, Varga J, Pope JE. 2013 classification criteria for systemic sclerosis: an American College of Rheumatology/European league against rheumatism collaborative initiative. Arthritis Rheum. 2013;65(11):2737–47.
7. Matucci-Cerinic M, Allanore Y, Czirják L, Tyndall A, Müller-Ladner U, Denton C, Valentini G, Distler O, Fligelstone K, Tyrrel-Kennedy A, Farge D, Kowal-Bielecka O, van den Hoogen F, Cutolo M, Sampaio-Barros PD, Nash P, Takehara K, Furst DE. The challenge of early systemic sclerosis for the EULAR scleroderma trial and research group (EUSTAR) community. It is time to cut the Gordian knot and develop a prevention or rescue strategy. Ann Rheum Dis. 2009;68(9):1377–80.
8. Kowal-Bielecka O, Fransen J, Avouac J, Becker M, Kulak A, Allanore Y, Distler O, Clements P, Cutolo M, Czirjak L, Damjanov N, Del Galdo F, Denton CP, Distler JHW, Foeldvari I, Figelstone K, Frerix M, Furst DE, Guiducci S, Hunzelmann N, Khanna D, Matucci-Cerinic M, Herrick AL, van den Hoogen F, van Laar JM, Riemekasten G, Silver R, Smith V, Sulli A, Tarner I, Tyndall A, Welling J, Wigley F, Valentini G, Walker UA, Zulian F, Müller-Ladner U, EUSTAR Coauthors. Update of EULAR recommendations for the treatment of systemic sclerosis. Ann Rheum Dis. 2017;76(8):1327–39. https://doi.org/10.1136/annrheumdis-2016-209909. Epub 2016 Nov 9.

Part II

Epidemiology, Genetics and Classification

Christopher P. Denton

Epidemiology, Environmental, and Infectious Risk Factors

2

Bochra Jandali, Luc Mouthon, and Maureen D. Mayes

Introduction

Systemic sclerosis (SSc) is an autoimmune connective tissue disease characterized by excessive collagen deposition in the skin and internal organs with associated vasculopathy and autoantibody production [1]. Classification of SSc is divided into two main groups: limited and diffuse cutaneous disease [2]. The limited form is characterized by skin thickening that is confined to areas distal to the elbows and knees and generally is associated with less severe internal organ involvement. The diffuse form involves skin thickening proximal to the elbows and/or knees as well as distal areas and is associated with more severe organ damage. It is important to categorize patients upon diagnosis as disease manifestations and outcomes vary between these two subtypes. A recent paper investigated skin, lung, and peripheral vasculopathy outcomes in patients with lcSSc and compared them to patients with dcSSc. It was observed that lcSSc patients have stable skin disease as compared to the diffuse form. However, interstitial lung disease (ILD) in lcSSc patients could be as progressive as in those with the diffuse subtype [3]. This chapter will focus on the epidemiology of systemic sclerosis including both limited and diffuse cutaneous forms.

B. Jandali · M. D. Mayes (✉)
Internal Medicine, Division of Rheumatology, University of Texas Health Science Center – Houston, Houston, TX, USA
e-mail: bochra.jandali@uth.tmc.edu; maureen.d.mayes@uth.tmc.edu

L. Mouthon
Internal Medicine, National Referral Center for Rare Autoimmune and Systemic Diseases, Universite Paris Descartes, Paris, France
e-mail: luc.mouthon@cch.aphp.fr

Incidence and Prevalence of SSc

Systemic sclerosis is a heterogeneous disease that can affect multiple organs with variable degrees of severity. This variability in the organs involved and its severity made systemic sclerosis a challenging disease in terms of classification and diagnosis. The available literature about systemic sclerosis reflects heterogeneous epidemiological data.

The incidence rates and prevalence estimates vary significantly depending on the year of the study, the geographic area, the method used for case ascertainment, and finally, the classification criteria used. It is worth noting that the first classification criteria officially addressed SSc were published in 1980 by the American Rheumatology Association [4] (ARA is now ACR*) and this resulted in higher reported incidence and prevalence when compared to studies published before 1980. All of these factors resulted in inconsistent epidemiological data regarding SSc incidence and prevalence worldwide. If we look at the incidence rates in the United States, we see a trend of increased incidence over time. The lowest rate was reported by Medsger et al. [5] between 1947 and 1968 at 2.8/million; whereas the highest rate was reported by Furst et al. [6] in 2012 at 56/million, in which insurance claims were used, which most probably reflected an overestimated incidence rate. A study done by Mayes et al. [7] reported SSc incidence to be 20/million in Michigan (1989–1991) with more recent studies showing similar incidence rates [8, 9]. If we look at incidences from different reports worldwide, we see tremendous heterogeneity with the lowest reported in Finland [10], Iceland [11], and Japan [12]. The highest incidence rates were seen in the United States [6, 7, 13], Australia [14–16], Spain [17], and Argentina [18] (please refer to Table 2.1). Similarly, the prevalence of SSc varied significantly worldwide and sometimes within the same region over time (please refer to Tables 2.2 and 2.3). It is reported to be low in the Dominican Republic [48], New Zealand [28], England [26], Japan [12], and Taiwan [45] and high in the United States [6–8], Canada [30, 34, 35], Spain [17], Italy [23, 24, 42, 46], and Australia

Y. Allanore et al. (eds.), *Scleroderma*, https://doi.org/10.1007/978-3-031-40658-4_2

Table 2.1 Variation of incidence of systemic sclerosis by time and region

Author	Region and population	Period	Incidence (total cases per million)	Female/male ratio	Case ascertainment
North America					
Medsger et al. [5]	US, 86 patients	1947–1968	2.7	1.5/1	Hospital record review
Michet et al. [19]	US, 13 patients	1950–1979	10	12/1	Diagnostic retrieval system
Steen et al. [13]	US 444	1963–1972 1973–1982 1963–1982	9.6 18.7 13.9	3/1	Hospital record review
Laing et al. [20]	US, 514 women	1985–1991	14.1	–	Multiple sources, capture–recapture analysis
Mayes et al. [7]	US, 706 patients	1989–1991	21	4.6/1	Multiple sources
Furst et al. [6]	US, 1529 patients	2003–2008	46	6.15/1	Medical claims and IDC-9
Bauer et al. [8]	US, 64 patients	1980–2010	14–24	8.1/1	Record linkage system
Fan et al. [9]	US, 8326 patients	2011–2016	16.4 (person-year)	–	The Optum Clinformatics Data Mart
Europe, Australia, New Zealand, and Japan					
Andreasson et al. [21]	Sweden, 94 patients	2006–2010	19	6/1	Medical record review and ICD-10
Alamanos et al. [22]	Greece, 109 patients	1981–2002	11	8.9/1	Multiple sources
Lo Monaco et al. [23]	Italy, 118	1991–2007	43	9.7/1	Hospital and outpatient record review
Ciaffi et al. [24]	Italy, 25,934,569	2016	18.5	7.8/1	Administrative health data from regional co-payment registries
Arias-Nunez et al. [17]	Spain, 78 patients	1988–2006	12–23	–	Two-stage hospital survey
Hoffmann-Vold et al. [13]	Norway, 269 patients	1999–2009	6–11	–	Survey
Vonk et al. [25]	The Netherlands, 98 patients	2005–2006	7.7	–	POEMAS Registry
Kaipiainen et al. [10]	Finland	1990	3.7	–	Multiple sources
Geirsson et al. [11]	Iceland	1975–1990	3.8	8/1	Multiple sources
Silman et al. [26]	England, 128	1986	3.7	–	Multiple sources
Wigley et al. [27]	New Zealand	1950–1973	1.96	–	Hospital record review
Eason et al. [28]	New Zealand, 50	1970–1979	6.3	3/1	Hospital records review and specialist practices
Eanglert et al. [16]	Australia	1974–1988	12	2.3/1	Hospital record review
Roberts-Thomson et al. [14]	Australia, 548	1993–1999	15.1–22.8	4/1	Multiple sources
Roberts-Thomson et al. [15]	Australia, 353	1993–2002	20.4	–	Multiple sources
Englert [16]	Australia	1947–1988	12	2.3/1	Multiple sources
Englert [29]	Australia	1986–1991	122	1/1	General Medical Practitioners and Rheumatologists
Tamaki et al. [12]	Japan, 629	1987	7.2	14/1	Public health system

Table 2.2 Variation of prevalence of systemic sclerosis in North America by time and region

Author	Region and population	Period	Prevalence (total cases per million)	Female to male ratio	Case ascertainment
Medsger et al. [5]	US, 86 patients	1947–1968	105	1.5/1	Hospital record review
Michet [19]	US	1980	138	12/1	Diagnostic retrieval system
Bauer et al. [8]	US, 64 patients	1980–2010	399	8.1/1	Record linkage system
Mayes et al. [7]	US, 706 patients	1989–1991	276	4.6/1	Multiple sources
Bernatsky [30]	Canada, population based	1989–2003	443	–	Hospital and physician billing database
Avina-Zubieta [31]	Canada, population based	1990–2007	213	–	Physician billing and hospitalization databases
Arnett et al. [32]	US, 21,255 (Choctaw Native Americans)	1990–1994	660	4.66/1	IHS database, hospital record review
Robinson Jr. et al. [33]	US, N:2,872,333	2001–2002	300	–	IMS Health and MarketScan databases + medical and drug claims
Furst et al. [6]	US, 2739 patients	2003–2008	135–184	6.15/1	Medical claims and ICD-9
Barnabe et al. [34]	Canada, population based	1994–2007	– 580 for females and 100 for males – 470 for First Nation – 330 for non-First Nation	5.8/1	Hospital and billing codes
Thompson et al. [35]	Sarina 72,738 Windsor: 197,694 Woodstock: 32,086	2001	96 71 280	6/1	Outpatient clinic
Gottschalk et al. [36]	Dominican Republic, 26 patients	2002–2013	9.3	2.7/1	Clinical records review

Table 2.3 Variation of systemic sclerosis prevalence in Europe, Australia, and Japan

Author	Region and population	Period	Prevalence (total cases per million)	Female to male ratio	Case ascertainment method
Allcock et al. [37]	Northeast England, 80 patients	2000	88	5.2/1	Multiple sources
Silman et al. [26]	England (West Midlands), 128 patients	1986	31	–	Multiple sources
Valter et al. [38]	Estonia (South), 13 cases	1996–1997	350 (for definite cases)	13/0	Multistage population survey
Alamanos et al. [22]	Northwest Greece, 75 patients	1981–2002	154	8.9/1	Multiple sources
Le Guern et al. [39]	France, 119 patients	2001	158	11/1	Multiple sources
El Adssi et al. [40]	France, 193 patients	2006	132	6.7/1	Capture Recapture
Radic et al. [41]	Croatia, 49 patients	2008	156	–	Medical records
Airo et al. [42]	Italy, 13 patients	2004	339	–	Public Hospital database and clinic records
Arias-Nunez et al. [17]	Spain, 78 patients	1988–2006	277	–	Two-stage hospital-based survey
Eaton et al. [43]	Denmark, population-based study 5,506,574	1977–2006	230–250	–	Public hospital database + ERS and outpatient clinics
Andreasson et al. [21]	Sweden, 302 patients	2006–2010	305	3.6/1	Register
Hoffmann-Vold et al. [44]	Norway, 269 patients	1999–2009	72–99	3.8/1	Survey
Vonk et al. [25]	The Netherlands, 1148 patients	2005–2006	89	–	POEMAS Registry
Kuo et al. [45]	Taiwan, 1479 patients	2002–2011	56.3	–	NHIRD database and National Death Registry

(continued)

Table 2.3 (continued)

Author	Region and population	Period	Prevalence (total cases per million)	Female to male ratio	Case ascertainment method
Sardu et al. [46]	Italy, 35 patients	2009	350	–	survey
LoMonaco et al. [23]	Italy, 118 patients	1991–2007	341	9.7/1	Hospital and outpatient record review
Rosa et al. [18]	Argentina, 26 patients (prospective cohort)	2011	296	15/1	Med care program
Eason et al. [28]	New Zealand, 47 patients	1970–1979	30	3/1	Hospital record review and specialist practices
Englert et al. [16]	Australia (Sydney), 715 identified patients and 960 estimated patients	1974–1988	45.2–86.2	2.3/1	Hospital record review
Englert et al. [29]	Australia, 6	1986–1991	610	1/1	General medical practitioners and rheumatologist
Roberts-Thomson et al. [14]	Australia, 548 patients	1993–1999	209	4/1	Multiple sources
Roberts-Thomson et al. [15]	Australia, 353 patients	1993–2002	232	–	Multiple sources
Minz et al. [47]	North India, 48 patients	2012	120	3/1	Medical records review
Geirsson et al. [11]	Iceland, 18 patients	1994	71	8/1	Multiple sources
Tamaki et al. [12]	Japan, 636 patients	1991	21–53	14/1	Public health system

[14, 15]. This large variation could be due to geographical differences and the influence of certain environmental factors on the population. Moreover, it is also thought that better recognition of the disease and improved survival affected prevalence numbers over time.

Temporal Changes in Incidence Rates

It is believed that the incidence of SSc has increased over time. This assumption is based on incidence reports from the United States, New Zealand, and Australia. Two studies from the United States were hospital based and showed doubling of SSc incidence during study periods. The first one showed an increase from 0.6 case/million/year for the years 1947–1952 to 4.5 case/million/year for the years 1953–1968 in Tennessee [5]. A later publication by Steen et al. showed doubling of SSc incidence in Pennsylvania from 9.6 case/million/year (1963–1972) to 18.7 case/million/year (1973–1982) [13].

Later studies showed similar numbers in the following years which suggested stable incidence figures after 1980 [7]. One relatively newer study by Furst et al. suggested otherwise, showing an incidence rate of 46 cases/million/year across the United States. In this report, the medical billing system was used to identify SSc cases and suspected cases were included in the analysis [6].

Similar data from New Zealand and Australia suggested an increased incidence over the years. The incidence in New Zealand increased [27] from 1.96 (1950–1973) to 6.3 in the 1970s [28]. Similarly, the incidence almost doubled from 15.1 (1993) to 22.8 (1999) in Australia [14].

Geographic Variations in SSc Occurrence

Higher prevalence figures have been consistently reported in North America and Australia as compared to Japan and Europe. Three recent US studies [7, 33, 49] covering the time period 1989–2002 have reported quite similar prevalence figures of 286, 276, and 300 cases/million, respectively, in spite of using dissimilar methods of case ascertainment. The South Carolina study [49] was population based and used a questionnaire with a physical exam done among the positive responders. This resulted in an estimated prevalence of 286 cases/million for systemic sclerosis (SSc) and an estimate of 3790 cases/million "scleroderma spectrum disease" in 1989. This latter prevalence figure is likely related to the inclusion of overlap syndromes and/or primary Raynaud's disease because the questionnaire focused on Raynaud's phenomenon symptoms. The Michigan study [7] used five different sources for case finding and used a capture–recapture method of analysis to adjust for incomplete case ascertainment. Based on fairly conservative assumptions for this model, the prevalence estimate was 276 cases/million as of 1991. A US population-based survey by Robinson et al. [33], which identified cases based on the International Classification of Diseases Version 9 (ICD-9) diagnostic codes as well as two medical and drug claims datasets, reported a prevalence of 300 cases/million in 2002.

In contrast to these three similar estimates, Bernatsky et al. [30] reported a considerably higher prevalence of 443 cases/million in 2003 in the province of Quebec, Canada, using physician billing and hospitalization databases and applying statistical modeling to address issues related to incomplete case ascertainment. Although the use of such administrative databases has value in epidemiology research, it is not yet clear that appropriate statistical models have been developed to provide reliable prevalence estimates.

Similar to the recent US figures noted above, studies from Australia have reported a prevalence of 200 cases/million and 233 cases/million for 1993 and 1999, respectively, using surveys conducted by the same group [14, 15]. However, an earlier study from Sydney [16] had reported a much lower prevalence of 45/million for 1975 and 86/million for 1988. This rather large difference may be explained by different methods of case finding as the earlier figures were based on hospital record review while the latter used multiple sources.

These figures are in marked contrast to incidence and prevalence figures reported in Japan. Tamaki et al. [12] conducted a survey based on a medical database and reported an incidence rate of 7.2 cases/million/year with a prevalence of 38–53 cases/million.

In the United Kingdom, two studies have reported prevalence estimates of 31 cases/million in 1986 [26] and 88 cases/million in 2000 [37].

Two Scandinavian studies have reported remarkably similar incidence rates of 3.8 cases/million/year in Iceland [11] and 3.7 in Finland [10]. Only the Icelandic study calculated a prevalence figure of 71 cases/million.

Three studies in Europe have reported occurrence figures, with similar prevalence estimates for France [39] and Greece [22] at 158 and 154 cases/million, respectively. A recent study in northwestern Spain [17] reported a prevalence of 277/million suggesting that there may be a geographic north–south gradient.

In addition, incidence and prevalence data from Northeastern Italy were found to be higher than reported in various geographical areas (UK, US, Australia) but similar to other Italian studies [23]. Similar results were found in a recent nationwide population-based study, which looked at SSc incidence, prevalence, and mortality, and the results were aligned with previous published research [24].

A study from the Dominican Republic [48] reported a significantly lower prevalence of 9.3 per million as compared to estimates reported in the United States and Canada as shown above.

Some of the geographic variance may be explained by unique features related to the population in the region. For example, Arnett et al. [32] reported a well-defined population of Choctaw Indians in Oklahoma with a high prevalence of SSc reported as 658.6 cases/million. The prevalence of SSc in the Choctaw group was higher than that reported in other Native Americans in Oklahoma. In addition, SSc disease expression was more uniform among these cases than in the general population, with most Choctaw cases having diffuse cutaneous disease and pulmonary fibrosis. No common exposure was found but a particular Amerindian histocompatibility locus antigen (HLA) haplotype was identified suggesting a genetic predisposition to disease. In addition to the Native Americans, a First Nations population in Alberta, Canada, also had a higher than expected prevalence reported at 580 cases/million [34]. Genetic studies have not been done in the First Nations group, but it is intriguing to speculate that shared genetic ancestry with a particular risk allele or alleles may be responsible.

Clusters

The phenomenon of clustering in epidemiology refers to a higher than expected number of cases in a specific subpopulation defined by shared geographic, occupational, or ethnic features. There have been multiple reports of SSc clustering.

A high SSc prevalence was reported in boroughs close to major airports near London [50], with an estimated prevalence of 150 cases/million in the three boroughs near the airports, compared to a prevalence of 30.8 cases/million in more distant areas. Although the clusters were seen near the airports, they did not involve airport employees and factors responsible for the clustering have not been identified.

Similarly, an increased prevalence of scleroderma was reported in the town of Woodstock, Ontario, Canada, compared to two nearby communities also in southwestern Ontario [35]. Explanatory factors in terms of occupation and health habits were not identified.

Two other clusters have been reported: one in Western Victoria, Australia [29] and one in rural Italy [51], but both involved a relatively small number of cases such that population estimates based on these figures may be unreliable.

Survival

Survival rates have recently been reported to have improved significantly compared to earlier published reports. According to Steen and Medsger [52], the 10-year cumulative survival rate improved in their Pittsburg cohort from 54% in the 1970s to 66% in the 1990s. Figure 2.1, adapted from Steen and Medsger, illustrates the changes in causes of systemic sclerosis-related deaths between 1972 and 2001.

Another study from a large Italian cohort showed similar improvement in survival rates, increasing from 60.6% in the period 1955–1985 to 78.6% during 1986–1999 [53]. This improvement in survival is likely related to earlier diagnosis and improvement in treatment, particularly the early detection and effective therapy of scleroderma renal crisis. Steen and Medsger [52] reported changes in organ-specific causes of mortality and found that pulmonary fibrosis and pulmonary hypertension had become the leading causes of SSc-related deaths as opposed to SSc renal crisis following the

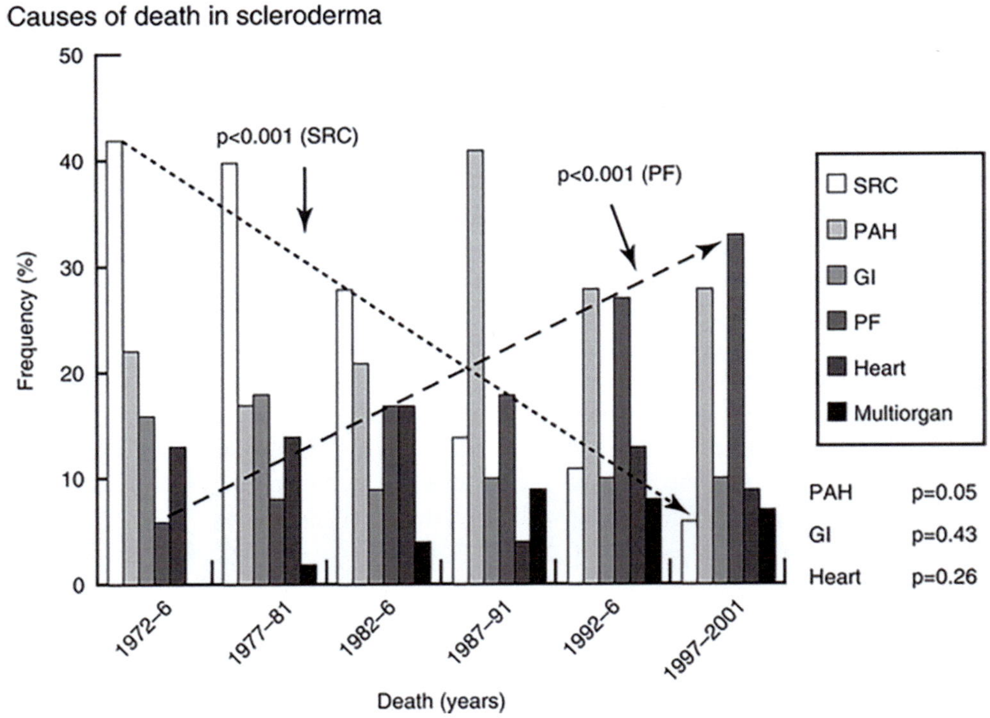

Fig. 2.1 Changes in causes of systemic sclerosis-related deaths between 1972 and 2001. *GI* gastrointestinal, *PAH* pulmonary arterial hypertension, *PF* pulmonary fibrosis, and *SRC* scleroderma renal crisis (with permission from Steen and Medsger [52])

introduction of treatment with angiotensin-converting enzyme inhibitors. Similarly, a study by Nihtyanova et al. [54] showed improved 5-year survival in the United Kingdom among dcSSc patients from 69% (1990–1993) to 84% (2000–2003), while no difference in 5-year survival in the lcSSc patients was observed.

Even with higher rates of survival found in these reports, the overall survival in SSc remains considerably less than that predicted for age-, sex-, and race-matched controls [7]. Multiple recent meta-analysis and systematic reviews studied mortality among SSc patients and confirmed this higher mortality. Elhai et al. [55] showed in their meta-analysis published in 2012 an SMR of 3.5. Similarly, Pokeerbux et al. [56] showed a similar result in their recent meta-analysis published in 2019 with an SMR of 3.45. In these two meta-analyses, there was no improvement in mortality with time. However, Komocsi et al. [57] showed different results in a meta-analysis published in 2012 with a trend for improvement in survival with lower SMR numbers in recent years. Similar trends were also observed in a recent epidemiological study that used the Center for Disease Control (CDC) Wonder Underlying Cause of Death database and its query system. This study showed that SSc-related mortality has decreased from 6.7/million in 1999 to 2.3/million in 2017 [58].

Survival: Prognostic Factors

In a recent 2010 analysis of 234 fatalities from the EUSTAR (EULAR Scleroderma Trials and Research) database, Tyndall et al. [59] reported the following independent risk factors for mortality: proteinuria, pulmonary arterial hypertension, restrictive pulmonary disease, dyspnea greater than New York Heart Association Class II, decreased pulmonary diffusing capacity, higher age at onset of Raynaud's phenomenon, and greater modified Rodnan skin score. A report by Domsic et al. in 2011 [60] found that a higher rate of progression of skin thickening (skin thickness progression rate) was a predictor of mortality and early internal organ involvement particularly the development of renal crisis.

In a 2012 Pennsylvania study, early mortality was seen in SSc patients with significant muscle and cardiac disease, anticentromere antibody negativity and time to first non-Raynaud's phenomenon symptoms [61]. Similar results were shown by Komocsi et al. in a meta-analysis published in 2012 [57]. It identified cardiac disease as the dominant cause of death in SSc followed by interstitial lung disease, pulmonary hypertension, and renal disease, respectively.

In a 2013 Norwegian cohort of SSc patients factors that trended toward a worse outcome included: pulmonary hypertension, male sex, diffuse disease, and interstitial lung disease [62]. There have been several studies that have found that lung disease was a main prognostic factor associated with death [59, 61–66].

Similar results have been reported in studies from South Australia [61], in a meta-analysis from cases from the United States, Europe, and Japan [67], in French Canadians [68], and in cases from the United Kingdom [69].

In 2014, a meta-analysis by Rubio-Rivas and colleagues [70] identified eight poor prognostic factors. These factors included ILD, pulmonary arterial hypertension (PAH), dcSSc, older age, kidney involvement, heart involvement, male gender, and high erythrocyte sedimentation rate (ESR). Similar findings were found in a French cohort reported by Elhai et al. [71] in 2017. Thirteen poor prognostic factors were identified as follows: age, male sex, dcSSc, elevated C-reactive protein (CRP), class II-IV dyspnea, ILD, low diffusion in liters of carbon monoxide (DLCO), low forced vital capacity (FVC), proteinuria, SRC, depressed left ventricular ejection fraction, digital ulcers, and joint involvement. Another report from a French cohort identified the following as poor prognostic factors: age at diagnosis greater than 60, dcSSc subtype, telangiectasia, SRC, severe dyspnea (New York Heart Association class III and IV), a shorter distance at the 6-min walk test, forced vital capacity <70% predicted, DLCO <70%, PAH, valvular disease, anemia, CRP >8 mg/L, and cancer [56]. The same group published a meta-analysis which included 36 studies and marked 11 poor prognostic factors. These factors were: age at disease onset, age at diagnosis, male sex, African origin, dcSSc subtype, anti-Scl70 antibodies, renal involvement, scleroderma renal crisis (SRC), ILD, cardiac involvement, PAH, and cancer.

With respect to race, African-American (AA) patients have higher mortality compared to their white counterparts [7, 72] believed due to more aggressive disease and perhaps due to health care disparities between these groups. A study in 2011 by Sharif et al. [73] found that African-American patients had a younger age of onset, higher frequency of digital ulcers, pericarditis, and more severe lower gastrointestinal involvement. There was also a high frequency of anti-fibrillarin antibody positivity (AFA) in the African-American patients. Those patients with AFA compared to African-Americans without AFA had less severe lung involvement. However, the presence of AFA did not change survival.

Although SSc has a higher prevalence in women, the risk of death was higher in male patients as seen in several studies [55–57]. In addition to gender, older age was identified as a predictor of mortality [55, 56, 59]. However, in a Barcelona study, after adjustment was made for population effects of age and sex, the standardized mortality ratio was found to be higher in younger patients [74].

In addition, a Japanese study has reported that SSc-gastrointestinal involvement was associated with a worse mortality [75]. Furthermore, other studies have found myositis to have an increase hazard ratio for mortality [76, 77].

With respect to pulmonary arterial hypertension (PAH) and mortality, Chung et al. found that severely reduced diffusing capacity for carbon monoxide and functional class IV at the time of PAH diagnosis were associated with a poorer prognosis [78]. In patients with SSc and interstitial lung disease (ILD), the extent of disease found on high-resolution computed topography was an independent variable that predicted both mortality and ILD progression [66]. Although monitoring for and treatment of SSc-PAH have become more common, data regarding a survival benefit from therapy are lacking. What is known, however, is that SSc patients being treated for PAH respond more poorly and have higher mortality rates than non-SSc patients with PAH [78].

Scleroderma-specific autoantibodies have been associated with both risk and survival benefit. For instance, anticentromere antibody positive patients had a better prognosis than those lacking this antibody [72, 76], while the anti-RNA polymerase III antibody was associated with scleroderma renal crisis and increased mortality [63, 79]. In another study, it was reported that antibodies to topoisomerase and U1 RNP negatively impacted survival [61]. As noted above, the anti-fibrilliarin antibody was associated with African-American SSc, but its presence did not affect survival [73].

Risk Factors for Susceptibility of SSc

Risk factors for the development of SSc include gender, race, age, family history, birth order, and environmental factors including occupational exposures and possibly infections.

Risk Factors: Female Gender

As reported in Table 2.1, all epidemiology studies that have reported gender have noted that women outnumber men with female to male ratios usually being 4:1–6:1. The reason for this female preponderance is not well understood. There is speculation that the difference may be related to hormones, pregnancy-related events, or gender-specific environmental exposures.

There are relatively few published reports that have investigated the relationship of pregnancy with development of SSc. A Swedish population-based study found that nulliparity was associated with an increased risk of SSc (OR = 1.37, 95% CI = 1.22–1.55), whereas increasing parity was associated with a decreased risk [80]. However, the increased risk with lower parity could also be explained by infertility due to subclinical or early disease. A more recent study by Cockrill et al. [81] compared pregnancy histories of SSc patients (n = 172) with that of their healthy sisters (n = 256) and found a positive association between gravidity and the risk of SSc (OR = 2.8, 95% CI 1.62–6.61). Furthermore, a systematic review by Russo et al. [82] showed no association between parity, birth order, age at first pregnancy, and the development of SSc.

The role of sex hormones was also proposed as a potential factor contributing to the higher prevalence of SSc among females, but data are still scarce. A recent systematic review by Ciaffi et al. [83] included 30 articles and looked at sex hormones in SSc patients. The report suggested that estrogen has a potential role through pro-fibrotic effects and a vasodilatory role in SSc, which could explain the higher prevalence of PAH and the skin loosening in postmenopausal women.

Microchimerism, the persistence of fetal cells in maternal tissues, with a subsequent immune response to non-self antigens, has been proposed as a trigger for scleroderma or other autoimmune diseases [84], and it has been suggested as an explanation for the increased female to male ratio in these diseases. However, the mechanism responsible for this association has not been identified.

Risk Factors: Race

In the Michigan study previously noted above, Mayes et al. [7] reported a higher prevalence among African-Americans compared to European-Americans with an adjusted prevalence ratio of 1.15 (95% CI 1.02–1.30). In addition, the proportion of diffuse disease was higher in black patients versus white and age at diagnosis was earlier (43.8 years for black patients vs. 55.5 years for white patients, $p < 0.001$). The same observation was also made by Gelber et al. in 2013 [85]. In another study, pulmonary fibrosis was more severe at diagnosis among African-Americans than in other ethnic groups [86].

Similar findings were described by Le Guern et al. [39] who reported a prevalence of SSc for non-Europeans (Northern and sub-Saharan African, Asians, and Caribbean ancestries) as 210.8 cases/million versus the prevalence for European Caucasians at 140.2 cases/million. In addition, as seen with prior studies, non-Europeans were more likely to have diffuse SSc (34% vs. 17%) and interstitial lung disease (53% vs. 33%).

Recent data published by Al-Sheikh et al. [87] showed variable disease manifestations among different ethnic groups (Europeans, Afro-Caribbean, South- and East-Asians, Hispanics, and Arabs) without a difference in short-term survival rates. Similar findings were reported from the data of two big randomized controlled trials suggesting that mortality did no't differ between African-American (AA) and non-AA in SSc patients with interstitial lung disease (ILD) when both groups were treated aggressively. Conversely, Chung et al. and her group reported in a recent retrospective study, conducted in US Kaiser Permanente adults, a higher mortality rate among Asian, Hispanic and black SSc patients compared to Whites.

Racial differences in disease susceptibility and expression can be a reflection of genetic differences among groups. Genetic risk factors are discussed in detail in another section of this book.

Risk Factors: Age at Onset

Systemic sclerosis is rare in childhood with a peak age of onset in the fifth to seventh decades [7]. A recent systematic review [88] included nine studies and reported disease onset at ages ranging between 33.5 and 59.8 years with the mean age of 46.1 [7] and 49.1 [8] in two studies done in North America. Moreover, data suggested that African-American patients were significantly younger at the time of diagnosis compared with European-American patients [7]. Figure 2.2 adapted from Mayes et al. [14] illustrates peak incidence by race and gender. The peak incidence occurred between the ages of 45 and 54 for African-American women, whereas the peak incidence among white women occurred in the 65–74-year age group. Peak incidence for African-American men was similar to that of African-American women. Among the European-American men, a gradually increasing incidence until the age of 75–84 years was observed.

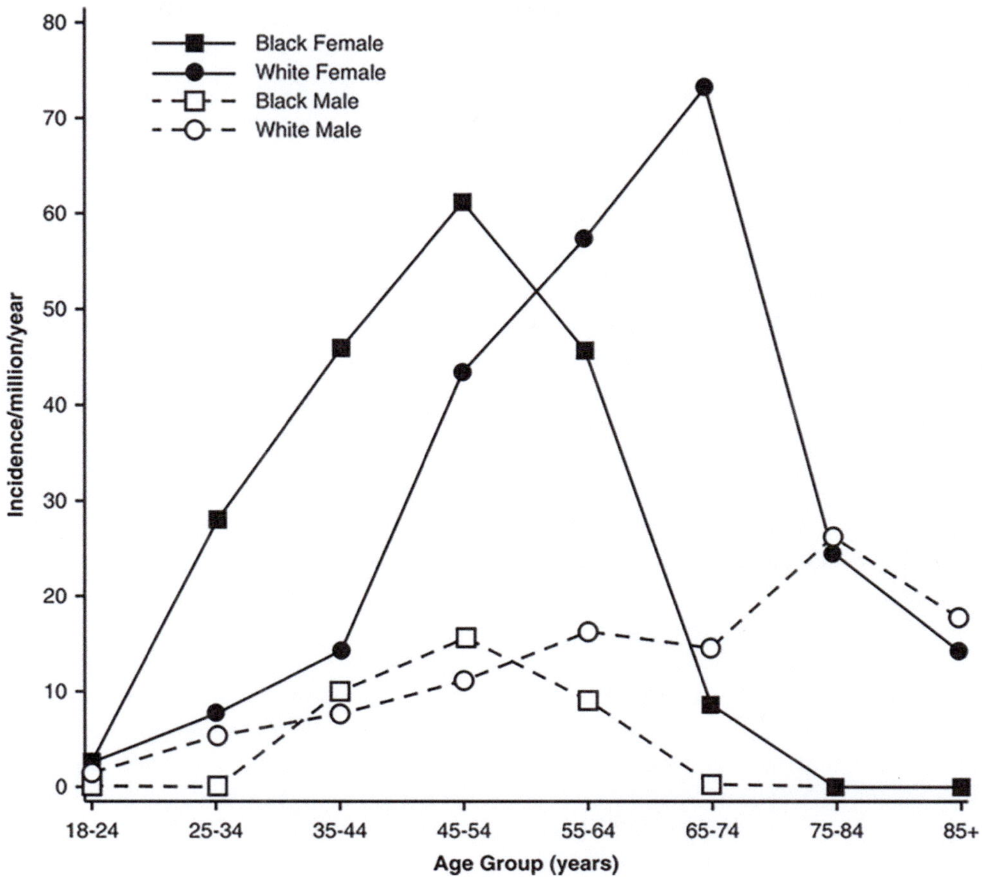

Fig. 2.2 Age-specific incidence of systemic sclerosis by race and sex (adapted with permission from Mayes et al. [7])

Familial Risk

In any discussion regarding heritability of disease, it is worthwhile to compare disease frequency between monozygotic (identical) and dizygotic (fraternal) twins in order to distinguish genetic from environmental factors. This is difficult to do in a rare disease and only one such twin study has been reported in SSc. Feghali-Bostwick et al. [89] studied 42 twin pairs (24 monozygotic twin pairs and 18 dizygotic pairs) in which at least 1 twin had SSc. They reported an overall concordance rate of 4.7% which did not differ between monozygotic and dizygotic twins. However, the number of twin pairs in this study was relatively small and may have underestimated the recurrence rate.

Although there are several reports of multicase SSc families, there are only four studies that have investigated heritability in a large case cohort. Most recently, Frech et al. [90] studied 1037 unique SSc cases and, linking the Utah Population Database and billing codes from the University of Utah Health Science Center Data Warehouse, reported a relative risk of SSc among first-degree relatives as 3.07 (95% CI 1.25–7.57, $p = 0.0148$). In addition, increased relative risks were found for multiple other autoimmune diseases. An Australian study [91] of 353 SSc cases reported a relative risk for SSc among first-degree family members of 14.3 (95% CI 5.9–34.5) which is remarkably similar to an earlier US study by Arnett et al. [92] of 703 families that found a relative risk of 13 (95% CI 2.9–48.6, $p < 0.001$) for SSc among first-degree family members. In addition, the relative risk among African-American families was greater than among whites in this study but this difference did not reach statistical significance. A fourth study using cases from Canada and Columbia [93] found increased frequency of multiple autoimmune disease in family members but did not find an increased relative risk for SSc.

To determine if familial scleroderma differed from spontaneously occurring disease, Assassi et al. [94] compared disease type, organ involvement, and autoantibody status among 18 familial SSc cases and 692 sporadic cases. SSc families tended to be concordant for SSc-specific autoantibodies and HLA haplotypes, but otherwise familial SSc did not appear to be a unique disease subset.

A recent systematic review looking at SSc risk factors identified family history as a positive risk factor. Seven studies showed positive association, with four of these studies suggesting that it is the strongest risk factor to develop SSc with odds ratio ranging between 10 and 16 [95].

Birth Order

Birth order has been found to be a risk factor for allergy and atopy [96] with first-born offspring more likely to have atopic disease than subsequent children in the family. The role of birth order in SSc susceptibility was reported by Cockrill et al. [81], who studied 974 sibships and found that the opposite situation held in scleroderma. The risk of SSc increased with increasing birth order with an odds ratio of 1.25 (95% CI 1.06–1.50) for birth order 2–5, an odds ratio of 2.22 (95% CI 1.57–3.15) for birth order 6–9, and an odds ratio of 3.53 (95% CI 1.68–7.45) for birth order 10–15. However, a study by Russo et al. did not find a statistically significant relationship between SSc and birth order for men or women, and no association with parity in females [82]. The inconsistency between these two reports is difficult to explain and must await further studies in multiple cohorts.

Risk Factors: Environmental Triggers

Table 2.4 summarizes the well-documented environmental associations with SSc and SSc-like illnesses. Although there have been several case reports of SSc occurring after exposure to various other agents that are not listed here, this table is meant to highlight the few exposures that have been reported in multiple studies and for which an association with SSc can be considered firm.

Table 2.4 Environmental exposures associated with SSc or SSc-like illnesses

Exposure	Disease	Evidence (reference)
Crystalline silica/ silica dust	SSc	Meta-analysis [95, 97, 98]
Solvents	SSc	Meta-analysis [95, 99]
Vinyl chloride monomer	Vinyl chloride disease	Investigation of outbreak [100]
Adulterated cooking oil	Toxic oil syndrome	Investigation of outbreak [101]
Tryptophan	Eosinophilic myalgia syndrome	Investigation of outbreak [102, 103]
Gadolinium	Nephrogenic systemic fibrosis	Multiple case series [104–106]
Drugs		
Bleomycin	Pulmonary fibrosis	Multiple observations [107, 108]
Pentazocine	Localized dermal fibrosis at injection site	Multiple observations [109, 110]

Silica

As noted above, numerous environmental factors have been associated with SSc in case reports and small case series, but few have been verified in case–control studies. One of the most frequently reported exposures to be associated with SSc is silica. Occupational exposure to particulate silica or silica dust occurs in professions such as mining, sandblasting, and pottery. In fact, silica has been associated as a risk factor for several autoimmune diseases including rheumatoid arthritis, systemic lupus erythematosus, and small vessel vasculitis [111] in addition to SSc. In a meta-analysis published by McCormic et al. [112], the relative risk of developing SSc after exposure to silica was elevated only for men at 3.02 (95% CI 1.24–7.35). This association was not seen in women with exposure to silica who had a minimal and insignificant elevation in relative risk of 1.03% (95% CI 0.74–1.44). Although this meta-analysis found considerable heterogeneity among the studies, it does indicate that silica exposure may be a true risk factor for developing SSc at least in some men. A prospective study to evaluate the association between SSc and occupation exposure by Marie et al. revealed that silica, white spirit, aromatic solvents, trichloroethylene, ketones, and welding fumes had increased odds ratio for development of SSc [97] but only in male patients. In female patients, an association was found with some of these exposures including white spirit, aromatic solvents, any solvents, and ketones. However, these exposures were only identified in a relatively small number of patients and still do not explain the vast majority of cases particularly in most women who comprise over 80% of SSc cases and men who have had no such exposure. Similar findings were reported in the systematic review by Abbot et al. [95], in which 14 studies examined silica as a risk factor for SSc. Nine studies reported positive association (OR 3.2–25) between exposure to silica and the development of SSc (both men and women) and two studies suggested increased risk in men only.

Although case reports suggested a possible association between silicone breast implants and SSc, multiple studies as described in a meta-analysis by Janowsky et al. [97, 98] have clearly disproved this association.

Solvents

Since 1957, there have been over 100 published articles on the possible association between exposure to various chemical solvents and the subsequent development of SSc. A meta-analysis of 11 case–control studies by Kettaneh et al. [99] involving 1291 cases and 3335 controls was performed. The conclusion from this meta-analysis is that there is indeed an increased risk of SSc both for men and women, and that this risk was greater for male cases than for female cases: for men the odds ratio for solvent exposure was 2.96 (95% CI 1.893–4.64, $p < 0.0001$) and for women the odds ratio was 1.75 (95% CI 1.48–2.09, $p < 0.0001$). The authors were unable to conduct separate analyses for specific solvent subtypes, due to the limited number of studies for each solvent category. The mechanism underlying this association is unclear, but it has been speculated that solvents could alter native molecules to generate self-antigens that would in turn initiate an autoimmune response.

The same results were replicated in Abbot's systematic review, in which organic solvents were found to be positively associated with the risk of developing SSc with odds ratios ranging between 2.07 and 2.91 [95].

Exposures and Scleroderma-Like Syndromes

In addition to case reports of SSc occurring after contact with various chemicals, the impetus to study environmental exposures has come from reports of scleroderma-like diseases that have occurred in an epidemic fashion and that have resulted from an identified source.

Vinyl Chloride Disease

In the mid-1960s, a syndrome was described in factory workers employed in the plastics industry involving exposure to vinyl chloride in the process of converting the monomer to the stable polyvinyl chloride form. The workers developed paresthesias, Raynaud's phenomenon, skin thickening, edema of the hands and forearms, pseudo-acropachy, and phalanx acro-osteolysis [100]. The risk of developing these symptoms was related to cumulative exposure over time. Once the association was identified and changes made in the manufacturing process to protect workers, this syndrome has virtually disappeared.

Toxic Oil Syndrome

A review by Posada de la Paz et al. [101] described an epidemic illness that occurred in 1981 in Spain that was a progressive multisystem disease affecting over 20,000 people and resulting in hundreds of deaths. The causative agent was traced to rapeseed oil that had been contaminated with aniline and illicitly sold as cooking oil. People who consumed this toxic oil developed pulmonary edema, myalgias, rash, cardiomyopathy, vasculopathy, and pulmonary hypertension. Once the causative agent was identified and removed from the market, the epidemic resolved.

L-Tryptophan and Eosinophilia-Myalgia Syndrome

Another scleroderma-like illness, the Eosinophilia-Myalgia Syndrome [102, 103], occurred in the United States in 1984–1989 and was traced to a nutritional supplement containing L-tryptophan that had a contaminant introduced in the manufacturing process. Characteristics of the illness included sclerodermatous skin thickening, sensorimotor polyneuropathy, proximal myopathy, severe myalgias, and peripheral eosinophilia. The prospective study by Marie et al. mentioned above did not find an association between L-tryptophan exposure and SSc [97].

Again, once the causal agent was identified and removed from the market in 1989, the syndrome essentially disappeared although sporadic cases are occasionally reported in the absence of use of nutritional supplements.

Gadolinium and Nephrogenic Systemic Fibrosis (see Chap. 13)

Nephrogenic Systemic Fibrosis (NSF, previously called Nephrogenic Fibrosing Dermopathy) was first reported by Cowper in 2000 [104] (for review see [105]) and characterized by rapidly progressive skin thickening with the early development of flexion contractures affecting the lower extremities more than upper extremities and typically sparing the face. Internal organ fibrosis affecting muscle, myocardium, and lung has also been reported. NSF typically occurred following administration of gadolinium contrast material for magnetic resonance imaging in the setting of renal compromise.

Prevention is the best approach, with the avoidance of gadolinium containing agents in at-risk patients, since treatment of established disease is unsatisfactory. Although the underlying pathogenic mechanism remains unclear, it is thought that fibrosis results from the activation of the transforming growth factor beta (TGF-beta) pathway [106].

Bleomycin and Pulmonary Fibrosis

Bleomycin is an antineoplastic antibiotic drug used for several types of cancer. A known side effect of this drug is pneumonitis which can be fatal [107, 108]. The central event is endothelial damage to the pulmonary vasculature and those who survive this complication usually recover completely with normalization of pulmonary function. There are several case reports that describe scleroderma or a scleroderma-like illness occurring after bleomycin therapy for neoplastic disease (for review see [104]).

This has led to the development of the bleomycin mouse model as an in vivo system to study pulmonary and lung fibrosis and to test potential agents for the treatment of human disease.

Pentazocine

Repeated injection of pentazocine, a synthetic narcotic analgesic, can cause a local fibrotic reaction affecting dermal, subcutaneous, and muscle layers in the area of administration that are suggestive of morphea rather than SSc [109]. This was first reported in 1975 [110] and since has been described in the setting of repetitive and prolonged use typically associated with narcotic abuse. The mechanism is not clear and the changes are usually irreversible.

Infection Risk

The hypothesis that infectious agents play a role in the pathogenesis of autoimmune disease has been extensively studied with mixed results. The following will review the current understanding of infections and their potential role in the development of SSc. It has been suggested that the production of SSc-specific antibodies results from an antigen-driven response due to molecular mimicry or events related to a break in immune tolerance [113]. In this review, parvovirus B19, cytomegalovirus (CMV), and *Helicobacter pylori* (*H. pylori*) are discussed.

Parvovirus B19 DNA was detected in the bone marrow of SSc patients ($n = 17/29$) and was not detected in healthy controls ($n = 0/10$) [114]. The SSc patients with bone marrow persistence of parvovirus B19 DNA had a shorter mean duration of SSc and showed more severe perivascular changes and active endothelial injury [115]. It has been suggested that parvovirus B19 viral components might play a role in activation of inflammatory pathways in monocytes, which could contribute to the development or progression of SSc-specific disease phenotypes [116]. However, since parvovirus B19 is frequently found in healthy individuals, it has been difficult to establish a causal link between this infection and disease.

CMV infection has also been postulated to contribute to SSc pathogenesis because of the virus' ability to infect endothelial and monocyte cells [115]. CMV can infect vascular endothelium leading to the development of intimal lesions as seen in mouse models. There is also a reported association with increased level of CMV-specific antibodies and SSc antibodies in patients [117] Again, there is difficulty in establishing a causal relationship between CMV infection and SSc since CMV infection is common (found in 60–90% of healthy adults), whereas SSc is a rare disease.

There has been an increased amount of interest in *Helicobacter pylori* (*H. pylori*) with respect to SSc. In one study of 26 patients that had primary Raynaud's phenomenon (RP), treatment and cure of *H. pylori* was associated with complete disappearance of RP in 17% of patients and reduction of symptoms in 72% of patients. In patients who were not cured of their *H. pylori* infection RP did not improve. There is conflicting data about *H. pylori* because other studies have not found a difference in SSc patients with and without the infection. A recent study about the effect of *H. pylori* and disease severity revealed that SSc patients with *H. pylori* infection had a higher severity score compared to those without the disease [118]. A recent meta-analysis by Yong and colleagues included 8 observational studies with a total of 1446 subjects. It was suggested that patients with SSc had an increased *H. pylori* infection as compared to healthy controls [119].

Several reports have implicated Epstein–Barr virus (EBV) in the pathogenesis of SSc. Similar to CMV virus, it is theorized that molecular mimicry leads to autoimmunity of SSc [120–122]. It has been reported that EBV is able to persistently infect human SSc fibroblast in vitro and produce an aberrant innate immune response [120]. It was also found that infectious EBV (the lytic form of EBV) is present in monocytes from SSc patient and can induce Toll-like Receptor 8 (TLR8) and interferon (IFN)-related innate immunity response, which suggests a novel mechanism in the inflammatory cascade mediated by monocytes in SSc [123]. However, EBV is also found in a large proportion of the healthy population suggesting that it may play a role but certainly is not the sole contributing factor to the development of SSc.

With respect to chlamydia infection, it has been postulated that persistent infection with this organism may play a role in SSc as it does for other inflammatory conditions. However, skin biopsies from 18 SSc patients as well as 26 controls were negative for DNA sequences for *C. trachomatis* and *C. pneumonia* [124]. In addition, a "pan-bacteria" PCR assay was used to detect a wide variety (but not all) of bacterial species and these were uniformly negative in patients and control skin.

Thus, several studies have linked various infectious diseases to SSc. These intriguing reports demonstrate associations but have failed to show a causal link. It is possible that the immune activation that occurs as part of the autoimmunity process, or even treatment of disease, may permit persistence of infections so that these organisms are the consequence of disease rather than the trigger.

Summary

Although incidence rates and prevalence estimates vary by region, these figures are fairly similar from recent reports for Europe, the United States, and Australia and suggest that prevalence is in the range of 150–300 cases/million with lower prevalence in Scandinavia, Japan, and the United Kingdom.

Incidence rates (number of new cases per year) have apparently increased from the 1940s to the present, but it is not clear if this represents a real increase in disease occurrence or if this is due to improved awareness and updated classification criteria permitting earlier diagnosis.

Survival in SSc has clearly improved over time, and this improvement is largely related to the introduction of angiotensin converting enzyme inhibitors for the treatment of scleroderma renal crisis. Interstitial lung disease and pulmonary vascular disease have replaced renal failure as the most common cause of SSc-related death. It is too early to tell if new therapies for ILD and/or earlier intervention for PAH will result in improved survival.

In terms of risk factors for disease susceptibility and severity, SSc is more common in women than in men with most reports of female to male ratios of 4:1–6:1. African ancestry as well as Choctaw Native American and Canadian First Nations ancestry are risk factors for the development of SSc, and African-Americans have more severe disease with an earlier age at onset and worst prognosis.

Familial clustering clearly suggests a genetic contribution and multiple recent studies, described elsewhere in this book, have begun to identify these factors. The finding that increasing birth order predisposes to SSc is intriguing and suggests that early exposure to infection and/or other agents may contribute to the development of SSc.

Although the evidence for an association between SSc and environmental exposure to particulate silica and chemical solvents is relatively well established, these exposures account for only a tiny percentage of all cases. Hence, the environmental trigger(s) for the majority of cases remains unknown.

Several agents have been associated with scleroderma-like illnesses, but the relevance to spontaneously occurring systemic sclerosis is unclear.

Finally, although numerous infectious agents have been implicated in the development of autoimmune disease, to date no clear relationship has been proven.

References

1. Bolster M, Silver RS. Clinical features of systemic sclerosis. Rheumatology. 2011;2:1373–86.
2. LeRoy EC, Black C, Fleischmajer R, Jablonska S, Krieg T, Medsger TA Jr, et al. Scleroderma (systemic sclerosis): classification, subsets and pathogenesis. J Rheumatol. 1988;15(2):202–5.
3. Frantz C, Huscher D, Avouac J, Hachulla E, Balbir-Gurman A, Riemekasten G, et al. Outcomes of limited cutaneous systemic sclerosis patients: results on more than 12,000 patients from the EUSTAR database. Autoimmun Rev. 2020;19(2):102452.
4. Preliminary criteria for the classification of systemic sclerosis (scleroderma). Subcommittee for scleroderma criteria of the American Rheumatism Association Diagnostic and Therapeutic Criteria Committee. Arthritis Rheum. 1980;23(5):581–90.
5. Medsger TA Jr, Masi AT. Epidemiology of systemic sclerosis (scleroderma). Ann Intern Med. 1971;74(5):714–21.
6. Furst DE, Fernandes AW, Iorga SR, Greth W, Bancroft T. Epidemiology of systemic sclerosis in a large US managed care population. J Rheumatol. 2012;39(4):784–6.
7. Mayes MD, Lacey JV Jr, Beebe-Dimmer J, Gillespie BW, Cooper B, Laing TJ, et al. Prevalence, incidence, survival, and disease characteristics of systemic sclerosis in a large US population. Arthritis Rheum. 2003;48(8):2246–55.
8. Bauer PR, Schiavo DN, Osborn TG, Levin DL, St Sauver J, Hanson AC, et al. Influence of interstitial lung disease on outcome in systemic sclerosis: a population-based historical cohort study. Chest. 2013;144(2):571–7.
9. Fan Y, Bender S, Shi W, Zoz D. Incidence and prevalence of systemic sclerosis and systemic sclerosis with interstitial lung disease in the United States. J Manag Care Spec Pharm. 2020;26(12):1539–47.
10. Kaipiainen-Seppänen O, Aho K. Incidence of rare systemic rheumatic and connective tissue diseases in Finland. J Intern Med. 1996;240(2):81–4.
11. Geirsson AJ, Steinsson K, Guthmundsson S, Sigurthsson V. Systemic sclerosis in Iceland. A nationwide epidemiological study. Ann Rheum Dis. 1994;53(8):502–5.
12. Tamaki T, Mori S, Takehara K. Epidemiological study of patients with systemic sclerosis in Tokyo. Arch Dermatol Res. 1991;283(6):366–71.
13. Steen VD, Oddis CV, Conte CG, Janoski J, Casterline GZ, Medsger TA Jr. Incidence of systemic sclerosis in Allegheny County, Pennsylvania. A twenty-year study of hospital-diagnosed cases, 1963-1982. Arthritis Rheum. 1997;40(3):441–5.
14. Roberts-Thomson PJ, Jones M, Hakendorf P, Kencana Dharmapatni AA, Walker JG, MacFarlane JG, et al. Scleroderma in South Australia: epidemiological observations of possible pathogenic significance. Intern Med J. 2001;31(4):220–9.
15. Roberts-Thomson PJ, Walker JG, Lu TY, Esterman A, Hakendorf P, Smith MD, et al. Scleroderma in South Australia: further epidemiological observations supporting a stochastic explanation. Intern Med J. 2006;36(8):489–97.
16. Englert H, Small-McMahon J, Davis K, O'Connor H, Chambers P, Brooks P. Systemic sclerosis prevalence and mortality in Sydney 1974-88. Aust NZ J Med. 1999;29(1):42–50.
17. Arias-Nunez MC, Llorca J, Vazquez-Rodriguez TR, Gomez-Acebo I, Miranda-Filloy JA, Martin J, et al. Systemic sclerosis in northwestern Spain: a 19-year epidemiologic study. Medicine (Baltimore). 2008;87(5):272–80.
18. Rosa JE, Soriano ER, Narvaez-Ponce L, del Cid CC, Imamura PM, Catoggio LJ. Incidence and prevalence of systemic sclerosis in a healthcare plan in Buenos Aires. J Clin Rheumatol. 2011;17(2):59–63.
19. Michet CJ Jr, McKenna CH, Elveback LR, Kaslow RA, Kurland LT. Epidemiology of systemic lupus erythematosus and other connective tissue diseases in Rochester, Minnesota, 1950 through 1979. Mayo Clin Proc. 1985;60(2):105–13.
20. Laing TJ, Gillespie BW, Toth MB, Mayes MD, Gallavan RH, Burns CJ, et al. Racial differences in scleroderma among women in Michigan. Arthritis Rheum. 1997;40(4):734–42.
21. Andréasson K, Saxne T, Bergknut C, Hesselstrand R, Englund M. Prevalence and incidence of systemic sclerosis in southern Sweden: population-based data with case ascertainment using the

1980 ARA criteria and the proposed ACR-EULAR classification criteria. Ann Rheum Dis. 2014;73(10):1788–92.
22. Alamanos Y, Tsifetaki N, Voulgari PV, Siozos C, Tsamandouraki K, Alexiou GA, et al. Epidemiology of systemic sclerosis in northwest Greece 1981 to 2002. Semin Arthritis Rheum. 2005;34(5):714–20.
23. Lo Monaco A, Bruschi M, La Corte R, Volpinari S, Trotta F. Epidemiology of systemic sclerosis in a district of northern Italy. Clin Exp Rheumatol. 2011;29(2 Suppl 65):S10–4.
24. Ciaffi J, Morabito MF, Ruscitti P, D'Angelo S, Mancarella L, Brusi V, et al. Incidence, prevalence and mortality of systemic sclerosis in Italy: a nationwide population-based study using administrative health data. Rheumatol Int. 2020;
25. Vonk MC, Broers B, Heijdra YF, Ton E, Snijder R, van Dijk AP, et al. Systemic sclerosis and its pulmonary complications in The Netherlands: an epidemiological study. Ann Rheum Dis. 2009;68(6):961–5.
26. Silman A, Jannini S, Symmons D, Bacon P. An epidemiological study of scleroderma in the West Midlands. Br J Rheumatol. 1988;27(4):286–90.
27. Wigley R, Borman B. Medical geography and the aetiology of the rare connective tissue diseases in New Zealand. Soc Sci Med Geogr. 1980;14(2):175–83.
28. Eason RJ, Tan PL, Gow PJ. Progressive systemic sclerosis in Auckland: a ten year review with emphasis on prognostic features. Aust NZ J Med. 1981;11(6):657–62.
29. Englert H, Joyner E, Bade R, Thompson M, Morris D, Chambers P, et al. Systemic scleroderma: a spatiotemporal clustering. Intern Med J. 2005;35(4):228–33.
30. Bernatsky S, Joseph L, Pineau CA, Belisle P, Hudson M, Clarke AE. Scleroderma prevalence: demographic variations in a population-based sample. Arthritis Rheum. 2009;61(3):400–4.
31. Avina-Zubieta A, Saure EC, Bernatsky S, Lehman AJ, Shoja K, Esdaile J, et al. Adult Prevalence of Systemic Autoimmune Rheumatic Diseases (SARDs) in British Columbia, Canada [Abstract]. Arthritis Rheum. 2011;63(suppl 10):S719.
32. Arnett FC, Howard RF, Tan F, Moulds JM, Bias WB, Durban E, et al. Increased prevalence of systemic sclerosis in a Native American tribe in Oklahoma. Association with an Amerindian HLA haplotype. Arthritis Rheum. 1996;39(8):1362–70.
33. Robinson D Jr, Eisenberg D, Nietert PJ, Doyle M, Bala M, Paramore C, et al. Systemic sclerosis prevalence and comorbidities in the US, 2001-2002. Curr Med Res Opin. 2008;24(4):1157–66.
34. Barnabe C, Joseph L, Belisle P, Labrecque J, Edworthy S, Barr SG, et al. Prevalence of systemic lupus erythematosus and systemic sclerosis in the First Nations population of Alberta, Canada. Arthritis Care Res (Hoboken). 2012;64(1):138–43.
35. Thompson AE, Pope JE. Increased prevalence of scleroderma in southwestern Ontario: a cluster analysis. J Rheumatol. 2002;29(9):1867–73.
36. Gottschalk P, Vasquez R, Lopez PD, Then J, Tineo C, Loyo E. Scleroderma in the Caribbean: characteristics in a Dominican case series. Reumatol Clin. 2014;10(6):373–9.
37. Allcock RJ, Forrest I, Corris PA, Crook PR, Griffiths ID. A study of the prevalence of systemic sclerosis in northeast England. Rheumatology (Oxford). 2004;43(5):596–602.
38. Valter I, Saretok S, Maricq HR. Prevalence of scleroderma spectrum disorders in the general population of Estonia. Scand J Rheumatol. 1997;26(6):419–25.
39. Le Guern V, Mahr A, Mouthon L, Jeanneret D, Carzon M, Guillevin L. Prevalence of systemic sclerosis in a French multi-ethnic county. Rheumatology (Oxford). 2004;43(9):1129–37.
40. El Adssi H, Cirstea D, Virion JM, Guillemin F, de Korwin JD. Estimating the prevalence of systemic sclerosis in the Lorraine region, France, by the capture-recapture method. Semin Arthritis Rheum. 2013;42(5):530–8.
41. Radic M, Martinovic Kaliterna D, Fabijanic D, Radic J. Prevalence of systemic sclerosis in Split-Dalmatia county in Southern Croatia. Clin Rheumatol. 2010;29(4):419–21.
42. Airo P, Tabaglio E, Frassi M, Scarsi M, Danieli E, Rossi M. Prevalence of systemic sclerosis in Valtrompia in northern Italy. A collaborative study of rheumatologists and general practitioners. Clin Exp Rheumatol. 2007;25(6):878–80.
43. Eaton WW, Pedersen MG, Atladottir HO, Gregory PE, Rose NR, Mortensen PB. The prevalence of 30 ICD-10 autoimmune diseases in Denmark. Immunol Res. 2010;47(1–3):228–31.
44. Hoffmann-Vold AM, Midtvedt O, Molberg O, Garen T, Gran JT. Prevalence of systemic sclerosis in south-east Norway. Rheumatology (Oxford). 2012;51(9):1600–5.
45. Kuo CF, See LC, Yu KH, Chou IJ, Tseng WY, Chang HC, et al. Epidemiology and mortality of systemic sclerosis: a nationwide population study in Taiwan. Scand J Rheumatol. 2011;40(5):373–8.
46. Sardu C, Cocco E, Mereu A, Massa R, Cuccu A, Marrosu MG, et al. Population based study of 12 autoimmune diseases in Sardinia, Italy: prevalence and comorbidity. PLoS One. 2012;7(3):e32487.
47. Minz RW, Kumar Y, Anand S, Singh S, Bamberi P, Verma S, et al. Antinuclear antibody positive autoimmune disorders in North India: an appraisal. Rheumatol Int. 2012;32(9):2883–8.
48. Gottschalk P, Vásquez R, López PD, Then J, Tineo C, Loyo E. Scleroderma in the Caribbean: characteristics in a Dominican case series. Reumatol Clin. 2014;10(6):373–9.
49. Maricq HR, Weinrich MC, Keil JE, Smith EA, Harper FE, Nussbaum AI, et al. Prevalence of scleroderma spectrum disorders in the general population of South Carolina. Arthritis Rheum. 1989;32(8):998–1006.
50. Silman AJ, Howard Y, Hicklin AJ, Black C. Geographical clustering of scleroderma in south and west London. Br J Rheumatol. 1990;29(2):93–6.
51. Valesini G, Litta A, Bonavita MS, Luan FL, Purpura M, Mariani M, et al. Geographical clustering of scleroderma in a rural area in the province of Rome. Clin Exp Rheumatol. 1993;11(1):41–7.
52. Steen VD, Medsger TA. Changes in causes of death in systemic sclerosis, 1972-2002. Ann Rheum Dis. 2007;66(7):940–4.
53. Ferri C, Valentini G, Cozzi F, Sebastiani M, Michelassi C, La Montagna G, et al. Systemic sclerosis: demographic, clinical, and serologic features and survival in 1,012 Italian patients. Medicine (Baltimore). 2002;81(2):139–53.
54. Nihtyanova SI, Tang EC, Coghlan JG, Wells AU, Black CM, Denton CP. Improved survival in systemic sclerosis is associated with better ascertainment of internal organ disease: a retrospective cohort study. QJM. 2010;103(2):109–15.
55. Elhai M, Meune C, Avouac J, Kahan A, Allanore Y. Trends in mortality in patients with systemic sclerosis over 40 years: a systematic review and meta-analysis of cohort studies. Rheumatology (Oxford). 2012;51(6):1017–26.
56. Pokeerbux MR, Giovannelli J, Dauchet L, Mouthon L, Agard C, Lega JC, et al. Survival and prognosis factors in systemic sclerosis: data of a French multicenter cohort, systematic review, and meta-analysis of the literature. Arthritis Res Ther. 2019;21(1):86.
57. Komocsi A, Vorobcsuk A, Faludi R, Pinter T, Lenkey Z, Kolto G, et al. The impact of cardiopulmonary manifestations on the mortality of SSc: a systematic review and meta-analysis of observational studies. Rheumatology (Oxford). 2012;51(6):1027–36.
58. Rodriguez-Pla A, Simms RW. Geographic Disparitis in Systemic Sclerosis Mortality in the United States: 1999 to 2017 [Abstract]. Arthritis Rheumatol. 2019; 71 (suppl 10).
59. Tyndall AJ, Bannert B, Vonk M, Airò P, Cozzi F, Carreira PE, et al. Causes and risk factors for death in systemic sclerosis: a study from the EULAR Scleroderma Trials and Research (EUSTAR) database. Ann Rheum Dis. 2010;69(10):1809–15.
60. Domsic RT, Rodriguez-Reyna T, Lucas M, Fertig N, Medsger TA Jr. Skin thickness progression rate: a predictor of mortality

and early internal organ involvement in diffuse scleroderma. Ann Rheum Dis. 2011;70(1):104–9.
61. Hissaria P, Lester S, Hakendorf P, Woodman R, Patterson K, Hill C, et al. Survival in scleroderma: results from the population-based South Australian Register. Intern Med J. 2011;41(5):381–90.
62. Hoffmann-Vold AM, Molberg Ø, Midtvedt Ø, Garen T, Gran JT. Survival and causes of death in an unselected and complete cohort of Norwegian patients with systemic sclerosis. J Rheumatol. 2013;40(7):1127–33.
63. Strickland G, Pauling J, Cavill C, Shaddick G, McHugh N. Mortality in systemic sclerosis-a single centre study from the UK. Clin Rheumatol. 2013;32(10):1533–9.
64. Sampaio-Barros PD, Bortoluzzo AB, Marangoni RG, Rocha LF, Del Rio AP, Samara AM, et al. Survival, causes of death, and prognostic factors in systemic sclerosis: analysis of 947 Brazilian patients. J Rheumatol. 2012;39(10):1971–8.
65. Foocharoen C, Mahakkanukrauh A, Suwannaroj S, Nanagara R. Clinical characteristics and mortality in systemic sclerosis: a comparison between early- and late-referred diseases. J Med Assoc Thail. 2014;97(1):28–35.
66. Winstone TA, Assayag D, Wilcox PG, Dunne JV, Hague CJ, Leipsic J, et al. Predictors of mortality and progression in scleroderma-associated interstitial lung disease: a systematic review. Chest. 2014;146(2):422–36.
67. Ioannidis JP, Vlachoyiannopoulos PG, Haidich AB, Medsger TA, Lucas M, Michet CJ, et al. Mortality in systemic sclerosis: an international meta-analysis of individual patient data. Am J Med. 2005;118(1):2–10.
68. Scussel-Lonzetti L, Joyal F, Raynauld JP, Roussin A, Rich E, Goulet JR, et al. Predicting mortality in systemic sclerosis: analysis of a cohort of 309 French Canadian patients with emphasis on features at diagnosis as predictive factors for survival. Medicine (Baltimore). 2002;81(2):154–67.
69. Bryan C, Knight C, Black CM, Silman AJ. Prediction of five-year survival following presentation with scleroderma: development of a simple model using three disease factors at first visit. Arthritis Rheum. 1999;42(12):2660–5.
70. Rubio-Rivas M, Royo C, Simeón CP, Corbella X, Fonollosa V. Mortality and survival in systemic sclerosis: systematic review and meta-analysis. Semin Arthritis Rheum. 2014;44(2):208–19.
71. Elhai M, Meune C, Boubaya M, Avouac J, Hachulla E, Balbir-Gurman A, et al. Mapping and predicting mortality from systemic sclerosis. Ann Rheum Dis. 2017;76(11):1897–905.
72. Mendoza F, Derk CT. Systemic sclerosis mortality in the United States: 1999-2002 implications for patient care. J Clin Rheumatol. 2007;13(4):187–92.
73. Sharif R, Fritzler MJ, Mayes MD, Gonzalez EB, McNearney TA, Draeger H, et al. Anti-fibrillarin antibody in African American patients with systemic sclerosis: immunogenetics, clinical features, and survival analysis. J Rheumatol. 2011;38(8):1622–30.
74. Alba MA, Velasco C, Simeón CP, Fonollosa V, Trapiella L, Egurbide MV, et al. Early- versus late-onset systemic sclerosis: differences in clinical presentation and outcome in 1037 patients. Medicine (Baltimore). 2014;93(2):73–81.
75. Hashimoto A, Tejima S, Tono T, Suzuki M, Tanaka S, Matsui T, et al. Predictors of survival and causes of death in Japanese patients with systemic sclerosis. J Rheumatol. 2011;38(9):1931–9.
76. Derk CT, Huaman G, Littlejohn J, Otieno F, Jimenez S. Predictors of early mortality in systemic sclerosis: a case-control study comparing early versus late mortality in systemic sclerosis. Rheumatol Int. 2012;32(12):3841–4.
77. Foocharoen C, Nanagara R, Kiatchoosakun S, Suwannaroj S, Mahakkanukrauh A. Prognostic factors of mortality and 2-year survival analysis of systemic sclerosis with pulmonary arterial hypertension in Thailand. Int J Rheum Dis. 2011;14(3):282–9.
78. Chung L, Farber HW, Benza R, Miller DP, Parsons L, Hassoun PM, et al. Unique predictors of mortality in patients with pulmonary arterial hypertension associated with systemic sclerosis in the REVEAL registry. Chest. 2014;146(6):1494–504.
79. Hesselstrand R, Scheja A, Wuttge DM. Scleroderma renal crisis in a Swedish systemic sclerosis cohort: survival, renal outcome, and RNA polymerase III antibodies as a risk factor. Scand J Rheumatol. 2012;41(1):39–43.
80. Lambe M, Bjornadal L, Neregard P, Nyren O, Cooper GS. Childbearing and the risk of scleroderma: a population-based study in Sweden. Am J Epidemiol. 2004;159(2):162–6.
81. Cockrill T, del Junco DJ, Arnett FC, Assassi S, Tan FK, McNearney T, et al. Separate influences of birth order and gravidity/parity on the development of systemic sclerosis. Arthritis Care Res (Hoboken). 2010;62(3):418–24.
82. Russo PA, Lester S, Roberts-Thomson PJ. Systemic sclerosis, birth order and parity. Int J Rheum Dis. 2014;17(5):557–61.
83. Ciaffi J, van Leeuwen NM, Schoones JW, Huizinga TWJ, de Vries-Bouwstra JK. Sex hormones and sex hormone-targeting therapies in systemic sclerosis: a systematic literature review. Semin Arthritis Rheum. 2019.
84. Adams Waldorf KM, Nelson JL. Autoimmune disease during pregnancy and the microchimerism legacy of pregnancy. Immunol Investig. 2008;37(5):631–44.
85. Gelber AC, Manno RL, Shah AA, Woods A, Le EN, Boin F, et al. Race and association with disease manifestations and mortality in scleroderma: a 20-year experience at the Johns Hopkins Scleroderma Center and review of the literature. Medicine (Baltimore). 2013;92(4):191–205.
86. McNearney TA, Reveille JD, Fischbach M, Friedman AW, Lisse JR, Goel N, et al. Pulmonary involvement in systemic sclerosis: associations with genetic, serologic, sociodemographic, and behavioral factors. Arthritis Rheum. 2007;57(2):318–26.
87. Al-Sheikh H, Ahmad Z, Johnson SR. Ethnic Variations in Systemic Sclerosis Disease Manifestations, Internal Organ Involvement, and Mortality. J Rheumatol. 2019;46(9):1103–8.
88. Bergamasco A, Hartmann N, Wallace L, Verpillat P. Epidemiology of systemic sclerosis and systemic sclerosis-associated interstitial lung disease. Clin Epidemiol. 2019;11:257–73.
89. Feghali-Bostwick C, Medsger TA Jr, Wright TM. Analysis of systemic sclerosis in twins reveals low concordance for disease and high concordance for the presence of antinuclear antibodies. Arthritis Rheum. 2003;48(7):1956–63.
90. Frech T, Khanna D, Markewitz B, Mineau G, Pimentel R, Sawitzke A. Heritability of vasculopathy, autoimmune disease, and fibrosis in systemic sclerosis: a population-based study. Arthritis Rheum. 2010;62(7):2109–16.
91. Chandran G, Smith M, Ahern MJ, Roberts-Thomson PJ. A study of scleroderma in South Australia: prevalence, subset characteristics and nailfold capillaroscopy. Aust NZ J Med. 1995;25(6):688–94.
92. Arnett FC, Cho M, Chatterjee S, Aguilar MB, Reveille JD, Mayes MD. Familial occurrence frequencies and relative risks for systemic sclerosis (scleroderma) in three United States cohorts. Arthritis Rheum. 2001;44(6):1359–62.
93. Hudson M, Rojas-Villarraga A, Coral-Alvarado P, López-Guzmán S, Mantilla RD, Chalem P, et al. Polyautoimmunity and familial autoimmunity in systemic sclerosis. J Autoimmun. 2008;31(2):156–9.
94. Assassi S, Arnett FC, Reveille JD, Gourh P, Mayes MD. Clinical, immunologic, and genetic features of familial systemic sclerosis. Arthritis Rheum. 2007;56(6):2031–7.
95. Abbot S, Bossingham D, Proudman S, de Costa C, Ho-Huynh A. Risk factors for the development of systemic sclerosis: a systematic review of the literature. Rheumatol Adv Pract. 2018;2(2):rky041.

96. McKeever TM, Lewis SA, Smith C, Collins J, Heatlie H, Frischer M, et al. Siblings, multiple births, and the incidence of allergic disease: a birth cohort study using the West Midlands general practice research database. Thorax. 2001;56(10):758–62.
97. Marie I, Gehanno JF, Bubenheim M, Duval-Modeste AB, Joly P, Dominique S, et al. Prospective study to evaluate the association between systemic sclerosis and occupational exposure and review of the literature. Autoimmun Rev. 2014;13(2):151–6.
98. Janowsky EC, Kupper LL, Hulka BS. Meta-analyses of the relation between silicone breast implants and the risk of connective-tissue diseases. N Engl J Med. 2000;342(11):781–90.
99. Kettaneh A, Al Moufti O, Tiev KP, Chayet C, Tolédano C, Fabre B, et al. Occupational exposure to solvents and gender-related risk of systemic sclerosis: a metaanalysis of case-control studies. J Rheumatol. 2007;34(1):97–103.
100. Nicholson WJ, Henneberger PK, Seidman H. Occupational hazards in the VC-PVC industry. Prog Clin Biol Res. 1984;141:155–75.
101. Posada de la Paz M, Philen RM, Borda AI. Toxic oil syndrome: the perspective after 20 years. Epidemiol Rev. 2001;23(2):231–47.
102. Kilbourne EM, Philen RM, Kamb ML, Falk H. Tryptophan produced by Showa Denko and epidemic eosinophilia-myalgia syndrome. J Rheumatol Suppl. 1996;46:81–8; discussion 9–91.
103. Kaufman LD, Seidman RJ. L-tryptophan-associated eosinophilia-myalgia syndrome: perspective of a new illness. Rheum Dis Clin N Am. 1991;17(2):427–41.
104. Cowper SE, Su LD, Bhawan J, Robin HS, LeBoit PE. Nephrogenic fibrosing dermopathy. Am J Dermatopathol. 2001;23(5):383–93.
105. Chen AY, Zirwas MJ, Heffernan MP. Nephrogenic systemic fibrosis: a review. J Drugs Dermatol. 2010;9(7):829–34.
106. Schieren G, Gambichler T, Skrygan M, Burkert B, Altmeyer P, Rump LC, et al. Balance of profibrotic and antifibrotic [corrected] signaling in nephrogenic systemic fibrosis skin lesions. Am J Kidney Dis. 2010;55(6):1040–9.
107. Sleijfer S. Bleomycin-induced pneumonitis. Chest. 2001;120(2):617–24.
108. Inaoki M, Kawabata C, Nishijima C, Yoshio N, Kita T. Case of bleomycin-induced scleroderma. J Dermatol. 2012;39(5):482–4.
109. Palestine RF, Millns JL, Spigel GT, Schroeter AL. Skin manifestations of pentazocine abuse. J Am Acad Dermatol. 1980;2(1):47–55.
110. Levin BE, Engel WK. Iatrogenic muscle fibrosis. Arm levitation as an initial sign. JAMA. 1975;234(6):621–4.
111. Makol A, Reilly MJ, Rosenman KD. Prevalence of connective tissue disease in silicosis (1985-2006)-a report from the state of Michigan surveillance system for silicosis. Am J Ind Med. 2011;54(4):255–62.
112. McCormic ZD, Khuder SS, Aryal BK, Ames AL, Khuder SA. Occupational silica exposure as a risk factor for scleroderma: a meta-analysis. Int Arch Occup Environ Health. 2010;83(7):763–9.
113. Radić M, Martinović Kaliterna D, Radić J. Infectious disease as aetiological factor in the pathogenesis of systemic sclerosis. Neth J Med. 2010;68(11):348–53.
114. Zakrzewska K, Corcioli F, Carlsen KM, Giuggioli D, Fanci R, Rinieri A, et al. Human parvovirus B19 (B19V) infection in systemic sclerosis patients. Intervirology. 2009;52(5):279–82.
115. Magro CM, Nuovo G, Ferri C, Crowson AN, Giuggioli D, Sebastiani M. Parvoviral infection of endothelial cells and stromal fibroblasts: a possible pathogenetic role in scleroderma. J Cutan Pathol. 2004;31(1):43–50.
116. Zakrzewska K, Arvia R, Torcia MG, Clemente AM, Tanturli M, Castronovo G, et al. Effects of parvovirus B19 in vitro infection on monocytes from patients with systemic sclerosis: enhanced inflammatory pathways by caspase-1 activation and cytokine production. J Invest Dermatol. 2019;139(10):2125–33.e1.
117. Neidhart M, Kuchen S, Distler O, Brühlmann P, Michel BA, Gay RE, et al. Increased serum levels of antibodies against human cytomegalovirus and prevalence of autoantibodies in systemic sclerosis. Arthritis Rheum. 1999;42(2):389–92.
118. Radić M, Kaliterna DM, Bonacin D, Vergles JM, Radić J, Fabijanić D, et al. Is Helicobacter pylori infection a risk factor for disease severity in systemic sclerosis? Rheumatol Int. 2013;33(11):2943–8.
119. Yong WC, Upala S, Sanguankeo A. Helicobacter pylori infection in systemic sclerosis: a systematic review and meta-analysis of observational studies. Clin Exp Rheumatol. 2018;36 Suppl 113(4):168–74.
120. Farina A, Cirone M, York M, Lenna S, Padilla C, McLaughlin S, et al. Epstein-Barr virus infection induces aberrant TLR activation pathway and fibroblast-myofibroblast conversion in scleroderma. J Invest Dermatol. 2014;134(4):954–64.
121. Grossman C, Dovrish Z, Shoenfeld Y, Amital H. Do infections facilitate the emergence of systemic sclerosis? Autoimmun Rev. 2011;10(5):244–7.
122. Dreyfus DH, Farina A, Farina GA. Molecular mimicry, genetic homology, and gene sharing proteomic "molecular fingerprints" using an EBV (Epstein-Barr virus)-derived microarray as a potential diagnostic method in autoimmune disease. Immunol Res. 2018;66(6):686–95.
123. Farina A, Peruzzi G, Lacconi V, Lenna S, Quarta S, Rosato E, et al. Epstein-Barr virus lytic infection promotes activation of Toll-like receptor 8 innate immune response in systemic sclerosis monocytes. Arthritis Res Ther. 2017;19(1):39.
124. Mayes MD, Whittum-Hudson JA, Oszust C, Gérard HC, Hudson AP. Lack of evidence for bacterial infections in skin in patients with systemic sclerosis. Am J Med Sci. 2009;337(4):233–5.

Influence of Ethnicity and Sex Bias in Systemic Sclerosis

3

Pravitt Gourh and Cosimo Bruni

Ethnicity in SSc

Ethnic and geographic differences in the prevalence and manifestations of SSc have been observed and are similar to differences in several non-rheumatologic autoimmune diseases [1, 2]. These differences could be driven by either ancestry or environment alone or a combination of gene–environment interactions leading to a higher disease burden. Several studies have proposed ethnicity as playing a pivotal role in SSc pathogenesis.

SSc Prevalence

SSc incidence and prevalence can vary widely in different epidemiological studies depending upon the ethnicity of the population being studied. The majority of these studies have reported individuals of European descent and a limited number of studies have included non-European individuals. The variation seen in these studies could be due to the genetic differences that exist in the different ethnic populations and these hereditary factors may be the drivers of increased disease susceptibility and severe phenotypic manifestations. Generally, the SSc prevalence is reported to be lower in populations from Europe and Japan as compared to Australia and North America [3].

The highest prevalence of SSc has been reported in the Native American populations in North America. Arnett et al. were the first to report Choctaw Native Americans in southeastern Oklahoma in the USA, as having the highest prevalence of SSc with 659 cases per million, going up to 4695 cases per million in full-blooded Choctaw; in this cohort, a founder effect was hypothesized [4]. SSc was 50 times more prevalent in the Choctaw group as compared to other non-Choctaw Native Americans in Oklahoma (95 cases per million) [5]. Similar to the Choctaw Native Americans, First Nations females in Alberta, Canada, had a high prevalence of SSc at 580 cases per million [6].

African American (AA) women in Michigan have been reported to have a higher incidence of SSc as compared to European American (EA) women (22.5 versus 12.8 cases per million per year) [7] and prevalence (315 cases per million in AAs versus 225 cases per million in EAs) [8]. From the few studies describing SSc prevalence in various parts of Africa, the SSc phenotype in Africans seems to be very similar to AAs and different from EAs [9, 10].

SSc prevalence in Europe is variable according to country, ranging from 71 cases per million in Iceland [11], 31 [12] to 88 cases/million in the UK [13], 94 cases per million in Poland [14], 154 cases per million in Greece [15], 158 cases per million in France [16], 277 cases per million in northwestern Spain [17] and, finally, 306 cases per million in Italy [18]. This variation in SSc prevalence in different parts of Europe has led to the proposition that there may be a north–south gradient with regard to SSc prevalence in Europe.

There is an obvious difference in the incidence and prevalence of SSc in different ethnicities in different parts of the world. These observed differences in SSc prevalence are likely driven by genetic factors that are specific to and arising from that ancestral population. For example, in Campo Grande in Brazil, Horimoto et al. reported an SSc prevalence of 106 cases per million [19], whereas in Buenos Aires in Argentina, Rosa et al. reported a prevalence of 296 cases per million [20]. In Japan, Tamaki et al. reported a prevalence of 53 cases per million [21]. Prevalence in New Zealand was 30 per million and in Australia has varied from 45 per million in 1975 to 200 per million in 1993 and 233 per million in 1999 [22–25]. In another study of patients with SSc from the

P. Gourh (✉)
Scleroderma Genomics and Health Disparities Unit, National Institute of Arthritis and Musculoskeletal and Skin Diseases, National Institutes of Health, Bethesda, MD, USA
e-mail: pravitt.gourh@nih.gov

C. Bruni
Department of Clinical and Experimental Medicine, Section of Rheumatology, University of Florence, Florence, Italy
e-mail: cosimo.bruni@unifi.it

Y. Allanore et al. (eds.), *Scleroderma*, https://doi.org/10.1007/978-3-031-40658-4_3

Cairns region of far North Queensland in Australia, SSc prevalence was 337 per million, higher than previously reported in South Australia [26].

Genetic Risk Factors

Numerous studies seeking to identify the genetic risk factors that contribute to SSc susceptibility have been conducted. These have led to the associations in the human leukocyte antigen (*HLA*) genes with SSc as one of the strongest and most consistent findings in SSc. *HLA* genes are highly polymorphic, and these *HLA* alleles define the variations in the antigen-binding grooves of the HLA molecules. Studies have shown that these *HLA* alleles are not just specific for ancestry but are also enriched in the autoantibody-positive subsets of SSc. In Choctaw Native Americans, the population with the highest prevalence of SSc, Tan et al. identified *HLA-DRB1*16:02/DQA1*05:01/DQB1*03:01/DPB1*13:01* extended haplotype increasing susceptibility for SSc [27]. Gourh et al. examining the Genome Research in African American Scleroderma Patients (GRASP) cohort, identified two predominantly African ancestral alleles, *HLA-DRB1*08:04* and *HLA-DRB1*11:02,* conferring a risk of 3.2-fold and 2.3-fold, respectively [28–30]. In AAs, the *HLA-DRB1*08:04/DQA1*05:01/DQB1*03:01* haplotype was even further enriched in the anti-fibrillarin antibody (AFA) positive subset of SSc. A previously unreported allele in SSc, *HLA-DQB1*06:09*, conferred a risk of 4.1-fold in the AFA+ subset, independent of the effect of *HLA-DRB1*08:04* [28]. In EAs, a susceptibility haplotype (*HLA-DRB1*11:04/DQA1*05:01/DQB1*03:01*) and a protective haplotype (*HLA-DRB1*07:01/DQA1*02:01/DQB1*02:02*) have been identified in SSc [28, 31]. Beretta et al. examined Italian and Spanish SSc cohorts and identified *DRB1*11:04/DQA1*05:01/DQB1*03:01* to be a susceptibility haplotype [32]. In Japanese, Thai and Korean populations, *HLA-DRB1*15:02* and *HLA-DQB1*0601* were identified as SSc risk alleles [33–35]. Rodriguez-Reyna et al. reported *HLA-DRB1*08:02* allele increased SSc susceptibility in the Mexican population [36]. Interestingly, the *HLA-DPB1*13:01* allele was identified as a risk allele in several ancestral populations and displayed a transancestry effect. The *HLA-DPB1*13:01* allele has a transancestral effect and its risk can be observed in several populations including AAs and EAs [28]. The Choctaw Native American SSc patients have a very uniform clinical phenotype with 95% anti-topoisomerase I antibody (ATA) positivity. They had an *HLA-DPB1*13:01* carrier frequency of 65% in the ATA-positive subset [5, 27]. The Choctaw native American SSc patients have the highest reported prevalence of SSc of any known population and simultaneously they also have the

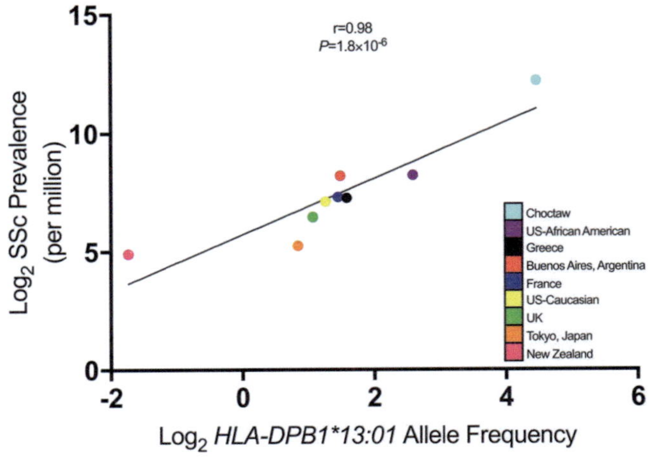

Fig. 3.1 Population frequency of the *HLA-DPB1*13:01* allele and SSc prevalence in various ethnic populations around the world [28]

highest population frequency of the *HLA-DPB1*13:01* allele (45%) [5, 27]. This led Gourh et al. to explore the relationship between SSc prevalence in any given population and the *HLA-DPB1*13:01* allele frequency in populations around the world (Fig. 3.1) [28]. This led to the identification of a direct correlation between the population frequency of the *HLA-DPB1*13:01* allele and the prevalence of SSc in that population, with a correlation coefficient of 0.98 and $P = 1.8 \times 10^{-6}$. This direct correlation of *HLA-DPB1*13:01* population frequency with SSc prevalence in various populations around the world suggests a distinct role of this allele in SSc pathogenesis.

HLA alleles are highly polymorphic and encode for the amino acids that define the antigen-binding grooves of the HLA molecules. The class II HLA molecules are responsible for presenting peptides to T helper cells and the antigen-binding grooves on the HLA molecules determine the binding affinity for specific peptides [37]. If a self-peptide is recognized by the class II HLA molecule on the antigen-presenting cells (APCs) then it can lead to the activation of autoreactive T helper cells. Activation of autoreactive T helper cells can lead to the activation of B cells, autoantibody formation and autoimmunity induction. Thus, SSc-associated HLA alleles coding for a specific antigen-binding groove sequence on the antigen-presenting cells will recognize a specific peptide causing the activation of T helper cells and production of autoantibodies. Gourh et al. identified several SSc-associated amino acid residues that were part of the peptide-binding groove in all of the class II HLA genes (Fig. 3.2) [28]. These peptide-binding groove residue changes might facilitate antigen presenting cell recognition of specific peptides that, upon presentation to T helper cells, lead to T helper cell activation and, in turn, B cell activation, ultimately resulting in autoimmunity. Amino acid leucine, at position 74, in the peptide-binding groove was specific to *HLA-DRB1*08:04*

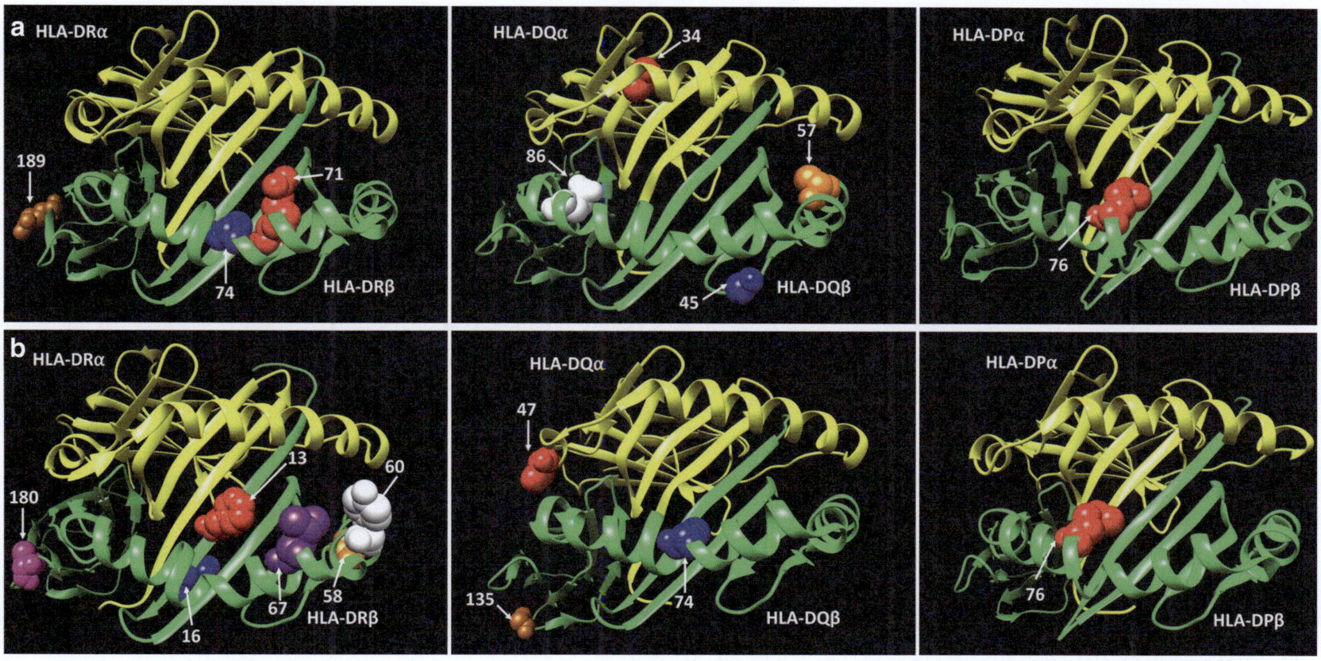

Fig. 3.2 Ribbon model of the HLA-DR, HLA-DQ and HLA-DP proteins with independently associated amino acid residues, based on PDB ID codes 6atf, 1s9v and 3lqz, respectively. (**a**) SSc-associated amino acid positions in AAs and (**b**) SSc-associated amino acid positions in EAs [28]

(the African-predominant allele) in AAs. Amino acid residue position 189 in AAs and residue 180 in EAs were outside of the peptide-binding groove and might be playing a role in altering the structure of the class II HLA molecule or, alternatively, in modifying the interaction of the class II HLA molecule with the T cell receptor. Interestingly, the transancestral allele *HLA-DPB1*13:01* encodes for amino acid position 76, isoleucine, in the HLA-DPβ peptide-binding groove in both the AA and EA populations, and hence could be playing an important role in disease pathogenesis.

SSc Onset

Age of onset of SSc is variable and has been proposed to be based on ethnicity of the population being studied. Peak incidence in AA women was reported to be between the ages of 45 and 54 years as compared to the 65–74-year age group for EA women [8]. Peak incidence for AA men was earlier than EA men and yet was similar to that for AA women. SSc in Africans manifests at an even earlier age than AAs [9, 10]. AA, African, and African ancestry patients in the European Scleroderma Trials and Research group (EUSTAR) cohort, Asian Americans and Asian patients in the EUSTAR cohort, and Choctaw Native Americans all have an earlier onset of SSc as compared to patients of European ancestry [2, 5, 38–42]. In a French study, African ancestry individuals were 10 years younger on average than European ancestry individuals [43].

Autoantibodies, Clinical Features and Internal Organ Involvement

Autoantibodies reported in SSc patients are usually mutually exclusive as well as specific for SSc. These SSc-specific autoantibodies are also associated with distinct patterns of cutaneous and internal organ involvement and are biomarkers of disease severity and mortality [28, 44].

Anti-centromere antibody (ACA) is associated with limited skin involvement and a lower frequency of interstitial lung disease (ILD) leading to a milder phenotype. Jaeger et al. reporting from the EUSTAR cohort, observed ACA in 42% of European ancestry individuals, 17% in Asian ancestry individuals and 10% in African ancestry individuals [42]. ACA is less frequently reported in African, AA, African Brazilians, Hispanic and Thai populations [1, 45–50]. Gelber et al. reported a threefold higher prevalence of ACA in EAs as compared to AA patients and a twofold higher prevalence of ATA in AA patients as compared to EA patients [2]. GRASP, the largest multicentre study of AA patients, reported autoantibody frequency of ACA at 8%, anti-Topoisomerase I antibody (ATA) at 30%, anti-U3-ribonucleoprotein antibody (fibrillarin, AFA) at 14% and anti-RNA polymerase III antibody (ARA) at 13% [29]. Africans with SSc have a predominantly diffuse skin involvement (dcSSc), along with the presence of nucleolar pattern on anti-nuclear antibody testing by immunofluorescence. They also develop ILD and have AFA and ATA similar to AAs [9, 10]. In the EUSTAR cohort, the prevalence of ATA was 35% in European, 47% in Asian and 34% in African ancestry patients [42]. ATA is associated with a more severe phenotype including dcSSc and ILD, and is seen in high frequency in the African, AA and Thai populations. Moreover, it is found with the highest frequency in the Choctaw Native American population [5]. AFA is more prevalent in AAs, African Brazilians and Native Americans as compared to individuals of European ancestry and has been independently associated with increased mortality [29, 50, 51]. Anti-U1-ribonucleoprotein antibody is more commonly seen in AAs and Chinese patients and is associated with overlap syndromes [2, 40, 41, 48, 52]. ARA was present in 20% of the EAs, compared to 12% in AAs as reported in a Hopkins study by Gelber et al. [2]. Nandiwada et al. studying a diverse cohort of SSc in the USA, reported ARA frequency of 14% in AAs, 17% in EAs, and 21% in Hispanic patients [53]. ARA frequency in the Asian ancestry individuals from the EUSTAR cohort was 8% [42]. Freire et al., reporting from a Spanish cohort of SSc patients, observed ACA frequency at 46%, ATA at 22% and ARA at 17% [54].

A higher prevalence of dcSSc has been reported in AAs and First Nations patients [2, 40, 41, 55]. Gelber et al. reported two-thirds of EA patients manifested the limited cutaneous disease, whereas the majority of AA patients manifested the dcSSc disease [2]. The GRASP study reported dcSSc in 57%, ILD prevalence at 68% and pulmonary hypertension in 30% of patients [29]. Asian patients in the EUSTAR cohort, had dcSSc present in 28%, ILD in 44% and pulmonary arterial hypertension (PAH) in 18% [42]. The African ancestry individuals from the same cohort had a higher dcSSc at 56%, ILD in 50% and PAH in 17% of patients [42]. Native North Americans and AAs are more likely to develop gastrointestinal manifestations [41, 56]. In African, AA, and Chinese SSc patients, myositis was more frequently observed than in European ancestry individuals [7, 41, 43, 52].

The presence of SSc-specific autoantibodies not only correlates with clinical manifestations of SSc and internal organ involvement but also correlates with the prevalence of SSc in any given ethnic group. In part, the increased prevalence of SSc-specific autoantibodies could help explain the severe disease manifestations seen in some populations around the world.

Mortality

SSc carries the highest case-based mortality among all rheumatic diseases, mostly led by the presence of ILD and PAH [57, 58]. African ancestry is reported to be an independent predictor of early pulmonary involvement and severe ILD. Higher mortality in SSc has been reported in AAs and Asians as compared to European ancestry individuals [41, 59, 60]. AA SSc patients have a 30–60% increased risk for mortality as compared to EA patients after controlling for age, gender, socioeconomic status, education and health insurance status [2, 8, 41, 61–64].

Pokeerbux et al. reported that African ancestry was associated with a hazard ratio of death of 1.38 based upon a meta-analysis of five cohorts [65]. A study comprised of cohorts from the United States and Japan, identified an increased rate of mortality among AAs and Japanese patients as compared to European ancestry individuals [66]. African ancestry has also been associated with increased mortality in African Brazilians and African ancestry patients of the EUSTAR cohort [42, 50]. Asian patients enrolled in the EUSTAR cohort also demonstrated higher mortality rates relative to European ancestry individuals [42]. In a pooled cohort study, Native North American and Australian Aboriginal ethnicities were associated with increased mortality [67].

Summary

There is clearly a strong role of ethnic disparities in SSc contributing to disease manifestations. SSc patients of African, Asian and Native American ethnicities experience a higher prevalence, earlier disease onset, diffuse cutaneous disease, increased pulmonary and renal involvement, and higher mortality, when compared with the European ancestry populations. This increased disease burden is partly due to the presence of SSc-specific autoantibodies, which are found in higher frequencies in these ethnic groups. This is presumably directed by genetic factors. Taken together, the increased disease burden and the presence of autoantibodies are both being driven by genetic factors of which *HLA* is the key player.

Sex Bias in SSc

Epidemiology and Etiopathogenesis

SSc manifests significantly more frequently among the female sex, and this has been demonstrated among many different cohorts, with the female:male ratio ranging from 3 to 8:1 [68–73].

In this light, different sex-related factors have been studied so far, including genetic, epigenetic and hormonal factors (Fig. 3.3) [74]. X-linked genes have been extensively studied among SSc patients: as a result of global DNA methylation, skewed X chromosome inactivation (occurring when there is a different level of inactivation of the X gene on one chromosome versus the other) was shown to be associated with autoantibody production [75]. Similarly, the methylation of other specific genes located on the X

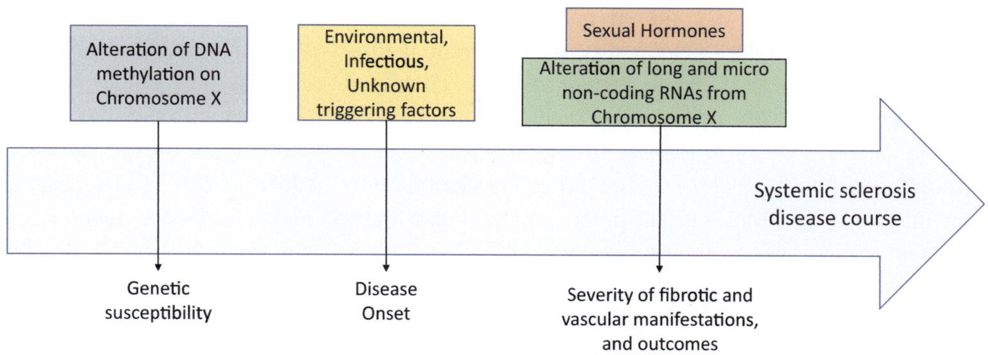

Fig. 3.3 X-linked pathogenetic factors and their clinical consequences in the SSc natural history

chromosome, such as *IL1RAPL2*, *CD40L* and *FOXP3*, is implicated with increased susceptibility to autoimmunity, including SSc and reduction of T regulatory cell activity [76]. On an RNA level, several X-linked molecules have been investigated in SSc patients. Among long non-coding RNAs, TSIX was found to be upregulated in fibroblast derived from SSc skin biopsies and in their sera, acting as a possible pro-fibrotic biomarker [77]. More information is available for micro non-coding RNA derived from chromosome X (miR), with evidence for increased profibrotic (such as miR-503-5p [78], miR-92a [79], miR-542-3p [80]) or decreased anti-fibrotic (i.e. miR-223-3p [78]) molecules.

Evidence of a pathogenetic role for female sexual hormones is still under debate, although the amount of data on this topic is substantial. Oestrogens have been demonstrated as both influencing vascular tone and enhancing a fibrotic environment: this was particularly based on comparing female patients in the pre-menopausal (normo-oestrogenic) and post-menopausal (hypo-oestrogenic) phases. Disease onset in the first phase is usually characterized by a higher fibrotic phenotype, with more frequent diffuse cutaneous involvement and interstitial lung disease [81]; conversely, the second phase carries higher numbers of cases with more severe vasculopathy, both peripheral and pulmonary [82]. In this light, the administration of female hormones to male subjects undergoing sexual transition has been described in the literature, with few cases of SSc onset during a hyper-oestrogenic status currently reported [83].

In theory, this is in contradiction to the clinical manifestation of SSc in men, which is frequently characterized by a more severe fibrotic cutaneous and pulmonary involvements (further discussed in the next section of this chapter; Table 3.1). These observations are also supported by pre-clinical research on a scleroderma mouse model in which oestrogens showed an inhibitory effect on the profibrotic transforming-growth-factor beta [84]. This might also explain the lack of therapeutic benefit from the drugs targeting the sexual hormones tested so far for the treatment of SSc [85].

Table 3.1 Summary of increased prevalence of systemic sclerosis manifestation among females and males

	Females	Males
More robust evidence	↑ Limited cutaneous subset	↑ Diffuse cutaneous subset ↑ Interstitial lung disease ↑ Scleroderma renal crisis ↑ Tendon friction rubs
Conflicting evidence	↑ PAH (in post-menopausal?)	↑ PAH at first presentation ↑ DU at first presentation ↑ Myositis in early disease ↑ Arthritis

Clinical Presentation and Disease Manifestations

The impact of sex on disease manifestations of SSc has been extensively studied in previous years and various, although somewhat conflicting, evidence are currently available [86].

Despite the epidemiological evidence showing higher prevalence in the female sex, women and men can already be distinguished in the first 3 years after disease onset (also called as “early disease”). A recent analysis on 650 early disease patients showed that males present with the diffuse skin subset more frequently [68]. As a counterpart, females are most frequently affected by the limited cutaneous subset, which tends to develop mildly over time and frequently has a slow progression to organ damage, several years after onset of Raynaud’s phenomenon (Table 3.1) [68]. As a possible consequence, males present to their first clinical consultation earlier than females and, therefore, receive an earlier diagnosis [69, 71–73]. Skin involvement, particularly with the diffuse distribution, may be the trigger for a rheumatology referral and, against epidemiological global prevalence of gender distribution of the disease, there is a significant higher frequency of diffuse cutaneous subset among men within both the EUSTAR database (61 versus 34%) [68] and in the Pittsburgh cohort (48 versus 37%) [73].

Possibly related to a common pro-fibrotic phenotype, males also manifest more frequently with interstitial lung disease (ILD) detectable on high-resolution computed tomography [87], with a prevalence range of 49–57% [70, 71, 73] versus 39–42% in females (Table 3.1) [70, 71, 73]. Similarly, despite the lack of a standardized uniform definition in data evaluation, cardiac involvement is also more prevalent among males, ranging from 7 to 18% [71, 73] versus 2.8 to 11% among women [71, 73]; this was particularly significant for conduction disturbances, as shown by the Spanish National Registry [71]. Finally, a higher number of patients with tendon friction rubs are also present in men [71, 73]. Still, in line with the inflammatory disease manifestations, there is also conflicting evidence regarding a higher incidence of muscular and articular SSc-related involvement, being more frequent among male patients [71, 73].

Vascular manifestations of SSc present the most conflicting data regarding the possible influence of sex. While the EUSTAR database showed that the prevalence of pulmonary arterial hypertension (PAH) was significantly higher among males at first clinical evaluation (1.2% versus 0.5%) [70], an opposite result was shown by the Spanish registry, in which this complication was more frequently manifest in females (7.0% versus 2.3%) [71], and no statistical difference was seen in the Pittsburgh database (Table 3.1) [73]. A similar debate is open for peripheral vasculopathy, in particular digital ulcers: while the EUSTAR database showed a higher prevalence of digital ulcers at baseline 41% versus 34% in EUSTAR [70] and the Spanish registry almost confirmed this prevalence (47% versus 40%, $p = 0.07$) [71], but was not confirmed by the Pittsburgh database [73]. The really strong evidence on vasculopathic manifestations comes from the higher prevalence of scleroderma renal crisis, which was confirmed for male sex among all available major cohorts [70, 71, 73].

Both sexes are similarly involved by other disease manifestations and currently data are controversial, both showing similar prevalence or conflicting results. This is the case in gastrointestinal manifestations, frequent in both sexes, as well as sexual discomfort/dysfunction and appearance concerns [88, 89]. Moreover, as a consequence of treatment with high-intensity immunosuppression with cyclophosphamide, both males and females may have an impairment of reproductive capacity, with impaired hormonal levels in men [90] and increased amenorrhoea in females [91].

Prognosis and Mortality

In addition to the overall higher disease burden in the early phase, male patients also carry an increased risk for the development of organ complication (with a more severe expression) during the disease course. Among the manifestations, male gender represents a significant predictive factor for the new occurrence of cardiac systolic dysfunction [70], PAH [70] and ILD progression [92]. As a probable consequence, male gender has also been identified as a predictive factor of mortality [70, 71, 73, 93]. In a recent meta-analysis, showing an overall standardized mortality ratio (SMR) 2.8 (95% CI 2.2–3.6) for SSc compared to general population, a higher SMR for male (3.5, 95% CI 2.9–4.2) versus female gender (2.9, 95% CI 2.5–33.4) was identified [94]. In addition, a different distribution of SSc-related cause of death has been noted among the two genders: males more frequently die as a consequence of interstitial lung disease, while females frequently die as a consequence of PAH-related complications [73].

References

1. Reveille JD. Ethnicity and race and systemic sclerosis: how it affects susceptibility, severity, antibody genetics, and clinical manifestations. Curr Rheumatol Rep. 2003;5(2):160–7. https://doi.org/10.1007/s11926-003-0045-1.
2. Gelber AC, Manno RL, Shah AA, Woods A, Le EN, Boin F, et al. Race and association with disease manifestations and mortality in scleroderma: a 20-year experience at the Johns Hopkins scleroderma center and review of the literature. Medicine (Baltimore). 2013;92(4):191–205. https://doi.org/10.1097/MD.0b013e31829be125.
3. Barnes J, Mayes MD. Epidemiology of systemic sclerosis: incidence, prevalence, survival, risk factors, malignancy, and environmental triggers. Curr Opin Rheumatol. 2012;24(2):165–70. https://doi.org/10.1097/BOR.0b013e32834ff2e8.
4. Harley JB, Neas BR. Oklahoma Choctaw and systemic sclerosis: the founder effect and genetic susceptibility. Arthritis Rheum. 1998;41(10):1725–8. https://doi.org/10.1002/1529-0131(199810)41:10<1725::AID-ART4>3.0.CO;2-N.
5. Arnett FC, Howard RF, Tan F, Moulds JM, Bias WB, Durban E, et al. Increased prevalence of systemic sclerosis in a native American tribe in Oklahoma. Association with an Amerindian HLA haplotype. Arthritis Rheum. 1996;39(8):1362–70. https://doi.org/10.1002/art.1780390814.
6. Barnabe C, Joseph L, Belisle P, Labrecque J, Edworthy S, Barr SG, et al. Prevalence of systemic lupus erythematosus and systemic sclerosis in the first nations population of Alberta, Canada. Arthritis Care Res (Hoboken). 2012;64(1):138–43. https://doi.org/10.1002/acr.20656.
7. Laing TJ, Gillespie BW, Toth MB, Mayes MD, Gallavan RH Jr, Burns CJ, et al. Racial differences in scleroderma among women in Michigan. Arthritis Rheum. 1997;40(4):734–42. https://doi.org/10.1002/art.1780400421.
8. Mayes MD, Lacey JV Jr, Beebe-Dimmer J, Gillespie BW, Cooper B, Laing TJ, et al. Prevalence, incidence, survival, and disease characteristics of systemic sclerosis in a large US population. Arthritis Rheum. 2003;48(8):2246–55. https://doi.org/10.1002/art.11073.
9. Adelowo OO, Oguntona S. Scleroderma (systemic sclerosis) among Nigerians. Clin Rheumatol. 2009;28(9):1121–5. https://doi.org/10.1007/s10067-009-1191-2.
10. Tager RE, Tikly M. Clinical and laboratory manifestations of systemic sclerosis (scleroderma) in black south Africans. Rheumatology (Oxford). 1999;38(5):397–400. https://doi.org/10.1093/rheumatology/38.5.397.
11. Geirsson AJ, Steinsson K, Guthmundsson S, Sigurthsson V. Systemic sclerosis in Iceland. A nationwide epidemiological

study. Ann Rheum Dis. 1994;53(8):502–5. https://doi.org/10.1136/ard.53.8.502.
12. Silman A, Jannini S, Symmons D, Bacon P. An epidemiological study of scleroderma in the west midlands. Br J Rheumatol. 1988;27(4):286–90. https://doi.org/10.1093/rheumatology/27.4.286.
13. Allcock RJ, Forrest I, Corris PA, Crook PR, Griffiths ID. A study of the prevalence of systemic sclerosis in Northeast England. Rheumatology (Oxford). 2004;43(5):596–602. https://doi.org/10.1093/rheumatology/keh124.
14. Kanecki K, Gorynski P, Tarka P, Wierzba W, Tyszko P. Incidence and prevalence of systemic sclerosis (SSc) in Poland—differences between rural and urban regions. Ann Agric Environ Med. 2017;24(2):240–4. https://doi.org/10.5604/12321966.1233570.
15. Alamanos Y, Tsifetaki N, Voulgari PV, Siozos C, Tsamandouraki K, Alexiou GA, et al. Epidemiology of systemic sclerosis in Northwest Greece 1981 to 2002. Semin Arthritis Rheum. 2005;34(5):714–20. https://doi.org/10.1016/j.semarthrit.2004.09.001.
16. Le Guern V, Mahr A, Mouthon L, Jeanneret D, Carzon M, Guillevin L. Prevalence of systemic sclerosis in a French multi-ethnic county. Rheumatology (Oxford). 2004;43(9):1129–37. https://doi.org/10.1093/rheumatology/keh253.
17. Arias-Nunez MC, Llorca J, Vazquez-Rodriguez TR, Gomez-Acebo I, Miranda-Filloy JA, Martin J, et al. Systemic sclerosis in northwestern Spain: a 19-year epidemiologic study. Medicine (Baltimore). 2008;87(5):272–80. https://doi.org/10.1097/MD.0b013e318189372f.
18. Ciaffi J, Morabito MF, Ruscitti P, D'Angelo S, Mancarella L, Brusi V, et al. Incidence, prevalence and mortality of systemic sclerosis in Italy: a nationwide population-based study using administrative health data. Rheumatol Int. 2020;41:129. https://doi.org/10.1007/s00296-020-04720-3.
19. Horimoto AMC, Matos ENN, Costa MRD, Takahashi F, Rezende MC, Kanomata LB, et al. Incidence and prevalence of systemic sclerosis in Campo Grande, State of Mato Grosso do Sul, Brazil. Rev Bras Reumatol Engl Ed. 2017;57(2):107–14. https://doi.org/10.1016/j.rbre.2016.09.005.
20. Rosa JE, Soriano ER, Narvaez-Ponce L, del Cid CC, Imamura PM, Catoggio LJ. Incidence and prevalence of systemic sclerosis in a healthcare plan in Buenos Aires. J Clin Rheumatol. 2011;17(2):59–63. https://doi.org/10.1097/RHU.0b013e31820e7e8d.
21. Tamaki T, Mori S, Takehara K. Epidemiological study of patients with systemic sclerosis in Tokyo. Arch Dermatol Res. 1991;283(6):366–71. https://doi.org/10.1007/BF00371817.
22. Englert H, Small-McMahon J, Davis K, O'Connor H, Chambers P, Brooks P. Systemic sclerosis prevalence and mortality in Sydney 1974-88. Aust NZ J Med. 1999;29(1):42–50. https://doi.org/10.1111/j.1445-5994.1999.tb01587.x.
23. Roberts-Thomson PJ, Jones M, Hakendorf P, Kencana Dharmapatni AA, Walker JG, MacFarlane JG, et al. Scleroderma in South Australia: epidemiological observations of possible pathogenic significance. Intern Med J. 2001;31(4):220–9. https://doi.org/10.1046/j.1445-5994.2001.00048.x.
24. Roberts-Thomson PJ, Walker JG, Lu TY, Esterman A, Hakendorf P, Smith MD, et al. Scleroderma in South Australia: further epidemiological observations supporting a stochastic explanation. Intern Med J. 2006;36(8):489–97. https://doi.org/10.1111/j.1445-5994.2006.01125.x.
25. Eason RJ, Tan PL, Gow PJ. Progressive systemic sclerosis in Auckland: a ten year review with emphasis on prognostic features. Aust NZ J Med. 1981;11(6):657–62. https://doi.org/10.1111/j.1445-5994.1981.tb03542.x.
26. Abbot S, McWilliams L, Spargo L, de Costa C, Ur-Rehman Z, Proudman S, et al. Scleroderma in Cairns: an epidemiological study. Intern Med J. 2020;50(4):445–52. https://doi.org/10.1111/imj.14376.
27. Tan FK, Stivers DN, Arnett FC, Chakraborty R, Howard R, Reveille JD. HLA haplotypes and microsatellite polymorphisms in and around the major histocompatibility complex region in a native American population with a high prevalence of scleroderma (systemic sclerosis). Tissue Antigens. 1999;53(1):74–80. https://doi.org/10.1034/j.1399-0039.1999.530108.x.
28. Gourh P, Safran SA, Alexander T, Boyden SE, Morgan ND, Shah AA, et al. HLA and autoantibodies define scleroderma subtypes and risk in African and European Americans and suggest a role for molecular mimicry. Proc Natl Acad Sci U S A. 2020;117(1):552–62. https://doi.org/10.1073/pnas.1906593116.
29. Morgan ND, Shah AA, Mayes MD, Domsic RT, Medsger TA Jr, Steen VD, et al. Clinical and serological features of systemic sclerosis in a multicenter African American cohort: analysis of the genome research in African American scleroderma patients clinical database. Medicine (Baltimore). 2017;96(51):e8980. https://doi.org/10.1097/MD.0000000000008980.
30. Gourh P, Remmers EF, Boyden SE, Alexander T, Morgan ND, Shah AA, et al. Brief report: whole-exome sequencing to identify rare variants and gene networks that increase susceptibility to scleroderma in African Americans. Arthritis Rheumatol. 2018;70(10):1654–60. https://doi.org/10.1002/art.40541.
31. Cockrill T, del Junco DJ, Arnett FC, Assassi S, Tan FK, McNearney T, et al. Separate influences of birth order and gravidity/parity on the development of systemic sclerosis. Arthritis Care Res (Hoboken). 2010;62(3):418–24. https://doi.org/10.1002/acr.20096.
32. Beretta L, Rueda B, Marchini M, Santaniello A, Simeon CP, Fonollosa V, et al. Analysis of class II human leucocyte antigens in Italian and Spanish systemic sclerosis. Rheumatology (Oxford). 2012;51(1):52–9. https://doi.org/10.1093/rheumatology/ker335.
33. Kuwana M, Inoko H, Kameda H, Nojima T, Sato S, Nakamura K, et al. Association of human leukocyte antigen class II genes with autoantibody profiles, but not with disease susceptibility in Japanese patients with systemic sclerosis. Intern Med. 1999;38(4):336–44. https://doi.org/10.2169/internalmedicine.38.336.
34. Kang SH, Park MH, Song EY, Kang SJ, Lee EB, Song YW, et al. Association of HLA class II genes with systemic sclerosis in Koreans. J Rheumatol. 2001;28(7):1577–83.
35. Louthrenoo W, Kasitanon N, Wichainun R, Wangkaew S, Sukitawut W, Ohnogi Y, et al. Association of HLA-DRB1*15:02 and DRB5*01:02 allele with the susceptibility to systemic sclerosis in Thai patients. Rheumatol Int. 2013;33(8):2069–77. https://doi.org/10.1007/s00296-013-2686-3.
36. Rodriguez-Reyna TS, Mercado-Velazquez P, Yu N, Alosco S, Ohashi M, Lebedeva T, et al. HLA class I and II blocks are associated to susceptibility, clinical subtypes and autoantibodies in Mexican systemic sclerosis (SSc) patients. PLoS One. 2015;10(5):e0126727. https://doi.org/10.1371/journal.pone.0126727.
37. Neefjes J, Jongsma ML, Paul P, Bakke O. Towards a systems understanding of MHC class I and MHC class II antigen presentation. Nat Rev Immunol. 2011;11(12):823–36. https://doi.org/10.1038/nri3084.
38. Moore DF, Steen VD. Racial disparities in systemic sclerosis. Rheum Dis Clin N Am. 2020;46(4):705–12. https://doi.org/10.1016/j.rdc.2020.07.009.
39. Greidinger EL, Flaherty KT, White B, Rosen A, Wigley FM, Wise RA. African-American race and antibodies to topoisomerase I are associated with increased severity of scleroderma lung disease. Chest. 1998;114(3):801–7. https://doi.org/10.1378/chest.114.3.801.
40. Nietert PJ, Mitchell HC, Bolster MB, Shaftman SR, Tilley BC, Silver RM. Racial variation in clinical and immunological manifestations of systemic sclerosis. J Rheumatol. 2006;33(2):263–8.
41. Steen V, Domsic RT, Lucas M, Fertig N, Medsger TA Jr. A clinical and serologic comparison of African American and Caucasian

patients with systemic sclerosis. Arthritis Rheum. 2012;64(9):2986–94. https://doi.org/10.1002/art.34482.
42. Jaeger VK, Tikly M, Xu D, Siegert E, Hachulla E, Airo P, et al. Racial differences in systemic sclerosis disease presentation: a European scleroderma trials and research group study. Rheumatology (Oxford). 2020;59(7):1684–94. https://doi.org/10.1093/rheumatology/kez486.
43. Steelandt A, Benmostefa N, Avouac J, Mouthon L, Allanore Y. Ethnic influence on the phenotype of French patients with systemic sclerosis. Joint Bone Spine. 2020;88:105081. https://doi.org/10.1016/j.jbspin.2020.09.013.
44. Steen VD. Autoantibodies in systemic sclerosis. Semin Arthritis Rheum. 2005;35(1):35–42. https://doi.org/10.1016/j.semarthrit.2005.03.005.
45. Pudifin DJ, Dinnematin H, Duursma J. Antinuclear antibodies in systemic sclerosis. Clinical and ethnic associations. S Afr Med J. 1991;80(9):438–40.
46. Panicheewa S, Chitrabamrung S, Verasertniyom O, Vanichaphantu M, Kraisit SO, Chiewsilp P, et al. Diffuse systemic sclerosis and related diseases in Thailand. Clin Rheumatol. 1991;10(2):124–9. https://doi.org/10.1007/BF02207649.
47. Davis P, Stein M, Ley H, Johnston C. Serological profiles in the connective tissue diseases in Zimbabwean patients. Ann Rheum Dis. 1989;48(1):73–6. https://doi.org/10.1136/ard.48.1.73.
48. Reveille JD, Fischbach M, McNearney T, Friedman AW, Aguilar MB, Lisse J, et al. Systemic sclerosis in 3 US ethnic groups: a comparison of clinical, sociodemographic, serologic, and immunogenetic determinants. Semin Arthritis Rheum. 2001;30(5):332–46. https://doi.org/10.1053/sarh.2001.20268.
49. Reveille JD, Solomon DH, American College of Rheumatology Ad Hoc Committee of Immunologic Testing G. Evidence-based guidelines for the use of immunologic tests: anticentromere, Scl-70, and nucleolar antibodies. Arthritis Rheum. 2003;49(3):399–412. https://doi.org/10.1002/art.11113.
50. Mendes C, Viana VST, Pasoto SG, Leon EP, Bonfa E, Sampaio-Barros PD. Clinical and laboratory features of African-Brazilian patients with systemic sclerosis. Clin Rheumatol. 2020;39(1):9–17. https://doi.org/10.1007/s10067-019-04575-5.
51. Tan FK, Arnett FC, Reveille JD, Ahn C, Antohi S, Sasaki T, et al. Autoantibodies to fibrillin 1 in systemic sclerosis: ethnic differences in antigen recognition and lack of correlation with specific clinical features or HLA alleles. Arthritis Rheum. 2000;43(11):2464–71. https://doi.org/10.1002/1529-0131(200011)43:11<2464::AID-ANR13>3.0.CO;2-F.
52. Low AH, Johnson SR, Lee P. Ethnic influence on disease manifestations and autoantibodies in Chinese-descent patients with systemic sclerosis. J Rheumatol. 2009;36(4):787–93. https://doi.org/10.3899/jrheum.080915.
53. Sarada L Nandiwada, Lisa K Peterson, Maureen D Mayes, Troy D Jaskowski, Elisabeth Malmberg, Shervin Assassi, Minoru Satoh, Anne E Tebo. Ethnic Differences in Autoantibody Diversity and Hierarchy: More Clues from a US Cohort of Patients with Systemic Sclerosis. J Rheumatol. 2016;43(10):1816–24. https://doi.org/10.3899/jrheum.160106. PMID: 27481902, Epub 2016 Aug 1.
54. Freire M, Rivera A, Sopena B, Tolosa Vilella C, Guillen-Del Castillo A, Colunga Arguelles D, et al. Clinical and epidemiological differences between men and women with systemic sclerosis: a study in a Spanish systemic sclerosis cohort and literature review. Clin Exp Rheumatol. 2017;35 Suppl 106(4):89–97.
55. Al-Sheikh H, Ahmad Z, Johnson SR. Ethnic variations in systemic sclerosis disease manifestations, internal organ involvement, and mortality. J Rheumatol. 2019;46(9):1103–8. https://doi.org/10.3899/jrheum.180042.
56. Bacher A, Mittoo S, Hudson M, Tatibouet S, Canadian Scleroderma Research G, Baron M. Systemic sclerosis in Canada's north American native population: assessment of clinical and serological manifestations. J Rheumatol. 2013;40(7):1121–6. https://doi.org/10.3899/jrheum.121212.
57. Denton CP, Khanna D. Systemic sclerosis. Lancet. 2017;390(10103):1685–99. https://doi.org/10.1016/S0140-6736(17)30933-9.
58. Poudel DR, Derk CT. Mortality and survival in systemic sclerosis: a review of recent literature. Curr Opin Rheumatol. 2018;30(6):588–93. https://doi.org/10.1097/BOR.0000000000000551.
59. McNearney TA, Reveille JD, Fischbach M, Friedman AW, Lisse JR, Goel N, et al. Pulmonary involvement in systemic sclerosis: associations with genetic, serologic, sociodemographic, and behavioral factors. Arthritis Rheum. 2007;57(2):318–26. https://doi.org/10.1002/art.22532.
60. Moore DF, Kramer E, Eltaraboulsi R, Steen VD. Increased morbidity and mortality of scleroderma in African Americans compared to non-African Americans. Arthritis Care Res (Hoboken). 2019;71(9):1154–63. https://doi.org/10.1002/acr.23861.
61. Mayes MD. Scleroderma epidemiology. Rheum Dis Clin N Am. 2003;29(2):239–54. https://doi.org/10.1016/s0889-857x(03)00022-x.
62. Krishnan E, Furst DE. Systemic sclerosis mortality in the United States: 1979-1998. Eur J Epidemiol. 2005;20(10):855–61. https://doi.org/10.1007/s10654-005-2210-5.
63. Steen VD, Medsger TA. Changes in causes of death in systemic sclerosis, 1972-2002. Ann Rheum Dis. 2007;66(7):940–4. https://doi.org/10.1136/ard.2006.066068.
64. Assassi S, Sharif R, Lasky RE, McNearney TA, Estrada YMRM, Draeger H, et al. Predictors of interstitial lung disease in early systemic sclerosis: a prospective longitudinal study of the GENISOS cohort. Arthritis Res Ther. 2010;12(5):R166. https://doi.org/10.1186/ar3125.
65. Pokeerbux MR, Giovannelli J, Dauchet L, Mouthon L, Agard C, Lega JC, et al. Survival and prognosis factors in systemic sclerosis: data of a French multicenter cohort, systematic review, and meta-analysis of the literature. Arthritis Res Ther. 2019;21(1):86. https://doi.org/10.1186/s13075-019-1867-1.
66. Kuwana M, Kaburaki J, Arnett FC, Howard RF, Medsger TA Jr, Wright TM. Influence of ethnic background on clinical and serologic features in patients with systemic sclerosis and anti-DNA topoisomerase I antibody. Arthritis Rheum. 1999;42(3):465–74. https://doi.org/10.1002/1529-0131(199904)42:3<465::AID-ANR11>3.0.CO;2-Y.
67. Mejia Otero C, Assassi S, Hudson M, Mayes MD, Estrada YMR, Pedroza C, et al. Antifibrillarin antibodies are associated with native north American ethnicity and poorer survival in systemic sclerosis. J Rheumatol. 2017;44(6):799–805. https://doi.org/10.3899/jrheum.160574.
68. Carreira PE, Carmona L, Joven BE, Loza E, Andreu JL, Riemekasten G, et al. Gender differences in early systemic sclerosis patients: a report from the EULAR scleroderma trials and research group (EUSTAR) database. Clin Exp Rheumatol. 2018;36 Suppl 113(4):68–75.
69. Delisle VC, Hudson M, Baron M, Thombs BD. And the Canadian scleroderma research group a. sex and time to diagnosis in systemic sclerosis: an updated analysis of 1,129 patients from the Canadian scleroderma research group registry. Clin Exp Rheumatol. 2014;32(6 Suppl 86):S-10–4.
70. Elhai M, Avouac J, Walker UA, Matucci-Cerinic M, Riemekasten G, Airò P, et al. A gender gap in primary and secondary heart dysfunctions in systemic sclerosis: a EUSTAR prospective study. Ann Rheum Dis. 2016;75(1):163–9. https://doi.org/10.1136/annrheumdis-2014-206386.
71. Freire M, Rivera A, Sopeña B, Tolosa Vilella C, Guillén-Del Castillo A, Colunga Argüelles D, et al. Clinical and epidemiologi-

cal differences between men and women with systemic sclerosis: a study in a Spanish systemic sclerosis cohort and literature review. Clin Exp Rheumatol. 2017;35 Suppl 106(4):89–97.
72. Hudson M, Thombs B, Baron M, Canadian Scleroderma Research G. Time to diagnosis in systemic sclerosis: is sex a factor? Arthritis Rheum. 2009;61(2):274–8. https://doi.org/10.1002/art.24284.
73. Peoples C, Medsger TA Jr, Lucas M, Rosario BL, Feghali-Bostwick CA. Gender differences in systemic sclerosis: relationship to clinical features, serologic status and outcomes. J Scleroderma Relat Disord. 2016;1(2):177–240. https://doi.org/10.5301/jsrd.5000209.
74. Saveria Fioretto B, Rosa I, Romano E, Wang Y, Guiducci S, Zhang G, et al. The contribution of epigenetics to the pathogenesis and gender dimorphism of systemic sclerosis: a comprehensive overview. Ther Adv Musculoskelet Dis. 2020;12:1759720X20918456. https://doi.org/10.1177/1759720x20918456.
75. Ozbalkan Z, Bagislar S, Kiraz S, Akyerli CB, Ozer HT, Yavuz S, et al. Skewed X chromosome inactivation in blood cells of women with scleroderma. Arthritis Rheum. 2005;52(5):1564–70. https://doi.org/10.1002/art.21026.
76. Selmi C, Feghali-Bostwick CA, Lleo A, Lombardi SA, De Santis M, Cavaciocchi F, et al. X chromosome gene methylation in peripheral lymphocytes from monozygotic twins discordant for scleroderma. Clin Exp Immunol. 2012;169(3):253–62. https://doi.org/10.1111/j.1365-2249.2012.04621.x.
77. Wang Z, Jinnin M, Nakamura K, Harada M, Kudo H, Nakayama W, et al. Long non-coding RNA TSIX is upregulated in scleroderma dermal fibroblasts and controls collagen mRNA stabilization. Exp Dermatol. 2016;25(2):131–6. https://doi.org/10.1111/exd.12900.
78. Wermuth PJ, Piera-Velazquez S, Jimenez SA. Exosomes isolated from serum of systemic sclerosis patients display alterations in their content of profibrotic and antifibrotic microRNA and induce a profibrotic phenotype in cultured normal dermal fibroblasts. Clin Exp Rheumatol. 2017;35 Suppl 106(4):21–30.
79. Sing T, Jinnin M, Yamane K, Honda N, Makino K, Kajihara I, et al. microRNA-92a expression in the sera and dermal fibroblasts increases in patients with scleroderma. Rheumatology (Oxford). 2012;51(9):1550–6. https://doi.org/10.1093/rheumatology/kes120.
80. Vahidi Manesh P, Farazmand A, Gharibdoost F, Vanaki N, Mostafaei S, Kavosi H, et al. Downregulation of miR-542-3p contributes to apoptosis resistance in dermal fibroblasts from systemic sclerosis patients via Survivin overexpression. Iran J Allergy Asthma Immunol. 2019;18(2):173–81.
81. Vinet E, Bernatsky S, Hudson M, Pineau CA, Baron M, Canadian Scleroderma Research G. Effect of menopause on the modified Rodnan skin score in systemic sclerosis. Arthritis Res Ther. 2014;16(3):R130. https://doi.org/10.1186/ar4587.
82. Scorza R, Caronni M, Bazzi S, Nador F, Beretta L, Antonioli R, et al. Post-menopause is the main risk factor for developing isolated pulmonary hypertension in systemic sclerosis. Ann N Y Acad Sci. 2002;966:238–46. https://doi.org/10.1111/j.1749-6632.2002.tb04221.x.
83. Campochiaro C, Host LV, Ong VH, Denton CP. Development of systemic sclerosis in transgender females: a case series and review of the literature. Clin Exp Rheumatol. 2018;36 Suppl 113(4):50–2.
84. Avouac J, Pezet S, Gonzalez V, Baudoin L, Cauvet A, Ruiz B, et al. Estrogens counteract the profibrotic effects of TGF-β and their inhibition exacerbates experimental dermal fibrosis. J Investig Dermatol. 2020;140(3):593–601.e7. https://doi.org/10.1016/j.jid.2019.07.719.
85. Ciaffi J, van Leeuwen NM, Schoones JW, Huizinga TWJ, de Vries-Bouwstra JK. Sex hormones and sex hormone-targeting therapies in systemic sclerosis: a systematic literature review. Semin Arthritis Rheum. 2020;50(1):140–8. https://doi.org/10.1016/j.semarthrit.2019.07.007.
86. Hughes M, Pauling JD, Armstrong-James L, Denton CP, Galdas P, Flurey C. Gender-related differences in systemic sclerosis. Autoimmun Rev. 2020;19(4):102494. https://doi.org/10.1016/j.autrev.2020.102494.
87. Hoffmann-Vold A-M, Maher TM, Philpot EE, Ashrafzadeh A, Barake R, Barsotti S, et al. The identification and management of interstitial lung disease in systemic sclerosis: evidence-based European consensus statements. Lancet Rheumatol. 2020;2(2):e71–83. https://doi.org/10.1016/S2665-9913(19)30144-4.
88. Jewett LR, Kwakkenbos L, Carrier ME, Malcarne VL, Bartlett SJ, Furst DE, et al. Examination of the association of sex and race/ethnicity with appearance concerns: a scleroderma patient-centered intervention network (SPIN) cohort study. Clin Exp Rheumatol. 2016;34 Suppl 100(5):92–9.
89. Bruni C, Raja J, Denton CP, Matucci-Cerinic M. The clinical relevance of sexual dysfunction in systemic sclerosis. Autoimmun Rev. 2015;14(12):1111–5. https://doi.org/10.1016/j.autrev.2015.07.016.
90. Arnaud L, Nordin A, Lundholm H, Svenungsson E, Hellbacher E, Wikner J, et al. Effect of corticosteroids and cyclophosphamide on sex hormone profiles in male patients with systemic lupus erythematosus or systemic sclerosis. Arthritis Rheumatol. 2017;69(6):1272–9. https://doi.org/10.1002/art.40057.
91. Bruni C, Tashkin DP, Steen V, Allanore Y, Distler O, Grotts J, et al. Intravenous versus oral cyclophosphamide for lung and/or skin fibrosis in systemic sclerosis: an indirect comparison from EUSTAR and randomised controlled trials. Clin Exp Rheumatol. 2020;38 Suppl 125(3):161–8.
92. Hoffmann-Vold AM, Allanore Y, Alves M, Brunborg C, Airo P, Ananieva LP, et al. Progressive interstitial lung disease in patients with systemic sclerosis-associated interstitial lung disease in the EUSTAR database. Ann Rheum Dis. 2020;80:219. https://doi.org/10.1136/annrheumdis-2020-217455.
93. Elhai M, Meune C, Boubaya M, Avouac J, Hachulla E, Balbir-Gurman A, et al. Mapping and predicting mortality from systemic sclerosis. Ann Rheum Dis. 2017;76(11):1897–905. https://doi.org/10.1136/annrheumdis-2017-211448.
94. Lee YH. Overall and sex- and disease subtype-specific mortality in patients with systemic sclerosis: an updated meta-analysis. Z Rheumatol. 2019;78(2):195–201. https://doi.org/10.1007/s00393-018-0492-8.

Genetic Factors

4

Shervin Assassi, Javier Martin, and Yannick Allanore

Introduction

Systemic sclerosis (SSc) is characterized by early vascular damage and immune dysregulation followed by tissue fibrosis affecting many organs, in particular, the skin, lungs, heart, kidneys, and digestive tract. The epidemiological data are consistent in defining SSc as an orphan disease. The combination of environmental and stochastic factors converging upon individuals of a particular genetic background seems to contribute to the development of this disease. Subtle combinations and interactions may also contribute to the heterogeneity of the disease that is a hallmark of this condition. We will begin by considering various genetic approaches that can be applied to the study of polygenic diseases and will then move on to the principal factors implicated in this disease, which will be considered in greater detail.

Genetic Approaches to the Study of Polygenic Diseases

There are several possible approaches to demonstrating the existence of a genetic component in the pathogenesis of a complex or polygenic disease. Genetic susceptibility to polygenic diseases is based on a combination of polymorphisms in several genes. These polymorphisms are variations of the coding (exons) and non-coding (introns) regions occurring at various frequencies in the general population. Genomic variations fall into three categories [1]: (1) single nucleotide polymorphisms (SNPs), which are single-base-pair changes in nucleotide sequences; (2) insertion and deletions of nucleotides from the DNA; (3) structural rearrangements that reshuffle the DNA sequence (e.g., Chromosome 9 and 22 translocation in Philadelphia gene predisposing to chronic myelogenous leukemia); and (4) copy number variation.

S. Assassi (✉)
University of Texas Health Science Centre at Houston, Houston, TX, USA
e-mail: Shervin.Assassi@uth.tmc.edu

J. Martin
Institute of Parasitology and Biomedicine López-Neyra, CSIC, Granada, Spain
e-mail: javiermartin@ipb.csic.es

Y. Allanore
Service de Rhumatologie A, Université Paris Descartes, Paris, France

Unité INSERM U1016, Université Paris Descartes, Institut Cochin, Paris, France

Single Nucleotide Polymorphism (SNP)

SNPs are biallelic, with a given individual carrying one allele inherited from each parent (Fig. 4.1). The nucleotide variations involved are classified as non-synonymous if they lead to the modification of the amino-acid sequence of the encoded protein. A SNP is considered "functional" if the function of the resulting protein is altered in some way. Such alterations, which may involve a gain or a loss of function, are much less frequent in polygenic diseases than in monogenic diseases and are generally not solely responsible for the phenotype in this context. However, such genetic variations may cause subtle differences in protein function or in the expression of the corresponding gene with biological implications. They may also contribute to the variability used to define the thresholds separating the normal and pathological ranges. These types of genetic variations are also known as quantitative trait loci. An example, relevant to rheumatic diseases, is the SNPs in urate transporter genes that affect serum uric acid concentrations [2].

There are about ten million SNPs in humans, and the rarest SNP alleles have a frequency of at least 1%. SNPs located in close proximity to each other on the chromosome tend to remain linked or inherited together "en bloc" during hereditary transmission. Such a group of associated SNP alleles inherited together as a group in a chromosomal region is known as a haplotype. In other words, these associated SNPs have a low frequency of recombination during meiosis. Most

Y. Allanore et al. (eds.), *Scleroderma*, https://doi.org/10.1007/978-3-031-40658-4_4

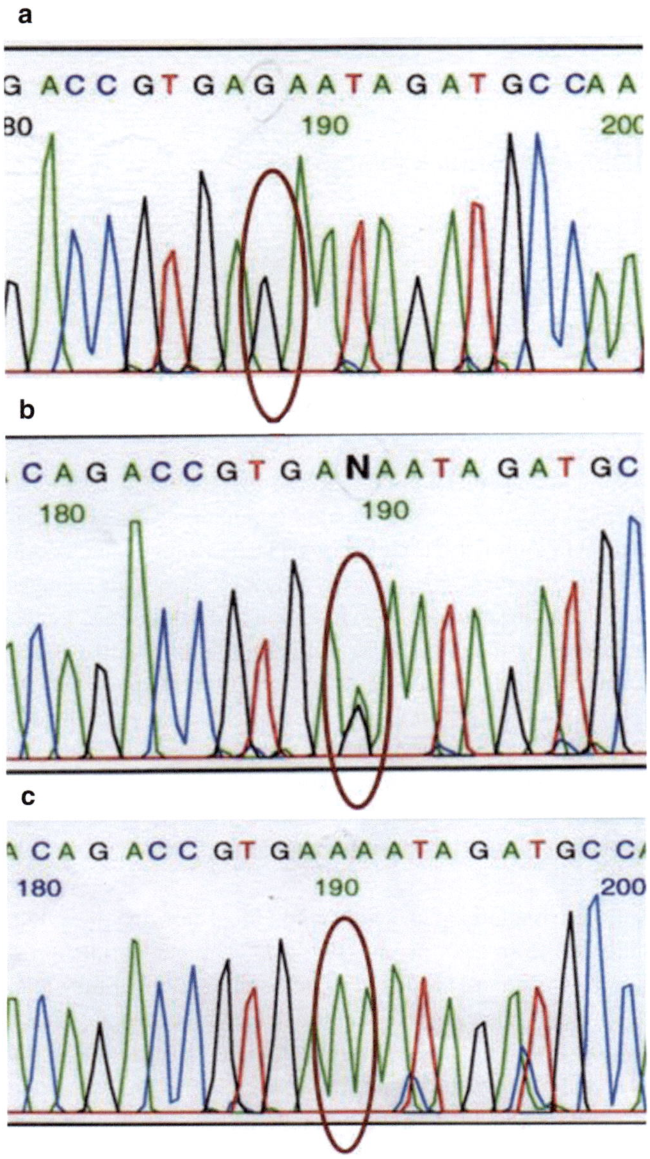

Fig. 4.1 Example of an SNP with the homozygous major allele profile (**a**), heterozygous (**b**), and homozygous (**c**) minor allele profiles

chromosomal regions have only a few common haplotypes (each with a frequency of at least 5%) accounting for most of the genetic diversity between the individuals of a population. A given chromosomal region may contain many SNPs, but the identification of only a few of these SNPs may be sufficient to capture the majority of the genetic variation in that region. These regions are called haploblocks.

General Approaches to Genetic Studies

The first type of analysis to be used when investigating the possible existence of a genetic component of a polygenic disease is the family association study. This involves checking for a larger number of cases among the first-degree relatives of patients than in the general population. It is then possible to establish the relative risk of a first-degree relative having the disease above the predicted risk for the general population. A higher frequency among monozygotic than among dizygotic twins may also be sought. Monozygotic twins are genetically identical, whereas dizygotic twins are only as genetically similar as their siblings. Their environment exposure during childhood may be considered identical, making it possible to attribute the resemblances or differences between mono- and dizygotic twins largely due to their genetic background.

Association studies are the most frequently used type of analysis in SSc. The association is sought either in so-called "case-control" studies or through a transmission disequilibrium test (TdT). In case–control studies, the frequency of the allele studied or of the genotype including the suspect allele is compared between patients and controls. Statistical tests are applied to compare the frequencies, after checking that the populations are in Hardy–Weinberg equilibrium (according to which the frequency of alleles and genotypes remains at equilibrium over successive generations). TdT tests require genetic material from both parents and the affected child (trios). It is rare for all these samples to be available in cases of SSc due to the late onset of the disease. This method compares the alleles transmitted to the affected child with the non-transmitted alleles used as controls. Table 4.1 summarizes the assumptions, advantages, and disadvantages of the above-mentioned study designs.

It is also recognized that differences in racial admixture (also known as population stratification) are a confounder that can lead to spurious associations. This is due to different degrees of recombination between genetic markers among

Table 4.1 Studies designs for genetic studies in systemic sclerosis

	Case–control	Trio (family studies)
Assumptions	Case and controls are recruited from the same population. Differences in allele frequencies relate to the disease rather than differences in the background population	Disease-related alleles are transmitted in excess of 50% to affected offspring from heterozygous parents
Advantages	Large numbers of case and control participants can be recruited in a relatively short period of time. Optimal for studying late-onset, rare diseases	Immune to population stratification. Does not require the phenotyping of parents
Disadvantages	Prone to biases arising from population stratification (systematic background differences) between case and control populations	Difficult to recruit both parents and offspring in disorders with older age of onset such as systemic sclerosis

the different racial groups. This concept is known as linkage disequilibrium (LD). For example, the extent of LD between groups of genetic markers in ancient populations such as African Yoruban is much lower than that of Northern European Caucasians. Therefore, many of the studies discussed examine subjects only from one racial group (e.g., Northern European whites), analyze each racial group separately, or utilize logistic regression models or other methods to account for differences in race. Moreover, since different races may experience different migration patterns and selection pressures, some associations may not cross ethnic barriers. Therefore, it is paramount that patients and controls are selected from the same population for genetic studies.

Genome-Wide Versus Candidate-Gene Studies

Genome-wide association studies (GWAS) use high-throughput genotyping platforms to examine hundreds of thousands common single-nucleotide polymorphisms (SNPs) at the same time [3]. The advantage of GWAS is that it allows the examination of common SNPs in the entire human genome. The genome-wide, non-hypothesis-driven nature of GWAS is an unprecedented opportunity to discover novel, disease related pathways in an unbiased manner. GWAS relies on the "common disease, common variant" hypothesis, which suggests that genetic influences in many common diseases will be at least in part explained by the limited number of allelic variants present in more than 1–5% of the general population. Common variants are either present directly on GWAS arrays or are covered by representative SNPs (tag SNPs) that are in linkage disequilibrium with them. Typically, variation in ten million common SNPs is captured in sufficient density by one million tag SNPs. However, the GWAS approach leads to a massive number of comparisons, raising the likelihood of false-positive results. Therefore, more stringent levels of significance are applied, and replication in an independent cohort is mandatory. Furthermore, it is possible that rare allelic variants (frequency < 1%) or other types of genetic variants contribute to the genetic susceptibility of disease. In addition to GWAS, the advent of next generation sequencing technology has enabled more cost-effective and timely sequencing of the human genome. The sequencing experiments can examine a specific area of the genome, human exome, or the entire genome [4].

Finally, association studies can be used as part of a "candidate-gene" approach. The candidate genes are identified on the basis of an understanding of, or hypotheses about, the physiopathology of the disease developed during or resulting from studies in vitro, in vivo, or based on animal models of SSc. The aim is to look for differences in frequency between certain polymorphisms of these genes encoding proteins of interest. While this approach is hypothesis-driven, it suffers from the major limitation that we have an incomplete or limited knowledge of disease processes. Nevertheless, based on similarities with other autoimmune connective tissue diseases, such as systemic lupus erythematosus (SLE) and rheumatoid arthritis (RA), this approach has been crucial in identifying multiple SSc associated genes.

A critical requirement for these genetic association studies is adequate sample size. For most non-HLA susceptibility genes that have been identified thus far in SSc, SLE, RA, and other autoimmune connective tissue diseases, the odds ratio conferred are usually modest (O.R. < 1.5), requiring sample sizes of several thousand subjects in order to detect significant associations.

Another fundamental notion in the genetic approach to complex diseases is the definition of a precise diagnostic profile (phenotype). This is of great importance when trying to optimize research on disease genes. The phenotype is the physical expression of the genotype (the genes responsible). Thus, the definition of genotypic variation depends on the correct definition of the phenotype. An imprecise definition increases the background noise in genetic analyses, limiting the likelihood of identifying genes involved in the disease. Furthermore, it is also important to point out that disease manifestations and characteristics (phenome) are only in part determined by genetic factors. Other factors, such as environment and stochastic events, have also an impact on the physiology and morphology of diseases.

Another potential approach would be to deconstruct a complex disease phenotype into a simpler variable as a proxy for the disease, which can be more precisely measured. This is readily applied to common disorders. For example, type II diabetes → hemoglobin A1C, or gout → serum uric acid level. This approach is known as quantitative trait loci analysis [5]. In this type of analysis, the phenotype is assumed to be a continuous variable, ideally normally distributed in the population. The SNPs being studied are considered covariates in a polygenic linear regression model.

Application of Genetic Approaches to Systemic Sclerosis

Family Association Studies

Analyses of three American cohorts including 703 families, 11 of which were multiplex for SSc, reported a risk for first-degree relatives of about 13 (10–16, depending on the cohort), with a recurrence rate of 1.6% versus 0.026% for the general population [6]. For brothers and sisters, the risk was estimated at 15 (10–27, depending on the cohort). This risk is the strongest risk factor for the disease established to date but, as concerns individuals, the risk of first-degree descendants having the disease is nonetheless below 1% [6]. A follow-up study showed that affected first degree relatives with SSc had significantly more concordance for the SSc related antibodies and class II HLA haplotypes than expected by chance [7].

Twin Studies

Only one twin study has been carried out to date [8]. This study was based on 42 pairs of twins (24 monozygotic twins) and showed poor concordance with clinical expression of the disease (4.7%). However, stronger concordance was observed for the presence of antinuclear antibodies: 40% for dizygotic twins and 90% for monozygotic twins. These results suggest that genetic predisposition alone is not sufficient for the development of this disease but that susceptibility could lead to a profile of autoantibody production. However, in a complementary study based on the same cohort, molecular concordance was found between the gene expression profiles of cultured dermal fibroblasts and a pro-fibrotic phenotype involving, in particular, the overexpression of genes regulated by TGF-beta, including *ACVR1B* (activin A receptor, type IB), *COL1A2* (alpha 2 chain of collagen I), *COL8A1* (alpha 1 chain of collagen VIII), *SPARC* (secreted protein acidic and rich in cysteine), *CTGF* (connective tissue growth factor) *THY1* (Thy-1 cell surface antigen), *AGTRL2* (angiotensin receptor-like 2), FHL2 (four and a half LIM domains 2), and *ARHB* (Ras homolog gene family, member B). The overexpression of *COL1A2, SPARC,* and *CTGF* was subsequently independently confirmed by RT-qPCR [9].

Genome Wide Association Studies (GWAS)

There are five GWA studies published so far based on Korean and US populations [10], European and US white populations [11]—see Fig. 4.2, European population [12]—see Fig. 4.3, Japanese population with transethnic meta-analysis with European population [13], and a large-scale metanalysis of European, US, and Australian white population (9095 SSc patients and 17,584 healthy controls) [14]—see Fig. 4.4. Their respective findings are discussed in section 3.4.

Candidate Gene Approach and Main Biological Pathways

Candidate gene studies have been conducted based on their relevance to SSc pathogenesis (i.e., inflammatory, fibrotic, or vascular pathways) or their relevance in other autoimmune diseases. Two Immunochip studies in SSc have been also completed, one investigated a large population of US/European white patients [15], and another one in an Australian white population [16]. Immunochip is an SNP microarray containing 195,806 SNPs and 718 insertion–deletion, which provides dense coverage for gene regions that were relevant in 11 distinct autoimmune and inflammatory diseases.

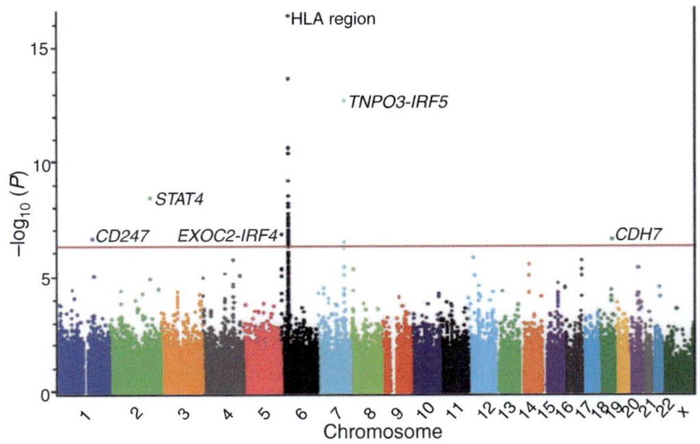

Fig. 4.2 Manhattan plot of the GWAS of 2346 white SSc cases and 5193 healthy controls. The $-\log_{10}$ of the Mantel–Haenszel test *P* value of 279,621 SNPs after genomic control correction is plotted against its physical chromosomal position. Chromosomes are shown in alternate colors. SNPs above the red line represent those with a genome-wide level of significance *P* value of $<5 \times 10^{-7}$. Note the considerable number of peaks that fall just below genome-wide significance. (Figure from Radstake et al, Nature Genetics 2010; 42:426–429, reproduced with permission from the author)

Gene Regions Associated with SSc

In this section, we will discuss a selection of gene regions that have been robustly associated with susceptibility to SSc in GWAS or candidate gene studies. As shown in Table 4.2 and Fig. 4.5, the vast majority of robustly replicated SSc susceptibility loci are involved in innate or adaptive immune systems. However, additional genes in apoptotic and fibrotic pathways are also emerging. For the non-HLA genes, we focused on a selected list of genetic loci that were associated with SSc, its clinical (limited vs diffuse) subtypes, or serological subtypes that fulfilled the following criteria:

1. The loci were verified in at least two independent cohorts (replication and confirmation cohorts) in one or more studies
2. The association was not contradicted by a larger subsequent study

Immune System Regulatory Genes

1. The Major Histocompatibility Complex (HLA) and Antigen Presentation

   The association between HLA molecules and SSc was established in the 1970s. SSc is associated with class II HLA molecules for which strong genotypic variation has

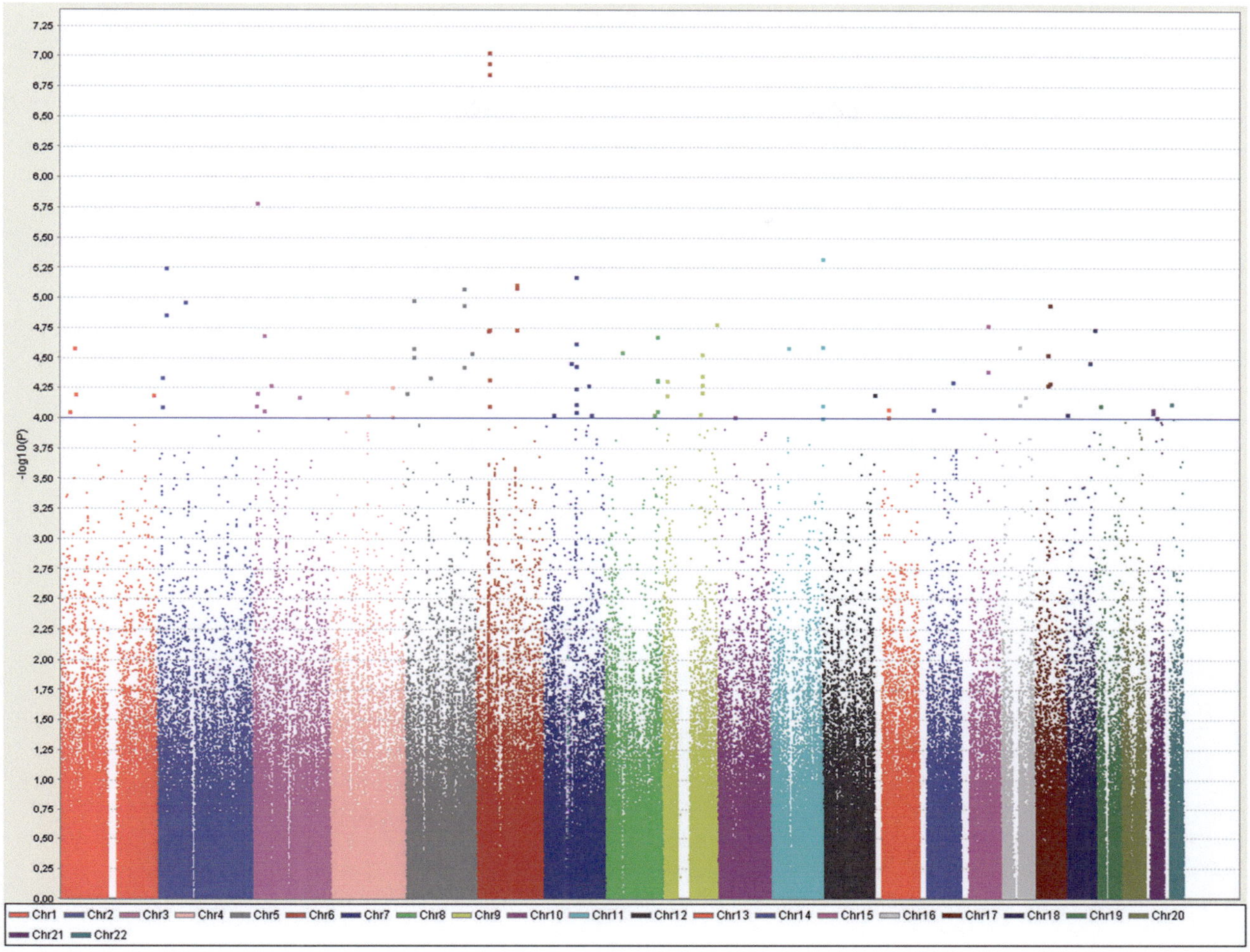

Fig. 4.3 Manhattan plot of the GWAS of 564 white SSc cases and 1776 healthy controls. (Figure from Allanore et al, PLoS Genet. 2011; e1002091, reproduced with permission from the author)

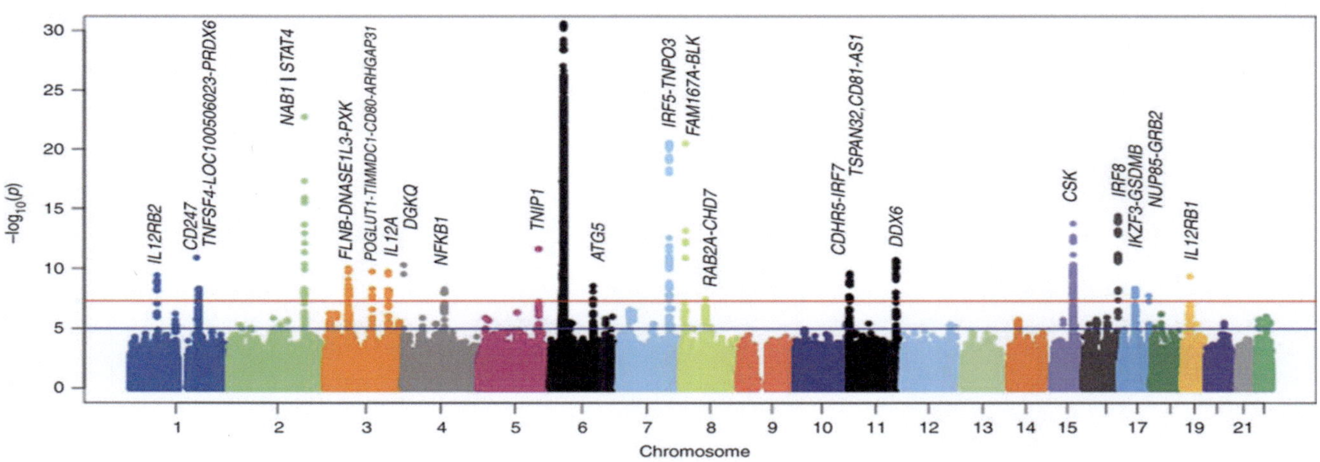

Fig. 4.4 Manhattan plot representing the meta-GWAS of 9095 patients with SSc and 17,584 controls. All study participants were white. This study identified 27 independent genome-wide associated signals, including 13 new risk loci. (Figure from Lopez-Isac et al. Nat Commun. 2019;10:4955, reproduced with permission from the author)

Table 4.2 Selected genetic susceptibility loci in systemic sclerosis

Gene	Chr	SNP	Type of study	Comments
TNFSF4 (OX40L)	1q25	rs1234314; rs2205960 rs844648	Candidate gene (American population)	Association particularly with autoantibody status; mainly limited cutaneous Scc
TNFSF4-PRDX6	1q25	rs2022449 rs1857066	Whole-genome	Regulatory region ncRNA intronic
PTPN22	1p13	rs2476601	Candidate gene (with replication in an independent population)	Limited to ACA+ or Topo+ patients
CD247	1q24	rs2056626	Whole-genome	
STAT4	2q32	rs7574865 rs3821236 rs4853458	Candidate gene and whole-genome	
BANK1	4q24	rs10516487 rs3733197 rs17266594	Candidate gene	Only the diffuse cutaneous subtype
NAB1	2q32	rs16832798	Whole-genome	
HLA class II	6	NA	Candidate gene and whole-genome	
TNFAIP3	6q23	rs5029939	Candidate gene (European white population)	Severe phenotype, causal variant not identified
IRF5	7q32	rs2004640, rs4728142 rs36073657, rs12155080	Candidate gene and whole-genome	Diffuse cutaneous form and pulmonary fibrosis SSc survival and risk of ILD
C8orf13/BLK	8p23-p22	rs2736340 rs13277113	Candidate gene (with replication in an independent population)	Higher risk if ACA+
IRF8	16q24	rs11117432; 11642873 rs11117420	Candidate gene Whole-genome	LcSSc
IRF7	11p1511p15	rs1131665	Candidate gene	ACA+
CDHR5 -IRF7	11p15	rs6598008	Whole-genome	
TLR2	4q32	rs5743704	Candidate gene	Topo+
CCR6	6q27	rs10946216	Candidate gene	Topo+
BANK1	4q24	rs10516487; 3733197	Candidate gene	DcSSc
BLK	8p23-p22	rs13277113; rs2736340	Candidate gene	
GRB10	7p12	rs12540874	Secondary analyses of GWAS	LcSSc
CAV1	7q31	rs959173	Candidate gene	
SOX5	12p12		Secondary analyses of GWAS	ACA+
CSK	15q24	rs1378942	Secondary analyses of GWAS	
DNASE1L3	3p14	rs35677470	Immunochip	ACA+
FLNB-DNASE1L3-PXK	3p14	rs7355798 rs4076852	Whole-genome	
DDX6	11q23	rs11217020	Whole-genome	
POGLUT1-TIMMDC1-CD80-ARHGAP31	3q13	rs9884090	Whole-genome	
DGKQ	4p16	Rs11724804	Whole-genome	
NFKB1	4q24	rs11724804	Whole-genome	
ATG5	6q21	rs9373839	Immunochip	
IL12RB2	1p31	rs3790567 rs3790567	Secondary analyses of GWAS Whole genome	
IL12RB1	19p13	rs2305743	Whole genome	
IL12A	3q25	rs589446	Whole-genome	ncRNA intronic
IL21	4q26	rs6822844	Candidate gene	
GSDMA	17q21	rs3894194	Multi-ethnic meta whole-genome	
IKZF3 -GSDMB	17q12	rs883770	Whole-genome	
PRDM1	6q21	rs4134466	Multi-ethnic meta whole-genome	
RAB2A-CHD7	8q12	rs685985	Whole-genome	
NUP85 -GRB2	17q25	rs1005714	Whole-genome	
IRAK1/MECP2	Xq28	IRAK1 rs1059702 MECP2 rs17435	Candidate gene	DcSSc, Topo+ ILD

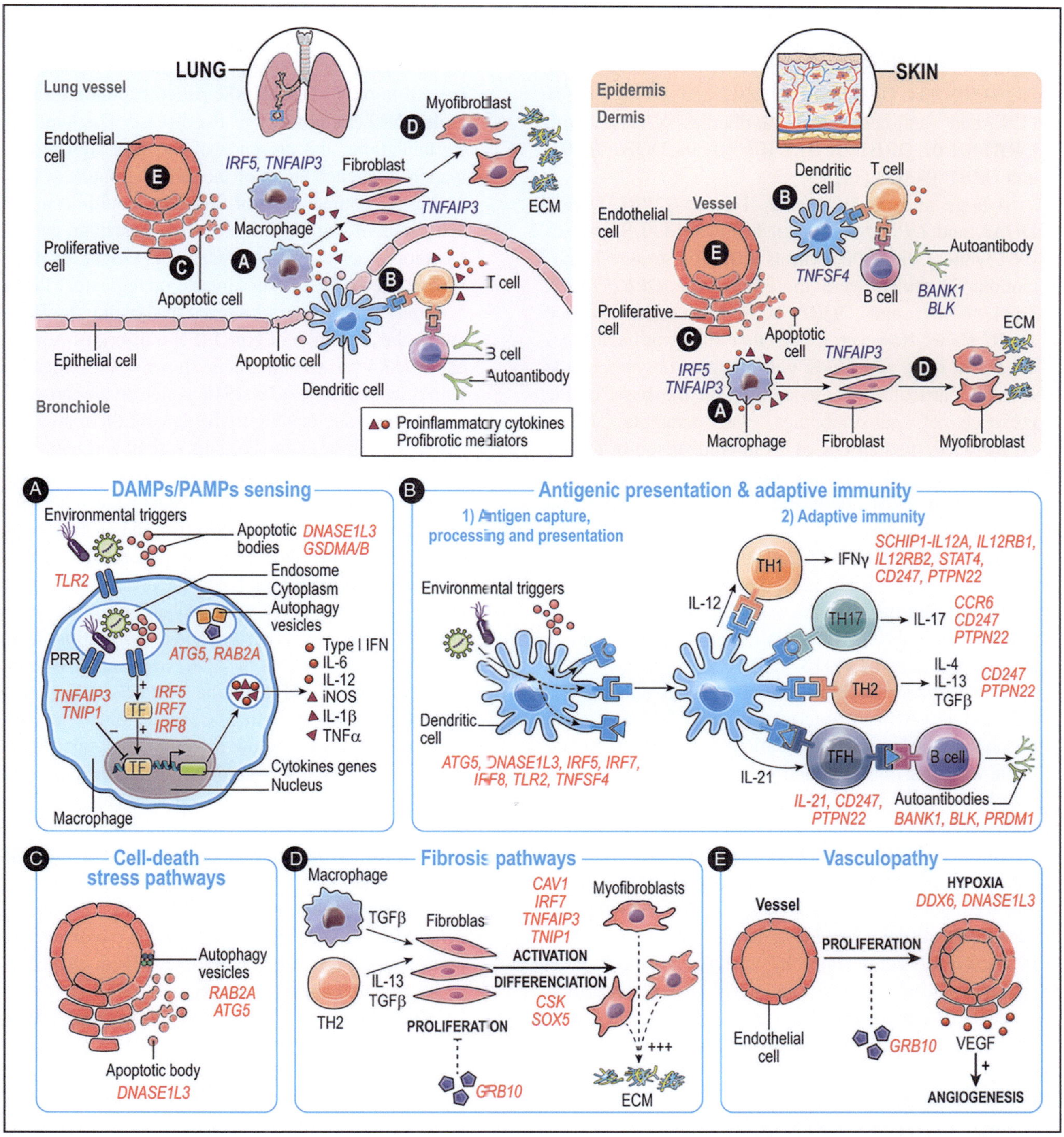

Fig. 4.5 Integration of SSc genetics in disease process. Susceptibility genes in red italic (located in each panel from A to E) and in blue italic (located in center panels) are, respectively, associated with SSc or with two severe forms of SSc: interstitial lung disease (ILD) and diffuse cutaneous sclerosis (dcSSc). Figure from Orvain et al. Curr Opin Rheumatol. 2020;32:505–514. Reproduced with permission from the author

been found between ethnic groups, as well as prominent associations with SSc related autoantibodies: anti-topoisomerase I (topo) with DRB1*11-*15:02 [17], DQB1*03-*04 [18], DPB1*13:01, and DPB1**09:01 [19] and anti-centromere antibodies (ACA) with DRB1*01:01, DRB1*01:04, DRB1*01:08, DQB1*05:01, and DPB1*04:02 ([17, 19].

A large study of HLA class II genes (*DRB1, DQB1, DQA1,* and *DPB1*) was carried out in 1300 SSc cases (961 whites) and 1000 controls [20]. The strongest associations identified were those with the *DRB1*11:04, DQA1*05:01,* and *DQB1*03:01* haplotypes and the *DQB1* allele. However, many other alleles or haplotypes have also been associated with certain subtypes of the disease, particularly those defined on the basis of the presence of autoantibodies. For example, HLA-*DPB1*13:01* had an OR of 14 in comparison of topo + SSc patients to controls. In a similar study, 944 white SSc patients and 1320 unaffected controls from Italy and Spain were examined. The association of *DRB1*11:04, DQA1*05:01,* and *DQB1*03:01* haplotype with SSc was confirmed in this study [21]. Recent GWAS data have confirmed that the strongest susceptibility locus in SSc was located in the class II HLA region on chromosome 6 (Figs. 4.1, 4.2, and 4.4) [10–12, 14].

A recent study in 662 African American patients with SSc and 946 African American controls [22] confirmed the previously described association of *HLA-DRB1*08:04* allele with anti-fibrillarin antibodies [23] and described a novel association of *HLA-DQB1*06:09* with this antibody subtype.

These findings also reflect the considerable differences in HLA genetic background between ethnic groups and the tremendous heterogeneity of the disease itself. Finally, the complex genetic structure of the HLA system in terms of LD complicates fine analyses and the identification of causal variants. The advent of next-generation sequencing technology demonstrates a unique opportunity to investigate this highly polymorphic genomic region.

2. Innate Immunity
   - Interferon pathway (*IRF5, IRF7,* and *IRF8*)

     Type I interferon (IFN) is a key mediator of innate immunity and the normal immune response triggered by microbial infection. IFN stimulates the maturation of monocytes to generate dendritic cells and plasmocytes, immunoglobulin class switching, the cytotoxic activity of natural killer cells and lymphocytes, and the synthesis of chemokines. Various studies, including some based-on transcriptomics, have shown a prominent IFN-regulated gene signature in circulating immune cells and skin in SSc [24–26]. Recent studies have generated consistent results but with several fine points of difference for SSc in terms of the magnitude and prevalence of the IFN signature in SSc compared to lupus patients [27]. In general, the IFN signature is present in only ~50% of SSc patients, pointing to the molecular heterogeneity of the disease. The hypothesis underlying the presence of the IFN signature is inappropriate activation of the innate immune system during the pathogenesis of SSc. This could occur via activation of pathogen-associated molecular pattern receptors, such as toll-like receptors (TLR) [28, 29].

The *IRF5* gene encodes interferon regulatory factor 5, a transcription factor involved in signaling by TLRs and in the activation of type I IFN transcripts. A number of *IFR5* variants have been shown to be associated with SSc, including rs2004640, which creates an alternative splice site leading to the generation of an alternative transcript (exon 1B). This variant was identified by a candidate gene approach [30], and the homozygous genotype was found to be associated with SSc-related pulmonary fibrosis. Multivariate analyses also showed this association to be significant for the allele and the homozygous genotype, suggesting a role in the severe pulmonary fibrosis phenotype. This finding was also replicated in an independent population from Japan [31]. In a GWAS of 2296 cases and 5014 controls [11], three SNPs in the *TNPO3-IRF5* region showed associations with SSc at a genome-wide significance level. In a follow-up study, the minor allele of one of those SNPs (rs4728142) was associated with longer survival and higher forced vital capacity. This gene variant was also associated with lower IRF5 transcript levels in monocytes of patients and controls [32]. Association of *IRF5* with SSc was also confirmed in the recent large-scale meta-GWAS [14]. These data definitively identify *IRF5* as one of the major susceptibility factors for SSc, playing a key role in type I IFN production and innate immunity.

IRF8 is another interferon regulatory factor that represents a risk locus in SSc. In a GWAS follow-up study examining the susceptibility loci of SSc serological and clinical subtypes, *IRF8* (rs11642873) was associated with limited cutaneous SSc (lcSSc) in the discovery and replication cohorts (OR = 0.75, $p = 2.32\text{E-}12$) [33].

These results were corroborated by another study, using an independent sample, and that showed an association between *IRF8* rs11117432 SNP and SSc susceptibility together with confirming, in a meta-analysis, the association signal for rs11642873 [34]. Haplotype analyses suggested a stronger association for rs11117432 for a subset of our patients, but a denser genotyping would be required to better narrow a potential causal variant. Furthermore, the latter report indicates that the variant *IRF8* rs11117432 increases IFN-γ, whereas decreases IFIT1 gene expression. IRF8 is a nuclear protein, which, upon stimulation by pathogen-associated molecular pattern molecules (PAMPs), moves into the cytoplasm and activates NF-κB and TLR signaling pathways, leading to cytokine production and regulating inflammatory responses. Moreover, an association of an additional *IRF8* SNP (rs11117420) with SSc was reported in the recently completed meta-GWAS [14].

Interferon regulatory factor 7 (IRF7) also represents a susceptibility locus for SSc, specifically for the ACA positive subgroup. A non-synonymous SNP (rs1131665) located in the exonic region of *IRF7* was associated with ACA positive SSc in US and European cohorts (overall OR = 0.78, $P_{FDR} = 6.14 \times 10^{-4}$—the minor allele is protective) [35]. This *IRF7* SNP is also associated with SLE in a concordant direction, and the disease associated variant was associated with higher *IRF7* activity [36] IRF7 is predicted to be among the top regulators of SSc skin and peripheral blood gene expression profile [27, 37]. It is also upregulated in SSc skin and dermal fibroblasts at transcript and protein levels. Importantly, IRF7 co-immunoprecipitated with SMAD3, a key mediator of transforming growth factor (TGF)-β signaling, and IRF7 knockdown reduced profibrotic factors in SSc fibroblasts. IRF7 knock out mice demonstrated attenuated dermal fibrosis compared with wild-type mice in response to bleomycin. An attenuated fibrotic response was also observed in IRF7 KO TSK/+mice [38]. *IRF7* was also confirmed as an SSc susceptibility locus in the recent meta GWAS [14].

- *Toll like receptor 2 (TLR2)*

  Toll like receptors as pattern recognition molecules are pivotal elements of innate immunity. A relatively rare, non-synonymous SNP in *TRL2* (rs5743704) was associated with anti-topo + SSc in two European patient cohorts (overall OR = 2.55, $P < 0.001$). The dendritic cells of SSc patients carrying the risk allele also showed increased IL6 and TNF-α production upon TLR-2 agonist stimulation [39]. The association of *TLR2* with SSc has not been confirmed in an independent study.
- *Interleukin 1 receptor associated kinase-1 (IRAK1) and methyl-CpG-binding protein 2 (MECP2)*
- SNPs in the *IRAK1* and *MECP2* have been linked to SSc. Both genes are located on the X-chromosome (Xq28 genomic region), which raises the possibility that these risk loci might contribute to female predilection in SSc. IRAK1 has an important immune modulatory function by modulating the IL1-induced activation of NF-κB in the TLR pathway whereas MECP2 encodes a nuclear protein that binds specifically to methylated DNA, playing a central role in the transcriptional regulation of methylation-sensitive genes. A non-synonymous SNP in the *IRAK1* (rs1059702) was associated with diffuse cutaneous SSc (dcSSc) and topo positive in female patients and controls recruited from French and follow-up German/Italian cohorts. Furthermore, this SNP was associated with SSc related fibrosing alveolitis in addition to dcSSc and topo positive SSc. These associations remained significant even in case–case comparisons (i.e., dcSSc versus lcSSc, topo- versus ACA-positive SSc, and SSc with- versus without fibrosing alveolitis) [40]. A follow-up study investigated the above *IRAK1* SNP and four additional SNPs on the *MECP2* gene. The *IRAK1* SNP rs1059702 and *MECP2* rs17435 were both associated specifically with dcSSc in female patients and controls recruited from Spain and follow-up European/US cohorts. However, conditional logistic regression analysis indicated that the association of *IRAK1* rs1059702 with dcSSc was explained by the effect of *MECP2* rs17435. These two SNPs were in moderate LD (r^2 0.6). However, only *IRAK1* SNP rs1059702 was associated with the presence of fibrosing alveolitis in case–control and case–case comparisons (OR = 1.3, $P_{FDR} = 0.039$; OR = 1.26, $p = 0.025$, respectively) [41].

3. Adaptive Immunity
   - CD247

     A SNP in the *CD247* gene (the rs2056626) was associated with SSc in the first white GWAS SSc Study (combined analysis: $P = 3.39E^{-9}$; OR 0.86; 95% CI 0.81–0.90) [11]. This gene encodes the zeta subunit of the T-cell receptor (TCR), which is involved in the formation of the TCR/CD3 complex. This finding was subsequently confirmed in a French independent cohort [42]. The recently completed meta GWAS confirmed the association of *CD247* rs2056626 with SSc and indicated that this intronic SNP is associated with regulatory elements for CD247 expression based on its strong H3K27ac HiChIP signal to CD247 promoter [14].
   - *Transcription factor signal transducer and activator of transcription 4 (STAT4)*

     The gene product of *STAT4* is a member of the STAT family that regulates the expression of many genes. Studies on STAT4 have focused particularly on T lymphocytes and have demonstrated that this molecule is activated by interleukins 12 and 23 and by type I interferon. STAT4 plays an important role in the orientation of T helper cells toward the Th1 and Th17 proinflammatory phenotypes. Several genetic studies have identified associations between variants of the *STAT4* gene and autoimmune diseases. Such an association has been identified, in particular, for an SNP within the third intron, rs7574865, which may induce alternative splicing or other changes to transcription, although its precise role remains to be established.

- Two large studies of European populations have independently demonstrated an association between this marker, rs7574865, and the disease [43, 44]. However, one of these studies found that the association was restricted to the limited cutaneous subtype [44], whereas the other found no restriction to a particular cutaneous subtype and instead showed an association with pulmonary fibrosis [43]. Complementary studies in North America [45] and Japan [46] provide support for an association between the *STAT4* gene and SSc, but the variants studied were principally susceptibility factors for the limited cutaneous form and for the presence of ACAs. As for *IRF5*, the association between *STAT4* and the disease has recently been confirmed by a whole-genome approach [11, 12, 14], definitively placing *STAT4* on the list of susceptibility factors for SSc.

  STAT4 is a genetic susceptibility factor not only in SSc but also in other autoimmune diseases. One very challenging question is the real impact of *STAT4* variants on the SSc phenotype. A first translational approach has been reported investigating the contribution of *STAT4* in the development of a fibrotic phenotype in two different mouse models of experimental dermal fibrosis [47]. Mice deficient for *stat4* (stat4(−/−)) and wildtype littermates (stat4(+/+)) were injected with bleomycin or NaCl, and the outcome of mice lacking *stat4* was also investigated in the tight-skin (tsk-1) mouse model. *Stat4*(−/−) mice appeared to be protected from bleomycin-induced dermal fibrosis with a reduction of dermal thickening (65 ± 3% reduction, $p = 0.03$), hydroxyproline content (68 ± 5% decrease, $p = 0.02$), and myofibroblast counts (71 ± 6% reduction, $p = 0.05$). Moreover, the number of infiltrating leukocytes, and especially T cells, was significantly decreased in the lesional skin of *stat4*(−/−) mice (63 ± 5% reduction of T-cell counts, $p = 0.02$). *Stat4*(−/−) mice also displayed decreased levels of inflammatory cytokines, such as TNFα, IL-6, IL-2, and IFNγ in the lesional skin. Consistent with the primary role of STAT4 in inflammation, STAT4 deficiency did not ameliorate fibrosis in *tsk-1* mice. These data demonstrate that the transcription factor STAT4 exerts potent profibrotic effects by controlling T-cell activation, proliferation, and cytokine release. These findings help validate the results of the genetic studies on the role of *STAT4* in the development of SSc and open new avenues for potential innovative therapies.

- *Tumor Necrosis Factor Ligand Superfamily, Member 4 (TNFSF4)*

  TNFSF4 encodes the OX40 antigen ligand, which is involved in interactions between T cells/antigen presentation and the activation of T and B cells. Variants of this gene are associated with lupus, and a case–control study of 1059 US white SSc cases and 698 controls revealed associations for several SNPs of this gene, with specific associations dependent on autoantibody status [48]. This finding was replicated in a study based on a total of eight European populations of white ancestry comprising 3014 patients with SSc and 3125 healthy controls [49]. A third study examined the association of *TNFSF4* SNPs in 1031 SSc patients and 1014 controls of French white ancestry and performed a meta-analysis of all three studies. The meta-analysis confirmed the overall association with SSc but also showed preferential association with the ACA+ subset. The strongest effect was seen with the *TNFSF4* SNP rs2205960 (OR 1.33, $p = 0.00013$) [50]. Association of *TNFSF4* with SSc was confirmed in the recent meta GWAS [14]. OX40L levels are increased in SSc skin, and serum OX40L levels were predictive of worsening pulmonary fibrosis. Moreover, both OX40L knock out and treatment with anti-OX40L mAb reduced bleomycin-induced dermal fibrosis in murine models. Furthermore, treatment anti-OX40L mAb reduced lung fibrosis and perivascular inflammation in the Fra-2 mouse model [51].

- *Protein tyrosine phosphatase, non-receptor type 22 (lymphoid) (PTPN22)*

  PTPN22 encodes the LYP protein, a tyrosine phosphatase expressed by lymphoid cell lines. This enzyme regulates T-lymphocyte activation by interacting with the effector kinases. It can down-regulate the negative selection of T cells in the thymus. The T allele of non-synonymous SNP rs2476601 (PTPN22*620W) induces a gain of function, which may prevent the deletion of autoreactive T cells in the thymus or may lead to insufficient activity of Treg cells. The PTPN22*620W allele is thus involved in various autoimmune diseases and has been shown to be associated, in particular, with type 1 diabetes, lupus, and rheumatoid factor-positive rheumatoid arthritis. An allelic association was found in North American multi-ethnic patients (905 patients and 656 controls) with topo and ACA antibodies [52]. Subsequently, seven SNPs were studied in a French sample of 659 patients and 504 healthy controls. In 8% of the patients, an autoimmune disease known to be associated with PTPN22 (e.g., thyroiditis) was discovered. These patients were excluded from the analysis. No allelic or genotype association was reported, but a haplotypic association was found: the disease was associated with the haplotype that carried the PTPN22*620W allele ($P = 1.52 \times 10^{-7}$) [53]. Finally, a meta-analysis study with the inclusion of the above studies and the addition of European Whites patients showed that PTPN22*620W was associated with SSc (OR = 1.15, $P_{FDR} = 0.03$) and ACA + SSc (OR = 1.22, $P_{FDR} = 0.02$) [54].

- *B cell-specific scaffold protein with ankyrin (BANK1)*

  Despite the specificity of certain autoantibodies in SSc, the role of B lymphocytes had not been clearly established. Genetic data confirm the probable role of these antibodies in the disease. The *BANK1* gene encodes the B cell-specific scaffold protein with ankyrin repeats, which act as a substrate of the LYN tyrosine, phosphorylating the inositol 1,4,5-triphosphate receptors. Two non-synonymous and functional SNPs of *BANK1* (rs10516487 and rs3733197) were associated with the diffuse cutaneous form of the disease in 1295 patients and 11,137 controls of French and German White ancestry [55] and in another European study of 2380 patients and 3270 controls [56].

- *Chemokine receptor 6 (CCR6):*

  CCR6 protein, the receptor of CCL20, is a surface marker for IL-17 producing TH17 cells. CCR6 is a key factor for recruiting TH17 into target tissue. *CCR6* rs10946216 was associated with topo+ SSc (OR = 1.32 Padj = 9E-5) in three European populations (France, Italy, and Germany) [57]. This genetic association has not been yet investigated in independent studies. This finding provides support for potential role of Th17 pathways in SSc pathogenesis.

- *B lymphocyte kinase (BLK):*

  The protein encoded by *BLK* transduces the downstream B-cell receptor (BCR) signal. Two variants of the *C8orf13-BLK* region (rs13277113 and rs2736340) were studied in 1050 white cases and 694 controls from the USA, and a replication study was carried out in 589 cases and 722 controls from Spain. In the pooled analyses, *BLK* SNP rs2736340 was associated with SSc and especially with the lcSSc and ACA+ subsets [58]. Furthermore, the SNP rs13277113 was found to be associated with SSc in a Japanese study [59]. In a meta-analysis that included the above studies and an additional 1031 patients and 1014 controls from France, this SNP was associated with SSc and especially with dcSSc [60]. *BLK* was also confirmed as an SSc susceptibility locus in the recent SSc meta GWAS [14].

- *IL12 signaling pathways*

  IL-12 levels are increased in the serum of SSc patients as well as in the alveolar lavage fluid from patients with SSc-associated interstitial lung disease. IL12 can trigger a pro-inflammatory cell-mediated immunity and Th1 response. Four genes in the IL12 signaling pathway were reported to be associated with SSc, implying an important role for this cytokine in SSc pathogenesis.

  IL12RB2 intronic SNP rs3790567 was associated with SSc in a GWAS follow-up study of US/European white patients (OR = 1.17, p = 2.82 E-9) [61]. Similarly, a SNP in the intergenic region of *SHIP1-IL12A* (rs7758790) was associated with SSc with a relatively high OR of 2.57 (p = 1.22 E-11) in the US/European white Immunochip study, providing further evidence for the importance of IL12 signaling in SSc [15]. Furthermore, an Immunochip follow-up study revealed that *IL12RB1* SNP rs436857 was associated with SSc (pooled OR = 0.81, p = 3.9 E-9) in combined US/European cohorts [62]. Lastly, *IL12RB1* SNP rs2305743 was associated with SSc (pooled OR = 0.83, p = 4.6 E-10) in the recent SSc meta GWAS [14]. The above associations in IL12 signaling pathways have not been yet replicated in independent studies.

- *Interleukin 21 (IL-21)*

  IL-21 protein is a potent regulatory cytokine that is expressed in Th2, Th17, and NK cells. The *IL-21* SNP rs6822844, which is located in the flanking 3′-untranslated region of *IL-21,* was associated with SSc in patients of European/US white descent (pooled OR = 0.86, p = 6.6E-04) [63]. This genetic association has not been yet replicated in independent studies.

NFκB Signaling

- *Tumor necrosis factor, alpha-induced protein 3 (TNFAIP3)*

  TNFAIP3 (6q23) encodes the A20 protein, a zinc-finger protein required for feedback control of the NFkB (nuclear factor–kB) signaling pathway. Furthermore, A20 can negatively regulate NLRP3 inflammasome activity [64], as well as Wnt/β-catenin signaling [65]. Three variants of this gene were genotyped in a European sample of 1656 patients and 1311 controls, and the rs5029939 (allele G) marker was identified as associated with the disease (OR 2.08; P = 1.16E-7) [66]. Strong associations have also been found with certain phenotypes, including, in particular, the diffuse cutaneous form of the disease (OR 2.71, P = 5.2E-9), pulmonary fibrosis (OR 2.26, P = 2.5E-6), and pulmonary arterial hypertension (OR 3.11, P = 1.3E-5), suggesting a possible role of TNFAIP3 in disease severity. The observed genetic association has not been yet investigated in independent studies, although another *TNFAIP3* SNP was associated with ACA+ SSc in the US/European Immunochip study [15]. In a study examining potential interaction between SSc susceptibility loci of environmental exposures, the *TNFAIP3* rs58905141 variant was associated with time–course and/or dose–response expression of MMP3 and MMP1 using an in-vitro model of fibroblasts stimulated by silica particles. In silico functional analysis revealed that rs58905141 might affect the binding activities of the transcription factors to TNFAIP3 [67].

- *TNFAIP3 interacting protein 1 (TNIP1)*

  TNIP1 protein down-regulates NFκB signaling in part by interacting with TNAIP3. *TNIP1* SNP rs2233287 was associated with SSc in the discovery and replication cohorts of the European GWAS (pooled OR: 1.31, $p = 4.7$E-09). Furthermore, TNIP1 levels were lower at protein and mRNA levels in the skin tissue of SSc patients compared to unaffected controls. Recombinant TNIP1 abrogated collagen ssynthesis in SSc and control fibroblasts, showing the relevance of this inflammatory molecule for fibrotic response [12]. The association of *TNIP1* with SSc was confirmed in an independent US/European study [68]. Furthermore, the recent SSc meta GWAS identified *TNIP1* rs3792783 as an SSc susceptibility locus [14].

- Nuclear factor–kB (NFκB)

  Further supporting the role of NFκB, an intronic SNP in NFκB gene region was found to be associated with SSc (pooled OR: 1.15, $p = 5.4$ E-09) in the recent meta GWAS [14].

Apoptosis and Autophagy

Several genes involved in apoptosis, and determination of cell fate have been associated with SSc and its clinical subtypes. The prominent role of dysregulated apoptosis in vascular and immune components of SSc pathogenesis raises the importance of the below genetic loci for follow-up mechanistic studies.

- *Autophagy-related 5 (ATG5)*

  ATG5 protein forms a complex with ATG12 and assists in autophagosomal elongation. Autophagy mediates pathogen degradation and allows cells to clear unwanted cytoplasmic material and recycle nutrients. It plays a pivotal role in adaptive and innate immunity. *ATG5* SNP rs9373839 was associated with SSc in the US/European white Immunochip study, linking SSc pathogenesis to autophagy (pooled OR = 1.19, $p = 3.75$ E-8) [15]. Moreover, another *ATG5* SNP (rs633724) was associated with SSc in the recent meta GWAS [14].

- *RAB2A*

  In the recent meta-GWAS, *RAB2A* sr68598 (pooled OR: 0.87, $p = 3.8$ E-08) was identified as an SSc susceptibility variant [14]. RAB2A is a member of the Rab family, a group of membrane-bound proteins, involved in vesicular fusion and trafficking. Specifically, RAB2A has been proposed to be a key factor in autophagosome clearance, further highlighting autophagy as a mechanism involved in SSc pathogenesis.

- *DDX6*

  DDX6 is another locus identified in the meta-GWAS (rs11217020; pooled OR = 0.84, $p = 2.08$ E-11) that is linked with autophagy where it could act as a suppressor [14]. This gene encodes a member of the DEAD box protein family. The protein is an RNA helicase found in P-bodies and stress granules, and functions in translation suppression and mRNA degradation. DDX6 regulates vascular endothelial growth factor under hypoxic conditions [69], which might be pertinent to vascular components of SSc pathogenesis.

- *Deoxyribonuclease I-like 3 (DNASEIL3)*

  DNASEIL3 protein plays an important role in vesicular DNA fragmentation during apoptosis and in the generation of resected double-strand breaks in immunoglobulin-encoding genes. The nonsynonymous *DNASEIL3* SNP rs35677470 was associated with SSc in the first SSc Immunochip study in patients of European/US white descent (pooled OR = 1.47, $p = 3.36$E-16). The association was strongest in the ACA$^+$ SSc (pooled OR = 2.03, $p = 4.25$ E-31) [15]. This gene variant results in an Arg-to-Cys amino acid substitution and loss of a hydrogen bond leading to diminished DNase activity. This genetic association was confirmed in subsequent Australian Immunochip study [16]. Although this SNP could not be investigated in the recently completed meta GWAS, two SNPs in the *FLNB-DNASE1L3-PXK* gene region were associated with SSc in this study [14].

- *SRY (sex determining region Y)-box 5 (SOX5)*

  SOX5 protein is a transcription factor involved in determination of cell fate. A *SOX5* SNP was associated with ACA+ SSc in a GWAS follow-up study in US/European White populations (pooled OR = 1.36, $P = 1.39$ E-7). This finding has not been investigated in independent studies.

- *GSDM A/B*

  A missense SNP in *GSDMA*, rs3894194, was associated with SSc in a Japanese and European population GWAS meta-analysis (overall OR 0.85, $P = 1.4$ E-10) [13]. GSDMA is highly expressed in the skin and is involved in the regulatory effect of gene expression in various cell types including skin fibroblasts. This association has not been yet independently confirmed. A GSDMB SNP (rs883770) was associated with SSc susceptibility (pooled OR: 1.13, $p = 4.79$ E-09) in the recent meta GWAS [14]. It encodes a member of the gasdermin-domain containing protein family. GSDMB variants have been associated with primary biliary cirrhosis. The functional mechanism of gasdermin proteins is not clearly understood, but GSDMA and GSDMB could have a role in pyroptosis, which is a programmed cell death associated with inflammation.

Fibrosis Pathways

Fibrosis is the ultimate end-product of SSc in several prominently affected organs, such as skin and lungs. Although the majority of SSc susceptibility loci belong to immune regulation pathways, genetic associations with few genes, prominently involved in fibrotic pathways, have been also reported.

- *c-Src tyrosine kinase (CSK)*

  CSK protein is involved in the regulation of myofibroblast differentiation in vitro and in mouse models by modulating the function of src kinase [70]. Src kinases are involved in fibrosis by regulating the transmission of integrin signaling upon the adhesion of fibroblasts to the extracellular matrix and their subsequent differentiation into myofibroblasts. *CSK* SNP rs1378942 was associated with SSc in a GWAS follow-up study in US/European white populations (pooled OR = 1.2, $P = 5.04E\text{-}12$) [71]. The association of this SNP with SSc was confirmed in the recent SSc meta GWAS [14].
- *Caveolin 1 (CAV1)*

  CAV1 protein is an inhibitor of tissue fibrosis, and decreased CAV1 expression has been thought to contribute to the fibrotic process in SSc. Based on its relevance to SSc pathogenesis, the SNPs with the highest association in *CAV1* in the GWAS of French SSc patients were investigated in an Italian white cohort. *CAV1* SNP rs959173 was associated with SSc (pooled OR 0.81, 95%, $p = 0.0018$). Indeed, *CAV1* protein expression levels were significantly higher in skin samples of both patients with SSc and controls carrying the allele that was protective for SSc (rs959173 C) in follow-up western blot and immunohistochemistry experiments [72]. The observed genetic association has not been yet investigated in independent studies.
- *Growth factor receptor-bound protein 10 (GRB10)*

  GRB10 protein interacts with a number of receptor tyrosine kinases and insulin-like growth factor receptors and regulates cell growth. Both tyrosine kinases and insulin-like growth factors have been implicated in SSc pathogenesis. *GRB10* SNP rs12540874 was associated with lc SSc in the GWAS follow-up study (OR = 1.15, $P = 1.27$ E-6) [33]. This finding has not been investigated in independent studies.

Conclusion

It is clear from these studies that there is a genetic component to the physiopathology of SSc, and major progress has been recently achieved in understanding the genetics of SSc susceptibility. Multi-center and transnational efforts have allowed the building of large cohorts, which are mandatory to investigate the genetic component in complex disorders. The majority of the risk loci that have been identified *and* replicated thus far are involved in autoimmune regulation. This finding provides further support for the hypothesis that the inciting immune dysregulations trigger and maintain the fibrotic manifestations of SSc. As in many polygenic diseases, the presence of several polymorphisms in a given individual probably contributes to the risk of the disease, with each polymorphism having only a minimal effect on its own. It is also possible that these genetic loci have a multiplicative effect on disease susceptibility by gene–gene or gene–environment interactions.

The most consistent results to date have been obtained for the autoimmune component, with replication in large studies identifying *HLA, IRF5, CD247 STAT4,* and so on as the principal genes involved (Table 4.2). Several of these genes are already well-established risk factors for other autoimmune diseases, raising the possibility of shared autoimmunity [73]. Several genetic factors of relatively small effect may cumulatively create a state of susceptibility to autoimmune diseases according to the quantitative threshold concept (reviewed in [74]). Self-reactive B and T cells are normal components of the immune system. However, they are usually kept in check by regulatory mechanisms in the thymus/bone marrow or peripheral blood. In the concept of quantitative threshold, the implicated shared genetic variations in autoimmune diseases lead cumulatively to an impairment of the necessary biological processes for the destruction of self-reactive immune cells, leading to autoimmunity. Although the disease manifestations of specific autoimmune diseases vary, the genetic basis for the occurrence of autoimmunity seems to overlap among them. It is possible that other triggers, such as environmental and stochastic factors, further contribute to the phenotypic manifestation of a specific autoimmune disease in a susceptible host.

Many of the reported susceptibility SNPs are located in non-coding regions (introns). It is possible that these loci are in LD with SNPs in coding regions. However, there is also increasing evidence that these loci might influence the transcription of regulatory RNAs, such as microRNAs or long-non-coding RNAs [75]. These regulatory RNAs might have important biological functions in SSc pathogenesis [76].

The identified susceptibility loci have individually only small to modest effect sizes for disease risk, raising the question of whether a combination of these risk loci can lead to a genetic risk score of higher effect size. In a recent study [77], a cumulative genetic risk score was developed based on the SSc meta GWAS data [14], and its diagnostic property for SSc was examined in an independent sample compromising 400 patients with SSc and 571 controls. The best fitting model combined the weighted effects of 33 susceptibility HLA and non-HLA SNPs was able to identify SSc patients with a diagnostic accuracy of an area under the receiver operating characteristic (ROC) curve (AUC) of 0.673. Individuals with genetic risk scores in the 95th percentile had 7.9-fold higher odds of having SSc than the reference group (40th–60th percentile). Although the resulting effect size is not sufficiently strong to make predictions about the individual person's risk for developing SSc in the clinical setting (as odds ratios in the range of 50 would be required [78]), this study represents a seminal work for future efforts focusing on multilevel models in which genetic risk factors are combined with other biological and clinical predictors to build a prediction tool of sufficient effect size. A recent study has indicated that genetic risk score calculation for inflammatory arthritis-causing diseases (rheumatoid arthritis, systemic lupus erythematosus, spondyloarthropathy, psoriatic arthritis, and gout) might be useful for improving the diagnostic efficiency during the initial clinical evaluation [79].

Last but not least, the highly complex puzzle of SSc genetics is not yet completely understood, and the so-called missing heritability is still challenging. This is a source of ongoing debate, and there are many potential contributors. Possible explanations are (1) Additional common variants with low genetic effects exist but current GWAS remain underpowered to identify such risk loci (Figs. 4.2, 4.3, and 4.4). (2) Rare variants might be involved that cannot be detected with the GWAS approach but direct association mapping through sequencing candidate genes, exomes, or entire genomes can be applied. (3) Genetic heterogeneity is also likely; genetic studies of clinically more homogeneous subforms of the disease may be targeted. (4) Interactions between genes or between genes and the environment are likely to contribute to the disease risk.

Key Points

- There is a familial risk of SSc, with the disease occurring more frequently in families in which cases have already been identified than in the general population.
- Clinical concordance between monozygotic twins is poor, but concordance rates are higher mainly for autoantibodies and fibrotic transcript profiles.
- International collaborations have enabled sufficiently powered, genome-wide association studies, leading to the discovery of robust and reproducible genetic susceptibility loci.
- The majority of SSc susceptibility loci are involved in innate and adaptive immunity, underscoring the role of immune dysregulation for the SSc pathogenesis.
- More recently, several genes involved in autophagy and apoptosis have been identified as SSc genetic risk loci.
- The majority of SSc susceptibility loci are located in the intronic areas, which might influence directly the transcription of non-coding regulatory RNAs or be in linkage disequilibrium with genetic variants in coding areas.

References

1. Feero WG, Guttmacher AE, Collins FS. Genomic medicine—an updated primer. N Engl J Med. 2010;362(21):2001–11.
2. Vitart V, Rudan I, Hayward C, Gray NK, Floyd J, Palmer CN, et al. SLC2A9 is a newly identified urate transporter influencing serum urate concentration, urate excretion and gout. Nat Genet. 2008;40(4):437–42.
3. Pearson TA, Manolio TA. How to interpret a genome-wide association study. JAMA. 2008;299(11):1335–44.
4. Kilpinen H, Barrett JC. How next-generation sequencing is transforming complex disease genetics. Trends Genet. 2013;29(1):23–30.
5. Plomin R, Haworth CM, Davis OS. Common disorders are quantitative traits. Nat Rev Genet. 2009;10(12):872–8.
6. Arnett FC, Cho M, Chatterjee S, Aguilar MB, Reveille JD, Mayes MD. Familial occurrence frequencies and relative risks for systemic sclerosis (scleroderma) in three United States cohorts. Arthritis Rheum. 2001;44(6):1359–62.
7. Assassi S, Arnett FC, Reveille JD, Gourh P, Mayes MD. Clinical, immunologic, and genetic features of familial systemic sclerosis. Arthritis Rheum. 2007;56(6):2031–7.
8. Feghali-Bostwick C, Medsger TA Jr, Wright TM. Analysis of systemic sclerosis in twins reveals low concordance for disease and high concordance for the presence of antinuclear antibodies. Arthritis Rheum. 2003;48(7):1956–63.
9. Zhou X, Tan FK, Xiong M, Arnett FC, Feghali-Bostwick CA. Monozygotic twins clinically discordant for scleroderma show concordance for fibroblast gene expression profiles. Arthritis Rheum. 2005;52(10):3305–14.
10. Zhou X, Lee JE, Arnett FC, Xiong M, Park MY, Yoo YK, et al. HLA-DPB1 and DPB2 are genetic loci for systemic sclerosis: a genome-wide association study in Koreans with replication in north Americans. Arthritis Rheum. 2009;60(12):3807–14.
11. Radstake TR, Gorlova O, Rueda B, Martin JE, Alizadeh BZ, Palomino-Morales R, et al. Genome-wide association study of systemic sclerosis identifies CD247 as a new susceptibility locus. Nat Genet. 2010;42(5):426–9.
12. Allanore Y, Saad M, Dieude P, Avouac J, Distler JH, Amouyel P, et al. Genome-wide scan identifies TNIP1, PSORS1C1, and RHOB as novel risk loci for systemic sclerosis. PLoS Genet. 2011;7(7):e1002091.
13. Terao C, Kawaguchi T, Dieude P, Varga J, Kuwana M, Hudson M, et al. Transethnic meta-analysis identifies GSDMA and PRDM1 as susceptibility genes to systemic sclerosis. Ann Rheum Dis. 2017;76(6):1150–8.
14. Lopez-Isac E, Acosta-Herrera M, Kerick M, Assassi S, Satpathy AT, Granja J, et al. GWAS for systemic sclerosis identifies multiple risk loci and highlights fibrotic and vasculopathy pathways. Nat Commun. 2019;10(1):4955.
15. Mayes MD, Bossini-Castillo L, Gorlova O, Martin JE, Zhou X, Chen WV, et al. Immunochip analysis identifies multiple susceptibility loci for systemic sclerosis. Am J Hum Genet. 2014;94(1):47–61.
16. Zochling J, Newell F, Charlesworth JC, Leo P, Stankovich J, Cortes A, et al. An Immunochip-based interrogation of scleroderma susceptibility variants identifies a novel association at DNASE1L3. Arthritis Res Ther. 2014;16(5):438.
17. Kuwana M, Inoko H, Kameda H, Nojima T, Sato S, Nakamura K, et al. Association of human leukocyte antigen class II genes with autoantibody profiles, but not with disease susceptibility in Japanese patients with systemic sclerosis. Intern Med. 1999;38(4):336–44.
18. Ueki A, Isozaki Y, Tomokuni A, Ueki H, Kusaka M, Tanaka S, et al. Different distribution of HLA class II alleles in anti-topoisomerase I autoantibody responders between silicosis and systemic sclerosis patients, with a common distinct amino acid sequence in the HLA-DQB1 domain. Immunobiology. 2001;204(4):458–65.

19. Gilchrist FC, Bunn C, Foley PJ, Lympany PA, Black CM, Welsh KI, et al. Class II HLA associations with autoantibodies in scleroderma: a highly significant role for HLA-DP. Genes Immun. 2001;2(2):76–81.
20. Arnett FC, Gourh P, Shete S, Ahn CW, Honey R, Agarwal SK, et al. Major histocompatibility complex (MHC) class II alleles, haplotypes, and epitopes which confer susceptibility or protection in the fibrosing autoimmune disease systemic sclerosis: analyses in 1300 Caucasian, African-American and Hispanic cases and 1000 controls. Ann Rheum Dis. 2009;69:822.
21. Beretta L, Rueda B, Marchini M, Santaniello A, Simeon CP, Fonollosa V, et al. Analysis of class II human leucocyte antigens in Italian and Spanish systemic sclerosis. Rheumatology (Oxford). 2012;51(1):52–9.
22. Gourh P, Safran SA, Alexander T, Boyden SE, Morgan ND, Shah AA, et al. HLA and autoantibodies define scleroderma subtypes and risk in African and European Americans and suggest a role for molecular mimicry. Proc Natl Acad Sci U S A. 2020;117(1):552–62.
23. Sharif R, Fritzler MJ, Mayes MD, Gonzalez EB, McNearney TA, Draeger H, et al. Anti-fibrillarin antibody in African American patients with systemic sclerosis: immunogenetics, clinical features, and survival analysis. J Rheumatol. 2011;38(8):1622–30.
24. Higgs BW, Liu Z, White B, Zhu W, White WI, Morehouse C, et al. Patients with systemic lupus erythematosus, myositis, rheumatoid arthritis and scleroderma share activation of a common type I interferon pathway. Ann Rheum Dis. 2011;70(11):2029–36.
25. Tan FK, Zhou X, Mayes MD, Gourh P, Guo X, Marcum C, et al. Signatures of differentially regulated interferon gene expression and vasculotrophism in the peripheral blood cells of systemic sclerosis patients. Rheumatology (Oxford). 2006;45(6):694–702.
26. York MR, Nagai T, Mangini AJ, Lemaire R, van Seventer JM, Lafyatis R. A macrophage marker, Siglec-1, is increased on circulating monocytes in patients with systemic sclerosis and induced by type I interferons and toll-like receptor agonists. Arthritis Rheum. 2007;56(3):1010–20.
27. Assassi S, Mayes MD, Arnett FC, Gourh P, Agarwal SK, McNearney TA, et al. Systemic sclerosis and lupus: points in an interferon-mediated continuum. Arthritis Rheum. 2010;62(2):589–98.
28. Farina GA, York MR, Di MM, Collins CA, Meller S, Homey B, et al. Poly(I:C) drives type I IFN- and TGFbeta-mediated inflammation and dermal fibrosis simulating altered gene expression in systemic sclerosis. J Invest Dermatol. 2010;130(11):2583–93.
29. Agarwal SK, Wu M, Livingston CK, Parks DH, Mayes MD, Arnett FC, et al. Toll-like receptor 3 upregulation by type I interferon in healthy and scleroderma dermal fibroblasts. Arthritis Res Ther. 2011;13(1):R3.
30. Dieude P, Guedj M, Wipff J, Avouac J, Fajardy I, Diot E, et al. Association between the IRF5 rs2004640 functional polymorphism and systemic sclerosis: a new perspective for pulmonary fibrosis. Arthritis Rheum. 2009;60(1):225–33.
31. Ito I, Kawaguchi Y, Kawasaki A, Hasegawa M, Ohashi J, Hikami K, et al. Association of a functional polymorphism in the IRF5 region with systemic sclerosis in a Japanese population. Arthritis Rheum. 2009;60(6):1845–50.
32. Sharif R, Mayes MD, Tan FK, Gorlova OY, Hummers LK, Shah AA, et al. IRF5 polymorphism predicts prognosis in patients with systemic sclerosis. Ann Rheum Dis. 2012;71:1197.
33. Gorlova O, Martin JE, Rueda B, Koeleman BP, Ying J, Teruel M, et al. Identification of novel genetic markers associated with clinical phenotypes of systemic sclerosis through a genome-wide association strategy. PLoS Genet. 2011;7(7):e1002178.
34. Arismendi M, Giraud M, Ruzehaji N, Dieude P, Koumakis E, Ruiz B, et al. Identification of NF-kappaB and PLCL2 as new susceptibility genes and highlights on a potential role of IRF8 through interferon signature modulation in systemic sclerosis. Arthritis Res Ther. 2015;17:71.
35. Carmona FD, Gutala R, Simeon CP, Carreira P, Ortego-Centeno N, Vicente-Rabaneda E, et al. Novel identification of the IRF7 region as an anticentromere autoantibody propensity locus in systemic sclerosis. Ann Rheum Dis. 2012;71(1):114–9.
36. Fu Q, Zhao J, Qian X, Wong JL, Kaufman KM, Yu CY, et al. Association of a functional IRF7 variant with systemic lupus erythematosus. Arthritis Rheum. 2011;63(3):749–54.
37. Assassi S, Swindell WR, Wu M, Tan FD, Khanna D, Furst DE, et al. Dissecting the heterogeneity of skin gene expression patterns in systemic sclerosis. Arthritis Rheumatol. 2015;67(11):3016–26.
38. Wu M, Skaug B, Bi X, Mills T, Salazar G, Zhou X, et al. Interferon regulatory factor 7 (IRF7) represents a link between inflammation and fibrosis in the pathogenesis of systemic sclerosis. Ann Rheum Dis. 2019;78(11):1583–91.
39. Broen JC, Bossini-Castillo L, Van BL, Vonk MC, Knaapen H, Beretta L, et al. A rare polymorphism in the gene for toll-like receptor 2 is associated with systemic sclerosis phenotype and increases the production of inflammatory mediators. Arthritis Rheum. 2012;64(1):264–71.
40. Dieude P, Bouaziz M, Guedj M, Riemekasten G, Airo P, Muller M, et al. Evidence of the contribution of the X chromosome to systemic sclerosis susceptibility: association with the functional IRAK1 196Phe/532Ser haplotype. Arthritis Rheum. 2011;63(12):3979–87.
41. Carmona FD, Cenit MC, Diaz-Gallo LM, Broen JC, Simeon CP, Carreira PE, et al. New insight on the Xq28 association with systemic sclerosis. Ann Rheum Dis. 2013;72:2032.
42. Dieude P, Boileau C, Guedj M, Avouac J, Ruiz B, Hachulla E, et al. Independent replication establishes the CD247 gene as a genetic systemic sclerosis susceptibility factor. Ann Rheum Dis. 2011;70:1695.
43. Dieude P, Guedj M, Wipff J, Ruiz B, Hachulla E, Diot E, et al. STAT4 is a genetic risk factor for systemic sclerosis having additive effects with IRF5 on disease susceptibility and related pulmonary fibrosis. Arthritis Rheum. 2009;60(8):2472–9.
44. Rueda B, Broen J, Simeon C, Hesselstrand R, Diaz B, Suarez H, et al. The STAT4 gene influences the genetic predisposition to systemic sclerosis phenotype. Hum Mol Genet. 2009;18(11):2071–7.
45. Gourh P, Agarwal SK, Divecha D, Assassi S, Paz G, Arora-Singh RK, et al. Polymorphisms in TBX21 and STAT4 increase the risk of systemic sclerosis: evidence of possible gene-gene interaction and alterations in Th1/Th2 cytokines. Arthritis Rheum. 2009;60(12):3794–806.
46. Tsuchiya N, Kawasaki A, Hasegawa M, Fujimoto M, Takehara K, Kawaguchi Y, et al. Association of STAT4 polymorphism with systemic sclerosis in a Japanese population. Ann Rheum Dis. 2009;68(8):1375–6.
47. Avouac J, Furnrohr BG, Tomcik M, Palumbo K, Zerr P, Horn A, et al. Inactivation of the transcription factor STAT-4 prevents inflammation-driven fibrosis in animal models of systemic sclerosis. Arthritis Rheum. 2011;63(3):800–9.
48. Gourh P, Arnett FC, Tan FK, Assassi S, Divecha D, Paz G, et al. Association of TNFSF4 (OX40L) polymorphisms with susceptibility to systemic sclerosis. Ann Rheum Dis. 2010;69(3):550–5.
49. Bossini-Castillo L, Broen JC, Simeon CP, Beretta L, Vonk MC, Ortego-Centeno N, et al. A replication study confirms the association of TNFSF4 (OX40L) polymorphisms with systemic sclerosis in a large European cohort. Ann Rheum Dis. 2011;70(4):638–41.
50. Coustet B, Bouaziz M, Dieude P, Guedj M, Bossini-Castillo L, Agarwal S, et al. Independent replication and Metaanalysis of association studies establish TNFSF4 as a susceptibility gene preferentially associated with the subset of Anticentromere-positive patients with systemic sclerosis. J Rheumatol. 2012;39(5):997–1003.
51. Elhai M, Avouac J, Hoffmann-Vold AM, Ruzehaji N, Amiar O, Ruiz B, et al. OX40L blockade protects against inflammation-driven fibrosis. Proc Natl Acad Sci U S A. 2016;113(27):E3901–10.

52. Gourh P, Tan FK, Assassi S, Ahn CW, McNearney TA, Fischbach M, et al. Association of the PTPN22 R620W polymorphism with anti-topoisomerase I- and anticentromere antibody-positive systemic sclerosis. Arthritis Rheum. 2006;54(12):3945–53.
53. Dieude P, Guedj M, Wipff J, Avouac J, Hachulla E, Diot E, et al. The PTPN22 620W allele confers susceptibility to systemic sclerosis: findings of a large case-control study of European Caucasians and a meta-analysis. Arthritis Rheum. 2008;58(7):2183–8.
54. Diaz-Gallo LM, Gourh P, Broen J, Simeon C, Fonollosa V, Ortego-Centeno N, et al. Analysis of the influence of PTPN22 gene polymorphisms in systemic sclerosis. Ann Rheum Dis. 2011;70(3):454–62.
55. Dieude P, Wipff J, Guedj M, Ruiz B, Melchers I, Hachulla E, et al. BANK1 is a genetic risk factor for diffuse cutaneous systemic sclerosis and has additive effects with IRF5 and STAT4. Arthritis Rheum. 2009;60(11):3447–54.
56. Rueda B, Gourh P, Broen J, Agarwal SK, Simeon C, Ortego-Centeno N, et al. BANK1 functional variants are associated with susceptibility to diffuse systemic sclerosis in Caucasians. Ann Rheum Dis. 2010;69(4):700–5.
57. Koumakis E, Bouaziz M, Dieude P, Ruiz B, Riemekasten G, Airo P, et al. A regulatory variant in CCR6 is associated with susceptibility to antitopoisomerase-positive systemic sclerosis. Arthritis Rheum. 2013;65(12):3202–8.
58. Gourh P, Agarwal SK, Martin E, Divecha D, Rueda B, Bunting H, et al. Association of the C8orf13-BLK region with systemic sclerosis in north-American and European populations. J Autoimmun. 2010;34(2):155–62.
59. Ito I, Kawaguchi Y, Kawasaki A, Hasegawa M, Ohashi J, Kawamoto M, et al. Association of the FAM167A-BLK region with systemic sclerosis. Arthritis Rheum. 2010;62(3):890–5.
60. Coustet B, Dieude P, Guedj M, Bouaziz M, Avouac J, Ruiz B, et al. C8orf13-BLK is a genetic risk locus for systemic sclerosis and has additive effects with BANK1: results from a large French cohort and meta-analysis. Arthritis Rheum. 2011;63(7):2091–6.
61. Bossini-Castillo L, Martin JE, Broen J, Gorlova O, Simeon CP, Beretta L, et al. A GWAS follow-up study reveals the association of the IL12RB2 gene with systemic sclerosis in Caucasian populations. Hum Mol Genet. 2012;21(4):926–33.
62. Lopez-Isac E, Bossini-Castillo L, Guerra SG, Denton C, Fonseca C, Assassi S, et al. Identification of IL12RB1 as a novel systemic sclerosis susceptibility locus. Arthritis Rheumatol. 2014;66(12):3521–3.
63. Diaz-Gallo LM, Simeon CP, Broen JC, Ortego-Centeno N, Beretta L, Vonk MC, et al. Implication of IL-2/IL-21 region in systemic sclerosis genetic susceptibility. Ann Rheum Dis. 2013;72(7):1233–8.
64. Vande Walle L, Van Opdenbosch N, Jacques P, Fossoul A, Verheugen E, Vogel P, et al. Negative regulation of the NLRP3 inflammasome by A20 protects against arthritis. Nature. 2014;512(7512):69–73.
65. Shao L, Oshima S, Duong B, Advincula R, Barrera J, Malynn BA, et al. A20 restricts wnt signaling in intestinal epithelial cells and suppresses colon carcinogenesis. PLoS One. 2013;8(5):e62223.
66. Dieude P, Guedj M, Wipff J, Ruiz B, Riemekasten G, Matucci-Cerinic M, et al. Association of the TNFAIP3 rs5029939 variant with systemic sclerosis in the European Caucasian population. Ann Rheum Dis. 2010;69(11):1958–64.
67. Wei P, Yang Y, Guo X, Hei N, Lai S, Assassi S, et al. Identification of an association of TNFAIP3 polymorphisms with matrix metalloproteinase expression in fibroblasts in an integrative study of systemic sclerosis-associated genetic and environmental factors. Arthritis Rheumatol. 2016;68(3):749–60.
68. Bossini-Castillo L, Martin JE, Broen J, Simeon CP, Beretta L, Gorlova OY, et al. Confirmation of TNIP1 but not RHOB and PSORS1C1 as systemic sclerosis risk factors in a large independent replication study. Ann Rheum Dis. 2013;72(4):602–7.
69. de Vries S, Naarmann-de Vries IS, Urlaub H, Lue H, Bernhagen J, Ostareck DH, et al. Identification of DEAD-box RNA helicase 6 (DDX6) as a cellular modulator of vascular endothelial growth factor expression under hypoxia. J Biol Chem. 2013;288(8):5815–27.
70. Skhirtladze C, Distler O, Dees C, Akhmetshina A, Busch N, Venalis P, et al. Src kinases in systemic sclerosis: central roles in fibroblast activation and in skin fibrosis. Arthritis Rheum. 2008;58(5):1475–84.
71. Martin JE, Broen JC, Carmona FD, Teruel M, Simeon CP, Vonk MC, et al. Identification of CSK as a systemic sclerosis genetic risk factor through genome wide association study follow-up. Hum Mol Genet. 2012;21(12):2825–35.
72. Manetti M, Allanore Y, Saad M, Fatini C, Cohignac V, Guiducci S, et al. Evidence for caveolin-1 as a new susceptibility gene regulating tissue fibrosis in systemic sclerosis. Ann Rheum Dis. 2012;71(6):1034–41.
73. Acosta-Herrera M, Kerick M, Gonzalez-Serna D, Myositis Genetics C, Scleroderma Genetics C, Wijmenga C, et al. Genome-wide meta-analysis reveals shared new loci in systemic seropositive rheumatic diseases. Ann Rheum Dis. 2019;78(3):311–9.
74. Cho JH, Gregersen PK. Genomics and the multifactorial nature of human autoimmune disease. N Engl J Med. 2011;365(17):1612–23.
75. Gardini A, Shiekhattar R. The many faces of long noncoding RNAs. FEBS J. 2015;282(9):1647–57.
76. Tsou PS, Sawalha AH. Unfolding the pathogenesis of scleroderma through genomics and epigenomics. J Autoimmun. 2017;83:73–94.
77. Bossini-Castillo L, Villanueva-Martin G, Kerick M, Acosta-Herrera M, Lopez-Isac E, Simeon CP, et al. Genomic risk score impact on susceptibility to systemic sclerosis. Ann Rheum Dis. 2021;80(1):118–27.
78. Manolio TA. Bringing genome-wide association findings into clinical use. Nat Rev Genet. 2013;14(8):549–58.
79. Knevel R, le Cessie S, Terao CC, Slowikowski K, Cui J, Huizinga TWJ, et al. Using genetics to prioritize diagnoses for rheumatology outpatients with inflammatory arthritis. Sci Transl Med. 2020;12(545)

Classification and Disease Subsets in Clinical Practice

5

Sindhu R. Johnson, Frank H. J. Van den Hoogen, and Robyn T. Domsic

Systemic sclerosis (SSc) is a rare connective tissue disease characterized by fibrosis of the skin and internal organs and a vasculopathy affecting the micro- and macro-vasculature. The pathogenesis of SSc involves the interplay between vascular injury and dysregulation of the immune response with resultant fibrosis of various target organs. More than 90% of patients with SSc suffer from the Raynaud phenomenon (RP), a reversible vasospastic disorder induced by cold or stress, which results in typical white, blue, and red color changes of the distal extremities from altered perfusion [1]. Cutaneous sclerosis is the hallmark of the disease; however, other clinical features that are common in patients include interstitial lung disease, gastrointestinal dysmotility, malabsorption, digital ulcerations, pulmonary hypertension, renal crisis, myopathy, arthritis, and cardiac involvement. There are two commonly recognized cutaneous subsets of SSc: limited cutaneous SSc and diffuse cutaneous SSc. The two subsets differ in their natural history with respect to both the presence and timing of skin and internal organ manifestations, as well as overall prognosis [2, 3]. Although disease-modifying therapies have demonstrated modest efficacy in SSc [3–6], several organ-specific therapies have emerged over the past couple of decades, resulting in improved survival and quality of life. These include angiotensin-converting enzyme (ACE) inhibitors for the treatment of scleroderma renal crisis (SRC) [7] and multiple agents for the treatment of pulmonary arterial hypertension (PAH), including prostacyclins, endothelin receptor antagonists, phosphodiesterase-5 inhibitors, and soluble guanylate cyclase stimulators [8, 9]. The development of successful disease-modifying therapies for SSc has been hindered by the heterogeneous clinical manifestations of this uncommon disease. Patients with early disease are more likely to respond to targeted therapies, when irreversible organ damage may be prevented. For studying the effects of potential disease-modifying drugs, and for a more successful treatment in clinical practice, it is of paramount importance to recognize the presence of SSc early in the disease process. This is equally important for the diagnosis in clinical practice as well as for classification criteria used to enroll patients in clinical studies. If patients who are classified with SSc are similar to patients who are diagnosed with the disease, then it is straightforward to generalize evidence from clinical studies to those patients who have been diagnosed in practice. Therefore, classification and diagnosis in SSc should be developed toward recognition of SSc early in the disease process. This chapter will review the clinical and serologic subsets of SSc, the current classification criteria for SSc, and ongoing and future projects for revising and improving classification criteria.

Classification and Diagnosis

Classification criteria are not synonymous with diagnostic criteria, but they almost always mirror the list of criteria that are used for diagnosis. A clinical diagnosis results from a clinical evaluation for features that suggest the presence (absence) of disease, which ultimately results in the physician making his/her mind up over the probability of the disease (SSc) being present. Therefore, classification according to diagnosis and the diagnostic process in practice are regarded as different. Classification typically has a yes/no form, while diagnosis involves the concept of probability. Since the function of classification criteria is to identify more homogeneous groups of patients (a narrower range of the

S. R. Johnson
Toronto Scleroderma Program, University of Toronto, Toronto, ON, Canada
e-mail: Sindhu.Johnson@uhn.ca

F. H. J. Van den Hoogen
Departments of Rheumatology, Radboud University, Nijmegen Medical Center and Sint Maartenskliniek, Nijmegen, The Netherlands
e-mail: Frank-reuma.vandenHoogen@radboudumc.nl

R. T. Domsic (✉)
University of Pittsburgh, Pittsburgh, PA, USA
e-mail: rtd4@pitt.edu

Y. Allanore et al. (eds.), *Scleroderma*, https://doi.org/10.1007/978-3-031-40658-4_5

disease spectrum), classification criteria may exclude some patients with the disease in question (SSc) [10]. However, if the classification criteria do not fully apply to the patients who are diagnosed with the disease in practice, evidence from studies using the criteria will not be applicable to all diagnosed patients. Classification of individuals should be determined at the time classification criteria are evaluated and met [11].

Clinical Cutaneous Subsets of Systemic Sclerosis

Original LeRoy Classification

In 1988, an international panel of scleroderma experts convened to define subsets of SSc that are clinically distinguishable [2]. The two subsets were termed diffuse cutaneous (dSSc) and limited cutaneous (lSSc) SSc, with the extent of cutaneous sclerosis as the primary differentiating feature. Patients with lSSc have skin involvement that is limited to distal to the knees and elbows but may include the face. Diffuse SSc patients have skin thickening proximal to the elbows and knees, and/or truncal involvement at any time in their disease course. There remains debate as to whether these subsets represent different diseases or a spectrum of the same disease. These two subsets follow different disease courses with particular organ manifestations [12, 13] and typically experience different outcomes, with poorer survival in patients with dSSc [14]. Patients with dSSc usually develop the Raynaud phenomenon within a year of the onset of skin changes, whereas patients with lSSc often experience symptoms of the Raynaud phenomenon for years before cutaneous or internal organ manifestations develop [12]. In dSSc, once the cutaneous disease begins, there is generally rapid progression with the majority of patients peaking their skin thickness score within 2 years. This can be accompanied by tendon friction rubs (a harbinger of active skin disease) and early finger and large joint contractures [2, 12]. Patients with dSSc are also more likely to develop severe interstitial lung disease (ILD), SRC, or myocardial involvement during the first few years of disease than those with lSSc, who typically have a later onset of pulmonary disease, particularly PAH [12].

These two cutaneous subsets are also distinguished serologically by SSc-associated autoantibodies, which will be detailed under serologic subsets below. Each cutaneous subset has specific SSc-associated antibodies associated with it. The CREST syndrome [15], an acronym for calcinosis, Raynaud phenomenon, esophageal dysmotility, sclerodactyly, and telangiectasias, has been considered a subset of lSSc because of the strong association with ACA [16, 17]. However, because patients with dSSc can present with any of the five features of CREST, the use of this term as a subset of lcSSc can be confusing [18]. *The classical two subset (dSSc vs. lSSc) classification scheme has been the most frequently cited and widely used in registries, clinical studies, and therapeutic trials* [19].

Systemic Sclerosis Sine Scleroderma

In 1986, Giordano et al. proposed a four-subset cutaneous classification with the inclusion of a group of patients who lacked any evidence of cutaneous sclerosis but had other systemic features of SSc [20]. This group of patients has been termed SSc sine scleroderma (ssSSc) and has since been further characterized [21]. The largest study of patients with ssSSc performed at the University of Pittsburgh defined these patients as follows: a clinical diagnosis of SSc with no skin thickening on physical examination and one or more of the following visceral involvements typical of SSc: distal esophageal or small bowel hypomotility, pulmonary fibrosis, PAH, cardiac involvement, or SRC [21]. In addition, Raynaud's phenomenon or a peripheral vascular equivalent (digital pitting scars, digital tip ulcers or gangrene, and abnormal nailfold capillaries), a positive anti-nuclear antibody (ANA), and the absence of another defined connective tissue disease were considered necessary for the diagnosis of ssSSc. This study compared 48 patients with ssSSc to 507 patients with lSSc as defined by LeRoy et al. No differences were found in the frequencies of individual internal organ involvements, laboratory features, SSc-specific autoantibodies, or survival between the groups. In this study, ssSSc patients were more likely to be ANA-positive with other non-SSc-specific autoantibodies than lSSc patients. The authors concluded that ssSSc patients should be considered a form of lSSc rather than a distinct subset [21].

Three-Subset Cutaneous Model of SSc

Three-subset models of SSc based on the extent of skin involvement have been proposed by at least four groups [20, 22–24]. The three-subset model described by Masi in 1988 included the following subsets: (1) lcSSc with sclerosis of fingers with or without sclerosis of the neck and/or face; (2) intermediate cutaneous SSc (icSSc) with sclerosis of the upper and lower limbs, neck, and face, without truncal involvement; and (3) dcSSc with truncal and acral involvement as described by LeRoy et al. [24]. Survival analysis in a cohort of Italian patients demonstrated that icSSc patients had survival rates that were midway between those of lcSSc and dcSSc [14]. However, a different study in a French-Canadian population showed no significant differences in survival between lcSSc and icSSc but did demonstrate a significant survival difference between patients with lcSSc and dcSSc [25]. In addition, anti-centromere antibodies have been found to perform best in predicting limited cutaneous involvement in SSc distal to the elbows and knees as opposed to fingers alone [16]. The icSSc subset becomes unnecessary when defining lcSSc more broadly and, therefore, the three-subset model has not been used in the majority of clinical studies [19]. However, the three-subset model highlights the prognostic value of skin involvement, even within lcSSc or dcSSc.

Early SSc Versus Undifferentiated Connective Tissue Disease

Early in the disease course, patients with SSc may present with some symptoms or signs suggestive of the disease, as well as serologic abnormalities, without fulfilling the classification criteria for SSc. These patients may be described as undifferentiated or unclassified connective tissue disease (UCTD). The definition of UCTD includes patients with clinical manifestations suggestive of any CTD and the presence of at least one non-organ-specific autoantibody, such as antinuclear antibodies (ANA) or anti-extractable nuclear antigen antibodies (ENA) [26, 27]. Although the majority of patients with UCTD remain undifferentiated or remit, up to one-third of patients may develop an established CTD within 5 years of follow-up [28]. Evolution into SSc occurs in 8–39% of those UCTD patients who develop a definite CTD [28, 29]. The most frequent symptom at the onset of UCTD is Raynaud's phenomenon, and 10% of patients with isolated Raynaud's phenomenon have been shown to progress to SSc [26, 28]. Sclerodactyly and esophageal dysfunction at the onset of UCTD have been identified as significant predictors for evolution into SSc [29]. Therefore, a subset of patients with UCTD may represent those with early SSc, particularly those with sclerodactyly and/or esophageal dysfunction.

Evolution of Mixed Connective Tissue Disease into SSc

Mixed connective tissue disease was initially described by Sharp et al. in 1972 as a disorder displaying clinical features of SLE, SSc, and PM/DM in association with the presence of a high titer of anti-U1-ribonucleoprotein (RNP) antibodies [30]. For many years, a debate existed as to whether MCTD represents a distinct disease entity or a variant of individual CTDs [31]. In more recent years, the consensus has been that it is a distinct clinical entity marked by specific serologic positivity. It is a challenge to diagnose, as individuals may accumulate disease features over time. It can present primarily as another CTD (such as lupus) or with SSc-predominant features. In observational cohort studies of SSc patients, anti-U1-RNP antibodies occur in approximately 7–21% of SSc patients, with different prevalence rates in different regions of the world. Patients with U1-RNP almost always have early development of the Raynaud phenomenon [30], and a nailfold capillary pattern that is the same as in SSc. The most commonly used diagnostic criteria with the highest sensitivity and specificity, by Alarcon-Segovia et al., require the presence of U1-RNP and three of the following: swollen hands, synovitis, myositis, Raynaud phenomenon, and acrosclerosis [32]. Patients with U1-RNP are susceptible to the development of pulmonary hypertension, which is the most frequent disease-associated cause of death [33].

American Rheumatism Association/American College of Rheumatology Classification Criteria

The intent of the 1980 American College of Rheumatology (ACR) classification criteria for SSc was "to establish a standard for definite or certain disease in order to permit comparison of groups of patients from different centers and to assist in the proper evaluation of the results of clinical investigation and therapeutic trials" [34]. These criteria were not designed to aid in the diagnosis of early disease but were based on patients who had a diagnosis of definite SSc that was made no longer than 2 years before entry into the study. The study included 264 cases of definite SSc and 413 comparison patients with systemic lupus erythematosus (SLE), polymyositis/dermatomyositis (PM/DM), and Raynaud's phenomenon. Twenty-nine rheumatology centers in the USA, Canada, and Mexico were involved in this multicenter effort [34]. Using univariate and multivariate analyses, the goal was to find the fewest items that yielded the highest sensitivity and specificity for SSc.

The original classification criteria are listed in Table 5.1 [34]. The major criterion of proximal scleroderma, defined

Table 5.1 1980 American Rheumatism Association criteria for the classification of systemic sclerosis [34][a]

Major criterion: proximal cutaneous sclerosis
Induration of the skin proximal to the metacarpophalangeal or metatarsophalangeal joints, affecting other parts of the extremities, face, neck, or trunk, usually bilateral, symmetrical, and almost always including sclerodactyly
Minor criteria
1. Sclerodactyly
2. Digital pitting scars of fingertips or loss of substance of the distal finger pad
3. Bibasilar pulmonary fibrosis

[a] One major criterion or two or more minor criteria provide a sensitivity of 97% and a specificity of 98% for definite systemic sclerosis

as "sclerodermatous involvement proximal to the digits, affecting parts of the extremities, the face, neck, or trunk," was found to be the most useful major criterion with a specificity of 99.8% differentiating SSc cases from comparison patients. Using multivariate analytic techniques, three minor criteria were identified: (1) sclerodactyly, (2) digital pitting scars of fingertips or loss of substance of the distal finger pad, and (3) bilateral basilar pulmonary fibrosis on chest x ray. Either the one major criterion or two minor criteria provided a sensitivity of 97% and a specificity of 98% [34]. The proposed criteria were then externally validated using more than 1300 case and comparison patients stored in the American Rheumatism Association Medical Information System (ARAMIS) database, yielding a sensitivity of 92% and a specificity of 96% [34].

Limitations

As mentioned above, the intent of the criteria was not specifically to identify patients with early SSc, and in fact, 35 patients with probable or early stage SSc were excluded from the analyses. Therefore, the population of patients with early disease who should be targeted for enrollment into clinical trials was not fully represented by these classification criteria. Several studies have verified the low sensitivity of the ACR classification criteria for early SSc. A study comparing 240 SSc patients from the USA and 87 SSc patients from France showed sensitivities of 83% and 87% in the two populations, respectively [35]. Nadashkevich et al. reported an even lower sensitivity of 70% due to the exclusion of patients with early disease who had SSc-specific serologic markers and rapidly progressive disease [36].

In addition to excluding patients with early SSc, the original ACR classification criteria exclude a substantial portion of patients with ssSSc or mild limited SSc. An initial evaluation of the ACR classification criteria in the Pittsburgh SSc cohort found that 41% of lcSSc did not fulfill the major criterion, and 20% did not fulfill either the major or two of the three minor criteria [37]. Maricq and Valter reported that only 53% of their cohort, which included patients with diffuse and intermediate cutaneous involvement, sclerodactyly only, sine sclerosis, UCTD, and CREST, fulfilled the ACR criteria [38]. Ninety-six percent (77/80) of patients in the latter three categories with more mild disease were excluded [38]. Hudson et al. studied a group of SSc patients from the Canadian Scleroderma Research Group who had skin involvement distal to the metacarpophalangeal joints only. Of 101 patients, only 68 (67%) met the ACR classification criteria [39]. Lonzetti et al. reported an even poorer sensitivity with only one-third of French Canadian patients with lcSSc as diagnosed by expert clinicians fulfilling the 1980 ACR classification criteria [40].

Importance of Revising the ACR Classification Criteria

There were several reasons why the revision of the ACR classification criteria was necessary and timely. As described above, the poor sensitivity of the original ACR Classification Criteria for patients with early SSc limits the identification of patients who may potentially have a greater response to treatment before irreversible damage ensues. The low sensitivity for patients with lcSSc may also result in patients with ILD or PAH being attributed to idiopathic causes, and the potential exclusion of these patients for consideration of specific therapies and clinical trials. However, most importantly, technological advances provided the opportunity to improve the sensitivity of the current classification criteria with the regular use of nailfold capillaroscopy and the widespread availability of tests for SSc-specific autoantibodies.

The Next Generation Classification Criteria for SSc

Multiple different classification criteria have been proposed for SSc over the past several decades [19].

LeRoy and Medsger Criteria

In 2001, LeRoy and Medsger proposed a classification system extending the criteria originally published by LeRoy in 1988 [41]. Taking advantage of the SSc-specific autoantibodies and nailfold capillaroscopy to detect vascular changes suggestive of connective tissue diseases, Leroy and Medsger suggested extending the classification criteria to include "early" cases of SSc still without skin manifestations. Criteria for limited SSc (lSSc or "pre-SSc" or "unclassifiable SSc") can be fulfilled by patients with Raynaud's phenomenon plus an SSc-type nailfold capillary pattern and/or SSc-specific autoantibodies (Table 5.4a) [41]. Patients with lSSc must have either (1) objective documentation of Raynaud's phenomenon (direct observation or direct measurement of response to cold) plus either abnormal widefield nailfold capillaroscopy or SSc-specific autoantibodies (ACA, anti-Scl-70, anti-fibrillarin, anti-PM-Scl, anti-fibrillin or anti-RNAP I or III in a titer of 1:100 or higher) or (2) subjective symptoms of Raynaud's phenomenon plus abnormal widefield nailfold capillaroscopy and SSc-specific autoantibodies [41]. Patients with lSSc can have overlap features, thus capturing patients with UCTD and MCTD who have prominent sclerodermatous features. Patients with lSSc who also have cutaneous manifestations of SSc are again subdivided into the limited cutaneous (lcSSc) and diffuse cutaneous (dcSSc) forms (Table 5.2) [41]. These subsets are differentiated from patients with diffuse fasciitis

Table 5.2 LeRoy and Medsger criteria for the classification of early systemic sclerosis (SSc)

A.	Proposed criteria for limited forms of SSc (lSSc)		
	Raynaud's phenomenon (RP), objectively documented by		
	1.	Direct observation of any two of	
		(a)	Pallor (well-demarcated whitening of acral skin)
		(b)	Cyanosis (dusky blueness, which disappears on rewarming)
		(c)	Suffusion (well-demarcated redness)
Or	2.	Direct measurement of response to cold by	
		(a)	Objective evidence of delayed recovery after cold challenge
		(b)	Nielsen test or equivalent
Plus	1.	Abnormal widefield nailfold capillaroscopy (dilation and/or avascular areas)	
Or	2.	SSc selective autoantibodies (anti-centromere, anti-Scl-70, antifibrillarin, anti-PM-Scl, anti-fibrillin, or anti-RNA polymerase I or III in a titer of 1:100 or higher)	
If RP is subjective only, both SSc capillary pattern and SSc selective autoantibodies (in titer >1:100) are required to define lSSc. LSSc can overlap with any other disease			
B.	Constellations of criteria for diagnosis of SSc		
	1.	LSSc: defined in A above	
	2.	LcSSc: criteria for lSSc + distal cutaneous changes	
	3.	DcSSc: criteria for lSSc + proximal cutaneous changes	
	4.	Diffuse fasciitis with eosinophilia (DFE): proximal cutaneous changes without criteria for lSSc or lcSSc	

Modified from [41]

and eosinophilia who have proximal cutaneous changes but do not have Raynaud's phenomenon, abnormal nailfold capillaries, autoantibodies, or distal cutaneous changes. A small retrospective Swiss study found that 33/49 (67%) of SSc patients fulfilled the ACR classification criteria for SSc [42]. When using the amended LeRoy and Medsger criteria, this improved to 80% [42]. The study by Lonzetti et al. also included a group of 152 lSSc patients with Raynaud's phenomenon, but these patients also had sclerodactyly [40]. When adding nailfold capillary abnormalities and positive ACA to the ACR classification criteria, the sensitivity for the diagnosis of SSc improved from 33.6 to 91.5% [40]. The amended LeRoy and Medsger criteria certainly improve the sensitivity of the ACR classification criteria but exclude a small percentage of patients with SSc who lack Raynaud's phenomenon. Studies indicate that approximately 10% of patients with SSc do not suffer from Raynaud's phenomenon [38]. Patients most likely to be excluded by these criteria are those who do not have sclerodactyly or cutaneous sclerosis but have internal organ disease consistent with SSc, and SSc-specific autoantibodies or nailfold capillary abnormalities.

Maricq and Valter Criteria

In 2004, Maricq and Valter proposed another set of classification criteria for SSc with six different categories (Table 5.3) [38]. The first three groups are divided based on the extent of cutaneous sclerosis. The fourth category includes patients with scleroderma sine sclerosis who have internal organ involvement and scleroderma-pattern nailfold capillary changes or pitting scars but no ACA or telangiectasias. The fifth group includes patients with UCTD with sclerodermatous features but no ACA or telangiectasias. The last category includes patients who fulfill the CREST criteria with telangiectasias plus one or more of the other acronyms or ACA plus two or more of the acronyms [38]. Using these classification criteria, Maricq and Valter were able to capture 77/165 (47%) patients with mild or early forms of SSc who were excluded from the ACR classification criteria [38]. Unlike the LeRoy and Medsger criteria, these criteria do not require the presence of Raynaud's phenomenon, thus increasing the sensitivity for SSc. However, the Maricq and Valter criteria only include the assessment of one SSc-specific autoantibody (ACA), which may compromise sensitivity. In addition, these criteria have not been externally validated and have been criticized for being too complicated.

Table 5.3 Maricq and Valter proposed a classification of scleroderma spectrum disorders

Group	Classification criteria definitions
I. Diffuse scleroderma disorder[a]	Skin involvement proximal to elbows/knees; includes trunk
II. Intermediate scleroderma disorder[a]	Skin involvement proximal to MCP/MTP, distal to elbows/knees; trunk not involved
III. Digital scleroderma disorder	Sclerodactyly only; meets ACR minor criteria but excludes those without skin involvement
IV. Scleroderma sine sclerosis	Scleroderma-capillary pattern or pitting scars and visceral involvement; no ACA; no telangiectasias
V. UCTD-scleroderma disorder	UCTD with scleroderma features; no ACA; no telangiectasias
VI. "CREST"	No skin involvement or sclerodactyly only; telangiectasias required with one or more other acronyms; or ACA is required with any two or more acronyms

Modified from [38]

MCP metacarpophalangeal, *MTP* metatarsophalangeal, *ACR* American College of Rheumatology, *ACA* anticentromere antibodies, *UCTD* undifferentiated connective tissue disease, and *CREST* calcinosis, Raynaud's phenomenon, esophageal dysmotility, sclerodactyly, telangiectasias

[a] Groups I and II were subdivided into two categories: (a) without and (b) with CREST features

Nadashkevich, Davis, and Fritzler Criteria

Nadashkevich et al. proposed another set of classification criteria in 2004 through a three-phase study [43]. The first phase involved 752 Ukrainian patients assessed between 1987 and 1994 who were diagnosed with SSc (n = 170, 38% dcSSc, 56% lcSSc, and 6% overlap), SLE (n = 170), RA (n = 170), PM/DM (n = 20), Sjogren's syndrome (n = 23), isolated Raynaud's phenomenon ($n = 88$), diabetes mellitus ($n = 100$), eosinophilic fasciitis ($n = 5$), and generalized morphea ($n = 6$). In this cohort, the sensitivity of the ACR classification criteria for SSc was only 71.2% [43]. In the proposed criteria, classification as SSc was based on the presence of Raynaud's phenomenon and/or sclerodactyly or non-pitting digital edema plus one of 13 other SSc-related clinical manifestations. This phase identified 8 of the 15 clinical criteria as sufficient to identify all patients with SSc if at least 3 of the 8 criteria were fulfilled. None of the controls had more than two of the clinical criteria. Phase IIA of the study validated the initial set of 8 clinical criteria in an independent cohort of 99 Canadian SSc patients and 138 controls with SLE, RA, PM/DM, and Sjogren's syndrome evaluated between 1995 and 1997 [43]. In the external validation study, the criteria had a sensitivity of 99% (compared with a sensitivity of 69.7% using ACR criteria) and a specificity of 100% for the diagnosis of SSc. In Phase IIB, various autoantibodies were assessed to add to the proposed criteria with the hopes of increasing sensitivity further. Ultimately, the presence of ACA (detected by indirect immunofluorescence), anti-Scl-70 antibodies (detected by double immunodiffusion), or antifibrillarin antibodies (detected by immunoprecipitation) was added as a final criterion [43]. Phase III of the study reviewed the SSc and isolated Raynaud's phenomenon patients in Phase I to develop the final set of classification criteria, requiring three or more criteria for a diagnosis of definite SSc (Table 5.4) [36]. Although the authors demonstrate good sensitivity and specificity of their proposed classification criteria, other independent validation studies have not been performed. Although this set of classification criteria does account for patients without Raynaud's phenomenon, abnormal nailfold capillaroscopic examination and other SSc-specific autoantibodies (i.e., Anti-RNAP III) were not included in the criteria.

Table 5.4 Nadashkevich, Davis, and Fritzler proposed criteria for systemic sclerosis (SSc)

Criterion	Comments
Autoantibodies	Anti-centromere, anti-Scl-70, or anti-fibrillarin
Bibasilar pulmonary fibrosis	Detected by chest radiograph
Contracture	Permanent limitation of joint motion
Dermal thickening proximal to wrists	Defined by the modified Rodnan skin score
Calcinosis cutis	Detected by x ray, crystallographic/chemical analysis
Raynaud's phenomenon	By patient's history or physician's observation
Esophageal distal hypomotility	Detected by cine/video barium esophagram or endoscopy
Sclerodactyly	Symmetric tightening of skin or nonpitting edema of digits
Telangiectasias	Common locations: digits, face, lips, tongue

Modified from [43]. Three or more of these criteria are necessary for a diagnosis of SSc

Criteria from the Canadian Scleroderma Research Group

In 2007, Hudson et al. proposed a revision to the ACR classification criteria using data from the Canadian Scleroderma Research Group (CSRG) [39]. The authors proposed the addition of nailfold capillary abnormalities as assessed by the handheld dermatoscope (dilated or giant capillary loops or avascular areas) plus visible mat-like telangiectasias to the ACR classification criteria. Using the proposed criteria, the sensitivity to identify SSc patients with skin involvement distal to the metacarpophalangeal joints improved from 67% to 99% [39]. However, this study did not include controls, and therefore, the specificity of the proposed criteria was not assessed. Since SSc-specific autoantibodies and Raynaud's phenomenon were not included, the specificity of this classification system may be lower than other proposed criteria.

Nailfold Capillaroscopy in the Diagnosis of SSc

Nailfold Capillaroscopic Patterns in SSc

Since the 1970s, patients with SSc have been known to demonstrate a distinct pattern of nailfold capillary abnormalities when examined microscopically compared with patients with primary Raynaud's phenomenon and other connective tissue diseases [44, 45]. Maricq et al. initially described the scleroderma pattern of capillary abnormalities using in vivo widefield capillaroscopic techniques. Enlarged and deformed capillary loops surrounded by relatively avascular areas were found in 82% of patients with SSc and 54% of patients with MCTD but only 2% of patients with SLE [45]. One of 11 patients with primary Raynaud's phenomenon showed these changes, but this patient developed SSc 5 months after the initial capillaroscopic examination. Another study found that the presence of the scleroderma pattern of capillary abnormalities predicted the development of SSc in five of ten patients with Raynaud's phenomenon within 9 months to 5 years of follow-up [46]. A more recent study found that approximately 14% of patients with UCTD had the scleroderma pattern on nailfold capillaroscopy and thus may be at higher risk of progressing to SSc or a related CTD [45].

During the past decade, nailfold videocapillaroscopic techniques have been used to describe three patterns of microangiopathy in SSc that correlate with disease duration: early, active, and late (Fig. 5.1) [47, 48]. The early pattern is characterized by few (fewer than four altered capillaries per

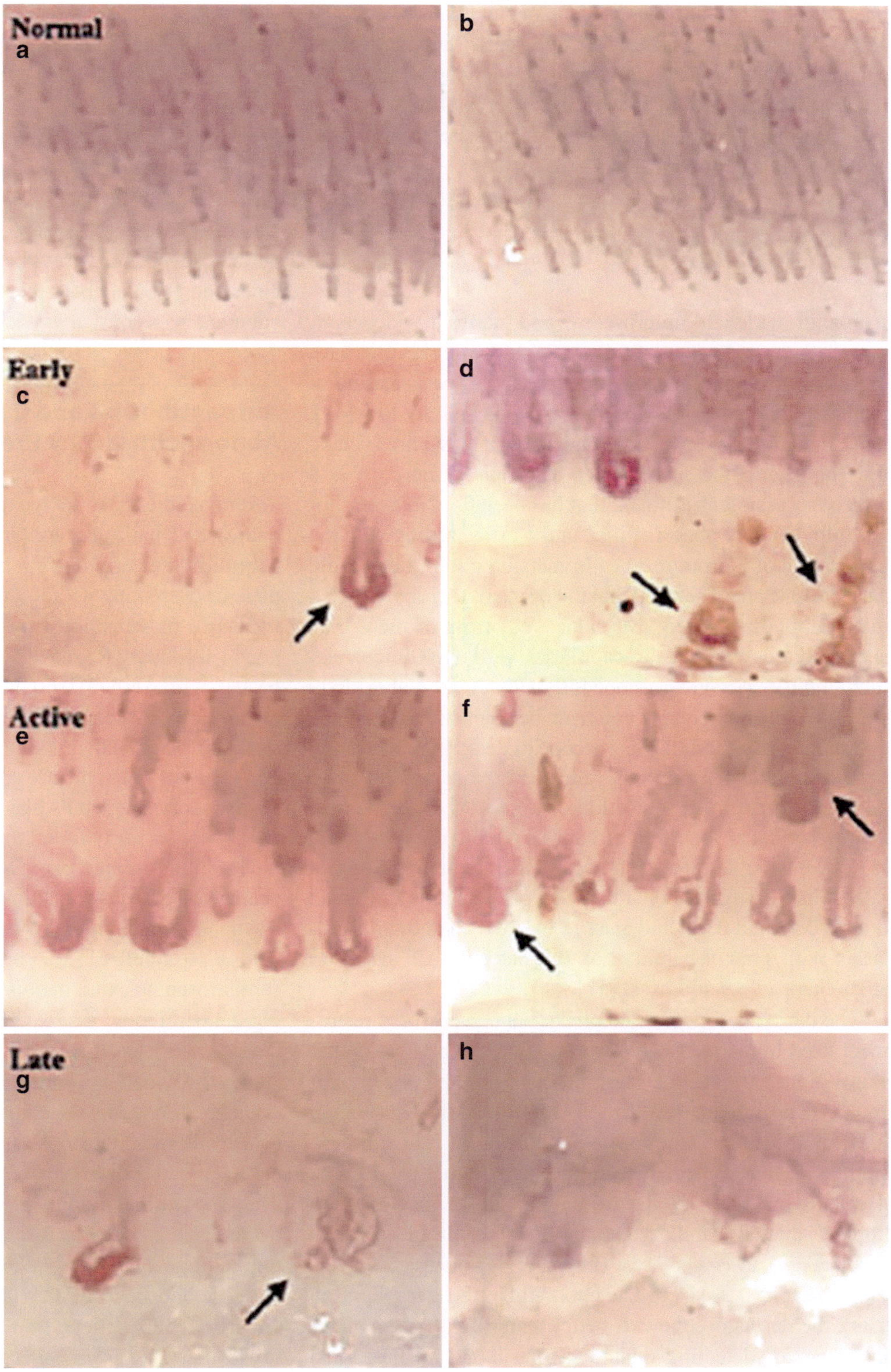

Fig. 5.1 Early, active, and late nailfold capillaroscopic patterns observed in systemic sclerosis. **a** and **b** are both 'normal'; **c** and **d** are both 'early', **e** and **f** are both 'active', and **g** and **h** are both 'late'

millimeter) enlarged or giant capillaries, few capillary hemorrhages, relatively well-preserved capillary distribution, and no evident loss of capillaries. The active pattern demonstrates frequent (more than six altered capillaries per millimeter) giant capillaries, frequent capillary hemorrhages, 20–30% loss of capillaries, mild (between four and six altered capillaries per millimeter) disorganization of the capillary architecture, and absent or mild ramified capillaries. The late pattern shows irregular enlargement of the capillaries, few or absent giant capillaries and hemorrhages, and 50–70% loss of capillaries with large avascular areas, disorganization of the normal capillary array, and ramified or bushy capillaries [47, 48]. The late pattern was shown to be associated with older age and longer duration of Raynaud's phenomenon and SSc when compared with the early and active patterns [48]. Therefore, the early capillaroscopic changes of enlarged and giant capillaries, along with hemorrhages, likely represent the earliest microvascular changes observed in patients with SSc or related diseases and may be useful in the early diagnosis of SSc.

Office Capillaroscopy

Although widefield microscopy and nailfold videocapillaroscopy provide detailed images of the nailfolds and have excellent inter- and intra-rater reliability in the detection of giant capillaries, microhemorrhages, and capillary loss [49], these modalities are not widely available and require specific training to use the instruments. The ophthalmoscope is a widely accessible instrument that has been used to assess for nailfold capillary abnormalities in the office setting with the application of a drop of oil or immersion gel to the nailfold surface. One study showed that the ophthalmoscope detected giant capillaries, severe avascular areas (loss of more than six capillaries), and bushy capillaries with a 100% correlation with the stereomicroscope [50]. However, another study showed only moderate agreement between the use of the ophthalmoscope and the microscope in detecting dilated and giant capillaries (kappa 0.63 and 0.52, respectively), with poor agreement in the detection of avascular areas (defined as any confluent area free of capillary loops) (kappa <0.1) [51]. The latter study also showed moderate inter- and intra-rater reliability for the ophthalmoscopic detection of dilated (kappa 0.43 and 0.61) and giant (kappa 0.54 and 0.56) capillaries with poor reliability for the detection of avascular areas (kappa 0.19 and 0.31) [51].

The dermatoscope is a handheld, battery-powered instrument used by dermatologists to assess pigmented and other skin lesions. The most current models use a polarized light source that eliminates reflection from the skin surface and, therefore, does not require the application of oil or immersion gel. When compared with the standard microscope, the dermatoscope has shown excellent agreement for the detection of dilated capillaries (kappa 0.93), megacapillaries (kappa 0.97), avascular areas (kappa 0.93), and microhemorrhages (kappa 0.94) [52]. The inter- and intra-rater reliability using the dermatoscope was better than that of the ophthalmoscope for detecting dilated (kappa 0.63 and 0.71) and giant (kappa 0.4 and 0.55) capillaries but was also poor for the detection of avascular areas (kappa 0.2 and 0.4) [51]. The dermatoscope is relatively inexpensive and easy to use with a mean capillaroscopic examination time of 4 min [52]. When used to differentiate patients with SSc from healthy controls, the presence of two or more enlarged capillaries in one or more fingers as detected by the dermatoscope showed a sensitivity of 83% and a specificity of 100% for the diagnosis of SSc [53]. Hudson et al. assessed the effect of the addition of capillaroscopic changes detected by the dermatoscope on the sensitivity of the ACR criteria in a population of SSc patients with skin involvement distal to the metacarpophalangeal joints (with or without face involvement) [39]. They found that the sensitivity improved from 67% to 91%, with further improvement to 99% if visible mat-like telangiectasias were added [39]. Capillaroscopic evaluation using the dermatoscope may provide a feasible technique for clinicians and researchers to assess patients with early microvascular changes consistent with the scleroderma pattern.

Autoantibodies and Capillaroscopic Abnormalities May Predict the Onset of SSc

Several studies have shown that the combination of autoantibodies and nailfold capillaroscopic abnormalities may be helpful in the early detection of SSc and related diseases in patients presenting with Raynaud's phenomenon. The annual incidence of transition from primary Raynaud's phenomenon to secondary Raynaud's phenomenon has been shown to be 1%, with ANA >1:160 at presentation increasing the risk of developing secondary Raynaud's phenomenon by more than 68-fold [47]. In this study, after a mean follow-up period of 11.2 ± 3.9 years, the prevalence of transition from primary to secondary Raynaud's phenomenon was in 14.9% of cases [54]. Another study found that the addition of serial nailfold videocapillaroscopic examinations identified a similar percentage of patients transitioning from primary to secondary Raynaud's phenomenon over a shorter follow-up time of 29.4 ± 10 months [55]. Therefore, the addition of nailfold capillaroscopic examination to standard evaluations, including autoantibody assessments, likely permits the earlier detection of secondary Raynaud's phenomenon. Another study of 152 patients with sclerodactyly and Raynaud's phenomenon found that the addition of dilated capillaries visualized by stereo microscope improved the sensitivity of ACR criteria for the diagnosis of SSc from 33.6 to 74.3% [40]. This was further improved to 82.9% with the addition of avascular areas detected by stereomicroscope, 88.8% with the addition of visible nailfold telangiectasias, and 91.5% with the addition of ACA [40]. A recent study evaluated a cohort of 586 patients with Raynaud's phenomenon and found that 12.6% (n = 74) of these patients progressed to definite SSc over a median follow-up time of 4.6 years [56]. Only 24 (32%) of these patients fulfilled the ACR criteria for SSc. The strongest independent predictors for the development of definite SSc were positive ANA, SSc-specific autoantibodies (anti-Scl-70, antiTh/To, ACA, or anti-RNAP III), and a scleroderma pattern on nailfold capillaroscopy using stereomicroscope [56]. The combination of the presence of abnormal findings on nailfold capillaroscopy and

SSc-specific autoantibody at baseline was associated with a 60-fold increased risk for the development of definite SSc, with a sensitivity of 47%. The presence of abnormal capillaroscopy and/or SSc-specific autoantibody at baseline improved the sensitivity to 89% with a negative predictive value of 98% [56]. In other words, patients with Raynaud's and normal findings on nailfold capillaroscopy and negative SSc-specific autoantibodies had a probability of only 1.6% to have SSc 10 years later; quite in contrast, patients with Raynaud's and SSc pattern on nailfold capllaroscopy and positive SSc-specific autoantibodies had a 73% probability to have developed SSc in the course of 10 years. This illustrates how the patient profile informs clinicians about the probability of SSc being present (becoming manifest). These studies support the usefulness of SSc-specific autoantibodies and nailfold capillaroscopic abnormalities in the early diagnosis of SSc and the revised classification criteria.

Autoantibodies and Subsets of SSc

SSc-Associated Autoantibodies have Diagnostic and Prognostic Value. Consideration of Serologic Subsets

Autoantibodies are detected in more than 95% of patients with SSc [57]. Ten SSc-specific autoantibodies have been described, although not all are widely clinically available (Fig. 5.2). These autoantibodies are rarely detected in patients with other CTDs and very infrequently observed in the general population [16]. These antibodies generally remain stable over time and are mutually exclusive in the majority of patients [16]. SSc-specific autoantibodies have been associated with the cutaneous subsets of SSc as well as different rates of internal organ involvement, therefore giving them prognostic use. Several SSc-associated autoantibodies have been shown to be associated with specific HLA alleles. A growing number of experts have proposed that serologic subsetting may augment the traditional clinical cutaneous classification scheme. It may allow for more personalized medicine with respect to both monitoring for early internal organ involvement and consideration of therapeutic aggressiveness. Finally, autoantibodies have also been shown to precede the onset of symptoms in SSc and other CTDs, such as SLE, and therefore, they are useful in the early diagnosis of disease [58, 59].

ANA and SSc-Associated Autoantibody Testing

A nucleolar staining pattern of ANA on indirect immunofluorescence can be observed when any of the following SSc-specific autoantibodies are present: anti-PM-Scl, anti-Th/To, anti-U3-RNP (antifibrillarin), and anti-RNA-polymerase (RNAP) I, II, and III. The anti-RNAP antibodies, and in particular anti-RNAP III, demonstrate nucleolar staining only 30–44% of the time [60, 61]; therefore, nucleolar staining on the ANA is not useful as a screening test for these autoantibodies, and they will be discussed separately. Immunodiffusion to detect anti-PM-Scl antibodies is commercially available, while the other nucleolar autoantibodies are typically detected by immunoprecipita-

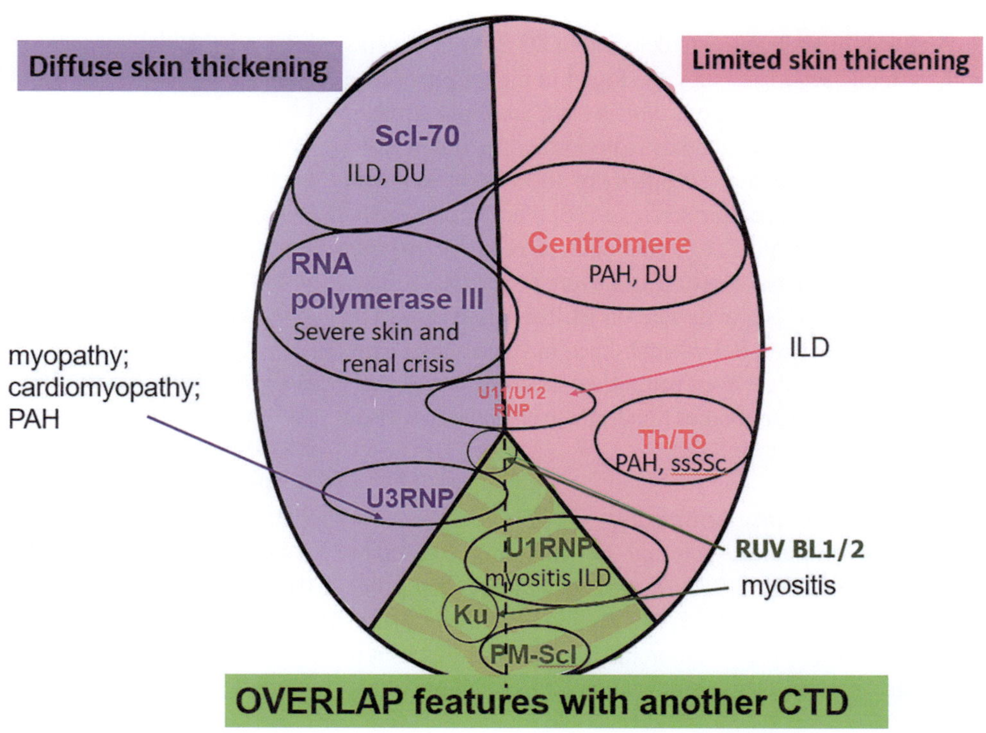

Fig. 5.2 SSc-associated antibodies and their associated cutaneous and SSc complications

tion performed only at certain centers. However, a new ELISA for the detection of antibodies to fibrillarin and PM-Scl was recently described [62]. When evaluated in 50 SSc patients who were negative for ACA and anti-Scl-70 compared with 122 controls (42 SSc positive for ACA or anti-Scl-70, 40 SLE, and 40 rheumatoid arthritis), the anti-fibrillarin ELISA had a sensitivity of 22% and a specificity of 92.5%, and the anti-PM-Scl antibody had a sensitivity of 8% and a specificity of 98.8% [62]. This study, however, did not compare the sensitivity and specificity of the ELISAs to immunoprecipitation.

Antibodies Associated with Diffuse Skin Thickening

Anti-Scl-70 Antibodies

Anti-Scl-70 (also known as anti-topoisomerase I) antibodies are classically associated with diffuse cutaneous disease; however, 31–36% of SSc patients with anti-Scl-70 antibodies present with limited skin thickening, although in long-term follow-up approximately 90% develop diffuse disease [63]. Ten percent of anti-Scl-70 positive patients will stay lcSSc [13]. Anti-Scl-70 positivity is associated with a higher prevalence of pulmonary fibrosis in up to 60% of severe heart diseases including conduction system involvement, tendon friction rubs, and joint complaints than other SSc-specific autoantibodies [57]. Results from an observational cohort study (DUO registry) identified patients with Scl-up as having a high prevalence of tip ulcers, gangrene, and digital tuft resorption [57]. Scl-70 positivity is associated with a higher prevalence of myocardial conduction block and diastolic dysfunction [13].

Anti-Scl-70 antibodies are detected in 20–35% of patients with systemic sclerosis. They are found in higher prevalence in European and Asian cohorts than in the USA. Gold standard testing for anti-scl70 antibodies is performed by immunodiffusion and has a very high specificity of 100% compared with normal controls or systemic sclerosis [16]. Further data on the diagnostic value of anti-Scl-70 antibodies detected by enzyme-linked immunosorbent assays (ELISA) are necessary, as many report a high false positivity rate on ELISA-based tests. The high specificity of anti-Scl-70 antibodies and the ability to predict organ involvement even better than the diffuse cutaneous subset makes these antibodies important to consider in revised classification criteria for SSc.

Anti-RNA-Polymerase Antibodies

Anti-RNAP antibodies detected by immunoprecipitation have been reported in 4–25% of patients with SSc depending on the population studied [35, 61]. Antibodies for RNA polymerase are much more common in US cohort studies than in European or Asian cohort studies. On indirect immunofluorescence, these antibodies typically display a fine-speckled nucleoplasmic stain with additional occasional bright dots, with or without concurrent punctate nucleolar staining [61]. Anti-RNAP II antibodies are associated with diffuse cutaneous disease and a high prevalence of SRC, but a low frequency of severe pulmonary fibrosis [57]. In recent years, anti-RNAP III antibodies have been detected by ELISA and have become more widely available. Compared with immunoprecipitation, the ELISA has a sensitivity of 91–96% and a specificity of 98–99% [61, 64]. As a diagnostic test for SSc, the sensitivity and specificity of the ELISA for anti-RNAP III have been reported as 11–17% and 98–99%, respectively [64, 65]. The relatively high sensitivity and specificity of anti-RNAP III antibodies for SSc, the strong predictive value of these antibodies for diffuse skin disease and SRC, and the increasing availability of the ELISA assay to test for these antibodies are all reasons that anti-RNAP III antibodies were included in the ACR/EULAR classification criteria. In more recent years there have been several papers reporting associations between RNA polymerase III and malignancy [66–69]. Studies from the Hopkins cohort reported that when malignancy within 36 months of SSc onset was examined, RNAP III antibody positive patients had a 5.83 times increased risk compared to other SSc patients. There is now a suggestion of a cancer-induced autoimmunity model in RNAP III antibody positive patients with particular antibody subunits [69].

Anti-U3-RNP (Fibrillin) Antibodies

Anti-U3-RNP antibodies are present in 8% of patients with SSc and are associated with African American race in more than one cohort study [70, 71]. These autoantibodies are associated with male gender and diffuse cutaneous disease in roughly half of patients [71]. SSc patients with these autoantibodies have higher rates of myopathy and gastrointestinal involvement [57, 70–72]. Three studies have not reported an association between anti-U3-RNP antibodies and pulmonary hypertension [57, 71]. The most recent study of 1365 patients found anti-U3-RNP patients to have the highest rate of pulmonary hypertension, although this study did not identify patients with anti-Th/To antibodies [73].

Anti-nucleolar Antibodies

Although anti-nucleolar antibodies have been reported in 15–40% of patients with SSc, few studies have reported the frequency of these autoantibodies in healthy controls or other CTDs [16]. One study indicated that anti-PM-Scl antibodies have a specificity of 96.9% for SSc when compared with healthy controls and other CTDs, but no patients with PM/DM were included in the comparison group [74]. Anti-Th/To antibodies have been shown to be 98.8% specific for SSc when compared with other CTDs [75]. However, one report evaluating antifibrillarin antibodies by radioimmunoassay found that these antibodies were present in a large percentage of patients with MCTD, SLE, rheumatoid arthritis, and Sjogren's syndrome in addition to patients with SSc [76]. The lack of specificity of the radioimmunoassay for antifibrillarin antibodies may not apply to immunoprecipitation methods. Although anti-nucleolar antibodies may be specific for SSc, the variable sensitivity and the lack of widespread commercially available assays for these autoantibodies make them less useful for classification criteria.

Anti-U11/U12 Antibodies

A more recently described autoantibody, just over half of the patients identified as having this autoantibody have a diffuse cutaneous disease. While it is not testable with an ELISA or immunoblot method at the time of this writing, this may evolve over time. Patients with these antibodies have high rates of ILD, at approximately 70% [77]. More recent work using the Hopkins cohort has identified an association with moderate to severe GI motility manifestations [78]. Until testing is easily available, it is unlikely to be adapted into classification criteria, and overall prevalence in SSc and specificity are difficult to establish.

Antibodies Associated with Limited Skin Thickening

Anticentromere Antibodies

ACA is detected by indirect immunofluorescence, although ELISA tests for available for the two components of the centromere complex: centromere a and centromere b. ACA presence has a high specificity for the limited cutaneous subset of SSc, with <5% of patients developing diffuse SSc over time in what appears to be a unique clinical subset [79]. ACA has been associated with delayed diagnosis, with a mean of 8.7 years since the first SSc symptom onset at the time of diagnosis [57]. Patients with ACA have a significantly higher prevalence of digital tip ulcers, gangrene, digital tuft resorption, and calcinosis than patients with other SSc-specific autoantibodies but a significantly lower prevalence of arthritis or muscle inflammation [57]. In addition, ACA is associated with the development of isolated pulmonary arterial hypertension or WHO Group 1 pulmonary hypertension [57, 80].

Anti-U1-RNP Antibodies

As described above, anti-U1-RNP antibodies are present in high titers in patients with MCTD, but they can also be detected in 7–21% of patients with SSc [35, 81] or MCTD with SSc predominant features. Clinical features associated with the presence of anti-U1-RNP antibodies in patients with SSc include younger age at disease onset, vasospasm, arthritis, muscle inflammation, and ILD [57, 81]. In patients with lcSSc, the presence of anti-U1-RNP antibodies predicts better survival when compared with other SSc-specific antibodies [57].

Anti-Th/To Antibodies

Anti-Th/To antibodies are highly specific for SSc, associated with the limited cutaneous subset, and have been reported in up to 24% of lcSSc patients compared with 2% of dcSSc patients [57]. Th/To patients do not infrequently present as ssSSc. Patients with these autoantibodies have a high prevalence of pulmonary hypertension in all three WHO groups, pulmonary fibrosis, as well as gastrointestinal involvement [57]. Long-term follow-up of >200 Th/To patients found that 42% had developed pulmonary hypertension as of the last follow-up. Of these, 27% had PAH and 14% had PH related to ILD (unpublished data Domsic 2021). Compared with ACA, lcSSc patients with anti-Th/To antibodies have more subtle skin disease, less severe digital vasculopathy, and a higher prevalence of ILD [82]. The presence of anti-Th/To antibodies in patients with lcSSc portends a poorer prognosis than other SSc-specific autoantibodies [57, 82], likely related to the high incidence of pulmonary hypertension.

Overlap Antibodies

Anti PM/Scl Antibodies

Anti-PM-Scl antibodies are detected in 3–12.5% of patients with SSc and are associated with a high prevalence of muscle inflammation [35, 74]. Patients with anti-PM-Scl antibodies also have a high prevalence of severe pulmonary fibrosis and digital ulcers with a lower frequency of PAH [57, 74].

Anti-RUV-BL1/2 Antibodies

Anti-RuvBL1/2 antibody was reported in 2014 to be exclusively detected in SSc patients. Compared to other SSc patients, those with anti-RuvBL1/2 displayed diffuse skin thickening and higher frequencies of myositis. They were also more frequently male and older at presentation [83, 84]. This antibody has been confirmed in other SSc cohorts. It is a rare antibody without available ELISA or immunoblot testing at the time of this writing.

Anti-Ku Antibodies

Anti-Ku antibodies were originally described by IP but now can be detected by line immunoassays and immunoblot assays [85]. Anti-Ku antibodies can occur alone or with other autoantibodies and are associated with a myositis overlap syndrome [86, 87]. A mutlicenter cohort study reported the associations of single-specificity anti-Ku antibodies with high rates of ILD (58%) and increased creatine kinase levels (11% vs. 1%) and during follow-up (10% vs. 2%) [88].

Modern Era of Classification Criteria

Very Early Diagnosis of Systemic Sclerosis (VEDOSS)

The very early diagnosis of systemic sclerosis (VEDOSS) project of the European League Against Rheumatism Scleroderma Trials and Research group (EUSTAR) aims at early diagnosis of SSc [89]. Their goal was to identify features that may precede characteristic skin thickening and internal organ involvement and facilitate earlier diagnosis. These criteria are provisional (Fig. 5.3) and need to be validated. In the VEDOSS cohort, patients are included with an increased probability of SSc; patients with Raynaud's phenomenon and/or puffy fingers who are positive for ANA are considered to be at risk (Fig. 5.4). The other items that were judged as most relevant for the diagnosis of SSc were sclerodactyly, abnormal capillaroscopy, positive ACA, and positive anti-Scl-70 antibodies (Table 5.5). The prevalence of these proposed diagnostic features was evaluated in a cohort of 469 patients with RP. Almost 90% of ANA-positive patients with RP and puffy swollen digits also had scleroderma-specific autoantibodies and/or a scleroderma pattern on nailfold capillaroscopy, fulfilling the VEDOSS preliminary criteria for early SSc.

ACR-EULAR Classification Criteria

The aim of the ACR-EULAR classification criteria for the SSc working group was to develop classification criteria for inclusion of patients in clinical studies, which met the demands of early recognition of SSc, include new knowledge gained over the preceding decades (e.g., importance of vascular manifestations, SSc-specific autoantibodies), and use a rigorous methodologic approach (Fig. 5.5) [90, 91]. Signs and symptoms (items) that should be considered to be included in the criteria were proposed through two independent Delphi exercises in Europe and North America; 168 items were scored for their importance. Low-scoring criteria were discarded, leaving 102 criteria [92, 93]. Through the use of a nominal group technique with 16 international experts, the proposed criteria were reduced to 23. Using cases and controls from databases from Madrid, Berlin, Toronto, Pittsburgh, Canadian Scleroderma Research Group, and 1000 Faces of Lupus cohorts, these criteria were found to have a face, discriminant, and construct validity [94]. The 23 candidate criteria were further reduced and weighted, and a threshold for classification was identified using multicriteria decision analysis [95].

– The presence of "Skin thickening sparing the fingers" was made an exclusionary criterion. If this is present, the clas-

Fig. 5.3 Algorithm to diagnose patients with very early systemic sclerosis

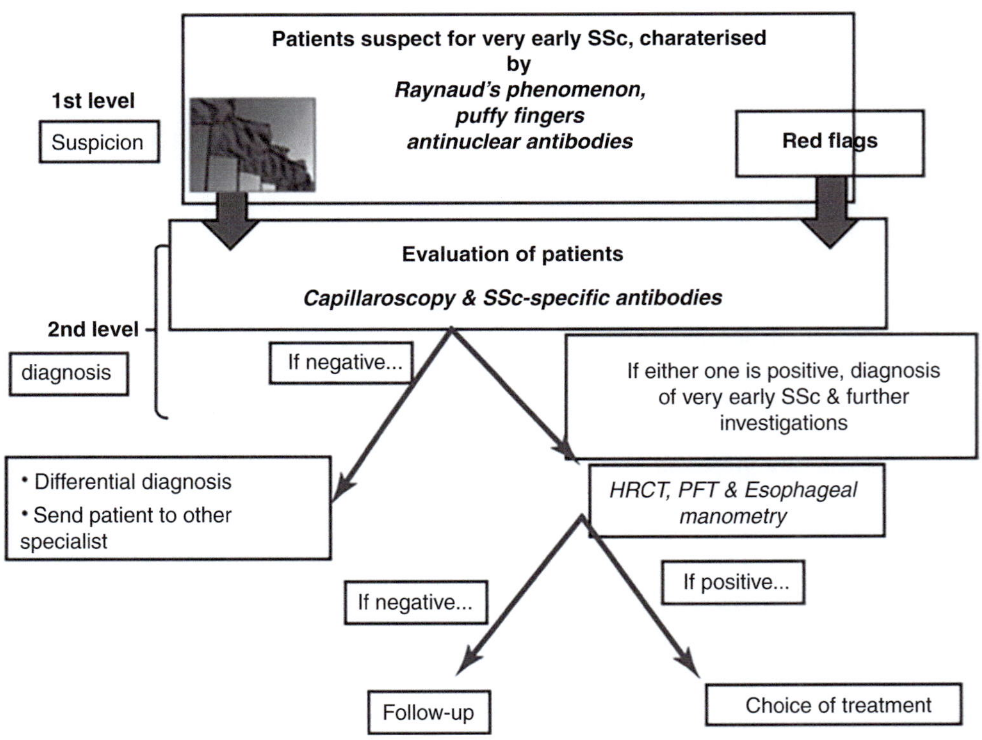

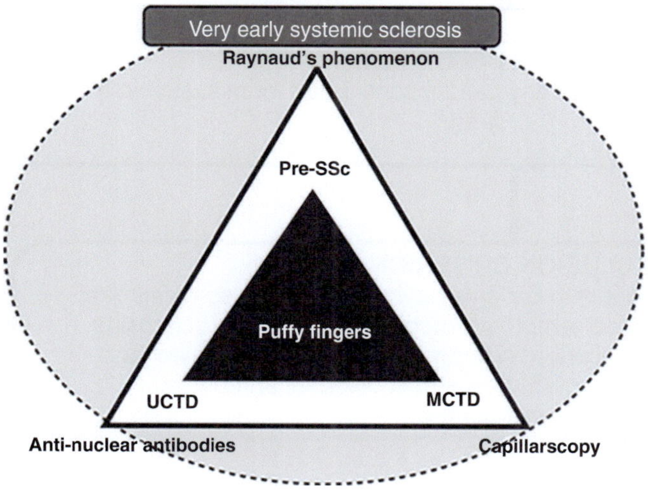

Fig. 5.4 Pyramid depiction of very early diagnosis of systemic sclerosis (SSc)

Table 5.5 Criteria for very early diagnosis of systemic sclerosis (SSc) determined by Delphi Consensus from EUSTAR[a]

	Criteria selected by experts
Criteria considered as having a high clinical relevance for the very early diagnosis of SSc	Raynaud's phenomenon
Criteria considered as leading to an early referral	Puffy swollen digits turning into sclerodactyly
	Abnormal capillaroscopy with scleroderma pattern
	Positive anticentromere antibodies
	Positive anti-topoisomerase I antibodies
	Raynaud's phenomenon
	Puffy fingers
	Positive antinuclear antibodies

Modified from [89]

[a] *EUSTAR* European League Against Rheumatism Scleroderma Trial and Research

sification criteria should not be applied, because if there is scleroderma that is not affecting the fingers, the presence of a similar disease not being SSc is far more likely.

- "Skin thickening of the fingers extending proximally to the metacarpophalangeal joints" was a sufficient criterion. If present, the individual can be classified as having systemic sclerosis.
- Acro-osteolysis, pitting scars, and digital ulcers were grouped under the heading "finger tip lesions."
- Systemic sclerosis-specific antibodies were also grouped under one criterion.
- Antinuclear antibody, esophageal reflux, digital pulp loss, forced vital capacity, dysphagia, and diffusing capacity were removed due to poor ability to distinguish cases from controls, minimal added value in classification (low weight), or insufficient reliability in the clinical setting. This methodologic approach facilitated a system of classification that produced a measure of the probability that an individual with certain features can be classified as having systemic sclerosis. The draft classification system and weights were then tested against a range of cases that reflected a low to high probability of having systemic sclerosis rated by experts. A total score of nine or more was identified as the threshold with the least misclassification [96].

The criteria set performance was tested in cases and controls from 10 European and 13 North American centers. The controls reflected conditions that could be confused with SSc and included scleromyxedema, graft versus host disease, undifferentiated connective tissue disease, dermatomyositis, nephrogenic sclerosing fibrosis, polymyositis, eosinophilic fasciitis, mixed connective tissue disease, and generalized morphea [96]. As they did not provide added value in sensitivity or specificity, esophageal dilation, calcinosis cutis, acro-osteolysis, finger flexion contractures, tendon or bursal friction rubs, and renal crisis were removed. The new criteria have improved sensitivity and specificity compared to the 1980 and LeRoy/Medsger criteria and classify more individuals with early and limited disease (Table 5.6) [96]. This has been independently replicated in other cohorts [97, 98].

The ACR-EULAR criteria have largely been lauded for their improved performance characteristics and large collaborative international effort. However, it is worth noting that it has also received some criticism [90]. Pragmatic criticisms are the use of a numeric additive point system requiring the use of "mental mathematics" and concerns that there remain too many criteria. Attempts to further reduce the number of criteria and simplify the weighting resulted in reduced sensitivity and specificity. The new SSc classification criteria reflect a tradeoff between a comprehensive system versus a feasible one that is easy to use [99]. An online tool is available to aid in the calculation of the score (http://rheuminfo.com/physician-tools/ssc-calculator).

A second criticism relates to the use of the criteria in individuals with mixed connective tissue disease [100]. The 1980 criteria investigators excluded MCTD patients from the derivation processes as they felt that it was "virtually impossible" to distinguish from SSc [100]. For the new criteria, the criteria testing, derivation, and validation cohorts included MCTD patients. Since many MCTD patients are SSc-predominant in their clinical features, it was decided that these criteria could be applied to MCTD when considering enrollment into an SSc study [96]. A Norwegian cohort of 178 MCTD patients reported that 10% fulfilled the new criteria [97]. However, this cohort study did not collect data on abnormal nailfold capillaries or telangiectasias, therefore 10% may be an underestimate [99].

Fig. 5.5 ACR-EULAR Classification Criteria for Systemic Sclerosis. (Adapted from van den Hoogen 2013, Johnson 2015)

ENTRY CRITERION:
These criteria are applicable to any patient considered for inclusion in a SSc study

↓

EXCLUSION CRITERION:
These criteria are not applicable to patients having a systemic sclerosis-like disorder better explaining their symptoms such as: nephrogenic sclerosing fibrosis, sclerodema diabeticorum, scleromyexedema, erythromylagia, porphyria, lichen sclerosis, graft versus host disease, and diabetic chierarthropathy

↓

EXCLUSION CRITERION:
Patients with skin thickening sparing the fingers are not classified as SSc
(*i.e. skin thickening elsewhere but not the fingers*)

↓

Items	**Sub-items**	**Weight**
Sufficient criterion		9
Skin thickening of the fingers of both hands extending proximal to the metacarpophalangeal joints		
Skin thickening of the fingers *(only count the highest score)*	Puffy fingers Whole Finger, distal to MCP	2 4
Finger tip lesions *(only count the highest score)*	Digital Tip Ulcers Pitting Scars	2 3
Telangiectasia		2
Abnormal nailfold capillaries		2
Pulmonary arterial hypertension and/or Interstitial lung Disease		2
Raynaud's phenomenon		3
Scleroderma related antibodies	(any of anti-centromere, anti-topoisomeraseI [anti-ScL 70], anti-RNA polymerase III)	3
	TOTAL SCORE:	
Patients having a total score of 9 or more are classified as having SSc		

Table 5.6 Performance characteristics of the ACR EULAR criteria compared to the 1980 criteria

Cohort	ACR EULAR criteria Sensitivity (95% CI)	ACR EULAR criteria Specificity (95% CI)	1980 criteria Sensitivity (95% CI)	1980 criteria Specificity (95% CI)
Internal validation				
Derivation cohort	95% (90%, 98%)	93% (86%, 97%)	80% (72%, 87%)	77% (68%, 84%)
Validation cohort	91% (87%, 94%)	92% (86%, 96%)	75% (70%, 80%)	72% (64%, 79%)
δ 3 years disease duration	91% (86%, 96%)	90% (70%, 99%)	75% (70%, 80%)	72% (63%, 79%)
External validation				
Alhajeri et al. 2015	98%	NA	88%	NA
Limited cutaneous SSc	99%	NA	86%	NA
δ 3 years disease duration	99%	NA	85%	NA
Hoffmann-Vold et al. 2015	96% (93%, 97%)	90% (85%, 94%)	75%	NA

Modified from Johnson SR. New ACR EULAR Guidelines for Systemic Sclerosis Classification. Curr Rheum Rev. 2015

Conclusions

It is clear that these hallmarks of the SSc pathogenic process play an important role in the recognition (diagnosis and classification) of SSc. Developed using a rigorous methodologic approach, the ACR-EULAR classification criteria for SSc emphasize the vasculopathic manifestations and include the early manifestation of puffy fingers. The new criteria have improved sensitivity and specificity, particularly among cases with early, mild, and/or limited disease. We may now include more individuals with SSc in clinical trials and are hopefully closer to achieving new goals of preventing disease progression and inducing remission.

The SSc subset criteria proposed by LeRoy in 1988 subdividing SSc into limited and diffuse subsets is widely accepted [2, 101] as they differ to a certain degree in their pathogenesis, clinical course, and prognosis. An international initiative is underway to update the system of subsetting SSc to reflect advances in our understanding of SSc, most notably in the area of autoantibodies [102, 103]. Recent scientific advances have shifted the way we think of the diagnosis and classification of SSc and its subsets, ushering in a new era.

References

1. Block JA, Sequeira W. Raynaud's phenomenon. Lancet. 2001;357(9273):2042–8. https://doi.org/10.1016/S0140-6736(00)05118-7.
2. LeRoy EC, Black C, Fleischmajer R, Jablonska S, Krieg T, Medsger TA Jr, et al. Scleroderma (systemic sclerosis): classification, subsets and pathogenesis. J Rheumatol. 1988;15(2):202–5.
3. Johnson SR, Feldman BM, Pope JE, Tomlinson GA. Shifting our thinking about uncommon disease trials: the case of methotrexate in scleroderma. J Rheumatol. 2009;36(2):323–9. https://doi.org/10.3899/jrheum.071169.
4. Pope JE, Bellamy N, Seibold JR, Baron M, Ellman M, Carette S, et al. A randomized, controlled trial of methotrexate versus placebo in early diffuse scleroderma. Arthritis Rheum. 2001;44(6):1351–8. https://doi.org/10.1002/1529-0131(200106)44:6<1351::AID-ART227>3.0.CO;2-I.
5. Tashkin DP, Elashoff R, Clements PJ, Goldin J, Roth MD, Furst DE, et al. Cyclophosphamide versus placebo in scleroderma lung disease. N Engl J Med. 2006;354(25):2655–66. https://doi.org/10.1056/NEJMoa055120.
6. Tashkin DP, Roth MD, Clements PJ, Furst DE, Khanna D, Kleerup EC, et al. Mycophenolate mofetil versus oral cyclophosphamide in scleroderma-related interstitial lung disease (SLS II): a randomised controlled, double-blind, parallel group trial. Lancet Respir Med. 2016;4(9):708–19. https://doi.org/10.1016/S2213-2600(16)30152-7.
7. Rhew EY, Barr WG. Scleroderma renal crisis: new insights and developments. Curr Rheumatol Rep. 2004;6(2):129–36. https://doi.org/10.1007/s11926-004-0057-5.
8. Mathai SC, Hassoun PM. Therapy for pulmonary arterial hypertension associated with systemic sclerosis. Curr Opin Rheumatol. 2009;21(6):642–8. https://doi.org/10.1097/BOR.0b013e3283307dc8.
9. Thenappan T, Al-Naamani N, Ghio S, Ghofrani HA, Hassoun PM, Pritzker M, et al. Effect of riociguat on pulmonary arterial compliance in the PATENT and CHEST studies. Pulm Circ. 2020;10(4):2045894020963836. https://doi.org/10.1177/2045894020963836.
10. Aggarwal R, Ringold S, Khanna D, Neogi T, Johnson SR, Miller A, et al. Distinctions between diagnostic and classification criteria? Arthritis Care Res (Hoboken). 2015;67(7):891–7. https://doi.org/10.1002/acr.22583.
11. Johnson SR, Laxer RM. Classification in systemic sclerosis. J Rheumatol. 2006;33(5):840–1.
12. Medsger TA Jr. Natural history of systemic sclerosis and the assessment of disease activity, severity, functional status, and psychologic Well-being. Rheum Dis Clin N Am. 2003;29(2):255–73, vi. https://doi.org/10.1016/s0889-857x(03)00023-1.
13. Walker UA, Tyndall A, Czirjak L, Denton CP, Farge BD, Kowal-Bielecka O, et al. Clinical risk assessment of organ manifestations in systemic sclerosis—a report from the EULAR scleroderma trials and research (EUSTAR) group data base. Ann RheumDis. 2007;66:754.
14. Ferri C, Valentini G, Cozzi F, Sebastiani M, Michelassi C, La Montagna G, et al. Systemic sclerosis: demographic, clinical, and serologic features and survival in 1,012 Italian patients. Medicine (Baltimore). 2002;81(2):139–53.
15. Winterbauer RH. Multiple telangiectasia, Raynaud's phenomenon, Sclerodactyly, and Subcutanious calcinosis: a syndrome mimicking hereditary hemorrhagic telangiectasia. Bull Johns Hopkins Hosp. 1964;114:361–83.

16. Reveille JD, Solomon DH, American College of Rheumatology Ad Hoc Committee of Immunologic Testing G. Evidence-based guidelines for the use of immunologic tests: anticentromere, Scl-70, and nucleolar antibodies. Arthritis Rheum. 2003;49(3):399–412. https://doi.org/10.1002/art.11113.
17. Tan EM, Rodnan GP, Garcia I, Moroi Y, Fritzler MJ, Peebles C. Diversity of antinuclear antibodies in progressive systemic sclerosis. Anti-centromere antibody and its relationship to CREST syndrome. Arthritis Rheum. 1980;23(6):617–25. https://doi.org/10.1002/art.1780230602.
18. Wigley FM. When is scleroderma really scleroderma? J Rheumatol. 2001;28(7):1471–3.
19. Johnson SR, Feldman BM, Hawker GA. Classification criteria for systemic sclerosis subsets. J Rheumatol. 2007;34(9):1855–63.
20. Giordano M, Valentini G, Migliaresi S, Picillo U, Vatti M. Different antibody patterns and different prognoses in patients with scleroderma with various extent of skin sclerosis. J Rheumatol. 1986;13(5):911–6.
21. Poormoghim H, Lucas M, Fertig N, Medsger TA Jr. Systemic sclerosis sine scleroderma: demographic, clinical, and serologic features and survival in forty-eight patients. Arthritis Rheum. 2000;43(2):444–51.
22. Barnett AJ, Coventry DA. Scleroderma. 1. Clinical features, course of illness and response to treatment in 61 cases. Med J Aust. 1969;1(19):992–1001.
23. Rodnan GP, Jablonska S, Medsger TA. Classification and nomenclature of progressive systemic sclerosis. Clin Rheumatic Dis. 1979;5(1):5–13.
24. Masi AT. Classification of systemic sclerosis (scleroderma): relationship of cutaneous subgroups in early disease to outcome and serologic reactivity. J Rheumatol. 1988;15(6):894–8.
25. Scussel-Lonzetti L, Joyal F, Raynauld JP, Roussin A, Rich E, Goulet JR, et al. Predicting mortality in systemic sclerosis: analysis of a cohort of 309 French Canadian patients with emphasis on features at diagnosis as predictive factors for survival. Medicine (Baltimore). 2002;81(2):154–67.
26. Williams HJ, Alarcon GS, Joks R, Steen VD, Bulpitt K, Clegg DO, et al. Early undifferentiated connective tissue disease (CTD). VI. An inception cohort after 10 years: disease remissions and changes in diagnoses in well established and undifferentiated CTD. J Rheumatol. 1999;26(4):816–25.
27. Mosca M, Tavoni A, Neri R, Bencivelli W, Bombardieri S. Undifferentiated connective tissue diseases: the clinical and serological profiles of 91 patients followed for at least 1 year. Lupus. 1998;7(2):95–100. https://doi.org/10.1191/096120398678919787.
28. Bodolay E, Csiki Z, Szekanecz Z, Ben T, Kiss E, Zeher M, et al. Five-year follow-up of 665 Hungarian patients with undifferentiated connective tissue disease (UCTD). Clin Exp Rheumatol. 2003;21(3):313–20.
29. Danieli MG, Fraticelli P, Salvi A, Gabrielli A, Danieli G. Undifferentiated connective tissue disease: natural history and evolution into definite CTD assessed in 84 patients initially diagnosed as early UCTD. Clin Rheumatol. 1998;17(3):195–201. https://doi.org/10.1007/BF01451046.
30. Sharp GC, Irvin WS, Tan EM, Gould RG, Holman HR. Mixed connective tissue disease—an apparently distinct rheumatic disease syndrome associated with a specific antibody to an extractable nuclear antigen (ENA). Am J Med. 1972;52(2):148–59. https://doi.org/10.1016/0002-9343(72)90064-2.
31. Venables PJ. Mixed connective tissue disease. Lupus. 2006;15(3):132–7. https://doi.org/10.1191/0961203306lu2283rr.
32. Alarcon-Segovia D, Cardiel MH. Comparison between 3 diagnostic criteria for mixed connective tissue disease. Study of 593 patients. J Rheumatol. 1989;16(3):328–34.
33. Burdt MA, Hoffman RW, Deutscher SL, Wang GS, Johnson JC, Sharp GC. Long-term outcome in mixed connective tissue disease: longitudinal clinical and serologic findings. Arthritis Rheum. 1999;42(5):899–909. https://doi.org/10.1002/1529-0131(199905)42:5<899::AID-ANR8>3.0.CO;2-L.
34. Preliminary criteria for the classification of systemic sclerosis (scleroderma). Subcommittee for scleroderma criteria of the American Rheumatism Association Diagnostic and Therapeutic Criteria Committee. Arthritis Rheum. 1980;23(5):581–90.
35. Meyer OC, Fertig N, Lucas M, Somogyi N, Medsger TA Jr. Disease subsets, antinuclear antibody profile, and clinical features in 127 French and 247 US adult patients with systemic sclerosis. J Rheumatol. 2007;34(1):104–9.
36. Nadashkevich O, Davis P, Fritzler MJ. Revising the classification criteria for systemic sclerosis. Arthritis Rheum. 2006;55(6):992–3.
37. Hachulla E, Launay D. Diagnosis and classification of systemic sclerosis. Clin Rev Allergy Immunol. 2011;40(2):78–83. https://doi.org/10.1007/s12016-010-8198-y.
38. Maricq HR, Valter I. A working classification of scleroderma spectrum disorders: a proposal and the results of testing on a sample of patients. Clin Exp Rheumatol. 2004;22(3 Suppl 33):S5–13.
39. Hudson M, Taillefer S, Steele R, Dunne J, Johnson SR, Jones N, et al. Improving the sensitivity of the American College of Rheumatology classification criteria for systemic sclerosis. Clin Exp Rheumatol. 2007;25(5):754–7.
40. Lonzetti LS, Joyal F, Raynauld JP, Roussin A, Goulet JR, Rich E, et al. Updating the American College of Rheumatology preliminary classification criteria for systemic sclerosis: addition of severe nailfold capillaroscopy abnormalities markedly increases the sensitivity for limited scleroderma. Arthritis Rheum. 2001;44(3):735–6.
41. LeRoy EC, Medsger TA Jr. Criteria for the classification of early systemic sclerosis. J Rheumatol. 2001;28(7):1573–6.
42. Ziswiler HR, Urech R, Balmer J, Ostensen M, Mierau R, Villiger PM. Clinical diagnosis compared to classification criteria in in a cohort of 54 patients with systemic sclerosis and associated disorders. Swiss Med Wkly. 2007;137(41–42):586–90.
43. Nadashkevich O, Davis P, Fritzler MJ. A proposal of criteria for the classification of systemic sclerosis. MedSciMonit. 2004;10(11):CR615–CR21.
44. Maricq HR, LeRoy EC. Patterns of finger capillary abnormalities in connective tissue disease by "wide-field" microscopy. Arthritis Rheum. 1973;16(5):619–28. https://doi.org/10.1002/art.1780160506.
45. Maricq HR, LeRoy EC, D'Angelo WA, Medsger TA Jr, Rodnan GP, Sharp GC, et al. Diagnostic potential of in vivo capillary microscopy in scleroderma and related disorders. Arthritis Rheum. 1980;23(2):183–9. https://doi.org/10.1002/art.1780230208.
46. Maricq HR, Weinberger AB, LeRoy EC. Early detection of scleroderma-spectrum disorders by in vivo capillary microscopy: a prospective study of patients with Raynaud's phenomenon. J Rheumatol. 1982;9(2):289–91.
47. Cutolo M, Sulli A, Pizzorni C, Accardo S. Nailfold videocapillaroscopy assessment of microvascular damage in systemic sclerosis. J Rheumatol. 2000;27(1):155–60.
48. Cutolo M, Pizzorni C, Tuccio M, Burroni A, Craviotto C, Basso M, et al. Nailfold videocapillaroscopic patterns and serum autoantibodies in systemic sclerosis. Rheumatology (Oxford). 2004;43(6):719–26. https://doi.org/10.1093/rheumatology/keh156.
49. Smith V, Pizzorni C, De Keyser F, Decuman S, Van Praet JT, Deschepper E, et al. Reliability of the qualitative and semi-quantitative nailfold videocapillaroscopy assessment in a systemic sclerosis cohort: a two-Centre study. Ann Rheum Dis. 2010;69(6):1092–6. https://doi.org/10.1136/ard.2009.115568.

50. Anders HJ, Sigl T, Schattenkirchner M. Differentiation between primary and secondary Raynaud's phenomenon: a prospective study comparing nailfold capillaroscopy using an ophthalmoscope or stereomicroscope. Ann Rheum Dis. 2001;60(4):407–9. https://doi.org/10.1136/ard.60.4.407.
51. Baron M, Bell M, Bookman A, Buchignani M, Dunne J, Hudson M, et al. Office capillaroscopy in systemic sclerosis. Clin Rheumatol. 2007;26(8):1268–74. https://doi.org/10.1007/s10067-006-0489-6.
52. Bauersachs RM, Lossner F. The poor man's capillary microscope. A novel technique for the assessment of capillary morphology. Ann Rheum Dis. 1997;56(7):435–7. https://doi.org/10.1136/ard.56.7.435.
53. Muroi E, Hara T, Yanaba K, Ogawa F, Yoshizaki A, Takenaka M, et al. A portable dermatoscope for easy, rapid examination of periungual nailfold capillary changes in patients with systemic sclerosis. Rheumatol Int. 2011;31(12):1601–6. https://doi.org/10.1007/s00296-010-1532-0.
54. Hirschl M, Hirschl K, Lenz M, Katzenschlager R, Hutter HP, Kundi M. Transition from primary Raynaud's phenomenon to secondary Raynaud's phenomenon identified by diagnosis of an associated disease: results of ten years of prospective surveillance. Arthritis Rheum. 2006;54(6):1974–81. https://doi.org/10.1002/art.21912.
55. Cutolo M, Pizzorni C, Sulli A. Identification of transition from primary Raynaud's phenomenon to secondary Raynaud's phenomenon by nailfold videocapillaroscopy: comment on the article by Hirschl et al. Arthritis Rheum. 2007;56(6):2102–3; author reply 3–4. https://doi.org/10.1002/art.22636.
56. Koenig M, Joyal F, Fritzler MJ, Roussin A, Abrahamowicz M, Boire G, et al. Autoantibodies and microvascular damage are independent predictive factors for the progression of Raynaud's phenomenon to systemic sclerosis: a twenty-year prospective study of 586 patients, with validation of proposed criteria for early systemic sclerosis. Arthritis Rheum. 2008;58(12):3902–12. https://doi.org/10.1002/art.24038.
57. Steen VD. Autoantibodies in systemic sclerosis. Semin Arthritis Rheum. 2005;35(1):35–42. https://doi.org/10.1016/j.semarthrit.2005.03.005.
58. Steen VD, Powell DL, Medsger TA Jr. Clinical correlations and prognosis based on serum autoantibodies in patients with systemic sclerosis. Arthritis Rheum. 1988;31(2):196–203. https://doi.org/10.1002/art.1780310207.
59. Arbuckle MR, McClain MT, Rubertone MV, Scofield RH, Dennis GJ, James JA, et al. Development of autoantibodies before the clinical onset of systemic lupus erythematosus. N Engl J Med. 2003;349(16):1526–33. https://doi.org/10.1056/NEJMoa021933.
60. Yamasaki Y, Honkanen-Scott M, Hernandez L, Ikeda K, Barker T, Bubb MR, et al. Nucleolar staining cannot be used as a screening test for the scleroderma marker anti-RNA polymerase I/III antibodies. Arthritis Rheum. 2006;54(9):3051–6. https://doi.org/10.1002/art.22043.
61. Parker JC, Burlingame RW, Webb TT, Bunn CC. Anti-RNA polymerase III antibodies in patients with systemic sclerosis detected by indirect immunofluorescence and ELISA. Rheumatology (Oxford). 2008;47(7):976–9. https://doi.org/10.1093/rheumatology/ken201.
62. Villalta D, Morozzi G, Tampoia M, Alpini C, Brusca I, Salgarolo V, et al. Antibodies to fibrillarin, PM-Scl and RNA polymerase III detected by ELISA assays in patients with systemic sclerosis. Clin Chim Acta. 2010;411(9–10):710–3. https://doi.org/10.1016/j.cca.2010.01.037.
63. Perera A, Fertig N, Lucas M, Rodriguez-Reyna TS, Hu P, Steen VD, et al. Clinical subsets, skin thickness progression rate, and serum antibody levels in systemic sclerosis patients with anti-topoisomerase I antibody. Arthritis Rheum. 2007;56(8):2740–6. https://doi.org/10.1002/art.22747.
64. Kuwana M, Okano Y, Pandey JP, Silver RM, Fertig N, Medsger TA Jr. Enzyme-linked immunosorbent assay for detection of anti-RNA polymerase III antibody: analytical accuracy and clinical associations in systemic sclerosis. Arthritis Rheum. 2005;52(8):2425–32. https://doi.org/10.1002/art.21232.
65. Satoh T, Ishikawa O, Ihn H, Endo H, Kawaguchi Y, Sasaki T, et al. Clinical usefulness of anti-RNA polymerase III antibody measurement by enzyme-linked immunosorbent assay. Rheumatology (Oxford). 2009;48(12):1570–4. https://doi.org/10.1093/rheumatology/kep290.
66. Moinzadeh P, Fonseca C, Hellmich M, Shah AA, Chighizola C, Denton CP, et al. Association of anti-RNA polymerase III autoantibodies and cancer in scleroderma. Arthritis Res Ther. 2014;16(1):R53. https://doi.org/10.1186/ar4486.
67. Shah AA, Rosen A, Hummers L, Wigley F, Casciola-Rosen L. Close temporal relationship between onset of cancer and scleroderma in patients with RNA polymerase I/III antibodies. Arthritis Rheum. 2010;62(9):2787–95. https://doi.org/10.1002/art.27549.
68. Joseph CG, Darrah E, Shah AA, Skora AD, Casciola-Rosen LA, Wigley FM, et al. Association of the autoimmune disease scleroderma with an immunologic response to cancer. Science. 2014;343(6167):152–7. https://doi.org/10.1126/science.1246886.
69. Shah AA, Laiho M, Rosen A, Casciola-Rosen L. Protective effect against cancer of antibodies to the large subunits of both RNA polymerases I and III in scleroderma. Arthritis & rheumatology. 2019;71(9):1571–9. https://doi.org/10.1002/art.40893.
70. Arnett FC, Reveille JD, Goldstein R, Pollard KM, Leaird K, Smith EA, et al. Autoantibodies to fibrillarin in systemic sclerosis (scleroderma). An immunogenetic, serologic, and clinical analysis. Arthritis Rheum. 1996;39(7):1151–60. https://doi.org/10.1002/art.1780390712.
71. Aggarwal R, Lucas M, Fertig N, Oddis CV, Medsger TA Jr. Anti-U3 RNP autoantibodies in systemic sclerosis. Arthritis Rheum. 2009;60(4):1112–8. https://doi.org/10.1002/art.24409.
72. Sharif R, Fritzler MJ, Mayes MD, Gonzalez EB, McNearney TA, Draeger H, et al. Anti-fibrillarin antibody in African American patients with systemic sclerosis: immunogenetics, clinical features, and survival analysis. J Rheumatol. 2011;38(8):1622–30. https://doi.org/10.3899/jrheum.110071.
73. Nihtyanova SI, Sari A, Harvey JC, Leslie A, Derrett-Smith EC, Fonseca C, et al. Using autoantibodies and cutaneous subset to develop outcome-based disease classification in systemic sclerosis. Arthritis Rheumatol. 2020;72(3):465–76. https://doi.org/10.1002/art.41153.
74. Hanke K, Bruckner CS, Dahnrich C, Huscher D, Komorowski L, Meyer W, et al. Antibodies against PM/Scl-75 and PM/Scl-100 are independent markers for different subsets of systemic sclerosis patients. Arthritis Res Ther. 2009;11(1):R22. https://doi.org/10.1186/ar2614.
75. Okano Y, Medsger TA Jr. Autoantibody to Th ribonucleoprotein (nucleolar 7-2 RNA protein particle) in patients with systemic sclerosis. Arthritis Rheum. 1990;33(12):1822–8. https://doi.org/10.1002/art.1780331210.
76. Kasturi KN, Hatakeyama A, Spiera H, Bona CA. Antifibrillarin autoantibodies present in systemic sclerosis and other connective tissue diseases interact with similar epitopes. J Exp Med. 1995;181(3):1027–36. https://doi.org/10.1084/jem.181.3.1027.
77. Fertig N, Domsic RT, Rodriguez-Reyna T, Kuwana M, Lucas M, Medsger TA Jr, et al. Anti-U11/U12 RNP antibodies in systemic sclerosis: a new serologic marker associated with pulmonary fibrosis. Arthritis Rheum. 2009;61(7):958–65. https://doi.org/10.1002/art.24586.

78. McMahan ZH, Domsic RT, Zhu L, Medsger TA, Casciola-Rosen L, Shah AA. Anti-RNPC-3 (U11/U12) antibodies in systemic sclerosis in patients with moderate-to-severe gastrointestinal dysmotility. Arthritis Care Res (Hoboken). 2019;71(9):1164–70. https://doi.org/10.1002/acr.23763.
79. Caetano J, Nihtyanova SI, Harvey J, Denton CP, Ong VH. Distinctive clinical phenotype of anti-centromere antibody-positive diffuse systemic sclerosis. Rheumatol Adv Pract. 2018;2(1):rky002. https://doi.org/10.1093/rap/rky002.
80. Simonneau G, Montani D, Celermajer DS, Denton CP, Gatzoulis MA, Krowka M, et al. Haemodynamic definitions and updated clinical classification of pulmonary hypertension. Eur Respir J. 2019;53(1):1801913. https://doi.org/10.1183/13993003.01913-2018.
81. Hesselstrand R, Scheja A, Shen GQ, Wiik A, Akesson A. The association of antinuclear antibodies with organ involvement and survival in systemic sclerosis. Rheumatology (Oxford). 2003;42(4):534–40. https://doi.org/10.1093/rheumatology/keg170.
82. Mitri GM, Lucas M, Fertig N, Steen VD, Medsger TA Jr. A comparison between anti-Th/to- and anticentromere antibody-positive systemic sclerosis patients with limited cutaneous involvement. Arthritis Rheum. 2003;48(1):203–9. https://doi.org/10.1002/art.10760.
83. Kaji K, Fertig N, Medsger TA Jr, Satoh T, Hoshino K, Hamaguchi Y, et al. Autoantibodies to RuvBL1 and RuvBL2: a novel systemic sclerosis-related antibody associated with diffuse cutaneous and skeletal muscle involvement. Arthritis Care Res (Hoboken). 2014;66(4):575–84. https://doi.org/10.1002/acr.22163.
84. Pauling JD, Salazar G, Lu H, Betteridge ZE, Assassi S, Mayes MD, et al. Presence of anti-eukaryotic initiation factor-2B, anti-RuvBL1/2 and anti-synthetase antibodies in patients with anti-nuclear antibody negative systemic sclerosis. Rheumatology (Oxford). 2018;57(4):712–7. https://doi.org/10.1093/rheumatology/kex458.
85. Hamaguchi Y, Kuwana M, Takehara K. Performance evaluation of a commercial line blot assay system for detection of myositis- and systemic sclerosis-related autoantibodies. Clin Rheumatol. 2020;39(11):3489–97. https://doi.org/10.1007/s10067-020-04973-0.
86. Ghirardello A, Borella E, Beggio M, Franceschini F, Fredi M, Doria A. Myositis autoantibodies and clinical phenotypes. Auto Immun Highlights. 2014;5(3):69–75. https://doi.org/10.1007/s13317-014-0060-4.
87. Cavazzana I, Fredi M, Taraborelli M, Quinzanini M, Tincani A, Franceschini F. A subset of systemic sclerosis but not of systemic lupus erythematosus is defined by isolated anti-Ku autoantibodies. Clin Exp Rheumatol. 2013;31(2 Suppl 76):118–21.
88. Hoa S, Hudson M, Troyanov Y, Proudman S, Walker J, Stevens W, et al. Single-specificity anti-Ku antibodies in an international cohort of 2140 systemic sclerosis subjects: clinical associations. Medicine (Baltimore). 2016;95(35):e4713. https://doi.org/10.1097/MD.0000000000004713.
89. Avouac J, Fransen J, Walker UA, Riccieri V, Smith V, Muller C, et al. Preliminary criteria for the very early diagnosis of systemic sclerosis: results of a Delphi consensus study from EULAR scleroderma trials and research group. Ann Rheum Dis. 2011;70(3):476–81. https://doi.org/10.1136/ard.2010.136929.
90. Johnson SR, New ACR. EULAR guidelines for systemic sclerosis classification. Curr Rheumatol Rep. 2015;17(5):32. https://doi.org/10.1007/s11926-015-0506-3.
91. Johnson SR. Progress in the clinical classification of systemic sclerosis. Curr Opin Rheumatol. 2017;29(6):568–73. https://doi.org/10.1097/BOR.0000000000000443.
92. Fransen J, Johnson SR, van den Hoogen F, Baron M, Allanore Y, Carreira PE, et al. Items for developing revised classification criteria in systemic sclerosis: results of a consensus exercise. Arthritis Care Res (Hoboken). 2012;64(3):351–7. https://doi.org/10.1002/acr.20679.
93. Coulter C, Baron M, Pope JE. A Delphi exercise and cluster analysis to aid in the development of potential classification criteria for systemic sclerosis using SSc experts and databases. Clin Exp Rheumatol. 2013;31(2 Suppl 76):24–30.
94. Johnson SR, Fransen J, Khanna D, Baron M, van den Hoogen F, Medsger TA Jr, et al. Validation of potential classification criteria for systemic sclerosis. Arthritis Care Res (Hoboken). 2012;64(3):358–67. https://doi.org/10.1002/acr.20684.
95. Johnson SR, Naden RP, Fransen J, van den Hoogen F, Pope JE, Baron M, et al. Multicriteria decision analysis methods with 1000Minds for developing systemic sclerosis classification criteria. J Clin Epidemiol. 2014;67(6):706–14. https://doi.org/10.1016/j.jclinepi.2013.12.009.
96. van den Hoogen F, Khanna D, Fransen J, Johnson SR, Baron M, Tyndall A, et al. 2013 classification criteria for systemic sclerosis: an American College of Rheumatology/European league against rheumatism collaborative initiative. Arthritis Rheum. 2013;65(11):2737–47. https://doi.org/10.1002/art.38098.
97. Hoffmann-Vold AM, Gunnarsson R, Garen T, Midtvedt O, Molberg O. Performance of the 2013 American College of Rheumatology/European league against rheumatism classification criteria for systemic sclerosis (SSc) in large, well-defined cohorts of SSc and mixed connective tissue disease. J Rheumatol. 2015;42(1):60–3. https://doi.org/10.3899/jrheum.140047.
98. Alhajeri H, Hudson M, Fritzler M, Pope J, Tatibouet S, Markland J, et al. The 2013 ACR/EULAR classification criteria for systemic sclerosis out-perform the 1980 criteria. Data from the Canadian Scleroderma Research Group. Arthritis Care Res (Hoboken). 2014;67(4):582–7. https://doi.org/10.1002/acr.22451.
99. Pope JE. Systemic sclerosis classification: a rose by any other name would smell as sweet? J Rheumatol. 2015;42(1):11–3. https://doi.org/10.3899/jrheum.141103.
100. Masi AT, Medsger TA Jr. Progress in the evolution of systemic sclerosis classification criteria and recommendation for additional comparative specificity studies. J Rheumatol. 2015;42(1):8–10. https://doi.org/10.3899/jrheum.141020.
101. Wollheim FA. Classification of systemic sclerosis. Visions Reality Rheumatol (Oxford). 2005;44(10):1212–6.
102. Johnson SR, Soowamber ML, Fransen J, Khanna D, Van Den Hoogen F, Baron M, et al. There is a need for new systemic sclerosis subset criteria. A content analytic approach. Scand J Rheumatol. 2018;47(1):62–70. https://doi.org/10.1080/03009742.2017.1299793.
103. Nevskaya T, Pope J, Turk M, Shu J, Marquardt A, van den Hoogen F, et al. Systematic analysis of the literature in search of defining systemic sclerosis subsets. J Rheumatol. 2021;48(11):1698–717.

6 Clustering and Evolving Concepts for Subclassification

Vincent Sobanski and Monique Hinchcliff

Systemic sclerosis (SSc) is the connective tissue disease with the highest morbidity and mortality. The mechanisms of the disease are complex, involving inflammation and autoimmunity, vascular involvement, and fibrosis [1]. SSc is characterized by significant heterogeneity in terms of clinical manifestations, organ involvement, serological profiles, and molecular signatures. This inter-individual variability strongly impacts the different evolutionary profiles and therapeutic responses, making it difficult to conduct clinical trials on a population of patients with this rare disease. The wide spectrum of clinical phenotypes has greatly influenced the design of different disease (sub)classifications and still represents a challenge to the inclusion of homogeneous patients in therapeutic trials [2]. This explains the important efforts in the last decades to design sub-classifications that allow to correctly represent the different subgroups of relatively homogeneous patients, if possible beyond the classical dichotomy of "limited" versus "diffuse" cutaneous forms [3, 4]. In this chapter, we will describe the concept of classification and its importance in heterogeneous conditions like SSc and review the different attempts to reach a new sub-classification of the disease. Then, we will approach the concept of unsupervised analysis, such as clustering techniques, and discuss the integration of heterogeneous data of variable dimensionality, in particular from high throughput technologies, toward a more global and integrative classification.

V. Sobanski (✉)
Univ. Lille, Inserm, CHU Lille, U1286 - INFINITE - Institute for Translational Research in Inflammation, Lille, France

Institut Universitaire de France (IUF), Lille, France
e-mail: vincent.sobanski@univ-lille.fr

M. Hinchcliff
Department of Internal Medicine, Section of Rheumatology, Allergy & Immunology, The Anlyan Center, Yale School of Medicine, New Haven, CT, USA
e-mail: monique.hinchcliff@yale.edu

Need for Classification and Subclassification in a Highly Heterogeneous Disease

The broad spectrum of clinical presentations has had a significant impact on the development of the various classification criteria for SSc. This term "classification" actually covers two concepts [3]. First, classification criteria establish criteria for classifying a disease in order to define homogeneous patient groups for clinical study inclusion (e.g., distinguishing between SSc and non-SSc patients). In SSc, the first set of criteria was developed by the *American College of Rheumatology (ACR)* in 1980 [5]. A revised set of criteria was adopted in 2013 by *EULAR (EUropean League Against Rheumatism)* and *ACR*, to allow the inclusion of patients with early and advanced disease [6]. Neither of these criteria intended to identify specific subgroups of SSc patients with different prognoses. Second, the concept of disease classification can be used to define subgroups of patients *within* a condition. Until now, the classification of SSc into subgroups has been mainly based on the criteria proposed by LeRoy et al. in 1988 and amended in 2001 [7, 8]. This (sub)classification defined two main forms according to the extent of skin fibrosis: the diffuse cutaneous form (dcSSc) where skin involvement includes the face, trunk, and proximal parts of the limbs, and the limited cutaneous form (lcSSc) where cutaneous fibrosis is limited to the hands, forearms, feet, legs, and face. Importantly, although a specific pattern of organ involvement associated with these two subgroups was initially provided, this subclassification was independent of the visceral manifestations since it was anchored solely on the extent of skin fibrosis [3].

As subgroup classification established on skin involvement was associated with significant survival differences, it was subsequently considered robust and clinically important [1]. Nevertheless, recent study results have shown that it is possible to identify subgroups based on other characteristics, such as the presence of serum autoantibodies, suggesting that more precise representations of different patient phenotypes can be achieved [4, 9–11].

Y. Allanore et al. (eds.), *Scleroderma*, https://doi.org/10.1007/978-3-031-40658-4_6

Exploring New SSc Classifications

Although it is well recognized that patients with dcSSc tend to have earlier organ damage and higher mortality than patients with lcSSc, results of recent studies with large sample sizes have demonstrated significant heterogeneity *within* these subgroups.

Studies Based on Skin, Organ Involvement, and Autoantibody Profiles

Nihtyanova et al. showed, in a population of about 400 consecutively followed patients, that the presence of organ involvement could be a powerful prognostic factor in both dcSSc and lcSSc. It was striking that survival curves were similar between the dcSSc/lcSSc groups when organ involvement was present [12]. While anti-topoisomerase I antibodies (ATA) are usually associated with dcSSc in contrast to the common association between anticentromere antibodies (ACA) and lcSSc, some studies analyzed groups of patients with lcSSc and ATA or dcSSc and ACA. There was a stronger association between the antibody profile and visceral involvement and survival compared to the extent of skin involvement [13–15]. In a more recent study, Nihtyanova et al. analyzed the associations between autoantibodies, clinical presentation, and outcomes in a cohort of 1325 SSc patients. By combining autoantibody profile and extent of skin involvement, the authors proposed a novel SSc classification scheme including seven groups (ACA+ lcSSc, anti-topo-I+ lcSSc, anti-topo-I+ dcSSc, anti-RNA polymerase 3+, anti-U3RNP+, other antibodies lcSSc and other antibodies dcSSc). This enabled a more precise risk stratification of patients than the historical dcSSc/lcSSc. It confirmed the strong association between ACA and low incidence rates of major organ-based complications and mortality. Yet, pulmonary hypertension (PH) was present with a similar incidence in the ACA+ group and the SSc cohort overall, challenging the classical association between ACA and PH [16].

Overlap Syndromes

Moinzadeh et al. studied the outcomes of 3240 patients from the German SSc registry. Patients with SSc overlapping with another connective tissue disease had a higher frequency of musculoskeletal involvement and earlier cardiac and lung involvement than lcSSc [17]. In another study, whole blood gene expression profiles were different between overlap syndromes and SSc [18].

Clinical Trajectories Over Time

The evolution of clinical variables over time has been studied in an attempt to isolate specific subgroups of patients. Ledoult et al. studied the trajectories of the modified Rodnan skin score (mRSS) in patients with early disease enrolled in the French SSc database. Using a latent class mixed model, they identified five distinct mRSS trajectories that were independent of SSc disease duration. Patients with mRSS trajectories that significantly changed over time had more internal organ involvement at baseline mRSS and increased morbimortality [19]. This methodology was also used to characterize the progression of SSc-ILD [20, 21].

High-Throughput Omics Technologies

New technological tools allowing high-throughput "omics" approaches have allowed important advances in the understanding of pathogenic mechanisms. These may also help to define new subgroups. Serum metabolomic profiles can differentiate SSc patients from healthy subjects and within SSc patients those with lcSSc or dcSSc [22]. Important work on transcriptomic signatures of skin biopsies has revealed "intrinsic" gene expression profiles in particular in patients with dcSSc [23]. Four gene expression signatures were frequently described: normal-like, inflammatory, fibroproliferative, and limited patterns, which may be stable over time. Importantly, (1) these subgroups did not seem to be associated with serological profiles; (2) even within these four groups, heterogeneity persisted and specific subgroups have been described; (3) other teams have suggested that a certain degree of overlap exists between these patterns since hierarchical clustering and cell type specific signature scores revealed that inflammatory and fibrosing signatures coexist in most patients [24]. However, in a recent phase II clinical trial evaluating abatacept in dcSSc, the 12-month mRSS decline discriminated treatment from placebo patients with inflammatory or normal-like profiles only [25]. This clinical trial was thus negative in the overall population, whereas a subgroup analysis using these finer profiles identified singular therapeutic responses. A pilot study similarly showed a trend toward skin score improvement at 24 weeks in patients with an inflammatory profile [26]. Moreover, results of new studies have been published proposing machine learning-assisted classifications to determine intrinsic molecular subgroups of patients based on transcriptomic analyses of skin biopsies [27]. These results suggest that the skin intrinsic genomic signature may reflect more systemic mechanistic processes. Thus, the skin molecular signature may represent, at least partially, the complete phenotype of a patient with SSc [4].

Radiomics

Because of the systemic nature of SSc and the host of radiographic studies that are used for diagnosis and disease monitoring, a broad array of radiographic data are available for analyses. Two recent examples of how radiographic data have been successfully leveraged for SSc research include analyses of chest high-resolution computed tomography (HRCT) exams for interstitial lung disease quantification and dual-energy computed tomography of the hands for calcinosis cutis assessment [28]. Chest HRCTs performed according to detailed protocols at baseline and 1-year follow-up for patients enrolled in the Scleroderma Lung Study I (SLSI) were subjected to quantitative image analysis to measure the extent of lung disease. Briefly, chest HRCT was divided into three lung zones/lung (upper, middle, and lower) and scored for the extent of ground glass opacification, pulmonary fibrosis, and honeycomb cysts using a Likert scale. Analysis of SLS II chest HRCT was performed using computer-aided quantitative image analysis whereby volumetric HRCT scans were scored for the degree of fibrosis (reticulations), ground glass opacifications, and honeycombing using a supervised texture classification model to generate a quantitative interstitial lung disease (QILD) score. This approach identified no significant differences in QILD changes between baseline and 24 months ($n = 80$ with paired HRCT) between patients who received 2 years of mycophenolate mofetil ($n = 48$) versus those treated with oral cyclophosphamide for 1 year followed by placebo for 1 year ($n = 32$) [29].

Machine learning algorithms have been developed to distinguish between patients with ILD and healthy controls [30], but the more clinically relevant questions in patients with SSc is to develop methods to inform whether ILD will be progressive or has progressed and whether a lung nodule is benign or cancerous. In terms of the first question, no machine learning radiomic algorithms have been developed to date to identify SSc patients who are likely to develop ILD. However, a recently published retrospective analysis of chest HRCT from 37 patients with SSc with no, mild, or severe ILD as assessed by three radiologists demonstrated a median Dice similarity coefficient for ILD contours of 0.74–0.75 between readers and the algorithm that exceeded the agreement between readers (0.68–0.71) [31]. Moreover, the whole lung disease burden as measured by the algorithm correlated with the diffusion lung capacity for carbon monoxide, total lung capacity, and forced vital capacity ($\rho = 0.76$, 0.70, and 0.62, respectively; $P < 0.001$ for all) showed that a deep learning algorithm was performed [31]. While these results are promising, the algorithm was developed using multiple HRCT images from the same patient, not independent images, thus there is the potential for overfitting the model. Additional studies using large independent curated datasets will be required in order to validate an algorithm appropriate for use in clinical settings and translational research. In terms of the second question, results of pathologic studies of lung nodules reveal increased heterogeneity within malignant nodules that are not visible in radiological studies with the naked eye but can be quantified with machine learning approaches [32]. One caveat is that a large number of images are required in order to train the computer to recognize differences in the appearance of malignant and benign nodules. There are many instances where models composed of image features (characteristics) were developed and tested and shown to perform well in one dataset; however, the prediction model performed poorly in independent datasets.

Using 156 SSc patients with ILD, Schniering et al. recently analyzed 1355 stable "radiomic" features extracted from chest HRCT allowing the description of several disease phenotypes with distinct prognoses in two independent cohorts. The authors proposed the first quantitative radiomic risk score to predict progression-free survival in SSc-ILD, outperforming current clinical stratification scores. This score appeared to correlate with genomic, proteomic, and histological profiles of lung biopsies suggesting that it may reflect pro-fibrotic remodeling processes [33].

How Can We Integrate Data from High-Throughput Technologies?

Integrating Between Study High-Dimensional Data

The goal of randomized clinical trials is to recruit patients who fulfill specific classification criteria and randomize them into groups with the goal of ensuring between-group homogeneity such that only the intervention differs. In this way, the effects of an intervention can be assessed. In time, once a sufficient number of studies that test a specific intervention have been published, a meta-analysis can be performed to determine treatment utility. This approach is laborious and expensive and decreases the number of agents that can be studied in parallel. Data scientists approach the problem of patient heterogeneity from a different angle. They examine all available data published for a specific disease agnostic to patient-specific factors. including demographic, treatment, disease duration differences, as well as analytic platform differences in order to find robust disease-specific signals [34].

Transcriptomics

In order to understand how transcriptomic data might be merged to gain insights into disease pathogenesis and heterogeneity, it is necessary to have a basic understanding of how the data are generated. As compared with DNA microarray (Fig. 6.1a), bulk-tissue and single-cell RNA sequencing (scRNA-seq) are newer methods for identifying differentially expressed genes. Bulk tissue RNA-seq, similar to DNA microarray, is less expensive than single-cell approaches and is typically used to determine gene expression differences across individuals (e.g., between SSc and healthy persons, or lcSSc vs. dcSSc). In scRNA-seq, the unit

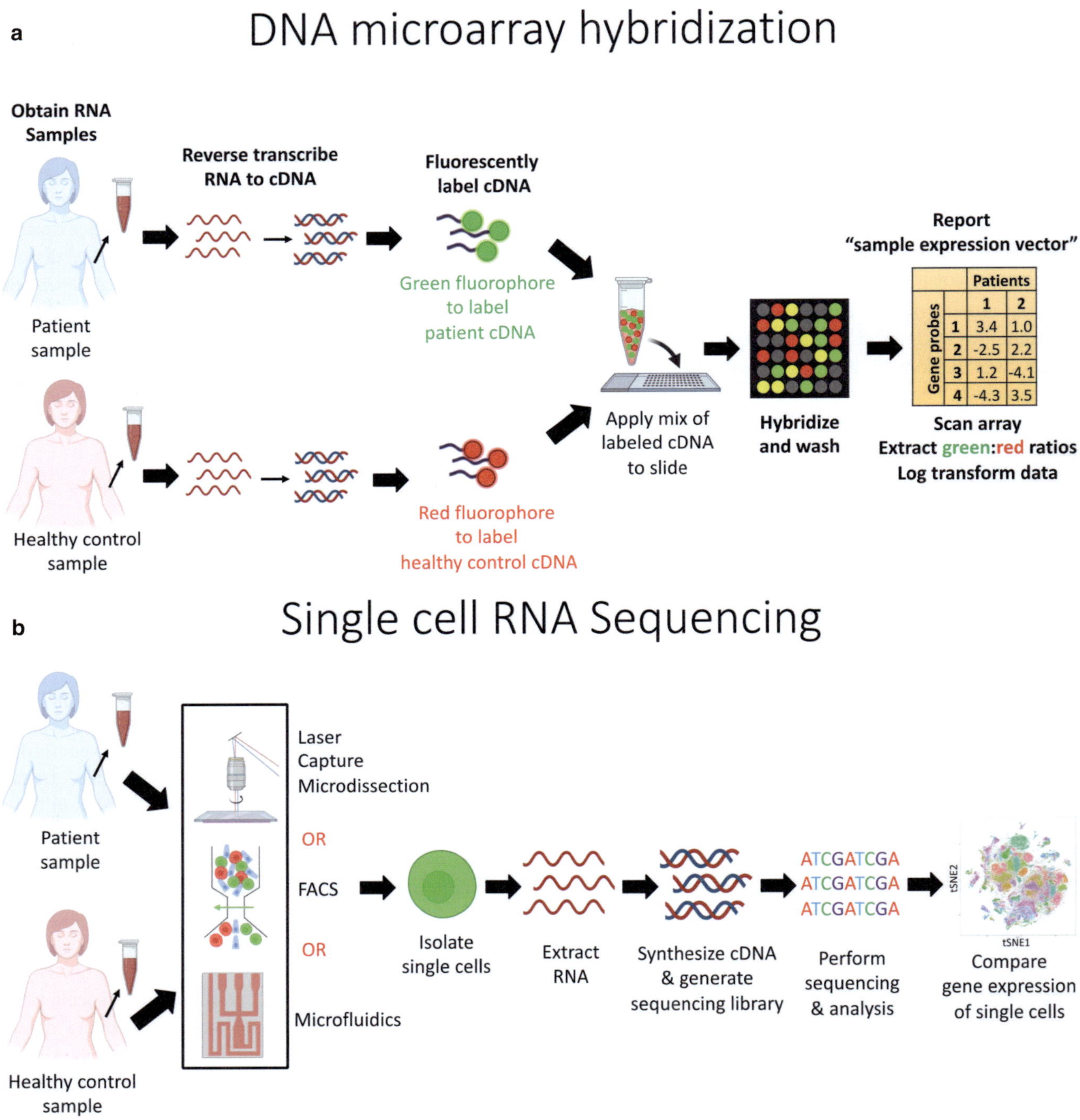

Fig. 6.1 Methods for assessing differential gene expression. (**a**) **Overview of DNA microarray.** DNA microarray is a technique whereby sample and universal reference RNA are labeled with fluorescent dyes, and the mixture is applied to a microarray containing gene probes on a slide. The binding of sample and control RNA is quantified using the fluorescent signal, and the measurements are depicted as a heat map where red generally represents overexpressed and green represents underexpressed genes compared to controls. (**b**) **RNA-seq work flow.** RNA from bulk tissue or single cells isolated using a variety of approaches is obtained, and mRNA is purified. cDNA is then generated and fragmented to permit sequencing. cDNA fragments are labeled with unique identifiers for each sample (molecular barcodes) and sequenced a known number of times. The sequence library is then demultiplexed (sequence reads are separated by sample) and compared to a reference sequence in order to determine the amount of mRNA in tissues/individual cells

of analysis is the cell rather than the tissue, so the generated gene expression signature applies to each cell. The steps utilized in a bulk-tissue and scRNA-seq experiment are similar consisting of three main parts: (1) cDNA library generation, (2) data processing, and (3) data analysis.

cDNA Library Generation

In RNA-seq approaches, the desired RNA is extracted based upon size or RNA type (e.g., mRNA) and converted into cDNA that is labeled with barcodes (unique short nucleotide tags attached to each fragment for identification), segmented (sometimes barcodes are ligated after segmentation), and amplified by PCR to generate libraries for sequencing [35]. Each step is performed with appropriate quality control measures to assess RNA integrity and cDNA concentration.

Data Processing

For RNA-seq experiments, quality control reports are used to assess contamination and distribution of base pairs. A demultiplexing step is required when multiple samples/experiments are pooled before sequencing. The main purpose of the computational pipeline is to align the reads to the genome and map them to specific genes. Some processing pipelines also include trimming whereby extraneous sequences introduced during library preparation are removed. Prior to the analysis of bulk RNA-seq data, data cleaning steps are performed on the samples including low-count filtering, establishing a noise threshold, and checking for potential outliers. In scRNA-seq experiments, data cleaning is applied at the cellular level, when barcodes that are (1) unbound to a cell (empty droplets), (2) bound to >1 cell (doublets), or (3) bound to cells with large numbers of unmapped reads or high percentages of mitochondrial gene products that indicate a dying cell are removed. Ambient RNA (mRNA molecules that have leaked into the cell suspension by stressed or dying cells) may also be a confounding variable in single-cell analysis. Next, data normalization to account for gene length, sequencing depth, and differences in the global distribution of gene expression may be performed [35]. The most up-to-date human reference genome denoted GRCh38 is composed of DNA from anonymous volunteers. Each update from the multinational Genome Reference Consortium (GRC) corrects errors and adds sequence including alternate loci. The output is an expression count table that shows the number of reads that align to the reference genome.

Data Analysis

The analysis of bulk-tissue RNA and scRNA-seq data is similar; however, the analysis of scRNA-seq data is more complex. Bulk RNA-seq analysis may include running appropriate statistical tests to identify DEGs, clustering of genes by expression pattern, and testing for gene ontology (GO) enrichment [35, 36]. Single-cell RNA-seq analyses typically revolve around clustering and visualizing cellular gene expression in order to annotate them as particular cell types.

Integrating Data Between Studies

RNA-seq data across studies can be integrated, but batch effects are the major issue to overcome. Thus, at this juncture, rather than merging datasets, it may be advantageous to compare results between them. For example, researchers could compare an experimental dataset to a cell atlas dataset in order to determine cell types, but this is an ongoing area of active research. Undoubtedly, computational strategies will continue to be developed to enable data from independent experiments to be more readily merged and analyzed.

A recent example of data integration is the paper by Lofgren and Hinchcliff et al., where skin gene expression data from seven DNA microarray datasets collected at six medical centers (515 biopsies) all previously analyzed independently were integrated, and a random-effects inverse variance model was used to identify a 415-gene SSc skin signature (Fig. 6.1a) that distinguished SSc patients from healthy control participants. An SSc Skin Severity Score (4S) for each biopsy was then defined as the difference between a mean of over-expressed genes and the mean of the under-expressed genes within the 415-gene signature [37]. There was a strong correlation between the 4S and the mRSS. More importantly, the change in the 4S in the first 12 months was significantly correlated with the change in mRSS between 12- and 24-months, suggesting 4S may have prognostic significance although additional validation is required. Another example is the paper by Franks et al. where a method for predicting the SSc intrinsic subset (fibroproliferative, inflammatory, limited, or normal-like) on a per-sample basis was developed in three skin gene expression datasets and externally validated in an additional three datasets [23, 27]. Identification of associated molecular pathways associated with each subset provides clues into pathogenesis and therapy.

Franks et al. performed an integrative analysis to permit the identification of the SSc intrinsic subset (fibroproliferative, inflammatory, limited, or normal-like) on a per patient basis [27]. The data integration was simplified because five of the six skin gene expression datasets were generated in one laboratory using an Agilent platform whereas only one dataset utilized an Illumina platform.

An integrative analysis of 955 patients with seven systemic autoimmune diseases including 200 SSc patients has been recently published using whole blood transcriptome and methylome data. It showed that a multidimensional analysis of patients with systemic autoimmune diseases can provide valuable results. Three stable clusters could be identified with specific molecular patterns. These patterns seemed stable overtime although the time points were limited (0, 6, and 14 months) with a significantly lower number of patients [38].

Pinal-Fernandez et al. performed bulk-tissue RNA-seq on 199 myositis patients and developed a support vector machine learning algorithm with >90% accuracy to classify muscle biopsies from patients with various forms of myositis [39]. Similarly, Hoffmann-Vold et al. demonstrated similar levels of PDGF, FGF, VEGF, and M-CSF in explanted lung tissue from 130 lung transplant recipients with various forms of ILD using wedge biopsies from 200 donor lungs as a control. The authors suggest that nintedanib (a tyrosine kinase receptor antagonist) may, therefore, be a useful ILD treatment regardless of the underlying cause [40].

Integrating Multiple Omic Datasets

As new methods are developed to quantify SSc heterogeneity (e.g., tissue transcriptomics, quantitative histology, echophenomics, and radiomics) and the cost for performing "omic" analyses (e.g., genome-wide association studies, DNA microarray, bulk tissue RNA-seq and scRNA-seq, proteomics, etc.) lessens, an increasing number of patients will have multi-omic profiles in need of integration in order to permit deep phenotyping [4]. These multidimensional datasets present a challenge for the number of variables vastly outnumbers the number of patients. To address this issue, new bioinformatics approaches will need to be developed, and clinicians will need to learn more about artificial intelligence, an ever-expanding scientific field.

Toward an Integrated and Comprehensive Classification

Beginning with the SSc classification based upon the mRSS [7], each subsequent proposed classification has made use of larger quantities of data [41]. Together with skin disease, serum autoantibodies are the best-studied biomarker in SSc, and their assessment has become the standard of clinical care [42]. Because of the systemic nature of SSc and the wide availability of diagnostic and screening tests (pulmonary function tests, echocardiograms, and chest HRCT), there is a wealth of data in addition to patient factors (e.g., demographic data and physical exam findings) and clinical laboratory assays (e.g., serum autoantibodies and erythrocyte sedimentation rate) that can be used to subset patients into potentially meaningful groups. In fact, the recent paper by Sobanski et al. demonstrated how unbiased machine learning approaches (clustering and the Jaccard Index) applied to clinical phenomic data that included PFT and radiographic data, laboratory results, as well as physical exam findings from 6927 SSc patients, was used to identify two novel patient groups [9]. One stable cluster (n = 3149; 46%) was primarily composed of patients with limited cutaneous SSc (81%), and most patients (>2/3) lacked severe organ damage (e.g., digital ulcers, intestinal symptoms, or muscle, joint, cardiac, or lung involvement) and had a lower risk of death. Moreover, 54% of patients manifested anticentromere antibodies while 21% had antibodies against anti-topoisomerase I. Patients in the second stable cluster (n = 3778; 55%) developed SSc at a younger age, 61% of the patients had diffuse cutaneous SSc, and most presented with digital ulcers, joint contractures, intestinal involvement, and ILD, as well as a higher risk of death compared to cluster 1 patients (HR 2.47 [95% CI 1.86–3.27]). These data suggest, not unsurprisingly, that patients with worse skin fibrosis and organ disease have worse outcomes than those with mild skin and less organ involvement. Importantly, they also demonstrate the feasibility and potential relevance of clinical phenomics.

With the age of "omics" upon us, we have an unprecedented opportunity to combine high-dimensional data with clinically assessed low-dimensional data for the purpose of improving prediction models and deepening our understanding of disease pathogenesis and heterogeneity. The ultimate goal is to be able to predict disease susceptibility and introduce preventive measures to avoid or reverse disease onset. Short of that, the ability to select the most effective drug with the least toxicity for an individual would be advantageous. The prerequisites for this new age of medicine will require large-scale investment from governments and private industry to pay for the generation and maintenance of high-dimensional datasets and associated health information including environmental exposure, medication and supplement utilization, physical activity data, etc. Publicly accessible data depots with deidentified yet detailed participant level data are required so that data scientists can mine the information in search of novel insights. Examples of potential areas of discovery include the identification of new risk factors, novel disease classification, repurposing of existing drugs, and deeper insights into disease pathogenesis. Until the age when disease development can be predicted based on an individual's DNA and environment, the medical research community will rely on accessible tools and select the most appropriate drug for an individual patient based on the genetic profile.

Acknowledgment The authors thank Ms. Shannon Teaw, BS for generating the figures.

References

1. Denton CP, Khanna D. Systemic sclerosis. Lancet (London, England). 2017;390(10103):1685–99.
2. Pope JE. The future of treatment in systemic sclerosis: can we design better trials? Lancet Rheumatol. 2020;2(3):e185–e94.

3. Sobanski V, Lescoat A, Launay D. Novel classifications for systemic sclerosis: challenging historical subsets to unlock new doors. Curr Opin Rheumatol. 2020;32(6):463–71.
4. Hinchcliff M, Mahoney JM. Towards a new classification of systemic sclerosis. Nat Rev Rheumatol. 2019;15(8):456–7.
5. Preliminary criteria for the classification of systemic sclerosis (scleroderma). Arthritis Rheumatol. 1980;23(5):581–90.
6. van den Hoogen F, Khanna D, Fransen J, Johnson SR, Baron M, Tyndall A, et al. 2013 classification criteria for systemic sclerosis: an American College of Rheumatology/European League against Rheumatism collaborative initiative. Arthritis Rheum. 2013;65(11):2737–47.
7. LeRoy EC, Black C, Fleischmajer R, Jablonska S, Krieg T, Medsger TA Jr, et al. Scleroderma (systemic sclerosis): classification, subsets and pathogenesis. J Rheumatol. 1988;15(2):202–5.
8. LeRoy EC, Medsger TA Jr. Criteria for the classification of early systemic sclerosis. J Rheumatol. 2001;28(7):1573–6.
9. Sobanski V, Giovannelli J, Allanore Y, Riemekasten G, Airo P, Vettori S, et al. Phenotypes determined by cluster analysis and their survival in the prospective European scleroderma trials and research cohort of patients with systemic sclerosis. Arthritis Rheumatol. 2019;71(9):1553–70.
10. Frantz C, Huscher D, Avouac J, Hachulla E, Balbir-Gurman A, Riemekasten G, et al. Outcomes of limited cutaneous systemic sclerosis patients: results on more than 12,000 patients from the EUSTAR database. Autoimmun Rev. 2020;19(2):102452.
11. Steen VD. Autoantibodies in systemic sclerosis. Semin Arthritis Rheum. 2005;35(1):35–42.
12. Nihtyanova SI, Schreiber BE, Ong VH, Rosenberg D, Moinzadeh P, Coghlan JG, et al. Prediction of pulmonary complications and long-term survival in systemic sclerosis. Arthritis Rheumatol. 2014;66(6):1625–35.
13. Kranenburg P, van den Hombergh WMT, Knaapen-Hans HKA, van den Hoogen FHJ, Fransen J, Vonk MC. Survival and organ involvement in patients with limited cutaneous systemic sclerosis and anti-topoisomerase-I antibodies: determined by skin subtype or auto-antibody subtype? A long-term follow-up study. Rheumatology. 2016;55(11):2001–8.
14. Srivastava N, Hudson M, Tatibouet S, Wang M, Baron M, Fritzler MJ, et al., editors. Thinking outside the box—the associations with cutaneous involvement and autoantibody status in systemic sclerosis are not always what we expect. Seminars in arthritis and rheumatism. Elsevier; 2015.
15. Patterson KA, Roberts-Thomson PJ, Lester S, Tan JA, Hakendorf P, Rischmueller M, et al. Interpretation of an extended autoantibody profile in a well-characterized Australian systemic sclerosis (scleroderma) cohort using principal components analysis. Arthritis Rheumatol. 2015;67(12):3234–44.
16. Nihtyanova SI, Sari A, Harvey JC, Leslie A, Derrett-Smith EC, Fonseca C, et al. Using autoantibodies and cutaneous subset to develop outcome-based disease classification in systemic sclerosis. Arthritis Rheumatol. 2020;72(3):465–76.
17. Moinzadeh P, Aberer E, Ahmadi-Simab K, Blank N, Distler JH, Fierlbeck G, et al. Disease progression in systemic sclerosis-overlap syndrome is significantly different from limited and diffuse cutaneous systemic sclerosis. Ann Rheum Dis. 2015;74(4):730–7.
18. Moinzadeh P, Frommolt P, Franitza M, Toliat MR, Becker K, Nürnberg P, et al. Whole blood gene expression profiling distinguishes systemic sclerosis-overlap syndromes from other subsets. J Eur Acad Dermatol Venereol. 2020;34(5):e236–e8.
19. Ledoult E, Launay D, Behal H, Mouthon L, Pugnet G, Lega JC, et al. Early trajectories of skin thickening are associated with severity and mortality in systemic sclerosis. Arthritis Res Ther. 2020;22(1):30.
20. Le Gouellec N, Duhamel A, Perez T, Hachulla AL, Sobanski V, Faivre JB, et al. Predictors of lung function test severity and outcome in systemic sclerosis-associated interstitial lung disease. PLoS One. 2017;12(8):e0181692.
21. Forestier A, Le Gouellec N, Behal H, Kramer GBG, Perez T, Sobanski V, et al. Evolution of high-resolution CT-scan in systemic sclerosis-associated interstitial lung disease: description and prognosis factors. Semin Arthritis Rheum. 2020;50:1406.
22. Murgia F, Svegliati S, Poddighe S, Lussu M, Manzin A, Spadoni T, et al. Metabolomic profile of systemic sclerosis patients. Sci Rep. 2018;8(1):7626.
23. Milano A, Pendergrass SA, Sargent JL, George LK, McCalmont TH, Connolly MK, et al. Molecular subsets in the gene expression signatures of scleroderma skin. PLoS One. 2008;3(7):e2696.
24. Assassi S, Swindell WR, Wu M, Tan FD, Khanna D, Furst DE, et al. Dissecting the heterogeneity of skin gene expression patterns in systemic sclerosis. Arthritis Rheumatol. 2015;67(11):3016–26.
25. Khanna D, Spino C, Johnson S, Chung L, Whitfield ML, Denton CP, et al. Abatacept in early diffuse cutaneous systemic sclerosis: results of a phase II investigator-initiated, multicenter, double-blind, randomized, placebo-controlled trial. Arthritis Rheumatol. 2020;72(1):125–36.
26. Chakravarty EF, Martyanov V, Fiorentino D, Wood TA, Haddon DJ, Jarrell JA, et al. Gene expression changes reflect clinical response in a placebo-controlled randomized trial of abatacept in patients with diffuse cutaneous systemic sclerosis. Arthritis Res Ther. 2015;17:159.
27. Franks JM, Martyanov V, Cai G, Wang Y, Li Z, Wood TA, et al. A machine learning classifier for assigning individual patients with systemic sclerosis to intrinsic molecular subsets. Arthritis. Rheumatol. 2019;71:1701.
28. Chandrasekaran A, Fu Z, Kraniski R, Wilson F, Cheng M, Wang A, et al. Computer vision applied to dual energy computed tomography images for precise calcinosis cutis quantification in patients with systemic sclerosis. Arthritis Res Ther. 2020; under revision.
29. Goldin JG, Kim GHJ, Tseng CH, Volkmann E, Furst D, Clements P, et al. Longitudinal changes in quantitative interstitial lung disease on computed tomography after immunosuppression in the scleroderma lung study II. Ann Am Thorac Soc. 2018;15(11):1286–95.
30. Yin N, Shen C, Dong F, Wang J, Guo Y, Bai L. Computer-aided identification of interstitial lung disease based on computed tomography. J Xray Sci Technol. 2019;27(4):591–603.
31. Chassagnon G, Vakalopoulou M, Régent A, Zacharaki EI, Aviram G, Martin C, et al. Deep learning–based approach for automated assessment of interstitial lung disease in systemic sclerosis on CT images. Radiol Artif Intell. 2020;2(4):e190006.
32. Ather S, Kadir T, Gleeson F. Artificial intelligence and radiomics in pulmonary nodule management: current status and future applications. Clin Radiol. 2020;75(1):13–9.
33. Schniering J, Maciukiewicz M, Gabrys HS, Brunner M, Blüthgen C, Meier C, et al. Computed tomography-based radiomics decodes prognostic and molecular differences in interstitial lung disease related to systemic sclerosis. Eur Respir J. 2021;59:2004503.
34. Longo DL, Drazen JM. Data Sharing. N Engl J Med. 2016;374(3):276–7.
35. Koch CM, Chiu SF, Akbarpour M, Bharat A, Ridge KM, Bartom ET, et al. A beginner's guide to analysis of RNA sequencing data. Am J Respir Cell Mol Biol. 2018;59(2):145–57.
36. Andrews TS, Kiselev VY, McCarthy D, Hemberg M. Tutorial: guidelines for the computational analysis of single-cell RNA sequencing data. Nat Protoc. 2021;16(1):1–9.
37. Lofgren S, Hinchcliff M, Carns M, Wood T, Aren K, Arroyo E, et al. Integrated, multicohort analysis of systemic sclerosis identifies robust transcriptional signature of disease severity. JCI insight. 2016;1(21):e89073.
38. Barturen G, Babaei S, Català-Moll F, Martínez-Bueno M, Makowska Z, Martorell-Marugán J, et al. Integrative analysis

reveals a molecular stratification of systemic autoimmune diseases. Arthritis Rheumatol. 2021;73(6):1073–85.
39. Pinal-Fernandez I, Casal-Dominguez M, Derfoul A, Pak K, Miller FW, Milisenda JC, et al. Machine learning algorithms reveal unique gene expression profiles in muscle biopsies from patients with different types of myositis. Ann Rheum Dis. 2020;79(9):1234–42.
40. Hoffmann-Vold AM, Weigt SS, Saggar R, Palchevskiy V, Volkmann ER, Liang LL, et al. Endotype-phenotyping may predict a treatment response in progressive fibrosing interstitial lung disease. EBioMedicine. 2019;50:379–86.
41. Hinchcliff M, Mahoney J. High-throughput quantitative histology in systemic sclerosis skin disease using computer vision. Nature reviews. Rheumatology. 2019;
42. Domsic RT, Medsger TA. Autoantibodies and their role in scleroderma clinical care. Curr Treatm Opt Rheumatol 2016;2(3):239–51. https://doi.org/10.1007/s40674-016-0050-y.

The Clinical Aspects of Autoantibodies

7

Masataka Kuwana and Jeska de Vries-Bouwstra

Introduction

Systemic sclerosis (SSc) is a systemic autoimmune disease characterized by microvascular abnormalities and excessive fibrosis of the skin and internal organs. One of the distinctive autoimmune features of SSc is the presence of circulating autoantibodies reactive with various cellular components, including nuclear antigens. In this case, they are termed antinuclear antibodies (ANAs). It has been shown that distinct autoantibody specificities are detected in SSc patients and are associated with unique disease manifestations. Since clinical presentation in SSc patients is highly heterogeneous, disease subgrouping and prediction of future organ involvement and prognosis are extremely important in the clinical setting. Therefore, autoantibodies are attractive biomarkers in routine rheumatology practice, owing to their high disease specificity, mutual exclusivity, persistence for the duration of illness, and, most importantly, strong associations with characteristic constellations of clinical features [1–3]. In addition, a new group of autoantibodies reactive with functional proteins, such as cell surface receptors and extracellular matrix (ECM) proteins, have been identified in SSc patients. This chapter covers the spectrum of autoantibody specificities reported in SSc patients, their detection methods, and their clinical utility.

M. Kuwana (✉)
Department of Allergy and Rheumatology, Nippon Medical School Graduate School of Medicine, Tokyo, Japan
e-mail: kuwanam@nms.ac.jp

J. de Vries-Bouwstra
Department of Rheumatology, Leiden University Medical Center, Leiden, The Netherlands
e-mail: J.K.de_Vries-Bouwstra@lumc.nl

SSc-Specific and SSc-Related Autoantibodies

ANAs detected by the indirect immunofluorescence (IIF) technique are a hallmark of SSc and are found in >95% of the patients. The majority of nuclear and cytoplasmic autoantigens specifically recognized by SSc sera have been already identified. As of this writing, at least 12 ANA specificities associated with SSc have been reported and well characterized, and >80% of SSc patients have one of these autoantibodies. Two classic autoantibodies discovered in the late 1970s are anti-Scl-70 or anti-topoisomerase I (topo I) antibody and anticentromere antibody (ACA). Another group of antibodies, including anti-U1 ribonucleoprotein (RNP), anti-Ku, and anti-PM-Scl antibodies, were first identified using the double immunodiffusion (DID) technique. The remaining ANA specificities, such as anti-RNA polymerase (RNAP) III, anti-U3 RNP, and anti-Th/To, were discovered using immunoprecipitation (IP) assays. SSc-specific autoantibodies target various nuclear or cytoplasmic components involved in essential cellular processes, such as cell division and transcription (Table 7.1). These autoantibodies are rarely seen in patients with other connective tissue diseases without SSc features and thus are important diagnostic markers. The detection of SSc-specific autoantibodies is clinically useful in classifying SSc patients into subtypes that are almost exclusively associated with characteristic clinical phenotypes (Table 7.2). SSc-specific autoantibodies are usually present at the onset of SSc symptoms, and patients do not switch from one antibody to another during the course of the disease. On the other hand, there is another group of autoantibodies, including anti-Ro52/tripartite motif-containing protein 21 (TRIM21) antibodies, which are detected not only in SSc patients but also in patients with various connective tissue diseases other than SSc. These SSc-related autoantibodies are useless for diagnostic pur-

Y. Allanore et al. (eds.), *Scleroderma*, https://doi.org/10.1007/978-3-031-40658-4_7

Table 7.1 Structure and function of molecules targeted by SSc-specific autoantibodies

Autoantibody specificity	Antigenic structure	Cellular localization	Main cellular function
Anticentromere (ACA)	Kinetochore complex containing CENP-A, CENP-B, and CENP-C	Chromatin	Separation of chromosome
Anti-topo I (Scl-70)	DNA topoisomerase I	Chromatin	Relaxation of supercoiled DNA
Anti-RNAP III	Multi-subunit components of RNA polymerase III, including RPC155	Nucleoplasm	Transcription of small nuclear RNAs
Anti-U3 RNP	U3 RNA and related components, including fibrillarin	Nucleoli	Processing of pre-ribosomal RNAs
Anti-Th/To	RNase P/RNase MRP	Nucleoli	Processing of transfer RNAs and other small RNAs
Anti-U11/U12 RNP	U11/U12 RNA and related components, including RNAC-3	Nucleoplasm	Regulation of mRNA splicing
Anticentriole	Centrosome	Cytoplasm	Cell division
Anti-eIF2B	Multi-subunit protein consisting of 5 subunits	Cytoplasm	Initiation of protein synthesis
Anti-PM-Scl	Exosome complex containing PM-Scl-100 and PM-Scl-75	Nucleoli	Processing and degradation of RNAs
Anti-Ku	Ku80 and Ku70	Nucleoplasm	DNA repair
Anti-RuvBL1/2	Double hexamer consisting of RuvBL1 and RuvBL2	Nucleoplasm	DNA repair and chromatin remodeling
Anti-U1 RNP	U1 RNA and related components including 70 K, A, and C proteins	Nucleoplasm	mRNA splicing

Table 7.2 Methods for detection and clinical associations with SSc-specific autoantibodies

Autoantibody specificity	Staining pattern on IF (ANA test)	Assay for detection	Disease subset	Clinical phenotype
Anticentromere (ACA)	Discrete speckled	IIF, IA, LB	lcSSc	PAH; severe peripheral vascular disease
Anti-topo I	Speckled (with or without nucleolar)	DID, IP, IA, LB	dcSSc	ILD; severe peripheral vascular disease
Anti-RNA polymerase III	Speckled (with or without nucleolar)	IP, IA, LB	dcSSc	Rapid progression of skin thickening; SRC; malignancy
Anti-U3 RNP	Clumpy nucleolar	IP, IA, LB	dcSSc/lcSSc	ILD, PAH, SRC, GI
Anti-Th/To	Homogeneous nucleolar	IP, LB	lcSSc	ILD, PAH
Anti-U11/U12 RNP	Speckled	IP	dcSSc/lcSSc	ILD
Anticentriole	Centriole	IIF	lcSSc	PAH
Anti-eIF2B	Fine cytoplasmic	IP	dcSSc	ILD
Anti-PM-Scl	Homogeneous nucleolar	DID, IP, IA, LB	lcSSc (myositis overlap)	Myositis (DM rash)
Anti-Ku	Speckled	DID, IP, LB	lcSSc (myositis overlap)	Myositis
Anti-RuvBL1/2	Speckled	IP	dcSSc (myositis overlap)	Myositis
Anti-U1 RNP	Course speckled	DID, IP, IA, LB	lcSSc ("MCTD")	Inflammatory arthritis, myositis, PAH

DID double immunodiffusion, *IA* immunoassay, *IIF* indirect immunofluorescence, *IP* immunoprecipitation, *LB* line-blot assay, *MCTD* mixed connective tissue disease, *PAH* pulmonary arterial hypertension, *ILD* interstitial lung disease, *SRC* scleroderma renal crisis, *GI* gastrointestinal tract involvement, and *DM* dermatomyositis

poses but are indeed useful in disease subsetting. SSc-specific autoantibodies and SSc-related autoantibodies typically remain detectable throughout the course of the disease, regardless of whether patients receive treatment or not. Patients rarely have two or more SSc-specific autoantibodies together, indicating mutual exclusiveness. SSc-related autoantibodies often coexist with SSc-specific autoantibodies.

SSc-Specific Autoantibodies

ACA

Moroi and colleagues were the first investigators to describe the presence of ACA originally associated with the CREST (calcinosis, Raynaud's phenomenon, esophageal dysmotility, sclerodactyly, and telangiectasia) variant of SSc [4]. The frequency of ACA in SSc patients has been reported to be 20–30% in many ethnic groups. ACA produces discrete speckled staining on IIF. The recognition of kinetochore proteins located at the centromeric regions of individual metaphase chromosomes is highly specific to ACA. ACA is sometimes detected in patients with primary Sjögren's syndrome or primary biliary cholangitis as well as in individuals without an apparent connective tissue disease, who are almost always elderly [5]. The natural history of ACA-positive SSc patients includes long-standing Raynaud's phenomenon followed by the appearance of puffy fingers after a variable period of time (months to 10 or more years). The presence of ACA in patients with Raynaud's phenomenon and/or nailfold capillary abnormalities is predictive of future development of SSc [6] and is now recognized as a very early diagnosis of SSc (VEDOSS) [7]. Patients with ACA are almost always classified as having limited cutaneous SSc (lcSSc) [8, 9], a term that has now replaced CREST. Severe interstitial lung disease (ILD), cardiomyopathy, or scleroderma renal crisis (SRC) are rare in ACA-positive patients, but some develop pulmonary arterial hypertension (PAH) later in the course of the disease. Recent cohort studies confirm a low incidence of major organ complications in ACA-positive patients, indicating that ACA-positivity carries a good prognosis [10].

Anti-Scl-70/Topo I Antibody

The Scl-70 antigen was originally isolated from rat liver extracts as a basic nonhistone chromosome protein [11], which was later identified as an enzyme that catalyzes the relaxation of supercoiled double-stranded DNA, termed topo I [12]. Anti-topo I antibody is detected in 20–30% of SSc patients in many ethnic groups. Approximately two-thirds of anti-topo I-positive patients have diffuse cutaneous SSc (dcSSc), but the progression of skin thickening is slower than in those with anti-RNAP III antibodies [13, 14]. Anti-topo I antibody is associated with a high risk for severe ILD, cardiomyopathy, and peripheral vascular complications, such as digital ulcers (DU) and gangrene, particularly early in the disease course [8, 9, 15]. Anti-topo I antibody is considered to be a marker for poor prognosis, and patients with severe ILD die of this complication at an average of 10 years after onset of SSc. The prevalence of ILD is comparable between dcSSc and lcSSc patients with anti-topo I, but survivals are worse in dcSSc than in lcSSc patients [10, 16]. Few studies have studied the anti-topo I antibody responses more thoroughly by evaluating anti-topo I antibody isotypes and titers over time. In SSc patients with anti-topo I, the concomitant presence of IgM isotype of anti-topo I antibodies is associated with subsequent disease progression [17].

Anti-RNAP III Antibody

SSc sera contain autoantibodies directed to the three forms of RNAPs: RNAP I, II, and III [18]. Anti-RNAP antibodies detected in SSc patients fall into four groups: those reactive with RNAP I, II, and III; those with RNAP I and III; those with RNAP III alone; and those with RNAP II alone [19]. Since antibodies to RNAP II alone are often found in association with anti-topo I antibodies in SSc patients and are also detected in patients without SSc [20], they are considered SSc-related autoantibodies. Instead, antibodies reactive with RNAP III, which are recognized by the remaining three specificity groups, are most often regarded as SSc-specific autoantibodies. Sera positive for anti-RNAP III antibody produces a speckled staining pattern on IIF but also produces nucleolar staining if anti-RNAP I antibody coexists. Anti-RNAP III is mutually exclusive to anti-topo I and ACA and is highly specific to SSc. The frequency of anti-RNAP III antibodies in SSc patients varies among ethnic groups. There is a higher frequency in North American Caucasian (24%) [21], Australian (15%) [22], and UK patients (11%) [10] in comparison with French, Dutch, or Japanese patients (<5%) [23–25]. Nearly all patients with this antibody have dcSSc with rapidly progressive skin thickening. In dcSSc patients with anti-RNAP III, modified Rodnan total skin thickness score (mRSS) was the highest and peaked earliest, compared with those without [26]. Patients with anti-RNAP III antibodies have the highest risk of developing SRC, but they seldom develop severe ILD [18, 21]. Skin thickening regresses over time even without treatment in many patients. In recent cohorts, survival in patients with anti-RNAP III is better than those with anti-topo I [10]. Long-term survival rates in patients with anti-RNAP III antibodies are comparable with those with ACA. Recently, it has been reported that there is an association with cancer among SSc patients with anti-RNAP III antibodies in a close temporal relationship to the onset of SSc, which suggests that SSc is a paraneoplastic phenomenon in this subset [27, 28].

Anti-U3 RNP Antibody

Anti-U3 RNP antibody produces clumpy nucleolar staining on IIF. Anti-U3 RNP antibody is found in 4–10% of patients with SSc and is most frequent in African Americans [29], followed by native North Americans [30]. Two-thirds of the patients have dcSSc, and noninflammatory skeletal myopathy is common. This autoantibody is associated with PAH, cardiomyopathy, SRC, and small bowel involvement with pseudo-obstruction and malabsorption [29, 30]. The prognosis in this subset is comparable to that in patients with anti-topo I antibodies. An unusual combination of SRC followed later by PAH is occasionally found in patients with dcSSc and anti-U3 RNP antibody [31].

Anti-Th/To Antibody

Anti-Th/To antibody occurs in patients with lcSSc, although its frequency overall in SSc patients is only 2–5%. Like ACA-positive patients, anti-Th/To-positive patients are predominantly Caucasians but tend to have a shorter duration of Raynaud's phenomenon before the onset of other symptoms such as puffy fingers. DU and digital gangrene are infrequent, but patients with anti-Th/To antibodies can have significant ILD or PAH, the latter often independent of ILD, which often occurs early in the disease course [32]. This increased frequency and severity of pulmonary complications result in decreased survival compared with lcSSc patients without this antibody.

Anti-U11/U12 RNP Antibody

Anti-U11/U12 RNP antibody is a rare antibody specificity found in 1–3% of patients with SSc [33]. This antibody recognizes RNA binding region containing 3 (RNPC-3) associated with U11/U12 RNA and produces speckled nuclear staining on IIF. Patients with this antibody are classified as having either dcSSc or lcSSc. A characteristic feature of patients with this antibody is a high frequency of ILD (~80%), which is often severe and progressive and associated with a 2.25-fold greater risk of death in comparison with anti-U11/U12 RNP-negative patients with ILD. A relationship between anti-U11/U12 RNP antibody and severe ILD has been replicated in an independent cohort, which has additionally found the association of this antibody with moderate-to-severe gastrointestinal (GI) involvement [34]. Recently, anti-U11/U12 RNP antibodies have been found in patients with cancer in a close temporal relationship to the onset of SSc [35].

Anticentriole Antibody

Anticentriole antibody is a rare autoantibody detected by IIF and shows a unique staining pattern: two distinct dots located at each of the spindle poles on mitotic cells [36]. A routine IIF gives a result of "a negative ANA" since the centriole is involved in the organization of the mitotic spindle in the cytoplasm. Anticentriole antibody is detected almost exclusively in patients with lcSSc or those with Raynaud's phenomenon alone [36]. A high prevalence of PAH is a unique feature of patients with anticentriole antibodies [37].

Anti-eIF2B Antibody

Autoantibody to eukaryotic initiation factor 2B (eIF2B) is a novel anti-cytoplasmic antibody identified by the IP assay in SSc sera negative for all known SSc-specific autoantibodies [38]. The prevalence was ~1% in the United Kingdom cohort [38] but 7% in the North American cohort [39]. The majority of patients with anti-eIF2B are classified as having dcSSc and ILD.

Anti-PM-Scl Antibody

Anti-PM-Scl antibody produces a homogenous nucleolar pattern and is rarely found in non-Caucasian patients [40]. Anti-PM-Scl-positive patients often present with subacute myositis but also have typical Raynaud's phenomenon and SSc skin changes, usually lcSSc [41]. They are most frequently diagnosed as having SSc-myositis overlap, but a significant proportion of the patients have rashes consistent with dermatomyositis. This antibody is found in more than 25% of SSc patients with myositis overlap but in only 2% of SSc patients overall. The anti-PM-Scl antibody is also associated with younger age at disease onset, calcinosis, ILD, cutaneous signs of dermatomyositis, and inflammatory arthritis, but the prevalence of ILD varies among studies probably due to the detection methods used [41, 42]. Serious internal organ involvement is rare, leading to a favorable prognosis. Myositis is usually mild and shows a good response to moderate-dose corticosteroids. In a recent large cross-sectional study of patients with idiopathic inflammatory myopathies, 9% had anti-PM-Scl antibodies in the absence of any SSc skin changes [43].

Anti-Ku Antibody

The prevalence of anti-Ku antibody in SSc patients is ~2% and is primarily detected in patients with SSc in overlap [44]. The majority of patients have typical Raynaud's phenomenon and SSc skin changes, usually lcSSc. Concomitant myositis is common, but some have additional features of lupus. Anti-Ku antibody is rarely detected in patients with systemic lupus erythematosus (SLE) or PM/DM without SSc features, but additional lupus-associated autoantibodies such as anti-DNA are always positive in the patients with SLE alone [45]. Disease onset is usually younger than age 50. Internal organ involvement is infrequent and usually mild if present, but arthritis is common. Anti-Ku antibody is associated with fewer vascular manifestations such as DU or telangiectasia [46]. An international cohort of 2140 SSc patients has shown associations of anti-Ku antibodies with myositis and ILD [47]. Myositis is usually mild and shows a good response to moderate-dose corticosteroids, leading to a favorable prognosis.

Anti-RuvBL1/2 Antibody

Anti-RuvBL1/2 antibody is a rare antibody specificity detected in 1–2% of patients with SSc and produces speckled nuclear staining with a high antibody titer on IIF [48]. Patients with this antibody are mostly males and have a unique combination of clinical features, including diffuse cutaneous involvement and myositis overlap. Internal organ involvement is mild in general, but some develop significant myocardial dysfunction.

Anti-U1 RNP Antibody

Anti-U1 RNP antibody, which produces a course-speckled pattern with a high antibody titer, is primarily detected in patients with SSc in the overlap. This antibody is preferentially found in African Americans and Orientals. Anti-U1 RNP antibody was first described as a serological marker for mixed connective tissue disease (MCTD) [49] but is also found in sera from patients with SSc, SLE, polymyositis/dermatomyositis, or Sjögren's syndrome alone. Disease onset is at a relatively young age. SSc patients with this antibody usually present with inflammatory symptoms, such as myositis and arthritis. Raynaud's phenomenon and puffy fingers occur early in the disease, but later, these patients develop typical manifestations of SSc. Most of them have lcSSc, although approximately 20% develop dcSSc. Serious complications are relatively uncommon, but pulmonary complications, including PAH and ILD, are sometimes life-threatening [50]. The prognosis is favorable, but PAH is the most common cause of death.

SSc-Related Autoantibodies

Anti-nucleolar antibodies, such as anti-nucleolar organizing region 90 (NOR-90) and anti-B23 antibodies, are SSc-related ANAs. Anti-NOR-90 antibody was first reported in patients with malignancy but later in individuals with connective tissue diseases, including SSc, Sjögren's syndrome, and rheumatoid arthritis [51]. Nearly, all SSc patients with this antibody have lcSSc, but detailed clinical characteristics have not been assessed [52]. Anti-B23 antibody is found not only in patients with malignancy but also occurs in ~11% of sera from SSc patients [53]. Anti-B23 reactivity is associated with PAH and often coexists with anti-U3 RNP or anti-U1 RNP antibodies. Anti-SSA/Ro and anti-SSB/La can occur in SSc patients but are usually associated with concomitant Sjögren's syndrome. The SSA/Ro autoantigen has two isoforms, Ro60 and Ro52/TRIM52. The latter is targeted independent of anti-SSA/Ro antibodies by sera from patients with various connective tissue diseases. A recent multicenter cohort study from the Canadian Scleroderma Research Group (CSRG) involving 963 patients with SSc has found that anti-Ro52/TRIM21 antibodies are present in 20% of SSc patients and coexist with other SSc-specific autoantibodies, including ACA, anti-topo I, anti-RNAP III, and anti-PM-Scl antibodies [54]. The presence of anti-Ro52/TRIM21 antibodies is associated with ILD and an increased risk of death [55]. Antibodies to interferon-inducible genes designated HIN-200, which encode evolutionarily related nuclear phosphoproteins (IFI16), are also detected in 30% of SSc patients in conjunction with anti-topo I or ACA [56]. Anti-IFI16 is found in patients with various connective tissue diseases, including SLE and Sjögren's syndrome, but is associated with digital gangrene in SSc patients, especially in those with ACA [57]. Autoantibodies to bicaudal D homolog 2 (BICD2), an intracellular protein involved in dynein and microtubule processes, are found in 26% of SSc patients, but the majority had concomitant SSc-specific ANAs, such as ACA and anti-U1 RNP [58]. Autoantibodies to cytoplasmic mitochondrial proteins are found in patients with SSc in conjunction with ACA and are associated with concomitant primary biliary cholangitis [59]. Recently, autoantibodies targeting telomerase and the shelterin proteins have been reported in SSc patients with severe ILD and short lymphocyte telomere length [60]. These autoantibodies are specific to SSc and idiopathic pulmonary fibrosis (IPF) and often coexist with anti-U1 RNP and anti-Ku.

ANA-Negative SSc

There is a small proportion of SSc patients who are negative for ANA by IIF. In a recent cohort study involving 3249 patients with SSc from a multicenter registry in North America, 6.4% were negative for ANA at a serum dilution of 1:80 [61]. ANA-negative SSc patients constitute a distinct subset with a greater proportion of males, less vasculopathy (PAH, DU, and telangiectasia), and more frequent lower GI involvement.

Screening of SSc-Specific Autoantibodies

A conventional screening method for ANA detection is IIF on cultured HEp-2 cell slides. This technique is recommended as the first ANA screening test because it is highly sensitive and provides additional information on the antibody titer and staining pattern. Speckled staining is often detected in patients with dcSSc and suggests the presence of anti-topo I in the case of a high titer (≥1:320) or anti-RNAP III in the case of a low titer (<1:160). Anti-U1 RNP and anti-RuvBL1/2 antibodies, which are associated with SSc in overlap, also produce a high-titer speckled pattern, while titers of anti-U11/U12 RNP antibodies vary among the positive sera. A nucleolar pattern is fairly specific to SSc, and the three major SSc-related anti-nucleolar antibodies are anti-U3 RNP, anti-Th/To, and anti-PM-Scl antibodies. Anti-RNAP III antibody also produces a nucleolar pattern when anti-RNAP I antibody coexists, but a concomitant speckled pattern is always present. A discrete speckled pattern is often detected in patients with lcSSc and suggests the presence of ACA, which recognizes a pair of dots located at the centromeric lesion of individual metaphase chromosomes (also called "centromere" pattern).

Solid-phase ANA assays have been commercially available since the early 1990s and might be viable alternatives to ANA detection on HEp-2 cells. This method has considerable potential, but it is of note that many SSc-specific ANAs, including anti-RNAP III and anti-nucleolar antibodies, are not identified by these assays and thus are reported as "a negative ANA." This is because the sensitivity ultimately depends on the choice of autoantigens used. In fact, one retrospective study of 238 SSc patients, which compared ANA by IIF with the multiplex bead assay from two commercial laboratories, concluded that the bead testing failed to identify 50% of the SSc patients, particularly those with anti-RNAP III or anti-nucleolar staining on IIF [62]. Therefore, it is our strong recommendation to use the conventional IIF for screening SSc-specific autoantibodies.

Methods for Detection of Individual SSc-Specific Autoantibodies

Identification of individual SSc-specific autoantibodies requires additional techniques, such as the DID, IP assay, and specific immunoassays including enzyme-linked immunosorbent assay (ELISA), chemiluminescence immunoassay (CIA), and fluorescence enzyme immunoassay (FEIA) (Table 7.2). The DID technique (Ouchterlony or counter-immune electrophoresis) has been used for more than 50 years and is still used in some clinical laboratories because it is inexpensive and specific. Immunoblots either in-house or commercially available may provide advantages in determining the detailed specificity of autoantigen recognition, e.g., the antigen recognition profile within a complex autoantigen. The multianalyte kine-blot (LB) assay is commercially available for simultaneous detection of a series of SSc-specific/related autoantibodies [63]. The IP assay of either protein or RNA components is a valuable detection method that is able to detect all SSc-specific ANAs except ACA and anticentriole antibodies. However, these conventional techniques are of limited use in routine clinical practice because they are labor-intensive, time-consuming, and limited in throughput.

The immunoassays have several advantages over other traditional techniques in terms of simplicity, reproducibility, speed, and ability to handle many samples at the same time. In addition, they provide semiquantitative results, and thus, there is the potential for more closer investigation of how autoantibody levels relate to disease activity and severity. The majority of commercially available immunoassays utilize recombinant autoantigens, which are expressed in the bacterial or eukaryotic system, while some assays still use native proteins purified from cellular extracts. However, the immunoassay requires the availability of highly purified autoantigens that contain the major epitopes recognized by virtually all sera positive for given SSc-specific autoantibodies. This is a critical limitation for developing immunoassays. For example, it is easy to prepare topo I as an antigenic source for immunoassays because the autoimmune target is a single molecule. However, the majority of autoantigens recognized by SSc-specific autoantibodies are multiprotein complexes consisting of many constituents and, in some cases, small RNAs. In this case, it is necessary to determine the antigenic subunit that is most commonly recognized by autoantibodies. For example, RNAP III exists as a multiprotein complex consisting of >12 subunits, requiring identification of the antigenic subunit recognized by all anti-RNAP III-positive sera. A series of experiments using individual subunits successfully identified the largest subunit RPC155 as the antigenic subunit, facilitating the development of a sensitive immunoassay [64]. Multiplex technologies, such as multibead arrays in combination with flow cytometry techniques, have been developed and used for the detection of multiple SSc-specific autoantibodies at the same time [65]. The multianalyte LB assay is becoming popular in some geographic areas because this system is able to screen <20 specificities at the same time. However, the LB assay sometimes gives false-positive and false-negative results [66, 67], probably because the denatured single antigens are used for detection.

Autoantibodies to Functional Molecules

There has been considerable interest in autoantibodies directed to cell surfaces or ECM proteins in SSc patients. However, the reproducibility of the published data is poor, probably because of the difficulty in reproducing antigenicity of the autoantigens with highly complicated conformation in the assays. This results in a lack of reliable commercial assay kits for the detection of these autoantibodies. Nevertheless, these autoantibodies are potentially relevant to the pathophysiology of SSc by modulating disease-related pathways, including those mediated by platelet-derived growth factor receptor [68], muscarinic-3 receptor [69, 70], angiotensin II type 1 receptor (AT1R), and endothelin-1 type A receptor (ETAR) [71]. There is a potential correlation between anti-muscarinic-3 receptor antibodies and severe GI involvement through inhibition of cholinergic neurotransmission [70]. Anti-AT1R and anti-ETAR antibodies have been associated with vascular complications, such as PAH and DU, but this observation needs to be confirmed [72, 73]. In addition, antibodies directed to fibrillin 1 may act to release active transforming growth factor (TGF)-β by blocking binding sites for the latent form [74]. Higher levels of autoantibodies reactive with CXCR3 and CXCR4 are shown to correlate with the severity of skin and lung fibrosis in SSc patients [75]. Despite the link to pathophysiology of these antibodies, the lack of commercially available kits that have been validated by multicenter studies complicates clinical application and feasibility. Pathogenic potentials of these autoantibodies are discussed in detail in another chapter.

Utility in SSc Diagnosis

SSc-specific autoantibodies are useful in support of the diagnosis of SSc because of their disease specificity. In cohorts of patients with established SSc and those with other connective tissue diseases, the specificity of anti-topo I and anti-RNAP III antibodies for SSc is >95%. ACA, anti-U3 RNP, anti-Th/To, and anti-U11/U12 RNP have specificity for SSc of approximately 90% but are sometimes found in patients with Raynaud's phenomenon alone, Sjögren's syndrome, or even in persons without apparent connective tissue disease. In contrast, anti-PM-Scl, anti-Ku, and anti-U1 RNP can be detected in patients with SLE or PM/DM without SSc features. In this regard, the presence of ACA, anti-topo I, or anti-RNAP III antibody is included in one of the criterion domains of a set of classification criteria for SSc, which has been proposed by the American College of Rheumatology (ACR) and the European League against Rheumatism (EULAR) [76]. The inclusion of these three antibodies was based on their high specificity for SSc and the availability of reliable assay kits worldwide.

In a prospective study involving a large cohort of patients who were referred for the evaluation of Raynaud's phenomenon, the presence of nailfold capillary abnormalities and/or SSc-specific autoantibodies, including ACA, anti-topo I, anti-RNAP III, and anti-Th/To, was found to be an independent predictor for developing SSc during follow-up [77]. To promote early detection and diagnosis of SSc, the EULAR Scleroderma Trials and Research group (EUSTAR) has proposed the term VEDOSS in patients with Raynaud's phenomenon who also have one of the following: an SSc-specific autoantibody, nailfold capillary abnormality, or puffy fingers [7].

Epidemiological Characteristics

Age at Onset

The distribution of SSc-specific autoantibodies varies according to age. In a series of 111 cases of childhood-onset SSc, there was a greater frequency of antibodies to anti-PM-Scl and anti-U1 RNP in comparison to adult-onset SSc [78, 79]. Accordingly, childhood SSc is associated with a much greater prevalence of myositis overlap. Anti-topo I antibody is commonly found in patients with childhood-onset and adult-onset SSc, but ACA and anti-RNAP III are almost lacking in childhood-onset SSc. Even in the adult SSc population, age at onset is older in patients with anti-RNAP III and anti-RuvBL1/2, while anti-U3 RNP, anti-PM-Scl, anti-Ku, and anti-U1 RNP are more common in younger patients.

Gender

The majority of patients with SSc are female, and hence, all autoantibodies are found more commonly in females than males. There are, however, gender-related differences in SSc-specific autoantibody specificities. ACA is particularly prominent in females (>95% of ACA-positive SSc patients are female).

Ethnicity

There are significant differences in the distribution of SSc-specific autoantibodies among ethnic groups (Table 7.3) [23, 24, 80, 81]. Interestingly, even in the United States, differences are observed between cohorts from the University of Pittsburgh, the University of Texas at Houston, and the University of Florida, likely owing to ethnic diversity. In this regard, there are also major differences in the antibody profile among SSc patients in different European countries. ACA is frequent in Caucasians but is found far less frequently in African American and Thai patients with SSc [82]. Anti-RNAP III is more common in North American Caucasians, UK, and Australian cohorts, compared with Japanese, French, Dutch, and Italian cohorts [25, 83, 84], although anti-topo I is commonly detected in many ethnic groups. A recent study using the EUSTAR cohort has shown that Asian patients have a faster and earlier disease onset with a high prevalence of anti-topo I [85]. A notable exception is that >80% of Oklahoma Choctaw Native Americans (an inbred population) with SSc have anti-topo I antibodies [86]. A greater frequency of anti-U3 RNP has been identified in African Americans with SSc compared with Caucasian populations. The anti-PM-Scl antibody has been barely reported in Japanese patients with SSc. Aanti-U1RNP anti-

Table 7.3 Frequencies (percent) of SSc-specific autoantibodies in various ethnic groups

	North American Caucasian			Hispanic	North American-African			French	Italian	Dutch	Australian	Japanese
Autoantibody specificity	Pittsburgh (*n* = 416)	Texas (*n* = 191)	Florida (*n* = 75)	Texas (*n* = 77)	Pittsburgh (*n* = 22)	Texas (*n* = 77)	Florida (*n* = 23)	Paris (*n* = 127)	Brescia (*n* = 216)	Leiden (*n* = 287)	All regions (*n* = 505)	Tokyo (*n* = 275)
References	[23]	[80]	[81]	[80]	[23]	[80]	[81]	[24]	[81]	[25]	[83]	[23]
ACA	19	32	17	18	8	4	0	18	31	37	41	15
Anti-topo I	21	13	15	19	13	16	35	35	38	24	18	26
Anti-RNAP III	23	ND	19	ND	13	ND	9	4	7	5	13	4
Anti-U3 RNP	4	4	3	7	42	17	30	2	0	4	<1	3
Anti-Th/To	4	ND	9	ND	0	ND	4	1	4	<1	<1	3
Anti-PM-Scl	3	ND	6	ND	0	ND	0	6	ND	3	2	0
Anti-Ku	1	ND	ND	ND	8	ND	ND	2	ND	1	<1	2
Anti-U1 RNP	8	5	13	11	33	29	30	9	ND	9	ND	34

Some patients have more than one SSc-specific autoantibodies
ND not determined

body is more prevalent in African American and Oriental SSc patients compared with Caucasians.

Disease Subset Classification

Classification of patients into dcSSc and lcSSc subsets according to the distribution of skin thickening is useful in predicting future organ involvement and prognosis, and more precise subgrouping is possible by also considering SSc-specific autoantibodies. In addition, SSc in overlap is a separate SSc subset, distinct from lcSSc and dcSSc, due to a different progression of the disease, different proportional distribution of specific autoantibodies, and different organ involvement [87]. It is often difficult to classify patients into dcSSc or lcSSc early in the course of the disease when skin thickness is restricted to the distal portion of extremities and face. In this case, information on SSc-specific autoantibodies is useful in predicting the future extent of skin involvement. Figure 7.1 illustrates the distribution of SSc-specific autoantibodies in association with disease classification.

lcSSc

ACA is the most common SSc-specific autoantibody in patients with lcSSc (~50%). Approximately 93% of patients with ACA are classified as having lcSSc [88]. Anti-Th/To is another antibody associated with lcSSc. Compared with ACA-positive patients with lcSSc, anti-Th/To-positive patients have more subtle cutaneous, vascular, and GI involvement but more often have PAH and ILD [32, 89]. It is of note that one-third of anti-topo I-positive patients are classified as having lcSSc, but the prevalence of ILD is comparable between dcSSc and lcSSc patients with anti-topo I [10, 16]. Other antibodies typically found in patients with lcSSc include anti-U11/U12 RNP, anticentriole, anti-U3 RNP, anti-PM-Scl, and anti-U1 RNP.

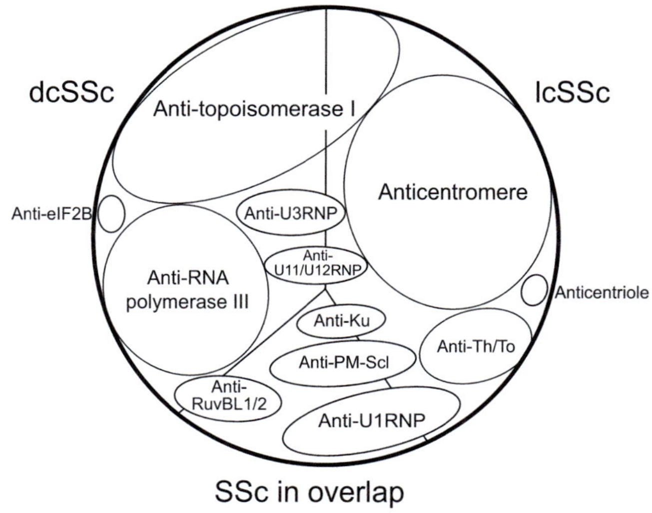

Fig. 7.1 Diagram showing SSc subsets stratified by SSc-specific autoantibodies. Areas of individual circles represent approximate proportions in the entire SSc patients

dcSSc

Almost two-thirds of patients with anti-topo I are classified as having dcSSc [16]. French patients with anti-topo I antibodies, however, are less likely to have dcSSc when compared with their US counterparts (38% versus 65%) [24]. Likewise, only 14% of French Canadians with dcSSc carry anti-topo I [90]. Anti-RNAP III antibody is also associated with dcSSc; over 80% of patients with this antibody have dcSSc [18, 21, 91]. The rate of progression of skin involvement also differs depending on antibody specificity [13]. In a recent series, all patients with anti-RNAP III had developed skin fibrosis within 6 months of the appearance of Raynaud's phenomenon in contrast to only 34% of those with anti-topo I [92]. Anti-U3 RNP is typically associated with dcSSc, particularly in African American patients. However, patients with dcSSc who carry anti-U3 RNP antibodies have been found to have a lower mRSS when compared with patients with dcSSc and other SSc-specific autoantibodies [29]. A rare anti-eIF2B antibody is also associated with dcSSc in case of fine cytoplasmic staining on IIF [38].

SSc in Overlap

Up to 20% of SSc patients have overlapping features of other connective tissue diseases. The most common SSc in overlap is SSc-myositis, often termed sclerodermatomyositis. In this group, anti-PM-Scl, anti-Ku, anti-RuvBL1/2, or anti-U1 RNP antibodies cover >70% of the patients. Of these, patients with anti-PM-Scl, anti-Ku, or anti-U1 RNP usually show limited cutaneous involvement, but those with anti-RuvBL1/2 frequently have diffuse cutaneous involvement [46, 48]. Patients with anti-U1 RNP often have additional lupus features, consistent with MCTD.

SSc Sine Scleroderma

It has been shown that SSc sine scleroderma should not be considered clinically distinct from SSc because organ manifestations and natural history of the disease are similar to those with lcSSc [93]. ACA was the most prevalent SSc-specific autoantibody in patients with SSc sine scleroderma, although 44% were positive for ANA but negative for known SSc-specific autoantibodies. In another series, anti-topo I was identified in 28% of such cases [94]. Anti-Th/To has also been identified in patients with idiopathic interstitial pneumonia in the absence of any SSc skin involvement [95, 96].

Prediction of Organ Manifestations

Clinical features in SSc patients are remarkably heterogeneous, and grouping patients based on autoantibody profiles is a useful approach in the clinical setting. Combining autoantibodies with the dcSSc/lcSSc cutaneous subset is useful for assessing organ involvement and mortality. However, subgroup analysis using hierarchical clustering has revealed that autoantibodies only partially contribute to risk stratification and clinical subsetting in SSc [97]. A recent clustering analysis has identified six clusters that differ with regard to their clinical features, autoantibody profile, and mortality [98]. Interestingly, some clusters resemble usual prototypes defined by ACA and anti-topo I antibodies, although others exhibit unique features independent of autoantibody status. Figure 7.2 shows SSc-specific autoantibodies found in patients with main organ-specific manifestations in the context of SSc cutaneous subsets.

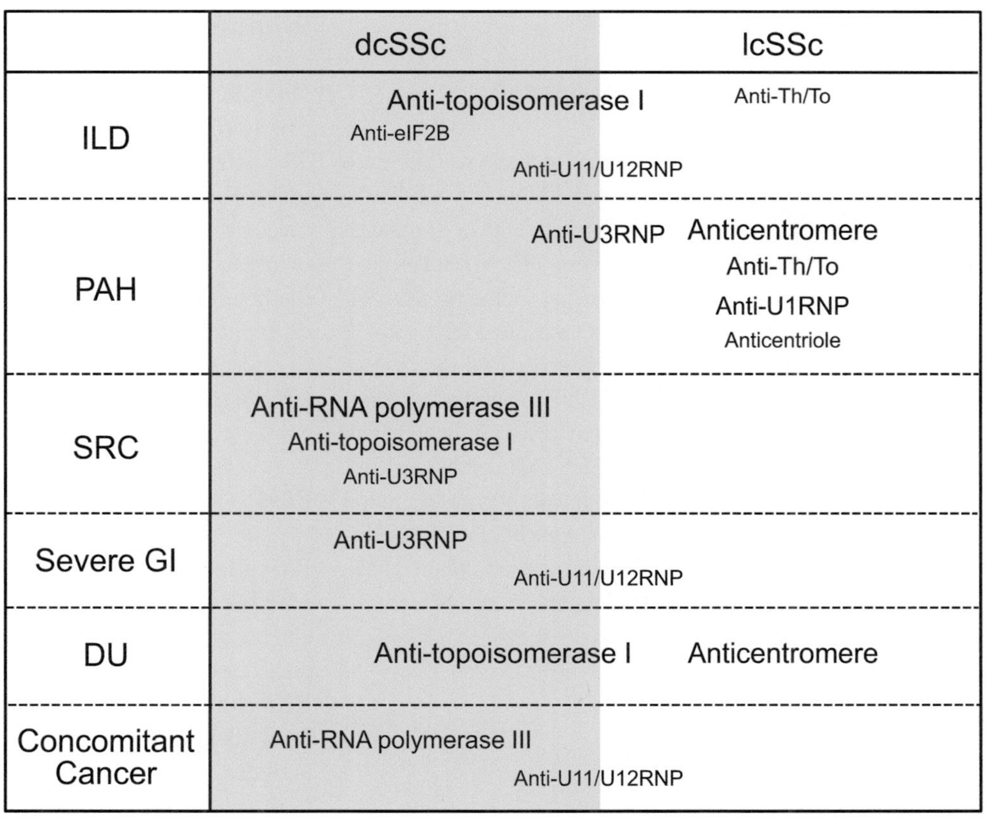

Fig. 7.2 SSc-specific autoantibodies found in patients with main organ-specific manifestations in the context of SSc cutaneous subsets. Letter sizes of individual autoantibodies represent approximate proportions in SSc patients with given organ manifestations. It is important to note, however, that these major clinical associations are not absolute, and organ-specific manifestations can occur in the presence of any autoantibody reactivity

Peripheral Vascular Manifestations

Raynaud's phenomenon is seen in virtually all patients with SSc, although the degree of peripheral vascular complication varies considerably between subgroups stratified by SSc-specific/related autoantibodies. Specifically, DU is commonly found in patients with ACA or anti-topo I. The lowest prevalence of DU is found in patients with either anti-Th/To or anti-RNAP III. Anti-IFI16 is associated with digital gangrene in SSc patients, especially in those with ACA [57]. High levels of anti-AT1R and anti-ETAR antibodies are shown to be useful in predicting the development of DU [73].

Joint Involvement

Up to two-thirds of patients with SSc experience joint pain, although a much smaller proportion have physical examination evidence of polyarthritis. Arthritis is seen commonly in SSc patients who carry antibodies associated with overlap features, such as anti-PM-Scl, anti-Ku, and anti-U1RNP. In contrast, joint involvement is less frequent in patients with ACA or anti-Th/To antibodies when compared with other SSc-specific autoantibodies. The majority of such patients have nonerosive arthritis, but some have erosive arthritis resembling rheumatoid arthritis. A meta-analysis has shown that the prevalence of anti-cyclic citrullinated peptide antibodies in SSc patients is 9.2%, and this antibody is associated with an increased risk for erosive arthritis [99].

GI Involvement

In terms of upper GI involvement, there is virtually no difference among patients stratified by SSc-related ANAs, but anti-Th/To and anti-PM-Scl antibodies are associated with a somewhat lower frequency of esophageal dysfunction [32, 41]. It has been reported that severe lower GI involvement, including psuedoileus and small bowel malabsorption, is associated with anti-U3 RNP antibody, especially in early the course of the disease (<2 years) [100, 101]. Anti-U11/U12 RNP is another autoantibody associated with moderate-to-severe lower GI involvement [34]. A case–control study using the EUSTAR database identified anti-RNAP III as one of the risk factors for gastric antral vascular ectasia (GAVE; "watermelon stomach") [102], and this correlation was replicated in a North American cohort [103]. Autoantibodies to muscarinic-3 acetylcholine receptors are associated with severe GI dysmotility [69].

Renal Crisis

In Northern Europe and North America, approximately 60% of all patients experiencing SRC carry anti-RNAP III [104]. SRC can also occur in the context of other SSc-specific autoantibodies, including anti-topo I and anti-U3 RNP, and antibody status has not been shown to influence outcomes following SRC in such patients. In SSc patients with anti-RNAP III antibodies, the coexistence of anti-RNAP II and a higher ELISA index is associated with a risk of developing SRC [105]. The lower incidence of SRC in Japan, French, and Mediterranean countries is thought to reflect the lower prevalence of anti-RNAP III antibodies within these populations when compared with the UK, Denmark, and North America [84]. Despite the lower prevalence of anti-RNAP III in French SSc patients, this antibody remains the most common serological marker for SRC [91]. In contrast, a study from Italy identified a much greater proportion of anti-topo I in patients with SRC [106]. SRC is rarely seen in the context of ACA or anti-PM-Scl. Interestingly, patients who survived SRC and then later developed PAH have been reported in the context of anti-RNAP III, anti-Th/To, and anti-U3 RNP [31]. Anti-RNAP III antibody has been detected in patients complicating acute renal failure mimicking SRC in the absence of SSc skin disease [107]. These patients might eventually develop progressive skin thickening. The presence of anti-RNAP III antibodies should alert the managing physician to the increased risk of SRC and appropriate monitoring of blood pressure for early detection of this complication since the prompt introduction of angiotensin-converting enzyme inhibitors can be lifesaving [108].

Primary Heart Involvement

Diastolic and systolic heart involvement potentially due to patchy fibrosis in the myocardium is relatively common in SSc patients, particularly in those with long-standing disease. There is no definitive association of primary heart involvement with SSc-specific autoantibodies, probably owing to the lack of a clear definition which is explained by the heterogeneous nature of the heart involvement, and the difficulty in distinguishing SSc-associated from other causes of myocardial and conduction system abnormalities, particularly in older adults.

PAH

PAH affects approximately 10% of patients with SSc and has now become a major cause of SSc-related mortality. PAH can occur in the context of several SSc-specific autoantibodies, including ACA, anti-U3 RNP, anti-Th/To, and anti-U1 RNP antibodies. The evidence-based DETECT algorithm for PAH identification of SSc patients at high risk for PAH includes ACA as one of the useful characteristics [109]., A high prevalence of PAH is also found in patients with antinucleolar antibodies, including anti-U3 RNP and anti-Th/To.

When comparing anti-U3 RNP with other antibody specificities, PAH was the most common cause of death, leading to increased mortality in this group of patients [29], and this may explain poor survival in patients with African American patients with SSc and PAH [110]. Coexistence with autoantibodies to another nucleolar protein, B23, further increases the PAH risk in patients with anti-U3 RNP [53]. The overall prevalence of PAH in anti-Th/To positivity is similar to that seen with ACA [32]. In addition, patients with anti-Th/To also develop pulmonary hypertension in the context of ILD. Among connective tissue disease-associated PAH, anti-U1 RNP-positive patients are younger and less functionally impaired and have better survival than anti-U1 RNP-negative patients [111]. Patients with anti-topo I rarely develop PAH but have pulmonary hypertension due to ILD and chronic hypoxia [112]. A systematic literature search of studies evaluating autoantibody profiles in patients with SSc-PAH has found half positive for ACA and one-fourth positive for anti-nucleolar antibodies such as anti-U3 RNP and anti-Th/To [113]. Aanti-AT1R and anti-ETAR antibodies are associated with PAH and serve as poor prognostic markers in SSc patients [72].

ILD

ILD is now a leading cause of SSc-related mortality. More than 70% of patients with anti-topo I have ILD, and ~25% develop severe disease, which requires oxygen supplementation [88]. Anti-topo I-positive patients have the highest incidence of ILD independent of dcSSc/lcSSc subsets [10]. A novel autoantibody targeting U11/U12 RNP is associated with severe ILD and decreased survival [33]. Other antibodies associated with ILD include anti-Th/To in case of a nucleolar pattern on IIF [32] and anti-eIF2B in case of a cytoplasmic pattern (a negative ANA) [38]. In the context of lcSSc with severe ILD, anti-U11/U12 RNP and anti-Th/To are the most common autoantibodies. In contrast, the presence of ACA is an independent protective factor for symptomatic ILD [114]. Severe ILD can occur in patients with anti-RNAP III but is infrequent in this patient subset [115]. The utility of autoantibodies as a prognostic biomarker to predict the future progression of ILD still remains controversial; one study has reported an association of anti-topo I positivity with a greater rate of decline in forced vital capacity over 3 years [116], but others have failed to replicate this association.

Cancer

A similar prevalence of anti-RNAP III, ACA, and anti-topo I is reported among patients with SSc and cancer, but the temporal relationship between cancer and SSc differed according to antibody status, with a median disease duration of 13.4 and 11.1 years for anti-topo I and ACA, respectively, in comparison to a nearly contemporaneous association between cancer and anti-RNAP III (median disease duration of 1.2 years) [27]. An association with cancer among SSc patients with anti-RNAP III antibodies in a close temporal relationship to the onset of SSc suggests that SSc is a paraneoplastic disorder in this patient subset [28]. Another large-scale cohort including 1044 patients with SSc found that anti-RNAP III is an independent marker of coincident cancer [117]. In the Johns Hopkins Scleroderma cohort, 8.6% of patients were diagnosed with cancer over 37,686 person-years, and the standardized incidence ratio (SIR) of cancer in anti-RNAP III-positive patients within 3 years of SSc diagnosis was 2.84 (95% CI 1.89–4.10). Interestingly, those patients with dcSSc had an increased breast cancer risk (SIR 5.14, 95% CI 2.66–8.98), whereas those with lcSSc had a high lung cancer risk (SIR 10.4, 95% CI 1.26–37.7) [118]. Based on these findings, cancer screening is recommended in anti-RNAP III-positive patients with newly diagnosed SSc [108, 119]. The coexistence of anti-RNAP I antibodies has a protective effect against cancer in patients with anti-RNAP III antibodies [120]. Recently, anti-U11/U12 RNP antibody has been identified as another SSc-specific autoantibody associated with a short-interval malignancy detection [35].

Survival

Several studies have identified an association between anti-topo I and a greater risk of mortality [8, 9]. Anti-RNAP III has been shown to be protective for 2-year mortality in one cohort enrolled after the introduction of angiotensin-converting enzyme inhibitor therapy [13]. Anti-U3 RNP is another SSc-specific antibody associated with increased mortality, particularly in relation to PAH [29]. In the largest study to date, using the Pittsburgh Scleroderma Databank of 1432 patients, anti-Th/To predicted the lowest 10-year survival among lcSSc (65% versus 88% and 75% with U1 RNP and ACA, respectively) [121]. In dcSSc, the best 10-year survival was identified in those carrying anti-RNAP III (75%) and the lowest survival with anti-U3 RNP (61%). In a recent study involving 1325 patients with SSc in the Royal Free hospital cohort, ACA-positive patients had the best survival rates, while the patients who were positive for ANA but were negative for the known SSc-specific autoantibodies had the lowest survival [10].

Autoantibody Titer and Disease Activity

There have been relatively few studies that have investigated whether autoantibody levels are useful in monitoring disease activity in SSc. The task is challenging, because the course of SSc is more indolent, and indices or biomarkers of disease activity are less developed. Most evidence for an association of autoantibody level with disease activity comes from studies of anti-topo I, where changing levels may correlate with the progression of skin thickness [122]. In contrast, patients who lose anti-topo I antibodies over time may have a more favorable outcome [123]. Anti-RNAP III antibody levels may also correlate with mRSS and the onset of SRC [124, 125]. Now that quantitative and semiquantitative laboratory tests are available, additional reports will help to clarify whether antibody levels will be helpful biomarkers in clinical practice or clinical trials.

Conclusions

In summary, circulating autoantibodies are the best diagnostic and prognostic biomarkers in SSc patients. Characterization of autoantibody status is an essential tool in clinical practice in the evaluation of patients who have SSc or are suspected to have this disease. Because of their specificity, they are highly useful in the diagnosis of SSc as well as in predicting future development to definite SSc in patients with Raynaud's phenomenon without any SSc skin changes. In addition, because of their strong clinical associations, they allow clinicians to predict future disease manifestations by combining them with the cutaneous subset. It is important to note, however, that these major clinical associations are not absolute, and organ-specific manifestations can occur in the presence of any autoantibody reactivity. Clinical decisions should be made based on comprehensive assessments, including physical findings, functional assessment, imaging studies, and autoantibodies.

References

1. Mehra S, Walker J, Patterson K, Fritzler MJ. Autoantibodies in systemic sclerosis. Autoimmun Rev. 2013;12(3):340–54.
2. Hamaguchi Y. Autoantibody profiles in systemic sclerosis: predictive value for clinical evaluation and prognosis. J Dermatol. 2010;37(1):42–53.
3. Kuwana M. Circulating anti-nuclear antibodies in systemic sclerosis: utility in diagnosis and disease subsetting. J Nippon Med Sch. 2017;84(2):56–63.
4. Moroi Y, Peebles C, Fritzler MJ, Steigerwald J, Tan EM. Autoantibody to centromere (kinetochore) in scleroderma sera. Proc Natl Acad Sci U S A. 1980;77(3):1627–31.
5. Gelber AC, Pillemer SR, Baum BJ, Wigley FM, Hummers LK, Morris S, et al. Distinct recognition of antibodies to centromere proteins in primary Sjogren's syndrome compared with limited scleroderma. Ann Rheum Dis. 2006;65(8):1028–32.
6. Senecal JL, Dieudé M, Koenig M. Predictive value of antinuclear autoantibodies: the lessons of the systemic sclerosis autoantibodies. Autoimmun Rev. 2008;7(8):588–93.
7. Matucci-Cerinic M, Allanore Y, Czirják L, Tyndall A, Müller-Ladner U, Denton C, et al. The challenge of early systemic sclerosis for the EULAR Scleroderma Trial and Research group (EUSTAR) community. It is time to cut the Gordian knot and develop a prevention or rescue strategy. Ann Rheum Dis. 2009;68(9):1377–80.
8. Steen VD, Powell DL, Medsger TA Jr. Clinical correlations and prognosis based on serum autoantibodies in patients with systemic sclerosis. Arthritis Rheum. 1988;31(2):196–203.
9. Kuwana M, Kaburaki J, Okano Y, Tojo T, Homma M. Clinical and prognostic associations based on serum antinuclear antibodies in Japanese patients with systemic sclerosis. Arthritis Rheum. 1994;37(1):75–83.
10. Nihtyanova SI, Sari A, Harvey JC, Leslie A, Derrett-Smith EC, Fonseca C, et al. Using autoantibodies and cutaneous subset to develop outcome-based disease classification in systemic sclerosis. Arthritis Rheumatol. 2020;72(3):465–76.
11. Douvas AS, Achten M, Tan EM. Identification of a nuclear protein (Scl-70) as a unique target of human antinuclear antibodies in scleroderma. J Biol Chem. 1979;254(20):10514–22.
12. Shero JH, Bordwell B, Rothfield NF, Earnshaw WC. High titers of autoantibodies to topoisomerase I (Scl-70) in sera from scleroderma patients. Science. 1986;231(4739):737–40.
13. Domsic RT, Rodriguez-Reyna T, Lucas M, Fertig N, Medsger TA Jr. Skin thickness progression rate: a predictor of mortality and early internal organ involvement in diffuse scleroderma. Ann Rheum Dis. 2011;70(1):104–9.
14. Wirz EG, Jaeger VK, Allanore Y, Riemekasten G, Hachulla E, Distler O, et al. Incidence and predictors of cutaneous manifestations during the early course of systemic sclerosis: a 10-year longitudinal study from the EUSTAR database. Ann Rheum Dis. 2016;75(7):1285–92.
15. Perera A, Fertig N, Lucas M, Rodriguez-Reyna TS, Hu P, Steen VD, Medsger TA Jr. Clinical subsets, skin thickness progression rate, and serum antibody levels in systemic sclerosis patients with anti-topoisomerase I antibody. Arthritis Rheum. 2007;56(8):2740–6.
16. Kranenburg P, van den Hombergh WM, Knaapen-Hans HK, van den Hoogen FH, Fransen J, Vonk MC. Survival and organ involvement in patients with limited cutaneous systemic sclerosis and anti-topoisomerase-I antibodies: determined by skin subtype or auto-antibody subtype? A long-term follow-up study. Rheumatology (Oxford). 2016;55(11):2001–8.
17. Boonstra M, Bakker JA, Grummels A, Ninaber MK, Ajmone Marsan N, et al. Association of anti-topoisomerase I antibodies of the IgM isotype with disease progression in anti-topoisomerase I-positive systemic sclerosis. Arthritis Rheumatol. 2020;72(11):1897–904.
18. Kuwana M, Kaburaki J, Mimori T, Tojo T, Homma M. Autoantibody reactive with three classes of RNA polymerases in sera from patients with systemic sclerosis. J Clin Invest. 1993;91(4):1399–404.
19. Kuwana M, Okano Y, Kaburaki J, Medsger TA Jr, Wright TM. Autoantibodies to RNA polymerases recognize multiple subunits and demonstrate cross-reactivity with RNA polymerase complexes. Arthritis Rheum. 1999;42(2):275–84.
20. Satoh M, Kuwana M, Ogasawara T, Ajmani AK, Langdon JJ, Kimpel D, et al. Association of autoantibodies to topoisomerase I and the phosphorylated (IIO) form of RNA polymerase II in Japanese scleroderma patients. J Immunol. 1994;153(12):5838–48.
21. Okano Y, Steen VD, Medsger TA Jr. Autoantibody reactive with RNA polymerase III in systemic sclerosis. Ann Intern Med. 1993;119(10):1005–13.
22. Nikpour M, Hissaria P, Byron J, Sahhar J, Micallef M, Paspaliaris W, et al. Prevalence, correlates and clinical usefulness of antibodies to RNA polymerase III in systemic sclerosis: a cross-sectional

analysis of data from an Australian cohort. Arthritis Res Ther. 2011;13(6):R211.
23. Kuwana M, Okano Y, Kaburaki J, Tojo T, Medsger TA Jr. Racial differences in the distribution of systemic sclerosis-related serum antinuclear antibodies. Arthritis Rheum. 1994;37(6):902–6.
24. Meyer OC, Fertig N, Lucas M, Somogyi N, Medsger TA Jr. Disease subsets, antinuclear antibody profile, and clinical features in 127 French and 247 US adult patients with systemic sclerosis. J Rheumatol. 2007;34(1):104–9.
25. Markusse IM, Meijs J, de Boer B, Bakker JA, Schippers HPC, Schouffoer AA, et al. Predicting cardiopulmonary involvement in patients with systemic sclerosis: complementary value of nailfold videocapillaroscopy patterns and disease-specific autoantibodies. Rheumatology (Oxford). 2017;56(7):1081–8.
26. Herrick AL, Peytrignet S, Lunt M, Pan X, Hesselstrand R, Mouthon L, et al. Patterns and predictors of skin score change in early diffuse systemic sclerosis from the European Scleroderma Observational Study. Ann Rheum Dis. 2018;77(4):563–70.
27. Shah AA, Rosen A, Hummers L, Wigley F, Casciola-Rosen L. Close temporal relationship between onset of cancer and scleroderma in patients with RNA polymerase I/III antibodies. Arthritis Rheum. 2010;62(9):2787–95.
28. Moinzadeh P, Fonseca C, Hellmich M, Shah AA, Chighizola C, Denton CP, Ong VH. Association of anti-RNA polymerase III autoantibodies and cancer in scleroderma. Arthritis Res Ther. 2014;16(1):R53.
29. Aggarwal R, Lucas M, Fertig N, Oddis CV, Medsger TA Jr. Anti-U3 RNP autoantibodies in systemic sclerosis. Arthritis Rheum. 2009;60(4):1112–8.
30. Mejia Otero C, Assassi S, Hudson M, Mayes MD, Estrada-Y-Martin R, Pedroza C, et al. Antifibrillarin antibodies are associated with native north American ethnicity and poorer survival in systemic sclerosis. J Rheumatol. 2017;44(6):799–805.
31. Gündüz OH, Fertig N, Lucas M, Medsger TA Jr. Systemic sclerosis with renal crisis and pulmonary hypertension: a report of eleven cases. Arthritis Rheum. 2001;44(7):1663–6.
32. Mitri GM, Lucas M, Fertig N, Steen VD, Medsger TA Jr. A comparison between anti-Th/To-and anticentromere antibody-positive systemic sclerosis patients with limited cutaneous involvement. Arthritis Rheum. 2003;48(1):203–9.
33. Fertig N, Domsic RT, Rodriguez-Reyna T, Kuwana M, Lucas M, Medsger TA Jr, et al. Anti-U11/U12 RNP antibodies in systemic sclerosis: a new serologic marker associated with pulmonary fibrosis. Arthritis Rheum. 2009;61(7):958–65.
34. McMahan ZH, Domsic RT, Zhu L, Medsger TA, Casciola-Rosen L, Shah AA. Anti-RNPC-3 (U11/U12) antibodies in systemic sclerosis in patients with moderate-to-severe gastrointestinal dysmotility. Arthritis Care Res (Hoboken). 2019;71(9):1164–70.
35. Shah AA, Xu G, Rosen A, Hummers LK, Wigley FM, Elledge SJ, et al. Anti-RNPC-3 antibodies as a marker of cancer-associated scleroderma. Arthritis Rheumatol. 2017;69(6):1306–12.
36. Moroi Y, Murata I, Takeuchi A, Kamatani N, Tanimoto K, Yokohari R. Human anticentriole autoantibody in patients with scleroderma and Raynaud's phenomenon. Clin Immunol Immunopathol. 1983;29(3):381–90.
37. Maki H, Kubota K, Hatano M, Minatsuki S, Amiya E, Yoshizaki A, et al. Characteristics of pulmonary arterial hypertension in patients with systemic sclerosis and anticentriole autoantibodies. Int Heart J. 2020;61(2):413–8.
38. Betteridge ZE, Woodhead F, Lu H, Shaddick G, Bunn CC, Denton CP, et al. Anti-eukaryotic initiation factor 2B autoantibodies are associated with interstitial lung disease in patients with systemic sclerosis. Arthritis Rheumatol. 2016;68(11):2778–83.
39. Pauling JD, Salazar G, Lu H, Betteridge ZE, Assassi S, Mayes MD, et al. Presence of anti-eukaryotic initiation factor-2B, anti-RuvBL1/2 and anti-synthetase antibodies in patients with anti-nuclear antibody negative systemic sclerosis. Rheumatology (Oxford). 2018;57(4):712–7.
40. Reimer G, Scheer U, Peters JM, Tan EM. Immunolocalization and partial characterization of a nucleolar autoantigen (PM-Scl) associated with polymyositis/scleroderma overlap syndromes. J Immunol. 1986;137(12):3802–8.
41. D'Aoust J, Hudson M, Tatibouet S, Wick J, Mahler M, Baron M, et al. Clinical and serologic correlates of anti-PM/Scl antibodies in systemic sclerosis: a multicenter study of 763 patients. Arthritis Rheumatol. 2014;66(6):1608–15.
42. Lazzaroni MG, Marasco E, Campochiaro C, De Vries-Bouwstra J, Gonzalez-Perez MI, Rojas-Serrano J, et al. The clinical phenotype of systemic sclerosis patients with anti-PM/Scl antibodies: results from the EUSTAR cohort. Rheumatology (Oxford). 2021;60:5028. https://doi.org/10.1093/rheumatology/keab152.
43. Brouwer R, Hengstman GJ, Vree Egberts W, Ehrfeld H, Bozic B, Ghirardello A, et al. Autoantibody profiles in the sera of European patients with myositis. Ann Rheum Dis. 2001;60(2):116–23.
44. Mimori T, Akizuki M, Yamagata H, Inada S, Yoshida S, Homma M. Characterization of a high molecular weight acidic nuclear protein recognized by autoantibodies in sera from patients with polymyositis-scleroderma overlap. J Clin Invest. 1981;68(3):611–20.
45. Cavazzana I, Fredi M, Taraborelli M, Quinzanini M, Tincani A, Franceschini F. A subset of systemic sclerosis but not of systemic lupus erythematosus is defined by isolated anti-Ku autoantibodies. Clin Exp Rheumatol. 2013;31(2 Suppl 76):118–21.
46. Rozman B, Cucnik S, Sodin-Semrl S, Czirjak L, Varju C, Distler O, et al. Prevalence and clinical associations of anti-Ku antibodies in patients with systemic sclerosis: a European EUSTAR-initiated multi-centre case-control study. Ann Rheum Dis. 2008;67(9):1282–6.
47. Hoa S, Hudson M, Troyanov Y, Proudman S, Walker J, Stevens W, et al. Single-specificity anti-Ku antibodies in an international cohort of 2140 systemic sclerosis subjects: clinical associations. Medicine (Baltimore). 2016;95(35):e4713.
48. Kaji K, Fertig N, Medsger TA Jr, Satoh T, Hoshino K, Hamaguchi Y, et al. Autoantibodies to RuvBL1 and RuvBL2: a novel systemic sclerosis-related antibody associated with diffuse cutaneous and skeletal muscle involvement. Arthritis Care Res (Hoboken). 2014;66(4):575–84.
49. Sharp GC, Irvin WS, Tan EM, Gould RG, Holman HR. Mixed connective tissue disease-an apparently distinct rheumatic disease syndrome associated with a specific antibody to an extractable nuclear antigen (ENA). Am J Med. 1972;52(2):148–59.
50. Gunnarsson R, Andreassen AK, Molberg Ø, Lexberg ÅS, Time K, Dhainaut AS, et al. Prevalence of pulmonary hypertension in an unselected, mixed connective tissue disease cohort: results of a nationwide, Norwegian cross-sectional multicentre study and review of current literature. Rheumatology (Oxford). 2013;52(7):1208–13.
51. Rodriguez-Sanchez JL, Gelpi C, Juarez C, Hardin JA. A new autoantibody in scleroderma that recognizes a 90-kDa component of the nucleolus-organizing region of chromatin. J Immunol. 1987;139(8):2579–84.
52. Dagher JH, Scheer U, Voit R, Grummt I, Lonzetti L, Raymond Y, et al. Autoantibodies to NOR 90/hUBF: longterm clinical and serological followup in a patient with limited systemic sclerosis suggests an antigen driven immune response. J Rheumatol. 2002;29(7):1543–7.
53. Ulanet DB, Wigley FM, Gelber AC, Rosen A. Autoantibodies against B23, a nucleolar phosphoprotein, occur in scleroderma and are associated with pulmonary hypertension. Arthritis Rheum. 2003;49(1):85–92.

54. Hudson M, Pope J, Mahler M, Tatibouet S, Steele R, Baron M, et al. Clinical significance of antibodies to Ro52/TRIM21 in systemic sclerosis. Arthritis Res Ther. 2012;14(2):R50.
55. Wodkowski M, Hudson M, Proudman S, Walker J, Stevens W, Nikpour M, et al. Monospecific anti-Ro52/TRIM21 antibodies in a tri-nation cohort of 1574 systemic sclerosis subjects: evidence of an association with interstitial lung disease and worse survival. Clin Exp Rheumatol. 2015;33(4 Suppl 91):S131–5.
56. Costa S, Mondini M, Caneparo V, Afeltra A, Airò P, Bellisai F, et al. Detection of anti-IFI16 antibodies by ELISA: clinical and serological associations in systemic sclerosis. Rheumatology (Oxford). 2011;50(4):674–81.
57. McMahan ZH, Wigley FM, Casciola-Rosen L. Risk of digital vascular events in scleroderma patients who have both anticentromere and anti-interferon-inducible protein 16 antibodies. Arthritis Care Res (Hoboken). 2017;69(6):922–6.
58. Fritzler MJ, Hudson M, Choi MY, Mahler M, Wang M, Bentow C, et al. Bicaudal D2 is a novel autoantibody target in systemic sclerosis that shares a key epitope with CENP-A but has a distinct clinical phenotype. Autoimmun Rev. 2018;17(3):267–75.
59. Cavazzana I, Ceribelli A, Taraborelli M, Fredi M, Norman G, Tincani A, et al. Primary biliary cirrhosis-related autoantibodies in a large cohort of Italian patients with systemic sclerosis. J Rheumatol. 2011;38(10):2180–5.
60. Adler BL, Boin F, Wolters PJ, Bingham CO, Shah AA, Greider C, et al. Autoantibodies targeting telomere-associated proteins in systemic sclerosis. Ann Rheum Dis. 2021;80:912–9. https://doi.org/10.1136/annrheumdis-2020-218918.
61. Salazar GA, Assassi S, Wigley F, Hummers L, Varga J, Hinchcliff M, et al. Antinuclear antibody-negative systemic sclerosis. Semin Arthritis Rheum. 2015;44(6):680–6.
62. Shanmugam VK, Swistowski DR, Saddic N, Wang H, Steen VD. Comparison of indirect immunofluorescence and multiplex antinuclear antibody screening in systemic sclerosis. Clin Rheumatol. 2011;30(10):1363–8.
63. Damoiseaux J, Boesten K, Giesen J, Austen J, Tervaert JW. Evaluation of a novel line-blot immunoassay for the detection of antibodies to extractable nuclear antigens. Ann N Y Acad Sci. 2005;1050(6):340–7.
64. Kuwana M, Kimura K, Kawakami Y. Identification of an immunodominant epitope on RNA polymerase III recognized by systemic sclerosis sera: application to enzyme-linked immunosorbent assay. Arthritis Rheum. 2002;46(10):2742–7.
65. Op De Beéck K, Vermeersch P, Verschueren P, Westhovens R, Mariën G, Blockmans D, et al. Antinuclear antibody detection by automated multiplex immunoassay in untreated patients at the time of diagnosis. Autoimmun Rev. 2012;12(2):137–43.
66. Hamaguchi Y, Kuwana M, Takehara K. Performance evaluation of a line blot assay system for detection of anti-PM-Scl antibody in Japanese patients with systemic sclerosis. Int J Rheum Dis. 2019;22(9):1746–51.
67. Hamaguchi Y, Kuwana M, Takehara K. Performance evaluation of a commercial line blot assay system for detection of myositis- and systemic sclerosis-related autoantibodies. Clin Rheumatol. 2020;39(11):3489–97.
68. Baroni SS, Santillo M, Bevilacqua F, Luchetti M, Spadoni T, Mancini M, et al. Stimulatory autoantibodies to the PDGF receptor in systemic sclerosis. N Engl J Med. 2006;354(25):2667–76.
69. Singh J, Mehendiratta V, Del Galdo F, Jimenez SA, Cohen S, et al. Immunoglobulins from scleroderma patients inhibit the muscarinic receptor activation in internal anal sphincter smooth muscle cells. Am J Physiol Gastrointest Liver Physiol. 2009;297(6):G1206–13.
70. Kawaguchi Y, Nakamura Y, Matsumoto I, Nishimagi E, Satoh T, Kuwana M, et al. Muscarinic-3 acetylcholine receptor autoantibody in patients with systemic sclerosis: contribution to severe gastrointestinal tract dysmotility. Ann Rheum Dis. 2009;68(5):710–4.
71. Riemekasten G, Philippe A, Näther M, Slowinski T, Müller DN, Heidecke H, et al. Involvement of functional autoantibodies against vascular receptors in systemic sclerosis. Ann Rheum Dis. 2011;70(3):530–6.
72. Becker MO, Kill A, Kutsche M, Guenther J, Rose A, Tabeling C, et al. Vascular receptor autoantibodies in pulmonary arterial hypertension associated with systemic sclerosis. Am J Respir Crit Care Med. 2014;190(7):808–17.
73. Avouac J, Riemekasten G, Meune C, Ruiz B, Kahan A, Allanore Y. Autoantibodies against endothelin 1 type a receptor are strong predictors of digital ulcers in systemic sclerosis. J Rheumatol. 2015;42(10):1801–7.
74. Tan FK, Arnett FC, Antohi S, Saito S, Mirarchi A, Spiera H, et al. Autoantibodies to the extracellular matrix microfibrillar protein, fibrillin-1, in patients with scleroderma and other connective tissue diseases. J Immunol. 1999;163(2):1066–72.
75. Weigold F, Günther J, Pfeiffenberger M, Cabral-Marques O, Siegert E, Dragun D, et al. Antibodies against chemokine receptors CXCR3 and CXCR4 predict progressive deterioration of lung function in patients with systemic sclerosis. Arthritis Res Ther. 2018;20(1):52.
76. van den Hoogen F, Khanna D, Fransen J, Johnson SR, Baron M, Tyndall A, et al. 2013 classification criteria for systemic sclerosis: an American College of Rheumatology/European League against Rheumatism collaborative initiative. Arthritis Rheum. 2013;65(11):2734–47.
77. Koenig M, Joyal F, Fritzler MJ, Roussin A, Abrahamowicz M, Boire G, et al. Autoantibodies and microvascular damage are independent predictive factors for the progression of Raynaud's phenomenon to systemic sclerosis: a twenty-year prospective study of 586 patients, with validation of proposed criteria for early systemic sclerosis. Arthritis Rheum. 2008;58(12):3902–12.
78. Scalapino K, Arkachaisri T, Lucas M, Fertig N, Helfrich DJ, Londino AV Jr, et al. Childhood onset systemic sclerosis: classification, clinical and serologic features, and survival in comparison with adult onset disease. J Rheumatol. 2006;33(5):1004–13.
79. Martini G, Foeldvari I, Russo R, Cuttica R, Eberhard A, Ravelli A, et al. Systemic sclerosis in childhood: clinical and immunologic features of 153 patients in an international database. Arthritis Rheum. 2006;54(12):3971–8.
80. Reveille JD, Fischbach M, McNearney T, Friedman AW, Aguilar MB, Lisse J, et al. Systemic sclerosis in 3 US ethnic groups: a comparison of clinical, sociodemographic, serologic, and immunogenetic determinants. Semin Arthritis Rheum. 2001;30(5):332–46.
81. Krzyszczak ME, Li Y, Ross SJ, Ceribelli A, Chan EK, Bubb MR, et al. Gender and ethnicity differences in the prevalence of scleroderma-related autoantibodies. Clin Rheumatol. 2011;30(10):1333–9.
82. Panicheewa S, Chitrabamrung S, Verasertniyom O, Vanichaphantu M, Kraisit SO, Chiewsilp P, et al. Diffuse systemic sclerosis and related diseases in Thailand. Clin Rheumatol. 1991;10(2):124–9.
83. Patterson KA, Roberts-Thomson PJ, Lester S, Tan JA, Hakendorf P, Rischmueller M, et al. Interpretation of an extended autoantibody profile in a well-characterized Australian systemic sclerosis (scleroderma) cohort using principal components analysis. Arthritis Rheumatol. 2015;67(12):3234–44.
84. Sobanski V, Dauchet L, Lefèvre G, Lambert M, Morell-Dubois S, Sy T, et al. Prevalence of anti-RNA polymerase III antibodies in systemic sclerosis: new data from a French cohort and a systematic review and meta-analysis. Arthritis Rheumatol. 2014;66(2):407–17.
85. Jaeger VK, Tikly M, Xu D, Siegert E, Hachulla E, Airò P, et al. Racial differences in systemic sclerosis disease presentation: a European scleroderma trials and research group study. Rheumatology (Oxford). 2020;59(7):1684–94.

86. Arnett FC, Howard RF, Tan F, Moulds JM, Bias WB, Durban E, et al. Increased prevalence of systemic sclerosis in a native American tribe in Oklahoma Association with an Amerindian HLA haplotype. Arthritis Rheum. 1996;39(8):1362–70.
87. Moinzadeh P, Aberer E, Ahmadi-Simab K, Blank N, Distler JH, Fierlbeck G, et al. Disease progression in systemic sclerosis-overlap syndrome is significantly different from limited and diffuse cutaneous systemic sclerosis. Ann Rheum Dis. 2015;74(4):730–7.
88. Reveille JD, Solomon DH. Evidence-based guidelines for the use of immunologic tests: anticentromere, Scl-70, and nucleolar antibodies. Arthritis Rheum. 2003;49(3):399–412.
89. Ceribelli A, Cavazzana I, Franceschini F, Airò P, Tincani A, Cattaneo R, et al. Anti-Th/To are common antinucleolar autoantibodies in Italian patients with scleroderma. J Rheumatol. 2010;37(10):2071–5.
90. Scussel-Lonzetti L, Joyal F, Raynauld JP, Roussin A, Rich E, Goulet JR, et al. Predicting mortality in systemic sclerosis: analysis of a cohort of 309 French Canadian patients with emphasis on features at diagnosis as predictive factors for survival. Medicine (Baltimore). 2002;81(2):154–67.
91. Meyer O, De Chaisemartin L, Nicaise-Roland P, Cabane J, Tubach F, Dieude P, Allanore Y, et al. Anti-RNA polymerase III antibody prevalence and associated clinical manifestations in a large series of French patients with systemic sclerosis: a cross-sectional study. J Rheumatol. 2010;37(1):125–30.
92. Cavazzana I, Angela C, Paolo A, Stefania Z, Angela T, Franco F. Anti-RNA polymerase III antibodies: a marker of systemic sclerosis with rapid onset and skin thickening progression. Autoimmun Rev. 2009;8(7):580–4.
93. Poormoghim H, Lucas M, Fertig N, Medsger TA Jr. Systemic sclerosis sine scleroderma: demographic, clinical, and serologic features and survival in forty-eight patients. Arthritis Rheum. 2000;43(2):444–51.
94. Toya SP, Tzelepis GE. The many faces of scleroderma sine scleroderma: a literature review focusing on cardiopulmonary complications. Rheumatol Int. 2009;29(8):861–8.
95. Fischer A, Pfalzgraf FJ, Feghali-Bostwick CA, Wright TM, Curran-Everett D, West SG, et al. Anti-th/to-positivity in a cohort of patients with idiopathic pulmonary fibrosis. J Rheumatol. 2006;33(8):1600–5.
96. Fischer A, Meehan RT, Feghali-Bostwick CA, West SG, Brown KK. Unique characteristics of systemic sclerosis sine scleroderma-associated interstitial lung disease. Chest. 2006;130(4):976–81.
97. Boonstra M, Mertens BJA, Bakker JA, Ninaber MK, Ajmone Marsan N, van der Helm-van Mil AHM, et al. To what extent do autoantibodies help to identify high-risk patients in systemic sclerosis? Clin Exp Rheumatol. 2018;36 Suppl 113(4):109–17.
98. Sobanski V, Giovannelli J, Allanore Y, Riemekasten G, Airò P, Vettori S, et al. Phenotypes determined by cluster analysis and their survival in the prospective European Scleroderma Trials and Research cohort of patients with systemic sclerosis. Arthritis Rheumatol. 2019;71(9):1553–70.
99. Laustriat G, Ruyssen-Witrand A, Constantin A, Barnetche T, Adoue D, Cantagrel A, et al. Anti-citrullinated peptides antibodies in systemic sclerosis: meta-analysis of frequency and meaning. Joint Bone Spine. 2018;85(2):147–53.
100. Sharif R, Fritzler MJ, Mayes MD, Gonzalez EB, McNearney TA, Draeger H, et al. Anti-fibrillarin antibody in African American patients with systemic sclerosis: immunogenetics, clinical features, and survival analysis. J Rheumatol. 2011;38(8):1622–30.
101. Nishimagi E, Tochimoto A, Kawaguchi Y, Satoh T, Kuwana M, Takagi K, et al. Characteristics of patients with early systemic sclerosis and severe gastrointestinal tract involvement. J Rheumatol. 2007;34(10):2050–5.
102. Ghrénassia E, Avouac J, Khanna D, Derk CT, Distler O, Suliman YA, et al. Prevalence, correlates and outcomes of gastric antral vascular ectasia in systemic sclerosis: a EUSTAR case-control study. J Rheumatol. 2014;41(1):99–105.
103. Serling-Boyd N, Chung MP, Li S, Becker L, Fernandez-Becker N, Clarke J, et al. Gastric antral vascular ectasia in systemic sclerosis: association with anti-RNA polymerase III and negative antinuclear antibodies. Semin Arthritis Rheum. 2020;50(5):938–42.
104. Penn H, Howie AJ, Kingdon EJ, Bunn CC, Stratton RJ, Black CM, et al. Scleroderma renal crisis: patient characteristics and long-term outcomes. QJM. 2007;100(8):485–94.
105. Hamaguchi Y, Kodera M, Matsushita T, Hasegawa M, Inaba Y, Usuda T, et al. Clinical and immunological predictors of scleroderma renal crisis for Japanese systemic sclerosis patients with anti-RNA polymerase III autoantibodies. Arthritis Rheumatol. 2015;67(4):1045–52.
106. Codullo V, Cavazzana I, Bonino C, Alpini C, Cavagna L, Cozzi F, et al. Serologic profile and mortality rates of scleroderma renal crisis in Italy. J Rheumatol. 2009;36(7):1464–9.
107. Bhavsar SV, Carmona R. Anti-RNA polymerase III antibodies in the diagnosis of scleroderma renal crisis in the absence of skin disease. J Clin Rheumatol. 2014;20(7):379–82.
108. Kuwana M. A to-do list at diagnosis of systemic sclerosis with positive anti-RNA polymerase III antibodies. J Rheumatol. 2017;44(5):550–2.
109. Coghlan JG, Denton CP, Grünig E, Bonderman D, Distler O, Khanna D, et al. Evidence-based detection of pulmonary arterial hypertension in systemic sclerosis: the DETECT study. Ann Rheum Dis. 2014;73(7):1340–9.
110. Blanco I, Mathai S, Shafiq M, Boyce D, Kolb TM, Chami H, et al. Severity of systemic sclerosis-associated pulmonary arterial hypertension in African Americans. Medicine (Baltimore). 2014;93(5):177–85.
111. Sobanski V, Giovannelli J, Lynch BM, Schreiber BE, Nihtyanova SI, Harvey J, et al. Characteristics and survival of anti-U1 RNP antibody-positive patients with connective tissue disease-associated pulmonary arterial hypertension. Arthritis Rheumatol. 2016;68(2):484–93.
112. Steen VD, Lucas M, Fertig N, Medsger TA Jr. Pulmonary arterial hypertension and severe pulmonary fibrosis in systemic sclerosis patients with a nucleolar antibody. J Rheumatol. 2007;34(11):2230–5.
113. Nunes JPL, Cunha AC, Meirinhos T, Nunes A, Araújo PM, Godinho AR, et al. Prevalence of auto-antibodies associated to pulmonary arterial hypertension in scleroderma—a review. Autoimmun Rev. 2018;17(12):1186–201.
114. McNearney TA, Reveille JD, Fischbach M, Friedman AW, Lisse JR, Goel N, et al. Pulmonary involvement in systemic sclerosis: associations with genetic, serologic, sociodemographic, and behavioral factors. Arthritis Rheum. 2007;57(2):318–26.
115. Hoffmann-Vold AM, Midtvedt Ø, Tennøe AH, Garen T, Lund MB, Aaløkken TM, et al. Cardiopulmonary disease development in anti-RNA polymerase III-positive systemic sclerosis: comparative analyses from an unselected, prospective patient cohort. J Rheumatol. 2017;44(4):459–65.
116. Assassi S, Sharif R, Lasky RE, McNearney TA, Estrada-Y-Martin RM, Draeger H, et al. Predictors of interstitial lung disease in early systemic sclerosis: a prospective longitudinal study of the GENISOS cohort. Arthritis Res Ther. 2010;12:R166.
117. Shah AA, Hummers LK, Casciola-Rosen L, Visvanathan K, Rosen A, Wigley FM. Examination of autoantibody status and clinical features that associate with cancer risk and cancer-associated scleroderma. Arthritis Rheumatol. 2015;67(4):1053–61.
118. Igusa T, Hummers LK, Visvanathan K, Richardson C, Wigley FM, Casciola-Rosen L, et al. Autoantibodies and scleroderma phenotype define subgroups at high-risk and low-risk for cancer. Ann Rheum Dis. 2018;77(8):1179–86.

119. Lazzaroni MG, Cavazzana I, Colombo E, Dobrota R, Hernandez J, Hesselstrand R, et al. Malignancies in patients with anti-RNA polymerase III antibodies and systemic sclerosis: analysis of the EULAR Scleroderma Trials and Research cohort and possible recommendations for screening. J Rheumatol. 2017;44(5):639–47.
120. Shah AA, Laiho M, Rosen A, Casciola-Rosen L. Protective effect against cancer of antibodies to the large subunits of both RNA polymerases I and III in scleroderma. Arthritis Rheumatol. 2019;71(9):1571–9.
121. Steen VD. Autoantibodies in systemic sclerosis. Semin Arthritis Rheum. 2005;35(1):35–42.
122. Hu PQ, Fertig N, Medsger TA Jr, Wright TM. Correlation of serum anti-DNA topoisomerase I antibody levels with disease severity and activity in systemic sclerosis. Arthritis Rheum. 2003;48(5):1363–73.
123. Kuwana M, Kaburaki J, Mimori T, Kawakami Y, Tojo T. Longitudinal analysis of autoantibody response to topoisomerase I in systemic sclerosis. Arthritis Rheum. 2000;43(5):1074–84.
124. Kuwana M, Okano Y, Pandey JP, Silver RM, Fertig N, Medsger TA Jr. Enzyme-linked immunosorbent assay for detection of anti-RNA polymerase III antibody: analytical accuracy and clinical associations in systemic sclerosis. Arthritis Rheum. 2005;52(8):2425–32.
125. Nihtyanova SI, Parker JC, Black CM, Bunn CC, Denton CP. A longitudinal study of anti-RNA polymerase III antibody levels in systemic sclerosis. Rheumatology (Oxford). 2009;48(10):1218–21.

Systemic Sclerosis Overlap Syndromes

8

Pia Moinzadeh and Christopher P. Denton

Definition/Classification

Systemic sclerosis (SSc) overlap syndrome is a term used to describe a very heterogeneous group of patients with features of different connective tissue diseases, combined with clinical signs of SSc [1–3].

Up to now, no firm classification criteria for SSc overlap syndromes have been established, but it is generally considered when musculoskeletal involvement or features of other rheumatic diseases are significantly greater than usually found in general SSc patients [4].

SSc as well as each of the other connective tissue disorders itself are already heterogeneous. SSc patients have been diagnosed in the past with established disease, using the American College of Rheumatology preliminary criteria (ACR), published in 1980 [5] and now based on the improved/amended EULAR/ACR criteria [6]. LeRoy et al. published, in 1988, the most widely used classification system for defining the major SSc forms, namely, those patients suffering from limited (lcSSc) and diffuse SSc (dcSSc), depending on the extent of skin thickening [7]. This classification system has been used in clinical practice and clinical trials and has been the basis for many patient registries worldwide [8].

Other autoimmune rheumatic disorders are classified depending on internationally accepted classification systems, including autoantibodies, such as anti-double stranded DNA (dsDNA) and anti-Smith antigen (Sm), for patients suffering from systemic lupus erythematosus (SLE) [2, 9], the detection of rheumatoid factor (RF) for rheumatoid arthritis [10, 11] and anti-smooth muscle antigen (SMA), and anti-liver/-kidney microsome bodies (LKM) for autoimmune hepatitis [2, 12].

Epidemiology

SSc overlap syndromes represent the third major subgroup of SSc, and epidemiological studies report divergent frequencies (incidence and prevalence rates are not reported yet) of overlap subgroups, ranging between 10 and 38% (see Table 8.2) [1–4, 18].

The most common SSc overlap syndromes are SSc/myositis (polymyositis (PM) or dermatomyositis (DM)), SSc/rheumatoid arthritis (RA), SSc/Sjogren's (SS), and SSc/systemic lupus erythematosus (SLE) overlap syndromes. SSc may also occur together with other organ-specific autoimmune diseases, such as autoimmune hepatitis/primary biliary cirrhosis (PBC), autoimmune thyroiditis, sarcoidosis, and antiphospholipid syndrome (see Table 8.2).

Pakozdi et al. reported recently that 20% of the patients attending the Centre for Rheumatology at the Royal Free Hospital had overlapping features with other rheumatologic diseases. Of these 43% overlapped with polymyositis/dermatomyositis, 8% with systemic lupus erythematosus (SLE), 17% with Sjogren's syndrome, and 32% with rheumatoid arthritis [4]. The German Network for Systemic Scleroderma (DNSS) has reported that 10% of the registered patients suffered from SSc-overlap syndromes [18].

A recent meta-analysis has revealed that the mean age at diagnosis of patients with SSc overlap syndromes was 47.6 (+2.6) years and that it was found more often in European patients than in patients from North America [19].

Balbir-Gurman reported that the overall mortality in their SSc overlap cohort did not differ from other SSc patients [3]. Depending on different geographical regions/centers, a wide range of frequencies of SSc Overlap syndromes have been reported (see Table 8.3).

P. Moinzadeh
Department of Dermatology and Venerology, University of Cologne, Cologne, Germany
e-mail: pia.moinzadeh@uk-koeln.de

C. P. Denton (✉)
Centre for Rheumatology, Royal Free Hospital, London, UK
e-mail: c.denton@ucl.ac.uk

Y. Allanore et al. (eds.), *Scleroderma*, https://doi.org/10.1007/978-3-031-40658-4_8

Pathogenesis

The pathogenesis of SSc-overlap syndromes is still not fully elucidated and likely to include generic mechanisms related to autoimmunity as well as those that are specific to systemic sclerosis or other rheumatic disorders that are intrinsic to the clinical phenotype. The question why some patients develop only one connective tissue disease and other patients a combination of clinical features of different rheumatic diseases has not been answered yet. Possibly, a common or overlapping genetic susceptibility plays an important role. Genetic studies have shown the existence of some susceptibility genes, which predispose to multiple other autoimmune diseases [19]. Koumakis has reported recently that a regulatory gene located in the TNFAIP3 region is associated with a higher risk of developing SSc with polyautoimmunity [19, 23]. A recent genome-wide meta-analysis provides powerful data supporting shared loci across seropositive rheumatic diseases [24].

While it is likely that there are shared pathogenic mechanisms between the constituents of the SSc overlap syndrome, there also appear to be specific molecular hallmarks based on studies of whole blood transcriptomics. This systematic study identified a gene set that was confined to overlap SSc as well as genes linked to SSc. This is notable because this could explain the basis of overlap susceptibility [25]. In addition, the delineation of a molecular phenotype differentiating overlap SSc offers potential for early case identification and stratification in management (see Fig. 8.1) Other published analyses using publicly available datasets have also highlighted potential differences for skin gene expression between clinical subgroups, and, in particular, a distinct gene expression pattern is associated with anti-U1-RNP [26].

In keeping with this, the shared nature of genetic associations across the autoimmune rheumatic diseases also highlights likely common mechanisms within the innate and adaptive immune systems.

An early study of mixed connective tissue disease was able to show that the class 2 MHC genotype was associated with a risk of progression and could predict whether cases were more likely to evolve into a more SSc-like phenotype over time or to SLE or RA [27].

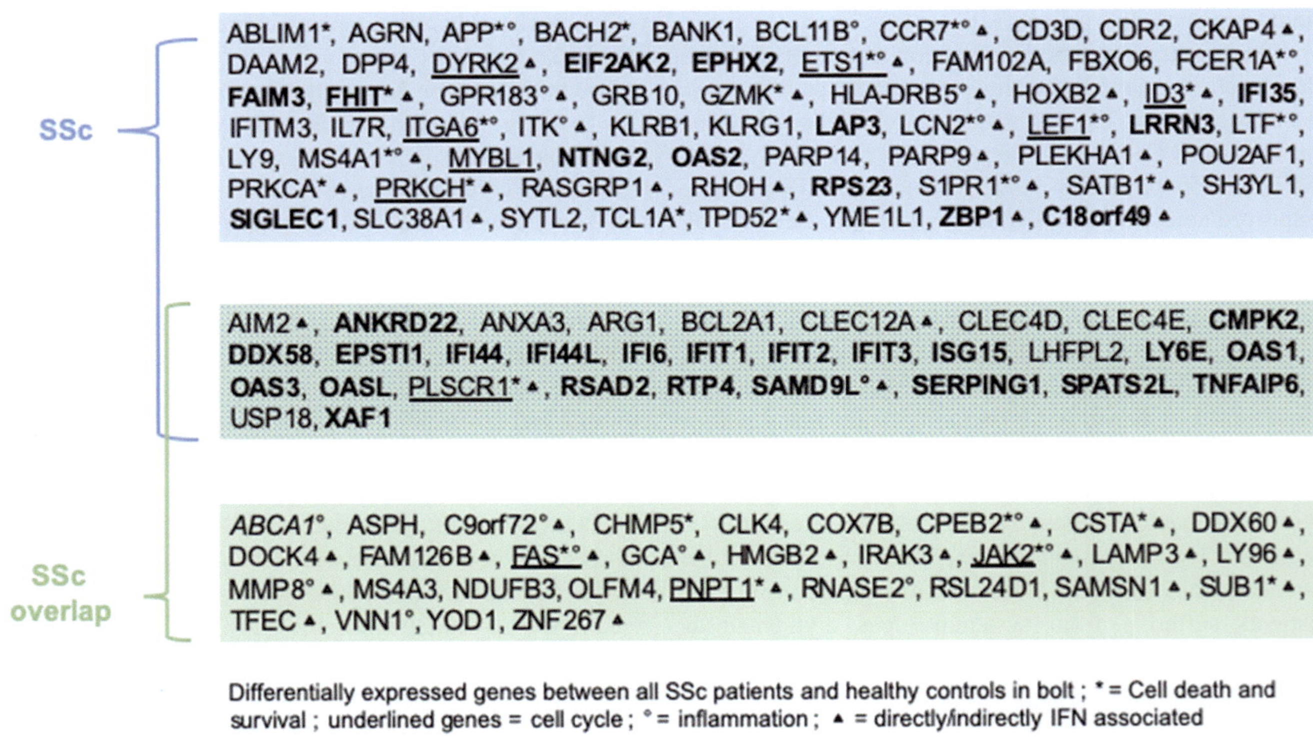

Fig. 8.1 Whole blood gene expression analysis differentiates overlap systemic sclerosis. A gene cluster discriminates overlap-SSc from non-overlap-SSc as shown and could form the basis of better molecular classification and stratification of patients. In addition, a cohort of differentially expressed genes is also associated with both the overlap and non-overlap subgroup of SSc, suggesting potentially shared pathogenic mechanisms that could have relevance to other autoimmune rheumatic diseases. Specific differentially expressed genes for SSc (blue box; FC > 1.5, FDR < 0.05) and SSc-overlap subsets (green box; FC > 2.0, FDR < 0.05) together with genes differentially expressed in both groups. (Figure reproduced from Moinzadeh P, et al. J Eur Acad Dermatol Venereol. 2020 May;34(5):e236–e238. doi: 10.1111/jdv.16198. Epub 2020 Feb 19. PMID: 31945216 [25])

SSc-Overlap Subgroups and Clinical Features

Clinical features of SSc-overlap syndrome patients are very heterogeneous; patients classified as SSc-overlap syndrome usually present with skin sclerosis typically for limited SSc, although organ manifestations clearly separate these patients as a distinct subset [18]. A German study showed that patients suffering from SSc overlap syndromes developed significantly earlier and more often an involvement of the musculoskeletal system than patients with the diffuse and limited form of SSc. Besides that, they interestingly developed lung fibrosis and heart involvement significantly earlier and more often than lcSSc patients, but still less frequently and later than dcSSc patients [18] (see Fig. 8.2).

Therefore, the identification of these patients is essential for clarifying prognosis and facilitating therapeutic options. The clinical signs include both cutaneous and extracutaneous features, depending on the overlapping connective tissue disease (CTD) and often overlap between the different overlap forms, especially regarding vasculopathy, gastrointestinal, and cardiopulmonary involvement. Recent expert guidelines for the management of fibrosing skin conditions have included specific recommendations for overlap syndromes that provide practical guidance in an area where experience and clinical expertise are valuable for clinical decision making in the absence of large clinical trial datasets [28].

Raynaud Phenomenon appears in more than 90% of SSc patients and is also a very common feature in patients with SSc-overlap syndromes (SS 20–50%, myositis 20–40%, SLE 20–30%, and RA <5%) [2]. It is usually caused by coldness and/or emotional stress and classically occurs as episodic pallor of the digits followed by cyanosis, suffusion, and/or pain and tingling. Some SSc-overlap patients also develop digital ulcerations but significantly less often compared to limited and diffuse SSc patients [18].

The Skin Sclerosis in patients with SSc-overlap syndromes can be generalized, similar to the diffuse SSc, but more frequently, it is only located below the elbow and knee joints, similar to the limited SSc form [4, 18]. The severity of the skin sclerosis, depending on the extension of thickened skin as well as the affected anatomic region, can cause all together a restricted mobility of extremities and especially joints (dermal contractures).

Calcinosis Cutis can be also observed in patients with SSc-overlap syndromes and occurs usually over pressure points (acral or next to joints). Nevertheless, patients with SSc overlap syndromes, although having limited skin sclerosis, have still a higher risk of developing severe internal organ manifestations [18]. Therefore, these patients should be seen as a separate SSc-subset.

The **Involvement of the Gastrointestinal Tract** is probably the most common internal organ system involved in patients suffering from SSc and SSc overlap syndromes (around 50–60%) [18, 22]. The clinical features include dysphagia, retrosternal discomfort due to reflux/esophagitis, and bowel disease with hypomotility. This all might lead to weight loss, cachexia, diarrhea, pseudo-obstruction, and malabsorption.

Lung Fibrosis and Myocardial Involvement is significantly less frequent than in patients with diffuse SSc but significantly more frequent than in patients diagnosed with the limited form of SSc [18]. The clinical features of cardiac and pulmonary involvement are very similar and overlapping. Distinguishing clinical features, such as dyspnea, nonproductive cough, disturbed diffusion capacity, and cyanosis, can be an important management challenge.

Pulmonary Arterial Hypertension (PAH) occurs less frequent in patients with SSc overlap syndromes, while

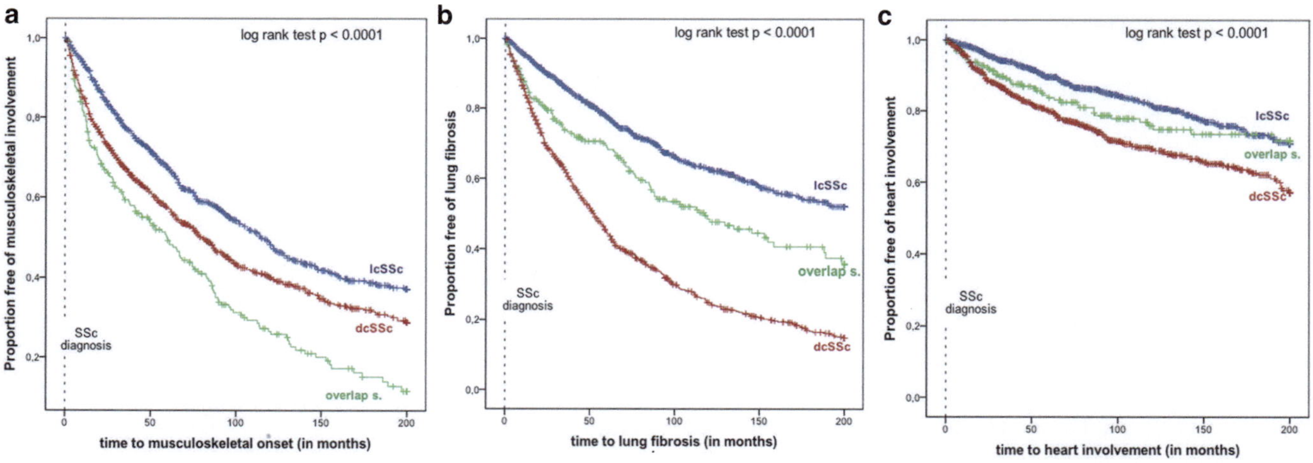

Fig. 8.2 Kaplan Meier curves indicate a clear difference between SSc overlap syndrome patients and patients with lcSSc or dcSSc, especially for musculoskeletal involvement (**a**), lung fibrosis (**b**), and heart involvement (**c**) [18]

lung fibrosis occurs less frequently in SSc overlap syndromes than in patients with diffuse SSc but clearly more often than in patients with limited SSc [18]. It is notable that patients with overlap syndromes who develop PAH may fall into the group of cases that benefit from immunosuppression alongside their specific PAH therapy. This has been shown in several studies [29]. A recent review of PAH patients with anti-U1-RNP identified those with an MCT phenotype (see below) as well as those with features of SSc or SLE. There were differences between the hemodynamic characteristics of these patient groups that reflect the associated CTD. It is considered that these cases will generally benefit from immunosuppressive therapy alongside targeted PAH treatments to secure the best long-term outcome, although as expected those with MCTD or SLE had better survival than those with a more typical SSc phenotype [30].

Further Organ Manifestation Depending on SSc Overlap Syndromes

Systemic Sclerosis and Myositis—Myositis is the most frequent systemic involvement in patients with SSc overlap syndromes (frequency ranging between 5.3 and 60.1%). In some SSc patients, muscle weakness, pain, and atrophy result from disuse secondary to joint contractures, skin contractures, or chronic disease. However, significantly more patients with SSc overlap syndromes present with musculoskeletal involvement, associated with poly- or dermatomyositis, characterized by myalgia, muscle weakness, and atrophy of muscles. Patients suffering from SSc/myositis overlap syndrome may develop myositis simultaneously, before or in already established SSc [3]. Additional main clinical features besides muscle involvement are arthralgia, RP, and sclerotic skin thickening [2].

The Raynaud phenomenon is present in 20–40% of SSc/myositis overlap patients [2]. A generalized extent of skin thickening is interestingly more often prevalent in patients with the SSc/myositis overlap syndrome, compared to other overlap forms [3, 4]. Comparing the limited and diffuse skin sclerosis within each overlap syndrome demonstrates that the limited extent of skin thickening is still the most frequent form [3, 4].

Recent studies have shown that an increased proportion of patients develop also lung fibrosis [18, 31]. Patients with SSc/myositis overlap syndromes have a higher risk of developing diffuse interstitial myocardial fibrosis, which may lead to diastolic dysfunctions as well as restricted contractibility of the myocardium. These patients typically present symptoms, such as cardiac arrhythmia, paroxysmal tachycardia, and incomplete or complete right-heart blocks, finally leading to heart insufficiency. The frequency of lung and gastrointestinal involvement varies among studies, ranging between 32.0 and 78.1% [1]. It is well established that patients suffering from the SSc/polymyositis overlap have a worse prognosis due to an increased risk of myocardial involvement, compared to patients with only SSc 32].

SSc myositis overlap syndromes may be associated with specific autoantibodies, including PmScl, anti-Ku, anti-U2RNP, and anti-U5snRNP [3, 32]. Patients carrying the antibody to PmScl usually are younger, have limited skin involvement, and suffer from arthritis and a benign course of interstitial lung disease (ILD) [3], which is also the reason for their better survival [15]. Positive antibodies against Ku are more characteristic for patients suffering from muscle involvement as well as severe ILD [33] (see Table 8.1).

Systemic sclerosis and Rheumatoid Arthritis (RA)—Inflammatory joint involvement is reported to be the second most frequent manifestation in patients with musculoskeletal involvement and overlap syndromes [4]. These patients often present with typical clinical symptoms (usually limited skin involvement) together with high titers of anti-cyclic citrullinated peptides (CCP/ACPA) and/or higher rheumatoid factors (RF). It is often very difficult to distinguish between SSc patients with mild, sero-negative arthralgia, and significant arthritis associated with SSc/RA-overlap syndrome. In 2012, Gheita and Hussein found significantly increased COMP levels in SSc patients with arthritis, indicating that COMP levels may become a marker for joint involvement in SSc patients [17].

Table 8.1 SSc overlap syndromes and associated autoantibodies

SSc overlap syndrome	Autoantibodies directed against
Mixed connective tissue disease	Anti-U1snRNP (specific), found in 75–90% of MCTD patients [13, 14]
SSc/Myositis overlap syndrome	Anti-PmScl (specific) [15] Anti-Ku, -U1RNP, -Scl70, -Jo1, -Ro/SSA, -U3RNP, -RNA-Polymerase have also been reported [1] Anti-RuvBL1/2 antibody is a new SSc-related autoantibody, associated with muscle involvement and diffuse skin thickening [16]
SSc/rheumatoid arthritis overlap syndrome	High titers of RF (60–72%), ACPA (prevalence of 64%) [1] ACPA is more frequent in patients with RA features in SSc patients [4] Anti-Scl-70 and anti-ACA antibodies have been reported [4] COMP level may become a nonspecific marker for joint involvement [17]
SSc/Sjogren's overlap syndrome	Anti-Ro/SSA and -La/SSB have been reported [1, 4] Clearly more often associated with anti-ACA [1, 4]
SSc/SLE overlap syndrome	Anti-dsDNA together with anti-Scl70 antibodies have been reported [1] Also, single cases with anti-ACA and -PmScl have been reported [1]

Table 8.2 Rare cases of SSc overlap syndromes [3]

SSc Overlap syndrome with	Definition
Antiphospholipid syndrome	• Incidence varies between 7 and 13% [3] • Presence of lupus anticoagulant, anti-cardiolipin, or anti-ß2-glycoprotein-1 antibodies has been reported in SSc patients [3] and has been associated with severe ischemia, PAH, digital loss, and thromboembolism
Sarcoidosis	• Rare variant of SSc overlap syndrome • Elevated temperature, weight loss, and biliary adenopathy have been shown in SSc sarcoidosis overlap syndromes • Lung and lymph node biopsy is necessary to define the disease [3]
PBC	• Prevalence ranges between 7 and 15% • Mostly associated with lcSSc • Positive ACA in PBC patients reveals a higher risk for lcSSc • Often clinically silent, but anti-mitochondrial antibodies, elevation of cholestatic enzymes as well as hyperglobulinemia is possible [3]

Table 8.3 Frequencies of different SSc overlap syndromes [1]

SSc overlap syndrome		Total
Patients with SSc	118 [20], 719 [21], 1483 [22], 165 [3], 1700 [4], 2425 [15]	6610 [1]
SSc overlap syndromes	32.2% [20], 38% [21], 10.9% [22], 24.2% [3], 20% [4], 9.2% [15]	16.2% [1]
SSc/PM or SSc/DM overlap syndrome	5.3% [20], 47.5% [3], 42.8% [4], 60.1% [15]	44.6% [1]
SSc/Sjogren's overlap syndrome	26.3% [20], 18% [21], 42.5% [3], 16.8% [4]	18.5% [1]
SSc/rheumatoid arthritis overlap syndrome	8% [20], 21.1% [21], 15.4% [3], 32% [4], 6.2% [15]	19.3% [1]

Systemic Sclerosis and Systemic Lupus Erythematosus (SLE)—This subtype is a very rare condition [34]. Patients often have a fatal course of the disease due to a higher risk of developing polyserositis, pancreatitis, avascular bone necrosis, PAH, lung involvement, lupus glomerulonephritis, skin rashes, and leukoencephalopathy [3]. It is also difficult to distinguish whether the patient suffers from a lupus nephritis or a scleroderma renal crisis. Depending on the reason for renal failure, patients need a different therapeutic strategy to improve renal function. Skin lesions can be a major esthetic disturbing factor, because of the predilection area, the face. In addition, oral lesions may reduce the quality of life, due to the pain of ulcerations and difficulties eating. Usually, these patients have a combination of SSc-associated antibodies and double-stranded DNA antibodies.

Systemic Sclerosis and Sjogren's Syndrome (SS)—This SSc overlap syndrome has been firstly described in 1965 by Bloch et al. [35]. Oral (xerostomia) and ocular sicca symptoms (xerophthalmia) are very common in patients suffering from SSc (68–83%), but only 14–20% of SSc patients really fulfill the criteria of Sjogren's syndrome [36], so that the diagnosis of SSc/SS overlap syndromes is always a challenge [37]. It is defined as a lymphocytic infiltration of the salivary glands. Patients with SSc/SS overlap syndrome show a limited form of skin involvement (83.6% versus 16.4%) and a very low frequency of lung involvement [3]. Antibodies against Ro are very likely in SSc/SS overlap syndromes, often together with ACA antibodies [4]. Anti-Ro and -La antibodies have been present in 38.8% of cases, but unfortunately, none of these antibodies can be used as a serological marker. One recent study has shown that ACA positivity allows the identification of SS overlap syndromes (not limited to SSc) [38]. It has more recently been suggested that ACA+ lcSSc can overlap with Sjogren's and represent a distinct grouping of patients at high risk of lymphoma [39].

Mixed-Connective Tissue Disease (MCTD)—First described by Sharp and colleagues in 1972 [40]. These patients present clinical symptoms typically found in patients with polymyositis/dermatomyositis, SLE, inflammatory arthritis (RA), and scleroderma (SSc). Typical for this condition are puffy fingers (50%), polyarthritis (65%), RP (53%), sclerodactyly (35%), muscle involvement and esophageal involvement [14, 41], and the occurrence of high ANA titers with high levels of U1snRNP antibodies, helping to differentiate the MCTD from other connective tissue diseases. Arthralgia occurs in approximately 60% of patients, while muscle disease is present in 80–90% of cases with proximal muscle involvement and elevation of serum creatine kinase levels (CK) [41]. Cardiovascular involvement (lung fibrosis and especially PAH) is less frequent but is the major contributor to a poor outcome/prognosis [14]. Immunogenetic studies have shown an association between the major histocompatibility complex (MHC), HLA-DR4, and -DR2 and the presence of U1snRNP antibodies [2, 42]. Paradowska-Gorycka et al. have shown in their study of 66 MCTD patients that Il-10 gene variants may be considered a genetic risk factor for MCTD susceptibility [43]. These patients also develop frequently the sicca syndrome. Many patients suffer from esophagus and lung involvement. There have recently been published expert recommendations on the management of MCTD that provide a clear template for investigation and treatment but also highlight the need for specific research to address unmet needs for patients in an area that has previously not received focus due to it falling outside single disease classification criteria [44] Recent well-conducted cohort studies from a large Australian registry of SSc [45]

Table 8.4 Autoantibodies associated with SSc overlap syndromes

Autoantibodies	Definition
U1snRNP	• Hallmark antibody for MCTD in high titers [32] • Patients with high titers evolve into MCTD usually over 2 years [32] • Positive in 75–90% of MCTD cases, compared to just 20–50% of SLE cases [14] • Seem to interact with the lung tissue, contributing to disease features [14]
PmScl	• Serological marker for SSc/polymyositis overlap syndrome [25] • Also found in other connective tissue diseases [25] • Directed predominantly against two molecules of 100 kDa and 75 kDa [4836] • Strongly associated with HLA-DQA1*0501, HLA-DQB1*02—DRB1*0301 [25] • Patients were younger and showed more frequently limited cutaneous involvement [15] • Overall survival was significantly better in PmScl-positive patients [15] • 33.1% of SSc/PM overlap syndrome carry this antibody [4]
Jo1	
Ku	• Heterodimer, including a 70 kDa and 80 kDa peptide bound to a 350 kDa AND-dependent protein kinase [35] • 2.3–55% of patients with SSc/PM OS were positive for Ku antibodies • Also found in other connective tissue diseases [35] • Not predictive for prognosis of the disease and also not associated with cancer risk
dsDNA	• In 70% of SLE patients but very rare in SSc patients [27] • In two cases patients with Scl70 and dsDNA antibodies have been reported [27, 47]
RuvBL1/ RuvBL2	• Novel SSc-associated antibody [16] • Associated with diffuse skin sclerosis and musculoskeletal involvement (myositis overlap) [16]

have highlighted the differences between patients fulfilling classification criteria for MCTD compared with other SSc overlap cases with demographic factors as well as outcome and frequency of major complications such as PAH being different. This highlights the importance of a better definition of cases and the potential value of molecular approaches to early differentiation of these subtypes of SSc [25].

Systemic Sclerosis and Vasculitis—Although vasculopathy is universal in systemic sclerosis, some patients develop additional features of vasculitis. This can occur in the context of overlap with SLE, rheumatoid arthritis, or Sjogren's syndrome when it manifests most often as a cutaneous vasculitis. However, a subset of patients demonstrates overlap with ANCA-associated vasculitis. This is reported in several case series. It is important in the context of acute kidney injury, which may be due to scleroderma renal crisis but also can occur due to ANCA-associated vasculitis, leading to glomerulonephritis or intra-renal arteritis. Most cases of SSc and AAV demonstrate an anti-myeloperoxidase p-ANCA pattern. These cases are especially associated with lung fibrosis. The c-ANCA staining pattern with proteinase-3 specificity on ELISA is much less frequent but can be associated with severe organ-based complications of vasculitis [46]. Cohort studies of pulmonary arterial hypertension in SSc have also highlighted that some overlap SSc patients have an inflammatory pulmonary vasculopathy that responds to immunosuppression. Thus, in those overlap syndromes that have features of SLE or MCTD (see above), immunosuppression should be given alongside PAH-specific therapy to secure the best long-term outcomes. This has been well illustrated in recent cohort studies [30]. The recent reports that SSc-PAH associated with ACA+ may benefit from treatment with rituximab are further indirect evidence that inflammatory vasculopathy is a component process in some cases of lcSSc. Table 8.4 summarizes autoantibody features of overlap SSc.

Diagnostics

Vasculopathy (Raynaud phenomenon)—To identify a secondary Raynaud Phenomenon (RP) and predict the further course of the disease, two simple and non-invasive procedures are essential, namely, the assessment of serum autoantibodies and the nailfold capillaroscopy [48, 49].

Skin Sclerosis—Careful mapping of the degree and extent of skin involvement is the single best clinical technique. This helps to suggest/predict the risk for further organ manifestations. The most widely used technique is the modified Rodnan Skin Score (mRSS), consisting of a 0–3 grading at 17 skin sites (maximum score 51) [50, 51].

Muscle Involvement (myositis/myopathy)—Elevation of serum creatine phosphokinase, ESR, possible changes on electromyography (EMG), and histological assessment of a muscle biopsy as well as an MRI of the affected muscles are helpful to identify muscle inflammation and/or atrophy [52, 53]. Typical histopathological features are perivascular inflammatory infiltrates with focal replacement of myofibrils with collagen and perimysial and epimysial fibrosis.

Involvement of the Gastrointestinal Tract—The presence of esophagitis can be determined by upper GI endoscopy with histological evaluations. Hypomotility can usually be diagnosed by esophagus scintigraphy or esophagogastrocolposcopy [53, 54].

Cardiopulmonary Involvement—All patients with systemic sclerosis and SSc-overlap syndromes should be followed up by using the pulmonary function test, echocardiography, 6-min walk test, and high-resolution computerized tomography (HRCT), to determine a possible cardio-pulmonary involvement. To detect fibrotic changes in the myocardium, non-invasive imaging techniques, such as MRI or spiral CT scanning, may be indicated, besides indirect clues of cardiac involvement, which may be deduced from ECG or echocardiographic studies [53]. Conduction defects are the most frequently observed disturbances, up to complete heart block necessitating pacemaker implantation. In addition, the use of N-terminal brain natriuretic peptide (NTproBNP) in patient serum is helpful in detecting right ventricular impairment [55].

Kidney Involvement—Creatinine clearance, urine sediments to control proteinuria and hematuria, as well as regular blood pressure tests, are necessary for the early identification of renal involvement [53, 56]. In the case of SSc-SLE overlap syndromes, it is sometimes necessary to take a kidney biopsy to distinguish between renal failures due to lupus nephritis [57] or scleroderma renal crisis [56].

Sicca Symptoms—Due to a reduced glandular function, especially patients with SSc-Sjogrens syndrome suffer from dry mouth (xerostomia) and dry eyes (xerophthalmia). Medical history, the assessment of ANAs (anti-Ro and anti-La antibodies) as well as the Schirmer test for ocular sicca symptoms together with a glandular biopsy can be helpful in defining a possible Sjogren's syndrome [58].

Joint Involvement—Joint involvement might be due to dermatogenous contractures but also due to inflammation. It is recommendable to examine the rheumatoid factor and CCP-antibodies in the serum of affected patients. An X ray of affected joints as well as MRI scans are helpful in identifying inflammation areas and damage to the joints [53].

Management of SSc-Overlap Syndromes

There have been major advances in treating many of the organ-specific complications of systemic sclerosis and overlapping diseases. Most of the patients are treated with standard drugs, which are usually used in specific rheumatic disorders. Sometimes shared clinical symptoms between SSc and other connective tissue diseases complicate the decision of treatment strategy. Treatment strategies are summarized in Table 8.5.

Systemic Glucocorticoids—Systemic glucocorticoids can be used for musculoskeletal involvement together with other immunosuppressive agents. It can be combined with other drugs or just as monotherapy. The use of high-dose corticosteroids has to be used with caution due to the increased risk in patients with diffuse extent of skin involvement to induce a renal crisis [1].

Table 8.5 SSc-associated therapeutic strategies, including disease-modifying drugs

Clinical feature	Therapeutic strategies
Raynaud phenomenon	• General recommendations: Avoid coldness, keep body warm, paraffin bath, heatable soles and gloves • Vitamins and supplements: Fish oil capsules, antioxidant vitamins, *Ginko biloba* • Oral treatments: Calcium channel blockers, angiotensin-II-receptor 1 blocker, or phosphodiesterase type 5 inhibitor (not licensed, trial in severe cases) • Topical treatment: GTN patches • Intravenous treatment: Prostacyclin infusion • Surgical treatment: Lumbar sympathectomy, radical microaretriolysis
Skin	
Skin thickening	• General recommendations: Skin care with moisturizing crème or ointments • Physical treatments: Lymphatic drainage/ physiotherapy, phototherapy • Topical treatment: Steroids or calcineurin inhibitors • Systemic treatment: Steroids usually short duration due to side effects and risk of renal crisis), methotrexate, Mycophenolate mofetil [68–72], or cyclophosphamide (trials have shown significant improvement in mRSS) CAVE: Side effects have to be balanced
Calcinosis cutis	• General recommendations: Improve blood flow and treat infection • Local corticosteroid injections, laser therapy, surgery, minocycline, or bisphosphonate p.o.
Teleangiectases	• Laser therapy and/or camouflage
Gastrointestinal involvement	
Reflux	• General recommendations: Bed head elevated during the night, small meals • Oral treatments: Proton pump inhibitors, prokinetics, and/or H_2 receptor antagonists
Dysphagia	• General recommendations: Change your habit of eating, small meals • Oral treatments: Prokinetics
GAVE	• Argon plasma coagulation
Diarrhea Constipation	• General recommendations: Change the habit of eating • Oral treatments: Prokinetics, antibiotics, and laxative
Scleroderma renal crisis	• Systemic treatments: ACE inhibitors (high-dosed) under blood pressure monitoring, Iloprost intravenous
Respiratory system	
Lung fibrosis	• Systemic treatments: Cyclophosphamide orally or intravenous, Glucocorticosteroids (short term), azathioprine orally, mycophenolate mofetil orally, and Nintedanib orally Oxygen (if needed)
PAH	• Systemic treatments: Endothelin receptor blockers (e.g., macitentan), NO stimulants (e.g., sildenafil and riociguat), and prostacyclin agonists (e.g., epoprostenol and selexipag) Oxygen (if needed)
Cardiac myopathy	• Systemic treatments: Cyclophosphamide orally or intravenous, glucocorticosteroids (short-dated), azathioprine orally, and mycophenolate mofetil orally Pacemaker (if needed)

Methotrexate—Methotrexate is a well-known immunosuppressive agent, which has been used in adults and children, with long experience of well-documented side effects. MTX is still a first-line therapy in many autoimmune diseases. It is the treatment of choice in patients with SSc/myositis and SSc/RA overlap syndromes [59, 60] but has to be used with caution in patients with alveolitis or patients with liver damage or alcohol use.

Mycophenolate Mofetil—MMF is a well-tolerated immunosuppressive agent, which is increasingly used for many autoimmune diseases. It is recommended as long-term therapy in scleroderma and has successfully been applied in several overlap syndromes, which respond well.

Azathioprine—*This immunosuppressive agent is usually well tolerated and has been used successfully in patients with MCTD as well as patients with SSc/SLE overlap. However, compared to MMF, side effects seem to be more pronounced and the response to the therapy is more limited.*

Cyclophosphamide—Often used for lung involvement in patients with SSc [61] and also SSc/myositis overlap or SSc/SLE overlap syndromes, in case of lupus nephritis. Cyclophosphamide should be used as a second-line immunosuppressive therapy after the others (MTX and MMF) have failed or cannot be used due to defined side effects. Similar to other autoimmune diseases, it can be used as i.v. pulse or oral treatment.

Specific Immunomodulatory Agents—For IVIG and anti-TNF therapy, only limited information is available for overlap syndromes. B-cell depletion by rituximab was initially described to be of only limited benefit in patients with scleroderma. More recent studies, however, have demonstrated better results, and there are several case reports demonstrating that rituximab can be successfully used in patients with overlap syndromes, especially if these are characterized by inflammatory muscle involvement. Certainly, long-term follow-ups of these patients are still missing, and no data are yet available for more potent B-cell depleting agents. However, a clear clinical classification of this heterogeneous group of patients is required to allow the appropriate clinical studies.

Nintedanib, a tyrosine kinase inhibitor, has shown antifibrotic and anti-inflammatory effects in preclinical models of SSc and other forms of ILD. The effect of nintedanib on SSc-associated ILD has been investigated within the SENCIS study and has shown that the annual rate of decline in FVC was lower with nintedanib than with placebo; however, there was no clinical benefit of nintedanib was observed for other manifestations of SSc [62].

Systemic Sclerosis and Myositis—In this group of patients, treatment is mainly directed against alveolitis, muscle inflammation, and skin sclerosis. Intravenous pulsed glucocorticoid therapy (not in patients with a higher risk for renal crisis), methotrexate (not in case of alveolitis), azathioprine, IVIG, and rituximab (in patients with uncontrolled myositis) may be helpful agents. Specifically in patients with PmScl-positive overlap syndrome, the mild form of myositis responds very well to low dosages of corticosteroids. Mycophenolate mofetil can be used in patients, in whom skin sclerosis is the predominant clinical feature, and cyclophosphamide is usually used in patients, in whom alveolitis causes the most severe symptoms. IVIG has also shown a clear benefit in patients with myositis and interestingly has also shown an improvement in skin and gastrointestinal involvement [3, 63]. Some case reports have shown that Rituximab was effective in patients with uncontrolled myositis and also helped to improve alveolitis and skin involvement [64, 65].

Systemic Sclerosis and Rheumatoid Arthritis—These patients are usually treated with methotrexate, anti-TNF agents as well as with tocilizumab. All these treatments have to be used with caution, especially regarding serious infections, tuberculosis, and fibrosis. Infliximab and etanercept have shown controversial results, partly improving and partly causing more problems, like lupus-like disease [3]. Due to increased Il6 levels in the serum of patients with rheumatoid arthritis and also in patients with SSc, tocilizumab has been approved for patients with rheumatoid arthritis and has been used in clinical trials of SSc.

Systemic Sclerosis and Systemic Lupus Erythematosus—The treatment of renal involvement differs between a lupus and a scleroderma-associated renal failure (cyclophosphamide versus vasoactive treatment with iloprost and ace inhibitors). SLE-driven PAH has to be treated with immunosuppressive agents, corticosteroids, or cytotoxic drugs, such as cyclophosphamide. Vasodilators, such as iloprost, endothelin receptor antagonists, or phosphodiesterase 5 inhibitors, are necessary to reduce pulmonary hypertension. Specifically in patients with a diffuse extent of skin involvement, the use and dosage of corticosteroids have to be considered very carefully due to the increased risk of triggering an SSc-related renal crisis.

Case studies have shown a positive effect of rituximab and MMF in SLE patients and should be considered for SSc-SLE overlap patients [3].

Mixed Connective Tissue Disease (MCTD)—Patients with MCTD usually respond well to systemic corticosteroid and immunosuppressive therapy with several classical agents. However, some long-term studies have shown that a group of patients with MCTD develops more severe organ manifestations and needs a more aggressive therapeutic strategy. Inflammatory features (elevated temperature, serositis, pleuritis, myositis, and arthritis) respond well to steroid treatment, while symptoms, such as sclerotic skin changes and cardiopulmonary involvement, need immunosuppressive/cytotoxic drugs [32, 66]. The most frequently used drugs are cyclophosphamide and methotrexate as well as hydroxychloroquine [32].

Systemic Sclerosis and Sjogren's Overlap Syndrome—Usually, clinical features, such as the xerostomia, can be improved by using various antiseptic mouth rinse as well as saliva substitutes. In addition, the xerophthalmia can be improved by using artificial tear drops [67]. Furthermore, it has been reported that patients with primary SS nonsteroidal anti-rheumatic drugs or low dosages of corticosteroids, as well as immunomodulatory drugs, such as hydroxychloroquine, azathioprine, methotrexate, and rituximab, have been effective in open-label studies, but data about Sc/SS overlap syndromes are lacking [66, 67].

References

1. Iaccarino L, Gatto M, Bettio S, et al. Overlap connective tissue disease syndromes. Autoimmun Rev. 2013;12:363–73. Epub 2012/06/30.
2. Jury EC, D'Cruz D, Morrow WJ. Autoantibodies and overlap syndromes in autoimmune rheumatic disease. J Clin Pathol. 2001;54:340–7. Epub 2001/05/01.
3. Balbir-Gurman A, Braun-Moscovici Y. Scleroderma overlap syndrome. Israel Med Assoc J. 2011;13:14–20. Epub 2011/03/31.
4. Pakozdi A, Nihtyanova S, Moinzadeh P, et al. Clinical and serological hallmarks of systemic sclerosis overlap syndromes. J Rheumatol. 2011;38:2406–9. Epub 2011/08/17.
5. Preliminary criteria for the classification of systemic sclerosis (scleroderma). Subcommittee for scleroderma criteria of the American Rheumatism Association Diagnostic and Therapeutic Criteria Committee. Arthritis Rheum. 1980;23:581–90. Epub 1980/05/01.
6. van den Hoogen F, Khanna D, Fransen J, et al. 2013 classification criteria for systemic sclerosis: an American College of Rheumatology/European league against rheumatism collaborative initiative. Arthritis Rheum. 2013;65:2737–47. Epub 2013/10/15.
7. LeRoy EC, Black C, Fleischmajer R, et al. Scleroderma (systemic sclerosis): classification, subsets and pathogenesis. J Rheumatol. 1988;15:202–5. Epub 1988/02/01.
8. Galluccio F, Walker UA, Nihtyanova S, et al. Registries in systemic sclerosis: a worldwide experience. Rheumatology (Oxford). 2011;50:60–8. Epub 2010/12/15.
9. Tan EM, Cohen AS, Fries JF, et al. The 1982 revised criteria for the classification of systemic lupus erythematosus. Arthritis Rheum. 1982;25:1271–7. Epub 1982/11/01.
10. Kay J, Upchurch KS. ACR/EULAR 2010 rheumatoid arthritis classification criteria. Rheumatology (Oxford). 2012;51 Suppl 6:vi5–9. Epub 2012/12/19.
11. Arnett FC, Edworthy SM, Bloch DA, et al. The American Rheumatism Association 1987 revised criteria for the classification of rheumatoid arthritis. Arthritis Rheum. 1988;31:315–24. Epub 1988/03/01.
12. Johnson PJ, McFarlane IG. Meeting report: International Autoimmune Hepatitis Group. Hepatology. 1993;18:998–1005. Epub 1993/10/01.
13. Habets WJ, de Rooij DJ, Salden MH, et al. Antibodies against distinct nuclear matrix proteins are characteristic for mixed connective tissue disease. Clin Exp Immunol. 1983;54:265–76. Epub 1983/10/01.
14. Tani C, Carli L, Vagnani S, et al. The diagnosis and classification of mixed connective tissue disease. J Autoimmun. 2014;48–49:46–9. Epub 2014/01/28.
15. Koschik RW 2nd, Fertig N, Lucas MR, et al. Anti-PM-Scl antibody in patients with systemic sclerosis. Clin Exp Rheumatol. 2012;30:S12–6. Epub 2012/01/21.
16. Kaji K, Fertig N, Medsger TA Jr, et al. Autoantibodies to RuvBL1 and RuvBL2: a novel systemic sclerosis-related antibody associated with diffuse cutaneous and skeletal muscle involvement. Arthritis Care Res. 2014;66:575–84. Epub 2013/09/12.
17. Gheita TA, Hussein H. Cartilage Oligomeric Matrix Protein (COMP) in systemic sclerosis (SSc): role in disease severity and subclinical rheumatoid arthritis overlap. Joint Bone Spine. 2012;79:51–6. Epub 2011/04/19.
18. Moinzadeh P, Aberer E, Ahmadi-Simab K, Blank N, Distler JHW, Fierlbeck G, Genth E, Guenther C, Hein R, Henes J, Herich L, Herrgott I, Koetter I, Kreuter A, Krieg T, Kuhr K, Lorenz H-M, Meier F, Melchers I, Mensing H, Mueller-Ladner U, Pfeiffer C, Riemekasten G, Sárdy M, Schmalzing M, Sunderkoetter C, Susok L, Tarner IH, Vaith P, Worm M, Wozel G, Zeidler G, Hunzelmann N. Disease progression in systemic sclerosis-overlap syndrome is significantly different from limited and diffuse cutaneous systemic sclerosis. Ann Rheum Dis. 2015;74:730–7. https://doi.org/10.1136/annrheumdis-2013-204487.
19. Elhai M, Avouac J, Kahan A, et al. Systemic sclerosis at the crossroad of polyautoimmunity. Autoimmun Rev. 2013;12:1052–7. Epub 2013/06/25.
20. Caramaschi P, Biasi D, Volpe A, et al. Coexistence of systemic sclerosis with other autoimmune diseases. Rheumatol Int. 2007;27:407–10. Epub 2006/10/19.
21. Hudson M, Rojas-Villarraga A, Coral-Alvarado P, et al. Polyautoimmunity and familial autoimmunity in systemic sclerosis. J Autoimmun. 2008;31:156–9. Epub 2008/07/23.
22. Hunzelmann N, Genth E, Krieg T, et al. The registry of the German Network for Systemic Scleroderma: frequency of disease subsets and patterns of organ involvement. Rheumatology (Oxford). 2008;47:1185–92. Epub 2008/06/03.
23. Koumakis E, Dieude P, Avouac J, et al. Familial autoimmunity in systemic sclerosis—results of a French-based case-control family study. J Rheumatol. 2012;39:532–8. Epub 2012/01/17.
24. Acosta-Herrera M, Kerick M, González-Serna D, Wijmenga C, Franke A, Gregersen PK, Padyukov L, Worthington J, Vyse TJ, Alarcón-Riquelme ME, Mayes MD, Martin J. Genome-wide meta-analysis reveals shared new loci in systemic seropositive rheumatic diseases. Ann Rheum Dis. 2019;78:311–9. https://doi.org/10.1136/annrheumdis-2018-214127.
25. Moinzadeh P, Frommolt P, Franitza M, Toliat MR, Becker K, Nürnberg P, Nihtyanova SI, Ahrazoglu M, Belz D, Hunzelmann N, Abraham D, Ong VH, Mouthon L, Hesselstrand R, Denton CP, Krieg T. Whole blood gene expression profiling distinguishes systemic sclerosis-overlap syndromes from other subsets. J Eur Acad Dermatol Venereol. 2020;34:e236–8. https://doi.org/10.1111/jdv.16198.
26. Inamo J. Association of differentially expressed genes and autoantibody type in patients with systemic sclerosis. Rheumatology (Oxford). 2021;60:929–39. https://doi.org/10.1093/rheumatology/keaa447.
27. Gendi NS, Welsh KI, Van Venrooij WJ, Vancheeswaran R, Gilroy J, Black CM. HLA type as a predictor of mixed connective tissue disease differentiation. Ten-year clinical and immunogenetic followup of 46 patients. Arthritis Rheum. 1995;38:259–66. https://doi.org/10.1002/art.1780380216.
28. Jais X, Launay D, Yaici A, Le Pavec J, Tchérakian C, Sitbon O, Simonneau G, Humbert M. Immunosuppressive therapy in lupus- and mixed connective tissue disease-associated pulmonary arterial hypertension: a retrospective analysis of twenty-three cases. Arthritis Rheum. 2008 Feb;58(2):521–31. https://doi.org/10.1002/art.23303.

29. Sobanski V, Giovannelli J, Lynch BM, Schreiber BE, Nihtyanova SI, Harvey J, Handler CE, Denton CP, Coghlan JG. Characteristics and survival of anti-U1 RNP antibody-positive patients with connective tissue disease-associated pulmonary arterial hypertension. Arthritis Rheumatol. 2016;68:484–93. https://doi.org/10.1002/art.39432.
30. Bhansing KJ, Lammens M, Knaapen HK, et al. Scleroderma-polymyositis overlap syndrome versus idiopathic polymyositis and systemic sclerosis: a descriptive study on clinical features and myopathology. Arthritis Res Ther. 2014;16:R111. Epub 2014/06/03.
31. Mahler M, Raijmakers R. Novel aspects of autoantibodies to the PM/Scl complex: clinical, genetic and diagnostic insights. Autoimmun Rev. 2007;6:432–7. Epub 2007/07/24.
32. Rigolet A, Musset L, Dubourg O, et al. Inflammatory myopathies with anti-Ku antibodies: a prognosis dependent on associated lung disease. Medicine. 2012;91:95–102. Epub 2012/03/07.
33. Lin HK, Wang JD, Fu LS. Juvenile diffuse systemic sclerosis/systemic lupus erythematosus overlap syndrome—a case report. Rheumatol Int. 2012;32:1809–11. Epub 2011/05/03.
34. Bloch KJ, Buchanan WW, Wohl MJ, et al. Sjoegren's syndrome. A clinical, pathological, and serological study of sixty-two cases. Medicine. 1965;44:187–231. Epub 1965/05/01.
35. Ramos-Casals M, Brito-Zeron P, Font J. The overlap of Sjogren's syndrome with other systemic autoimmune diseases. Semin Arthritis Rheum. 2007;36:246–55. Epub 2006/09/26.
36. Avouac J, Sordet C, Depinay C, et al. Systemic sclerosis-associated Sjogren's syndrome and relationship to the limited cutaneous subtype: results of a prospective study of sicca syndrome in 133 consecutive patients. Arthritis Rheum. 2006;54:2243–9. Epub 2006/06/28.
37. Salliot C, Gottenberg JE, Bengoufa D, et al. Anticentromere antibodies identify patients with Sjogren's syndrome and autoimmune overlap syndrome. J Rheumatol. 2007;34:2253–8. Epub 2007/10/17.
38. Baldini C, Mosca M, Della Rossa A, Pepe P, Notarstefano C, Ferro F, Luciano N, Talarico R, Tani C, Tavoni AG, Bombardieri S. Overlap of ACA-positive systemic sclerosis and Sjögren's syndrome: a distinct clinical entity with mild organ involvement but at high risk of lymphoma. Clin Exp Rheumatol. 2013;31:272–80.
39. Sharp GC, Irvin WS, Tan EM, et al. Mixed connective tissue disease—an apparently distinct rheumatic disease syndrome associated with a specific antibody to an extractable nuclear antigen (ENA). Am J Med. 1972;52:148–59. Epub 1972/02/01.
40. Ortega-Hernandez OD, Shoenfeld Y. Mixed connective tissue disease: an overview of clinical manifestations, diagnosis and treatment. Best Pract Res Clin Rheumatol. 2012;26:61–72. Epub 2012/03/20.
41. Hoffman RW, Greidinger EL. Mixed connective tissue disease. Curr Opin Rheumatol. 2000;12:386–90. Epub 2000/09/16.
42. Paradowska-Gorycka A, Jurkowska M, Czuszynska Z, et al. IL-10, IL-12B and IL-17 gene polymorphisms in patients with mixed connective tissue disease. Modern Rheumatol. 2014:1–3. Epub 2014/08/28.
43. Chaigne B, Scirè CA, Talarico R, Alexander T, Amoura Z, Avcin T, Beretta L, Doria A, Guffroy A, Guimarães V, Hachulla É, Krieg T, Launay D, Lepri G, Moinzadeh P, Müller-Ladner U, Rednic S, Rodrigues A, Tas SW, van Vollenhoven RF, Vieira A, Bombardieri S, Fonseca JE, Galetti I, Schneider M, Smith V, Cutolo M, Mosca M, Fischer-Betz R. Mixed connective tissue disease: state of the art on clinical practice guidelines. RMD Open. 2018;4:e000783. https://doi.org/10.1136/rmdopen-2018-000783.
44. Fairley JL, Hansen D, Proudman S, Sahhar J, Ngian G-S, Walker J, Strickland G, Wilson M, Morrisroe K, Ferdowsi N, Major G, Roddy J, Stevens W, Nikpour M. Clinical characteristics and survival in systemic sclerosis-mixed connective tissue disease and systemic sclerosis-overlap syndrome. Arthritis Care Res (Hoboken). 2020;73:732. https://doi.org/10.1002/acr.24167.
45. Derrett-Smith EC, Nihtyanova SI, Harvey J, Salama AD, Denton CP. Revisiting ANCA-associated vasculitis in systemic sclerosis: clinical, serological and immunogenetic factors. Rheumatology (Oxford). 2013a;52:1824–31. https://doi.org/10.1093/rheumatology/ket213.
46. Sordet C, Goetz J, Sibilia J. Contribution of autoantibodies to the diagnosis and nosology of inflammatory muscle disease. Joint Bone Spine. 2006;73:646–54. Epub 2006/11/18.
47. Cutolo M, Matucci Cerinic M. Nailfold capillaroscopy and classification criteria for systemic sclerosis. Clin Exp Rheumatol. 2007;25:663–5. Epub 2007/12/15.
48. Cutolo M, Sulli A, Secchi ME, et al. The contribution of capillaroscopy to the differential diagnosis of connective autoimmune diseases. Best Pract Res Clin Rheumatol. 2007;21:1093–108. Epub 2007/12/11.
49. Valentini G, D'Angelo S, Della Rossa A, et al. European scleroderma study group to define disease activity criteria for systemic sclerosis. IV. Assessment of skin thickening by modified Rodnan skin score. Ann Rheumatic Diseases. 2003;62:904–5. Epub 2003/08/19.
50. Czirjak L, Nagy Z, Aringer M, et al. The EUSTAR model for teaching and implementing the modified Rodnan skin score in systemic sclerosis. Ann Rheum Dis. 2007;66:966–9. Epub 2007/01/20.
51. Akesson A, Fiori G, Krieg T, et al. Assessment of skin, joint, tendon and muscle involvement. Clin Exp Rheumatol. 2003;21:S5–8. Epub 2003/08/02.
52. Hunzelmann N, Genth E, Krieg T, et al. Organspezifische Diagnostik von Patienten mit systemischer Sklerodermie: Empfehlungen des Deutschen Netzwerkes fur Systemische Sklerodermie (DNSS). [Organ-specific diagnosis in patients with systemic sclerosis: recommendations of the German Network for Systemic Sclerosis (DNSS)]. Zeitschrift fur Rheumatologie 2008;67:334–6, 7–40. Epub 2008/04/18.
53. Jaovisidha K, Csuka ME, Almagro UA, et al. Severe gastrointestinal involvement in systemic sclerosis: report of five cases and review of the literature. Semin Arthritis Rheum. 2005;34:689–702. Epub 2005/02/05.
54. Thakkar V, Stevens W, Prior D, et al. The inclusion of N-terminal pro-brain natriuretic peptide in a sensitive screening strategy for systemic sclerosis-related pulmonary arterial hypertension: a cohort study. Arthritis Res Ther. 2013;15:R193. Epub 2013/11/20.
55. Steen VD, Mayes MD, Merkel PA. Assessment of kidney involvement. Clin Exp Rheumatol. 2003;21:S29–31. Epub 2003/08/02.
56. Kistler AD. Therapeutische Umschau revue therapeutique 2015;72:171–7. Epub 2015/02/28.
57. Santiago ML, Seisdedos MR, Garcia Salinas RN, et al. Utilidad de los anticuerpos y de la biopsia de glandula salival menor en el estudio del complejo sicca en la practica diaria. [Usefulness of antibodies and minor salivary gland biopsy in the study of sicca sindrome in daily clinical practice]. Reumatologia Clinica 2015;11:156. Epub 2015/01/13.
58. Kowal-Bielecka O, Distler O. Use of methotrexate in patients with scleroderma and mixed connective tissue disease. Clin Exp Rheumatol. 2010;28:S160–3. Epub 2010/11/26.
59. Fendler C, Braun J. Use of methotrexate in inflammatory myopathies. Clin Exp Rheumatol. 2010;28:S164–7. Epub 2010/11/26.
60. Walker KM, Pope J. Expert agreement on EULAR/EUSTAR recommendations for the management of systemic sclerosis. J Rheumatol. 2011;38:1326–8. Epub 2011/04/05.
61. Highland KB, Distler O, Kuwana M, Allanore Y, Assassi S, Azuma A, Bourdin A, Denton CP, Distler JHW, Hoffmann-Vold AM, Khanna D, Mayes MD, Raghu G, Vonk MC, Gahlemann M, Clerisme-Beaty E, Girard M, Stowasser S, Zoz D, Maher TM, SENSCIS trial investigators. Efficacy and safety of nintedanib

in patients with systemic sclerosis-associated interstitial lung disease treated with mycophenolate: a subgroup analysis of the SENSCIS trial. Lancet. Respir Med. 2021;9(1):96–106. https://doi.org/10.1016/S2213-2600(20)30330-1.
62. Raja J, Nihtyanova SI, Murray CD, Denton CP, Ong VH. Sustained benefit from intravenous immunoglobulin therapy for gastrointestinal involvement in systemic sclerosis. Rheumatology (Oxford). 2016;55(1):115–9. https://doi.org/10.1093/rheumatology/kev318. Epub 2015 Aug 28.65.
63. Levine TD. Rituximab in the treatment of dermatomyositis: an open-label pilot study. Arthritis Rheum. 2005;52:601–7. Epub 2005/02/05.
64. Mok CC, Ho LY, To CH. Rituximab for refractory polymyositis: an open-label prospective study. J Rheumatol. 2007;34:1864–8. Epub 2007/08/28.
65. Lundberg IE. The prognosis of mixed connective tissue disease. Rheum Dis Clin N Am. 2005;31:535–47, vii–viii. Epub 2005/08/09.
66. Feltsan T, Stanko P, Mracna J. Sjogren s syndrome in present. Bratislavske lekarske listy. 2012;113:514–6. Epub 2012/08/18.
67. van den Hoogen FH, Boerbooms AM, Swaak AJ, et al. Comparison of methotrexate with placebo in the treatment of systemic sclerosis: a 24 week randomized double-blind trial, followed by a 24 week observational trial. Br J Rheumatol. 1996;35:364–72. Epub 1996/04/01.

Juvenile Localized and Systemic Scleroderma

9

Lauren V. Graham, Amy S. Paller, and Ivan Foeldvari

Juvenile Localized Scleroderma

Pediatric localized scleroderma comprises a group of conditions in which the skin and subcutaneous tissues become fibrotic. Lesions range from very small plaques to extensive indurated lesions that cause significant functional impairment and cosmetic deformity. Localized scleroderma also is called morphea. Pediatric localized scleroderma has been divided into five subtypes: circumscribed morphea, linear scleroderma, generalized morphea, pansclerotic morphea, and a mixed subtype with a combination of two or more subtypes (15% of patients) (Table 9.1) [1, 2].

Table 9.1 Proposed preliminary classification criteria for juvenile localized scleroderma (Consensus Conference, Padua (Italy) 2004) [2]

Main group	Subtype	Description
1. Circumscribed morphea	(a) Superficial	Oval or round circumscribed areas of induration limited to the epidermis and dermis, often with altered pigmentation and violaceous, erythematous halo (lilac ring). Lesions can be single or multiple
	(b) Deep	Oval or round circumscribed deep induration of the skin involving subcutaneous tissue extending to fascia and may involve underlying muscle. Lesions can be single or multiple
		Subcutaneous tissue may be the primary site of involvement without involvement of the overlying skin
2. Linear scleroderma	(a) Trunk/limbs	Linear induration involving the dermis, the subcutaneous tissue, and, sometimes, underlying muscle and bone and affecting the limbs and/or trunk
	(b) Head	En coup de sabre (ECDS). Linear induration that affects the face and/or the scalp and sometimes underlying muscle and bone
		Parry-Romberg or progressive hemifacial atrophy. Loss of tissue on one side of the face that may involve the dermis, subcutaneous tissue, muscle, and bone. The skin is mobile
3 . Generalized morphea		Induration of the skin starts as individual plaques (four or more and larger than 3 cm) that become confluent and involve at least two anatomic sites
4. Pansclerotic morphea		Circumferential involvement of limb(s) affects the skin, subcutaneous tissue, muscle, and bone. Lesions may involve more than one body area but do not affect internal organs
5. Mixed type morphea		Combination of two or more of the previous subtypes. The order of the concomitant subtypes, specified in brackets, will follow their predominant representation in the individual patient (i.e., mixed (linear circumscribed))

L. V. Graham
Department of Dermatology, Northwestern University, McGraw Medical Center, Chicago, IL, USA

A. S. Paller
Department of Dermatology, Northwestern University Feinberg School of Medicine, Chicago, IL, USA

I. Foeldvari (✉)
Hamburg Centre for Pediatric Rheumatology, Head of the Juvenile Scleroderma Working Group (JSScWG), Hamburger Zentrum Für Kinder- und Jugendrheumatologie, Hamburg, Germany
e-mail: sprechstunde@kinderrheumatologie.de

Y. Allanore et al. (eds.), *Scleroderma*, https://doi.org/10.1007/978-3-031-40658-4_9

Epidemiology

Although pediatric localized scleroderma is an orphan disease, it is at least ten times more common than systemic sclerosis in childhood [3]. Girls predominate with the female/male ratio estimated at 1.9–2.7:1 [1, 3, 4]. The mean age at disease onset is 7.3–8.3 years of age [5, 6]. Less than 1% of cases are present at birth (congenital localized scleroderma) [6]. Linear scleroderma is the most common subtype seen in children; in one recent study, the overall incidence of localized scleroderma was 3.4 cases per million children per year with 2.7 cases per million per year of linear scleroderma [3]. Early-onset disease and more severe forms (linear scleroderma, generalized morphea, pansclerotic morphea) are risk factors for extracutaneous manifestations [4, 7].

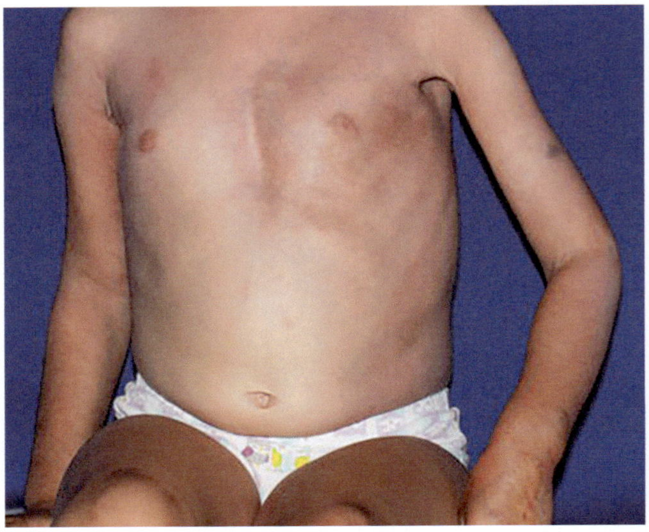

Fig. 9.2 Generalized morphea in this 4-year-old girl. Shown are sites of involvement on the left side of the trunk, left arm and hand, and right upper arm. The face, neck, and legs were also involved with circumscribed morphea lesions. Note the increased visibility of veins on the left side of the chest because of cutaneous atrophy

Clinical Manifestations

Circumscribed morphea (CM) is characterized by oval or round circumscribed areas of induration surrounded by a violaceous halo (Fig. 9.1). Superficial circumscribed morphea is confined to the dermis with only occasional involvement of the superficial panniculus. Circumscribed morphea is most commonly seen on the trunk and includes 15–37% of pediatric localized scleroderma [1, 4, 5]. Guttate morphea (numerous small plaques) and localized scleroderma that resemble the atrophoderma of Pasini and Pierini or lichen sclerosus et atrophicus are included in the circumscribed morphea subset. Deep morphea is another subset of circumscribed morphea, which can extend to the fascia and muscle and is more recalcitrant to intervention.

The diagnosis is *generalized morphea* (GM) when there are four or more plaques, often with plaque confluence, that are larger than 3 cm and involve at least two of seven anatomic sites (head-neck, right upper extremity, left upper extremity, right lower extremity, left lower extremity, anterior trunk, and posterior trunk) (Fig. 9.2). Overall, 7–9% of children with localized scleroderma have the generalized type [1, 4, 5]. Unilateral GM has been proposed as an uncommon variant, usually beginning in childhood [8].

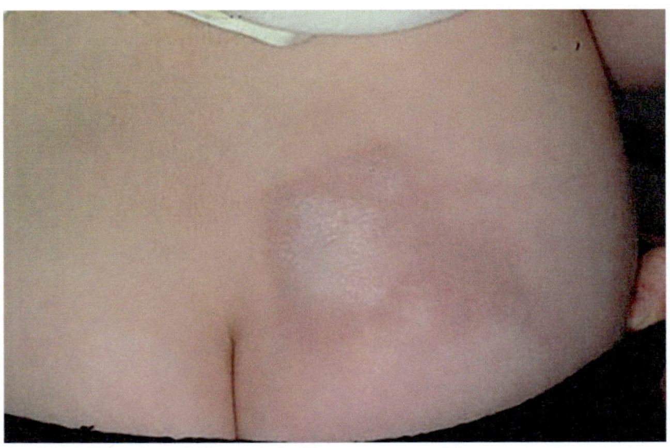

Fig. 9.1 Circumscribed localized scleroderma of the buttock area, characterized by an area of induration with waxy consistency (ivory color at center), surrounded by an inflammatory edge. Note the cutaneous atrophy, characterized by fine wrinkling and shininess

Linear scleroderma is the most common subtype in children and adolescents, representing 42–65% of cases of pediatric localized scleroderma [1, 4, 5, 9]. Linear scleroderma occurs more often in children than adults [10]. Linear scleroderma is characterized by one or more linear streaks that can extend through the dermis, subcutaneous tissue, and muscle to the underlying bone, often causing significant deformity (Fig. 9.3). In one study, 25.6% of patients with linear morphea involving an extremity developed contractures and 32.6% developed limb undergrowth [4]. The *en coup de sabre* (ECDS) variety is linear localized scleroderma of the face and scalp. ECDS often affects the forehead unilaterally (Fig. 9.4) and can be associated with "white" anterior uveitis, alopecia, neurological, and/or ocular signs [7]. If involving the lower face, ECDS can be associated with dental and tongue abnormalities [11–14]. The presentation of ECDS on the forehead can be subtle and resemble a port-wine stain [15, 16]. The Parry-Romberg syndrome (PRS) is characterized by hemifacial atrophy with mild or absent involvement of the superficial skin and can involve the underlying fat, muscle, cartilage, or bone. It is considered the severe end of the spectrum of ECDS [11].

Pansclerotic morphea, an extremely rare but severe subtype, is characterized by generalized full-thickness involvement of the skin of the trunk, extremities, face, and/or scalp.

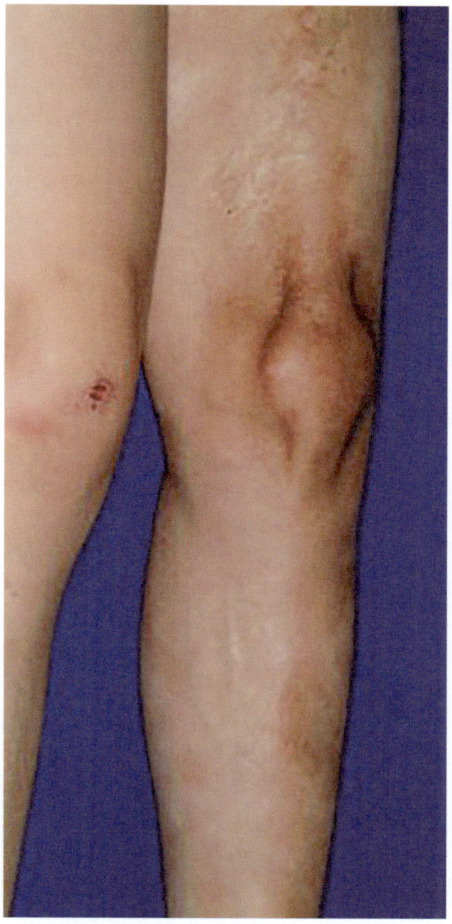

Fig. 9.3 Linear scleroderma. The lesion tracks down the anterior aspect of the left thigh to the lower leg. Not shown are the involvement of the ankle and dorsal aspect of the foot. Note the irregular dyschromia (hypo- and hyperpigmentation) on the thigh and the prominent veins on the shin

It is more common in children than adults. Chronic ulcers may develop and evolve into squamous cell carcinoma [17–20]. Other complications are site-specific: joint contractures, reduction of chest expansion, lagophthalmos and ectropion, gastrointestinal reflux, cicatricial alopecia, and thrombosis of the foot leading to amputation [21].

Up to 40% of the patients have extracutaneous manifestations, most commonly individuals with linear scleroderma, generalized morphea, or pansclerotic morphea [4, 7, 22]. Arthralgias and arthritis are the most frequent findings (23%) [4]. Children who develop arthritis often have a lesion that crosses over the joint, but some of them develop arthritis in joints without skin involvement. Gastroesophageal reflux is the only gastrointestinal complication reported so far in pediatric localized scleroderma [1, 23, 24], but it is not more common than expected in the pediatric population. Extracutaneous

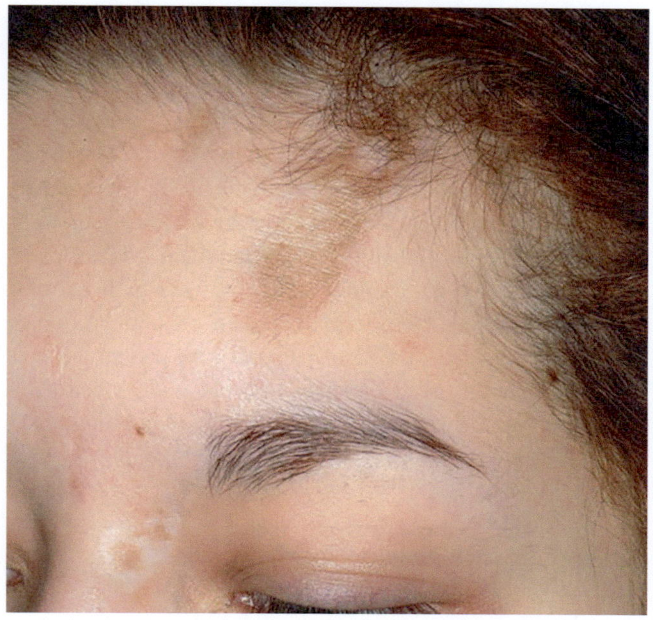

Fig. 9.4 En coup de sabre morphea. Note the old hyperpigmented streak on the left side of the forehead; the active, newer area on the left side of the upper nose; and the loss of the medial eyebrow

manifestations of ECDS are not uncommon. Migraine and non-migraine headaches can precede the development of cutaneous findings [25, 26], and seizures, behavioral changes, and learning disabilities have also been described [22, 27]. Abnormalities on magnetic resonance imaging (MRI), such as calcifications, white matter changes, vascular malformations, and vasculitis, may be associated, even without clinical evidence of neurological manifestations [28, 29]. Although most of the imaging abnormalities have little clinical relevance, biopsy findings have shown sclerosis, fibrosis, gliosis, as well as vasculitis [29, 30]. Ocular involvement has been found in 3.2–8.3% of patients with ECDS linear scleroderma [22, 31]. Ocular involvement most commonly includes "white" anterior uveitis, eyelid and eyelash abnormalities, episcleritis, CNS abnormalities, glaucoma, papilledema, or xerophthalmia [22, 31]. The Parry-Romberg syndrome can be associated with vascular changes (i.e., Raynaud's phenomenon and deep vein thrombosis), seizures, brain atrophy, and intracranial vascular malformation [32].

The concurrence of other autoimmune disorders is less common in children (3–10%) than in adults, although children with localized scleroderma are more likely to have a family history of autoimmune disease than adults with localized scleroderma [9]. These include juvenile idiopathic arthritis, systemic lupus erythematosus, autoimmune thyroid disease, Raynaud's syndrome, vitiligo, celiac disease, and alopecia areata [7, 22].

Autoantibodies

Antinuclear antibodies (ANA) have been reported in 30–40% of patients with pediatric localized scleroderma [1, 9]. This frequency is lower than in adults with localized scleroderma [33] but is significantly higher than in the normal population. Having a positive ANA does not correlate with any particular subtype or disease course [1, 34]. Rheumatoid factor (RF) has been detected at low titer in 16% of the patients with pediatric localized scleroderma [1]. Anti-histone antibodies (AHA) are detected in 47% of patients with pediatric localized scleroderma, most often in patients with generalized and linear localized scleroderma and rarely in circumscribed localized scleroderma [33, 34].

Diagnosis and Disease Assessment

There has been a recent validation of a clinical assessment tool for localized scleroderma, the modified localized scleroderma skin severity index (mLoSSI). The mLoSSI is easily applicable without any additional instruments besides clinical examination and is the summation of 18 anatomical sites evaluated for erythema, skin thickness, and new lesion/extension of lesions [35, 36]. The score changes with the activity of the disease. It does not assess extracutaneous manifestations. Additional objective measures such as ultrasound, infrared thermography, durometry, computerized skin score, and magnetic resonance imaging (MRI) promise to improve the clinical evaluation of localized scleroderma. However, all of these measures need validation to differentiate between activity and "scar" of the disease. In a pediatric population, the mLoSSI and physician's global assessment of disease activity were found to be sensitive to clinical change [37]. A validated quality-of-life assessment is not yet available.

The computerized skin score, which is only available in some centers, involves the demarcation of hyperemic and indurated borders of the lesions onto an adhesive transparent film. The film is transferred over cardboard, scanned, and the affected area is calculated by computing software [38]. Although objective calculations increase reliability, the dyspigmentation of inactive lesions can be misinterpreted as disease activity.

High-frequency ultrasonography (18 MHz) has been used to detect clinical disease activity as assessed by dermal thickness, increased blood flow (inflammation), and increased echogenicity (atrophy, fibrosis) [39, 40]. Ultrasonography should be performed using a standardized protocol [41, 42]. Infrared thermography can detect disease activity based on increased temperature caused by the inflammatory process [43], but is rarely available. This noninvasive technique has shown high reproducibility, but yields false-positive results in assessing old lesions that are characterized by marked atrophy of the skin and subcutaneous tissues; the clinical examination can complement to distinguish old atrophic lesions. Durometry has been used for detecting the induration/hardness of skin in systemic sclerosis and correlates with the modified Rodnan skin score and ultrasound thickness [44, 45]. MRI can be valuable in the assessment of CNS abnormalities, limb discrepancies, arthritis, or eye involvement [46]. However, given the need for sedation in younger patients, the cost and the presence of possible artifacts, MRI is not a reasonable assessment tool for everyday practice.

Treatment

Treatment options are shown in Fig. 9.5. Localized scleroderma can lead to significant disability. Systemic treatment is suggested in cases of contractures or for lesions that (i) cross joint lines; (ii) are overlying the spine, which can cause severe scoliosis; (iii) affect the face because of the concern for cosmetic changes; (iv) course down the extremities, which can cause limb shortening and dysfunction of hands and feet; and (v) occur in other cosmetically sensitive areas. All of these can significantly influence the quality of life. The consensus meeting of the Pediatric Rheumatology European Society (PreS) made clear suggestions for the indications of systemic treatment (paper submitted).

Local treatment for circumscribed morphea is reserved for lesions small and not leading to any kind of disability. Local treatment is generally restricted to the application of vitamin D analogues (calcipotriene or calcitriol) with or without topical corticosteroids. Calcipotriene and calcitriol are used twice daily, usually with the evening dose under occlusion [47, 48]. Newer studies have suggested that topical tacrolimus or imiquimod may be of benefit, but these are used less often. In a double-blind, placebo-controlled pilot study in adults, tacrolimus 0.1% ointment twice daily was superior to placebo in decreasing skin hardness measured by a durometer (not a validated measure) and improving clinical features (measuring erythema, induration, dyspigmentation, and atrophy) [49]. One case study described the improvement of generalized morphea in an adult with tacrolimus 0.1% ointment, applied twice daily for 8 weeks [50]. In a prospective, open-label, double-blind study of nine children, topical imiquimod 5% cream, applied three times weekly for 1 month and then five times weekly for 32 weeks, led to an improvement of induration/dermal thickness [51]. An open phase II clinical trial in adults suggests that topical pirfenidone, a molecule shown to have anti-fibrotic activity, led to improvement in the mLoSSI in 100% of the patients after being used three times daily for 6 months [52].

Phototherapy with UVA1 represents another possible therapeutic choice for pediatric localized scleroderma [29, 30, 32], but requires long-term therapy. The relapse rate after UVA1 phototherapy in a study of both adults and children

Fig. 9.5 Management of localized scleroderma

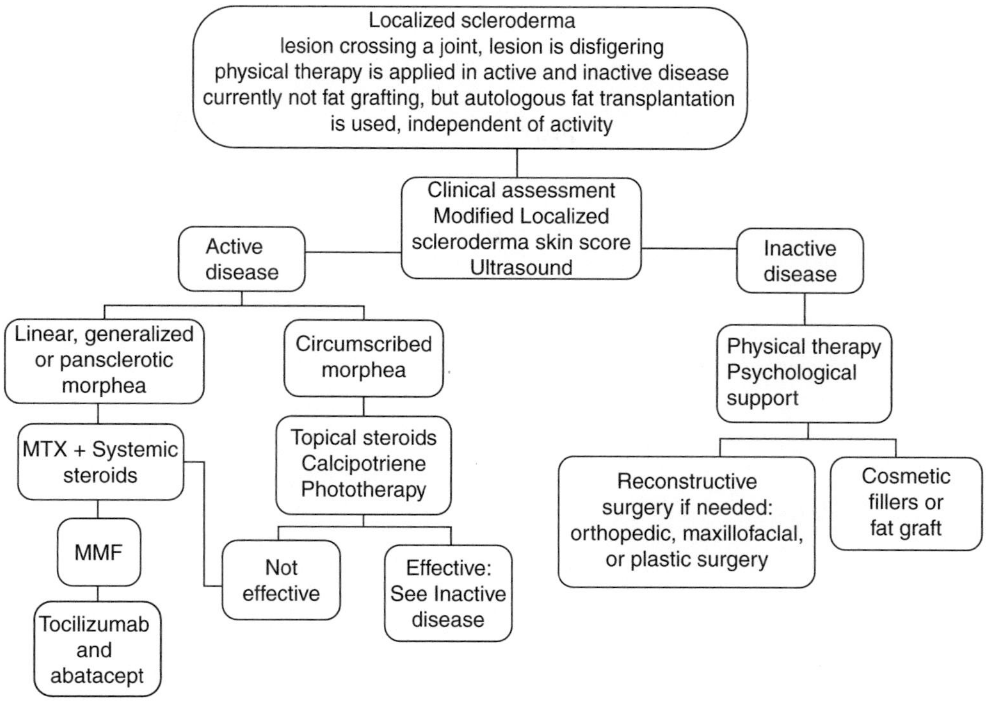

was 44% and 48%, respectively, 2 and 3 years after discontinuation [53]. Recurrence was increased with older lesions, emphasizing the importance of early detection and treatment. Lack of long-term safety data with the use of UVA1 and adherence difficulties in young children (who need to sit in a light box for 20–30 min) are limitations. Given its potential long-term side effects, psoralen with UVA (PUVA) is not usually recommended for children.

In addition to topical vitamin D analogs, systemic vitamin D analogs have also been used. In an open prospective study, the daily administration of oral calcitriol for 4–6 months improved skin induration, joint mobility, and skin extensibility [54]; however, oral calcitriol was not more effective than placebo in a controlled trial [55] and is associated with the risk of hypercalciuria and renal stones.

First-line systemic therapy is methotrexate, initiated with oral or pulsed intravenous corticosteroids [56–62], which has been found to be effective in 73.8% of patients [63] (Table 9.2). The Childhood Arthritis and Rheumatology Research Alliance [5] recommended three treatment plans (without steroid, with oral steroid, with IV pulsed steroid), each with a dose of methotrexate of 1 mg/kg/week s.c. [64] based on 15 published studies with A ($n = 1$) and B ($n = 3$) levels of evidence. However, the suggested dose based on the only controlled trial [62] is 15 mg/m^2 body surface once a week (0.3 mg/kg/week) administered subcutaneously (maximum, 25 mg/week), and other reports suggest that 0.3–0.5 mg/kg/week given orally or subcutaneously is successful [4, 58]. During the first 2–3 months of therapy, a course of glucocorticoids may be used as adjunctive bridge therapy. The corticosteroid regimen can be (1) methylprednisolone IV 30 mg/kg/dose with a schedule of one dose/week × 12 weeks, (2) three consecutive daily doses/month × 3 months, or (3) oral prednisone 2 mg/kg/day (maximum dose of 60 mg) for a minimum of 2 weeks but a maximum of 4 weeks. Success has also been described with oral prednisone at 1 mg/kg/day, either used for 1 month and then decreased to 0.5 mg/kg/day for 1–2 months or used continuously for 3 months and then tapered [4, 60, 62]. Weaning off methotrexate should be tried after 12–24 months of remission.

However, the suggested dose based on the only controlled trial (62) is 15 mg/m^2 body surface once a week (0.3 mg/kg/wk) administered subcutaneously (maximum, 25 mg/wk) and other reports suggest that 0.3–0.5 mg/kg/week given orally or subcutaneously is successful [4, 58].

Side effects of methotrexate have been described in up to 48.3% of children, but are generally mild and do not require discontinuation of therapy. Nausea is most common and can be mitigated by switching from oral to s.c. or the manipulation of the folate dosing. All patients should receive folic acid supplementation, but whether to give folate 1 mg (most common dosing) daily or for 6 days, skipping the day of methotrexate administration, or whether a single dose of 5 mg folate (e.g., on the day after the methotrexate) remains controversial [65].

If a patient does not respond to methotrexate and corticosteroids, mycophenolate mofetil (MMF) can be added, although sometimes it is effective as a single agent. A retrospective review of ten patients with pediatric localized scleroderma who failed methotrexate and/or corticosteroids described the clinical response to MMF [66]. Six of the

Table 9.2 Treatment with methotrexate in localized scleroderma

Author (year)	Study design	Regimen	No. of patients (children)	Follow-up	Result	Assessment
Seyger (1998)	Retrospective	MTX 15 mg/week orally	9 (0)	24 weeks	Effective (67%)	Skin score Durometer Patient's judgment (VAS)
Uziel (2000)	Retrospective	MTX 0.3–0.6 mg/kg/week orally or s.c. + MPDN 30 mg/kg/day pulse for 3 days/month for 3 months	10 (10)	8–30 weeks	Effective (90%)	Clinical judgment
Kreuter (2005)	Pilot, uncontrolled	MTX 15 mg/week orally + MPDN 1000 mg/day pulse for 3 days/month for 6 months	15 (0)	6–25 months	Effective (93%)	Skin score Patient's judgment (VAS) USG, histopathology
Fitch (2006)	Retrospective	MTX 0.4–1.0 mg/kg/week os or sc ± PDN 1 mg/kg/day or every other day for 3–6 months	17 (17)	6–60 months	Effective (94%)	Clinical judgment Telephone questionnaire
Wiebel (2006)	Retrospective	MTX 10 mg/m^2/week ± PDN 1 mg/kg/day or every other day for 3–6 months	34 (34)	24 months	Effective (74%)	Clinical judgment, thermography
Christen-Zaech (2008)	Retrospective chart review	MTX 0.3–0.5 mg/kg/week starting dose + PDN 1 mg/kg/day for 1 month and then decreased to 0.5 mg/kg/day		1 month–17 years	Effective	Clinical judgment
Zulian (2011)	Double-blind randomized controlled trial	MTX 15 mg/m^2/week for 12 months + PDN 1 mg/kg/day for 3 months versus	70 (70)	12 months	Effective (MTX 67%)	Clinical judgment Clinical judgment thermography
		Placebo for 12 months + PDN 1 mg/kg/day for 3 months			(PLAC 29%)	Computerized skin score
Koch (2013)	Retrospective chart review	MTX 5–17.5 mg/week ± PDN 10–20 mg daily	17 (all subjects <25 years of age)	Average of 6.6 years	100% had improvement but 54% required a second course of MTX	Clinical judgment

MPDN methylprednisolone, *MTX* methotrexate, *PDN* prednisolone, *USG* ultrasonography

patients who responded were concurrently administered methotrexate and corticosteroids, two patients were concurrently using corticosteroids, and two patients were administered only MMF. The CARRA consensus recommended treatment dosing with MMF 600 mg/m^2 twice daily for patients <1.25 m^2, 750 mg twice daily for 40–50 kg weight, and 1000 mg twice daily for patients over 50 kg [64].

A 3-year-old girl with generalized morphea was successfully treated with MTX 0.5 mg/m^2/week, prednisolone 1 mg/kg/day (tapered after 3 months), and imatinib 235 mg/m^2/day with nearly complete resolution of her skin lesions after 1 year [67]. However, trials of imatinib in generalized morphea or systemic sclerosis have not shown changes in skin involvement as measured by the modified Rodnan skin score or dermal thickness measured by skin biopsies [68, 69].

Rituximab, tocilizumab [70], abatacept [70, 71], and intravenous immunoglobulin (IVIG) are treatments that have been tried in refractory cases of adult systemic sclerosis and may be considered in severe cases of pediatric localized scleroderma. In adult patients, rituximab administration improved the skin score after two treatments given 6 months apart [72, 73]. An 11-year-old boy with ulcerating plaques of sclerotic skin and severe ankyloses improved with IVIG treatment [74].

Surgical reconstruction may be required if the disease has not been adequately controlled. Surgery should only be performed after the active phase of the disease has abated and when the child's growth is complete [75]. Facial recontouring is a surgical treatment option that may improve the quality of life in adolescents with facial asymmetry due to en coup de sabre linear scleroderma [76]. A recent study in patients with the Parry-Romberg syndrome found that fat graft assisted by bone marrow-derived mesenchymal stem cells required fewer injections to reach a satisfactory cosmetic outcome than fat graft treatment alone [77]. This technology requires larger studies but may be a viable treatment option in the future.

Quality of Life

There are no prospectively validated quality-of-life instruments for localized scleroderma. Localized scleroderma shows a moderate effect on quality of life [78]. Pain, itch, and tightness and especially cosmetic changes have been associated with a poorer quality of life in affected children [79].

Prognosis

Information on the long-term outcome of children with pediatric localized scleroderma is increasing. A retrospective review of 52 patients with linear scleroderma, seen over a span of 20 years, showed that 31% of patients with a disease duration of ≥10 years still had active disease [80]. A case of reactivation after 20 years was also reported. With an average of 5 years of follow-up time, 98% of patients reported residual dyspigmentation, atrophy, or both [80]. A larger study of 344 patients showed disease recurrence in 27% of pediatric-onset localized scleroderma as compared to 17% recurrence for adult-onset [81]. The median time between remission and first recurrence was similar in both groups (26–27 months). This new data confirm the importance of long-term follow-up in this patient population.

Juvenile Systemic Sclerosis

Juvenile systemic sclerosis (jSSc) is a rare multisystem connective tissue disease [82]. Approximately 5–10% of all adults with systemic sclerosis (SSc) report the onset of the disease during childhood. It has a variety of clinical manifestations and the distribution of diffuse versus limited forms, and the proportion of patients with overlap features differs from the adult form. Mixed connective tissue disease (MCTD) and overlap syndromes have features of jSSc and sometimes even fulfill the criteria of jSSc [83]. Localized scleroderma is a separate disorder and does not evolve into systemic sclerosis, although some children develop some of the features of systemic disease, such as dysphagia or abnormal pulmonary function tests [4, 84].

jSSc is characterized by pathologic thickening and tethering of the skin. It is thought that the fibrosis is a consequence of a vasculopathy of the small vessel system, associated with altered endothelial cell function [85], which leads to fibrotic changes of the skin and other organs. Alterations of the immune system and genetic and environmental factors are part of the pathogenesis. Several recent publications review this topic extensively [85–89]. The triggers of the disease are still unclear. A positive family history of SSc is one of the strongest known risk factors for SSc [90, 91]. This chapter will be focused on the clinical characteristics and outcome of jSSc in childhood and on the clinical presentation and outcome of jSSc patients in adult cohorts of SSc patients. The specific clinical features of jSSc will be compared to adult-onset systemic sclerosis (aSSc). Unfortunately, there is still no evidence-based data regarding the treatment of jSSc patients. Most of the therapeutic suggestions are derived from the adult literature and the therapeutic recommendations of the EULAR/EUSTAR [92, 93], which summarizes the state of evidence-based expert opinion on SSc management.

Clinical Presentation of Patients with Juvenile Systemic Scleroderma

The first, large cross-sectional cohort based on a multinational survey of pediatric rheumatologists was published in 2000 [94]. A recently initiated prospective registry with standardized assessment of jSSc patients includes more than 70 patients to date (www.juvenile-scleroderma.com). In this prospective cohort, disease subset distribution differs from that of affected adults. The youngest patient enrolled is 2 years of age and the mean is 6.1 years of age; 77% are female; and the mean age of onset of Raynaud's symptoms was 9.2 years old (range, 2–16 years). The mean age at the onset of symptoms other than Raynaud's was 9.7 years (range, 3–16 years). The diffuse subtype was recognized in 74% and overlap symptoms in 38% (submitted for publication, Foeldvari et al.); these data are consistent with previous survey data [10, 94].

In the large, multicenter cross-sectional case collection [94] of 135 jSSc patients followed for a mean of 5 years, the mean age of the disease onset was 8.8 years, significantly younger than previously expected. The male/female ratio of 1:2.85 showed less of a female preponderance than the adult cohort. In one other multicenter cross-sectional study of 153 patients [95], the mean age at disease onset was 8.1 years. Organ involvement in these patients is presented in Table 9.3. Taken together, these two studies showed that 63.5–79% of patients have joint involvement, 65–69% have gastrointestinal involvement, and 41.8–50% have pulmonary involvement. Renal involvement is relatively infrequent (9.8–13%). In the cohort of Foeldvari et al., 16% of the patients had central nervous system involvement, which seems to be unique [94]. In the cohort of Martini et al., 90.8% of the patients showed a diffuse subtype, which was consistent with the few (7.1%) patients with anti-centromere antibodies [95]. In the cohort of Foeldvari et al., no patient had anti-centromere antibodies, despite typical pitting fingertip scars that are reminiscent of a CREST pattern of limited scleroderma in adult patients (Fig. 9.6). Only one patient in either cohort had

Table 9.3 Organ involvement of the patients in the two pediatric multicenter cross-sectional studies

Organ involvement	Foeldvari et al. $n = 135$ (%)	Martini et al. $n = 153$ (%)
Skin	135 (100)	116 (75.8)[a]
Joints	106 (79)	97(63.5)
GI tract	88 (65)	106(69)
Only esophageal	63 (47)	47(31)
Pulmonary	68 (50)	64 (41.8)
Cardiovascular	60 (44)	44(28.8)
CNS	21 (16)	4 (3)
Renal	17 (13)	15 (9.8)
Muscular	13 (10)	37(24.2)
Raynaud's	97 (72)	128(83.7)
Calcinosis	36 (27)	28(18.3)
Sjögren's syndr.	7 (5)	?
CREST	1	?

[a] 75.8% skin induration; 66% sclerodactyly; and 44.1% edema.

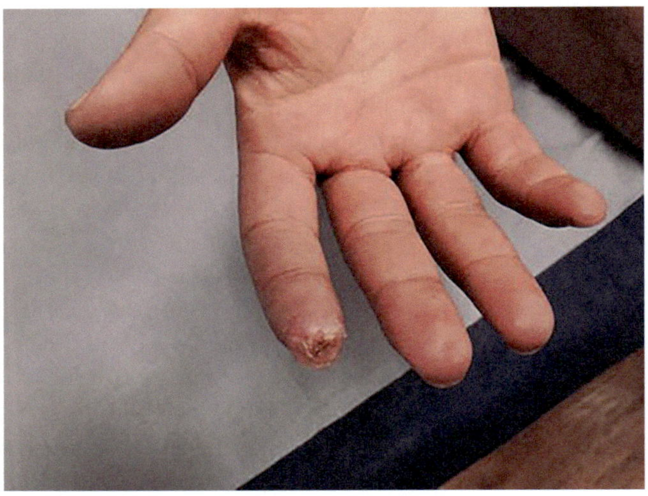

Fig. 9.6 Scarring on the fingertips associated with severe secondary Raynaud's in jSSc

CREST syndrome, part of the limited subtype spectrum. In the prospective cohort, 68% (34/50) of the patients have diffuse subset.

Note, these studies represent retrospective multicenter data, with overlapping cohorts and evaluation of organ involvement that was not standardized. However, results are comparable between the two, as well as with other published single-center case series from Japan (61 patients) [96], South America (23 cases) [97], and Asia (23 cases) [98]. Ethnic differences in the East Indian population may explain the 39% of patients with the limited subtype [98]; in all other case series, the diffuse subtype affected 90.9–100% of patients. The prevalence of the anti-centromere antibody positivity was from 0 to 7.1%.

Incidence and Prevalence of Juvenile Systemic Sclerosis

Juvenile systemic sclerosis (jSSc) is an orphan autoimmune disease, and data regarding incidence and prevalence are rare. In a study from Finland in 1994 [91, 99], where nationwide, prospective, hospital-based assessments during a 4-year period were conducted and supplemented with data from the National Hospital Discharge Register, an annual incidence rate was found to be 0.05 per 100,000 with a population at risk of 1.02 million. According to a recent cross-sectional study from Herrick et al. [82], the incidence rate of patients younger than 16 years of age with abnormal skin thickening consistent with SSc or linear scleroderma was 0.27 (95% confidence interval 0.1–0.5) per million children. The mean age of these patients was 12.1 years. No prevalence data have been published. In a German Pediatric Rheumatology Registry, 19 patients were recorded among 14 million children under the age of 18 years (1.36 cases per one million children; Dr. Kirsten Minden, personal communication).

Classification

The first classification criteria specific to jSSc were published in 2007 [83]. The patient has to fulfill one major and two minor criteria. Major criteria are proximal sclerosis and induration of the skin from the metacarpophalangeal joint or metatarsophalangeal joint. The established eight minor criteria domains are listed in Table 9.4 and are organ-specific [83]. These proposed criteria have 90% sensitivity and 96% specificity, although prospective validation is pending.

Adult rheumatologists also have a consensus classification [100] with organ-specific scores. A score of 9 is required for the diagnosis of SSc. Skin involvement proximal to the metacarpophalangeal joint or metatarsophalangeal joint is sufficient to make the diagnosis. These criteria are currently

Table 9.4 The provisional classification criteria for juvenile systemic sclerosis [83]

Major criteria	Minor criteria
Induration/sclerosis	Vascular changes
	Pulmonary involvement
	Gastrointestinal involvement
	Renal involvement
	Cardiovascular involvement
	Musculoskeletal involvement
	Neurologic involvement
	Serology

in the process of validation testing in the adult SSc population. All children who meet pediatric criteria also meet the adult criteria.

Diagnosis and Assessment of the Patient

A key clinical goal is earlier detection and diagnosis of jSSc. The typical facial appearance of a child with juvenile-onset systemic scleroderma is shown in Fig. 9.7. Raynaud's phenomenon is the presenting symptom in 75% of the patients at the time of diagnosis [95], and sclerodactyly is another key feature at onset, but is present only in 37% [95]. Capillaroscopy is not prospectively validated in jSSc patients, although it is used to diagnose SSc and specifically Raynaud's in adults. In the largest retrospective pediatric study [95], only 10% of patients had capillary changes at disease onset and 25% at diagnosis of jSSc. However, it is unclear how many reporting centers reviewed capillary changes routinely and what kind of capillaroscopy they used. Normal capillaries behave differently in children vs. adults, and capillary dimension needs to be age-adjusted, since arterial and venous dimensions increase with age and tortuous capillaries can appear in healthy children [101–104]. Video capillaroscopy is the most sensitive for detecting changes. The handheld dermatoscope or ophthalmoscope can visualize changes, but these devices are inadequate to gauge quantitative change [105]. The Pediatric Rheumatology European Society (PreS) Juvenile Scleroderma Working Group recommends that patients with Raynaud's and pathologic nail fold capillary changes be followed at least every 6 months (paper submitted for publication).

The modified Rodnan skin score, which has been validated in adults, is not necessarily applicable to pediatric patients. The skin score in healthy children depends on Tanner's stage and body mass index (BMI) [106]. The durometer, a handheld device, can differentiate between healthy and sclerotic skin but does not work well if a bony structure directly underlies the skin, like in the fingers, face, and dorsal foot.

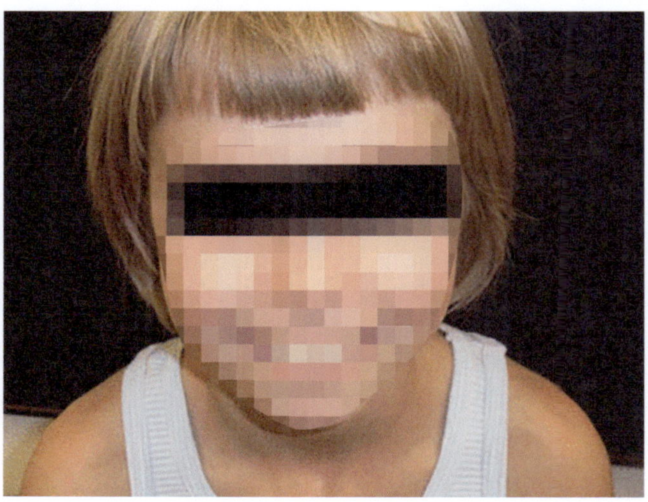

Fig. 9.7 Classical facial appearance of a child with juvenile-onset systemic scleroderma

The 6-min walk test (6MWT) is a well-established primary outcome measure in adult treatment studies for pulmonary hypertension but is not validated in jSSc patients. Two studies looked at normal values of 6MWT in children [107, 108], but the range for age groups in the two studies differs significantly, making analysis difficult. The length of the lap and the physical condition correlate with the distance that can be walked in 6 min and establish a percentile curve for normal values (paper submitted). Pulmonary function is one of the main dominators of the walk distance in jSSc patients. Pulmonary function tests in jSSc patients correlate well with the high-resolution computed tomography findings [109].

There is no specific antibody to prove the diagnosis. Because most pediatric patients have a diffuse subset, anti-Scl70 is more frequent, occurring in ~34% [95]. Anti-centromere antibodies are detected in 0–7% of children [94, 95, 110]. Inflammatory markers, such as sedimentation rate or CRP, are elevated in only 34–38% and 12.6% of patients, respectively.

Biologic markers of general disease or organ involvement may facilitate the diagnosis and serial evaluation of organ involvement or disease activity noninvasively [111–115]. In a pilot study, jSSc children with interstitial lung disease had higher levels of anti-KL6 than healthy children or children with jSSc without lung disease [116]. There are also studies regarding the prognostic value of B-type natriuretic peptides in children with pulmonary hypertension [117–119].

Differential Diagnosis

In scleroderma-like disorders, the distribution and characteristics of skin involvement seem to be "atypical" as compared to classic SSc, and the acral skin involvement and typical antibody pattern are usually missing. Exposure to certain chemicals or drugs may also suggest the presence of a scleroderma-like disease. These exposures are in the pediatric population less frequent than in the adult population. Lack of Raynaud's phenomenon, scleroderma-specific antinuclear antibodies, scleroderma capillary pattern on nail fold capillaroscopy, and typical internal organ manifestations may also indicate the presence of a scleroderma-like disorder. A skin biopsy may be valuable in considering the differential diagnosis.

Scleroderma-like disorders include diseases with mucin deposition (scleromyxedema, scleredema, etc.). Some disorders show papulonodular skin changes with or without dermal deposition of materials (amyloid, mucin deposition; fibroblastic rheumatism, etc.). Diseases with monoclonal gammopathy (scleromyxedema, POEMS syndrome, myeloma with scleroderma-like skin changes) also belong to the large group of scleroderma-like diseases. Some disorders are characterized by eosinophilia (diffuse fasciitis with eosinophilia, eosinophilia-myalgia syndrome, toxic oil syndrome), metabolic/biochemical abnormalities (IDDM, nephrogenic fibrosing dermopathy), and endocrine abnormalities (POEMS syndrome, hypo-/hyperthyroidism with mucin deposition, diabetes). Chronic graft-versus-host disease (cGVHD) may also show scleroderma-like skin changes.

Scleroderma-like disorders can be induced by drugs or chemicals (eosinophilia-myalgia syndrome, toxic oil syndrome, vinyl chloride disease; cytostatic agents (docetaxel, paclitaxel, gemcitabine, bleomycin, peplomycin, melphalan, capecitabine, and uracyl-tegafur); appetite suppressants; and physical injury (trauma, vibration stress, radiation injury). Inherited progeroid syndromes with early aging (e.g., Werner syndrome) and a large heterogeneous group of hereditary disorders with either skin thickening (porphyria, phenylketonuria) or skin atrophy/tightening (restrictive dermopathy, scleroatrophic and keratotic dermatosis of the limbs, etc.) should also be considered in the differential diagnosis of scleroderma-like disorders. These categories are not mutually exclusive, because the remarkably different scleroderma-like diseases show overlapping features.

Management

There are no controlled studies or specific recommendations for the treatment of pediatric disease. Therefore, therapeutic suggestions are based on publications in adult systemic sclerosis patients. Some of the medications used in adults are not available for children, there is no pediatric dosing for some drugs, and there is growing evidence that pediatric patients have higher or lower dosing requirements than adults. EULAR/EUSTAR, representing specialized centers for children, published its last therapeutic guidelines in 2009 [120].

There is no curative treatment for SSc. Autologous bone marrow transplantation is the most effective treatment with an effect on all organ systems if conducted early in the disease course in carefully selected, rapidly progressing patients [121]. If used as rescue therapy late in the disease course, transplantation has a high mortality rate [84]. There are only case reports regarding the effect of bone marrow transplantation in children.

Certain drugs have led to organ-specific improvements, such as the ameliorative effect of methotrexate on skin, joints, muscle, or interstitial lung disease. Most experts prefer methotrexate for pediatric SSc (15 mg/m^2) [122], but some prefer mycophenolate mofetil as first-line treatment. No comparative studies have been performed. Cyclophosphamide led to disease stabilization in two large adult studies [123, 124], but showed no significant effect after 12 months in a meta-analysis [125] and has higher toxicity. Several reports suggest some efficacy of biologics for skin and organ involvement, including rituximab [126–128], tocilizumab [70], abatacept [70], and tumor necrosis factor (TNF) inhibitors. TNF inhibitors are particularly effective for the associated arthritis [129, 130]. Several controlled studies are currently underway in adults with SSc. Because they increase the risk of renal hypertension in adult SSc, medium to high-dose glucocorticoids are avoided, but to date, there is no pediatric data regarding this increased risk.

Several "palliative" drugs influence the effect of disease without having a direct effect on the autoimmune process. Examples include proton pump inhibitors for reflux; calcium and anti-endothelin antagonists, phosphodiesterase blocking agents, and prostacyclins for Raynaud's phenomenon and associated ulceration; and prokinetics for obstipation. ACE inhibitors are the treatment of choice for renal crisis but are not used prophylactically.

Comparison of the Largest Pediatric Cohort of jSSc with a Large Adult Cohort with Diffuse Subset jSSc

In comparison with the 1349 adult patients with diffuse aSSc from the EUSTAR cohort (Table 9.5) [131], jSSc patients had fewer digital infarcts, pulmonary involvement, gastrointestinal involvement, hypertension, muscle weakness, and tendon friction rub. It is unlikely that the difference in disease duration (mean 7.4 years in adults vs. 3.9 years in the pediatric cohort) accounted for these different features since most new-onset organ involvement evolves during the first 4 years. The prevalence of anti-centromere antibodies was similar (6% in the adult diffuse population).

There is scarce data regarding quality-of-life assessment in children with jSSc and no SSc-specific quality-of-life instrument has been validated in jSSc. A pilot study with four patients showed an impairment of quality of life compared to a healthy population [78].

Table 9.5 Comparison of the largest pediatric cohort with the EUSTAR adult cohort

	Pediatric cohort [95]	EUSTAR-diffuse subtype [131]
Skin		
Edema	43.8	
Sclerodactyly	66.0	
Skin induration	75.8	100
Calcinosis	18.3	
Peripheral vascular system		
Raynaud's phenomenon	83.7	96
Digital infarcts	28.6	43
Digital pitting	37.9	
Abnormal nail fold capillaries	39.9	
Positive capillaroscopy	51.0	
Respiratory system		
Dyspnea	17.7	45
Abnormal chest X-rays	28.8	53
Abnormal chest HRCT	23.5	
Reduced DLCO	27.5	64
Reduced FVC	41.8	
Cardiac involvement		
Pericarditis/arrhythmias	9.8	13
Heart failure	7.2	17
Pulmonary hypertension	7.2	22
Musculoskeletal system		
Muscle weakness	24.2	37
Arthritis	27.5	21
Arthralgia	36.0	
Tendon friction rubs	10.5	22
Gastrointestinal system		
Dysphagia	24.2	68
Gastroesophageal reflux	30.1	68
Diarrhea	10.5	
Weight loss	27.5	
Renal system		
Raised creatinine/ proteinuria	4.6	9
Renal crisis	0.7	4
Hypertension	2.6	19
Nervous system		
Seizures	2.6	
Peripheral neuropathy	1.3	
Abnormal brain MRI	2.6	

Outcome of the Patients in Two Pediatric Cohorts

In both cohorts [95, 106], survival of the patients after 5 years of the disease was between 90 and 95%. The eight deaths during the first 2 years of disease in the cohort of Foeldvari et al. [106] resulted from multisystem involvement with pulmonary (75%), cardiovascular (100%), central nervous system (38%), and renal (50%) involvement. The male-to-female ratio was 1:1 and the median age at disease onset was 10.5 years, but the ratio of fatality in the cohort of Martini et al. [95] was male/female 1:2.2 with a 10.4 years mean age of disease onset. The mean time until death was 4.6 years after diagnosis. Patients with fatal outcomes had higher rates of pulmonary, gastrointestinal, and cardiac involvement. All had the diffuse subtype of jSSc. The patients who died had a significantly shorter time interval to diagnosis (8.8 months vs. 23 months in patients who survived).

Special Issues in the Care for Children with jSSc

Patients and parents/caregivers can have different fears and hopes regarding the side effects of the treatment and side effects of the disease. Understanding of the treatment by the patient is essential.

Outcome of Pediatric-Onset Juvenile Systemic Sclerosis Patients into Adulthood

Three studies in adult SSc cohorts including patients with juvenile onset have evaluated the long-term prognosis of jSSc [110, 132, 133]. In Table 9.6, the characteristics of adult patients with juvenile-onset SSc are compared to juvenile patients in a jSSc cohort. As noted above, the preponderance of females increases in the adult cohort (male/female ratio of 1:5–10 compared to 1:3.6 in the pediatric-aged cohort), and the subset distribution at the adult age of juvenile-onset patients changed to the adult pattern with 35–40% the diffuse subtype and 46.7–61% the limited subtype. In the Royal Free Cohort, a large percentage of the patients showed overlap features [132], which seemed to offer a survival advantage. The prevalence of anti-centromere antibodies remained low (5–6.5%), consistent with better survival with more limited disease. The percentage of patients with pulmonary hypertension is lower than expected compared to the EUSTAR population (20% in EUSTAR). Unfortunately, not all organ involvement is described in detail in the different populations, so it is not possible to have a complete comparison.

Table 9.6 Comparison of characteristics in adults with SSc whose disease started during childhood vs. characteristics of children with jSSc (right column)

	jSSc in EUSTAR (*n* = 60)	jSSc Royal Free (*n* = 57)	jSSc Pittsburgh (*n* = 57)	jSSc PRESS (*n* = 153)
Mean age at disease onset	12.4 (2–15.9)	13.06 (5–16)	?	8.1 (0.4–15.6)
Disease duration	17.64 (1.8–54.8)	21.15 (3–58)	17.2	3.9 (0.2–18.1)
Sex (male/female)	5/55	11/35	19/92	33/120
Disease subtype diffuse (%)	40	39	35	90.9
Disease subtype limited (%)	46.7	61	40	9.1
Overlap features	NN	43.5	NN	NN
Outcome	59 (98%)	97%/15Y//93%/20Y)//83%25Y	(89(5y)//74(20Y)	112/127(88) 15/127(12) 26
Lost to follow-up (%)	1(2%)	NN	NN	(17%)
ANA positive	90%		97	80.7%
Anti-Scl 70 positive	40%	26	23	34%
Anti-centromere positive	5%	6.5	0	7.1%
Raynaud's phenomenon (%)	95	NN	96	83.7
Pulmonary hypertension (%)	13.3	15	3.6	7.2
Pulmonary fibrosis (%)	23.3	47	9	23.5
Renal crisis (%)	0	2	3.6	0.7

Summary

In summary, juvenile localized scleroderma and juvenile systemic sclerosis are a group of heterogeneous diseases. Both can cause significant morbidity in children. While there are treatment options for both disease groups, more research is needed to develop the best therapies for children.

References

1. Zulian F, Athreya BH, Laxer R, Nelson AM, Feitosa de Oliveira SK, Punaro MG, et al. Juvenile localized scleroderma: clinical and epidemiological features in 750 children. An international study. Rheumatology. 2006;45(5):614–20.
2. Laxer R, Zulian F. Localized scleroderma. Curr Opin Rheumatol. 2006;18(6):606–13.
3. Herrick AL, Ennis H, Bhushan M, Silman AJ, Baildam EM. Incidence of childhood linear scleroderma and systemic sclerosis in the UK and Ireland. Arthritis Care Res. 2010;62(2):213–8.
4. Christen-Zaech S, Hakim MD, Afsar FS, Paller AS. Pediatric morphea (localized scleroderma): review of 136 patients. J Am Acad Dermatol. 2008;59(3):385–96.
5. Wu E, Li S, Torok K, Virkud Y, Fuhlbrigge R, Rabinovich C, et al. A28: description of the juvenile localized scleroderma subgroup of the CARRA registry. Arthritis Rheumatol. 2014;66(S3):S43–4.
6. Zulian F, Vallongo C, de Oliveira SKF, Punaro MG, Ros J, Mazur-Zielinska H, et al. Congenital localized scleroderma. J Pediatr. 2006;149(2):248–51.
7. Pequet MS, Holland KE, Zhao S, Drolet BA, Galbraith SS, Siegel DH, et al. Risk factors for morphoea disease severity: a retrospective review of 114 paediatric patients. Br J Dermatol. 2014;170(4):895–900.
8. Peterson LS, Nelson AM, Su WPD. Classification of morphea (localized scleroderma). Mayo Clin Proc. 1995;70(11):1068–76.
9. Leitenberger JJ, Cayce RL, Haley RW, Adams-Huet B, Bergstresser PR, Jacobe HT. Distinct autoimmune syndromes in morphea: a review of 245 adult and pediatric cases. Arch Dermatol. 2009;145(5):545–50.
10. Marzano A, Menni S, Parodi A, Borghi A, Fuligni A, Fabbri P, et al. Localized scleroderma in adults and children. Clinical and laboratory investigations on 239 cases. Eur J Dermatol. 2003;13(2):171–6.
11. Jablonska S, Blaszczyk M. Long-lasting follow-up favours a close relationship between progressive facial hemiatrophy and scleroderma en coup de sabre*. J Eur Acad Dermatol Venereol. 2005;19(4):403–4.
12. Menni S, Marzano A, Passoni E. Neurologic abnormalities in two patients with facial hemiatrophy and sclerosis coexisting with morphea. Pediatr Dermatol. 1997;14(2):113–6.
13. Blaszczyk M, Jablonska S. Linear scleroderma en coup de sabre. Relationship with progressive facial hemiatrophy. Adv Exp Med Biol. 1999;455:101–4.
14. Sommer A, Gambichler T, Bacharach-Buhles M, von Rothenburg T, Altmeyer P, Kreuter A. Clinical and serological characteristics of progressive facial hemiatrophy: a case series of 12 patients. J Am Acad Dermatol. 2006;54(2):227–33.
15. Kakimoto C, Ross V, Uebelhoer N. En coup de sabre presenting as a port-wine stain previously treated with pulsed dye laser. Dermatol Surg. 2009;35(1):165–7.
16. Kim HS, Lee JY, Kim HO, Park YM. En coup de sabre presenting as a port-wine stain initially treated with a pulsed dye laser. J Dermatol. 2011;38(2):209–10.
17. Petrov I, Gantcheva M, Miteva L, Vassileva S, Pramatarov K. Lower lip squamous cell carcinoma in disabling pansclerotic morphea of childhood. Pediatr Dermatol. 2009;26(1):59–61.
18. Wollina U, Buslau M, Weyers W. Squamous cell carcinoma in pansclerotic morphea of childhood. Pediatr Dermatol. 2002;19(2):151–4.
19. Parodi PC, Riberti C, Draganic Stinco D, Patrone P, Stinco G. Squamous cell carcinoma arising in a patient with long-standing pansclerotic morphea. Br J Dermatol. 2001;144(2):417–9.
20. Maragh SH, Davis MDP, Bruce AJ, Nelson AM. Disabling pansclerotic morphea: clinical presentation in two adults. J Am Acad Dermatol. 2005;53(2, Supplement):S115–9.
21. Kura M, Jidai S. Disabling pansclerotic morphea of childhood with extracutaneous manifestations. Indian J Dermatol. 2013;58(2):159.
22. Zulian F, Vallongo C, Woo P, Russo R, Ruperto N, Harper J, et al. Localized scleroderma in childhood is not just a skin disease. Arthritis Rheum. 2005;52(9):2873–81.

23. Weber P, Ganser G, Frosch M, Roth J, Hulskamp G, Zimmer K. Twenty-four hour intraesophageal pH monitoring in children and adolescents with scleroderma and mixed connective tissue disease. J Rheumatol. 2000;27(11):2692–5.
24. Guariso G, Conte S, Galeazzi F, Vettorato M, Martini G, Zulian F. Esophageal involvement in juvenile localized scleroderma: a pilot study. Clin Exp Rheumatol. 2007;25(5):786–9.
25. Polcari I, Moon A, Mathes EF, Gilmore ES, Paller AS. Headaches as a presenting symptom of linear morphea en coup de sabre. Pediatrics. 2014;134(6):e1715–9.
26. Kraus V, Lawson EF, Scheven EV, Tihan T, Garza J, Nathan RG, et al. Atypical cases of scleroderma en coup de sabre. J Child Neurol. 2014;29(5):698–703.
27. Blaszczyk M, Królicki L, Krasu M, Glinska O, Jablonska S. Progressive facial hemiatrophy: central nervous system involvement and relationship with scleroderma en coup de sabre. J Rheumatol. 2003;30(9):1997–2004.
28. DeFelipe J, Segura T, Arellano JI, Merchán A, DeFelipe-Oroquieta J, Martín P, et al. Neuropathological findings in a patient with epilepsy and the Parry–Romberg syndrome. Epilepsia. 2001;42(9):1198–203.
29. Flores-Alvarado DE, Esquivel-Valerio JA, Garza-Elizondo M, Espinoza LR. Linear scleroderma en coup de sabre and brain calcification: is there a pathogenic relationship? J Rheumatol. 2003;30(1):193–5.
30. Holland KE, Steffes B, Nocton JJ, Schwabe MJ, Jacobson RD, Drolet BA. Linear scleroderma en coup de sabre with associated neurologic abnormalities. Pediatrics. 2006;117(1):e132–6.
31. Zannin ME, Martini G, Athreya BH, Russo R, Higgins G, Vittadello F, et al. Ocular involvement in children with localised scleroderma: a multi-Centre study. Br J Ophthalmol. 2007;91(10):1311–4.
32. El-Kehdy J, Abbas O, Rubeiz N. A review of parry-Romberg syndrome. J Am Acad Dermatol. 2012;67(4):769–84.
33. Takehara K, Sato S. Localized scleroderma is an autoimmune disorder. Rheumatology. 2005;44(3):274–9.
34. Warner Dharamsi J, Victor S, Aguwa N, et al. Morphea in adults and children cohort iii: nested case-control study—the clinical significance of autoantibodies in morphea. JAMA Dermatol. 2013;149(10):1159–65.
35. Arkachaisri T, Pino S. Localized scleroderma severity index and global assessments: a pilot study of outcome instruments. J Rheumatol. 2008;35(4):650–7.
36. Arkachaisri T, Vilaiyuk S, Li S, O'Neil KM, Pope E, Higgins GC, et al. The localized scleroderma skin severity index and physician global assessment of disease activity: a work in progress toward development of localized scleroderma outcome measures. J Rheumatol. 2009;36(12):2819–29.
37. Kelsey C, Torok K. The localized scleroderma assessment tool: responsiveness to change in a pediatric clinical population. JAAD. 2013;69(2):214–20.
38. Zulian F, Meneghesso D, Grisan E, Vittadello F, Belloni Fortina A, Pigozzi B, et al. A new computerized method for the assessment of skin lesions in localized scleroderma. Rheumatology. 2007;46(5):856–60.
39. Nezafati KA, Cayce RL, Susa JS, et al. 14-mhz ultrasonography as an outcome measure in morphea (localized scleroderma). Arch Dermatol. 2011;147(9):1112–5.
40. Porta F, Kaloudi O, Garzitto A, Prignano F, Nacci F, Falcini F, et al. High frequency ultrasound can detect improvement of lesions in juvenile localized scleroderma. Mod Rheumatol. 2014;24(5):869–73.
41. Li SC, Liebling MS, Haines KA, Weiss JE, Prann A. Initial evaluation of an ultrasound measure for assessing the activity of skin lesions in juvenile localized scleroderma. Arthritis Care Res (Hoboken). 2011;63(5):735–42.
42. Li SC, Liebling MS, Haines KA. Ultrasonography is a sensitive tool for monitoring localized scleroderma. Rheumatology. 2007;46(8):1316–9.
43. Martini G, Murray KJ, Howell KJ, Harper J, Atherton D, Woo P, et al. Juvenile-onset localized scleroderma activity detection by infrared thermography. Rheumatology. 2002;41(10):1178–82.
44. Kissin EY, Schiller AM, Gelbard RB, Anderson JJ, Falanga V, Simms RW, et al. Durometry for the assessment of skin disease in systemic sclerosis. Arthritis Care Res. 2006;55(4):603–9.
45. Kuwahara Y, Shima Y, Kawai M, Hagihara K, Hirano T, Arimitsu J, et al. What kind of durometer is best suited for the assessment of skin disease in systemic sclerosis? Comment on the article by Kissin et al. Arthritis Care Res. 2008;59(4):601.
46. Liu P, Uziel Y, Chuang S, Silverman E, Krakfchik B, Laxer R. Localized scleroderma: imaging features. Pediatr Radiol. 1994;24(3):207–9.
47. Dytoc MT, Kossintseva I, Ting PT. First case series on the use of calcipotriol–betamethasone dipropionate for morphoea. Br J Dermatol. 2007;157(3):615–8.
48. Cunningham BB, Landells IDR, Langman C, Sailer DE, Paller AS. Topical calcipotriene for morphea/linear scleroderma. J Am Acad Dermatol. 1998;39(2):211–5.
49. Kroft E, Groeneveld T, Seyger M, Jong ED. Efficacy of topical tacrolimus 0.1% in active plaque morphea. Am J Clin Dermatol. 2009;10(3):181–7.
50. Cantisani C, Miraglia E, Richetta A, Mattozzi C, Calvieri S. Generalized morphea successfully treated with tacrolimus 0.1% ointment. J Drugs Dermatol. 2013;12(1):14–5.
51. Pope E, Doria AS, Theriault M, Mohanta A, Laxer RM. Topical imiquimod 5% cream for pediatric plaque morphea: a prospective, multiple-baseline open-label pilot study. Dermatology. 2011;223(4):363–9.
52. Rodriquez-Castellanos M, Tlacuilo-Parra A, Sanchez-Enriquez S, Velez-Gomez E, Guevara-Gutierrez E. Pirfenidone gel in patients with localized scleroderma: a phase II study. Arthritis Res Ther. 2014;16(6):510.
53. Vasquez R, Jabbar A, Khan F, Buethe D, Ahn C, Jacobe H. Recurrence of morphea after successful ultraviolet A1 phototherapy: a cohort study. J Am Acad Dermatol. 2014;70(3):481–8.
54. Caca-Biljanovska N, Vickova-Laskoska M, Dervendi D, Pesic N, Laskoski D. Treatment of generalized morphea with oral 1,25-dihydroxyvitamin D3. Adv Exp Med Biol. 1999;455:299–304.
55. Hulshof M, Bavinck JB, Bergman W, Masclee A, Heickendorff L, Breedveld F, et al. Double-blind, placebo-controlled study of oral calcitriol for the treatment of localized and systemic scleroderma. J Am Acad Dermatol. 2000;43(6):1017–23.
56. Koch SB, Cerci FB, Jorizzo JL, Krowchuk DP. Linear morphea: a case series with long-term follow-up of young, methotrexate-treated patients. J Dermatol Treat. 2013;24(6):435–8.
57. Seyger MMB, van den Hoogen FHJ, de Boo T, de Jong EMGJ. Low-dose methotrexate in the treatment of widespread morphea. J Am Acad Dermatol. 1998;39(2):220–5.
58. Uziel Y, Feldman BM, Krafchik BR, Yeung RSM, Laxer RM. Methotrexate and corticosteroid therapy for pediatric localized scleroderma. J Pediatr. 2000;136(1):91–5.
59. Kreuter A, Gambichler T, Breuckmann F, et al. Pulsed high-dose corticosteroids combined with low-dose methotrexate in severe localized scleroderma. Arch Dermatol. 2005;141(7):847–52.
60. Fitch PG, Rettig P, Burnham JM, Finkel TH, Yan AC, Akin E, et al. Treatment of pediatric localized scleroderma with methotrexate. J Rheumatol. 2006;33(3):609–14.
61. Weibel L, Sampaio MC, Visentin MT, Howell KJ, Woo P, Harper JI. Evaluation of methotrexate and corticosteroids for the treatment of localized scleroderma (morphoea) in children. Br J Dermatol. 2006;155(5):1013–20.

62. Zulian F, Martini G, Vallongo C, Vittadello F, Falcini F, Patrizi A, et al. Methotrexate treatment in juvenile localized scleroderma: a randomized, double-blind, placebo-controlled trial. Arthritis Rheum. 2011;63(7):1998–2006.
63. Zulian F, Vallongo C, Patrizi A, Belloni-Fortina A, Cutrone M, Alessio M, et al. A long-term follow-up study of methotrexate in juvenile localized scleroderma (morphea). J Am Acad Dermatol. 2012;67(6):1151–6.
64. Li SC, Torok KS, Pope E, Dedeoglu F, Hong S, Jacobe HT, et al. Development of consensus treatment plans for juvenile localized scleroderma: a roadmap toward comparative effectiveness studies in juvenile localized scleroderma. Arthritis Care Res. 2012;64(8):1175–85.
65. Amarilyo G, Rullo OJ, McCurdy DK, Woo JM, Furst DE. Folate usage in MTX-treated juvenile idiopathic arthritis (JIA) patients is inconsistent and highly variable. Rheumatol Int. 2013;33(9):2437–40.
66. Martini G, Ramanan AV, Falcini F, Girschick H, Goldsmith DP, Zulian F. Successful treatment of severe or methotrexate-resistant juvenile localized scleroderma with mycophenolate mofetil. Rheumatology. 2009;48(11):1410–3.
67. Inamo Y, Ochiai T. Successful combination treatment of a patient with progressive juvenile localized scleroderma (morphea) using imatinib, corticosteroids, and methotrexate. Pediatr Dermatol. 2013;30(6):e191–3.
68. Prey S, Ezzedine K, Doussau A, Grandoulier AS, Barcat D, Chatelus E, et al. Imatinib mesylate in scleroderma-associated diffuse skin fibrosis: a phase II multicentre randomized double-blinded controlled trial. Br J Dermatol. 2012;167(5):1138–44.
69. Fraticelli P, Gabrielli B, Pomponio G, Valentini G, Bosello S, Riboldi P, et al. Low-dose oral imatinib in the treatment of systemic sclerosis interstitial lung disease unresponsive to cyclophosphamide: a phase II pilot study. Arthritis Res Ther. 2014;16(4):R144.
70. Elhai M, Meunier M, Matucci-Cerinic M, Maurer B, Riemekasten G, Leturcq T, et al. Outcomes of patients with systemic sclerosis-associated polyarthritis and myopathy treated with tocilizumab or abatacept: a EUSTAR observational study. Ann Rheum Dis. 2013;72(7):1217–20.
71. Stausbol-Gron B, Olesen AB, Deleuran B, Deleuran MS. Abatacept is a promising treatment for patients with disseminated morphea profunda: presentation of two cases. Acta Derm Venereol. 2011;91(6):686–8.
72. Smith V, Piette Y, van Praet JT, Decuman S, Deschepper E, Elewaut D, et al. Two-year results of an open pilot study of a 2-treatment course with rituximab in patients with early systemic sclerosis with diffuse skin involvement. J Rheumatol. 2013;40(1):52–7.
73. Jordan S, Distler JHW, Maurer B, Huscher D, van Laar JM, Allanore Y, et al. Effects and safety of rituximab in systemic sclerosis: an analysis from the European scleroderma trial and research (EUSTAR) group. Ann Rheum Dis. 2015;74(6):1188–94.
74. Wollina U, Looks A, Schneider R, Maak B. Disabling morphoea of childhood—beneficial effect of intravenous immunoglobulin therapy. Clin Exp Dermatol. 1998;23(6):292–3.
75. Lapiere J-C, Aasi S, Cook B, Montalvo A. Successful correction of depressed scars of the forehead secondary to trauma and morphea en coup de sabre by en bloc autologous dermal fat graft. Dermatol Surg. 2000;26(8):793–7. https://doi.org/10.1046/j.524-4725.2000.00073.x.
76. Palmero MLH, Uziel Y, Laxer RM, Forrest CR, Pope E. En coup de sabre scleroderma and parry-Romberg syndrome in adolescents: surgical options and patient-related outcomes. J Rheumatol. 2010;37(10):2174–9.
77. Zhao J, Chenggang Y, Binglun L, Yan H, Li Y, Xianjie M, et al. Autologous fat graft and bone marrow-derived mesenchymal stem cells assisted fat graft for treatment of parry-Romberg syndrome. Ann Plast Surg. 2014;73(Suppl 1):S99–103.
78. Baildam EM, Ennis H, Foster HE, Shaw L, Chieng AS, Kelly J, et al. Influence of childhood scleroderma on physical function and quality of life. J Rheumatol. 2011;38(1):167–73.
79. Das S, Bernstein I, Jacobe H. Correlates of self-reported quality of life in adults and children with morphea. J Am Acad Dermatol. 2014;70(5):904–10.
80. Piram M, McCuaig CC, Saint-Cyr C, Marcoux D, Hatami A, Haddad E, et al. Short- and long-term outcome of linear morphoea in children. Br J Dermatol. 2013;169(6):1265–71.
81. Mertens JS, Seyger MMB, Kievit W, Hoppenreijs EPAH, Jansen TLTA, van de Kerkhof PCM, et al. Disease recurrence in localized scleroderma: a retrospective analysis of 344 patients with pediatric or adult-onset disease. Br J Dermatol. 2015;172(3):722–8.
82. Herrick AL, Ennis H, Bhushan M, Silman AJ, Baildam EM. Incidence of childhood linear scleroderma and systemic sclerosis in the UK and Ireland. Arthritis Care Res (Hoboken). 2010;62(2):213–8.
83. Zulian F, Woo P, Athreya BH, Laxer RM, Medsger TA Jr, Lehman TJ, et al. The pediatric rheumatology European society/American College of Rheumatology/European league against rheumatism provisional classification criteria for juvenile systemic sclerosis. Arthritis Rheum. 2007;57(2):203–12.
84. Tyndall A, Furst D. Adult stem cell treatment of scleroderma. Curr Opin Rheumatol. 2007;19(6):604–10.
85. Matucci-Cerinic M, Kahaleh B, Wigley FM. Review: evidence that systemic sclerosis is a vascular disease. Arthritis Rheum. 2013;65(8):1953–62.
86. Reiff A, Weinberg KI, Triche T, Masinsin B, Mahadeo KM, Lin CH, et al. T lymphocyte abnormalities in juvenile systemic sclerosis patients. Clin Immunol. 2013;149(1):146–55.
87. Abraham DJ, Krieg T, Distler J, Distler O. Overview of pathogenesis of systemic sclerosis. Rheumatology (Oxford). 2009;48 Suppl 3:iii3–7.
88. Halper J, Kjaer M. Basic components of connective tissues and extracellular matrix: elastin, fibrillin, fibulins, fibrinogen, fibronectin, laminin, tenascins and thrombospondins. Adv Exp Med Biol. 2014;802:31–47.
89. Castelino FV, Varga J. Emerging cellular and molecular targets in fibrosis: implications for scleroderma pathogenesis and targeted therapy. Curr Opin Rheumatol. 2014;26(6):607–14.
90. Romano E, Manetti M, Guiducci S, Ceccarelli C, Allanore Y, Matucci-Cerinic M. The genetics of systemic sclerosis: an update. Clin Exp Rheumatol. 2011;29(2 Suppl 65):S75–86.
91. Mayes MD, Trojanowska M. Genetic factors in systemic sclerosis. Arthritis Res Ther. 2007;9(Suppl 2):S2–5.
92. Romano E, Manetti M, Guiducci S, Ceccarelli C, Allanore Y, Matucci-Cerinic M. The genetics of systemic sclerosis: an update. Clin Exp Dermatol. 2011;29(2 Suppl 65):S75–86.
93. Mayes M, Trojanowska M. Genetic factors in systemic sclerosis. Arthritis Res Ther. 2007;9(Suppl 2):S5.
94. Foeldvari I, Zhavania M, Birdi N, Cuttica RJ, de Oliveira SH, Dent PB, et al. Favourable outcome in 135 children with juvenile systemic sclerosis: results of a multi-national survey. Rheumatology (Oxford). 2000;39(5):556–9.
95. Martini G, Foeldvari I, Russo R, Cuttica R, Eberhard A, Ravelli A, et al. Systemic sclerosis in childhood: clinical and immunologic features of 153 patients in an international database. Arthritis Rheum. 2006;54(12):3971–8.
96. Aoyama K, Nagai Y, Endo Y, Ishikawa O. Juvenile systemic sclerosis: report of three cases and review of Japanese published work. J Dermatol. 2007;34(9):658–61.
97. Russo R, Katsicas M. Clinical characteristics of children with juvenile systemic sclerosis: follow-up of 23 patients in a single tertiary center. Pediatr Rheumatol Online J. 2007;5:6.
98. Misra R, Singh G, Aggarwal P, Aggarwal A. Juvenile onset systemic sclerosis: a single center experience of 23 cases from Asia. Clin Rheumatol. 2007;26(8):1259–62.

99. Pelkonen PM, Jalanko HJ, Lantto RK, Makela AL, Pietikainen MA, Savolainen HA, et al. Incidence of systemic connective tissue diseases in children: a nationwide prospective study in Finland. J Rheumatol. 1994;21(11):2143–6.
100. van den Hoogen F, Khanna D, Fransen J, Johnson SR, Baron M, Tyndall A, et al. 2013 classification criteria for systemic sclerosis: an American college of rheumatology/European league against rheumatism collaborative initiative. Ann Rheum Dis. 2013;72(11):1747–55.
101. Terreri MT, Andrade LE, Puccinelli ML, Hilario MO, Goldenberg J. Nail fold capillaroscopy: normal findings in children and adolescents. Semin Arthritis Rheum. 1999;29(1):36–42.
102. Ingegnoli F, Herrick AL. Nailfold capillaroscopy in pediatrics. Arthritis Care Res (Hoboken). 2013;65(9):1393–400.
103. Herrick ML, Moore T, Hollis S, Jayson MIV. The influence of age on nailfold capillary dimension in childhood. J Rheumatol. 2000;27:797–800.
104. Dolezalova P, Young SP, Bacon PA, Southwood TR. Nailfold capillary microscopy in healthy children and in childhood rheumatic diseases: a prospective single blind observational study. Ann Rheum Dis. 2003;62:444–9.
105. Herrick AL, Cutolo M. Clinical implications from capillaroscopic analysis in patients with Raynaud's phenomenon and systemic sclerosis. Arthritis Rheum. 2010;62(9):2595–604.
106. Foeldvari I, Wierk A. Healthy children have a significantly increased skin score assessed with the modified Rodnan skin score. Rheumatology. 2006;45:76–8.
107. Li AM, Yin J, Au JT, So HK, Tsang T, Wong E, et al. Standard reference for the six-minute-walk test in healthy children aged 7 to 16 years. Am J Respir Crit Care Med. 2007;176(2):174–80.
108. Lammers AE, Hislop AA, Flynn Y, Haworth SG. The 6-minute walk test: normal values for children of 4–11 years of age. Arch Dis Child. 2008;93(6):464–8.
109. Panigada S, Ravelli A, Silvestri M, Granata C, Magni-Manzoni S, Cerveri I, et al. HRCT and pulmonary function tests in monitoring of lung involvement in juvenile systemic sclerosis. Pediatr Pulmonol. 2009;44(12):1226–34.
110. Scalapino K, Arkachaisri T, Lucas M, Fertig N, Helfrich DJ, Londino AV Jr, et al. Childhood onset systemic sclerosis: classification, clinical and serologic features, and survival in comparison with adult onset disease. J Rheumatol. 2006;33(5):1004–13.
111. Lanteri A, Sobanski V, Langlois C, Lefevre G, Hauspie C, Sanges S, et al. Serum free light chains of immunoglobulins as biomarkers for systemic sclerosis characteristics, activity and severity. Autoimmun Rev. 2014;13(9):974–80.
112. van Bon L, Affandi AJ, Broen J, Christmann RB, Marijnissen RJ, Stawski L, et al. Proteome-wide analysis and CXCL4 as a biomarker in systemic sclerosis. N Engl J Med. 2014;370(5):433–43.
113. Castelino FV, Varga J. Current status of systemic sclerosis biomarkers: applications for diagnosis, management and drug development. Expert Rev Clin Immunol. 2013;9(11):1077–90.
114. Kolto G, Vuolteenaho O, Szokodi I, Faludi R, Tornyos A, Ruskoaho H, et al. Prognostic value of N-terminal natriuretic peptides in systemic sclerosis: a single centre study. Clin Exp Rheumatol. 2014;32(Suppl 86 (6)):75–81.
115. Abignano G, Cuomo G, Buch MH, Rosenberg WM, Valentini G, Emery P, et al. The enhanced liver fibrosis test: a clinical grade, validated serum test, biomarker of overall fibrosis in systemic sclerosis. Ann Rheum Dis. 2014;73(2):420–7.
116. Vesely R, Vargova V, Ravelli A, et al. Serum level of KL-6 as a marker of interstitial lung disease in patients with juvenile systemic scleroderma. J Rheumatol. 2004;31:795–800.
117. Lammers AE, Hislop AA, Haworth SG. Prognostic value of B-type natriuretic peptide in children with pulmonary hypertension. Int J Cardiol. 2009;135(1):21–6.
118. Van Albada ME, Loot FG, Fokkema R, Roofthooft MT, Berger RM. Biological serum markers in the management of pediatric pulmonary arterial hypertension. Pediatr Res. 2008;63(3):321–7.
119. Bernus A, Wagner BD, Accurso F, Doran A, Kaess H, Ivy DD. Brain natriuretic peptide levels in managing pediatric patients with pulmonary arterial hypertension. Chest. 2009;135(3):745–51.
120. Kowal-Bielecka O, Landewé R, Avouac J, Chwiesko S, Miniati I, Czirjak L, et al. EULAR recommendations for the treatment of systemic sclerosis: a report from the EULAR Scleroderma Trials and Research Group (EUSTAR). Ann Rheum Dis. 2009;68(5):620–8.
121. van Laar JM, Farge D, Sont JK, et al. Autologous hematopoietic stem cell transplantation vs intravenous pulse cyclophosphamide in diffuse cutaneous systemic sclerosis: a randomized clinical trial. JAMA. 2014;311(24):2490–8.
122. Lehman T. Methotrexate for the treatment of early diffuse scleroderma: comment on the article by Pope et al. Arthritis Rheum. 2002;46(3):845.
123. Tashkin DP, Elashoff R, Clements PJ, Roth MD, Furst DE, Silver RM, et al. Effects of 1-year treatment with cyclophosphamide on outcomes at 2 years in scleroderma lung disease. Am J Respir Crit Care Med. 2007;176(10):1026–34.
124. Clements PJ, Roth MD, Elashoff R, Tashkin DP, Goldin J, Silver RM, et al. Scleroderma lung study (SLS): differences in the presentation and course of patients with limited versus diffuse systemic sclerosis. Ann Rheum Dis. 2007;66(12):1641–7.
125. Poormoghim H, Moradi Lakeh M, Mohammadipour M, Sodagari F, Toofaninjed N. Cyclophosphamide for scleroderma lung disease: a systematic review and meta-analysis. Rheumatol Int. 2012;32(8):2431–44.
126. Smith V, Van Praet JT, Vandooren B, Van der Cruyssen B, Naeyaert JM, Decuman S, et al. Rituximab in diffuse cutaneous systemic sclerosis: an open-label clinical and histopathological study. Ann Rheum Dis. 2010;69(1):193–7.
127. Daoussis D, Liossis S, Tsamandas A, Kalogeropoulou C, Paliogianni F, Sirinian C, et al. Effect of long-term treatment with rituximab on pulmonary function and skin fibrosis in patients with diffuse systemic sclerosis. Clin Exp Dermatol. 2012;30(2 Suppl 71):S17–22.
128. Daoussis D, Liossis SN, Tsamandas AC, Kalogeropoulou C, Paliogianni F, Sirinian C, et al. Effect of long-term treatment with rituximab on pulmonary function and skin fibrosis in patients with diffuse systemic sclerosis. Clin Exp Rheumatol. 2012;30(2 Suppl 71):S17–22.
129. Distler J, Jordan S, Airo P, Alegre-Sancho J, Allanore Y, Gurman AB, et al. Is there a role for TNFalpha antagonists in the treatment of SSc? EUSTAR expert consensus development using the Delphi technique. Clin Exp Rheumatol. 2011;29(2 Suppl 65):S40–5.
130. Denton CP, Engelhart M, Tvede N, Wilson H, Khan K, Shiwen X, et al. An open-label pilot study of infliximab therapy in diffuse cutaneous systemic sclerosis. Ann Rheum Dis. 2009;68(9):1433–9.
131. Walker UA, Tyndall A, Czirják L, Denton C, Farge-Bancel D, Kowal-Bielecka O, et al. Clinical risk assessment of organ manifestations in systemic sclerosis: a report from the EULAR scleroderma trials and research group database. Ann Rheum Dis. 2007;66(6):754–63.
132. Foeldvari I, Nihtyanova SI, Wierk A, Denton CP. Characteristics of patients with juvenile onset systemic sclerosis in an adult single-center cohort. J Rheumatol. 2010;37:2422–6.
133. Foeldvari I, Tyndall A, Zulian F, Muller-Ladner U, Czirjak L, Denton C, et al. Juvenile and young adult-onset systemic sclerosis share the same organ involvement in adulthood: data from the EUSTAR database. Rheumatology (Oxford). 2012;51:1832–7.

Morphea (Localized Scleroderma)

10

Noelle M. Teske and Heidi T. Jacobe

Classification and Epidemiology of Morphea

Morphea, also called localized scleroderma, is a chronic autoimmune disease characterized by inflammation and sclerosis of the skin. Morphea, such as scleroderma, is characterized as a sclerosing skin disorder, due to characteristic histological findings shared by both disorders, including sclerosis of the dermis and sometimes subcutis in the absence of fibroblast proliferation. However, morphea differs from scleroderma demographically and clinically. In contrast to scleroderma, the involvement of internal organs in morphea is unusual and very different from that in scleroderma, and the diagnosis does not carry the same implications in terms of morbidity and increased mortality. Thus, it is the opinion of the authors that the term "localized scleroderma" should be avoided to limit unnecessary evaluation and anxiety for patients, and confusion among providers. In this chapter, we will exclusively use the term "morphea."

The clinical features of morphea are single or multiple sclerotic or indurated cutaneous plaques that are often dyspigmented (hypo- or hyperpigmented) and may have an erythematous border, depending on their stage of evolution. These plaques vary in appearance, depending on the subtype of morphea (Table 10.1) and the activity of the disease (see *Assessment of disease activity in morphea* and *Stages of morphea lesions*). Notably, cutaneous features of scleroderma, including Raynaud's phenomenon, mat-like telangiectasias, sclerodactyly, acrosclerosis, decreased oral aperture, and nail fold capillary changes, are not seen in morphea.

The major subtypes of morphea include circumscribed or plaque-type, linear, generalized, pansclerotic, and mixed forms. Clinical images of the morphea subtypes are pre-

N. M. Teske (✉)
Department of Dermatology, Oregon Health & Science University, OR, USA
e-mail: tesken@ohsu.edu

H. T. Jacobe
Department of Dermatology, University of Texas Southwestern Medical Center, Dallas, TX, USA
e-mail: Heidi.Jacobe@UTSouthwestern.edu

Y. Allanore et al. (eds.), *Scleroderma*, https://doi.org/10.1007/978-3-031-40658-4_10

Table 10.1 Classification of morphea

Morphea subtype	Modifiers	Clinical
Circumscribed	Superficial	Single or multiple oval/round lesions; pathology limited to the dermis
	Deep	Single or multiple oval/round lesions involving the dermis and subcutaneous tissue, fascia, or muscle
Linear	Trunk/limbs	Linear lesions; possible primary site of involvement in the subcutaneous tissue without involvement of the dermis; may involve the subcutaneous tissue, muscle, and/or bone
	Head	En coup de sabre (ECDS), progressive hemifacial atrophy (PHA), linear lesions of the face and scalp (may involve the underlying bone)
Generalized		
1. Coalescent plaque		≥4 plaques in at least two of seven anatomic sites (head-neck, right/left upper extremity, right/left lower extremity, anterior/posterior trunk); Isomorphic pattern: coalescent plaques inframammary fold, waistline, lower abdomen, proximal thighs; symmetric pattern: symmetric plaque circumferential around the breasts, umbilicus, arms, and legs
2. Pansclerotic[a]		Circumferential involvement of the majority of body surface area (sparing the fingertips and toes), affecting the skin, subcutaneous tissue, muscle, or bone; no internal organ involvement characteristic of scleroderma
Mixed		Combination of any above subtype: linear—circumscribed

[a]While Zulian and Laxer categorized pansclerotic morphea separately, it is the opinion of the authors that this subtype can be classified under the broader heading of generalized morphea, as the features of pansclerotic morphea fulfill the criteria for generalized morphea in terms of the extent of involvement. The classification was further modified by the authors from the original by clarifying the level of pathology of the various subtypes (adapted with permission from Laxer and Zulian [110]).

sented in Fig. 10.1. The classification scheme presented herein was developed by the Committee on Classification Criteria for Juvenile Systemic Sclerosis, composed of members of the Pediatric Rheumatology European Society (PRES), the American College of Rheumatology (ACR), and the European League Against Rheumatism (ELAR) [1] (Table 10.1). Although there are many reported classifications of morphea, the authors have found this to be the most clinically relevant. The classification of morphea is based on the morphology of the skin lesions, as histopathology is similar in all the forms of morphea, and there are no known biomarkers for morphea subtypes. Histology is useful, however, in excluding other entities in the differential diagnosis (see *Differential diagnosis of morphea*).

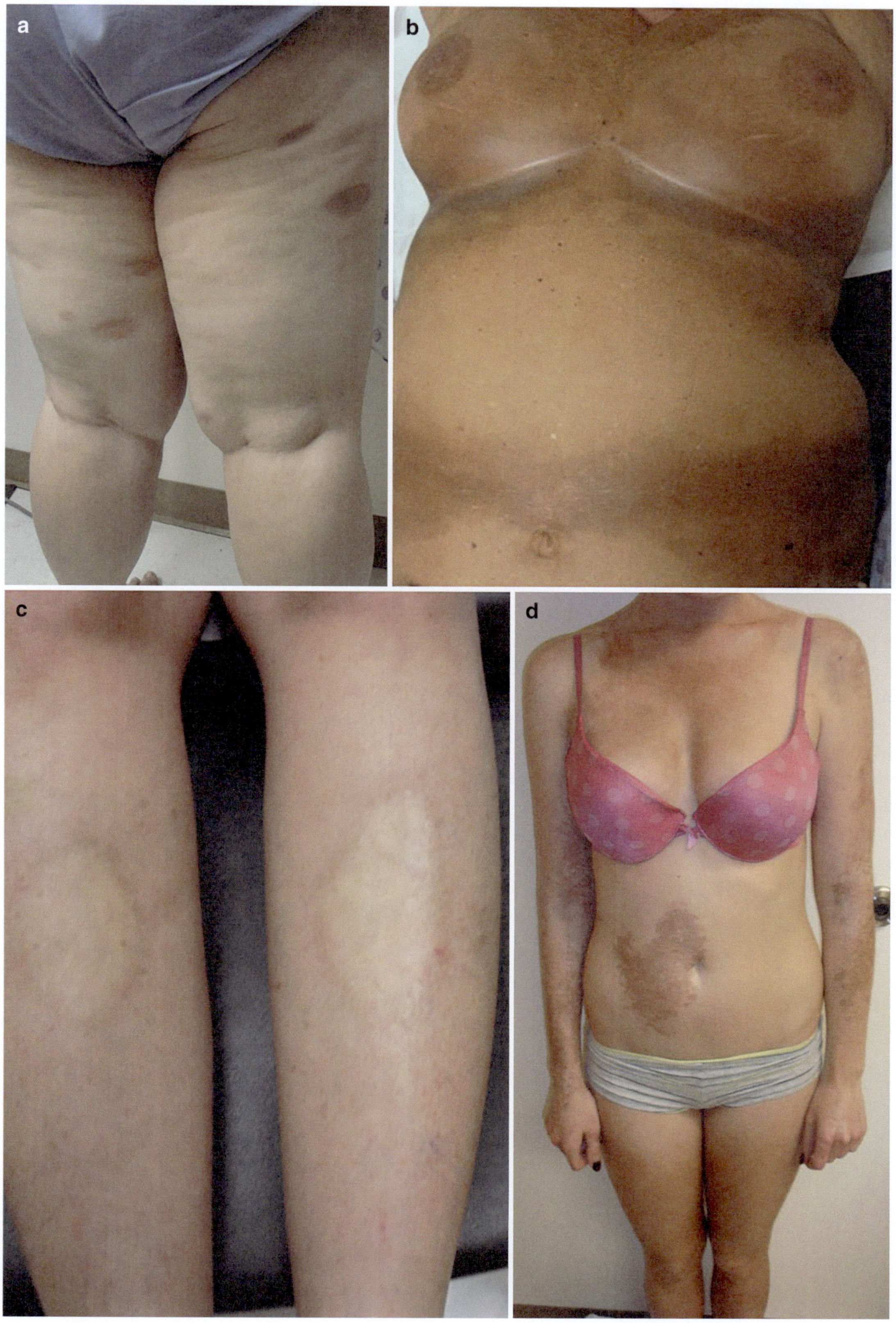

Fig. 10.1 (**a**) *Plaque-type morphea*. Circumscribed hyperpigmented plaques are present on the posterior legs of this patient with morphea. (**b**) *Generalized morphea on the trunk*. Hyperpigmented sclerotic plaques are present on the chest and abdomen. (**c**) *Generalized morphea on the extremities*. Symmetric, hypopigmented, sclerotic plaques are present on the legs of this patient with generalized morphea. (**d**) *Linear morphea*. Linear lesions of both the extremity and trunk are seen in this patient. Note that early linear lesions may not completely coalesce and may be confused with plaque-type morphea if not carefully examined. Note that on the trunk, linear lesions characteristically obey the midline. (**e**, **f**) *Pansclerotic morphea*. Note sheets of contiguous sclerosis, encompassing the majority of the body surface area (**e**) and characteristically sparing the fingertips, stopping at the metacarpophalangeal joints (**f**)

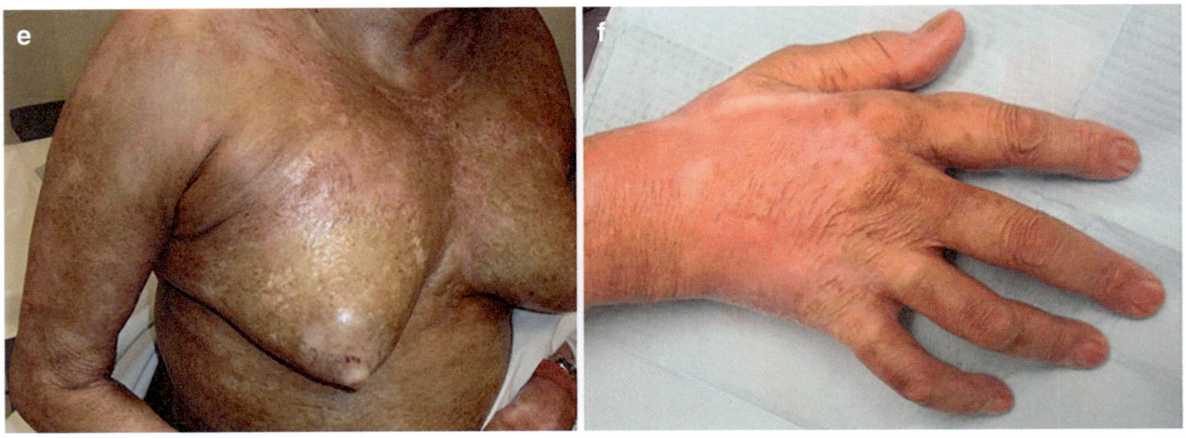

Fig. 10.1 (continued)

Variants and Related Entities

When linear morphea occurs on the upper face, especially the paramedian forehead, it is often called en coup de sabre (ECDS) (Fig. 10.2a, b). When it involves the lower face or produces hemifacial atrophy of deeper tissues, it is called progressive hemifacial atrophy (PHA), also known as the Parry-Romberg syndrome (PRS) (Fig. 10.2c–f). Whether these conditions represent an entity different from morphea has been a subject of considerable debate, but recent literature suggests that they are part of the morphea disease spectrum [2] in the sense that PHA represents a deep involvement of the facial tissues with resultant residual atrophy.

Overlying lichen sclerosus, changes may be seen in morphea lesions of all subtypes (Fig. 10.3). This observation has led to controversy over whether these represent two independent processes or whether changes similar to lichen sclerosus occur in morphea. Eosinophilic fasciitis (EF) has also been considered by some to be a variant of morphea, as about a third of patients with EF have findings typical of classic plaque-type morphea [3].

Other entities, such as bullous morphea and guttate morphea, have been described in case reports and case series [4–13]. Examination of reports of bullous morphea reveals that bullae were largely present in areas of dense sclerosis in dependent areas [7]. This suggests that the bulla is a secondary change related to edema in dependent areas or lymphatic obstruction due to sclerotic changes in the skin, rather than a primary process [7, 11, 14]. Therefore, it is the opinion of the authors that bullae should not warrant a designation as a separate subtype. Similarly, guttate lesions likely represent a variant of circumscribed morphea.

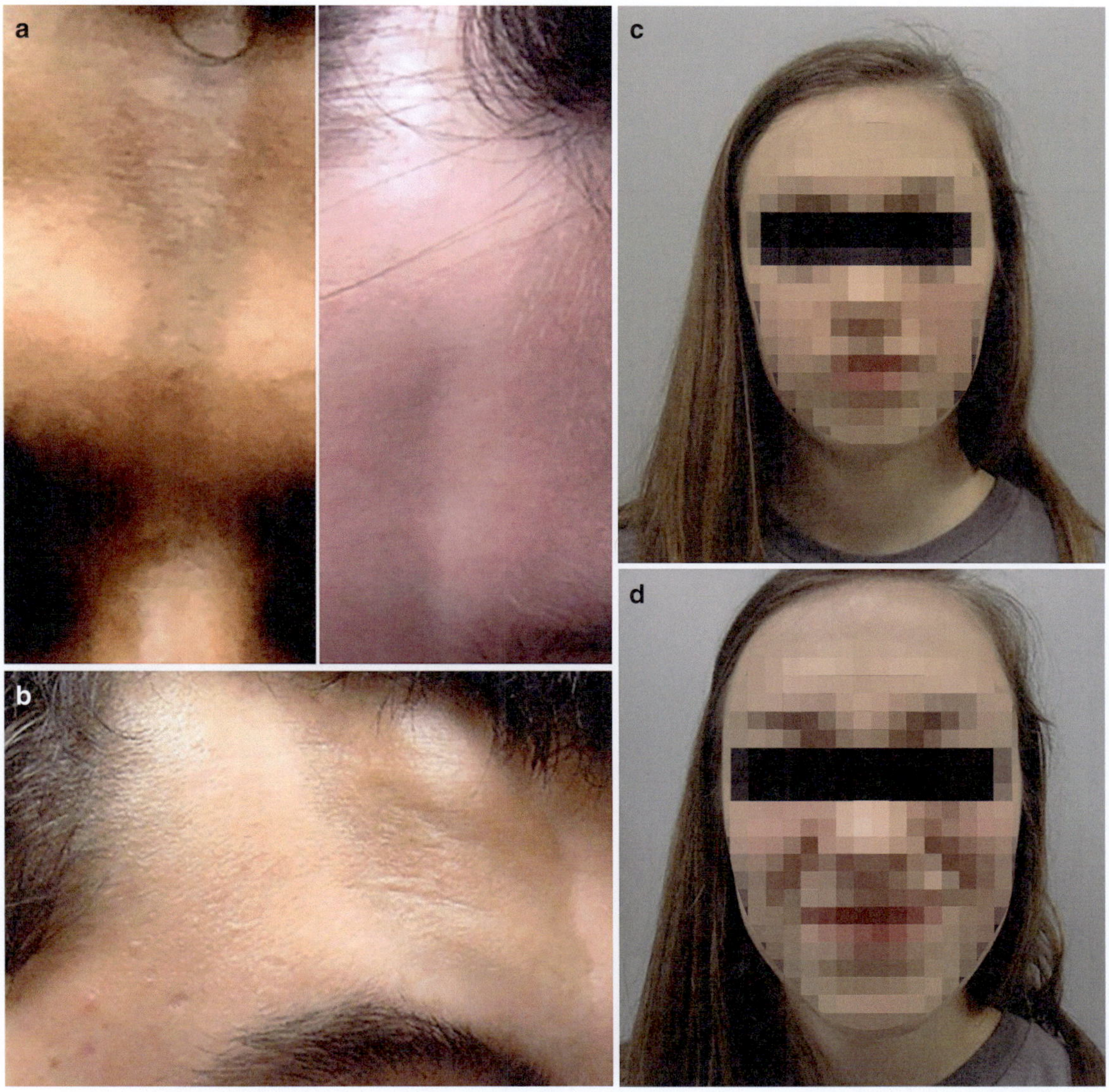

Fig. 10.2 (**a**, **b**) *En coup de sabre morphea*. Depressed linear plaques are present on the foreheads of these patients. These lesions are often dyspigmented and may have more obvious dermal changes (**a**) or change predominantly in the subcutis. Interestingly, years after this initial period of activity on the forehead, this patient (**b**) also developed tenosynovitis. (**c–f**) *Progressive hemifacial atrophy* also known as the Parry-Romberg Syndrome may be subtle (**c**), requiring additional exam maneuvers to detect. Asymmetry can sometimes be better appreciated using different facial expressions (**d**). When progressive, hemifacial atrophy may lead to more obvious lesions, as seen here on the chin, mandible, neck and tongue (**e–f**)

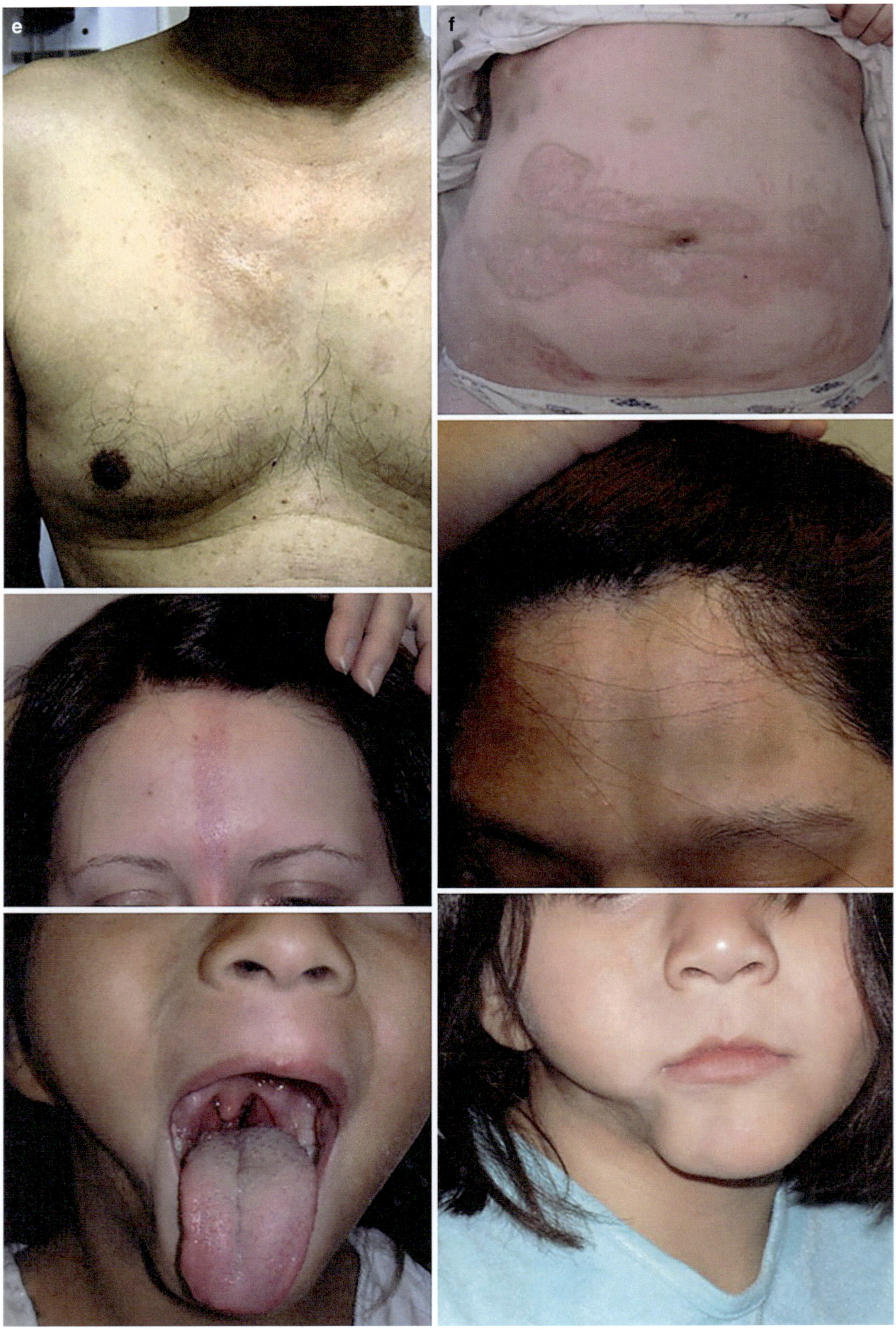

Fig. 10.2 (continued)

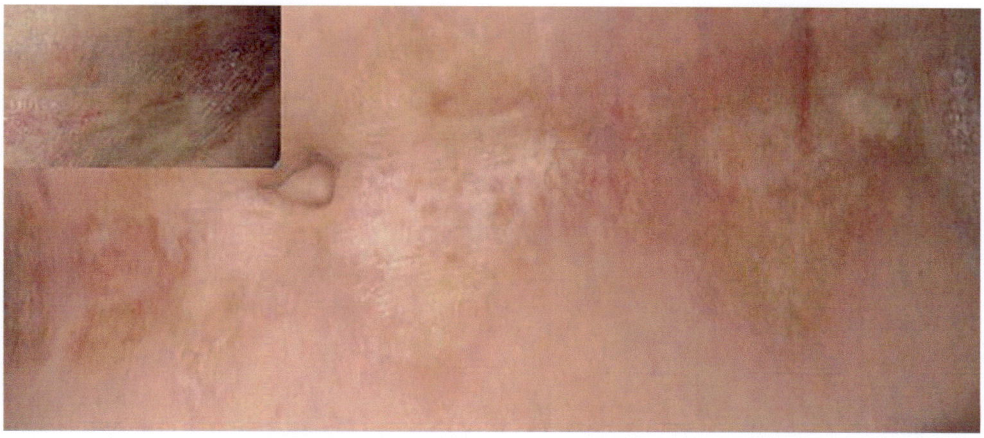

Fig. 10.3 *Morphea and lichen sclerosus*. Sclerotic lesions of morphea with overlying areas of fine, hypopigmented, wrinkled skin are present. This lesion also has features of active inflammatory morphea with an erythematous border

Epidemiology and Clinical Course

Morphea has an estimated incidence of 2.7/10000 with a female to male ratio of 2–3:1 [15]. Existing studies suggest that morphea occurs most frequently in Caucasians, though population-based studies are needed to confirm this finding [16–18]. The reported frequency of different subtypes varies likely due to differing classification systems. However, linear morphea is more common in the pediatric population [15, 19], while the generalized and plaque subtypes predominate in adults. The clinical course is not well described, with periods of disease activity ranging from 3 to 6 years, and reactivation occurring after periods of remission in some patients [20]. Patients with pediatric-onset disease may also experience persistent disease and/or recurrences in adulthood [21, 22]. A retrospective evaluation of long-term outcomes of adults with pediatric-onset morphea from the Morphea in Adults and Children (MAC) cohort revealed that 89% of patients (24/27) developed new or expanding lesions over time, suggesting that patients may need lifelong evaluation and repeated courses of treatment to prevent morbidity [21] (Fig. 10.4).

Studies examining recurrence rates after the treatment with methotrexate and/or systemic steroids report recurrence in 6–19 months after the discontinuation of therapy in 10–44% of patients [23–26]. Studies evaluating long-term outcomes after the methotrexate therapy vary greatly in methods and duration of follow-up, so comparison of recurrence is difficult [23, 27]. Recurrence has also been described in patients after successful treatment with UVA-1 phototherapy at rates as high as 46%, which may exceed those rates described with methotrexate. Median time to recurrence ranges from 10 months up to 20–30 months for those treated with UVA-1 and methotrexate, respectively [22, 23, 27–29]. These findings emphasize the need for regular monitoring of patients with morphea for signs of new disease activity even after successful treatment (see *Assessment of disease activity in morphea*).

Factors associated with recurrence in previous studies have included a longer duration of disease before treatment [28], older age of onset in the pediatric population [25], and the presence of linear morphea of the limbs [25, 30]. However, these associations have not always been replicated across studies. Prognostic markers have not yet been identified for recurrent or chronic disease in the form of prospective longitudinal studies, but retrospective reviews and cross-sectional studies have implicated that an increased duration of disease before treatment may be associated with the increased likelihood of recurrent disease [28]. The preliminary analysis from the prospective MAC cohort has revealed similar recurrence rates between pediatric and adult patients and across subtypes of morphea. The only variable associated with recurrence in this cohort has been disease duration, in that patients with a longer disease duration have been more likely to recur.

Etiology and Pathogenesis of Morphea

The etiology and pathogenesis of morphea are not well understood. Most pathological events ascribed to morphea have been extrapolated from research in scleroderma, as the two disorders are assumed to arise from a similar etiology [31]. Morphea, like other autoimmune disorders, likely arises from a genetic background of increased immune disease susceptibility, combined with other causative factors, such as trauma or environmental exposures, which modulate the expression of disease.

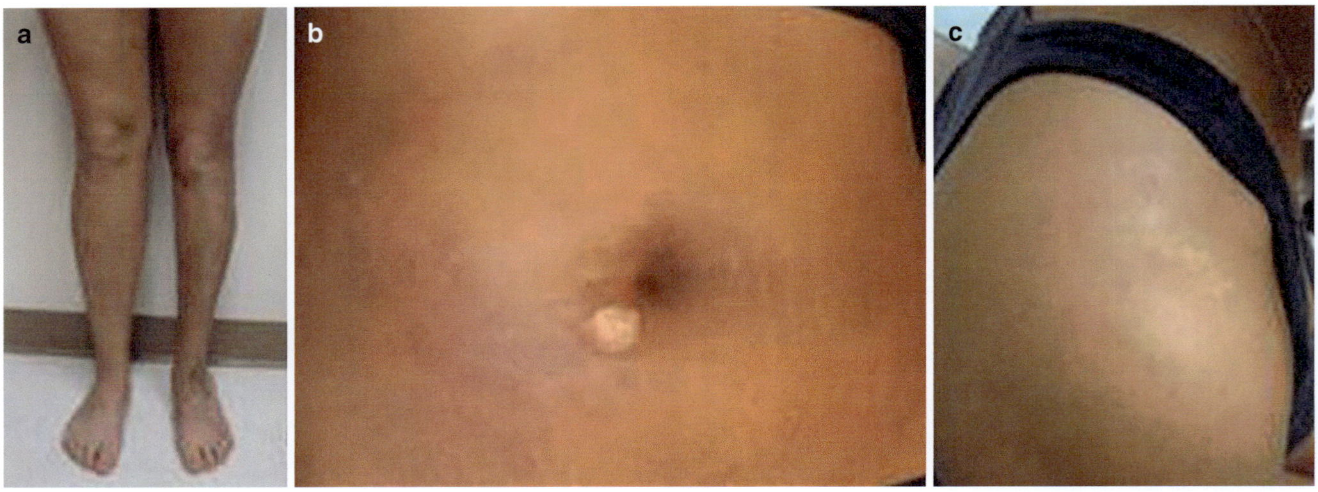

Fig. 10.4 *Chronic nature of morphea and sequelae*. Lesions began on the right leg at age five in this patient. Note muscle atrophy, limb length discrepancy, and pes planus foot deformity (**a**). In adulthood, the same patient had a recurrence of morphea in the form of active inflammatory lesions of the trunk, seen here on the abdomen (**b**), as well as a plaque that appeared on the shoulder (**c**)

Genetics and Autoimmunity in Morphea

Like many autoimmune connective tissue diseases, morphea is likely a complex genetic disease. Familial clustering has been reported, although rarely [18, 32, 33], and morphea is also associated with higher than expected rates of familial autoimmune disorders [18, 21, 34]. In retrospective studies, morphea patients have demonstrated concomitant autoimmune disease, including psoriasis, systemic lupus erythematosus, multiple sclerosis, and vitiligo, at higher than expected frequency when compared with published population-based prevalence estimates [18, 34–36]. A population-based study examining a rheumatoid arthritis population in Sweden reported a higher risk of morphea among these patients with a reported standardized incidence ratio (SIR) of 2.40 [35]. A similar population-based study in Sweden also reported a higher risk of morphea among siblings of patients with multiple sclerosis with an SIR of 1.72 [36]. Morphea has been reported, in case studies, to coexist with other autoimmune diseases, including inflammatory bowel disease [37], autoimmune thyroid disease [38, 39], alopecia areata, type I diabetes mellitus [37], antiphospholipid syndrome [40], and necrotizing vasculitis [68]. Other types of inflammatory skin disorders can also be associated with morphea, such as psoriasis [41] and lichen planopilaris [42].

Of interest, the risk for morphea has been associated with the presence of specific HLA class I and II alleles, further implicating a possible underlying genetic predisposition for the disease. A large case–control association study of patients from the MAC cohort revealed strong associations with specific HLA class I and II alleles, including, most significantly, HLA-B*37, as well as another, DRB1*04:04, in common with a risk allele previously identified for systemic sclerosis [43]. Alleles conferring the greatest risk included HLA DRB1*04:04 and HLAB37 [43]. Risk alleles identified in this case–control study have also been associated with the risk of rheumatoid arthritis and autoimmune thyroid disease [44, 45], implying that there may be a common genetic susceptibility to these disorders.

Increasing evidence supports immune dysregulation as an important pathogenic event early in the course of morphea. Early morphea lesions are characterized by the influx of large amounts of mononuclear lymphocytes (usually activated T-lymphocytes), plasma cells, and eosinophils [31]. This is likely the result of autoimmunity, as there is widespread autoimmune reactivity in morphea patients including elevated ANAs (see *Laboratory findings in morphea*), cytokines, and adhesion molecules [18, 21, 46]. Vessel damage and upregulation of adhesion molecules (ICAM-1, VCAM 1, and E-selectin) occur related to the inflammatory cell infiltrate in morphea, which facilitates local monocyte recruitment [47]. These adhesion molecules also facilitate the recruitment of T-lymphocytes that are capable of producing pro-fibrotic cytokines (IL-4, IL-6, and TGF-beta) and may contribute to the development of sclerosis [31, 48]. Of note, increased levels of these vascular adhesion molecules have been detected in serum from patients with morphea [49]. These adhesion molecules are upregulated by cytokines classically associated with a Th2 immune response (IL-4, IL-1, and TNFs). Cytokines found in increased concentration in the sera and skin of morphea patients include IL-4, IL-6, and IL-8 [47, 50]. These cytokines, especially IL-4, upregulate TGF-beta, initiating a cascade of events that results in the increased production of collagen and other extracellular matrix components via the induction of connective tissue growth factor, platelet-derived growth factor, and matrix metalloproteinases. Chimerism or nonself cells may also play a role in the pathogenesis of morphea by initiating a local inflammatory reaction [51].

In a recent study of 69 pediatric patients with morphea, interferon-gamma-inducible protein 10 (IP-10) levels were significantly elevated in the plasma of morphea patients when compared with healthy controls. Immunohistochemistry staining of IP-10 was also present in the dermal infiltrate of a subset of morphea patients who had available skin biopsies. IP-10 levels were significantly elevated in those with active versus inactive disease and correlated with standardized disease outcome measures of activity, further suggesting that IP-10 may be a potential biomarker for the activity of disease in morphea [52].

Although large-scale studies examining gene expression profiles in morphea are lacking, Milano et al. [53] have used gene expression array analysis to establish gene expression signatures for scleroderma skin subsets as compared to unaffected skin of the same patient. In their first study, they included the skin of three patients with morphea. They identified five significantly different gene expression clusters: diffuse proliferation, inflammatory, limited, and normal-like in scleroderma. Gene expression profiles from all three biopsies of morphea skin fell into the inflammatory category, which was characterized by markers for an increase in immune response, response to a pathogen, humoral defense, lymphocyte proliferation, chemokine binding, and chemokine receptor activity, and response to virus. These findings provide further evidence for an important role of immune dysregulation in morphea.

Taken together and extrapolating from research in scleroderma, these studies implicate an important role for interferons and Th1-skewed immune responses in early morphea, while Th2 cell lineages may become dominant in later disease as sclerosis predominates. Studies of this sort are necessary to identify pathways relevant to the pathogenesis of morphea and to pave the way for the identification of biomarkers and therapeutic targets.

Histopathology of Morphea

Histopathological changes in morphea evolve over the duration of individual lesions. The histopathological changes have been divided into indeterminate (early), inflammatory, mixed inflammatory and sclerotic, and sclerotic (late) stage morphea [54] (Figs. 10.5 and 10.6). Increased numbers of T cells are present in the inflammatory stage compared with normal skin. As in scleroderma, the inflammatory stage of morphea is characterized by dermal edema and by lymphocytic and histiocytic inflammatory cell infiltrates with plasma cells in a perivascular, periadnexal, and interstitial pattern. Eosinophils, mast cells, and macrophages may also be present. One finding particularly characteristic of morphea is the presence of an inflammatory cell infiltrate in the junction between the dermis and subcutaneous fat. From there, the inflammatory cell infiltrate may stream down the septa of the subcutaneous fat (Fig. 10.6c, d).

Recently, a cross-sectional study of the MAC cohort revealed a predilection for the inflammatory cell infiltrate to occur in the border between the subcutis and the dermis. This was particularly true in cases where sclerosis followed a bottom-heavy pattern, characterized by hyalinized collagen bundles in the deep dermis and subcutis, sparing the papillary through the mid-dermis, a pattern that was typical of those with morphea profunda [55] (Fig. 10.6b). A biopsy with such changes, even in the absence of sclerosis, should alert providers to the possibility of early inflammatory morphea profunda. In contrast, in this same study, a top-heavy pattern, characterized by collagen bundles exclusively in the papillary to superficial reticular dermis, was typical of those with lichen sclerosus overlap. Patterns of sclerosis varied equally in those with linear and plaque-type morphea between top-heavy, bottom-heavy, and full thickness patterns, with thickened collagen bundles throughout the dermis. Interestingly, among patients with generalized morphea, those with isomorphic patterns of distribution in patterns of chronic friction more often had top-heavy patterns of sclerosis, while bottom-heavy patterns predominated among those with symmetric patterns of distribution in generalized morphea. When inflammation was present, it consisted most often of lymphocytes (83/91, 91%) and plasma cells (68/91, 75%), but eosinophils were also noted with some frequency (17/91, 19%).

The later sclerotic stage of morphea is characterized histopathologically by thickened, acellular, homogenized-appearing collagen bundles that may involve all levels of dermis and/or subcutis (where collagen bundles stream downward through the septa) (Fig. 10.6e, f). The adnexal structures (hair, eccrine glands) are surrounded by dense fibrosis with loss of fat around the eccrine glands in chronic disease (Fig. 10.6g). In specimens from morphea profunda, the deep reticular dermis, subcutis, and/or fascia also show sclerotic changes. It is not uncommon for inflammation and sclerosis to coexist (Fig. 10.6a). The atrophic stage is characterized by loss of inflammatory cell infiltrate, decreasing sclerosis, and an absence of appendageal structures. Telangiectasia may be evident.

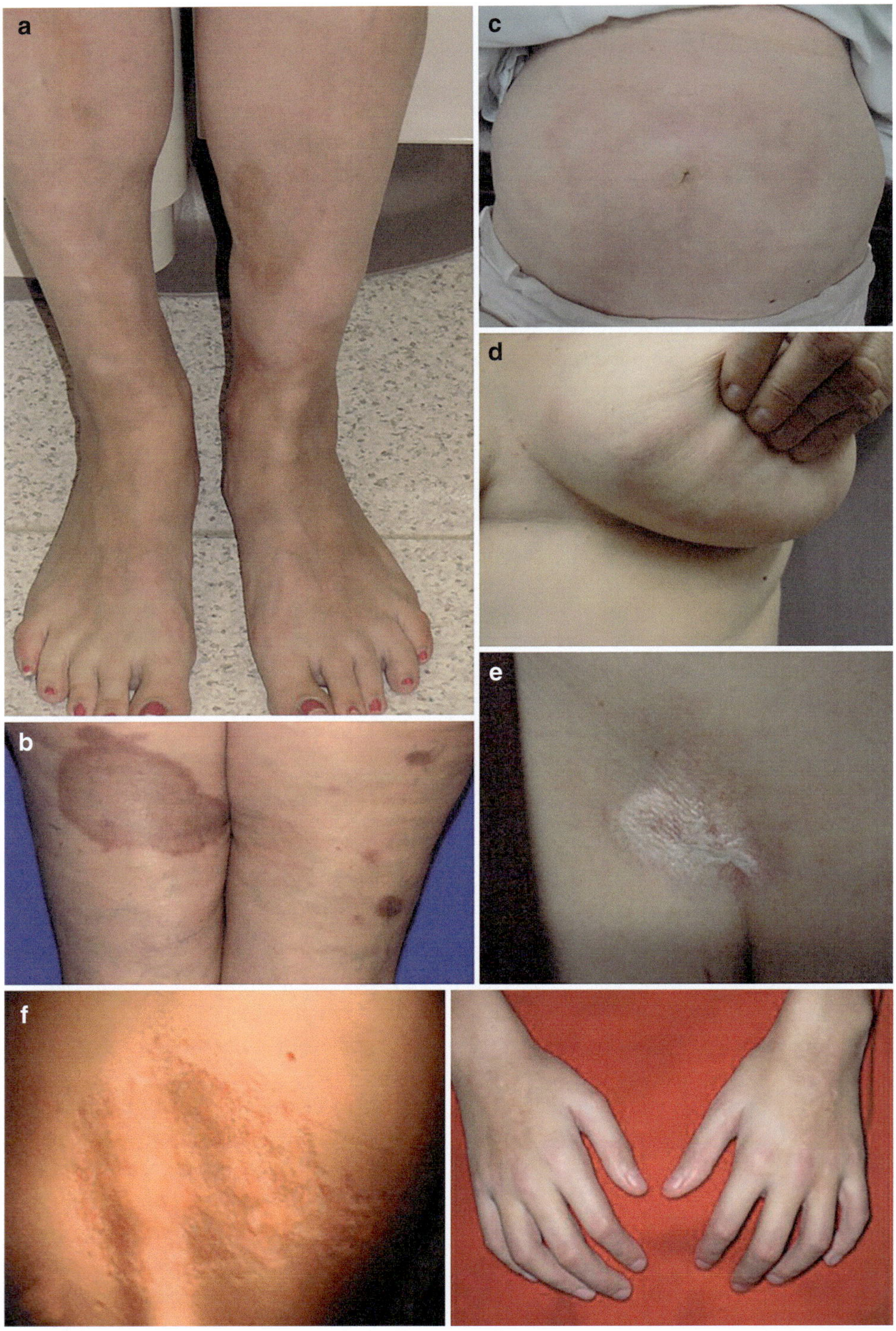

Fig. 10.5 *Disease features in morphea.* (**a**) *Deep morphea.* The areas affected by deep morphea, also known as morphea profunda, may have a cobblestone appearance with subcutaneous atrophy. (**b–d**) *Inflammatory morphea.* An active plaque in the inflammatory stage is present on the left leg of this patient (**b**) note the violaceous border. There are also multiple early lesions present on the right. (**c**) Early morphea lesions may be subtle, as seen here on the patient's abdomen, where ill-defined indurated plaques with peripheral erythema indicate active inflammatory morphea. (**d**) This well-circumscribed plaque on the patient's breast exemplifies the erythematous border and central sclerosis typical of an early evolving morphea lesion. (**e**) *Sclerotic morphea.* This lesion demonstrates exuberant sclerosis centrally with surrounding hypopigmentation and erythema, likely indicating that the lesion is transitioning toward a more inactive state. Also note telangiectasias, which can occur in the surrounding atrophy and should not be mistaken for erythema indicating inflammation. (**f**) *Atrophoderma of Pasini and Pierini.* Preadolescent girl with several-year history of a large plaque and small patches of atrophy on the lumbar back. The lesions have a sharp drop-off with a "punched out" appearance and are not indurated clinically. (**g**) *Atrophy.* Severe subcutaneous atrophy is present in this patient with linear morphea in the atrophic stage, as well as postinflammatory hyperpigmentation changes and limb length discrepancy. (**h, i**) *Linear morphea of the extremity associated with disabling contractures.* Note contractures of the hands in children with long-standing linear morphea. Contractures can be a manifestation of damage occurring most commonly in linear lesions crossing joints, but may also be a component of other subtypes, including generalized morphea, when distributed over the joints

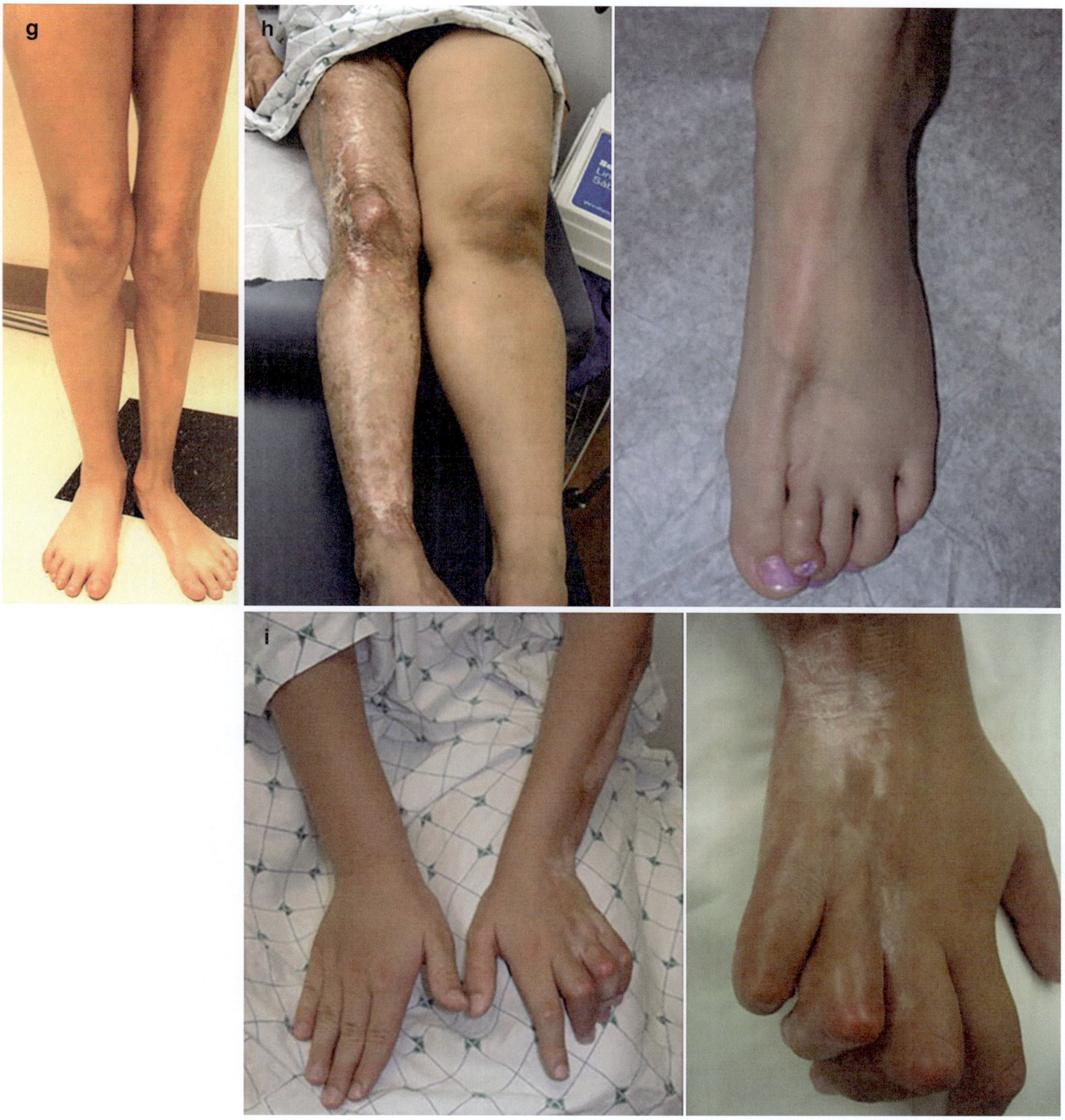

Fig. 10.5 (continued)

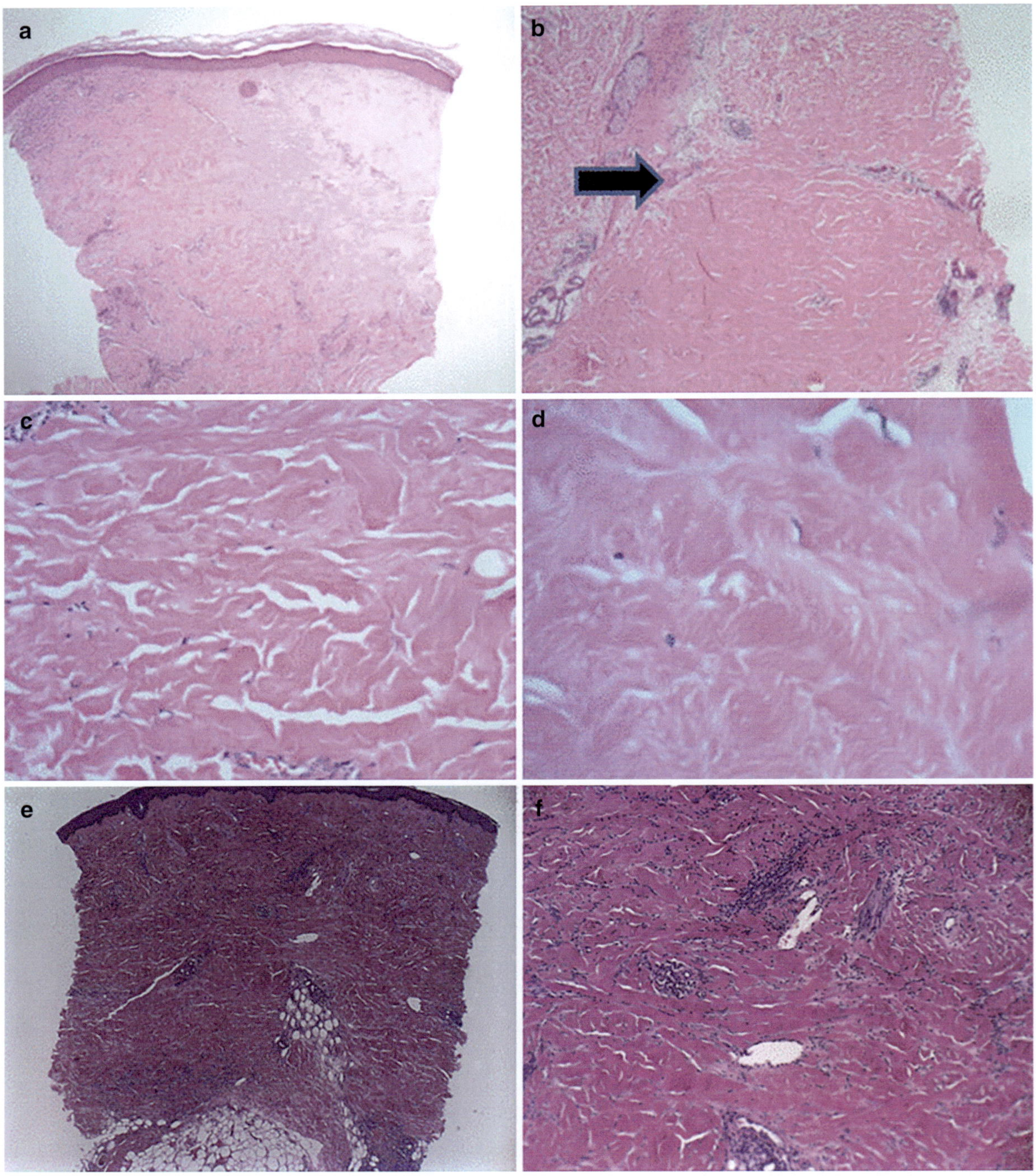

Fig. 10.6 (**a**) Skin biopsies of morphea have a characteristic "squared-off" shape because of the dense dermal sclerosis. There are patchy perivascular mononuclear cell infiltrates of lymphocytes, histiocytes, and occasional plasma cells, but otherwise the dermis is acellular compared with the normal skin. Flattening and atrophy of the epidermis are associated with underlying sclerosis. Hair follicles and sebaceous glands normally seen in a skin biopsy of hair-bearing skin are absent (magnification = 2.5×). (**b**) This specimen shows a pattern of "bottom-up" sclerosis that can be seen in morphea before the entire dermis is involved. The sclerotic collagen is in the *lower half* of dermis, while the normal collagen is in the *upper half*. Dense collagen has replaced normal collagen from the *arrow down*. The *left upper corner* of the image also shows the edge of an atrophic hair follicle (magnification = 5×). Sclerosis can also occur from the top down or may encompass the entire dermis, even extending into the subcutis and beyond in some cases. (**c**, **d**) Biopsies of active inflammatory morphea reveal perivascular, periadnexal, and interstitial inflammatory infiltrate. Also note the inflammatory cell infiltrate in the junction between the dermis and subcutaneous fat, streaming down through the septa of the subcutaneous fat. Though difficult to appreciate at this power, inflammatory infiltrate is typically composed of lymphocytes, plasma cells, and, occasionally, eosinophils. (**e**, **f**) Higher-power views of the non-sclerotic (**e**) and sclerotic (**f**) dermal areas show that the collagen in the sclerotic area has lost the fine fibrillar texture of normal collagen (magnification = 40×). (**g**) Encasement of adnexal structures by dense collagen with loss of the fat around eccrine glands is shown. Eventually, atrophy of hair follicles, sebaceous glands, and eccrine glands (*arrow*) occurs in long-standing morphea (Magnification = 20×)

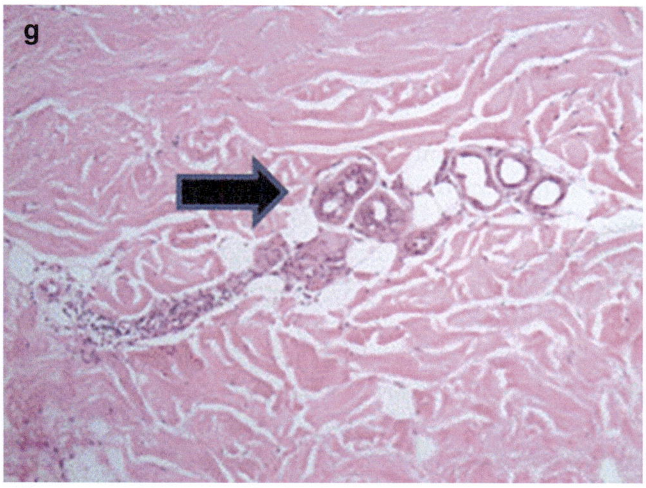

Fig. 10.6 (continued)

Triggers and Precipitating Factors

The emergence of morphea following exposure to environmental exposures is intriguing and may provide clues for the pathophysiology of morphea. While there are no definitive associations, the development of morphea lesions has been linked to local tissue trauma including radiation, surgery, insect bites, and intramuscular injections [56]. Although controversial, infectious agents have also been linked to pathogenesis. Studies in Europe had implicated a role for *Borrelia* infection in the pathogenesis of morphea, but this association has been largely discounted.

Increasing evidence, however, exists for the role of trauma in the development of morphea lesions. In a study of 26 patients with severe juvenile localized scleroderma, four (15%) reported a history of trauma to the area, and one had a history of dental extraction ipsilateral to the area in which morphea developed [57]. There are many examples in the literature of injection-site morphea [56, 58], including the onset of morphea at the site of vaccinations as well as at the site of an insulin pump placement, observed by the authors. In a cross-sectional analysis of 329 patients in the MAC cohort, 52 (16%) had trauma-associated lesions at the onset of disease, most commonly chronic friction (isomorphic) and surgery/isotopic triggers [59]. These findings, if confirmed in future studies, might suggest that elective procedures and skin trauma or friction be avoided in morphea patients. However, necessary and lifesaving surgery, radiation, or other procedures should not be avoided merely due to the diagnosis of morphea.

Clinical Features of Morphea

Assessment of Disease Activity in Morphea

The assessment of disease activity in morphea is important to clinical decision-making, as most treatments with proven efficacy are directed at the inflammatory stage of disease and will not be effective in predominantly sclerotic or atrophic lesions. The risk–benefit assessment of pursuing treatment for morphea lesions depends on the potential for functional or cosmetic impairment and symptom burden due to active lesions. It is therefore important to make an accurate assessment of lesion activity in each clinical examination, including clinical photographs to compare lesions to prior visits, since active disease may warrant intervention, while inactive disease may be carefully observed over time (see Fig. 10.10). Though imaging modalities such as ultrasound can be useful for assessing disease activity (see *Imaging methods*), active morphea lesions can usually be distinguished from inactive lesions by clinical features. Signs of disease activity (which have been established by expert consensus and validated) include new lesions, lesions that have expanded in size from previous visits, the presence of an erythematous or violaceous border around lesions, and possibly increased patient symptomology such as pain or itch at the site of lesions [60, 61].

Stages of Morphea Lesions

Morphea of all subtypes can begin as erythematous patches or plaques and may be preceded by pain or itch. Later, hypopigmentation with skin thickening, which is a manifestation of sclerosis, begins to develop at the center of lesions. These lesions typically have an erythematous/violaceous border indicative of active inflammation and expansion (inflammatory phase) (Fig. 10.5b–d). Sclerosis develops centrally and may lead to a shiny white-yellow color, with surrounding hyperpigmentation, as lesions stop expanding (sclerotic phase) (Fig. 10.5e). The loss of hair follicles can lead to alopecia in areas of morphea.

As activity subsides, these sclerotic plaques will soften over the course of months to years and become atrophic with hyper- or hypopigmentation (atrophic phase). Sclerosis can lead to contractures and limitations in range of motion and may impede growth in the pediatric population, leading to limb length discrepancies. Limitations in range of motion may actually improve as the lesions progress from sclerosis into atrophy.

Atrophy produces varying features depending on the level of skin involvement: cigarette-paper atrophy (papillary dermis), cliff-drop atrophy (dermis), or deep indentations that alter the contour of the affected site (subcutis). Atrophoderma of Pasini and Pierini (Fig. 10.5f) is thought to be the residua of plaque-type morphea involving dermal atrophy, as the borders of these lesions are characterized by the cliff-drop appearance. When morphea affects the subcutis or deeper, long-term sequelae may include limb length discrepancies, limitations in range of motion, and contractures (Fig. 10.5g–i).

Depth of Involvement

Assessment of the level of involvement in morphea is important to recognize potential comorbidities as well as to guide treatment (see Fig. 10.10). Morphea involving the superficial to the mid-dermis may be amenable to topical or phototherapy. Deep morphea, or morphea profunda, on the other hand, which involves the deep dermis, subcutaneous tissue, fascia, and/or muscle, will require systemic therapy to suppress disease activity when lesions are widespread or threaten function or cosmesis.

Deep involvement can occur with any subtype of morphea. Hemifacial atrophy, previously known as the Parry-Romberg syndrome, represents deep morphea (morphea profunda) of the face that may or may not be accompanied by a more dermal linear or en coup de sabre (ECDS) lesion. Similar changes are seen in other anatomic sites with deep involvement (morphea profunda). Lesions in which the pathology is predominantly located in the deep dermis/subcutis are poorly circumscribed and may be accompanied by changes such as cobblestoning and altered contour in the sclerotic phase, as the skin becomes tacked down by sclerosis to the underlying fascia (Fig. 10.5a). A "groove" sign or depression may be present at the site of tendons and ligaments, and deep tissue loss may result in the atrophic phase. However, as deep involvement can occur without obvious superficial changes, it may be more reliably detected with careful palpation, biopsy, and/or imaging than by visual exam alone (see Figs. 10.9 and 10.10).

Data are lacking on the correlation between depth and involvement and the amount of damage in morphea. However, a preliminary analysis of the MAC cohort revealed that the vast majority of patients who had functional abnormalities (including limited range of motion, contractures, limb length discrepancies in morphea-involved areas) also had deep involvement of their disease (80/86, 93%). These results imply a possible connection between the depth of disease and the potential for damage and further emphasize the importance of assessment of the level of involvement as part of the clinical evaluation of the patient with morphea (Fig. 10.10) [62].

Morbidity in Morphea

Quality-of-life assessments show that individuals with morphea have better outcomes than those with disabling severe atopic dermatitis, with the exception of children and adolescents with the more severe forms of morphea affecting the face and limbs [63]. However, large cross-sectional studies of the MAC cohort have demonstrated that morphea patients do experience impairment of health-related quality of life that is greater than those with nonmelanoma skin cancer, vitiligo, and alopecia [64]. Notably, symptoms of pruritus and pain have been significantly associated with impaired quality of life in morphea, contrary to conventional wisdom that morphea is an asymptomatic disorder [64, 65].

A variety of internal disorders are reported to occur in patients with morphea, more frequently in the linear [34] and generalized or mixed subtypes [18], though they are different than the internal organ manifestations of scleroderma. The most commonly associated disorders include musculoskeletal and deep soft tissue abnormalities and neurologic and ophthalmologic problems. Malignancy is a rarely associated morbidity and may include squamous cell carcinoma in long-standing pansclerotic morphea [66]. Few systematic studies have been performed because of the infrequency of morphea and even more infrequent coexisting morbidities, so relatively little is known about the course and treatment of these disorders in the context of morphea [57].

- *Musculoskeletal and soft tissue complications.* The most common extracutaneous finding in morphea patients is arthritis/arthralgias, which have been reported in 12% of pediatric patients with morphea (Fig. 10.7a) [34]. Both articular and soft tissue/bony abnormalities are typically associated with linear morphea. Other musculoskeletal complications include joint swelling, myalgia, and limb contractures [18] (Fig. 10.4a). Individuals with facial linear morphea can have dental abnormalities [66] including gingival involvement (Fig. 10.7b) and even ipsilateral tongue hypoplasia. Musculoskeletal changes including fascial thickening and enhancement, articular synovitis, tenosynovitis, perifascial enhancement, and myositis have been detected using MRI in morphea patients, particularly those with pansclerotic morphea, and have been observed in some cases even when involvement was not expected based on the exam [67]. However, the clinical significance of such findings has yet to be determined, and the authors would not recommend routine imaging in morphea patients without signs or symptoms of musculoskeletal involvement.
- *Neurologic complications.* Neurologic involvement was reported in 4% of pediatric patients with morphea [34] and is more common in patients with linear morphea of the head. Complications include seizures, headache, and

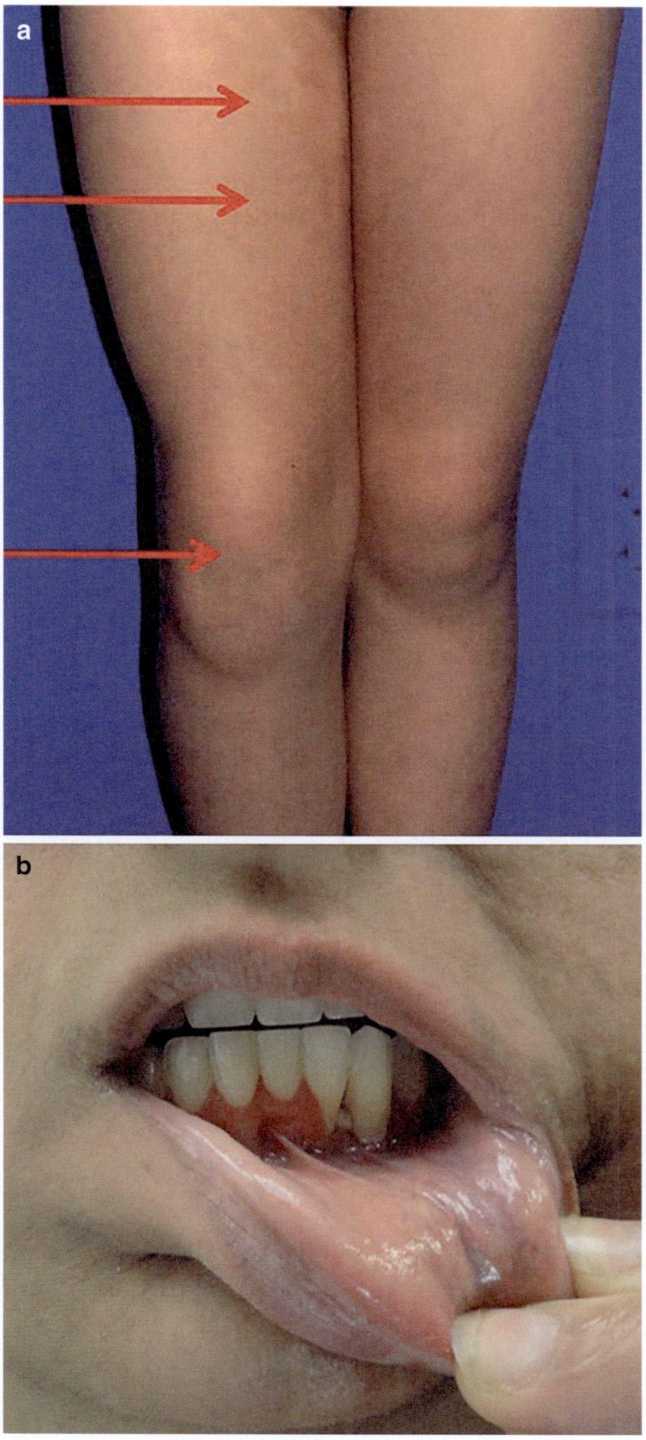

Fig. 10.7 *Morbidity in* morphea. (**a**) *Arthritis in morphea*. A swollen right knee with effusion (*lowest arrow*) is present in this patient with morphea (*upper areas*). Notably, this patient also had spondyloarthropathy. (**b**) *Gingival changes in morphea*. Gingival changes, in the form of a kind of destructive gingivitis, are seen in this patient with linear morphea of the face. Referral to oral maxillofacial surgery may be warranted to determine the need for intervention once lesions are inactive

peripheral neuropathy among others. Intractable partial seizures [68], epileptic encephalopathy [69], status migrainosus [70], and central nervous system vasculitis [71, 72] have all been reported in association with morphea. Kistger et al. reviewed 54 patients with craniofacial scleroderma who also had neuroimaging (head CT or MRI) for neurologic symptoms. They found some common atypical features on imaging including atrophy, calcifications, and T2 hyperintensities. Others have described abnormal MRI results in patients with the Parry-Romberg syndrome [73]. The clinical significance of such abnormal findings has yet to be determined, and at the current time, there is not sufficient evidence to recommend imaging in the morphea population in the absence of neurologic manifestations by history or physical examination.

- *Ophthalmologic complications*. Ocular involvement was reported in 2% of pediatric patients with morphea [34]. Ocular involvement in morphea is also more common in patients with linear morphea that affects the face, although it has also been reported to occur in patients without facial lesions [74]. Associated ophthalmologic abnormalities may include enophthalmos, anterior uveitis, episcleritis, glaucoma, xerophthalmia, keratitis, and strabismus [74].
- *Other manifestations*. Genital involvement has been reported in association with morphea, particularly the generalized subtype, though to date, the frequency of such changes is not well described. Patients with genital involvement will often complain of pruritus, as well as dyspareunia, dysuria, and pain with defecation. Importantly, patients will not typically volunteer these symptoms without specific inquiry by providers [75, 76]. From the literature, the most common changes in the genital area include lichen sclerosus changes of porcelain-like polygonal macules, as well as more typical classical plaque-type morphea lesions with areas of waxy induration, and even labial fusion [75–78]. Patients with reported genital involvement have typically been postmenopausal women with the generalized subtype of morphea, though lichen sclerosus changes have also been reported with some frequency in plaque-type morphea [75, 78]. Review of the MAC cohort database revealed genital changes were present in 3.5% of all participants (14/433), though this represented almost 10% of patients with the generalized subtype of morphea (13/149, 8.7%). Similar to reports in the literature, those affected were all women and were typically postmenopausal (13/14, 92.8%). Similar to previous reports, genital involvement in the MAC cohort was primarily seen in patients with the generalized subtype of morphea, typically with features of lichen sclerosus overlap (13/14, 92.8%).

- *Malignancy.* Rare cases of malignancy are reported in morphea lesions, such as squamous cell carcinoma of the lip that developed in an individual with pansclerotic disabling morphea [66]. The etiology is likely similar to carcinoma developing in chronic venous insufficiency ulcerations and burn scars. Providers should take care to exclude cutaneous metastasis in lesions of morphea involving the breast (see *Differential diagnosis of morphea*).

Laboratory Findings in Morphea

Individuals with all subtypes of morphea, particularly those with deep involvement, may have peripheral eosinophilia and the presence of markers of inflammation and autoimmunity (though this is relatively uncommon). The most common of these markers are positive antinuclear antibody (ANA) and/or rheumatoid factor and the presence of anti-ssDNA and antihistone antibodies (AHAs), which suggest a predisposition to autoimmunity, but do not reliably correlate with disease activity or severity [16, 37, 38]. In one nested case–control study, morphea patients had a higher prevalence of ANA (63/187, 34%) and AHA positivity (22/187, 22%) as compared to matched healthy controls. There was a similar prevalence of ssDNA antibodies in cases (15/187, 8%) and controls (10/149, 7%). Of those morphea patients with positive ANA, most had the speckled pattern (52/63, 81%) at a high titer (>1:1280), though few patients with ANA positivity had extractable nuclear antigen (ENA) antibodies (7/63, 11%), implying the possible presence of an unidentified antigen in morphea. The presence of these autoantibodies, however, has not reliably correlated with any measures of clinical activity. Thus ANAs and AHAs have limited clinical utility except in linear morphea, where their presence may be associated with greater disease burden and functional impairment [79].

There are no laboratory tests that confirm the diagnosis of morphea, which is made on clinical features with confirmatory histopathology. Biomarkers predictive of activity or prognosis are also lacking. Thus, clinical assessment remains the mainstay of diagnosis and evaluation.

Differential Diagnosis of Morphea

Many morphea patients experience a delay in the diagnosis and treatment because providers fail to recognize this relatively rare disease [80]. The development of morphea can be insidious and subtle, and initial misdiagnosis, particularly by nondermatologists, occurs frequently [80]. Morphea can mimic other cutaneous diseases, including atrophic conditions, vascular lesions, dyspigmentation disorders, and even more common skin lesions such as bruises and scars (see Table 10.2) [81–83]. Early morphea lesions have been periodically confused with port-wine stains in the pediatric population [83, 84], because early lesions may present as erythematous linear patches with minimal sclerosis. Histology can be useful to distinguish these entities, and lesions should also be monitored for changes over time, as induration, atrophy, and sclerosis may develop over time and reveal the correct diagnosis [83].

Providers should consider common entities in their differential diagnosis, including lipodermatosclerosis and trauma-induced fat necrosis. Steroid atrophy can mimic morphea, as subcutaneous atrophy may result at the site of steroid and other intramuscular injections, and injection of the scalp to treat other skin conditions can actually mimic linear morphea of the scalp. These entities can usually be differentiated from morphea by a careful history and physical examination, and, when necessary, a biopsy. Providers should also make sure to exclude more dangerous entities such as metastatic carcinoma in the appropriate settings (for instance, of lesions on the breast, overlying the site of known prior carcinoma). Post-radiation morphea can mimic radiation dermatitis, infection, or recurrent breast carcinoma (Fig. 10.8), and

Table 10.2 Differential Diagnosis of Morphea

Most likely
1. Scleroderma (systemic sclerosis)
2. Lipodermatosclerosis
3. Eosinophilic fasciitis (may be a related process)
4. Trauma-induced fat necrosis (intramuscular injections)
5. Nephrogenic systemic fibrosis
6. Chronic graft-versus-host disease
7. Steroid atrophy
Consider
1. Lichen sclerosus (may be a related process)
2. Pretibial myxedema
3. Connective tissue nevi
4. Morpheaform basal cell carcinoma
5. Chemical-mediated sclerosing skin conditions (toxic oil syndrome, rapeseed oil)
6. Lyme disease (acrodermatitis atrophicans)
7. Phenylketonuria
8. Scleromyxedema
9. Pretibial myxedema
10. POEMS syndrome
11. Drug-induced sclerosing skin conditions: taxanes, IM injections, interferon-alpha
12. Lupus profundus
13. Port-wine stain
Always rule out
1. Carcinoma of the breast metastatic to the skin (*carcinoma en cuirase*)
2. Porphyria cutanea tarda
3. Dermatofibrosarcoma protuberans

POEMS polyneuropathy, organomegaly, endocrinopathy, *M* protein, and skin changes. (Reproduced with permission from: Saxton-Daniels and Jacobe [111].)

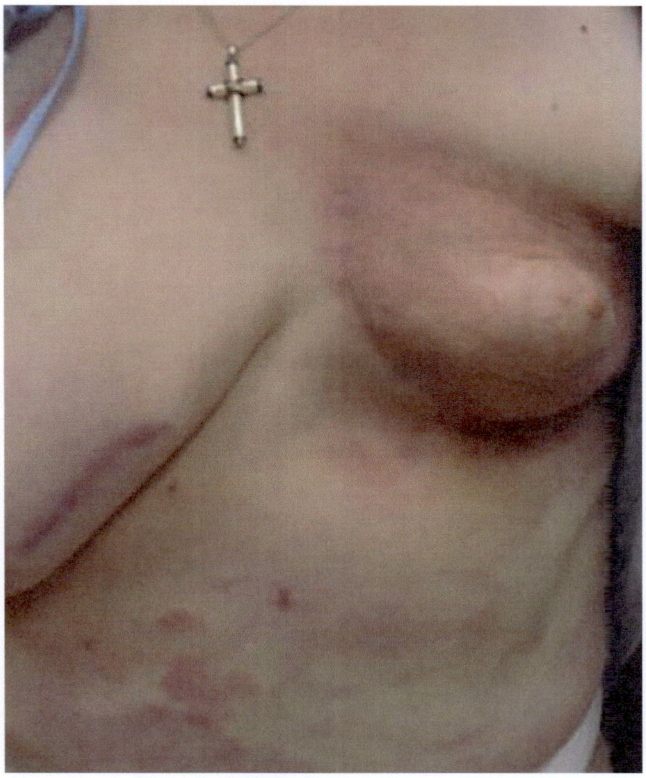

Fig. 10.8 *Postirradiation morphea on the breast.* Morpheaform changes occurred after breast reconstruction and radiation therapy in this patient with a history of breast cancer. Note the importance of a wider skin examination to differentiate this process from radiation dermatitis or recurrent carcinoma, as multiple morphea lesions are present on the trunk as well. Biopsy would be warranted in this case to rule out malignancy. Though postirradiation morphea has been reported, patients should not avoid necessary radiation or other lifesaving treatments due to a diagnosis of morphea

differentiating morphea from radiation dermatitis will depend on both clinical and histopathological features [85]. Special care should also be taken to distinguish morphea from scleroderma based on clinical features already described. Patients will often confuse the two entities, and misplaced concern over systemic disease damage to internal organs may impact negatively on patient quality of life [64].

The diagnosis of morphea is made clinically, but biopsy and histological examination may be useful to aid decision-making based on the depth of involvement (see Fig. 10.9). Biopsy should also be done to exclude potential malignancy and in cases in which history and physical examination findings are not definitive, and pathology is needed to exclude disorders other than squamous cell carcinoma. Given the lack of accepted biomarkers, laboratory-based tests are not currently recommended for the evaluation of morphea in the absence of specific signs or symptoms that would otherwise prompt them (see *Laboratory findings in morphea*). Imaging is not recommended routinely for diagnosis but may be useful to evaluate for depth of involvement or to monitor disease activity (see *Imaging methods* and Fig. 10.9).

Approach to the Evaluation of the Patient with Morphea

Approach to the patient with morphea depends on a number of factors, including disease subtype, disease activity, and depth of involvement, as well as patient symptomatology and the potential for cosmetic or functional impairment. Patients may benefit from a multidisciplinary approach to address functional and cosmetic issues as well as comorbidities when present (Fig. 10.9). As noted earlier, there are no widely accepted biomarkers for morphea, so laboratory-based tests are not routinely recommended for the evaluation of morphea in the absence of specific signs or symptoms that would otherwise warrant them. Depending on features found on clinical examination or on patient complaints (muscle pain, limited range of motion, neurologic symptoms or deficits, etc.), imaging may be warranted to evaluate the depth of lesions and involvement of underlying structures (see *Imaging methods*).

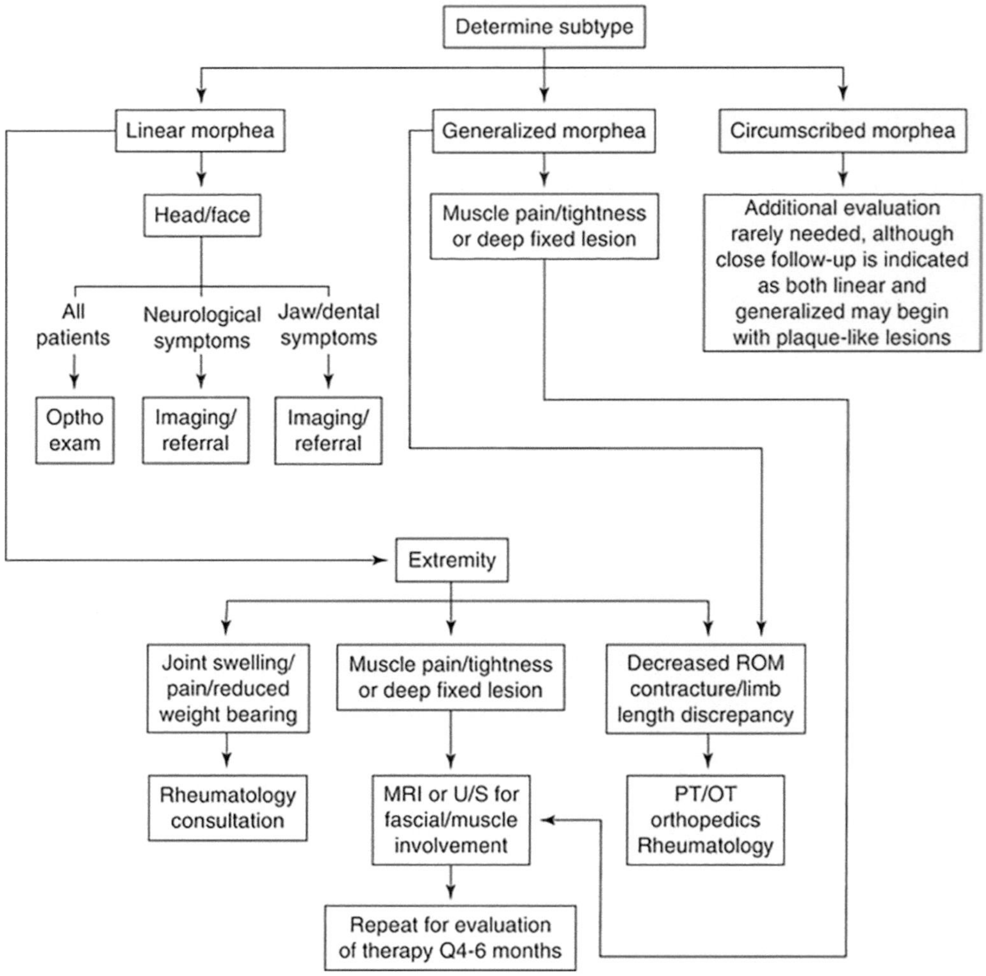

Fig. 10.9 Algorithm for the evaluation of patients with morphea (reproduced with permission from: Jacobe H. Treatment of morphea (localized scleroderma) in adults. In: UpToDate, Post TW (Ed), UpToDate, Waltham, MA. (Accessed on 19 Dec 2014.) Copyright © 2014 UpToDate, Inc. For more information visit www.uptodate.com)

Imaging Methods

- *Ultrasound* [86–89]. The most reliable assessment uses 20–25 MHz ultrasound (US). Ultrasound at 10–15 MHz—which is more readily available in the United States—is also useful [86, 87]. This modality has been more extensively used in making the diagnosis of morphea, but has been used more recently for measuring disease activity based on the increased cutaneous blood flow and increased subcutaneous tissue echogenicity, and has been found to be a sensitive tool for monitoring localized scleroderma in the pediatric population [86, 90, 91]. However, the ultrasound assessment is operator dependent and lacks standardization.
- *Magnetic resonance imaging* (MRI) [67, 92]. Although the MRI findings in morphea can overlap with other soft tissue abnormalities such as fibromatoses and myofibromatoses, the experienced radiologist can distinguish features of morphea including thickening of the dermis and increased signal intensity during the inflammatory stages, as well as changes in signal in the bone marrow with deeper involvement. MRI is particularly useful for the evaluation of the depth of infiltration in morphea and sequential analysis of disease activity [92]. MRI has also been used to detect musculoskeletal involvement, including fascial thickening and enhancement, articular synovitis, and tenosynovitis, in patients with morphea, even some in whom musculoskeletal involvement was not suspected based on the history and exam [67] However, the clinical significance of such findings has yet to be determined, and at this point there is no evidence for pan imaging in the patient diagnosed with morphea without signs or symptoms concerning for musculoskeletal involvement. Imaging is best done after conferring with a radiologist to optimize the methods in which the patient is imaged and to ensure attention to possible features of morphea.

Therapeutic Options for Morphea

A majority of morphea patients experience a delay in diagnosis of greater than 6 months, as well as quite varied treatment that appears to depend more on provider specialty than on disease characteristics or evidence for treatment modalities [80]. However, there are a number of therapeutic options with proven efficacy in morphea (Table 10.3). Each of these may be considered depending on disease subtype, activity, depth of involvement, and other patient considerations. The authors recommend using the evidence-based algorithm below when considering therapeutic options for patients with morphea (Fig. 10.10).

It is important to note that, contrary to conventional wisdom, morphea can be successfully treated with proper therapy and patient selection. However, providers should remember, and emphasize to patients, that the therapeutic end point in morphea is not the complete resolution of lesions but rather the loss of features of activity (reduction of erythema, halting progression of lesions, or development of new lesions). Disease damage may actually increase for a time with treatment as lesions transition from inflammatory to atrophic or sclerotic stages (though skin thickening is likely to soften over time, even after treatment cessation). Providers should make sure to distinguish features of damage, such as dyspigmentation or atrophy, which can result in more visible blood vessels and apparent erythema, from true erythema mediated by inflammation (this may be accomplished by examining areas of erythema with magnification and looking for the induration that accompanies inflammation).

Table 10.3 Treatments for morphea by the level of evidence

Treatment	Level of evidence
BB UVA	1, 2
UVA-1	1, 2
Calcitriol, oral (inefficacy 1)	1, 2
MTX plus oral/IV corticosteroids	1, 2
IFN-gamma (inefficacy 1)	1
PUVA bath	2
PUVA cream	2
ECP	2
Calcipotriene, topical	2
MTX monotherapy	2
PCMT	2
Tacrolimus, topical	2
Corticosteroids, oral	2
Hydroxychloroquine, mycophenolate mofetil, cyclosporine, bosentan, infliximab, imiquimod, antimicrobials, D-penicillamine, 585 nm long-pulse laser, wide surgical resection, orthopedic surgery, Apligraf	Minimal evidence (≥level 3)

BB broadband, *IFN* interferon, *ECP* extracorporeal photochemotherapy, *MTX* methotrexate

Level of evidence: *1*, indicates randomized controlled trial; *2*, uncontrolled trial, *3*, case report, case series (adapted from content in Jacobe H. Treatment of morphea (localized scleroderma) in adults. In: UpToDate, Post TW (Ed), UpToDate, Waltham, MA. (Accessed on 19 Dec 2014.) Copyright © 2014 UpToDate, Inc. For more information visit www.uptodate.com)

The approach to the patient with morphea depends on the assessment of disease activity, depth of involvement, and the presence of other sequelae, which is typically based on clinical examination. Careful clinical photographs should be taken at each visit to monitor patient's lesions, as subtle changes indicative of disease activity may otherwise be missed. Clinical scoring measures, such as the LOSCAT, may also be useful for quantifying and monitoring the progression of disease or the efficacy of therapy [60, 93]. Histological examination may aid in initial therapeutic decision-making, as it can be difficult to determine the depth of involvement by clinical exam alone. In these cases, biopsy of the advancing edge of a lesion can be undertaken to provide insight into both activity and depth of morphea (see *Histopathology of morphea*).

Phototherapy

There is substantial evidence for the efficacy of phototherapy in morphea, particularly for broadband UVA, narrowband UVB, and UVA-1 [94–99] (Table 10.3). UVB is more appropriate for lesions restricted to the superficial dermis, which are relatively thin on palpation and, on biopsy, have sclerosis and inflammation in the papillary and superficial reticular dermis. UVA-based treatments can penetrate to a greater depth and are therefore more effective for deeper dermal lesions. UVA-1, in particular, has been shown to normalize dermal collagen and reduce inflammation in morphea and thus may be effective for disease in either the inflammatory or sclerotic phase [95]. There is also evidence in the literature for the efficacy of broadband UVA phototherapy, which can be an appropriate alternative when UVA-1 is not available [94]. Improvement in disease, noted by the halting of lesion progression and the reduction of erythema, should be seen after 10–20 treatments. A trial can usually be discontinued after 20–30 treatments if improvement is not seen in that period. Treatments are usually given three to five times weekly for a period of several weeks until this number of total treatments has been reached. Evidence suggests that patients may continue to improve even after the cessation of therapy, leading some to suggest an even greater number of treatments (30–50) for further therapeutic benefit. Optimum doses and the regimen for UVA-1 phototherapy have yet to be determined; however, one randomized controlled trial has suggested that both low-dose (20 J per square centimeter) UVA-1 and medium-dose (50 J per square centimeter) UVA-1 are equally effective, while medium-dose UVA-1 is more effective than narrow band UVB [96]. Phototherapy is

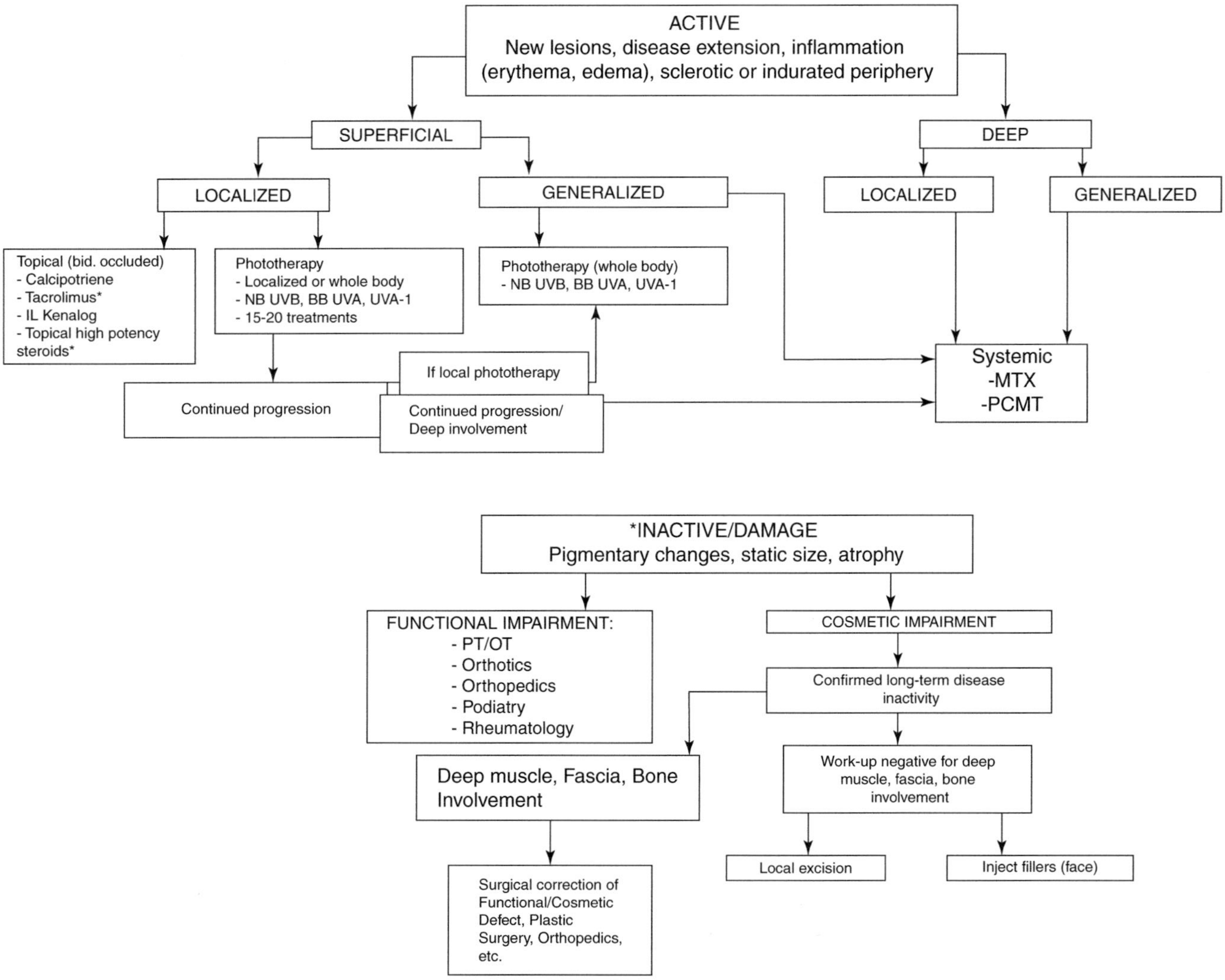

Fig. 10.10 Therapeutic algorithm for morphea based on existing evidence. Histological examination and/or MRI are encouraged to evaluate lesions for the depth of involvement and, likewise, determine appropriate treatment as well as evaluation of therapeutic efficacy. Superficial involvement is defined by histological evidence of papillary dermal involvement. Deep involvement is defined as sclerosis or inflammation of the deep dermis, subcutis, fascia, or muscle (reproduced with permission from: Jacobe H. Treatment of morphea (localized scleroderma) in adults. In: UpToDate, Post TW (Ed), UpToDate, Waltham, MA. (Accessed on [19 Dec 2014].) Copyright © 2014 UpToDate, Inc. For more information visit www.uptodate.com). *There is very little evidence for any therapy addressing disease damage in morphea. The risk of disease reactivation is also unknown, but possible with the use of invasive procedures. Therefore, surgery and the like should only be undertaken after prolonged inactivity of disease. + There is no evidence for efficacy in the literature

not likely to be effective for lesions with deep involvement of the subcutis, fascia, or muscle, and therefore should not be considered a primary therapy for such disease.

Vitamin D Derivatives

Only one study provides level-1 evidence on the effect of vitamin D derivatives in morphea and actually showed no difference between oral calcitriol and placebo, with both groups improving equally [100] (Table 10.3). The authors also point out that this study was underpowered, making definitive conclusions about the efficacy of oral calcitriol difficult. Various uncontrolled trials and case reports have shown improvement in patients using topical vitamin D derivatives applied under occlusion. However, this improvement took place over a period of several months, during which time lesions might be expected to improve independently.

Immunomodulators

- *Methotrexate with or without corticosteroids*. The use of methotrexate monotherapy and methotrexate combined with systemic corticosteroids has been shown to be effective based on multiple prospective trials [2, 26, 29, 101–103] (Table 10.3). One double-blind randomized controlled trial has also shown that pediatric morphea patients treated with 15–20 mg weekly of methotrexate for 12 months, after induction with 1 mg/kg/day oral prednisone for 3 months, had lower clinical disease scores, decreased lesion temperature, and lower rates of relapse than those treated with prednisone induction alone (plus placebo) [29]. Relapse occurred within 12 months in 15 patients treated with methotrexate in addition to corticosteroids (32.6%) versus 17 of those treated with placebo only after steroids (70.8%). More specifically, new lesions developed in three methotrexate-treated patients (6.5%) versus four placebo-treated patients (16.7%) within 3–9 months. As the primary end point in the study was response to treatment within 12 months, it is difficult to determine the actual time for effect of this medication regimen. Similarly, optimum dose, route, and indications for the additions of corticosteroids to methotrexate, as well as the duration of therapy, have not been definitively established. In most studies with combined therapy, including the randomized trial described, corticosteroids are used for induction therapy either orally or via intravenous pulse (IV methylprednisolone 30 mg/kg/day for 3 days/month or 1 mg/kg/day prednisone) over the first 3 months. Methotrexate is used as a steroid-sparing agent and initiated simultaneously (0.6 mg/kg/week in children or 15–25 mg/week for adults), then maintained for a prolonged period (1–2 years) and gradually tapered. Consensus treatment plans for pediatric morphea have recently been established that detail these monotherapy and combined therapy approaches [61]. As evidence to date has not suggested a difference in disease processes between pediatric and adult morphea, it is likely that adults will respond similarly to this regimen. From the literature, most patients will respond in a mean of 2–5 months with this approach, with patients early in their disease course typically responding best. Importantly, relapse has been noted frequently after the cessation of therapy (see *Epidemiology and clinical course*), indicating that therapy suppresses disease activity but is not curative [27].

- *Other immunomodulators*. Level 2 evidence supports the use of topical tacrolimus 0.1% ointment under occlusion for active, inflammatory superficial plaque-type morphea [104] (Table 10.3). Recent case series using oral mycophenolate mofetil indicate possible efficacy in patients who are refractory to methotrexate or have intolerable side effects [105]. Mycophenolate mofetil also may be effective as a treatment adjunct in children with morphea; in one retrospective analysis, ten patients with severe or methotrexate-resistant pediatric morphea experienced clinical improvement with mycophenolate mofetil that resulted in withdrawal or reduction of doses of corticosteroids and methotrexate [106]. Retrospective case reports on the use of oral cyclosporine, bosentan, infliximab, and topical imiquimod have reported some efficacy, but definitive studies are lacking (Table 10.3).

Antimicrobials

Despite the widespread use of antimicrobials in morphea, including antibiotics and antimalarials, no published clinical trials of these agents exist [107]. Literature supporting the use of antimalarials is limited to a case series in which two patients improved with hydroxychloroquine, while simultaneously receiving methotrexate and corticosteroids [108]. In one retrospective review, 7 out of 11 patients had persistently active disease 3–153 months after initiating therapy with hydroxychloroquine [16]. At this time, the use of these agents in severe morphea is not indicated, pending more definitive evidence for their efficacy (Table 10.3).

Treatments Not Supported by Current Evidence

The efficacy of the most commonly used treatment for morphea, topical corticosteroids, has never been formally evaluated [62, 80]. There have also been no studies investigating the use of intralesional steroids. In the authors' experience, intralesional steroids have been effective in treating circumscribed plaques of morphea or as an adjuvant for recalcitrant areas in patients receiving phototherapy or systemic treatment. Current evidence does not support the use of interferon-gamma in morphea [109], and the risks of penicillamine, including toxicities, outweigh its potential benefits, which have not been well established. At this time, there is no sufficient evidence to support the use of these agents, especially in moderate-to-severe morphea, when other agents have proven efficacy (unless contraindications exist to their use) (Table 10.3).

Adjunctive Therapy

A significant number of patients with morphea suffer irreversible sequelae that persist even after disease activity has subsided. Patients should be carefully evaluated for limitations in range of motion, contractures, limb length discrepancies, or other functional impairments. Treatment modalities may include physical therapy techniques for improving the range of motion of affected limbs, stretching exercises for contractures, orthotics, or shoe inserts to adjust for limb length discrepancies and to compensate for loss of subcutaneous fat, or even tendon release in some cases [16]. Referral to specialists, such as rheumatologists, physical therapists, orthopedists, oral maxillofacial surgeons, or plastic surgeons, may be helpful to maximize cosmesis and function and to minimize further damage. Importantly, studies to date are completely lacking in addressing this type of damage due to morphea.

Surgical Therapies

There is limited evidence to support the use of surgical therapies for morphea. Importantly, these therapies should only be considered when morphea has been inactive, and a patient has been off treatment for a number of years. Patients should be monitored closely with serial examinations for reactivation, and collaboration with an experienced plastic surgeon is vital.

Summary

Morphea is a relatively uncommon idiopathic inflammatory disorder that leads to the development of sclerotic plaques in the skin. Though morphea may share common histopathological features with scleroderma, the disease differs demographically and clinically. The involvement of internal organs in morphea is unusual and very different from that in scleroderma. Morphea occurs in adults and children and preferentially affects females. The pathogenesis of morphea is not well understood but is likely to involve autoimmunity, as well as genetic and environmental factors. Lesions typically begin as inflammatory patches that evolve into firm, sclerotic plaques. Involvement may be limited to the dermis or may extend to underlying subcutaneous fat, muscle, or bone. Atrophic changes often remain after the resolution of lesion activity.

Morphea has a variety of clinical presentations. Circumscribed and generalized morphea occurs more frequently in adults, while linear morphea predominates in children. The identification of characteristic clinical findings often is sufficient for the diagnosis of morphea, but biopsy may be performed to exclude other entities or to obtain information on the depth of disease. Antinuclear antibody (ANA) levels are elevated in some patients with morphea; however, routine testing for autoantibodies is not indicated. Magnetic resonance imaging (MRI) or ultrasound can be used to assess the extent of involvement, in those patients for whom clinical examination suggests involvement deeper than the dermis, and may be useful for following disease activity during treatment.

The assessment of disease activity and depth of involvement guides therapeutic decision-making in morphea. Because of the self-limited nature of morphea, patients with limited plaque disease may elect to defer therapy. For patients with superficial (dermal) circumscribed disease who desire treatment, but do not have access to or prefer to avoid the frequent visits required for phototherapy, treatment options include high-potency topical corticosteroids, intralesional corticosteroids, a topical vitamin D analog, topical tacrolimus, or imiquimod. For patients with superficial (dermal) forms of morphea who are able to receive phototherapy, treatment with UVA-1 is preferred; alternatives include broadband UVA, narrow band UVB, or PUVA. Phototherapy is unlikely to be effective for morphea involving the subcutaneous tissue, muscle, or bone. Rapidly progressive, severe, disabling disease requires systemic therapy, involving a combination of methotrexate and systemic corticosteroids. Morphea may cause joint contractures and other functional impairments secondary to deep tissue sclerosis. All patients should be clinically assessed for the development of these findings. Physical therapy is essential for patients who are at risk of or who show evidence of functional impairments.

Acknowledgments The authors wish to thank Rose Ann Cannon for her support in the preparation of this manuscript.

References

1. Zulian F, Woo P, Athreya BH, Laxer RM, Medsger TA Jr, Lehman TJ, et al. The pediatric rheumatology European Society/American College of Rheumatology/European league against rheumatism provisional classification criteria for juvenile systemic sclerosis. Arthritis Rheum. 2007;57(2):203–12.
2. Tollefson MM, Witman PM. En coup de sabre morphea and parry-Romberg syndrome: a retrospective review of 54 patients. J Am Acad Dermatol. 2007;56(2):257–63.
3. Pinal-Fernandez I, Selva-O'Callaghan A, Grau JM. Diagnosis and classification of eosinophilic fasciitis. Autoimmun Rev. 2014;13(4–5):379–82.
4. Su WP, Greene SL. Bullous morphea profunda. Am J Dermatopathol. 1986;8(2):144–7.
5. Rencic A, Goyal S, Mofid M, Wigley F, Nousari HC. Bullous lesions in scleroderma. Int J Dermatol. 2002;41(6):335–9.
6. Trattner A, David M, Sandbank M. Bullous morphea: a distinct entity? Am J Dermatopathol. 1994;16(4):414–7.
7. Daoud MS, Su WP, Leiferman KM, Perniciaro C. Bullous morphea: clinical, pathologic, and immunopathologic evaluation of thirteen cases. J Am Acad Dermatol. 1994;30(6):937–43.
8. Kobayasi T, Willeberg A, Serup J, Ullman S. Generalized morphea with blisters. A case report. Acta Derm Venereol. 1990;70(5):454–6.
9. Blaya B, Gardeazabal J, de Lagran ZM, Diaz-Perez JL. Patient with generalized guttate morphea and lichen sclerosus et atrophicus. Actas Dermosifiliogr. 2008;99(10):808–11.
10. Yamanaka M, Ishikawa O. Guttate morphea in a scleroderma spectrum disorder patient with anticentromere antibody. Eur J Dermatol. 2009;19(6):630–1.
11. Synkowski DR, Lobitz WC Jr, Provost TT. Bullous scleroderma. Arch Dermatol. 1981;117(3):135–7.

12. Rencic A, Brinster N, Nousari CH. Keloid morphea and nodular scleroderma: two distinct clinical variants of scleroderma? J Cutan Med Surg. 2003;7(1):20–4.
13. Fernandez-Flores A, Gatica-Torres M, Tinoco-Fragoso F, Garcia-Hidalgo L, Monroy E, Saeb-Lima M. Three cases of bullous morphea: histopathologic findings with implications regarding pathogenesis. J Cutan Pathol. 2015;42(2):144–9.
14. Kavala M, Zindanci I, Demirkesen C, Beyhan EK, Turkoglu Z. Intertriginous bullous morphea: a clue for the pathogenesis? Indian J Dermatol Venereol Leprol. 2007;73(4):262–4.
15. Peterson LS, Nelson AM, Su WP, Mason T, O'Fallon WM, Gabriel SE. The epidemiology of morphea (localized scleroderma) in Olmsted County 1960–1993. J Rheumatol. 1997;24(1):73–80.
16. Christen-Zaech S, Hakim MD, Afsar FS, Paller AS. Pediatric morphea (localized scleroderma): review of 136 patients. J Am Acad Dermatol. 2008;59(3):385–96.
17. Sehgal VN, Srivastava G, Aggarwal AK, Behl PN, Choudhary M, Bajaj P. Localized scleroderma/morphea. Int J Dermatol. 2002;41(8):467–75.
18. Leitenberger JJ, Cayce RL, Haley RW, Adams-Huet B, Bergstresser PR, Jacobe HT. Distinct autoimmune syndromes in morphea: a review of 245 adult and pediatric cases. Arch Dermatol. 2009;145(5):545–50.
19. Vierra E, Cunningham BB. Morphea and localized scleroderma in children. Semin Cutan Med Surg. 1999;18(3):210–25.
20. Marzano AV, Menni S, Parodi A, Borghi A, Fuligni A, Fabbri P, et al. Localized scleroderma in adults and children. Clinical and laboratory investigations on 239 cases. Eur J Dermatol. 2003;13(2):171–6.
21. Saxton-Daniels S, Jacobe HT. An evaluation of long-term outcomes in adults with pediatric-onset morphea. Arch Dermatol. 2010;146(9):1044–5.
22. Condie D, Grabell D, Jacobe H. Comparison of outcomes in adults with pediatric-onset morphea and those with adult-onset morphea: a cross-sectional study from the morphea in adults and children cohort. Arthritis Rheum. 2014;66(12):3496–504.
23. Kroft EB, Creemers MC, van den Hoogen FH, Boezeman JB, de Jong EM. Effectiveness, side-effects and period of remission after treatment with methotrexate in localized scleroderma and related sclerotic skin diseases: an inception cohort study. Br J Dermatol. 2009;160(5):1075–82.
24. Cox D, O'Regan G, Collins S, Byrne A, Irvine A, Watson R. Juvenile localised scleroderma: a retrospective review of response to systemic treatment. Ir J Med Sci. 2008;177(4):343–6.
25. Mirsky L, Chakkittakandiyil A, Laxer RM, O'Brien C, Pope E. Relapse after systemic treatment in paediatric morphoea. Br J Dermatol. 2012;166(2):443–5.
26. Weibel L, Sampaio MC, Visentin MT, Howell KJ, Woo P, Harper JI. Evaluation of methotrexate and corticosteroids for the treatment of localized scleroderma (morphoea) in children. Br J Dermatol. 2006;155(5):1013–20.
27. Zulian F, Vallongo C, Patrizi A, Belloni-Fortina A, Cutrone M, Alessio M, et al. A long-term follow-up study of methotrexate in juvenile localized scleroderma (morphea). J Am Acad Dermatol. 2012;67(6):1151–6.
28. Vasquez R, Jabbar A, Khan F, Buethe D, Ahn C, Jacobe H. Recurrence of morphea after successful ultraviolet A1 phototherapy: a cohort study. J Am Acad Dermatol. 2014;70(3):481–488.
29. Zulian F, Martini G, Vallongo C, Vittadello F, Falcini F, Patrizi A, et al. Methotrexate treatment in juvenile localized scleroderma: a randomized, double-blind, placebo-controlled trial. Arthritis Rheum. 2011;63(7):1998–2006.
30. Mertens JS, Seyger MM, Kievit W, Hoppenreijs EP, Jansen TL, van de Kerkhof PC, et al. Disease recurrence in localized scleroderma: a retrospective analysis of 344 patients with paediatric- or adult-onset disease. Br J Dermatol. 2015;172(3):722–8.
31. Badea I, Taylor M, Rosenberg A, Foldvari M. Pathogenesis and therapeutic approaches for improved topical treatment in localized scleroderma and systemic sclerosis. Rheumatology. 2009;48(3):213–21.
32. Wadud MA, Bose BK, Al NT. Familial localised scleroderma from Bangladesh: two case reports. Bangladesh Med Res Counc Bull. 1989;15(1):15–9.
33. Rees RB, Bennett J. Localized scleroderma in father and daughter. AMA Arch Dermatol Syphilol. 1953;68(3):360.
34. Zulian F, Vallongo C, Woo P, Russo R, Ruperto N, Harper J, et al. Localized scleroderma in childhood is not just a skin disease. Arthritis Rheum. 2005;52(9):2873–81.
35. Hemminki K, Li X, Sundquist J, Sundquist K. Familial associations of rheumatoid arthritis with autoimmune diseases and related conditions. Arthritis Rheum. 2009;60(3):661–8.
36. Hemminki K, Li X, Sundquist J, Hillert J, Sundquist K. Risk for multiple sclerosis in relatives and spouses of patients diagnosed with autoimmune and related conditions. Neurogenetics. 2009;10(1):5–11.
37. Firoz EF, Kamino H, Lehman TJ, Orlow SJ. Morphea, diabetes mellitus type I, and celiac disease: case report and review of the literature. Pediatr Dermatol. 2010;27(1):48–52.
38. Dervis E, Acbay O, Barut G, Karaoglu A, Ersoy L. Association of vitiligo, morphea, and Hashimoto's thyroiditis. Int J Dermatol. 2004;43(3):236–7.
39. Hiremath NC, Madan Mohan NT, Srinivas C, Sangolli PM, Srinivas K, Vrushali VD. Juvenile localized scleroderma with autoimmune thyroid disorder. Indian J Dermatol. 2010;55(3):308–9.
40. Hasegawa M, Fujimoto M, Hayakawa I, Matsushita T, Nishijima C, Yamazaki M, et al. Anti-phosphatidylserine-prothrombin complex antibodies in patients with localized scleroderma. Clin Exp Rheumatol. 2006;24(1):19–24.
41. Slimani S, Hounas F, Ladjouze-Rezig A. Multiple linear sclerodermas with a diffuse parry-Romberg syndrome. Joint Bone Spine: Rev Rhum. 2009;76(1):114–6.
42. Saleh Z, Arayssi T, Saleh Z, Ghosn S. Superficial morphea: 20-year follow up in a patient with concomitant psoriasis vulgaris. J Cutan Pathol. 2009;36(10):1105–8.
43. Jacobe H, Ahn C, Arnett FC, Reveille JD. Major histocompatibility complex class I and class II alleles may confer susceptibility to or protection against morphea: findings from the morphea in adults and children cohort. Arthritis Rheum. 2014;66(11):3170–7.
44. Simmonds MJ, Gough SC. Unravelling the genetic complexity of autoimmune thyroid disease: HLA, CTLA-4 and beyond. Clin Exp Immunol. 2004;136(1):1–10.
45. Weyand CM, Hicok KC, Conn DL, Goronzy JJ. The influence of HLA-DRB1 genes on disease severity in rheumatoid arthritis. Ann Intern Med. 1992;117(10):801–6.
46. Takehara K, Moroi Y, Nakabayashi Y, Ishibashi Y. Antinuclear antibodies in localized scleroderma. Arthritis Rheum. 1983;26(5):612–6.
47. Gruschwitz MS, Hornstein OP, von Den Driesch P. Correlation of soluble adhesion molecules in the peripheral blood of scleroderma patients with their in situ expression and with disease activity. Arthritis Rheum. 1995;38(2):184–9.
48. Fett N, Werth VP. Update on morphea: part I. epidemiology, clinical presentation, and pathogenesis. J Am Acad Dermatol. 2011;64(2):217–28. quiz 29–30.
49. Yamane K, Ihn H, Kubo M, Yazawa N, Kikuchi K, Soma Y, et al. Increased serum levels of soluble vascular cell adhesion molecule 1 and E-selectin in patients with localized scleroderma. J Am Acad Dermatol. 2000;42(1 Pt 1):64–9.
50. Ihn H, Sato S, Fujimoto M, Kikuchi K, Takehara K. Demonstration of interleukin-2, interleukin-4 and interleukin-6 in sera from patients with localized scleroderma. Arch Dermatol Res. 1995;287(2):193–7.

51. McNallan KT, Aponte C, El-Azhary R, Mason T, Nelson AM, Paat JJ, et al. Immunophenotyping of chimeric cells in localized scleroderma. Rheumatology. 2007;46(3):398–402.
52. Magee KE, Kelsey CE, Kurzinski KL, Ho J, Mlakar LR, Feghali-Bostwick CA, et al. Interferon-gamma inducible protein-10 as a potential biomarker in localized scleroderma. Arthritis Res Ther. 2013;15(6):R188.
53. Milano A, Pendergrass SA, Sargent JL, George LK, McCalmont TH, Connolly MK, et al. Molecular subsets in the gene expression signatures of scleroderma skin. PLoS One. 2008;3(7):e2696.
54. Uziel Y, Feldman BM, Krafchik BR, Laxer RM, Yeung RS. Increased serum levels of TGFbeta1 in children with localized scleroderma. Pediatr Rheumatol Online J. 2007;5:22.
55. Walker D, Susa JS, Karai L, Currimbhoy S, Jacobe H. Histopathological changes in morphea and their clinical correlates: results from the Morphea in Adults and Children Cohort (MAC) V. J Am Acad Dermatol. 2017;76(6):1124–30.
56. Torrelo A, Suarez J, Colmenero I, Azorin D, Perera A, Zambrano A. Deep morphea after vaccination in two young children. Pediatr Dermatol. 2006;23(5):484–7.
57. Beltramelli M, Vercellesi P, Frasin A, Gelmetti C, Corona F. Localized severe scleroderma: a retrospective study of 26 pediatric patients. Pediatr Dermatol. 2010;27(5):476–80.
58. Ueda T, Niiyama S, Amoh Y, Katsuoka K. Linear scleroderma after contusion and injection of mepivacaine hydrochloride. Dermatol Online J. 2010;16(5):11.
59. Grabell D, Hsieh C, Andrew R, Martires K, Kim A, Vasquez R, et al. The role of skin trauma in the distribution of morphea lesions: a cross-sectional survey of the Morphea in adults and children cohort IV. J Am Acad Dermatol. 2014;71(3):493–8.
60. Arkachaisri T, Vilaiyuk S, Torok KS, Medsger TA Jr. Development and initial validation of the localized scleroderma skin damage index and physician global assessment of disease damage: a proof-of-concept study. Rheumatology. 2010;49(2):373–81.
61. Li SC, Torok KS, Pope E, Dedeoglu F, Hong S, Jacobe HT, et al. Development of consensus treatment plans for juvenile localized scleroderma: a roadmap toward comparative effectiveness studies in juvenile localized scleroderma. Arthritis Care Res. 2012;64(8):1175–85.
62. Strickland NSA, Fett N, Connolly MK, Hansen C, Jacobe H. Current practices in the evaluation and treatment of morphea. 2016.
63. Orzechowski NM, Davis DM, Mason TG 3rd, Crowson CS, Reed AM. Health-related quality of life in children and adolescents with juvenile localized scleroderma. Rheumatology. 2009;48(6):670–2.
64. Klimas NK, Shedd AD, Bernstein IH, Jacobe H. Health-related quality of life in morphea. Br J Dermatol. 2015;172(5):1329–37.
65. Das S, Bernstein I, Jacobe H. Correlates of self-reported quality of life in adults and children with morphea. J Am Acad Dermatol. 2014;70(5):904–10.
66. Petrov I, Gantcheva M, Miteva L, Vassileva S, Pramatarov K. Lower lip squamous cell carcinoma in disabling pansclerotic morphea of childhood. Pediatr Dermatol. 2009;26(1):59–61.
67. Schanz S, Fierlbeck G, Ulmer A, Schmalzing M, Kummerle-Deschner J, Claussen CD, et al. Localized scleroderma: MR findings and clinical features. Radiology. 2011;260(3):817–24.
68. Chiang KL, Chang KP, Wong TT, Hsu TR. Linear scleroderma "en coup de sabre": initial presentation as intractable partial seizures in a child. Pediatr Neonatol. 2009;50(6):294–8.
69. Rigante D, Battaglia D, Contaldo I, La Torraca I, Avallone L, Gaspari S, et al. Longstanding epileptic encephalopathy and linear localized scleroderma: two distinct pathologic processes in an adolescent. Rheumatol Int. 2008;28(9):925–9.
70. Menascu S, Padeh S, Hoffman C, Ben-Zeev B. Parry-Romberg syndrome presenting as status migrainosus. Pediatr Neurol. 2009;40(4):321–3.
71. Holl-Wieden A, Klink T, Klink J, Warmuth-Metz M, Girschick HJ. Linear scleroderma 'en coup de sabre' associated with cerebral and ocular vasculitis. Scand J Rheumatol. 2006;35(5):402–4.
72. Bonilla-Abadia F, Munoz-Buitron E, Ochoa CD, Carrascal E, Canas CA. A rare association of localized scleroderma type morphea, vitiligo, autoimmune hypothyroidism, pneumonitis, autoimmune thrombocytopenic purpura and central nervous system vasculitis. Case report. BMC Res Notes. 2012;5:689.
73. Moseley BD, Burrus TM, Mason TG, Shin C, Neurological picture. Contralateral cutaneous and MRI findings in a patient with parry-Romberg syndrome. J Neurol Neurosurg Psychiatry. 2010;81(12):1400–1.
74. Zannin ME, Martini G, Athreya BH, Russo R, Higgins G, Vittadello F, et al. Ocular involvement in children with localised scleroderma: a multi-centre study. Br J Ophthalmol. 2007;91(10):1311–4.
75. Lutz V, Frances C, Bessis D, Cosnes A, Kluger N, Godet J, et al. High frequency of genital lichen sclerosus in a prospective series of 76 patients with morphea: toward a better understanding of the spectrum of morphea. Arch Dermatol. 2012;148(1):24–8.
76. Schlosser BJ, Practice gaps. Missing genital lichen sclerosus in patients with morphea: don't ask? Don't tell?: comment on "High frequency of genital lichen sclerosus in a prospective series of 76 patients with morphea". Arch Dermatol. 2012;148(1):28–9.
77. Farrell AM, Marren PM, Wojnarowska F. Genital lichen sclerosus associated with morphoea or systemic sclerosis: clinical and HLA characteristics. Br J Dermatol. 2000;143(3):598–603.
78. Kreuter A, Wischnewski J, Terras S, Altmeyer P, Stucker M, Gambichler T. Coexistence of lichen sclerosus and morphea: a retrospective analysis of 472 patients with localized scleroderma from a German tertiary referral center. J Am Acad Dermatol. 2012;67(6):1157–62.
79. Dharamsi JW, Victor S, Aguwa N, Ahn C, Arnett F, Mayes MD, et al. Morphea in adults and children cohort III: nested case-control study—the clinical significance of autoantibodies in morphea. JAMA Dermatol. 2013;149(10):1159–65.
80. Johnson W, Jacobe H. Morphea in adults and children cohort II: patients with morphea experience delay in diagnosis and large variation in treatment. J Am Acad Dermatol. 2012;67(5):881–9.
81. Sung JJ, Chen TS, Gilliam AC, McCalmont TH, Gilliam AE. Clinicohistopathological correlations in juvenile localized scleroderma: studies on a subset of children with hypopigmented juvenile localized scleroderma due to loss of epidermal melanocytes. J Am Acad Dermatol. 2011;65(2):364–73.
82. Kakimoto CV, Victor Ross E, Uebelhoer NS. En coup de sabre presenting as a port-wine stain previously treated with pulsed dye laser. Dermatol Surg Off Publ Am Soc Dermatol Surg. 2009;35(1):165–7.
83. Nijhawan RI, Bard S, Blyumin M, Smidt AC, Chamlin SL, Connelly EA. Early localized morphea mimicking an acquired port-wine stain. J Am Acad Dermatol. 2011;64(4):779–82.
84. Kim HS, Lee JY, Kim HO, Park YM. En coup de sabre presenting as a port-wine stain initially treated with a pulsed dye laser. J Dermatol. 2011;38(2):209–10.
85. Schaffer JV, Carroll C, Dvoretsky I, Huether MJ, Girardi M. Postirradiation morphea of the breast presentation of two cases and review of the literature. Dermatology. 2000;200(1):67–71.
86. Cosnes A, Anglade MC, Revuz J, Radier C. Thirteen-megahertz ultrasound probe: its role in diagnosing localized scleroderma. Br J Dermatol. 2003;148(4):724–9.
87. Bendeck SE, Jacobe HT. Ultrasound as an outcome measure to assess disease activity in disorders of skin thickening: an example of the use of radiologic techniques to assess skin disease. Dermatol Ther. 2007;20(2):86–92.

88. Li SC, Liebling MS. The use of Doppler ultrasound to evaluate lesions of localized scleroderma. Curr Rheumatol Rep. 2009;11(3):205–11.
89. Li SC, Feldman BM, Higgins GC, Haines KA, Punaro MG, O'Neil KM. Treatment of pediatric localized scleroderma: results of a survey of north American pediatric rheumatologists. J Rheumatol. 2010;37(1):175–81.
90. Wortsman X, Wortsman J, Sazunic I, Carreno L. Activity assessment in morphea using color Doppler ultrasound. J Am Acad Dermatol. 2011;65(5):942–8.
91. Li SC, Liebling MS, Haines KA. Ultrasonography is a sensitive tool for monitoring localized scleroderma. Rheumatology. 2007;46(8):1316–9.
92. Horger M, Fierlbeck G, Kuemmerle-Deschner J, Tzaribachev N, Wehrmann M, Claussen CD, et al. MRI findings in deep and generalized morphea (localized scleroderma). AJR Am J Roentgenol. 2008;190(1):32–9.
93. Kelsey CE, Torok KS. The localized scleroderma cutaneous assessment tool: responsiveness to change in a pediatric clinical population. J Am Acad Dermatol. 2013;69(2):214–20.
94. El-Mofty M, Mostafa W, Esmat S, Youssef R, Bousseila M, Nagi N, et al. Suggested mechanisms of action of UVA phototherapy in morphea: a molecular study. Photodermatol Photoimmunol Photomed. 2004;20(2):93–100.
95. El-Mofty M, Zaher H, Bosseila M, Yousef R, Saad B. Low-dose broad-band UVA in morphea using a new method for evaluation. Photodermatol Photoimmunol Photomed. 2000;16(2):43–9.
96. Kreuter A, Hyun J, Stucker M, Sommer A, Altmeyer P, Gambichler T. A randomized controlled study of low-dose UVA1, medium-dose UVA1, and narrowband UVB phototherapy in the treatment of localized scleroderma. J Am Acad Dermatol. 2006;54(3):440–7.
97. de Rie MA, Enomoto DN, de Vries HJ, Bos JD. Evaluation of medium-dose UVA1 phototherapy in localized scleroderma with the cutometer and fast Fourier transform method. Dermatology. 2003;207(3):298–301.
98. Kerscher M, Meurer M, Sander C, Volkenandt M, Lehmann P, Plewig G, et al. PUVA bath photochemotherapy for localized scleroderma. Evaluation of 17 consecutive patients. Arch Dermatol. 1996;132(11):1280–2.
99. Grundmann-Kollmann M, Behrens S, Gruss C, Gottlober P, Peter RU, Kerscher M. Chronic sclerodermic graft-versus-host disease refractory to immunosuppressive treatment responds to UVA1 phototherapy. J Am Acad Dermatol. 2000;42(1 Pt 1):134–6.
100. Hulshof MM, Bouwes Bavinck JN, Bergman W, Masclee AA, Heickendorff L, Breedveld FC, et al. Double-blind, placebo-controlled study of oral calcitriol for the treatment of localized and systemic scleroderma. J Am Acad Dermatol. 2000;43(6):1017–23.
101. Uziel Y, Feldman BM, Krafchik BR, Yeung RS, Laxer RM. Methotrexate and corticosteroid therapy for pediatric localized scleroderma. J Pediatr. 2000;136(1):91–5.
102. Seyger MM, van den Hoogen FH, de Boo T, de Jong EM. Low-dose methotrexate in the treatment of widespread morphea. J Am Acad Dermatol. 1998;39(2 Pt 1):220–5.
103. Kreuter A, Gambichler T, Breuckmann F, Rotterdam S, Freitag M, Stuecker M, et al. Pulsed high-dose corticosteroids combined with low-dose methotrexate in severe localized scleroderma. Arch Dermatol. 2005;141(7):847–52.
104. Mancuso G, Berdondini RM. Localized scleroderma: response to occlusive treatment with tacrolimus ointment. J Am Acad Dermatol. 2005;152(1):180–2.
105. Schlaak M, Friedlein H, Kauer F, Renner R, Rogalski C, Simon JC. Successful therapy of a patient with therapy recalcitrant generalized bullous scleroderma by extracorporeal photopheresis and mycophenolate mofetil. J Eur Acad Dermatol Venereol. 2008;22(5):631–3.
106. Martini G, Ramanan AV, Falcini F, Girschick H, Goldsmith DP, Zulian F. Successful treatment of severe or methotrexate-resistant juvenile localized scleroderma with mycophenolate mofetil. Rheumatology. 2009;48(11):1410–3.
107. Mohrenschlager M, Jung C, Ring J, Abeck D. Effect of penicillin G on corium thickness in linear morphea of childhood: an analysis using ultrasound technique. Pediatr Dermatol. 1999;16(4):314–6.
108. Maragh SH, Davis MD, Bruce AJ, Nelson AM. Disabling pansclerotic morphea: clinical presentation in two adults. J Am Acad Dermatol. 2005;53(2 Suppl 1):S115–9.
109. Hunzelmann N, Anders S, Fierlbeck G, Hein R, Herrmann K, Albrecht M, et al. Double-blind, placebo-controlled study of intralesional interferon gamma for the treatment of localized scleroderma. J Am Acad Dermatol. 1997;36(3 Pt 1):433–5.
110. Laxer R, Zulian F. Localized scleroderma. Curr Opin Rheumatol. 2006;18:606–3.
111. Saxton-Daniels S, Jacobe H. Morphea. In: Goldsmith L, et al., editors. Fitzpatrick's dermatology in general medicine. 8th ed. Chicago: McGraw-Hill; 2012.

Scleroderma Mimics

11

Laura K. Hummers and Alan Tyndall

Differential Diagnosis of the Raynaud Phenomenon

Cold sensitivity, color changes, and ischemic injury of the digits are one of the cardinal features of scleroderma but may also be presenting features of other systemic, toxic, or infectious etiologies. When a patient presents with features typical of the Raynaud phenomenon with or without ischemic digital lesions, one needs to consider the broad differential of potential etiologies that include other rheumatic diseases, structural vessel abnormalities, embolic phenomena, or cold-precipitating circulating proteins.

Primary Raynaud phenomenon is common in the general population and presents without signs of structural vessel abnormalities or ischemic damage to tissues [2–5]. Primary Raynaud phenomenon typically begins in those younger than 30 and is more common in women (female/male ratio approximately 4:1). Primary Raynaud phenomenon is characterized by symmetric, episodic, cold-induced color changes in the fingers and/or toes on a normal physical examination and no signs of tissue damage such as ulceration of the skin or digital pitting. The blood vessel structure is normal as evidenced by nailfold capillaries that are thin, hairpin-like parallel vessels evenly distributed across the nailfold. Patients with the primary form of Raynaud phenomenon should have normal lab values, no evidence of autoimmunity (antinuclear antibody (ANA) negative), and normal inflammatory markers. Treating physicians must determine whether the presence of the Raynaud phenomenon is an early symptom of a secondary illness or is due to other causes such as medications, anatomic vessel changes, or other inflammatory conditions such as vasculitis (Table 11.1). There are several key points in the history and physical examination that should help clarify etiology. A history should explore vasoactive medications, toxins, trauma, or other associated medical issues that may point to a secondary cause. Physical examination should focus on several key findings including distal and proximal pulses, including provocative maneuvers for possible thoracic outlet syndrome (Adson's test), nailfold capillary examination, the presence and location of ischemic injury, and other evidence of a systemic disease (rashes, synovitis, muscle weakness). Key history and exam features of some more common etiologies of Raynaud-like diseases are included in Table 11.1. Large prospective studies have demonstrated that abnormal nailfold capillaries or the presence of autoantibodies are each associated with a significant risk of future development of definite scleroderma and may be appropriately classified as early scleroderma when both nailfold capillaroscopy (NFC) abnormalities and scleroderma-specific autoantibodies are present [6]. However, the 2013 ACR/EULAR classification of systemic sclerosis would require at least one additional feature to support the diagnosis, such as telangiectasia, sclerodactyly, or lung disease [1]. Alternatively, those patients with Raynaud alone and normal nailfold capillaries and negative serologies (including ANA) will only rarely progress to definite scleroderma [6]. While the majority of the 12% of those patients with the Raynaud phenomenon who went on to develop secondary disease do develop scleroderma, other connective tissue diseases may share Raynaud as a common feature. These would include particularly systemic lupus erythematosus (prevalence of 20%, including infrequent cases of digital gangrene) [7], dermatomyositis (prevalence as high as 65% in some subsets) [8, 9], and mixed connective tissue disease (85% prevalence, often with scleroderma-like nailfold capillary patterns), so a careful review of associated symptoms and appropriate serologic evaluation are warranted for patients exhibiting features of these diseases. Of note a 2022 meta-analysis of NFC changes in idiopathic inflammatory myopathy patients notes that scleroderma-like changes are more notable amongst patients

L. K. Hummers (✉)
Department of Medicine, Division of Rheumatology, Johns Hopkins University, Baltimore, MD, USA
e-mail: lhummers@jhmi.edu

A. Tyndall
Department of Rheumatology, University Hospital Basel, Basel, Switzerland

Y. Allanore et al. (eds.), *Scleroderma*, https://doi.org/10.1007/978-3-031-40658-4_11

Table 11.1 Differential diagnosis of the Raynaud phenomenon

		History/physical examination	Laboratory findings
Small artery disease	Systemic lupus erythematosus	Arthritis, rash	+ANA, +Sm, +dsDNA, +RNP
	Dermatomyositis	Rash, muscle weakness	+MDA-5, +TIF1gamma >anti-synthetase
	Antiphospholipid antibody syndrome	Arterial/venous clots; splinter hemorrhage	Elevated PTT or RVTT; anticardiolipin or B2 glycoprotein-1 antibodies
	Small vessel vasculitis	Sinusitis, pulmonary hemorrhage, petechiae	ANCA, hypocomplementemia, HCV antibodies
	Cryoglobulinemia	Petechiae, distal ischemia	+ Cryoglobulins, low C4, HCV antibodies
	Cryofibrinogenemia	Distal punctate lesions on toes	+ Cryofibrinogens
	Cold agglutinin disease	Recent infection; livedo reticularis	Anemia; (MGUS)
	Polycythemia	Pruritus; erythromelalgia; clots	Elevated WBC, RBC, platelets
	Thromboangiitis obliterans	Tobacco exposure; distal ischemia	None
	Chilblains (pernio), COVID toes	Erythematous plaques or nodules	None
Structural vasculopathy	Thoracic outlet syndrome	Positional symptoms; + Adson test	None
	Carpal tunnel syndrome	Positional symptoms; + Tinel test	None
	Atherosclerosis	Diminished distal pulses; claudication	Elevated lipids
Abnormal vasomotion	Primary Raynaud phenomenon	Normal nailfold capillaries; no ulcers	None
	Acrocyanosis	Painless persistent color changes	None
Medications/toxins	Sympathomimetics	Exposure to offending medication	None
	Polyvinyl chloride	Distal ischemia	None
	Nicotine	Tobacco exposure	None
	Cocaine	Exposure	+ Urinary toxin screening

with dermatomyositis, shows changes consistent with the "early" pattern of scleroderma NFC, and may normalize after therapy [9].

Other potential causes of the Raynaud-like phenomenon include mechanical obstruction (thoracic outlet syndrome), neurovascular compression (carpal tunnel syndrome), and cold-precipitating agglutination processes (cold agglutinins, cryoglobulins). In addition, other circulating proteins may cause small vessel occlusion such as antiphospholipid antibodies, paraproteinemias (IgM typically), and cryofibrinogenemia. Medications, particularly sympathomimetics, may induce Raynaud-like vasospasm and certain chemotherapeutic agents or toxins that may induce direct vascular injury (bleomycin, polyvinyl chloride, nicotine, levamisole) [10, 11]. Other forms of vascular damage may also lead to clinical syndromes including digital ischemia that may mimic the Raynaud phenomenon (cutaneous polyarteritis nodosa, thromboangiitis obliterans, cryoglobulinemic vasculitis). These vasculitic syndromes often will be accompanied by tissue ischemia that is profound and threatens major distal tissue loss.

Differential Diagnosis of Skin Thickening

Scleroderma-like disorders often show features that are quite similar to systemic sclerosis, but the diagnostic evaluation, risk for internal organ complications, and treatment options are distinct, and a careful diagnostic evaluation is warranted when the diagnosis is unclear. A delay in diagnosis can impede access to potentially effective therapy or avoid toxic therapies that may not be needed. Several key clinical features early in the presentation help distinguish these diseases and can prompt expedient screening for associated complications and facilitate treatment and appropriate referral to a speciality center.

Several diseases can present with thickening of the skin and mimic diffuse scleroderma. Such diseases include scleromyxedema, nephrogenic systemic fibrosis (NSF), eosinophilic fasciitis (EF), scleredema, toxic exposure-induced syndromes (eosinophilia-myalgia syndrome (EMS) and toxic oil syndrome (TOS)), and generalized subsets of localized scleroderma. These syndromes can be differenti-

Table 11.2 Differentiating features of scleroderma-like disorders and scleroderma

Disorder	Distribution of tight skin	Quality of the skin	Systemic features/ associated conditions	Laboratory abnormalities	Raynaud phenomenon/ nailfold capillaries
Eosinophilic fasciitis	Extremities and trunk; face, hands and feet spared	Woody induration deeper than the superficial dermis	Can overlap with plaque morphea; hematologic conditions; preceding intense exercise or trauma	Peripheral eosinophilia	Uncommon/ normal
Nephrogenic systemic fibrosis	Extremities and trunk; face spared	Nodular, indurated plaques with brawny hyperpigmentation	Marked flexion contractures; renal failure and/or insufficiency; exposure to gadolinium	Renal failure/ insufficiency (may be transient)	Rare/normal
Pansclerotic morphea	Extremities and trunk; hands spared	Thick induration similar to that of diffuse scleroderma; plaques	Contractures; no systemic features of scleroderma	None	Uncommon/ normal
Scleredema	The neck, back and proximal arms, face; and hands spared	Doughy induration	Discomfort in areas of involvement Poorly controlled diabetes Recent streptococcal infection Monoclonal gammopathy (MGUS)	Hyperglycemia; MGUS	None
Scleroderma	Hands and face common; diffuse subset involves proximal extremities and trunk; mid-back spared	Thick, smooth, shiny induration	Gastroesophageal reflux; dysphagia; interstitial lung disease; pulmonary hypertension	Positive antinuclear antibody; scleroderma-specific autoantibodies	Universal/ common
Scleromyxedema	Scleroderma distribution with prominent findings around the glabella, ears, and posterior neck	Cobblestone induration with 2–3 mm waxy papules	Dysphagia; musculoskeletal pain; neurologic involvement (seizures, coma)	MGUS	Uncommon/ normal

ated from systemic sclerosis by the pattern of distribution of skin changes, the texture and quality of the skin changes, and the presence and type of associated systemic manifestations, including the Raynaud phenomenon and lab abnormalities (Table 11.2). These disorders have very diverse etiologies and often an unclear pathogenic mechanism. Distinct clinical characteristics, skin histology, and systemic and laboratory associations distinguish these conditions from scleroderma and from each other. A prompt diagnosis is important to spare the patients from ineffective treatments, to facilitate appropriate diagnostic evaluations, and to allow for accurate determination of prognosis.

There is a long list of disorders that may mimic scleroderma by having cutaneous fibrosis or mucin deposition and includes other immune-mediated diseases (eosinophilic fasciitis, graft-versus-host disease), deposition disorders (scleromyxedema, scleredema, nephrogenic systemic fibrosis, systemic amyloidosis), and toxic exposures including occupational and iatrogenic (aniline-denatured rapeseed oil, contaminated L-tryptophan, polyvinyl chloride, bleomycin, carbidopa), and genetic syndromes (progeroid disorders, stiff skin syndrome). A carefully performed clinical history and physical examination may distinguish these conditions from scleroderma and each other. The distribution and the quality of skin involvement, the presence of Raynaud or abnormal nailfold capillary microscopy, and the association with particular concurrent diseases or specific laboratory parameters can be of substantial help in refining the diagnosis. In some cases, a full-thickness skin biopsy is helpful to confirm the clinical suspicion. Effective therapies are available for some of these conditions, whereas others are more refractory. For this reason, a prompt diagnosis is important to guide treatment decisions wisely. We will discuss some of the conditions most often confused with scleroderma either by the nature of the skin involvement or the presence of systemic features which may also mimic scleroderma. We will not include some other conditions that resemble scleroderma, but where the diagnosis is clear based on other clinical features, such as graft-versus-host disease (in those posttransplant) or genetic conditions (progeroid syndromes which occur in the very young often with other complications).

Toxin-Associated Scleroderma-Like Disorders

We will only briefly review some scleroderma-like diseases that are mostly of historical interest (i.e., toxic oil syndrome, eosinophilia-myalgia syndrome). These conditions may be a paradigm for possible future similar outbreaks. There are infrequent instances where exposure to agents such as aerosolized silica dust (as in coal miners and sandblasters) causes a syndrome indistinguishable from systemic sclerosis [12]. However, other clusters of scleroderma-like diseases occurred in outbreaks that were linked to a specific toxic exposure.

Toxic Oil Syndrome (TOS) and Eosinophilia Myalgia Syndrome (EMS)

The two classic examples of this type of event are the epidemic of the eosinophilia-myalgia syndrome associated with contaminated L-tryptophan supplements and the toxic oil syndrome from tainted rapeseed oil in Spain in 1981. The eosinophilia-myalgia syndrome (EMS) was identified in 1989 and determined to be related to a single impurity by a single manufacturer of L-tryptophan, which was marketed as a sleep aid [13]. The syndrome consists of peripheral eosinophilia with prominent myalgias with induration of the skin in the upper and lower extremities. The skin involvement is distinct from scleroderma in that it spares the hands and feet, and the induration of the skin is deeper with a "woody" quality (similar to eosinophilic fasciitis). The muscles (myalgia and myoclonus) and peripheral nerves (axonal polyneuropathy) may be involved [14]. Toxic oil syndrome (TOS) was another acute epidemic that occurred in Spain in 1981 related to an adulterated rapeseed oil that had been denatured with aniline. The syndrome affected >20,000 patients who were noted to have long-term health consequences [15]. The acute syndrome was manifested by interstitial pulmonary infiltrates and pleural effusions, myalgias, and peripheral eosinophilia. Associated features included skin itching and rash, peripheral sensory neuropathy, dysphagia, and pulmonary hypertension. Later manifestations included progressive fibrosing disease of the skin and lung [16, 17]. When the skin was involved, it seemed to have a clear progression from a more toxic-allergic presentation with distinct urticarial lesions to edema to fibrosis. While we are unlikely to see new patients with these specific syndromes, there may be other similar outbreaks in the future related to yet-to-be-defined toxins, so having an appropriate level of awareness of these prior experiences is important and may give us insight into the pathogenesis of similar syndromes with unknown etiology such as systemic sclerosis [18].

Nephrogenic Systemic Fibrosis

A more recent exposure-associated scleroderma mimicker or nephrogenic systemic fibrosis (NSF) (previously named nephrogenic fibrosing dermopathy) was first reported in 2000 [19]. A new entity was initially described among patients receiving renal dialysis and ultimately linked to the use of high doses of linear-chelated gadolinium-based contrast agents (GBCA) for MRI studies among those with stage IV and V chronic kidney disease, although some patients are unaware of gadolinium exposure [20]. The connection with exposure to gadolinium-based contrast agents (GBCA) was recognized around 2006, and case rates subsequently dropped [21]. In the United States, NSF cases are tracked by the FDA via the MedWatch program (https://www.fda.gov/safety/medwatch-fda-safety-information-and-adverse-event-reporting-program) and over 3000 cases have been reported in this system (as of 5/2022). There are now also consensus statements by nephrology and radiologic societies on the use of GBCA in patients with kidney disease [22].

Illness is characterized by the rapid development of edema followed by fibrotic skin induration with associated nodular plaques, hyperpigmentation of the skin, and marked flexion contractures of the extremities. The skin lesions of NSF usually develop subacutely shortly after gadolinium exposure (mean of 47 days) and subsequently assume a progressive course, rapidly developing joint contractures. The distribution is often symmetrical, commonly involving the extremities up to the knees and elbows. The hands and the trunk may be involved but typically spares the face. The texture of the skin is different than scleroderma in that the skin has a lumpy-nodular thickening with a tendency to form indurated irregularly shaped plaques with reticular discoloration varying from violaceous to brawny hyperpigmentation. A deeper subcutaneous fibrotic process leads to severe flexion contractures (particularly hands, wrists, ankles, and knees) which cause significant disability. Nerve conduction studies seem to confirm the presence of a true peripheral neuropathy, further complicating the management of the underlying pain syndrome, which is usually very difficult to control. NSF may be further distinguished from scleroderma by the absence of Raynaud phenomenon or nailfold capillary abnormalities. In addition, antinuclear antibodies and scleroderma-specific autoantibodies are negative. Tissue pathology is notable for the increased presence of CD34+ fibroblasts, mononuclear cell infiltrates and an increase in collagen (dermis into the subcutaneous structures) and variable mucin deposition. Treatment has been largely unsatisfactory, although case reports highlight possible benefits with tyrosine kinase inhibitors (imatinib), thalidomide, phototherapy, extracorporeal photopheresis, and plasmapheresis.

Scleredema

Scleredema is a condition associated with the deposition of collagen and mucin in the dermis and occurs in three specific conditions: (1) poorly controlled diabetes, (2) monoclonal gammopathies, and (3) postinfectious, particularly streptococcal pharyngitis. In a case series of 44 patients, 30 were related to diabetes, 5 were related to monoclonal gammopathies, and the others were unclear [23]. Scleredema of any etiology causes scleroderma-like skin changes but in a distribution distinct from systemic sclerosis. It has been estimated that as many as 1–14% of diabetics have scleredema in some cross-sectional studies, so it is thought that this may be underreported [24, 25]. Diabetic patients with scleredema are commonly poorly controlled and insulin requiring and have evidence of diabetic complications, specifically microangiopathy and retinopathy. There is an association between elevated hemoglobin A1C and the presence of scleredema [25]. The pathology of scleredema is notable for marked thickening of the upper and lower dermis, and mucin deposition between thickened collagen bundles. Scleredema causes a non-pitting, doughy induration of the skin that characteristically involves the neck, back, interscapular region, face, and chest. Typically the fingers and feet are spared and, in contrast with scleroderma, the mid back is almost always involved (Fig. 11.1). Involvement of the face can cause ocular muscle palsy, diminished oral aperture, and periorbital edema. Systemic involvement has been only infrequently reported, but some case reports highlight the involvement of the tongue, pharynx, and upper esophagus leading to dysphagia as a potentially reported systemic symptom [26]. Patients with infection-related disease are noted to have a rapid onset of symptoms days to months after the infection (often termed scleredema fulminans) with a course that typically resolves in several months to 2 years. Patients with diabetes and (MGUS)-associated scleredema have a very insidious onset with a gradual progression of symptoms over many years. Treatment may be symptomatic only (with physical therapy), particularly in those with an expected self-limited course (postinfectious). Treatments for diabetes and monoclonal protein-associated scleredema include phototherapy, corticosteroids, intravenous immunoglobulin (IVIG), thalidomide, or bortezomib (for paraprotein-associated) [23, 27–29].

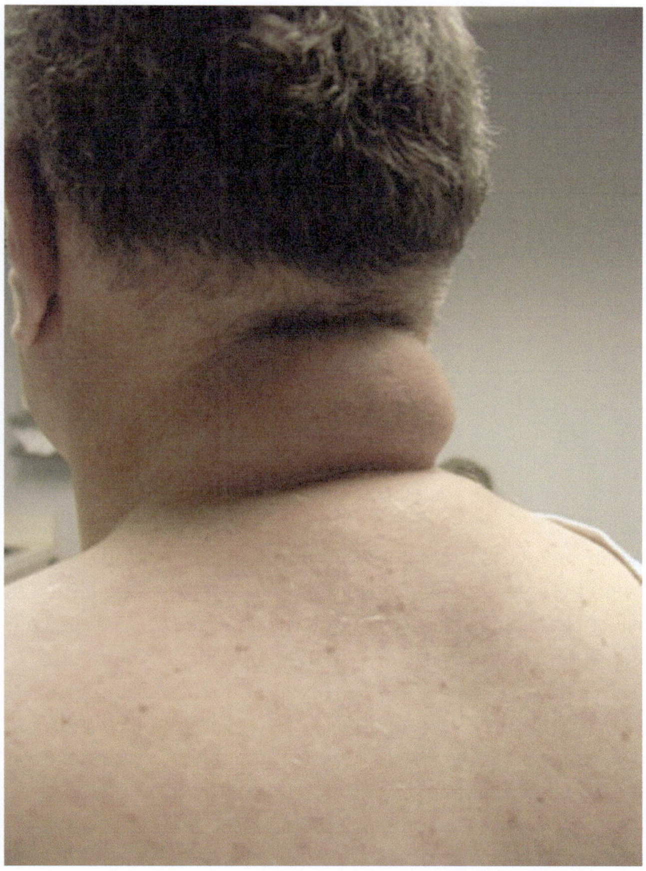

Fig. 11.1 Posterior neck in a patient with (MGUS)-associated scleredema

Scleromyxedema

Scleromyxedema (papular mucinosis) is a condition of mucinous deposition in the skin associated with a presence of a (MGUS) characterized by a diffuse, papular skin eruption. The average age of onset is around 50–55 years with a roughly equal gender distribution but this has not been reported in children. Diagnosis requires the presence of characteristic skin involvement, diagnostic biopsy (extensive interstitial mucin, thickened collagen bundles, and increased number of spindled fibroblast-like cells), and the presence of a monoclonal protein (typically IgG either kappa or lambda). More limited skin forms with restricted distribution (localized papular mucinosis) may not be associated with monoclonal gammopathies. The skin in scleromyxedema is indurated and papular in quality with a cobblestone feel, and its involvement occurs in a characteristic distribution with the glabellum, posterior auricular area, and neck being most commonly affected (Fig. 11.2). Other areas include the back and extremities and may be quite similar in distribution to scleroderma. Similar to scleredema, the midportion of the back is commonly affected in scleromyxedema and is almost

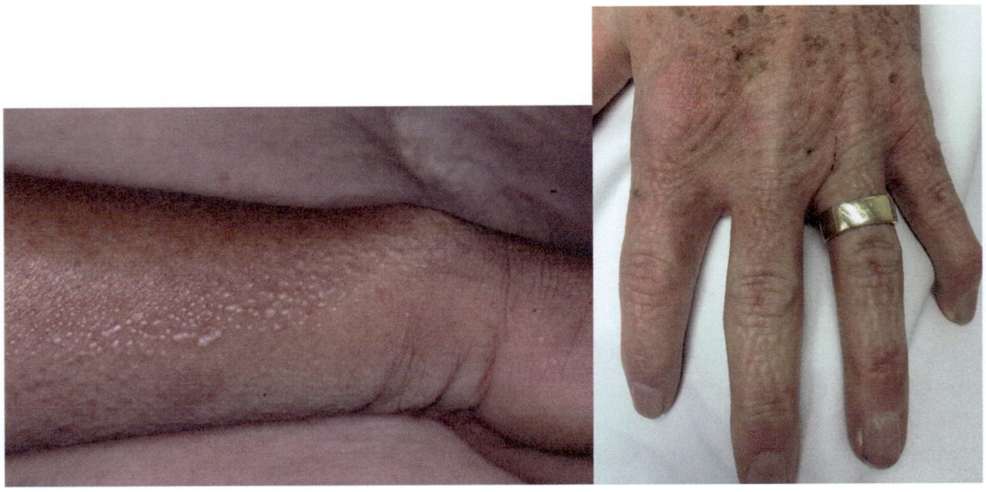

Fig. 11.2 The posterior forearm and hand in two patients with scleromyxedema

never involved in scleroderma patients. Sclerodactyly is often present and appears identical to scleroderma, although it is often subtly papular in quality. In addition to skin findings, patients may have organ involvement that seems to mimic scleroderma as well. Raynaud phenomenon, esophageal dysmotility, and myopathy have been reported [30, 31]. Less common but potentially life-threatening complications may involve the neurological system in the form of encephalopathy, seizures, coma, and psychosis [32, 33]. The natural history of this disease has not been well defined, but fatal cases have been reported, most commonly due to neurologic complications [34]. Several studies have highlighted cytometric and transcriptomic features of scleromyxedema suggesting possible roles of T cells and TGF-beta in scleromyxedema pathogenesis [33, 35, 36]. The most commonly reported effective treatment has been intravenous immunoglobulin (IVIG) and this is considered to be first-line therapy. Other treatments reported to be of benefit in some have included thalidomide/thalidomide analogues, autologous hematopoietic stem cell transplant, and corticosteroids [33, 37, 38].

Eosinophilic Fasciitis

Eosinophilic fasciitis was first described in 1974 by Schulman who reported two patients with scleroderma-like skin changes, painful induration of subcutaneous tissues with marked peripheral eosinophilia, and histological evidence of a diffuse fasciitis [39]. EF has a slight male predominance and has been reported more in Caucasians than other groups with cases occurring across the age spectrum. Dominant laboratory features include peripheral blood and tissue eosinophilia, hypergammaglobulinemia, and elevated inflammatory markers [40]. The classic histopathologic changes in EF are dermal-hypodermic sclerosis associated with fibrotic thickening of the subcutaneous adipose lobular septa, superficial fascia, and perimysium, and there is no mucin. The epidermis is usually spared. Eosinophils can be enriched within affected tissues but are not likely to be present when biopsies are obtained after the initiation of corticosteroid therapy. Given the similar appearance of EF to the toxin-associated epidemic syndromes (TOS and EMS), exposure histories have been examined for EF. The only clear historical association has been with an antecedent history of vigorous exercise or trauma which is found in about half of the described cases [40]. There are reported associations between EF and a number of hematologic conditions (malignant and non-malignant) and up to 30% of patients overlap with localized forms of scleroderma (morphea) [40]. More recently, there have been a number of case reports describing EF occurring after the initiation of immune checkpoint inhibitors [41, 42]. The onset and distribution of EF are very similar to NSF which is usually subacute symmetric thickening predominantly over the distal extremities within a short period of time (typically weeks). The trunk or neck can be involved but typically spares the hands and face. Early on, the skin is edematous with a "peau de orange" appearance (Fig. 11.3). This is followed by a progressive "woody" induration of subcutaneous tissues leading to skin puckering and the "venous groove sign." Importantly, the superficial dermis is usually spared allowing an examiner to be able to pinch the skin, which may be a helpful distinguishing feature from scleroderma and other scleroderma-like disorders. Deeper involvement and fibrosis of periarticular structures can cause flexion contractures as well as disturbances secondary to peripheral nerve compression, such as carpal tunnel syndrome. Raynaud phenomenon is infrequently present, but the nailfold capillary microscopy examination is normal and systemic features are absent except in cases where the extensive fibrosis around the chest or neck may lead to chest wall restriction or dysphagia. Common laboratory features include peripheral eosinophilia, hypergammaglobulinemia, and elevated inflammatory markers, but have low specificity to this condition compared with scleroderma and other scleroderma-like disorders. However, monoclonal gammopathies and autoantibodies are typically absent. The standard treatment for EF is corticosteroids, which are often intentionally avoided in scleroderma, making this diagnostic distinction particularly important. Pulse doses of steroids may be particularly beneficial and associated with higher rates of complete remission [34]. Refractory cases may be treated with methotrexate, mycophenolate mofetil, IVIG, and JAK inhibitors [43, 44]. In addition, the natural history is typically of remission with excellent prognosis. MRI (showing hyperintensity of the fascia on fluid-sensitive and contrasted sequences) may help establish the diagnosis and may help monitor disease activity and treatment response [45]. Ultrasonography may also be useful and aldolase may be a possible biomarker [46, 47].

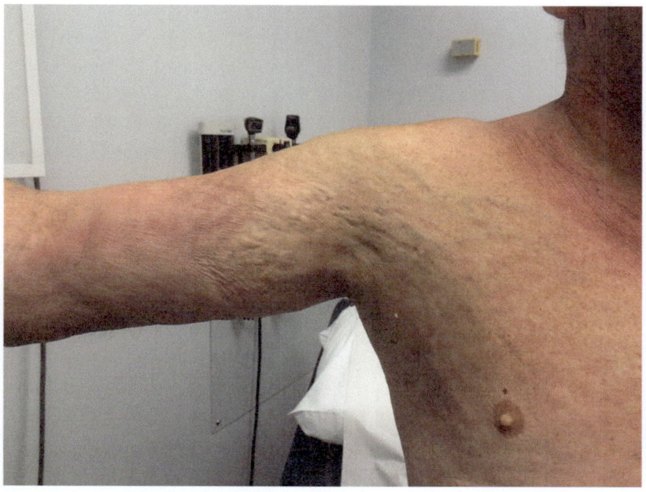

Fig. 11.3 The upper arm of a patient with eosinophilic fasciitis with a "peau de orange" appearance and venous groove sign

Localized Scleroderma

Most forms of localized scleroderma are more prevalent in children and quite distinct in appearance from systemic disease. These include plaque morphea and linear (en coup de sabre) variants of localized scleroderma. However, some forms, such as generalized morphea and pansclerotic morphea, may be difficult to distinguish from diffuse cutaneous systemic sclerosis and require special mention. Generalized morphea refers to multiple patches of scleroderma skin involvement that evolve into discrete lesions. The lesions are typically circular with a violaceous or erythematous border (when active) and then often develop a white, fibrotic center. Some patients have extensive involvement of the skin which typically involves the trunk (back > chest) and may linearly extend down one or more extremities (linear morphea) but spares the fingers in all of these cases. Pansclerotic morphea (severe form known as disabling pansclerotic morphea of childhood) typically spreads homogeneously over large areas of the skin typically involving the whole trunk and proximal extremities almost always sparing of hands, fingers, and distal forearms; however the feet are often deeply and characteristically involved (Fig. 11.4). Histological examination reveals fibrosis that extends through all layers of the dermis and subcutaneous tissues and may extend deeper into muscles and around tendons. Occasionally patients with morphea have antinuclear antibodies but typically do not have scleroderma-specific autoantibodies, Raynaud phenomenon, or abnormal nailfold capillaries [48]. The distribution of skin involvement is differentiated from diffuse cutaneous systemic sclerosis, the typical sparing of the fingers and hands and the plaque-like distribution of skin lesions. This condition may or may not involve the back so the lack of back involvement may not be helpful in distinguishing it from systemic sclerosis as it is with scleredema,

Fig. 11.4 The feet and face of a patient with severe pansclerotic morphea

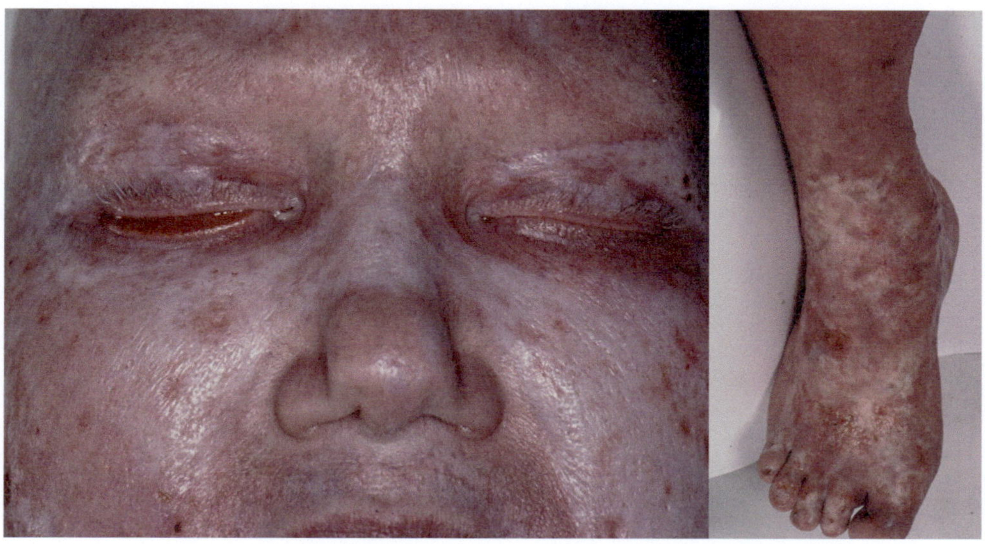

scleromyxedema, and generalized morphea. The most commonly utilized treatment modalities include phototherapy and methotrexate and other systemic immunosuppressants in more severe forms such as pansclerotic morphea where topical and UV-based therapy are unlikely to be effective [49].

Treatment Differences

There is no clinical trial data to guide therapy in any of the scleroderma mimics and very little in systemic sclerosis. These conditions are rare but need to be included in the differential when evaluating a patient with suspected scleroderma, so an internal organ disease screening may be performed, appropriate treatments may be suggested, and a more clear prognosis may be given. The therapeutic choices for someone with a "skin-only" disease may be markedly different than ones with potential for severe systemic involvement (scleroderma, scleromyxedema). Some conditions, such as infection-associated scleredema, eosinophilic fasciitis, and plaque morphea may be self-limited conditions that require short term or even no treatment, whereas others may require prolonged courses of immunosuppression and chronic management of complications (scleroderma, scleromyxedema, NSF). Table 11.3 includes common therapies and internal organ complication-screening strategies for each of the conditions discussed in this chapter.

Table 11.3 Screening algorithms and treatment options for scleroderma and related disorders

	Screening test in all patients	Treatment options
Scleroderma	Pulmonary function tests	Immunosuppression for skin or lung fibrosis
	Echocardiogram	Vasodilators for Raynaud
	Ambulatory blood pressure monitoring	Acid suppression for gastroesophageal reflux disease (GERD)
		Vasodilators for pulmonary hypertension
Nephrogenic systemic fibrosis	None	Intravenous immunoglobulin
		Tyrosine kinase inhibitors
		Physical therapy
Eosinophilic fasciitis	Complete blood counts	Prednisone Methotrexate Mycophenolate Mofetil
Scleromyxedema	Serum protein electrophoresis with immunofixation	Intravenous immunoglobulin
		Thalidomide/thalidomide analogues
Scleredema	Serum protein electrophoresis with immunofixation	UV light-based therapy IVIG
	Fasting blood glucose; hemoglobin A1C	Strict diabetes control UV light-based therapy
Pansclerotic morphea	ANA and scleroderma-specific antibodies	Immunosuppression (methotrexate, MMF)
		UV light-based therapy

References

1. van den Hoogen F, Khanna D, Fransen J, Johnson SR, Baron M, Tyndall A, et al. 2013 classification criteria for systemic sclerosis: an American college of rheumatology/European league against rheumatism collaborative initiative. Ann Rheum Dis. 2013;72(11):1747–55.
2. Gelber AC, Wigley FM, Stallings RY, Bone LR, Barker AV, Baylor I, et al. Symptoms of Raynaud's phenomenon in an inner-city African-American community: prevalence and self-reported cardiovascular comorbidity. J Clin Epidemiol. 1999;52(5):441–6.
3. Jones GT, Herrick AL, Woodham SE, Baildam EM, Macfarlane GJ, Silman AJ. Occurrence of Raynaud's phenomenon in children ages 12-15 years: prevalence and association with other common symptoms. Arthritis Rheum. 2003;48(12):3518–21.
4. Voulgari PV, Alamanos Y, Papazisi D, Christou K, Papanikolaou C, Drosos AA. Prevalence of Raynaud's phenomenon in a healthy Greek population. Ann Rheum Dis. 2000;59(3):206–10.
5. Maricq HR, Carpentier PH, Weinrich MC, Keil JE, Palesch Y, Biro C, et al. Geographic variation in the prevalence of Raynaud's phenomenon: a 5 region comparison. J Rheumatol. 1997;24(5):879–89.
6. Koenig M, Joyal F, Fritzler MJ, Roussin A, Abrahamowicz M, Boire G, et al. Autoantibodies and microvascular damage are independent predictive factors for the progression of Raynaud's phenomenon to systemic sclerosis: a twenty-year prospective study of 586 patients, with validation of proposed criteria for early systemic sclerosis. Arthritis Rheum. 2008;58(12):3902–12.
7. Liu A, Zhang W, Tian X, Zhang X, Zhang F, Zeng X. Prevalence, risk factors and outcome of digital gangrene in 2684 lupus patients. Lupus. 2009;18(12):1112–8.
8. Kalluri M, Sahn SA, Oddis CV, Gharib SL, Christopher-Stine L, Danoff SK, et al. Clinical profile of anti-PL-12 autoantibody. Cohort study and review of the literature. Chest. 2009;135(6):1550–6.
9. Piette Y, Reynaert V, Vanhaecke A, Bonroy C, Gutermuth J, Sulli A, et al. Standardised interpretation of capillaroscopy in autoimmune idiopathic inflammatory myopathies: a structured review on behalf of the EULAR study group on microcirculation in rheumatic diseases. Autoimmun Rev. 2022;21(6):103087.
10. Glendenning JL, Barbachano Y, Norman AR, Dearnaley DP, Horwich A, Huddart RA. Long-term neurologic and peripheral vascular toxicity after chemotherapy treatment of testicular cancer. Cancer. 2010;116(10):2322–31.
11. Maricq HR, Johnson MN, Whetstone CL, LeRoy EC. Capillary abnormalities in polyvinyl chloride production workers. Examination by in vivo microscopy. Jama. 1976;236(12):1368–71.
12. Rustin MH, Bull HA, Ziegler V, Mehlhorn J, Haustein UF, Maddison PJ, et al. Silica-associated systemic sclerosis is clinically, serologically and immunologically indistinguishable from idiopathic systemic sclerosis. Br J Dermatol. 1990;123(6):725–34.
13. Belongia EA, Hedberg CW, Gleich GJ, White KE, Mayeno AN, Loegering DA, et al. An investigation of the cause of the eosinophilia-myalgia syndrome associated with tryptophan use. N Engl J Med. 1990;323(6):357–65.
14. Kaufman LD, Krupp LB. Eosinophilia-myalgia syndrome, toxic-oil syndrome, and diffuse fasciitis with eosinophilia. Curr Opin Rheumatol. 1995;7(6):560–7.
15. Posada de la Paz M, Díaz-Guerra E, Alonso-Ferreira V, Villaverde-Hueso A, Arias-Merino G, Garrido-Estepa M. Toxic oil syndrome: health-related quality-of-life assessment using the SF-36 health survey. Int J Epidemiol. 2022;51(2):491–500.

16. Kilbourne EM, Posada de la Paz M, Abaitua Borda I, Diez Ruiz-Navarro M, Philen RM, Falk H. Toxic oil syndrome: a current clinical and epidemiologic summary, including comparisons with the eosinophilia-myalgia syndrome. J Am Coll Cardiol. 1991;18(3):711–7.
17. Fonseca E, Contreras F. Cutaneous mucinosis in the toxic oil syndrome. J Am Acad Dermatol. 1987;16(1 Pt 1):139–40.
18. Piera-Velazquez S, Wermuth PJ, Gomez-Reino JJ, Varga J, Jimenez SA. Chemical exposure-induced systemic fibrosing disorders: novel insights into systemic sclerosis etiology and pathogenesis. Semin Arthritis Rheum. 2020;50(6):1226–37.
19. Cowper SE, Robin HS, Steinberg SM, Su LD, Gupta S, LeBoit PE. Scleromyxoedema-like cutaneous diseases in renal-dialysis patients. Lancet. 2000;356(9234):1000–1.
20. Bennett CL, Qureshi ZP, Sartor AO, Norris LB, Murday A, Xirasagar S, et al. Gadolinium-induced nephrogenic systemic fibrosis: the rise and fall of an iatrogenic disease. Clin Kidney J. 2012;5(1):82–8.
21. Bennett CL, Starko KM, Thomsen HS, Cowper S, Sartor O, Macdougall IC, et al. Linking drugs to obscure illnesses: lessons from pure red cell aplasia, nephrogenic systemic fibrosis, and Reye's syndrome. A report from the southern network on adverse reactions (SONAR). J Gen Intern Med. 2012;27(12):1697–703.
22. Weinreb JC, Rodby RA, Yee J, Wang CL, Fine D, McDonald RJ, et al. Use of intravenous gadolinium-based contrast media in patients with kidney disease: consensus statements from the American College of Radiology and the National Kidney Foundation. Kidney Med. 2021;3(1):142–50.
23. Rongioletti F, Kaiser F, Cinotti E, Metze D, Battistella M, Calzavara-Pinton PG, et al. Scleredema. A multicentre study of characteristics, comorbidities, course and therapy in 44 patients. J Eur Acad Dermatol Venereol. 2015;29(12):2399–404.
24. Cole GW, Headley J, Skowsky R. Scleredema diabeticorum: a common and distinct cutaneous manifestation of diabetes mellitus. Diabetes Care. 1983;6(2):189–92.
25. Ghosh A, Shah SV, Dave JN, Vora NS, Roy K, Cardoso BJ. Scleredema. Indian J Dermatol Venereol Leprol. 1995;61(5):324–5.
26. Wright RA, Bernie H. Scleredema adultorum of Buschke with upper esophageal involvement. Am J Gastroenterol. 1982;77(1):9–11.
27. Barnes M, Kumar V, Le TH, Nabeel S, Singh J, Rana V, et al. A case of paraproteinemia-associated scleredema successfully treated with thalidomide. JAAD Case Rep. 2020;6(10):1039–41.
28. Mark PB, Dekkers I, Blankestijn PJ, Leiner T, Roditi G. Letter on 'European dermatology forum S1-guideline on the diagnosis and treatment of sclerosing diseases of the skin, part 2: Scleromyxedema, scleredema and nephrogenic systemic fibrosis'. J Eur Acad Dermatol Venereol. 2018;32(2):e84–e5.
29. Eastham AB, Femia AN, Velez NF, Smith HP, Vleugels RA. Paraproteinemia-associated scleredema treated successfully with intravenous immunoglobulin. JAMA Dermatol. 2014;150(7):788–9.
30. Dinneen AM, Dicken CH. Scleromyxedema. J Am Acad Dermatol. 1995;33(1):37–43.
31. Blum M, Wigley FM, Hummers LK. Scleromyxedema: a case series highlighting long-term outcomes of treatment with intravenous immunoglobulin (IVIG). Medicine (Baltimore). 2008;87(1):10–20.
32. Berger JR, Dobbs MR, Terhune MH, Maragos WF. The neurologic complications of scleromyxedema. Medicine (Baltimore). 2001;80(5):313–9.
33. Mahévas T, Arnulf B, Bouaziz JD, Livideanu CB, Osio A, Servy A, et al. Plasma cell-directed therapies in monoclonal gammopathy-associated scleromyxedema. Blood. 2020;135(14):1101–10.
34. Sala AC, Cunha PR, Pinto CA, Alves CA, Paiva IB, Araujo AP. Scleromyxedema: clinical diagnosis and autopsy findings. An Bras Dermatol. 2016;91(5 suppl 1):48–50.
35. Kalli F, Cioni M, Parodi A, Altosole T, Ferrera F, Barra G, et al. Increased frequency of interleukin-4 and reduced frequency of interferon-γ and IL-17-producing CD4+ and CD8+ cells in scleromyxedema. J Eur Acad Dermatol Venereol. 2020;34(5):1092–7.
36. Mecoli CA, Talbot CC Jr, Fava A, Cheadle C, Boin F, Wigley FM, et al. Clinical and molecular phenotyping in Scleromyxedema pretreatment and posttreatment with intravenous immunoglobulin. Arthritis Care Res (Hoboken). 2020;72(6):761–7.
37. Rongioletti F, Merlo G, Cinotti E, Fausti V, Cozzani E, Cribier B, et al. Scleromyxedema: a multicenter study of characteristics, comorbidities, course, and therapy in 30 patients. J Am Acad Dermatol. 2013;69(1):66–72.
38. Mahevas T, Arnulf B, Bouaziz JD, Livideanu CB, Osio A, Servy A, et al. Plasma cell-directed therapies in monoclonal gammopathy-associated scleromyxedema. Blood. 2020;135(14):1101–10.
39. Shulman LE. Diffuse fasciitis with eosinophilia: a new syndrome? Trans Assoc Am Phys. 1975;88:70–86.
40. Lakhanpal S, Ginsburg WW, Michet CJ, Doyle JA, Moore SB. Eosinophilic fasciitis: clinical spectrum and therapeutic response in 52 cases. Semin Arthritis Rheum. 1988;17(4):221–31.
41. Salamaliki C, Solomou EE, Liossis SC. Immune checkpoint inhibitor-associated scleroderma-like syndrome: a report of a pembrolizumab-induced "eosinophilic fasciitis-like" case and a review of the literature. Rheumatol Ther. 2020;7(4):1045–52.
42. Chan KK, Magro C, Shoushtari A, Rudin C, Rotemberg V, Rossi A, et al. Eosinophilic fasciitis following checkpoint inhibitor therapy: four cases and a review of literature. Oncologist. 2020;25(2):140–9.
43. Cao XY, Zhao JL, Hou Y, Wang FD, Lu ZH. Janus kinase inhibitor tofacitinib is a potential therapeutic option for refractory eosinophilic fasciitis. Clin Exp Rheumatol. 2020;38(3):567–8.
44. Lebeaux D, Francès C, Barete S, Wechsler B, Dubourg O, Renoux J, et al. Eosinophilic fasciitis (Shulman disease): new insights into the therapeutic management from a series of 34 patients. Rheumatology (Oxford). 2012;51(3):557–61.
45. Primitivo A, Madeira N, Lopez D, Afonso D. Eosinophilic fasciitis (Shulman disease) with clinical, imaging and pathological correlation. BMJ Case Rep. 2021;14(12).
46. Mango RL, Bugdayli K, Crowson CS, Drage LA, Wetter DA, Lehman JS, et al. Baseline characteristics and long-term outcomes of eosinophilic fasciitis in 89 patients seen at a single center over 20 years. Int J Rheum Dis. 2020;23(2):233–9.
47. Nashel J, Steen V. The use of an elevated aldolase in diagnosing and managing eosinophilic fasciitis. Clin Rheumatol. 2015;34(8):1481–4.
48. Li SC, Higgins GC, Chen M, Torok KS, Rabinovich CE, Stewart K, et al. Extracutaneous involvement is common and associated with prolonged disease activity and greater impact in juvenile localized scleroderma. Rheumatology (Oxford). 2021;60(12):5724–33.
49. Ulc E, Rudnicka L, Waśkiel-Burnat A, Warszawik-Hendzel O, Niemczyk A, Olszewska M. Therapeutic and reconstructive management options in scleroderma (morphea) en coup de sabre in children and adults. A systematic literature review. J Clin Med. 2021;10(19):4517.

Part III

The Biological Basis of Systemic Sclerosis

John Varga

Introduction: The Etiopathogenesis of Systemic Sclerosis—An Integrated Overview

12

Carol Feghali-Bostwick, David J. Abraham, and John Varga

Abbreviations

DC	Dendritic cells
EMT	Epithelial-to-mesenchymal transition
Endo-MT	Endothelial-to-mesenchymal transition
FGF	Fibroblast growth factor family
Fibro	Fibroblasts
IFN	Interferon
Mo	Monocytes
MyoF	Myofibroblasts
NETs	Neutrophil extra-cellular traps
ROS	Reactive oxygen species
SiO_2	Crystallin silica
Tfh	T-follicular helper
Th	T-helper

Introduction

Systemic sclerosis (SSc) is a heterogeneous chronic multisystem disease with global distribution and a strong female predominance. Multiple genes have been linked with susceptibility to SSc or to particular endophenotypes. The genetic architecture is dominated by the HLA locus and shows considerable overlap with other autoimmune diseases including systemic lupus erythematosus, inflammatory bowel disease, psoriasis, and others. The variable and unpredictable disease course, high burden of mortality and morbidity, and lack of safe and effective therapies make SSc a top research priority in the rheumatic disease space.

A global view of SSc suggests the following integrated paradigm for disease pathogenesis, supported by current data presented in the chapters that follow: initial trigger (repeated injury) in an individual harboring a permissive genetic background (combination of genetic risk variants) initiates a series of complex and sustained interactions among vascular and immune cells in a variety of tissues. Oxidative stress, immune cell activation, and autoantibody generation ensue, and a panoply of soluble and matrix-associated signals are generated that initiate and sustain mesenchymal cell activation, transdifferentiation, and survival, leading to extracellular matrix production and accumulation. The altered extracellular environment in turn further amplifies these processes, culminating in progressive and intractable multi-organ fibrosis. Details of this process are described in the following chapters and are schematically summarized in Fig. 12.1.

C. Feghali-Bostwick (✉)
Division of Rheumatology and Immunology, Department of Medicine, Medical University of South Carolina, Charleston, SC, USA
e-mail: feghalib@musc.edu

D. J. Abraham
Division of Medicine, Department of Inflammation, UCL Centre for Rheumatology, University College London, London, UK
e-mail: david.abraham@ucl.ac.uk

J. Varga
Division of Rheumatology, Department of Internal Medicine, University of Michigan, Ann Arbor, MI, USA
e-mail: vargaj@umich.edu

Y. Allanore et al. (eds.), *Scleroderma*, https://doi.org/10.1007/978-3-031-40658-4_12

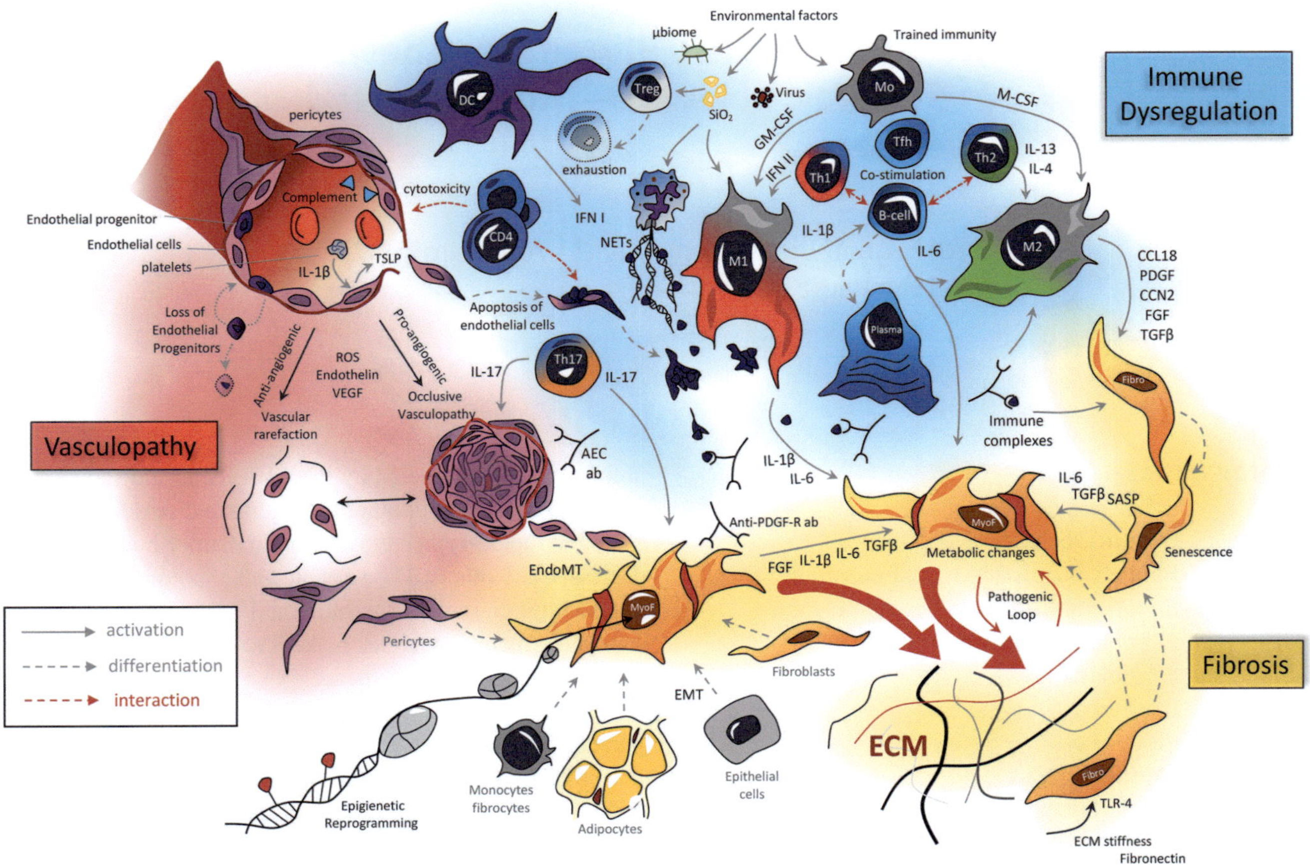

Fig. 12.1 Current integrated understanding of the pathogenesis of systemic sclerosis (SSc). SSc is characterized by a triad of intermediate "pathophenotypes," including widespread microvascular abnormalities (red), immune dysregulation (blue), and excessive scarring leading to fibrosis (yellow) of the skin and internal organs. SSc-associated vasculopathy is considered as one of the earliest events in the pathogenesis of the disease. The unregulated production of proangiogenic factors leads to an uncontrolled proliferation of endothelial cells and pericytes with a subsequent narrowing of the vascular lumen and tissue ischemia. Hypoxia and ROS production may exacerbate this process and, in parallel, may induce a loss of endothelial progenitors with progressive vascular rarefaction. Several factors contribute to endothelial dysfunction such as complement activation, platelet-derived mediators (IL-1β), and cytotoxicity induced by CD4 Tl ymphocytes. The excess of endothelial apoptosis and the production of NETs by activated neutrophils could represent a source of nuclear autoantigens. A defect in pro-resolving properties of macrophages such as efferocytosis, i.e., the phagocytosis of cellular debris, could favor the persistence of such autoantigens that could be targeted by autoantibodies produced by adaptive immunity. The exact mechanisms leading to the activation of innate and adaptive immunity in SSc are still to be determined but several environmental factors such as crystalline silica exposure could participate in this immune dysregulation. In early SSc, dendritic cells and Th1 lymphocytes produce IFN type I and II participating in the activation of macrophages into pro-inflammatory M1 macrophages characterized by altered efferocytosis capacities. T-reg exhaustion and Th17 activation could also perpetuate this proinflammatory milieu. Th2 lymphocytes produce IL-4 and IL-13 that can orientate macrophage polarization toward an M2 profibrotic phenotype leading to the production of key cytokines and growth factors responsible for myofibroblast activation. Adaptive immunity also plays a major role in the disease process as co-stimulation and B cell activation cascade leads to the production of autoantibodies (ab) with potential direct functional properties (anti-endothelin receptor ab or anti-PDGF-R ab with agonist effects). Autoantibodies can also participate in the formation of immune complexes that can notably activate myofibroblasts, the key integrators of profibrotic signals in SSc and the major producers of extracellular matrix (ECM) in fibrotic tissues. Myofibroblasts can notably derive from fibroblasts, epithelial cells (notably in the lung), adipocytes, monocytes (also called fibrocytes in this context), pericytes, or endothelial cells, through a process called endothelial to mesenchymal transition. Myofibroblasts in SSc are characterized by a mesenchymal phenotype with altered metabolism and acquired resistance to apoptosis potentially mediated by epigenetic regulations. The senescence of fibroblasts can also participate in myofibroblast activation notably as this senescence-associated secretory phenotype (SASP) is associated with the production of IL-6, TGF-β, or IL-1β. ECM stiffness and associated components such as fibronectin can also directly activate myofibroblasts in a TLR-4 dependent manner, leading to a sustained activation loop. Figure developed with the assistance of Dr Alain Lescoat (created by Dr Alain Lescoat)

Intermediate Pathophenotypes (the Triad), Disease Heterogeneity, and the Role of Heredity

The distinctive features of SSc are widespread microvascular abnormalities, immune dysregulation with inflammation and cellular and humoral autoimmunity, and excessive scarring leading to fibrosis of the skin and internal organs. These three distinct yet intricately linked dynamic processes can be labeled "intermediate pathophenotypes" that constitute the characteristic triad of SSc and underlie its clinical presentation or phenotype. The tissues affected by these processes, the relative impact and activity of these individual processes in a given patient at a given point in the disease course, and their rates of progression or regression vary widely across patients. This heterogeneity in the phenotypic expression of SSc, no doubt determined in part by individual host genetic factors and their epistatic interactions, accounts for the exceptional variability of SSc, and the challenge of accurately predicting treatment responses, natural history, and outcomes. Progress has been made in understanding ethnicity-related genetic differences in SSc as well as features of disease in pediatric SSc. Understanding the genetic, molecule and cellular bases of disease heterogeneity and identifying tractable markers for their classification represent perhaps the major current unmet need in the field of scleroderma research.

The genetic basis of SSc is complex and incompletely understood [1]. A growing number of genetic loci are recognized to be associated with SSc across multiple ethnic cohorts, and in aggregate underscore the important role that immune processes play in disease susceptibility. However, a great deal of the heritability of SSc remains unaccounted for, and the genetic associations recognized to date carry only a modest risk. The complex role of heredity in disease susceptibility is highlighted by an SSc twin study, which reveals a low concordance rate for disease in both monozygotic and dizygotic twin pairs, but a very high concordance rate for anti-nuclear antibody (ANA) positivity [2]. Environmental stimuli elicit both transient effects, as well as durable changes in gene expression (the transcriptome) due to epigenetic modifications (imprinting). The three principal epigenetic modifications, namely, histone acetylation, DNA and histone methylation, and non-coding RNAs (micro-RNAs and long non-coding RNAs) together drive environmentally induced heritable changes in gene expression that are not due to changes in the DNA sequence. The epigenome, which represents a record of accrued environmental influences, has received increasing attention in SSc. Novel insights have been reported on the levels of roles of epigenome-modifying enzymes in angiogenesis, fibrosis, and immune cell function [3–6]. Epigenetic differences have also been reported in twins discordant for SSc [7]. More recently, active DNA regulatory elements were identified in different skin types in the skin with the greatest SSc-associated chromatin accessibility noted in skin-resident dendritic cells [8]. While the studies to date have been informative, additional functional implications of these changes are needed. The identification of microRNA and non-coding RNA alterations has contributed additional insights into the epigenome in SSc. Additionally, random (stochastic) events, together with biological aging, may cause somatic mutations and further modulate the epigenome, particularly in cells of the immune system, resulting in a break in immune tolerance. Gene–environment interactions therefore are likely to be of paramount significance in disease risk and progression, but the environmental and stochastic events contributing to the etiopathogenesis of SSc remain virtually unknown [9].

Heterogeneity in both clinical, pathological, and molecular features of disease and evolution over time is a notable hallmark of SSc [10]. Nevertheless, despite varying clinical manifestations, internal organ involvement, autoantibody profiles, disease progression, and outcomes, patients with SSc share certain key features in common. In particular, all patients with SSc display the triad of intermediate pathophenotypes affecting multiple tissues and organs (Fig. 12.2): vascular injury, immune abnormalities, and fibrosis. Consequently, a staggering diversity of cell types, progenitor cells, and cell lineages play important roles in pathogenesis. These include immune cells, vascular and stromal cells, and multipotent stem cells (Table 12.1), with considerable plasticity to differentiate into alternate cell fates.

There is currently no cure, nor effective disease-modifying or prevention therapies, for SSc, and there is unlikely to be a "one size fits all" therapy. Consequently, research in the field seeks to gain a detailed understanding of the genetic and environmental risk factors for and the pathogenesis of SSc and its various subsets or "endophenotypes," the development and validation of preclinical in vivo and ex vivo models of disease, identification of tools to precisely stratify patients into subsets, and discovery of key mediators and mechanisms for the development of targeted therapies [10].

This brief introductory chapter aims to provide a birds' eye view of the etiopathogenesis of SSc that attempts to synthesize and integrate current evidence. We highlight key themes that are discussed in detail in the chapters in the pathogenesis section that follows.

The Scleroderma Triad of Intermediate Pathophenotypes

The pathogenesis of SSc is complex, multifactorial, and incompletely understood. Evidence of a characteristic triad of intermediate pathophenotypes can be detected in virtually every patient with SSc. These processes are interlinked and

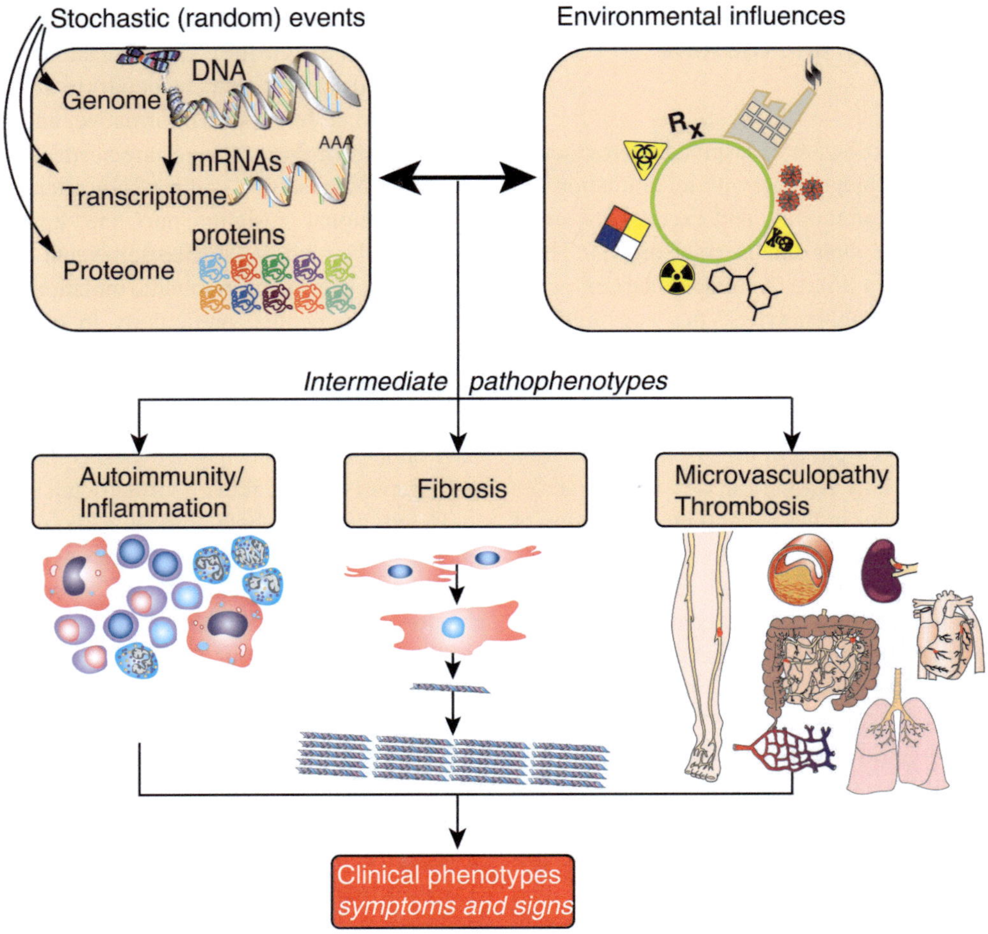

Fig. 12.2 The etiopathogenesis of SSc: triad of intermediate pathophenotypes. Illustrated are the reciprocal interactions of genetic and environmental influences and events that underlie the development of SSc, and the impact of random (stochastic) events, on the triad of cardinal biological processes termed "intermediate pathophenotypes" that form the pathogenic triad of SSc. The dynamic interplay of these intermediate pathophenotypes underlies the protean and fluctuating clinical manifestations of the disease. For example, variations in the timing and intensity of the intermediate pathophenotypes in affected tissues determine the unique clinical presentations of SSc among different individuals and different time-points during the evolution of the disease. The three intermediate pathophenotypes of SSc share traits such as impaired autophagy, endoplasmic reticulum stress and oxidative stress, reduced cell-intrinsic cytoprotective mechanisms, loss of immune self-tolerance, disruption of circadian rhythms, and failure to replenish injured cells and regenerate damaged structures. It does not escape our attention that these same traits are hallmarks of biological aging, suggesting mechanistic parallels between biological aging and SSc [Modified after Barabasi and Loscalzo [22]]

Table 12.1 Cell types prominently implicated in the pathogenesis of SSc

Immune	Monocytes/macrophages
	Dendritic cells
	B lymphocytes, plasma cells
	T lymphocytes, subsets
	Innate lymphoid cells
	NK cells
	Mast cells
Vascular	Endothelial cells
	Vascular smooth muscle cells
	Pericytes
	Platelets
Stromal cells	Mesenchymal stem cells
	Epithelial cells
	Fibroblasts/myofibroblasts
	Adipocytes
	Telocytes

dynamically modulated in each other in a cascade of events that culminate in the overall clinical disease phenotype and endophenotype (Fig. 12.2). Research on SSc has been hampered by disease complexity and the lack of appropriate animal models, since no single animal model faithfully phenocopies the full ensemble of cardinal features or recapitulates the organ-based manifestations or temporal evolution and chronicity of the human disease.

Primacy of Vascular Injury and Damage

Vascular injury and consequent blood vessel damage are prominent, and perhaps primary events in the pathogenesis of SSc [11]. Widespread vascular abnormalities in virtually every organ, a distinguishing hallmark of SSc, manifest clinically as the Raynaud phenomenon, distorted nailfold capillary architecture, myocardial perfusion abnormalities, mucocutaneous telangiectasias, ischemic digital ulcers, gastric antral vascular ectasia, PAH, and microangiopathic scleroderma renal crisis [12]. Vascular abnormalities are almost universal and frequently the earliest clinical manifestations of SSc and typically precede recognizable immune abnormalities and fibrosis. Vascular injury may be triggered by toxic, autoimmune, metabolic, or infectious factors, and is initially associated with largely reversible functional changes in the blood vessels, such as the recurrent spasms in the Raynaud phenomenon. However, these early aberrations progress and lead to irreversible structural vascular alterations impact on endothelial cells, vascular smooth muscle cells, adventitial cells, and perivascular supporting cells called pericytes. Progressive vascular damage leads to neointima formation, luminal narrowing, perivascular fibrosis, and obliteration of small- and medium-sized arteries in multiple vascular beds. Endothelial cells exhibit markers of vascular injury, activation and altered angiogenesis, increased oxidative stress, and dysregulated expression of cell-adhesion molecules, which facilitates the extravasation of immune cells into inflamed tissues. Perivascular inflammation is common and plays an important role in vasculopathy, particularly that underlying pulmonary artery hypertension and enhancing pulmonary vascular remodeling. Platelet aggregation and activation of thrombotic and coagulation cascades ensue. Compromised vascular blood supply leads to chronic tissue hypoxia, ischemic complications, and the development of tissue necrosis.

Critical drivers of vascular dysfunction in SSc include endothelial cell injury and release of reactive oxygen species, thromboxane and anti-angiogenic factors, and generation of anti-endothelial cell antibodies, although the specific nature of the injurious agents remains elusive. Additional triggering factors implicated in SSc vascular disease include a marked imbalance in vasoactive factors promoting vasodilation versus vasoconstriction, including angiotensin, nitric oxide, and endothelin-1, as well as the development of functional autoantibodies that are directed against surface receptors present on endothelial cells. Additional evidence highlighting a profound vasculopathy in SSc indicates that vasculogenesis, the formation of new blood vessels to replace lost and damaged ones, is impaired in SSc. Despite tissue ischemia and elevated levels of angiogenic factors that normally serve as potent stimuli for vasculogenesis, in SSc the number and function of endothelial progenitor cells (EPCs) are reduced. Prompting discussions around therapeutic strategies to enhance the production of EPCs or their direct use to repair the vasculature. Pericytes, which are key in maintaining endothelial cell function and the structural environment of small blood vessels, are found dysfunctional in SSc, further aggravating the loss of vasculature and provide a functional link between vessel integrity and remodeling. Additionally, both pericytes and adventitial fibroblasts are activated and have the capacity to transdifferentiate into myofibroblast-like cells contributing to perivascular and interstitial tissue fibrosis. The sequence of microvascular injury, vascular damage, and ensuing fibrosis leading to capillary rarefaction in the skin and other organs is partially phenocopied in several mouse models including the Fra-2 transgenic mice, as well as in Fli1 and uPAR knockout mice. These genetically engineered mouse models provide further evidence to support the notion that microangiopathy is prominently associated with tissue fibrosis (Table 12.2).

Table 12.2 Prominent mouse models used to explore the pathogenesis of SSc and to test new therapies

Primarily vasculopathy[a]	Fra-2 transgenic
	VEGF transgenic
	uPAR null
	Fli1 null
	Topoisomerase1 induced
Primarily immune	Inducible: injection of bleomycin, hypochlorous acid
	Mouse cGVHD
	PSGL null (also develop vasculopathy)
Primarily fibrotic	TSK1 and TSK2 spontaneous mutants
	Wnt10 transgenic
	Fibrillin mutant transgenic (stiff skin)
	PDGFR transgenic
	Relaxin model
	CTGF transgenic model
	TGF-beta receptor transgenic models
	Caveolin null
	Fli-1 null
	Angiotensin II model
	Srt3 null

cGVHD chronic graft-versus-host disease; *uPAR* urokinase-type plasminogen activator receptor; and *PSGL* P-selectin glycoprotein ligand-1
[a] Each of these models is associated with prominent fibrotic features in the skin.

The Immune System: Inflammation, Innate Immunity, Adaptive Immunity, and Autoimmunity

In view of the near-universal presence of ANA and a range of specific autoantibodies, as well as evidence of immune cell activation in both the circulation and in affected target tissues, SSc has been traditionally viewed as an inflammatory autoimmune disease. However, the modest efficacy of glucocorticoids and other immunosuppressive therapies has led to questions regarding the importance of autoimmunity in pathogenesis. On the other hand, the remarkable efficacy of hematopoietic stem cell therapy, which is thought to “reset” the immune system, in some patients with SSc, has been viewed as further evidence in support of the autoimmune nature of the disease. Whether immune dysregulation is a primary pathogenic event in SSc, is secondary to vascular injury and tissue damage, or co-exist as key drivers of pathology remains a subject of intense debate and the focus of much research. Nevertheless, insights from genetic studies unequivocally point to a fundamental role of altered immune processes in disease susceptibility, and, together with the presence of circulating autoantibodies, the "interferon signature" in immune cells and of inflammatory gene signatures in the lesional tissue in our opinion justify the classification of SSc as an autoimmune disease. Abnormalities in the numbers, distribution, and function of cells of the immune system are prevalent in all forms of SSc. Local and systemic changes in cytokine, chemokine and growth factor levels, and activation, migration, and differentiation of T cells, B cells, monocytes, macrophages, NK cells, and dendritic cells, and their functional sub-sets have been documented [13]. T lymphocytes show a pronounced skewing toward a Th2 pattern, and in recent studies have implicated Th17 cells which promotes an inflammatory-fibrosis-prone milieu. An important role for B cells and defined B cell sub-sets in SSc in generating autoantibodies as well as IL-6 and other pathogenic cytokines is emerging and provides the therapeutic rationale for the use of B cell depletion, as well as therapies targeting the IL-6 axis and its downstream cellular signaling pathways. Genome wide analysis of SSc skin and lung tissue-derived transcriptomes and single cell RNA analysis reveals robust and consistent inflammatory signature, indicating the activation of immune/inflammatory cellular signaling within lesional tissues. These observations lead to a plausible scenario for the development of inflammation and autoimmunity in SSc: innate immune responses in dendritic cells, NK cells, and monocytes/macrophages trigger adaptive immunity, including skewing the T cell response toward a Th2 predominant pattern. Since immune cells must exit the circulation in order to accumulate within the lesional tissue, leukocyte interaction with the damaged endothelium mediated via endothelial and leukocyte adhesion molecules plays an important role in SSc, a notion supported by the observation that mice deficient in the leukocyte adhesion receptor PSGL-1 spontaneously develop age-dependent skin fibrosis. The interplay between the microbiome and the immune system is garnering attention, although the exact role of the microbiome and dysbiosis in the pathophenotypes characteristic of SSc remains obscure.

Highlighting the role of immune mechanisms in the pathogenesis of SSc is the profound effect of immune cells and their secreted factors on other structural cells and connective tissues including endothelial cells, epithelial cells, and fibroblasts. Innate immunity is increasingly recognized as having a key role in pathogenesis. Type I interferon, produced in response to activation of toll-like receptors (TLRs) and other pattern recognition receptors, contributes to systemic inflammation and tissue damage. TLRs are expressed on both immune cells, such as dendritic cells and monocytes, as well as non-immune tissue-resident cells including endothelial and epithelial cells and fibroblasts. A key arm of innate immunity is the inflammasome, which by generating active IL-1, contributes to the proinflammatory and profibrotic cellular milieu in SSc. Multiple studies in mice have established an indispensable role for both TLRs and the inflammasome in experimental fibrosis and recent studies in SSc highlight an activated NLRP3 inflammasome in the lesional tissue.

Autoantibodies in SSc: Markers of Autoimmunity—And Drivers of Disease?

An intriguing facet of SSc is the presence of one of the nine SSc-associated autoantibodies that are observed to correlate with internal organ involvement. SSc-associated autoantibodies are typically mutually exclusive and while their direct role (if any) in disease pathogenesis remains to be demonstrated, they can serve as important and informative tools for patient stratification. These antibodies target self-antigens including Scl-70 (topoisomerase I), centromere, RNA polymerase, U1 RNP, U3 RNP, U11/U12 RNP, Th/To, Ku, and PM-Scl. Beyond their clinical utility in diagnosis, prognosis, and patient stratification, SSc-associated autoantibodies may play a direct role in disease pathogenesis. In particular, accumulating evidence suggests that SSc-associated autoantibodies directly activate monocytes and stimulate the generation of monocyte-derived secreted factors, potentiate immune responses, and TLR activation, and thereby amplify pathological immune responses. The mechanisms responsible for generating a highly specific humoral immune response to self-antigens in SSc remain elusive. One intriguing clue has recently emerged from the study of cancer associated with SSc. This study revealed an association between oncogenic mutations in the gene encoding RNA polymerase III, anti-RNA polymerase III antibodies, and the near-contemporaneous onset of cancer and SSc in a sub-group of patients [14]. These observations suggest that the origin of (at least some) SSc-associated autoantibodies might lie in an anti-tumor immune response targeting oncogenic tumor mutations. In addition to these SSc-associated autoantibodies, an increasing number of functional antibodies with agonistic activity for vascular receptors have been described in SSc. Targets include a variety of cellular receptors, including the endothelin-1 receptor and the angiotensin II receptor on endothelial cells. The pathogenic role of functional autoantibodies in SSc is being elucidated, with recent data suggesting that these autoantibodies exert biological effects via the activation of receptor-dependent cell signaling pathways, contributing to disease pathogenesis. They may serve as new biomarkers for assessment of disease risk and progression.

Multisystem Fibrosis: The Distinguishing Hallmark of SSc

Fibrosis as a predominant pathophenotype distinguishes SSc from other autoimmune diseases. A truly remarkable and puzzling feature of SSc is that fibrosis synchronously affects multiple organs; in addition to the skin, the lungs, heart, gastrointestinal tract, and kidneys exhibit connective tissue fibrosis [15]. Within affected organs, fibrosis due to SSc exhibits similarities to organ-specific forms of fibrosis such as idiopathic pulmonary fibrosis (IPF). Notably, however, the genetic loci implicated in SSc-associated lung disease versus idiopathic lung fibrosis show no overlap; as an example, the MUC5B variant strongly linked to lung fibrosis associated with IPF has not been detected in patients with SSc-associated lung fibrosis. It is suggested that diverse etiopathogenic processes may converge on a generic intermediate pathophenotype such as fibrosis [16].

Fibrosis results when extracellular matrix (ECM) homeostasis is disrupted and the dynamic balance between ECM synthesis and turnover is perturbed. Numerous soluble factors, biomechanical forces, and progenitor and resident cell lineages have been implicated in the process. Cytokines, chemokines, growth factors, bioactive lipids, coagulation factors, hypoxia, reactive oxygen species (ROS), and biomechanical forces generated within a stiff matrix provide signals triggering fibroblast activation. Transforming growth factor-β is the master regulator of fibrogenesis, and much evidence implicates TGF-β and associated pathways in the pathogenesis of SSc. The source of excessive TGF-β is not well established, but activated platelets, tissue macrophages, and T lymphocytes are all candidates that contribute to the production and release of TGF-β. In addition, the aberrant activation of tissue-sequestered latent TGF-β by fibroblasts expressing surface integrins such as αvβ3 and αvβ8 has been documented in SSc; moreover, this process is accentuated in a mechanically stressed microenvironment such as in the scar tissue. A variety of developmental morphogen pathways are deregulated in patients with SSc and are increasingly implicated in the pathogenesis of fibrosis. Bone morphogenic proteins, Wnt, Notch, and sonic hedgehog regulate embryonic development, and are tightly regulated in healthy adults, but become aberrantly expressed during sustained inflammation and tissue injury. In the case of Wnt signaling, deregulation of the pathway in SSc reflects epigenetic silencing of Wnt repressors such as DKK1. Mice with overexpression of the Wnt ligand and other developmental pathways spontaneously develop age-dependent organ fibrosis. While targeting morphogen pathways in experimental animal models of fibrosis is associated with the amelioration of the process, translation of these successful strategies into clinical therapies for SSc remains a major challenge.

Increasingly recognized for their role in triggering and maintaining the fibrotic process are endogenous TLR ligands collectively termed DAMPs (damage-associated molecular patterns). DAMPs include proteins, peptides, glycoproteins and lipids, as well as nucleic acids and cellular components such as HMGB1 and S100A4 that are generated or released at sites of tissue injury and cell death. Many DAMPs, particularly when secreted in alternately spiced variants or having undergone post-translational modifications, accumulate in affected tissues where they contribute to the "matrisome." Fibronectin-EDA, tenascin C, proteoglycans, and SLRPs are ECM-related endogenous TLR ligands that act as "danger signals" alerting the host to tissue damage. In response, TLRs on resident stromal cells initiate a self-limited tissue repair process. While regulated TLR activation is beneficial under normal conditions, deregulated TLR activation by uncontrolled accumulation of DAMPs, as can be seen in the skin and lungs in patients with SSc, is deleterious, and is a major factor responsible for maintaining sustained fibroblast activation [17].

Cellular Mediators of Fibrosis

The key effector cell in fibrosis, in both SSc and other fibrotic diseases is the fibroblast and its activated progeny the myofibroblast. Myofibroblasts are transitional cells that display features of both fibroblasts and smooth muscle cells, contributing to both the biochemical and biomechanical attributes of tissue fibrosis by copious collagen and other ECM protein production as well as connective tissue contraction. Myofibroblasts within the lesional tissue are a key hallmark of SSc and distinguish affected versus unaffected skin. A number of cell types exhibit considerable functional and morphological plasticity that allows them to undergo "phenotypic transitions" such as "epithelial mesenchymal transition" and "endothelial mesenchymal transition". These processes may contribute to the expansion of the myofibroblast pool in SSc. Additional sources for activated myofibroblasts in the lesional dermis include Sox2-expressing skin progenitor cells and intradermal preadipocytes, which undergo transdifferentiation under the influence of TGF-β, PDGF, Wnts, and other profibrotic ligands. There is also evidence that bone marrow-derived monocytes and fibrocytes differentiate into myofibroblasts in SSc. Targeting myofibroblasts has proven to be an effective strategy for ameliorating fibrosis in murine models of the disease [18]. However, despite experimental support for the role of such processes in fibrosis, primarily from studies in mice, the occurrence, extent, and pathogenic significance of such cell fate changes in patients with SSc remain to be validated.

Fibroblasts established from SSc patient biopsies exhibit cell-autonomous alterations that persist in serial ex vivo culture. "Scleroderma fibroblasts" show constitutive ECM production, spontaneous generation of both mitochondrial and cytosolic ROS, focal prominent alpha smooth muscle actin-positive intracellular stress fiber networks, adhesion assembly, and FAK activation. Moreover, these cells show diminished autophagic flux and additional metabolic alterations with reduced fatty acid oxidation and increased glycolysis that are reminiscent of cancer-associated and aged fibroblasts [19]. The evasion of apoptosis, inherent adhesive and contractile properties, impaired cytoprotective mechanisms, altered miR29 expression, and other epigenomic changes, along with a variety of other abnormalities, persist even when SSc fibroblasts are removed from their in vivo milieu. This suggests that fibroblast activators in SSc induce sustained and heritable cellular changes driving fibrosis. Such changes are likely to involve epigenetic mechanisms that modulate the transcription of genes encoding key transcription factors and signaling molecules, including DNA methylation, histone modifications, microRNAs, and long noncoding RNAs involved in myofibroblast differentiation. This area also represents a fertile landscape for drug development focused at modulating the epigenetic alterations (20). Recent studies deploying transcriptome analysis at the single-cell scale in skin and lung tissues indicate that fibroblasts and myofibroblasts comprise multiple distinct subsets of cell populations identified by distinct gene expression signatures and cell surface markers. These studies suggest that certain fibroblast subpopulations in the skin are more likely to contribute to fibrosis than other fibroblast subpopulations, and the presence of different subtypes of cells such as pericytes opens the door toward the development of highly targeted approaches to selectively eliminate the pathogenic fibroblast populations.

The Interplay of the Triad of Intermediate Pathophenotypes in the Pathogenesis of SSc

The dynamic interplay between the vascular, immune, and fibrosis-promoting processes illustrated in Fig. 12.2 underlies the protean and fluctuating manifestations of SSc, and their evolution during the course of the disease. It is difficult to ascertain which of these processes is primal; however, the observation that the Raynaud phenomenon is very commonly the initial disease manifestation of SSc suggests that vascular changes are early and likely to precede, and may be and important initiating event for other disease manifestations. Furthermore, based on current data, vascular changes are likely to be responsible for triggering inflammation and innate immune and ischemic responses that might be linked to the initiation and maintenance of the deregulated wound repair process underlying fibrosis. Nevertheless, in a given individual with SSc, the vascular, immune, and fibrotic processes generally exist contemporaneously, while their activity and impact fluctuate during the course of the disease, and even across affected organs. The coexistence of inflammatory and fibrotic processes within the same tissue is underscored by transcriptome analyses of skin biopsies in longitudinally followed patient cohorts [20]. Accordingly, effective therapies will need to address the predominant pathomechanism driving the disease at a given point in time, which will vary form one patient to another, and within the same patient with temporal evolution of the disease. Emerging tools of precision medicine hold the promise of therapeutic interventions that selectively target the process or processes most prominent in a given patient at a specific point along their disease trajectory, thereby maximizing efficacy while minimizing unwanted side effects. Biomarkers, and in particular tissue-based genomic and epigenomic analyses and peripheral blood proteomics and cell type profiling, are likely to emerge as powerful weapons in the fight against SSc [21].

References

1. Korman BD, Criswell LA. Recent advances in the genetics of systemic sclerosis: toward biological and clinical significance. Curr Rheumatol Rep. 2015;17:21.
2. Feghali-Bostwick C, Medsger TA Jr, Wright TM. Analysis of systemic sclerosis in twins reveals low concordance for disease and high concordance for the presence of antinuclear antibodies. Arthritis Rheum. 2003;48:1956–63.
3. Tsou PS, Wren JD, Amin MA, Schiopu E, Fox DA, Khanna D, Sawalha AH. Histone deacetylase 5 is overexpressed in scleroderma endothelial cells and impairs angiogenesis via repression of proangiogenic factors. Arthritis Rheumatol. 2016;68:2975–85.
4. Tsou PS, Campbell P, Amin MA, Coit P, Miller S, Fox DA, Khanna D, Sawalha AH. Inhibition of EZH2 prevents fibrosis and restores normal angiogenesis in scleroderma. Proc Natl Acad Sci U S A. 2019;116:3695–702.
5. Tsou PS, Coit P, Kilian NC, Sawalha AH. EZH2 modulates the DNA methylome and controls T cell adhesion through junctional adhesion molecule a in lupus patients. Arthritis Rheumatol. 2018;70:98–108.
6. He Y, Tsou PS, Khanna D, Sawalha AH. Methyl-CpG-binding protein 2 mediates antifibrotic effects in scleroderma fibroblasts. Ann Rheum Dis. 2018;77:1208–18.
7. Ramos PS, Zimmerman KD, Haddad S, Langefeld CD, Medsger TA Jr, Feghali-Bostwick CA. Integrative analysis of DNA methylation in discordant twins unveils distinct architectures of systemic sclerosis subsets. Clin Epigenetics. 2019;11:58.
8. Liu Q, Zaba LC, Satpathy AT, Longmire M, Zhang W, Li K, Granja J, Guo C, Lin J, Li R, Tolentino K, Kania G, Distler O, Fiorentino D, Chung L, Qu K, Chang HY. Chromatin accessibility landscapes of skin cells in systemic sclerosis nominate dendritic cells in disease pathogenesis. Nat Commun. 2020;11:5843.
9. Roberts-Thomson PJ, Walker JG. Stochastic processes in the aetiopathogenesis of scleroderma. Intern Med J. 2012;42:235–42.
10. Varga J, Hinchcliff M. Connective tissue diseases: systemic sclerosis: beyond limited and diffuse subsets? Nat Rev Rheumatol. 2014;10:200–2.
11. Matucci-Cerinic M, Kahaleh B, Wigley FM. Review: evidence that systemic sclerosis is a vascular disease. Arthritis Rheum. 2013;65:1953–62.

12. Trojanowska M. Cellular and molecular aspects of vascular dysfunction in systemic sclerosis. Nat Rev Rheumatol. 2010;6:453–60.
13. Greenblatt MB, Aliprantis AO. The immune pathogenesis of scleroderma: context is everything. Curr Rheumatol Rep. 2013;15:297.
14. Joseph CG, Darrah E, Shah AA, Skora AD, Casciola-Rosen LA, Wigley FM, Boin F, Fava A, Thoburn C, Kinde I, Jiao Y, Papadopoulos N, Kinzler KW, Vogelstein B, Rosen A. Association of the autoimmune disease scleroderma with an immunologic response to cancer. Science. 2014;343:152–7.
15. Varga J, Abraham D. Systemic sclerosis: a prototypic multisystem fibrotic disorder. J Clin Invest. 2007;117:557–67.
16. Herzog EL, Mathur A, Tager AM, Feghali-Bostwick C, Schneider F, Varga J. Review: interstitial lung disease associated with systemic sclerosis and idiopathic pulmonary fibrosis: how similar and distinct? Arthritis Rheumatol. 2014;66:1967–78.
17. Bhattacharyya S, Tamaki Z, Wang W, Hinchcliff M, Hoover P, Getsios S, White ES, Varga J. Fibronectin EDA promotes chronic cutaneous fibrosis through toll-like receptor signaling. Sci Transl Med. 2014;6:232ra250.
18. Yazdani A, Bansal R, Prakash J. Drug targeting to myofibroblasts: implications for fibrosis and cancer. Adv Drug Deliv. 2017;121:101–16.
19. Zhao X, Psarianos P, Ghoraie LS, Yip K, Goldstein D, Gilbert R, Witterick I, Pang H, Hussain A, Lee JH, Williams J, Bratman SV, Ailles L, Haibe-Kains B, Liu FF. Metabolic regulation of dermal fibroblasts contributes to skin extracellular matrix homeostasis and fibrosis. Nat Metab. 2019;1(1):147–57.
20. Mahoney JM, Taroni J, Martyanov V, Wood TA, Greene CS, Pioli PA, Hinchcliff ME, Whitfield ML. Systems level analysis of systemic sclerosis shows a network of immune and profibrotic pathways connected with genetic polymorphisms. PLoS Comput Biol. 2015;11:e1004005.
21. Castelino FV, Varga J. Current status of systemic sclerosis biomarkers: applications for diagnosis, management and drug development. Expert Rev Clin Immunol. 2013;9:1077–90.
22. Loscalzo J, Kohane I, Barabasi AL. Human disease classification in the postgenomic era: a complex systems approach to human pathobiology. Mol Syst Biol. 2007;3:124.

13 Pathology of Systemic Sclerosis

Lisa M. Rooper and Frederic B. Askin

Introduction

Although the clinical syndrome of systemic sclerosis (SSc) was described as early as the seventeenth century, a detailed characterization of its associated pathologic findings was not published until the middle of the twentieth century [1]. Autopsy studies played a vital role in initially characterizing the many visceral manifestations of this disease [2–5]. Despite recent advances in imaging and laboratory diagnosis of SSc, pathologic examination remains essential to the diagnosis and management of affected patients today. Skin biopsy is frequently employed in the initial evaluation of SSc patients, lung and kidney biopsies are utilized to diagnose its most deadly visceral manifestations, and GI biopsy aids in the investigation of many disabling complications. Moreover, the autopsy of SSc patients still may be the most comprehensive way to directly visualize the protean manifestations of this devastating disease.

While the specific pathologic manifestations of SSc vary widely across anatomic sites, several common features can be identified irrespective of the organ system. Indeed, the hallmark pathophysiologic triad of vascular damage, immune dysfunction, and tissue remodeling with fibrosis discussed elsewhere in this book is reflected in the pathologic findings in SSc [6]. Most obviously, vascular pathology, including thrombotic microangiopathy and luminal obliteration, can be recognized in virtually every organ affected by SSc, especially the skin, lungs, kidneys, gastrointestinal tract, and placenta. Tissue remodeling, represented histologically as fibrosis, also is a key finding, particularly in the skin, cardiovascular, gastrointestinal, and musculoskeletal systems. Lastly, inflammation serves as a direct microscopic correlate for immune dysregulation, being most consistently seen in the lungs and cardiovascular system. This chapter will describe the most common and distinctive pathologic findings in SSc across these organ systems.

L. M. Rooper
Department of Pathology, Johns Hopkins Hospital, Baltimore, MD, USA
e-mail: rooper@jhmi.edu

F. B. Askin (✉)
Department of Pathology, Johns Hopkins University School of Medicine, Baltimore, MD, USA
e-mail: faskin@jhmi.edu

Skin

The namesake skin thickening was the first reported clinical manifestation of SSc, and the pathological findings in the skin remain one of this disease's most characteristic histologic features. Although the 2013 American College of Rheumatology/European League Against Rheumatism (ACR/EULAR) criteria do not require skin biopsy for diagnosis of SSc [7], it is often performed to support the diagnosis in seronegative patients or to differentiate SSc from other skin thickening disorders, including stiff skin syndrome, eosinophilic fasciitis, graft versus host disease, scleromyxedema, amyloidosis, nephrogenic systemic fibrosis, and overlap syndromes with other collagen vascular diseases [8]. Moreover, a histologic examination of skin specimens also helps characterize the many other skin lesions associated with SSc. Skin in SSc commonly demonstrates morpheaform thickening, telangiectasias, ulceration, and calcinosis cutis. Less commonly, livedoid vasculopathy and lipodystrophy can also be seen.

Even though the clinical appearance of skin thickening in SSc is so classic that biopsy is rarely performed, the equally distinctive histologic appearance can go far to resolve any diagnostic uncertainty [9]. At low power, skin biopsies demonstrate characteristic squared-off edges, in contrast to the irregular borders seen in most conditions. The dermis is thickened by broad, elongated bundles of homogenized collagen that are oriented parallel to the surface epithelium (Fig. 13.1a). Adnexal glands appear atrophic with loss of the periadnexal adipose tissue (Fig. 13.1b). This appearance contrasts sharply with the irregular collagen bundles and the abundant periadnexal adipose tissue in normal skin (Fig. 13.1c, d). In rare cases of nodular SSc, abnormal collagen can also appear as keloidal nodules [10] (Fig. 13.2).

Y. Allanore et al. (eds.), *Scleroderma*, https://doi.org/10.1007/978-3-031-40658-4_13

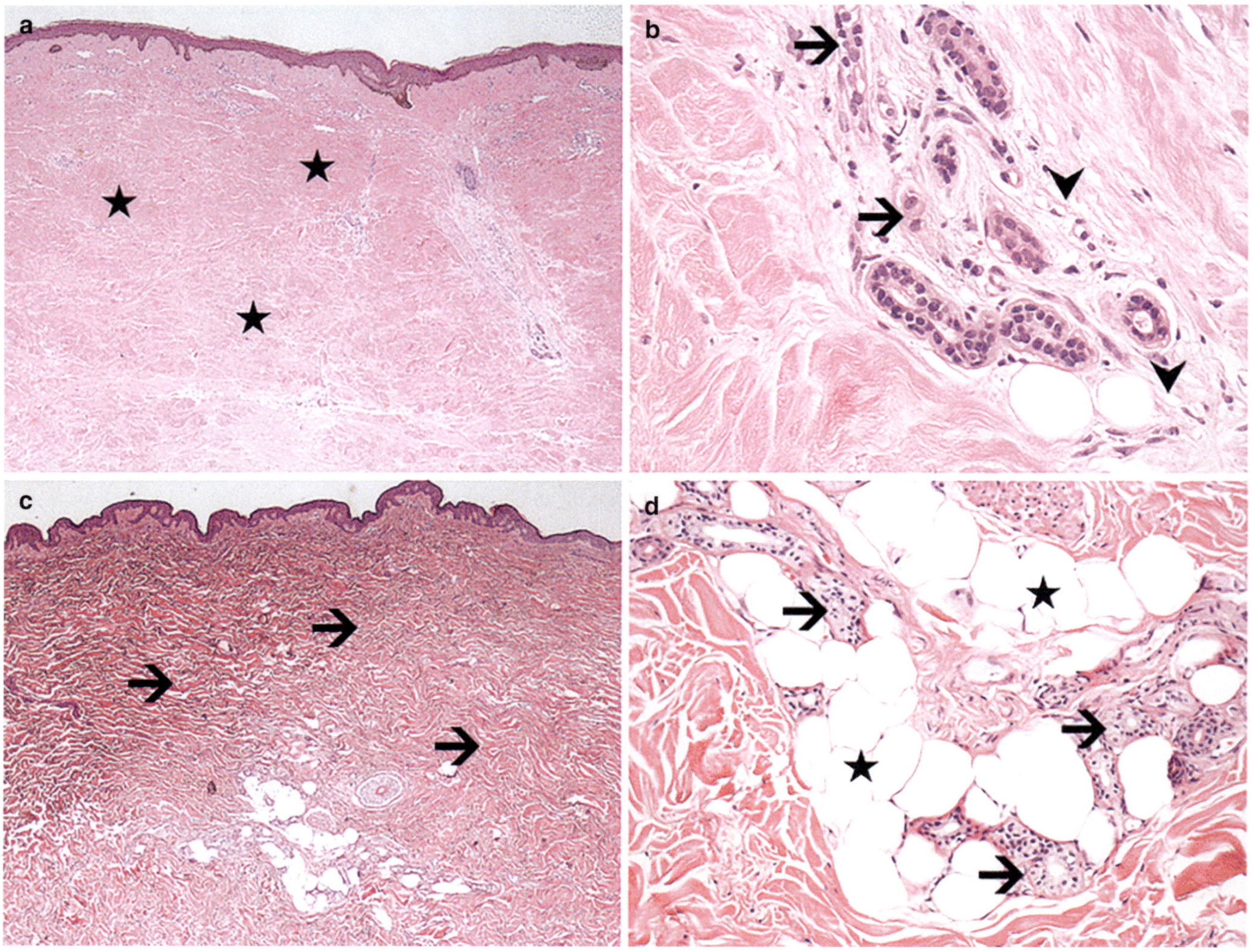

Fig. 13.1 Comparison of skin in SSc to normal. Skin in SSc has broad bundles of homogenized collagen (⋆) running parallel to the epidermis (**a**). Adnexal glands are atrophic (→) and show loss of periadnexal adipose tissue (▼) (**b**). In contrast, normal skin demonstrates irregular collagen bundles (→) (**c**) and abundant adipose tissue (⋆) surrounding plump apocrine glands (→) (**d**)

Arteries in the dermis and subcutis demonstrate intimal thickening and medial hypertrophy with occasional complete occlusion (Fig. 13.3a, b). A mononuclear cell infiltrate can be seen around blood vessels in early disease, but established lesions tend to lack chronic inflammation. While histologic skin thickening correlates closely with the clinically modified Rodnan skin score [11], it is rarely quantitated in clinical practice. The findings in SSc are histologically indistinguishable from those of localized SSc, or morphea, and are thus frequently described as morpheaform [12].

Beyond the diagnostic skin thickening, several other characteristic skin lesions are frequently seen in SSc. Telangiectasias are one common finding that are present in almost all SSc patients and are included in the ACR/EULAR 2013 criteria for the diagnosis of SSc [7]. While they are also rarely biopsied, telangiectasias can easily be identified histologically as dilated blood vessels in the superficial dermis (Fig. 13.4a). In contrast to vascular abnormalities seen in

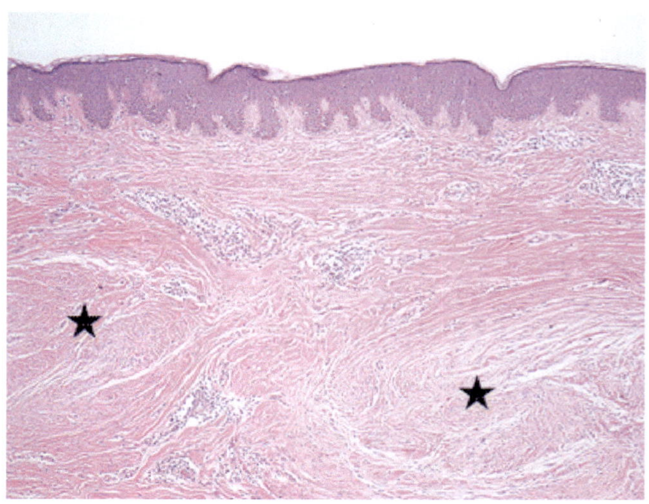

Fig. 13.2 Nodular scleroderma. In this rare variant of SSc, the collagen maintains a morpheaform homogenized appearance but is organized in keloidal nodules (⋆)

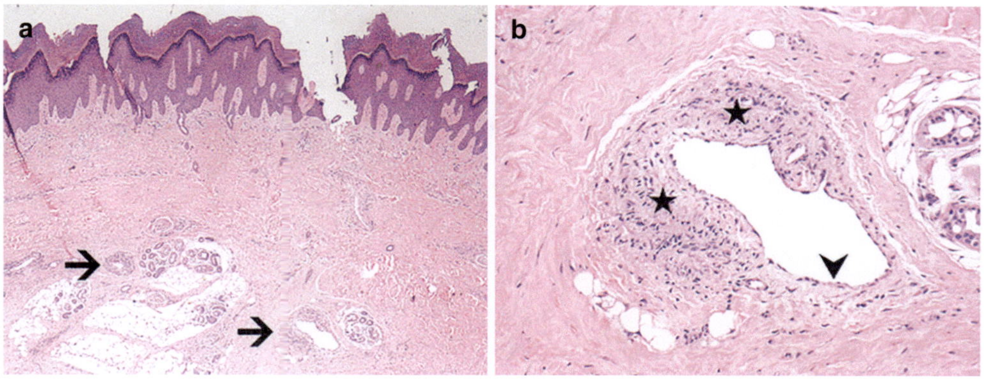

Fig. 13.3 Cutaneous blood vessel remodeling. Blood vessels in the dermis and subcutis of SSc patients show marked intimal and medial hypertrophies (→) with resultant luminal narrowing (**a**). A partially affected vessel allows a direct comparison of normal wall thickness (▼) to that seen after remodeling (⋆) (**b**)

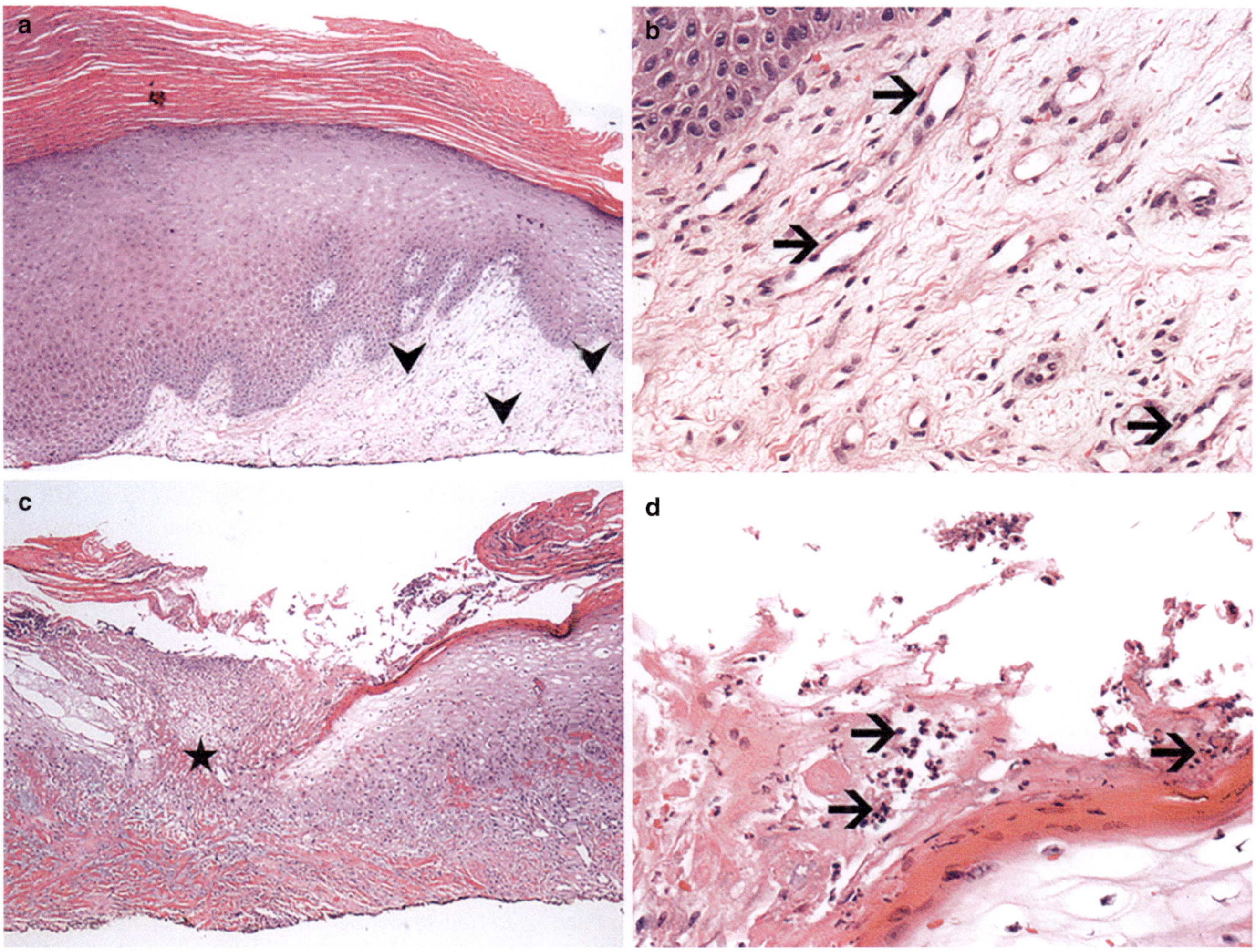

Fig. 13.4 Common dermatologic findings. SSc patients almost universally have telangiectasias with diffusely dilated dermal blood vessels (▼) (**a**). These blood vessels are thin-walled (→), without endothelial proliferation (**b**). In digital ulceration, the skin shows erosion of the epidermis (⋆) and underlying dermal tissue (**c**). Many neutrophils (→) can be seen in the associated fibrinopurulent inflammatory infiltrate (**d**). Deep subcutaneous arterioles in an amputation specimen demonstrate intimal and medial proliferation and fibrosis (▼) (**e**). The blood vessel shows complete luminal occlusion with associated hemosiderin deposition (→) (**f**). Calcinosis cutis demonstrates acellular deposition of purple calcified material (⋆) in the dermis and subcutis (**g**). Calcinosis cutis can have associated fibrosis and foreign body giant cell reaction (▼) (**h**)

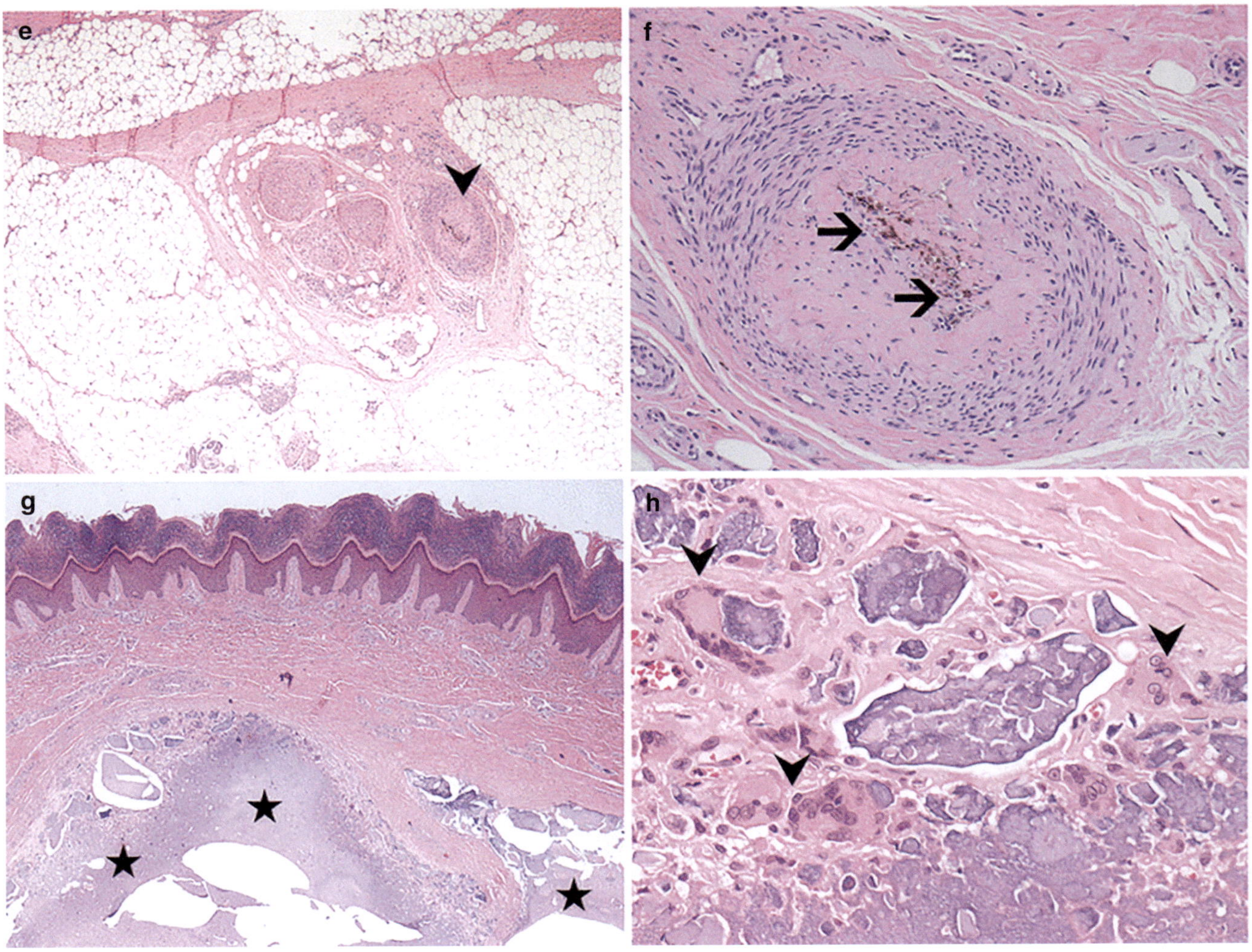

Fig. 13.4 (continued)

other diseases, telangiectasias in SSc do not represent vascular malformation or neovascularization but instead are simple dilations of the postcapillary venules of the upper dermal plexus [13]. As such, they lack endothelial proliferation or an organized growth pattern (Fig. 13.4b). They likely occur secondary to abnormalities in downstream blood flow [14].

Fingertip ulceration is another skin lesion that occurs frequently in SSc; it also counts toward the ACR/EULAR 2013 criteria for diagnosis [7]. Digital ulcers are more likely to occur in patients who present at a younger age and have more extensive skin involvement, and they are linked to an earlier development of visceral organ involvement [14, 15]. Histologic sections show erosion of the epidermis and superficial dermis (Fig. 13.4c) with an overlying fibrinopurulent exudate (Fig. 13.4d). Ultimately, ulceration reflects tissue ischemia due to underlying vasculopathy. Affected vessels demonstrate intimal thickening, medial hypertrophy, and luminal occlusion (Fig. 13.4e, f). In 5.9% of cases, resultant ischemia progresses beyond ulceration and culminates in digital amputation [16]. Gross examination of such fingers show black discoloration; gangrenous necrosis can be confirmed microscopically.

Approximately 25% of limited cutaneous SSc patients develop calcinosis cutis, which frequently occurs ten years or more after their diagnosis [17]. Although the exact mechanism is still unknown, calcinosis cutis is thought to arise when cellular injury provides a nidus for ectopic calcification in a setting of altered extracellular proteins [18]. Histologic sections show large mass-like deposits as well as smaller irregular accumulations of extracellular calcium in the dermis and subcutaneous tissue (Fig. 13.4g). Ulceration of the overlying epidermis and surrounding foreign body giant cell reaction, inflammation, or fibrosis may be seen in association with these lesions (Fig. 13.4h). Calcinosis cutis must be differentiated from other syndromes of aberrant calcification, including tumoral calcinosis, metastatic calcification, and calciphylaxis. While calcinosis cutis is classically associated with limited cutaneous SSc, it also occurs in the setting of diffuse cutaneous disease as well as several other autoimmune diseases [19].

In addition to the common skin findings described above, several rarer skin lesions have been associated with SSc. Livedoid vasculopathy, with a resultant development of atro-

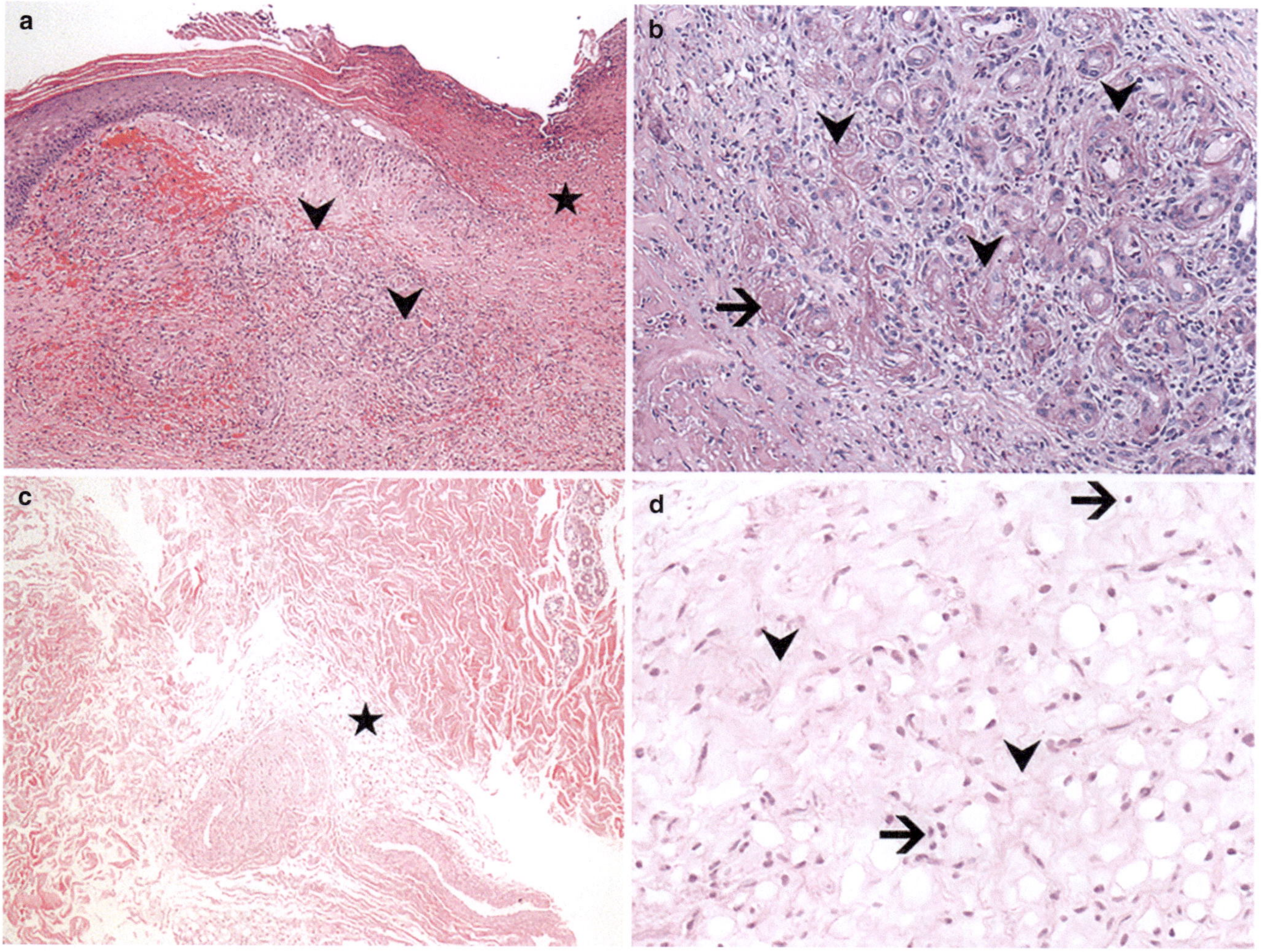

Fig. 13.5 Uncommon dermatologic complications. Livedoid vasculopathy is characterized by thickened and damaged dermal blood vessels (▼); it frequently leads to ulceration (★) of the overlying epithelium (**a**). A Periodic-Acid Schiff (PAS) stain highlights the fibrin deposition in the blood vessel walls (▼) and focal fibrin thrombi (→) (**b**). In lipodystrophy, the lipid mass (★) is decreased in the subcutaneous adipose tissue (**c**). There is hyalinization of the adipose cells (▼) with rare interspersed lymphocytes (→) (**d**)

phie blanche, is one such uncommon complication [20]. Although early livedoid vasculopathy can have various clinical appearances, the histologic appearance is distinct with fibrin deposition within the lumens and walls of dermal blood vessels in the absence of inflammatory cells (Fig. 13.5a, b). As lesions progress, segmental infarction and hyalinization of the vessel walls develop. Older lesions are labeled atrophie blanche because of the distinctive ivory-white plaques seen on physical examination and microscopically show dermal sclerosis, scarring, epidermal atrophy, and dilated lymphatics. Livedoid vasculopathy is not unique to SSc and has been linked with a wide range of diseases that cause endothelial injury, including other autoimmune diseases and coagulopathies [21].

A final uncommon and nonspecific skin finding associated with SSc is lipodystrophy, which is thought to arise because of the local mechanical effects of fibrosis [22]. In a small series of SSc patients with limb ischemia, the prevalence of lipodystrophy was 50% [23]. In this condition, the subcutaneous adipose tissue becomes atrophic (Fig. 13.5c), with loss of lipid volume, hyalinization of fibrous septae, and occasional mononuclear cell infiltrates (Fig. 13.5d). Other cases can demonstrate cystic structures lined by amorphous PAS-positive, diastase-resistant eosinophilic membranes [24]. Lipodystrophy can also be seen in isolation as a rare genetic disease, in various collagen vascular diseases, and as a consequence of chronic circulatory disturbance.

Pulmonary

Pulmonary complications currently represent the predominant cause of death among SSc patients, accounting for 33–60% of disease-specific mortality [25–28]. Clinically, pulmonary disease in SSc tends to be classified as either interstitial fibrosis or pulmonary arterial hypertension (PAH), both of which are included in the ACR/EULAR 2013 criteria for diagnosis of SSc [7]. However, three distinct patterns of lung damage can be identified histologically: interstitial pneumonitis, pulmonary vascular damage, and bronchiolitis. All of these patterns of damage are thought to have their origins in similar pathways of inflammatory injury and microvascular remodeling [29, 30]. Although open lung biopsy is not always carried out in SSc patients because of high surgical risk and acceptable surrogate clinical studies, pathological evaluation can be useful to help evaluate the extent of disease and the presence of overlapping histologic patterns [31].

Early autopsy studies found evidence of pulmonary fibrosis in 100% of SSc patients [5, 32], while more recent series using high-resolution CT scans demonstrate some changes in 90% (Solomon 2013). Overall, interstitial lung disease appears to be responsible for 19% of SSc deaths [28]. Many of these end-stage lesions are best diagnosed as honeycomb change, which is characterized grossly and microscopically by extensive interstitial fibrosis with peripheral cyst formation. However, more distinctive pathologic findings can be seen in early lesions. On pathologic evaluation, between 50 and 77% of interstitial pneumonitis cases in SSc demonstrate a nonspecific interstitial pneumonia (NSIP) pattern [33–35]. Histologically, NSIP is characterized by temporally uniform lung damage with minimal to moderate interstitial fibrosis and interspersed chronic inflammation (Fig. 13.6a, c, e). It lacks the heterogeneity of the usual interstitial pneumonia (UIP) pattern described below. A minority of cases can be classified within the fibrotic subtype of NSIP, which demonstrates fibrosis with only minimal inflammation.

SSc-associated interstitial lung disease can also manifest in a UIP pattern, although these findings are seen in less than 10% of cases [35]. UIP is a nonspecific but distinctive pattern of lung damage characterized by spatial and temporal heterogeneity (Fig. 13.6b). Histologic sections demonstrate simultaneous areas of acute lung injury with inflammation or diffuse alveolar damage, fibroblast foci reflecting ongoing subacute organizing injury, and old fibrosis (Fig. 13.6d, f). In contrast to patients with a clinical diagnosis of idiopathic pulmonary fibrosis, UIP that occurs in the setting of SSc tends to have more germinal centers and inflammation and fewer fibroblast foci [36, 37]. While patients with UIP have worse outcomes than NSIP in the general population and in some series of SSc patients [38], other investigators have observed that the outcome in SSc interstitial lung disease is more closely linked to disease severity at presentation than histologic pattern [35].

The estimated prevalence of PAH in SSc ranges from 8% at cardiac catheterization to 49% using echocardiography [39]. PAH is responsible for approximately 14% of deaths in SSc [28]. In pathologic materials, lesions of pulmonary hypertension can show a spectrum of histologic changes that are graded from least (grade I) to most severe (grade VI) using the modified Heath and Edwards classification [40]. Early lesions show medial then intimal hypertrophy, subsequent subintimal fibrosis in an onion-skin pattern, and eventual reduplication of the internal elastic lamina (Fig. 13.7a). Later disease demonstrates plexiform and glomeruloid nodules in small arteries with fibrin thrombi formation (Fig. 13.7b). Rarely, acute necrotizing arteritis with fibrinoid necrosis can be seen. It may be difficult to separate PAH in SSc from pulmonary hypertension associated with vascular and alveolar remodeling (honeycomb change) in patients with advanced interstitial lung disease; the latter patients have a markedly worse prognosis [41]. Nevertheless, there is clearly a subset of patients, mostly with limited SSc, who have pulmonary artery disease without interstitial lung disease [42].

Interestingly, patients with systemic sclerosis-associated PAH have also been shown to have a worse prognosis than idiopathic PAH [39]. Recent pathological studies have linked such outcomes to the almost uniform additional presence of veno-occlusive disease in SSc patients [43, 44]. Histologically, such venous pathology can be identified as fibrosis and intimal proliferation of preseptal venules and veins (Fig. 13.7c). Systemic sclerosis patients also can have coexisting interstitial pneumonitis and PAH, which not only complicates the diagnosis as described above, but also contributes to worse outcomes by decreasing pulmonary reserve [44]. Moreover, SSc patients also have a high risk of pulmonary thromboembolism, which can still further compound vascular disease (Fig. 13.8).

Finally, perhaps the least well-recognized pulmonary manifestation of SSc is constrictive and/or lymphocytic bronchiolitis. Between 13% and 25% of SSc patients are estimated to demonstrate small airway disease [45]. Although most patients are asymptomatic, the resultant decrease in the maximal mid-expiratory flow rate can come to clinical attention in patients with other pulmonary pathologies [45]. Histologic sections of SSc-associated bronchiolitis show a chronic inflammatory infiltrate involving the submucosa of terminal and respiratory bronchioles. Affected airways may demonstrate luminal constriction, fibrosis, and smooth muscle proliferation (Fig. 13.9a, b). Similar microscopic findings can be seen in other autoimmune diseases, particularly the Sjogren syndrome, as well as in drug reactions [45]. Such constrictive or obliterative bronchiolitis must be separated both morphologically and semantically from the intraluminal fibrosis seen in bronchiolitis obliterans organizing pneumonia (BOOP) [46].

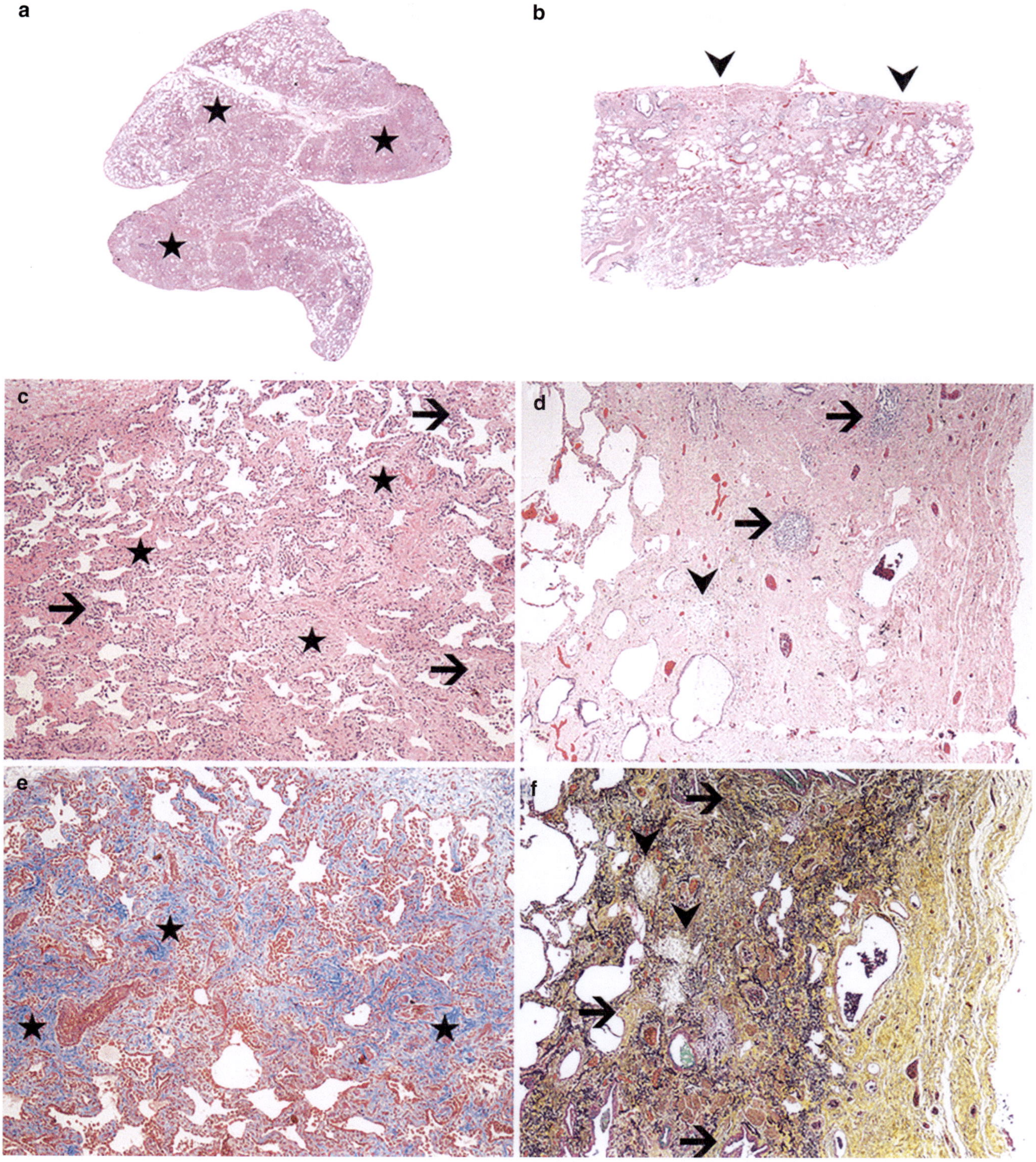

Fig. 13.6 Interstitial lung disease. At low power, non-specific interstitial fibrosis (NSIP) shows homogenous involvement with similar degrees of fibrosis in most areas (⋆) of the lung (**a**) while usual interstitial pneumonitis (UIP) has subpleural (▾) accentuation (**b**). At higher power, NSIP demonstrates moderate interstitial fibrosis (⋆) with interspersed chronic inflammatory cells (→) (**c**). A Masson trichrome (Masson) stain highlights the fibrosis in blue (⋆) (**e**). UIP demonstrates more lymphoid aggregates (→) and fewer fibroblast foci (▾) in SSc than would be expected in idiopathic pulmonary fibrosis (**d**). A Movat pentachrome stain emphasizes the temporal and spatial heterogeneity, with fibroblast foci staining light blue (▾) and old fibrosis staining yellow (→) (**f**)

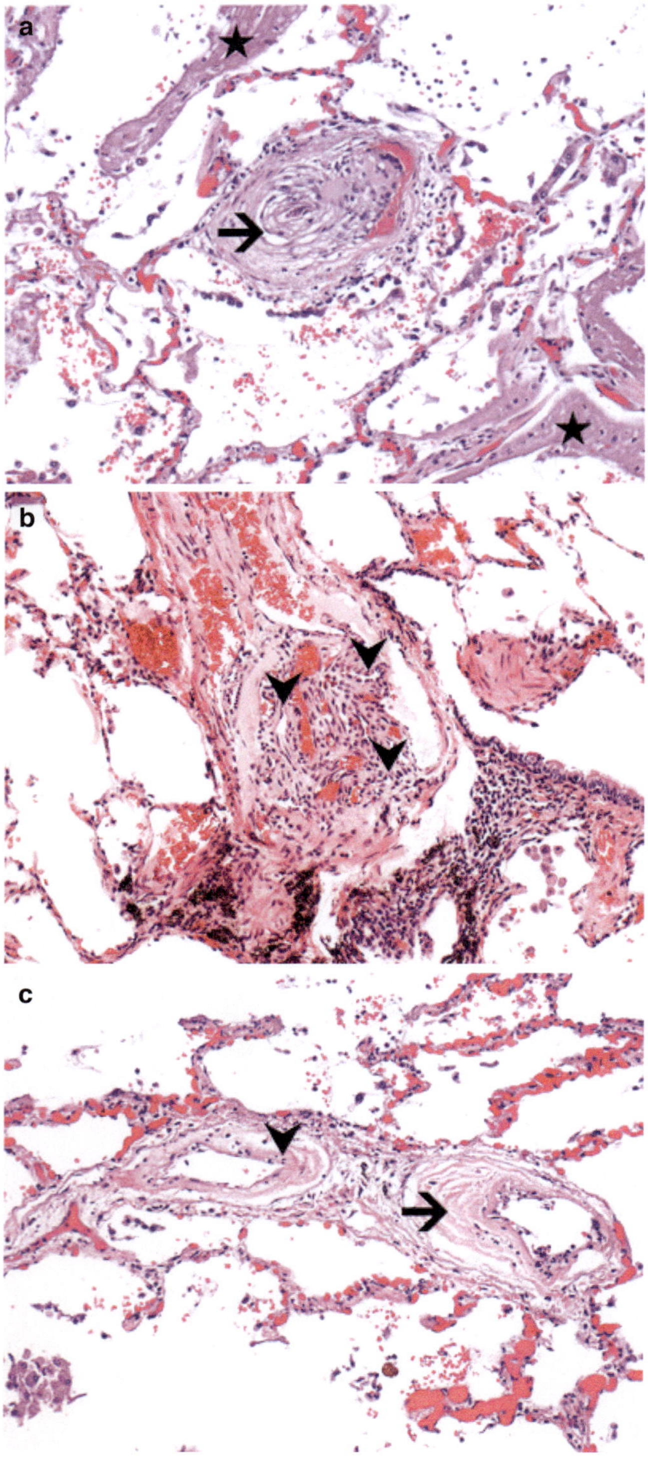

Fig. 13.7 Pulmonary vascular disease. Early lesions of pulmonary artery hypertension (PAH) in SSc demonstrate intimal hypertrophy with onion-skin fibrosis (→) of the vessel wall. In this case, the surrounding lung also demonstrates diffuse alveolar damage with hyaline membranes (⋆) (**a**). Later lesions of PAH have plexiform vascular proliferation with many small vascular channels (▾) in a previously obstructed vessel (**b**). PAH in SSc also shows veno-occlusive disease with intimal proliferation (→) and fibrosis (▾) of preseptal venules (**c**)

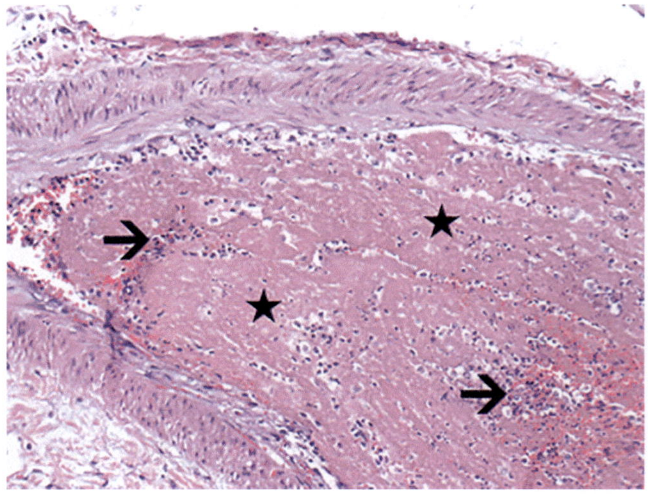

Fig. 13.8 Organizing thromboembolus with intermixed fibrin (⋆) and inflammatory cells (→). Pulmonary thromboembolism can complicate PAH in SSc patients

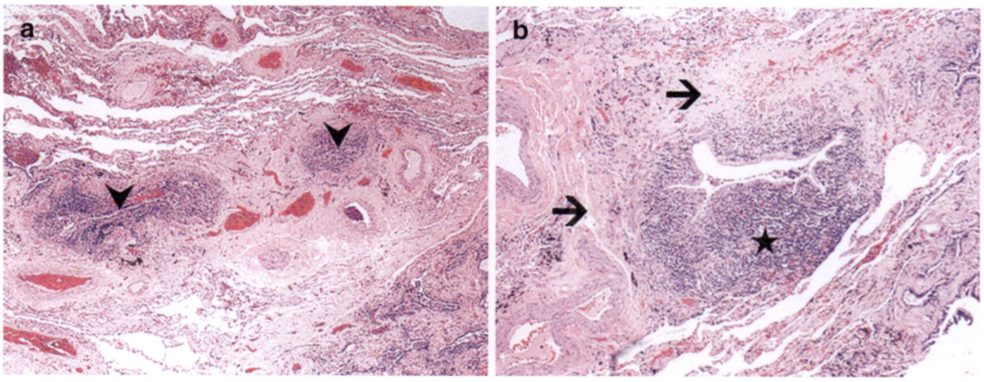

Fig. 13.9 Follicular and constrictive bronchiolitis. At low power, the bronchial lumen (▼) is largely obliterated (**a**). Peribronchial fibrosis (→) and a prominent lymphoid aggregate (★) are highlighted at higher power (**b**)

Renal

While the historically high mortality rate of scleroderma renal crisis meant that renal disease was once responsible for 42% of deaths in SSc patients, the use of angiotensin converting enzyme inhibitors has decreased the death rate from renal complications to less than 6% in recent years [25, 47, 48]. However, the existence of highly effective treatments makes it all the more essential to diagnose this condition in an accurate and timely manner. Although appropriate clinical findings can strongly favor scleroderma renal crisis, kidney biopsy is required to definitively differentiate it from overlap syndromes or other unrelated conditions; it also can provide important prognostic information. Moreover, histological examination is essential in the 10% of renal crisis patients who are normotensive at presentation [49]. It is also important to note that scleroderma renal crisis is not the only manifestation of SSc in the kidneys; chronic kidney disease and inflammatory conditions are also seen histologically.

Scleroderma renal crisis occurs in up to 15% of SSc patients [49]. If examined grossly, affected kidneys demonstrate multiple surface petechial hemorrhages and wedge-shaped cortical infarcts. In early disease, histologic sections show the accumulation of myxoid material in the intima of interlobular arteries (Fig. 13.10a, b), while afferent arterioles demonstrate fibrinoid necrosis (Fig. 13.10c, d). Later on, vessels undergo intimal proliferation in an onion-skin pattern (Fig. 13.10e, f), while glomeruli develop ischemic changes with collapse and wall thickening (Fig. 13.10g, h). These findings are identical to those seen in malignant hypertension but are distinguishable from other thrombotic microangiopathies because of the predominance of small vessel involvement over glomerular changes [50]. Patients with extensive vascular thrombosis, severe glomerular ischemic collapse, and peritubular capillary C4d deposits at biopsy have been shown to have an increased risk of irreversible renal failure and death [51].

Other evidence of chronic kidney disease can also be identified histologically in SSc patients. Even patients who never demonstrated symptoms of scleroderma renal crisis can show some of the characteristic vascular changes, particularly vascular fibrosis and the accumulation of extracellular matrix material [5, 50] (Fig. 13.11a, b). Less specific evidence of chronic vasculopathy and surrounding renal parenchymal damage is frequently seen as well, including intimal fibrosis, tubulointerstitial fibrosis, tubular atrophy, and interstitial chronic inflammation [52] (Fig. 13.11c, d). In contrast to most other autoimmune diseases, underlying chronic renal disease does not correlate with prognosis in scleroderma renal crisis, and some investigators postulate that it is somehow protective against the more damaging acute injury [53].

Finally, inflammatory renal disease is another rare complication of SSc. Parenchymal inflammation is not classically associated with scleroderma renal crisis but is not uncommon in acute episodes. A wide range of different inflammatory findings have also been reported in SSc outside of renal crisis, including focal segmental glomerulonephritis, mesangioproliferative glomerulonephritis, and diffuse membranous glomerulonephritis [54]. Several cases of ANCA-associated vasculitis, including granulomatosis with polyangiitis, microscopic polyangiitis, and Churg-Strauss syndrome, have been reported in association with SSc and may represent an uncommon overlap syndrome [55, 56]. Histologic findings in these cases include crescentic glomerulonephritis.

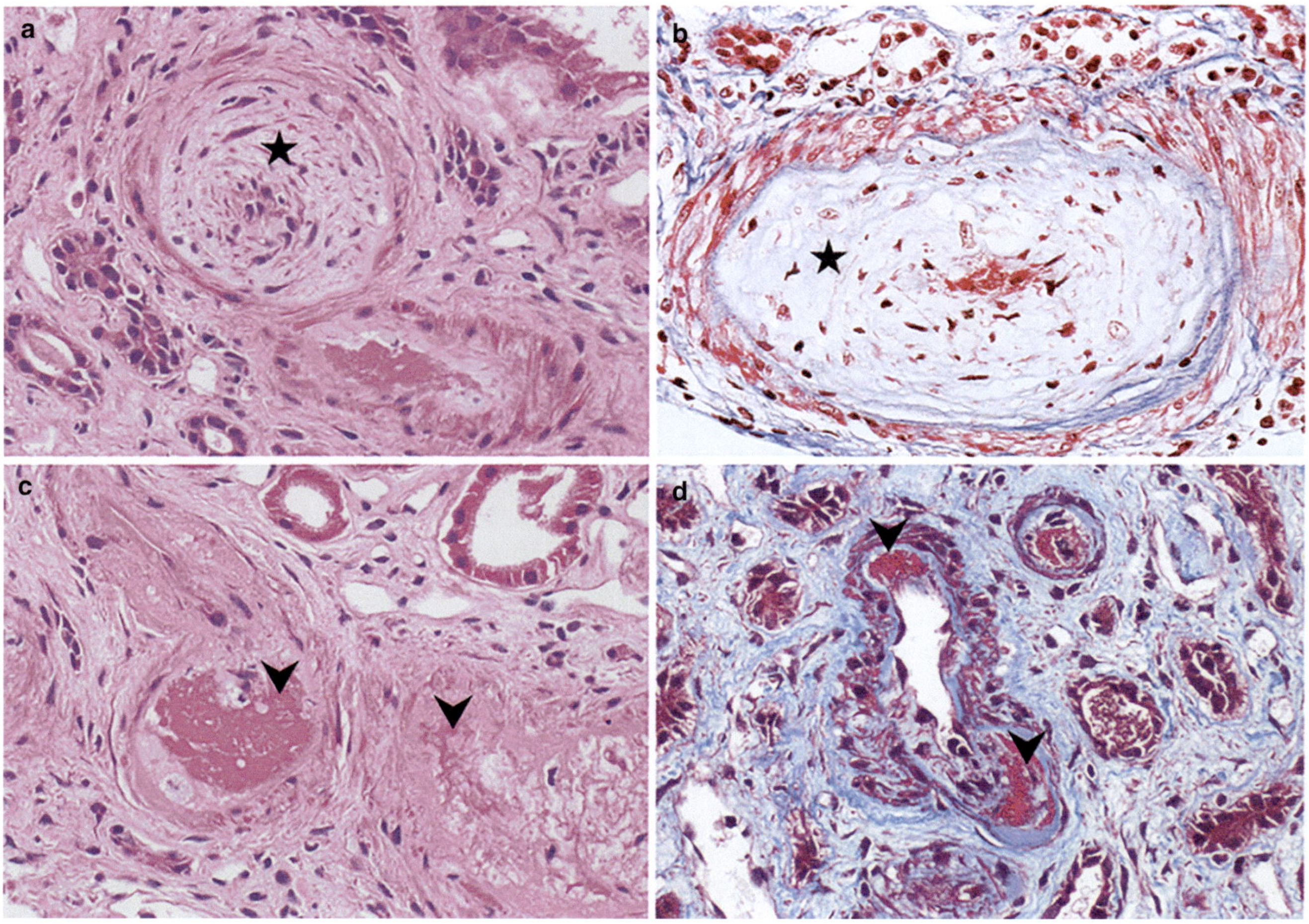

Fig. 13.10 Scleroderma renal crisis. In early scleroderma renal crisis, the myxoid material is deposited in the intima (⋆) of interlobular arteries (**a**). A Masson stain highlights the gray-blue myxoid material (⋆) in the intima surrounded by red muscle fibers in the media (**b**). Fibrinoid necrosis of afferent arterioles with red blood cells in vessel walls (▾) is also characteristic of early changes in scleroderma renal crisis (**c**). On trichrome, the fibrinoid necrosis appears bright red (▾) (**d**). Chronic changes in scleroderma renal crisis include onion-skin change (→) in renal blood vessels (**e**). A VVG emphasizes the reduplication of elastic fibers (→) in the vessel media (**f**). A PAS stain highlights thickening (▾) and wrinkling (→) of glomerular capillary loops (→) (**g**). Capillary wall collapse and thickening (→) are emphasized on a PAS-Methamine Silver stain (**h**)

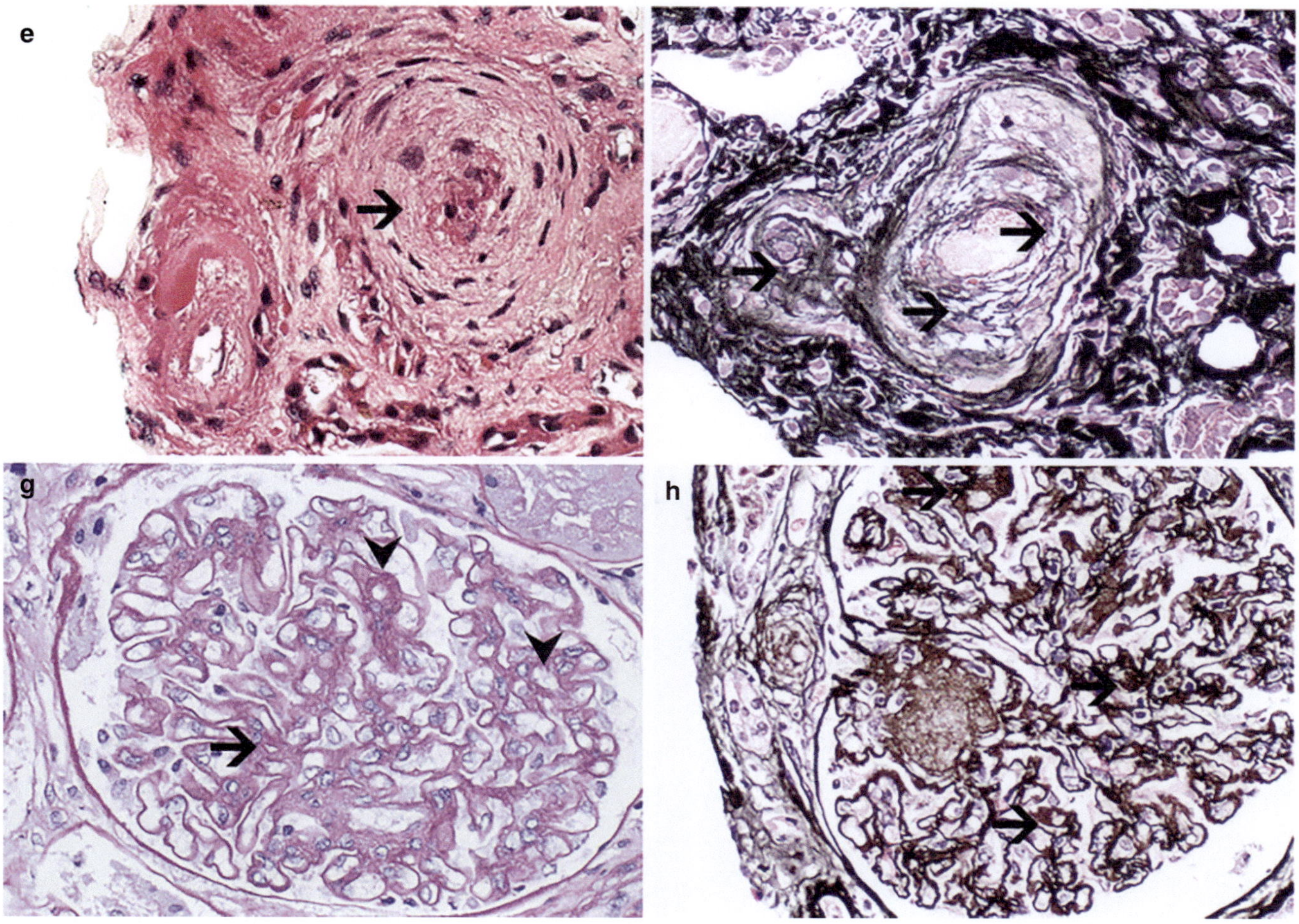

Fig. 13.10 (continued)

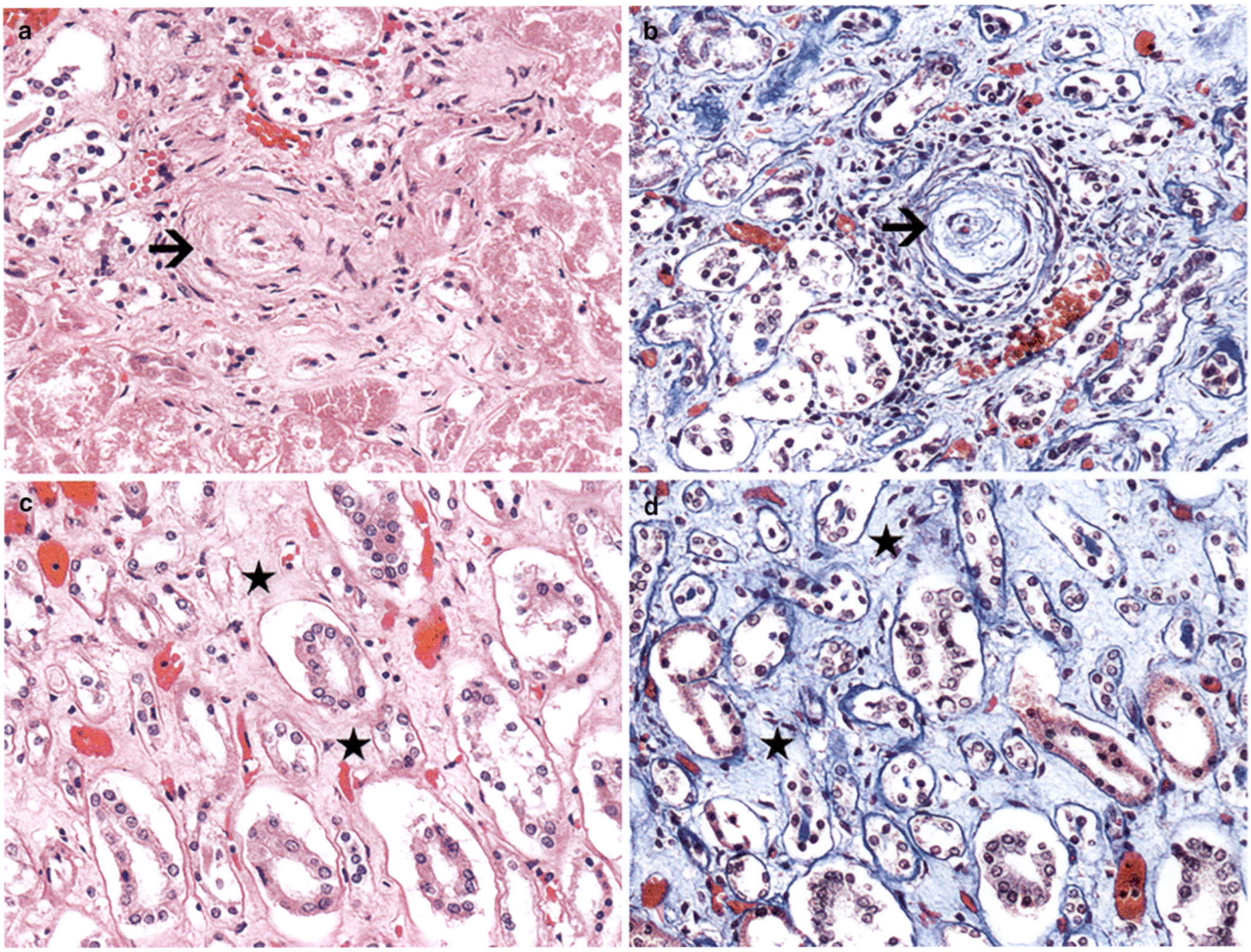

Fig. 13.11 Chronic kidney disease. Even patients with no history of scleroderma renal crisis can show onion-skin changes (→) in renal vessel walls (**a**). A Masson stain emphasizes accompanying fibrosis (→) of the vessel walls (**b**). Kidneys also demonstrate interstitial scarring (★) (**c**). A Masson stain highlights the interstitial fibrosis (★) (**d**)

Cardiovascular

Cardiovascular disease is the cause of death in 14–36% of all SSc cases [28, 47, 48, 57], a proportion that is similar to the recognized incidence of clinically symptomatic cardiovascular disease in these patients [58]. However, both radiologic and autopsy studies have reported much higher rates of cardiac involvement, with subclinical disease identified in up to 100% of patients in some series [5, 59, 60]. Although myocardial biopsy is occasionally performed on these patients, the heart is rarely assessed pathologically in SSc outside the autopsy setting. Nevertheless, a wide range of cardiac manifestations can be identified in pathologic material from SSc patients, including myocardial fibrosis, microvascular disease, atherosclerotic coronary artery disease, pericarditis, and secondary cor pulmonale.

The hallmark histologic lesion of SSc is patchy myocardial fibrosis, which contributes to the cardiac arrhythmias and impaired contractility that are appreciated clinically. As in other organ systems affected by SSc, this fibrosis is thought to arise secondary to microvascular abnormalities [61]. At autopsy, scarring is grossly visible within the myocardium of SSc patients in only a few cases. However, the patchy replacement of cardiac myocytes with acellular collagenous material can be seen microscopically throughout the heart (Fig. 13.12a, b). Unlike the myocardial fibrosis characteristic of atherosclerotic cardiovascular disease, that seen in SSc can affect the immediate subendocardial layer and tends to lack associated hemosiderin deposition [5, 60]. Rarely, fibrosis extends directly into the endocardium and even involves cardiac valves (Fig. 13.13).

Despite the central role of microvascular pathology in precipitating the aforementioned fibrosis, it is uncommon to see histologic evidence of actual microcirculatory obstruction in SSc patients. Instead, autopsy studies have documented a

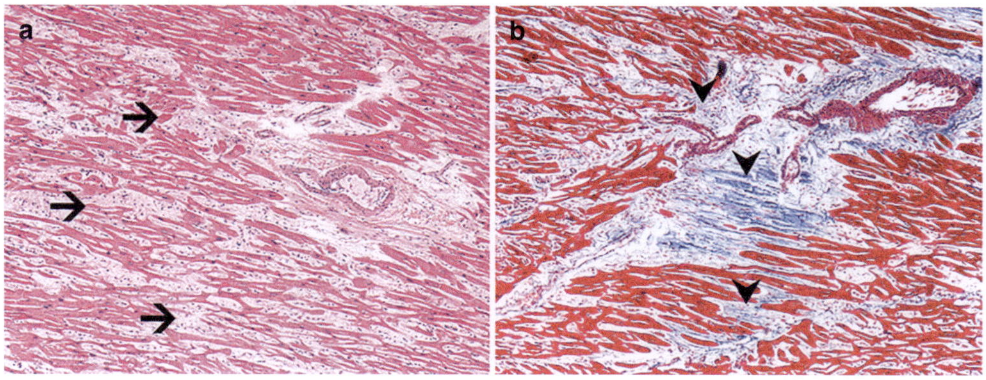

Fig. 13.12 Myocardial fibrosis. Patients with SSc demonstrate patchy myocardial fibrosis (→) throughout the heart (**a**). A Masson stain highlights the replacement of red cardiac myocytes with blue-staining fibrosis (▼) (**b**)

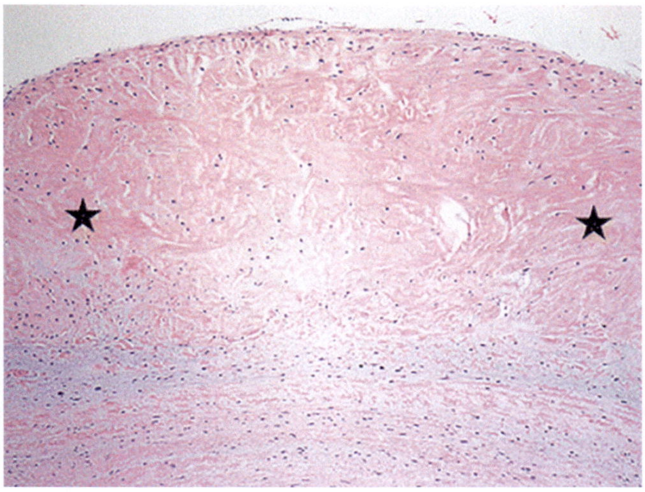

Fig. 13.13 Valve fibrosis. The aortic valve from a scleroderma patient shows increased fibrosis (⋆)

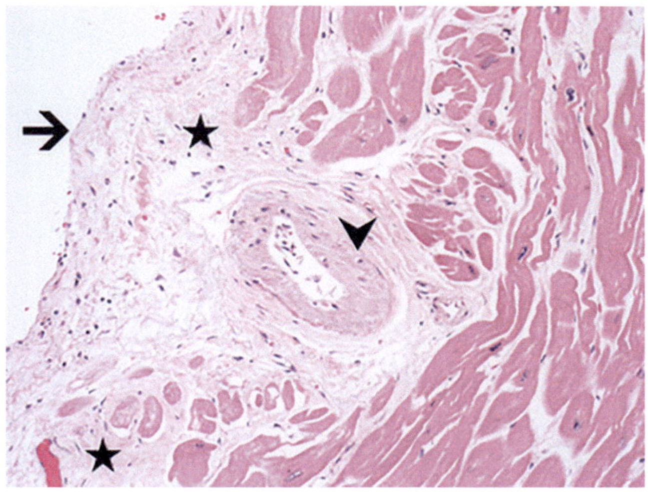

Fig. 13.14 Myocardial blood vessel remodeling. The cardiac microcirculation in SSc can demonstrate thickening of the tunica media (▼). Surrounding fibrosis (▼), which can extend into the endothelium (→) as well as the myocardium, suggests periodic ischemia

wide range of underlying vascular abnormalities in coronary arteries of <1 mm in size, including fibrinoid necrosis, mural fibrosis, intimal proliferation, and medial hyperplasia, with rare identification of luminal obstruction by platelet-fibrin clots (Fig. 13.14) [62]. The more frequently reported indication of microvascular obstruction is contraction band necrosis in the absence of atherosclerotic coronary vascular disease [5, 63]. Overall, these changes reflect decreased reserve capacity in the cardiac microvasculature, precipitating intermittent ischemia, and eventually fibrosis [64].

The question of systemic large-vessel involvement in SSc is also not entirely resolved. While older autopsy studies reported that the rates of atherosclerotic cardiovascular disease in SSc were no higher than that in the unaffected population [5, 60], more recent imaging studies have demonstrated that some SSc patients do experience accelerated atherosclerosis, similar to that seen in other systemic inflammatory diseases [61, 65]. Regardless of specific etiology, the atherosclerosis seen in SSc patients appears identical to that arising from more frequent causes. Affected arteries have thickened intima and occlusion by atheromatous plaques containing abundant foamy macrophages and cholesterol clefts with an overlying fibrous cap.

Pericardial disease is another common pathologic finding in systemic sclerosis. Large autopsy studies have suggested that up to 62% of SSc patients show evidence of acute pericarditis [5, 60, 63], even though reviews identify clinical symptoms in only 5–16% of patients [65]. Grossly, the affected pericardium appears dull and roughened. Microscopic sections demonstrate a fibrinous exudate on the pericardial surface with intermixed acute and chronic inflammatory cells (Fig. 13.15). Patients frequently develop a pericardial effusion in association with pericarditis, although pericardial tamponade is rare. Cytologic examination of the pericardial fluid generally demonstrates reactive mesothelial cells, histiocytes, and variable numbers of acute and chronic inflammatory cells.

Finally, cardiovascular pathology can also arise secondary to the aforementioned pulmonary complications of SSc. Most notably, heart failure is a common consequence of pulmonary arterial hypertension and is thought to be a determining factor in the prognosis of affected patients [66]. Pathologically, the

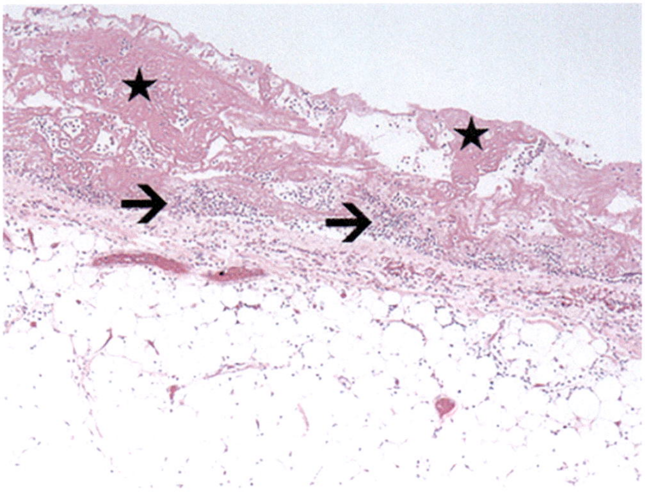

Fig. 13.15 Fibrinous pericarditis. SSc patients commonly have a pericardial exudate with fibrin deposition (★) and a prominent acute inflammatory infiltrate (→)

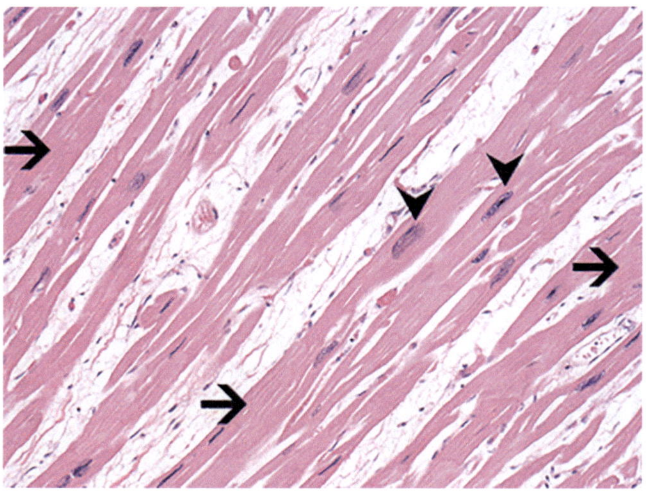

Fig. 13.16 Myocyte hypertrophy. The right ventricle shows marked hypertrophy with nuclear (▼) and cytoplasmic (→) enlargement secondary to pulmonary hypertension

findings in cor pulmonale in SSc are indistinguishable from those in patients without underlying autoimmune disease. At gross examination, the heart demonstrates hypertrophy and dilation of both the right atrium and ventricle, with normal to increased wall thickness and enlarged cardiac chambers. Microscopically, individual cardiac myocytes also demonstrate marked hypertrophy, with simultaneous nuclear and cytoplasmic enlargement (Fig. 13.16).

Gastrointestinal

Although gastrointestinal (GI) complications are responsible for fewer than 10% of SSc-related deaths, they affect more than 90% of SSc patients and represent a considerable source of morbidity and decreased quality of life [67, 68]. GI biopsy can be very helpful in SSc patients to differentiate complications of the disease from more treatable conditions such as *Helicobacter pylori* infection or drug reactions. Other GI manifestations of SSc can be seen pathologically when surgical resection is employed in management. While many of the GI complications of SSc have similar appearances throughout the GI tract, other manifestations are site specific. Findings include fibrosis of the muscularis propria, gastroesophageal reflux, mucosal ulceration, thermal injury, telangiectasias, and gastric antral vascular ectasia.

As in the myocardium, muscular fibrosis is the pathognomonic lesion of SSc in the GI tract. In one large autopsy series, 74% of patients with SSc demonstrated fibrosis or atrophy of the esophageal muscularis propria, while 48% and 39%, respectively, demonstrated such changes in the small and large bowel [5]. Grossly, these organs are characterized by stiff, thin walls and can have wide-mouthed diverticula [69]. Microscopic sections demonstrate collagenous replacement of the muscularis propria, often with associated wall thinning and flattening of the overlying epithelium (Fig. 13.17a–d). Perforation is a common complication of this process. As in other organ systems, vasculopathy is thought to be the underlying cause of fibrosis [70], and intimal thickening of muscularis propria vessels is frequently observed histologically (Fig. 13.18).

The impaired smooth muscle motility that results from such fibrosis can lead to additional complications for SSc patients. While obstruction, malabsorption, delayed gastric emptying, and constipation are primarily clinical diagnoses [71], defects in motility often lead to direct mucosal injury that can be appreciated pathologically. The most common such injury is gastroesophageal reflux. On biopsy, the esophageal mucosa demonstrates basal cell hyperplasia, elongation of the lamina propria into the upper third of the epithelium, and scattered intraepithelial eosinophils (Fig. 13.19a). Prolonged reflux underlies the propensity to develop Barrett esophagus in SSc patients, with an estimated incidence of 6.8–12.7% and an attendant increased risk of esophageal adenocarcinoma [71]. A biopsy of Barrett lesions shows distinctive incomplete intestinal metaplasia of the esophageal mucosa. Reflux also has a strong association with the development of interstitial lung disease [72].

Other forms of mucosal injury can also be seen in SSc patients. Mucosal erosion and ulceration can result from a number of causes throughout the GI tract, including bacterial overgrowth, obstruction, and mechanical trauma [69]. Similar to sampling of skin ulcerations, biopsies of these lesions demonstrate a loss of surface epithelium with associated fibrinopurulent inflammatory exudate (Fig. 13.19b). A more specific injury pattern occurs in the esophagus when impaired esophageal peristalsis allows hot substances to have prolonged contact with the mucosal surfaces, leading to

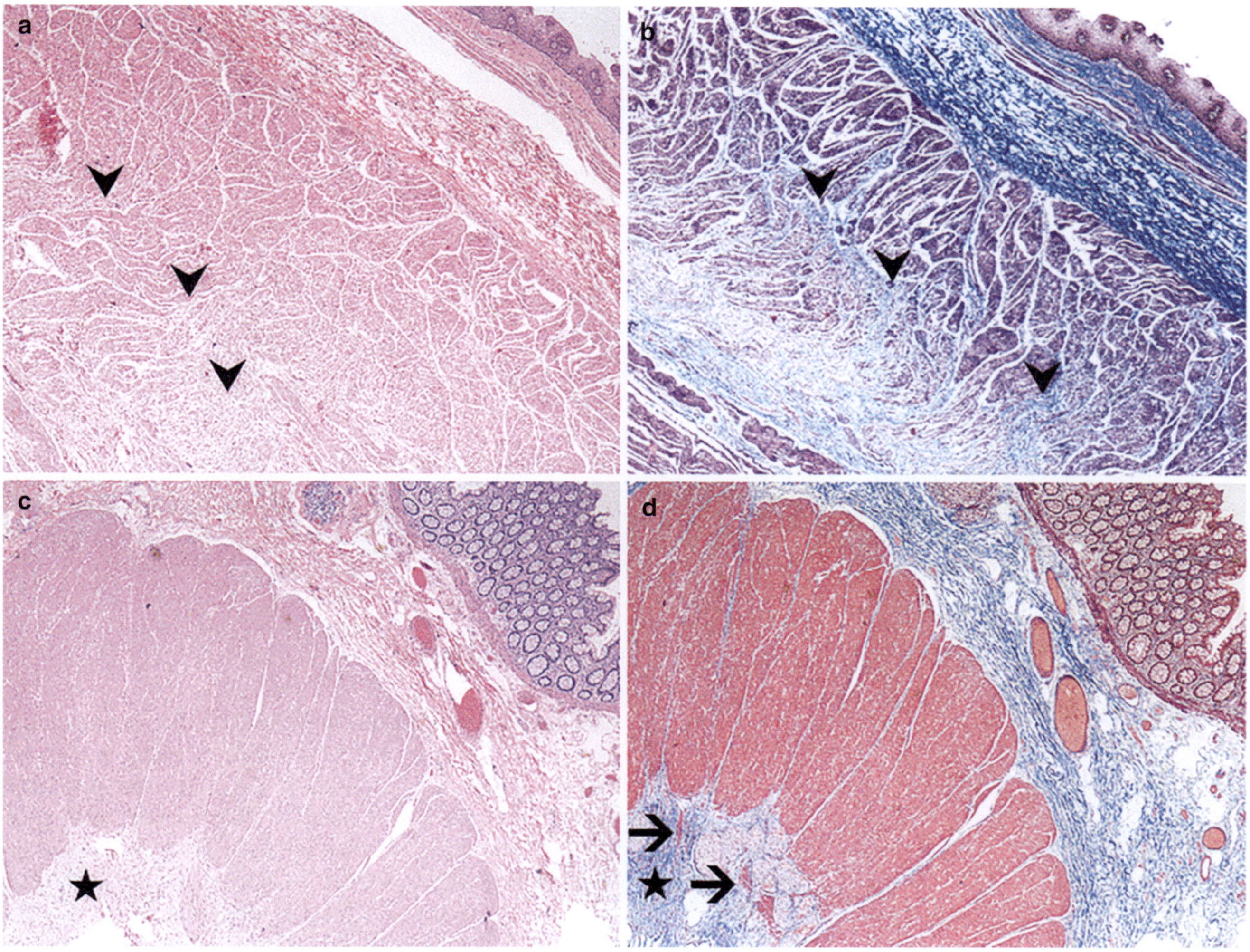

Fig. 13.17 Gastrointestinal smooth muscle fibrosis. A section of esophagus demonstrates partial fibrosis of the inner circular layer of the muscularis propria, barely visible as areas of pale pink collagen on H&E (▼) (**a**). A Masson stain highlights the fibrils of collagen in blue (▼) interdigitating between red muscle fibers. Likewise, there is almost complete replacement of the outer longitudinal muscle of this colon with pale pink fibrosis (★) (**c**). A Masson stain highlights the complete fibrosis in blue (★) with only rare remaining red muscle fibers (→) (**d**)

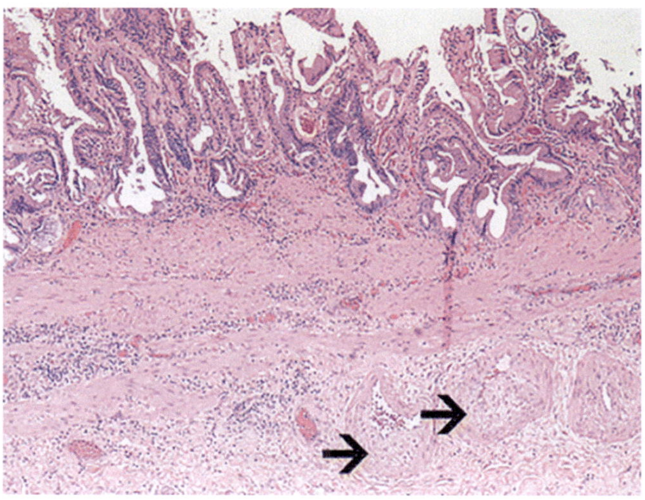

Fig. 13.18 Gastrointestinal blood vessel remodeling. Asymmetric intimal and medial hypertrophy (→) is seen in blood vessels within the gallbladder muscularis propria of an SSc patient

thermal damage. Histologically, this appears as mummification of the upper third of the epithelium with coagulative necrosis, loss of nuclear basophilia, and separation from the underlying layers of cells (Fig. 13.19c).

Vascular pathology is also common within the GI mucosa in SSc. Indeed, 15% of SSc patients experience GI hemorrhage at some point during their illness [69]. Telangiectasias are the most common source of GI bleeding but are rarely biopsied. Histologically, they appear as dilated blood vessels in the lamina propria, similar to those seen in the skin. Another rare source of GI bleeding frequently linked to SSc is gastric antral vascular ectasia (GAVE) [73]. This condition is colloquially known as watermelon stomach because dilated blood vessels in the antrum grossly appear as parallel red stripes, similar to a watermelon rind. Biopsies show dilated vessels in the lamina propria plugged by fibrin thrombi, reactive changes in surrounding epithelial cells, and smooth muscle hyperplasia of the lamina propria (Fig. 13.20).

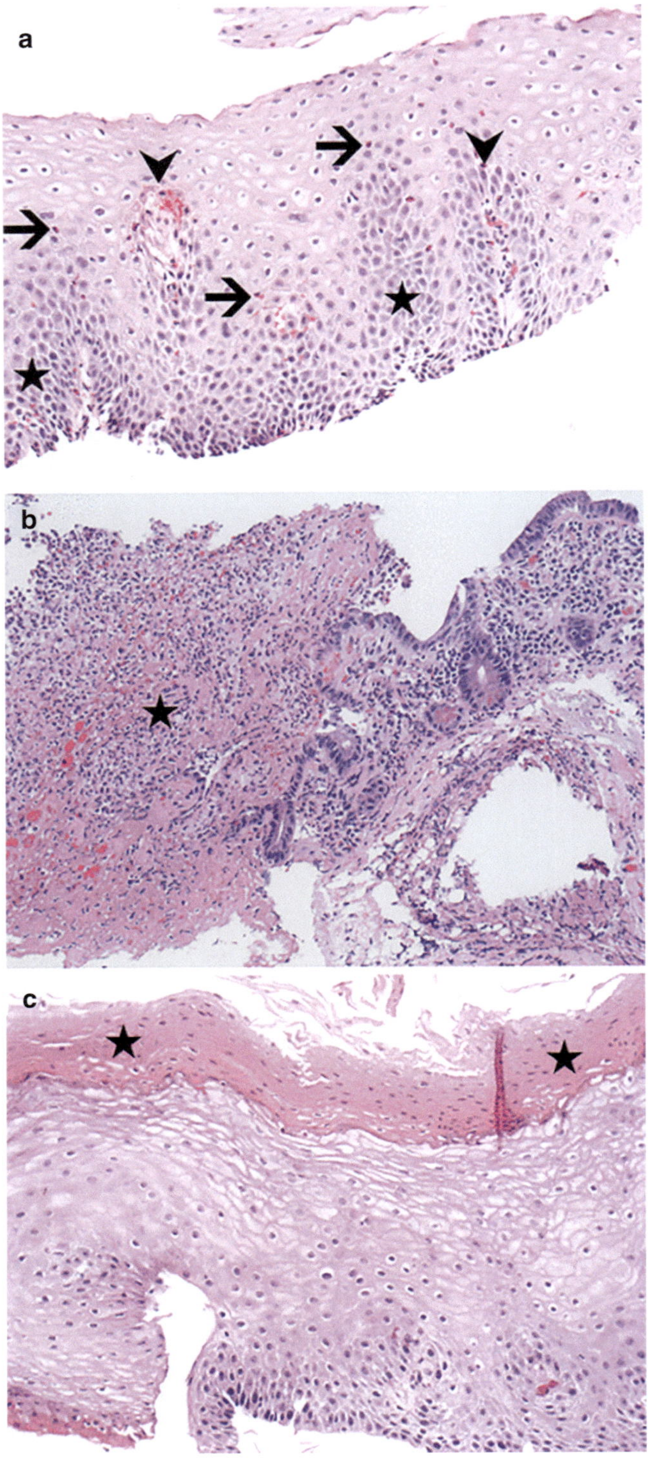

Fig. 13.19 Gastrointestinal mucosal injury. In reflux esophagitis, the epithelium displays basal cell hyperplasia (★), elongation of the rete ridges into the upper third of the epithelium (→), and intraepithelial eosinophils (→) (**a**). Colonic ulceration results in loss of surface epithelium and lamina propria with associated fibrinopurulent exudate (★) (**b**). Thermal injury in the esophagus demonstrates coagulative necrosis of the upper third of the epithelium (→) (**c**)

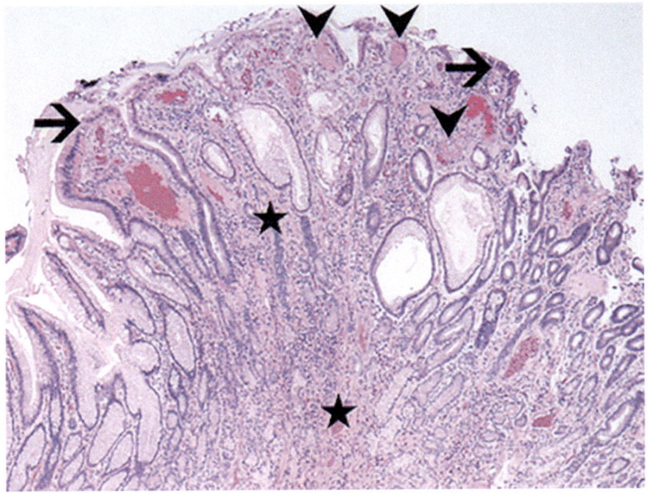

Fig. 13.20 Gastric antral vascular ectasia. There are fibrin thrombi in lamina propria vessels (▼), reactive epithelial changes (→), and foveolar hyperplasia with prominent smooth muscle bundles (★)

Musculoskeletal

Although musculoskeletal involvement is not as widely recognized in SSc as in other autoimmune diseases, it also represents a significant source of disability and decreased quality of life for affected patients [68]. Approximately 24% of SSc patients demonstrate proximal limb weakness [16], and 20–86% report muscle or joint pain [74]. Although histologic assessment of muscle and joint tissue is rarely made in clinical practice, these tissues do demonstrate characteristic pathologic findings. Musculoskeletal involvement includes skeletal muscle inflammation and fibrosis, tendon fibrosis, and synovitis.

Muscular involvement in SSc has two main manifestations: atrophy and inflammation. Histologically, 41% of SSc patients demonstrate skeletal muscular atrophy at autopsy, while 8% show myositis with chronic inflammation [5]. Sections of the skeletal muscle demonstrate a wide range of nonspecific findings. Myocyte atrophy can be identified with loss of contractile fibers, perimysial and epimysial fibrosis, fibrous replacement of muscle cells, rare necrosis, and variable degrees of regeneration (Fig. 13.21). Inflammation tends to consist of a mild mononuclear cell infiltrate involving the muscle parenchyma. Overall, the muscular findings in SSc are indistinguishable from patients with polymyositis and dermatomyositis [74].

In addition to direct involvement of the skeletal muscle, SSc also can affect tendons. Clinically, tendon disease is measured by the presence of tendon friction rubs, defined as a rubbing sensation upon the movement of the tendon. Such

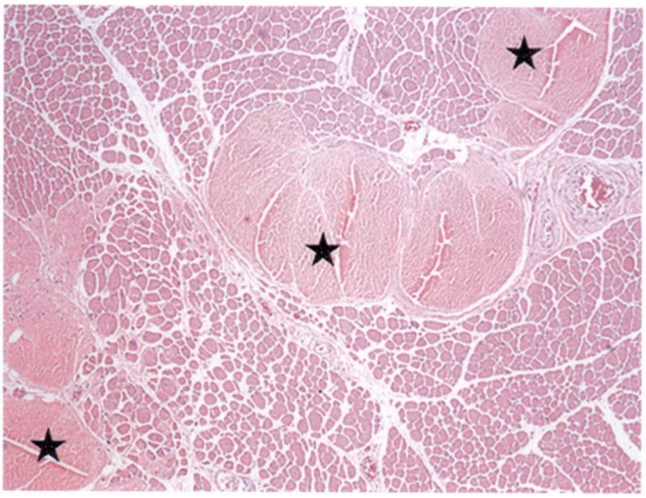

Fig. 13.21 Skeletal muscle fibrosis. At autopsy, a section of the skeletal muscle demonstrates loss of myocytes with fibrous replacement (⋆)

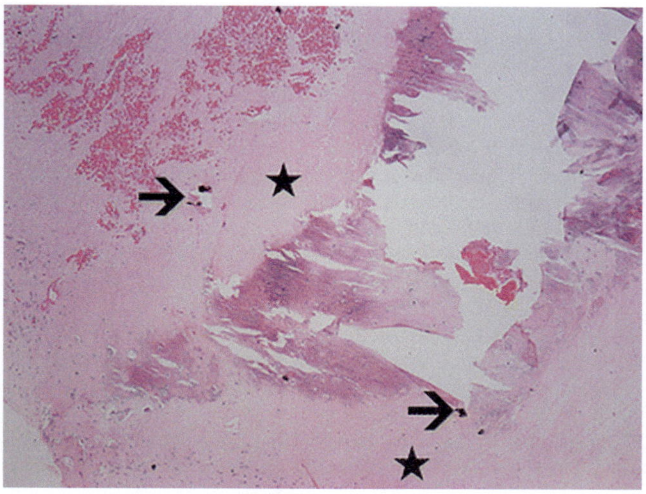

Fig. 13.22 Tendon rupture. A biceps tendon from a scleroderma patient shows fibrosis (⋆), calcification (→), and disruption

rubs have a strong association with visceral involvement and disease progression [75]. Imaging studies have suggested that tendon friction rubs reflect fibrous remodeling of the tendon rather than an active inflammatory process [76]. Histologically, tendons from SSc confirm the presence of fibrosis with occasional calcifications (Fig. 13.22). Blood vessels with intimal proliferation and luminal obliteration can occasionally be noted in the tendon sheath [1]. Tendon rupture is a rare late complication of this finding.

Joint synovitis is another common finding in SSc that has been reported in anywhere between 18 and 60% of patients [1, 75]. This finding seems to be independent from tendon involvement but is also a strong predictor of disease progression [75]. Most studies of synovitis rely on imaging findings, but a few cases have been studied histologically [77]. Cases of acute synovitis demonstrate focal to diffuse lymphoplasmacytic inflammation in the synovium with variable associated fibrin deposition. In contrast to rheumatoid arthritis, SSc joint disease is not associated with pannus formation or bone resorption. Chronic synovitis histologically is characterized by vascular obliteration and synovial atrophy.

Placenta

While careful clinical monitoring can allow for successful pregnancies in SSc, an overall higher rate of adverse pregnancy outcomes is well documented in these patients [78]. Although studies have differed regarding whether the rate of miscarriage in SSc patients is significantly higher than that of normal controls, they do highlight a uniformly elevated frequency of preterm births of up to 29% in pregnancies of affected mothers [78, 79]. Women with SSc also have a higher rate of delivering low-birth weight infants even at term [80]. Pathologic examination of the placenta is frequently carried out in cases with such pregnancy complications, and several histologic abnormalities strongly correlate with the aforementioned clinical findings.

The most significant lesion identified in placentas from SSc pregnancies is decidual vasculopathy, which has been identified in up to 38% of placentas and associated with poor perinatal outcomes and fetal death [81]. Decidual vasculopathy is a broad term that encompasses several abnormalities of the placental vasculature, including fibrinoid necrosis of the vascular wall, subendothelial and intramural accumulation of macrophages, and thickening of the muscular wall of small blood vessels (Fig. 13.23a). These findings can occur focally or may diffusely involve the decidual blood vessels. Decidual vasculopathy is not specific for SSc and, indeed, is most commonly seen in preeclampsia; it has also been documented in a wide range of autoimmune diseases [81].

Placentas from SSc pregnancies have also been shown to demonstrate several other abnormalities that arise secondary to the previously described vascular compromise. Placental infarcts can be visible both grossly and microscopically [81] (Fig. 13.23b), reflecting complete loss of blood flow to all or part of the placenta. Gross examination reveals pale induration of the placental parenchyma with a granular cut surface, corresponding histologically to an area of coagulative necrosis with architectural collapse of villi, increased fibrin deposition, villous agglutination, and loss of nuclear basophilia. The placental villi can also show abnormal growth patterns for gestational age, including fibrosis; distal villous hypoplasia with long, avascular villi; and increased syncytial knotting (Fig. 13.23c) [82]. Placental mesenchymal dysplasia, including stem villi with mesenchymal proliferation, foci of myxoid degeneration, and large stromal macrophages, has also been rarely reported [83].

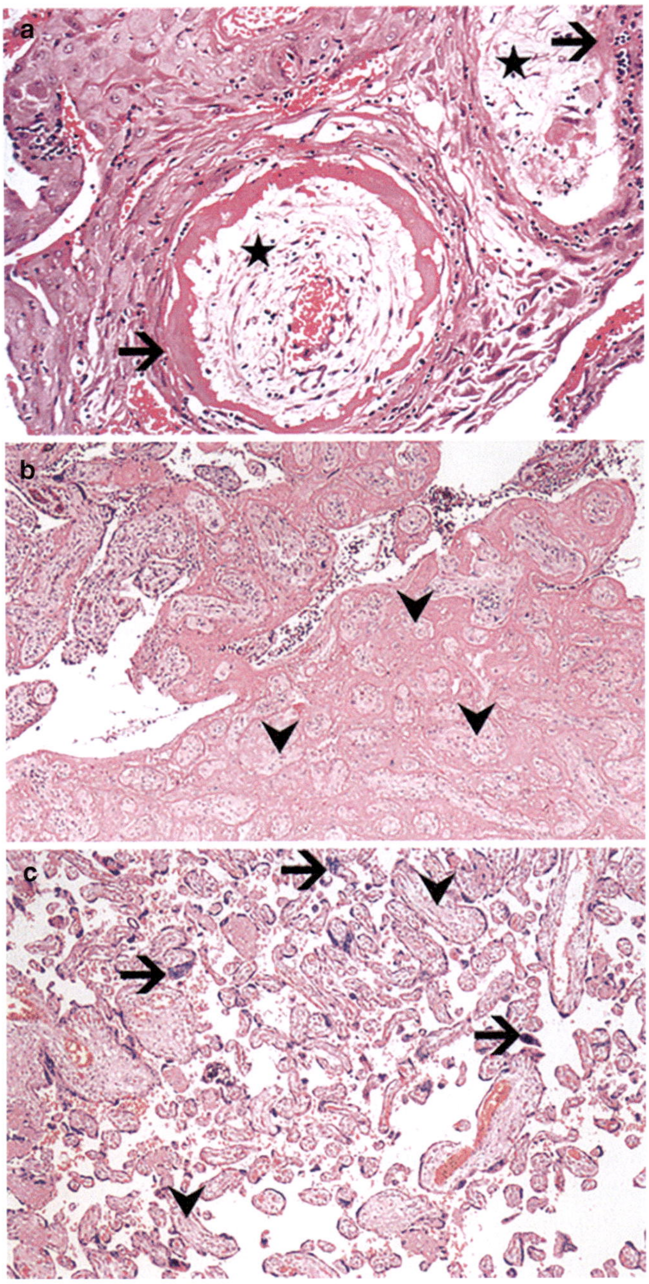

Fig. 13.23 Placental changes. In decidual vasculopathy, maternal decidual blood vessels undergo acute atherosis with an accumulation of foamy macrophages (★) and associated fibrinoid necrosis of the vessel walls (→) (**a**). This vascular compromise often leads to placental infarct, with the condensation of villi and complete loss of nuclear basophilia (▼) (**b**). Viable placental tissue can demonstrate distal villous hypoplasia with elongated, avascular villi (▼) and increased numbers of syncytial knots (→) for gestational age (**c**)

References

1. Gardner DL. In: Gardner DL, editor. Pathological basis of the connective tissue diseases. 2nd ed. Philadelphia: Lea & Febiger; 1992.
2. Piper WN, Helwig EB. Progressive systemic sclerosis; visceral manifestations in generalized scleroderma. AMA Arch Dermatol. 1955;72(6):535–46.
3. Klemperer P, Pollack AD, Baehr G. Landmark article may 23, 1942: diffuse collagen disease. Acute disseminated lupus erythematosus and diffuse scleroderma. By Paul Klemperer, Abou D. Pollack and George Baehr. JAMA. 1984;251(12):1593–4.
4. Kinder RR, Fleischmajer R. Systemic scleroderma: a review of organ systems. Int J Dermatol. 1974;13(6):382–95.
5. D'Angelo WA, Fries JF, Masi AT, Shulman LE. Pathologic observations in systemic sclerosis (scleroderma). A study of fifty-eight autopsy cases and fifty-eight matched controls. Am J Med. 1969;46(3):428–40.
6. Rockey DC, Bell PD, Hill JA. Fibrosis–a common pathway to organ injury and failure. N Engl J Med. 2015;373(1):96.
7. van den Hoogen F, Khanna D, Fransen J, Johnson SR, Baron M, Tyndall A, et al. 2013 classification criteria for systemic sclerosis: an American College of Rheumatology/European league against rheumatism collaborative initiative. Arthritis Rheum. 2013;65(11):2737–47.
8. Tyndall A, Fistarol S. The differential diagnosis of systemic sclerosis. Curr Opin Rheumatol. 2013;25(6):692–9.
9. Calonje JE. In: Brenn T, Lazar A, PH MK, editors. McKee's pathology of the skin with clinical correlations. 4th ed. Saint Louis: Elsevier/Saunders; 2012.
10. Wriston CC, Rubin AI, Elenitsas R, Crawford GH. Nodular scleroderma: a report of 2 cases. Am J Dermatopathol. 2008;30(4):385–8.
11. Verrecchia F, Laboureau J, Verola O, Roos N, Porcher R, Bruneval P, et al. Skin involvement in scleroderma—where histological and clinical scores meet. Rheumatology (Oxford). 2007;46(5):833–41.
12. Fett N, Werth VP. Update on morphea: part I. epidemiology, clinical presentation, and pathogenesis. J Am Acad Dermatol 2011;64(2):217–28; quiz 29–30.
13. Braverman IM. Ultrastructure and organization of the cutaneous microvasculature in normal and pathologic states. J Invest Dermatol. 1989;93(2 Suppl):2S–9.
14. Sticherling M. Systemic sclerosis-dermatological aspects. Part 1: pathogenesis, epidemiology, clinical findings. J Dtsch Dermatol Ges. 2012;10(10):705–18. quiz 16
15. Sunderkötter C, Herrgott I, Brückner C, Moinzadeh P, Pfeiffer C, Gerss J, et al. Comparison of patients with and without digital ulcers in systemic sclerosis: detection of possible risk factors. Br J Dermatol. 2009;160(4):835–43.
16. Muangchan C, Baron M, Pope J, Canadian Scleroderma Research G. The 15% rule in scleroderma: the frequency of severe organ complications in systemic sclerosis. A systematic review. J Rheumatol. 2013;40(9):1545–56.
17. Gutierrez A Jr, Wetter DA. Calcinosis cutis in autoimmune connective tissue diseases. Dermatol Ther. 2012;25(2):195–206.
18. Reiter N, El-Shabrawi L, Leinweber B, Berghold A, Aberer E. Calcinosis cutis: part I. Diagnostic pathway. J Am Acad Dermatol. 2011;65(1):1–12; quiz 3–4.
19. Boulman N, Slobodin G, Rozenbaum M, Rosner I. Calcinosis in rheumatic diseases. Semin Arthritis Rheum. 2005;34(6):805–12.
20. Alavi A, Hafner J, Dutz JP, Mayer D, Sibbald RG, Criado PR, et al. Atrophie blanche: is it associated with venous disease or livedoid vasculopathy? Adv Skin Wound Care. 2014;27(11):518–24.
21. Criado PR, Rivitti EA, Sotto MN, de Carvalho JF. Livedoid vasculopathy as a coagulation disorder. Autoimmun Rev. 2011;10(6):353–60.
22. Varga J. In: Denton CP, Wigley FM, editors. Scleroderma from pathogenesis to comprehensive management. 1st ed. Boston: Springer US; 2012.
23. Machinami R. Incidence of membranous lipodystrophy-like change among patients with limb necrosis caused by chronic arterial obstruction. Arch Pathol Lab Med. 1984;108(10):823–6.
24. Snow JL, Su WP, Gibson LE. Lipomembranous (membranocystic) changes associated with morphea: a clinicopathologic review of three cases. J Am Acad Dermatol. 1994;31(2 Pt 1):246–50.

25. Steen VD, Medsger TA. Changes in causes of death in systemic sclerosis, 1972–2002. Ann Rheum Dis. 2007;66(7):940–4.
26. Akter T, Silver RM, Bogatkevich GS. Recent advances in understanding the pathogenesis of scleroderma-interstitial lung disease. Curr Rheumatol Rep. 2014;16(4):411.
27. Solomon JJ, Olson AL, Fischer A, Bull T, Brown KK, Raghu G. Scleroderma lung disease. Eur Respir Rev. 2013;22(127):6–19.
28. Nikpour M, Baron M. Mortality in systemic sclerosis: lessons learned from population-based and observational cohort studies. Curr Opin Rheumatol. 2014;26(2):131–7.
29. du Bois RM. Mechanisms of scleroderma-induced lung disease. Proc Am Thorac Soc. 2007;4(5):434–8.
30. Farkas L, Kolb M. Pulmonary microcirculation in interstitial lung disease. Proc Am Thoracic Soc. 2011;8(6):516–21.
31. Wagenvoort CA. Lung biopsy specimens in the evaluation of pulmonary vascular disease. Chest. 1980;77(5):614–25.
32. Weaver AL, Divertie MB, Titus JL. Pulmonary scleroderma. Dis Chest. 1968;54(6):490–8.
33. Fujita J, Yoshinouchi T, Ohtsuki Y, Tokuda M, Yang Y, Yamadori I, et al. Non-specific interstitial pneumonia as pulmonary involvement of systemic sclerosis. Ann Rheum Dis. 2001;60(3): 281–3.
34. Fischer A, Meehan RT, Feghali-Bostwick CA, West SG, Brown KK. Unique characteristics of systemic sclerosis sine scleroderma-associated interstitial lung disease. Chest. 2006;130(4):976–81.
35. Bouros D, Wells A, Nicholson A, Colby T, Polychronopoulos V, Pantelidis P, et al. Histopathologic subsets of fibrosing alveolitis in patients with systemic sclerosis and their relationship to outcome. Am J Respir Crit Care Med. 2002;165(12):1581–6.
36. Song JW, Do KH, Kim MY, Jang SJ, Colby TV, Kim DS. Pathologic and radiologic differences between idiopathic and collagen vascular disease-related usual interstitial pneumonia. Chest. 2009;136(1):23–30.
37. Herzog EL, Mathur A, Tager AM, Feghali-Bostwick C, Schneider F, Varga J. Review: interstitial lung disease associated with systemic sclerosis and idiopathic pulmonary fibrosis: how similar and distinct? Arthritis Rheumatol. 2014;66(8):1967–78.
38. Fischer A, Swigris JJ, Groshong SD, Cool CD, Sahin H, Lynch DA, et al. Clinically significant interstitial lung disease in limited scleroderma: histopathology, clinical features, and survival. Chest. 2008;134(3):601–5.
39. Hassoun PM. Lung involvement in systemic sclerosis. Presse Med. 2011;40(1 Pt 2):e3–17.
40. Heath D, Edwards JE. The pathology of hypertensive pulmonary vascular disease; a description of six grades of structural changes in the pulmonary arteries with special reference to congenital cardiac septal defects. Circulation. 1958;18(4 Part 1):533–47.
41. Launay D, Humbert M, Berezne A, Cottin V, Allanore Y, Couderc LJ, et al. Clinical characteristics and survival in systemic sclerosis-related pulmonary hypertension associated with interstitial lung disease. Chest. 2011;140(4):1016–24.
42. Yousem SA. The pulmonary pathologic manifestations of the CREST syndrome. Hum Pathol. 1990;21(5):467–74.
43. Overbeek MJ, Vonk MC, Boonstra A, Voskuyl AE, Vonk-Noordegraaf A, Smit EF, et al. Pulmonary arterial hypertension in limited cutaneous systemic sclerosis: a distinctive vasculopathy. Eur Respir J. 2009;34(2):371–9.
44. Dorfmüller P, Humbert M, Perros F, Sanchez O, Simonneau G, Müller KM, et al. Fibrous remodeling of the pulmonary venous system in pulmonary arterial hypertension associated with connective tissue diseases. Hum Pathol. 2007;38(6):893–902.
45. Breit SN, Thornton SC, Penny R. Lung involvement in scleroderma. Clin Dermatol. 1994;12(2):243–52.
46. Urisman A, Jones KD. Pulmonary pathology in connective tissue disease. Semin Respirat Crit Care Med. 2014;35(2):201–12.
47. Steen VD, Medsger TA Jr. Severe organ involvement in systemic sclerosis with diffuse scleroderma. Arthritis Rheum. 2000;43(11):2437–44.
48. Ferri C, Sebastiani M, Lo Monaco A, Iudici M, Giuggioli D, Furini F, et al. Systemic sclerosis evolution of disease pathomorphosis and survival. Our experience on Italian patients' population and review of the literature. Autoimmun Rev. 2014;13(10):1026–34.
49. Bose N, Chiesa-Vottero A, Chatterjee S. Scleroderma renal crisis. Semin Arthritis Rheum. 2005;44(6):687–94.
50. Batal I, Domsic RT, Medsger TA, Bastacky S. Scleroderma renal crisis: a pathology perspective. Int J Rheumatol. 2010;2010:543704.
51. Batal I, Domsic RT, Shafer A, Medsger TA Jr, Kiss LP, Randhawa P, et al. Renal biopsy findings predicting outcome in scleroderma renal crisis. Hum Pathol. 2009;40(3):332–40.
52. Lee S, Sharma K. The pathogenesis of fibrosis and renal disease in scleroderma: recent insights from glomerulosclerosis. Curr Rheumatol Rep. 2004;6(2):141–8.
53. Penn H, Howie AJ, Kingdon EJ, Bunn CC, Stratton RJ, Black CM, et al. Scleroderma renal crisis: patient characteristics and long-term outcomes. Qjm-Int J Med. 2007;100(8):485–94.
54. Scheja A, Bartosik I, Wuttge DM, Hesselstrand R. Renal function is mostly preserved in patients with systemic sclerosis. Scand J Rheumatol. 2009;38(4):295–8.
55. Shanmugam VK, Steen VD. Renal disease in scleroderma: an update on evaluation, risk stratification, pathogenesis and management. Curr Opin Rheumatol. 2012;24(6):669–76.
56. Kao L, Weyand C. Vasculitis in systemic sclerosis. Int J Rheumatol. 2010;2010:385938.
57. Elhai M, Meune C, Avouac J, Kahan A, Allanore Y. Trends in mortality in patients with systemic sclerosis over 40 years: a systematic review and meta-analysis of cohort studies. Rheumatology (Oxford). 2012;51(6):1017–26.
58. Kahan A, Coghlan G, McLaughlin V. Cardiac complications of systemic sclerosis. Rheumatology (Oxford). 2009;48 Suppl 3:iii45–8.
59. Rodriguez-Reyna TS, Morelos-Guzman M, Hernandez-Reyes P, Montero-Duarte K, Martinez-Reyes C, Reyes-Utrera C, et al. Assessment of myocardial fibrosis and microvascular damage in systemic sclerosis by magnetic resonance imaging and coronary angiotomography. Rheumatology (Oxford). 2015;54(4):647–54.
60. Bulkley BH, Ridolfi RL, Salyer WR, Hutchins GM. Myocardial lesions of progressive systemic sclerosis. A cause of cardiac dysfunction. Circulation. 1976;53(3):483–90.
61. Allanore Y, Meune C. Primary myocardial involvement in systemic sclerosis: evidence for a microvascular origin. Clin Exp Rheumatol. 2010;28(5 Suppl 62):S48–53.
62. James TN. De subitaneis mortibus. VIII. Coronary arteries and conduction system in scleroderma heart disease. Circulation. 1974;50(4):844–56.
63. McWhorter JE, LeRoy EC. Pericardial disease in scleroderma (systemic sclerosis). Am J Med. 1974;57(4):566–75.
64. Parks JL, Taylor MH, Parks LP, Silver RM. Systemic sclerosis and the heart. Rheum Dis Clin N Am. 2014;40(1):87–102.
65. Lambova S. Cardiac manifestations in systemic sclerosis. World J Cardiol. 2014;6(9):993–1005.
66. Lefevre G, Dauchet L, Hachulla E, Montani D, Sobanski V, Lambert M, et al. Survival and prognostic factors in systemic sclerosis-associated pulmonary hypertension: a systematic review and meta-analysis. Arthritis Rheum. 2013;65(9):2412–23.
67. Klein-Weigel P, Opitz C, Riemekasten G. Systemic sclerosis—a systematic overview: part 1—disease characteristics and classification, pathophysiologic concepts, and recommendations for diagnosis and surveillance. Vasa. 2011;40(1):6–19.
68. Johnson SR, Glaman DD, Schentag CT, Lee P. Quality of life and functional status in systemic sclerosis compared to other rheumatic diseases. J Rheumatol. 2006;33(6):1117–22.

69. Ebert EC. Gastric and enteric involvement in progressive systemic sclerosis. J Clin Gastroenterol. 2008;42(1):5–12.
70. Di Ciaula A, Covelli M, Berardino M, Wang DQ, Lapadula G, Palasciano G, et al. Gastrointestinal symptoms and motility disorders in patients with systemic scleroderma. BMC Gastroenterol. 2008;8:7.
71. Forbes A, Marie I. Gastrointestinal complications: the most frequent internal complications of systemic sclerosis. Rheumatology. 2009;48:36–9.
72. Christmann RB, Wells AU, Capelozzi VL, Silver RM. Gastroesophageal reflux incites interstitial lung disease in systemic sclerosis: clinical, radiologic, histopathologic, and treatment evidence. Semin Arthritis Rheumatism. 2010;40(3): 241–9.
73. Watson M, Hally RJ, McCue PA, Varga J, Jimenez SA. Gastric antral vascular ectasia (watermelon stomach) in patients with systemic sclerosis. Arthritis Rheum. 1996;39(2):341–6.
74. Lóránd V, Czirják L, Minier T. Musculoskeletal involvement in systemic sclerosis. Presse Med. 2014;43(10 Pt 2):e315–28.
75. Avouac J, Walker UA, Hachulla E, Riemekasten G, Cuomo G, Carreira PE, et al. Joint and tendon involvement predict disease progression in systemic sclerosis: a EUSTAR prospective study. Ann Rheum Dis. 2016;75(1):103–9.
76. Elhai M, Guerini H, Bazeli R, Avouac J, Freire V, Drapé JL, et al. Ultrasonographic hand features in systemic sclerosis and correlates with clinical, biologic, and radiographic findings. Arthritis Care Res (Hoboken). 2012;64(8):1244–9.
77. Rodnan GP. The nature of joint involvement in progressive systemic sclerosis (diffuse scleroderma). Ann Intern Med. 1962;56:422–39.
78. Steen VD. Pregnancy in scleroderma. Rheum Dis Clin N Am. 2007;33(2):345–58. vii
79. Steen VD. Pregnancy in women with systemic sclerosis. Obstet Gynecol. 1999;94(1):15–20.
80. Steen VD, Conte C, Day N, Ramsey-Goldman R, Medsger TA Jr. Pregnancy in women with systemic sclerosis. Arthritis Rheum. 1989;32(2):151–7.
81. Doss BJ, Jacques SM, Mayes MD, Qureshi F. Maternal scleroderma: placental findings and perinatal outcome. Hum Pathol. 1998;29(12):1524–30.
82. Ibba-Manneschi L, Manetti M, Milia AF, Miniati I, Benelli G, Guiducci S, et al. Severe fibrotic changes and altered expression of angiogenic factors in maternal scleroderma: placental findings. Ann Rheum Dis. 2010;69(2):458–61.
83. Papakonstantinou K, Hasiakos D, Kondi-Paphiti A. Clinicopathology of maternal scleroderma. Int J Gynaecol Obstet. 2007;99(3):248–9.

14 Inflammation and Immunity in Systemic Sclerosis

Francesco Boin, Armando Gabrielli, and Carlo Chizzolini

T Cells

Histological examination of early SSc-skin lesions demonstrates that an inflammatory infiltrate precedes fibrosis and development of vascular disease, including ultrastructural changes affecting endothelial cells (Fig. 14.1) [1]. Of interest, collagen synthesis determined by in situ localization of procollagen I mRNA appears to be higher in fibroblasts adjacent to inflammatory cells [2, 3]. These findings support the hypothesis that inflammatory cells and in particular T cells can provide important stimuli that drive collagen synthesis in fibroblasts, in addition to the development of abnormalities involving endothelial cells. Cutaneous mononuclear cell infiltrates are notably pronounced early on, during the edematous-inflammatory phase of the disease and then tend to disappear with transition to the sclerotic phase. Consistently, the majority of infiltrating T cells in SSc skin lesions express activation markers and secrete products of activated T cells such as soluble CD25 (the soluble form of the high-affinity IL-2 receptor chain), which have been found in fluid obtained from the suction skin blister of SSc patients with early cutaneous disease [4].

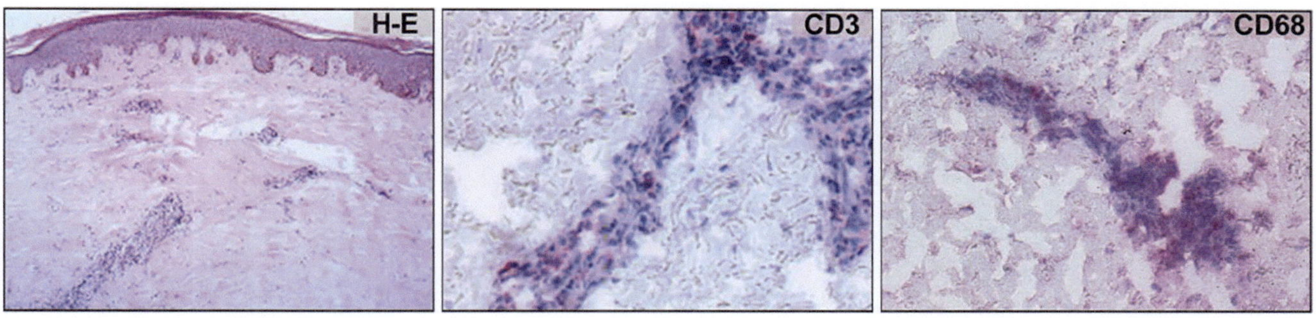

Fig. 14.1 Representative immunohistological analysis of the inflammatory infiltrate characteristic of early skin involvement in SSc. Left panel: (low-magnification) hematoxylin-eosin staining showing thickened dermis with increased collagen deposition and perivascular inflammatory infiltrate. Middle panel: (high-power magnification) T-cell infiltrates identified by anti-CD3 monoclonal antibody. Right panel: (high-power magnification) macrophages are identified by anti-CD68 monoclonal antibody. Of note, some studies have shown by in situ hybridization that type I collagen mRNA is abundantly expressed by fibroblasts present in the dermal region adjacent to the inflammatory infiltrate [2, 3]. This suggests an important pro-fibrotic role of the cells present in the inflammatory infiltrate, including T cells

F. Boin (✉)
Division of Rheumatology, Department of Medicine, Cedars-Sinai Medical Center, Los Angeles, CA, USA
e-mail: francesco.boin@cshs.org

A. Gabrielli
Fondazione di Medicina Molecolare e Terapia Cellulare, Università Politecnica delle Marche, Ancona, Italy
e-mail: a.gabrielli@staff.univpm.it

C. Chizzolini
Department of Pathology and Immunology, Centre Médical Universitaire, Geneva University, Geneva, Switzerland
e-mail: carlo.chizzolini@unige.ch

Y. Allanore et al. (eds.), *Scleroderma*, https://doi.org/10.1007/978-3-031-40658-4_14

Polarized T-Cell Subsets in SSc

T cells are tremendously heterogeneous in terms of T-cell receptor (TcR) expression which determines their antigen specificity and function. They can be classified according to the expression of the accessory molecules expressed in CD4+ helper and CD8+ cytolytic T cellular subsets, the chains composing the TcR (α/β or γ/δ), and the pattern of cytokines produced. CD4+ T helper cells have been categorized into the Th1, Th2, Th9, Th17, Th22, Tregs, T regulatory 1 (Tr1), T follicular helper (TFH), and T peripheral helper (TPH) cells mostly according to the set of cytokines they produce [5, 6]. To a lesser extent, also CD8+ T cells can produce polarized sets of cytokines. Vice versa CD4+ T cells may be endowed with cytolytic functions. Of major importance for the fate determination of T cells is the cytokine milieu where T-cell activation takes place. Major polarizing cytokines and master transcription factors involved in the polarization of Th cells are summarized in Fig. 14.2. Abnormalities in almost all these Th subsets have been described in SSc, with contributing roles to the pathogenic process that vary with time during the disease course. Interestingly, some T-cell subpopulations have been specifically identified in SSc skin and they are represented in Fig. 14.3.

T-Cell Cytokines in Animal Models of Fibrosis

Transcriptome analyses in animal models performed before the identification of Th17 cells have shown that genes involved in wound healing and fibrosis are associated with Th2 polarized responses and are characterized by the production of IL-4, IL-5, IL-13, and IL-21 as opposed to IFNγ. Considerable evidence indicates that type 2 polarized responses are indeed important for fibrosis development [7]. Interestingly, IL-4 and IL-13 have been shown to enhance collagen synthesis by fibroblasts while IFNγ has an inhibitory effect. The in vivo relevance of IL-4 in fibrogenesis has been documented in several animal models including among others TSK-1 mice, where a targeted mutation of the IL-4 receptor α-chain or IL-4 gene can prevent the development of fibrosis. Additional data indicate that IL-13 interaction with the IL-13Rα2 receptor induces in macrophages the pro-

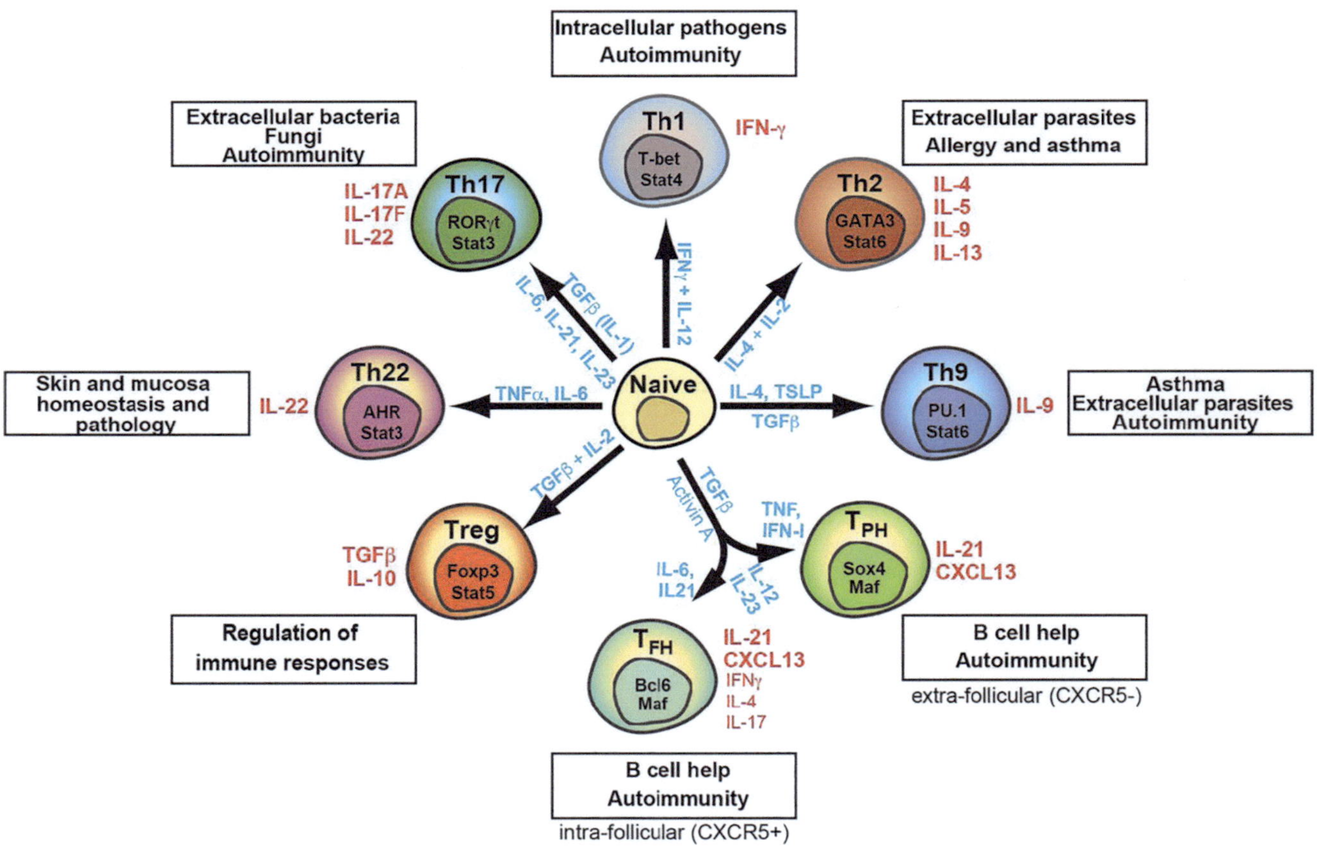

Fig. 14.2 T helper subsets are identified based on the cytokines important for their differentiation from naïve CD4+ T cells (blue), their master transcription factors and key intracellular signaling molecules, their cytokine secretion profile (red), and their prevalent effector function (black boxes). Figure author, Dr. Nicolò C Brembilla. *IFNγ* interferon γ; *TFH* follicular helper T cell; *Th* T helper cell; *TPH* peripheral helper T cell; *Treg* regulatory T cell; *TGF* transforming growth factor; and *TSLP* thymic stroma lymphopoietin

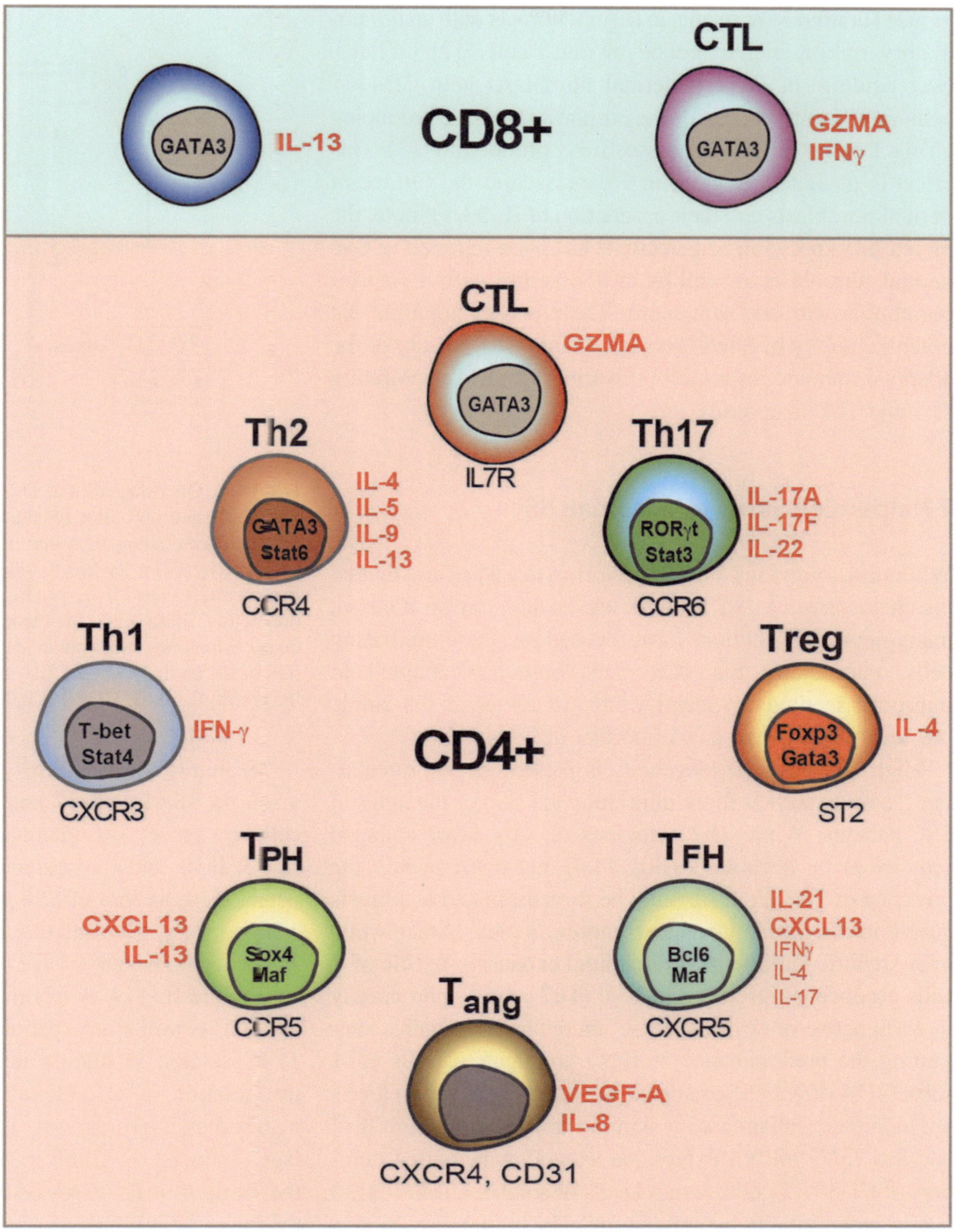

Fig. 14.3 SSc-specific polarized T-cell subsets are identified in the peripheral blood and involved tissues, particularly the skin, of SSc patients. These T cells drive effector functions through the secretion of specific soluble factors (red) and expression of unique surface receptors (black) which mediate selective homing capabilities. Figure author: Dr. Nicolò C Brembilla. *CTL* cytolytic T cells; *GZMA* granzyme-A; *ST2* receptor for IL-33; *Tang* T angiogenic; *TFH* follicular T helper cell; *Th* T helper cell; *TPH* peripheral helper T cell; *Treg* regulatory T cell; *TGF* transforming growth factor; *TSLP* thymic stroma lymphopoietin; and *VEGF-A* vascular endothelial growth factor A

duction of TGFβ and drives enhanced collagen synthesis and fibrosis. Therefore, the dichotomous view of the adaptive immune response condensed in the Th1 and Th2 paradigm can appropriately be translated in the field of fibrosis as Th2/Tc2 cells being profibrotic and Th1/Tc1 cells being antifibrotic. More recently, a predominant role for IL-17A in conjunction with IL-1β has been defined in bleomycin-induced lung fibrosis [8]. Furthermore, Th17-polarized responses mediate lung fibrosis in a model of chronic hypersensitivity and IL-17A deficiency attenuates skin thickness in tight skin-1 (TSK-1/+) mice [9]. Consistently, IL-17 increases TGFβ, CTGF, and collagen production by mouse skin fibroblasts, and promotes collagen production and epithelial–mesenchymal transition in mouse alveolar epithelial cells in a TGFβ-dependent manner [10]. Taking a different approach, dermal fibrosis induced by bleomycin has been assessed in mice deficient or sufficient in STAT-4, a transcription factor whose polymorphism has been associated with autoimmunity including SSc and is important for Th1 polarized responses. Strikingly, STAT-4 deficient mice were protected against bleomycin-induced fibrosis, thus suggesting that the inflammatory response induced by bleomycin could enhance fibrosis through a Th1-like response [11]. It should be noted, however, that the fibrotic reaction observed in response to bleomycin treatment may develop in the absence of functioning T cells, thus an unequivocal interpretation of these results is not at hand. It has been demonstrated recently that Friend leukemia virus integration 1 (Fli1) deficiency in mouse keratinocytes results in dermal fibrosis with an inflammatory infiltrate rich in monocytes and T cells [12]. Of interest, coculture of Fli1+/− dermal fibroblasts with CD4+ T cells significantly increases the proportion of IL-4-producing CD4+ T cells while it suppresses IFNγ production [13]. This effect is mediated by galectin 9 expressed at the surface of dermal fibroblasts and their production of IL-33. Of note, the increased expression of galectin-9 has been reported in SSc dermal fibroblasts as well as in SSc serum with a positive correlation with the skin score. These results highlight the potential ability of SSc fibroblasts to shape the quality of the adaptive immune response by favoring Th2 while inhibiting Th1 and Th17 responses.

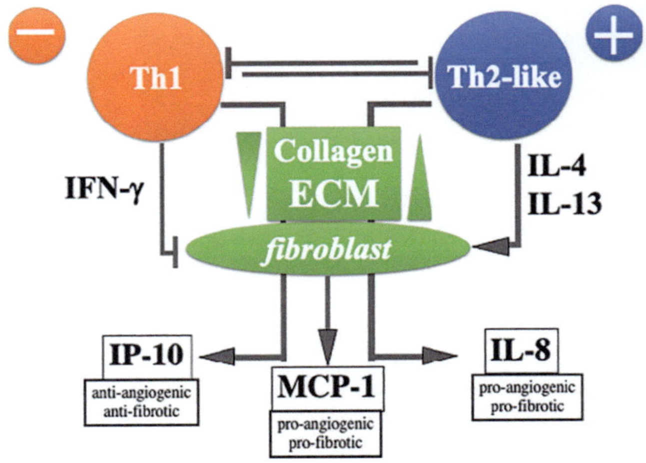

Fig. 14.4 Opposing roles of Th1 and Th2-like cells in respect of ECM deposition and fibroblast inflammatory responses. *Arrows* and *arrowheads* indicate stimulation and *blunted ends* indicate inhibition. IFNγ produced by Th1 cells directly inhibits collagen secretion by fibroblasts. In contrast, IL-4 and IL-13 produced by Th2 cells directly favor collagen production. Illustrated is the capacity of fibroblasts to differentially produce chemokines under polarized stimulation. IFNγ favors the production of the antifibrotic CXCL10 and IL4/IL13 favors the production of the profibrotic IL-8. MCP-1 is induced by both Th1 and Th2 cells

T Helper Cell Subsets in Human SSc

While most previous studies performed in SSc investigated the characteristics of T cells present in the peripheral blood, many novel contributions have focused on tissue infiltrating cells, particularly the skin. This approach coupled to improved methods to identify functionalities at the single cell level is providing new important insights.

High functional heterogeneity is present among circulating T cells as well as those infiltrating the skin or the lungs in SSc patients. While Th2 cytokines directly favor collagen production by fibroblasts (Fig. 14.4) and consequently the presence of Th2-like cells may be directly linked to fibrosis development, the reality appears more complex. In fact, while many reports indicate the preferential expansion in SSc of T cells producing high levels of IL-4 (Th2 subset), particularly in early active or severe disease, there are also studies suggesting the predominance of IFNγ producing T cells (Th1 subset) [14–17]. In SSc patients, IL-4 and IL-13 serum levels are increased; inflammatory skin infiltrates exhibit high IL-4 and low IFNγ mRNA expression as well as increased numbers of CD30+ T cells; serum levels of soluble CD30 (CD30 being preferentially expressed by Th2 cells) are higher. Furthermore, the frequency in the peripheral blood of IL-13-producing CD8+ T cells expressing the GATA3 transcription factor is associated with severity of skin fibrosis, while that of IL-4-producing CD8+ T cells quantitatively predicts a faster decline in lung function [17–19]. In addition, microchimeric T cells of male origin recovered from the blood and skin of SSc-affected women preferentially produce IL-4 [16]. Finally, the enhanced expression of IL-31 by SSc dermal fibroblasts appears to promote increased collagen production as well as the secretion of Th2 cytokines [20]. In contrast, a higher frequency of circulating Th1 cells and increased serum levels of IL-12, a cytokine favoring Th1 cell differentiation, have also been reported in SSc patients [21]. Interestingly, these findings were more evident in subjects at later disease stages when fibrosis tends to regress [22, 23].

Adding to the complexity, consolidated findings indicate a role in SSc for IL-17 and the cytokines promoting Th17 cellular subset differentiation and expansion, including IL-23, IL-6, and IL-1. Increased levels of IL-17 have been detected in the sera of SSc patients. The frequency of Th17 cells appears to be increased in the peripheral blood, skin, and bronchoalveolar lavage fluid from SSc-ILD subjects [24, 25]. While IL-17A is reported to induce IL-6 and IL-8 production, as well as intercellular adhesion molecule 1 (ICAM-1) expression in human fibroblasts, and to enhance their proliferation, it also directly enhances the production of matrix metalloproteinase-1 (MMP-1) and inhibits type I collagen induced by TGFβ in these cells [26, 27]. In addition, the number of IL-17A+ cells inversely correlates with skin thickness [25]. Similarly, Th17 cells expressing CD146 (vascular adhesion molecule) are reported to be increased in SSc and their numbers inversely correlate with the extent of lung fibrosis [28]. Serum levels of semaphorin A4 are elevated and its expression in monocytes and CD4+ cells is increased in SSc patients compared to healthy controls [29]. This regulatory molecule can drive Th17 polarization and IL-17A production, to directly enhance collagen production by dermal fibroblasts. Lastly, using a novel organotypic culture system where human skin is submitted to the influence of profibrotic stimuli, IL-17A is shown to counteract the collagen enhancing effects of TGFβ most likely by inhibiting the Wnt/βcatenin signaling pathway [30]. In aggregate, these findings raise the possibility that at variance with animal models of fibrosis, in humans the increased production of IL-17 conjugates a proinflammatory as well as an antifibrotic effect. In

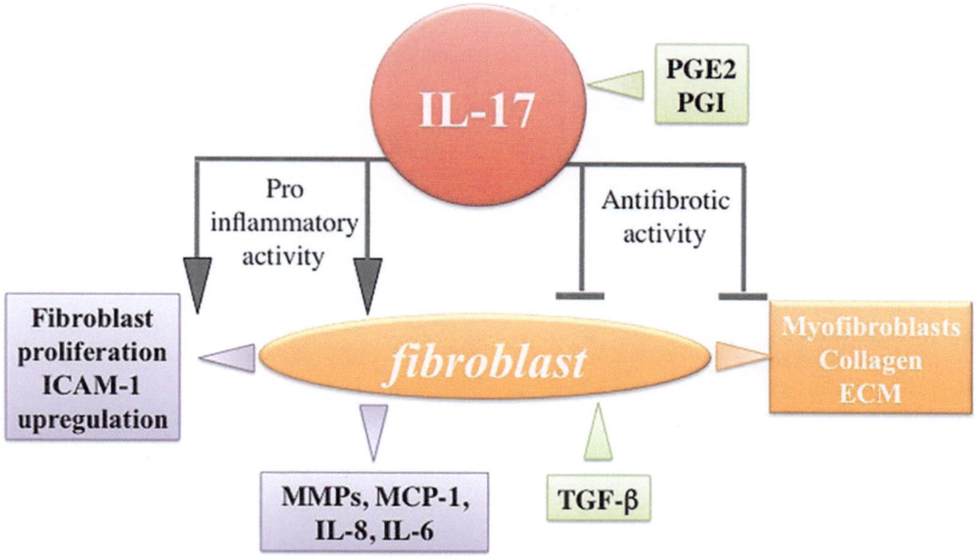

Fig. 14.5 IL-17 exerts a wide array of different functions on human fibroblasts, which may vary according to the context in which they take place. *Arrows* and *arrowheads* indicate stimulation and *blunted-ends* indicate inhibition. *Green boxes*: endogenous and exogenous mediators that modify the context. Thus, PGE2 and PGI enhance IL-17 production by Th17. The anti-fibrotic potential of IL-17A is illustrated by the capacity of this cytokine to inhibit the profibrotic activity of TGFβ

this respect, it is worth mentioning that prostanoids currently used to treat SSc vasculopathy, including prostaglandin I2 (PGI2), increase in vivo the number of Th17 cells, thus implying their additional ability to specifically modulate key features of the profibrotic inflammatory response in SSc [31]. An integrated view of IL-17 function and its modulatory effect on the fibrotic process are shown in Fig. 14.5.

Increased frequency of Th22 cells has also been reported in SSc and IL-22 has shown the ability to enhance fibroblast responses to other inflammatory cytokines [32–34].

Fibroblasts carry CD40 on their surface and can respond upon engagement with its ligand CD40L (CD154) expressed on activated T cells. Interestingly, CD40 is upregulated on SSc fibroblasts, and T cells from SSc patients exhibit a higher expression of CD40L. In addition, serum levels of both soluble CD40 and CD40L molecules are increased in SSc [35]. All these findings, together with the fact that blockade of the CD40-CD40L interaction attenuates fibrosis in the TSK-1 mouse model, indicate a possible role for this biologic axis in fibrogenesis [36].

T Follicular Helper Cells in SSc

T follicular helper (TFH) cells are characterized by the expression of CXCR5 which allows their recruitment into lymphoid follicles in response to CXCL13 as well as of the inducible T-cell co-stimulator (ICOS or CD278) and the inhibitory molecule programmed death-1 (PD1). These cells can secrete different cytokines including IFNγ, IL-4, and IL-17A, but most distinctly they produce IL-21. TFH cells are increased in SSc peripheral blood and in the skin where their number correlates with the extent of skin fibrosis. They present an activated phenotype, with high expression of Bcl-6, increased capacity to produce IL-21, and higher capacity to stimulate the differentiation of CD19+CD27+CD38hi B cells and their secretion of IgG and IgM through the IL-21 pathway compared to healthy controls. In a murine model of sclerodermatous graft vs host disease (sGVHD), the blockade of IL-21 or of inducible T-cell co-stimulator ICOS resulted in decreased skin fibrosis establishing a link between TFH cells and the underlying immune-mediated fibrotic reaction [37, 38].

Of major interest, a study based on single cell RNAseq has identified eight distinct T-cell clusters, of which one uniquely present in the skin of SSc patients compared to healthy controls [39]. This CD4+ T-cell subset is characterized by the expression of CXCL13 and secretion of IL-21 in addition to a gene expression signature recapitulating the phenotype of the recently identified peripheral T helper subset (TPH), which appears to be poised to promote B-cell responses within the inflamed skin of SSc patients (Fig. 14.3) [40].

Cytotoxic CD4+ and CD8+ T Cells in SSc

Under certain conditions CD4+ T cells may exhibit cytotoxic capabilities. Limited but intriguing evidence, obtained by employing a novel quantitative microscopy-based image analysis to visualize and measure all major CD4+T cell subsets in the skin of untreated patients with early dcSSc, suggests that activated CD4+ T cells with the cytolytic function are clonally expanded in SSc skin in association with tissue damage [41]. Interestingly, these cytotoxic T cells were able to target directly endothelial cells, driving apoptosis. This study showed that the majority of skin-infiltrating T cells belong to this CD4+ cytolytic subset. Other studies have shown that infiltrating, perivascular CD8+ T

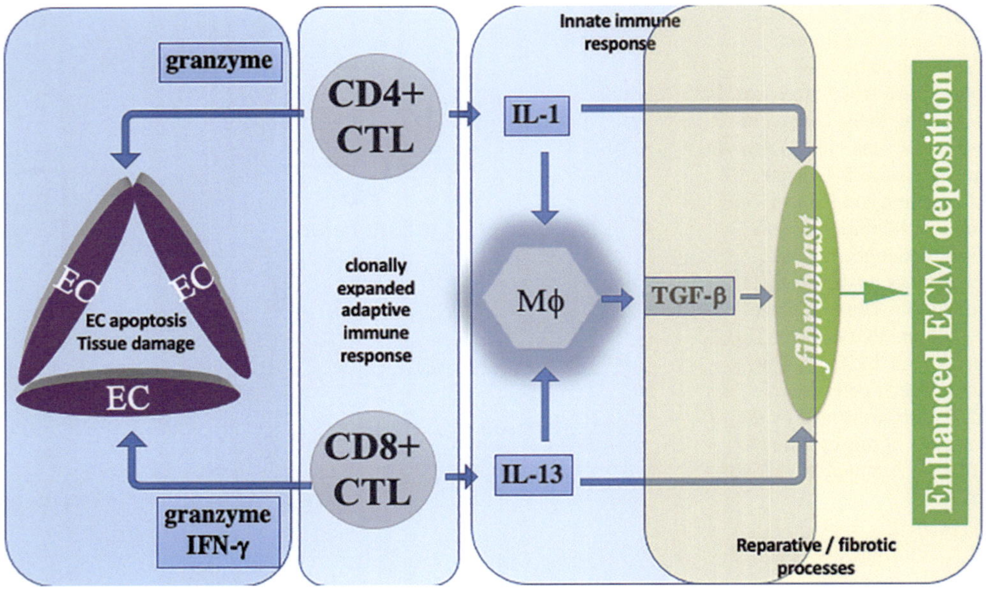

Fig. 14.6 Role of cytotoxic T cells in SSc. Cytolytic CD4+ and CD8+ T cells may participate in the pathophysiology of vasculopathy and fibrosis in SSc. The partially overlapping rectangles represent distinct pathophysiologic events. CTL, cytolytic; EC, endothelial cells; ECM, extracellular matrix; IFNγ, interferon-gamma; IL, interleukin; MØ, macrophage; TGFβ, transforming growth factor-beta

cells present in SSc dermis express abnormal levels of CD226 (also known as DNAM-1) with enhanced cytolytic activity against endothelial cells and a preferential production of IL-13 [42]. Therefore, both these studies on cytolytic T cells highlight the possible direct connection between adaptive immune responses and SSc vasculopathy (Figs. 14.3, 14.4, 14.5, and 14.6).

Angiogenetic T Cells in SSc

A T-cell subset with documented capacity to drive angiogenesis has been described almost a decade ago and named Tang. Tang cells, characterized by the surface expression of CD31 and CXCR4, produce VEGF and G-CSF, driving enhanced endothelial cell proliferation and activation (Fig. 14.5). Two distinct groups have shown that Tang is expanded in the circulation of SSc patients with severe peripheral vascular complications including "late" nailfold capillary patterns, digital ulcers, and pulmonary artery hypertension. Proportion of circulating Tang was also positively associated with VEGF levels [43, 44]. These observations suggest that Tang may be involved in reparative vascular processes in SSc.

Regulatory T Cells

Regulatory T cells (Tregs) are thought to be critical in maintaining immunologic self-tolerance and preventing autoimmunity. Their ability to limit potentially dangerous immune responses and to regulate the function of other T cells is exerted by a variety of mechanisms including the production of immunosuppressive cytokines (TGFβ, IL-10, IL-35), the inhibition by contact via surface molecules such as CTLA-4, the depletion of IL-2, or the expression of enzymes such as indoleamine 2,3-deoxygenase, which by reducing the availability of the essential amino acid tryptophan drives potent anti-proliferative effects [45]. At least two main subsets of Tregs are recognized: the natural Tregs (nTreg) and the inducible Tregs (iTreg). nTregs are CD4+ T cells generated in the thymus during the process of negative selection which allows the retention of cells bearing TcR with an intermediate affinity for self-antigens in association with a developmental program leading to a regulatory phenotype [46]. iTregs develop from naïve, mature CD4+ T cells after encountering their nominal antigen within secondary lymphoid organs in the presence of TGFβ and high levels of IL-2. Markers used for their identification include the intracellular expression of the transcription factor FoxP3, the high surface expression of CD25, the combination of CD45 isoforms with the above molecules, and the decreased expression of CD127 as well as the decreased expression of CD49d [47]. In humans, the phenotypic and functional identification of Treg is still imprecisely defined, explaining in part the inconsistencies of study results reported in SSc. Some authors have found that while the number of Tregs is increased in all clinical SSc phenotypes, these Tregs exhibit a diminished capacity to control CD4 T-cell effector function [48]. Furthermore, this defective function seems to correlate with lower expression of CD69 and TGFβ. Others have found a quantitative reduction of Tregs in the skin and peripheral blood of affected patients [33, 49]. Mathian et al. have reported that "activated" Treg (CD4 CD45RA − FoxP3brightCD25bright) are decreased in SSc patients at any disease stage, while "resting" Treg (CD4 CD45RA + FOXP3 + CD25+) frequency declines in late phases of SSc [33]. Their data also show that both subsets retain an intact suppressive function, supporting the possibility that activation and proliferation of autoreactive T cells may be driven by the overall quantitative Tregs deficit. A small prospective study conducted in seven SSc patients with diffuse skin phenotype has found that depressed Treg number and function can be restored after autologous hematopoietic stem cell transplantation [50]. Aberrant epigenetic modifications such as hypermethylation of FoxP3 gene detected in SSc Tregs indicated as a possible cause for decreased FoxP3 expression and lower circulating levels of this cell type [51]. Further, lower FoxP3 expression and less efficient suppressor activity in CD25+ high Treg cells have been associated with skewed X chromosome inactivation patterns in SSc [52]. An intriguing twist to the understanding of Tregs function in SSc has been brought by the demonstration that FoxP3-positive cells with high IL-4 and IL-13 production are enriched in the skin of SSc patients compared to normal controls [53]. The authors concluded that these FoxP3+ T cells may indeed be Tregs with a functional Th2-like phenotype, able to enhance profibrotic responses in dermal fibroblasts. Of interest, this study also found that skin-infiltrating FoxP3+ T cells express high levels of the IL-33 receptor ST2 and that the number of IL-13-producing FoxP3+ T cells is increased by culturing SSc skin biopsies in the presence of IL-33. This, together with the fact that only skin but not peripheral blood FoxP3+ T cells manifested this aberrant Th2-like behavior, further supports the possibility that in SSc patients the skin provides the appropriate environment for trans differentiation of Tregs toward an effector Th2-like phenotype with the consequent amplification of a pro-fibrotic loop. In mice, studies have shown that skin homing Tregs already express Th2-related genes, notably GATA3, the Th2 master transcription factor (Fig. 14.5). These Tregs that co-express FoxP3 and GATA3 exert a direct control over fibroblast activation and their reduction results in overt skin fibrosis. Interestingly, their deficiency is also associated with enhanced IL-13 and IL-4 production by skin residing Th2 cells [54]. While these results strongly support a direct role of skin-tissue-resident T cells in controlling fibrosis, confirmation in human studies will be needed to establish their relevance.

Molecules with inhibitory properties contribute to regulate and balance adaptive immune responses, thus limiting pathogenic immune activation and tissue damage. Their chronic expression and upregulation have been linked to the concept of T-cell exhaustion, which is characterized by aberrant cellular functions including loss of effector activity. Programmed death-1 (PD-1) and its ligands PDL1 and PDL2, as well as CTLA-4, TIGIT (T-cell immunoglobulin and ITIM domain), LAG3 (lymphocyte activation gene 3), and TIM3 (T-cell immunoglobulin and mucin domain 3) are part of this system. Limited but important evidence suggests that in SSc, CD4+ T cells (including Tregs) show increased expression of PD1 and TIGIT compared to healthy subjects and that the blockade of this molecule significantly impacts disease-specific T-cell cytokine production [55]. Soluble forms of PD1 and its ligands are increased in SSc serum and correlate with the extent of skin fibrosis [56]. In mouse models of fibrosis, the blockade of PD1 has favorable effects on the disease course [57]. Thus, it is possible to hypothesize that PD1 expression and activity may be associated with profibrotic T-cell responses and that its careful inhibition can be considered to achieve therapeutic benefit in SSc. Notably, the use in cancer patients of nivolumab and pembrolizumab (which block the PD1-PD1R interaction) has been associated with the development of scleroderma [58].

Autoantigen-Specific T-Cell Responses in SSc

The detection of expanded oligoclonal T-cell subsets in affected skin, lungs (BALF), and blood of SSc patients supports the notion that an antigen-driven, T-cell-dependent process may be involved in SSc pathogenesis [41, 59–61]. Along similar lines, high-throughput sequencing of CD4+ and CD8+ TCRβ chains on longitudinal samples obtained from four SSc patients has shown that CD4+ and CD8+ T cells are highly persistent in SSc patients over time, and that this persistence likely results from antigenic selection [62].

T cells recognizing SSc-specific autoantigens such as topoisomerase-1 (Topo-1) or RNA polymerase III (RNApol3) have been documented in SSc [63–68]. A close temporal association between the onset of SSc and the detection of cancer has been described in a subset of patients positive for anti-RNA polymerase III antibodies [69]. This observation led to the discovery that mutated autoantigens (RNApol3) are expressed in the tumors obtained from these patients and that these drive mutant-specific T-cell immune responses as well as production of cross-reactive autoantibodies [70]. These findings support the possibility that, at least in some patients, an abnormal (mutated) cancer antigen may be the initial trigger for an autoimmune T-cell activation in SSc. Animal models have also been used to test whether the generation of autoimmune responses against known SSc autoantigen (i.e., Topo-1) could drive a pathological phenotype resembling SSc. The immunization of mice prone to autoimmunity with human recombinant Topo-1 can induce protein-specific T-cell responses and antibodies, but do not drive any SSc clinical or pathologic features [71]. In contrast, when C57BL/6 mice are repeatedly immunized with human Topo-1 in the presence of complete Freund's adjuvant, skin and lung fibroses in addition to autoimmune manifestations can be generated [72]. Of interest, these pathologic manifestations are associated with increased production of IL-6 and IL-17 as well as higher levels of circulating Th17 cells. This report indicates that besides an autoimmune background, a second trigger may be needed to drive the immune response toward a pro-fibrotic process, such as the one provided by repeated stimulation of the innate immune system by complete Freund's adjuvant.

The observation that a higher proportion of SSc women compared to healthy controls have circulating male cells and that these can be found particularly in tissues undergoing fibrosis, suggests the possibility that alloantigens may be driving pathogenetic immune responses in SSc [73, 74]. The hypothesis that microchimerism may be mechanistically relevant in SSc has also been supported by the close similarity between fibrotic skin lesions observed in SSc and chronic graft-versus-host disease (GVHD), a known condition of chimerism developing after allogeneic bone marrow transplantation. In fact, murine models of fibrosis have been developed based on chimerism and GVHD [75]. An interesting interaction between exposure to vinyl chloride (an agent that increases the risk of developing human SSc) and multiple pregnancies in murine models results in enhanced scleroderma associated with increased microchimerism [76].

Overall, these data support the concept that T cells upon nominal antigen recognition may initiate an inflammatory process ultimately resulting in tissue fibrosis. It remains however possible that T cells may be only activated bystanders with functional characteristics depending on and not causing the underlying disease process. Furthermore, the possibility that T cells, at least in certain phases of the disease, may restrain rather than favor fibrosis cannot be disregarded.

B Cells

The participation of B cells to the immune response is not exclusively mediated by antibody production but includes other key activities such as antigen presentation, cytokine secretion, modulation of T cell, and dendritic cell activation (Fig. 14.7) [77]. B-cell responses are mainly determined by signaling thresholds through the B-cell receptor (BcR) complex and are regulated by specific cell surface and cytoplasmic molecules. These "response regulators" concurrently contribute to the amplification (i.e., CD19, CD21, CD45) or suppression (i.e., CD22, CD72, FcγRIIB) of the BcR signal and modulate the resulting B-cell activity.

Several genome-wide association studies (GWAS) have identified multiple B-cell genes associated with increased susceptibility for SSc, including BANK1, BLK, CSK, PTPN22, CD19, and IRF8 [78, 79]. A single nucleotide polymorphism (SNP) in the upstream region of CD19 gene is associated with higher expression of this molecule in circulating B cells and the loss of CD19 expression attenuates skin and lung fibrosis in the bleomycin-induced SSc mouse model [80]. Increased proportions of polyreactive as well as autoantigen-reactive emigrant/transitional B cells have been found in SSc, indicating that defective central and peripheral B-cell tolerance checkpoints can drive the accumulation of

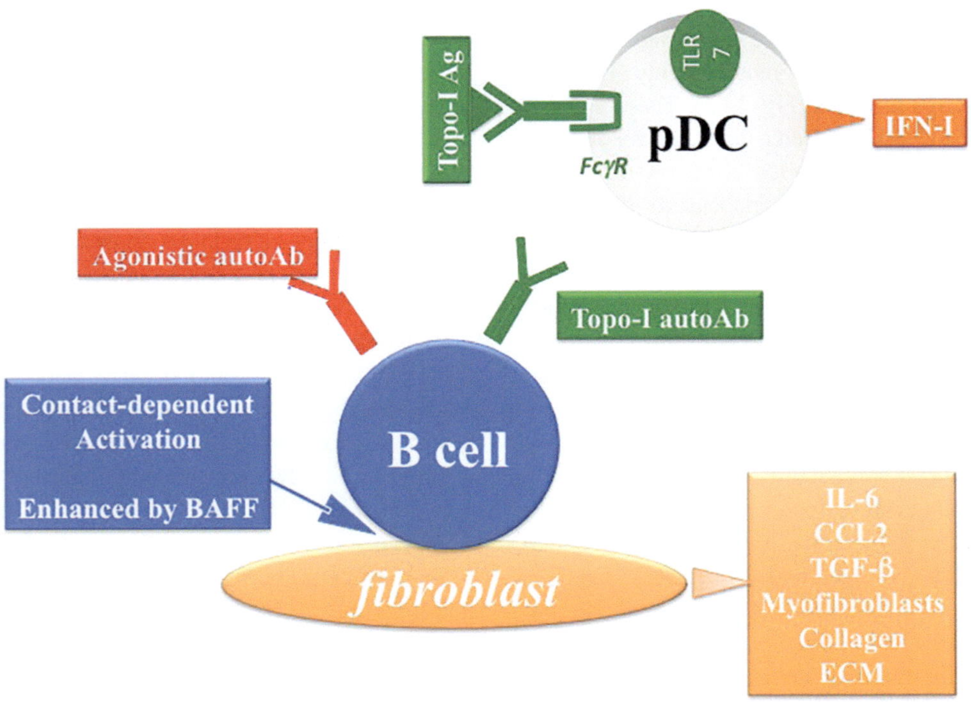

Fig. 14.7 B cells play multiple roles in systemic sclerosis. Autoantibody directed against ubiquitous autoantigens (green) may form immune complexes, which may be captured by pDC through Fcg-receptors, internalized in endosomal compartments where they may interact with TLR and induce an interferon response. Autoantibodies (red) against surface receptors such as TLR, endothelin-1 receptors, and angiotensin-receptors may display agonistic activity resulting in the activation of cells bearing such receptors. B cells may directly interact with fibroblasts in a cell–cell dependent manner and favor pro-fibrotic responses augmented by BAFF. The capacity of B cells to produce regulatory IL-10, a property decreased in SSc, is not here represented

autoreactive cells [81]. Affected SSc skin demonstrates prominent B-cell infiltration, with upregulation of B cell and plasma cell gene signatures correlating with the severity of mRSS [82–85]. Of note, B-cell infiltrates are also more pronounced in early diffuse skin lesions and in association with progressive skin fibrosis [86]. Analysis of circulating B-cell repertoire in SSc patients indicates the expansion of the (CD27−) naïve B-cell subset and the concurrent decline of memory B-cell and plasmacellular components [84, 87]. Interestingly, the expression of positive B-cell response regulators such as CD19 and the associated molecule CD21 (complement receptor type 2) is increased in both subsets, while that of CD22 is decreased, supporting the possibility that an abnormal balance between stimulatory and inhibitory receptors could contribute to aberrant B-cell activation in SSc [84, 88, 89]. Mavroupolos et al. report that in SSc patients both CD19 + CD24highCD38high immature/transitional B cells and CD19 + CD24highCD27+ memory B cells are significantly decreased and functionally impaired, to a greater extent in dcSSc and ILD patients [90]. These cellular subsets are also identified as B regulatory cell (Bregs) and exhibit the ability of suppressing inflammatory responses through robust IL-10 secretion. Aravena et al. have found that most IL-10 producing Bregs express T-cell Ig and mucin domain protein 1 (TIM-1) and that this subset is significantly decreased in SSc patients, exhibiting impaired suppressive function compared to healthy individuals [91]. Bregs levels correlate negatively with anti-topo I and anti-centromere antibody titers. In addition, Breg counts are lower in the most severe forms of the disease and increase significantly in dcSSc patients after treatment [90, 92]. Other two studies have confirmed a lower frequency of circulating memory B cells in SSc patients, but also have reported that, compared to healthy individuals, these cells are activated (i.e., upregulation of CD95, CD69, CD86), secrete proinflammatory (IL-6) and profibrotic (TGFβ) cytokines, and produce less IL-10 [87, 93]. Recent investigations have addressed the presence in SSc of the so-called ABC (age-associated B cells or autoimmune-associated B cells), also dubbed by the acronym of Double Negative (DN) B cells based on the joint negativity of IgD and CD27 on the surface of CD19+ B cells. Evidence is provided that the CD19 + CD21lo/neg subset of these DN B cells is expanded on SSc-ILD and infiltrates affected lung parenchyma [94]. DN B cells also exhibit an exquisite sensitivity to TLR7 activation and may play important roles the production of autoantibodies as well as proinflammatory cytokines [95].

Few studies have addressed the ability of B cells to activate dermal fibroblasts. Francois et al. demonstrated that peripheral blood B cells can stimulate IL-6, TGFβ, CCL2, and collagen secretion, as well as α-SMA, TIMP1, and MMP9 expression in dermal fibroblasts isolated from SSc patients [96]. Importantly, this induction was dependent on cell–cell contact and the addition of BAFF to these cocultures enhanced fibroblast activation. The role of BAFF, in conjunction with IL-17, in favoring fibrosis development, has been documented also in a model of bleomycin-induced SSc lung disease [96]. Some of these findings have been confirmed by Dumoitier et al. showing that the supernatant of SSc B cells stimulated with CpG- (TLR9 ligand) significantly enhances activation and phenotypic switch into myofibroblasts of fibroblasts from both healthy controls and involved SSc skin [93].

A proliferation-inducing ligand (APRIL) and B-cell activating factor (BAFF) are members of the tumor necrosis factor (TNF) superfamily exerting important homeostatic functions on B cells such as maturation, activation, and survival (anti-apoptotic) [97]. Serum levels of BAFF and APRIL are increased in SSc patients compared to controls and are associated with extent of skin involvement (BAFF) and the presence of pulmonary fibrosis (APRIL) [98, 99]. Secretion of APRIL from PBMCs is significantly higher in SSc patients compared to controls and is associated with diffuse skin phenotype, presence of ILD, and anti-Topo-1 positivity [100]. Interestingly, BAFF serum levels are increased in the tight-skin (TSK/+) mouse, and blockade of the BAFF/BAFF-receptor interaction can prevent the development of skin fibrosis, inhibit autoantibody generation, and increase the production of anti-fibrotic cytokines (i.e., IFNγ) [101]. BAFF expression enhances the production of IL-6 but decreases that of IL-10 from B cells inhibition, and its inhibition in the bleomycin-induced SSc mouse model results in the attenuation of skin and lung fibrosis [102]. All these data indicate that B-cell activation and overactivity are important features of the immune response in SSc and that an imbalance of B-cell homeostasis and function may contribute to the amplification of the inflammatory as well as fibrotic process in this disease. This hypothesis is supported in part by recent data indicating some clinical benefit from CD20+ B-cell depletion (rituximab) in SSc patients [103–105].

Concluding Remarks

The immune system and its tightly intertwined inflammatory response are deeply involved in the pathophysiological processes underlying SSc. An abnormal immune activation involving humoral as well as cellular immune adaptive events appears to be a fundamental step both for disease initiation as well as disease amplification. The perturbed function of adaptive immune effectors contribute significantly to the disease process. We have learned that T helper cells exhibit a skewed functional repertoire, which may vary along disease progression. While type 2 responses may contribute to the development of fibrosis in SSc with the expansion of the ILC2/Th2/Tc2 cell differentiation programs, experimental evidence based on single cell RNAseq technology indicates that unique T-cell subsets are present in SSc skin, with features and effector phenotype distinguishing SSc from other SADs. Specific autoantibodies detected in SSc exhibit agonistic activities on fibroblasts and endothelial cells, which by far exceed their role as markers of disease. Finally, adding to the knowledge that T cells with restricted T-cell receptor (TcR) usage are present and persist in blood, skin, and lungs of SSc patients, indicating an antigen-driven process, new studies provide evidence that cancer immunoediting may be a possible mechanism leading to loss of tolerance to self-antigens. The complex and pleiotropic nature of the immune response in SSc constitutes a great challenge. The identification of SSc-specific cellular and molecular immune effectors not only can shed new light on SSc pathogenesis but also can provide new rationale to develop more selective and effective therapeutic strategies. Admittedly, a major gap still exists between the pace of the scientific advancement and its clinical application. The integration of "omics" approaches with sophisticated system biology analyses will hopefully contribute to the refinement of our understanding of key mechanisms underpinning SSc pathogenesis and support the development of therapeutic interventions directed to patient subsets exhibiting greater biological affinity and targeting disease-specific pathogenetic mechanisms.

References

1. Prescott RJ, Freemont AJ, Jones CJ, Hoyland J, Fielding P. Sequential dermal microvascular and perivascular changes in the development of scleroderma. J Pathol. 1992;166:255–63.
2. Kahari VM, Sandberg M, Kalimo H, Vuorio T, Vuorio E. Identification of fibroblasts responsible for increased collagen production in localized scleroderma by in situ hybridization. J Invest Dermatol. 1988;90:664–70.
3. Scharffetter K, Lankat-Buttgereit B, Krieg T. Localization of collagen mRNA in normal and scleroderma skin by in-situ hybridization. Eur J Clin Investig. 1988;18:9–17.
4. Sondergaard K, Stengaard-Pedersen K, Zachariae H, Heickendorff L, Deleuran M, Deleuran B. Soluble intercellular adhesion molecule-1 (sICAM-1) and soluble interleukin-2 receptors (sIL-2R) in scleroderma skin. Br J Rheumatol. 1998;37:304–10.
5. Zhu J, Paul WE. CD4 T cells: fates, functions, and faults. Blood. 2008;112:1557–69.
6. Zhu X, Zhu J. CD4 T Helper Cell Subsets and Related Human Immunological Disorders. Int J Mol Sci. 2020;21:1–26.
7. Wynn TA. Fibrotic disease and the T(H)1/T(H)2 paradigm. Nat Rev Immunol. 2004;4:583–94.
8. Wilson MS, Madala SK, Ramalingam TR, Gochuico BR, Rosas IO, Cheever AW, et al. Bleomycin and IL-1beta-mediated pulmonary fibrosis is IL-17A dependent. J Exp Med. 2010;207:535–52.
9. Okamoto Y, Hasegawa M, Matsushita T, Hamaguchi Y, Huu DL, Iwakura Y, et al. Potential roles of interleukin-17A in the development of skin fibrosis in mice. Arthritis Rheum. 2012;64:3726–35.
10. Mi S, Li Z, Yang HZ, Liu H, Wang JP, Ma YG, et al. Blocking IL-17A promotes the resolution of pulmonary inflammation and fibrosis via TGF-beta1-dependent and -independent mechanisms. J Immunol. 2011;187:3003–14.
11. Avouac J, Fürnrohr BG, Tomcik M, Palumbo K, Zerr P, Horn A, et al. Inactivation of the transcription factor STAT-4 prevents inflammation-driven fibrosis in animal models of systemic sclerosis. Arthritis Rheum. 2011;63:800–9.
12. Takahashi T, Asano Y, Sugawara K, Yamashita T, Nakamura K, Saigusa R, et al. Epithelial Fli1 deficiency drives systemic autoimmunity and fibrosis: possible roles in scleroderma. J Exp Med. 2017;214:1129–51.
13. Saigusa R, Asano Y, Taniguchi T, Hirabayashi M, Nakamura K, Miura S, et al. Fli1-haploinsufficient dermal fibroblasts promote skin-localized transdifferentiation of Th2-like regulatory T cells. Arthritis Res Ther. 2018;20:1–11.
14. Mavalia C, Scaletti C, Romagnani P, Carossino AM, Pignone A, Emmi L, et al. Type 2 helper T-cell predominance and high CD30 expression in systemic sclerosis. Am J Pathol. 1997;151:1751–8.
15. Atamas SP, Yurovsky V, Wise R, Wigley FM, Goter Robinson CJ, Henry P, et al. Production of type 2 cytokines by CD8+ lung cells is associated with greater decline in pulmonary function in patients with systemic sclerosis. Arthritis Rheum. 1999;42:1168–78.
16. Scaletti C, Vultaggio A, Bonifacio S, Emmi L, Torricelli F, Maggi E, et al. Th2-oriented profile of male offspring T cells present in women with systemic sclerosis and reactive with maternal major histocompatibility complex antigens. Arthritis Rheum. 2002;46:445–50.
17. Parel Y, Aurrand-Lions M, Scheja A, Dayer JM, Roosnek E, Chizzolini C. Presence of CD4+CD8+ double-positive T cells with very high interleukin-4 production potential in lesional skin of patients with systemic sclerosis. Arthritis Rheum. 2007;56:3459–67.
18. Fuschiotti P, Larregina AT, Ho J, Feghali-Bostwick C, Medsger TA Jr. Interleukin-13-producing CD8+ T cells mediate dermal fibrosis in patients with systemic sclerosis. Arthritis Rheum. 2013;65:236–46.
19. Cascio S, Medsger TA, Hawse WF, Watkins SC, Milcarek C, Moreland LW, et al. 14-3-3z sequesters cytosolic T-bet, upregulating IL-13 levels in T C 2 and CD8 + lymphocytes from patients with scleroderma. J Allergy Clin Immunol. 2018;142:109–119.e6.
20. Kuzumi A, Yoshizaki A, Matsuda KM, Kotani H, Norimatsu Y, Fukayama M, et al. Interleukin-31 promotes fibrosis and T helper 2 polarization in systemic sclerosis. Nat Commun. 2021:12.
21. Sato S, Hanakawa H, Hasegawa M, Nagaoka T, Hamaguchi Y, Nishijima C, et al. Levels of interleukin 12, a cytokine of type 1 helper T cells, are elevated in sera from patients with systemic sclerosis. J Rheumatol. 2000;27:2838–42.
22. Valentini G, Baroni A, Esposito K, Naclerio C, Buommino E, Farzati A, et al. Peripheral blood T lymphocytes from systemic sclerosis patients show both Th1 and Th2 activation. J Clin Immunol. 2001;21:210–7.
23. Matsushita T, Hasegawa M, Hamaguchi Y, Takehara K, Sato S. Longitudinal analysis of serum cytokine concentrations in systemic sclerosis: association of interleukin 12 elevation with spontaneous regression of skin sclerosis. J Rheumatol. 2006;33:275–84.
24. Radstake TR, van Bon L, Broen J, Wenink M, Santegoets K, Deng Y, et al. Increased frequency and compromised function of T regulatory cells in systemic sclerosis (SSc) is related to a diminished CD69 and TGFbeta expression. PLoS One. 2009;4:e5981.
25. Truchetet ME, Brembilla NC, Montanari E, Lonati P, Raschi E, Zeni S, et al. Interleukin-17A+ Cell Counts Are Increased in Systemic Sclerosis Skin and Their Number Is Inversely Correlated With the Extent of Skin Involvement. Arthritis Rheum. 2013;65:1347–56.
26. Kurasawa K, Hirose K, Sano H, Endo H, Shinkai H, Nawata Y, et al. Increased interleukin-17 production in patients with systemic sclerosis. Arthritis Rheum. 2000;43:2455–63.
27. Nakashima T, Jinnin M, Yamane K, Honda N, Kajihara I, Makino T, et al. Impaired IL-17 Signaling Pathway Contributes to the

Increased Collagen Expression in Scleroderma Fibroblasts. J Immunol. 2012;188:3573–83.
28. Gabsi A, Heim X, Dlala A, Gati A, Sakhri H, Abidi A, et al. TH17 cells expressing CD146 are significantly increased in patients with Systemic sclerosis. Sci Rep. 2019;9:1–8.
29. Carvalheiro T, Affandi AJ, Malvar-Fernández B, Dullemond I, Cossu M, Ottria A, et al. Induction of inflammation and fibrosis by semaphorin 4A in systemic sclerosis. Arthritis Rheumatol. 2019;71:1711–22.
30. Dufour AM, Borowczyk-Michalowska J, Alvarez M, Truchetet ME, Modarressi A, Brembilla NC, et al. IL-17A dissociates inflammation from fibrogenesis in systemic sclerosis. J Investig Dermatol. 2020;140:103–112.e8.
31. Truchetet ME, Allanore Y, Montanari E, Chizzolini C, Brembilla NC. Prostaglandin I2 analogues enhance already exuberant Th17 cell responses in systemic sclerosis. Ann Rheum Dis. 2012;71:2044–50.
32. Truchetet ME, Brembilla NC, Montanari E, Allanore Y, Chizzolini C. Increased frequency of circulating Th22 in addition to Th17 and Th2 lymphocytes in systemic sclerosis: association with interstitial lung disease. Arthritis Res Ther. 2011;13:R166.
33. Mathian A, Parizot C, Dorgham K, Trad S, Arnaud L, Larsen M, et al. Activated and resting regulatory T cell exhaustion concurs with high levels of interleukin-22 expression in systemic sclerosis lesions. Ann Rheum Dis. 2012;71:1227–34.
34. Brembilla NC, Dufour AM, Alvarez M, Hugues S, Montanari E, Truchetet ME, et al. IL-22 capacitates dermal fibroblast responses to TNF in scleroderma. Ann Rheum Dis. 2016;75:1697–705.
35. Fukasawa C, Kawaguchi Y, Harigai M, Sugiura T, Takagi K, Kawamoto M, et al. Increased CD40 expression in skin fibroblasts from patients with systemic sclerosis (SSc): role of CD40-CD154 in the phenotype of SSc fibroblasts. Eur J Immunol. 2003;33:2792–800.
36. Komura K, Fujimoto M, Hasegawa M, Ogawa F, Hara T, Muroi E, et al. Increased serum interleukin 23 in patients with systemic sclerosis. J Rheumatol. 2008;35:120–5.
37. Ricard L, Jachiet V, Malard F, Ye Y, Stocker N, Rivière S, et al. Circulating follicular helper T cells are increased in systemic sclerosis and promote plasmablast differentiation through the IL-21 pathway which can be inhibited by ruxolitinib. Ann Rheum Dis. 2019;78:539–50.
38. Taylor DK, Mittereder N, Kuta E, Delaney T, Burwell T, Dacosta K, et al. T follicular helper-like cells contribute to skin fibrosis. Sci Transl Med. 2018:10.
39. Gaydosik AM, Tabib T, Domsic R, Khanna D, Lafyatis R, Fuschiotti P. Single-cell transcriptome analysis identifies skin-specific T-cell responses in systemic sclerosis. Ann Rheum Dis. 2021;80:1453.
40. Rao DA, Gurish MF, Marshall JL, Slowikowski K, Fonseka CY, Liu Y, et al. Pathologically expanded peripheral T helper cell subset drives B cells in rheumatoid arthritis. Nature. 2017;542:110–4.
41. Maehara T, Kaneko N, Perugino CA, Mattoo H, Kers J, Allard-Chamard H, et al. Cytotoxic CD4+ T lymphocytes may induce endothelial cell apoptosis in systemic sclerosis. J Clin Invest. 2020;130:2451–64.
42. Ayano M, Tsukamoto H, Kohno K, Ueda N, Tanaka A, Mitoma H, et al. Increased CD226 expression on CD8 + T cells is associated with upregulated cytokine production and endothelial cell injury in patients with systemic sclerosis. J Immunol. 2015;195:892–900.
43. Manetti M, Pratesi S, Romano E, Bellando-Randone S, Rosa I, Guiducci S, et al. Angiogenic T cell expansion correlates with severity of peripheral vascular damage in systemic sclerosis. PLoS One. 2017;12:e0183102.
44. Lv T, Yang F, Zhang K, Lv M, Zhang Y, Zhu P. The risk of circulating angiogenic T cells and subsets in patients with systemic sclerosis. Int Immunopharmacol. 2020;81:106282.
45. Sakaguchi S, Miyara M, Costantino CM, Hafler DA. FOXP3+ regulatory T cells in the human immune system. Nat Rev Immunol. 2010;10:490–500.
46. Ohkura N, Kitagawa Y, Sakaguchi S. Development and maintenance of regulatory T cells. Immunity. 2013;38:414–23.
47. Frantz C, Auffray C, Avouac J, Allanore Y. Regulatory T cells in systemic sclerosis. Front Immunol. 2018;9:2356.
48. Radstake TR, van Bon L, Broen J, Hussiani A, Hesselstrand R, Wuttge DM, et al. The pronounced Th17 profile in systemic sclerosis (SSc) together with intracellular expression of TGFbeta and IFNgamma distinguishes SSc phenotypes. PLoS One. 2009;4:e5903.
49. Antiga E, Quaglino P, Bellandi S, Volpi W, Del Bianco E, Comessatti A, et al. Regulatory T cells in the skin lesions and blood of patients with systemic sclerosis and morphoea. Br J Dermatol. 2010;162(1056–63):1056.
50. Baraut J, Grigore EI, Jean-Louis F, Khelifa SH, Durand C, Verrecchia F, et al. Peripheral blood regulatory T cells in patients with diffuse systemic sclerosis (SSc) before and after autologous hematopoietic SCT: a pilot study. Bone Marrow Transplant. 2014;49:349–54.
51. Wang YY, Wang Q, Sun XH, Liu RZ, Shu Y, Kanekura T, et al. DNA hypermethylation of the forkhead box protein 3 (FOXP3) promoter in CD4+ T cells of patients with systemic sclerosis. Br J Dermatol. 2014;171:39–47.
52. Broen JC, Wolvers-Tettero IL, Geurts-van Bon L, Vonk MC, Coenen MJ, Lafyatis R, et al. Skewed X chromosomal inactivation impacts T regulatory cell function in systemic sclerosis. Ann Rheum Dis. 2010;69(12):2213–6.
53. MacDonald KG, Dawson NAJ, Huang Q, Dunne J, v, Levings MK, Broady R. Regulatory T cells produce profibrotic cytokines in the skin of patients with systemic sclerosis. J Allergy Clin Immunol. 2015;135:946–955.e9.
54. Kalekar LA, Rosenblum MD. Regulatory T cells in inflammatory skin disease: from mice to humans. Int Immunol. 2019;31:457–63.
55. Fleury M, Belkina AC, Proctor EA, Zammitti C, Simms RW, Lauffenburger DA, et al. Increased expression and modulated regulatory activity of coinhibitory receptors PD-1, TIGIT, and TIM-3 in lymphocytes from patients with systemic sclerosis. Arthritis Rheumatol. 2018;70:566–77.
56. Fukasawa T, Yoshizaki A, Ebata S, Nakamura K, Saigusa R, Miura S, et al. Contribution of soluble forms of programmed death 1 and programmed death ligand 2 to disease severity and progression in systemic sclerosis. Arthritis Rheumatol. 2017;69: 1879–90.
57. Ni K, Liu M, Zheng J, Wen L, Chen Q, Xiang Z, et al. PD-1/PD-L1 pathway mediates the alleviation of pulmonary fibrosis by human mesenchymal stem cells in humanized mice. Am J Respir Cell Mol Biol. 2018;58:684–95.
58. Terrier B, Humbert S, Preta LH, Delage L, Razanamahery J, Laurent-Roussel S, et al. Risk of scleroderma according to the type of immune checkpoint inhibitors. Autoimmun Rev. 2020;19:102596.
59. Yurovsky V, Wigley FM, Wise RA, White B. Skewing of the CD8+ T-cell repertoire in the lungs of patients with systemic sclerosis. Hum Immunol. 1996;48:84–97.
60. Sakkas LI, Xu B, Artlett CM, Lu S, Jimenez SA, Platsoucas CD. Oligoclonal T cell expansion in the skin of patients with systemic sclerosis. J Immunol. 2002;168:3649–59.
61. Farge D, Henegar C, Carmagnat M, Daneshpouy M, Marjanovic Z, Rabian C, et al. Analysis of immune reconstitution after autologous bone marrow transplantation in systemic sclerosis. Arthritis Rheum. 2005;52:1555–63.
62. Servaas NH, Zaaraoui-Boutahar F, Wichers CGK, Ottria A, Chouri E, Affandi AJ, et al. Longitudinal analysis of T-cell receptor repertoires reveals persistence of antigen-driven CD4 +

and CD8 + T-cell clusters in systemic sclerosis. J Autoimmun. 2021;117:102574.
63. Kuwana M, Medsger TA Jr, Wright TM. T cell proliferative response induced by DNA topoisomerase I in patients with systemic sclerosis and healthy donors. J Clin Invest. 1995;96:586–96.
64. Kuwana M, Feghali CA, Medsger TA, Wright TM. Autoreactive T cells to topoisomerase I in monozygotic twins discordant for systemic sclerosis. Arthritis Rheum. 2001;44:1654–9.
65. Boin F, Wigley FM, Schneck JP, Oelke M, Rosen A. Evaluation of topoisomerase-1-specific CD8+ T-cell response in systemic sclerosis. Ann N Y Acad Sci. 2005;1062
66. Hu PQ, Oppenheim JJ, A. Jr MT, Wright TM. T cell lines from systemic sclerosis patients and healthy controls recognize multiple epitopes on DNA topoisomerase I. J Autoimmun. 2006;26:258–67.
67. Fava A, Cimbro R, Wigley FM, Liu QR, Rosen A, Boin F. Frequency of circulating topoisomerase-I-specific CD4 T cells predicts presence and progression of interstitial lung disease in scleroderma. Arthritis Res Ther. 2016;18
68. Tiniakou E, Fava A, McMahan ZH, Guhr T, O'Meally RN, Shah AA, et al. Definition of naturally processed peptides reveals convergent presentation of autoantigenic topoisomerase I epitopes in scleroderma. Arthritis Rheumatol. 2020;72:1375–84.
69. Shah AA, Rosen A, Hummers L, Wigley F, Casciola-Rosen L. Close temporal relationship between onset of cancer and scleroderma in patients with RNA polymerase I/III antibodies. Arthritis Rheum. 2010;62:2787–95.
70. Joseph CG, Darrah E, Shah A, Skora AD, Casciola-Rosen L, Wigley FM, et al. Association of the autoimmune disease scleroderma with an immunologic response to cancer. Science. 1979;2014(343):152–7.
71. Hu PQ, Hurwitz AA, Oppenheim JJ. Immunization with DNA topoisomerase I induces autoimmune responses but not scleroderma-like pathologies in mice. J Rheumatol. 2007;34:2243–52.
72. Yoshizaki A, Yanaba K, Ogawa A, Asano Y, Kadono T, Sato S. Immunization with DNA topoisomerase I and complete Freund's adjuvant induces skin and lung fibrosis and autoimmunity via interleukin-6 signaling. Arthritis Rheum. 2011; submitted
73. Artlett CM, Smith JB, Jimenez SA. Identification of fetal DNA and cells in skin lesions from women with systemic sclerosis. N Engl J Med. 1998;338:1186–91.
74. Nelson JL, Furst DE, Maloney S, Gooley T, Evans PC, Smith A, et al. Microchimerism and HLA-compatible relationships of pregnancy in scleroderma. Lancet. 1998;351:559–62.
75. Zhang Y, McCormick LL, Desai SR, Wu C, Gilliam AC. Murine sclerodermatous graft-versus-host disease, a model for human scleroderma: cutaneous cytokines, chemokines, and immune cell activation. J Immunol. 2002;168:3088–98.
76. Christner PJ, Artlett CM, Conway RF, Jimenez SA. Increased numbers of microchimeric cells of fetal origin are associated with dermal fibrosis in mice following injection of vinyl chloride. Arthritis Rheum. 2000;43:2598–605.
77. Lipsky PE. Systemic lupus erythematosus: an autoimmune disease of B cell hyperactivity. Nat Immunol. 2001;2:764–6.
78. Tsuchiya N, Kuroki K, Fujimoto M, Murakami Y, Tedder TF, Tokunaga K, et al. Association of a functional CD19 polymorphism with susceptibility to systemic sclerosis. Arthritis Rheum. 2004;50:4002–7.
79. Wu M, Mohan C. B-cells in systemic sclerosis: emerging evidence from genetics to phenotypes. Curr Opin Rheumatol. 2015;27:537–41.
80. Yoshizaki A, Iwata Y, Komura K, Ogawa F, Hara T, Muroi E, et al. CD19 regulates skin and lung fibrosis via Toll-like receptor signaling in a model of bleomycin-induced scleroderma. Am J Pathol. 2008;172:1650–63.
81. Glauzy S, Olson B, May CK, Parisi D, Massad C, Hansen JE, et al. Defective early B cell tolerance checkpoints in patients with systemic sclerosis allow the production of self antigen-specific clones. Arthritis Rheumatol. 2022;74:307–17.
82. Whitfield ML, Finlay DR, Murray JI, Troyanskaya OG, Chi JT, Pergamenschikov A, et al. Systemic and cell type-specific gene expression patterns in scleroderma skin. Proc Natl Acad Sci U S A. 2003;100:12319–24.
83. Streicher K, Sridhar S, Kuziora M, Morehouse CA, Higgs BW, Sebastian Y, et al. Baseline plasma cell gene signature predicts improvement in systemic sclerosis skin scores following treatment with inebilizumab (MEDI-551) and correlates with disease activity in systemic lupus erythematosus and chronic obstructive pulmonary disease. Arthritis Rheumatol. 2018;70:2087–95.
84. Sato S, Fujimoto M, Hasegawa M, Takehara K. Altered blood B lymphocyte homeostasis in systemic sclerosis: expanded naive B cells and diminished but activated memory B cells. Arthritis Rheum. 2004;50:1918–27.
85. Lafyatis R, O'Hara C, Feghali-Bostwick CA, Matteson E. B cell infiltration in systemic sclerosis-associated interstitial lung disease. Arthritis Rheum. 2007;56:3167–8.
86. Bosello S, Angelucci C, Lama G, Alivernini S, Proietti G, Tolusso B, et al. Characterization of inflammatory cell infiltrate of scleroderma skin: B cells and skin score progression. Arthritis Res Ther. 2018;20:1–11.
87. Forestier A, Guerrier T, Jouvray M, Giovannelli J, Lefèvre G, Sobanski V, et al. Altered B lymphocyte homeostasis and functions in systemic sclerosis. Autoimmun Rev. 2018;17:244–55.
88. Melissaropoulos K, Liossis SN. Decreased CD22 expression and intracellular signaling aberrations in B cells of patients with systemic sclerosis. Rheumatol Int. 2018;38:1225–34.
89. Sato S, Hasegawa M, Fujimoto M, Tedder TF, Takehara K. Quantitative genetic variation in CD19 expression correlates with autoimmunity. J Immunol (Baltimore, Md: 1950). 2000;165:6635–43.
90. Mavropoulos A, Simopoulou T, Varna A, Liaskos C, Katsiari CG, Bogdanos DP, et al. Breg cells are numerically decreased and functionally impaired in patients with systemic sclerosis. Arthritis Rheumatol. 2016;68:494–504.
91. Aravena O, Ferrier A, Menon M, Mauri C, Aguillón JC, Soto L, et al. TIM-1 defines a human regulatory B cell population that is altered in frequency and function in systemic sclerosis patients. Arthritis Res Ther. 2017;19:1–13.
92. Matsushita T, Hamaguchi Y, Hasegawa M, Takehara K, Fujimoto M. Decreased levels of regulatory B cells in patients with systemic sclerosis: association with autoantibody production and disease activity. Rheumatology (Oxford). 2015;55(2):263–7.
93. Dumoitier N, Chaigne B, Régent A, Lofek S, Mhibik M, Dorfmüller P, et al. Scleroderma peripheral B lymphocytes secrete interleukin-6 and transforming growth factor β and activate fibroblasts. Arthritis Rheumatol. 2017;69:1078–89.
94. Wilfong EM, Vowell KN, Bunn KE, Rizzi E, Annapureddy N, Dudenhofer RB, et al. CD19 + CD21 lo/neg cells are increased in systemic sclerosis-associated interstitial lung disease. Clin Exp Med. 2021;22(2):209–20.
95. Jenks SA, Cashman KS, Zumaquero E, Marigorta UM, Patel A, Wang X, et al. Distinct effector B cells induced by unregulated toll-like receptor 7 contribute to pathogenic responses in systemic lupus erythematosus. Immunity. 2018;49:725–739.e6.
96. Francois A, Chatelus E, Wachsmann D, Sibilia J, Bahram S, Alsaleh G, et al. B lymphocytes and B-cell activating factor promote collagen and profibrotic markers expression by dermal fibroblasts in systemic sclerosis. Arthritis Res Ther. 2013;15:R168.
97. Mackay F, Schneider P, Rennert P, Browning J. BAFF AND APRIL: a tutorial on B cell survival. Annu Rev Immunol. 2003;21:231–64.

98. Matsushita T, Fujimoto M, Hasegawa M, Matsushita Y, Komura K, Ogawa F, et al. BAFF antagonist attenuates the development of skin fibrosis in tight-skin mice. J Invest Dermatol. 2007;127:2772–80.
99. Matsushita T, Hasegawa M, Yanaba K, Kodera M, Takehara K, Sato S. Elevated serum BAFF levels in patients with systemic sclerosis: enhanced BAFF signaling in systemic sclerosis B lymphocytes. Arthritis Rheum. 2006;54:192–201.
100. Bielecki M, Kowal K, Lapinska A, Bernatowicz P, Chyczewski L, Kowal-Bielecka O. Increased production of a proliferation-inducing ligand (APRIL) by peripheral blood mononuclear cells is associated with antitopoisomerase I antibody and more severe disease in systemic sclerosis. J Rheumatol. 2010;37:2286–9.
101. Matsushita T, Fujimoto M, Hasegawa M, Tanaka C, Kumada S, Ogawa F, et al. Elevated serum APRIL levels in patients with systemic sclerosis: distinct profiles of systemic sclerosis categorized by APRIL and BAFF. J Rheumatol. 2007;34:2056–62.
102. Matsushita T, Kobayashi T, Mizumaki K, Kano M, Sawada T, Tennichi M, et al. BAFF inhibition attenuates fibrosis in scleroderma by modulating the regulatory and effector B cell balance. Sci Adv. 2018;4:9944–55.
103. Jordan S, Distler JH, Maurer B, Huscher D, van Laar JM, Allanore Y, et al. Effects and safety of rituximab in systemic sclerosis: an analysis from the European Scleroderma Trial and Research (EUSTAR) group. Ann Rheum Dis. 2015;74:1188–94.
104. Bosello SL, de Luca G, Rucco M, Berardi G, Falcione M, Danza FM, et al. Long-term efficacy of B cell depletion therapy on lung and skin involvement in diffuse systemic sclerosis. Semin Arthritis Rheum. 2015;44:428–36.
105. Zamanian RT, Badesch D, Chung L, Domsic RT, Medsger T, Pinckney A, et al. Safety and efficacy of B-cell depletion with rituximab for the treatment of systemic sclerosis-associated pulmonary arterial hypertension: a multicenter, double-blind, randomized, placebo-controlled trial. Am J Respir Crit Care Med. 2021;204:209–21.

Autoantibodies as Markers and Possible Mediators of Scleroderma Pathogenesis

15

Christopher A. Mecoli, Kimberly Doering Maurer, Antony Rosen, and Livia Casciola-Rosen

Introduction

Scleroderma or systemic sclerosis is a systemic autoimmune disease characterized by a proliferative vasculopathy associated with skin thickening and fibrosis within internal organs and is associated with a unique autoimmune response. While vascular damage is almost universal in scleroderma, disease expression is heterogeneous in terms of phenotypic characteristics and disease course. Nevertheless, clear clinical subtypes can be discerned. The limited cutaneous form of scleroderma is characterized by skin thickening on the distal limbs, face, and sometimes chest and an increased prevalence of isolated pulmonary hypertension and ischemic digital loss. In contrast, the diffuse form of the disease involves more proximal skin and more often affects visceral organs, including the lungs, heart, gastrointestinal tract, skeletal muscle, and kidneys, with attendant negative effects on mortality. There are striking associations between specific autoantibodies and the distinct phenotypic subsets of scleroderma. These clinically useful associations suggest that the different autoantibodies report on specific circumstances which underlie disease propagation in different tissues. It is also possible that specific autoantibodies play a direct pathogenic role in the propagation and amplification of autoimmune reactions and pathology in scleroderma. This chapter reviews some of the interesting insights that autoantibodies and their specificity provide into scleroderma pathogenesis.

C. A. Mecoli · A. Rosen · L. Casciola-Rosen (✉)
Division of Rheumatology, Johns Hopkins University, Baltimore, MD, USA
e-mail: cmecoli1@jhmi.edu; arosen@jhmi.edu; lcr@jhmi.edu

K. D. Maurer
Department of Radiology, Duke University Health System, Durham, NC, USA

Autoantibody Profiles as Markers of Pathogenic Events

Although the role of disease-specific autoantibodies in systemic autoimmune diseases remains controversial, the specificity of these antibodies provides a critical clue to understanding their origin. Each systemic autoimmune disease (e.g., scleroderma, systemic lupus erythematosus (SLE), rheumatoid arthritis, idiopathic inflammatory myositis) is characterized by the elaboration of a distinct group of autoantibodies that target a limited number of ubiquitously expressed autoantigens. Within the scleroderma spectrum, autoantibody profiles are associated with specific disease phenotypes, making serological tests helpful in diagnosis and prognosis. The major clinical subsets of scleroderma have distinct serological associations, with topoisomerase-1 and RNA polymerase antibodies associated with the diffuse form of the disease, and centromere autoantibodies enriched in the limited form. Many of these scleroderma-specific autoantibodies are mutually exclusive, a finding that has been conclusively established over the past 25 years [1–3]. In one study of 5423 patients, only 26 (0.52%) had the coexistence of anti-topoisomerase-1 and anti-centromere antibodies [4].

The existence of significant phenotypic differences between limited and diffuse forms of scleroderma has led some to propose that these are discrete disease processes, and thus the distinct autoantibody profiles in the two subsets are not surprising. However, distinct autoantibody patterns with specific target tissue involvement, even within the diffuse disease spectrum, suggest that autoantibody specificity might reflect unique amplification pathways within specific tissues. For example, while antibodies to topoisomerase-1 and RNA polymerases are both associated with a more aggressive form of diffuse skin disease in scleroderma, anti-topoisomerase is associated with interstitial lung disease and RNA polymerase I/III antibodies are not. The latter autoantibodies occur in patients with rapidly progressive, severe skin disease, as well as renal crisis [5, 6]. Additionally, patients

Y. Allanore et al. (eds.), *Scleroderma*, https://doi.org/10.1007/978-3-031-40658-4_15

with scleroderma in overlap with other autoimmune diseases express antibodies to "overlap" antigens, including anti-PM-Scl antibodies with myositis [7] or anti-U1-RNP antibodies with SLE [5, 6]. Taken together, the observation of specific autoantibody associations with distinct tissue injury patterns, and the tendency for autoantibody subsets to be non-overlapping, suggests that target tissue and immune response interact and both participate in antigen selection, tissue damage, and disease manifestations.

Although there is widespread agreement that autoimmunity is an important participant in scleroderma pathogenesis, ~10% of patients with classical scleroderma phenotypes lack both ANAs and scleroderma-specific autoantibodies. This subgroup is extremely interesting, as these patients may shed light on critical mechanisms of tissue damage that are not evident from studying the autoantibodies to ubiquitously expressed antigens (see below).

Some Autoantibody Titers Can Change Over Time: Association with Disease Severity and Activity

Since the autoantibody response in various autoimmune rheumatic diseases has been noted to be antigen-driven and T-cell dependent, there have been numerous attempts to determine whether an association exists between autoantibody titers and disease activity/severity in scleroderma [8–10]. This is a particularly difficult task in scleroderma, where quantitation of disease activity and severity are insensitive compared to other rheumatic processes like RA. In some studies, topoisomerase-1 autoantibody titers in scleroderma appear to be positively correlated with total skin score measurements [11]. Additionally, the rate of deterioration in lung function tests (forced vital capacity and carbon monoxide diffusing capacity) was greater in patients whose anti-topoisomerase antibodies were sustained over time [9]. However, the dynamic range of changes in anti-toposiomerase-1 titers is quite limited, and changes in titers of other autoantibodies (CENP or RNA polymerase) do not appear to be associated with clinically significant variation in disease activity [12]. Therefore, the available data suggests that the levels of defined autoantibody specificities in scleroderma do not vary in clinically meaningful ways. The implications of this conclusion may include the following scenarios, depicted in Fig. 15.1. (1) Although the generation of autoantibodies might be initiated after exposure of these specific antigens during early events in the disease, they may be driven by events not directly on the pathogenic pathway. The specific autoantigens themselves may be released in a disease-nonspecific way during homeostasis, becoming markers of damage. Other antigens, unrelated to the disease, may be present and continue to drive a cross-reactive antibody response. (2) There have been studies showing that antibody effector function can be modified by Fc posttranslational modification like sialylation, where antibody titers do not reflect inflammatory properties [13]. (3) All of the autoantigens discussed above are intracellular and ubiquitously expressed, making it unlikely that autoantibodies to these antigens have easy access to the relevant antigens. Using the antibodies to identify important antigen specificities, and then prospectively quantifying antigen-specific T cells recognizing these scleroderma autoantigens over time, may better allow associations to be defined between the magnitude of immune response to specific antigens and rate

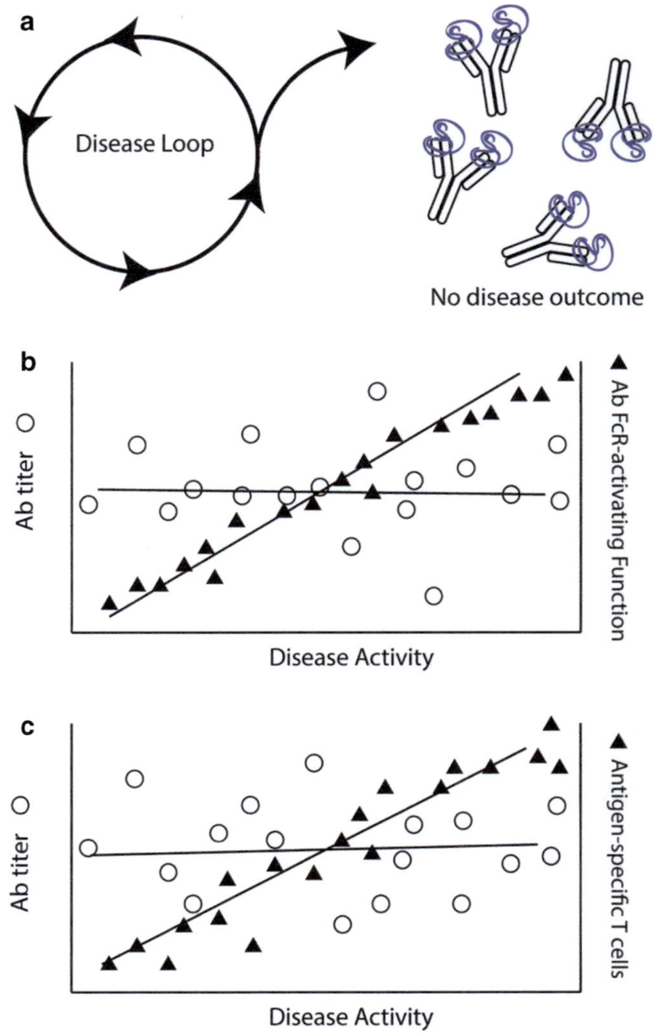

Fig. 15.1 Possible reasons that autoantibody titers do not correlate with disease activity. (**a**) Autoantibodies may simply be markers of tissue damage and not play a role in disease propagation. (**b**) Total antibody titers may not correlate with disease activity because only a subset of autoantibodies bind to activating FcRs and therefore mediate effector functions (e.g., non-sialylated Fc sugars). The extent of Ig sialylation, therefore, may correlate with disease activity or severity. (**c**) Autoantibody specificity may be significantly impacted by intra- and intermolecular epitope spreading and therefore be driven by the specific disease-associated epitopes as well as cross-reactive antigens

of phenotypic changes. Consistent with this, Fava et al. recently quantified anti-toposiomerase-1 specific CD4-positive T cells by flow cytometry and reported that this cell population predicts the progression of interstitial lung disease in scleroderma patients [14]. Notably, the titer of anti-topoisomerase-1 antibodies did not correlate with the percentage of topoisomerase-1-positive CD4 T cells ($r = 0.17$, $P = 0.554$). (4) The fact that anti-topoisomerase-1 antibodies do change in association with severity and activity suggests that disease activity in some organs may be associated with antigen exposure or release, contributing to the autoimmune response. This would suggest the existence of an auto-amplifying loop, where antigen expression, immune response, and tissue damage are all components of the mechanism driving the increased autoantibody titers. Defining the components of such a loop and the sites at which this occurs is of great importance and can only be accomplished in vivo in scleroderma patients.

Finally, recent data documents the presence of scleroderma-specific/associated autoantibodies (including centromere A, PM-Scl, and RNA polymerase) up to 20 years before diagnosis of scleroderma and its complications [15]. These data imply that autoantibodies alone are insufficient to cause tissue damage, and/or that damage/immune dysregulation occurs subclinically for a longer period than previously appreciated.

Autoantigens in Target Tissues: Partners in Propagation

The frequently targeted autoantigens in scleroderma are all ubiquitously expressed molecules, participating in numerous important cellular processes. In spite of ubiquitous expression, the immune response to these autoantigens is associated with distinct phenotypes, often enriching for damage of a specific tissue. For example, scleroderma patients with anti-topoisomerase-1 antibodies frequently have interstitial lung disease. These associations have the potential to greatly clarify pathogenesis. One possible explanation is that unique features of autoantigens in specific microenvironments participate in their selection as autoantigens (Fig. 15.2). These features could include novel autoantigen forms that alter autoantigen structure and processing (e.g., novel isoforms, proteolytic cleavage, posttranslational modifications; see below), increased antigen expression levels [16, 17], and microenvironment-specific modifications which allow autoantigens themselves to activate the innate immune system [18, 19]. Recent studies have furthered our understanding of the serologic-clinical phenotypic relationship. McMahan et al. reported that autoantibodies against centromere and interferon-gamma-induced protein 16 (IFI-16) are associated with digital lesions: Scleroderma patients positive for both anti-centromere and anti-IFI-16, OR 3.55 (95% CI 1.1–

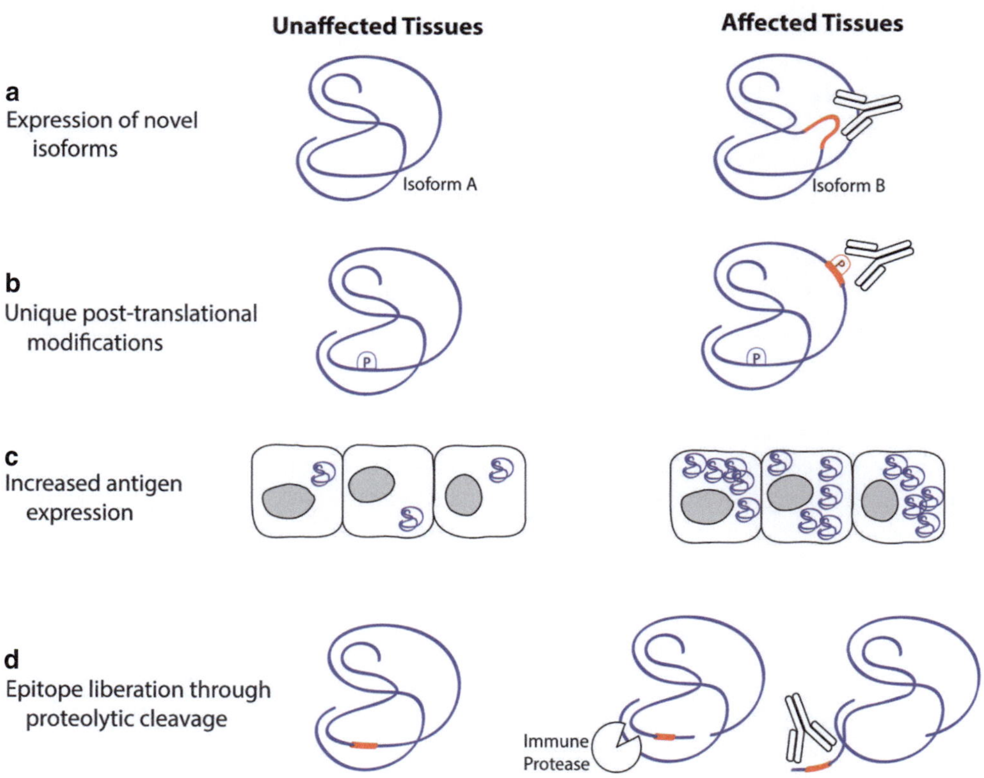

Fig. 15.2 Possible mechanisms underlying association of specific immune responses with distinct patterns of tissue damage in scleroderma. (**a**) Autoantibodies may recognize a polypeptide sequence expressed in protein isoforms restricted to a particular tissue. (**b**) Affected tissue may express an antigen with a unique posttranslational modification. (**c**) Affected tissue may express higher amounts of antigen. (**d**) Proteolytic cleavage may reveal an autoantibody epitope typically hidden within the molecule

11.3, $P = 0.03$) after adjusting for age, disease duration, smoking and cutaneous subtype. Interestingly, the same autoantigens were found to be enriched in endothelial cells ($CD31^+$ embryoid bodies, vascular progenitors, and mature endothelial cells), potentially explaining the association between certain autoantibodies and clinical characteristics [20, 21]. Furthermore, anti-IFI-16 antibody titers correlated with the severity of digital lesions, with the highest titers present in patients with digital gangrene, and progressively lower titers found in patients with digital ulcers, digital pits, and Raynaud's phenomenon.

Although studies of autoantigen levels and conformation in target tissues would be optimal, data from such studies is not yet available. However, multiple studies have shown that scleroderma autoantigens are particularly susceptible to structural modifications by pathways induced during scleroderma tissue damage. For example, data from numerous studies has shown that cytotoxic T lymphocyte (CTL) granule-mediated killing results in the generation of altered forms of self-antigens (Fig. 15.2d). Granzyme B (GrB), a protease contained within the cytotoxic granules released by CTLs and NK cells, cleaves 80% of autoantigens targeted in systemic autoimmune diseases to generate novel fragments [16, 22]. Several scleroderma autoantigens (including topoisomerase-1, CENPs B and C, RNA polymerases, U1-RNP, PM-Scl, fibrillarin, and B23) are all cleaved by GrB [16, 23]. Interestingly, sera from 84.2% of patients with ischemic digital loss (IDL) recognized GrB-cleaved antigens [24]. This was in contrast to only 40% of patients without IDL. Some IDL sera preferentially recognize the cleaved fragment of the centromere protein CENP-C, but not the intact CENP-C molecule, suggesting that GrB might unmask a cryptic B-cell epitope in this molecule and potentially play a pathogenic role in the IDL process [24].

The state of the cell being killed by CTLs may also play an important role in providing altered forms of autoantigens. Indeed, scleroderma autoantigens are not all equally susceptible to cleavage by GrB during cytotoxic cell killing. Although B23 is a sensitive substrate for GrB in vitro, it is poorly cleaved in numerous intact cells. Since the immune response to B23 is associated with pulmonary hypertension, Ulanet et al. examined B23 cleavage in vascular smooth muscle (VSM) cells in distinct differentiation states. They found that B23 was poorly cleaved in undifferentiated vascular smooth muscle cells, but was exquisitely sensitive to cleavage when these cells are differentiated toward the contractile phenotype, suggesting the presence of a unique form of B23 in this cell population [25].

Autoantibodies as Clues to the Scleroderma-Cancer Interface

The association between scleroderma and cancer [26, 27] is intriguing. Shah et al. have made several observations which demonstrate that cancers can express scleroderma autoantigens at high levels and serve as an initiating stimulus for autoimmunity in patients who develop scleroderma. To address whether autoantibody status was associated with the temporal relationship between cancer and scleroderma, they examined autoantibody responses in patients that had both scleroderma and cancer. Interestingly, while the mean duration of scleroderma at cancer diagnosis among 23 scleroderma patients was 7.2 ± 10.4 years, patients positive for anti-RNA polymerase I/III antibodies had a significantly lower duration of −1.2 years. The investigators then examined the expression of RNA polymerases in tumor specimens from these patients. Most of the cancer sections from RNA polymerase III antibody-positive patients showed distinct, nucleolar staining with the anti-RNA polymerase III antibody. In contrast, this pattern was not seen in the cancer tissue of patients negative for this antibody. These observations suggested that the form of RNA polymerase III in cancer tissue might be distinctly immunogenic, capable of initiating an antitumor immune response, and potentially cross-reacting with RNA polymerase III in other tissues (e.g., blood vessels, skin), generating tissue damage characteristic of scleroderma [28]. Evidence supporting this hypothesis was subsequently provided by Joseph et al. [19]. Characterization of tumors from patients with RNA polymerase III-antibody-positive scleroderma and cancer identified somatic mutations in the *POLR3A* gene. Mutations in the *POLR3A* gene were not present in cancers from scleroderma patients with any other autoantibody specificity.

Interestingly, patients with antibodies recognizing RNA polymerase III also had striking loss of heterozygosity (LOH) at the *POLR3A* locus. In these patients, LOH was not evident at chromosomal regions containing either the *TOP1* or *CENP-B* genes, demonstrating a striking association between the target of the immune response and the target of LOH, and indicating that these two phenomena are likely mechanistically related. In two of three patients with somatic tumor mutations, the mutations generated peptides predicted to bind with high affinity to one of the patient's MHC class II alleles. Studies directly showed specific CD4 T cell responses recognizing the mutated epitope. There was also evidence in one patient of a distinct population of CD4 T cells responding specifically to the wild-type antigen, suggesting that the mutant-specific immune response spreads to recognize the wild-type version and cross-reacts with normal tissue, possibly through a B-cell-dependent mechanism (Fig. 15.2a). Interestingly, the accompanying autoantibody response was cross-reactive and could not distinguish between mutant and wild-type antigen. The reason that specific normal tissues might be targeted by the immune response may relate to tissue-specific expression of autoantigens either in the baseline or the damaged state. Understanding in vivo antigen expression in different tissues under different perturbed states will likely provide important insights. The observation that only 20% of scleroderma patients with RNA polymerase III antibodies have a malignancy diagnosed, together with findings of RNA polymerase-specific T cells and frequent LOH at the POLR3A locus, strongly suggests the existence of immunoediting of cancers in scleroderma patients. The authors proposed that scleroderma patients with RNA polymerase III autoantibodies may have successfully cleared an occult malignancy [19]. In follow-up studies, Shah et al. demonstrated that in RNA polymerase III-positive scleroderma patients, the concomitant presence of antibodies to the large subunit of RNA polymerase I (RPA194) is enriched in patients without cancer. One interpretation of this intruiging finding is that development of orthogonal immune responses may influence the clinical emergence of cancer in scleroderma patients [29].

Autoantibodies as Possible Mediators of Scleroderma Pathogenesis

The data demonstrating that autoantibodies are serological markers of a specific disease phenotype in scleroderma is extremely strong, but the mechanistic implications of such observations remain uncertain. The use of transformed cell lines as an antigen source to identify all intracellular autoantigens defined to date raises important cautions about whether all relevant autoantibodies have been identified. Important questions that remain to be addressed include: (1) Do phenotype-specific antibodies themselves play a role in the generation of that phenotype? (2) Are there antibodies which might participate directly in generating the phenotype, potentially through ligation of antigens which are exposed extracellularly? Potential pathogenic roles for scleroderma autoantibodies can be divided into two categories: amplification of the immune response and direct pathogenicity (see below). A summary of antibodies discussed in this chapter can be found in Table 15.1.

Table 15.1 Summary of autoantibodies with pathogenic potential

I. Amplification of immune responses		
Anti-topoisomerase-1	Recruitment and activation of immune cells	[1, 30]
	Induction of type I IFN secretion from pDCs	[31]
Anti-centromere B	Induction of pro-fibrotic activation of human dermal fibroblasts	[32]
II. Direct pathogenicity		
A. Antibodies against unidentified cell surface molecules		
Anti-endothelial cell antibodies (specific antigens unknown)	Endothelial cell apoptosis	[6, 33]
Anti-fibroblast antibodies (specific antigens unknown)	Pro-adhesive phenotype in fibroblasts and cytokine modulation	[10]
	Upregulation of pro-fibrotic and pro-angiogenic transcriptional programs in fibroblasts	[34]
B. Antibodies against extracellular matrix components		
Anti-fibrillin	Regulation of extracellular matrix components and TGFβ signaling (controversial; see text)	[2, 35]
Anti-matrix metalloproteinases 1 and 3	Inhibition of ECM turnover	[23, 25]
C. Antibodies stimulating receptor signaling		
Antiplatelet-derived growth factor receptor	Generation of cellular smooth muscle and fibroblast lesions and upregulation of collagen production (controversial; see text)	[36]
Anti-M3 muscarinic receptor	Inhibition of muscle contraction	[37]
Anti-angiotensin II type 1 receptor (AT_1R)	Induction of proinflammatory chemokines including IL-8 and CXCL8 from endothelial cells and PBMCs	[38, 39]
Anti-endothelin-1 type A receptor (ET_AR)	Induction of proinflammatory chemokines including IL-8 and CXCL8 from endothelial cells and PBMCs	[38, 39]

Amplification of Immune Responses

Although many of the defined autoantigens in scleroderma are intracellular, such antigens may become re-localized during cell damage or death and potentially during other physiological processes such as protein moonlighting—that is, a single protein having multiple functions in different regions throughout the cell [40]. Such re-localization may allow autoantibodies to access these antigens, with pro-inflammatory consequences. Cells that have a special tendency to bind the antigen may therefore become targets of a redirected immune effector pathway. Antibodies to topoisomerase-1 appear to be relevant in this regard. Henault et al. demonstrated that anti-topoisomerase-1 antibodies bind the surface of fibroblasts, but not smooth muscle or endothelial cells. In a tissue culture-based cell adhesion assay, they showed that the binding of anti-topoisomerase-1 antibodies to fibroblasts was dose-dependent and saturable [41]. This phenomenon was facilitated by purified topoisomerase protein or topoisomerase protein released from apoptotic endothelial cells. Bound anti-topoisomerase-1 antibodies enhanced the adhesion and activation of THP1 human monocytes [42]. It is important to note the limited power of such a "redirected" effector pathway to explain self-sustaining, amplifying, tissue-specific phenotypes. Additional parameters still to be defined include whether topoisomerase-1 binding to the surface of a bystander cell induces damage of the bystander, thus supplying additional autoantigen to further drive immune response and bystander injury, as well as whether the specificity of surface binding directs the amplifying effects to particular cells and tissues.

This general mechanism is supported by findings showing that antibodies against CENP-B (an autoantigen associated with limited cutaneous scleroderma) can ligate and activate signaling through CCR3 [43]. Furthermore, both centromere and topoisomerase-1 autoantibodies have been shown to induce pro-fibrotic activation of human dermal fibroblasts. In a study of 10 patients with limited cutaneous anti-centromere scleroderma and 10 patients with diffuse cutaneuous anti-topoisomerase-1 scleroderma, Corallo et al. showed that stimulation with both anti-centromere and topoisomerase-1 IgG statistically increased profibrotic markers (ACTA2, COL1A1, and TAGLN) in cultured dermal fibroblasts [32].

The "trans" effects of anti-topoisomerase-1 on inflammatory signaling in the setting of released nuclear topoisomerase-1 antigen have also been demonstrated. Kim et al. showed that anti-topoisomerase-1-positive sera, but not sera containing other well-characterized scleroderma autoantibodies, could induce the secretion of high levels of interferon α (IFNα) in PBMC preparations when supplied with nuclear cell extracts [44]. This group went on to show that the observed production of IFNα was as a result of suspected immune complexes (containing likely anti-topoisomerase-1 IgG antibodies, nuclear cell extracts of protein and nucleic acids) which are able to bind FCγ receptor and TLRs in plasmacytoid dendritic cells (pDCs), potent producers of type I interferons. Interestingly, the induction of IFNα was more prominent in patients with diffuse disease compared to limited scleroderma (multivariable analysis, however, was not performed to determine whether this was accounted for by increased titers of anti-topoisomerase-1 antibodies). Perhaps even more interesting was the observation that increased IFNα secretion was associated with interstitial lung disease, with a median IFN secretion almost threefold higher in those with lung fibrosis [44]. Of note, since the number of patients studied in this way to date is very small, these observations and their clinical associations need to be confirmed. However, the potential association of increased activation of the IFN pathway with clinical phenotype is very intriguing, as it implies that specific autoantibodies might exert feedforward properties which do not require binding to autoantigen in unperturbed cells. Raschi et al. [45] further investigated the role of scleroderma-Ig immune complexes and their functional consequences on human fibroblasts. Immune complexes from 16 scleroderma patients with different scleroderma autoantibody specificities (topoisomerase-1, centromere, RNA polymerase III, and Th/To as determined using a line blot assay) were measured, and evidence of vascular dysfunction (increased endothelin-1), inflammation (increased cytokines/chemokine levels such as IL6, IL8, MCP1) and fibrosis (increase in TGFbeta and procollagen1alpha1) was reported. The authors also posited the role of TLRs when discussing how the immune complexes may be exerting their effects [45]. Studies to date that highlight the potential role of immune complexes in scleroderma have not yet reconciled the absence of other immune complex-mediated clinical signs such as glomerulonephritis and palpable purpura. Thus, the impact that immune complexes have on the pathophysiology of scleroderma has yet to be fully determined.

Additionally, B lymphocytes are also suspected to be a driving force of scleroderma pathogenesis, as they are increased in scleroderma affected skin [46] and several reports have reported the efficacy of B-cell depleting therapies for both skin and lung involvement [47, 48]. B cells in scleroderma populations display multiple aberrancies including decreased levels of regulatory B cells [49] and increased levels of CD19 on their peripheral blood B cells, the presence of which may have a role in promoting fibrosis [34, 50]. Furthermore, human in vitro studies have reported on the pathogenic potential of aberrant B cell activity, demonstrating the ability to produce a pro-fibrotic phenotype and increased collagen secretion upon culturing B cells with human dermal fibroblasts [51, 52]. Together, these studies suggest that B cells play a role in fibrosis, although the mechanisms whereby they may be contributing remain unclear. Their contributions certainly include increasing autoantibody titers, antigen presentation, and providing help to T cells. Any of these functions could contribute to the self-reinforcing nature of T- and B-cell interactions, which Schlomchik et al. have proposed could be a major driving force behind systemic autoimmune disease [53].

Direct Pathogenicity

An important requirement for antibodies to exert direct pathogenic effects on intact cells is availability of accessible antigen on the surface of the target cell. One of the major challenges in this area is careful molecular definition of these autoantigens, which are, with some exceptions, poorly characterized. Defining membrane and extracellular autoantigens is a notoriously difficult task, with challenges of solubility, affinity, and posttranslational modifications. Nevertheless, it is likely that directly pathogenic autoantibodies do exist in this disease and can contribute to ongoing tissue damage and dysfunction. Defining the key antigens is critical.

Antibodies Recognizing Unidentified Cell Surface Molecules

Anti-endothelial cell antibodies (AECA), although not specific for scleroderma, are observed in 25–85% of scleroderma patients and may define a subgroup of patients that have a high incidence of vascular involvement [54]. These antibodies are thought to induce endothelial apoptosis in scleroderma [55]. Endothelial cell death and dysfunction may play direct roles in thwarting normal vessel function in scleroderma [56]. Dying cells might also constitute a source of autoantigens, which, through binding to bystander cells, could contribute to pathogenicity [42]. A proposed model illustrating how some of these antibodies may contribute to an auto-amplifying loop of immune activation, vasculopathy, and fibrosis is shown in Fig. 15.3. This hypothetical model depicts potential ways that antibodies with proposed pathogenic roles in scleroderma could collaborate to sustain disease processes.

Antibodies recognizing fibroblasts have also been identified by many groups of investigators. Reported frequency of these anti-fibroblast antibodies (AFA) range from 26–58% of scleroderma patients [35, 41, 57–60]. In one study, 58–69% patients were found to be positive for AFA, and

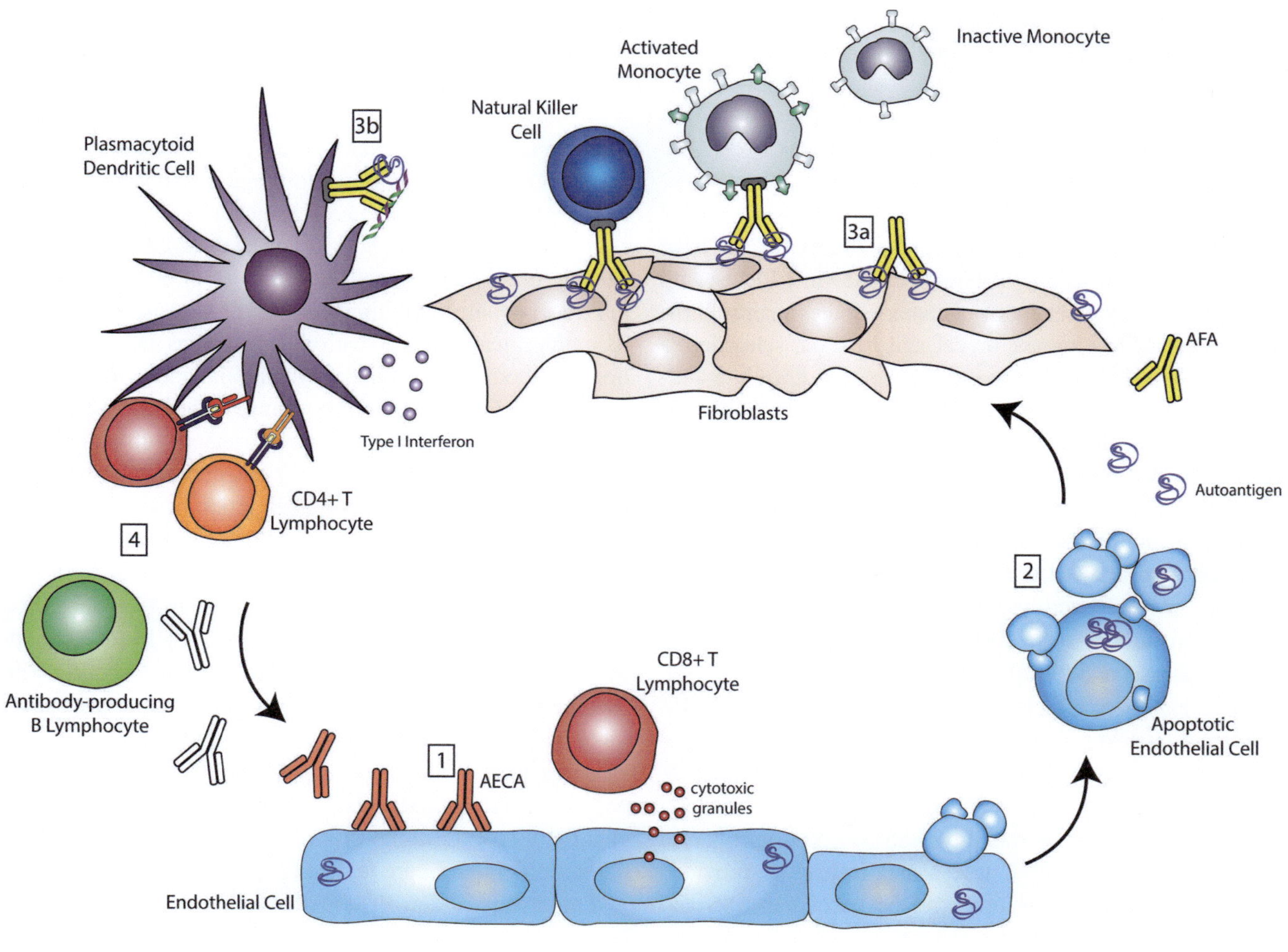

Fig. 15.3 Hypothetical model of immune-mediated vascular damage, highlighting potential opportunities of antibody-assisted disease propagation. (*1*) AECA and likely cytotoxic T cells can cause endothelial cell apoptosis. (*2*) Apoptotic endothelial cells may be a cause of vascular dysfunction and a source of ongoing antigen to drive the immune response. (*3*) Since it has been proposed that antigen (e.g., topoisomerase-1) can preferentially bind to fibroblasts, anti-topoisomerase-1 antibodies might recruit immune effector cells (such as monocytes and NK cells) to sites of tissue damage and amplify the destruction (*3a*). Additionally, immune complexes containing anti-topoisomerase-1 antibodies may contribute to pathogenesis via their ability to stimulate IFN production from pDCs (*3b*). (*4*) Activation and stimulation of the adaptive immune response perpetuates these cycles through further augmenting antibody, T cell, cytokine, and tissue damage pathways

these sera promoted a pro-adhesive phenotype in fibroblasts, induced upregulation of the adhesion molecule, ICAM-1, and enhanced mRNA expression of the cytokines IL-1α, IL-1β, and IL-6 [57]. Further evidence for the presence and effects of AFAs continues to accumulate. For example, in a study where 40% of patients with scleroderma were positive for AFA, microarrays containing probes for 112 human chemokines and receptors were used to interrogate the transcriptional program triggered by incubation of fibroblasts with AFA [58]. Compared to control sera, AFA-positive sera upregulated the expression of a number of pro-fibrotic and pro-angiogenic genes, such as CCL2 and CXCL8. This response was partially dependent on signaling through TLR4 as shown by use of selective inhibitors, TLR4-deficient mouse cells, and an antagonistic anti-TLR4 antibody. The specific molecular targets of these antibodies, the cell type-specific expression of such molecules, and the in vivo effects of such antibodies in scleroderma remain to be defined. If pathologic in nature, such antibodies could initiate and/or amplify vascular inflammation and fibrosis in scleroderma.

Autoantibodies Affecting Extracellular Matrix and Its Components

Several components of the extracellular matrix (ECM) have been shown to be targets of autoantibodies in patients with scleroderma. There are reports of autoantibodies against fibrillin-1 in the TSK/+ mouse model and in some scleroderma patient cohorts [61–65]. Demonstration of anti-fibrillin-1 antibodies in scleroderma has not, however, been broadly confirmed [66]. While the reasons for this remain unclear, it is noteworthy that fibrillin-1 is challenging to assay because it is large, and its recognition by antibodies is influenced by whether it is in the disulfide-bonded or reduced state, and the presence of posttranslational modifications [36, 37]. Although fibrillin-1 may be controversial in terms of the presence and role of autoantibodies, the fibrillin family has interesting functions in fibrosis and TGFβ binding. Studies of families with multiple members afflicted with stiff skin syndrome (SSS) have shed interesting insights into the role of ECM components in scleroderma. SSS is an autosomal dominant, noninflammatory disorder characterized by hard, thick skin and subsequent limited joint mobility. SSS has been ascribed to mutations in fibrillin [67]. Loeys and colleagues provided important evidence suggesting that the fibrosis in SSS and scleroderma may share similar mechanisms. Mutations in fibrillin decreased binding to integrins, caused aberrant ECM accumulation and TGFβ signaling, and increased the number of cells expressing α-smooth muscle cell actin, indicative of cells recruited to assist in tissue remodeling. Whether autoimmunity to matrix components can have similar consequences to those observed in SSS skin is of significant interest.

Autoantibodies against matrix metalloproteinase-1 (MMP-1), an enzyme that degrades collagen types I and III, have been found in sera of up to 75% of patients with diffuse scleroderma [68]. Anti-MMP-1 IgG titers were higher in patients with diffuse disease than in those with limited disease ($P < 0.001$) and correlated with the extent of fibrosis in the lung (vital capacity, $r = 0.36$, $P < 0.01$ and diffusion capacity for carbon monoxide, $r = 0.43$, $P < 0.005$), skin (total skin score, $r = 0.06$, $P < 0.002$), and renal blood vessels (pulsatility index, $r = 0.52$, $P < 0.001$). Serum IgG fractions were also able to inhibit MMP-1 collagenase activity by 77% as compared to normal control IgG ($P < 0.001$). Similar findings have been presented for autoantibodies targeting MMP-3 [31]. The authors speculate that anti-MMP antibodies might disrupt the balance between collagen synthesis and degradation, ultimately promoting excessive extracellular matrix deposition and fibrosis in scleroderma.

Autoantibodies Stimulating Receptor Signaling

The identification of platelet-derived growth factor receptor (PDGFR) as a target of the autoimmune response in scleroderma patients has generated significant interest and discussion [69]. The investigators found anti-PDGFR antibodies capable of stimulating cells specifically through ligation of this receptor and initiating a series of downstream effects including increased reactive oxygen species (ROS) generation, Ras activation, collagen production, and myofibroblast conversion [69]. The presence of autoantibodies appeared to be a very frequent finding in scleroderma patients and did not associate with the disease phenotype. An attractive aspect of the proposed model was that such antibodies could participate directly in generating cellular smooth muscle and fibroblast lesions. However, PDGFR autoantibodies have not been found in other studies, using different techniques for identification and functional activity [30, 70]. More recently, Moroncini et al. described multiple autoantibody PDGFR specificities based on variable light chains. While one specificity was non-agonistic and present in other rheumatic diseases as well as healthy controls, another specificity was both agonistic and scleroderma-specific. If validated in larger cohorts, this work could provide a potential explanation of the discordant literature to date [71].

The effects of anti-PDGFR have been further studied in mouse models. Luchetti et al. described a skin-SCID chimeric mouse model of scleroderma and demonstrated that pooled scleroderma Ig can induce scleroderma-like changes in the engrafted skin. They further demonstrated that anti-PDGFR monoclonal antibodies generated from pooled scleroderma B cells induce activation of fibrosis in healthy control skin-humanized mice. While of interest, the use of pooled serum and IgG is a limitation of the study. Furthermore, as has been pointed out by others, the notion that autoantibodies directed against a single target such as PDFGR could explain the incredible diversity of disease phenotype seems counterintuitive [72]. In this context, it will be important to further investigate what role(s) additional and/or orthogonal immune responses and mechanisms play in the observed clinical disease heterogeneity.

In addition to anti-PDGFR, autoantibodies against the angiotensin II type 1 receptor (AT_1R) and endothelin-1 type A receptor (ET_AR) have been found in scleroderma patients, and have been shown to have functional effects on endothelial cells [39]. Of note, these autoantibodies were not specific to scleroderma, correlated highly with each other ($r > 0.9$), and resulted in increased TGFB gene expression through interaction with their native receptors via ERK1/2 phosphorylation. Higher levels of either autoantibody associated with clinical outcomes including PAH, diffuse disease, ILD, and digital ulcers. The same group studied effects of pooled IgG from scleroderma patients positive for either AT_1R and ET_AR on human endothelial cells, and reported increased levels of proinflammatory chemokines including IL-8 and CXCL8 as well as increased mRNA levels of vascular cell adhesion molecule-1 (VCAM-1). Beyond human endothelial cells, both AT_1R and ET_AR are expressed on human PBMCs [38], including T cells, B cells, and monocytes. Upon combining IgG from scleroderma patients positive for either AT_1R and ET_AR with human PBMCs, increased production of IL-8 and CCL18 was observed compared to Ig from healthy donors. These effects were attenuated (but not eliminated) by selective AT_1R and ET_AR antagonists. Given that the majority of scleroderma patients tested were positive for these autoantibodies, the question of how a single specificity can explain such a spectrum of clinical features and trajectories is uncertain. It is worth exploring whether multiple specificities (scleroderma-specific and scleroderma-associated) in different combinations and strengths can account for clinically-relevant subgroups.

Research findings over the last 20 years have suggested that functional antibodies may underlie GI dysmotility in scleroderma patients [73, 74]. Autoantibodies against the muscarinic-3-receptor (M3R), which is found on both smooth muscle cells and myenteric cholinergic neurons, have been proposed in scleroderma as well as other rheumatic diseases with GI dysmotility (e.g. Sjogren's syndrome). Pooled IgG from scleroderma patients with severe GI dysmotility co-localized with the M3R on immunohistochemistry in rat colon [75]. This pooled serum was subsequently demonstrated to block cholinergic stimulation at both neural and muscular levels, inhibiting smooth muscle contraction. Interestingly, IVIG has been demonstrated to attenuate/disrupt these effects in vitro via an anti-idiotype mechanism [76]. Further studies to define the prevalence, phenotypic associations, and functional consequences of anti-M3R and similar antibodies are a priority, both in terms of identifying novel pathogenic mechanisms and potentially therapeutically amenable pathways.

Conclusions

Autoimmunity in scleroderma may play important pathogenic roles in the disease. The striking specificity of this immune response and its association with distinct clinical phenotypes has provided important diagnostic and predictive markers in this disease. The value of these specific immune responses as markers (and potentially mediators) of disease initiation and propagation in scleroderma cannot be overstated. With time, such immune responses likely will have utility for monitoring disease activity and response to therapy in the clinic, as well as translate to scleroderma-specific therapies.

References

1. Maes L, Blockmans D, Verschueren P, Westhovens R, De Beeck KO, Vermeersch P, et al. Anti-PM/Scl-100 and anti-RNA-polymerase III antibodies in scleroderma. Clin Chim Acta. 2010;411(13–14):965–71.
2. Steen VD, Powell DL, Medsger TA Jr. Clinical correlations and prognosis based on serum autoantibodies in patients with systemic sclerosis. Arthritis Rheum. 1988;31(2):196–203.
3. Weiner ES, Earnshaw WC, Senecal JL, Bordwell B, Johnson P, Rothfield NF. Clinical associations of anticentromere antibodies and antibodies to topoisomerase I. a study of 355 patients. Arthritis Rheum. 1988;31(3):378–85.
4. Dick T, Mierau R, Bartz-Bazzanella P, Alavi M, Stoyanova-Scholz M, Kindler J, et al. Coexistence of antitopoisomerase I and anticentromere antibodies in patients with systemic sclerosis. Ann Rheum Dis. 2002;61(2):121–7.
5. Harvey GR, McHugh NJ. Serologic abnormalities in systemic sclerosis. Curr Opin Rheumatol. 1999;11(6):495–502.
6. Rothfield NF. Autoantibodies in scleroderma. Rheum Dis Clin N Am. 1992;18(2):483–98.
7. Reimer G, Steen VD, Penning CA, Medsger TA Jr, Tan EM. Correlates between autoantibodies to nucleolar antigens and clinical features in patients with systemic sclerosis (scleroderma). Arthritis Rheum. 1988;31(4):525–32.
8. Henry PA, Atamas SP, Yurovsky VV, Luzina I, Wigley FM, White B. Diversity and plasticity of the anti-DNA topoisomerase I autoantibody response in scleroderma. Arthritis Rheum. 2000;43(12):2733–42.
9. Kuwana M, Kaburaki J, Mimori T, Kawakami Y, Tojo T. Longitudinal analysis of autoantibody response to topoisomerase I in systemic sclerosis. Arthritis Rheum. 2000;43(5):1074–84.
10. Sato S, Hamaguchi Y, Hasegawa M, Takehara K. Clinical significance of anti-topoisomerase I antibody levels determined by ELISA in systemic sclerosis. Rheumatology (Oxford). 2001;40(10):1135–40.
11. Hu PQ, Fertig N, Medsger TA Jr, Wright TM. Correlation of serum anti-DNA topoisomerase I antibody levels with disease severity and activity in systemic sclerosis. Arthritis Rheum. 2003;48(5):1363–73.

12. Nihtyanova SI, Parker JC, Black CM, Bunn CC, Denton CP. A longitudinal study of anti-RNA polymerase III antibody levels in systemic sclerosis. Rheumatology (Oxford). 2009;48(10):1218–21. https://doi.org/10.1093/rheumatology/kep215. Epub 2009 Aug 20.
13. Anthony RM, Ravetch JV. A novel role for the IgG fc glycan: the anti-inflammatory activity of sialylated IgG fcs. J Clin Immunol. 2010;30(Suppl 1):S9–14.
14. Fava A, Cimbro R, Wigley FM, Liu QR, Rosen A, Boin F. Frequency of circulating topoisomerase-I-specific CD4 T cells predicts presence and progression of interstitial lung disease in scleroderma. Arthritis Res Ther. 2016;18(1):99. https://doi.org/10.1186/s13075-016-0993-2.
15. Burbelo PD, Gordon SM, Waldman M, Edison JD, Little DJ, Stitt RS, Bailey WT, Hughes JB, Olson SW. Autoantibodies are present before the clinical diagnosis of systemic sclerosis. PLoS One. 2019;14(3):e0214202.
16. Casciola-Rosen L, Andrade F, Ulanet D, Wong WB, Rosen A. Cleavage by granzyme B is strongly predictive of autoantigen status: implications for initiation of autoimmunity. J Exp Med. 1999;190(6):815–26.
17. Zhou X, Tan FK, Xiong M, Milewicz DM, Feghali CA, Fritzler MJ, et al. Systemic sclerosis (scleroderma): specific autoantigen genes are selectively overexpressed in scleroderma fibroblasts. J Immunol (Baltimore, Md: 1950). 2001;167(12):7126–33.
18. Howard OM, Dong HF, Yang D, Raben N, Nagaraju K, Rosen A, et al. Histidyl-tRNA synthetase and asparaginyl-tRNA synthetase, autoantigens in myositis, activate chemokine receptors on T lymphocytes and immature dendritic cells. J Exp Med. 2002;196(6):781–91.
19. Joseph CG, Darrah E, Shah AA, Skora AD, Casciola-Rosen LA, Wigley FM, Boin F, Fava A, Thoburn C, Kindle I, Jiao Y, Papadopoulos N, Kinzler KW, Vogelstein B, Rosen A. Association of the autoimmune disease scleroderma with an immunological response to cancer. Science. 2014;343:152–7.
20. McMahan ZH, Cottrell TR, Wigley FM, Antiochos B, Zambidis ET, Park TS, Halushka MK, Gutierrez-Alamillo L, Cimbro R, Rosen A, Casciola-Rosen L. Enrichment of scleroderma vascular disease-associated autoantigens in endothelial lineage cells. Arthritis Rheumatol. 2016;68(10):2540–9. https://doi.org/10.1002/art.39743.
21. McMahan ZH, Wigley FM, Casciola-Rosen L. Risk of digital vascular events in scleroderma patients who have both Anticentromere and anti-interferon-inducible protein 16 antibodies. Arthritis Care Res (Hoboken). 2017;69(6):922–6. https://doi.org/10.1002/acr.22978.
22. Andrade F, Roy S, Nicholson D, Thornberry N, Rosen A, Casciola-Rosen L. Granzyme B directly and efficiently cleaves several downstream caspase substrates: implications for CTL-induced apoptosis. Immunity. 1998;8(4):451–60.
23. Ulanet DB, Torbenson M, Dang CV, Casciola-Rosen L, Rosen A. Unique conformation of cancer autoantigen B23 in hepatoma: a mechanism for specificity in the autoimmune response. Proc Natl Acad Sci U S A. 2003;100(21):12361–6.
24. Schachna L, Wigley FM, Morris S, Gelber AC, Rosen A, Casciola-Rosen L. Recognition of granzyme B-generated autoantigen fragments in scleroderma patients with ischemic digital loss. Arthritis Rheum. 2002;46(7):1873–84.
25. Ulanet DB, Flavahan NA, Casciola-Rosen L, Rosen A. Selective cleavage of nucleolar autoantigen B23 by granzyme B in differentiated vascular smooth muscle cells: insights into the association of specific autoantibodies with distinct disease phenotypes. Arthritis Rheum. 2004;50(1):233–41.
26. Rosenthal AK, McLaughlin JK, Gridley G, Nyren O. Incidence of cancer among patients with systemic sclerosis. Cancer. 1995;76(5):910–4.
27. Rosenthal AK, McLaughlin JK, Linet MS, Persson I. Scleroderma and malignancy: an epidemiological study. Ann Rheum Dis. 1993;52(7):531–3.
28. Shah AA, Rosen A, Hummers L, Wigley F, Casciola-Rosen L. Close temporal relationship between onset of cancer and scleroderma in patients with RNA polymerase I/III antibodies. Arthritis Rheum. 2010;62(9):2787–95.
29. Shah AA, Laiho M, Rosen A, Casciola-Rosen L. Protective effect against cancer of antibodies to the large subunits of both RNA polymerases I and III in scleroderma. Arthritis Rheumatol. 2019;71(9):1571–9. https://doi.org/10.1002/art.40893. Epub 2019 Aug 1.
30. Loizos N, Lariccia L, Weiner J, Griffith H, Boin F, Hummers L, et al. Lack of detection of agonist activity by antibodies to platelet-derived growth factor receptor alpha in a subset of normal and systemic sclerosis patient sera. Arthritis Rheum. 2009;60(4):1145–51.
31. Nishijima C, Hayakawa I, Matsushita T, Komura K, Hasegawa M, Takehara K, et al. Autoantibody against matrix metalloproteinase-3 in patients with systemic sclerosis. Clin Exp Immunol. 2004;138(2):357–63.
32. Corallo C, Cheleschi S, Cutolo M, Soldano S, Fioravanti A, Volpi N, Franci D, Nuti R, Giordano N. Antibodies against specific extractable nuclear antigens (ENAs) as diagnostic and prognostic tools and inducers of a profibrotic phenotype in cultured human skin fibroblasts: are they functional? Arthritis Res Ther. 2019;21(1):152. https://doi.org/10.1186/s13075-019-1931-x.
33. Saito E, Fujimoto M, Hasegawa M, Komura K, Hamaguchi Y, Kaburagi Y, et al. CD19-dependent B lymphocyte signaling thresholds influence skin fibrosis and autoimmunity in the tight-skin mouse. J Clin Invest. 2002;109(11):1453–62.
34. Sato S, Hasegawa M, Fujimoto M, Tedder TF, Takehara K. Quantitative genetic variation in CD19 expression correlates with autoimmunity. J Immunol (Baltimore, Md: 1950). 2000;165(11):6635–43.
35. Tamby MC, Humbert M, Guilpain P, Servettaz A, Dupin N, Christner JJ, et al. Antibodies to fibroblasts in idiopathic and scleroderma-associated pulmonary hypertension. Eur Respir J. 2006;28(4):799–807.
36. Wallis DD, Tan FK, Kielty CM, Kimball MD, Arnett FC, Milewicz DM. Abnormalities in fibrillin 1-containing microfibrils in dermal fibroblast cultures from patients with systemic sclerosis (scleroderma). Arthritis Rheum. 2001;44(8):1855–64.
37. Yuan X, Downing AK, Knott V, Handford PA. Solution structure of the transforming growth factor beta-binding protein-like module, a domain associated with matrix fibrils. EMBO J. 1997;16(22):6659–66.
38. Günther J, Kill A, Becker MO, Heidecke H, Rademacher J, Siegert E, Radić M, Burmester GR, Dragun D, Riemekasten G. Angiotensin receptor type 1 and endothelin receptor type A on immune cells mediate migration and the expression of IL-8 and CCL18 when stimulated by autoantibodies from systemic sclerosis patients. Arthritis Res Ther. 2014;16(2):R65. https://doi.org/10.1186/ar4503.
39. Riemekasten G, Philippe A, Näther M, Slowinski T, Müller DN, Heidecke H, Matucci-Cerinic M, Czirják L, Lukitsch I, Becker M, Kill A, van Laar JM, Catar R, Luft FC, Burmester GR, Hegner B, Dragun D. Involvement of functional autoantibodies against vascular receptors in systemic sclerosis. Ann Rheum Dis. 2011;70(3):530–6. https://doi.org/10.1136/ard.2010.135772. Epub 2010 Nov 15.
40. Henderson B, Martin AC. Protein moonlighting: a new factor in biology and medicine. Biochem Soc Trans. 2014;42(6):1671–8. https://doi.org/10.1042/BST20140273.
41. Henault J, Tremblay M, Clement I, Raymond Y, Senecal JL. Direct binding of anti-DNA topoisomerase I autoantibodies to the cell

surface of fibroblasts in patients with systemic sclerosis. Arthritis Rheum. 2004;50(10):3265–74.
42. Henault J, Robitaille G, Senecal JL, Raymond Y. DNA topoisomerase I binding to fibroblasts induces monocyte adhesion and activation in the presence of anti-topoisomerase I autoantibodies from systemic sclerosis patients. Arthritis Rheum. 2006;54(3):963–73.
43. Robitaille G, Christin MS, Clement I, Senecal JL, Raymond Y. Nuclear autoantigen CENP-B transactivation of the epidermal growth factor receptor via chemokine receptor 3 in vascular smooth muscle cells. Arthritis Rheum. 2009;60(9):2805–16.
44. Kim D, Peck A, Santer D, Patole P, Schwartz SM, Molitor JA, et al. Induction of interferon-alpha by scleroderma sera containing autoantibodies to topoisomerase I: association of higher interferon-alpha activity with lung fibrosis. Arthritis Rheum. 2008;58(7):2163–73.
45. Raschi E, Chighizola CB, Cesana L, Privitera D, Ingegnoli F, Mastaglio C, Meroni PL, Borghi MO. Immune complexes containing scleroderma-specific autoantibodies induce a profibrotic and proinflammatory phenotype in skin fibroblasts. Arthritis Res Ther. 2018;20(1):187. https://doi.org/10.1186/s13075-018-1689-6.
46. Bosello S, Angelucci C, Lama G, Alivernini S, Proietti G, Tolusso B, Sica G, Gremese E, Ferraccioli G. Characterization of inflammatory cell infiltrate of scleroderma skin: B cells and skin score progression. Arthritis Res Ther. 2018;20(1):75. https://doi.org/10.1186/s13075-018-1569-0.
47. Daoussis D, Melissaropoulos K, Sakellaropoulos G, Antonopoulos I, Markatseli TE, Simopoulou T, Georgiou P, Andonopoulos AP, Drosos AA, Sakkas L, Liossis SN. A multicenter, open-label, comparative study of B-cell depletion therapy with rituximab for systemic sclerosis-associated interstitial lung disease. Semin Arthritis Rheum. 2017;46(5):625–31. https://doi.org/10.1016/j.semarthrit.2016.10.003. Epub 2016 Oct 13.
48. Jordan S, Distler JH, Maurer B, Huscher D, van Laar JM, Allanore Y, Distler O, EUSTAR Rituximab Study Group. Effects and safety of rituximab in systemic sclerosis: an analysis from the European Scleroderma Trial and Research (EUSTAR) group. Ann Rheum Dis. 2015;74(6):1188–94. https://doi.org/10.1136/annrheumdis--2013-204522. Epub 2014 Jan 17.
49. Matsushita T, Hamaguchi Y, Hasegawa M, Takehara K, Fujimoto M. Decreased levels of regulatory B cells in patients with systemic sclerosis: association with autoantibody production and disease activity. Rheumatology (Oxford). 2016;55(2):263–7. https://doi.org/10.1093/rheumatology/kev331. Epub 2015 Sep 8.
50. Komura K, Yanaba K, Horikawa M, Ogawa F, Fujimoto M, Tedder TF, Sato S. CD19 regulates the development of bleomycin-induced pulmonary fibrosis in a mouse model. Arthritis Rheum. 2008;58(11):3574–84. https://doi.org/10.1002/art.23995.
51. Dumoitier N, Chaigne B, Régent A, Lofek S, Mhibik M, Dorfmüller P, Terrier B, London J, Bérezné A, Tamas N, Varin-Blank N, Mouthon L. Scleroderma peripheral B lymphocytes secrete interleukin-6 and transforming growth factor β and activate fibroblasts. Arthritis Rheumatol. 2017;69(5):1078–89. https://doi.org/10.1002/art.40016.
52. François A, Chatelus E, Wachsmann D, Sibilia J, Bahram S, Alsaleh G, Gottenberg JE. B lymphocytes and B-cell activating factor promote collagen and profibrotic markers expression by dermal fibroblasts in systemic sclerosis. Arthritis Res Ther. 2013;15(5):R168. https://doi.org/10.1186/ar4352.
53. Shlomchik MJ, Craft JE, Mamula MJ. From T to B and back again: positive feedback in systemic autoimmune disease. Nat Rev Immunol. 2001;1(2):147–53.
54. Renaudineau Y, Revelen R, Levy Y, Salojin K, Gilburg B, Shoenfeld Y, et al. Anti-endothelial cell antibodies in systemic sclerosis. Clin Diagn Lab Immunol. 1999;6(2):156–60.
55. Worda M, Sgonc R, Dietrich H, Niederegger H, Sundick RS, Gershwin ME, et al. In vivo analysis of the apoptosis-inducing effect of anti-endothelial cell antibodies in systemic sclerosis by the chorioallantoic membrane assay. Arthritis Rheum. 2003;48(9):2605–14.
56. Sgonc R, Gruschwitz MS, Dietrich H, Recheis H, Gershwin ME, Wick G. Endothelial cell apoptosis is a primary pathogenetic event underlying skin lesions in avian and human scleroderma. J Clin Invest. 1996;98(3):785–92.
57. Chizzolini C, Raschi E, Rezzonico R, Testoni C, Mallone R, Gabrielli A, et al. Autoantibodies to fibroblasts induce a proadhesive and proinflammatory fibroblast phenotype in patients with systemic sclerosis. Arthritis Rheum. 2002;46(6):1602–13.
58. Fineschi S, Goffin L, Rezzonico R, Cozzi F, Dayer JM, Meroni PL, et al. Antifibroblast antibodies in systemic sclerosis induce fibroblasts to produce profibrotic chemokines, with partial exploitation of toll-like receptor 4. Arthritis Rheum. 2008;58(12):3913–23.
59. Ronda N, Raschi E, Testoni C, Borghi MO, Gatti R, Dayer JM, et al. Anti-fibroblast antibodies in systemic sclerosis. Israel Med Assoc J. 2002;4(11 Suppl):858–64.
60. Terrier B, Tamby MC, Camoin L, Guilpain P, Broussard C, Bussone G, et al. Identification of target antigens of antifibroblast antibodies in pulmonary arterial hypertension. Am J Respir Crit Care Med. 2008;177(10):1128–34.
61. Jimenez SA, Christner PJ. Murine animal models of systemic sclerosis. Curr Opin Rheumatol. 2002;14(6):671–80.
62. Kodera T, Tan FK, Sasaki T, Arnett FC, Bona CA. Association of 5′-untranslated region of the fibrillin-1 gene with Japanese scleroderma. Gene. 2002;297(1–2):61–7.
63. Tan FK, Arnett FC, Antohi S, Saito S, Mirarchi A, Spiera H, et al. Autoantibodies to the extracellular matrix microfibrillar protein, fibrillin-1, in patients with scleroderma and other connective tissue diseases. J Immunol (Baltimore, Md: 1950). 1999;163(2):1066–72.
64. Tan FK, Arnett FC, Reveille JD, Ahn C, Antohi S, Sasaki T, et al. Autoantibodies to fibrillin 1 in systemic sclerosis: ethnic differences in antigen recognition and lack of correlation with specific clinical features or HLA alleles. Arthritis Rheum. 2000;43(11):2464–71.
65. Tan FK, Wang N, Kuwana M, Chakraborty R, Bona CA, Milewicz DM, et al. Association of fibrillin 1 single-nucleotide polymorphism haplotypes with systemic sclerosis in Choctaw and japanese populations. Arthritis Rheum. 2001;44(4):893–901.
66. Brinckmann J, Hunzelmann N, El-Hallous E, Krieg T, Sakai LY, Krengel S, et al. Absence of autoantibodies against correctly folded recombinant fibrillin-1 protein in systemic sclerosis patients. Arthritis Res Ther. 2005;7(6):R1221–6.
67. Loeys BL, Gerber EE, Riegert-Johnson D, Iqbal S, Whiteman P, McConnell V, et al. Mutations in fibrillin-1 cause congenital scleroderma: stiff skin syndrome. Sci Transl Med. 2010;2(23):23ra20.
68. Sato S, Hayakawa I, Hasegawa M, Fujimoto M, Takehara K. Function blocking autoantibodies against matrix metalloproteinase-1 in patients with systemic sclerosis. J Invest Dermatol. 2003;120(4):542–7.
69. Baroni SS, Santillo M, Bevilacqua F, Luchetti M, Spadoni T, Mancini M, et al. Stimulatory autoantibodies to the PDGF receptor in systemic sclerosis. N Engl J Med. 2006;354(25):2667–76.
70. Classen JF, Henrohn D, Rorsman F, Lennartsson J, Lauwerys BR, Wikstrom G, et al. Lack of evidence of stimulatory autoantibodies to platelet-derived growth factor receptor in patients with systemic sclerosis. Arthritis Rheum. 2009;60(4):1137–44.
71. Moroncini G, Grieco A, Nacci G, Paolini C, Tonnini C, Pozniak KN, Cuccioloni M, Mozzicafreddo M, Svegliati S, Angeletti M, Kazlauskas A, Avvedimento EV, Funaro A, Gabrielli A. Epitope specificity determines pathogenicity and detectability of anti-platelet-derived growth factor receptor α autoantibodies in systemic sclerosis. Arthritis Rheumatol. 2015;67(7):1891–903. https://doi.org/10.1002/art.39125.
72. Fritzler MJ, Choi MY. Editorial: are autoantibodies involved in the pathogenesis of systemic sclerosis? Arthritis Rheumatol. 2016;68(9):2067–70. https://doi.org/10.1002/art.39727.

73. Eaker EY, Kuldau JG, Verne GN, Ross SO, Sallustio JE. Myenteric neuronal antibodies in scleroderma: passive transfer evokes alterations in intestinal myoelectric activity in a rat model. J Lab Clin Med. 1999;133(6):551–6. https://doi.org/10.1016/s0022-2143(99)90184-1.
74. Goldblatt F, Gordon TP, Waterman SA. Antibody-mediated gastrointestinal dysmotility in scleroderma. Gastroenterology. 2002;123(4):1144–50.
75. Singh J, Cohen S, Mehendiratta V, Mendoza F, Jimenez SA, Dimarino AJ, Rattan S. Effects of scleroderma antibodies and pooled human immunoglobulin on anal sphincter and colonic smooth muscle function. Gastroenterology. 2012;143(5):1308–18. https://doi.org/10.1053/j.gastro.2012.07.109. Epub 2012 Aug 1.
76. Kumar S, Singh J, Kedika R, Mendoza F, Jimenez SA, Blomain ES, DiMarino AJ, Cohen S, Rattan S. Role of muscarinic-3 receptor antibody in systemic sclerosis: correlation with disease duration and effects of IVIG. Am J Physiol Gastrointest Liver Physiol. 2016;310(11):G1052–60. https://doi.org/10.1152/ajpgi.00034.2016. Epub 2016 May 12.

Mechanisms of Vascular Disease

16

Mirko Manetti and Bashar Kahaleh

Introduction

Scleroderma (systemic sclerosis (SSc)) is to a large degree identified by the vascular features which may precede the onset of tissue fibrosis by months or even years. Abnormalities in microvessel morphology and vascular dysfunction occur early during the disease course and evolve into a distinctive fibroproliferative and destructive microvasculopathy that relentlessly advances in nearly all affected organs. This evidence suggests that endothelial cells (ECs) are the primary target in SSc and that multiple interactions of ECs with other cell types and pathways, including cells of both the innate and adaptive immune systems and autoantibodies, platelets and coagulation factors, vascular smooth muscle cells (VSMCs), and fibroblasts, are likely crucial to the disease pathogenesis. In SSc, vascular injury includes persistent EC activation/damage and apoptosis, intimal thickening, and microvessel obliteration. These profound vascular changes lead to vascular tone dysfunction and reduced capillary blood flow, with consequent chronic tissue ischemia. The resulting tissue hypoxia triggers complex cellular and molecular mechanisms in the attempt to compensate for altered EC functions and to insure adequate tissue perfusion. Nonetheless, the evidence for significant compensatory angiogenesis in SSc is lacking, and the disease evolves toward irreversible structural changes in multiple microvascular beds culminating in substantial loss of the peripheral capillary network and further aggravating tissue ischemia. A critical imbalance between proangiogenic and antiangiogenic factors may be largely responsible for the lack of vascular repair and regeneration in SSc. Besides insufficient angiogenesis, it appears that defective vasculogenesis with altered numbers and functional impairment of bone marrow-derived endothelial progenitor cells (EPCs) may further prevent vascular recovery in SSc. Furthermore, the recently described process of endothelial-to-mesenchymal transition (EndoMT) adds to endothelial loss, promotes vessel wall fibrosis, and contributes to perivascular tissue fibrosis.

Clinically, the vascular manifestations in SSc include Raynaud's phenomenon (RP), the early edematous puffy hands, telangiectasias, digital ulcers, gastric antral vascular ectasia (GAVE), pulmonary arterial hypertension (PAH), myocardial dysfunction, and scleroderma renal crisis. Therapeutically, the use of angiotensin-converting enzyme inhibitors for scleroderma renal crisis, endothelin receptor antagonists for PAH, and phosphodiesterase inhibitors for PAH, RP, and digital ulcers have significantly improved the care of SSc patients over the last two decades. However, despite this symptomatic improvement, regression of the vascular lesions has been difficult to achieve.

The Vascular Problem

Vascular involvement in SSc includes a spectrum of changes that affect predominantly the microcirculation, mainly the capillaries and the small arterioles. The pathologic changes in the microvascular tree range from EC activation with increased expression of adhesion molecules to EC injury and apoptosis, capillary necrosis, intimal proliferation, and luminal occlusion that result in tissue ischemia and contribute to organ failure together with concomitant perivascular and interstitial fibrosis. The current hypotheses in SSc vascular pathogenesis mainly implicate a possible, yet unidentified, microbial trigger and an immune-mediated mechanism that results in vascular injury possibly through recognition of a putative vascular or perivascular autoantigen and the induction of autoantibodies. This chapter will review the current knowledge of the morphologic and functional features of SSc vasculopathy with special emphasis on the cellular and

M. Manetti (✉)
Section of Anatomy and Histology, Department of Experimental and Clinical Medicine, University of Florence, Florence, Italy
e-mail: mirko.manetti@unifi.it

B. Kahaleh
Division of Rheumatology, Allergy and Immunology, University of Toledo Medical Center, Toledo, OH, USA
e-mail: bashar.kahaleh@utoledo.edu

Y. Allanore et al. (eds.), *Scleroderma*, https://doi.org/10.1007/978-3-031-40658-4_16

molecular mechanisms and pathologic sequences of vascular injury and defective vascular repair and regeneration.

The Vascular Lesion

The prominent vascular abnormalities in SSc are typically observed in the capillaries and the small blood vessels [1, 2]. Swelling and proliferation of the intima with mononuclear cell infiltration are seen in the small arterioles. In the capillary network, the vascular disease is characterized by distorted and irregular capillary loops in all involved organs including the skin, kidneys, lungs, heart, and muscles, reflecting the diffuse nature of the microvascular disorder in SSc, even in sites not affected by fibrosis [1–3]. At the ultrastructural level, the earliest vascular changes in the edematous stage of the disease consist of vascular leaking with opening of EC tight junctions, vacuolization of cytoplasm with increase in the number of basal lamina-like layers, and occasional entrapment of lymphocytes and cellular vesicles in the vessel wall [1, 4]. Further signs of nuclear injury in association with EC membrane disruption occur in more advanced disease. Ghost vessels consisting of an intact basal lamina with remnants of ECs are occasionally noted in association with perivascular cellular infiltrates that consist of macrophages and T and B cells, with predominance of $CD4^+$ T cells [5]. EC apoptosis was first described on ultrastructural examination of SSc skin biopsies in the early inflammatory stages of the disease, suggesting a causal association [5]. It was later noted in the University of California at Davis (UCD) lines 200/206 chickens that spontaneously develop a systemic disease that closely resembles human SSc [6]. Apoptosis of ECs is not unique to SSc vasculopathy and is frequently observed in diseases with prominent vascular involvement, such as early atherosclerotic lesions, graft rejection, thrombotic thrombocytopenic purpura, and the hemolytic uremic syndrome, suggesting that EC apoptosis may be a common prerequisite for a variety of vascular disorders [7, 8]. The fate of apoptotic ECs in SSc is not well examined. A possible defect in the orderly removal of apoptotic cells may lead to phagocytosis by dendritic cells and macrophages and subsequent presentation of cellular antigens to $CD8^+$ T cells [9], leading to immune recognition of vascular antigens. Moreover, apoptotic ECs can activate the alternative complement and coagulation cascades leading to vascular microthrombosis and further tissue compromise [10, 11]. Typical ultrastructural SSc microvascular changes are shown in Fig. 16.1.

Increased EC thymidine labeling has been reported in SSc, particularly in the indurated phase of the disease [12]. EC thymidine labeling is seen only in the involved "fibrotic" skin, suggesting that EC changes in the uninvolved skin represent cellular activation but not true injury. Significant intimal proliferation and accumulation of proteoglycans in the arterioles and small-sized arteries are common in SSc [13]. Moreover, abnormality of the vessel wall is likely to result from increased synthesis of extracellular matrix (ECM) by intimal and adventitial fibroblasts. Transdifferentiation of ECs into profibrotic myofibroblasts via the process of EndoMT may contribute further to vascular wall fibrosis [14].

The presence of vascular pathology at one site does not necessarily indicate similar pathology at other sites; for instance, the presence of vascular pulmonary pathology clinically manifesting as PAH may not be associated with vascular pathology in the kidneys nor is there any relationship between vascular changes in the gastrointestinal tract (i.e., GAVE) and vascular changes in either the lungs or the kidneys. Milder degrees of vascular changes can be seen in clinically uninvolved skin, mainly in the papillary dermal layer in association with platelets adhering to the vessel walls of the dermal microvasculature [5]. It is not known if these changes precede the development of tissue fibrosis or are independent of it. In contrast to small arterioles, large-sized vessel occlusion in SSc is unusual; however, it can occur particularly in the ulnar arteries in patients with the limited cutaneous form of SSc in association with anticentromere antibodies [15]. In the arteries, intimal proliferation of a uniform and symmetrical nature leads to the formation of a neointima indistinguishable from that seen in other autoimmune diseases, chronic homograft rejection, and accelerated atherosclerosis such as restenosis after coronary bypass [16]. The medial layers are usually thinned, except in hypertensive patients where medial hypertrophy and fibrinoid deposition can be seen [17]. The capillary changes in SSc are most visible in the nailfolds.

Nailfold capillaroscopy: The first description of capillary abnormalities in SSc was published in 1925 by Brown and O'Leary who employed a simple technique to describe capillary changes typical of the microvasculature involvement in SSc [18]. In the 1970s–1980s, the seminal work by Maricq and colleagues popularized the use of wide-field capillary microscopy and described specific "SSc patterns" of capillary changes [19–24] (Fig. 16.2).

Nailfold capillaroscopy has great diagnostic value in the early stages of the disease. It is the technique of choice for the identification of patients with RP who are at risk for developing SSc [25–27].

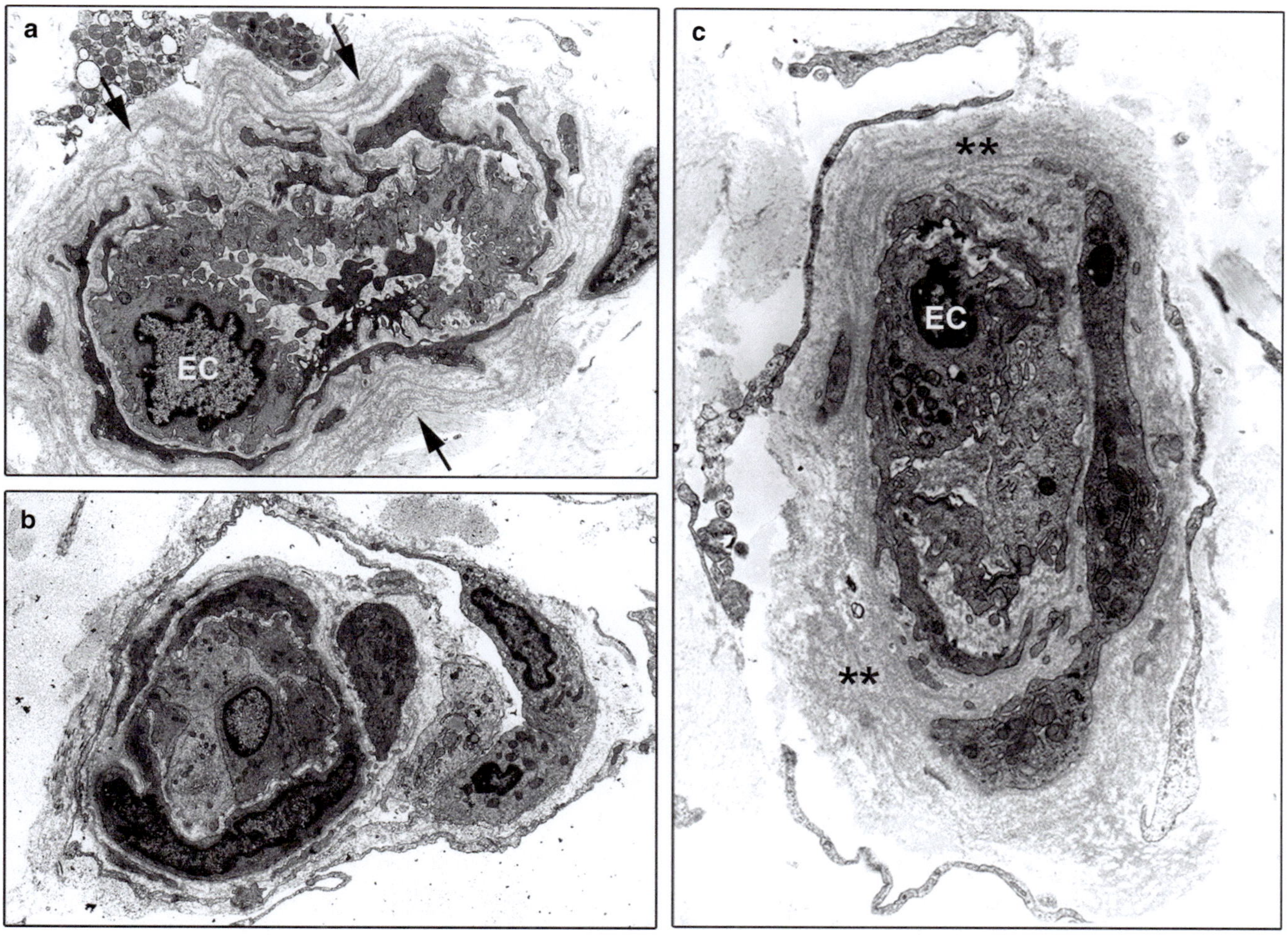

Fig. 16.1 (**a–c**) Representative transmission electron microscopy (TEM) photomicrographs of SSc dermal microvessels. (**a**) Microvessel shows apoptosis of ECs and reduplication of the basal lamina (arrows). Apoptotic ECs display plasma membrane blebbing with release of apoptotic bodies. (**b**) Swollen ECs occluding microvessel's lumen. (**c**) Microvessel with an occluded lumen shows thickened basal lamina (asterisks). *EC* endothelial cell. TEM; original magnification: ×6000

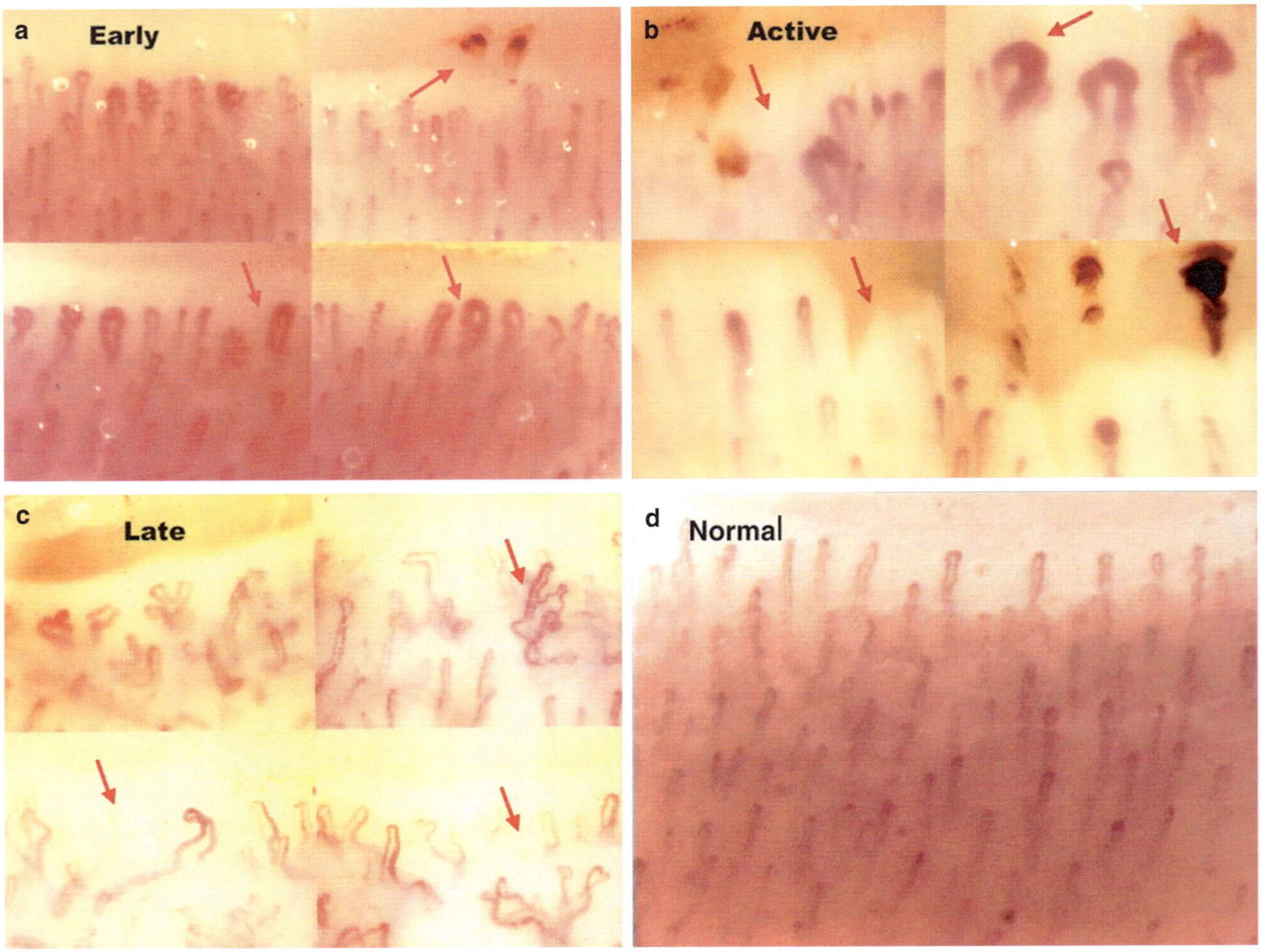

Fig. 16.2 Nailfold capillaroscopy. (**a**) Early scleroderma pattern shows well-preserved capillary architecture and density and presence of dilated and giant capillaries. (**b**) Active scleroderma pattern shows frequent giant capillaries and hemorrhages, moderate loss of capillaries, and disorganization of capillary architecture. (**c**) Late scleroderma pattern shows severe capillary architecture disorganization with dropouts, presence of arborized capillaries, and absence of giant capillaries. (**d**) Normal nailfold capillaroscopic pattern. (Courtesy of Cutolo et al. [24], published by Oxford University Press. With permission)

Vascular Dysfunction in Scleroderma

The normal vascular endothelium is a single-cell thick layer that is endowed with remarkably diverse functions. ECs regulate coagulation and fibrinolysis, vascular permeability, vascular tone, and metabolism and nutrition of surrounding cells. Injury to the endothelium in SSc leads to profound vascular dysfunction that is prominent in the early stages of the disease and progressively worsens over time [2, 4, 5, 28]. ECs also regulate vascular tone by producing vasoconstrictive and vasodilatory molecules. Endothelial dysfunction is typically associated with an imbalance favoring the production of vasoconstrictors and represses the production of vasodilators resulting in vasospasm and reduced blood flow. This is particularly true in SSc where overexpression of the potent vasoconstrictor endothelin-1 (ET-1) and reduced production of the vasodilators nitric oxide (NO) and prostacyclin are seen.

Endothelin-1

ET-1 is a powerful dose-dependent vasoconstrictor. At low concentrations, ET-1 is vasodilator, while at higher concentrations, it mediates vasoconstriction and reduction of blood flow [29]. ET-1 is overexpressed in the skin of SSc patients [30, 31]. Moreover, the circulating levels of ET-1 and tissue concentrations of ET-1 in the lungs, kidneys, and liver are elevated in SSc [32–35].

Early studies showed that ET-1 induces fibroblast proliferation and collagen synthesis in a dose-dependent manner, potentially linking vascular dysfunction to tissue fibrosis.

ET-1 acts through the endothelin receptors type A (ETAR) and type B (ETBR) that are expressed in various cell types. An imbalanced expression of ETAR and ETBR has been reported in SSc patients [36, 37]. The role of endogenous ET-1 in EC dysfunction was examined in tight-skin mice (TSK1), a mouse model of SSc [38]. The mesenteric arteries of TSK1 mice showed decreased responses to acetylcholine, suggesting impaired NO-independent, and prostaglandin-mediated relaxation that was partially restored by the dual endothelin receptor antagonist (ERA) bosentan [39], suggesting a role for ET1 in the impaired vasodilation.

ET-1 also stimulates VSMC proliferation and contraction, possibly contributing to remodeling of the vascular wall and vasculopathic manifestations characteristic of SSc, such as PAH and digital ulcers. Indeed, clinical studies have shown that ERAs may be effective in the treatment of SSc-related PAH and in the prevention of digital ulcers [40, 41]. Treatment with the ERA bosentan may also improve peripheral microcirculation in SSc patients, as demonstrated by the shifting from the "late" to the "active" nailfold videocapillaroscopy pattern after therapy [42]. In another study, long-term treatment with bosentan in combination with iloprost reduced the progression of nailfold microvascular damage in SSc patients over a 3-year follow-up period [43]. Conversely, another study reported that treatment with the ERA macitentan did not reduce the development of new digital ulcers over 16 weeks in SSc patients with active ischemic digital ulcers [44].

Nitric Oxide

NO can play a dual role in the endothelium, depending on which NO synthase (NOS) catalyzes its synthesis from L-arginine. Mammals produce three NOS isoforms. Two are expressed in the endothelium; endothelial NO synthase (eNOS) is expressed in ECs, whereas inducible NO synthase (iNOS) is expressed in ECs, VSMCs, fibroblasts, macrophages, and other cell types [45]. Endothelial NOS plays a crucial role in maintaining vasorelaxation and in controlling vascular tone, blood pressure, and thrombosis [46]. Disruption of the endothelium reduces NO synthesis and release with significant consequences to the vasculature. Deficient endothelial-dependent relaxation in SSc is suggested by impaired maximal responses to endothelial-dependent vasodilators and normal responses to endothelial-independent dilators [47–50].

Despite the expectation that NO production would be reduced in a dysfunctional endothelium, NOx (NO and NO_2) and nitrated protein levels appear to be elevated in SSc patients [51]. This is probably related to the upregulation of iNOS expression in association with increased levels of immunodetectable nitrotyrosine, a marker of NO-mediated free radical injury, as shown by immunohistochemical studies on skin biopsies [52]. Still, endothelial dysfunction in SSc is in part attributable to reduced constitutive release of NO due to repressed eNOS expression.

Nature of the Endothelial Injury

The triggers for vascular injury and dysfunction in SSc are largely unknown. However, infectious agents, EC cytotoxicity, activation and apoptosis, autoantibodies, shear stress, and ischemia/reperfusion are among the potential contributors. Current hypotheses in the pathogenesis of SSc vascular disease implicate a possible, yet unidentified, microbial trigger and an immune-mediated activation that lead to vascular injury and the generation of progressive occlusive arteriolar disease (Fig. 16.3).

Microbial Triggers

Infectious agents may be part of the etiology of SSc, but the evidence is indirect. In one study, patients with RP were treated with triple antibiotics to eliminate Helicobacter pylori infection, a gastric bacterium associated with other vascular diseases [53]. The treatment regimen resulted in the disappearance of RP in 17% of the patients and reduced symptoms in 72% [54]. Other studies evaluated the incidence of Helicobacter pylori infection in SSc patients [55]; one study showed a higher correlation, while others showed none [56, 57].

Cytomegalovirus (CMV) infection may play a role in the pathogenesis of SSc vasculopathy. CMV infects ECs and monocytes/macrophages leading to dysregulation of the immune system and upregulation of fibrogenic cytokines [16, 58], events that are also characteristic of SSc. Indirect evidence supporting a role for CMV includes the presence of CMV antibodies in serum from SSc patients that could potentially interact with autoantigens [58, 59]. Rat and mouse models show that CMV infection leads to formation of intimal lesions [60, 61]. An immune-suppressed mouse model of CMV-induced neointima development has many characteristics of SSc including EC apoptosis, myofibroblast differentiation, and increased expression of transforming growth factor-β (TGF-β) and platelet-derived growth factor (PDGF). However, a significant difference between this model and human SSc is that the vascular lesions develop in the main abdominal vessels, while in SSc, the lesions occur in the microvasculature [62].

Parvovirus B19 has also been implicated in the pathogenesis of SSc. Parvovirus B19 is much more commonly found as an active infection in SSc patients (4%) than the general population (0.6%) [63]. Parvovirus B19 was detected in bone marrow biopsies from a high percentage of SSc patients (57%), who did not have an active B19 infection [64]. Further

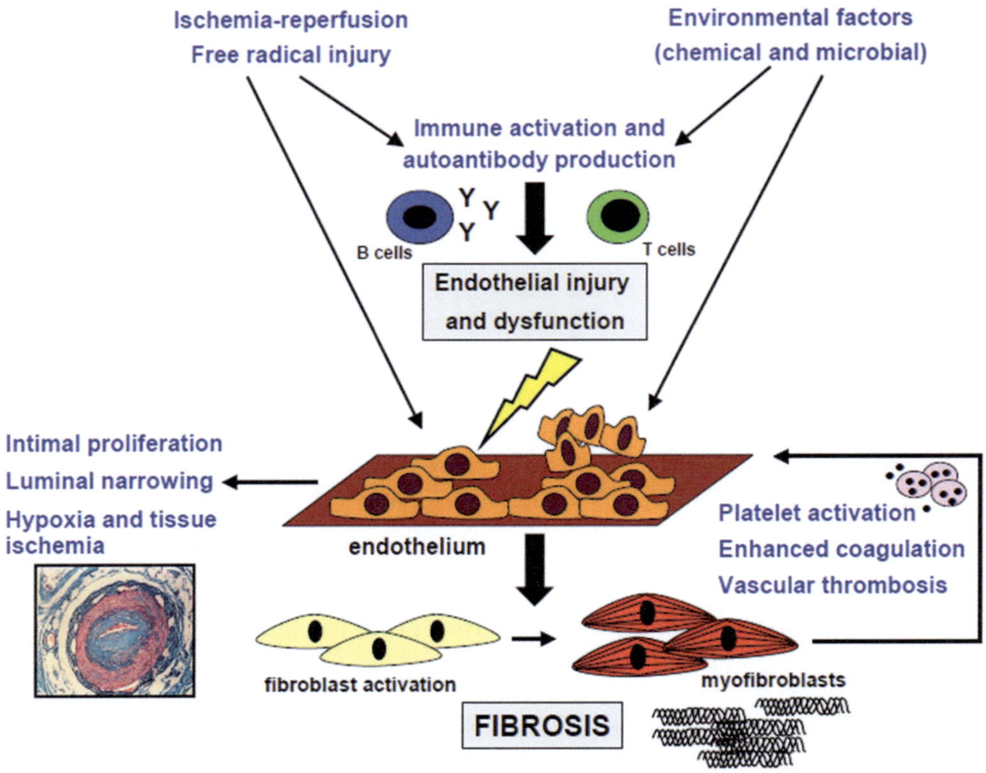

Fig. 16.3 Pathogenesis of SSc vasculopathy. Endothelial injury and dysfunction are initiated by the actions of free radicals and environmental, chemical, or microbial agents that injure the endothelium either directly or indirectly by the induction of immune activation and the generation of autoantibodies and activated cellular immunity. The vascular injury leads to the activation of platelet and coagulation pathways that result in vascular microthrombosis. The resulting vasculopathy is associated with intimal hyperplasia in the small arterioles, and the ensuing luminal narrowing results in tissue hypoxia and the generation of the state of chronic ischemia. Released vascular products, in association with hypoxia and ischemia, collectively contribute to the activation of resident fibroblasts that transdifferentiate into profibrotic myofibroblasts and, in turn, perpetuate the vasculopathy by triggering vascular wall fibrosis

studies found a correlation between B19 expression levels and the severity of endothelial dysfunction in SSc [65]. In a recent study, parvovirus B19 was found to activate in vitro normal human dermal fibroblasts [66]. In particular, B19 infection significantly increased both fibroblast migration and invasiveness, along with mRNA expression of different profibrotic genes, some genes associated with the inflammasome platform, and genes for matrix metalloproteinases (MMPs) such as MMP-12, whose upregulation is implicated in SSc-related microvasculopathy and defective angiogenesis [66]. This suggests a potential role for this virus in SSc pathogenesis.

Endothelial Cell Cytotoxicity, Apoptosis, and Activation

The evidence of EC injury in SSc patients prompted studies to investigate the presence of potential cytotoxic factors in their serum. Some studies suggest that the cytotoxic effect of SSc plasma on ECs is antibody-dependent [67–69]. Sgonc et al. showed that activated natural killer (NK) cells are required for antiendothelial cell antibody (AECA)-dependent apoptosis in human dermal microvascular ECs (MVECs) [70]. Two different cytotoxic mechanisms can be stimulated by NK cells: a granzyme/perforin synergistic mechanism and Fas/FasL interaction [71].

Kahaleh et al. reported a circulating proteolytic EC cytotoxic factor in plasma of SSc patients [72]. In a later study, they identified a granular enzyme, thought to be granzyme A that significantly inhibited EC growth [73].

Granzyme B (GrB), a serine protease found in cytoplasmic granules of NK cells and T lymphocytes, is protective against various pathogens [74, 75]. Some studies demonstrate that GrB cleaves vitronectin, fibronectin, and laminin, three proteins that have a primary role in ECM function, and consequently inhibits cell migration, spreading, and invasion [76]. Other studies have shown that the proteolytic activity of GrB and other proteases contained in T-cell granules cleaves plasminogen and plasmin into angiostatin fragments [77], which have multiple consequences in the ECM. Indeed, plasminogen cleavage in the kringle domains produces antiangiogenic angiostatin, the pool of plasminogen that can be converted to plasmin is reduced, and subsequently, plasmin activity and its effects on regulating ECM composition become limited. Evidence indicates that this mechanism may be enhanced in SSc plasma contributing to increased levels of angiostatin [77].

A number of ECM cleavage products are inhibitors of angiogenesis; they all induce EC apoptosis. These antiangiogenic fragments include the collagen XV and XVIII breakdown product endostatin [78], collagen IV breakdown product tumstatin [79] and canstatin [80], plasminogen breakdown product angiostatin [77, 81], and 18-kDa prolactin fragment [82][83]. Under normal conditions, antiangiogenic factors are tightly regulated to maintain a balance with proangiogenic factors. In addition to elevated circulating angiostatin levels [77], in SSc, there is evidence of elevated levels of endostatin [84–86], which suggests an imbalance that favors angiogenesis inhibitors with proapoptotic activity. Of note, an in vitro study employing human dermal MVECs challenged with sera from SSc patients revealed that treatment with the immunosuppressive drug cyclophosphamide (CYC) may significantly reduce EC apoptosis and improve angiogenesis by rebalancing dysregulated antiangiogenic factors, including angiostatin, endostatin, pentraxin 3 (PTX3), and MMP-12 [86].

Antibody-Dependent Cellular Cytotoxicity

Autoimmunity is a major component of SSc. Interestingly, all autoantigens are redistributed and clustered in blebs or apoptotic bodies on the cell surface of apoptotic cells despite their varied functions, structures, and cellular localization [87]. This led Casciola-Rosen et al. to propose that reactive oxygen species (ROS) in the blebs and apoptotic bodies may produce fragments of autoantigens which expose cryptic epitopes recognized by T cells [87]. This hypothesis has been supported by others showing that posttranslational protein alterations expose cryptic cleavage sites with significance in selection of autoantigens [88, 89]. The role of GrB cleavage of autoantigens is suggested by the presence of autoantibodies that recognize GrB-generated autoantigen fragments particularly in limited SSc (lSSc) patients with ischemic digital loss [90–92].

Antiendothelial Cell Antibodies (AECAs)

Circulating autoantibodies to ECs (AECAs) are found in 44–84% of SSc patients in clinical trials [93, 94]. A greater incidence of AECAs is found in patients with digital ischemia or PAH [95, 96]. Interestingly, AECAs bind distinctly different micro- and macrovascular EC antigens in SSc patients with associated PAH and in patients with idiopathic PAH as compared to SSc patients without PAH [97]. The variant affinities could potentially be used as a predictor of more advanced vascular disease in SSc patients.

The role of AECAs in the induction of EC apoptosis is suggested by findings in the avian model of SSc (UCD-200/206 chickens) [6]. EC apoptosis was noted following the transfer of AECAs into normal chick embryos [98]; however, apoptosis was also noted in other cell types making it difficult to determine if apoptosis results directly from AECAs binding or if it is part of normal embryogenesis.

SSc sera containing autoantibodies were shown to induce EC apoptosis [99]. A caspase inhibitor could only partially inhibit the apoptosis, suggesting that additional factors are involved in the induction of apoptosis. One such factor may be the ECM microfibrillar protein fibrillin-1. Autoantibodies to fibrillin-1 are found in a large proportion of SSc patients [100]. Fibrillin-1 expression was detected in apoptotic ECs (identified in the blebs and apoptotic bodies) exposed to SSc serum containing AECAs. These data suggest that AECAs found in SSc serum may induce fibrillin-1 expression and EC apoptosis, but the evidence is indirect.

Besides apoptosis, more recently, it has been reported that AECAs may play an important role in activating ECs [101]. Arends et al. demonstrated that immunoglobulins G (IgG) from AECA-positive SSc patients, patients with idiopathic PAH, and patients with systemic lupus erythematosus activate MVECs with increased expression of intercellular adhesion molecule-1 (ICAM-1) [101]. However, disease specificity for this observation is not established. Moreover, Wolf et al. reported significant elevation of anti-ICAM-1 IgM antibodies in the sera of both lSSc and diffuse SSc (dSSc) patients, while elevated anti-ICAM-1 IgG antibodies were found only in lSSc patients [102]. Moreover, anti-ICAM-1 IgG antibodies bind to ECs leading to a significant increase in ROS production [102].

Shear Stress and SSc Vascular Disease

Intimal hypertrophy and vascular remodeling are major contributors to vascular complications and mortality in SSc [103–105]. Key factors that contribute to vascular wall remodeling are shear stress, chronic hypoxia, and inflammation.

Increased shear stress impacts many aspects of the vascular wall. It can enhance EC and VSMC proliferation, increase levels of inflammatory molecules such as interleukin-8 (IL-8, also known as CXCL8), promote ROS and collagen production, and inhibit eNOS levels and EC repair.

Increased cyclic stretch, which accompanies shear stress, plays an important role in regulating EC phenotype and gene expression by inducing ROS production. This leads to increased permeability, production of vascular endothelial growth factor (VEGF) and fibroblast growth factor (FGF), apoptosis and cytoskeletal remodeling and increased production of ECM, matrix-degrading enzymes, and inflammation [106, 107]. In this manner, increased cyclic stretch could partially explain the increased formation of ECM in disorders such as SSc. Cyclic stretch causes a much greater loss of endothelial barrier function in response to VEGF stimulation compared to no stretch controls; this effect is partially ameliorated by adding a ROS scavenger to the cells [106].

Reperfusion and Oxidative Injury

The concept that ischemia/reperfusion generates ROS was reported by McCord in 1985 [108]. Ischemia/reperfusion associated with RP leads to ROS generation that may contribute to vascular endothelial damage. Reactive oxygen and nitrogen species can contribute to vascular damage through peroxidation of lipids, oxidation of proteins, or a flawed antioxidant defense system such as that described for NO. Thus, significant decrease in total plasma antioxidant capacity was noted in SSc patients [109]. Moreover, antioxidant levels inversely correlated with the severity of RP and with capillary loss, suggesting that oxidative stress worsens in advanced microvasculature disease. In addition, increased levels of oxidative stress markers were reported and correlated with the overall severity of the disease [110]. A role for autoantibodies in deficient oxidative stress defense was suggested by the presence of autoantibodies that inhibit the oxidative stress repair enzyme methionine sulfoxide reductase A and B (MSRA and MSRB [111–113]) in SSc patients [114]. The antibody titer correlated with renal vascular damage and inversely correlated with pulmonary function [114].

Agonistic Autoantibodies to the Platelet-Derived Growth Factor Receptor and Generation of ROS

Baroni et al. identified autoantibodies in the sera of SSc patients that interact with and activate the receptor for platelet-derived growth factor (PDGFR), resulting in ROS accumulation in target cells that can potentially account for tissue injury [115]. Furthermore, these antibodies are capable of upregulating the expression of α-smooth muscle actin (α-SMA) and type I collagen in fibroblasts. Of note, these genes are characteristically overexpressed in SSc fibroblasts. However, other studies were unable to confirm the presence of stimulatory anti-PDGFR autoantibodies in SSc sera [116]. Moroncini et al. subsequently developed novel assays for detection of serum anti-PDGFR autoantibodies, showing that epitope specificity is crucial in determining the pathogenicity and detectability of these antibodies in SSc [117]. In particular, they found that agonistic anti-PDGFR autoantibodies are enriched in SSc sera and recognize specific conformational epitopes that can be used to discriminate agonistic from nonagonistic antibodies [117]. In another study, the same authors investigated the biologic effect of agonistic anti-PDGFR autoantibodies from SSc patients on human pulmonary VSMCs demonstrating that they may contribute to the pathogenesis of intimal hyperplasia [118]. Indeed, pulmonary VSMCs acquired a synthetic phenotype characterized by higher proliferation rate, migratory activity, gene expression of type I collagen α1 chain, and reduced expression of markers characteristic of the contractile phenotype (i.e., smooth muscle myosin heavy chain and smooth muscle calponin) when stimulated with anti-PDGFR autoantibodies, but not with normal IgG [118]. Of note, these effects appeared to be mediated by increased generation of ROS and expression of NOX4 and mammalian target of rapamycin (mTOR)C1 [118]. Besides the abovementioned effects on VSMCs, whether agonistic anti-PDGFR autoantibodies may contribute to EC injury in SSc has yet to be determined.

Autoantibodies to Angiotensin and Endothelin Receptors

Circulating autoantibodies directed against vascular receptors, namely the angiotensin II type 1 receptor (AT1R) and ETAR, have been associated with characteristic disease features including vascular, inflammatory, and fibrotic complications of SSc patients [119]. Kill et al. demonstrated that anti-AT1R and anti-ETAR autoantibody-positive IgG from SSc patients foster the activation of human MVECs in vitro by inducing the overexpression of the proinflammatory chemokine IL-8 and vascular cell adhesion molecule-1, with consequent increase in neutrophil migration through an endothelial layer and activation of ROS [119]. Moreover, SSc-IgG decreased MVEC wound repair [119]. Anti-AT1R and anti-ETAR autoantibodies were found to be more frequent in SSc-associated PAH, as well as in PAH associated with other connective tissue diseases compared with other forms of pulmonary hypertension, and could serve as predictive and prognostic biomarkers in SSc-associated PAH [120]. In vivo experiments further demonstrated that in SSc both autoantibodies may contribute to the development of PAH via increased vascular endothelial reactivity and induction of pulmonary vasculopathy [120]. In addition, Avouac et al. reported that anti-ETAR autoantibodies are strong predictors of digital ulcers in SSc [121]. Therefore, anti-AT1R and anti-ETAR autoantibodies could represent novel targets for therapeutic intervention in the treatment of SSc vasculopathy.

Epigenetics and SSc Vasculopathy

The basis for EC dysfunction and altered cellular phenotype in SSc has not been determined, but primary metabolic abnormalities, responses to abnormal environmental signals, and clonal selection have all been hypothesized to play a role [122]. Still, it is known that SSc cellular abnormalities persist in multiple generations in vitro. The persistence of dysfunctional phenotype outside the disease environment suggests the possibility of an in vivo imprinting of disease phenotype that is inherited and is transmitted from one generation to the next. The term epigenetics describes all inherited changes in gene expression that are not coded in the DNA sequence itself. The three major mechanisms that are known to mediate epigenetic alterations are DNA methylation, histone modification, and microRNAs (miRNAs), the latter contributing to gene expression through posttranscriptional mechanisms [123].

Methylation of the CpG dinucleotides has long been recognized as a major epigenetic modification of the mammalian genome and is implicated in imprinting, X chromosome inactivation, embryonic development, defense against retroviral sequences, transcriptional repression of certain genes, and carcinogenesis [124, 125]. CpG islands are stretches of DNA located within the promoter regions of about 40% of mammalian genes. The methylation of CpG islands leads to a stable, heritable repression of transcription of the affected gene. DNA methylation is the most widely studied epigenetic mechanism in autoimmune diseases and is considered the core epigenetic control mechanism. DNA methylation is accomplished by the de novo DNA methyltransferases (DNMTs) DNMT3a and DNMT3b, while an existing methylation pattern is maintained during cell division and thus inherited in proliferating cells by DNMT1 [126].

There is emerging evidence suggesting that alteration of DNA methylation profiles at global or gene-specific levels may contribute to SSc pathogenesis. Endothelial nitric oxide synthase gene (NOS3) expression is reduced in SSc skin and cultured ECs [127]. Data suggest that heavy methylation of the CpG sites in the promoter region of NOS3 gene leads to gene repression and that the addition of DNMT1 inhibitor 5-azacytidine leads to normalization of NOS3 expression. The significance of underexpression of NOS3 is illustrated by the fact that NOS3-null mice are characterized by systemic and pulmonary hypertension, impaired wound healing and angiogenesis, as well as impaired mobilization of stem and endothelial precursors, leading to failure of neovascularization [128, 129]. Another endothelial gene that appears to be regulated by epigenetic control is bone morphogenic protein receptor II (BMPRII). BMPs are members of the TGF-β superfamily of proteins that coordinate cell proliferation, differentiation, and survival. The latter is particularly true for ECs, since BMP signaling through BMPRII favors EC survival and apoptosis resistance. An inactivating mutation in the BMPRII gene has been linked to primary pulmonary hypertension suggesting a crucial role in the development of PAH-related vasculopathy [130]. In SSc, significant decrease in the expression levels of BMPRII in ECs and skin was described [131]. This was shown to be associated with enhanced responses of SSc ECs to apoptotic signals, including serum starvation and oxidation injury. Sequencing the BMPRII promoter region after bisulfite conversion demonstrated heavy methylation of CpG sites in BMPRII promoter in SSc ECs. BMPRII expression levels and the enhanced EC apoptotic responses were normalized by the addition of 5-azacytidine. These data suggest that epigenetic repression of BMPRII gene may play a central role in EC vulnerability to apoptosis and that impaired BMPRII signaling in SSc ECs may contribute to the pathogenesis of SSc vasculopathy [131].

Tsou et al. reported that the antiangiogenic histone deacetylase 5 (HDAC5) is overexpressed in SSc ECs compared to healthy control ECs [132]. Of note, silencing of HDAC5 in SSc ECs restored normal angiogenesis. Indeed, HDAC5 knockdown followed by an assay for transposase-accessible chromatin using sequencing (ATAC-seq) in SSc ECs identified several novel HDAC5-regulated target genes associated with impaired angiogenesis, including CYR61, PVRL2, and FSTL1 [132]. Overexpression of these genes individually led to an increase in tube formation as assessed by Matrigel assay, suggesting that endothelial HDAC5 overexpression impairs angiogenesis via epigenetic repression of proangiogenic factors in SSc [132]. In a subsequent study, the same authors showed that overexpression of CYR61 in SSc ECs induces increased production of VEGF and that the proangiogenic effects of CYR61 are mediated by signaling through $\alpha v\beta 3$ receptors and downstream activation of AMP-activated protein kinase, AKT, and the eNOS/NO pathway system [133]. Therapeutic intervention to promote CYR61 activity or increase CYR61 levels might therefore be of benefit in SSc vasculopathy.

The histone methyltransferase enhancer of zeste homolog 2 (EZH2) mediates trimethylation of lysine 27 of histone 3 (H3K27me3), which acts as a repressive epigenetic mark. Both EZH2 and H3K27me3 were found to be elevated in SSc dermal ECs compared with healthy dermal ECs [134]. In SSc ECs, inhibition of EZH2 restored normal angiogenesis via activating the Notch pathway, specifically by upregulating the Notch ligand DLL4. Thus, overexpression of EZH2 in SSc ECs appears to be antiangiogenic and targeting EZH2 or EZH2-regulated genes might represent a novel therapeutic strategy for the treatment of SSc vasculopathy [134].

The exact nature of epigenetic triggers in SSc is not known, but both hypoxia and oxidation injury are suggested triggers, as well as nutrients and other environmental factors [135, 136].

Defective Vascular Repair and Regeneration in SSc

The vasculopathy in SSc is systemic, progressive, and often irreversible. This fact suggests that the structural changes resulting in the diffuse obliteration and loss of the microvasculature are not balanced and repaired by compensatory growth of new vessels from existing vessels (angiogenesis) or by de novo formation of new vessels (vasculogenesis). Both defective angiogenic pathways and abnormalities in the release and function of bone marrow-derived progenitor cells, which have the potential to initiate vascular repair, have been identified in SSc patients.

Defective Angiogenesis: The Proangiogenic to Antiangiogenic Switch

Tissue ischemia and hypoxia are usually the main triggers for angiogenesis through the upregulation of proangiogenic factors, which then initiate angiogenic sprouting from preexisting microvessels by inducing vasodilation, proliferation, and migration of ECs, invasion of the surrounding extracellular matrix, and formation and stabilization of the vascular lumen of newly formed capillary vessels [137]. However, despite chronic tissue ischemia and progressive loss of microvessels in multiple vascular beds, compensatory angiogenesis is dysregulated and insufficient, and it does not allow vascular recovery in the course of SSc [138, 139].

Cumulative evidence indicates that a dysregulated expression of a large array of proangiogenic and antiangiogenic factors may be largely responsible for impaired angiogenic response in SSc [138, 139]. The nailfold capillaroscopic changes observed in the course of SSc may be explained by the action of different factors on angiogenesis. In the early stages of the disease, a proinflammatory state and an increased production of proangiogenic factors may stimulate angiogenesis. As a result, capillaroscopic analysis of the nailfold bed demonstrates the presence of microhemorrhages and tortuous, giant capillary loops, which are immature and instable microvessels presumably formed during an uncontrolled angiogenic response. This short proangiogenic response is followed by a dramatic impairment of the angiogenic process that might in part be explained by the action of several antiangiogenic factors, ultimately resulting in reduced capillary density and widespread avascular areas. Thus, the dramatic switch from proangiogenic to antiangiogenic characteristics suggests that the angiogenic process becomes impaired.

However, the functional role of angiogenic mediators in the disease pathogenesis is still poorly understood. Interestingly, while both several proangiogenic and antiangiogenic factors are overexpressed in SSc [138, 139], there appears to be an imbalance in the ratio of these mediators, favoring inhibition of angiogenesis and progressive vascular disease (Table 16.1).

Table 16.1 Dysregulated proangiogenic and antiangiogenic mediators in SSc

Proangiogenic	Antiangiogenic
VEGF	Endostatin
FGF-2	Angiostatin
Platelet-derived growth factor	Pentraxin 3
Interleukin-8/CXCL8	$VEGF_{165}b$
Stromal cell-derived factor 1/CXCL12	IP-10/CXCL10
Interleukin-6	MIG/CXCL9
CXCL16	Angiopoietin 2
Gro-γ/CXCL3	Interleukin-4
GCP-2/CXCL6	Platelet factor 4
EGFL7	Soluble endoglin
Kallikrein 1, 9, 11, and 12	Thrombospondin 1
Fractalkine/CX3CL1	Kallikrein 3
Soluble α-Klotho	Semaphorin 3E
CCN3	Slit2

Among the proangiogenic factors, VEGF is considered one of the most potent regulators of physiologic and pathologic angiogenesis and is overexpressed in most angiogenic conditions. Surprisingly, several studies have demonstrated enhanced expression of VEGF in both the skin and the circulation of SSc patients throughout different disease stages [138, 140–144]. The paradox is that VEGF levels, rather than being associated with evidence of angiogenesis, actually correlate with progressive microvascular loss and disease progression. In fact, a positive correlation was found between VEGF levels and the severity of nailfold capillary loss as well as with the extent of skin fibrosis measured by Rodnan skin thickness score [143]. Moreover, VEGFR-1 and VEGFR-2 are also upregulated on dermal ECs in SSc-affected skin [142, 144]. Nevertheless, there is also evidence suggesting that VEGF receptor signaling may be impaired in SSc based on the observation that dermal MVECs isolated from SSc patients show impaired response to VEGF in vitro [145, 146]. In particular, Tsou et al. have shown that activation of the thromboxane A2 receptor (TXAR) by 8-isoprostane, an oxidized lipid created by oxidative stress that is elevated in SSc plasma and SSc EC-conditioned media, inhibits the proangiogenic effect of VEGF [146]. Indeed, SSc EC-conditioned media inhibited EC tube formation, whereas addition of vitamin E, by reducing 8-isoprostane, increased tube formation. VEGF did not induce angiogenesis in SSc ECs displaying increased TXAR expression, but vitamin E or TXAR inhibition could restore its effect [146].

As an explanation for the "VEGF paradox," it has been shown that VEGF-A primary transcript can be alternatively spliced in its terminal exon, producing two distinct mRNA splice variants that are translated to the proangiogenic

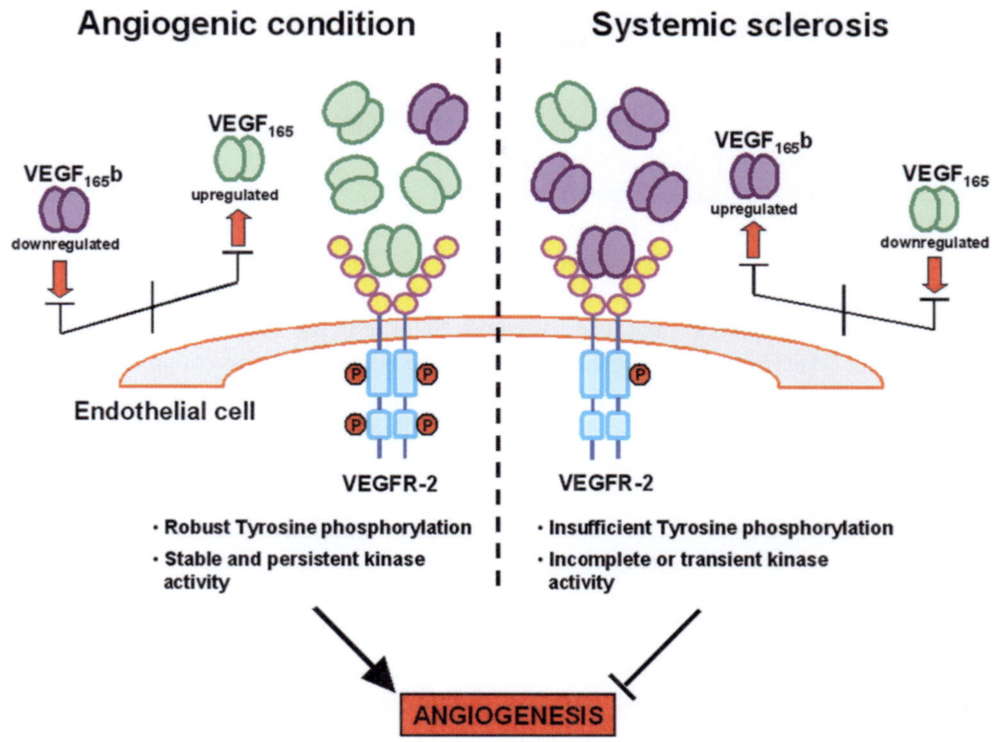

Fig. 16.4 In most angiogenic conditions, such as cancers, proangiogenic $VEGF_{165}$ predominates, whereas in deficient angiogenic conditions, such as SSc, the balance shifts to favor the expression of the $VEGF_{165}b$ antiangiogenic isoform. The two isoforms bind to VEGFR-2 with the same affinity, but binding of $VEGF_{165}b$ results in an insufficient tyrosine phosphorylation/activation of VEGFR-2 and incomplete or transient downstream signaling, which lead to impaired angiogenic response

$VEGF_{165}$ and antiangiogenic $VEGF_{165}b$ isoforms. Of interest, Manetti et al. reported that the increase in VEGF in SSc skin was the result of a significant increase in the antiangiogenic $VEGF_{165}b$ isoform instead of $VEGF_{165}$ [147]. Moreover, they provided evidence that circulating levels of $VEGF_{165}b$ were raised in SSc and that these increased levels were both early and persistent features of the disease. In addition, MVECs isolated from SSc skin constitutively expressed and released higher levels of $VEGF_{165}b$ than did MVECs from healthy individuals [147]. Interestingly, $VEGF_{165}$ and $VEGF_{165}b$ isoforms bind to the tyrosine kinase receptor VEGFR-2 with the same affinity, but binding of $VEGF_{165}b$ results in an insufficient tyrosine phosphorylation/activation of VEGFR-2 and incomplete or transient downstream signaling, which leads to an impaired angiogenic response [140]. Accordingly, SSc MVECs expressed higher levels of VEGFR-2 but also showed impaired phosphorylation/activation of this receptor, reduced activation of extracellular signal-regulated kinase (ERK)1/2, and impaired capillary morphogenesis in vitro [147]. Of note, treatment with recombinant $VEGF_{165}b$, as well as with conditioned media from SSc MVECs, inhibited $VEGF_{165}$-mediated VEGFR-2 phosphorylation, ERK1/2 signaling, and capillary morphogenesis in healthy MVECs, and these antiangiogenic effects could be abrogated by the administration of anti-$VEGF_{165}b$ neutralizing antibodies. The angiogenic potential of SSc MVECs is significantly impaired, but can be restored by the addition of combination of high-dose recombinant $VEGF_{165}$ and anti-$VEGF_{165}b$-blocking antibodies [147]. Finally, it is interesting to note that the switch from proangiogenic to antiangiogenic VEGF isoforms may be driven by TGF-β and the SRp55 splicing factor [147]. In a subsequent study, Manetti et al. [148] have reported that plasma levels of the antiangiogenic $VEGF_{165}b$ isoform correlated with the severity of capillary architectural loss and derangement, further suggesting that $VEGF_{165}b$ may participate in the loss of microvessels in SSc (Fig. 16.4). Of note, Hirigoyen et al. reported that $VEGF_{165}b$ is the main factor implicated in the inhibition of angiogenesis by platelets in SSc patients [149]. Indeed, in SSc platelet releasates, $VEGF_{165}b$ was significantly higher and the $VEGF_{165}b$/VEGF ratio was increased compared with that of control subjects, and incubation of healthy dermal MVECs with SSc platelet releasates resulted in a significant inhibition of capillary-like tube formation on Matrigel [149].

A dysregulated expression of different chemokines and their receptors has also been linked to disturbed angiogenesis in SSc. In particular, antiangiogenic chemokines lacking the enzyme-linked receptor (ELR) motif, such as monokine induced by interferon-γ (IFN-γ) (MIG/CXCL9) and IFN-inducible protein 10 (IP-10/CXCL10), are elevated in SSc serum, whereas the expression of their receptor CXCR3 is downregulated on SSc dermal ECs [150]. In contrast, proangiogenic CXCL16 and its receptor CXCR6 are elevated in SSc serum and on SSc dermal ECs, respectively [150]. Thus, these findings may suggest that angiogenic chemokine receptor expression is likely regulated in an effort to promote angiogenesis. Interestingly, an in vitro study employing EC chemotaxis assay demonstrated that SSc ECs are unable to migrate toward growth-regulated protein-γ (Gro-γ/CXCL3), granulocyte chemotactic protein 2 (GCP-2/CXCL6) or

CXCL16 proangiogenic chemokines, as well as toward VEGF [151]. The signaling pathways stimulated by these chemokines were also dysregulated in SSc ECs [151]. The expression of the proangiogenic transcription factor inhibitor of DNA-binding protein 1 (Id-1) in SSc ECs was lower compared with normal ECs, and overexpression of Id-1 in SSc ECs increased their ability to migrate toward VEGF and CXCL16 [151].

Elevated levels of antiangiogenic PTX3, a multifunctional pattern recognition protein that can suppress fibroblast growth factor 2 (FGF-2) proangiogenic function, have been associated with vascular manifestations of SSc [152]. Circulating PTX3 and FGF-2 levels were significantly higher in SSc patients than in healthy subjects. Moreover, circulating levels of PTX3 are elevated in SSc patients with digital ulcers or PAH, while FGF-2 is reduced in SSc patients with PAH. Multivariate analysis identified elevated PTX3 as an independent parameter associated with the presence of digital ulcers and PAH, and PTX3 levels were a useful predictor of future occurrences of digital ulcers. Reduced FGF-2 was independently associated with the presence of PAH [152].

In another study, Manetti et al. investigated the possible involvement of epidermal growth factor-like domain 7 (EGFL7), a unique proangiogenic molecule which is predominantly expressed and secreted by ECs and their progenitors and controls vascular development and integrity [153]. Circulating levels and dermal expression of EGFL7 were significantly decreased in SSc patients. Remarkably, the decrease of serum EGFL7 levels in SSc patients correlated with the severity of nailfold capillary abnormalities and presence of digital ulcers. In contrast to constitutive endothelial expression of EGFL7 in healthy skin, EGFL7 was found to be strongly reduced or even undetectable in SSc dermal microvessels. Furthermore, EGFL7 protein was found to be significantly downregulated in vitro in dermal MVECs obtained from SSc patients compared with control cells. Thus, it has been suggested that the loss of EGFL7 expression might contribute to the development and progression of peripheral microvascular damage and defective vascular repair process in SSc patients [153].

Since there is clinical evidence that the therapeutic use of ERAs may induce the regeneration of the peripheral microcirculatory network in SSc, Romano et al. investigated in vitro whether the ERA bosentan may counteract the antiangiogenic effects of SSc sera on healthy dermal MVECs [154]. Remarkably, the administration of bosentan to MVECs challenged with SSc sera effectively increased cell viability, chemoinvasion, and capillary-like tube formation, suggesting that ET-1 signaling blockade with ERAs may contribute to restore angiogenesis in SSc [154].

Experimental evidence indicates that soluble α-Klotho (sKl), a pleiotropic molecule with multiple effects on ECs, including antioxidant and vasculoprotective activities, may act as a protective factor to improve angiogenesis in SSc ECs [155]. On the EC surface, sKl interacts with VEGFR-2 and transient receptor potential canonical-1 (TRPC-1) cation channel to control EC homeostasis. A reduced expression of α-Klotho has been detected in dermal microvessels and cultured dermal MVECs from SSc patients compared to controls [155]. The administration of sKl was capable to improve angiogenesis maintaining over time capillary-like tube formation in vitro by SSc MVECs [155]. Mechanistically, stimulation of SSc MVECs with sKl resulted in the upregulation of the proliferation marker Ki67 in parallel with the downregulation of proapoptotic active caspase-3 [155]. Moreover, the expression of TRPC-1 was significantly decreased, while that of VEGFR-2 and antiangiogenic $VEGF_{165}b$ was significantly increased in SSc MVECs compared with healthy MVECs, and challenge with sKl both significantly upregulated TRPC-1 and downregulated $VEGF_{165}b$ in SSc MVECs [155].

Increasing evidence supports the notion that ECs express receptors for axon guidance molecules, including Ephrin family receptor tyrosine kinases, neuropilins, plexins, Roundabout receptors (Robos), and UNC5B that are able to respond to their soluble neuroendothelial trophic ligands, such as semaphorins and slits, to guide the sprouting of endothelial tip cells during the angiogenic process [156]. In this context, a series of recent studies have revealed an emerging role of members of semaphorin/plexin/neuropilin and slit/Robo families in SSc-related peripheral microvasculopathy and defective angiogenesis [156]. Neuropilin-1 (NRP1) is a receptor for both class-3 semaphorins (Sema3s) and VEGF-A that is required for optimal VEGF-A/VEGFR-2 signaling [157]. Serum levels of soluble NRP1 were significantly reduced both in patients with SSc and in patients with a very early diagnosis of SSc (VEDOSS) compared with controls [157, 158]. Moreover, decreased serum levels of soluble NRP1 were associated with the presence of active and late nailfold videocapillaroscopy patterns and digital ulcers in SSc patients [157]. NRP1 was significantly decreased in SSc MVECs, as well as in healthy MVECs challenged with SSc sera [157]. Molecular analyses further revealed that the transcription factor Friend leukemia integration-1 (Fli1) occupies the NRP1 gene promoter, and Fli1 gene silencing may reduce NRP1 expression in healthy MVECs [157]. Of note, NRP1 gene silencing in healthy MVECs resulted in a significantly impaired angiogenic capacity comparable to that of cells treated with SSc sera, which suggests that NRP1 deficiency may be an additional factor in the perturbed VEGF-A/VEGFR-2 system contributing to peripheral microvasculopathy and defective angiogenesis in SSc [157]. Another study reported that the Plexin-D1/Sema3E pathway may contribute to dysregulation of vascular tone control and defective angiogenesis in SSc patients [159]. Sema3E is a natural antiangiogenic molecule that acts through the Plexin-D1 receptor inhibiting cell adhesion through the disruption of integrin-mediated adhesive structures and causing filopodial retraction in ECs [159]. Serum levels of Sema3E were found to be increased both in SSc patients and in subjects with primary RP compared with controls [159]. In SSc skin, Sema3E was overexpressed in the microvascular endothelium [159]. Furthermore, cultured SSc MVECs showed higher phosphorylated Plexin-D1 and Sema3E expression than healthy MVECs, and stimulation with SSc sera increased phosphorylated Plexin-D1 and Sema3E levels in healthy MVECs [159]. The antiangiogenic effect of SSc sera on healthy MVECs was significantly attenuated by targeting the Plexin-D1/Sema3E pathway with a Sema3E-binding Plexin-D1 soluble peptide [159]. In a recent investigation, Romano et al. demonstrated that also the Slit2/Robo4 axis may make a substantial contribution to EC dysfunction and angiogenesis disturbance in SSc since the very early disease phase [160]. Indeed, circulating levels of Slit2 were significantly increased in SSc and VEDOSS patients compared with healthy controls [160]. In particular, serum Slit2 levels were raised in patients with VEDOSS with nailfold videocapillaroscopy abnormalities, while they were similar in VEDOSS with a normal nailfold videocapillaroscopy pattern and controls [160]. Slit2 and Robo4 expression was upregulated in SSc skin and explanted MVECs respect to controls [160]. In healthy MVECs, angiogenesis was strongly inhibited by challenge with recombinant human Slit2 or SSc sera, and these inhibitory effects were significantly attenuated when SSc sera were preincubated with an anti-Slit2 blocking antibody [160]. Defective angiogenesis was significantly ameliorated by Slit2 neutralization or ROBO4 gene silencing in SSc MVECs, suggesting that the Slit2/Robo4 axis might represent a novel target in the treatment of SSc microvasculopathy [160].

Finally, a very recent study provided evidence that the expression of the proangiogenic factor CCN3, a member of the CCN family of ECM proteins, is systematically decreased in the dermis of SSc patients compared with healthy controls, particularly in dermal blood vessels [161]. Moreover, CCN3 downregulation was maintained in vitro in SSc ECs, which resulted in a profound impairment of cell migration and angiogenesis [161]. In light of these findings, it has been suggested that CCN3 may represent a promising therapeutic target for SSc patients presenting with severe vascular involvement [161].

Defective Vasculogenesis

Defective neovessel formation in SSc is not only related to impaired angiogenesis, but is also linked to impaired vasculogenesis (i.e., the generation of new blood capillary vessels by endothelial precursors) and vascular repair as shown by altered numbers and functional defects of circulating EPCs [138, 162]. In fact, new blood vessels can be formed in the adult not only by the sprouting of fully differentiated ECs but also by recruitment of circulating progenitor cells, independently of the preexisting vasculature [163]. In particular, a subset of bone marrow-derived CD34$^+$ progenitor cells can acquire the characteristics of mature ECs, express EC markers, and incorporate into new capillary vessels at sites of ischemia [163]. Postnatal vasculogenesis contributes to vascular healing in response to vascular injury through the processes of rapid re-endothelialization of denuded vessels and collateral vessel formation in ischemic tissues. In this process, EPCs (identified as CD34$^+$/CD133$^+$/VEGFR-2$^+$ cells) are mobilized from their bone marrow niches into the circulation in response to stress- and/or damage-related signals and migrate through the bloodstream and home to the sites of vascular injury, where they extravasate through the endothelium and contribute to the formation of neovessels and the repair of damaged vasculature working in concert with preexisting mature ECs.

Several studies have analyzed the levels of circulating EPCs in the peripheral blood of SSc patients in comparison with healthy controls and/or other rheumatic conditions [138, 162, 164, 165]. Although conflicting results have been reported, a possible correlation between reduction in the number of EPCs and severity of peripheral vascular manifestations has been demonstrated [166]. Moreover, it has been shown that SSc serum may induce EPC apoptosis and that this may account, at least in part, for the decreased numbers of circulating EPCs in SSc patients [167]. AECAs may also be directly responsible for apoptosis of EPCs in SSc [168]. In another study, EPC (defined as CD34$^+$/CD133$^+$/CD309$^+$) counts were significantly lower in SSc patients with digital ulcers or PAH and correlated negatively with circulating levels of antiangiogenic PTX3 [152]. Interestingly, PTX3 inhibited the differentiation of EPCs in vitro [152]. Moreover, EPCs from SSc patients exhibited an impaired in vivo neovascularization capacity in a model of cotransplantation of immunomagnetically sorted circulating EPCs and murine colon carcinoma CT-26 cells beneath the skin of severe combined immunodeficiency (SCID) mice [169].

Angiogenic T (Tang) cells (defined as CD3$^+$/CD31$^+$/CXCR4$^+$) have been proposed to play an important role in the repair of damaged endothelium by secreting proangiogenic factors and working in concert with EPCs [170]. In SSc peripheral blood, Tang cell counts were shown to be inversely correlated to those of CD34$^+$/CD133$^+$/VEGFR-2$^+$ EPCs, suggesting that Tang cell expansion may be an ineffective attempt to compensate the need for increased angiogenesis and vasculogenesis [170].

In addition to CD34$^+$ EPCs, it has been proposed that bone marrow-derived CD14$^+$ monocytes can serve as a subset of EPCs because of their expression of endothelial markers and ability to promote neovascularization in vitro and in vivo [171]. However, the current consensus is that monocytic cells do not give rise to ECs in vivo, but rather function as support cells, by promoting vascular formation and repair through their recruitment to the site of vascular injury, secretion of proangiogenic factors, and differentiation into mural cells (VSMCs and pericytes). These CD14$^+$ monocytes that function in a supporting role in vascular repair are now termed monocytic proangiogenic hematopoietic cells (PHCs) [171]. Yamaguchi et al. showed that in patients with SSc, circulating monocytic PHCs increase dramatically in association with enhanced angiogenic potency, suggesting that these compensatory effects may be induced in response to defective vascular repair machinery [171].

Cipriani et al. examined the in vitro capacity of bone marrow-derived mesenchymal stem cells (MSCs) to differentiate toward the EC lineage [172]. In SSc patients, the percentage of VEGFR-2$^+$ and CXCR4$^+$ MSCs and endothelial-like MSCs was significantly lower than in controls. Accordingly, both SSc MSCs and endothelial-like MSCs displayed impaired responses to VEGF- and stromal cell-derived factor-1 (SDF-1)-induced migration, invasion, and capillary-like structure formation on Matrigel, as well as an early senescence [172]. These data collectively suggest that endothelial repair may be affected in SSc starting from bone marrow stem niches. However, despite an impaired commitment toward the endothelial phenotype, Guiducci et al. [173] demonstrated that SSc bone marrow-derived MSCs exhibit an intact, or even potentiated, proangiogenic paracrine machinery that is suitable for autologous therapeutic approaches. Indeed, SSc MSCs overexpress different proangiogenic growth factors and are able to promote dermal EC sprouting angiogenesis in vitro [173]. In agreement with these findings, the same authors reported that intravenous infusion of culture-expanded autologous bone marrow-derived MSCs could regenerate the peripheral vascular network in a case of SSc complicated by acute gangrene of the extremities [174]. Other observations have provided support for the efficacy of MSCs in treating intractable digital ulcers, where autologous injection of MSCs led to a reduction in the size of the ulcers, an increase in blood flow, and the formation of new capillaries [2]. Besides MSCs, autologous adipose-derived stem cells (ADSCs) residing in the stromal vascular fraction of white adipose tissue have shown promising results for the treatment of both fibrotic and vascular features of SSc [175]. Of note, in vitro expanded ADSCs from SSc patients were found to retain the ability to stimulate angiogenesis through paracrine mechanisms, though functional assays revealed reduced potential compared to healthy ADSCs [176].

The Plasminogen Activator Pathway

The plasminogen activator (PA) pathway plays key roles in angiogenesis. Plasminogen is a precursor of proangiogenic plasmin [177] and a precursor of antiangiogenic angiostatin [81]; therefore, it plays a complicated role in the regulation of vascular homeostasis. Plasminogen can be cleaved at the carboxy terminus by PA to produce plasmin, a proteolytic and fibrinolytic protease. Its proteolytic activity activates many key proangiogenic factors including VEGF [178], TGF-β [179], and MMPs [180]. Plasminogen can also be cleaved within its amino terminus kringle domains by a number of proteases [181, 182]. The cleaved kringle domain fragments are angiostatin of various sizes with different antiangiogenic activity. Thus, alterations in plasminogen processing can have a profound effect on angiogenic homeostasis.

Plasmin activity is reduced in SSc, while the amount of circulating angiostatin is increased [77]. This proangiogenic/antiangiogenic imbalance was manifested by reduced migration and proliferation of normal human dermal MVECs when exposed to SSc patients' plasma. Interestingly, exposure of normal dermal MVECs to angiostatin in amounts similar to those detected in SSc plasma resulted in a significant impairment of cell migration and ability to form vascular structures in collagen gels [77].

The PA pathway is further implicated in SSc by studies that examined the importance of urokinase plasminogen activator receptor (uPAR) in ECs isolated from SSc patients' skin biopsies. uPAR plays an important role in cell motility, adhesion, and matrix invasion through its binding interactions with urokinase plasminogen activator (uPA) [183], vitronectin [184], and intracellular signaling mediators, such as the integrin receptors [185]. D'Alessio et al. have shown that in dermal MVECs isolated from SSc skin, uPAR undergoes truncation between domains 1 and 2, a cleavage that is known to impair uPAR functions [145]. The uPAR cleavage in SSc MVECs was associated with the overexpression of MMP-12 [145]. Indeed, overproduction of MMP-12 by SSc dermal MVECs and fibroblasts accounts for endothelial uPAR cleavage leading to impaired uPA-induced MVECs migration, invasion, proliferation, and capillary morphogenesis on Matrigel [145]. Strikingly, treatment with an anti-MMP-12 monoclonal antibody was able to restore the angiogenic activity of normal MVECs treated with conditioned media from SSc MVECs [145, 186]. Furthermore, uPAR cleavage in SSc MVECs results in loss of integrin-mediated uPAR connection with the actin cytoskeleton [186]. The uncoupling of cleaved uPAR from β2 integrins impairs the activation of the small Rho GTPases Rac and Cdc42 and thus inhibits uPAR-dependent cytoskeletal rearrangement and cell motility, ultimately resulting in impaired angiogenesis [186]. In a subsequent study, the same authors reported that MMP-12 gene silencing could in part restore the ability of SSc MVECs to produce capillary structures in vitro [187]. Moreover, elevated levels of MMP-12 in the circulation of SSc patients were associated with the severity of nailfold capillary abnormalities and the presence of digital ulcers [188]. Interestingly, elevated MMP-12 may suppress angiogenesis not only through the cleavage and subsequent inactivation of uPAR [145] but also through the proteolysis of plasminogen and generation of angiostatin [189]. In SSc, the cleavage of uPAR by MMP-12 has also been implicated in the EndoMT process of dermal MVECs, suggesting that it may represent a crucial process underlying both peripheral microvasculopathy and tissue fibrosis [190]. Finally, it has been reported that plasma levels of soluble uPAR are increased in SSc patients compared to controls and correlate both with parameters of fibrosis and presence of microvascular lesions, such as RP, nailfold capillaroscopic abnormalities, and digital ulcers [191].

Microarray and Single-Cell RNA Sequencing Studies Revealing Altered Balance of Proangiogenic and Antiangiogenic Factors in SSc

Gene expression levels of proangiogenic and antiangiogenic factors have been analyzed in microarray studies which compared the transcriptome profiling of dermal MVECs isolated from skin biopsies from normal individuals and SSc patients [192, 193]. One microarray gene expression study detected important differences between normal and SSc MVECs in the kallikrein gene family [192]. Proangiogenic kallikreins 9, 11, and 12 were downregulated in SSc MVECs, whereas antiangiogenic kallikrein 3 was upregulated. The microarray data were further validated in experiments using normal MVECs treated with antibodies against kallikreins 9, 11, and 12 and subsequently analyzed in migration, proliferation, and capillary morphogenesis functional assays. All three antibodies were able to block angiogenesis in healthy MVECs [192]. Among the multiple kallikrein family members, tissue kallikrein (also known as kallikrein 1 or "true" tissue kallikrein) is a serine protease that cleaves kininogen and thereby regulates the kininogen–kinin pathway. Tissue kallikrein synthetized at the blood vessels acts through kinins which modulate a broad spectrum of vascular functions, playing an important role in the regulation of vascular homeostasis and angiogenesis [194–196]. Del Rosso et al. found that tissue kallikrein circulating levels are increased in SSc, particularly in patients with signs of early and active vascular disease, suggesting a role in the development of SSc microvascular abnormalities [197].

A second microarray gene expression study examined the expression of 14,000 genes in MVECs from skin biopsies obtained from normal subjects and dSSc patients [193]. Genes were categorized into functional groups based on gene ontology. Of those 14,000 genes, SSc MVECs overexpressed a number of proangiogenic transcripts but also a variety of genes that have a negative effect on angiogenesis [193]. Conversely, several genes that promote cell migration and adhesion to the ECM were downregulated in SSc MVECs, suggesting an anti-invasive phenotype of these cells [193]. In particular, the angiogenesis inhibitor PTX3, which is known to inhibit the proangiogenic effects of FGF-2, was strongly upregulated in SSc MVECs compared with normal MVECs [193]. Interestingly, in a subsequent study, Margheri et al. reported that silencing of PTX3 in SSc MVECs significantly increased their invasion in Matrigel and could in part restore their ability to produce capillary tubes in vitro [187]. Moreover, the 14,000 gene microarray study reported a reduced expression of desmoglein-2 (DSG2) in SSc MVECs [193]. Thus, to identify the role of DSG2 downregulation in the defective angiogenesis characteristic of SSc, Giusti et al. [198] studied the effect of silencing DSG2 in normal MVECs using DSG2-siRNA. The authors reported impaired actin stress fiber formation and diminished capillary morphogenesis in vitro. Of note, transfection of DSG2 into SSc MVECs restored their angiogenic properties in vitro to normal levels [198].

Avouac et al. investigated the gene expression profile of circulating EPC-derived ECs in normal and hypoxic conditions [199]. Their data revealed important gene expression changes in EPC-derived ECs from SSc patients, characterized by a proadhesive, proinflammatory, and activated phenotype [199].

The gene array study of Tinazzi et al. showed that circulating ECs from SSc patients display an altered expression of genes involved in the control of apoptosis and angiogenesis which may be modified by iloprost infusion [200].

Finally, Apostolidis et al. have recently carried out the first single-cell RNA sequencing (scRNA-seq) study to identify EC markers and signature pathways associated with vascular injury in SSc skin [201]. Interestingly, scRNA-seq followed by differential gene expression and pathway analysis revealed that dermal ECs from SSc patients show a discrete pattern of gene expression associated with vascular injury and activation, extracellular matrix generation, and negative regulation of angiogenesis [201]. HSPG2 and APLNR were identified as two of the top markers of EC injury in SSc patients [201].

Role of Perivascular Cells

Pericytes are located on the abluminal side of ECs in capillaries, precapillary arterioles, and postcapillary venules [202–204]. They are in close spatial proximity to and provide partial coverage for ECs [202]. Pericyte cell bodies and ECs are contained within the same basement membrane [205]. Vascular stabilization or maturation requires maintenance of established vessels and EC coverage by pericytes or VSMCs around the endothelial layer during angiogenesis [206].

Pericytes are contractile cells [207] which enable them to participate in hemodynamic regulation of microvascular blood flow and permeability by modifying (increase or decrease) inflammatory leakage at EC junctions. Additionally, pericytes contract in response to vasoactive mediators; ET-1, norepinephrine, angiotensin II, and bradykinin stimulate pericyte contraction, while NO, adenosine, adrenergic antagonists, and lipopolysaccharide induce pericyte relaxation [208–211].

Vascular permeability can be regulated by the extent of EC coverage by pericytes or by the extent of pericyte contraction that modifies EC intercellular junctions [212–215]. Pericyte coverage of EC junctions prevents leakage of proteins and cells from the vessel wall [204].

Pericytes are considered to be progenitor cells with the potential to differentiate into different cell types such as fibroblasts and myofibroblasts [216–219]; thus, they may link vascular injury to tissue fibrosis. Microvascular pericytes express PDGF receptors in wound healing and dermal scarring tissue [220, 221], as well as in early stages of SSc [222–224]. In another study [225], myofibroblasts were found in SSc skin biopsies, but not in normal skin. Two markers of myofibroblast differentiation were expressed in both pericytes and myofibroblasts in SSc but not in control biopsies [225], suggesting that pericytes may represent a source of myofibroblasts during dermal fibrosis. Asano et al. reported a decreased pericyte coverage of dermal capillaries in SSc [226].

Besides fibroblasts, myofibroblasts, and pericytes, recent evidence indicates that other stromal cell types may be implicated in the pathophysiology of SSc. Telocytes, formerly called interstitial Cajal-like cells and also referred to as $CD34^+$ stromal cells, are a distinct population of stromal cells that are characterized by very long cytoplasmic processes [227, 228]. Telocytes act as supporting cells by forming a scaffold that defines the correct three-dimensional organization of tissues/organs during prenatal life and during tissue repair/renewal in postnatal life. It has been suggested that telocytes are involved in intercellular signaling that could influence the transcriptional activity of neighboring cells, either directly, by cell-to-cell contacts, or indirectly, by shedding microvesicles and exosomes or by secreting paracrine signaling molecules, including miRNAs [227, 228]. Manetti et al. reported that telocytes display severe ultrastructural damage suggestive of ischemia-induced cell degeneration and are progressively lost from clinically affected SSc skin [229]. The authors proposed that, in SSc skin, the progressive loss of telocytes contributes to the altered three-dimensional organization of the ECM and may reduce the control of fibroblast and myofibroblast activity, thus favoring the fibrotic process [229]. Since telocytes are abundant in perivascular location, where they intimately surround the vessel basement membrane and produce proangiogenic factors and participate in vascular stability [227], presumably their loss may even be linked to microvascular abnormalities in SSc. Immunofluorescence and transmission electron microscopy photomicrographs of telocytes and microvessels in healthy and SSc skin are shown in Fig. 16.5.

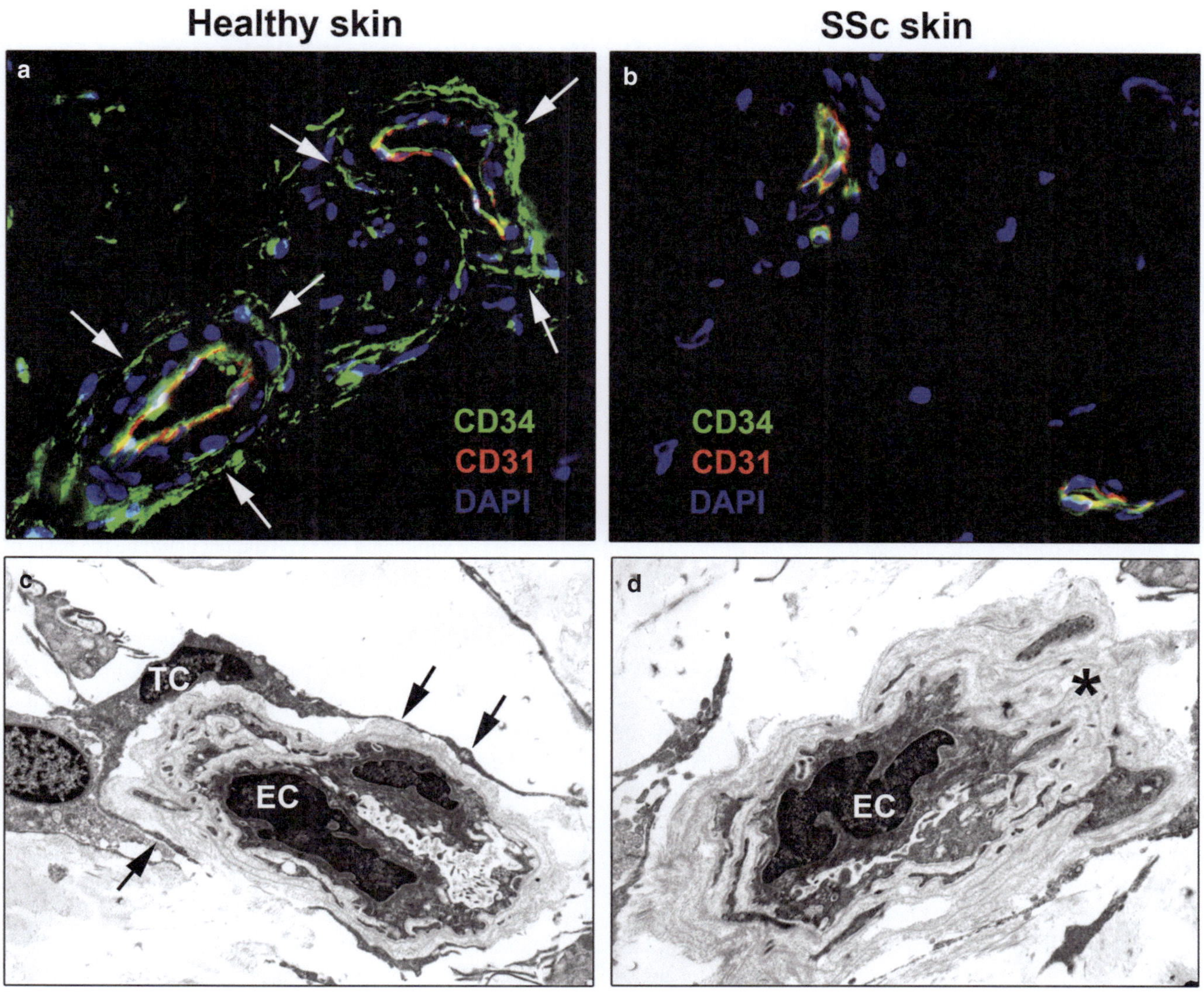

Fig. 16.5 (**a, b**) Representative photomicrographs of skin sections from healthy controls and SSc patients double immunostained for CD34 (*green*) and CD31 (*red*) and counterstained with DAPI (*blue*) to identify the nuclei. Telocytes are identified as CD34-positive/CD31-negative stromal cells, while endothelial cells are CD34/CD31 double positive. (**a**) Telocytes are numerous in healthy dermis, where they surround the microvessels (*arrows*). (**b**) No telocytes can be observed in SSc-affected dermis. Original magnification: ×40. (**c, d**) Representative transmission electron microscopy (TEM) photomicrographs of healthy and SSc skin. (**c**) Healthy skin. The thin and long varicose processes of a perivascular telocyte (TC) encircle the basal lamina of a blood microvessel (*arrows*). (**d**) SSc skin. Telocytes are not identifiable around an occluded microvessel. Only a few cell debris are observed. The vessel basal lamina is thickened (*asterisk*). *EC* endothelial cell. TEM; original magnification: ×6000

Vascular Wall Remodeling in SSc

Vascular remodeling follows microvascular injury and damage. Intimal and medial thickening and adventitial fibrosis are the common forms of remodeling found in SSc [2]. Intimal lesions change the vessel function and alter the composition and organization of the ECM. VSMCs are likely responsible for generating the fibrotic intimal lesions [2]. Under normal conditions, they assume a contractile or differentiated phenotype and regulate vessel diameter and blood flow. In pathological conditions, VSMCs become synthetic or dedifferentiated and generate intimal lesions through their secretion of ECM proteins in the absence of their contractile function [230–232]. Dysfunctional ECs, infiltrating leukocytes, and altered ECM in SSc provide the cues for intimal VSMCs to proliferate and form a fibrotic vascular lesion. Arts et al. demonstrated that a unique SSc-IgG may induce growth and profibrotic state in VSMCs through the activation of the epidermal growth factor receptor signaling cascade [233]. Anti-PDGFR autoantibodies may also contribute to the altered phenotype of VSMCs and development of intimal hyperplasia in SSc [118].

Another theory is that transdifferentiation of ECs via the process of TGF-β-induced EndoMT may preferentially lead to subendothelial accumulation of myofibroblasts and fibrotic tissue with subsequent neointimal thickening, leading to a fibroproliferative obliterative vasculopathy [14, 190, 234, 235]. Indeed, transitional ECs coexpressing endothelial markers (e.g., CD31, von Willebrand factor, vascular endothelial-cadherin) and mesenchymal markers (e.g., α-SMA, fibroblast-specific protein 1/S100A4, type I collagen) have been detected both in SSc skin and lung of patients with SSc-associated PAH, as well as in mouse models of skin fibrosis and PAH [190, 234, 235]. Of note, treatment of healthy dermal MVECs either with SSc sera or TGF-β resulted in the acquisition of a myofibroblast-like morphology and contractile phenotype and downregulation of endothelial markers in parallel with the induction of mesenchymal markers [190]. Similarly, stimulation of pulmonary artery ECs with TGF-β and proinflammatory cytokines IL-1β and tumor necrosis factor-α led to actin cytoskeleton reorganization and the development of a mesenchymal morphology, together with failure to form viable biological barriers and increased secretion of proinflammatory mediators accompanied by sustained immune cell transendothelial migration [234].

The ECM and basement membrane provide a support scaffold that is essential for blood vessel stability. Adhesion of ECs to the ECM enables them to undergo migration, proliferation, and morphogenesis, which are all necessary for neovascularization [236]. Degradation of the ECM/basement membrane leads to vessel collapse/regression [237–240]. Proteases that degrade the ECM/basement membrane play a key role in matrix remodeling during normal wound healing as well as in vascular diseases such as SSc.

The proteolytic activity of plasmin modifies many aspects of the ECM. It is the primary protease that degrades fibrin [239, 240], an ECM protein that forms a supportive scaffold for angiogenic vessels [241–243]. Fibrin, the major constituent of provisional matrix, enables ECs to adhere, spread, and proliferate [244, 245]. Fibrin or accumulated fibrinogen can be broken down by plasmin to negatively regulate angiogenesis [246, 247]. Reduced plasmin in SSc patients has been reported [77].

In addition to its own proteolytic activity, plasmin contributes to matrix remodeling by activating numerous MMPs [248, 249]. Of those, MMP-1, MMP-3, MMP-9, MMP-10, and MMP-13 promote capillary network regression followed by EC apoptosis [250, 251]. Several laboratories have examined plasma from SSc patients for the presence of various MMPs. One study reported that MMP-9 was downregulated in SSc patients, particularly those with PAH [252]. In another study, MMP-9 concentrations were greater in SSc plasma than in controls [253]. Gene expression profiling of EPC-derived ECs identified MMP-10 as a novel candidate gene in SSc-associated pulmonary hypertension [254]. In fact, MMP-10 was found to be overexpressed in the serum and pulmonary arteries of patients with SSc-associated pulmonary hypertension, and its blockade alleviated pulmonary vascular remodeling in the Fos-related antigen (Fra-2) transgenic mouse model [254].

Vascular Hypoxia in the Pathogenesis of SSc

Capillary rarefaction and disturbed blood flow, as well as excessive ECM accumulation, cause chronic tissue hypoxia in SSc. It was postulated that the avascular antiangiogenic areas visible in nailfold beds may result from tissue hypoxia and that the enlargement of capillaries may be a localized compensatory proangiogenic response to tissue hypoxia [138, 142]. In fact, intradermal skin oxygenation measurements verified hypoxic conditions in SSc patients with more advanced disease as compared to those with early disease and controls. Interestingly, expression of HIF-1α, a hypoxia-inducible transcriptional factor that upregulates VEGF, in the skin of SSc patients was lower than in controls. Additionally, HIF-1α expression did not correlate with VEGF expression pattern. Thus, it was concluded that increased VEGF expression in SSc patients is not stimulated by hypoxia, but could be the basis of megacapillaries [142]. However, subsequent studies demonstrated that the increase in VEGF expression in SSc skin was mainly the result of a significant increase in the antiangiogenic $VEGF_{165}b$ isoform instead of proangiogenic $VEGF_{165}$ [147].

The expression levels of VEGF, VEGFR-1, and VEGFR-2 have been examined also in late-outgrowth EPCs isolated from SSc patients and normal controls [255]. This study showed reduced mRNA and protein expression of VEGFR-1 in SSc EPCs under hypoxic conditions. Serum levels of soluble VEGFR-1 were significantly lower in SSc patients compared to controls, while soluble VEGF levels were elevated in SSc patients [255].

Thickened skin in SSc may lead to hypoxia, as suggested by oxygen measurement in SSc skin [142, 256]. In both studies, the lowest oxygen levels were found in the thickened fibrotic skin. DNA microarray studies in human pulmonary arterial ECs exposed to normoxic or hypoxic conditions and in ECs infected with a constitutively active HIF-1α or β-galactosidase and exposed to nonhypoxic conditions showed that genes upregulated by HIF-1α regulate collagen biosynthesis [257]. The list includes COL1A2, COL4A1, COL4A2, COL5A1, COL9A1, COL18A1, procollagen prolyl hydroxylases, lysyl oxidase, and lysyl hydroxylases [257]. Thus, hypoxia could actively contribute to the fibroproliferative vasculopathy with intimal thickening characteristic of SSc.

Makarenko et al. [258] demonstrated that exposing human MVECs to intermittent hypoxia induces cell dysfunction associated with an increase in ROS formation and ERK phosphorylation. Of note, inhibition of the ERK signaling pathway and the use of antioxidants prevented the effect of intermittent hypoxia on MVECs [258]. This observation argues for a possible role for antioxidants in prevention of MVEC dysfunction mediated by intermittent hypoxia in vascular disorders such as SSc.

Relationship of Vasculopathy to Fibrosis

SSc is a connective tissue disease with markedly increased levels of collagen deposition that causes tissue fibrosis. Fibroblasts acquire abnormal characteristics that include increased proliferation, a switch to the activated state (myofibroblasts), and synthesis of abnormally high levels of collagen and other ECM components [259]. Excessive ECM deposition and accumulation in the heart, lung, vessels, skin, and kidney result in uncontrolled organ fibrosis and organ dysfunction, which are a major part of the SSc pathology. Despite the abnormal fibroblast activities that lead to the fibrotic state in SSc patients, the defective vasculature response to injury is considered to occur before fibrosis [2]. There are various hypotheses as to the mechanism by which the vascular system may contribute to fibrosis. One theory proposes that cytokines secreted by activated ECs form a gradient that attracts fibroblasts to the blood vessels which, in turn, stimulate fibroblast proliferation, activation, as well as synthesis and secretion of collagen. In support of this hypothesis, the deposition of ECM appears mostly clustered in perivascular regions in early fibrotic lesions. Another proposed mechanism is that ECs become permeable, which results in interstitial secretion of factors that stimulate fibroblast proliferation, activation, and production of collagen [259].

Two factors that have been implicated in the link between SSc vasculopathy and fibrosis are TGF-β and connective tissue growth factor (CTGF/CCN2). The TGF-β-dependent mechanism is linked to EC apoptosis and myofibroblast differentiation. Apoptotic ECs recruit phagocytes, particularly macrophages that engulf the apoptotic cells. This event stimulates upregulation of TGF-β, which promotes profibrotic myofibroblast differentiation and apoptosis resistance [260]. Another proposed mechanism is centered on CTGF and is independent of TGF-β pathway [261]. CTGF is a fibrinogenic protein that is constitutively expressed in dermal fibroblasts isolated from dSSc patients [262, 263]. Furthermore, CTGF injected subcutaneously into neonatal NIH Swiss mice stimulates tissue fibrosis without TGF-β upregulation. Further delineation of this mechanism was performed in C3H mice injected subcutaneously with serum-free medium conditioned by apoptotic murine aortic ECs. The mice that received the apoptotic ECs developed thickening of the skin with elevated expression of α-SMA, vimentin, and collagen and myofibroblast differentiation. Myofibroblast differentiation was reversed when caspase-3 expression was inhibited in ECs. CTGF was identified as the sole fibrinogenic protein whose expression was upregulated in mice treated with apoptotic ECs [261].

The notion that MVECs may play a central role in the pathogenesis of SSc, including activation of the fibrotic program, was reemphasized recently by a report from Serratì et al. [264], who demonstrated that conditioned media obtained from cultured SSc MVECs, but not control MVECs, evoked fibroblast activation as suggested by the overexpression of α-SMA, vimentin, and type I collagen. Moreover, the activated fibroblasts exhibited an aggressive mesenchymal cell behavior by upregulating MMP-2 and MMP-9 expression and acquiring the ability to invade Matrigel. The effect of SSc MVEC-conditioned media on fibroblasts was mediated by elevated CTGF/CCN2, which in turn activates TGF-β. Interestingly, the use of CTGF/CCN2 inhibitor and TGF-β inhibitor peptides reversed fibroblast activation induced by SSc MVEC-conditioned media [264].

EndoMT may also play a fundamental role in the pathogenesis of tissue fibrosis in SSc [190, 235]. Indeed, while in arterioles/small arteries EndoMT may contribute to the development of fibroproliferative vasculopathy through the accumulation of profibrotic myofibroblasts within the vessel wall, when affecting capillaries it may instead generate myofibroblasts that migrate into the perivascular space with consequent tissue fibrosis and microvessel rarefaction (i.e., destructive vasculopathy) [235] (Fig. 16.6). ECs isolated from clinically involved SSc skin and from lung tissue of patients with SSc-associated interstitial lung disease have been shown to exhibit a spindle-shaped morphology, coexpress endothelial and myofibroblast markers, and display a profibrotic phenotype [190, 235, 265]. Besides ECs, it has been suggested that bone marrow-derived circulating EPCs might also transdifferentiate toward a myofibroblast-like phenotype in SSc [235].

Vascular injury can also activate platelets to release serotonin and other profibrotic mediators, which ensures efficient and self-limited wound healing under physiologic conditions. By contrast, chronic vasculopathy may cause persistent increase in serotonin levels and perpetuate profibrotic tissue repair processes, thus linking vascular disease and fibrosis in SSc [266]. Indeed, serotonin stimulates fibroblasts to release excessive amounts of ECM proteins. The profibrotic effects of serotonin are exclusively mediated via $5HT_{2B}$ receptors which are overexpressed in SSc, suggesting an increased sensitivity of SSc fibroblasts to the profibrotic effects of serotonin [266].

An important link between vasculopathy and fibrosis in SSc pathogenesis may also be represented by chronic overexpression of VEGF. In fact, Maurer et al. reported that double (+/+) VEGF transgenic mice spontaneously develop significant skin fibrosis, indicating profibrotic effect of VEGF in a gene-dosing manner [267]. Moreover, in vitro analysis revealed that VEGF is able to directly induce collagen synthesis in dermal fibroblasts [267]. Finally, it has been demonstrated that profibrotic TGF-β may suppress angiogenesis in SSc through decreased fibroblast caveolin-1 expression and subsequent secretion of pigment epithelium-derived factor [268].

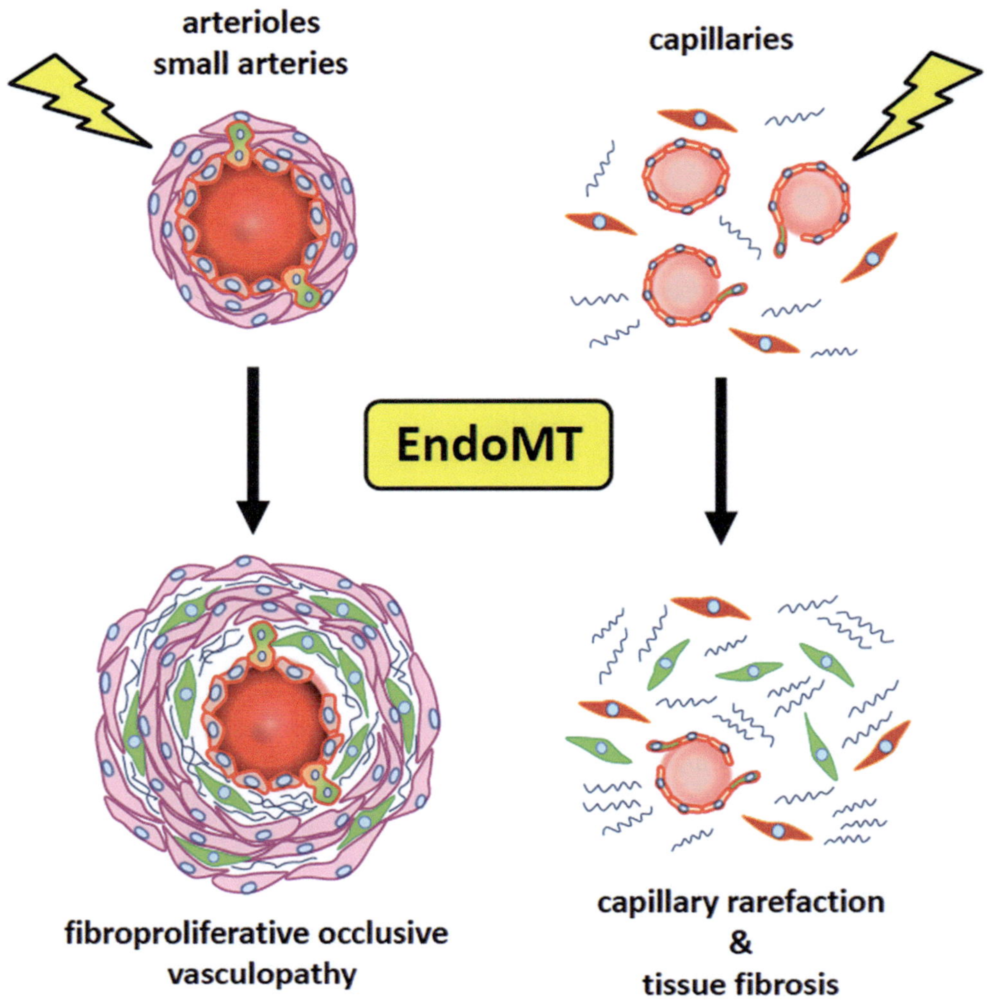

Fig. 16.6 In arterioles and small arteries, EndoMT may contribute to the development of fibroproliferative occlusive vasculopathy through the accumulation of profibrotic myofibroblasts in the vessel intima and media, resulting in progressive thickening of the vessel wall and occlusion of the vascular lumen. In capillaries, EndoMT may instead generate profibrotic myofibroblasts that migrate into the perivascular space with consequent tissue fibrosis and microvessel rarefaction (destructive vasculopathy). *EndoMT* endothelial-to-mesenchymal transition

Animal Models of SSc Vasculopathy

Animal models provided invaluable tools for unraveling the cellular and molecular events that drive the development of tissue fibrosis. All SSc models were discovered because of their fibrotic phenotype [269, 270]. However, only few animal models of SSc replicate the full spectrum of the human disease, including the fibrotic, vascular, inflammatory, and autoimmune features. Endothelial dysfunction occurs in various models [270, 271]; however, it is not clear if EC dysfunction is a primary or secondary event in animals with chronic hypoxia and intense tissue fibrosis.

UCD-200/206 Chickens

This chicken model manifests the entire spectrum of the clinical, histopathological, and serological features of SSc. EC apoptosis, induced by AECA-dependent cellular cytotoxicity, is considered to be a primary event in this model [272]. Other immunologic features include the presence of antinuclear antibodies, anticardiolipin antibodies, and rheumatoid factors [272]. A recent study demonstrated that the molecular profile and vascular changes occurring in UCD-200 chickens strongly resemble the early phase of human SSc, as testified by increased levels of SDF-1, CXCR4, VEGF-A, VEGFR-1, VEGFR-2, ET-1, ETAR, ETBR, PDGF-BB, and PDGFR [273]. In another study using the UCD-206 chickens, cell-demanded release of $VEGF_{121}$ from fibrin matrix was able to control angiogenesis by differential regulation of VEGFR-1 and VEGFR-2 expression, shifting the balance toward the proangiogenic VEGFR-2 and improving ischemic lesions [274]. These findings suggested the potential of covalently conjugated VEGF–fibrin matrices for the therapy of ischemic lesions such as fingertip ulcers in SSc patients [274]. However, it has been rather difficult to use this model because of the high variability of disease course, the long generation time of chicken, the challenges in housing chicken, and the lack of easy availability of chicken reagents.

Chronic Graft-Versus-Host Disease (GVHD)

This model is produced by the transplantation of immunologically incompatible spleen and bone marrow cells in a susceptible host. Tissue fibrosis is noted after host tissue infiltration by donor T cells and monocytes/macrophages. A very interesting chronic GVHD model, avoiding the need for irradiation, has been produced using the Rag-2 mouse, an immune-deficient mouse secondary to the loss of ability to rearrange immunoglobulin and T-cell receptor genes [275]. In this model, not only fibrosis is noted but also vasoconstriction and intimal hyperplasia in both skin and kidney are noted. In addition, there is an increase in ET-1 and adhesion molecule expression with circulating antinuclear antibodies and anti-Scl-70 antibodies in more than 90% of these mice [275].

Endothelial Fli1-Deficient Mouse and Bleomycin-Treated Fli1-Haploinsufficient (+/−) Mouse

Fli1 is a member of the Ets family of transcription factors that represses the transcription of collagen genes via Sp1-dependent pathway. Embryonic fibroblasts from Fli1-deficient mice exhibit significantly increased type I collagen expression levels in association with increased CTGF and decreased MMP-1 expression. Interestingly, a mouse model with a conditional deletion of Fli1 in ECs (Fli1 ECKO) develops disorganized dermal vascular network with greatly compromised vessel integrity and markedly increased vessel permeability [226]. Downregulation of VE-cadherin and CD31/platelet-endothelial cell adhesion molecule 1, impaired development of basement membrane, and decreased pericyte coverage in dermal microvessels were also noted [226]. This phenotype is consistent with a role of Fli1 as a regulator of vessel maturation and stabilization. Importantly, a reduced expression level of Fli1 in SSc ECs was noted suggesting that Fli1 may play a critical role in the development of SSc vasculopathy [226]. Accordingly, silencing of Fli1 in human dermal MVECs was found to profoundly disturb the angiogenic process [276]. In another study, the same authors showed that Fli-1-haploinsufficient (+/−) mice treated with bleomycin develop fibrosis, vascular activation, and immune abnormalities closely resembling human SSc [277].

Klf5 and Fli1 Gene Double Heterozygous (Klf5+/−;Fli1+/−) Mouse

A new murine model which recapitulates the three cardinal features of SSc (i.e., fibrosis, vasculopathy, and autoimmunity) has been recently established by simultaneous haploinsufficiency of Krüppel-like factor 5 (Klf5) and Fli1 genes, both of which are epigenetically suppressed in SSc dermal fibroblasts [278, 279]. In addition to enhanced dermal thickness, these mice closely resemble dermal fibrosis of SSc at the ultrastructural level. Furthermore, these mice simulate altered vascular structure in the skin and lungs and B-cell activation with autoantibody production characteristic of SSc [278, 279]. In vitro, dermal MVECs, bone marrow-derived MSCs, and EPCs from Klf5+/−; Fli1+/− mice exhibit impaired neovascularization/angiogenesis and vascular maturation very similar to those observed in human SSc [280].

Fra-2 Transgenic Mouse

Fra-2 belongs to the activator protein 1 (AP1) family of transcription factors. Fra-2 is overexpressed in SSc tissues and is shown to act as a novel downstream mediator of the profibrotic effects of TGF-β and PDGF. Mice with ectopic expression of Fra-2 in various organs develop generalized fibrosis and inflammation that is most pronounced in the lungs. Moreover, Fra-2 transgenic mice develop severe loss of small blood vessels in the skin that is paralleled by progressive skin fibrosis [281]. Fra-2 transgenic mice display various features of SSc vasculopathy with decreased dermal capillary density and early EC apoptosis [281]. Interestingly, dermal EC apoptosis appears to occur before the onset of tissue fibrosis. The suppression of Fra-2 by small interfering RNA prevents EC apoptosis and improves parameters of EC angiogenic potential. However, no proliferative vasculopathy was detectable in the skin [281]. Conversely, Fra-2 transgenic mice have been reported to develop proliferative vasculopathy in the lungs closely resembling SSc-related PAH [282], as well as typical manifestations of SSc-related cardiomyopathy [283]. Thus, Fra-2 transgenic mice may be a potentially useful model for the investigation of the link between vasculopathy and fibrosis and for the exploration of the mechanisms of vasculopathy in different organs.

uPAR-Deficient Mouse

The cleavage/inactivation of uPAR is a crucial step in fibroblast-to-myofibroblast transition and has been implicated in SSc peripheral microvasculopathy [145, 186, 284]. Therefore, Manetti et al. investigated whether uPAR gene knockout in mice could result in fibrosis and peripheral microvasculopathy resembling human SSc [285]. The skin of uPAR-deficient mice displays most of the typical pathological features of SSc. Dermal thickness, collagen content, and myofibroblast counts were significantly greater in uPAR-deficient mice than in wild-type mice. Similar to SSc, the skin of uPAR-deficient mice was characterized by the presence of thickened, closely packed and irregularly distributed collagen bundles, abundant perivascular fibrosis, and partial replacement of subcutaneous fat with connective tissue [285]. Moreover, in the dermis of uPAR-deficient mice, there was a marked overexpression of the SSc-related profibrotic factors TGF-β, CTGF/CCN2, and ET-1. Of note, in uPAR-deficient mice, dermal fibrosis was paralleled by EC apoptosis and severe loss of microvessels similar to what is seen in SSc peripheral microvasculopathy [285]. EndoMT was detected in dermal microvessels of these mice [190]. In addition, uPAR-deficient mice also develop progressive lung fibrosis resembling the nonspecific interstitial pneumonia pattern of SSc [285]. However, no evidence of vessel intima-media proliferation was reported either in the skin or the lungs [285]. In a subsequent study, the same authors have shown that uPAR-deficient mice mimic typical histopathological features of SSc-related cardiomyopathy, including myocardial fibrosis paralleled by EC apoptosis and reduced capillary density [286]. Further studies are required to ascertain whether uPAR-deficient mice may develop SSc-like features in other internal organs. In this regard, it was reported that uPAR deficiency accelerates renal fibrosis in obstructive nephropathy [287].

Transgenic Mouse with Endothelial Cell-Specific Inducible Expression of Constitutively Active TGF-β Receptor I

This mouse model was generated by intercrossing mice harboring a constitutively active TGF-β receptor I with a mouse strain containing the EC-specific Cdh5 gene promoter directing the tamoxifen-inducible expression of the Cre-ER^{T2} cassette [288]. Administration of tamoxifen to these mice results in constitutive TGF-β activation and signaling restricted to ECs. Constitutive TGF-β signaling in ECs resulted in skin and visceral fibrosis with prominent fibrotic involvement of the lungs and severe perivascular and subendothelial fibrosis of small arterioles [288]. These mice also displayed increased expression of fibrosis-associated genes and of genes indicative of myofibroblast activation, as well as induction of EndoMT in pulmonary vessels [288].

Conclusions

The pathogenesis of the vascular disease in SSc appears to involve many cell types and signaling pathways. A complex interaction between ECs, immune cells, VSMCs, fibroblasts, pericytes, and the ECM is likely to contribute to the vascular reactivity, remodeling, and occlusive disease of SSc. EC activation/injury is an early and probably initiating event in disease pathogenesis. The exact mechanism for the widespread vascular disease in SSc is still unknown, but EC injury induced by an infectious agent, immune-mediated cytotoxicity, AECAs, and/or ischemia–reperfusion have all been suggested. Moreover, substantial evidence indicates that angiogenic and vasculogenic repair machineries are profoundly impaired and do not allow vascular recovery. In this context, EndoMT may further aggravate SSc vascular disease providing a unique link between vasculopathy and fibrosis. The downstream effects of vascular dysfunction adversely affect organ function and determine clinical outcomes. Understanding the cellular and molecular mechanisms underlying these processes provides the rationale for novel therapeutic strategies and specific targeted therapy. The definition of prefibrotic vascular lesions may have future therapeutic and preventive implications for SSc. The development of means to quantify endothelial injury and the activity of the vascular lesions are essential for the monitoring of therapies designed to block further vascular injury.

References

1. Fleischmajer R, Perlish JS, Shaw KV, Pirozzi DJ. Skin capillary changes in early systemic scleroderma. Electron microscopy and "in vitro" autoradiography with tritiated thymidine. Arch Dermatol. 1976;112(11):1553–7.
2. Matucci-Cerinic M, Kahaleh B, Wigley FM. Review: evidence that systemic sclerosis is a vascular disease. Arthritis Rheum. 2013;65(8):1953–62.
3. Grassi W, Core P, Carlino G, Blasetti P, Cervini M. Labial capillary microscopy in systemic sclerosis. Ann Rheum Dis. 1993;52(8):564–9.
4. Bruni C, Frech T, Manetti M, Rossi FW, Furst DE, De Paulis A, Rivellese F, Guiducci S, Matucci-Cerinic M, Bellando-Randone S. Vascular leaking, a pivotal and early pathogenetic event in systemic sclerosis: should the door be closed? Front Immunol. 2018;9:2045.
5. Fleischmajer R, Perlish JS. Capillary alterations in scleroderma. J Am Acad Dermatol. 1980;2(2):161–70.
6. Sgonc R, Gruschwitz MS, Dietrich H, Recheis H, Gershwin ME, Wick G. Endothelial cell apoptosis is a primary pathogenetic event underlying skin lesions in avian and human scleroderma. J Clin Invest. 1996;98(3):785–92.
7. Chen F, Eriksson P, Kimura T, Herzfeld I, Valen G. Apoptosis and angiogenesis are induced in the unstable coronary atherosclerotic plaque. Coron Artery Dis. 2005;16(3):191–7.
8. Laurence J, Mitra D, Steiner M, Staiano-Coico L, Jaffe E. Plasma from patients with idiopathic and human immunodeficiency virus-associated thrombotic thrombocytopenic purpura induces apoptosis in microvascular endothelial cells. Blood. 1996;87(8):3245–54.
9. Albert ML, Pearce SF, Francisco LM, Sauter B, Roy P, Silverstein RL, Bhardwaj N. Immature dendritic cells phagocytose apoptotic cells via alphavbeta5 and CD36, and cross-present antigens to cytotoxic T lymphocytes. J Exp Med. 1998;188(7):1359–68.
10. Greeno EW, Bach RR, Moldow CF. Apoptosis is associated with increased cell surface tissue factor procoagulant activity. Lab Invest. 1996;75(2):281–9.
11. Tsuji S, Kaji K, Nagasawa S. Activation of the alternative pathway of human complement by apoptotic human umbilical vein endothelial cells. J Biochem. 1994;116(4):794–800.
12. Fleischmajer R, Perlish JS. [3H]Thymidine labeling of dermal endothelial cells in scleroderma. J Invest Dermatol. 1977;69(4):379–82.
13. Rodnan GP, Myerowitz RL, Justh GO. Morphologic changes in the digital arteries of patients with progressive systemic sclerosis (scleroderma) and Raynaud phenomenon. Medicine (Baltimore). 1980;59(6):393–408.
14. Manetti M, Guiducci S, Matucci-Cerinic M. The origin of the myofibroblast in fibroproliferative vasculopathy: does the endothelial cell steer the pathophysiology of systemic sclerosis? Arthritis Rheum. 2011;63(8):2164–7.
15. Youssef P, Englert H, Bertouch J. Large vessel occlusive disease associated with CREST syndrome and scleroderma. Ann Rheum Dis. 1993;52(6):464–6.
16. Pandey JP, LeRoy EC. Human cytomegalovirus and the vasculopathies of autoimmune diseases (especially scleroderma), allograft rejection, and coronary restenosis. Arthritis Rheum. 1998;41(1):10–5.

17. Cannon PJ, Hassar M, Case DB, Casarella WJ, Sommers SC, LeRoy EC. The relationship of hypertension and renal failure in scleroderma (progressive systemic sclerosis) to structural and functional abnormalities of the renal cortical circulation. Medicine (Baltimore). 1974;53(1):1–46.
18. Brown GE, O'Leary PA. Skin capillaries in scleroderma. Arch Intern Med. 1925;36:73–88.
19. Anderson ME, Allen PD, Moore T, Hillier V, Taylor CJ, Herrick AL. Computerized nailfold video capillaroscopy—a new tool for assessment of Raynaud's phenomenon. J Rheumatol. 2005;32(5):841–8.
20. Maricq HR, LeRoy EC. Patterns of finger capillary abnormalities in connective tissue disease by "wide-field" microscopy. Arthritis Rheum. 1973;16(5):619–28.
21. Blann AD, Illingworth K, Jayson MI. Mechanisms of endothelial cell damage in systemic sclerosis and Raynaud's phenomenon. J Rheumatol. 1993;20(8):1325–30.
22. Carpentier PH, Maricq HR. Microvasculature in systemic sclerosis. Rheum Dis Clin N Am. 1990;16(1):75–91.
23. Bukhari M, Herrick AL, Moore T, Manning J, Jayson MI. Increased nailfold capillary dimensions in primary Raynaud's phenomenon and systemic sclerosis. Br J Rheumatol. 1996;35(11):1127–31
24. Cutolo M, Sulli A, Secchi ME, Paolino S, Pizzorni C. Nailfold capillaroscopy is useful for the diagnosis and follow-up of autoimmune rheumatic diseases. A future tool for the analysis of microvascular heart involvement? Rheumatology (Oxford). 2006;45 Suppl 4:iv43–6.
25. Meli M, Gitzelmann G, Koppensteiner R, Amann-Vesti BR. Predictive value of nailfold capillaroscopy in patients with Raynaud's phenomenon. Clin Rheumatol. 2006;25(2):153–8.
26. Miniati I, Guiducci S, Conforti ML, Rogai V, Fiori G, Cinelli M, Saccardi R, Guidi S, Bosi A, Tyndall A, Matucci-Cerinic M. Autologous stem cell transplantation improves microcirculation in systemic sclerosis. Ann Rheum Dis. 2009;68(1):94–8.
27. Albrecht HP, Hiller D, Hornstein OP, Bühler-Singer S, Mück M, Gruschwitz M. Microcirculatory functions in systemic sclerosis: additional parameters for therapeutic concepts? J Invest Dermatol. 1993;101(2):211–5.
28. Prescott RJ, Freemont AJ, Jones CJ, Hoyland J, Fielding P. Sequential dermal microvascular and perivascular changes in the development of scleroderma. J Pathol. 1992;166(3):255–63.
29. Lippton HL, Hauth TA, Summer WR, Hyman AL. Endothelin produces pulmonary vasoconstriction and systemic vasodilation. J Appl Physiol (1985). 1989;66(2):1008–12.
30. Vancheeswaran R, Azam A, Black C, Dashwood MR. Localization of endothelin-1 and its binding sites in scleroderma skin. J Rheumatol. 1994;21(7):1268–76.
31. Vancheeswaran R, Magoulas T, Efrat G, Wheeler-Jones C, Olsen I, Penny R, Black CM. Circulating endothelin-1 levels in systemic sclerosis subsets; a marker of fibrosis or vascular dysfunction? J Rheumatol. 1994;21(10):1838–44.
32. Cambrey AD, Harrison NK, Dawes KE, Southcott AM, Black CM, du Bois RM, Laurent GJ, McAnulty RJ. Increased levels of endothelin-1 in bronchoalveolar lavage fluid from patients with systemic sclerosis contribute to fibroblast mitogenic activity in vitro. Am J Respir Cell Mol Biol. 1994;1 (4): 439–45.
33. Kawaguchi Y, Suzuki K, Hara M, Hidaka T, Ishizuka T, Kawagoe M, Nakamura H. Increased endothelin-1 production in fibroblasts derived from patients with systemic sclerosis. Ann Rheum Dis. 1994;53(8):506–10.
34. Morelli S, Ferri C, Di Francesco L, Baldoncini R, Carlesimo M, Bottoni U, Properzi G, Santucci A. Plasma endothelin-1 levels in patients with systemic sclerosis: influence of pulmonary or systemic arterial hypertension. Ann Rheum Dis. 1995;54(9):730–4.
35. Morelli S, Ferri C, Polettini E, Bellini C, Gualdi GF, Pittoni V, Valesini G, Santucci A. Plasma endothelin-1 levels, pulmonary hypertension, and lung fibrosis in patients with systemic sclerosis. Am J Med. 1995;99(3):255–60.
36. Abraham D, Distler O. How does endothelial cell injury start? The role of endothelin in systemic sclerosis. Arthritis Res Ther. 2007;9(Suppl 2):S2.
37. Frommer KW, Müller-Ladner U. Expression and function of ETA and ETB receptors in SSc. Rheumatology (Oxford). 2008;47(Suppl 5):v27–8.
38. Kasturi KN, Shibata S, Muryoi T, Bona CA. Tight-skin mouse an experimental model for scleroderma. Int Rev Immunol. 1994;11(3):253–71.
39. Richard V, Solans V, Favre J, Henry JP, Lallemand F, Thuillez C, Marie I. Role of endogenous endothelin in endothelial dysfunction in murine model of systemic sclerosis: tight skin mice 1. Fundam Clin Pharmacol. 2008;22(6):649–55.
40. Cozzi F, Pigatto E, Rizzo M, Favaro M, Zanatta E, Cardarelli S, Riato L, Punzi L. Low occurrence of digital ulcers in scleroderma patients treated with bosentan for pulmonary arterial hypertension: a retrospective case-control study. Clin Rheumatol. 2013;32(5):679–83.
41. Matucci-Cerinic M, Denton CP, Furst DE, Mayes MD, Hsu VM, Carpentier P, Wigley FM, Black CM, Fessler BJ, Merkel PA, Pope JE, Sweiss NJ, Doyle MK, Hellmich B, Medsger TA Jr, Morganti A, Kramer F, Korn JH, Seibold JR. Bosentan treatment of digital ulcers related to systemic sclerosis: results from the RAPIDS-2 randomised, double-blind, placebo-controlled trial. Ann Rheum Dis. 2011;70(1):32–8.
42. Guiducci S, Bellando Randone S, Bruni C, Carnesecchi G, Maresta A, Iannone F, Lapadula G, Matucci CM. Bosentan fosters microvascular de-remodelling in systemic sclerosis. Clin Rheumatol. 2012;31(12):1723–5.
43. Cutolo M, Zampogna G, Vremis L, Smith V, Pizzorni C, Sulli A. Long-term effects of endothelin receptor antagonism on microvascular damage evaluated by nailfold capillaroscopic analysis in systemic sclerosis. J Rheumatol. 2013;40(1):40–5.
44. Khanna D, Denton CP, Merkel PA, Krieg T, Le Brun FO, Marr A, Papadakis K, Pope J, Matucci-Cerinic M, Furst DE. DUAL-1 investigators; DUAL-2 investigators. Effect of macitentan on the development of new ischemic digital ulcers in patients with systemic sclerosis: DUAL-1 and DUAL-2 randomized clinical trials. JAMA. 2016;315(18):1975–88.
45. Ignarro LJ. Biosynthesis and metabolism of endothelium-derived nitric oxide. Annu Rev Pharmacol Toxicol. 1990;30:535–60.
46. Ignarro LJ. Endothelium-derived nitric oxide: actions and properties. FASEB J. 1989;3(1):31–6.
47. Agostoni A, Marasini B, Biondi ML, Bassani C, Cazzaniga A, Bottasso B, Cugno M. L-arginine therapy in Raynaud's phenomenon? Int J Clin Lab Res. 1991;21(2):202–3.
48. Cailes J, Winter S, du Bois RM, Evans TW. Defective endothelially mediated pulmonary vasodilation in systemic sclerosis. Chest. 1998;114(1):178–84.
49. Livi R, Teghini L, Generini S, Matucci-Cerinic M. The loss of endothelium-dependent vascular tone control in systemic sclerosis. Chest. 2001;119(2):672–3.
50. Matucci-Cerinic M, Pietrini U, Marabini S. Local venomotor response to intravenous infusion of substance P and glyceryl trinitrate in systemic sclerosis. Clin Exp Rheumatol. 1990;8(6):561–5.
51. Dooley A, Gao B, Bradley N, Abraham DJ, Black CM, Jacobs M, Bruckdorfer KR. Abnormal nitric oxide metabolism in systemic sclerosis: increased levels of nitrated proteins and asymmetric dimethylarginine. Rheumatology (Oxford). 2006;45(6):676–84.
52. Cotton SA, Herrick AL, Jayson MI, Freemont AJ. Endothelial expression of nitric oxide synthases and nitrotyrosine in systemic sclerosis skin. J Pathol. 1999;189(2):273–8.
53. Mendall MA, Goggin PM, Molineaux N, Levy J, Toosy T, Strachan D, Camm AJ, Northfield TC. Relation of Helicobacter pylori infection and coronary heart disease. Br Heart J. 1994;71(5): 437–9.

54. Gasbarrini A, Massari I, Serricchio M, Tondi P, De Luca A, Franceschi F, Ojetti V, Dal Lago A, Flore R, Santoliquido A, Gasbarrini G, Pola P. Helicobacter pylori eradication ameliorates primary Raynaud's phenomenon. Dig Dis Sci. 1998;43(8):1641–5.
55. Aragona P, Magazz G, Macchia G, Bartolone S, Di Pasquale G, Vitali C, Ferreri G. Presence of antibodies against Helicobacter pylori and its heat-shock protein 60 in the serum of patients with Sjögren's syndrome. J Rheumatol. 1999;26(6):1306–11.
56. Savarino V, Sulli A, Zentilin P, Raffaella Mele M, Cutolo M. No evidence of an association between Helicobacter pylori infection and Raynaud phenomenon. Scand J Gastroenterol. 2000;35(12):1251–4.
57. Sulli A, Seriolo B, Savarino V, Cutolo M. Lack of correlation between gastric Helicobacter pylori infection and primary or secondary Raynaud's phenomenon in patients with systemic sclerosis. J Rheumatol. 2000;27(7):1820–1.
58. Vaughan JH, Shaw PX, Nguyen MD, Medsger TA Jr, Wright TM, Metcalf JS, Leroy EC. Evidence of activation of 2 herpesviruses, Epstein-Barr virus and cytomegalovirus, in systemic sclerosis and normal skins. J Rheumatol. 2000;27(3):821–3.
59. Neidhart M, Kuchen S, Distler O, Brühlmann P, Michel BA, Gay RE, Gay S. Increased serum levels of antibodies against human cytomegalovirus and prevalence of autoantibodies in systemic sclerosis. Arthritis Rheum. 1999;42(2):389–92.
60. Presti RM, Pollock JL, Dal Canto AJ, O'Guin AK, Virgin HW 4th. Interferon gamma regulates acute and latent murine cytomegalovirus infection and chronic disease of the great vessels. J Exp Med. 1998;188(3):577–88.
61. Zhou YF, Shou M, Harrell RF, Yu ZX, Unger EF, Epstein SE. Chronic non-vascular cytomegalovirus infection: effects on the neointimal response to experimental vascular injury. Cardiovasc Res. 2000;45(4):1019–25.
62. Hamamdzic D, Harley RA, Hazen-Martin D, LeRoy EC. MCMV induces neointima in IFN-gammaR/mice: intimal cell apoptosis and persistent proliferation of myofibroblasts. BMC Musculoskelet Disord. 2001;2:3.
63. Ferri C, Longombardo G, Azzi A, Zakrzewska K. Parvovirus B19 and systemic sclerosis. Clin Exp Rheumatol. 1999;17(2):267–8.
64. Magro CM, Nuovo G, Ferri C, Crowson AN, Giuggioli D, Sebastiani M. Parvoviral infection of endothelial cells and stromal fibroblasts: a possible pathogenetic role in scleroderma. J Cutan Pathol. 2004;31(1):43–50.
65. Zakrzewska K, Corcioli F, Carlsen KM, Giuggioli D, Fanci R, Rinieri A, Ferri C, Azzi A. Human parvovirus B19 (B19V) infection in systemic sclerosis patients. Intervirology. 2009;52(5):279–82.
66. Arvia R, Margheri F, Stincarelli MA, Laurenzana A, Fibbi G, Gallinella G, Ferri C, Del Rosso M, Zakrzewska K. Parvovirus B19 activates in vitro normal human dermal fibroblasts: a possible implication in skin fibrosis and systemic sclerosis. Rheumatology (Oxford). 2020;59(11):3526–32.
67. Drenk F, Deicher HR. Pathophysiological effects of endothelial cytotoxic activity derived from sera of patients with progressive systemic sclerosis. J Rheumatol. 1988;15(3):468–74.
68. Holt CM, Lindsey N, Moult J, Malia RG, Greaves M, Hume A, Rowell NR, Hughes P. Antibody-dependent cellular cytotoxicity of vascular endothelium: characterization and pathogenic associations in systemic sclerosis. Clin Exp Immunol. 1989;78(3):359–65.
69. Penning CA, Cunningham J, French MA, Harrison G, Rowell NR, Hughes P. Antibody-dependent cellular cytotoxicity of human vascular endothelium in systemic sclerosis. Clin Exp Immunol. 1984;57(3):548–56.
70. Sgonc R, Gruschwitz MS, Boeck G, Sepp N, Gruber J, Wick G. Endothelial cell apoptosis in systemic sclerosis is induced by antibody-dependent cell-mediated cytotoxicity via CD95. Arthritis Rheum. 2000;43(11):2550–62.
71. Trapani JA. Dual mechanisms of apoptosis induction by cytotoxic lymphocytes. Int Rev Cytol. 1998;182:111–92.
72. Kahaleh MB, Leroy EC. Endothelial injury in scleroderma. A protease mechanism. J Lab Clin Med. 1983;101(4):553–60.
73. Kahaleh MB, Fan PS. Mechanism of serum-mediated endothelial injury in scleroderma: identification of a granular enzyme in scleroderma skin and sera. Clin Immunol Immunopathol. 1997;83(1):32–40.
74. Müllbacher A, Waring P, Tha Hla R, Tran T, Chin S, Stehle T, Museteanu C, Simon MM. Granzymes are the essential downstream effector molecules for the control of primary virus infections by cytolytic leukocytes. Proc Natl Acad Sci U S A. 1999;96(24):13950–5.
75. Müller U, Sobek V, Balkow S, Hölscher C, Müllbacher A, Museteanu C, Mossmann H, Simon MM. Concerted action of perforin and granzymes is critical for the elimination of Trypanosoma cruzi from mouse tissues, but prevention of early host death is in addition dependent on the FasL/Fas pathway. Eur J Immunol. 2003;33(1):70–8.
76. Buzza MS, Zamurs L, Sun J, Bird CH, Smith AI, Trapani JA, Froelich CJ, Nice EC, Bird PI. Extracellular matrix remodeling by human granzyme B via cleavage of vitronectin, fibronectin, and laminin. J Biol Chem. 2005;280(25):23549–58.
77. Mulligan-Kehoe MJ, Drinane MC, Mollmark J, Casciola-Rosen L, Hummers LK, Hall A, Rosen A, Wigley FM, Simons M. Antiangiogenic plasma activity in patients with systemic sclerosis. Arthritis Rheum. 2007;56(10):3448–58.
78. Sasaki T, Larsson H, Tisi D, Claesson-Welsh L, Hohenester E, Timpl R. Endostatins derived from collagens XV and XVIII differ in structural and binding properties, tissue distribution and anti-angiogenic activity. J Mol Biol. 2000;301(5):1179–90.
79. Maeshima Y, Sudhakar A, Lively JC, Ueki K, Kharbanda S, Kahn CR, Sonenberg N, Hynes RO, Kalluri R. Tumstatin, an endothelial cell-specific inhibitor of protein synthesis. Science. 2002;295(5552):140–3.
80. Kamphaus GD, Colorado PC, Panka DJ, Hopfer H, Ramchandran R, Torre A, Maeshima Y, Mier JW, Sukhatme VP, Kalluri R. Canstatin, a novel matrix-derived inhibitor of angiogenesis and tumor growth. J Biol Chem. 2000;275(2):1209–15.
81. Cao Y, Ji RW, Davidson D, Schaller J, Marti D, Söhndel S, SG MC, O'Reilly MS, Llinás M, Folkman J. Kringle domains of human angiostatin. Characterization of the anti-proliferative activity on endothelial cells. J Biol Chem. 1996;271(46):29461–7.
82. Ferrara N, Clapp C, Weiner R. The 16K fragment of prolactin specifically inhibits basal or fibroblast growth factor stimulated growth of capillary endothelial cells. Endocrinology. 1991;129(2):896–900.
83. Staton CA, Lewis CE. Angiogenesis inhibitors found within the haemostasis pathway. J Cell Mol Med. 2005;9(2):286–302.
84. Hebbar M, Peyrat JP, Hornez L, Hatron PY, Hachulla E, Devulder B. Increased concentrations of the circulating angiogenesis inhibitor endostatin in patients with systemic sclerosis. Arthritis Rheum. 2000;43(4):889–93.
85. Hummers LK, Hall A, Wigley FM, Simons M. Abnormalities in the regulators of angiogenesis in patients with scleroderma. J Rheumatol. 2009;36(3):576–82.
86. Borghini A, Manetti M, Nacci F, Bellando-Randone S, Guiducci S, Matucci-Cerinic M, Ibba-Manneschi L, Weber E. Systemic sclerosis sera impair angiogenic performance of dermal microvascular endothelial cells: therapeutic implications of cyclophosphamide. PLoS One. 2015;10(6):e0130166.
87. Casciola-Rosen LA, Anhalt G, Rosen A. Autoantigens targeted in systemic lupus erythematosus are clustered in two populations of surface structures on apoptotic keratinocytes. J Exp Med. 1994;179(4):1317–30.
88. Sercarz EE, Lehmann PV, Ametani A, Benichou G, Miller A, Moudgil K. Dominance and crypticity of T cell antigenic determinants. Annu Rev Immunol. 1993;11:729–66.
89. Zhou Z, Ménard HA. Autoantigenic posttranslational modifications of proteins: does it apply to rheumatoid arthritis? Curr Opin Rheumatol. 2002;14(3):250–3.

90. Andrade F, Roy S, Nicholson D, Thornberry N, Rosen A, Casciola-Rosen L. Granzyme B directly and efficiently cleaves several downstream caspase substrates: implications for CTL-induced apoptosis. Immunity. 1998;8(4):451–60.
91. Casciola-Rosen L, Andrade F, Ulanet D, Wong WB, Rosen A. Cleavage by granzyme B is strongly predictive of autoantigen status: implications for initiation of autoimmunity. J Exp Med. 1999;190(6):815–26.
92. Schachna L, Wigley FM, Morris S, Gelber AC, Rosen A, Casciola-Rosen L. Recognition of Granzyme B-generated autoantigen fragments in scleroderma patients with ischemic digital loss. Arthritis Rheum. 2002;46(7):1873–84.
93. Youinou P, Revelen R, Bordron A. Is antiendothelial cell antibody the murder weapon in systemic sclerosis? Clin Exp Rheumatol. 1999;17(1):35–6.
94. Hill MB, Phipps JL, Cartwright RJ, Milford Ward A, Greaves M, Hughes P. Antibodies to membranes of endothelial cells and fibroblasts in scleroderma. Clin Exp Immunol. 1996;106(3):491–7.
95. Negi VS, Tripathy NK, Misra R, Nityanand S. Antiendothelial cell antibodies in scleroderma correlate with severe digital ischemia and pulmonary arterial hypertension. J Rheumatol. 1998;25(3):462–6.
96. Garcia de la Pena-Lefebvre P, Chanseaud Y, Tamby MC, Reinbolt J, Batteux F, Allanore Y, Kahan A, Meyer O, Benveniste O, Boyer O, Guillevin L, Boissier MC, Mouthon L. IgG reactivity with a 100-kDa tissue and endothelial cell antigen identified as topoisomerase 1 distinguishes between limited and diffuse systemic sclerosis patients. Clin Immunol. 2004;111(3):241–51.
97. Tamby MC, Chanseaud Y, Humbert M, Fermanian J, Guilpain P, Garcia-de-la-Pena-Lefebvre P, Brunet S, Servettaz A, Weill B, Simonneau G, Guillevin L, Boissier MC, Mouthon L. Anti-endothelial cell antibodies in idiopathic and systemic sclerosis associated pulmonary arterial hypertension. Thorax. 2005;60(9):765–72.
98. Worda M, Sgonc R, Dietrich H, Niederegger H, Sundick RS, Gershwin ME, Wick G. In vivo analysis of the apoptosis-inducing effect of anti-endothelial cell antibodies in systemic sclerosis by the chorioallantoic membrane assay. Arthritis Rheum. 2003;48(9):2605–14.
99. Bordron A, Dueymes M, Levy Y, Jamin C, Leroy JP, Piette JC, Shoenfeld Y, Youinou PY. The binding of some human antiendothelial cell antibodies induces endothelial cell apoptosis. J Clin Invest. 1998;101(10):2029–35.
100. Tan FK, Arnett FC, Reveille JD, Ahn C, Antohi S, Sasaki T, Nishioka K, Bona CA. Autoantibodies to fibrillin 1 in systemic sclerosis: ethnic differences in antigen recognition and lack of correlation with specific clinical features or HLA alleles. Arthritis Rheum. 2000;43(11):2464–71.
101. Arends SJ, Damoiseaux JG, Duijvestijn AM, Debrus-Palmans L, Boomars KA, Brunner-La Rocca HP, Cohen Tervaert JW, van Paassen P. Functional implications of IgG anti-endothelial cell antibodies in pulmonary arterial hypertension. Autoimmunity. 2013;46(7):463–70.
102. Wolf SI, Howat S, Abraham DJ, Pearson JD, Lawson C. Agonistic anti-ICAM-1 antibodies in scleroderma: activation of endothelial pro-inflammatory cascades. Vasc Pharmacol. 2013;59(1–2):19–26.
103. Al-Dhaher FF, Pope JE, Ouimet JM. Determinants of morbidity and mortality of systemic sclerosis in Canada. Semin Arthritis Rheum. 2010;39(4):269–77.
104. Steen VD, Medsger TA. Changes in causes of death in systemic sclerosis, 1972–2002. Ann Rheum Dis. 2007;66(7):940–4.
105. Mathai SC, Hummers LK, Champion HC, Wigley FM, Zaiman A, Hassoun PM, Girgis RE. Survival in pulmonary hypertension associated with the scleroderma spectrum of diseases: impact of interstitial lung disease. Arthritis Rheum. 2009;60(2):569–77.
106. Birukov KG. Cyclic stretch, reactive oxygen species, and vascular remodeling. Antioxid Redox Signal. 2009;11(7):1651–67.
107. Grote K, Flach I, Luchtefeld M, Akin E, Holland SM, Drexler H, Schieffer B. Mechanical stretch enhances mRNA expression and proenzyme release of matrix metalloproteinase-2 (MMP-2) via NAD(P)H oxidase-derived reactive oxygen species. Circ Res. 2003;92(11):e80–6.
108. McCord JM. Oxygen-derived free radicals in postischemic tissue injury. N Engl J Med. 1985;312(3):159–63.
109. Riccieri V, Spadaro A, Fuksa L, Firuzi O, Saso L, Valesini G. Specific oxidative stress parameters differently correlate with nailfold capillaroscopy changes and organ involvement in systemic sclerosis. Clin Rheumatol. 2008;27(2):225–30.
110. Valko M, Leibfritz D, Moncol J, Cronin MT, Mazur M, Telser J. Free radicals and antioxidants in normal physiological functions and human disease. Int J Biochem Cell Biol. 2007;39(1):44–84.
111. Kuschel L, Hansel A, Schönherr R, Weissbach H, Brot N, Hoshi T, Heinemann SH. Molecular cloning and functional expression of a human peptide methionine sulfoxide reductase (hMsrA). FEBS Lett. 1999;456(1):17–21.
112. Ogawa F, Sander CS, Hansel A, Oehrl W, Kasperczyk H, Elsner P, Shimizu K, Heinemann SH, Thiele JJ. The repair enzyme peptide methionine-S-sulfoxide reductase is expressed in human epidermis and upregulated by UVA radiation. J Invest Dermatol. 2006;126(5):1128–34.
113. Prentice HM, Moench IA, Rickaway ZT, Dougherty CJ, Webster KA, Weissbach H. MsrA protects cardiomyocytes against hypoxia/reoxygenation induced cell death. Biochem Biophys Res Commun. 2008;366(3):775–8.
114. Ogawa F, Shimizu K, Hara T, Muroi E, Komura K, Takenaka M, Hasegawa M, Fujimoto M, Takehara K, Sato S. Autoantibody against one of the antioxidant repair enzymes, methionine sulfoxide reductase A, in systemic sclerosis: association with pulmonary fibrosis and vascular damage. Arch Dermatol Res. 2010;302(1):27–35.
115. Baroni SS, Santillo M, Bevilacqua F, Luchetti M, Spadoni T, Mancini M, Fraticelli P, Sambo P, Funaro A, Kazlauskas A, Avvedimento EV, Gabrielli A. Stimulatory autoantibodies to the PDGF receptor in systemic sclerosis. N Engl J Med. 2006;354(25):2667–76.
116. Classen JF, Henrohn D, Rorsman F, Lennartsson J, Lauwerys BR, Wikström G, Rorsman C, Lenglez S, Franck-Larsson K, Tomasi JP, Kämpe O, Vanthuyne M, Houssiau FA, Demoulin JB. Lack of evidence of stimulatory autoantibodies to platelet-derived growth factor receptor in patients with systemic sclerosis. Arthritis Rheum. 2009;60(4):1137–44.
117. Moroncini G, Grieco A, Nacci G, Paolini C, Tonnini C, Pozniak KN, Cuccioloni M, Mozzicafreddo M, Svegliati S, Angeletti M, Kazlauskas A, Avvedimento EV, Funaro A, Gabrielli A. Epitope specificity determines pathogenicity and detectability of anti-platelet-derived growth factor receptor α autoantibodies in systemic sclerosis. Arthritis Rheumatol. 2015;67(7):1891–903.
118. Svegliati S, Amico D, Spadoni T, Fischetti C, Finke D, Moroncini G, Paolini C, Tonnini C, Grieco A, Rovinelli M, Funaro A, Gabrielli A. Agonistic anti-PDGF receptor autoantibodies from patients with systemic sclerosis impact human pulmonary artery smooth muscle cells function in vitro. Front Immunol. 2017;8:75.
119. Kill A, Tabeling C, Undeutsch R, Kühl AA, Günther J, Radic M, Becker MO, Heidecke H, Worm M, Witzenrath M, Burmester GR, Dragun D, Riemekasten G. Autoantibodies to angiotensin and endothelin receptors in systemic sclerosis induce cellular and systemic events associated with disease pathogenesis. Arthritis Res Ther. 2014;16(1):R29.
120. Becker MO, Kill A, Kutsche M, Guenther J, Rose A, Tabeling C, Witzenrath M, Kühl AA, Heidecke H, Ghofrani HA, Tiede H, Schermuly RT, Nickel N, Hoeper MM, Lukitsch I, Gollasch M, Kuebler WM, Bock S, Burmester GR, Dragun D, Riemekasten G. Vascular receptor autoantibodies in pulmonary arterial hyper-

tension associated with systemic sclerosis. Am J Respir Crit Care Med. 2014;190(7):808–17.
121. Avouac J, Riemekasten G, Meune C, Ruiz B, Kahan A, Allanore Y. Autoantibodies against endothelin 1 type A receptor are strong predictors of digital ulcers in systemic sclerosis. J Rheumatol. 2015;42(10):1801–7.
122. Derk CT, Jimenez SA. Systemic sclerosis: current views of its pathogenesis. Autoimmun Rev. 2003;2(4):181–91.
123. Reinhart BJ, Slack FJ, Basson M, Pasquinelli AE, Bettinger JC, Rougvie AE, Horvitz HR, Ruvkun G. The 21-nucleotide let-7 RNA regulates developmental timing in Caenorhabditis elegans. Nature. 2000;403(6772):901–6.
124. Razin A, Cedar H. DNA methylation and gene expression. Microbiol Rev. 1991;55(3):451–8.
125. Herman JG, Baylin SB. Gene silencing in cancer in association with promoter hypermethylation. N Engl J Med. 2003;349(21):2042–54.
126. Richardson B. Primer: epigenetics of autoimmunity. Nat Clin Pract Rheumatol. 2007;3(9):521–7.
127. Romero LI, Zhang DN, Cooke JP, Ho HK, Avalos E, Herrera R, Herron GS. Differential expression of nitric oxide by dermal microvascular endothelial cells from patients with scleroderma. Vasc Med. 2000;5(3):147–58.
128. Huang PL, Huang Z, Mashimo H, Bloch KD, Moskowitz MA, Bevan JA, Fishman MC. Hypertension in mice lacking the gene for endothelial nitric oxide synthase. Nature. 1995;377(6546):239–42.
129. Lee PC, Salyapongse AN, Bragdon GA, Shears LL 2nd, Watkins SC, Edington HD, Billiar TR. Impaired wound healing and angiogenesis in eNOS-deficient mice. Am J Phys. 1999;277(4):H1600–8.
130. Rabinovitch M. Molecular pathogenesis of pulmonary arterial hypertension. J Clin Invest. 2012;122(12):4306–13.
131. Wang Y, Kahaleh B. Epigenetic repression of bone morphogenetic protein receptor II expression in scleroderma. J Cell Mol Med. 2013;17(10):1291–9.
132. Tsou PS, Wren JD, Amin MA, Schiopu E, Fox DA, Khanna D, Sawalha AH. Histone deacetylase 5 is overexpressed in scleroderma endothelial cells and impairs angiogenesis via repression of proangiogenic factors. Arthritis Rheumatol. 2016;68(12):2975–85.
133. Tsou PS, Khanna D, Sawalha AH. Identification of cysteine-rich angiogenic inducer 61 as a potential antifibrotic and proangiogenic mediator in scleroderma. Arthritis Rheumatol. 2019;71(8):1350–9.
134. Tsou PS, Campbell P, Amin MA, Coit P, Miller S, Fox DA, Khanna D, Sawalha AH. Inhibition of EZH2 prevents fibrosis and restores normal angiogenesis in scleroderma. Proc Natl Acad Sci U S A. 2019;116(9):3695–702.
135. Altorok N, Almeshal N, Wang Y, Kahaleh B. Epigenetics, the holy grail in the pathogenesis of systemic sclerosis. Rheumatology (Oxford). 2015;54(10):1759–70.
136. Ramahi A, Altorok N, Kahaleh B. Epigenetics and systemic sclerosis: an answer to disease onset and evolution? Eur J Rheumatol. 2020;7(Suppl 3):S147–56.
137. Carmeliet P. Mechanisms of angiogenesis and arteriogenesis. Nat Med. 2000;6(4):389–95.
138. Manetti M, Guiducci S, Ibba-Manneschi L, Matucci-Cerinic M. Mechanisms in the loss of capillaries in systemic sclerosis: angiogenesis versus vasculogenesis. J Cell Mol Med. 2010;14(6A):1241–54.
139. Rabquer BJ, Koch AE. Angiogenesis and vasculopathy in systemic sclerosis: evolving concepts. Curr Rheumatol Rep. 2012;14(1):56–63.
140. Manetti M, Guiducci S, Ibba-Manneschi L, Matucci-Cerinic M. Impaired angiogenesis in systemic sclerosis: the emerging role of the antiangiogenic VEGF(165)b splice variant. Trends Cardiovasc Med. 2011;21(7):204–10.
141. Distler O, Del Rosso A, Giacomelli R, Cipriani P, Conforti ML, Guiducci S, Gay RE, Michel BA, Brühlmann P, Müller-Ladner U, Gay S, Matucci-Cerinic M. Angiogenic and angiostatic factors in systemic sclerosis: increased levels of vascular endothelial growth factor are a feature of the earliest disease stages and are associated with the absence of fingertip ulcers. Arthritis Res. 2002;4(6):R11.
142. Distler O, Distler JH, Scheid A, Acker T, Hirth A, Rethage J, Michel BA, Gay RE, Müller-Ladner U, Matucci-Cerinic M, Plate KH, Gassmann M, Gay S. Uncontrolled expression of vascular endothelial growth factor and its receptors leads to insufficient skin angiogenesis in patients with systemic sclerosis. Circ Res. 2004;95(1):109–16.
143. Choi JJ, Min DJ, Cho ML, Min SY, Kim SJ, Lee SS, Park KS, Seo YI, Kim WU, Park SH, Cho CS. Elevated vascular endothelial growth factor in systemic sclerosis. J Rheumatol. 2003;30(7):1529–33.
144. Mackiewicz Z, Sukura A, Povilenait D, Ceponis A, Virtanen I, Hukkanen M, Konttinen YT. Increased but imbalanced expression of VEGF and its receptors has no positive effect on angiogenesis in systemic sclerosis skin. Clin Exp Rheumatol. 2002;20(5):641–6.
145. D'Alessio S, Fibbi G, Cinelli M, Guiducci S, Del Rosso A, Margheri F, Serratì S, Pucci M, Kahaleh B, Fan P, Annunziato F, Cosmi L, Liotta F, Matucci-Cerinic M, Del Rosso M. Matrix metalloproteinase 12-dependent cleavage of urokinase receptor in systemic sclerosis microvascular endothelial cells results in impaired angiogenesis. Arthritis Rheum. 2004;50(10):3275–85.
146. Tsou PS, Amin MA, Campbell PL, Zakhem G, Balogh B, Edhayan G, Ohara RA, Schiopu E, Khanna D, Koch AE, Fox DA. Activation of the thromboxane A2 receptor by 8-isoprostane inhibits the pro-angiogenic effect of vascular endothelial growth factor in scleroderma. J Invest Dermatol. 2015;135(12):3153–62.
147. Manetti M, Guiducci S, Romano E, Ceccarelli C, Bellando-Randone S, Conforti ML, Ibba-Manneschi L, Matucci-Cerinic M. Overexpression of VEGF165b, an inhibitory splice variant of vascular endothelial growth factor, leads to insufficient angiogenesis in patients with systemic sclerosis. Circ Res. 2011;109(3):e14–26.
148. Manetti M, Guiducci S, Romano E, Bellando-Randone S, Lepri G, Bruni C, Conforti ML, Ibba-Manneschi L, Matucci-Cerinic M. Increased plasma levels of the VEGF165b splice variant are associated with the severity of nailfold capillary loss in systemic sclerosis. Ann Rheum Dis. 2013;72(8):1425–7.
149. Hirigoyen D, Burgos PI, Mezzano V, Duran J, Barrientos M, Saez CG, Panes O, Mezzano D, Iruretagoyena M. Inhibition of angiogenesis by platelets in systemic sclerosis patients. Arthritis Res Ther. 2015;17:332.
150. Rabquer BJ, Tsou PS, Hou Y, Thirunavukkarasu E, Haines GK 3rd, Impens AJ, Phillips K, Kahaleh B, Seibold JR, Koch AE. Dysregulated expression of MIG/CXCL9, IP-10/CXCL10 and CXCL16 and their receptors in systemic sclerosis. Arthritis Res Ther. 2011;13(1):R18.
151. Tsou PS, Rabquer BJ, Ohara RA, Stinson WA, Campbell PL, Amin MA, Balogh B, Zakhem G, Renauer PA, Lozier A, Arasu E, Haines GK 3rd, Kahaleh B, Schiopu E, Khanna D, Koch AE. Scleroderma dermal microvascular endothelial cells exhibit defective response to pro-angiogenic chemokines. Rheumatology (Oxford). 2016;55(4):745–54.
152. Shirai Y, Okazaki Y, Inoue Y, Tamura Y, Yasuoka H, Takeuchi T, Kuwana M. Elevated levels of pentraxin 3 in systemic sclerosis: associations with vascular manifestations and defective vasculogenesis. Arthritis Rheumatol. 2015;67(2):498–507.
153. Manetti M, Guiducci S, Romano E, Avouac J, Rosa I, Ruiz B, Lepri G, Bellando-Randone S, Ibba-Manneschi L, Allanore Y, Matucci-Cerinic M. Decreased expression of the endothelial cell-derived factor EGFL7 in systemic sclerosis: potential contribution to impaired angiogenesis and vasculogenesis. Arthritis Res Ther. 2013;15(5):R165.
154. Romano E, Bellando-Randone S, Manetti M, Bruni C, Lepri G, Matucci-Cerinic M, Guiducci S. Bosentan blocks the antiangio-

genic effects of sera from systemic sclerosis patients: an in vitro study. Clin Exp Rheumatol. 2015;33(4 Suppl 91):S148–52.
155. Mazzotta C, Manetti M, Rosa I, Romano E, Blagojevic J, Bellando-Randone S, Bruni C, Lepri G, Guiducci S, Ibba-Manneschi L, Matucci-Cerinic M. Proangiogenic effects of soluble alpha-Klotho on systemic sclerosis dermal microvascular endothelial cells. Arthritis Res Ther. 2017;19(1):27.
156. Romano E, Rosa I, Fioretto BS, Guiducci S, Manetti M, Matucci-Cerinic M. A new avenue in the pathogenesis of systemic sclerosis: the molecular interface between the endothelial and the nervous systems. Clin Exp Rheumatol. 2019;37(Suppl 119(4)):133–40.
157. Romano E, Chora I, Manetti M, Mazzotta C, Rosa I, Bellando-Randone S, Blagojevic J, Soares R, Avouac J, Allanore Y, Ibba-Manneschi L, Matucci-Cerinic M, Guiducci S. Decreased expression of neuropilin-1 as a novel key factor contributing to peripheral microvasculopathy and defective angiogenesis in systemic sclerosis. Ann Rheum Dis. 2016;75(8):1541–9.
158. Chora I, Romano E, Manetti M, Mazzotta C, Costa R, Machado V, Cortez A, Bruni C, Lepri G, Guiducci S, De Paulis A, Soares R, Matucci-Cerinic M. Evidence for a derangement of the microvascular system in patients with a very early diagnosis of systemic sclerosis. J Rheumatol. 2017;44(8):1190–7.
159. Mazzotta C, Romano E, Bruni C, Manetti M, Lepri G, Bellando-Randone S, Blagojevic J, Ibba-Manneschi L, Matucci-Cerinic M, Guiducci S. Plexin-D1/Semaphorin 3E pathway may contribute to dysregulation of vascular tone control and defective angiogenesis in systemic sclerosis. Arthritis Res Ther. 2015;17(1):221.
160. Romano E, Manetti M, Rosa I, Fioretto BS, Ibba-Manneschi L, Matucci-Cerinic M, Guiducci S. Slit2/Robo4 axis may contribute to endothelial cell dysfunction and angiogenesis disturbance in systemic sclerosis. Ann Rheum Dis. 2018;77(11):1665–74.
161. Henrot P, Moisan F, Laurent P, Manicki P, Kaulanjan-Checkmodine P, Jolivel V, Rezvani HR, Leroy V, Picard F, Boulon C, Schaeverbeke T, Seneschal J, Lazaro E, Taïeb A, Truchetet ME, Cario M. Decreased CCN3 in systemic sclerosis endothelial cells contributes to impaired angiogenesis. J Invest Dermatol. 2020;140(7):1427–34.e5.
162. Del Papa N, Pignataro F. The role of endothelial progenitors in the repair of vascular damage in systemic sclerosis. Front Immunol. 2018;9:1383.
163. Asahara T, Murohara T, Sullivan A, Silver M, van der Zee R, Li T, Witzenbichler B, Schatteman G, Isner JM. Isolation of putative progenitor endothelial cells for angiogenesis. Science. 1997;275(5302):964–7.
164. Kuwana M, Okazaki Y, Yasuoka H, Kawakami Y, Ikeda Y. Defective vasculogenesis in systemic sclerosis. Lancet. 2004;364(9434):603–10.
165. Allanore Y, Batteux F, Avouac J, Assous N, Weill B, Kahan A. Levels of circulating endothelial progenitor cells in systemic sclerosis. Clin Exp Rheumatol. 2007;25(1):60–6.
166. Avouac J, Juin F, Wipff J, Couraud PO, Chiocchia G, Kahan A, Boileau C, Uzan G, Allanore Y. Circulating endothelial progenitor cells in systemic sclerosis: association with disease severity. Ann Rheum Dis. 2008;67(10):1455–60.
167. Zhu S, Evans S, Yan B, Povsic TJ, Tapson V, Goldschmidt-Clermont PJ, Dong C. Transcriptional regulation of Bim by FOXO3a and Akt mediates scleroderma serum-induced apoptosis in endothelial progenitor cells. Circulation. 2008;118(21):2156–65.
168. Del Papa N, Quirici N, Scavullo C, Gianelli U, Corti L, Vitali C, Ferri C, Giuggioli D, Manfredi A, Maglione W, Onida F, Colaci M, Bosari S, Lambertenghi DG. Antiendothelial cell antibodies induce apoptosis of bone marrow endothelial progenitors in systemic sclerosis. J Rheumatol. 2010;37(10):2053–63.
169. Kuwana M, Okazaki Y. Brief report: impaired in vivo neovascularization capacity of endothelial progenitor cells in patients with systemic sclerosis. Arthritis Rheumatol. 2014;66(5):1300–5.
170. Manetti M, Pratesi S, Romano E, Bellando-Randone S, Rosa I, Guiducci S, Fioretto BS, Ibba-Manneschi L, Maggi E, Matucci-Cerinic M. Angiogenic T cell expansion correlates with severity of peripheral vascular damage in systemic sclerosis. PLoS One. 2017;12(8):e0183102.
171. Yamaguchi Y, Kuwana M. Proangiogenic hematopoietic cells of monocytic origin: roles in vascular regeneration and pathogenic processes of systemic sclerosis. Histol Histopathol. 2013;28(2):175–83.
172. Cipriani P, Guiducci S, Miniati I, Cinelli M, Urbani S, Marrelli A, Dolo V, Pavan A, Saccardi R, Tyndall A, Giacomelli R, Cerinic MM. Impairment of endothelial cell differentiation from bone marrow-derived mesenchymal stem cells: new insight into the pathogenesis of systemic sclerosis. Arthritis Rheum. 2007;56(6):1994–2004.
173. Guiducci S, Manetti M, Romano E, Mazzanti B, Ceccarelli C, Dal Pozzo S, Milia AF, Bellando-Randone S, Fiori G, Conforti ML, Saccardi R, Ibba-Manneschi L, Matucci-Cerinic M. Bone marrow-derived mesenchymal stem cells from early diffuse systemic sclerosis exhibit a paracrine machinery and stimulate angiogenesis in vitro. Ann Rheum Dis. 2011;70(11):2011–21.
174. Guiducci S, Porta F, Saccardi R, Guidi S, Ibba-Manneschi L, Manetti M, Mazzanti B, Dal Pozzo S, Milia AF, Bellando-Randone S, Miniati I, Fiori G, Fontana R, Amanzi L, Braschi F, Bosi A, Matucci-Cerinic M. Autologous mesenchymal stem cells foster revascularization of ischemic limbs in systemic sclerosis: a case report. Ann Intern Med. 2010;153(10):650–4.
175. Rosa I, Romano E, Fioretto BS, Matucci-Cerinic M, Manetti M. Adipose-derived stem cells: pathophysiologic implications vs therapeutic potential in systemic sclerosis. World J Stem Cells. 2021;13:30–48.
176. Velier M, Simoncini S, Abellan M, Francois P, Eap S, Lagrange A, Bertrand B, Daumas A, Granel B, Delorme B, Dignat George F, Magalon J, Sabatier F. Adipose-derived stem cells from systemic sclerosis patients maintain pro-angiogenic and antifibrotic paracrine effects in vitro. J Clin Med. 2019;8(11):1979.
177. Pepper MS. Role of the matrix metalloproteinase and plasminogen activator-plasmin systems in angiogenesis. Arterioscler Thromb Vasc Biol. 2001;21(7):1104–17.
178. Keck RG, Berleau L, Harris R, Keyt BA. Disulfide structure of the heparin binding domain in vascular endothelial growth factor: characterization of posttranslational modifications in VEGF. Arch Biochem Biophys. 1997;344(1):103–13.
179. Ihn H. The role of TGF-beta signaling in the pathogenesis of fibrosis in scleroderma. Arch Immunol Ther Exp. 2002;50(5):325–31.
180. Jinnin M, Ihn H, Mimura Y, Asano Y, Yamane K, Tamaki K. Effects of hepatocyte growth factor on the expression of type I collagen and matrix metalloproteinase-1 in normal and scleroderma dermal fibroblasts. J Invest Dermatol. 2005;124(2):324–30.
181. Lijnen HR, Ugwu F, Bini A, Collen D. Generation of an angiostatin-like fragment from plasminogen by stromelysin-1 (MMP-3). Biochemistry. 1998;37(14):4699–702.
182. O'Reilly MS, Wiederschain D, Stetler-Stevenson WG, Folkman J, Moses MA. Regulation of angiostatin production by matrix metalloproteinase-2 in a model of concomitant resistance. J Biol Chem. 1999;274(41):29568–71.
183. Vassalli JD, Baccino D, Belin D. A cellular binding site for the Mr 55,000 form of the human plasminogen activator, urokinase. J Cell Biol. 1985;100(1):86–92.
184. Wei Y, Waltz DA, Rao N, Drummond RJ, Rosenberg S, Chapman HA. Identification of the urokinase receptor as an adhesion receptor for vitronectin. J Biol Chem. 1994;269(51):32380–8.
185. Ragno P. The urokinase receptor: a ligand or a receptor? Story of a sociable molecule. Cell Mol Life Sci. 2006;63(9):1028–37.
186. Margheri F, Manetti M, Serratì S, Nosi D, Pucci M, Matucci-Cerinic M, Kahaleh B, Bazzichi L, Fibbi G, Ibba-Manneschi L, Del Rosso M. Domain 1 of the urokinase-type plasminogen activator receptor is required for its morphologic and functional, beta2 integrin-mediated connection with actin cytoskeleton in human

microvascular endothelial cells: failure of association in systemic sclerosis endothelial cells. Arthritis Rheum. 2006;54(12):3926–38.
187. Margheri F, Serratì S, Lapucci A, Chillà A, Bazzichi L, Bombardieri S, Kahaleh B, Calorini L, Bianchini F, Fibbi G, Del Rosso M. Modulation of the angiogenic phenotype of normal and systemic sclerosis endothelial cells by gain-loss of function of pentraxin 3 and matrix metalloproteinase 12. Arthritis Rheum. 2010;62(8):2488–98.
188. Manetti M, Guiducci S, Romano E, Bellando-Randone S, Conforti ML, Ibba-Manneschi L, Matucci-Cerinic M. Increased serum levels and tissue expression of matrix metalloproteinase-12 in patients with systemic sclerosis: correlation with severity of skin and pulmonary fibrosis and vascular damage. Ann Rheum Dis. 2012;71(6):1064–72.
189. Xu Z, Shi H, Li Q, Mei Q, Bao J, Shen Y, Xu J. Mouse macrophage metalloelastase generates angiostatin from plasminogen and suppresses tumor angiogenesis in murine colon cancer. Oncol Rep. 2008;20(1):81–8.
190. Manetti M, Romano E, Rosa I, Guiducci S, Bellando-Randone S, De Paulis A, Ibba-Manneschi L, Matucci-Cerinic M. Endothelial-to-mesenchymal transition contributes to endothelial dysfunction and dermal fibrosis in systemic sclerosis. Ann Rheum Dis. 2017;76(5):924–34.
191. Legány N, Toldi G, Distler JH, Beyer C, Szalay B, Kovács L, Vásárhelyi B, Balog A. Increased plasma soluble urokinase plasminogen activator receptor levels in systemic sclerosis: possible association with microvascular abnormalities and extent of fibrosis. Clin Chem Lab Med. 2015;53(11):1799–805.
192. Giusti B, Serratì S, Margheri F, Papucci L, Rossi L, Poggi F, Magi A, Del Rosso A, Cinelli M, Guiducci S, Kahaleh B, Matucci-Cerinic M, Abbate R, Fibbi G, Del Rosso M. The antiangiogenic tissue kallikrein pattern of endothelial cells in systemic sclerosis. Arthritis Rheum. 2005;52(11):3618–28.
193. Giusti B, Fibbi G, Margheri F, Serratì S, Rossi L, Poggi F, Lapini I, Magi A, Del Rosso A, Cinelli M, Guiducci S, Kahaleh B, Bazzichi L, Bombardieri S, Matucci-Cerinic M, Gensini GF, Del Rosso M, Abbate R. A model of anti-angiogenesis: differential transcriptosome profiling of microvascular endothelial cells from diffuse systemic sclerosis patients. Arthritis Res Ther. 2006;8(4):R115.
194. Bhoola KD, Figueroa CD, Worthy K. Bioregulation of kinins: kallikreins, kininogens, and kininases. Pharmacol Rev. 1992;44(1):1–80.
195. Plendl J, Snyman C, Naidoo S, Sawant S, Mahabeer R, Bhoola KD. Expression of tissue kallikrein and kinin receptors in angiogenic microvascular endothelial cells. Biol Chem. 2000;381(11):1103–15.
196. Emanueli C, Madeddu P. Targeting kinin receptors for the treatment of tissue ischaemia. Trends Pharmacol Sci. 2001;22(9):478–84.
197. Del Rosso A, Distler O, Milia AF, Emanueli C, Ibba-Manneschi L, Guiducci S, Conforti ML, Generini S, Pignone A, Gay S, Madeddu P, Matucci-Cerinic M. Increased circulating levels of tissue kallikrein in systemic sclerosis correlate with microvascular involvement. Ann Rheum Dis. 2005;64(3):382–7.
198. Giusti B, Margheri F, Rossi L, Lapini I, Magi A, Serratì S, Chillà A, Laurenzana A, Magnelli L, Calorini L, Bianchini F, Fibbi G, Abbate R, Del Rosso M. Desmoglein-2-integrin Beta-8 interaction regulates actin assembly in endothelial cells: deregulation in systemic sclerosis. PLoS One. 2013;8(7):e68117.
199. Avouac J, Cagnard N, Distler JH, Schoindre Y, Ruiz B, Couraud PO, Uzan G, Boileau C, Chiocchia G, Allanore Y. Insights into the pathogenesis of systemic sclerosis based on the gene expression profile of progenitor-derived endothelial cells. Arthritis Rheum. 2011;63(11):3552–62.
200. Tinazzi E, Dolcino M, Puccetti A, Rigo A, Beri R, Valenti MT, Corrocher R, Lunardi C. Gene expression profiling in circulating endothelial cells from systemic sclerosis patients shows an altered control of apoptosis and angiogenesis that is modified by iloprost infusion. Arthritis Res Ther. 2010;12(4):R131.
201. Apostolidis SA, Stifano G, Tabib T, Rice LM, Morse CM, Kahaleh B, Lafyatis R. Single cell RNA sequencing identifies HSPG2 and APLNR as markers of endothelial cell injury in systemic sclerosis skin. Front Immunol. 2018;9:2191.
202. Allt G, Lawrenson JG. Pericytes: cell biology and pathology. Cells Tissues Organs. 2001;169(1):1–11.
203. Sima AA, Chakrabarti S, Garcia-Salinas R, Basu PK. The BB-rat; an authentic model of human diabetic retinopathy. Curr Eye Res. 1985;4(10):1087–92.
204. Sims DE. Recent advances in pericyte biology—implications for health and disease. Can J Cardiol. 1991;7(10):431–43.
205. Mandarino LJ, Sundarraj N, Finlayson J, Hassell HR. Regulation of fibronectin and laminin synthesis by retinal capillary endothelial cells and pericytes in vitro. Exp Eye Res. 1993;57(5):609–21.
206. Hirschi KK, D'Amore PA. Control of angiogenesis by the pericyte: molecular mechanisms and significance. EXS. 1997;79:419–28.
207. Herman IM, D'Amore PA. Microvascular pericytes contain muscle and nonmuscle actins. J Cell Biol. 1985;101(1):43–52.
208. Edelman DA, Jiang Y, Tyburski J, Wilson RF, Steffes C. Pericytes and their role in microvasculature homeostasis. J Surg Res. 2006;135(2):305–11.
209. Hirschi KK, Rohovsky SA, D'Amore PA. PDGF, TGF-beta, and heterotypic cell-cell interactions mediate endothelial cell-induced recruitment of 10T1/2 cells and their differentiation to a smooth muscle fate. J Cell Biol. 1998;141(3):805–14.
210. Kelley C, D'Amore P, Hechtman HB, Shepro D. Microvascular pericyte contractility in vitro: comparison with other cells of the vascular wall. J Cell Biol. 1987;104(3):483–90.
211. Tilton RG, Kilo C, Williamson JR. Pericyte-endothelial relationships in cardiac and skeletal muscle capillaries. Microvasc Res. 1979;18(3):325–35.
212. Cuevas P, Gutierrez-Diaz JA, Reimers D, Dujovny M, Diaz FG, Ausman JI. Pericyte endothelial gap junctions in human cerebral capillaries. Anat Embryol (Berl). 1984;170(2):155–9.
213. Miller FN, Sims DE. Contractile elements in the regulation of macromolecular permeability. Fed Proc. 1986;45(2):84–8.
214. Murphy DD, Wagner RC. Differential contractile response of cultured microvascular pericytes to vasoactive agents. Microcirculation. 1994;1(2):121–8.
215. Shepro D, Morel NM. Pericyte physiology. FASEB J. 1993;7(11):1031–8.
216. Carmeliet P. Blood vessels and nerves: common signals, pathways and diseases. Nat Rev Genet. 2003;4(9):710–20.
217. Louissaint A Jr, Rao S, Leventhal C, Goldman SA. Coordinated interaction of neurogenesis and angiogenesis in the adult songbird brain. Neuron. 2002;34(6):945–60.
218. Palmer TD, Willhoite AR, Gage FH. Vascular niche for adult hippocampal neurogenesis. J Comp Neurol. 2000;425(4):479–94.
219. Ronnov-Jessen L, Petersen OW, Koteliansky VE, Bissell MJ. The origin of the myofibroblasts in breast cancer. Recapitulation of tumor environment in culture unravels diversity and implicates converted fibroblasts and recruited smooth muscle cells. J Clin Invest. 1995;95(2):859–73.
220. Sundberg C, Ivarsson M, Gerdin B, Rubin K. Pericytes as collagen-producing cells in excessive dermal scarring. Lab Invest. 1996;74(2):452–66.
221. Sundberg C, Ljungström M, Lindmark G, Gerdin B, Rubin K. Microvascular pericytes express platelet-derived growth factor-beta receptors in human healing wounds and colorectal adenocarcinoma. Am J Pathol. 1993;143(5):1377–88.
222. Rajkumar VS, Sundberg C, Abraham DJ, Rubin K, Black CM. Activation of microvascular pericytes in autoimmune Raynaud's phenomenon and systemic sclerosis. Arthritis Rheum. 1999;42(5):930–41.

223. Jelaska A, Korn JH. Role of apoptosis and transforming growth factor beta1 in fibroblast selection and activation in systemic sclerosis. Arthritis Rheum. 2000;43(10):2230–9.
224. Sappino AP, Masouy I, Saurat JH, Gabbiani G. Smooth muscle differentiation in scleroderma fibroblastic cells. Am J Pathol. 1990;137(3):585–91.
225. Rajkumar VS, Howell K, Csiszar K, Denton CP, Black CM, Abraham DJ. Shared expression of phenotypic markers in systemic sclerosis indicates a convergence of pericytes and fibroblasts to a myofibroblast lineage in fibrosis. Arthritis Res Ther. 2005;7(5):R1113–23.
226. Asano Y, Stawski L, Hant F, Highland K, Silver R, Szalai G, Watson DK, Trojanowska M. Endothelial Fli1 deficiency impairs vascular homeostasis: a role in scleroderma vasculopathy. Am J Pathol. 2010;176(4):1983–98.
227. Cretoiu SM, Popescu LM. Telocytes revisited. Biomol Concepts. 2014;5(5):353–69.
228. Romano E, Rosa I, Fioretto BS, Lucattelli E, Innocenti M, Ibba-Manneschi L, Matucci-Cerinic M, Manetti M. A two-step immunomagnetic microbead-based method for the isolation of human primary skin telocytes/CD34+ stromal cells. Int J Mol Sci. 2020;21(16):5877.
229. Manetti M, Guiducci S, Ruffo M, Rosa I, Faussone-Pellegrini MS, Matucci-Cerinic M, Ibba-Manneschi L. Evidence for progressive reduction and loss of telocytes in the dermal cellular network of systemic sclerosis. J Cell Mol Med. 2013;17(4):482–96.
230. Frid MG, Dempsey EC, Durmowicz AG, Stenmark KR. Smooth muscle cell heterogeneity in pulmonary and systemic vessels. Importance in vascular disease. Arterioscler Thromb Vasc Biol. 1997;17(7):1203–9.
231. Gittenberger-de Groot AC, DeRuiter MC, Bergwerff M, Poelmann RE. Smooth muscle cell origin and its relation to heterogeneity in development and disease. Arterioscler Thromb Vasc Biol. 1999;19(7):1589–94.
232. Owens GK. Molecular control of vascular smooth muscle cell differentiation. Acta Physiol Scand. 1998;164(4):623–35.
233. Arts MR, Baron M, Chokr N, Fritzler MJ, Canadian Scleroderma Research Group (CSRG), Servant MJ. Systemic sclerosis immunoglobulin induces growth and a pro-fibrotic state in vascular smooth muscle cells through the epidermal growth factor receptor. PLoS One. 2014;9(6):e100035.
234. Good RB, Gilbane AJ, Trinder SL, Denton CP, Coghlan G, Abraham DJ, Holmes AM. Endothelial to mesenchymal transition contributes to endothelial dysfunction in pulmonary arterial hypertension. Am J Pathol. 2015;185(7):1850–8.
235. Rosa I, Romano E, Fioretto BS, Manetti M. The contribution of mesenchymal transitions to the pathogenesis of systemic sclerosis. Eur J Rheumatol. 2020;7(Suppl 3):S157–64.
236. Rhodes JM, Simons M. The extracellular matrix and blood vessel formation: not just a scaffold. J Cell Mol Med. 2007;11(2):176–205.
237. Davis GE, Saunders WB. Molecular balance of capillary tube formation versus regression in wound repair: role of matrix metalloproteinases and their inhibitors. J Investig Dermatol Symp Proc. 2006;11(1):44–56.
238. Davis GE, Senger DR. Endothelial extracellular matrix: biosynthesis, remodeling, and functions during vascular morphogenesis and neovessel stabilization. Circ Res. 2005;97(11):1093–107.
239. Senger DR. Molecular framework for angiogenesis: a complex web of interactions between extravasated plasma proteins and endothelial cell proteins induced by angiogenic cytokines. Am J Pathol. 1996;149(1):1–7.
240. Vernon RB, Sage EH. Between molecules and morphology. Extracellular matrix and creation of vascular form. Am J Pathol. 1995;147(4):873–83.
241. Dvorak HF, Nagy JA, Berse B, Brown LF, Yeo KT, Yeo TK, Dvorak AM, van de Water L, Sioussat TM, Senger DR. Vascular permeability factor, fibrin, and the pathogenesis of tumor stroma formation. Ann N Y Acad Sci. 1992;667:101–11.
242. Dvorak HF, Senger DR, Dvorak AM. Fibrin as a component of the tumor stroma: origins and biological significance. Cancer Metastasis Rev. 1983;2(1):41–73.
243. Nagy JA, Brown LF, Senger DR, Lanir N, Van de Water L, Dvorak AM, Dvorak HF. Pathogenesis of tumor stroma generation: a critical role for leaky blood vessels and fibrin deposition. Biochim Biophys Acta. 1989;948(3):305–26.
244. Cheresh DA, Berliner SA, Vicente V, Ruggeri ZM. Recognition of distinct adhesive sites on fibrinogen by related integrins on platelets and endothelial cells. Cell. 1989;58(5):945–53.
245. Suehiro K, Gailit J, Plow EF. Fibrinogen is a ligand for integrin alpha-5beta1 on endothelial cells. J Biol Chem. 1997;272(8):5360–6.
246. Sahni A, Altland OD, Francis CW. FGF-2 but not FGF-1 binds fibrin and supports prolonged endothelial cell growth. J Thromb Haemost. 2003;1(6):1304–10.
247. Sahni A, Francis CW. Plasmic degradation modulates activity of fibrinogen-bound fibroblast growth factor-2. J Thromb Haemost. 2003;1(6):1271–7.
248. Bobik A, Tkachuk V. Metalloproteinases and plasminogen activators in vessel remodeling. Curr Hypertens Rep. 2003;5(6):466–72.
249. Garcia-Touchard A, Henry TD, Sangiorgi G, Spagnoli LG, Mauriello A, Conover C, Schwartz RS. Extracellular proteases in atherosclerosis and restenosis. Arterioscler Thromb Vasc Biol. 2005;25(6):1119–27.
250. Davis GE, Pintar Allen KA, Salazar R, Maxwell SA. Matrix metalloproteinase-1 and -9 activation by plasmin regulates a novel endothelial cell-mediated mechanism of collagen gel contraction and capillary tube regression in three-dimensional collagen matrices. J Cell Sci. 2001;114(Pt 5):917–30.
251. Saunders WB, Bayless KJ, Davis GE. MMP-1 activation by serine proteases and MMP-10 induces human capillary tubular network collapse and regression in 3D collagen matrices. J Cell Sci. 2005;118(Pt 10):2325–40.
252. Giannelli G, Iannone F, Marinosci F, Lapadula G, Antonaci S. The effect of bosentan on matrix metalloproteinase-9 levels in patients with systemic sclerosis-induced pulmonary hypertension. Curr Med Res Opin. 2005;21(3):327–32.
253. Kim WU, Min SY, Cho ML, Hong KH, Shin YJ, Park SH, Cho CS. Elevated matrix metalloproteinase-9 in patients with systemic sclerosis. Arthritis Res Ther. 2005;7(1):R71–9.
254. Avouac J, Guignabert C, Hoffmann-Vold AM, Ruiz B, Dorfmuller P, Pezet S, Amar O, Tu L, Van Wassenhove J, Sadoine J, Launay D, Elhai M, Cauvet A, Subramaniam A, Resnick R, Hachulla E, Molberg Ø, Kahan A, Humbert M, Allanore Y. Role of stromelysin 2 (matrix metalloproteinase 10) as a novel mediator of vascular remodeling underlying pulmonary hypertension associated with systemic sclerosis. Arthritis Rheumatol. 2017;69(11):2209–21.
255. Avouac J, Wipff J, Goldman O, Ruiz B, Couraud PO, Chiocchia G, Kahan A, Boileau C, Uzan G, Allanore Y. Angiogenesis in systemic sclerosis: impaired expression of vascular endothelial growth factor receptor 1 in endothelial progenitor-derived cells under hypoxic conditions. Arthritis Rheum. 2008;58(11):3550–61.
256. Silverstein JL, Steen VD, Medsger TA Jr, Falanga V. Cutaneous hypoxia in patients with systemic sclerosis (scleroderma). Arch Dermatol. 1988;124(9):1379–82.
257. Manalo DJ, Rowan A, Lavoie T, Natarajan L, Kelly BD, Ye SQ, Garcia JG, Semenza GL. Transcriptional regulation of vascular endothelial cell responses to hypoxia by HIF-1. Blood. 2005;105(2):659–69.
258. Makarenko VV, Usatyuk PV, Yuan G, Lee MM, Nanduri J, Natarajan V, Kumar GK, Prabhakar NR. Intermittent hypoxia-induced endothelial barrier dysfunction requires ROS-dependent MAP kinase activation. Am J Physiol Cell Physiol. 2014;306(8):C745–52.
259. Kahaleh MB. The role of vascular endothelium in fibroblast activation and tissue fibrosis, particularly in scleroderma (systemic

sclerosis) and pachydermoperiostosis (primary hypertrophic osteoarthropathy). Clin Exp Rheumatol. 1992;10(Suppl 7):51–6.

260. Tomasek JJ, Gabbiani G, Hinz B, Chaponnier C, Brown RA. Myofibroblasts and mechano-regulation of connective tissue remodelling. Nat Rev Mol Cell Biol. 2002;3(5):349–63.
261. Lauber K, Bohn E, Kröber SM, Xiao YJ, Blumenthal SG, Lindemann RK, Marini P, Wiedig C, Zobywalski A, Baksh S, Xu Y, Autenrieth IB, Schulze-Osthoff K, Belka C, Stuhler G, Wesselborg S. Apoptotic cells induce migration of phagocytes via caspase-3-mediated release of a lipid attraction signal. Cell. 2003;113(6):717–30.
262. Holmes A, Abraham DJ, Chen Y, Denton C, Shi-wen X, Black CM, Leask A. Constitutive connective tissue growth factor expression in scleroderma fibroblasts is dependent on Sp1. J Biol Chem. 2003;278(43):41728–33.
263. Shi-Wen X, Leask A, Abraham D. Regulation and function of connective tissue growth factor/CCN2 in tissue repair, scarring and fibrosis. Cytokine Growth Factor Rev. 2008;19(2):133–44.
264. Serratì S, Chillà A, Laurenzana A, Margheri F, Giannoni E, Magnelli L, Chiarugi P, Dotor J, Feijoo E, Bazzichi L, Bombardieri S, Kahaleh B, Fibbi G, Del Rosso M. Systemic sclerosis endothelial cells recruit and activate dermal fibroblasts by induction of a connective tissue growth factor (CCN2)/transforming growth factor β-dependent mesenchymal-to-mesenchymal transition. Arthritis Rheum. 2013;65(1):258–69.
265. Mendoza FA, Piera-Velazquez S, Farber JL, Feghali-Bostwick C, Jiménez SA. Endothelial cells expressing endothelial and mesenchymal cell gene products in lung tissue from patients with systemic sclerosis-associated interstitial lung disease. Arthritis Rheumatol. 2016;68(1):210–7.
266. Dees C, Akhmetshina A, Zerr P, Reich N, Palumbo K, Horn A, Jüngel A, Beyer C, Krönke G, Zwerina J, Reiter R, Alenina N, Maroteaux L, Gay S, Schett G, Distler O, Distler JH. Platelet-derived serotonin links vascular disease and tissue fibrosis. J Exp Med. 2011;208(5):961–72.
267. Maurer B, Distler A, Suliman YA, Gay RE, Michel BA, Gay S, Distler JH, Distler O. Vascular endothelial growth factor aggravates fibrosis and vasculopathy in experimental models of systemic sclerosis. Ann Rheum Dis. 2014;73(10):1880–7.
268. Liakouli V, Elies J, El-Sherbiny YM, Scarcia M, Grant G, Abignano G, Derrett-Smith EC, Esteves F, Cipriani P, Emery P, Denton CP, Giacomelli R, Mavria G, Del Galdo F. Scleroderma fibroblasts suppress angiogenesis via TGF-beta/caveolin-1 dependent secretion of pigment epithelium-derived factor. Ann Rheum Dis. 2018;77(3):431–40.
269. Smith GP, Chan ES. Molecular pathogenesis of skin fibrosis: insight from animal models. Curr Rheumatol Rep. 2010;12(1):26–33.
270. Yue X, Yu X, Petersen F, Riemekasten G. Recent advances in mouse models for systemic sclerosis. Autoimmun Rev. 2018;17(12):1225–34.
271. Marangoni RG, Varga J, Tourtellotte WG. Animal models of scleroderma: recent progress. Curr Opin Rheumatol. 2016;28(6):561–70.
272. Sgonc R. The vascular perspective of systemic sclerosis: of chickens, mice and men. Int Arch Allergy Immunol. 1999;120(3):169–76.
273. Cipriani P, Di Benedetto P, Dietrich H, Ruscitti P, Liakouli V, Carubbi F, Pantano I, Berardicurti O, Sgonc R, Giacomelli R. Searching for a good model for systemic sclerosis: the molecular profile and vascular changes occurring in UCD-200 chickens strongly resemble the early phase of human systemic sclerosis. Arch Med Sci. 2016;12(4):828–43.
274. Allipour Birgani S, Mailänder M, Wasle I, Dietrich H, Gruber J, Distler O, Sgonc R. Efficient therapy of ischaemic lesions with VEGF121-fibrin in an animal model of systemic sclerosis. Ann Rheum Dis. 2016;75(7):1399–406.
275. Ruzek MC, Jha S, Ledbetter S, Richards SM, Garman RD. A modified model of graft-versus-host-induced systemic sclerosis (scleroderma) exhibits all major aspects of the human disease. Arthritis Rheum. 2004;50(4):1319–31.
276. Toyama T, Asano Y, Miyagawa T, Nakamura K, Hirabayashi M, Yamashita T, Saigusa R, Miura S, Ichimura Y, Takahashi T, Taniguchi T, Yoshizaki A, Sato S. The impact of transcription factor Fli1 deficiency on the regulation of angiogenesis. Exp Dermatol. 2017;26(10):912–8.
277. Taniguchi T, Asano Y, Akamata K, Noda S, Takahashi T, Ichimura Y, Toyama T, Trojanowska M, Sato S. Fibrosis, vascular activation, and immune abnormalities resembling systemic sclerosis in bleomycin-treated Fli-1-haploinsufficient mice. Arthritis Rheumatol. 2015;67(2):517–26.
278. Asano Y. Double heterozygous mice for Klf5 and Fli1 genes: a new animal model of systemic sclerosis recapitulating its three cardinal pathological features. Med Mol Morphol. 2015;48(3):123–8.
279. Noda S, Asano Y, Nishimura S, Taniguchi T, Fujiu K, Manabe I, Nakamura K, Yamashita T, Saigusa R, Akamata K, Takahashi T, Ichimura Y, Toyama T, Tsuruta D, Trojanowska M, Nagai R, Sato S. Simultaneous downregulation of KLF5 and Fli1 is a key feature underlying systemic sclerosis. Nat Commun. 2014;5:5797.
280. Nakamura K, Taniguchi T, Hirabayashi M, Yamashita T, Saigusa R, Miura S, Takahashi T, Toyama T, Ichimura Y, Yoshizaki A, Trojanowska M, Fujiu K, Nagai R, Sato S, Asano Y. Altered properties of endothelial cells and mesenchymal stem cells underlying the development of scleroderma-like vasculopathy in Klf5(+/−);Fli-1(+/−) mice. Arthritis Rheumatol. 2020;72(12):2136–46.
281. Maurer B, Busch N, Jüngel A, Pileckyte M, Gay RE, Michel BA, Schett G, Gay S, Distler J, Distler O. Transcription factor fos-related antigen-2 induces progressive peripheral vasculopathy in mice closely resembling human systemic sclerosis. Circulation. 2009;120(23):2367–76.
282. Maurer B, Reich N, Juengel A, Kriegsmann J, Gay RE, Schett G, Michel BA, Gay S, Distler JH, Distler O. Fra-2 transgenic mice as a novel model of pulmonary hypertension associated with systemic sclerosis. Ann Rheum Dis. 2012;71(8):1382–7.
283. Venalis P, Kumánovics G, Schulze-Koops H, Distler A, Dees C, Zerr P, Palumbo-Zerr K, Czirják L, Mackevic Z, Lundberg IE, Distler O, Schett G, Distler JH. Cardiomyopathy in murine models of systemic sclerosis. Arthritis Rheumatol. 2015;67(2):508–16.
284. Bernstein AM, Twining SS, Warejcka DJ, Tall E, Masur SK. Urokinase receptor cleavage: a crucial step in fibroblast-to-myofibroblast differentiation. Mol Biol Cell. 2007;18(7):2716–27.
285. Manetti M, Rosa I, Milia AF, Guiducci S, Carmeliet P, Ibba-Manneschi L, Matucci-Cerinic M. Inactivation of urokinase-type plasminogen activator receptor (uPAR) gene induces dermal and pulmonary fibrosis and peripheral microvasculopathy in mice: a new model of experimental scleroderma? Ann Rheum Dis. 2014;73(9):1700–9.
286. Manetti M, Rosa I, Fazi M, Guiducci S, Carmeliet P, Ibba-Manneschi L, Matucci-Cerinic M. Systemic sclerosis-like histopathological features in the myocardium of uPAR-deficient mice. Ann Rheum Dis. 2016;75(2):474–8.
287. Zhang G, Kim H, Cai X, López-Guisa JM, Alpers CE, Liu Y, Carmeliet P, Eddy AA. Urokinase receptor deficiency accelerates renal fibrosis in obstructive nephropathy. J Am Soc Nephrol. 2003;14(5):1254–71.
288. Wermuth PJ, Carney KR, Mendoza FA, Piera-Velazquez S, Jimenez SA. Endothelial cell-specific activation of transforming growth factor-β signaling in mice induces cutaneous, visceral, and microvascular fibrosis. Lab Invest. 2017;97(7):806–18.

Biomarkers in Systemic Sclerosis

17

Francesco Del Galdo, Elizabeth R. Volkmann, and Robert Lafyatis

Introduction

Over the past decades, biomarkers science has progressed from a rarely considered subject of scientific inquiry to a crucial aspect of stratified and personalized medicine. Biomarkers carry the enormous potential to improve the performance of clinical trials as well as the efficiency of clinical management, while simultaneously creating a bridge to understanding disease pathogenesis. Strong correlations between biomarkers and disease activity suggest direct roles in pathogenesis for the biomarker; the stronger the correlation is, the more likely a biomarker is implicated in pathogenesis. Thus, biomarkers provide unique opportunities to understand disease mechanisms. Biomarkers are also particularly valuable in clinical setting where the disease is hard to measure using clinical outcomes, as is the case for virtually all SSc manifestations. However, the most exciting aspect of biomarkers is the interface between clinical and translational medicine. The effect of drug treatment on biomarkers can lead to exciting insights into the roles of drug-targeted pathways in pathogenesis.

Biomarkers already permeate clinical care as commonly used laboratory tests. In the clinical setting, biomarkers are useful in several different contexts. In their most basic application, biomarkers are used in diagnosis of diseases or disease complications. Such laboratory tests are used in countless ways in diagnostics from TSH levels for thyroid disease to CK levels to assess the occurrence of muscle injury and myocardial infarction. However, biomarkers have several other utilities that have been increasingly explored, which are particularly important in clinical trials. They can be used to track the progression or regression of disease, to select patients more likely to show progressive disease, and to predict which patients are most likely to respond to a given treatment. Utilizing biomarkers in such settings is also increasingly entering routine clinical care, paving the way for personalized medicine, in which care and drug therapy can be based on molecular characters of individual patients.

The FDA has laid out categories of biomarkers, and the nomenclature they have established will be used here in referring to different types of biomarkers; see [1] and Figs. 17.1, 17.2, and 17.3.

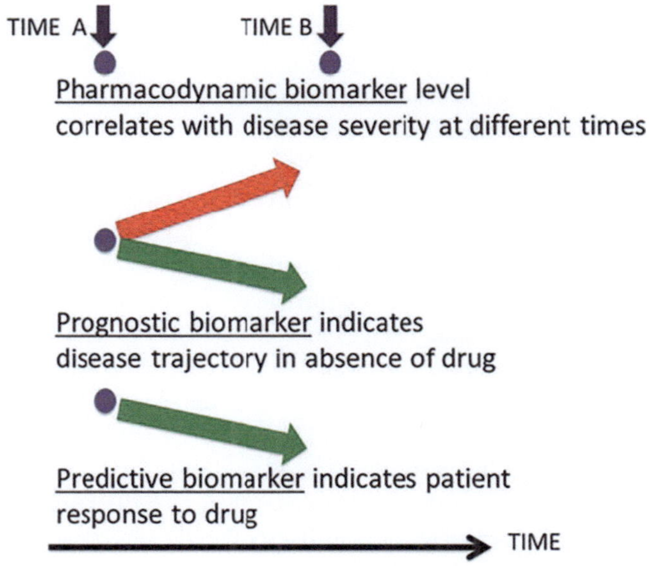

Fig. 17.1 Pharmacodynamic, prognostic, and predictive biomarkers. Pharmacodynamic biomarkers change with disease activity. Prognostic biomarkers indicate the disease trajectory in an untreated state. Predictive biomarkers indicate which patients will respond to a given drug treatment

F. Del Galdo (✉)
Scleroderma Programme, NIHR Biomedical Research Centre and Leeds Institute of Rheumatic and Musculoskeletal Medicine, University of Leeds, Leeds, UK
e-mail: F.DelGaldo@leeds.ac.uk

E. R. Volkmann
Division of Rheumatology, Department of Medicine, David Geffen School of Medicine, University of California, Los Angeles, Los Angeles, CA, USA
e-mail: EVolkmann@mednet.ucla.edu

R. Lafyatis
Division of Rheumatology and Clinical Immunology, Department of Medicine, Scleroderma Center, University of Pittsburgh Medical Center, Pittsburgh, PA, USA
e-mail: lafyiatis@pitt.edu

Y. Allanore et al. (eds.), *Scleroderma*, https://doi.org/10.1007/978-3-031-40658-4_17

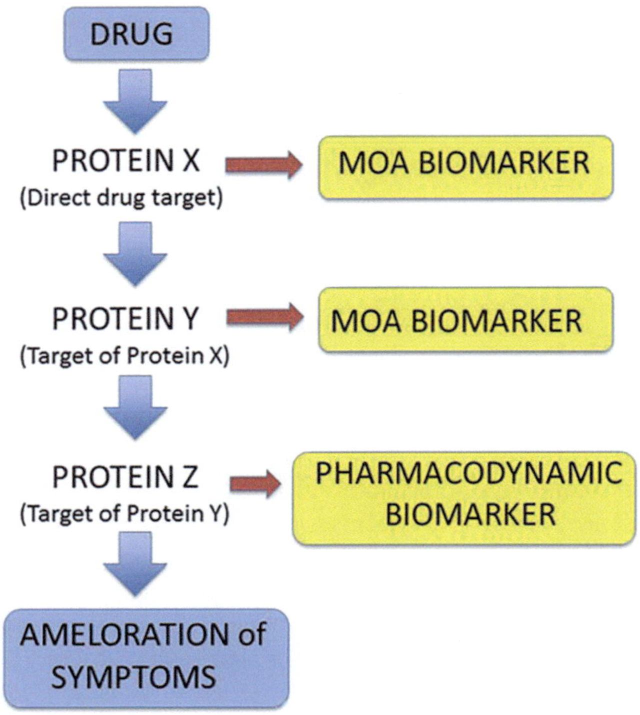

Fig. 17.2 Pharmacodynamic biomarkers. Pharmacodynamic biomarkers can serve to detect a drug's mechanisms of action (*MOA*). Typically, these MOA biomarkers are identified on the basis of known targets of the drug. Pharmacodynamic biomarkers that serve as surrogate outcome measures are typically defined by a high association with the clinical outcome and are tightly associated with the pathogenic biochemical events leading to that outcome

A clinical outcome is typically used to anchor a pharmacodynamic biomarker. For SSc, the most obvious anchors would be the MRSS or, in patients with interstitial lung disease (ILD), the forced vital capacity (FVC). The biomarker should thus change as the clinical outcome changes. If skin disease gets worse, then the biomarker should change proportionately. Pharmacodynamic biomarkers are particularly useful for clinical trials, where they can supplement a clinical outcome. However, pharmacodynamic biomarkers could also be useful for clinicians as a way of following disease severity. Pharmacodynamic biomarkers that meet certain criteria can graduate to become surrogate outcome measures.

Pharmacodynamic biomarkers can also serve to detect the expected mechanism of action of the therapeutic, if known. This is particularly important in early drug development when the proper dose of drug may not be known. These "mechanism of action (MOA)" biomarkers are easiest to identify for drugs with known discrete targets, for example, IL-6 or CRP levels in patients after treatment with anti-IL-6 or B-cell levels in patients treated with anti-CD20. Although these biomarkers seem trivial for approved therapeutics, they are key for assessing target engagement for early drug development. Such MOA should be used in combination with a pharmacodynamic biomarker that is more closely associated with a clinical outcome measure to detect the likely drug effect on the disease (Fig. 17.2).

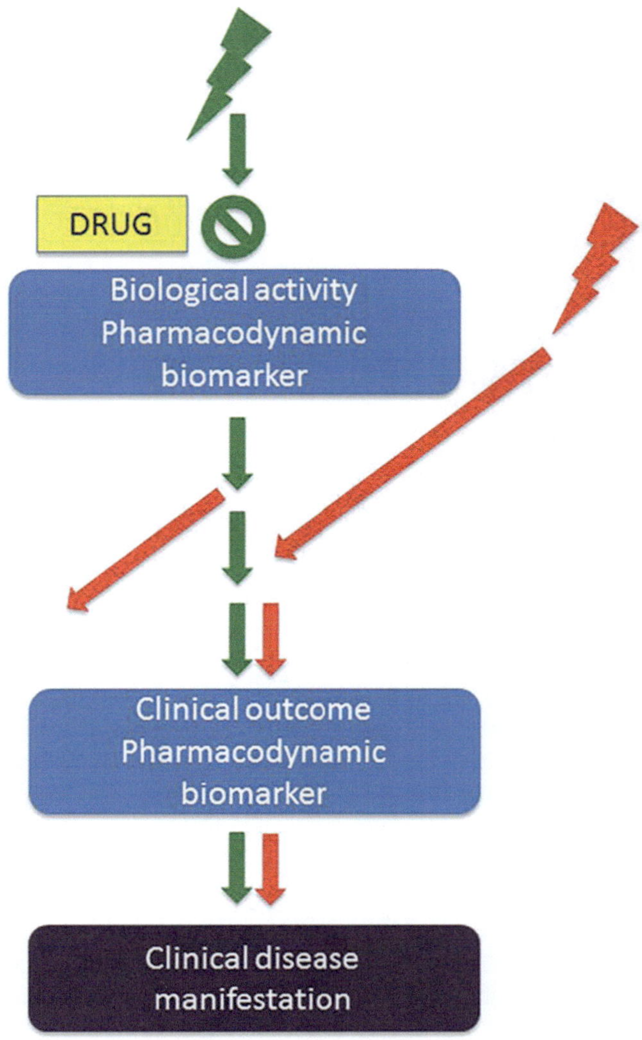

Fig. 17.3 Drug biological activity and clinical outcome pharmacodynamic biomarkers. The *green* lightning bolt and *arrows* indicate a drug that is successfully targeting a key pathogenic pathway. An effect of the drug on the biological activity biomarker indicates that the drug has successfully engaged a known biological target of the drug. The clinical response biomarker indicates that the drug is having an effect on the clinical outcome. The *red* lightning bolt and *arrows* indicate a pathogenic pathway in which the drug is unsuccessful. The drug may still succeed at blocking biological activity, but since this pathway is not involved in the pathogenic process, the clinical outcome biomarker is not affected. Note that it is important that the clinical outcome biomarker reflects biological processes directly in the route of pathogenesis and that it is proximal to the clinical outcome. If not, then a clinical outcome biomarker might respond like a drug biological activity biomarker; i.e., it might improve toward normal with drug treatment, but not reflect an improvement in clinical disease

Biomarkers as Surrogate Outcome Measures

Surrogate outcome measures are pharmacodynamic biomarkers or other nonclinical outcomes that have achieved a status such that they can be used for drug approval, a feature generally given only to clinical outcomes. Clinical outcome measures are defined as a finding that reflects how a patient feels, functions, or survives. Several biomarkers have been found suitable for drug approval, such as LDL cholesterol and HbA1C. Neither of these directly measures patient symptoms, but both are tied to survival. Thus approval of biomarkers as surrogate outcomes must meet several criteria. They must be strongly associated with a relevant clinical outcome, but in addition they must be directly implicated in the pathogenic pathway of the disease.

The FDA has provided a mechanism for approval (referred to as qualification) of biomarkers meeting stringent criteria as surrogate outcome measures, making them approvable outcomes for a disease. However, the FDA expects that pharmacodynamic biomarkers will be most often used to guide drug development rather than as a basis for regulatory approval ([1], Appendix 2, Drug Development Tools). This conservative approach to qualification of biomarkers as surrogate outcomes is due to failures of past biomarkers to accurately reflect clinical outcomes. For example, biomarkers that reflect a drug's mechanism of action may not reflect a clinical response (Fig. 17.3).

Mechanism of Action (MOA) Biomarkers

Although increasingly drugs are designed to block or activate a specific molecular target, this may be far removed from the anticipated effect on the disease. This latter effect is better assessed with a pharmacodynamic biomarker and/or clinical outcome. All intervening steps in drug activation might be assessed by MOA biomarkers. In cases where the action of the drug is proximal to the effect on clinical markers, then pharmacodynamic and MOA biomarkers may be the same.

Prognostic Biomarkers

In contrast to pharmacodynamic biomarkers, which measure disease severity at a point in time, prognostic biomarkers measure where the disease is going. As such, they measure future disease trajectory. Will the skin get worse or better? Will ILD progress or stabilize? A particular challenge in identifying prognostic biomarkers is that they must be evaluated on an untreated patient population or be adjusted for treatment effects. As SSc patients are often treated with medications of unknown efficacy, prognostic biomarkers are particularly difficult to identify in SSc. Prognostic biomarkers in SSc include autoantibodies and genetic studies.

The highly variable clinical course of SSc makes prognostic biomarkers particularly important. In addition, they can be used effectively in clinical trial settings to help stratify patients for entry who are likely to show progressive disease.

Predictive Biomarkers

Predictive biomarkers tell whether a patient will respond to a given drug or other therapy. A prominent example of these is molecular markers used for patients with breast cancer [2]. These biomarkers have been widely embraced by both the FDA and the pharmaceutical industry. They are often identified during early phases of clinical development, where they can subsequently be used in Phase 3 trials to identify patients likely to respond to a given treatment. The identification of serum periostin in asthma as a predictive biomarker for response to anti-IL13 is a notable recent example of this approach [3]. Two recent randomized clinical trials have adopted CRP as biomarker for biological target enrichment in early diffuse SSc. Both the phase 2 and phase 3 trials of tocilizumab in SSc have in fact adopted elevated CRP as inclusion criteria to identify patients with higher probability of responding to the drug. The success of this trial design is witnessed by the recent FDA approval of tocilizumab for the treatment of early diffuse SSc interstitial lung disease (REFS). Incidentally, the analysis of the rate of progression of ILD, as measured by the cumulative proportion of patients with negative change in FVC at 12 months, has also informed the value of elevated CRP as a biomarker of worse clinical outcome in SSc-ILD. This latter notion is a very cogent example of how a biomarker of biological target activation such as CRP for the IL-6 pathway activation has informed, through a targeted therapy trial, the value of this pathway in the pathogenesis and progression of tissue damage in SSc.

Toxicity Biomarkers

Biomarkers of drug toxicity are of considerable importance for drug development, but will not be discussed further here.

Developing Biomarkers for Clinical Applications

Sources of Biomarker Information

Biomarkers can be assessed in many ways, including various measures of physiology such as EKG changes, blood pressure or hemodynamic monitoring, radiographic studies, as well as biochemical measures: protein and lipid mediator levels, mRNA expression, and DNA allelism. The best biomarker for a given application depends on the biology of the disease or disease complication. However, high-throughput technologies, particularly microarray analyses of gene expression and emerging proteomics, appear to be favoring mRNA and proteins.

The relationship between a biomarker and disease pathogenesis is important in defining the best biomarker. If a disease is primarily genetic, then genetic markers would be expected to prove most useful. If driven by immune mediators or lipids, then interleukins or lipid mediators might, respectively, be more informative. Thus, one's bias about SSc pathogenesis might lead one investigator to focus more on genetic biomarkers, while another investigator focuses more on autoantibodies. In many cases, the best biomarker measure will not be known and must be discovered empirically. Practical and innovative approaches based on clinical observations may prove particularly fruitful, such as assessing nailfold vascular changes. However, reproducibility and ease of applying a biomarker in a clinical setting may ultimately decide biomarker utility.

Generally speaking, getting as close as possible to the diseased tissue is likely to be most rewarding. When the diseased tissue is accessible, such as is often the case for tumor biomarkers and skin in SSc, it will typically be most informative. Skin is particularly attractive for analysis because of the ability to biopsy and re-biopsy. Major organs involved in SSc such as lungs and kidneys are much less accessible and so require other approaches.

Diseased Tissues

The advantage of analyzing diseased tissue is self-evident. Repeated sampling is currently only practical for skin. Because lung biopsy is not generally needed for diagnosis, tissue is rarely now available from patients with ILD. This may represent a significant loss for patients, as the biomarker information that could be obtained now from biopsies might have provided biomarkers that could guide therapy. However, studies discussed below have not yet identified a biomarker that provides a strong enough motive for obtaining biopsies to guide clinical care. Thus, most lung tissues have and will be obtained from patients at the time of transplant—of very limited value in terms of identifying clinically useful biomarkers.

Blood Biomarkers

Serum and plasma have been mainstays of biomarker studies. The obvious advantages are that blood circulates through all organs, so it samples disease at multiple sites. The ease of procurement and the ability to repetitively sample are also clear advantages of blood and blood element biomarkers. The main disadvantage of blood biomarkers is that they rely on what is discharged into the blood, which may or may not accurately represent what is happening in the diseased tissue. Although historically assessed mainly for proteins, blood also contains immune cells, microparticles, and other apparent "debris" possibly originating from cell turnover. Thus, recent novel approaches to biomarker discovery include measurements of mRNA, miRNA, and DNA.

Circulating miRNAs

Following the recent demonstration of the presence of nucleic acids in plasma and serum, and the highly productive NIH initiative providing strong support to study the role of extracellular RNA, there have been numerous publications describing the functional effects of extracellular RNA [4]. Most of these publications have focused on microRNAs (miRNAs) and in their potential utility as biomarkers of various disease processes [5]. MicroRNAs are small (~22 nucleotides), evolutionarily conserved noncoding RNA, which play important roles in the regulation of expression of a large number of protein-coding genes at the posttranscriptional level [6, 7]. Although the role of miRNA in malignant disorders has been extensively studied [8, 9], recent interest has been devoted to elucidating their participation in tissue fibrosis and fibrotic diseases [10–14]. Several miRNA have been shown to be involved in SSc tissue fibrosis, displaying either profibrotic or antifibrotic effects [15–21]. Furthermore, relevant targets of these miRNA are translated mRNAs involved in the pathogenesis of SSc-associated tissue fibrosis including collagens, matrix metalloproteinases, Smad signaling proteins, and even TGF-β [10, 12, 14]. One of the most extensively studied miRNA involved in SSc is miRNA-29, which was found to be markedly decreased in SSc dermal fibroblasts and skin [15, 16]. Overexpression of miR-29 in SSc fibroblasts decreased the levels of type I and type III collagens demonstrating a potent antifibrotic effect in vitro. Similar reduction of miR-29 was observed in fibrotic processes affecting other organs, including the heart, kidney, and lung. It was also shown that profibrotic stimuli including TGF-β, PDGF-B, and IL-4 reduced the levels of miR-29 in normal fibroblasts to levels similar to those observed in SSc fibroblasts, and a marked reduction in its levels was observed in the bleomycin model of skin fibrosis [15].

Besides the strong recent interest in the study of the functional role of miRNA in the regulation of important molecular pathways, the potential of circulating miRNAs as biomarkers has been extensively investigated in recent years [4, 5, 22]. MicroRNA were first detected in the blood plasma and serum in 2008 and have subsequently been shown to be present in other body fluids including urine, saliva, tears, and breast milk and thus rendering them quite accessible for initial and serial determinations. Other reasons that render miRNAs excellent biomarker candidates include their remarkable stability in body fluids and the fact that they can be easily measured with high sensitivity since they are amplifiable employing widely available PCR methods. The changes in circulating miRNA levels have been extensively used as diagnostic biomarkers for various types of cancer and numerous other clinical conditions [4, 5, 22]. However, their use as biomarkers for SSc is just becoming recognized.

Radiographic Studies

Radiographic tests provide a particularly rich opportunity for biomarker and biomarker development. CT scan, MRI, ultrasound, and PET scanning have each been applied to SSc with varying success. Newer technologies, particularly in quantitative CT and PET scanning, might yield much more informative biomarkers than those currently available.

Genetic Studies

Genetic associations with disease complications might be prognostic or predictive biomarkers. These biomarkers will be discussed in Chap. 3 on SSc Genetics.

Autoantibodies

Autoantibodies have emerged as very useful markers for subsets of SSc patients. These disease subsets are associated with different disease complications and prognosis.

Titers of anti-RNA pol3 have been reported to correlate with the extent of skin disease. Generally, autoantibody titers are relatively stable, so that their main value as biomarkers is as prognostic biomarkers of the risk of disease complications and perhaps in some cases of disease severity. These are discussed more fully in Chap. 15 on Autoantibodies.

Other Biomarker Sources

Nailfold capillaroscopy, urine biomarkers, and digital plethysmography are examples of other modalities that might be utilized as biomarkers. This chapter will largely focus on biochemical biomarkers.

Biomarkers and High-Throughput Technologies

High-throughput technologies are increasingly driving biomarker studies as they permit nonhypothesis-driven identification of biomolecules. High-throughput mRNA technologies are well established. Microarrays can economically assess expression of all mRNAs in a single sample. However, RNA sequencing is rapidly supplanting microarrays. This technology is able to look at noncoding RNAs and alternatively spliced mRNA that are not typically targeted on microarrays. Depending on the number of transcripts sequenced, RNA-seq can also be more sensitive than microarrays.

High-throughput proteomics has been more challenging particularly when applied to serum or plasma samples. Mass spectrometry is the most robust method for agnostically examining proteins in a biological sample. However, the utility of direct mass spectrometry measurements is restricted by the large dynamic range of serum proteins from abundant proteins such as albumins and immunoglobulins in blood (5–100 g/L) to rare cytokines (<1 fg/L) [23]. These proteins make it very difficult to see rarer (but potentially more informative) protein biomarkers in blood. Technologies aimed at depleting serum proteins before analysis have only partially mitigated this problem. New technologies, such as top-down proteomics [24] and SISCAPA [25], are beginning to show promise in translational research as well. Other technologies, such as Luminex and Somascan, use capture antibodies or aptamers to quantify proteins. These technologies can now permit identification or 200–1000 proteins in a single sample, providing rich high-throughput methodologies for quantification of potential new protein biomarkers in serum and plasma.

Metabolomics provides another source of biomarker identification, though the value of this in biomarker identification is less proven. Single-cell studies connect biomarkers to specific aberrant cellular function in SSc. One challenge for many biomarkers is connecting them to disease pathogenesis, i.e., what cell is expressing or secreting the biomarker gene or protein. The most exciting aspect of single-cell studies is that they have enabled us to capture the molecular state of human disease without manipulation other than tissue digestion. Even this latter step is now being overcome with the advent of increasingly refined spatial transcriptomics. In this rapidly emerging field, the application to biomarkers and clinical care has only begun.

The first exciting and still enduring advance in single-cell analyses came through the large-scale capture of single-cell transcriptomes using droplet-based technology. The first step in single-cell RNA sequencing (scRNA-seq) is carried out on single cells captured in droplets "reaction chambers," in which the primers for reverse transcription contain nucleic acid sequence identifier "bar codes." Thus, a cell-specific bar code is added to each mRNA transcript. After cDNA library preparation and sequencing, the bar code identifies the cell source for each mRNA, providing information on the transcriptome of each cell. Typically, 2000–4000 cells are analyzed, giving a rich cross section of the cells within a tissue. This technology has been applied to skin from SSc patients showing that specific fibroblast populations express the biomarker genes, such as THBS1 and COMP, previously shown to correlate with the MRSS. Applied to SSc-ILD lung explants scRNA-seq has shown that biomarkers CCL18/PARC and SPP1/osteopontin are upregulated on a specific subpopulation of macrophages, while POSTN/periostin is expressed mainly by myofibroblasts. Such ongoing analyses and insights promise to solidify our understandings of the link between biomarkers and pathogenic disease mechanisms.

Other more recent single-cell technologies are providing insights into proteins: cellular indexing of transcriptomes and epitopes by sequencing (CITE-seq) and changes in chromatin structure—single-cell sequencing assay for transposase-accessible chromatin (scATAC-seq) at single-cell resolution. As for scRNA-seq, the dramatic impact on understanding disease is related to the ability for these technologies to examine cell molecular biology directly from tissue (or blood). CITE-seq extends scRNA-seq using nucleic acid and bar-coded antibodies to identify surface proteins. It thus can provide similar information to flow cytometry but on hundreds of proteins and simultaneous information on transcriptomes from the same cells. The unprecedented molecular characterization that can be applied equally to tissues or blood promises future biomarker discovery. ScATAC-seq examines open chromatin in single cells. This exciting technology, while informative about alterations driving differentiation of pathogenic cells, may have less immediate relevance for biomarker discovery.

Spatial transcriptomics is the latest technology that is now rapidly entering translational science and may soon impact our approach to disease biomarkers. This technology essentially applies scRNA-seq to tissue sections. It could thus be applied to archival tissues, as well as patient skin biopsies in clinical care or clinical trial settings. The exhaustive molecular phenotypes provided by each of these technologies will have to be balanced by both cost and analytical capabilities. The overload of data will not necessarily translate into better clinical care until we understand more completely how to extract the useful and actionable information into quantifiable measures of disease.

Biomarker Performance: Correlations, Models, and ROC Curves

Biomarker utility is closely tied to how robustly they associate with the outcome they are modeling. Weak associations may tie the gene or protein marker to disease pathogenesis, but are unlikely to have much clinical utility. In some cases biomarkers weakly associated with a clinical outcome might be combined to provide more robust biomarkers. Developing biomarker models and evaluating biomarker performance depends on the type of biomarkers and, in particular, whether it is modeling a discrete or continuous variable.

Continuous variables are typically assessed using correlations or linear regression. Does the biomarker correlate with the MRSS or the FVC or other clinical measure? Multiple linear regression can be used to assess the value of using several analytes in a model. Methodologies for selecting analytes for models that include multiple analytes, such as forward selection and backward elimination and stepwise regression, have grown more complex [26]. More sophisticated statistical approaches are required to examine longitudinal changes in biomarkers and how these relate to longitudinal changes in clinical outcomes. General estimating equation or mixed models permit such analyses and also allow multiple analytes to be included in models.

Discrete variables include the presence or absence of disease or complication, i.e., diagnostic biomarkers. Does the patient have diffuse or limited SSc? Does the patient have ILD or PAH? Prognostic and predictive biomarkers can also be modeled as discrete variables. Is the patient going to show progressive or stable/regressive lung disease? Is the patient going to respond (or not respond) to a medication? Models of discreet variables can be developed using logistic regression and multiple logistic regression. Sensitivity and specificity of discrete variables can be assessed using receiver-operator characteristic (ROC) curves, plotting the sensitivity on the y-axis and 1-specificity on the x-axis. The area under the curve (AUC) of a ROC provides a global measure of performance and can be used for comparing biomarker performance, with AUC of 0.90–1 considered excellent, 0.80–0.90 considered good, 0.7–0.8 considered fair, 0.6–0.7 considered poor, and 0.5–0.06 considered without value. Various methods can be applied to choose the best threshold level of the biomarker to maximize sensitivity and specificity [27].

Other statistical methodologies can be applied to prognostic or predictive biomarkers, patients can be divided into various trajectories and biomarkers used to predict which trajectory is most likely. Regardless of the model developed, validation using an independent dataset is critical. Models developed using a "discovery" dataset will almost always be less robust in a "validation" dataset. The more variables added to models and the less strong the independent associations, the more likely the model will not be robust.

Biomarkers of Disease Target Organs in SSc

Skin

Because of its easy accessibility and uniform involvement in patients with dcSSc, several groups have studied skin biomarkers. As the only tissue that can be easily biopsied and re-biopsied, skin biomarkers are particularly valuable for monitoring therapy as pharmacodynamic biomarkers.

Generally biomarkers of skin disease have been examined in patients with dcSSc. Skin can also be used for assessing whether a drug is effectively engaging its target by examining expression of known drug targets. mRNA expression in skin has also been examined for biomarkers predictive of clinical responses and has been used to develop a classifier of skin disease. A gene classifier based on broad changes in gene expression has been developed that permits the division of patients into subsets of disease.

Pharmacodynamic Biomarkers of Skin

mRNA Biomarkers

Skin gene expression has provided the most robust pharmacodynamic biomarker of skin disease. Although skin shows many changes in gene expression, only a subset of these genes correlates with the MRSS. Several years ago, a pharmacodynamic biomarker of skin disease was described [28]. This biomarker was composed of a combination of genes: two genes known to be regulated by TGF-β (THBS1 and COMP) and two other genes known to be regulated by interferons (SIGLEC1 and IFI44). These genes were combined into a "four-gene biomarker" using multiple linear regression. This biomarker correlated highly with the MRSS in a cross-sectional study. However, utility of a pharmacodynamic biomarker requires movement of the biomarker over time with disease severity, in this case assessed by MRSS. Only five patients were examined longitudinally using the four-gene biomarker.

More recently, Rice et al. systematically examined the best genes to use as pharmacodynamic biomarkers by examining microarray data [29]. The key step in identifying a more robust pharmacodynamic biomarker was focusing on the correlation between the longitudinal change in gene expression with the longitudinal change in MRSS. Using a general estimating equation, two genes (THBS1 and MS4A4A) were found in combination to most closely change with change in MRSS. This "2GSSc skin biomarker" has been applied to samples from two open-label clinical trials. The biomarker changed dramatically in patients treated with anti-TGF-β, fresolimumab, whereas it did not change in patients treated with the c-abl inhibitor, nilotinib, providing valuable objective data for clinical efficacy of fresolimumab [30]. These studies show the promise of robust pharmacodynamic biomarkers, as they can provide an objective signal in early-phase clinical trials.

In 2008, Milano et al. described the first molecular classification of SSc, suggesting 4 intrinsic signatures of biomarker genes within patients with SSc [31]. Interestingly, this signature has been used retrospectively to assess whether treatment with specific drugs may have a different effect in patients with distinct molecular signatures. Hinchcliff et al. have shown that treatment with the immune suppressive drug mycophenolate was more effective in patients with an 'inflammatory" skin signature, suggesting a potential use of this approach to stratify for best treatment [32]. Consistently with these data, patients with fibroproliferative signature had instead a better response to antifibrotic drug imatinib mesylate [33].

Complementary to this approach, Clark et al. have recently shown that patients with different autoantibody profiles have specific skin transcriptome (and proteomic) signatures, further suggesting the importance of skin transcriptome as potential biomarker window in scleroderma [34].

Serum and Plasma Biomarkers

Many serum and plasma biomarkers have been identified for dSSc skin disease. Some of these proteins appear to be markers of fibrosis and/or are regulated by TGF-β. Serum cartilage oligomeric protein 1 (COMP) is increased in sera from SSc patients and correlates moderately well with the MRSS ($r = 0.57$) [35]. In one report, serum COMP levels changed longitudinally with a change in the MRSS, indicating possible utility of COMP as a pharmacodynamic biomarker. Most other studies of dSSc skin biomarkers are cross-sectional. Plasma levels of osteopontin correlate, but only weakly, with the MRSS ($r = 0.3$; $P = 0.05$) [36]. Two other TGF-β-regulated proteins, thrombospondin-1 (TSP-1) and matrix metalloproteinase 9 (MMP9), are increased in SSc sera [37]. Serum MMP-9 concentrations correlate relatively well with the MRSS ($r = 0.425$) [38]. Carboxy-terminal telopeptide of type I collagen (PICP) is elevated in patients with dSSc [39], and one study correlated highly with the skin score, $r = 0.646$ [40]. In contrast, aminoterminal procollagen I (P1NP) did not correlate with the skin score in this study [40]. Aminoterminal III procollagen (PIIINP) levels are also higher in dcSSc patients and in one study were prognostic of poor survival [36, 41]. However, in the CAT-192 study, where collagen propeptides were used as biomarkers, although both PINP and PIIINP levels were elevated in dSSc patients, only PINP levels showed statistically significant changes that correlated with the MRSS ($r = 0.37$) [42]. Tissue inhibitor of metalloproteinases-1 (TIMP-1) is also higher in dSSc than lSSc [43]. Lysyl oxidase (LOX) levels were shown to trend toward a weak correlation with the MRSS in a small dSSc group of patients ($r = 0.374$). Periostin levels were found in one study to correlate highly with the MRSS in SSc patients; however, most of the patients had lSSc ($r = 0.79$) [44].

The relationship between inflammation and fibrosis is strongly supported by the co-upregulation of profibrotic and proinflammatory biomarkers. Sato showed that IL-6 and IL-10 correlate highly with the MRSS in SSc ($r = 0.625$, and

$r = 0.663$, respectively) [45]. SSc patients express higher levels of IL-1RA and IL-13 CCL2, CCL3, CCL4, and CXCL8, but no clear associations were seen with the MRSS or other clinical parameters [46]. CCL2 was shown to correlate with MRSS in one study but most of the patients in this study had lSSc [47].

Interestingly, a composite biomarker including the concentration of PIIINP, TIMP1, and hyaluronic acid fragments (HA) has been shown to correlate in two very large cross-sectional cohorts including more than 500 patients with both mRSS and FVC, further confirming the importance of these biomarkers in the fibrogenesis process [48, 49].

Pentraxin 3, a protein closely related to C-reactive protein, correlates weakly with the MRSS ($r = 0.34$) [50]. sCD30, a member of the TNF receptor family (TNFR8), is an inflammatory marker elevated in many diseases. sCD30 levels have been shown to correlate moderately with the MRSS ($r = 0.53$) [51]. Elevated sCD30 and IL-6, particularly in patients with dSSc, were confirmed by Scala [52]. Markers of both B-cell activation and B-cell activating factor (BAFF), and T-cell activation and soluble cytotoxic lymphocyte antigen 4 (CTLA-4) also correlate with the MRSS ($r = 0.41$ and $r = 0.37$, respectively) [53, 54].

Several biomarkers that may reflect vascular injury are elevated in SSc patients. A vascular marker, L-selectin, correlates negatively with the MRSS [55]. Endostatin is elevated in SSc compared to controls and was higher in patients with more diffuse skin disease [56, 57], though not shown to correlate directly with the MRSS longitudinally. Endothelin-1 and von Willebrand factor are also elevated in patients with SSc [58]. Adiponectin, an adipokine released by fat, correlates inversely with the MRSS [59].

The large number of serum biomarkers for skin disease in dSSc patients suggests that combining measures, particularly measures that are capturing different aspects of pathogenesis, might provide a successful approach for finding a serum biomarker of skin disease robust enough for utilization as a surrogate outcome measure in clinical trials.

Circulating miRNA Biomarkers

Several recent studies have already demonstrated that the levels of selected miRNAs were altered in the serum of SSc patients [60–63]. One of the most extensive studies examined 95 miRNA that were predicted by in silico analyses to target SSc-related genes including IL-4, TGF-β, CTGF, PDGF-B, PDGF receptor (PDGFR) α/β, and COL1A2. The expression of these miRNA was measured by quantitative PCR in sera of SSc patients and healthy controls [62]. The results showed that 19 miRNAs were significantly downregulated in the serum of SSc patients as compared with healthy controls. Among them, miR-30b and the let-7 and miR-302 families of miRNAs were uniformly reduced in SSc patients. Other miRNA that were also significantly decreased in SSc patients included miR-19a, miR-26a, miR-106b, miR-181a, miR-181b, miR-191, miR-203, miR-376a, miR-409-3p, miR-410, miR-484, and miR-549. Consistent with previous reports, the levels of miR-29a and miR-142-3p tended to be higher in SSc patients. Of substantial interest were the results of comparison of miRNA levels in the serum of patients with limited (lcSSc) and diffuse (dcSSc) subsets of SSc patients. These showed that among the 19 miRNAs that were significantly lower in the serum of SSc patients, miR30b was decreased more profoundly in dcSSc than in lcSSc and its levels were inversely correlated with the modified Rodnan skin score. However, although the levels of miR30b in lcSSc patients are less decreased than in the sera of dcSSc patients, they were still significantly lower than in healthy controls.

Other miRNA that have been studied as potential SSc biomarkers include miR-142-3p that was shown to be elevated in serum from SSc patients compared to patients with systemic lupus erythematosus and were also significantly different compared to the levels in serum from normal individuals and from patients with SSc-spectrum disorder [60]. The levels of miR-150 were found to be decreased in the serum of SSc patients compared to healthy controls and lower levels correlated with more severe clinical manifestations. Furthermore, patients with lower miR-150 levels had a higher ratio of dcSSc to lcSSc, a higher modified Rodnan skin score, and higher incidence of Scl-70 antibodies when compared with patients with normal serum miR-150 levels [19]. A similar correlation was observed for miR-196a, showing that patients with lower serum miR-196a levels had significantly higher ratio of dcSSc to lcSSc and higher extent and severity of skin involvement and showed higher prevalence of pitting scars [18]. Other studies demonstrated that the serum levels of miR-30b [62] and let-7a [21] were markedly decreased in SSc patients compared with healthy controls and levels of both miRNAs were more profoundly decreased in patients with dcSSc than in patients with lcSSc, and both were inversely correlated with the modified Rodnan skin score [60, 62]. In contrast, other studies showed that serum levels of miR-92a [61] and miR-142-3p [60] were markedly higher in SSc patients when compared to healthy controls or to systemic lupus erythematosus, dermatomyositis, and SSc-spectrum disorder patients.

Another recent study analyzed differences in extracellular miRNA in the plasma of a Swedish cohort of 95 SSc patients and identified four miRNA (miRNA-223, miR-181b, miRNA-342-3p, and miRNA-184) that differed between the lcSSc and dcSSc subsets [63]. Also, these authors found that the levels of 10 miRNA displayed statistically significant differences between different autoantibody subgroups and that miRNA-233 correlated with the presence of anticentromere antibodies. Thus, the authors suggested that miRNA played a role in SSc pathogenesis and clinical manifestations because specific miRNAs were found in significant association with distinct SSc autoantibody profiles and clinical SSc subsets.

Although the studies that examined circulating miRNA in SSc are relatively few and despite problems with the specificity and reproducibility [22], the studies published clearly indicate that the assessment of microRNA in the serum of SSc patients may provide valuable and reliable biomarkers for SSc diagnosis and for assessment of its clinical subsets, extent of organ involvement, and clinical course and potential outcomes.

Prognostic and Predictive Biomarkers of SSc Skin Disease

Prognostic mRNA biomarkers of SSc skin disease have generally been harder to identify. This may be biological, related to the variable and changing progression of the disease, or it may represent difficulty in assembling datasets from untreated patients. However, levels of one prognostic biomarker, skin CD14 mRNA levels, are prognostic for progressive disease in SSc patients [64]. As more skin RNA datasets become available from controlled trials, we might anticipate that other prognostic biomarkers will be identified.

Several predictive biomarkers have been identified for SSc skin disease. However, none of these have been identified for proven therapeutics, which arguably have not been found for SSc skin disease. In a study of anti-TGFβ, THBS1 was shown to predict patients more likely to respond to the study medication [30].

Biomarkers for SSc-ILD

Genetic and Epigenetic Factors

Several studies have identified associations between specific genetic variants (e.g., *HLA-DRB1*3*, *CTGF rs6918698*) and risk of ILD in patients with SSc [65]. However, the majority of these studies are small and lack validation cohorts. Few studies have evaluated the relationship between genetic variants and progression of ILD. A common gain-of-function variant rs3570595016 in the promoter of *MUC5B* has been associated with ILD risk in patients with rheumatoid arthritis (RA) [66], but studies in SSc have failed to demonstrate an association between the *MUC5B* variant and ILD presence [67–69] and ILD progression [70].

Epigenetic factors likely play a role in the pathogenesis of SSc-ILD as genome-wide studies have reported underexpression of methylation-regulated genes (*F2R*, *FYN*, *APG1*, *PRKCH*) in peripheral blood mononuclear cells in SSc patients with ILD compared with SSc patients without ILD [71]. Moreover, microRNA (miRNA) gene expression is altered in both the lung tissue and peripheral blood mononuclear cells in patients with SSc-ILD [72]. Because miRNA can be reliably measured in the blood, they represent important candidate biomarkers for this disease state.

Autoantibodies

The presence of antitopoisomerase I antibodies, or anti-scl-70, is associated with a progressive SSc-ILD phenotype, while the presence of the anticentromere antibody is associated with a stable SSc-ILD phenotype [73]. These associations are discussed further in the autoantibody chapter.

Serum/Plasma

A number of studies have now investigated the relationship between serum/plasma proteins and SSc-ILD progression, including interleukin (IL)-6 [74], C-reactive protein (CRP) [75], CCL-18 [76, 77], CXCL4 [78], and Krebs von den Lungen-6 (KL-6) [79–81]. Among these candidate biomarkers, both KL-6 and CCL-18 have emerged as the leading predictors of SSc-ILD progression across multiple cohorts [76, 77] 79–81]. In contrast to general inflammatory markers (e.g., CRP, IL-6), these two pneumoproteins are specifically associated with parenchymal lung injury [82] and thus may be less susceptible to the effects of extrapulmonary processes. Observational studies have demonstrated that high KL-6 [79, 80, 83] and high CCl-18 [76, 77, 84, 85] individually predict worse outcomes in patients with SSc-ILD. A recent study of a SSc-ILD clinical trial cohort (Scleroderma Lung Study II comparing cyclophosphamide versus mycophenolate) demonstrated that patients with high KL-6 and CCL-18 at baseline experienced increased ILD progression despite treatment with immunosuppression [81]. Conceivably, these biomarkers may play a role in not only predicting ILD progression, but also in identifying patients with treatment-resistant phenotypes. For example, measurement of serum CCL18 helped to differentiate the effects of tocilizumab versus placebo on FVC% predicted in early SSc-ILD patients [86].

Additional biomarkers under clinical investigation include mediators of matrix remodeling, including the matrix metallopeptidases (MMP). Prior studies have demonstrated increased genetic expression of MMP-7 [87] and increased levels of MMP-7 [88] in the peripheral blood in patients with SSc-ILD. Moreover, higher peripheral blood levels of both MMP-7 and MMP-12 were observed in SSc patients with extensive ILD compared with limited ILD [88]. Collectively, these findings reaffirm the importance of matrix remodeling in SSc-ILD pathogenesis and future studies are needed to determine whether analysis of specific MMPs helps to predict response to specific ILD therapies (i.e., immunosuppressive versus antifibrotic).

The chemokines, MCP-1 (CCL-2) and MCP-3 (CCL-7), have been implicated as biomarkers of SSc-ILD; both are considered proinflammatory and contribute to tissue fibrosis by activating the synthesis of extracellular matrix proteins in fibroblasts. Observational studies have demonstrated that levels of peripheral MCP-1 are higher in SSc patients with ILD [52, 89] and that increased MCP-1 is associated with accelerated ILD progression [90]. While MCP-3 is closely related to MCP-1, MCP-3 has chemotactic effects not only for monocytes, but also for dendritic cells and granulocytes [91]. Serum levels of MCP-3 were elevated in SSc patients with ILD and associated with more severe restriction on pulmonary function testing [92]. The chemokine (C-X-C motif ligand 4, aka CXCL4) has also been found to correlate with the presence of ILD (van Bon 2014). Moreover, studies have demonstrated that increased decline in CXCL4 levels in response to immunosuppression predicted greater improvement in lung function over time [93]. Understanding the dynamic nature of biomarkers in relation to treatment will undoubtedly uncover new therapeutic targets and help to advance precision medicine in this field.

Bronchoalveolar Lavage Biomarkers of ILD

While bronchoalveolar lavage (BAL) fluid provides a source for biomarkers that may more closely approximate intrinsic pulmonary pathology, BAL is not currently routinely performed in patients with SSc-ILD. Early studies demonstrated that SSc-ILD patients with evidence of active alveolitis in BAL fluid had more extensive ILD on HRCT of the chest [94, 95]. For example, among patients enrolled in the Scleroderma Lung Study I (cyclophosphamide versus placebo for SSc-ILD) [96], increased polymorphonuclear leukocytes and/or eosinophils in BAL fluid was associated with more extensive quantitative ground glass opacity and fibrosis scores based on semiquantitative analysis of radiographic ILD [95]. These findings are consistent with those of a more recent single-center study that demonstrated that patients with a higher eosinophil count in BAL fluid had increased extent of ground glass opacity and fibrosis by semiquantitative assessment [97]. Interestingly, this study also found that the concentration of certain BAL proteins correlated with the extent of GGO (e.g., KL-6), while other BAL proteins correlated with the extent of fibrosis (e.g., CXCL8) [97]. The latter observation suggests that unique biological pathways may mediate the development of pulmonary interstitial inflammation and fibrosis in SSc-ILD.

Radiographic Studies of SSc-ILD

Objectively quantifying the radiographic extent of ILD represents a direct assessment of parenchymal lung disease burden in SSc. Increased radiographic extent of ILD at baseline predicts an increased risk of mortality in SSc [98], as well as responsiveness to immunosuppressive therapy [99, 100]. In addition, clinical trials have demonstrated that radiographic ILD endpoints are sensitive to change in SSc-ILD patients undergoing treatment [101–104]. A recent study demonstrated that short-term changes in the quantitative radiographic extent of SSc-ILD predicted long-term mortality in two clinical trial cohorts [105].

Novel molecular imaging techniques are under investigation in SSc. For example, Bergmann and colleagues [106] foundation increased uptake of a gallium-labeled selective inhibitor of fibroblast activation protein (Ga-FAPI-04 PET/CT) associated with more extensive ILD in a small number of patients in SSc. Molecular imaging offers the promise of distinguishing areas of active fibrotic remodeling from those with active inflammation and could potentially be used in the future to guide treatment decisions.

Clinical and Biochemical Biomarkers of Pulmonary Arterial Hypertension

Many studies have examined clinical and serum/plasma biomarkers of idiopathic and SSc-associated pulmonary arterial hypertension (iPAH and SSc-PAH) (reviewed in [107]). Pulmonary arterial hypertension is defined by hemodynamic pressures measured on right heart catheterization (RHC): a mean pulmonary arterial pressure (PAP) of $\geq$25 mmHg, a pulmonary vascular resistance of >3, and Wood units and pulmonary capillary wedge pressure of $\leq$15 [108]. Early diagnosis in SSc-PAH may lead to better outcomes [109], so diagnostic biomarkers indicating the need for right heart catheterization (RHC) might improve survival.

Echocardiographic assessment of systolic PAP (sPAP) by assessing tricuspid velocity has been the most robust clinical biomarker to date, showing a good correlation with PAH on RHC (90% sensitivity and specificity of 75%) [110]. Numerous studies have shown the value, but also the limitations, of echocardiography (see [111]). Subsequent studies have shown enhanced detection of PAH using echocardiographic sPAP in combination with other measures. Echocardiographic sPAP in combination with the DLCO and proNT-BNP more accurately predicts the development of SSc-PAH [112]. Echocardiographic sPAP is a prominent component of recent algorithms for PAH diagnosis [113, 114]. The latter of these, the DETECT study, devises a complex, two-step algorithm based on a large prospective study designed to determine the best clinical and biochemical biomarkers for SSc-PAH [114]. DLCO %predicted/FVC %predicted, current/past telangiectasia, anticentromere antibody, NTpro-BNP, serum urate, and right axis deviation on electrocardiogram define patients needing echocardiography, and right atrial area and tricuspid velocity echocardiographic features define which patients should have RHC. Another echocardiographic measure, tricuspid annular plane systolic excursion (TAPSE), a measure that reflects right ventricular function, is prognostic for survival in SSc-PAH in one study [115].

Many biochemical measures have been shown to be diagnostic of PAH or prognostic of survival in patients with PAH. However, often studies of biochemical biomarkers of PAH do not include SSc-PAH patients or group SSc with other connective tissue disease (CTD) patients. SSc-PAH compared to iPAH is associated with increased mortality and shows higher BNP levels and lower DLCO %predicted [116]. Thus, it is important that biomarkers of iPAH are evaluated discretely also in SSc-PAH patients. PAH biomarkers in SSc patients are also potentially confounded by co-morbid disease complications, including ILD and cardiac fibrosis. In SSc-ILD patients, PAH might also be secondary to hypoxia from ILD. However, this distinction has been rarely assessed in SSc-PAH biomarkers. Even biomarkers of pure SSc-PAH might reflect different pathogenic processes. Biomarkers might reflect the effect of PAH on vascular remodeling, affecting endothelial or vascular smooth muscle cells, or they might measure inflammation, right heart failure, or hypoxia.

By far the most studied and only clinically available PAH biomarkers are markers of heart strain/failure: brain natriuretic peptide (BNP) and N-terminal fragment of pro-brain natriuretic peptide (NT-proBNP). These appear to have similar diagnostic accuracy [117]. In one study, NT-proBNP had a diagnostic specificity for SSc-PAH of 95.1% and a sensitivity of 55.9% [118]. This is consistent with other PAH studies, indicating that BNP and NT-proBNP are generally specific for PH but lack sensitivity. NT-proBNP also correlates with mPAP, PVR, and survival. In patients with iPAH, BNP and NT-proBNP are also both predictive of survival.

Inflammatory biomarkers have also shown some utility in PAH. Elevated CRP is associated with mortality, and in thromboembolic disease decreases with treatment, suggesting it may act as both a prognostic and PD biomarker [119]. More recently, human pentraxin 3 was shown to be another inflammatory biomarker for PAH and CTD-PAH [120]. Pentraxin 3 was much more robust than CRP for distinguishing CTD-PAH from CTD patients ($ROC_{AUC} = 0.866$ compared to CRP $ROC_{AUC} = 0.516$ and BNP $ROC_{AUC} = 0.670$).

However, only 59% of the patients in the CTD and control groups had SSc. Using a proteomic approach, another study confirmed and extended inflammatory markers, showing that CRP, IL1, IL8, and TNFa are all increased in SSc-PAH compared to SSc-PAH [121]. This study included only patients with lSSc and most patients did not have ILD; thus, it appears these markers are truly associated with SSc-PAH and no other disease manifestations. Urinary 15-F_{2t}-isoprostane, a marker of lipid peroxidation and oxidative stress, is also highly prognostic of survival in PAH. In this study 15-F_{2t}-isoprostane was more highly prognostic of survival than NT-proBNP or big ET-1 [122].

Several markers of vascular disease are elevated in SSc-PAH. In an early study, endothelin-1 (ET-1) levels were elevated in SSc-PAH but did not correlate with survival or PAP [123]. However, subsequent studies have shown that ET-1 levels correlate with PAP in PAH patients [124, 125] and big ET-1 levels are shown to correlate with survival in PAH [126]. Endoglin levels are elevated in PAH and correlate with survival [127]. A proteomic approach showed that intercellular adhesion molecule-1 (ICAM-1), vascular cell adhesion molecular-1 VCAM, von Willebrand factor (vWF), and vascular endothelial cell growth factor (VEGF) are all elevated in lSSc-PAH patients compared to lSSc patients [121].

Several other biomarkers have been described for PAH. Osteopontin levels correlate with NT-BNP and survival in patients with iPAH [128]; osteopontin levels are also elevated in patients with SSc-ILD or SSc-PAH [129]. Provirus integration site for Moloney murine leukemia virus (Pim-1) has also been shown to be associated with iPAH, CTD-PAH, and SSc-PAH [130]. Pim-1 is also highly prognostic of survival. The SSc patients in this, as most PAH biomarker studies, were not phenotyped as to the presence of ILD and for the main analysis were grouped with other CTD patients. In contrast to what is seen in the skin, adiponectin levels are elevated in patients with PAH [131].

Digital Ischemia, Digital Ulcers

Several vascular biomarkers correlate with digital ulcers (DU) in SSc [132]. sICAM-1 is elevated in SSc patients with DUs, but did not correlate with the MRSS [133]. Increased endoglin is associated with DUs and decreased DLCO [134]. Elevated endothelin-1 is associated with DUs as well as PAH [135, 136]. sCD36 correlates with PAH on echocardiogram and with DLCO and is elevated in lSSc [137], but not in dSSc patients. PDGF-BB and PECAM1 were both found to be elevated in SSc patients with DU [138]. More recently, PIGF and sVCAM have been shown to be elevated in patients with DUs, and PIGF levels strongly prognostic of future DUs [139].

In other studies, IL-33 levels were found to correlate with DU [140] and microangiopathic changes [141]. IL-33 induces fibrosis dependent on the type 2 cytokines, IL-13 [142], suggesting a potential important role in SSc pathogenesis.

Biomarkers of Overall Disease in SSc

Although everyone agrees that the most exciting therapeutic advance would be discovery of a drug that treats overall disease of SSc patients, biomarker discovery in this area has been limited. The only widely accepted current methodology for assessing overall clinical disease activity is the European Scleroderma Study Group activity index (ESSGAI) [143, 144]. The anchor for this index was expert assessment of disease activity. An ongoing study based on validation of longitudinal data, the combined response index for systemic sclerosis (CRISS), may prove a more robust measure of overall disease [145]. Microhemorrhages and giant capillaries on capillaroscopy correlate with the ESSGAI [146].

Angiopoietin-2 levels correlate with ESSGAI ($r = 0.403$) [147], as do levels of GDF-15 [148] ($r = 0.338$). GDF-15 levels were also shown to be associated with the change in ESSGAI over time [148]. Borrowing from biomarkers discovered for liver fibrosis, the enhanced liver fibrosis score was shown to correlate with the ESSGAI [48] as well as the MRSS. Although highly statistically significant, these correlations are relatively low ($r = 0.28$–0.23, respectively). Leptin levels were found in a small study to be lower in active patients [149]. Elevated CRP is associated with ESSGAI, skin disease, and decreased FVC, though these correlations are all quite low [150]. CRP was also found to be weakly prognostic for long-term survival. Elevated COMP levels are associated with increased mortality [151]. Both clinical and biomarker approaches are underway to better classify SSc patients into subsets. Limited compared to diffuse skin disease has provided very useful information about prognosis of many disease complications. Using skin gene expression, Dr. Whitfield's group has developed methodologies for distinguishing patients with different patterns of skin gene expression that appear to reflect activation of different pathogenic pathways. This is described more completely elsewhere in this text.

Conclusion

Many biomarkers of SSc and its complications have already been identified. However, very few of these have been validated in multiple datasets and/or applied in a clinical setting. The burgeoning number of new therapeutics that might be tried for SSc patients makes the application of biomarkers to clinical trials increasingly important. Biomarkers help bridge our understanding of animal models to human disease. Pathways leading to fibrosis in mice may not be similar to those leading to fibrosis in human SSc. Biomarkers can indicate the vascular, fibrotic, and immunologic pathways most likely to be contributing to SSc pathogenesis and thus help in selecting drugs most likely to show efficacy. Biomarkers can also help in testing the effect of targeted therapeutics, as well as in patient selection. They will serve increasing roles in all aspects of medicine as we reach for a future of targeted therapeutics and precision medicine.

References

1. Qualification process for drug development tools. Food and drug administration-draft document. 2010. www.fdagov/downloads/Drugs//Guidances/UCM230597pdf.
2. Stopeck AT, Brown-Glaberman U, Wong HY, Park BH, Barnato SE, Gradishar WJ, et al. The role of targeted therapy and biomarkers in breast cancer treatment. Clin Exp Metastasis. 2012;29(7):807–19.
3. Corren J, Lemanske RF, Hanania NA, Korenblat PE, Parsey MV, Arron JR, et al. Lebrikizumab treatment in adults with asthma. N Engl J Med. 2011;365(12):1088–98.
4. Etheridge A, Gomes CP, Pereira RW, Galas D, Wang K. The complexity, function and applications of RNA in circulation. Front Genet. 2013;4:115.
5. Etheridge A, Lee I, Hood L, Galas D, Wang K. Extracellular microRNA: a new source of biomarkers. Mutat Res. 2011;717(1–2):85–90.
6. Bartel DP. MicroRNAs: genomics, biogenesis, mechanism, and function. Cell. 2004;116(2):281–97.
7. Eulalio A, Huntzinger E, Izaurralde E. Getting to the root of miRNA-mediated gene silencing. Cell. 2008;132(1):9–14.
8. Iorio MV, Croce CM. MicroRNA dysregulation in cancer: diagnostics, monitoring and therapeutics. A comprehensive review. EMBO Mol Med. 2012;4(3):143–59.
9. Lages E, Ipas H, Guttin A, Nesr H, Berger F, Issartel JP. MicroRNAs: molecular features and role in cancer. Front Biosci. 2012;17:2508–40.
10. Babalola O, Mamalis A, Lev-Tov H, Jagdeo J. The role of microRNAs in skin fibrosis. Arch Dermatol Res. 2013;305(9):763–76.
11. Bowen T, Jenkins RH, Fraser DJ. MicroRNAs, transforming growth factor beta-1, and tissue fibrosis. J Pathol. 2013;229(2):274–85.
12. Jiang X, Tsitsiou E, Herrick SE, Lindsay MA. MicroRNAs and the regulation of fibrosis. FEBS J. 2010;277(9):2015–21.
13. Patel V, Noureddine L. MicroRNAs and fibrosis. Curr Opin Nephrol Hypertens. 2012;21(4):410–6.
14. Vettori S, Gay S, Distler O. Role of MicroRNAs in fibrosis. Open Rheumatol J. 2012;6:130–9.
15. Maurer B, Stanczyk J, Jungel A, Akhmetshina A, Trenkmann M, Brock M, et al. MicroRNA-29, a key regulator of collagen expression in systemic sclerosis. Arthritis Rheum. 2010;62(6):1733–43.
16. Peng WJ, Tao JH, Mei B, Chen B, Li BZ, Yang GJ, et al. MicroRNA-29: a potential therapeutic target for systemic sclerosis. Expert Opin Ther Targets. 2012;16(9):875–9.
17. Zhu H, Li Y, Qu S, Luo H, Zhou Y, Wang Y, et al. MicroRNA expression abnormalities in limited cutaneous scleroderma and diffuse cutaneous scleroderma. J Clin Immunol. 2012;32(3):514–22.
18. Honda N, Jinnin M, Kajihara I, Makino T, Makino K, Masuguchi S, et al. TGF-beta-mediated downregulation of microRNA-196a contributes to the constitutive upregulated type I collagen expression in scleroderma dermal fibroblasts. J Immunol. 2012;188(7):3323–31.
19. Honda N, Jinnin M, Kira-Etoh T, Makino K, Kajihara I, Makino T, et al. miR-150 down-regulation contributes to the constitutive type I collagen overexpression in scleroderma dermal fibroblasts via the induction of integrin beta3. Am J Pathol. 2013;182(1):206–16.

20. Li H, Yang R, Fan X, Gu T, Zhao Z, Chang D, et al. MicroRNA array analysis of microRNAs related to systemic scleroderma. Rheumatol Int. 2012;32(2):307–13.
21. Makino K, Jinnin M, Hirano A, Yamane K, Eto M, Kusano T, et al. The downregulation of microRNA let-7a contributes to the excessive expression of type I collagen in systemic and localized scleroderma. J Immunol. 2013;190(8):3905–15.
22. Witwer KW. Circulating microRNA biomarker studies: pitfalls and potential solutions. Clin Chem. 2015;61(1):56–63.
23. Mitchell P. Proteomics retrenches. Nat Biotechnol. 2010;28(7):665–70.
24. Kelleher NL, Thomas PM, Ntai I, Compton PD, LeDuc RD. Deep and quantitative top-down proteomics in clinical and translational research. Expert Rev Proteomics. 2014;11(6):649–51.
25. Weiss F, van den Berg BH, Planatscher H, Pynn CJ, Joos TO, Poetz O. Catch and measure-mass spectrometry-based immunoassays in biomarker research. Biochim Biophys Acta. 2014;1844(5):927–32.
26. Slinker BK, Glantz SA. Multiple linear regression: accounting for multiple simultaneous determinants of a continuous dependent variable. Circulation. 2008;117(13):1732–7.
27. Froud R, Abel G. Using ROC curves to choose minimally important change thresholds when sensitivity and specificity are valued equally: the forgotten lesson of pythagoras. Theoretical considerations and an example application of change in health status. PLoS One. 2014;9(12):e114468.
28. Farina G, Lafyatis D, Lemaire R, Lafyatis R. A four-gene biomarker predicts skin disease in patients with diffuse cutaneous systemic sclerosis. Arthritis Rheum. 2010;62(2):580–8.
29. Rice LM, Ziemek J, Stratton EA, McLaughlin S, Padilla CM, Mathes AL, et al. A longitudinal biomarker for the extent of skin disease in patients with diffuse cutaneous systemic sclerosis. Arthritis Rheumatol. 2015;67:3004.
30. Rice LM, Padilla CM, McLaughlin SR, Mathes A, Ziemek J, Goummih S, et al. Fresolimumab treatment decreases biomarkers and improves clinical symptoms in systemic sclerosis patients. J Clin Invest. 2015;125(7):2795–807.
31. Milano A, Pendergrass SA, Sargent JL, George LK, McCalmont TH, Connolly MK, et al. Molecular subsets in the gene expression signatures of scleroderma skin. PLoS One. 2008;3(7):e2696.
32. J Invest Dermatol. 2013;133(8):1979–89. https://doi.org/10.1038/jid.2013.130. Epub 2013;14.
33. Chung L, Fiorentino DF, Benbarak MJ, Adler AS, Mariano MM, Paniagua RT, et al. Molecular framework for response to imatinib mesylate in systemic sclerosis. Arthritis Rheum. 2009;60(2):584–91.
34. Clark KEN, Campochiaro C, Csomor E, Taylor A, Nevin K, Galwey N, Morse MA, Singh J, Teo YV, Ong VH, Derrett-Smith E, Wisniacki N, Flint SM, Denton CP. Molecular basis for clinical diversity between autoantibody subsets in diffuse cutaneous systemic sclerosis. Ann Rheum Dis. 2021;80(12):1584–93. https://doi.org/10.1136/annrheumdis-2021-220402.
35. Hesselstrand R, Kassner A, Heinegard D, Saxne T. COMP: a candidate molecule in the pathogenesis of systemic sclerosis with a potential as a disease marker. Ann Rheum Dis. 2008;67(9):1242–8.
36. Horslev-Petersen K, Ammitzboll T, Engstrom-Laurent A, Bentsen K, Junker P, Asboe-Hansen G, et al. Serum and urinary aminoterminal type III procollagen peptide in progressive systemic sclerosis: relationship to sclerodermal involvement, serum hyaluronan and urinary collagen metabolites. J Rheumatol. 1988;15(3):460–7.
37. Macko RF, Gelber AC, Young BA, Lowitt MH, White B, Wigley FM, et al. Increased circulating concentrations of the counter adhesive proteins SPARC and thrombospondin-1 in systemic sclerosis (scleroderma). Relationship to platelet and endothelial cell activation. J Rheumatol. 2002;29(12):2565–70.
38. Kim WU, Min SY, Cho ML, Hong KH, Shin YJ, Park SH, et al. Elevated matrix metalloproteinase-9 in patients with systemic sclerosis. Arthritis Res Ther. 2005;7(1):R71–9.
39. Kikuchi K, Ihn H, Sato S, Igarashi A, Soma Y, Ishibashi Y, et al. Serum concentration of procollagen type I carboxyterminal propeptide in systemic sclerosis. Arch Dermatol Res. 1994;286(2):77–80.
40. Hunzelmann N, Risteli J, Risteli L, Sacher C, Vancheeswaran R, Black C, et al. Circulating type I collagen degradation products: a new serum marker for clinical severity in patients with scleroderma? Br J Dermatol. 1998;139(6):1020–5.
41. Nagy Z, Czirjak L. Increased levels of amino terminal propeptide of type III procollagen are an unfavourable predictor of survival in systemic sclerosis. Clin Exp Rheumatol. 2005;23(2):165–72.
42. Denton CP, Merkel PA, Furst DE, Khanna D, Emery P, Hsu VM, et al. Recombinant human anti-transforming growth factor beta1 antibody therapy in systemic sclerosis: a multicenter, randomized, placebo-controlled phase I/II trial of CAT-192. Arthritis Rheum. 2007;56(1):323–33.
43. Kikuchi K, Kubo M, Sato S, Fujimoto M, Tamaki K. Serum tissue inhibitor of metalloproteinases in patients with systemic sclerosis. J Am Acad Dermatol. 1995;33(6):973–8.
44. Yamaguchi Y, Ono J, Masuoka M, Ohta S, Izuhara K, Ikezawa Z, et al. Serum periostin levels are correlated with progressive skin sclerosis in patients with systemic sclerosis. Br J Dermatol. 2013;168(4):717–25.
45. Sato S, Hasegawa M, Takehara K. Serum levels of interleukin-6 and interleukin-10 correlate with total skin thickness score in patients with systemic sclerosis. J Dermatol Sci. 2001;27(2):140–6.
46. Codullo V, Baldwin HM, Singh MD, Fraser AR, Wilson C, Gilmour A, et al. An investigation of the inflammatory cytokine and chemokine network in systemic sclerosis. Ann Rheum Dis. 2011;70(6):1115–21.
47. Bandinelli F, Del Rosso A, Gabrielli A, Giacomelli R, Bartoli F, Guiducci S, et al. CCL2, CCL3 and CCL5 chemokines in systemic sclerosis: the correlation with SSc clinical features and the effect of prostaglandin E1 treatment. Clin Exp Rheumatol. 2012;30(2 Suppl 71):S44–9.
48. Abignano G, Cuomo G, Buch MH, Rosenberg WM, Valentini G, Emery P, et al. The enhanced liver fibrosis test: a clinical grade, validated serum test, biomarker of overall fibrosis in systemic sclerosis. Ann Rheum Dis. 2014;73(2):420–7.
49. Heuck A, Reiser M, Rupp N, Lehner K, Erlemann R. [Imaging of femur head necrosis using MR tomography]. Rofo. 1987;146(2):191–5.
50. Iwata Y, Yoshizaki A, Ogawa F, Komura K, Hara T, Muroi E, et al. Increased serum pentraxin 3 in patients with systemic sclerosis. J Rheumatol. 2009;36(5):976–83.
51. Giacomelli R, Cipriani P, Lattanzio R, Di Franco M, Locanto M, Parzanese I, et al. Circulating levels of soluble CD30 are increased in patients with systemic sclerosis (SSc) and correlate with serological and clinical features of the disease. Clin Exp Immunol. 1997;108(1):42–6.
52. Scala E, Pallotta S, Frezzolini A, Abeni D, Barbieri C, Sampogna F, et al. Cytokine and chemokine levels in systemic sclerosis: relationship with cutaneous and internal organ involvement. Clin Exp Immunol. 2004;138(3):540–6.
53. Matsushita T, Hasegawa M, Yanaba K, Kodera M, Takehara K, Sato S. Elevated serum BAFF levels in patients with systemic sclerosis: enhanced BAFF signaling in systemic sclerosis B lymphocytes. Arthritis Rheum. 2006;54(1):192–201.
54. Sato S, Fujimoto M, Hasegawa M, Komura K, Yanaba K, Hayakawa I, et al. Serum soluble CTLA-4 levels are increased in diffuse cutaneous systemic sclerosis. Rheumatology (Oxford). 2004;43(10):1261–6.

55. Dunne JV, van Eeden SF, Keen KJ. L-selectin and skin damage in systemic sclerosis. PLoS One. 2012;7(9):e44814.
56. Hebbar M, Peyrat JP, Hornez L, Hatron PY, Hachulla E, Devulder B. Increased concentrations of the circulating angiogenesis inhibitor endostatin in patients with systemic sclerosis. Arthritis Rheum. 2000;43(4):889–93.
57. Farouk HM, Hamza SH, El Bakry SA, Youssef SS, Aly IM, Moustafa AA, et al. Dysregulation of angiogenic homeostasis in systemic sclerosis. Int J Rheum Dis. 2013;16(4):448–54.
58. Vancheeswaran R, Magoulas T, Efrat G, Wheeler-Jones C, Olsen I, Penny R, et al. Circulating endothelin-1 levels in systemic sclerosis subsets—a marker of fibrosis or vascular dysfunction? J Rheumatol. 1994;21(10):1838–44.
59. Lakota K, Wei J, Carns M, Hinchcliff M, Lee J, Whitfield ML, et al. Levels of adiponectin, a marker for PPAR-gamma activity, correlate with skin fibrosis in systemic sclerosis: potential utility as biomarker? Arthritis Res Ther. 2012;14(3):R102.
60. Makino K, Jinnin M, Kajihara I, Honda N, Sakai K, Masuguchi S, et al. Circulating miR-142-3p levels in patients with systemic sclerosis. Clin Exp Dermatol. 2012;37(1):34–9.
61. Sing T, Jinnin M, Yamane K, Honda N, Makino K, Kajihara I, et al. microRNA-92a expression in the sera and dermal fibroblasts increases in patients with scleroderma. Rheumatology. 2012;51(9):1550–6.
62. Tanaka S, Suto A, Ikeda K, Sanayama Y, Nakagomi D, Iwamoto T, et al. Alteration of circulating miRNAs in SSc: miR-30b regulates the expression of PDGF receptor beta. Rheumatology. 2013;52(11):1963–72.
63. Wuttge DM, Carlsen AL, Teku G, Steen SO, Wildt M, Vihinen M, et al. Specific autoantibody profiles and disease subgroups correlate with circulating micro-RNA in systemic sclerosis. Rheumatology. 2015;54(11):2100–7.
64. Stifano G, Affandi AJ, Mathes AL, Rice LM, Nakerakanti S, Nazari B, et al. Chronic toll-like receptor 4 stimulation in skin induces inflammation, macrophage activation, transforming growth factor beta signature gene expression, and fibrosis. Arthritis Res Ther. 2014;16(4):R136.
65. Stock CJW, Renzoni EA. Genetic predictors of systemic sclerosis-associated interstitial lung disease: a review of recent literature. Eur J Hum Genet. 2018;26:765–77.
66. Juge P-A, Lee JS, Ebstein E, Furukawa E, Dobrinskikh E, Gazal S, et al. MUC5B promoter variant and rheumatoid arthritis with interstitial lung disease. N Engl J Med. 2018;379:2209-19.
67. Stock CJ, Sato H, Fonseca C, Banya WAS, Molyneaux PL, Adamali H, et al. Mucin 5B promoter polymorphism is associated with idiopathic pulmonary fibrosis but not with development of lung fibrosis in systemic sclerosis or sarcoidosis. Thorax. 2013;68:436-41.
68. Peljto AL, Steele MP, Fingerlin TE, Hinchcliff ME, Murphy E, Podlusky S, et al. The pulmonary fibrosis-associated MUC5B promoter polymorphism does not influence the development of interstitial pneumonia in systemic sclerosis. Chest. 2012;142:1584-8.
69. Borie R, Crestani B, Sieude P, Nunes H, Allanore Y, Kannengiesser C, et al. The MUC5B variant is associated with idiopathic pulmonary fibrosis but not with systemic sclerosis interstitial lung disease in the European Caucasian population. PLOS ONE. 2013;8:e70621.
70. Volkmann ER, Tashkin DP, Roth MD, Li N, Charles J, Mayes M, Kim G, Goldin J, Pourzand L, Clements PJ, Furst DE, Khanna D, Elashoff RM, Assassi S. The MUC5B promoter variant does not predict progression of interstitial lung disease in systemic sclerosis. Semin Arthritis Rheum. 2020;50:963-67.
71. Zhu H, Zhu C, Mi W, Chen T, Zhao H, Zuo X, et al. Integration of genome-wide DNA methylation and transcription uncovered aberrant methylation-regulated genes and pathways in the peripheral blood mononuclear cells of systemic sclerosis. Int J Rheumatol. 2018;2018:7342472.
72. Christmann RB, Wooten A, Sampaio-Barros P, Borges CL, Carvalho CR, Kairalla RA, et al. miR-155 in the progression of lung fibrosis in systemic sclerosis. Arthritis Res Ther. 2016;18:155
73. Ho KT, Reveille JD. The clinical relevance of autoantibodies in scleroderma. Arthritis Res Ther. 2003;5:80–93.
74. De Lauretis A, Sestini P, Pantelidis P, Hoyles R, Hansell DM, Goh NS, et al. Serum interleukin 6 is predictive of early functional decline and mortality in interstitial lung disease associated with systemic sclerosis. J Rheumatol. 2013;40(4):435–46.
75. Liu X, Mayes MD, Pedroza C, Draeger HT, Gonzalez EB, Harper BE, et al. Does C-reactive protein predict the long-term progression of interstitial lung disease and survival in patients with early systemic sclerosis? Arthritis Care Res. 2013;65:1375-80.
76. Schupp J, Becker M, Günther J, Muller-Quernheim J, Riemekasten G, Prasse A. Serum CCL18 is predictive for lung disease progression and mortality in systemic sclerosis. Eur Respir J. 2014;43:1530-2.
77. Tiev KP, Hua-Huy T, Kettaneh A, Gain M, Duong-Quy S, Toledano C, et al. Serum CC chemokine ligand-18 predicts lung disease worsening in systemic sclerosis. Eur Respir J. 2011;38:1355-60.
78. van Bon L, Affandi AJ, Broen J, Christmann RBm Marijnissen RJ, Stawski L, et al. Proteome-wide analysis and CXCL4 as a biomarker in systemic sclerosis. N Engl J Med. 2014;370:433-43.
79. Kuwana M, Shirai Y, Takeuchi T. Elevated serum Krebs von den Lungen-6 in early disease predicts subsequent deterioration of pulmonary function in patients with systemic sclerosis and interstitial lung disease. J Rheumatol. 2016;43:1825-31.
80. Salazar GA, Kuwana M, Wu M, Estrada-Y-Martin RM, Ying J, Charles J, et al. KL-6 but not CCL-18 is a predictor of early progression of systemic sclerosis-related interstitial lung disease. J Rheumatol. 2018;45:1153-8.
81. Volkmann ER, Tashkin DP, Kuwana M, Li N, Roth MD, Charles J, Hant FN, Bogatkevich GS, Akter T, Kim G, Goldin J, Khanna D, Clements PJ, Furst DE, Elashoff RM, Silver RM, Assassi S. Progression of Interstitial Lung Disease in Systemic Sclerosis: The Importance of Pneumoproteins Krebs von den Lungen 6 and CCL18. Arthritis Rheumatol. 2019;71:2059-67.
82. Nukiwa T. The role of biomarkers in management of interstitial lung disease: implications of biomarkers derived from type II pneumocytes. European Respiratory Monograph. 2009;46:47-66.
83. Sumida H, Asano Y, Tamaki Z, Aozasa N, Taniguchi T, Toyama T, et al. Prediction of therapeutic response before and during IV cyclophosphamide pulse therapy for interstitial lung disease in systemic sclerosis: A longitudinal observational study. J Dermatol. 2018;45:1425-33.
84. Hoffmann-Vold AM, Tennoe AH, Garen T, Midtvedt O, Abraityte A, Aalokken TM, et al. High level of chemokine CCL18 is associated with pulmonary function deterioration, lung fibrosis progression, and reduced survival in systemic sclerosis. Chest. 2016;150:299-306.
85. Elhaj M, Charles J, Pedroza C, Liu X, Zhou X, Estrada YMRM, et al. Can serum surfactant protein D or CC-chemokine ligand 18 predict outcome of interstitial lung disease in patients with early systemic sclerosis? J Rheumatol. 2013;40(7):1114–20.
86. Khanna D, Denton CP, Jahreis A, van Laar JM, Frech TM, Anderson ME, et al. Safety and efficacy of subcutaneous tocilizumab in adults with systemic sclerosis (faSScinate): a phase 2, randomised, controlled trial. Lancet. 2016;387:2630–2640.
87. Xu Z, Chen W, Chen C. Matrix metalloproteinase 7 is a candidate biomarker in systemic sclerosis-associated interstitial lung disease. Acta Reumatol Port. 2020;45:191-200.
88. Stock C, De Lauretis AD, Visca D, Daccord C, Kokosi M, Alfieri V, et al. Serum biomarkers in SSc-ILD: association with presence, severity and prognosis. Europ Resp J. 2019;54:Suppl. 63, PA5198.
89. Carulli MT, Handler C, Coghlan JG, Black CM, Denton CP. Can CCL2 serum levels be used in risk stratification or to moni-

tor treatment response in systemic sclerosis? Ann Rheum Dis. 2008;67:105–9.
90. Wu M, Baron M, Pedroza C, Salazar GA, Ying J, Charles J, Agarwal SK, Hudson M, Pope J, Zhou X, Reveille JD, Fritzler MJ, Mayes MD, Assassi S. CCL2 in the Circulation Predicts Long-Term Progression of Interstitial Lung Disease in Patients With Early Systemic Sclerosis: Data From Two Independent Cohorts. Arthritis Rheumatol. 2017;69:1871–8.
91. Proost P, Wuyts A, Van Damme J. Human monocyte chemotactic proteins-2 and -3: structural and functional comparison with MCP-1. J Leukoc Biol 1996;59:67-74.
92. Yanaba K, Komura K, Kodera M, Matsushita T, Hasegawa M, Takehara K, Sato S. Serum levels of monocyte chemotactic protein-3/CCL7 are raised in patients with systemic sclerosis: association with extent of skin sclerosis and severity of pulmonary fibrosis. Ann Rheum Dis. 2006;65:124-6.
93. Volkmann ER, Tashkin DP, Roth MD, Clements PJ, Khanna D, Furst DE, Mayes M, Charles J, Tseng CH, Elashoff RM, Assassi S. Changes in plasma CXCL4 levels are associated with improvements in lung function in patients receiving immunosuppressive therapy for systemic sclerosis-related interstitial lung disease. Arthritis Res Ther. 2016;18:305.
94. Volpinari S, La Corte R, Bighi S, Ravenna F, Prandini N, Lo Monaco A, Trotta F. Bronchoalveolar lavage in systemic sclerosis with lung involvement: role and correlations with functional, radiological and scintigraphic parameters. Rheumatol Int. 2011;31:1183-8.
95. Strange C, Bolster MB, Roth MD, Silver RM, Theodore A, Goldin J, Clements P, Chung J, Elashoff RM, Suh R, Smith EA, Furst DE, Tashkin DP; Scleroderma Lung Study Research Group. Bronchoalveolar lavage and response to cyclophosphamide in scleroderma interstitial lung disease. Am J Respir Crit Care Med. 2008;177:91-8.
96. Tashkin DP, Elashoff R, Clements PJ, Goldin J, Roth MD, Furst DE, Arriola E, Silver R, Strange C, Bolster M, Seibold JR, Riley DJ, Hsu VM, Varga J, Schraufnagel DE, Theodore A, Simms R, Wise R, Wigley F, White B, Steen V, Read C, Mayes M, Parsley E, Mubarak K, Connolly MK, Golden J, Olman M, Fessler B, Rothfield N, Metersky M; Scleroderma Lung Study Research Group. Cyclophosphamide versus placebo in scleroderma lung disease. N Engl J Med. 2006;354:2655-66.
97. Hesselstrand R, Wildt M, Bozovic G, Andersson-Sjöland A, Andréasson K, Scheja A, Westergren-Thorsson G, Bjermer L, Wuttge DM. Biomarkers from bronchoalveolar lavage fluid in systemic sclerosis patients with interstitial lung disease relate to severity of lung fibrosis. Respir Med. 2013;107:1079-86
98. Goh NS, Desai SR, Veeraraghavan S, Hansell DM, Copley SJ, Maher TM, Corte TJ, Sander CR, Ratoff J, Devaraj A, Bozovic G, Denton CP, Black CM, du Bois RM, Wells AU. Interstitial lung disease in systemic sclerosis: a simple staging system. Am J Respir Crit Care Med. 2008;77:1248-54.
99. Khanna D, Nagaraja V, Tseng CH, Abtin F, Suh R, Kim G, Wells A, Furst DE, Clements PJ, Roth MD, Tashkin DP, Goldin J. Predictors of lung function decline in scleroderma-related interstitial lung disease based on high-resolution computed tomography: implications for cohort enrichment in systemic sclerosis-associated interstitial lung disease trials. Arthritis Res Ther. 2015;17:372.
100. Roth MD, Tseng CH, Clements PJ, Furst DE, Tashkin DP, Goldin JG, Khanna D, Kleerup EC, Li N, Elashoff D, Elashoff RM; Scleroderma Lung Study Research Group. Predicting treatment outcomes and responder subsets in scleroderma-related interstitial lung disease. Arthritis Rheum. 2011;63:2797-808.
101. Kim HJ, Tashkin DP, Chong S, Brown M, Gjertson DW Kleerup E, Abtin F, Roth M, Elashoff R, Tseng C, Khanna D, Belperio J, Goldiin JG. Transitions to different patterns of interstitial lung disease in scleroderma with and without treatment. Ann Rheum Dis. 2016; 75:1367-71.
102. Goldin JG, Kim GH, Volkmann ER, Clements P, Tseng C-H, Furst DE, Brown M, Roth M, Tashkin DP. Longitudinal changes in quantitative lung disease on CT after immunosuppression in the Scleroderma Lung Study II. Ann Am Thorac Soc 2018;15:1286-95.
103. Khanna D, Lin CJF, Furst DE, Goldin J, Kim G, Kuwana M, Allanore Y, Matucci-Cerinic M, Distler O, Shima Y, van Laar JM, Spotswood H, Wagner B, Siegel J, Jahreis A, Denton CP; focuSSced investigators. Tocilizumab in systemic sclerosis: a randomised, double-blind, placebo-controlled, phase 3 trial. Lancet Respir Med. 2020;8:963-74.
104. Kim HJ, Brown MS, Elashoff F, Li G, Gjertson DW, Lynch DA, et al. Quantitative texture-based assessment of one-year changes in fibrotic reticular patterns on HRCT in scleroderma lung disease treated with oral cyclophosphamide. Eur Radiol. 2011;21(12):2455–65.
105. Volkmann ER, Tashkin DP, Roth MD, Goldin J, Kim G. Short-term changes in the radiographic extent of interstitial lung disease predict long-term mortality in systemic sclerosis [Abstract]. Ann Rheum Dis. 2021;80:162-3.
106. Bergmann C, Distler JHW, Treutlein C, et al. 68Ga-FAPI-04 PET-CT for molecular assessment of fibroblast activation and risk evaluation in systemic sclerosis-associated interstitial lung disease: a single-centre, pilot study. Lancet Rheumatol. 2021;3:e185-e194.
107. Foris V, Kovacs G, Tscherner M, Olschewski A, Olschewski H. Biomarkers in pulmonary hypertension: what do we know? Chest. 2013;144(1):274–83.
108. Hoeper MM, Bogaard HJ, Condliffe R, Frantz R, Khanna D, Kurzyna M, et al. Definitions and diagnosis of pulmonary hypertension. J Am Coll Cardiol. 2013;62(25 Suppl):D42–50.
109. Humbert M, Yaici A, de Groote P, Montani D, Sitbon O, Launay D, et al. Screening for pulmonary arterial hypertension in patients with systemic sclerosis: clinical characteristics at diagnosis and long-term survival. Arthritis Rheum. 2011;63(11):3522–30.
110. Denton CP, Cailes JB, Phillips GD, Wells AU, Black CM, Bois RM. Comparison of Doppler echocardiography and right heart catheterization to assess pulmonary hypertension in systemic sclerosis. Br J Rheumatol. 1997;36(2):239–43.
111. McGoon M, Gutterman D, Steen V, Barst R, McCrory DC, Fortin TA, et al. Screening, early detection, and diagnosis of pulmonary arterial hypertension: ACCP evidence-based clinical practice guidelines. Chest. 2004;126(1 Suppl):14S–34.
112. Allanore Y, Borderie D, Avouac J, Zerkak D, Meune C, Hachulla E, et al. High N-terminal pro-brain natriuretic peptide levels and low diffusing capacity for carbon monoxide as independent predictors of the occurrence of precapillary pulmonary arterial hypertension in patients with systemic sclerosis. Arthritis Rheum. 2008;58(1):284–91.
113. Galie N, Hoeper MM, Humbert M, Torbicki A, Vachiery JL, Barbera JA, et al. Guidelines for the diagnosis and treatment of pulmonary hypertension: the Task Force for the Diagnosis and Treatment of Pulmonary Hypertension of the European Society of Cardiology (ESC) and the European Respiratory Society (ERS), endorsed by the International Society of Heart and Lung Transplantation (ISHLT). Eur Heart J. 2009;30(20):2493–537.
114. Coghlan JG, Denton CP, Grunig E, Bonderman D, Distler O, Khanna D, et al. Evidence-based detection of pulmonary arterial hypertension in systemic sclerosis: the DETECT study. Ann Rheum Dis. 2014;73(7):1340–9.
115. Mathai SC, Sibley CT, Forfia PR, Mudd JO, Fisher MR, Tedford RJ, et al. Tricuspid annular plane systolic excursion is a robust outcome measure in systemic sclerosis-associated pulmonary arterial hypertension. J Rheumatol. 2011;38(11):2410–8.
116. Chung L, Liu J, Parsons L, Hassoun PM, McGoon M, Badesch DB, et al. Characterization of connective tissue disease-associated pulmonary arterial hypertension from REVEAL: identifying systemic sclerosis as a unique phenotype. Chest. 2010;138(6): 1383–94.

117. Cavagna L, Caporali R, Klersy C, Ghio S, Albertini R, Scelsi L, et al. Comparison of brain natriuretic peptide (BNP) and NT-proBNP in screening for pulmonary arterial hypertension in patients with systemic sclerosis. J Rheumatol. 2010;37(10):2064–70.
118. Williams MH, Handler CE, Akram R, Smith CJ, Das C, Smee J, et al. Role of N-terminal brain natriuretic peptide (N-TproBNP) in scleroderma-associated pulmonary arterial hypertension. Eur Heart J. 2006;27(12):1485–94.
119. Quarck R, Nawrot T, Meyns B, Delcroix M. C-reactive protein: a new predictor of adverse outcome in pulmonary arterial hypertension. J Am Coll Cardiol. 2009;53(14):1211–8.
120. Tamura Y, Ono T, Kuwana M, Inoue K, Takei M, Yamamoto T, et al. Human pentraxin 3 (PTX3) as a novel biomarker for the diagnosis of pulmonary arterial hypertension. PLoS One. 2012;7(9):e45834.
121. Pendergrass SA, Hayes E, Farina G, Lemaire R, Farber HW, Whitfield ML, et al. Limited systemic sclerosis patients with pulmonary arterial hypertension show biomarkers of inflammation and vascular injury. PLoS One. 2010;5(8):e12106.
122. Dromparis P, Michelakis ED. F2-isoprostanes: an emerging pulmonary arterial hypertension biomarker and potential link to the metabolic theory of pulmonary arterial hypertension? Chest. 2012;142(4):816–20.
123. Morelli S, Ferri C, Polettini E, Bellini C, Gualdi GF, Pittoni V, et al. Plasma endothelin-1 levels, pulmonary hypertension, and lung fibrosis in patients with systemic sclerosis. Am J Med. 1995;99(3):255–60.
124. Ciurzynski M, Bienias P, Irzyk K, Kostrubiec M, Bartoszewicz Z, Siwicka M, et al. Serum endothelin-1 and NT-proBNP, but not ADMA, endoglin and TIMP-1 levels, reflect impaired right ventricular function in patients with systemic sclerosis. Clin Rheumatol. 2014;33(1):83–9.
125. Rubens C, Ewert R, Halank M, Wensel R, Orzechowski HD, Schultheiss HP, et al. Big endothelin-1 and endothelin-1 plasma levels are correlated with the severity of primary pulmonary hypertension. Chest. 2001;120(5):1562–9.
126. Cracowski JL, Degano B, Chabot F, Labarere J, Schwedhelm E, Monneret D, et al. Independent association of urinary F2-isoprostanes with survival in pulmonary arterial hypertension. Chest. 2012;142(4):869–76.
127. Malhotra R, Paskin-Flerlage S, Zamanian RT, Zimmerman P, Schmidt JW, Deng DY, et al. Circulating angiogenic modulatory factors predict survival and functional class in pulmonary arterial hypertension. Pulm Circ. 2013;3(2):369–80.
128. Lorenzen JM, Nickel N, Kramer R, Golpon H, Westerkamp V, Olsson KM, et al. Osteopontin in patients with idiopathic pulmonary hypertension. Chest. 2011;139(5):1010–7.
129. Lorenzen JM, Kramer R, Meier M, Werfel T, Wichmann K, Hoeper MM, et al. Osteopontin in the development of systemic sclerosis—relation to disease activity and organ manifestation. Rheumatology (Oxford). 2010;49(10):1989–91.
130. Renard S, Paulin R, Breuils-Bonnet S, Simard S, Pibarot P, Bonnet S, et al. Pim-1: a new biomarker in pulmonary arterial hypertension. Pulm Circ. 2013;3(1):74–81.
131. Santos M, Reis A, Goncalves F, Ferreira-Pinto MJ, Cabral S, Torres S, et al. Adiponectin levels are elevated in patients with pulmonary arterial hypertension. Clin Cardiol. 2013;37:21.
132. Chora I, Guiducci S, Manetti M, Romano E, Mazzotta C, Bellando-Randone S, et al. Vascular biomarkers and correlation with peripheral vasculopathy in systemic sclerosis. Autoimmun Rev. 2015;14(4):314–22.
133. Sfikakis PP, Tesar J, Baraf H, Lipnick R, Klipple G, Tsokos GC. Circulating intercellular adhesion molecule-1 in patients with systemic sclerosis. Clin Immunol Immunopathol. 1993;68(1):88–92.
134. Wipff J, Avouac J, Borderie D, Zerkak D, Lemarechal H, Kahan A, et al. Disturbed angiogenesis in systemic sclerosis: high levels of soluble endoglin. Rheumatology (Oxford). 2008;47(7):972–5.
135. Sulli A, Soldano S, Pizzorni C, Montagna P, Secchi ME, Villaggio B, et al. Raynaud's phenomenon and plasma endothelin: correlations with capillaroscopic patterns in systemic sclerosis. J Rheumatol. 2009;36(6):1235–9.
136. Kim HS, Park MK, Kim HY, Park SH. Capillary dimension measured by computer-based digitalized image correlated with plasma endothelin-1 levels in patients with systemic sclerosis. Clin Rheumatol. 2010;29(3):247–54.
137. Bassyouni IH, Gheita TA, Talaat RM. Clinical significance of serum levels of sCD36 in patients with systemic sclerosis: preliminary data. Rheumatology (Oxford). 2011;50(11):2108–12.
138. Riccieri V, Stefanantoni K, Vasile M, Macri V, Sciarra I, Iannace N, et al. Abnormal plasma levels of different angiogenic molecules are associated with different clinical manifestations in patients with systemic sclerosis. Clin Exp Rheumatol. 2011;29(2 Suppl 65):S46–52.
139. Avouac J, Meune C, Ruiz B, Couraud PO, Uzan G, Boileau C, et al. Angiogenic biomarkers predict the occurrence of digital ulcers in systemic sclerosis. Ann Rheum Dis. 2012;71(3):394–9.
140. Terras S, Opitz E, Moritz RK, Hoxtermann S, Gambichler T, Kreuter A. Increased serum IL-33 levels may indicate vascular involvement in systemic sclerosis. Ann Rheum Dis. 2013;72(1):144–5.
141. Manetti M, Guiducci S, Ceccarelli C, Romano E, Bellando-Randone S, Conforti ML, et al. Increased circulating levels of interleukin 33 in systemic sclerosis correlate with early disease stage and microvascular involvement. Ann Rheum Dis. 2011;70(10):1876–8.
142. Rankin AL, Mumm JB, Murphy E, Turner S, Yu N, McClanahan TK, et al. IL-33 induces IL-13-dependent cutaneous fibrosis. J Immunol. 2010;184(3):1526–35.
143. Valentini G, Bencivelli W, Bombardieri S, D'Angelo S, Della Rossa A, Silman AJ, et al. European Scleroderma Study Group to define disease activity criteria for systemic sclerosis. III. Assessment of the construct validity of the preliminary activity criteria. Ann Rheum Dis. 2003;62(9):901–3.
144. Valentini G, Della Rossa A, Bombardieri S, Bencivelli W, Silman AJ, D'Angelo S, et al. European multicentre study to define disease activity criteria for systemic sclerosis. II. Identification of disease activity variables and development of preliminary activity indexes. Ann Rheum Dis. 2001;60(6):592–8.
145. Khanna D, Distler O, Avouac J, Behrens F, Clements PJ, Denton C, et al. Measures of response in clinical trials of systemic sclerosis: the Combined Response Index for Systemic Sclerosis (CRISS) and Outcome Measures in Pulmonary Arterial Hypertension related to Systemic Sclerosis (EPOSS). J Rheumatol. 2009;36(10):2356–61.
146. Sambataro D, Sambataro G, Zaccara E, Maglione W, Polosa R, Afeltra AM, et al. Nailfold videocapillaroscopy microhaemorrhage and giant capillary counting as an accurate approach for a steady state definition of disease activity in systemic sclerosis. Arthritis Res Ther. 2014;16(5):462.
147. Michalska-Jakubus M, Kowal-Bielecka O, Chodorowska G, Bielecki M, Krasowska D. Angiopoietins-1 and -2 are differentially expressed in the sera of patients with systemic sclerosis: high angiopoietin-2 levels are associated with greater severity and higher activity of the disease. Rheumatology (Oxford). 2011;50(4):746–55.
148. Lambrecht S, Smith V, De Wilde K, Coudenys J, Decuman S, Deforce D, et al. Growth differentiation factor 15, a marker of lung involvement in systemic sclerosis, is involved in fibrosis

development but is not indispensable for fibrosis development. Arthritis Rheumatol. 2014;66(2):418–27.
149. Budulgan M, Dilek B, Dag SB, Batmaz I, Yildiz I, Sariyildiz MA, et al. Relationship between serum leptin level and disease activity in patients with systemic sclerosis. Clin Rheumatol. 2014;33(3):335–9.
150. Muangchan C, Harding S, Khimdas S, Bonner A, Canadian Scleroderma Research Group, Baron M, et al. Association of C-reactive protein with high disease activity in systemic sclerosis: results from the Canadian Scleroderma Research Group. Arthritis Care Res. 2012;64(9):1405–14.
151. Hesselstrand R, Andreasson K, Wuttge DM, Bozovic G, Scheja A, Saxne T. Increased serum COMP predicts mortality in SSc: results from a longitudinal study of interstitial lung disease. Rheumatology (Oxford). 2012;51(5):915–20.

Further Reading

Rimar D, Rosner I, Nov Y, Slobodin G, Rozenbaum M, Halasz K, et al. Brief report: lysyl oxidase is a potential biomarker of fibrosis in systemic sclerosis. Arthritis Rheumatol. 2014;66(3): 726–30.

Asano Y, Ihn H, Yamane K, Yazawa N, Kubo M, Fujimoto M, et al. Clinical significance of surfactant protein D as a serum marker for evaluating pulmonary fibrosis in patients with systemic sclerosis. Arthritis Rheum. 2001;44(6):1363–9.

Hant FN, Ludwicka-Bradley A, Wang HJ, Li N, Elashoff R, Tashkin DP, et al. Surfactant protein D and KL-6 as serum biomarkers of interstitial lung disease in patients with scleroderma. J Rheumatol. 2009;36(4):773–80.

Yanaba K, Hasegawa M, Takehara K, Sato S. Comparative study of serum surfactant protein-D and KL-6 concentrations in patients with systemic sclerosis as markers for monitoring the activity of pulmonary fibrosis. J Rheumatol. 2004;31(6):1112–20.

Kumanovics G, Gorbe E, Minier T, Simon D, Berki T, Czirjak L. Follow-up of serum KL-6 lung fibrosis biomarker levels in 173 patients with systemic sclerosis. Clin Exp Rheumatol. 2014;32(6 Suppl 86):S-138–44.

Song JW, Do KH, Jang SJ, Colby TV, Han S, Kim DS. Blood biomarkers MMP-7 and SP-A: predictors of outcome in idiopathic pulmonary fibrosis. Chest. 2013;143(5):1422–9.

Moinzadeh P, Krieg T, Hellmich M, Brinckmann J, Neumann E, Muller-Ladner U, et al. Elevated MMP-7 levels in patients with systemic sclerosis: correlation with pulmonary involvement. Exp Dermatol. 2011;20(9):770–3.

Manetti M, Guiducci S, Romano E, Bellando-Randone S, Conforti ML, Ibba-Manneschi L, et al. Increased serum levels and tissue expression of matrix metalloproteinase-12 in patients with systemic sclerosis: correlation with severity of skin and pulmonary fibrosis and vascular damage. Ann Rheum Dis. 2012;71(6):1064–72.

Jenkins RG, Simpson JK, Saini G, Bentley JH, Russell AM, Braybrooke R, et al. Longitudinal change in collagen degradation biomarkers in idiopathic pulmonary fibrosis: an analysis from the prospective, multicentre PROFILE study. Lancet Respir Med. 2015;3(6):462–72.

Doyle TJ, Patel AS, Hatabu H, Nishino M, Wu G, Osorio JC, et al. Detection of rheumatoid arthritis-interstitial lung disease is enhanced by serum biomarkers. Am J Respir Crit Care Med. 2015;191(12):1403–12.

Lota HK, Renzoni EA. Circulating biomarkers of interstitial lung disease in systemic sclerosis. Int J Rheumatol. 2012;2012:121439.

Prasse A, Pechkovsky DV, Toews GB, Schafer M, Eggeling S, Ludwig C, et al. CCL18 as an indicator of pulmonary fibrotic activity in idiopathic interstitial pneumonias and systemic sclerosis. Arthritis Rheum. 2007;56(5):1685–93.

Kodera M, Hasegawa M, Komura K, Yanaba K, Takehara K, Sato S. Serum pulmonary and activation-regulated chemokine/CCL18 levels in patients with systemic sclerosis: a sensitive indicator of active pulmonary fibrosis. Arthritis Rheum. 2005;52(9):2889–96.

Wuttge DM, Wildt M, Geborek P, Wollheim FA, Scheja A, Akesson A. Serum IL-15 in patients with early systemic sclerosis: a potential novel marker of lung disease. Arthritis Res Ther. 2007;9(5):R85.

Lee CG, Hartl D, Lee GR, Koller B, Matsuura H, Da Silva CA, et al. Role of breast regression protein 39 (BRP-39)/chitinase 3-like-1 in Th2 and IL-13-induced tissue responses and apoptosis. J Exp Med. 2009;206(5):1149–66.

Nordenbaek C, Johansen JS, Halberg P, Wiik A, Garbarsch C, Ullman S, et al. High serum levels of YKL-40 in patients with systemic sclerosis are associated with pulmonary involvement. Scand J Rheumatol. 2005;34(4):293–7.

Lee CG, Herzog EL, Ahangari F, Zhou Y, Gulati M, Lee CM, et al. Chitinase 1 is a biomarker for and therapeutic target in scleroderma-associated interstitial lung disease that augments TGF-beta1 signaling. J Immunol. 2012;189(5):2635–44.

Hasegawa M, Asano Y, Endo H, Fujimoto M, Goto D, Ihn H, et al. Serum adhesion molecule levels as prognostic markers in patients with early systemic sclerosis: a multicentre, prospective, observational study. PLoS One. 2014;9(2):e88150.

Ogawa F, Shimizu K, Muroi E, Hara T, Hasegawa M, Takehara K, et al. Serum levels of 8-isoprostane, a marker of oxidative stress, are elevated in patients with systemic sclerosis. Rheumatology (Oxford). 2006;45(7):815–8.

Volpe A, Biasi D, Caramaschi P, Mantovani W, Bambara LM, Canestrini S, et al. Levels of F2-isoprostanes in systemic sclerosis: correlation with clinical features. Rheumatology (Oxford). 2006;45(3):314–20.

Stuart BD, Lee JS, Kozlitina J, Noth I, Devine MS, Glazer CS, et al. Effect of telomere length on survival in patients with idiopathic pulmonary fibrosis: an observational cohort study with independent validation. Lancet Respir Med. 2014;2(7):557–65.

Schmidt K, Martinez-Gamboa L, Meier S, Witt C, Meisel C, Hanitsch LG, et al. Bronchoalveoloar lavage fluid cytokines and chemokines as markers and predictors for the outcome of interstitial lung disease in systemic sclerosis patients. Arthritis Res Ther. 2009;11(4):R111.

Stewart NJ, Leung G, Norquay G, Marshall H, Parra-Robles J, Murphy PS, et al. Experimental validation of the hyperpolarized Xe chemical shift saturation recovery technique in healthy volunteers and subjects with interstitial lung disease. Magn Reson Med. 2014;74:196.

Hashefi M, Curiel R. Future and upcoming non-neoplastic applications of PET/CT imaging. Ann N Y Acad Sci. 2011;1228:167–74.

Morita Y, Kuwagata S, Kato N, Tsujimura Y, Mizutani H, Suehiro M, et al. 18F-FDG PET/CT useful for the early detection of rapidly progressive fatal interstitial lung disease in dermatomyositis. Intern Med. 2012;51(12):1613–8.

Owada T, Maezawa R, Kurasawa K, Okada H, Arai S, Fukuda T. Detection of inflammatory lesions by f-18 fluorodeoxyglucose positron emission tomography in patients with polymyositis and dermatomyositis. J Rheumatol. 2012;39(8): 1659–65.

Cellular and Molecular Mechanisms of Fibrosis in Systemic Sclerosis

18

Maria Trojanowska, John Varga, and David Lagares

Introduction: Cellular Determinants of Repair and Fibrosis

Fibrosis is characterized by excessive accumulation of connective tissue in parenchymal organs and replacement of normal tissue architecture with stiff collagen-rich matrix, resulting in failure of the affected organs. Fibrosis in the skin and multiple visceral organs is the hallmark of systemic sclerosis (SSc), in common with a diverse group of chronic human diseases (Fig. 18.1). While in the latter conditions fibrosis is typically confined to a single target organ such as the lungs or kidney, in scleroderma fibrosis can occur synchronously in the skin and multiple internal organs and musculoskeletal structures.

In fibrotic conditions, fibrosis is the end result of a complex cascade of vascular and immune-mediated responses to environmental injury in a genetically predisposed individual [1]. As illustrated in Fig. 18.2, injured or activated vascular, epithelial, and immune cells produce profibrotic mediators including cytokines and growth factors, autoantibodies, and reactive oxygen species (ROS) that can serve as paracrine cues to trigger the activation, differentiation, and persistent survival of stromal cells such as fibroblasts. Myofibroblast is the cell type that is ultimately accountable for excessive ECM deposition, tissue remodeling, and stiffening in all forms of fibrosis. Established fibrosis progresses via a variety of self-sustaining amplification mechanisms including mechanical activation of myofibroblasts by matrix stiffness, durable epigenetic modifications, matrikines, and the acquisition of an apoptosis-resistant senescent phenotype, ultimately leading to chronic tissue damage and organ failure.

M. Trojanowska (✉)
Arthritis and Autoimmune Diseases Center, Boston University School of Medicine, Boston, MA, USA
e-mail: trojanme@bu.edu

J. Varga
Division of Rheumatology, Department of Internal Medicine, University of Michigan, Ann Arbor, MI, USA
e-mail: vargaj@med.umich.edu

D. Lagares
Division of Pulmonary and Critical Care Medicine, Massachusetts General Hospital, Harvard Medical School, Boston, MA, USA
e-mail: dlagares@mgh.harvard.edu

Y. Allanore et al. (eds.), *Scleroderma*, https://doi.org/10.1007/978-3-031-40658-4_18

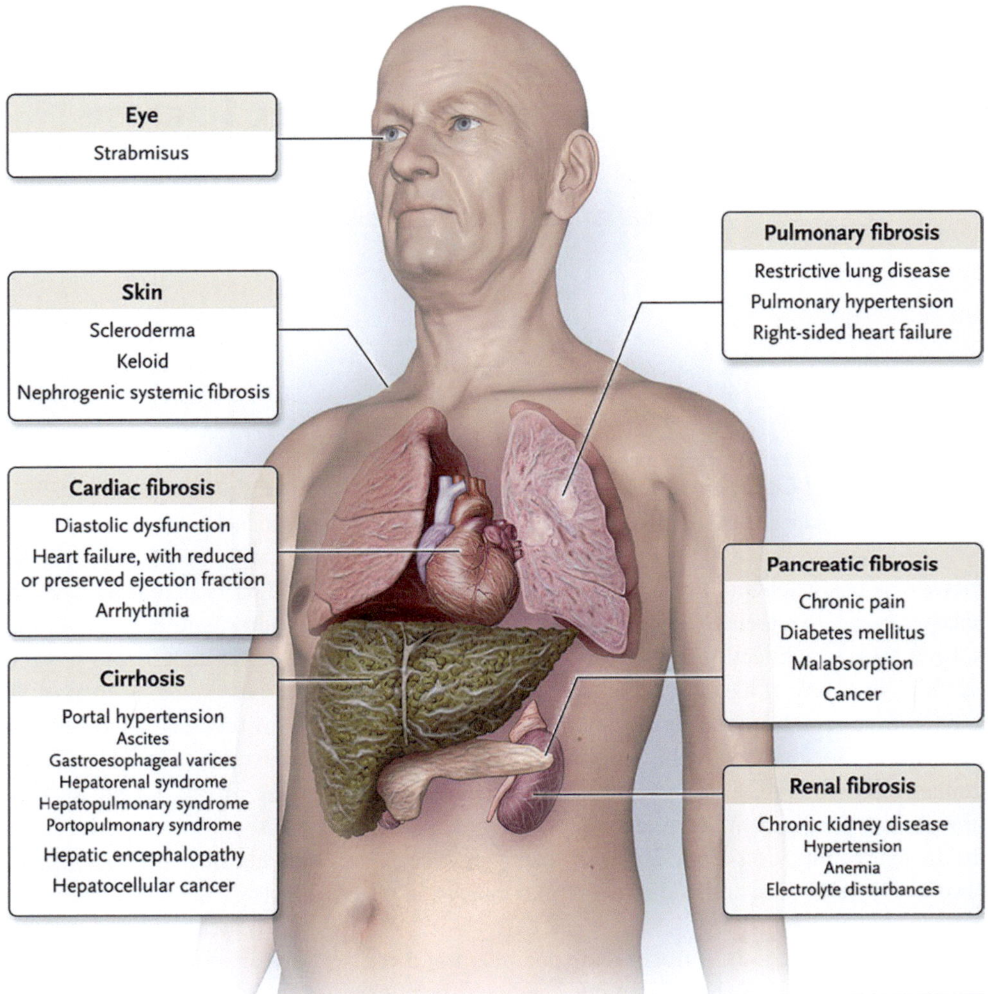

Fig. 18.1 Human fibrotic diseases. Pathological scarring occurs in multiple organs, leading to loss of function. Fibrosis in the bone marrow, heart, intestinal tract, kidney, liver, and lungs together contributes to more than one-third of all deaths worldwide. The stroma of solid tumors also represents a fibrotic lesion. Effective therapies to prevent, or halt the progression, or promote regression, of fibrosis are not yet available. (With permission, Rockey et al. [1])

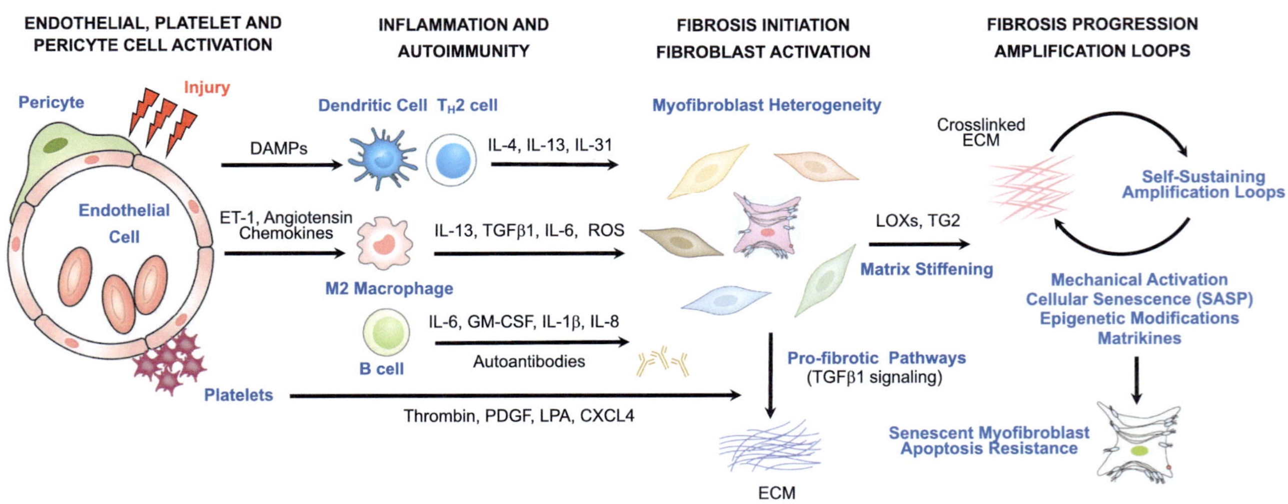

The Extracellular Matrix

The ECM is a complex and dynamic tissue composed of collagens and other large structural proteins such as proteoglycan, fibrillin, fibronectin, and elastin. In addition to its role as a structural scaffold, the biochemical and biophysical properties of the ECM also play a dynamic role in instructing the behavior (differentiation, proliferation, migration, adhesion, biosynthetic capacity, and survival) of stromal cells including fibroblasts. Moreover, the ECM serves as a major reservoir for sequestering growth factors and matricellular proteins. In SSc, excessive connective tissue accumulation results from its overproduction by fibroblasts activated in response to soluble factors, hypoxia and ROS, biochemical and mechanical signals from the surrounding ECM, or via cell–cell interactions [2]. Impaired matrix degradation and turnover and expansion of the pool of ECM-producing stromal cells similarly contribute to the development of persistent and progressive fibrosis.

Collagen Synthesis and Its Regulation

The collagen family comprises over two dozen structural proteins with critical roles in organ development, growth, and differentiation. The ECM of the skin, bones, and tendons is composed largely of type I collagen, with smaller amounts of associated type III collagen. In contrast, type II collagen is found mainly in articular cartilage. Type VI collagen, made primarily by macrophages and adipocytes, is a widely distributed heterotrimer. Enzymatic cleavage of its α3 chain gives rise to endotrophin, which has profibrotic activity. The characteristic triple helix structure of the fibrillar collagens is made possible by the presence of a glycine at every third residue of a repeating Gly-X-Y sequence, where X is a proline and Y is a hydroxyproline. During their biosynthesis, fibrillar collagens undergo extensive enzymatic modifications both inside the cell and additional processing following their secretion. Covalent cross-linking catalyzed by enzymes such as lysyl oxidase-like 2 (LOXL2) and transglutaminase 2 (TG2) stabilizes the collagen fiber network in the extracellular space and impedes matrix turnover.

Type I collagen synthesis is regulated by a number of cues including cytokines and other soluble extracellular factors, ROS, and cell–cell and cell–matrix contact (Table 18.1). Environmental cues allow fibroblasts to respond to dynamic tissue requirements during development and tissue repair [3]. The genes encoding the various collagens harbor cis-acting conserved regulatory elements that are recognized by DNA-binding transcription factors. Among these, Sp1, Ets1, Smad2/3, Egr-1, and CCAAT-binding factor (CBF) stimulate and C/EBP, YB1, c-Krox, and Fli-1 suppress transcription [4]. These transcription factors interact with one another as well as with non-DNA-binding cofactors, scaffold proteins, and chromatin-modifying enzymes such as p300/CBP, PCAF, sirtuins, and histone deacetylases (HDACs). The activities and interactions of transcription factors and cofactors are controlled by extracellular cues. Chromatin-modifying enzymes such as acetyltransferases and HDACs facilitate the access of DNA-binding factors to cognate cis-acting regulatory DNA sequences and enhance transcription [5]. Alterations in the levels, intracellular compartmentaliza-

Fig. 18.2 Pathogenesis of fibrosis in systemic sclerosis: an integrated schematic view. Vascular injury triggers endothelial cell activation and perivascular inflammation, intravascular platelet activation, altered fibrinolysis, and reduced blood flow [2]. Consequent tissue hypoxia and oxidative stress lead to generation of reactive oxygen species (ROS), which directly activates fibroblasts. Activated endothelial cells and platelets secrete endothelin-1, platelet-derived growth factors, thrombin, CXCL4, and LPA, each of which can further activate fibroblasts. Inflammation is associated with secretion of TGF-β1, IL-4, IL-6, IL-13, and IL-31 that drive further activation of fibroblasts and their differentiation into contractile myofibroblasts, which are a heterogeneous population of fibrogenic cells. Myofibroblasts produce large amounts of type I collagen and other matrix components, leading to the initiation of tissue fibrogenesis [8]. Once fibrosis is established, it progresses through multiple self-sustaining amplification loops: (**a**) The matrix undergoes remodeling via matrix cross-linking enzymes such as lysyl oxidases (LOXs) and transglutaminases (TG2), resulting in increased mechanical stiffness. Stiff matrix promotes fibroblast mechanoactivation via mechanotransduction pathways and activation of matrix-bound latent TGF-β via integrin-mediated traction forces [94]; (**b**) myofibroblast persists in the tissue by acquiring a senescent apoptosis-resistant phenotype [194], which is regulated by epigenetic mechanisms; and (**c**) damage-associated matricellular proteins or matrikines such as the alternately spliced EDA-fibronectin, tenascin C, and hyaluronic acid (HA) are sensed by fibroblasts via toll-like receptors (TLRs) and elicit activation [219]. Self-sustaining and cell-autonomous persistent fibroblast activation results in the progression of fibrosis and formation of an intractable scar. Studies with animal models of fibrosis indicate that organ fibrosis is potentially reversible

Table 18.1 Selected extracellular signals that contribute to fibrosis in scleroderma

	Cellular source	Putative role in scleroderma
Growth factors		
TGF-β[a]	Inflammatory cells, platelets, fibroblasts, macrophages, ECM	Promotes myofibroblast differentiation via multiple downstream mechanisms
PDGF	Platelets, macrophages, fibroblasts, endothelium	Stimulates fibroblast proliferation and matrix synthesis
F9/FGFR3	Fibroblasts, γδT cells	Promotes myofibroblast differentiation
CTGF/CCN2	Fibroblasts, endothelium	Promotes myofibroblast differentiation
IGF1/IGBP-3, -5	Fibroblasts	Stimulates expression of profibrotic genes
Ephrin-B2	Endothelial and smooth muscle cells	Soluble EphB2 released by ADAM10 promotes myofibroblast differentiation
Cytokines		
IL-6	Macrophages, B cells, T cells, fibroblasts	Induces collagen expression via JAK/STAT3 and Gremlin-1 pathway
Oncostatin M	Macrophages, T cells, dendritic cells, fibroblasts	Stimulates fibroblast proliferation, migration, and collagen synthesis
IL-31	Th2 cells	Induces collagen via STAT3 pathway
IL-1α	Keratinocytes	Profibrotic, induces macrophages and ILC2 to produce TGF-β and IL-6
IL-1β	Monocytes via inflammasome	Profibrotic via induction of TGF-β and IL-6
IL-33	Immune cells fibroblasts epithelial and endothelial cells	Secreted IL-33 promotes inflammation Nuclear IL-33 regulates Smad3
IL-4	Th2 lymphocytes, mast cells	Stimulates fibroblast proliferation, chemotaxis, and collagen synthesis
IL-13	$CD8^+$ T cells	Promotes collagen synthesis via JAK/STAT6 pathway
IL-35 (p35, EBI3)	Fibroblasts, perivascular inflammatory cells	Promotes myofibroblast differentiation
Chemokines		
MCP1 (CCL2)	Fibroblasts, endothelium, keratinocytes, monocytes	Stimulates collagen production, induces TGF-β
MCP-3 (CCL7)	Keratinocytes, fibroblasts mononuclear cells	Promotes monocyte and T-cell recruitment and stimulates collagen
MIP-1α (CCL3) MIP-1β (CCL4)	Monocytes	Recruit inflammatory cells
Fractalkine (CX3CL1)	Endothelium	Promotes pulmonary hypertension
PF4 (CXCL4)	Megakaryocytes, pDCs	Potent angiostatic factor, a marker of fibrosis and PAH
Peptides		
Angiotensin II	Liver, circulation	Induces TGF-β and collagen Induces vasoconstriction
Endothelin 1	Endothelium, platelets	Mediates some of the profibrotic effects of TGF-β and induces vasoconstriction
Serotonin	Platelets, endothelial cells	Stimulates fibroblast proliferation and collagen synthesis
Proteases		
Thrombin	Circulation	Thrombin via PAR-1 promotes myofibroblast differentiation
Cathepsin B	Circulation	Promotes myofibroblast differentiation
Lipids		
S1P	Platelets, red blood cells	Promotes fibroblast proliferation and myofibroblast differentiation
LPA	Circulation	Induces myofibroblast differentiation
Leukotriene B_4	Myofibroblasts, endothelium, macrophages, T cells	Promotes myofibroblast differentiation via PI3K/Akt/mTOR pathway
ECM components		
Tenascin C Fibronectin EDA	Fibroblasts	TLR4 ligands, which promote myofibroblast differentiation and enhance TGF-β signaling

[a] All factors listed in this table are expressed at elevated levels in scleroderma

tion, activities, or interactions among the various transcription factors, cofactors, and chromatin-modifying enzymes contribute to persistent fibroblast activation in SSc.

Effector Cells of Scleroderma Fibrosis: Fibroblasts and Myofibroblasts

Fibroblasts are versatile stromal cells residing in virtually all tissues that are capable of synthesis, degradation, and remodeling of the ECM. Markers in common use as research tools to identify all fibroblasts include α-smooth muscle actin (α-SMA), vimentin, FSP1, desmin, fibroblast activation protein (FAP), and prolyl hydroxylase. However, no unique markers that specifically identify fibroblasts have been described to date, and the developmental origins of these specialized cells remain unsettled.

Under homeostasis, fibroblasts adhere to, synthesize, degrade, and remodel the ECM in response to minor changes in the biomechanical state, integrity, and biochemical composition of the ECM. However, in the context of chronic tissue injury, fibroblasts become activated and differentiate into professional tissue repair cells named myofibroblasts, which secrete large amounts of ECM macromolecules, cytokines, and growth factors that regulate the physiological wound-healing program. α-SMA+ myofibroblasts also promote ECM contraction and remodeling, ultimately promoting wound closure. Together, these biosynthetic, proinflammatory, contractile, and adhesive functions enable myofibroblasts to execute their primary function, which is rapid and effective wound healing [6]. Whereas under physiologic conditions the fibroblast repair program is tightly regulated and self-limited via diverse mechanisms including apoptosis (programmed cell death), pathological fibrosis is characterized by uncontrolled fibroblast activation and evasion of apoptosis, and persistent ECM accumulation and remodeling, culminating in scarring in the skin, lungs, kidneys, heart, and other organs [7, 8].

Myofibroblast Origin and Heterogeneity

Fibroblasts explanted from lesional skin or fibrotic lungs of patients with SSc represent a heterogeneous and poorly defined cell population. In mass culture, these fibroblasts display relatively stable phenotypic alterations that persist during their serial passage in vitro. Hallmarks of the so-called scleroderma fibroblast phenotype include the following: constitutively enhanced ECM synthesis, adhesion and contraction, secretion of profibrotic cytokines and chemokines, resistance to apoptosis and insensitivity to IFN-γ, and other inhibitory signals. Additionally, SSc fibroblasts spontaneously generate both mitochondrial and Nox4-dependent ROS.

Genome-wide DNA microarray studies reveal that skin fibroblasts explanted from different anatomic locations differ markedly in their pattern of gene expression, suggesting that fibroblasts at different positions in the body axis could be considered distinct differentiated cell types [9, 10]. The apparent fibroblast "positional memory" is governed by epigenetic mechanisms via imprinting by the homeobox (HOX) family transcription factors for the "hox code." Lineage tracing studies in transgenic mice are providing a nuanced and increasingly complex picture of the developmental origins, lineage specificities, and diversity of dermal fibroblasts. These studies reveal that fibroblasts residing within the dermis arise from at least two distinct lineages. One lineage gives rise to the cells of the papillary (upper) dermis, including dermal papilla, whereas the other lineage gives rise to cells in the lower dermis, including reticular fibroblasts, preadipocytes, and adipocytes [11]. A remarkable series of recent studies further illuminate the lineage specificity of cells responsible for fibrosis in the dermis. A fibroblast lineage defined by the embryonic expression of *Engrailed-1* (En1) within the dermis appears to be almost exclusively responsible for the synthesis of connective tissue during skin fibrogenesis [12]. The fibrogenic En1 dermal fibroblasts express the CD26/dipeptidyl peptidase-4 (DPP4) cell surface marker. Ablation of CD26-positive fibroblasts in mice results in mitigated scar formation and diminished experimental skin fibrosis, identifying CD26 as a potential target for antifibrotic therapy [12].

In fibrotic tissues, the pool of biosynthetically activated stromal cells is expanded not only by proliferation of resident fibroblasts, which is not robust, but also by transdifferentiation from other cell lineages, as well as the influx of bone marrow-derived myeloid cells and mesenchymal progenitor cells. Recent advances in cell fate mapping approaches in mice facilitate increasingly accurate characterization of the origin of activated fibroblasts in fibrotic lesions. Several recent studies point to perivascular mesenchymal stem cells called pericytes as the main precursors of collagen-producing cells in fibrosis [13]. Pericytes are mesenchymal stromal cells in the walls of small blood vessels that are normally in intimate contact with the underlying endothelium. Their primary physiologic function is to regulate vascular homeostasis [14]. Such profibrotic precursors were further characterized as a progeny of perivascular PDGFRα^{+}/ADAM12^{+} cells during acute skin and muscle injury [15]. In SSc patients, a marked increase in microvascular pericyte compartment and increased expression of PDGF receptors has been reported. It has been demonstrated that activated pericytes can give rise to collagen-producing myofibroblasts, thus linking microvascular injury and fibrosis [16].

Interestingly, analyses of lung and kidney fibrosis implicated a heterogeneous origin of activated fibroblasts/myofibroblasts. For example, in a mouse model of kidney fibrosis, ~50% of myofibroblasts originated from resident fibroblasts through proliferation, while the rest were derived through differentiation from bone marrow progenitors, with a small proportion originating from endothelial or epithelial cells through endothelial/epithelial-to-mesenchymal transition [17]. Expansion of PDGFRα-positive, collagen-producing local fibroblasts was also observed in bleomycin-induced lung fibrosis [18]. Another major population of collagen-producing myofibroblasts in this model is derived from the FoxD1+ PDGFRα+ NG2+ pericytes [18]. Expansion of PDGFRα-positive cells during organ fibrosis is consistent with the phenotype of transgenic mice expressing activated PDGFRα, which develop fibrosis in multiple organs [19]. Lineage tracing studies of dermal fibrosis support the existence of multiple profibrotic precursor cells. One study showed that Sox2-positive progenitor cells residing within dermal papillae give rise to myofibroblasts accumulating in the fibrotic dermis in response to bleomycin injury [20]. Furthermore, endogenous connective tissue growth factor (CTGF/CCN2) was required for the expansion of these progenitor cells. A more recent study using lineage tracing in a mouse model of SSc indicated that the majority of myofibroblasts in the fibrotic dermis arise from intradermal adipocyte progenitors [21]. These studies need to be interpreted with caution as the precise markers to identify specific cell populations are still lacking. Furthermore, the relevance of the findings from models of experimental injury using lineage tracing transgenic mice to the respective human disease conditions remains to be established and will continue to be a significant challenge.

Myofibroblasts, characterized by expression of cytoskeletal protein α-SMA, synthesize collagens, tissue inhibitors of metalloproteinases (TIMPs), and most other ECM components, are a major source of transforming growth factor beta (TGF-β) secretion and activation during the fibrotic response [22]. Myofibroblasts can originate from resident fibroblasts upon stimulation by TGF-β, a process that also requires the presence of alternately spliced fibronectin (EDA), as well as mechanical tension. Under certain conditions, epithelial cells can undergo transformation into fibroblasts. This process, referred to as epithelial–mesenchymal transition (EMT), plays a vital role during vertebrate embryonic development. Upon stimulation, epithelial cells lose characteristic markers of cell–cell adhesion such as E-cadherin, acquire fibroblast markers such as alpha-smooth muscle actin, desmin, and podoplanin, and display fibroblast features such as collagen synthesis and contractility. Pathological EMT occurs prominently in cancer and is potentially implicated in renal fibrosis, cirrhosis, and idiopathic pulmonary fibrosis [23]. Recent studies suggest that chronic epithelial cell injury is associated with endoplasmic reticulum stress, which may contribute to epithelial cell apoptosis or transdifferentiation [24]. Similar to epithelial cells, vascular endothelial cells can, upon injury, also undergo a transition to fibroblasts. This process, called endothelial–mesenchymal transition (EndMT), has been demonstrated in the liver and other organs in various forms of experimentally induced fibrosis. Both EMT and EndMT processes are triggered by TGF-β and Notch, via Snail, and both appear to be implicated in the generation of tissue fibrosis in SSc [25].

Notwithstanding major advances in our understanding of the cellular origins of myofibroblasts in fibrosis, it is still unclear whether distinct profibrotic cell types carry out specific functions during tissue fibrogenesis. Recent studies using single-cell RNA sequencing (scRNA-seq) have revealed unprecedented insights into the heterogeneity of fibroblasts in healthy and fibrotic skin and other tissues. These studies indicate the presence of heterogeneous fibroblast populations with distinct gene expression profiles in SSc skin and other fibrotic tissues [26–30], suggesting that myofibroblasts may indeed originate from different lineages or exhibit remarkable plasticity, which may actually represent different cellular states. It is tempting to speculate that spatial and temporal accumulation of particular myofibroblast subpopulations or their persistence in specific fibrogenic states contributes to the development of organ fibrosis, a hypothesis that deserves further investigation. Further, loss of specific fibroblastic populations in fibrotic tissue has been also implicated as a potential mechanism in fibrosis in SSc. In particular, it has been reported that a peculiar dermal cell population of CD34+ stromal cells with long dendritic processes, known as telocytes, disappears as skin fibrosis progresses. More recent work suggests that CD34+ telocytes may transition into podoplanin+, CD90+ myofibroblasts in the upper dermis in SSc, further underscoring the plasticity of dermal fibroblasts in response to tissue injury [31].

Pathways Regulating Myofibroblast Activation

Myofibroblast differentiation and activation are regulated by a myriad of profibrotic growth factors, cytokines, and signaling pathways that promote uncontrolled ECM synthesis and remodeling. These mediators show aberrant expression or activity in SSc (Table 18.1, Fig. 18.3) and are known to contribute to fibrosis in mouse models of disease, therefore potentially representing both biomarkers and druggable therapeutic targets. More recent studies have shed light on alternative mechanisms promoting persistent activation of myofibroblasts not only during the initiation but also progression of fibrosis in SSc. These novel mechanisms include cell-autonomous self-amplifying activation loops such as fibroblast mechanoactivation, matrikines, epigenetic mechanisms, and cellular senescence (Fig. 18.2). The following

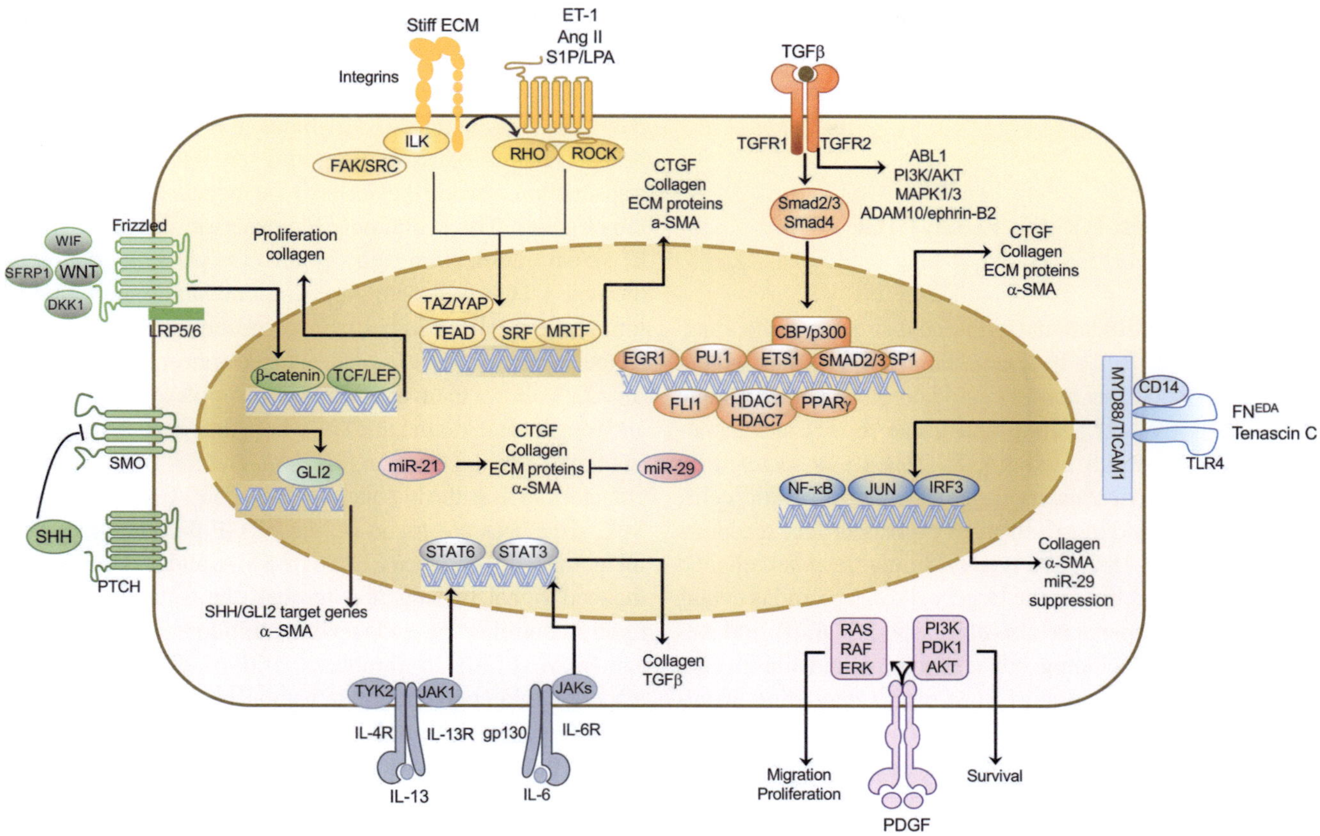

Fig. 18.3 Molecular mechanisms of fibroblast activation in systemic sclerosis. Fibroblast activation and their transdifferentiation into myofibroblasts are regulated by various paracrine and/or autocrine molecules and mechanical stimuli, and this process involves a highly complex and interconnected intracellular signaling cascade. Transforming growth factor-β (TGF-β) signaling has a central role by inducing profibrotic gene expression through activation of canonical SMAD2/3 and SMAD4-dependent and noncanonical pathways and through crosstalk with other intracellular signaling pathways. SMAD2/3 cooperates with other transcriptional activators (e.g., ETS1) to induce the expression of connective tissue growth factor (CTGF), collagen, and other profibrotic genes [220–222]. PU.1 is an activator of the fibrotic phenotype by functioning as a central hub of the network of the profibrotic transcription factors, including TEAD, SMAD3, and AP1 [130]. Transcription activators recruit co-activators, such as p300 and CBP, which relax chromatin structure by catalyzing histone acetylation, with recruitment of the basal transcription machinery and increasing activator-dependent transcription. Levels of p300 are constitutively elevated in SSc fibroblasts [128]. In addition, TGF-β signaling promotes profibrotic gene expression by inactivating the transcriptional repressors Friend leukemia integration 1 (FLI1) and peroxisome proliferator-activated receptor-γ (PPARγ) [207, 223]. Noncanonical TGF-β signaling pathways with relevance to fibrosis include focal adhesion kinase (FAK), ABL1, phosphatidylinositol 3-kinase (PI3K), mitogen-activated protein kinase 1 (MAPK1)–MAPK3 (MAPK1/3), p38, endoglin, ADAM10/ephrin-B2 [224], and SMAD1 pathways [225]. The ABL1 pathway, for example, regulates the profibrotic transcription factor early growth response 1 (EGR1) [226]. Mechanical stress, sensed by integrins, also has a pivotal role in the formation of myofibroblasts through induction of α-smooth muscle actin (α-SMA), CTGF, and tenascin C, among others. Mechanical stimulation activates integrin-linked protein kinase (ILK), RhoA, and F-actin formation. Moreover, the profibrotic effects of CTGF are mediated through the integrin/SRC pathway in dermal fibroblasts [227]. Two known transcriptional regulatory pathways mediate the cellular response to mechanical signals: myocardin-related transcription factors, MKL/myocardin-like protein 1 (MKL1), MKL2, and serum response factor (SRF) and the components of the Hippo pathway, YAP, and WW domain-containing transcription regulator protein 1 (WWTR1) [45, 77]. Alternatively, this pathway can be stimulated by RHO small GTPase and F-actin signaling, which is activated by endothelin 1, angiotensin II, and sphingosine 1 phosphate/lysophosphatidic acid (S1P/LPA). The developmental pathways, Hedgehog and WNT, promote fibrosis through the crosstalk with the TGF-β signaling pathway. These pathways are found to be hyperactivated in fibrotic lesions [83, 91]. TGF-β inhibits expression of WNT signaling inhibitors, SFRP1 and DKK1 [122]. WNT inhibitory factor 1 (WIF1) is a ROS target and is constitutively downregulated in fibroblasts derived from patients with systemic sclerosis [228]. Connective tissue molecules, such as an alternately spliced variant of fibronectin (Fn^{EDA}) and tenascin C, which are induced by TGF-β and constitutively upregulated in systemic sclerosis, represent damage-associated molecular patterns (DAMPs) that serve as endogenous ligands of toll-like receptor 4 (TLR4) [229]. The TLR4-mediated profibrotic pathway is not yet fully understood, but it might involve suppression of antifibrotic microRNA-29 (miR-29) [134, 135]. Of note, miR-21 is suggested to be involved in promoting the fibrotic response by suppressing an inhibitor of the TGF-β noncanonical pathway, SMAD7 [133]. IL-6 and IL-13 are pleiotropic cytokines, which directly or indirectly through TGF-β, drive collagen production, and promote fibrotic matrix deposition [158, 230]. Finally, platelet-derived growth factor (PDGF) signaling stimulates fibroblast migration, proliferation, survival, and matrix gene expression [231]

section discusses established and emerging mechanisms responsible for promoting myofibroblast activation and persistence during the initiation and progression of tissue fibrosis.

Growth Factors: TGF-β1, PDGF, CTGF

TGF-β1

TGF-β1 is a multifunctional cytokine that belongs the transforming growth factor beta superfamily. TGF-β1 is widely considered to be the master regulator of both physiologic fibrogenesis (wound healing and tissue repair) and pathological fibrosis in all organs [32]. TGF-β1 is secreted by platelets, monocytes/macrophages, T cells, dendritic cells, and fibroblasts, and most cell types express surface receptors for TGF-β1 (Fig. 18.2). The type of cellular response elicited by TGF-β1 is specific for the target cell lineage and is exquisitely context-dependent. In fibroblasts, TGF-β1 induces ECM synthesis including collagen type I and fibronectin, suppresses the production of most matrix-degrading metalloproteinases, promotes ECM contraction via induction of α-SMA and fibroblast resistance to apoptosis, all features of the so-called myofibroblast phenotype. In endothelial and epithelial cells, TGF-β1 also elicits EMT and EndMT, resulting in the formation of more myofibroblasts derived from these cells types [33]. A recent study suggests that adipocytic progenitor cells also undergo a similar myofibroblast transition in response to TGF-β1. Importantly, TGF-β1 is also a potent immunosuppressor by inhibiting immune cell proliferation and function, which has limited the efficacy of anti-TGF-β neutralizing antibodies for the treatment of systemic sclerosis due to on-target proinflammatory side effects.

Importantly, TGF-β1 is secreted and stored within the ECM in a latent form bound to fibronectin and fibrillin through latency-associated peptide (LAP) and latent TGF-β-binding proteins (LTBPs). This mechanism allows cells to activate TGF-β1 in precisely localized areas following tissue injury. The activation of latent TGF-β1 is a complex process controlled in part by fibrillin-1 and is mediated by surface integrins including αvβ6 (on epithelial cells), αvβ8 (on dendritic cells), αvβ5 (on fibroblasts), and potentially additional integrins expressed in cell type-specific manner; thrombospondins, and proteolytic enzymes such as MMP14, thrombin, and plasmin. These findings highlight the fact that TGF-β1 bioavailability and activity are regulated primarily through its spatially and temporally restricted activation from the latent form, and deregulation of this complex process is implicated in diseases such as systemic sclerosis and other fibrotic diseases. Small molecules and neutralizing antibodies targeting integrins involved in TGF-β1 activation are currently being investigating in multiple clinical trials for the treatment of fibrotic diseases [34].

Once activated, TGF-β1 signaling induces fibroblast-to-myofibroblast differentiation through Smad-dependent (canonical) and Smad-independent (noncanonical) signaling pathways (Fig. 18.3). TGF-β1 binds to its type II cell membrane receptor (ALK5), triggering an intracellular signal transduction cascade that leads to the induction of profibrotic target genes. The evolutionarily conserved canonical TGF-β1 signal transduction pathway involves phosphorylation of the type I TGF-β receptor, a serine-threonine kinase that in turn phosphorylates downstream cytosolic signal transducers called Smads [35]. Ligand-induced phosphorylation of Smad2/3 allows them to form heterocomplexes with Smad4 and translocate into the nucleus where they bind to a consensus Smad-binding element (SBE) and recruit transcriptional cofactors such as the histone acetylase p300/CBP. Conserved SBE sequences are found in many TGF-β-inducible genes, including type I collagens, PAI-1, α-SMA, and CTGF. Ligand-induced signal transduction through the Smad pathway is tightly controlled by endogenous inhibitors such as Smad7 and BAMBI [36]. In fibroblasts, TGF-β1 elicits profibrotic responses via concomitant activation of the so-called non-Smad (noncanonical) pathways, which include non-receptor protein tyrosine kinases such as c-Abl [37], p38 [38] and JNK, focal adhesion kinase (FAK) [39], ROCK [40], and TGF-β-activated kinase (TAK1) [41]. Additional mechanisms implicate metalloproteinases such as ADAM10, which activates profibrotic factors such as ephrin-B2 via proteolytic cleavage [42], lipid kinases such as PI3 kinase and its downstream target Akt [38], the calcium-dependent phosphatase calcineurin, and NADPH oxidase 4 (NOX4) [43]. Moreover, transcriptional co-activators such as Yes-associated protein (YAP), transcriptional co-activator with PDZ binding motif, WWTR1 (TAZ) [44], and myocardin-related transcription factors (MRTFs) [45] have also been implicated in pathological fibrosis. Multiple agents for therapeutic targeting of non-Smad signaling pathways have shown promising antifibrotic effects in preclinical disease models (Fig. 18.3).

Platelet-Derived Growth Factors (PDGFs)

Platelet-derived growth factors are disulfide-bonded heterodimeric proteins that act mainly on stromal cells and regulate the wound-healing process. Originally isolated from platelets, PDGF isoforms are also secreted from macrophages, endothelial cells, and fibroblasts. PDGF, signaling via the alpha and beta receptors, acts as a potent mitogen and chemoattractant for fibroblasts. Moreover, in fibroblasts, PDGF induces ROS generation and stimulates the synthesis of collagen, fibronectin, proteoglycans, and the secretion of TGF-β1, MCP-1, and IL-6 [46]. Transgenic mice expressing a constitutively active mutant PDGF alpha receptor (PDGFRα) develop progressive fibrosis in the skin and multiple organs [19]. Lesional skin fibroblasts explanted from SSc patients show elevated expression of both PDGF and

PDGF beta receptor [47, 48], and PDGF levels are increased in the bronchoalveolar lavage fluid. In some SSc patients, functional circulating antibodies targeting the PDGF receptor have been described [49]. These serum autoantibodies induce fibroblast activation and ROS generation in vitro; however, they are not specific for SSc and have also been detected in patients with graft-versus-host disease.

Connective Tissue Growth Factor (CTGF/CCN2)

CTGF is a 40 kDa cysteine-rich member of the CCN early-response gene family increasingly implicated, along with TGF-ß, in all forms of pathological fibrosis. This matricellular growth factor is involved in normal angiogenesis, wound healing, and development Mice lacking CCN2 die at birth. Normal tissues have undetectable levels of CTGF, but its expression is markedly elevated in fibrotic conditions. Serum levels of CTGF correlate with the extent of skin and pulmonary fibrosis in SSc patients. The expression of CTGF is readily induced in normal fibroblasts by TGF-β, IL-4, and VEGF, whereas tumor necrosis factor-α (TNF-α) and iloprost block stimulation. Transgenic mice overexpressing CTGF develop SSc-like skin fibrosis and microvascular pathology [50]. Further support for the pathogenic role of CTGF in fibrosis was provided by a study that showed that ablation of *CCN2* in the fibroblast precursor cells attenuated the development of bleomycin-induced in mice [20]. In vitro, CTGF exerts multiple profibrotic effects in normal fibroblasts. Because many of these CTGF effects parallel those induced by TGF-β, it has been suggested that TGF-β responses are mediated through endogenous CTGF. However, the nature of the cellular CTGF receptors and the mechanism underlying CTGF profibrotic responses remain incompletely characterized.

Bioactive Lipids: LPA and LTB4

Lysophosphatidic Acid (LPA)

LPA, generated locally via the hydrolysis of membrane phospholipids, exerts multiple biological activities via G-protein-coupled transmembrane receptors. LPA was shown to induce fibroblast chemotaxis and CTGF production [51, 52]. Significantly, levels of LPA are elevated in the lungs of patients with pulmonary fibrosis [53, 54]. Moreover, *LPA1* knockout mice are protected from bleomycin-induced skin and lung fibrosis. Studies have shown that LPA induces avβ6 integrin-mediated activation of latent TGF-β in epithelial cells, contributing to sustained autocrine and paracrine TGF-β signaling [52]. An LPA_1 orally selective receptor antagonist SAR100842 was shown to reverse myofibroblast differentiation in cultured SSc fibroblasts and reduce skin collagen content and Wnt pathway activation in Tsk1 model [55]. A double-blind, randomized, placebo-controlled phase IIa study of SAR100842 showed good safety and tolerability, as well as some promising clinical and biological changes in patients with SSc [56].

Leukotriene B4 (LTB4)

The leukotrienes are a family of arachidonic acid-derived lipid mediators with proinflammatory properties. Levels of leukotriene B4 (LTB4) and LTE4 are significantly elevated in bronchoalveolar lavage (BAL) fluids of patients with SSc-ILD [57]. Similarly, serum levels of LTB4 are elevated in SSc patients and correlate with disease severity and ILD [58]. Moreover, increased expression of LTB4 hydrolase (LTB4H) and a LTB4 receptor BLT1 is present in affected skin and lungs of SSc patients, including strong expression in myofibroblasts and endothelial cells [58]. Mechanistically, the LTB4-BLT1 axis promotes myofibroblast differentiation and endothelial-to-mesenchymal transition via activation of the mTOR/PI3K pathway, independent of TGF-β. Serum levels of LTB4 are also elevated in patients with CTD-PAH [59].

Vasoactive Peptides: Angiotensin II and Endothelin 1

Angiotensin II (Ang II)

Ang II, a key component of the renin–angiotensin system (RAS), is a vasoactive peptide that regulates vascular constriction, salt, and water retention and increases vascular blood pressure [60]. Recent studies have demonstrated that Ang II is also a potent profibrotic molecule that induces kidney, liver, heart, and skin fibrosis in animal models [61]. Ang II signals through two receptors, angiotensin receptor 1 (AT_1R) and angiotensin receptor 2 (AT_2R). Locally, AT_1R activation stimulates many of the signaling pathways including tyrosine kinases, c-Src, FAK, and PI3K, as well as RhoA/Rho kinase and MAP kinase families [60]. The fibrogenic effects of Ang II are also mediated through activation of TGF-β signaling, as well as through the upregulation of NOX-4 and subsequent generation of ROS. The role of AT_2R in pathogenesis is less known, and some studies suggest that it may have a protective and antifibrotic function by counteracting many AT_1R-mediated effects. Other components of the "protective arm" of RAS include the newly described Ang-derived small peptides Ang (1–7), which signal through the G protein-coupled receptor Mas, as well as angiotensin-converting enzyme 2 (ACE2) that selectively degrades Ang II and generates Ang (1–7). Studies in rodent models of pulmonary and dermal fibrosis demonstrated that blockade of the Ang II/AT_1R axis has beneficial therapeutic effects [62, 63]. A different strategy of upregulating the ACE2/Ang-(1–7)/Mas axis similarly prevented lung fibrosis and pulmonary hypertension [64, 65].

Endothelin 1 (ET-1)

ET-1 signaling network consists of a family of three vasoactive peptides, ET1, ET2, and ET3, which signal through two distinct G protein-coupled receptors, ET_AR and ET_BR. ET1; the best characterized isoform is known for its pleiotropic biological effects, including a well-documented role in tissue fibrosis [66]. ET-1 is induced by TGF-β in dermal fibroblasts and mediates some of its profibrotic effects [67]. Potent profibrotic effects of ET-1 were confirmed in vivo either by overexpressing ET-1 in murine skin or lungs or by blocking ET-1 signaling in bleomycin-induced pulmonary or dermal fibrosis [67–69]. Expression of ET-1 and its receptors is elevated in SSc skin [70]. Moreover, functional and pathogenic antibodies directed against AT_1R and ET_AR were identified in patients with SSc and linked to increased prevalence of SSc-related vascular and fibrotic complications and higher risk for SSc-induced mortality [71, 72].

Developmental Pathways Implicated in Fibrosis: Hippo, Wnt, Jagged/Notch, and Hedgehog

Hippo

The Hippo pathway is an evolutionarily conserved intracellular signaling cascade important in regulating cell proliferation, apoptosis, and differentiation [73–75]. The core Hippo signaling pathway consists of serine/threonine protein kinases MST1/2 (the sterile 20-like kinases) and LATS1/2 (large tumor suppressor like kinases 1 and 2) that regulate the phosphorylation of transcriptional co-activators YAP/TAZ (Fig. 18.3). In SSc fibroblasts, both TGF-β and mechanical signaling have been shown to promote YAP/TAZ phosphorylation, ultimately driving their translocation to the nucleus where they function as transcriptional co-activators by interacting with their primary partner TEAD, as well as a number of other transcription factors, including Smads, Egr1, and Runx to regulate specific subsets of profibrotic genes [76]. Expression of TAZ and YAP is increased in fibroblasts in SSc skin [77].

Wingless-Related Integration Site (Wnt)

The Wnt pathway plays fundamental roles in normal embryogenesis, and their deregulation is implicated in various disorders including fibrosis and SSc [78]. The Wnts comprise a family of poorly soluble glycoproteins with dual roles in cell–cell adhesion and transcriptional regulation. Transcription of a large number of profibrotic genes is induced by Wnt ligands through β-catenin and YAP/TAZ, which act as components of the β-catenin destruction complex (Fig. 18.3) [79]. On the other hand, TAZ/YAP can also dampen Wnt responses by sequestering β-catenin in the cytoplasm. The functional outcomes of the interplay between these two signaling pathways depend on the activation status of each pathway and the cellular context [80]. In mice, transgenic overexpression of Wnt10b, or a constitutively active mutant β-catenin, leads to exuberant wound-healing responses, the development of SSc-like dermal fibrosis, and increased collagen accumulation in the skin [81–83]. In humans, lungs from patients with idiopathic and SSc-associated pulmonary fibrosis show increased nuclear β-catenin accumulation at fibrotic foci [84, 85]. Transcriptome profiling of SSc skin biopsies shows elevated expression of multiple Wnt ligands, Wnt receptors, and Wnt targets. In a pilot randomized, placebo-controlled trial, treatment with a topical inhibitor of β-catenin/CBP complex, promoted regeneration of adipocytes, and sebocytes without affecting fibrosis [86].

Notch

Notch is a transmembrane receptor that is activated by its ligand Jagged. The Jagged–Notch axis has fundamental roles in embryonic development, wound healing, and tissue repair. Notch signaling via Snail regulates endothelial cell responses including myofibroblast differentiation through the process of endothelial–mesenchymal transition (EndMT), which links vascular injury and fibrosis in SSc. A mouse model of SSc was shown to exhibit activated Notch signaling in the skin and lungs, and expression of ADAM-17, a proteinase induced by TGF-β and ROS that initiates Notch signal transduction, was elevated in SSc skin biopsies [87].

Hedgehog

The Hedgehog (Hh) family of ligands plays key role in developmental processes and is also important in tissue repair and regeneration in adults [88]. It is noteworthy that like Notch and other morphogens, HH signaling is also regulated at the level of the primary cilia. Sonic hedgehog (Shh), the most widely expressed and best characterized member of the HH ligand family in mammalian tissues, binds to its transmembrane receptor Patched 1 (Ptch1). Once HH is bound to Ptch1, it relieves repression of smoothened (Smo) and triggers intracellular signaling cascades downstream from Smo. The transcription factors Gli1, Gli2, and Gli3 mediate HH target gene expression. The primary cilia play a fundamental but incompletely understood complex role in the regulation of canonical and noncanonical HH signaling, and aberrant primary cilia formation or function may be linked to various forms of fibrosis. Accumulating evidence links aberrant HH signaling to pathological fibrosis in the liver, kidney, and lungs [89]. Aberrant activation of the Hh signaling has also been implicated in SSc. For instance, serum levels of SHH are elevated in diffuse SSc patients and correlate with fibrotic and vascular manifestations [90]. Several components of the Hh signaling pathway, including SHH, Gli-1, Gli-2, and Hh acetyltransferase (HHAT), are upregulated in SSc skin [91, 92]. Both TGF-ß and canonical Wnt signaling stimulated SHH expression in dermal fibroblasts. In fibroblasts, treatment with SHH stimulated collagen gene expression and myofibroblast transdifferentiation. In vivo studies confirmed the profibrotic role of the Hh pathway in dermal fibrosis [91, 92].

Although Wnt, Hippo, Notch, and Hh developmental pathways are attractive as potential targets for antifibrotic therapies, due to their important physiologic role in stem cell function, long-term blockade of these morphogens may be associated with substantial toxicity, especially in tissues with high cell turnover. However, therapeutic effects with minimal toxicity were achieved by low doses of combined Hedgehog/Wnt or Hedgehog/Notch inhibitors. Combination therapies demonstrated additive antifibrotic effects in preventive as well as therapeutic regimes and were well-tolerated [93].

Feedback Amplification Loops

Once activated, myofibroblasts persist within fibrotic tissues through multiple self-sustaining amplification loops including (a) fibroblast mechanoactivation by matrix stiffness, (b) epigenetic mechanisms, and (c) matrikines (Fig. 18.2). Cell-autonomous persistent fibroblast activation results in the progression of fibrosis and ultimately organ failure.

Mechanical Factors: Matrix Stiffness

The hallmark of fibrotic diseases including SSc is pathological ECM deposition, remodeling, and stiffening. Compelling evidence suggests that increased matrix stiffness, traditionally thought to simply be a consequence of pathological fibrosis, is in fact also a major contributing factor to its pathogenesis [94]. Recent studies indicate that the mechanical properties of the ECM directly trigger fibroblast mechanoactivation, ECM synthesis, and survival [8, 95]. These findings have led to the emergence of a novel fibrosis paradigm: That matrix rigidity and tension are themselves responsible for promoting, amplifying, and sustaining the pathological fibrotic process [94, 96]. Matrix stiffness increases from 0.5–2 kilopascals (kPa) in healthy tissues up to 25–100 kPa in fibrotic organs affected in SSc such as the skin, lungs, and heart [34, 94]. Noteworthy, recent studies have also shown that increased matrix stiffness precedes the formation of myofibroblasts and the development of fibrosis, indicating that matrix stiffness may indeed drive fibrogenic processes including fibroblast activation [97]. In vitro studies show that explanted fibroblasts plated on substrates of increasing rigidity promote stiffness-dependent upregulation of profibrotic genes including type I collagen and α-SMA, supporting a major role for mechanical forces at promoting myofibroblast formation [44, 96, 98]. In addition to fibrosis initiation, matrix stiffening has been proposed as a mechanism that promotes fibrosis progression by locking myofibroblasts in a mechanical positive feedback loop [34, 94]. In this mechanism, stiffness-activated fibroblasts further promote pathologic ECM remodeling and progressive matrix stiffening, ultimately promoting a self-reinforcing vicious cycle of fibrosis by driving mechanoactivation of surrounding quiescent fibroblasts (Fig. 18.2).

The precise mechanisms whereby change in matrix stiffness drives mechanoactivation of fibroblasts are not well understood but certainly involve the activation of mechanotransduction signaling pathways. These cellular pathways enable fibroblasts to convert biophysical cues such as matrix stiffness into biochemical signaling pathways that ultimately regulate gene expression programs and cell behavior [99]. Fibroblast mechanotransduction pathways are initiated by cell surface integrins and matrix receptors that mechanically link the actin cytoskeleton to the ECM via focal adhesions [94]. The composition and activity of integrin adhesion complexes are regulated by matrix stiffness by controlling the extent of traction forces produced by cells. For instance, cell-generated traction forces directly modulate the activity of focal adhesion proteins such as FAK by promoting force-dependent stretching of FAK, which exposes and activates its catalytic domain [100]. On soft matrices, the resistance of the ECM is low and therefore cell-generated traction forces are not able to promote FAK stretching and activation. On the contrary, stiff matrices enable higher traction forces by cells through integrin-based adhesions, leading to FAK stretching, activation, and the initiation of mechanochemical signaling via downstream phosphorylation of FAK targets [101]. Recent work has identified ROCK as a major downstream mediator of FAK signaling in fibroblasts [102]. ROCK activation drives actomyosin contractions and the formation of actin stress fibers, which promote cytoplasmic-to-nuclear translocation of transcriptional co-activators YAP/TAZ and MRTFs [44, 45, 103–106]. Accordingly, disruption of F-actin or inhibition of the small GTPase RhoA results in YAP/TAZ inactivation [106, 107]. Studies in lung fibroblasts have confirmed the role of YAP/TAZ as sensors of matrix stiffness and revealed that YAP/TAZ regulates profibrotic gene expression, including PAI-I and type I collagen in a TGF-β-independent manner in vitro [44]. However, mechanical YAP/TAZ signaling directly interacts with several other signaling pathways such as TGF-β/Smad, Wnt/β-catenin, and GPCRs to coordinate inputs from the intracellular signaling network with the cues from the cell's environment, ultimately controlling full activation of myofibroblasts [76, 80, 108] (Fig. 18.3). YAP and, especially, TAZ are prominently expressed in fibrotic, but not in healthy lung tissues [44]. MRTFs represent another group of mechanosensitive transcription activators regulated by matrix stiffness; however, the mode of their activation appears to be distinct from that of YAP/TAZ [109]. MRTF-A is sequestered in the cytoplasm by monomeric G-actin and is released upon Rho-induced actin polymerization [109]. MRTF-A promotes a myofibroblast phenotype by inducing α-SMA and collagen expression [110]. Integrin, FAK, ROCK, YAP/TAZ, and MRTF expression levels and activation states have been reported upregulated in SSc and other fibrotic disorders, and pharmacological inhibition of these mechanotransducers mitigates fibrosis in preclinical models [34]. In addition to fibroblast mechanoactivation, matrix stiffness has been shown to promote evasion of apoptosis in myofibroblasts [8, 98] and self-activation of matrix-bound latent TGF-β [111], further promoting a persistent activated myofibroblast phenotype and progression of organ fibrosis. Understanding the mechanotransductive pathways that couple alterations in matrix stiffness to fibroblast activation and survival might identify novel strategies to control fibrosis [34, 94].

Epigenetic Reprogramming and Noncoding RNAs in Fibrosis

Cell type-specific epigenetic alterations in SSc are associated with persistent and heritable acquired changes in fibroblast function. Although not fully understood, TGF-β and other inflammatory cytokines secreted by inflammatory cells during early stages of SSc are among the factors implicated in the reprogramming of resident stromal cells into metabolically active, matrix-producing myofibroblasts [112, 113]. Indeed, activation of the major profibrotic programs, including TGF-β, WNT, and NOTCH pathways, in SSc fibroblasts involves epigenetic modifications including DNA and histone methylation, additional histone modifications, and noncoding RNAs [114–116].

DNA methylation is the most widely studied epigenetic modification in SSc. A genome-wide DNA methylation analysis of fibroblasts revealed a large number of differentially methylated CpG sites in SSc [117]. The majority of the differentially methylated genes were hypomethylated in both lcSSc and dcSSc fibroblasts. Although lcSSc and dcSSc show largely distinct methylation patterns, a subgroup of genes, including genes with known profibrotic roles such as ADAM12, and transcription factors RUNX1, RUNX2, and RUNX3, were present in both SSc subsets. Moreover, components of the WNT/β-catenin pathway were among the hypomethylated genes in both SSc subsets. Conversely, increased DNA methylation was associated with silencing endogenous negative regulators of collagen gene expression in SSc owing to increased levels of the enzymes involved in DNA methylation: DNA methyltransferase 3A (DNMT3A) and DNMT1 and a protein that binds methylated DNA and mediates transcriptional repression, called methyl cap-binding protein 2 (MeCP2) expressed in SSc fibroblasts [118, 119]. Studies demonstrated that two transcription factors shown to inhibit fibrotic gene expression, KLF5 and FLI1, were simultaneously repressed at the epigenetic level through the increased promoter methylation and silencing [120, 121]. Likewise, reduced expression of the endogenous antagonists of the WNT pathway, Dickkopf-related protein 1 (DKK1) and secreted frizzled-related protein 1 (SFRP1), has been associated with the hypermethylation of their promoters, while another WNT pathway inhibitor Wnt inhibitory factor 1 (WIF1) was silenced by promoter histone deacetylation [46, 122].

Posttranslation modifications of histones, including methylation and acetylation, represent another major epigenetic mechanism [116]. One such modification is trimethylation of lysine 27 of histone 3 (H3K27me3), which is mediated by the histone methyltransferase enhancer of zeste homolog 2 (EZH2). Both H3K27me3 and EZH2 are elevated in SSc fibroblasts and promote fibrotic phenotype [123]. Further studies showed that EZH2/H3K27me3 contributes to activation of the NOTCH pathway by downregulating miR-34a, an inhibitor of the NOTCH pathway-related genes [124]. Interestingly, another epigenetic mediator, long noncoding RNA HOX transcript antisense RNA (HOTAIR), which is upregulated in SSc fibroblasts, was identified as an upstream regulator of the EZH2/H3K27me3/miR-34a/Notch pathway [125]. Although levels of histone deacetylases (HDACs) have been reported to be either elevated or reduced in SSc, pharmacological HDAC inhibition in healthy subject fibroblasts resulted in suppression of fibrotic responses [126, 127]. The levels of p300, a histone acetyltransferase, are elevated in SSc fibroblasts, and p300 promotes fibrotic responses by enhancing stimulation of collagen gene transcription [128]. SSc fibroblasts spontaneously produce excessive amounts of TGF-β2, which is mediated by the p300-dependent histone acetylation of the TGF-β2 enhancer [129]. The sustained activity of the TGF-β2 enhancer also requires NF-κB and the bromodomain-containing protein 4 (BRD4) [129].

Epigenetic mechanisms also underlie the aberrant expression of transcription factor PU.1 (*SPI1*), a member of the ETS family of transcription factors. PU.1 plays a central role in regulating the switch between the profibrotic and the proinflammatory phenotypes in dermal fibroblasts [130]. Overexpression of PU.1 in resting fibroblasts was sufficient to induce profibrotic genes, while inhibition of PU.1 repressed this phenotype. Induction of the proinflammatory phenotype required inhibition of miR-155, in addition to the silencing of PU.1. Although, not yet fully investigated, EZH2-dependent methylation was implicated in suppression of PU.1 in resting fibroblasts [130].

To assess the global epigenetic landscape of various cell types contributing to SSc, H. Chang and colleagues used the assay of transposase accessible chromatin (ATAC-seq) approach to investigate the active DNA elements of resident cell types isolated from healthy controls and clinically affected and unaffected SSc skin [131]. The study revealed the pivotal role of dendritic cells (DCs), and especially conventional DCs, as a major epigenetic driver in the pathogenesis of SSc. DCs displayed the greatest disease-associated changes in chromatin accessibility and the highest enrichment of SSc-associated single-nucleotide polymorphisms (SNPs). Increased cDC infiltrates were present in SSc skin, and DC signature genes were most significantly correlated with skin fibrosis. As DCs remain relatively understudied in SSc, further investigations of the novel pathways identified in this study are needed to better understand the consequences of defective communication between the epigenetically altered DCs and skin resident cells during progression of pathological processes in SSc.

The ATAC-seq approach also revealed reduction of chromatin accessibility in endothelial cells and fibroblasts cultured from SSc skin [132]. Interestingly, the differentially accessible chromosome loci in both endothelial cells and fibroblasts were enriched in pathways and ontology terms related to the nervous system, including axon guidance pathways and synaptic-related genes. Among the functionally validated differentially expressed genes in endothelial cells were neurexin 1 (NRXN1) and an ETS family member ETV2, as well as snail (SNAI1), suggesting that these pathways may directly contribute to the defective angiogenesis in SSc.

A very large family of noncoding RNAs (ncRNA), including microRNAs (miRNA) and long ncRNAs, emerged as critical regulators of gene expression in SSc fibrosis. Of particular interest are miR-21 and miR-29. Both microRNAs show aberrant expression in patients with SSc, and may contribute to pathogenesis. On one hand, miR-21, the level of which is elevated in SSc fibroblasts, suppresses the expression of antifibrotic Smad7, thereby promoting expression of profibrotic genes [133]. On the other hand, miR-29, the level of which is reduced in SSc fibroblasts and which is suppressed by fibrotic stimuli, has inhibitory effects on fibrotic gene expression [134, 135]. Many other miRNAs with regulatory roles in SSc fibrosis have been uncovered to date, reviewed in [116].

The less studied lncRNAs can reside in different cellular compartments, where they can interact with nucleic acids or proteins, suggesting their diverse roles in regulating cellular function [136]. Indeed, several lncRNAs, including HOTAIR, XIST, and H19X, have already been implicated in regulation of the fibrotic programs in SSc [125, 137, 138]. Of interest is a human-specific nuclear lncRNA H19X. H19X is upregulated in SSc and other fibrotic diseases and is required for matrix remodeling, as well as survival of myofibroblasts [137]. H19X exerts its profibrotic effects by repressing transcription of the damage-inducible transcript 4-like protein (DDITL4), which functions as an inhibitor of the TGF-β pathway. Remarkably, ncRNAs can be detected in the circulation and exert biological activities when incorporated into microvesicles. Although much remains to be learned about the full spectrum, regulation, and mechanism of action of aberrant miRNAs in SSc, these noncoding RNAs may serve as both biomarkers and therapeutic targets in the future.

Matrikines and Toll-Like Receptor (TLR) Signaling

Damage-associated molecular patterns (DAMPs) are biologically active molecules generated at sites of tissue injury in response to mechanical damage, inflammation, autoimmunity, and oxidative stress (Fig. 18.2). The DAMPs shape biological responses in immune and stromal cells via activation of Toll-like receptors (TLRs). TLRs are located at the cell surface (TLR2 and TLR4) or on endosomal membranes (TLR3, TLR7 and TLR9) in most cell types. The expression of both TLR3 and TLR4 is elevated in SSc skin and lung biopsies, and levels correlate with disease severity and progression. In addition, the expression levels of endogenous "damage-associated molecular pattern" TLR4 ligands such as alternatively spliced form of fibronectin containing an extra domain A (fibronectin EDA), and tenascin C, are similarly upregulated in the skin and lungs of patients with SSc and serve as markers of tissue fibrosis. These molecules represent damage-associated matricellular proteins, also known as matrikines. In vitro, activation of TLR4 signaling via profibrotic matrikines drives myofibroblast activation and increases sensitivity of fibroblasts to profibrotic effects of TGF-β1 (Fig. 18.3). In vivo, mice lacking either TLR4, or endogenous TLR4 ligands fibronectin EDA or Tenascin C exhibit reduced skin, lung, and cardiac fibrosis when challenged with bleomycin or angiotensin II. TLR9, expressed on endosomes, recognizes nucleic acids, primarily unmethylated CpG-containing bacterial and viral DNA. While TLR9 stimulation on fibroblasts elicits fibrotic responses in vitro, the precise role of TLR9 in fibrosis and SSc remains to be clarified. The TLR3 ligand poly(I:C) causes dramatic induction of type I IFN, as well as IL-6 and other inflammatory cytokines in normal fibroblasts, and blocks TGF-β-induced fibrotic responses [139].

Paracrine Mediators Released by Immune Cells, Keratinocytes, and Endothelial Cells

Immune cells are the primary source of paracrine mediators that contribute to activation of the stromal cells leading to excessive extracellular matrix production (Fig. 18.2).

Immune cell infiltrates consisting of M1 and M2 macrophages, CD8+ and CD4+ T cells, and B cells, are frequently found in the perivascular areas during early stages of the disease suggesting that these cells may play key roles in disease initiation [140, 141]. The section below discusses how molecular signals between immune cells and fibroblasts mutually regulate fibrosis. While the immune cells are considered the main producers of the proinflammatory and profibrotic mediators, other tissue-resident cells, including keratinocytes and endothelial cells, also become activated providing additional source of mediators contributing to fibroblast activation.

Monocytes/Macrophages

Activated monocytes and macrophages (MΦ) have emerged as central mediators of inflammation and fibrosis in SSc. As a result of their plasticity and heterogeneity, MΦ exert a wide range of proinflammatory and profibrotic responses. In SSc, both circulating undifferentiated monocytes and in vitro differentiated MΦ display surface markers consisting of a mix of classically (M1) and alternatively (M2) activated MΦ [142, 143]. Patients with lung involvement have a higher proportion of M2 and mixed M1/M2 MΦ populations [144]. Molecular characterization of M-CSF monocyte-derived macrophages (MDM) obtained from SSc patients demonstrated altered expression of a large number of genes including downregulation of IFN-γ related genes and upregulation of genes related to glycolysis, MTORC1 signaling, and oxidative phosphorylation [145]. In addition to interferon-related genes, SSc monocytes are also characterized by an increased expression of profibrotic cytokines [146–148].

Undifferentiated SSc monocytes were shown to secrete increased amounts of CCL2, IL-6, and TGF-β [149]. Notably, exposure to SSc plasma conferred SSc immunophenotype to healthy donor monocytes, and conversely incubation of SSc monocytes with plasma from healthy donors reduced this phenotype, suggesting that activation of monocytes may be induced by the mediators present in circulation of SSc patients. Furthermore, monocytes differentiated in SSc plasma acquired profibrotic characteristics and induced expression of α-SMA in co-culture with fibroblasts [149]. These findings are consistent with the concept of "trained immunity" that proposes long-term changes in innate immune cells in response to antigenic challenge through epigenetic and metabolic reprogramming [150]. Indeed, it was found that a large number of SSc monocyte genes, including interferon and inflammatory genes undergo epigenetic reprograming [151]. Further supporting this concept, studies in SSc twins found enrichment of DNAse I hypersensitive sites in SSc myeloid cells [152]. It was also reported that circulating SSc monocytes express low levels of the Friend leukemia integration 1 transcription factor (FLI1) [153]. In vitro deletion of FLI1 in MΦ stimulated collagen and periostin expression in co-cultures with fibroblasts. Another characteristic of SSc monocytes is an increased migratory capacity owing to the elevated expression of functional chemokine receptors, CCR1, CCR2, and CCR3 [154].

In addition to producing soluble mediators, MΦ are capable of activating fibroblasts more directly through a formation of cell–cell contacts. Such contacts have been shown to be mediated by cadherin-11 (CDH11), a transmembrane adhesion molecule that is expressed on MΦ and fibroblasts in fibrotic skin and lung tissues [155]. CDH11 junctions allow for close proximity of MΦ and myofibroblasts facilitating integrin-mediated activation of MΦ-derived latent TGF-β and subsequent induction of TGF-β signaling in fibroblasts [156]. Interestingly, contracting fibroblasts can attract MΦ by inducing deformation fields in fibrillar collagen matrix that can be sensed by MΦ over a relatively large distance to migrate toward contracting fibroblasts [157].

T Cells

Activated T cells are an important source of profibrotic cytokines such as IL-4, IL-5, IL-13, IL-21, IL-31, as well as antifibrotic cytokines, including IFN-γ and IL-12. Cytotoxic T cells constitute the major T-cell subsets identified in SSc skin lesions [140, 158–160]. Cytotoxic CD4+ is characterized by a highly cytotoxic profile and enhanced metabolic activity. T cells co-expressing CD4+ CTL marker SLAMF7 and granzyme A colocalize with apoptotic endothelial cells, suggesting their direct involvement in endothelial and peri-endothelial cell death [140]. CD4+ T cells also express profibrotic cytokines TGF-β and IL-1, but their role in direct fibroblast activation has not yet been tested. CD8+ T cells produce high levels of IL-13 and have been shown to exert profibrotic effects on SSc and healthy subject fibroblasts [158, 159].

Despite substantial literature implicating various T-cell subsets in the pathogenesis of SSc, in comparison to cytotoxic T cells, other T-cell subsets are relatively sparse in early SSc skin [140]. Nonetheless, they may contribute to tissue fibrosis in later stages of disease or in a subset of SSc patients. The involvement of Th2 cells has been primarily described in mouse models of fibrosis, but there is less evidence for the role of these cells in human SSc. However, a Th2 cytokine IL-31 was present at high levels in plasma and in immune infiltrates in fibrotic skin and lungs in about 10% of SSc patients [161]. IL-31 induced collagen production in dermal fibroblasts, in a TGF-β-independent manner via activation of STAT3 pathway. Another T-cell population increased in SSc skin was characterized as CD4 + ICOS+ T cells with a follicular helper cell (T_{FH})-like phenotype [162]. Increased presence of ICOS$^+$ T_{FH}-like cells correlated with dermal fibrosis and clinical disease status. ICOS$^+$ T_{FH}-like cells were also increased in the skin of graft-versus-host disease (GVDH) SSc mice and contributed to fibrosis via an IL-21-driven mechanism [162]. In SSc, circulating T_{regs} were found to be functionally impaired resulting in a lower production of inhibitory cytokines or suppression of effector T cells [163]. Interestingly, T_{regs} present in the skin of SSc patients produced higher amounts of IL-4 and IL-13 [162]. This differentiation of T_{regs} to the Th2-like cells was induced by IL-33 via ST2 receptor expressed on T_{regs}.

B Cells

B cells contribute to SSc fibrosis by secreting proinflammatory and profibrotic cytokines and by producing pathogenic autoantibodies [164]. Pathogenic autoantibodies directed against PDGFRα, endothelin, and angiotensin receptors have been described in a significant proportion of SSc patients [165]. These autoantibodies can interact with the cognate receptors mimicking stimulation by the native ligands; however, their contribution to the disease process in SSc requires further study. Circulating activated B cells producing IL-6, GM-CSF, IL-1β, and IL-8 have been reported in SSc patients [166]. The presence of B cells in SSc biopsies has also been documented in several studies, although with a lesser frequency than T cells and macrophages [141, 167, 168]. B cells co-cultured with SSc fibroblasts induced fibroblasts to produce collagen in a TGF-β-dependent manner [169].

Dendritic Cells

Dendritic cells (DC) encompass heterogeneous population of cells including myeloid DC (mDC) and plasmacytoid DC (pDC). Accumulating evidence implicates pDCs in the pathogenesis of SSc. Although pDC are decreased in patient blood, they accumulate in the skin and lungs and are also increased in animal models of SSc [170–172]. Circulating SSc pDCs have an activated phenotype and are characterized by the epigenetic downregulation of the Runt-related transcription factor 3 (RUNX3) [173]. RUNX3 is also downregulated in the skin and lungs of SSc patients. Furthermore, ablation of Runx3 in dendritic cells leads to exaggerated bleomycin-induced fibrosis [173]. Activated pDCs in SSc skin spontaneously secrete IFN-γ and CXCL4 [170]. TLR8 signaling promoted IFN-γ and CXCL4 secretion in SSc fibroblasts, but not in healthy subject fibroblasts. The specific mechanism linking the TLR8-CXCL4-IFN-γ axis to fibrosis is not entirely clear; however, depletion of pDCs reduced inflammation, as well as skin and lung fibrosis in the bleomycin model of SSc [170, 171]. Furthermore, overexpression of TLR8 exacerbated fibrosis in the bleomycin model [170].

Keratinocytes

The epidermis plays an important role in maintaining skin homeostasis and disruption of this homeostasis leads to various pathological changes in the skin, including fibrosis [174]. Keratinocytes and fibroblasts are engaged in a cross-talk via secretion of soluble mediators that regulate healthy skin homeostasis; however, both cell types are phenotypically altered in SSc patients contributing to their pathological mutual activation [174]. SSc epidermal layers exhibit activated wound-healing characteristics manifested by production of the proinflammatory and profibrotic mediators including IL-1β, CTGF, and S100A9 [175, 176]. Keratinocytes also secrete oncostatin M (OSM) upon stimulation with keratinocyte growth factor (KGF), which is overexpressed in SSc fibroblasts [177]. Activation of SSc keratinocytes may be in part mediated by abnormally low expression of transcription factor FLI1 [178]. Depletion of FLI1 in healthy keratinocytes led to upregulation of CTGF and IL-1β. Mice carrying keratin 14 (K14) deletion of Fli1 spontaneously developed dermal and lung fibrosis.

Endothelial Cells and Pericytes

Injured endothelial cells in SSc acquire a proinflammatory and a profibrotic phenotype and may contribute to activation of fibroblasts in the perivascular area. Media conditioned by SSc dermal endothelial cells induced CTGF-dependent fibroblast Matrigel invasion and promoted fibroblast-to-myofibroblast differentiation by activating the endogenous TGF-β/TGF-β receptor pathway in fibroblasts [179]. Endothelial cells may also contribute to fibrosis by undergoing transdifferentiation to mesenchymal-like cells through the process of EndMT [180, 181]. Additionally vascular mural cells called pericytes have also been shown to undergo myofibroblast differentiation upon injury and represent an alternate cellular source for myofibroblasts in fibrosis.

Pathways Regulating Myofibroblast Survival and Apoptosis Evasion in SSc

Whereas our understanding of the mechanisms that induce myofibroblast activation has grown exponentially over the last decades, the mechanisms that promote myofibroblast persistence in fibrotic tissues remain poorly understood. Myofibroblasts evade programmed cell death or apoptosis by activating pro-survival pathways in response to mechanical and biochemical cues from the fibrotic microenvironment. Abnormal activation of these survival pathways reflects the need to block concomitant activation of pro-apoptotic signaling [8], which normally limits fibrosis by promoting myofi-

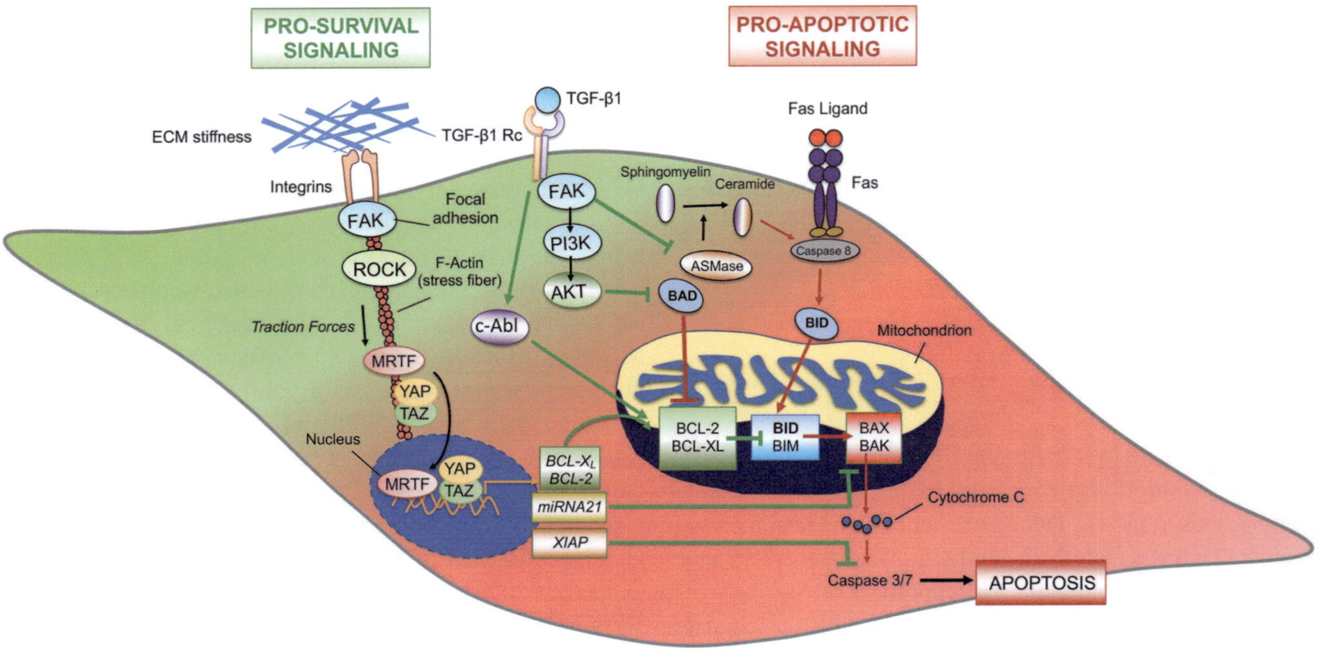

Fig. 18.4 Molecular mechanisms of fibroblast survival and apoptosis evasion in systemic sclerosis. Mitochondria in activated myofibroblasts are loaded with pro-apoptotic factors, which force these cells to activate pro-survival pathways to ensure survival. Myofibroblast survival is jointly controlled by mechanical and biochemical cues, which activate pro-survival signaling pathways that inhibit programmed cell death or apoptosis [8]. The noncanonical TGF-β/FAK pathway blocks the extrinsic pathway of apoptosis by inhibiting sphingomyelinase (ASMase) [190], an enzyme that controls FAS-dependent apoptosis by generating ceramide from sphingomyelin. TGF-β also blocks the intrinsic mitochondrial pathway of apoptosis by inhibiting the pro-apoptotic protein BCL-2-associated death promoter (BAD) via FAK–PI3K–AKT signaling and protects cells from apoptosis by increasing levels of pro-survival BCL-2 and BCL-X_L via activation of c-Abl [232]. Matrix stiffness similarly inhibits intrinsic apoptosis via activation of the mechanotransduction pathways FAK–YAP/TAZ–BCL-X_L and ROCK–MRTF–BCL-2 [98, 233]. In addition, mechanical signaling induces expression of the microRNAs miR-21 and miR-29a, which promote the survival of myofibroblasts by increasing levels of BCL-2 proteins. Both matrix stiffness and TGF-β can also inhibit programmed cell death by increasing levels of X-linked inhibitor of apoptosis protein (XIAP), a direct caspase 3/7 inhibitor

broblast apoptosis during physiological tissue repair. Thus, myofibroblasts are primed for death and depend on continual activation of pro-survival signaling to evade apoptosis [98] (Fig. 18.4). This knowledge has paved the way to the design of new antifibrotic therapies based on inducing myofibroblast apoptosis by targeting pro-survival signaling pathways, a therapeutic strategy that could lead to reversion of established fibrosis [8, 182].

Biochemical, Mechanical, and Metabolic Factors

In normal wound healing, myofibroblasts are detected transiently in the early granulation tissue and then progressively disappear via apoptosis. Timely elimination of myofibroblasts is a crucial step in successful wound resolution and requires withdrawal of pro-survival factors including TGF-β or PDGF [183]. In pathological fibrogenesis, myofibroblasts persist in lesioned tissues, resulting in excessively contracted and mechanically stressed matrix characteristic of chronic scar [184]. Persistent TGF-β and ET-1 signaling has been shown to promote myofibroblast resistance to apoptosis by activating pro-survival pathways including protein kinase B (PKB, also known as AKT) and FAK [69, 185–187]. In addition, mechanical activation of FAK by stiff matrices has been also shown to promote myofibroblast resistance to apoptosis, a mechanism dependent on β1 integrin signaling [98]. Accordingly, inhibition of β1 integrin, FAK, or AKT signaling promotes myofibroblast apoptosis and treats fibrosis in experimental models [39, 94]. Mechanistically, biochemical and mechanical pro-survival signaling has been shown to upregulate expression of anti-apoptotic BCL-X_L and BCL-2 proteins in SSc fibroblasts (Fig. 18.4). Accordingly, direct inhibition of BCL-X_L/BCL-2 with the ABT-263 drug activates the mitochondrial apoptotic pathway in SSc fibroblasts and reverses established skin fibrosis in experimental models [98, 182]. Similarly, TGF-β and matrix stiffness have been shown to prevent activation of the extrinsic pathway of apoptosis in SSc fibroblasts by inhibiting sphingomyelinase, thereby protecting these cells from apoptosis induced by Fas ligand (Fig. 18.4) [188–190]. Of note, treatment with PGE2, a lipid mediator derived from the metabolism of arachidonic acid, restores Fas ligand-induced myofibroblast apoptosis by inhibiting TGF-β-induced FAK/AKT signaling [191]. In this regard, metabolic reprogramming is increasingly implicated in governing myofibroblast sensitivity to apoptosis by yet poorly understood mechanisms. Myofibroblasts are characterized by activating aerobic glycolysis (Warburg effect) in order to sustain their high-energy status, which is associated with fragmented mitochondria and impaired activation of the mitochondrial apoptosis pathway [192]. Pharmacological activation of the energy sensor AMP-activated protein kinase (AMPK) with metformin induces mitochondrial biogenesis and restores sensitivity of myofibroblasts to apoptosis [193]. Additionally, intermediate metabolites generated during the TCA cycle themselves have potent effects on fibroblast behavior. The metabolic dysregulation of fibroblasts during fibrosis represents an emerging area of research with high potential for therapeutic applications.

Cellular Senescence

In addition to escaping apoptotic signaling, myofibroblasts can persist in fibrotic tissues by acquiring a senescent cellular phenotype characterized by irreversible cell cycle arrest and a senescence-associated secretory phenotype (SASP) (Fig. 18.2). A growing body of evidence implicates accumulation of profibrotic senescent myofibroblasts in fibrotic diseases including SSc and pulmonary fibrosis [194]. The SASP of senescent myofibroblasts is comprised of proinflammatory cytokines and growth factors involved in tissue fibrosis including IL-1α, IL-1β, IL-8, TGF-β, PDGF, and IL-6 as well as ECM proteins such as fibronectin, collagens, and MMPs, and is thought to promote progressive fibrosis by spreading profibrotic signaling to immune and stromal cells. The mechanisms driving the acquisition of this senescent phenotype in myofibroblasts are poorly understood, but appear to be TGF-β-independent. Based on this emerging biology, novel studies have shown that elimination of senescent myofibroblasts with the use of "senolytic" agents could treat SSc fibrosis. Senolytic drugs including dasatinib and inhibitors of the anti-apoptotic proteins BCL-X_L/BCL-2 such as ABT-263 have been shown to target senescent myofibroblasts for apoptosis and reduce established fibrosis in mouse models of SSc [8, 98]. A recent open-label clinical trial of the senolytic agent dasatinib in patients with SSc-ILD showed improvement in radiological measures of lung fibrosis that was accompanied by a reduction in the senescence signature [195]. Similarly, novel immunotherapeutic approaches such as engineered T cells have been shown to treat organ fibrosis by targeting fibroblasts for apoptosis [196]. In addition, targeting myofibroblast senescence with the so-called senomorphic agents, which modulate the activities of senescence cells including their SASP, has been shown to modulate tissue fibrogenesis. For instance, pharmacological inhibition of the JAK/STAT pathway has been shown to ameliorate SASP-induced tissue injury and fibrosis in SSc fibroblasts [197, 198]. Additionally, expression of the antiaging histone deacetylases SIRT1 and SIRT3 is significantly reduced in SSc patients, and genetic inhibition of these enzymes results in aggravated development of organ fibrosis in experimental models [199, 200]. Mechanistically, this is linked to depletion of NAD+, which in turn is largely due to increased expression of the NAD hydrolase CD38 in SSc skin biopsies. Accordingly, CD38-deficient mice showed protection from fibrosis via boosting NAD+ levels [201]. Thus, NAD metabolism appears to play an important and previously unknown role in modulating physiological and pathological tissue repair. The biological mechanism promoting aged myofibroblast clearance remains poorly understood. Recent studies suggest that targeting CD47, a molecule that prevents macrophages from targeting diseased fibroblasts, reversed skin fibrosis in mice and led to the rapid elimination of ectopically transplanted SSc cells [202].

Pathways Promoting Myofibroblast Deactivation

To avoid excessive matrix accumulation and scarring in response to injury, redundant control mechanisms have evolved. Fibroblasts are equipped with a plethora of cell-intrinsic mechanisms for negatively regulating ECM gene expression, myofibroblast accumulation, and TGF-β stimulation. For example, Smad7 blocks TGF-β signaling by accelerating TGF-β receptor degradation. Functional impairment of Smad7 was demonstrated in SSc fibroblasts. There are a number of additional cell-intrinsic endogenous repressors of collagen synthesis that might have a role in preventing fibrosis. The list includes the transcription factors Sp3, Fli-1, p53, Ras, and Nrf2 and cofactors such as Nab2 and HDACs, microRNAs, and several nuclear receptors. Itaconate, an intermediate metabolite of the TCA cycle, is a potent endogenous inducer of Nrf2, and represses collagen production. Impaired expression, regulation, or function of these endogenous inhibitors may contribute to failure to limit fibroblast activation in SSc.

Interferon-γ

The inflammatory cytokine interferon-γ, produced primarily by Th1 lymphocytes, is a major negative regulator of fibroblast activation. IFN-γ represses collagen gene expression and abrogates stimulation induced by TGF-β [203]. IFN-γ is also a potent inhibitor of fibroblast proliferation and migration, fibroblast-mediated matrix contraction, and myofibroblast transdifferentiation. However, IFN-γ may have an indirect profibrotic effect by stimulating TGF-β and ET1 synthesis in microvascular endothelial cells and inducing endothelial-to-mesenchymal transition [204]. Significantly, some studies have shown that fibroblasts explanted from SSc patients are relatively resistant to the inhibitory effects of IFN-γ. Clinical trials of IFN-γ in SSc have demonstrated modest and inconsistent improvement in skin fibrosis, but a large randomized trial in idiopathic pulmonary fibrosis showed no benefit [205, 206].

Nuclear Receptors: PPAR-γ, VDR, and NR4A1

Peroxisome Proliferator-Activated Receptor-γ (PPAR-γ)

PPAR-γ is a type-2 orphan nuclear receptor present in adipocytes, but also detected in macrophages, fibroblasts, and other cell types. PPAR-γ modulates TGF-β signaling and mesenchymal stromal cell plasticity and is implicated in fibrosis. Originally identified as a key regulator of adipogenesis and lipid metabolism, PPAR-γ is a dual-function molecule acting as both a nuclear receptor and ligand-inducible transcription factor in diverse tissues. Various lipid moieties and electrophilic prostanoids such as 15d-prostaglandin J_2 (15d-PGJ_2) serve as endogenous ligands for PPAR-γ. Insulin-sensitizing drugs such as rosiglitazone or pioglitazone were found to be potent pharmacological PPAR-γ agonists. Many target genes positively regulated by PPAR-γ play key roles in adipogenesis, including adiponectin. PPAR-γ also controls a plethora of vascular and immune processes, and abnormal PPAR-γ function is implicated in lipodystrophy, atherosclerosis, PAH, and inflammatory diseases. In skin and lung fibroblasts, 15d-PGJ_2 or pharmacological PPAR-γ ligands caused virtual abrogation of TGF-β-induced collagen production, myofibroblast transdifferentiation, EMT, and other Smad3-dependent profibrotic responses [207]. These antifibrotic effects include both direct transrepression, as well as negative regulation mediated through adiponectin, which activates AMP kinase and disrupts focal adhesion assembly and FAK activation. The expression and activity of PPAR-γ in the skin are impaired in patients with SSc and scarring alopecia. Both candidate gene and GWA studies have identified SNPs in *PPARG* associated with SSc, but the functional consequences of these genetic polymorphisms and their contribution to disease manifestations such as fibrosis and PAH remain to be elucidated. Recent studies have indicated that expression of adipogenic genes and peroxisomal biogenesis are compromised in patients with pulmonary fibrosis. Additionally, circulating levels of adiponectin, a direct transcriptional target of PPAR-γ and a marker for its activity, are reduced in SSc patients and correlate with disease severity [208]. Furthermore, PPAR-γ expression in lesional tissue shows an inverse relationship with TGF-β signaling. Of note, many factors implicated in fibrosis including TGF-β, Wnt ligands, IL-13, hypoxia, LPA, and CTGF potently inhibit PPAR-γ expression or function [209]. Compromised PPAR-γ expression and function in SSc and other fibrotic conditions of the skin and lungs may be an important pathogenic factor that contributes to the persistence and progression of fibrosis as well as vascular damage [210].

Vitamin D Receptor (VDR)

Vitamin D_3 is a steroidal hormone synthesized in the skin with a primary role in regulating bone metabolism and calcium homeostasis. In addition to its primary endocrine function, vitamin D_3 and its non-calcemic derivatives have anti-inflammatory, anti-proliferative, and antifibrotic effects. A widely expressed vitamin D receptor (VDR), a member of the nuclear receptor family, functions as a ligand-inducible transcription factor that stimulates target gene expression in a cell-specific manner by binding to the vitamin D-responsive element (VDRE). Activated VDR negatively regulates TGF-β/SMAD by forming a protein–protein complex with SMAD3 and preventing its binding to the DNA [211]. The mRNA and protein levels of VDR are decreased in SSc skin and in the bleomycin model of skin fibrosis [212]. SSc patients have reduced levels of vitamin D with the lowest levels in diffuse SSc [213].

Nuclear Receptor Subfamily 4, Group A, Member 1 (NR4A1)

NR4A1, also known as *Nur77*, is an orphan nuclear receptor expressed in many cell types, where it is involved in regulating diverse cellular processes including proliferation, apoptosis, cellular stress, inflammation, and glucose and lipid metabolism. The regulation of these processes occurs through both nuclear and non-genomic functions. During physiological tissue repair, NR4A1 is induced by TGF-β and functions as an endogenous inhibitor of TGF-β signaling. TGF-β promotes assembly of the transcription factor SP1 with the SIN3A/HDAC1 repressor complex resulting in the inhibition of the TGF-β target genes through the SP1-dependent *trans*repression [214]. In contrast, prolonged stimulation with TGF-β epigenetically silences NR4A1 or renders NR4A1 functionally impaired by inducing its phosphorylation. Experimentally, deficiency of Nr4a1 exacerbates skin and lung fibrosis, while treatment with the NR4A1 agonist Csn-B ameliorates fibrosis in the preclinical models. Thus, although NR4A1 accumulates in SSc and other fibrotic diseases, impairment of the NR4A1 negative feedback leads to persistent TGF-β signaling and enhanced fibrogenesis.

Soluble Guanylate Cyclase

The intracellular receptor for nitric oxide soluble guanylate cyclase (sGC) controls important physiological responses, including smooth muscle relaxation, platelet aggregation, and hemostasis. Decreased NO bioavailability is associated with cardiovascular diseases and pulmonary and systemic hypertension. The sGC also functions as an antifibrotic agent by inhibiting TGF-β/ERK signaling and mitigating experimental organ fibrosis [215]. However, the antifibrotic sGC-sGMP-PKG signaling pathway is dysregulated in SSc fibroblasts [216]. Despite the elevated expression of its key mediators, protein kinase G1 (PKG1) and G2 in SSc biopsies, and explanted fibroblast, the sGMP-PKG signaling is impaired due to the greatly reduced levels of sGC that hampers efficient production of sGMP and activation of PKG. The prolonged TGF-β stimulation induces defective sGC-sGMP-PKG signaling observed in SSc fibroblasts, suggesting that TGF-β may contribute to the inactivation of the sGC pathway in SSc. An FDA-approved sGC stimulator Riociguat sensitizes sGC to NO and stabilizes sGC-NO binding. Riociguat has beneficial effects in patients with PAH, including CTD-PAH, which are refractory to the PDE-5i therapy [217]. However, the randomized, double-blind, placebo-controlled trial of Riociguat in patients with early diffuse SSc failed to meet the primary endpoint of change in mRSS, but some secondary end points showed potential efficacy signals [218].

References

1. Rockey DC, Bell PD, Hill JA. Fibrosis—a common pathway to organ injury and failure. N Engl J Med. 2015;372:1138–49. https://doi.org/10.1056/NEJMra1300575.
2. Ho YY, Lagares D, Tager AM, Kapoor M. Fibrosis—a lethal component of systemic sclerosis. Nat Rev Rheumatol. 2014;10:390–402. https://doi.org/10.1038/nrrheum.2014.53.
3. Rosenbloom J, Mendoza FA, Jimenez SA. Strategies for anti-fibrotic therapies. Biochim Biophys Acta. 2013;1832:1088–103. https://doi.org/10.1016/j.bbadis.2012.12.007.
4. Ramirez F, Tanaka S, Bou-Gharios G. Transcriptional regulation of the human alpha2(I) collagen gene (COL1A2), an informative model system to study fibrotic diseases. Matrix Biol. 2006;25:365–72. https://doi.org/10.1016/j.matbio.2006.05.002.
5. Ghosh AK, Wei J, Wu M, Varga J. Constitutive Smad signaling and Smad-dependent collagen gene expression in mouse embryonic fibroblasts lacking peroxisome proliferator-activated receptor-gamma. Biochem Biophys Res Commun. 2008;374:231–6. https://doi.org/10.1016/j.bbrc.2008.07.014.
6. Watsky MA, Weber KT, Sun Y, Postlethwaite A. New insights into the mechanism of fibroblast to myofibroblast transformation and associated pathologies. Int Rev Cell Mol Biol. 2010;282:165–92. https://doi.org/10.1016/S1937-6448(10)82004-0.
7. Bhattacharyya S, Wei J, Varga J. Understanding fibrosis in systemic sclerosis: shifting paradigms, emerging opportunities. Nat Rev Rheumatol. 2012;8:42–54. https://doi.org/10.1038/nrrheum.2011.149.
8. Hinz B, Lagares D. Evasion of apoptosis by myofibroblasts: a hallmark of fibrotic diseases. Nat Rev Rheumatol. 2020;16:11–31. https://doi.org/10.1038/s41584-019-0324-5.
9. Chang HY, et al. Diversity, topographic differentiation, and positional memory in human fibroblasts. Proc Natl Acad Sci U S A. 2002;99:12877–82. https://doi.org/10.1073/pnas.162488599.
10. Rinn JL, Bondre C, Gladstone HB, Brown PO, Chang HY. Anatomic demarcation by positional variation in fibroblast gene expression programs. PLoS Genet. 2006;2:e119. https://doi.org/10.1371/journal.pgen.0020119.
11. Driskell RR, et al. Distinct fibroblast lineages determine dermal architecture in skin development and repair. Nature. 2013;504:277–81. https://doi.org/10.1038/nature12783.
12. Rinkevich Y, et al. Skin fibrosis. Identification and isolation of a dermal lineage with intrinsic fibrogenic potential. Science. 2015;348:aaa2151. https://doi.org/10.1126/science.aaa2151.
13. Greenhalgh SN, Iredale JP, Henderson NC. Origins of fibrosis: pericytes take centre stage. F1000prime Rep. 2013;5:37. https://doi.org/10.12703/P5-37.
14. Schrimpf C, Duffield JS. Mechanisms of fibrosis: the role of the pericyte. Curr Opin Nephrol Hypertens. 2011;20:297–305. https://doi.org/10.1097/MNH.0b013e328344c3d4.
15. Dulauroy S, Di Carlo SE, Langa F, Eberl G, Peduto L. Lineage tracing and genetic ablation of ADAM12(+) perivascular cells identify a major source of profibrotic cells during acute tissue injury. Nat Med. 2012;18:1262–70. https://doi.org/10.1038/nm.2848.
16. Rajkumar VS, et al. Shared expression of phenotypic markers in systemic sclerosis indicates a convergence of pericytes and fibroblasts to a myofibroblast lineage in fibrosis. Arthritis Res Ther. 2005;7:R1113–23. https://doi.org/10.1186/ar1790.
17. LeBleu VS, et al. Origin and function of myofibroblasts in kidney fibrosis. Nat Med. 2013;19:1047–53. https://doi.org/10.1038/nm.3218.
18. Hung C, et al. Role of lung pericytes and resident fibroblasts in the pathogenesis of pulmonary fibrosis. Am J Respir Crit Care Med. 2013;188:820–30. https://doi.org/10.1164/rccm.201212-2297OC.
19. Olson LE, Soriano P. Increased PDGFRalpha activation disrupts connective tissue development and drives systemic fibrosis. Dev Cell. 2009;16:303–13. https://doi.org/10.1016/j.devcel.2008.12.003.
20. Liu S, Shi-Wen X, Abraham DJ, Leask A. CCN2 is required for bleomycin-induced skin fibrosis in mice. Arthritis Rheum. 2011;63:239–46. https://doi.org/10.1002/art.30074.
21. Marangoni RG, et al. Myofibroblasts in cutaneous fibrosis originate from adiponectin-positive intradermal progenitors. Arthritis Rheumatol. 2014; https://doi.org/10.1002/art.38990.
22. Hinz B. The myofibroblast: paradigm for a mechanically active cell. J Biomech. 2010;43:146–55. https://doi.org/10.1016/j.jbiomech.2009.09.020.
23. Kalluri R, Neilson EG. Epithelial-mesenchymal transition and its implications for fibrosis. J Clin Invest. 2003;112:1776–84. https://doi.org/10.1172/JCI20530.
24. Korfei M, et al. Epithelial endoplasmic reticulum stress and apoptosis in sporadic idiopathic pulmonary fibrosis. Am J Respir Crit Care Med. 2008;178:838–46. https://doi.org/10.1164/rccm.200802-313OC.
25. Li Z, Jimenez SA. Protein kinase Cdelta and c-Abl kinase are required for transforming growth factor beta induction of endothelial-mesenchymal transition in vitro. Arthritis Rheum. 2011;63:2473–83. https://doi.org/10.1002/art.30317.
26. Guerrero-Juarez CF, et al. Single-cell analysis reveals fibroblast heterogeneity and myeloid-derived adipocyte progenitors in murine skin wounds. Nat Commun. 2019;10:650. https://doi.org/10.1038/s41467-018-08247-x.
27. Tabib T, Morse C, Wang T, Chen W, Lafyatis R. SFRP2/DPP4 and FMO1/LSP1 define major fibroblast populations in human skin. J Invest Dermatol. 2018;138:802–10. https://doi.org/10.1016/j.jid.2017.09.045.
28. Farbehi N, et al. Single-cell expression profiling reveals dynamic flux of cardiac stromal, vascular and immune cells in health and injury. Elife. 2019;8 https://doi.org/10.7554/eLife.43882.

29. Valenzi E, et al. Single-cell analysis reveals fibroblast heterogeneity and myofibroblasts in systemic sclerosis-associated interstitial lung disease. Ann Rheum Dis. 2019;78:1379–87. https://doi.org/10.1136/annrheumdis-2018-214865.
30. Xie T, et al. Single-cell deconvolution of fibroblast heterogeneity in mouse pulmonary fibrosis. Cell Rep. 2018;22:3625–40. https://doi.org/10.1016/j.celrep.2018.03.010.
31. Nazari B, et al. Altered dermal fibroblasts in systemic sclerosis display podoplanin and CD90. Am J Pathol. 2016;186:2650–64. https://doi.org/10.1016/j.ajpath.2016.06.020.
32. Varga J, Pasche B. Transforming growth factor beta as a therapeutic target in systemic sclerosis. Nat Rev Rheumatol. 2009;5:200–6. https://doi.org/10.1038/nrrheum.2009.26.
33. Iwano M. EMT and TGF-beta in renal fibrosis. Front Biosci. 2010;2:229–38.
34. Tschumperlin DJ, Lagares D. Mechano-therapeutics: targeting mechanical signaling in fibrosis and tumor stroma. Pharmacol Ther. 2020;212:107575. https://doi.org/10.1016/j.pharmthera.2020.107575.
35. Feng XH, Derynck R. Specificity and versatility in tgf-beta signaling through Smads. Annu Rev Cell Dev Biol. 2005;21:659–93. https://doi.org/10.1146/annurev.cellbio.21.022404.142018.
36. Briones-Orta MA, Tecalco-Cruz AC, Sosa-Garrocho M, Caligaris C, Macias-Silva M. Inhibitory Smad7: emerging roles in health and disease. Curr Mol Pharmacol. 2011;4:141–53.
37. Bhattacharyya S, et al. A non-Smad mechanism of fibroblast activation by transforming growth factor-beta via c-Abl and Egr-1: selective modulation by imatinib mesylate. Oncogene. 2009;28:1285–97. https://doi.org/10.1038/onc.2008.479.
38. Horowitz JC, et al. Activation of the pro-survival phosphatidylinositol 3-kinase/AKT pathway by transforming growth factor-beta1 in mesenchymal cells is mediated by p38 MAPK-dependent induction of an autocrine growth factor. J Biol Chem. 2004;279:1359–67.
39. Lagares D, et al. Inhibition of focal adhesion kinase prevents experimental lung fibrosis and myofibroblast formation. Arthritis Rheum. 2012;64:1653–64. https://doi.org/10.1002/art.33482.
40. Akhmetshina A, et al. Rho-associated kinases are crucial for myofibroblast differentiation and production of extracellular matrix in scleroderma fibroblasts. Arthritis Rheum. 2008;58:2553–64. https://doi.org/10.1002/art.23677.
41. Kim SI, Choi ME. TGF-beta-activated kinase-1: new insights into the mechanism of TGF-beta signaling and kidney disease. Kidney Res Clin Pract. 2012;31:94–105. https://doi.org/10.1016/j.krcp.2012.04.322.
42. Lagares D, et al. ADAM10-mediated ephrin-B2 shedding promotes myofibroblast activation and organ fibrosis. Nat Med. 2017;23:1405–15. https://doi.org/10.1038/nm.4419.
43. Hecker L, et al. Reversal of persistent fibrosis in aging by targeting Nox4-Nrf2 redox imbalance. Sci Transl Med. 2014;6:231ra247. https://doi.org/10.1126/scitranslmed.3008182.
44. Liu F, et al. Mechanosignaling through YAP and TAZ drives fibroblast activation and fibrosis. Am J Physiol Lung Cell Mol Physiol. 2015;308:L344–57. https://doi.org/10.1152/ajplung.00300.2014.
45. Shiwen X, et al. A role of myocardin related transcription factor-A (MRTF-A) in scleroderma related fibrosis. PLoS One. 2015;10:e0126015. https://doi.org/10.1371/journal.pone.0126015.
46. Svegliati S, et al. Platelet-derived growth factor and reactive oxygen species (ROS) regulate Ras protein levels in primary human fibroblasts via ERK1/2. Amplification of ROS and Ras in systemic sclerosis fibroblasts. J Biol Chem. 2005;280:36474–82. https://doi.org/10.1074/jbc.M502851200.
47. Klareskog L, Gustafsson R, Scheynius A, Hallgren R. Increased expression of platelet-derived growth factor type B receptors in the skin of patients with systemic sclerosis. Arthritis Rheum. 1990;33:1534–41.
48. Yamakage A, Kikuchi K, Smith EA, LeRoy EC, Trojanowska M. Selective upregulation of platelet-derived growth factor alpha receptors by transforming growth factor beta in scleroderma fibroblasts. J Exp Med. 1992;175:1227–34.
49. Baroni SS, et al. Stimulatory autoantibodies to the PDGF receptor in systemic sclerosis. N Engl J Med. 2006;354:2667–76. https://doi.org/10.1056/NEJMoa052955.
50. Sonnylal S, et al. Selective expression of connective tissue growth factor in fibroblasts in vivo promotes systemic tissue fibrosis. Arthritis Rheum. 2010;62:1523–32. https://doi.org/10.1002/art.27382.
51. Rancoule C, et al. Lysophosphatidic acid-1-receptor targeting agents for fibrosis. Expert Opin Investig Drugs. 2011;20:657–67. https://doi.org/10.1517/13543784.2011.566864.
52. Xu MY, et al. Lysophosphatidic acid induces alphavbeta6 integrin-mediated TGF-beta activation via the LPA2 receptor and the small G protein G alpha(q). Am J Pathol. 2009;174:1264–79. https://doi.org/10.2353/ajpath.2009.080160.
53. Castelino FV, et al. Amelioration of dermal fibrosis by genetic deletion or pharmacologic antagonism of lysophosphatidic acid receptor 1 in a mouse model of scleroderma. Arthritis Rheum. 2011;63:1405–15. https://doi.org/10.1002/art.30262.
54. Tager AM, et al. The lysophosphatidic acid receptor LPA1 links pulmonary fibrosis to lung injury by mediating fibroblast recruitment and vascular leak. Nat Med. 2008;14:45–54. https://doi.org/10.1038/nm1685.
55. Ledein L, et al. Translational engagement of lysophosphatidic acid receptor 1 in skin fibrosis: from dermal fibroblasts of patients with scleroderma to tight skin 1 mouse. Br J Pharmacol. 2020;177:4296–309. https://doi.org/10.1111/bph.15190.
56. Allanore Y, et al. Lysophosphatidic acid receptor 1 antagonist SAR100842 for patients with diffuse cutaneous systemic sclerosis: a double-blind, randomized, eight-week placebo-controlled study followed by a sixteen-week open-label extension study. Arthritis Rheumatol. 2018;70:1634–43. https://doi.org/10.1002/art.40547.
57. Kowal-Bielecka O, et al. Elevated levels of leukotriene B4 and leukotriene E4 in bronchoalveolar lavage fluid from patients with scleroderma lung disease. Arthritis Rheum. 2003;48:1639–46. https://doi.org/10.1002/art.11042.
58. Liang M, et al. Promotion of myofibroblast differentiation and tissue fibrosis by the leukotriene B4-leukotriene B4 receptor axis in systemic sclerosis. Arthritis Rheumatol. 2020;72:1013–25. https://doi.org/10.1002/art.41192.
59. Tian W, et al. Blocking macrophage leukotriene b4 prevents endothelial injury and reverses pulmonary hypertension. Sci Transl Med. 2013;5:200ra117. https://doi.org/10.1126/scitranslmed.3006674.
60. Montezano AC, Nguyen Dinh Cat A, Rios FJ, Touyz RM. Angiotensin II and vascular injury. Curr Hypertens Rep. 2014;16:431. https://doi.org/10.1007/s11906-014-0431-2.
61. Stawski L, Haines P, Fine A, Rudnicka L, Trojanowska M. MMP-12 deficiency attenuates angiotensin II-induced vascular injury, M2 macrophage accumulation, and skin and heart fibrosis. PLoS One. 2014;9:e109763. https://doi.org/10.1371/journal.pone.0109763.
62. Marut W, et al. Amelioration of systemic fibrosis in mice by angiotensin II receptor blockade. Arthritis Rheum. 2013;65:1367–77. https://doi.org/10.1002/art.37873.
63. Tanaka J, et al. Preventive effect of irbesartan on bleomycin-induced lung injury in mice. Respir Investig. 2013;51:76–83. https://doi.org/10.1016/j.resinv.2012.12.005.
64. Meng Y, et al. Angiotensin-converting enzyme 2/angiotensin-(1-7)/Mas axis protects against lung fibrosis by inhibiting the MAPK/NF-kappaB pathway. Am J Respir Cell Mol Biol. 2014;50:723–36. https://doi.org/10.1165/rcmb.2012-0451OC.

65. Shenoy V, et al. The angiotensin-converting enzyme 2/angiogenesis-(1-7)/Mas axis confers cardiopulmonary protection against lung fibrosis and pulmonary hypertension. Am J Respir Crit Care Med. 2010;182:1065–72. https://doi.org/10.1164/rccm.200912-1840OC.
66. Rodriguez-Pascual F, Busnadiego O, Gonzalez-Santamaria J. The profibrotic role of endothelin-1: is the door still open for the treatment of fibrotic diseases? Life Sci. 2014;118:156–64. https://doi.org/10.1016/j.lfs.2013.12.024.
67. Lagares D, et al. Endothelin 1 contributes to the effect of transforming growth factor beta1 on wound repair and skin fibrosis. Arthritis Rheum. 2010;62:878–89. https://doi.org/10.1002/art.27307.
68. Makino K, et al. Knockout of endothelial cell-derived endothelin-1 attenuates skin fibrosis but accelerates cutaneous wound healing. PLoS One. 2014;9:e97972. https://doi.org/10.1371/journal.pone.0097972.
69. Lagares D, Busnadiego O, Garcia-Fernandez RA, Lamas S, Rodriguez-Pascual F. Adenoviral gene transfer of endothelin-1 in the lung induces pulmonary fibrosis through the activation of focal adhesion kinase. Am J Respir Cell Mol Biol. 2012;47:834–42. https://doi.org/10.1165/rcmb.2011-0446OC.
70. Abraham DJ, et al. Increased levels of endothelin-1 and differential endothelin type A and B receptor expression in scleroderma-associated fibrotic lung disease. Am J Pathol. 1997;151:831–41.
71. Kill A, et al. Autoantibodies to angiotensin and endothelin receptors in systemic sclerosis induce cellular and systemic events associated with disease pathogenesis. Arthritis Res Ther. 2014;16:R29. https://doi.org/10.1186/ar4457.
72. Riemekasten G, et al. Involvement of functional autoantibodies against vascular receptors in systemic sclerosis. Ann Rheum Dis. 2011;70:530–6. https://doi.org/10.1136/ard.2010.135772.
73. Halder G, Dupont S, Piccolo S. Transduction of mechanical and cytoskeletal cues by YAP and TAZ. Nat Rev Mol Cell Biol. 2012;13:591–600. https://doi.org/10.1038/nrm3416.
74. Moroishi T, Hansen CG, Guan KL. The emerging roles of YAP and TAZ in cancer. Nat Rev Cancer. 2015;15:73–9. https://doi.org/10.1038/nrc3876.
75. Varelas X. The Hippo pathway effectors TAZ and YAP in development, homeostasis and disease. Development. 2014;141:1614–26. https://doi.org/10.1242/dev.102376.
76. Mauviel A, Nallet-Staub F, Varelas X. Integrating developmental signals: a Hippo in the (path)way. Oncogene. 2012;31:1743–56. https://doi.org/10.1038/onc.2011.363.
77. Toyama T, et al. Therapeutic targeting of TAZ and YAP by dimethyl fumarate in systemic sclerosis fibrosis. J Invest Dermatol. 2018;138:78–88. https://doi.org/10.1016/j.jid.2017.08.024.
78. Rao TP, Kuhl M. An updated overview on Wnt signaling pathways: a prelude for more. Circ Res. 2010;106:1798–806. https://doi.org/10.1161/CIRCRESAHA.110.219840.
79. Azzolin L, et al. Role of TAZ as mediator of Wnt signaling. Cell. 2012;151:1443–56. https://doi.org/10.1016/j.cell.2012.11.027.
80. Piccolo S, Dupont S, Cordenonsi M. The biology of YAP/TAZ: hippo signaling and beyond. Physiol Rev. 2014;94:1287–312. https://doi.org/10.1152/physrev.00005.2014.
81. Atit R, et al. Beta-catenin activation is necessary and sufficient to specify the dorsal dermal fate in the mouse. Dev Biol. 2006;296:164–76. https://doi.org/10.1016/j.ydbio.2006.04.449.
82. Cheon S, et al. Prolonged beta-catenin stabilization and tcf-dependent transcriptional activation in hyperplastic cutaneous wounds. Lab Invest. 2005;85:416–25. https://doi.org/10.1038/labinvest.3700237.
83. Wei J, et al. Canonical Wnt signaling induces skin fibrosis and subcutaneous lipoatrophy: a novel mouse model for scleroderma? Arthritis Rheum. 2011;63:1707–17. https://doi.org/10.1002/art.30312.
84. Konigshoff M, Eickelberg O. WNT signaling in lung disease: a failure or a regeneration signal? Am J Respir Cell Mol Biol. 2010;42:21–31. https://doi.org/10.1165/rcmb.2008-0485TR.
85. Lam AP, et al. Nuclear beta-catenin is increased in systemic sclerosis pulmonary fibrosis and promotes lung fibroblast migration and proliferation. Am J Respir Cell Mol Biol. 2011;45:915–22. https://doi.org/10.1165/rcmb.2010-0113OC.
86. Lafyatis R, et al. Inhibition of beta-catenin signaling in the skin rescues cutaneous adipogenesis in systemic sclerosis: a randomized, double-blind, placebo-controlled trial of C-82. J Invest Dermatol. 2017;137:2473–83. https://doi.org/10.1016/j.jid.2017.06.032.
87. Kavian N, et al. Targeting ADAM-17/notch signaling abrogates the development of systemic sclerosis in a murine model. Arthritis Rheum. 2010;62:3477–87. https://doi.org/10.1002/art.27626.
88. Yao E, Chuang PT. Hedgehog signaling: From basic research to clinical applications. J Formosan Med Assoc (Taiwan yi zhi). 2015; https://doi.org/10.1016/j.jfma.2015.01.005.
89. Hu L, Lin X, Lu H, Chen B, Bai Y. An overview of hedgehog signaling in fibrosis. Mol Pharmacol. 2015;87:174–82. https://doi.org/10.1124/mol.114.095141.
90. Beyer C, et al. Elevated serum levels of sonic hedgehog are associated with fibrotic and vascular manifestations in systemic sclerosis. Ann Rheum Dis. 2018;77:626–8. https://doi.org/10.1136/annrheumdis-2016-210834.
91. Horn A, et al. Hedgehog signaling controls fibroblast activation and tissue fibrosis in systemic sclerosis. Arthritis Rheum. 2012;64:2724–33. https://doi.org/10.1002/art.34444.
92. Liang R, et al. Acyltransferase skinny hedgehog regulates TGFbeta-dependent fibroblast activation in SSc. Ann Rheum Dis. 2019;78:1269–73. https://doi.org/10.1136/annrheumdis-2019-215066.
93. Distler A, et al. Combined inhibition of morphogen pathways demonstrates additive antifibrotic effects and improved tolerability. Ann Rheum Dis. 2014;73:1264–8. https://doi.org/10.1136/annrheumdis-2013-204221.
94. Santos A, Lagares D. Matrix stiffness: the conductor of organ fibrosis. Curr Rheumatol Rep. 2018;20:2. https://doi.org/10.1007/s11926-018-0710-z.
95. Hinz B. Formation and function of the myofibroblast during tissue repair. J Invest Dermatol. 2007;127:526–37. https://doi.org/10.1038/sj.jid.5700613.
96. Liu F, et al. Feedback amplification of fibrosis through matrix stiffening and COX-2 suppression. J Cell Biol. 2010;190:693–706. https://doi.org/10.1083/jcb.201004082.
97. Georges PC, et al. Increased stiffness of the rat liver precedes matrix deposition: implications for fibrosis. Am J Physiol Gastrointest Liver Physiol. 2007;293:G1147–54. https://doi.org/10.1152/ajpgi.00032.2007.
98. Lagares D, et al. Targeted apoptosis of myofibroblasts with the BH3 mimetic ABT-263 reverses established fibrosis. Sci Transl Med. 2017;9 https://doi.org/10.1126/scitranslmed.aal3765.
99. Humphrey JD, Dufresne ER, Schwartz MA. Mechanotransduction and extracellular matrix homeostasis. Nat Rev Mol Cell Biol. 2014;15:802–12. https://doi.org/10.1038/nrm3896.
100. Frame MC, Patel H, Serrels B, Lietha D, Eck MJ. The FERM domain: organizing the structure and function of FAK. Nat Rev Mol Cell Biol. 2010;11:802–14. https://doi.org/10.1038/nrm2996.
101. Solon J, Levental I, Sengupta K, Georges PC, Janmey PA. Fibroblast adaptation and stiffness matching to soft elastic substrates. Biophys J. 2007;93:4453–61. https://doi.org/10.1529/biophysj.106.101386.
102. Bei Y, et al. RhoA/Rho-kinase activation promotes lung fibrosis in an animal model of systemic sclerosis. Exp Lung Res. 2016;42:44–55. https://doi.org/10.3109/01902148.2016.1141263.

103. Panciera T, Azzolin L, Cordenonsi M, Piccolo S. Mechanobiology of YAP and TAZ in physiology and disease. Nat Rev Mol Cell Biol. 2017;18:758–70. https://doi.org/10.1038/nrm.2017.87.
104. Seo J, Kim J. Regulation of Hippo signaling by actin remodeling. BMB Rep. 2018;51:151–6. https://doi.org/10.5483/bmbrep.2018.51.3.012.
105. Velasquez LS, et al. Activation of MRTF-A-dependent gene expression with a small molecule promotes myofibroblast differentiation and wound healing. Proc Natl Acad Sci U S A. 2013;110:16850–5. https://doi.org/10.1073/pnas.1316764110.
106. Aragona M, et al. A mechanical checkpoint controls multicellular growth through YAP/TAZ regulation by actin-processing factors. Cell. 2013;154:1047–59. https://doi.org/10.1016/j.cell.2013.07.042.
107. Dupont S, et al. Role of YAP/TAZ in mechanotransduction. Nature. 2011;474:179–83. https://doi.org/10.1038/nature10137.
108. Yu FX, et al. Regulation of the Hippo-YAP pathway by G-protein-coupled receptor signaling. Cell. 2012;150:780–91. https://doi.org/10.1016/j.cell.2012.06.037.
109. Janmey PA, Wells RG, Assoian RK, McCulloch CA. From tissue mechanics to transcription factors. Differentiation. 2013;86:112–20. https://doi.org/10.1016/j.diff.2013.07.004.
110. Luchsinger LL, Patenaude CA, Smith BD, Layne MD. Myocardin-related transcription factor-A complexes activate type I collagen expression in lung fibroblasts. J Biol Chem. 2011;286:44116–25. https://doi.org/10.1074/jbc.M111.276931.
111. Wipff PJ, Rifkin DB, Meister JJ, Hinz B. Myofibroblast contraction activates latent TGF-beta1 from the extracellular matrix. J Cell Biol. 2007;179:1311–23. https://doi.org/10.1083/jcb.200704042.
112. Querfeld C, Eckes B, Huerkamp C, Krieg T, Sollberg S. Expression of TGF-beta 1, -beta 2 and -beta 3 in localized and systemic scleroderma. J Dermatol Sci. 1999;21:13–22. https://doi.org/10.1016/s0923-1811(99)00008-0.
113. Sfikakis PP, et al. Immunohistological demonstration of transforming growth factor-beta isoforms in the skin of patients with systemic sclerosis. Clin Immunol Immunopathol. 1993;69:199–204. https://doi.org/10.1006/clin.1993.1170.
114. Angiolilli C, et al. New insights into the genetics and epigenetics of systemic sclerosis. Nat Rev Rheumatol. 2018;14:657–73. https://doi.org/10.1038/s41584-018-0099-0.
115. Bergmann C, Distler JH. Epigenetic factors as drivers of fibrosis in systemic sclerosis. Epigenomics. 2017;9:463–77. https://doi.org/10.2217/epi-2016-0150.
116. Tsou PS, Sawalha AH. Unfolding the pathogenesis of scleroderma through genomics and epigenomics. J Autoimmun. 2017;83:73–94. https://doi.org/10.1016/j.jaut.2017.05.004.
117. Altorok N, Tsou PS, Coit P, Khanna D, Sawalha AH. Genome-wide DNA methylation analysis in dermal fibroblasts from patients with diffuse and limited systemic sclerosis reveals common and subset-specific DNA methylation aberrancies. Ann Rheum Dis. 2014; https://doi.org/10.1136/annrheumdis-2014-205303.
118. Dees C, et al. TGF-beta-induced epigenetic deregulation of SOCS3 facilitates STAT3 signaling to promote fibrosis. J Clin Invest. 2020;130:2347–63. https://doi.org/10.1172/JCI122462.
119. Henderson J, et al. Methyl cap binding protein 2: a key epigenetic protein in systemic sclerosis. Rheumatology (Oxford). 2019;58:527–35. https://doi.org/10.1093/rheumatology/key327.
120. Noda S, et al. Simultaneous downregulation of KLF5 and Fli1 is a key feature underlying systemic sclerosis. Nat Commun. 2014;5:5797. https://doi.org/10.1038/ncomms6797.
121. Wang Y, Fan PS, Kahaleh B. Association between enhanced type I collagen expression and epigenetic repression of the FLI1 gene in scleroderma fibroblasts. Arthritis Rheum. 2006;54:2271–9. https://doi.org/10.1002/art.21948.
122. Dees C, et al. The Wnt antagonists DKK1 and SFRP1 are downregulated by promoter hypermethylation in systemic sclerosis. Ann Rheum Dis. 2014;73:1232–9. https://doi.org/10.1136/annrheumdis-2012-203194.
123. Tsou PS, et al. Inhibition of EZH2 prevents fibrosis and restores normal angiogenesis in scleroderma. Proc Natl Acad Sci U S A. 2019;116:3695–702. https://doi.org/10.1073/pnas.1813006116.
124. Kwon H, et al. Epigenetic silencing of miRNA-34a in human cholangiocarcinoma via EZH2 and DNA methylation: impact on regulation of notch pathway. Am J Pathol. 2017;187:2288–99. https://doi.org/10.1016/j.ajpath.2017.06.014.
125. Wasson CW, et al. Long non-coding RNA HOTAIR drives EZH2-dependent myofibroblast activation in systemic sclerosis through miRNA 34a-dependent activation of NOTCH. Ann Rheum Dis. 2020;79:507–17. https://doi.org/10.1136/annrheumdis-2019-216542.
126. Ghosh AK, Mori Y, Dowling E, Varga J. Trichostatin A blocks TGF-beta-induced collagen gene expression in skin fibroblasts: involvement of Sp1. Biochem Biophys Res Commun. 2007;354:420–6. https://doi.org/10.1016/j.bbrc.2006.12.204.
127. Huber LC, et al. Trichostatin A prevents the accumulation of extracellular matrix in a mouse model of bleomycin-induced skin fibrosis. Arthritis Rheum. 2007;56:2755–64. https://doi.org/10.1002/art.22759.
128. Ghosh AK, et al. p300 is elevated in systemic sclerosis and its expression is positively regulated by TGF-beta: epigenetic feed-forward amplification of fibrosis. J Invest Dermatol. 2013;133:1302–10. https://doi.org/10.1038/jid.2012.479.
129. Shin JY, et al. Epigenetic activation and memory at a TGFB2 enhancer in systemic sclerosis. Sci Transl Med. 2019;11 https://doi.org/10.1126/scitranslmed.aaw0790.
130. Wohlfahrt T, et al. PU.1 controls fibroblast polarization and tissue fibrosis. Nature. 2019;566:344–9. https://doi.org/10.1038/s41586-019-0896-x.
131. Liu Q, et al. Chromatin accessibility landscapes of skin cells in systemic sclerosis nominate dendritic cells in disease pathogenesis. Nat Commun. 2020;11:5843. https://doi.org/10.1038/s41467-020-19702-z.
132. Tsou PS, Palisoc PJ, Ali M, Khanna D, Sawalha AH. Genome-wide reduction in chromatin accessibility and unique transcription factor footprints in endothelial cells and fibroblasts in scleroderma skin. Arthritis Rheumatol. 2021; https://doi.org/10.1002/art.41694.
133. Zhu H, et al. MicroRNA-21 in scleroderma fibrosis and its function in TGF-beta-regulated fibrosis-related genes expression. J Clin Immunol. 2013;33:1100–9. https://doi.org/10.1007/s10875-013-9896-z.
134. Bhattacharyya S, et al. Toll-like receptor 4 signaling augments transforming growth factor-beta responses: a novel mechanism for maintaining and amplifying fibrosis in scleroderma. Am J Pathol. 2013;182:192–205. https://doi.org/10.1016/j.ajpath.2012.09.007.
135. Maurer B, et al. MicroRNA-29, a key regulator of collagen expression in systemic sclerosis. Arthritis Rheum. 2010;62:1733–43. https://doi.org/10.1002/art.27443.
136. Messemaker TC, et al. Antisense long non-coding RNAs are deregulated in skin tissue of patients with systemic sclerosis. J Invest Dermatol. 2018;138:826–35. https://doi.org/10.1016/j.jid.2017.09.053.
137. Pachera E, et al. Long noncoding RNA H19X is a key mediator of TGF-beta-driven fibrosis. J Clin Invest. 2020;130:4888–905. https://doi.org/10.1172/JCI135439.
138. Wang Z, et al. Long non-coding RNA TSIX is upregulated in scleroderma dermal fibroblasts and controls collagen mRNA stabilization. Exp Dermatol. 2016;25:131–6. https://doi.org/10.1111/exd.12900.
139. Fang F, et al. A synthetic TLR3 ligand mitigates profibrotic fibroblast responses by inducing autocrine IFN signaling. J Immunol. 2013;191:2956–66. https://doi.org/10.4049/jimmunol.1300376.

140. Maehara T, et al. Cytotoxic CD4+ T lymphocytes may induce endothelial cell apoptosis in systemic sclerosis. J Clin Invest. 2020;130:2451–64. https://doi.org/10.1172/JCI131700.
141. Skaug B, et al. Global skin gene expression analysis of early diffuse cutaneous systemic sclerosis shows a prominent innate and adaptive inflammatory profile. Ann Rheum Dis. 2020;79:379–86. https://doi.org/10.1136/annrheumdis-2019-215894.
142. Lescoat A, et al. M1/M2 polarisation state of M-CSF blood-derived macrophages in systemic sclerosis. Ann Rheum Dis. 2019;78:e127. https://doi.org/10.1136/annrheumdis-2018-214333.
143. Soldano S, et al. Increase in circulating cells coexpressing M1 and M2 macrophage surface markers in patients with systemic sclerosis. Ann Rheum Dis. 2018;77:1842–5. https://doi.org/10.1136/annrheumdis-2018-213648.
144. Trombetta AC, et al. A circulating cell population showing both M1 and M2 monocyte/macrophage surface markers characterizes systemic sclerosis patients with lung involvement. Respir Res. 2018;19:186. https://doi.org/10.1186/s12931-018-0891-z.
145. Moreno-Moral A, et al. Changes in macrophage transcriptome associate with systemic sclerosis and mediate GSDMA contribution to disease risk. Ann Rheum Dis. 2018;77:596–601. https://doi.org/10.1136/annrheumdis-2017-212454.
146. Brkic Z, et al. The interferon type I signature is present in systemic sclerosis before overt fibrosis and might contribute to its pathogenesis through high BAFF gene expression and high collagen synthesis. Ann Rheum Dis. 2016;75:1567–73. https://doi.org/10.1136/annrheumdis-2015-207392.
147. Mathai SK, et al. Circulating monocytes from systemic sclerosis patients with interstitial lung disease show an enhanced profibrotic phenotype. Lab Invest. 2010;90:812–23. https://doi.org/10.1038/labinvest.2010.73.
148. York MR, et al. A macrophage marker, Siglec-1, is increased on circulating monocytes in patients with systemic sclerosis and induced by type I interferons and toll-like receptor agonists. Arthritis Rheum. 2007;56:1010–20. https://doi.org/10.1002/art.22382.
149. Bhandari R, et al. Profibrotic activation of human macrophages in systemic sclerosis. Arthritis Rheumatol. 2020;72:1160–9. https://doi.org/10.1002/art.41243.
150. Netea MG, et al. Trained immunity: a program of innate immune memory in health and disease. Science. 2016;352:aaf1098. https://doi.org/10.1126/science.aaf1098.
151. van der Kroef M, et al. Histone modifications underlie monocyte dysregulation in patients with systemic sclerosis, underlining the treatment potential of epigenetic targeting. Ann Rheum Dis. 2019;78:529–38. https://doi.org/10.1136/annrheumdis-2018-214295.
152. Ramos PS, et al. Integrative analysis of DNA methylation in discordant twins unveils distinct architectures of systemic sclerosis subsets. Clin Epigenetics. 2019;11:58. https://doi.org/10.1186/s13148-019-0652-y.
153. Bujor AM, El Adili F, Parvez A, Marden G, Trojanowska M. Fli1 downregulation in scleroderma myeloid cells has profibrotic and proinflammatory effects. Front Immunol. 2020;11:800. https://doi.org/10.3389/fimmu.2020.00800.
154. Lee R, et al. Enhanced chemokine-receptor expression, function, and signaling in healthy African American and scleroderma-patient monocytes are regulated by caveolin-1. Fibrogenesis Tissue Repair. 2015;8:11. https://doi.org/10.1186/s13069-015-0028-7.
155. To S, Agarwal SK. Macrophages and cadherins in fibrosis and systemic sclerosis. Curr Opin Rheumatol. 2019;31:582–8. https://doi.org/10.1097/BOR.0000000000000657.
156. Lodyga M, et al. Cadherin-11-mediated adhesion of macrophages to myofibroblasts establishes a profibrotic niche of active TGF-beta. Sci Signal. 2019;12 https://doi.org/10.1126/scisignal.aao3469.
157. Pakshir P, et al. Dynamic fibroblast contractions attract remote macrophages in fibrillar collagen matrix. Nat Commun. 2019;10:1850. https://doi.org/10.1038/s41467-019-09709-6.
158. Fuschiotti P, Larregina AT, Ho J, Feghali-Bostwick C, Medsger TA Jr. Interleukin-13-producing CD8+ T cells mediate dermal fibrosis in patients with systemic sclerosis. Arthritis Rheum. 2013;65:236–46. https://doi.org/10.1002/art.37706.
159. Fuschiotti P, Medsger TA Jr, Morel PA. Effector CD8+ T cells in systemic sclerosis patients produce abnormally high levels of interleukin-13 associated with increased skin fibrosis. Arthritis Rheum. 2009;60:1119–28. https://doi.org/10.1002/art.24432.
160. Li G, et al. Skin-resident effector memory CD8(+)CD28(−) T cells exhibit a profibrotic phenotype in patients with systemic sclerosis. J Invest Dermatol. 2017;137:1042–50. https://doi.org/10.1016/j.jid.2016.11.037.
161. Yaseen B, et al. Interleukin-31 promotes pathogenic mechanisms underlying skin and lung fibrosis in scleroderma. Rheumatology. 2020;59:2625–36. https://doi.org/10.1093/rheumatology/keaa195.
162. Taylor DK, et al. T follicular helper-like cells contribute to skin fibrosis. Sci Transl Med. 2018;10 https://doi.org/10.1126/scitranslmed.aaf5307.
163. Frantz C, Auffray C, Avouac J, Allanore Y, Regulatory T. Cells in systemic sclerosis. Front Immunol. 2018;9:2356. https://doi.org/10.3389/fimmu.2018.02356.
164. Worrell JC, O'Reilly S. Bi-directional communication: conversations between fibroblasts and immune cells in systemic sclerosis. J Autoimmun. 2020;113:102526. https://doi.org/10.1016/j.jaut.2020.102526.
165. Moroncini G, Svegliati Baroni S, Gabrielli A. Agonistic antibodies in systemic sclerosis. Immunol Lett. 2018;195:83–7. https://doi.org/10.1016/j.imlet.2017.10.007.
166. Taher TE, et al. Association of defective regulation of autoreactive interleukin-6-producing transitional B lymphocytes with disease in patients with systemic sclerosis. Arthritis Rheumatol. 2018;70:450–61. https://doi.org/10.1002/art.40390.
167. Bosello S, et al. Characterization of inflammatory cell infiltrate of scleroderma skin: B cells and skin score progression. Arthritis Res Ther. 2018;20:75. https://doi.org/10.1186/s13075-018-1569-0.
168. Whitfield ML, et al. Systemic and cell type-specific gene expression patterns in scleroderma skin. Proc Natl Acad Sci U S A. 2003;100:12319–24. https://doi.org/10.1073/pnas.1635114100.
169. Francois A, et al. B lymphocytes and B-cell activating factor promote collagen and profibrotic markers expression by dermal fibroblasts in systemic sclerosis. Arthritis Res Ther. 2013;15:R168. https://doi.org/10.1186/ar4352.
170. Ah Kioon MD, et al. Plasmacytoid dendritic cells promote systemic sclerosis with a key role for TLR8. Sci Transl Med. 2018;10 https://doi.org/10.1126/scitranslmed.aam8458.
171. Kafaja S, et al. pDCs in lung and skin fibrosis in a bleomycin-induced model and patients with systemic sclerosis. JCI Insight. 2018;3 https://doi.org/10.1172/jci.insight.98380.
172. van Bon L, et al. Proteome-wide analysis and CXCL4 as a biomarker in systemic sclerosis. N Engl J Med. 2014;370:433–43. https://doi.org/10.1056/NEJMoa1114576.
173. Affandi AJ, et al. Low RUNX3 expression alters dendritic cell function in patients with systemic sclerosis and contributes to enhanced fibrosis. Ann Rheum Dis. 2019;78:1249–59. https://doi.org/10.1136/annrheumdis-2018-214991.
174. Russo B, Brembilla NC, Chizzolini C. Interplay between keratinocytes and fibroblasts: a systematic review providing a new angle for understanding skin fibrotic disorders. Front Immunol. 2020;11:648. https://doi.org/10.3389/fimmu.2020.00648.

175. Aden N, et al. Epithelial cells promote fibroblast activation via IL-1alpha in systemic sclerosis. J Invest Dermatol. 2010;130:2191–200. https://doi.org/10.1038/jid.2010.120.
176. Nikitorowicz-Buniak J, Shiwen X, Denton CP, Abraham D, Stratton R. Abnormally differentiating keratinocytes in the epidermis of systemic sclerosis patients show enhanced secretion of CCN2 and S100A9. J Invest Dermatol. 2014;134:2693–702. https://doi.org/10.1038/jid.2014.253.
177. Canady J, Arndt S, Karrer S, Bosserhoff AK. Increased KGF expression promotes fibroblast activation in a double paracrine manner resulting in cutaneous fibrosis. J Invest Dermatol. 2013;133:647–57. https://doi.org/10.1038/jid.2012.389.
178. Takahashi T, et al. Epithelial Fli1 deficiency drives systemic autoimmunity and fibrosis: possible roles in scleroderma. J Exp Med. 2017;214:1129–51. https://doi.org/10.1084/jem.20160247.
179. Serrati S, et al. Systemic sclerosis endothelial cells recruit and activate dermal fibroblasts by induction of a connective tissue growth factor (CCN2)/transforming growth factor beta-dependent mesenchymal-to-mesenchymal transition. Arthritis Rheum. 2013;65:258–69. https://doi.org/10.1002/art.37705.
180. Jimenez SA, Piera-Velazquez S. Endothelial to mesenchymal transition (EndoMT) in the pathogenesis of systemic sclerosis-associated pulmonary fibrosis and pulmonary arterial hypertension. Myth or reality? Matrix Biol. 2016;51:26–36. https://doi.org/10.1016/j.matbio.2016.01.012.
181. Rosa I, Romano E, Fioretto BS, Manetti M. The contribution of mesenchymal transitions to the pathogenesis of systemic sclerosis. Eur J Rheumatol. 2020;7:S157–64. https://doi.org/10.5152/eurjrheum.2019.19081.
182. Kuehl T, Lagares D. BH3 mimetics as anti-fibrotic therapy: unleashing the mitochondrial pathway of apoptosis in myofibroblasts. Matrix Biol. 2018;68-69:94–105. https://doi.org/10.1016/j.matbio.2018.01.020.
183. Jun JI, Lau LF. The matricellular protein CCN1 induces fibroblast senescence and restricts fibrosis in cutaneous wound healing. Nat Cell Biol. 2010;12:676–85. https://doi.org/10.1038/ncb2070.
184. Chan MW, Hinz B, McCulloch CA. Mechanical induction of gene expression in connective tissue cells. Methods Cell Biol. 2010;98:178–205. https://doi.org/10.1016/S0091-679X(10)98008-4.
185. Jun JB, et al. Scleroderma fibroblasts demonstrate enhanced activation of Akt (protein kinase B) in situ. J Invest Dermatol. 2005;124:298–303. https://doi.org/10.1111/j.0022-202X.2004.23559.x.
186. Horowitz JC, et al. Combinatorial activation of FAK and AKT by transforming growth factor-beta1 confers an anoikis-resistant phenotype to myofibroblasts. Cell Signal. 2007;19:761–71. https://doi.org/10.1016/j.cellsig.2006.10.001.
187. Kulasekaran P, et al. Endothelin-1 and transforming growth factor-beta1 independently induce fibroblast resistance to apoptosis via AKT activation. Am J Respir Cell Mol Biol. 2009;41:484–93. https://doi.org/10.1165/rcmb.2008-0447OC.
188. Santiago B, Galindo M, Rivero M, Pablos JL. Decreased susceptibility to Fas-induced apoptosis of systemic sclerosis dermal fibroblasts. Arthritis Rheum. 2001;44:1667–76. https://doi.org/10.1002/1529-0131(200107)44:7<1667::AID-ART291>3.0.CO;2-Y.
189. Jelaska A, Korn JH. Role of apoptosis and transforming growth factor beta1 in fibroblast selection and activation in systemic sclerosis. Arthritis Rheum. 2000;43:2230–9. https://doi.org/10.1002/1529-0131(200010)43:10<2230::AID-ANR10>3.0.CO;2-8.
190. Samuel GH, Lenna S, Bujor AM, Lafyatis R, Trojanowska M. Acid sphingomyelinase deficiency contributes to resistance of scleroderma fibroblasts to Fas-mediated apoptosis. J Dermatol Sci. 2012;67:166–72. https://doi.org/10.1016/j.jdermsci.2012.06.001.
191. Huang SK, et al. Prostaglandin E(2) induces fibroblast apoptosis by modulating multiple survival pathways. FASEB J. 2009;23:4317–26. https://doi.org/10.1096/fj.08-128801.
192. Bernard K, et al. Metabolic reprogramming is required for myofibroblast contractility and differentiation. J Biol Chem. 2015;290:25427–38. https://doi.org/10.1074/jbc.M115.646984.
193. Rangarajan S, et al. Metformin reverses established lung fibrosis in a bleomycin model. Nat Med. 2018;24:1121–7. https://doi.org/10.1038/s41591-018-0087-6.
194. Merkt W, Bueno M, Mora AL, Lagares D. Senotherapeutics: Targeting senescence in idiopathic pulmonary fibrosis. Semin Cell Dev Biol. 2020;101:104–10. https://doi.org/10.1016/j.semcdb.2019.12.008.
195. Martyanov V, et al. Novel lung imaging biomarkers and skin gene expression subsetting in dasatinib treatment of systemic sclerosis-associated interstitial lung disease. PLoS One. 2017;12:e0187580. https://doi.org/10.1371/journal.pone.0187580.
196. Aghajanian H, et al. Targeting cardiac fibrosis with engineered T cells. Nature. 2019;573:430–3. https://doi.org/10.1038/s41586-019-1546-z.
197. Dees C, et al. JAK-2 as a novel mediator of the profibrotic effects of transforming growth factor beta in systemic sclerosis. Arthritis Rheum. 2012;64:3006–15. https://doi.org/10.1002/art.34500.
198. Deverapalli SC, Rosmarin D. The use of JAK inhibitors in the treatment of progressive systemic sclerosis. J Eur Acad Dermatol Venereol. 2018;32:e328. https://doi.org/10.1111/jdv.14876.
199. Akamata K, et al. SIRT3 is attenuated in systemic sclerosis skin and lungs, and its pharmacologic activation mitigates organ fibrosis. Oncotarget. 2016;7:69321–36. https://doi.org/10.18632/oncotarget.12504.
200. Wei J, et al. The histone deacetylase sirtuin 1 is reduced in systemic sclerosis and abrogates fibrotic responses by targeting transforming growth factor beta signaling. Arthritis Rheumatol. 2015;67:1323–34. https://doi.org/10.1002/art.39061.
201. Shi B, Wang W, Korman B, Kai L, Wang Q, Wei J, Bale S, Marangoni RG, Bhattacharyya S, Miller S, Xu D, Akbarpour M, Cheresh P, Proccissi D, Gursel D, Espindola-Netto JM, Chini CCS, de Oliveira GC, Gudjonsson JE, Chini EN, Varga J. Targeting CD38-dependent NAD+ metabolism to mitigate multiple organ fibrosis. iScience. 2020;24(1):101902. https://doi.org/10.1016/j.isci.2020.101902. eCollection 2021 Jan 22. PMID: 33385109.
202. Lerbs T, et al. CD47 prevents the elimination of diseased fibroblasts in scleroderma. JCI Insight. 2020;5 https://doi.org/10.1172/jci.insight.140458.
203. Varga J, et al. Interferon-gamma reverses the stimulation of collagen but not fibronectin gene expression by transforming growth factor-beta in normal human fibroblasts. Eur J Clin Investig. 1990;20:487–93.
204. Chrobak I, Lenna S, Stawski L, Trojanowska M. Interferon-gamma promotes vascular remodeling in human microvascular endothelial cells by upregulating endothelin (ET)-1 and transforming growth factor (TGF) beta2. J Cell Physiol. 2013;228:1774–83. https://doi.org/10.1002/jcp.24337.
205. King TE Jr, et al. Effect of interferon gamma-1b on survival in patients with idiopathic pulmonary fibrosis (INSPIRE): a multicentre, randomised, placebo-controlled trial. Lancet. 2009;374:222–8. https://doi.org/10.1016/S0140-6736(09)60551-1.
206. Varga J. Recombinant cytokine treatment for scleroderma. Can the antifibrotic potential of interferon-gamma be realized clinically? Arch Dermatol. 1997;133:637–42.
207. Ghosh AK, et al. Peroxisome proliferator-activated receptor-gamma abrogates Smad-dependent collagen stimulation by targeting the p300 transcriptional coactivator. FASEB J. 2009;23:2968–77. https://doi.org/10.1096/fj.08-128736.
208. Wei J, et al. PPARgamma downregulation by TGFss in fibroblast and impaired expression and function in systemic sclerosis: a novel mechanism for progressive fibrogenesis. PLoS One. 2010;5:e13778. https://doi.org/10.1371/journal.pone.0013778.

209. Wei J, Bhattacharyya S, Varga J. Peroxisome proliferator-activated receptor gamma: innate protection from excessive fibrogenesis and potential therapeutic target in systemic sclerosis. Curr Opin Rheumatol. 2010;22:671–6. https://doi.org/10.1097/BOR.0b013e32833de1a7.
210. Oruqaj G, et al. Compromised peroxisomes in idiopathic pulmonary fibrosis, a vicious cycle inducing a higher fibrotic response via TGF-beta signaling. Proc Natl Acad Sci U S A. 2015; https://doi.org/10.1073/pnas.1415111112.
211. Ito I, et al. A nonclassical vitamin D receptor pathway suppresses renal fibrosis. J Clin Invest. 2013;123:4579–94. https://doi.org/10.1172/JCI67804.
212. Zerr P, et al. Vitamin D receptor regulates TGF-beta signalling in systemic sclerosis. Ann Rheum Dis. 2015;74:e20. https://doi.org/10.1136/annrheumdis-2013-204378.
213. An L, Sun MH, Chen F, Li JR. Vitamin D levels in systemic sclerosis patients: a meta-analysis. Drug Des Dev Ther. 2017;11:3119–25. https://doi.org/10.2147/DDDT.S144860.
214. Palumbo-Zerr K, et al. Orphan nuclear receptor NR4A1 regulates transforming growth factor-beta signaling and fibrosis. Nat Med. 2015;21:150–8. https://doi.org/10.1038/nm.3777.
215. Beyer C, et al. Stimulation of the soluble guanylate cyclase (sGC) inhibits fibrosis by blocking non-canonical TGFbeta signalling. Ann Rheum Dis. 2015;74:1408–16. https://doi.org/10.1136/annrheumdis-2013-204508.
216. Matei AE, et al. Protein kinases G are essential downstream mediators of the antifibrotic effects of sGC stimulators. Ann Rheum Dis. 2018;77:459. https://doi.org/10.1136/annrheumdis-2017-212489.
217. Humbert M, et al. Riociguat for the treatment of pulmonary arterial hypertension associated with connective tissue disease: results from PATENT-1 and PATENT-2. Ann Rheum Dis. 2017;76:422–6. https://doi.org/10.1136/annrheumdis-2015-209087.
218. Khanna D, et al. Riociguat in patients with early diffuse cutaneous systemic sclerosis (RISE-SSc): randomised, double-blind, placebo-controlled multicentre trial. Ann Rheum Dis. 2020;79:618–25. https://doi.org/10.1136/annrheumdis-2019-216823.
219. Volkmann ER, Varga J. Emerging targets of disease-modifying therapy for systemic sclerosis. Nat Rev Rheumatol. 2019;15:208–24. https://doi.org/10.1038/s41584-019-0184-z.
220. Asano Y, Trojanowska M. Fli1 represses transcription of the human alpha2(I) collagen gene by recruitment of the HDAC1/p300 complex. PLoS One. 2013;8:e74930. https://doi.org/10.1371/journal.pone.0074930.
221. Koinuma D, et al. Chromatin immunoprecipitation on microarray analysis of Smad2/3 binding sites reveals roles of ETS1 and TFAP2A in transforming growth factor beta signaling. Mol Cell Biol. 2009;29:172–86. https://doi.org/10.1128/MCB.01038-08.
222. Van Beek JP, Kennedy L, Rockel JS, Bernier SM, Leask A. The induction of CCN2 by TGFbeta1 involves Ets-1. Arthritis Res Ther. 2006;8:R36. https://doi.org/10.1186/ar1890.
223. Kubo M, et al. Persistent down-regulation of Fli1, a suppressor of collagen transcription, in fibrotic scleroderma skin. Am J Pathol. 2003;163:571–81. https://doi.org/10.1016/S0002-9440(10)63685-1.
224. Wu B, Rockel JS, Lagares D, Kapoor M. Ephrins and Eph receptor signaling in tissue repair and fibrosis. Curr Rheumatol Rep. 2019;21:23. https://doi.org/10.1007/s11926-019-0825-x.
225. Nakerakanti S, Trojanowska M. The role of TGF-beta receptors in fibrosis. Open Rheumatol J. 2012;6:156–62. https://doi.org/10.2174/1874312901206010156.
226. Bhattacharyya S, Fang F, Tourtellotte W, Varga J. Egr-1: new conductor for the tissue repair orchestra directs harmony (regeneration) or cacophony (fibrosis). J Pathol. 2013;229:286–97. https://doi.org/10.1002/path.4131.
227. Nakerakanti SS, Bujor AM, Trojanowska M. CCN2 is required for the TGF-beta induced activation of Smad1-Erk1/2 signaling network. PLoS One. 2011;6:e21911. https://doi.org/10.1371/journal.pone.0021911.
228. Svegliati S, et al. Oxidative DNA damage induces the ATM-mediated transcriptional suppression of the Wnt inhibitor WIF-1 in systemic sclerosis and fibrosis. Sci Signal. 2014;7:ra84. https://doi.org/10.1126/scisignal.2004592.
229. Bhattacharyya S, et al. Fibronectin EDA promotes chronic cutaneous fibrosis through Toll-like receptor signaling. Sci Transl Med. 2014;6:232ra250. https://doi.org/10.1126/scitranslmed.3008264.
230. O'Reilly S, Ciechomska M, Cant R, Hugle T, van Laar JM. Interleukin-6, its role in fibrosing conditions. Cytokine Growth Factor Rev. 2012;23:99–107. https://doi.org/10.1016/j.cytogfr.2012.04.003.
231. Trojanowska M. Role of PDGF in fibrotic diseases and systemic sclerosis. Rheumatology. 2008;47(Suppl 5):v2–4. https://doi.org/10.1093/rheumatology/ken265.
232. Karimizadeh E, et al. c-Abl silencing reduced the inhibitory effects of TGF-beta1 on apoptosis in systemic sclerosis dermal fibroblasts. Mol Cell Biochem. 2015;405:169–76. https://doi.org/10.1007/s11010-015-2408-0.
233. Zhou Y, et al. Inhibition of mechanosensitive signaling in myofibroblasts ameliorates experimental pulmonary fibrosis. J Clin Invest. 2013;123:1096–108. https://doi.org/10.1172/JCI66700.

Overview of Animal Models

19

Yoshihide Asano and Jörg H. W. Distler

Introduction

The ability to sample fibrotic tissue in SSc by performing skin biopsy has been a major strength in trying to understand the pathobiology of this disease in comparison to other forms of organ-based fibrosis. It has permitted the identification of cardinal histological features of scleroderma and has defined key phases of the pathology in a temporal sequence so that there is now a clear understanding that as the disease develops, the first changes occur at the level of the dermal microcirculation followed by the development of inflammation that first involves cells of the innate immune and later adaptive immune system. Finally, there is the fibrotic stage of the disease that results in the replacement of specialized structures with rather vascular fibrotic connective tissue. The final component is the most important in determining the morbidity and mortality of SSc as it occurs in all target tissues. It is noteworthy that the activated pathways are largely overlapping with the biological responses during normal wound healing, but, in contrast to physiological tissue responses to injury, are not effectively terminated, but become chronically activated. In addition to defining these components of the SSc disease process, skin biopsy material has also proven valuable as a starting point to identify deregulated signaling cascades and to generate novel hypotheses. To test the importance of a candidate pathway, process, or mediator, it is necessary to explore the relevance experimentally. While experiments on cellular components isolated from affected tissues such as primary fibroblasts are essential to provide the first proof of concept, there is a pressing need to further validate the results in vivo. Animal models of SSc are crucially required to close the gap between in vitro studies and clinical trials.

However, this translation from bench to bedside has long been hindered by a paucity of suitable animal models, as well as insufficient characterization of the existing models; however, this has changed over the last years. Several promising animal models of SSc have recently been described. Moreover, intensive characterization of the existing models greatly improved our understanding of the strengths and limitations of preexisting models.

Traditionally, murine models of SSc have been considered primarily in the context of skin fibrosis. As skin fibrosis is seen in the vast majority of patients, this is a reasonable starting point. However, as our understanding of the disease process has evolved, the breadth of animal models addressing these pathogenic mechanisms has also evolved. In particular, models of immunity and inflammation, and vascular injury, as well as pathogenic processes in other organ systems, particularly the lungs, need to be considered as models of SSc. Unfortunately, no current animal model manifests the whole range of pathological features seen in patients. Instead, in most models, only a fraction of disease manifestations are modeled, reflecting the limitations of our understanding of underlying pathogenesis. Thus, a comprehensive description of mouse models of SSc requires consideration of a vast array of animal models of fibrosis, inflammation, autoimmunity, and vascular injury. This chapter describes traditional models of SSc in more detail, but also provides a more comprehensive review of models, including emerging

The current version is based on a previous version of the chapter by:
Christopher P. Denton PhD, FRCP, Professor of Experimental Rheumatology[3,a*]; Robert Lafyatis MD[4,b]
[3] Department of Inflammation, Division of Medicine, Centre for Rheumatology and Connective Tissue Diseases, UCL Medical School, London, UK
[4] Department of Medicine, Rheumatology Section, Boston University School of Medicine, Boston, MA, USA
[a] Email: c.denton@medsch.ucl.ac.uk
[b] Email: lafyatis@bu.edu

Y. Asano (✉)
Department of Dermatology, Tohoku University, Graduate School of Medicine, Sendai, Japan
e-mail: yasano@derma.med.tohoku.ac.jp

J. H. W. Distler
Department of Rheumatology and Hiller Research Center, University Hospital Düsseldorf, Heinrich-Heine University, Düsseldorf, Germany
e-mail: joerg.distler@med.uni-duesseldorf.de

Y. Allanore et al. (eds.), *Scleroderma*, https://doi.org/10.1007/978-3-031-40658-4_19

disease models. We will outline strengths and weaknesses of each model. Models will be somewhat arbitrarily divided into models with fibrosis as predominant clinical feature, models with immune and inflammatory deregulation and subsequent, inflammation-dependent fibrosis, and models with SSc-like vascular disease. We will demonstrate that there is not the one perfect model of SSc that resembles all features of human SSc [1]. However, we aim to highlight that a wise combination of complimentary models can booster our understanding of the molecular pathogenesis of SSc and might support the development of novel targeted therapies.

Models of SSc with Fibrosis as Predominant Clinical Feature

Although fibrosis is a feature of several organs in SSc, the predominantly affected sites are skin, seen in most patients, and lungs, seen in many patients and one of the major causes of morbidity and mortality.

The Tight-Skin 1 Mouse (Tsk-1)

One of the best-characterized and most widely used genetic mouse models for SSc is the tight-skin 1 mouse (Tsk-1). This strain, originally identified as a spontaneous mutant, shows diffusely tethered skin that can be detected shortly after birth, but is more easily appreciated as tightening over the intercapsular skin as the mice age [2]. A stable mouse strain was derived and through backcross linked to the pallid locus for skin color. A series of elegant genetic mapping studies identified fibrillin 1 as the responsible gene, and sequencing of this gene showed that an in-frame tandem partial reduplication was the mutation responsible for the phenotype [3] (Fig. 19.1). Heterozygous mice manifest the phenotype, while homozygous mutant mice die in utero at ~day 8. Skin pathology causing skin tethering is due to thickening of the fascial layers of the skin rather than the dermis. Histologically, this manifests as thickening of the so-called hypodermis without major collagen accumulation in the dermis. However, this process may be relevant to the subcutaneous fascia hyperplasia seen in SSc skin. Of interest, fibroblasts isolated from Tsk-1 display an activated phenotype in vitro with increased release of collagen, thus resembling the endogenous activation of SSc fibroblasts in culture. In addition to skin fibrosis, Tsk-1 mice show more widespread effects linked to the central structural role fibrillin plays in microfibrils and elastic fibers, including muscle fascia and tendon hyperplasia, skeletal overgrowth, and pulmonary emphysema. The mutant fibrillin-1 protein leads to altered microfibril structure, stability and turnover, and altered depositions of other fibrillin-associated microfibril proteins [4, 5]. The molecular pathways activated by mutant fibrillin in Tsk-1 mice resemble those in SSc with activation of central profibrotic pathways including TGF-β, canonical Wnt, and AP-1 signaling [6–8].

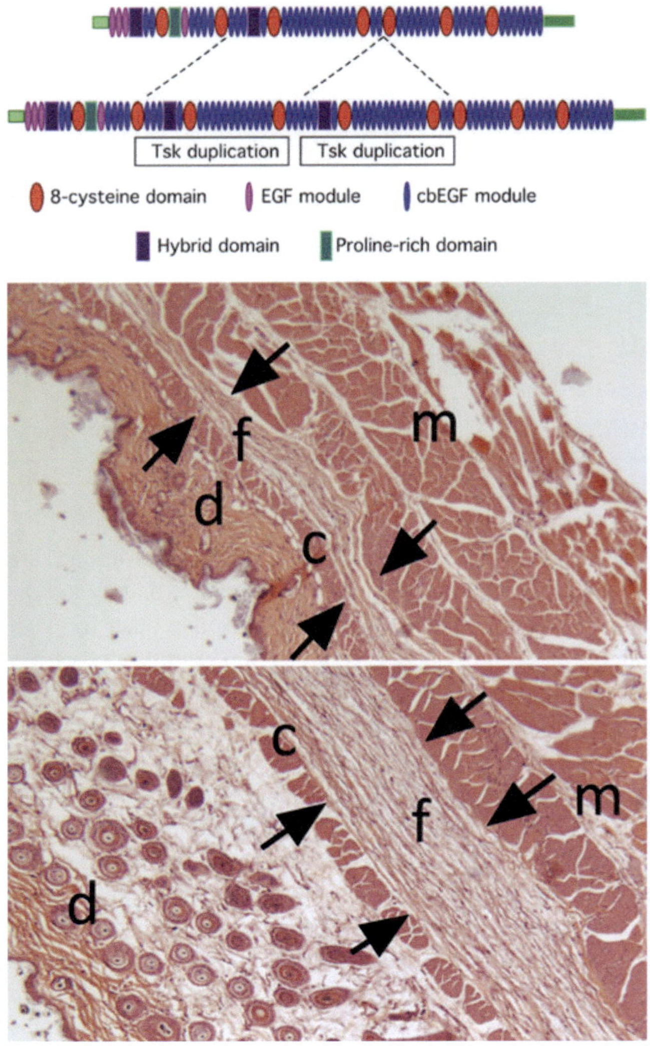

Fig. 19.1 Mutant fibrillin in Tsk-1 mice leads to fascia hyperplasia. *Upper panel*: protein structure resulting from the in-frame duplication seen in Tsk-1 mice. *Middle and lower panels*: cross section of skin to body wall from control (*middle panel*) and Tsk-1 (*lower panel*) mice showing increased fascia thickness (*f*, marked with *arrows*), dermis (*d*), panniculus carnosus (*c*), and skeletal muscle (*m*), hematoxylin, and eosin stain. Proper measurement of fascia thickness requires full-thickness biopsy including subcutaneous muscle in this model. The increased subcutaneous fat seen here in Tsk-1 skin is not a feature of these mouse, but an irregular feature of mouse skin depending on the location of the skin and weight/age of them mouse

Inflammatory infiltrates are absent in Tsk-1 mice. However, several publications demonstrate that B cells are activated in Tsk-1 mice and that inhibition of B-cell function ameliorates the Tsk-1 phenotype [9, 10]. Indeed, Tsk-1 mice display autoantibodies [11, 12], and passive transfer of Tsk1 immune cells partially reproduces the Tsk-1 phenotype [13, 14]. Contrary, the tsk-1 phenotype has been reported to be largely preserved in RAG-deficient mice [15, 16].

The Tight-Skin 2 Mouse (Tsk-2)

The Tsk2 mouse strain was a product of chemical mutagenesis using ethylnitrosourea that led to a similar phenotype in the skin as Tsk-1 [17]. Tsk2/+ mouse fibrotic phenotype has recently been shown to be due to a gain-of-function mutation in the PIIINP segment of the Col3a1 gene [18]. It has been reported to be some histological and serological differences in this phenotype compared to Tsk-1, such as a more generalized fibrotic phenotype associated with inflammatory change in the skin and a high prevalence of SSc-associated autoantibodies. In an intriguing experiment, Tsk-1 and Tsk-2 strains were intercrossed and a mouse with more marked skin tightness was produced. The Tsk-2 strain has not been extensively validated, and so, the validity or utility of this strain cannot be concluded.

TGF-ß Mediated Models of Fibrosis

The overwhelming evidence supporting a role of enhanced TGF-β signaling in human SSc led to the development of mouse strains in which there is a more defined abnormality of TGF-β activity.

Inducible Expression of Activated TGF-βRI

Expression of a mutated, constitutively active form of the type I TGF-β receptor (TGF-βRI^{CA}) offers the possibility for sustained ligand-independent activation of TGF-β signaling. Two different strategies are currently employed to overexpress TGF-βRI^{CA}: an elegant compound genetic strategy with fibroblast-specific overexpression of TGF-βRI^{CA} and overexpression with adeno-associated viral vectors. In the genetic approach, TGF-βRI^{CA} was conditionally expressed by insertion after a floxed STOP cassette. When these mice were bred to estrogen-inducible Cre recombinase mice and challenged with tamoxifen, the stop codon was excised and TGFβRI^{CA} expression was selectively activated in fibroblasts. This proved very effective, and mice demonstrated severe skin fibrosis and abnormalities in multiple organs [19] (Fig. 19.2). Replication-deficient type V adeno-associated viral vectors encoding for TGFβRI^{CA}

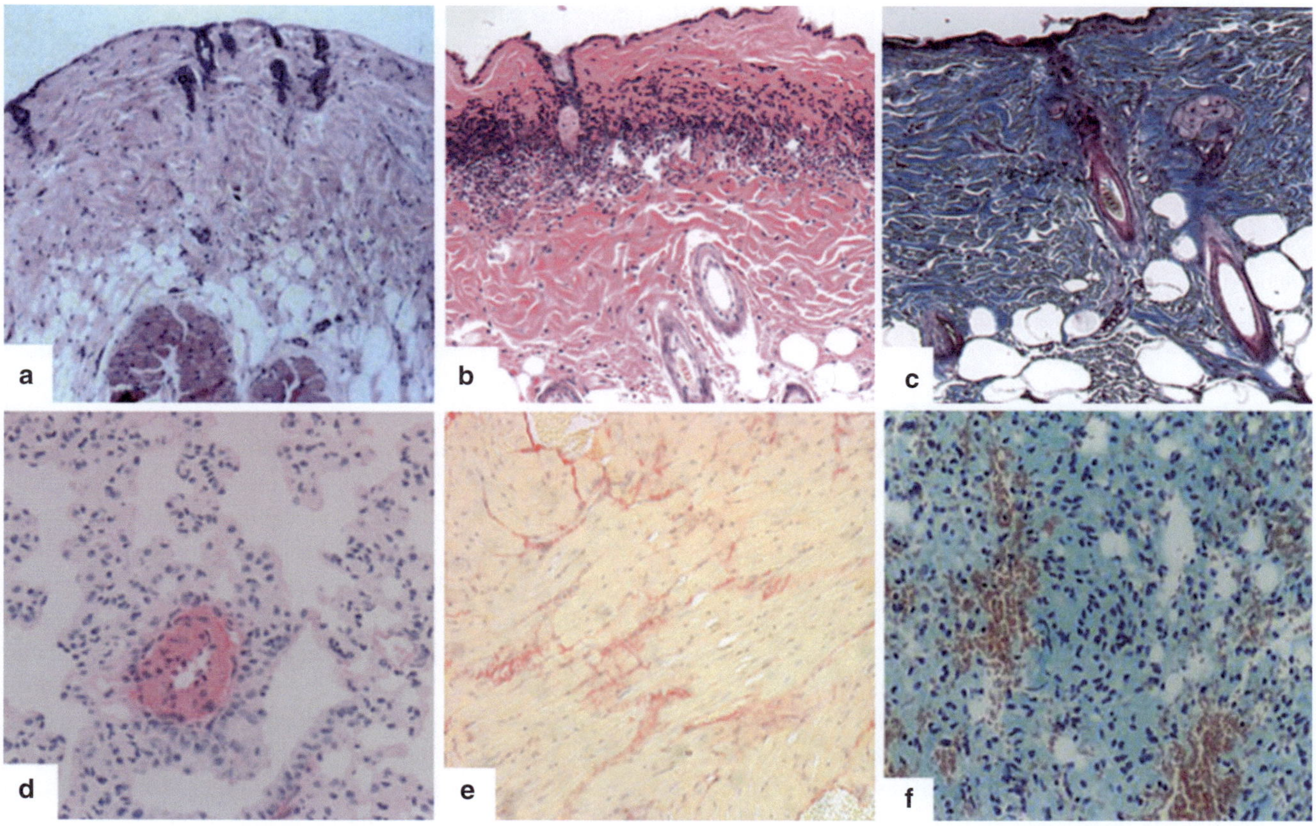

Fig. 19.2 Genetic models of SSc with directed activation of TGF-β signaling. Two complementary mouse models with fibroblast-specific activation of TGF-β signaling are shown. Both express mutated TGF-β receptors. Panels (**a–c**) show skin fibrosis. The strain TβRIIΔk-fib has a mutant form of TβRII and develops mild skin fibrosis (**a**). The strain TβRI-CA-fib expresses a constitutively active TβRI receptor and has high-level activation of TGF-β signaling. There is marked fibrosis in the skin shown by H&E stain (**b**) and Masson's trichrome (**c**). The TβRIIΔk-fib strain also shows susceptibility to relevant organ-based features of scleroderma including pulmonary vasculopathy (**d**), cardiac fibrosis (**e**), and, in a minority of cases, lung fibrosis (**f**)

offer a technically less complex approach to locally overexpress TGFβRI^{CA} in tissues of interest. Both approaches have been extensively used to study TGF-β signaling in vivo [20–23].

Fibroblast-Specific Deletion of the TGF-βRII-Kinase Domain-TβRIIΔk

Another mouse model with aberrant TGF-β signaling was developed by fibroblast-specific overexpression of a non-signaling mutant type II TGF-β receptor using the same promoter construct as in TGFβRI^{CA} mice [24] lacking in the intracellular kinase domain. Although this construct had been shown to operate as a dominant negative inhibitor of TGF-β signaling in tissue culture, in vivo paradoxical upregulation of TGF-β signaling was observed and mice developed fibrosis [24]. Lungs of TGF-βRII-kinase domain-TβRIIΔk-fib mice treated with intratracheal saline, a treatment not resulting in any pathology in normal mice, or bleomycin, showed epithelial injury or increased epithelial injury and fibrosis, respectively. The strain provided the first evidence that upregulated fibroblast TGF-β activity leads to perivascular fibrosis [25]. Moreover, this strain is more sensitive to SU5416-induced PAH (inhibitor of the Flk-1/KDR VEGF receptor tyrosine kinase, a common model of PAH) with pulmonary arteriolar luminal obliteration caused by proliferating endothelial cells [26] (Fig. 19.2). One potential limitation of this strain is the relatively mild nature of baseline fibrosis, and its future probably lies in studies aiming to better understand the interplay between TGF-β and other candidate pathways and in understanding second events in the pathogenesis of organ-based disease in SSc.

Fibroblast-Specific Transgenic Overexpression of Connective Tissue Growth Factor (CTGF)

The matricellular protein connective tissue growth factor (CTGF), a member of the CCN family of proteins (CCN2), is a common target gene of TGF-β and mediates in part the profibrotic effects of TGF-β. Although its profibrotic effects on cultured fibroblasts are modest, CTGF is expressed at sustained high levels in SSc tissues and by explanted SSc fibroblasts. A similar approach to the experiments examining TGF-β signaling has been employed to overexpress CTGF in fibroblasts. Fibroblast-specific CTGF-overexpressing mice develop fibrosis in the skin and internal organs [27]. This model may be an elegant tool to study CTGF signaling in vivo.

Models of Fibrosis Induced by Activation of Canonical Wnt Signaling

Wnt-10b Transgenic Mice

Transgenic mice with overexpression of Wnt10b under control of the adipocyte promoter FABP4 develop massive skin fibrosis with up to fivefold increase in dermal thickness and up to tenfold increase in hydroxyproline content and prominent hypodermal atrophy with replacement of subcutaneous fat by collagen as in SSc [28]. Consistent with these in vivo effects, Wnt overexpression in vitro in fibroblasts and pre-adipocytes shows blockade of adipogenesis and upregulated profibrotic gene expression. These effects are similar to changes seen in SSc skin and suggest that Wnts might contribute to fibrosis in SSc by activating resident fibroblasts and through altered developmental programming of pre-adipocytes [20, 29].

Fibroblast-Specific Overexpression of a Constitutively Active β-Catenin

Another model with selective activation of canonical Wnt signaling is the β-catenin^{CA} Fib model. In this model, an exon 3-deficient mutant of β-catenin that is resistant to phosphorylation and subsequent degradation of β-catenin is overexpressed in an inducible manner selectively in fibroblasts using the same Col1a2 CreER line as described for TGFβRI^{CA} mice [30]. These mice rapidly develop skin fibrosis within 2–4 weeks. However, other features of SSc such as vasculopathy have not been studied in those mice.

Caveolin-1-Deficient Mice

Caveolin-1 deficiency in mice leads to a complex phenotype partially resembling SSc with both vascular and fibrotic features, including lung fibrosis, cardiomyopathy, and pulmonary hypertension [31–37]. While data on the effects of caveolin-1 vascular permeability are conflicting, several lines of evidence suggest that caveolin-1 regulates vasoreaction. Aortic rings of caveolin-1 deficient mice show enhanced relaxation to acetylcholine challenge. Aortic endothelial cells isolated from caveolin-deleted mice produce increased levels of NO, possibly due to disruption of the normal inhibitory interaction of caveolin with eNOS. In addition, small arteries in caveolin-deficient mice show decreased vascular smooth muscle cell-dependent endothelin-1 or angiotensin II-elicited vasoconstriction. Notably, these mice also show marked changes in lung morphology with large areas of the lungs displaying markedly thickened septa, increased immunostaining for Flk1-positive cells, a marker of endothelial and hematopoietic progenitors, increased extracellular matrix, and hypertrophy of type II pneumocytes. Increased matrix is also seen in the dermis of these mice fibrotic, possibly related to enhanced TGF-β activity as caveolin-1 overexpression inhibits TGF-β signaling [36, 38].

Xenograft Model of SSc Skin in SCID Mice

In other areas of experimental medicine, the use of models in which disease tissue is grafted onto immunodeficient mice has been fruitful in understanding aspects of the human disease. This approach has been applied in a limited way to SSc by transplanting skin onto severe combined immunodeficiency (SCID) mice that lack most components of a competent immune system [39, 40]. The skin survives and 30 days after transplant shows increased intranuclear phospho-Smad 2 and -3 and decreased Smad 7 staining, compared to control skin, a similar pattern of expression as seen in untransplanted skin. The extent to which this adds to studies of tissue samples or from cultured cells or tissue equivalent models derived from these skin biopsies is unclear. Moreover, standardization of this model is challenging. However, this is a promising area for future evaluation and deserves further exploration.

VEGF tg Mice

Mice with transgenic insertion of a keratin 14 promoter expression cassette containing the gene for murine VEGF164 [41] were recently studied as a novel mouse model of SSc. The keratin 14 promoter cassette selectively targets VEGF164 expression to basal epidermal keratinocytes, resulting in a selective upregulation of VEGF164 in the epidermis and dermis of transgenic mice. Mice carrying two copies of the expression cassette (VEGF+/+), but not mice with only one expression cassette and one normal allele (VEGF+/−), spontaneously developed skin fibrosis with increased dermal thickness, collagen deposition, and fibroblast-to-myofibroblast transition, indicating profibrotic effect of VEGF on the skin in a gene-dosing manner. Moreover, transgenic overexpression of VEGF also rendered mice more susceptible to fibrosis induced by other stimuli. The profibrotic effect of bleomycin became more pronounced with induction of skin fibrosis in VEGF+/− tg mice and even more enhanced fibrosis in VEGF+/+ tg mice. Moreover, analysis in TSK1/VEGF+/+ mice showed similar profibrotic effects of VEGF also under noninflammatory in vivo conditions. In addition, the authors described an inverse gene-dosing effect on the number of microvessels in the skin, with a higher number of microvessels in VEGF+/− tg mice than in VEGF+/+ tg mice. However, further studies are required to determine whether these microvascular changes are reminiscent of the ones in SSc patients and whether VEGF tg mice may serve as a model for microvascular disease in SSc.

PTEN-Deficient Mice

Phosphatase and tensin homolog (PTEN) is a dual-specific lipid and protein phosphatase, regulating a broad range of biological activities such as tumor progression and tissue repair. As a lipid phosphatase, PTEN dephosphorylates phosphatidylinositol-3, 4, 5-phosphate (PIP3) and reduces the level of PIP3, a critical second messenger mediating the signals of fibrosis and inflammation. In SSc dermal fibroblasts, decreased PTEN expression and increased Akt phosphorylation are observed, suggesting that impaired PTEN-dependent suppression of the phosphatidylinositol 3-kinase (PI3K)/Akt pathway may contribute to fibroblast activation [42]. Supporting this idea, fibroblast-specific PTEN knockout mice develop fibrosis spontaneously in the skin and lungs in parallel with elevated Akt phosphorylation and increased expression of CTGF in dermal fibroblasts [42, 43]. The inhibition of the PI3K/Akt pathway reduces the overexpression of collagen and CCN2 in PTEN-deficient fibroblasts, while overexpression of PTEN reduces the excessive expression of type I collagen and CCN2 in SSc fibroblasts [42]. Thus, PTEN appears to be a potential in vivo master regulator of fibrogenesis. Given that PTEN is implicated in the pathogenesis of pulmonary arterial hypertension and cardiac fibrosis [44, 45], PTEN deficiency may be a critical driver of multiple organ fibrosis. Further characterization of conditional PTEN knockout mice may help us understand the role of PTEN in multiple organ fibrosis of SSc.

Models of SSc with Immune and Inflammatory Deregulation and Subsequent Fibrosis

Mice have provided a powerful experimental system for immunology research. It is not surprising that this has led to the development of immunologically based mouse models for SSc. In some cases, this has been through genetic modification of other strains, but the best-characterized immune models are those based upon transplantation of splenocyte with or without bone marrow cells with minor HLA mismatches and subsequent chronic graft-versus-host disease (cGvHD). Like some of the models described above, these models not only provide mimics of the disease and a platform to explore potential targeted therapies, but also shed important light upon possible key immunopathology relevant to human SSc.

Murine Sclerodermatous Chronic Graft-Versus-Host Disease (cGvHD)

Many forms of cGvHD have been described in mice with the common theme of transfer of immune cells, typically splenocytes and/or bone marrow cells from a donor animal to a recipient with minor histocompatibility mismatch (Fig. 19.3). cGvHD models of SSc have several appeals: the similarity to human chronic graft-versus host disease, which sometimes manifests sclerodermatous skin changes in addition to other autoimmune feature; moreover, cGvHD is clearly immune driven and further thought to require adaptive immunity, representing the only available models requiring the adaptive immune system.

Several chronic GVHD models, a subset of the large number of GVHD models, have been described (reviewed in [46]). Models strains mismatched for minor histocompatibility differences more typically drive a chronic immunological activation reminiscent of SSc, while models utilizing mismatched MHC donors and recipients more typically lead to SLE-like disease. The most common strain combination for SSc-GVHD utilizes splenocytes and bone marrow cells from B10. D2 (H-2^d) into irradiated BALB/c (H-2^d) hosts (B10.D2 (H-2^d) → BALB/c (H-2^d) model) [47–52]. The phenotype is observed in the skin and some viscera, including the lungs, persists for some time and then usually undergoes some degree of spontaneous resolution after very long follow-up. The histological characteristics show a mononuclear cell infiltrate with T cells and monocyte-macrophage cells that resemble some of the features of human GVHD and SSc. In general, there is activation of dermal connective tissue synthesis and thickened fibrosis of affected tissues, although the degree of persistent cellular infiltrate is rather more than is typical of human SSc.

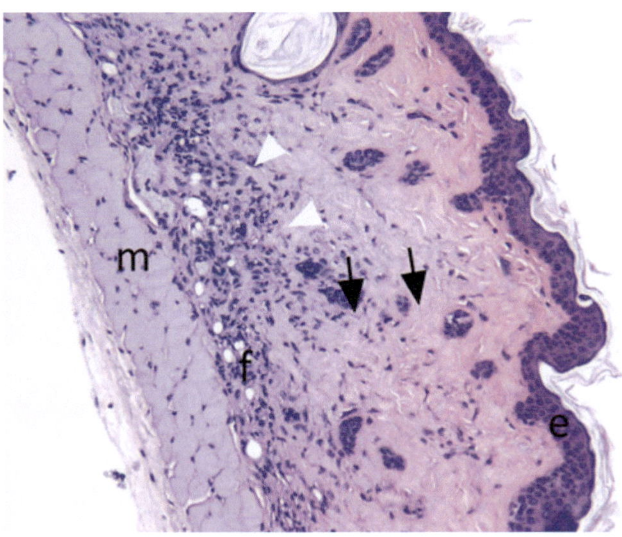

Fig. 19.3 Graft-versus-host disease-induced skin fibrosis. Skin pathology, hematoxylin, and eosin stain, 4 weeks after B10. D2 splenocyte injection into BalbC RAG2−/− mice, showing intact hypodermal muscle (*m*, panniculus carnosus), fat largely replaced by inflammatory cell infiltrate (*f*) epidermal hyperplasia (*e*), collagen deposition (*black arrows*), and dermal inflammation (*white arrowheads*)

A further modification of this model was the use of a genetically immunodeficient mouse that lacks any adaptive immune system due to the genomic deletion of both copies of the critical recombination activation gene-2 (RAG2) that encodes for an enzyme which is essential for T- and B-lymphocyte maturation by combining constituent genes to assemble T-cell receptor and immunoglobulin. RAG2-deleted mice develop several features of SSc including autoantibodies, vascular disease, and skin and intestinal fibrosis. These mice lack lung fibrosis described in the irradiated model. They apparently develop more robust skin disease due to a radio-resistant host $CD4^+CD25^+$ cell population possibly representing regulatory T cells (Fig. 19.3). The development of disease in this model requires either donor or host APCs, $CD4^+$T cells, and CD80/86-dependent costimulation [53, 54].

Another common model for sclerodermatous cGvHD is the LP/J (H-2^b) → C57Bl/6 (H-2^b) model. In this model, cGvHD is induced by transplantation of spenocytes from LP/J (H-2^b) donor mice into C57Bl/6 (H-2^b) mice after sublethal irradiation. Allogeneically transplanted mice develop systemic inflammation and subsequent fibrosis as described for the B10.D2 (H-2^d) → BALB/c (H-2^d) model. The onset of inflammation is more acute and severe as in the B10.D2 (H-2^d) → BALB/c (H-2^d) model. However, the major advantage is C57Bl/6 serves as recipients. As most genetically modified strains are available on a C57Bl/6 background, those strains are accessible for evaluation in this model.

Bleomycin-Induced Inflammation and Fibrosis

Bleomycin is a cancer chemotherapeutic that has established itself as a potent initiator of tissue injury and fibrosis. It has become associated with two models that have become a cornerstone of experimental biology that is highly relevant to studies of SSc. Bleomycin can be given intravenous, intraperitoneal, subcutaneous, or intratracheal routes to initiate lung fibrosis. This only occurs in certain susceptible mouse strains, the basis of this susceptibility defined genetically by the expression levels of the inactivating enzyme. The mechanisms for bleomycin-induced tissue injury and fibrosis are complex, including profibrotic mediators such as TGF-β, Wnt, Notch, Hedgehog and its activator αvβ6 integrin; innate immune and inflammasome mediators such as IL-1, IL-6, HMGB1; and the lipid mediator lysophosphatidic acid [20, 55–63] This may represent one of the strengths of this model, as it is likely to replicate some of the complexity of fibrotic initiation in human disease. As a consequence of tissue damage, there is inflammation and subsequent activation of myofibroblasts.

In wild-type mice challenged intratracheally with bleomycin, fibrosis can be lethal, but if mice survive, there is generally slow resolution of the fibrotic pathology. This is in contrast to most human lung pathology but is an important reminder that fibrosis may be reversible under some circumstances. Being a well-established model for lung fibrosis, there has been considerable use of bleomycin as an inducer of skin changes that reflect SSc (Fig. 19.4). The model of bleomycin-induced skin fibrosis has become one of the most widely used models for pathogenetic studies of SSc and has been very widely used to explore candidate therapies for SSc that may address the inflammatory as well as the fibrotic phase of the disease. However, one has to be aware of the limitations of this approach: Bleomycin-induced fibrosis is dependent on an initial phase of inflammation. In preventive set-ups, treatments that interfere with this early inflammatory phase will also prevent the development of fibrosis. Bleomycin-induced fibrosis is thus hyper-responsive to anti-inflammatory treatment, in particular with preventive dosing schedules. Models of bleomycin-induced fibrosis are thus suited for therapeutic evaluation of the antifibrotic effects of drugs with anti-inflammatory mode of action Nevertheless, the bleomycin skin model tests facets of the pathogenic process that may not be included in genetically determined models and has a number of practical advantages in terms of ease of use. Another advantage of this model is that it can be used in various genetically manipulated mice to explore the relationship between inflammatory and fibrotic pathways.

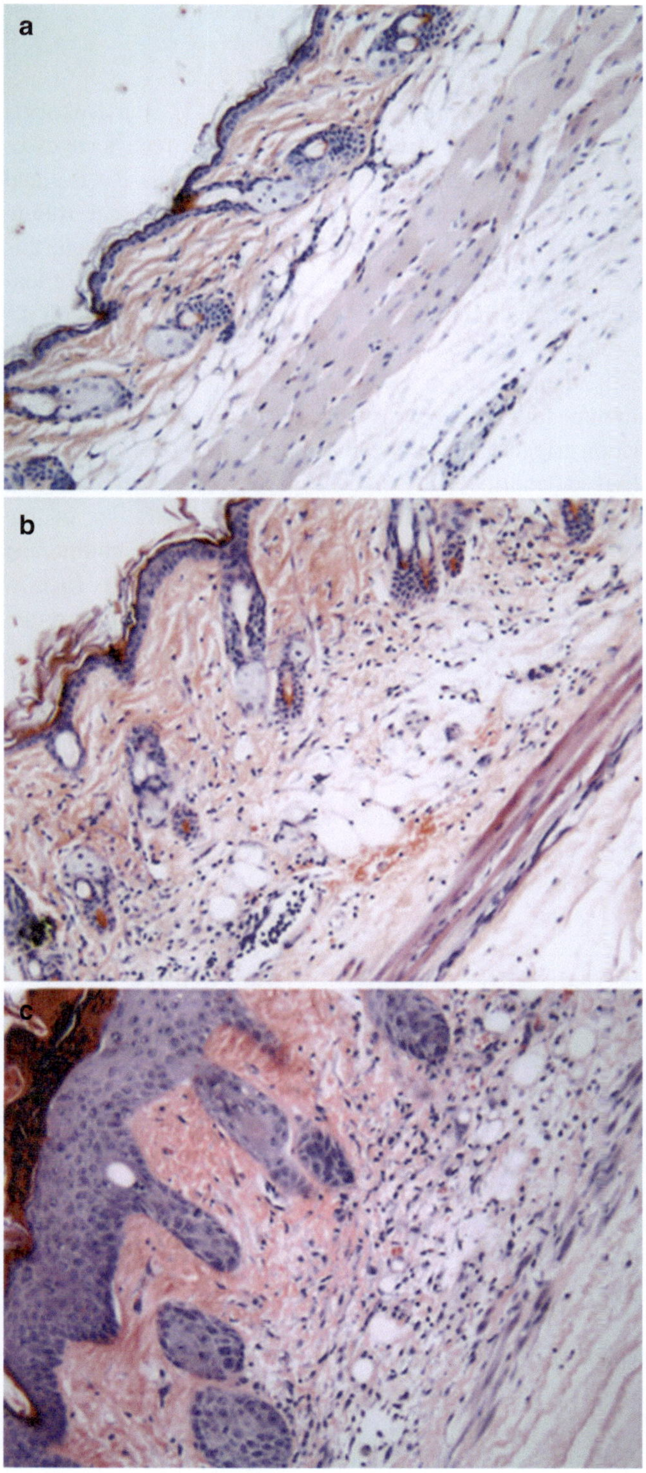

Fig. 19.4 Bleomycin-induced skin fibrosis. Intradermal bleomycin injected daily for 21 days induces inflammation and fibrosis (panels **b** and **c**), and epidermal hyperplasia (panel **c**) compared to control skin (panel **a**), hematoxylin and eosin stain

Models of Reactive Oxygen Species in SSc

In the recent decade, hypochlorous acid (HOCl)-treated mice are widely recognized as a new inducible murine model of SSc [64]. A 4–6-week daily subcutaneous injection of HOCl induces extensive fibrosis of the skin, lungs, and heart along with the production of anti-topoisomerase I (topo-I) antibody [64, 65]. This model also displays intima-media thickening with reduced lumen diameter in the aorta and small renal arteries [66, 67]. In contrast to localized skin involvement around the injection site in BLM-treated mice, HOCl-treated mice develop diffuse cutaneous involvement. Fibrosis pathway proteins, such as TGF-β, NF-kB, Smad3, p-Smad3, STAT3, p-STAT3, AKT and Wnt/β-catenin, and the infiltration of $CD4^+$ T cells, $CD8^+$ T cells, $CD20^+$ B cells, $CD11c^+$ DC, $CD11b^+$ myeloid cells, and myofibroblasts, are significantly elevated in the skin and lungs of HOCl-treated mice. mRNA expression of fibrosis mediators, such as IL-1β, IL-4, IL-13, IL-6, IL-17, IL-33, TNF-α, and CTGF, is also upregulated in the skin and/or lungs. An early expansion of transitional B cells is evident, followed by a late expansion of mature naïve B cells and a decrease in plasmablasts and memory B cells. B cells reveal IL-6 overproduction and IL-10 reduction at the early inflammatory phase, while expressing profibrotic cytokines (TGF-β and IL-6) at the late fibrotic phase [68–71]. Overall, HOCl-treated mice demonstrate fibrosis, vasculopathy, and systemic immune cell activation similar to those of SSc. This model provides a clear definition of the importance of reactive oxygen species in SSc pathogenesis.

Topo-I Immunization Model

Disease-specific autoantibodies against topo-I, centromere, and RNA polymerase III antigens are associated with clinical subsets of SSc. Accumulating data have shown that anti-topo-I antibody levels are positively correlated with disease severity and are predictive for certain clinical features, suggesting that autoimmunity against the topo-I antigen may contribute to the development of SSc. Indeed, anti-topo-I antibody is detectable in bleomycin-treated mice. Based on these backgrounds, a topo-I immunization murine model of SSc was established [72]. Four-time subcutaneous injection of recombinant human topo-I protein emulsified in complete Freund's adjuvant at an interval of 2 weeks induces dermal and pulmonary fibrosis along with the induction of anti-topo-I antibody and the skewed Th17/Treg balance toward Th17. Reminiscent of SSc and the upregulation of a number of proinflammatory and profibrotic cytokines are detected in this model, including IL-4, IL-6, IL-10, TGF-β1, TNF-α, and IL-17. Especially, IL-6 plays a critical part because the majority of symptoms are largely attenuated by IL-6 depletion. Importantly, IL-6 induced by complete Freund's adjuvant shifts topo-I immunization-dependent immune response from Treg responses toward pathogenic Th17 responses. Thus, this model supports the role of topo-I as a pathogenic autoantigen in SSc. However, the exact role of anti-topo-I antibody in the pathogenesis of SSc remains to be elucidated.

Type V Collagen Immunization Model

The induction of SSc-like disease by immunization of type V collagen (COLV) was first reported in rabbits, characterized by vascular remodeling and fibrosis of the skin and lungs [73, 74]. Then, a murine model was developed by the same researchers [75]. In human SSc, COLV is upregulated in the skin and lungs, especially correlating with the severity of interstitial lung disease [76–78]. Importantly, the nasal tolerance induction with COLV attenuated dermal and pulmonary fibrosis in a COLV-immunized rabbit SSc model, supporting the participation of COLV in autoimmunity and SSc development [79]. A COLV-immunized murine SSc model was generated by immunization twice with subcutaneous injections of human placental COLV emulsified with complete Freund's adjuvant at an interval of 4 weeks, followed by two other boosters with intramuscular injection of human placental COLV emulsified with incomplete Freund's adjuvant at 15 days' intervals. The development of SSc-like disease was confirmed 60 days after the last immunization. The deposition of fibrillar collagen was increased in the skin and lungs of COLV-immunized mice. The lungs histologically represented a nonspecific interstitial pneumonia along with the thickening of the small and medium intrapulmonary arteries [80]. Furthermore, apoptotic endothelial cells were evident, while endothelial expression of VEGF and endothelin-1 was increased in the lungs. In addition to anti-COLV antibody, antinuclear antibodies and antibodies against type III and type IV collagens were detected in sera of COLV-immunized mice. Thus, SSc-like cutaneous, vascular, and pulmonary remodeling is mimicked in this model.

PSGL-1-Deficient Mouse

P-selectin glycoprotein ligand 1 (PSGL-1) is a leukocyte receptor regulating the initial contacts between leukocytes and endothelial cells. PSGL-1 interacts with P-, E-, and L-selectin and promotes leukocyte tethering and rolling before extravasation to the inflammatory foci. As well, this interaction controls the homeostatic homing and entry of leukocytes into different tissues and organs. Homeostatic PSGL-1-selectin interaction during leukocyte recirculation and tissue replenishment is a critical step in the regulation of immune tolerance. For instance, the PSGL-1-P-selectin interaction triggers a tolerogenic program in human monocyte-derived dendritic cells, which drive Treg cell generation [81]. *Psgl1*$^{-/-}$ mice present the constitutive activation of the immune system and spontaneously develop an autoimmune syndrome which shares multiple features with SSc, such as autoantibody production, skin fibrosis, interstitial lung disease, pulmonary arterial hypertension, decreased dermal small vessels, and renal arteriolar stenosis [82, 83]. Importantly, interferon-γ-producing *Psgl1*$^{-/-}$ T cells and B cells are expanded, and regulatory T cells are decreased [83]. Since deregulated PSGL-1 expression in B cells and dendritic cells seems to be implicated in SSc development [84], further studies with *Psgl1*$^{-/-}$ mice would provide us with a useful clue to better understand the immunological aspect of SSc.

Models with SSc-Like Vascular Disease

Although several promising models have been described in the last years, murine models with SSc-like vascular disease are still very limited and often not generally available. However, given the prominent vascular features of SSc and the high risk of serious vascular complications in SSc patients, effective model systems are crucially required to improve our understanding of the vascular pathogenesis of SSc.

Models of Pulmonary Arterial Hypertension (PAH)

Several methods are used for detecting features of PAH, including endothelial injury, perivascular muscular hyperplasia, perivascular inflammation, and right heart hypertrophy. However, most of those models resemble idiopathic PAH rather than SSc/CTD-PAH. Those models have been extensively reviewed elsewhere and will not be discussed here.

Vascular Hyperplasia and Fibrosis in Fra-2 Transgenic Mice

Fra2 is a member of the AP-1 family of transcription factors. AP-1 signaling has been shown to be activated by profibrotic mediators such as TGF-β and hedgehog signaling in SSc, resulting in a prominent overexpression of Fra2 in SSc patients. Mice with transgenic, nonconditional overexpression of Fra2 (Fra2 tg) recapitulate the major vascular and fibrotic manifestations of SSc [85–87]. Fra2 tg mice demonstrate a major pulmonary phenotype that includes fibrosis and vasculopathy with a marked proliferative pattern. Neointimal hyperplasia induced by proliferation of vascular smooth muscle cells and obliteration of pulmonary arteries accompanied by perivascular inflammation appears first [85]. This is followed by interstitial inflammation and progressive collagen deposition. In addition to lung disease, these mice develop a similar process in the skin, also showing endothelial cell apoptosis followed by loss of capillaries and fibrosis, thus replicating the pathological cascade of human SSc (Fig. 19.5). Moreover, other organ manifestations of SSc such as cardiac and intestinal involvement also occur in Fra2 tg mice. First studies indicate that Fra2 tg mice may provide an novel platform for interventional studies for vasomodulatory and antifibrotic therapies.

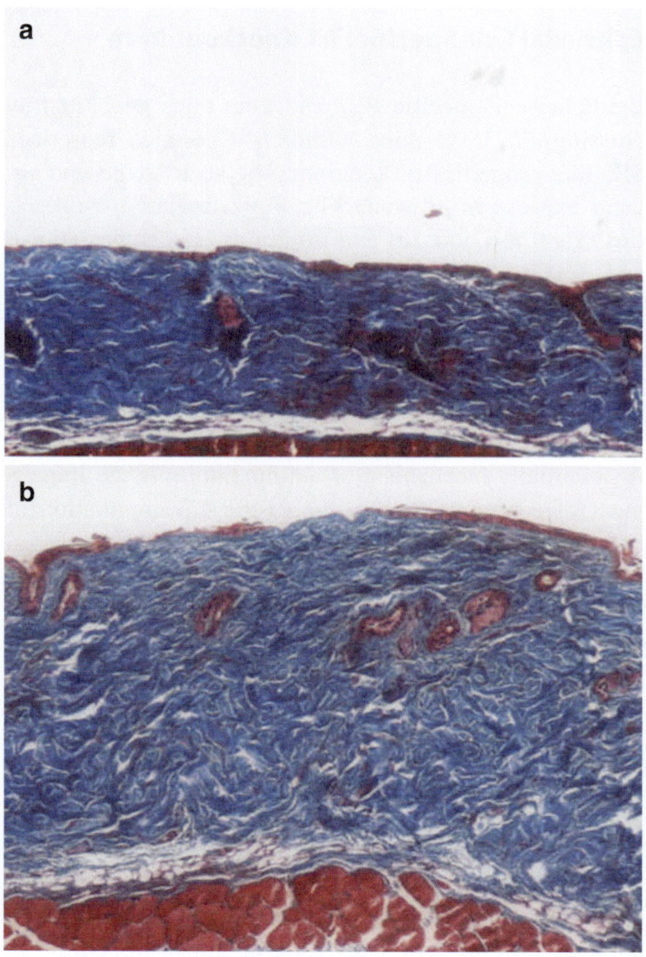

Fig. 19.5 Skin pathology in Fra-2 transgenic mice. Fra-2 transgenic mice show increased dermal thickness (panel **b**) compared to control skin (panel **a**), trichrome stain, collagen stains *blue*

Urokinase-Type Plasminogen Activator Receptor (uPAR) Deficient Mice

Another exciting new model with vascular and fibrotic features of SSc is urokinase-type plasminogen activator receptor (uPAR)-deficient mice. uPAR is a key component of the fibrinolytic system and is also involved in extracellular matrix remodeling and angiogenesis. Full-length uPAR is downregulated in fibrotic skin of SSc patients, and this downregulation may contribute to fibroblast activation. uPAR-deficient mice present with endothelial cell apoptosis, loss of microvessels, and collagen accumulation in the skin [88]. This strain also displays pulmonary disease with nonspecific interstitial pneumonia-like features, inflammation, and thickening of the alveolar septae. Further studies to investigate other organs and to determine the chronology of the pathologic findings are ongoing. However, uPAR-deficient mice may also be an exciting model to study the interplay between vascular manifestations and fibrosis in SSc.

Allograft Arteriopathy

Vascular occlusion is frequently the main pathogenic process limiting allograft survival in late allograft failure. These vascular lesions are similar to SSc vascular changes with smooth muscle cell hyperplasia and associated perivascular extracellular matrix accumulation and inflammation [89, 90]. Heterotopic cardiac or intraaortic transplants are most widely used and several different host and donor strains, having more severe mismatches, require immunosupression for survival. Though cellular immunity mediated by $CD4^+$ T cells is mainly responsible for initiating allo-reactivity, macrophages and releasing a variety of mediators, including IFN-γ, are thought to mediate vascular injury [91]. Notably, in addition to inflammatory cells, a portion of neointimal cells in murine aortic arteriopathy are host-derived. In rats, allogeneic aorta transplants revealed increased TGF-β-signaling protein, phospho-Smad2 [92]. Thus, this model provides further evidence that TGF-β is an important mediator of vascular damage. A major challenge of these models is the surgical skill required for successful transplants.

UCD200 Chicken

The best characterization of the non-mouse models of SSc is the UCD200 chicken model [93]. There is evidence of endothelial cell apoptosis and microvascular damage, and this is associated with some areas of localized skin fibrosis i.p. at the crown [94, 95]. Those manifestations seem to be triggered by skin traumata. Some very elegant studies using this chicken strain have been undertaken, and the model has value in testing interventions that may influence early vascular changes in SSc. However, the practical challenge of working with chickens and the limited genetic and functional biological data to apply to these studies hinder widespread use of this model.

New Murine SSc Models with *Fli1* Deficiency

SSc is believed to be a multifactorial disease caused by the complex interplay between hereditary and environmental factors [96]. Various combinations of predisposing factors may explain the disease heterogeneity and a variety of organ involvement in this disease. Transcription factor Friend leukemia virus integration 1 (Fli1), a member of the Ets transcription factor family, may represent such a predisposing factor for the development of SSc. Fli1 expression is constitutively suppressed in dermal fibroblasts, dermal microvascular endothelial cells, keratinocytes, and perivascular inflammatory cells in the lesional and non-lesional skin of SSc patients [97], which is likely to be mediated by both genetic and epigenetic mechanisms. Extended repeat alleles of *FLI1* (GA)*n* microsatellite are associated with lower *FLI1* mRNA levels in the peripheral blood and susceptibility to human SSc [98]. Epigenetic suppression of *Fli1* gene is clearly proved by the increased methylation of CpG island and the decreased acetylation of histones H3 and H4 in the *Fli1* promoter using genomic DNA isolated from bulk skin and/or cultivated dermal fibroblasts of SSc patients [99]. Although Fli1 deficiency induces SSc-like phenotypes in dermal fibroblasts, dermal microvascular endothelial cells, keratinocytes, and inflammatory cells at molecular levels [97, 100–103], *Fli1*$^{+/-}$ mice do not spontaneously develop apparent clinical symptoms characteristic of SSc [104]. Therefore, *Fli1* haploinsufficiency is not enough to induce clinical features of SSc in vivo, suggesting that additional factors are required to generate genetic animal models of SSc. Based on this idea, three genetic animal models were generated, endothelial cell-specific *Fli1* knockout mice, epithelial cell-specific *Fli1* knockout mice, and double heterozygous mice for *Fli1* and *Klf5* genes. The former two mice reproduce a part of SSc-related pathological features, and the last mice recapitulate immune abnormalities, vasculopathy, and tissue fibrosis of SSc [100, 105].

Endothelial Cell-Specific *Fli1* Knockout Mice

Endothelial cell-specific *Fli1* knockout (*Fli1* EcKO) mice generated by crossing *Fli1*$^{flox/flox}$ mice with *Tie2*-Cre transgenic mice mimic the structural and functional abnormalities of SSc vasculopathy, such as stenosis of arterioles, dilation of capillaries, and increased vascular permeability of small vessels. This vascular phenotype is largely attributable to the altered expression of several molecules regulating vascular integrity, such as the decreased expression of VE-cadherin, PECAM1, PDGF-B and $S1P_1$ receptor and the increased expression of MMP-9. The reduction of VE-cadherin and PECAM1 expression results in a weak endothelial cell–cell interaction. Increased expression of MMP-9 leads to altered remodeling of vascular basement membrane, such as loss of type IV collagen and compensatory increase of proteoglycans. Furthermore, downregulation of VE-cadherin, PDGF-B, and $S1P_1$ receptor causes the loss of endothelial cell–mural cell interaction. Importantly, the expression profile of these molecules is identical to that seen in dermal small vasculature of SSc lesional skin [100]. Thus, *Fli1* EcKO mice recapitulate the vascular phenotype of SSc, suggesting the involvement of endothelial Fli1 deficiency in the pathogenesis of SSc vasculopathy.

Epithelial Cell-Specific *Fli1* Knockout Mice

Epithelial cell-specific *Fli1* knockout mice generated by crossing *Fli1*$^{flox/flox}$ mice with *K14*-Cre mice reproduce SSc-like properties of keratinocytes, such as the upregulated expression of wound healing-associated cytokeratins (keratin 6 and 16) and profibrotic molecules (IL-1α and CTGF). *Fli1*$^{flox/flox}$; *K14*-Cre mice spontaneously develop dermal and esophageal fibrosis and interstitial lung disease similar to those of SSc. These mice produce antinuclear antibodies but do not show vascular abnormalities, indicating the reproduction of SSc-like tissue fibrosis and immune abnormalities without vasculopathy. A potentially mechanism of autoimmunity is the impairment of central tolerance due to the downregulation of autoimmune regulatory in medullary thymic epithelial cells which express keratin 14. Of interest, adoptive transfer of splenic NK1.1$^-$CD3$^+$ T cells from *Fli1*$^{flox/flox}$; *K14*-Cre mice to *Rag1*$^{-/-}$ mice results in the development of interstitial lung disease in recipient mice, while *Rag1*$^{-/-}$; *Fli1*$^{flox/flox}$; *K14*-Cre mice reveal dermal and esophageal fibrosis without interstitial lung disease [101]. Therefore, epithelial cells, such as keratinocytes and esophageal squamous epithelia, induce dermal and esophageal fibrosis independent of immune activation, while autoreactive T cells cause interstitial lung disease in this animal model. This animal model provided us with a new insight into the potential role of epithelial cells in the pathogenesis of SSc, which may explain the cause of organ selectivity and the origin of autoimmunity in this disease.

Klf5$^{+/-}$; *Fli1*$^{+/-}$ Mice

Krüppel-like factor 5 (KLF5) is a member of the SP/KLF transcription factor family [106]. *KLF5* gene expression is downregulated in SSc skin [107], and *Klf5* haploinsufficiency alters the fibrotic response following experimental tissue damage in the heart and kidney [108, 109]. In addition, the increased methylation of CpG island and the decreased acetylation of histones H3 and H4 are noted in the *KLF5* promoter of SSc dermal fibroblasts [110]. Therefore, the downregulated expression of *KLF5* gene is likely to be a potential predisposing factor for SSc and the suppression of *FLI1* gene expression. Consistent with this notion, double heterozygous mice for *Klf5* and *Fli1* genes spontaneously develop three cardinal features of SSc such as immune abnormalities, vasculopathy, and extensive tissue fibrosis of the skin and lungs. *Klf5*$^{+/-}$; *Fli1*$^{+/-}$ mice develop inflammation and vascular changes such as stenosis of arterioles and dilation of capillaries in the skin around 4 weeks of age and autoantibody production and the decrease of vascular beds around 8 weeks of age. Dermal and pulmonary fibrosis becomes apparent around 3 and 4 months of age, respectively. Abnormal collagen fibril assembly similar to SSc is also induced after 2 months of age and tissue hypoxia and decreased blood flow velocity are noted around 4 months of age in the skin. In the lungs, diffuse uniform expansion of alveolar septa with patchy septal lymphocytic infiltration is present, reminiscent of human nonspecific interstitial pneumonia, while the pathological findings indicating usual interstitial pneumonia, honeycombing or fibroblastic foci, are rarely seen. Pulmonary vascular changes characteristic of pulmonary arterial hypertension, and pulmonary veno-occlusive disease become remarkable around 8 months of age. *Klf5*$^{+/-}$; *Fli1*$^{+/-}$ mice also exhibit CD19 upregulation in B cells, which has been shown to largely contribute to the pathogenesis of SSc [111]. In addition, the properties of dermal microvascular endothelial cells, bone marrow-derived endothelial progenitor cells, and bone marrow-derived mesenchymal stem cells, a precursor of pericytes, are reminiscent of those cells derived from SSc patients [112]. A series of studies with *Klf5*$^{+/-}$; *Fli1*$^{+/-}$ mice suggests a novel concept that the downregulation of these two transcription factors may be the primary event triggering the three major manifestations in SSc [105]. These findings support the idea that environmental factors determine the clinical phenotype of SSc, while genetic factors contribute to the susceptibility to and the severity of this disease [113, 114].

Myocardial Disease in Mouse Models

Myocardial involvement is a major cause of death in SSc and may account for up to one-third of deaths in SSc patients [115–118]. Cardiac involvement is believed to occur in the majority, if not all SSc patients, although it is often clinically occult [119, 120]. Abnormal vasoreactivity and structural defects of small arterioles and capillaries in the myocardium lead to repeated local hypoperfusion, which subsequently could trigger myocardial fibrosis, which is often patchy and affects both ventricles [121, 122].

Despite its clinical relevance, only few studies analyzed myocardial alterations in murine models of SSc so far. A recent study compared myocardial changes in Tsk-1, B10.D2 (H-2d) → BALB/c (H-2d) cGvHD model and Fra2 tg mice to those of SSc patients [123]. Tsk-1 mice and mice with cGvHD mimicked only few features of SSc-associated cardiomyopathy and were not considered as suitable models of SSc-related cardiomyopathy. However, heart involvement of Fra-2 tg mice resembled all major histopathological features of SSc-associated myocardial disease with apoptosis of endothelial cells and decreased capillary counts, perivascular inflammatory infiltrates, and activation of fibroblasts with subsequent accumulation of collagen. Fra-2 tg mice may indeed share a similar molecular pathophysiology, as Fra-2 is also overexpressed in the heart of SSc patients and the expression pattern of Fra-2 in SSc patients resembled the one in Fra-2 tg mice with predominant expression in capillaries. Caveolin-1 knockout mice have been shown to suffer from severe biventricular hypertrophy with systolic and diastolic severe heart failure [124]. Although caveolin-1 is not expressed in cardiomyocytes, caveolin-1 knockout mice are characterized by a severe eNOS-hyperactivation yielding increased systemic NO levels, which are thought to mediate the cardiac phenotype of caveolin-1 knockout mice [125]. However, no microvascular alterations have been reported in caveolin-1-deficient mice. A fibrotic cardiomyopathy has also been described in TβRIIΔk fib mice and HOCl-treated mice, whereas other histopathologic findings of myocardial disease in humans were not noted [24, 65]. Conclusive data on other mouse models of SSc are not yet available. However, it would be of major interest to study the myocardial involvement in particular other systemic models of SSc.

What Have We Learned from Analyzing Animal Models?

It can clearly be observed that there is no lack of interesting animal models for SSc and there has been a major increase in the number and type of models used in recent studies (Table 19.1). It has become commonplace to use gene-targeted mice to help to understand facet of the disease and inducible models for SSc such as the bleomycin skin or lung models are central to this. There must, however, be caution. No single model reflects the entire pathology of human SSc in its complexity and chronicity, and so, each model needs to be considered carefully on its merits

Table 19.1 Key features of common animal models of SSc

	Fibrosis: skin/internal organs	SSc-like vasculopathy	Inflammation	Autoimmunity
Bleomycin-induced skin fibrosis	+++/(+)	Ø	+++	+
HOCl-induced fibrosis	+++/++	+	+++	+++
cGvHD models	+++/+	Ø	++	+
Tsk-1 mice	+++/Ø	Ø	(+)	++
Tsk-2 mice	+++/Ø	Ø	(+)	++
Fra2 tg mice	+++/+++	+++	++	Ø
uPAR$^{-/-}$ mice	+++/+++	++	++	?
Cav1$^{-/-}$ mice	+++/++	(+)	++	Ø
TβRI^{CA} mice	+++/Ø or (+)[a]	Ø	Ø	Ø
TβRIIΔk × Col1a2; CreER mice	+++/++	++	Ø	Ø
CTGF × Col1a2; CreER mice	+++/++	?	Ø	?
Wnt10 tg mice	+++/Ø	?	Ø	Ø
β-catenin$^{\Delta Exon3}$ × Col1a2; CreER mice	+++/(+)[a]	Ø	Ø	Ø
Fli1$^{flox/flox}$ × Tie2; Cre mice	Ø	+++	Ø	Ø
Fli1$^{flox/flox}$ × K14; Cre mice	++/++	Ø	++	++
Klf5$^{+/-}$; *Fli1*$^{+/-}$ mice	+++/+++	+++	+++	+
UCD200/206 chicken	++/++	+++	+	+
VEGF tg mice	++/ Ø	+	Ø	Ø
PTEN × Col1a2; CreER mice	++/++	Ø	Ø	Ø
Psgl1$^{-/-}$ mice	++/++	++	++	++
Topo-I-immunized mice	++/++	Ø	++	++
COLV-immunized mice	++/++	++	+	+

Among these animal models, Fra2 tg mice, uPAR$^{-/-}$ mice, and *Klf5*$^{+/-}$; *Fli1*$^{+/-}$ mice mimic the histology of nonspecific interstitial pneumonia and pulmonary vascular changes characteristic of SSc

and the strengths and weaknesses that it can bring to any study. It is of critical importance to test any hypothesis in several complementary models before drawing firm conclusions.

The use of conditional genetic strategies has substantially increased the power and relevance of many experiments that use mouse models of SSc. The advantages of some of these approaches are that genes can be turned on or off in selected cell lineages at particulate timer points. This allows molecular triggering events to be replicated, and the impact of gene expression changes at defined time points in experimental pathology to be explored (e.g., treatment or reversal rather than prevention). Also, genes that are lethal in germline manipulation or even conventional lineage-specific disruption can be investigated. This has been a fruitful area and one that is set to continue to be productive and informative in the immediate future.

References

1. Beyer C, Schett G, Distler O, Distler JH. Animal models of systemic sclerosis: prospects and limitations. Arthritis Rheum. 2010;62(10):2831–44.
2. Green MC, Sweet HO, Bunker LE. Tight-skin, a new mutation of the mouse causing excessive growth of connective tissue and skeleton. Am J Pathol. 1976;82(3):493–512.
3. Siracusa LD, McGrath R, Ma Q, Moskow JJ, Manne J, Christner PJ, et al. A tandem duplication within the fibrillin 1 gene is associated with the mouse tight skin mutation. Genome Res. 1996;6(4):300–13.
4. Kielty CM, Raghunath M, Siracusa LD, Sherratt MJ, Peters R, Shuttleworth CA, et al. The Tight skin mouse: demonstration of mutant fibrillin-1 production and assembly into abnormal microfibrils. J Cell Biol. 1998;140(5):1159–66.
5. Lemaire R, Farina G, Kissin E, Shipley JM, Bona C, Korn JH, et al. Mutant fibrillin 1 from tight skin mice increases extracellular matrix incorporation of microfibril-associated glycoprotein 2 and type I collagen. Arthritis Rheum. 2004;50(3):915–26.
6. Bayle J, Fitch J, Jacobsen K, Kumar R, Lafyatis R, Lemaire R. Increased expression of Wnt2 and SFRP4 in Tsk mouse skin: role of Wnt signaling in altered dermal fibrillin deposition and systemic sclerosis. J Invest Dermatol. 2008;128(4):871–81.
7. Dees C, Akhmetshina A, Zerr P, Reich N, Palumbo K, Horn A, et al. Platelet-derived serotonin links vascular disease and tissue fibrosis. J Exp Med. 2011;208(5):961–72.
8. Avouac J, Palumbo K, Tomcik M, Zerr P, Dees C, Horn A, et al. Inhibition of activator protein 1 signaling abrogates transforming growth factor beta-mediated activation of fibroblasts and prevents experimental fibrosis. Arthritis Rheum. 2012;64(5):1642–52.
9. Komura K, Fujimoto M, Yanaba K, Matsushita T, Matsushita Y, Horikawa M, et al. Blockade of CD40/CD40 ligand interactions attenuates skin fibrosis and autoimmunity in the tight-skin mouse. Ann Rheum Dis. 2008;67(6):867–72.
10. Saito E, Fujimoto M, Hasegawa M, Komura K, Hamaguchi Y, Kaburagi Y, et al. CD19-dependent B lymphocyte signaling thresholds influence skin fibrosis and autoimmunity in the tight-skin mouse. J Clin Invest. 2002;109(11):1453–62.
11. Murai C, Saito S, Kasturi KN, Bona CA. Spontaneous occurrence of anti-fibrillin-1 autoantibodies in tight-skin mice. Autoimmunity. 1998;28(3):151–5.
12. Shibata S, Muryoi T, Saitoh Y, Brumeanu TD, Bona CA, Kasturi KN. Immunochemical and molecular characterization of anti-

RNA polymerase I autoantibodies produced by tight skin mouse. J Clin Invest. 1993;92(2):984–92.
13. Walker MA, Harley RA, DeLustro FA, LeRoy EC. Adoptive transfer of tsk skin fibrosis to +/+ recipients by tsk bone marrow and spleen cells. Proc Soc Exp Biol Med (New York, NY). 1989;192(2):196–200.
14. Phelps RG, Daian C, Shibata S, Fleischmajer R, Bona CA. Induction of skin fibrosis and autoantibodies by infusion of immunocompetent cells from tight skin mice into C57BL/6 Pa/Pa mice. J Autoimmun. 1993;6(6):701–18.
15. Siracusa LD, McGrath R, Fisher JK, Jimenez SA. The mouse tight skin (Tsk) phenotype is not dependent on the presence of mature T and B lymphocytes. Mammal Genome. 1998;9(11):907–9.
16. Kasturi KN, Hatakeyama A, Murai C, Gordon R, Phelps RG, Bona CA. B-cell deficiency does not abrogate development of cutaneous hyperplasia in mice inheriting the defective fibrillin-1 gene. J Autoimmun. 1997;10(6):505–17.
17. Christner PJ, Peters J, Hawkins D, Siracusa LD, Jimenez SA. The tight skin 2 mouse. An animal model of scleroderma displaying cutaneous fibrosis and mononuclear cell infiltration. Arthritis Rheum. 1995;38(12):1791–8.
18. Long KB, Li Z, Burgwin CM, Choe SG, Martyanov V, Sassi-Gaha S, et al. The Tsk2/+ mouse fibrotic phenotype is due to a gain-of-function mutation in the PIIINP segment of the Col3a1 gene. J Invest Dermatol. 2015;135(3):718–27.
19. Sonnylal S, Denton CP, Zheng B, Keene DR, He R, Adams HP, et al. Postnatal induction of transforming growth factor beta signaling in fibroblasts of mice recapitulates clinical, histologic, and biochemical features of scleroderma. Arthritis Rheum. 2007;56(1):334–44.
20. Akhmetshina A, Palumbo K, Dees C, Bergmann C, Venalis P, Zerr P, et al. Activation of canonical Wnt signalling is required for TGF-beta-mediated fibrosis. Nat Commun. 2012;3:735.
21. Beyer C, Zenzmaier C, Palumbo-Zerr K, Mancuso R, Distler A, Dees C, et al. Stimulation of the soluble guanylate cyclase (sGC) inhibits fibrosis by blocking non-canonical TGFbeta signalling. Ann Rheum Dis. 2015;74:1408.
22. Tomcik M, Zerr P, Pitkowski J, Palumbo-Zerr K, Avouac J, Distler O, et al. Heat shock protein 90 (Hsp90) inhibition targets canonical TGF-beta signalling to prevent fibrosis. Ann Rheum Dis. 2014;73(6):1215–22.
23. Zerr P, Vollath S, Palumbo-Zerr K, Tomcik M, Huang J, Distler A, et al. Vitamin D receptor regulates TGF-beta signalling in systemic sclerosis. Ann Rheum Dis. 2015;74:e20.
24. Denton CP, Zheng B, Evans LA, Shi-wen X, Ong VH, Fisher I, et al. Fibroblast-specific expression of a kinase-deficient type II transforming growth factor beta (TGFbeta) receptor leads to paradoxical activation of TGFbeta signaling pathways with fibrosis in transgenic mice. J Biol Chem. 2003;278(27):25109–19.
25. Derrett-Smith EC, Dooley A, Khan K, Shi-Wen X, Abraham D, Denton CP. Systemic vasculopathy with altered vasoreactivity in a transgenic mouse model of scleroderma. Arthritis Res Ther. 2010;12(2):R69.
26. Derrett-Smith EC, Dooley A, Gilbane AJ, Trinder SL, Khan K, Baliga R, et al. Endothelial injury in a transforming growth factor beta-dependent mouse model of scleroderma induces pulmonary arterial hypertension. Arthritis Rheum. 2013;65(11):2928–39.
27. Sonnylal S, Shi-Wen X, Leoni P, Naff K, Van Pelt CS, Nakamura H, et al. Selective expression of connective tissue growth factor in fibroblasts in vivo promotes systemic tissue fibrosis. Arthritis Rheum. 2010;62(5):1523–32.
28. Longo KA, Wright WS, Kang S, Gerin I, Chiang SH, Lucas PC, et al. Wnt10b inhibits development of white and brown adipose tissues. J Biol Chem. 2004;279(34):35503–9.
29. Wei J, Melichian D, Komura K, Hinchcliff M, Lam AP, Lafyatis R, et al. Canonical Wnt signaling induces skin fibrosis and subcutaneous lipoatrophy: a novel mouse model for scleroderma? Arthritis Rheum. 2011;63(6):1707–17.
30. Beyer C, Schramm A, Akhmetshina A, Dees C, Kireva T, Gelse K, et al. Beta-catenin is a central mediator of pro-fibrotic Wnt signaling in systemic sclerosis. Ann Rheum Dis. 2012;71(5):761–7.
31. Castello-Cros R, Whitaker-Menezes D, Molchansky A, Purkins G, Soslowsky LJ, Beason DP, et al. Scleroderma-like properties of skin from caveolin-1-deficient mice: implications for new treatment strategies in patients with fibrosis and systemic sclerosis. Cell Cycle (Georgetown, Tex). 2011;10(13):2140–50.
32. Del Galdo F, Sotgia F, de Almeida CJ, Jasmin JF, Musick M, Lisanti MP, et al. Decreased expression of caveolin 1 in patients with systemic sclerosis: crucial role in the pathogenesis of tissue fibrosis. Arthritis Rheum. 2008;58(9):2854–65.
33. Le Saux O, Teeters K, Miyasato S, Choi J, Nakamatsu G, Richardson JA, et al. The role of caveolin-1 in pulmonary matrix remodeling and mechanical properties. Am J Physiol Lung Cell Mol Physiol. 2008;295(6):L1007–17.
34. Tourkina E, Richard M, Gooz P, Bonner M, Pannu J, Harley R, et al. Antifibrotic properties of caveolin-1 scaffolding domain in vitro and in vivo. Am J Physiol Lung Cell Mol Physiol. 2008;294(5):L843–61.
35. Tourkina E, Richard M, Oates J, Hofbauer A, Bonner M, Gooz P, et al. Caveolin-1 regulates leucocyte behaviour in fibrotic lung disease. Ann Rheum Dis. 2010;69(6):1220–6.
36. Wang XM, Zhang Y, Kim HP, Zhou Z, Feghali-Bostwick CA, Liu F, et al. Caveolin-1: a critical regulator of lung fibrosis in idiopathic pulmonary fibrosis. J Exp Med. 2006;203(13):2895–906.
37. Yamaguchi Y, Yasuoka H, Stolz DB, Feghali-Bostwick CA. Decreased caveolin-1 levels contribute to fibrosis and deposition of extracellular IGFBP-5. J Cell Mol Med. 2011;15(4):957–69.
38. Del Galdo F, Lisanti MP, Jimenez SA. Caveolin-1, transforming growth factor-beta receptor internalization, and the pathogenesis of systemic sclerosis. Curr Opin Rheumatol. 2008;20(6):713–9.
39. Dong C, Zhu S, Wang T, Yoon W, Li Z, Alvarez RJ, et al. Deficient Smad7 expression: a putative molecular defect in scleroderma. Proc Natl Acad Sci U S A. 2002;99(6):3908–13.
40. Distler JH, Jungel A, Kowal-Bielecka O, Michel BA, Gay RE, Sprott H, et al. Expression of interleukin-21 receptor in epidermis from patients with systemic sclerosis. Arthritis Rheum. 2005;52(3):856–64.
41. Detmar M, Brown LF, Schön MP, Elicker BM, Velasco P, Richard L, et al. Increased microvascular density and enhanced leukocyte rolling and adhesion in the skin of VEGF transgenic mice. J Invest Dermatol. 1998;111(1):1–6.
42. Parapuram SK, Shi-wen X, Elliott C, Welch ID, Jones H, Baron M, et al. Loss of PTEN expression by dermal fibroblasts causes skin fibrosis. J Invest Dermatol. 2011;131(10):1996–2003.
43. Parapuram SK, Thompson K, Tsang M, Hutchenreuther J, Bekking C, Liu S, et al. Loss of PTEN expression by mouse fibroblasts results in lung fibrosis through a CCN2-dependent mechanism. Matrix Biol. 2015;43:35–41.
44. Liu Y, Cao Y, Sun S, Zhu J, Gao S, Pang J, et al. Transforming growth factor-beta1 upregulation triggers pulmonary artery smooth muscle cell proliferation and apoptosis imbalance in rats with hypoxic pulmonary hypertension via the PTEN/AKT pathways. Int J Biochem Cell Biol. 2016;77(Pt A):141–54.
45. Oudit GY, Kassiri Z, Zhou J, Liu QC, Liu PP, Backx PH, et al. Loss of PTEN attenuates the development of pathological hypertrophy and heart failure in response to biomechanical stress. Cardiovasc Res. 2008;78(3):505–14.
46. Chu YW, Gress RE. Murine models of chronic graft-versus-host disease: insights and unresolved issues. Biol Blood Marrow Transpl. 2008;14(4):365–78.
47. Huu DL, Matsushita T, Jin G, Hamaguchi Y, Hasegawa M, Takehara K, et al. FTY720 ameliorates murine sclerodermatous

chronic graft-versus-host disease by promoting expansion of splenic regulatory cells and inhibiting immune cell infiltration into skin. Arthritis Rheum. 2013;65(6):1624–35.
48. McCormick LL, Zhang Y, Tootell E, Gilliam AC. Anti-TGF-beta treatment prevents skin and lung fibrosis in murine sclerodermatous graft-versus-host disease: a model for human scleroderma. J Immunol (Baltimore, Md : 1950). 1999;163(10):5693–9.
49. Zhang Y, McCormick LL, Desai SR, Wu C, Gilliam AC. Murine sclerodermatous graft-versus-host disease, a model for human scleroderma: cutaneous cytokines, chemokines, and immune cell activation. J Immunol (Baltimore, Md : 1950). 2002;168(6):3088–98.
50. Zerr P, Distler A, Palumbo-Zerr K, Tomcik M, Vollath S, Dees C, et al. Combined inhibition of c-Abl and PDGF receptors for prevention and treatment of murine sclerodermatous chronic graft-versus-host disease. Am J Pathol. 2012;181(5):1672–80.
51. Zerr P, Palumbo-Zerr K, Distler A, Tomcik M, Vollath S, Munoz LE, et al. Inhibition of hedgehog signaling for the treatment of murine sclerodermatous chronic graft-versus-host disease. Blood. 2012;120(14):2909–17.
52. Ruzek MC, Jha S, Ledbetter S, Richards SM, Garman RD. A modified model of graft-versus-host-induced systemic sclerosis (scleroderma) exhibits all major aspects of the human disease. Arthritis Rheum. 2004;50(4):1319–31.
53. Anderson BE, McNiff JM, Matte C, Athanasiadis I, Shlomchik WD, Shlomchik MJ. Recipient CD4+ T cells that survive irradiation regulate chronic graft-versus-host disease. Blood. 2004;104(5):1565–73.
54. Anderson BE, McNiff JM, Jain D, Blazar BR, Shlomchik WD, Shlomchik MJ. Distinct roles for donor- and host-derived antigen-presenting cells and costimulatory molecules in murine chronic graft-versus-host disease: requirements depend on target organ. Blood. 2005;105(5):2227–34.
55. Akhmetshina A, Venalis P, Dees C, Busch N, Zwerina J, Schett G, et al. Treatment with imatinib prevents fibrosis in different preclinical models of systemic sclerosis and induces regression of established fibrosis. Arthritis Rheum. 2009;60(1):219–24.
56. Beyer C, Huang J, Beer J, Zhang Y, Palumbo-Zerr K, Zerr P, et al. Activation of liver X receptors inhibits experimental fibrosis by interfering with interleukin-6 release from macrophages. Ann Rheum Dis. 2015;74:1317.
57. Beyer C, Reichert H, Akan H, Mallano T, Schramm A, Dees C, et al. Blockade of canonical Wnt signalling ameliorates experimental dermal fibrosis. Ann Rheum Dis. 2013;72(7):1255–8.
58. Dees C, Zerr P, Tomcik M, Beyer C, Horn A, Akhmetshina A, et al. Inhibition of Notch signaling prevents experimental fibrosis and induces regression of established fibrosis. Arthritis Rheum. 2011;63(5):1396–404.
59. Palumbo K, Zerr P, Tomcik M, Vollath S, Dees C, Akhmetshina A, et al. The transcription factor JunD mediates transforming growth factor {beta}-induced fibroblast activation and fibrosis in systemic sclerosis. Ann Rheum Dis. 2011;70(7):1320–6.
60. Gasse P, Mary C, Guenon I, Noulin N, Charron S, Schnyder-Candrian S, et al. IL-1R1/MyD88 signaling and the inflammasome are essential in pulmonary inflammation and fibrosis in mice. J Clin Invest. 2007;117(12):3786–99.
61. Horan GS, Wood S, Ona V, Li DJ, Lukashev ME, Weinreb PH, et al. Partial inhibition of integrin alpha(v)beta6 prevents pulmonary fibrosis without exacerbating inflammation. Am J Respir Crit Care Med. 2008;177(1):56–65.
62. Tager AM, LaCamera P, Shea BS, Campanella GS, Selman M, Zhao Z, et al. The lysophosphatidic acid receptor LPA1 links pulmonary fibrosis to lung injury by mediating fibroblast recruitment and vascular leak. Nat Med. 2008;14(1):45–54.
63. Avouac J, Elhai M, Tomcik M, Ruiz B, Friese M, Piedavent M, et al. Critical role of the adhesion receptor DNAX accessory molecule-1 (DNAM-1) in the development of inflammation-driven dermal fibrosis in a mouse model of systemic sclerosis. Ann Rheum Dis. 2013;72(6):1089–98.
64. Servettaz A, Goulvestre C, Kavian N, Nicco C, Guilpain P, Chéreau C, et al. Selective oxidation of DNA topoisomerase 1 induces systemic sclerosis in the mouse. J Immunol. 2009;182(9):5855–64.
65. Bagnato GL, Irrera N, Pizzino G, Santoro D, Roberts WN, Bagnato G, et al. Dual αvβ3 and αvβ5 blockade attenuates fibrotic and vascular alterations in a murine model of systemic sclerosis. Clin Sci (Lond). 2018;132(2):231–42.
66. Bagnato G, Bitto A, Pizzino G, Roberts WN, Squadrito F, Altavilla D, et al. Propylthiouracil modulates aortic vasculopathy in the oxidative stress model of systemic sclerosis. Vasc Pharmacol. 2015;71:79–83.
67. Bitto A, Bagnato GL, Pizzino G, Roberts WN, Irrera N, Minutoli L, et al. Simvastatin prevents vascular complications in the chronic reactive oxygen species murine model of systemic sclerosis. Free Radic Res. 2016;50(5):514–22.
68. Raker VK, Ook KY, Haub J, Lorenz N, Schmidt T, Stegemann A, et al. Myeloid cell populations and fibrogenic parameters in bleomycin- and HOCl-induced fibrosis. Exp Dermatol. 2016;25(11):887–94.
69. Sanges S, Jendoubi M, Kavian N, Hauspie C, Speca S, Crave JC, et al. B cell homeostasis and functional properties are altered in an hypochlorous acid-induced murine model of systemic sclerosis. Front Immunol. 2017;8:53.
70. Maria ATJ, Toupet K, Maumus M, Rozier P, Vozenin MC, Le Quellec A, et al. Fibrosis development in HOCl-induced systemic sclerosis: a multistage process hampered by mesenchymal stem cells. Front Immunol. 2018;9:2571.
71. Meng M, Tan J, Chen W, Du Q, Xie B, Wang N, et al. The fibrosis and immunological features of hypochlorous acid induced mouse model of systemic sclerosis. Front Immunol. 2019;10:1861.
72. Yoshizaki A, Yanaba K, Ogawa A, Asano Y, Kadono T, Sato S. Immunization with DNA topoisomerase I and Freund's complete adjuvant induces skin and lung fibrosis and autoimmunity via interleukin-6 signaling. Arthritis Rheum. 2011;63(11):3575–85.
73. Teodoro WR, Velosa AP, Witzel SS, Garippo AL, Farhat C, Parra ER, et al. Architectural remodelling in lungs of rabbits induced by type V collagen immunization: a preliminary morphologic model to study diffuse connective tissue diseases. Pathol Res Pract. 2004;200(10):681–91.
74. Callado MR, Viana VS, Vendramini MB, Leon EP, Bueno C, Velosa AP, et al. Autoantibody profile in the experimental model of scleroderma induced by type V human collagen. Immunology. 2007;122(1):38–46.
75. Teodoro WR, de Jesus Queiroz ZA, Dos Santos LA, Catanozi S, Dos Santos FA, Bueno C, et al. Proposition of a novel animal model of systemic sclerosis induced by type V collagen in C57BL/6 mice that reproduces fibrosis, vasculopathy and autoimmunity. Arthritis Res Ther. 2019;21(1):278.
76. Martin P, Teodoro WR, Velosa AP, de Morais J, Carrasco S, Christmann RB, et al. Abnormal collagen V deposition in dermis correlates with skin thickening and disease activity in systemic sclerosis. Autoimmun Rev. 2012;11(11):827–35.
77. Parra ER, Aguiar AC Jr, Teodoro WR, de Souza R, Yoshinari NH, Capelozzi VL. Collagen V and vascular injury promote lung architectural changes in systemic sclerosis. Clin Respir J. 2009;3(3):135–42.
78. Parra ER, Teodoro WR, de Morais J, Katayama ML, de Souza R, Yoshinari NH, et al. Increased mRNA expression of collagen

V gene in pulmonary fibrosis of systemic sclerosis. Eur J Clin Investig. 2010;40(2):110–20.
79. Velosa AP, Teodoro WR, dos Anjos DM, Konno R, Oliveira CC, Katayama ML, et al. Collagen V-induced nasal tolerance downregulates pulmonary collagen mRNA gene and TGF-beta expression in experimental systemic sclerosis. Respir Res. 2010;11(1):1.
80. Marangoni RG, Korman BD, Parra ER, Velosa APP, Barbeiro HV, Martins V, et al. Pathological pulmonary vascular remodeling is induced by type V collagen in a model of scleroderma. Pathol Res Pract. 2021;220:153382.
81. Urzainqui A, Martínez del Hoyo G, Lamana A, de la Fuente H, Barreiro O, Olazabal IM, et al. Functional role of P-selectin glycoprotein ligand 1/P-selectin interaction in the generation of tolerogenic dendritic cells. J Immunol. 2007;179(11):7457–65.
82. Pérez-Frías A, González-Tajuelo R, Núñez-Andrade N, Tejedor R, García-Blanco MJ, Vicente-Rabaneda E, et al. Development of an autoimmune syndrome affecting the skin and internal organs in P-selectin glycoprotein ligand 1 leukocyte receptor-deficient mice. Arthritis Rheumatol. 2014;66(11):3178–89.
83. Gonzalez-Tajuelo R, de la Fuente-Fernandez M, Morales-Cano D, Munoz-Callejas A, Gonzalez-Sanchez E, Silvan J, et al. PSGL1-deficient mice develop spontaneous pulmonary hypertension associated to systemic sclerosis. Arthritis Rheumatol. 2019; https://doi.org/10.1002/art.41100.
84. Silván J, González-Tajuelo R, Vicente-Rabaneda E, Pérez-Frías A, Espartero-Santos M, Muñoz-Callejas A, et al. Deregulated PSGL-1 expression in B cells and dendritic cells may be implicated in human systemic sclerosis development. J Invest Dermatol. 2018;138(10):2123–32.
85. Maurer B, Busch N, Jungel A, Pileckyte M, Gay RE, Michel BA, et al. Transcription factor fos-related antigen-2 induces progressive peripheral vasculopathy in mice closely resembling human systemic sclerosis. Circulation. 2009;120(23):2367–76.
86. Maurer B, Distler JH, Distler O. The Fra-2 transgenic mouse model of systemic sclerosis. Vasc Pharmacol. 2013;58(3):194–201.
87. Reich N, Maurer B, Akhmetshina A, Venalis P, Dees C, Zerr P, et al. The transcription factor Fra-2 regulates the production of extracellular matrix in systemic sclerosis. Arthritis Rheum. 2010;62(1):280–90.
88. Manetti M, Rosa I, Milia AF, Guiducci S, Carmeliet P, Ibba-Manneschi L, et al. Inactivation of urokinase-type plasminogen activator receptor (uPAR) gene induces dermal and pulmonary fibrosis and peripheral microvasculopathy in mice: a new model of experimental scleroderma? Ann Rheum Dis. 2014;73(9):1700–9.
89. Mitchell RN. Graft vascular disease: immune response meets the vessel wall. Annu Rev Pathol. 2009;4:19–47.
90. Mitchell RN, Libby P. Vascular remodeling in transplant vasculopathy. Circ Res. 2007;100(7):967–78.
91. Nagano H, Mitchell RN, Taylor MK, Hasegawa S, Tilney NL, Libby P. Interferon-gamma deficiency prevents coronary arteriosclerosis but not myocardial rejection in transplanted mouse hearts. J Clin Invest. 1997;100(3):550–7.
92. Dong C, Zhu S, Wang T, Yoon W, Goldschmidt-Clermont PJ. Upregulation of PAI-1 is mediated through TGF-beta/Smad pathway in transplant arteriopathy. J Heart Lung Transpl. 2002;21(9):999–1008.
93. Wick G, Andersson L, Hala K, Gershwin ME, Selmi C, Erf GF, et al. Avian models with spontaneous autoimmune diseases. Adv Immunol. 2006;92:71–117.
94. Gruschwitz MS, Moormann S, Kromer G, Sgonc R, Dietrich H, Boeck G, et al. Phenotypic analysis of skin infiltrates in comparison with peripheral blood lymphocytes, spleen cells and thymocytes in early avian scleroderma. J Autoimmun. 1991;4(4):577–93.
95. Sgonc R, Gruschwitz MS, Dietrich H, Recheis H, Gershwin ME, Wick G. Endothelial cell apoptosis is a primary pathogenetic event underlying skin lesions in avian and human scleroderma. J Clin Invest. 1996;98(3):785–92.
96. Asano Y, Sato S. Animal models of scleroderma: current state and recent development. Curr Rheumatol Rep. 2013;15(12):382.
97. Kubo M, Czuwara-Ladykowska J, Moussa O, Markiewicz M, Smith E, Silver RM, et al. Persistent down-regulation of Fli1, a suppressor of collagen transcription, in fibrotic scleroderma skin. Am J Pathol. 2003;163(2):571–81.
98. Yamashita K, Kawasaki A, Matsushita T, Furukawa H, Kondo Y, Okiyama N, et al. Association of functional (GA)n microsatellite polymorphism in the FLI1 gene with susceptibility to human systemic sclerosis. Rheumatology (Oxford). 2020;59:3553.
99. Wang Y, Fan PS, Kahaleh B. Association between enhanced type I collagen expression and epigenetic repression of the FLI1 gene in scleroderma fibroblasts. Arthritis Rheum. 2006;54(7):2271–9.
100. Asano Y, Stawski L, Hant F, Highland K, Silver R, Szalai G, et al. Endothelial Fli1 deficiency impairs vascular homeostasis: a role in scleroderma vasculopathy. Am J Pathol. 2010;176(4):1983–98.
101. Takahashi T, Asano Y, Sugawara K, Yamashita T, Nakamura K, Saigusa R, et al. Epithelial Fli1 deficiency drives systemic autoimmunity and fibrosis: possible roles in scleroderma. J Exp Med. 2017;214(4):1129–51.
102. Saigusa R, Asano Y, Taniguchi T, Hirabayashi M, Nakamura K, Miura S, et al. Fli1-haploinsufficient dermal fibroblasts promote skin-localized transdifferentiation of Th2-like regulatory T cells. Arthritis Res Ther. 2018;20(1):23.
103. Taniguchi T, Miyagawa T, Toyama S, Yamashita T, Nakamura K, Saigusa R, et al. CXCL13 produced by macrophages due to Fli1 deficiency may contribute to the development of tissue fibrosis, vasculopathy and immune activation in systemic sclerosis. Exp Dermatol. 2018;27(9):1030–7.
104. Taniguchi T, Asano Y, Akamata K, Noda S, Takahashi T, Ichimura Y, et al. Fibrosis, vascular activation, and immune abnormalities resembling systemic sclerosis in bleomycin-treated Fli-1-haploinsufficient mice. Arthritis Rheumatol (Hoboken, NJ). 2015;67(2):517–26.
105. Noda S, Asano Y, Nishimura S, Taniguchi T, Fujiu K, Manabe I, et al. Simultaneous downregulation of KLF5 and Fli1 is a key feature underlying systemic sclerosis. Nat Commun. 2014;5:5797.
106. Dong JT, Chen C. Essential role of KLF5 transcription factor in cell proliferation and differentiation and its implications for human diseases. Cell Mol Life Sci. 2009;66(16):2691–706.
107. Whitfield ML, Finlay DR, Murray JI, Troyanskaya OG, Chi JT, Pergamenschikov A, et al. Systemic and cell type-specific gene expression patterns in scleroderma skin. Proc Natl Acad Sci U S A. 2003;100(21):12319–24.
108. Takeda N, Manabe I, Uchino Y, Eguchi K, Matsumoto S, Nishimura S, et al. Cardiac fibroblasts are essential for the adaptive response of the murine heart to pressure overload. J Clin Invest. 2010;120(1):254–65.
109. Fujiu K, Manabe I, Nagai R. Renal collecting duct epithelial cells regulate inflammation in tubulointerstitial damage in mice. J Clin Invest. 2011;121(9):3425–41.
110. Kavian N, Servettaz A, Mongaret C, Wang A, Nicco C, Chereau C, et al. Targeting ADAM-17/notch signaling abrogates the development of systemic sclerosis in a murine model. Arthritis Rheum. 2010;62(11):3477–87.
111. Sato S, Fujimoto M, Hasegawa M, Takehara K, Tedder TF. Altered B lymphocyte function induces systemic autoimmunity in systemic sclerosis. Mol Immunol. 2004;41(12):1123–33.
112. Nakamura K, Taniguchi T, Hirabayashi M, Yamashita T, Saigusa R, Miura S, et al. Altered properties of endothelial cells and mesenchymal stem cells underlying the development of scleroderma-like vasculopathy in KLF5(+/−);Fli-1(+/−) mice. Arthritis Rheumatol. 2020;72(12):2136–46.

113. Feghali-Bostwick C, Medsger TA Jr, Wright TM. Analysis of systemic sclerosis in twins reveals low concordance for disease and high concordance for the presence of antinuclear antibodies. Arthritis Rheum. 2003;48(7):1956–63.
114. Sharif R, Mayes MD, Tan FK, Gorlova OY, Hummers LK, Shah AA, et al. IRF5 polymorphism predicts prognosis in patients with systemic sclerosis. Ann Rheum Dis. 2012;71(7):1197–202.
115. Ferri C, Valentini G, Cozzi F, Sebastiani M, Michelassi C, La Montagna G, et al. Systemic sclerosis: demographic, clinical, and serologic features and survival in 1,012 Italian patients. Medicine. 2002;81(2):139–53.
116. Ioannidis JP, Vlachoyiannopoulos PG, Haidich AB, Medsger TA Jr, Lucas M, Michet CJ, et al. Mortality in systemic sclerosis: an international meta-analysis of individual patient data. Am J Med. 2005;118(1):2–10.
117. Steen VD, Medsger TA Jr. Severe organ involvement in systemic sclerosis with diffuse scleroderma. Arthritis Rheum. 2000;43(11):2437–44.
118. Ferri C, Valentini G, Cozzi F, Sebastiani M, Michelassi C, La Montagna G, et al. Systemic sclerosis: demographic, clinical, and serologic features and survival in 1,012 Italian patients. Medicine (Baltimore). 2002;81(2):139–53.
119. Allanore Y, Meune C. Primary myocardial involvement in systemic sclerosis: evidence for a microvascular origin. Clin Exp Rheumatol. 2010;28(5 Suppl 62):S48–53.
120. Hachulla AL, Launay D, Gaxotte V, de Groote P, Lamblin N, Devos P, et al. Cardiac magnetic resonance imaging in systemic sclerosis: a cross-sectional observational study of 52 patients. Ann Rheum Dis. 2009;68(12):1878–84.
121. Bulkley BH, Ridolfi RL, Salyer WR, Hutchins GM. Myocardial lesions of progressive systemic sclerosis. A cause of cardiac dysfunction. Circulation. 1976;53(3):483–90.
122. Tzelepis GE, Kelekis NL, Plastiras SC, Mitseas P, Economopoulos N, Kampolis C, et al. Pattern and distribution of myocardial fibrosis in systemic sclerosis: a delayed enhanced magnetic resonance imaging study. Arthritis Rheum. 2007;56(11): 3827–36.
123. Venalis P, Kumanovics G, Schulze-Koops H, Distler A, Dees C, Zerr P, et al. Cardiomyopathy in murine models of systemic sclerosis. Arthritis Rheumatol (Hoboken, NJ). 2015;67(2):508–16.
124. Zhao YY, Liu Y, Stan RV, Fan L, Gu Y, Dalton N, et al. Defects in caveolin-1 cause dilated cardiomyopathy and pulmonary hypertension in knockout mice. Proc Natl Acad Sci U S A. 2002;99(17):11375–80.
125. Wunderlich C, Schober K, Lange SA, Drab M, Braun-Dullaeus RC, Kasper M, et al. Disruption of caveolin-1 leads to enhanced nitrosative stress and severe systolic and diastolic heart failure. Biochem Biophys Res Commun. 2006;340(2): 702–8.

Part IV

Cardiovascular Manifestations and Management

Masataka Kuwana

Raynaud's Phenomenon, Digital Ulcers and Nailfold Capillaroscopy

20

Michael Hughes and Marco Matucci-Cerinic

Raynaud's Phenomenon

Clinical Features

Patients with RP report episodic colour change (Fig. 20.1) of the extremities (fingers and toes), although other vascular beds including the nose, lips and ears can also be affected. Typical triggers for attacks of RP are exposure to cold and/or emotional stress. The skin progresses through a classical series of colour changes (physiological mechanisms in parentheses) from pallor (vasoconstriction or occlusion of pre-capillary arterioles) to blue (cyanosis from the deoxygenation of sequestered blood) and finally red (from hyperaemia). However, patients may only experience one- or two-colour changes. Attacks of RP can be overtly painful and/or associated with intrusive neurosensory symptoms (e.g. paraesthesia and dysaesthesia), in particular, during the rewarming (hyperaemic) phase. Irrespective of the underlying cause, RP has a major impact on patient's quality of life and function.

Diagnosis and Classification of Raynaud's Phenomenon

RP can be considered as a 'symptom' complex akin to 'chest pain' and 'shortness of breath' and always requires full elucidation of the underlying aetiology. The majority (80–90%) of patients have primary RP (PRP) [1]. However, there are a broad range of underlying secondary causes of RP, which can result in digital vascular compromise (Table 20.1). The diagnosis of RP is based on clinical grounds with a strong reliance on patient-reported symptoms of episodic digital symptoms in response to cold exposure. A number of criteria have been proposed to diagnose and classify RP [2–6]. In general, these have been based on patient-reported episodic digital symptoms requiring at least two-colour changes in response to cold exposure. The proposed criteria for PRP by LeRoy and Medsger are presented in Table 20.2.

M. Hughes (✉)
Department of Rheumatology, Salford Care Organisation, Northern Care Alliance NHS Foundation Trust, Salford, UK

Division of Musculoskeletal and Dermatological Sciences, Faculty of Biology, Medicine and Health, The University of Manchester, Manchester, UK
e-mail: Michael.hughes-6@postgrad.manchester.ac.uk

M. Matucci-Cerinic
Department of Experimental and Clinical Medicine, University of Florence, Florence, Italy

Division of Rheumatology, AOUC, Florence, Italy

Unit of Immunology, Rheumatology, Allergy and Rare Diseases (UniRAR), IRCCS San Raffaele Hospital, Milan, Italy
e-mail: marco.matuccicerinic@unifi.it

Y. Allanore et al. (eds.), *Scleroderma*, https://doi.org/10.1007/978-3-031-40658-4_20

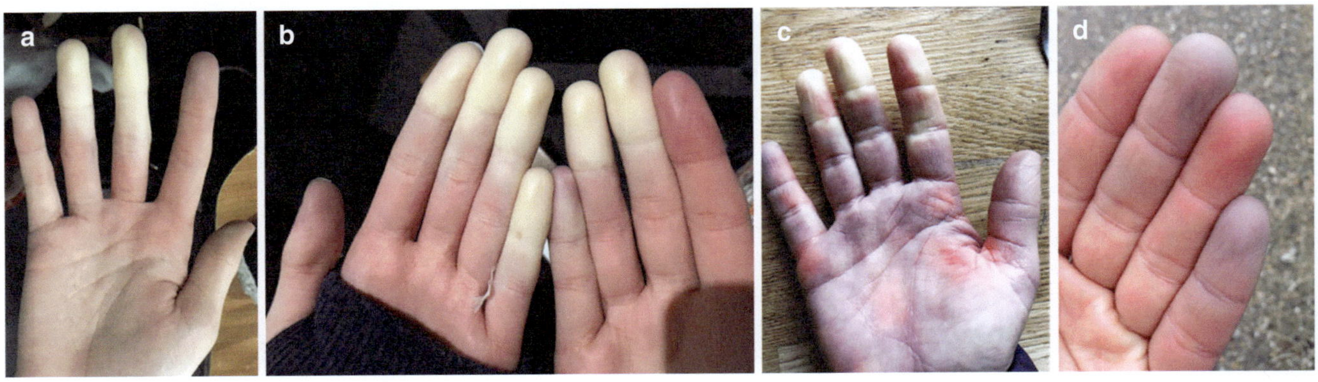

Fig. 20.1 Raynaud's phenomenon. Mobile phone photographs of RP attacks in patients with PRP (**a**, **b**) and limited cutaneous SSc (**c**, **d**). There is sparing of the thumb in PRP unlike in SSc-associated RP. Marked pallor in the patient with PRP (**a**, **b**), whereas there is more notable cyanosis in SSc-RP (**c**, **d**)

Table 20.1 Secondary causes of Raynaud's phenomenon (reproduced from [134]). POEMS syndrome: Polyneuropathy, Organomegaly, Endocrinopathy, Monoclonal gammopathy, and Skin abnormalities

Cause of RP	Underlying aetiology	Clinical findings/investigations aiding diagnosis
Large vessel (usually proximal large-vessel disease, often unilateral symptoms)	Compressive (e.g. cervical rib) Neurogenic (thoracic outlet obstruction) Inflammatory vascular disease (e.g. thromboangiitis obliterans [Buerger's disease] or large-vessel vasculitis) Atherosclerosis	Careful clinical examination of the peripheral pulses Large-vessel imaging (e.g. angiography)
Autoimmune rheumatic diseases	Systemic sclerosis Systemic lupus erythematosus Sjogren's syndrome Mixed connective tissue disease/overlap syndromes Undifferentiated connective tissue disease Idiopathic inflammatory Myopathies Vasculitis	History and careful physical examination Targeted investigations as indicated by clinical assessment (e.g. autoantibodies and nailfold capillaroscopy)
Occupational	Hand–arm vibration syndrome (vibration white finger)	Obtaining a detailed occupational history (e.g. use of vibratory tools)
Drug/chemical-related	Amphetamines Beta blockers Bleomycin Cisplatin Clonidine Cyclosporine Interferons Methysergide Polyvinyl chloride	Eliciting a relevant drug/medication history including exploring chemical exposures
Vaso-occlusive disease	Cold agglutinin disease Cryoglobulinaemia Cryofibrinogenaemia Paraproteinaemia Malignancy (including as a paraneoplastic phenomenon)	Clinical assessment and targeted investigations as appropriate towards any suspected cause of vaso-occlusive disease (e.g. detection of cryoglobulins or cryofibrinogen)
Other causes and associations	Carpal tunnel syndrome Frostbite Hypothyroidism POEMS syndrome Fibromyalgia syndrome	Clinical assessment and investigation to identify other causes and associations (e.g. nerve conduction studies for carpal tunnel syndrome)

Table 20.2 Proposed criteria for primary Raynaud's phenomenon by LeRoy and Medsger [2]

Episodic attacks of acral pallor or cyanosis
Strong and symmetric peripheral pulses
No evidence of digital pitting scars, ulcerations or gangrene
Normal nailfold capillaries
Negative antinuclear antibody
Normal erythrocyte sedimentation rate

Epidemiology of Raynaud's Phenomenon

The reported prevalence of RP is around 3–5% [1]. However, there is wide variation in the reported literature with the prevalence of PRP ranging from 2% to 12% in women and 1% to 12% in men [1]. Differences in such disparities likely include geographical location and differences in study design (e.g. RP definition used and methods of case ascertainment) [1, 7]. As a generalisation, PRP tends to develop before the age of 30 and SRP over 40 years of age [1]. Therefore, although 'isolated' PRP can potentially develop at any age, the likelihood of an underlying secondary cause is significantly more likely [1, 8]. However, progression to secondary forms of RP, almost invariably connective tissue disease (CTD) (e.g. definitive SSc) has been reported to be 12.6% [9, 10]. Risk factors for PRP include (but are not limited to) female sex, family history of RP and manual work/occupational exposure to vibration [1, 7]. Vibration white finger is characterised by uniphasic digital blanching with similar triggers to RP but is limited to areas (i.e. the extremities of the upper limb) that have been exposed to excessive vibration [1, 11]. There are a number of reports describing that patients with RP have increased mortality, which could suggest that in some patients RP is a manifestation of subclinical cardiovascular disease [12, 13].

Summary of the Pathogenesis of Raynaud's Phenomenon

A detailed appraisal of the complex RP pathogenesis is beyond the scope of this chapter; however, by understanding the major factors involved this can help to rationalise the therapeutic strategy. In summary, the pathogenesis of RP is currently incompletely understood, but an imbalance between the normal regulation of vasoconstriction and vasodilation of cutaneous vessels is postulated. Vascular reactivity is regulated by both intrinsic vascular mediators and extrinsic factors including the neural control of vascular tone and the influence of circulating mediators that affect thermoregulatory vessels [14–16]. A complex interaction of these regulators creates a delicate balance that provides important physiological responses including regulating regional blood flow and maintaining normal core body temperature [16]. RP is an exaggeration of the normal responses to our environmental temperatures. In SSc, abnormal vasoreactivity and RP are caused by the disease process disrupting digital and thermoregulatory vessels and usual neurovascular control [14–16]. Furthermore, in SSc there are progressive obliterative microangiopathy and intravascular factors (e.g. impaired fibrinolysis and platelet activation), which also contribute to impaired digital perfusion [14, 15].

Raynaud's Phenomenon in Systemic Sclerosis

RP is almost universally (~97%) observed in patients with SSc and is usually the first manifestation of the disease [17]. This is reflected through the inclusion of RP in the American College of Rheumatology/European League Against Rheumatism (ACR/EULAR) classification criteria for SSc [18]. RP can occur many years (even decades) before the onset of other disease-associated manifestations (e.g. skin sclerosis) in the limited subset of the disease [19], whereas, in patients with diffuse cutaneous SSc, RP develops in close proximity to a year, either before or after the development of skin involvement [19]. Cyanosis (without blanching) has been reported to be more common in SSc (e.g. compared to PRP), and hyperaemia is less common [4, 20]. Patients with SSc-RP (unlike PRP) invariably experience symptoms throughout the course of the year, presumably due to a lower cold sensitivity. Patients with SSc identify that RP is a major source of disease-associated morbidity including its impact on quality of life [21–23]. For example, in a Canadian-based survey of 464 persons with SSc, out of 69 symptoms, RP was the second highest-rated symptom in terms of both frequency (86%) and moderate-to-severe impact on daily activities (67%) [24]. RP has a major impact on hand function in patients with SSc and has also been reported to be associated with DUs [21, 25].

Assessment of the Patient with Raynaud's Phenomenon

Patients presenting with RP require a comprehensive clinical assessment (history and physical examination) including requesting investigations. The clinician should seek to answer these two key questions:

1. What is the underlying aetiology of RP, and in particular, is there evidence of an underlying secondary cause including connective tissue disease (CTD), in particular, SSc?
2. How severe is the patient's RP including the presence of other digital vasculopathic complications (e.g. DUs)?

Clinicians should be actively aware of and consider the very early diagnosis of SSc (VEDOSS), which seeks to identify patients in the very earliest phase of the disease before the onset of irreversible tissue fibrosis and organ dysfunction. VEDOSS should be considered in the presence of RP, puffy fingers and antinuclear antibody positivity, and is confirmed by the presence of SSc-type capillaroscopic abnormalities and/or SSc-associated autoantibodies [26, 27].

History and Examination

History

Patient-reported symptoms in keeping with RP, including colour changes, triggers of attacks and distribution, should be explored. Patients are increasingly using mobile phone cameras to capture attacks of RP, and this can be helpful in the clinical setting. Thumb involvement can be seen in both patients with PRP and SRP; however, relative sparing of the thumb has been reported in PRP [28]. The functional impact of RP should be explored including the activities of daily living including occupation and the development of digital ischaemic complications (e.g. DUs). A full systematic review should be undertaken including features, which could suggest the presence of an underlying CTD (e.g. UV photosensitivity and gastrointestinal motility issues).

Physical Examination

Significant attention must be paid to the examination of the hands including to establish evidence of irreversible ischaemic tissue loss (e.g. digital pitting scars), active digital ischaemia (e.g. DUs), functional impairment and cutaneous manifestations of CTDs including SSc (e.g. telangiectases and calcinosis). The peripheral pulses should be strong and symmetrical, and abnormalities suggest the presence of significant proximal (large) vessel disease and require prompt investigation (e.g. by arterial Doppler ultrasound). A cardiorespiratory examination should include elicitation of features of pulmonary hypertension and/or interstitial lung disease.

Investigations

Key investigations are requesting autoantibodies and performing capillaroscopy, both of which are independent predictors of progression from isolated RP to a secondary disorder, in particular, SSc [9, 10]. This is recognised through their inclusion in both the ACR EULAR SSc classification and VEDOSS criteria. 'Minimal' investigations when the history and examination strongly suggest PRP consist of full blood count, ESR or CRP, antinuclear antibody and nailfold capillaroscopy [29]. Further investigations requested by clinicians often include urea and electrolytes, liver function tests, bone biochemistry, thyroid function tests, creatine kinase, immunoglobulins with serum protein electrophoresis (when there is clinical suspicion of paraproteinaemia), complements C3 and C4, and a chest (or thoracic outlet) radiograph to exclude a cervical rib [29].

Antibodies

Autoantibodies play a major role in establishing the diagnosis of SSc and the likely prognosis including the development of major organ-based complications [18, 30]. The majority (95%) of patients with SSc are antinuclear antibody-positive [17, 31], and the primary method of detection is usually by indirect immunofluorescence. In SSc, there are a wide range of disease-specific autoantibodies directed towards a range of intracellular antigens [31]. Examples include anticentromere, anti-Scl-70, anti-RNA polymerase (I–III), anti-U3RNP and anti-Th/To ribonucleoprotein [31]. SSc can also overlap with other CTDs (e.g. anti-PM/Scl with myositis). Anti-SSA/Ro60 and anti-Ro52 antibodies are not uncommon in SSc and can be a marker of overlap features (e.g. interstitial lung disease) [32]. SSc-spectrum disorders can sometimes occur in the presence of anti-synthetase (e.g. anti-Jo-1) antibodies [33].

Capillaroscopy

Capillaroscopy provides a non-invasive 'window' in which the microcirculation can be examined *in situ*. Nailfold capillaroscopic abnormalities are predicative of a severe disease course including the development of internal organ-based complications and DUs. Capillaroscopy is performed at the nailfold where the capillaries lie parallel to the surface of the skin, and therefore, the capillaries of the distal row can be visualised in their entirety. Both low-magnification (e.g. dermatoscope or USB-microscopy) and high-magnification (e.g. videocapillaroscopy) devices can be used. Low magnification provides a wide-field overview of the whole nailfold area and allows normality to be distinguished from abnormality, whereas higher magnification enables a detailed examination of individual capillaries and semi-quantitative and quantitative measurements to be performed (e.g. capillary density). The increasing availability of low-cost, low-magnification USB-microscope devices should help to expand access to capillaroscopy in non-specialist centres [34, 35].

Normal capillaries have a regular, homogeneous, 'hairpin-like appearance' (Fig. 20.2). In SSc-spectrum disorders, capillaroscopic abnormalities include enlarged (and even 'giant') capillaries, microhaemorrhages, capillary loss ('drop-out') and a failed aberrant attempt at restorative neoangiogenesis. Cutolo et al. [36] propose division into three groups based on the morphological nailfold videocapillaroscopy patterns observed: 'early', 'active' and 'late'. Furthermore, they highlight that the *early* appearance of giant capillaries and haemorrhages is of great relevance to the early diagnosis of SSc, and these abnormalities are even more evident in the *active* phase of the disease [36]. *Late* morphological alterations are the loss of capillaries, vascular architectural disorganisation and the presence of ramified or bushy capillaries [36]. A 'fast track algorithm' to differentiate between a 'non-scleroderma' and a 'scleroderma' pattern has been proposed with excellent reported inter-rater reliability [37]. A recent international effort has developed a checklist of 33 items to provide guidance on how to improve and standardise nailfold capillaroscopy methodology in future clinical research studies [38].

The 'severity' of capillaroscopic abnormalities (e.g. reduced density or more advanced appearance) have been reported to be associated with a more severe disease course, including DU (discussed later) and internal organ complications (e.g. pulmonary hypertension) [39, 40].

Other Imaging Techniques

Laser-based imaging techniques (e.g. laser Doppler imaging and laser speckle contrast imaging) allow evaluation and quantification of skin blood flow, including to investigate the pathogenesis of RP and SSc and to assess treatment response to intervention (e.g. drug therapies). Thermography uses a thermal camera to assess skin temperature, which is an indirect measure of perfusion of both small and large vessels. Infrared thermography can successfully distinguish between PRP and SRP (e.g. the fingertips are cooler than the dorsum of the hand in the latter), and some protocols also advocate dynamic assessment (e.g. through administration of a cold challenge). However, the current use of thermography is

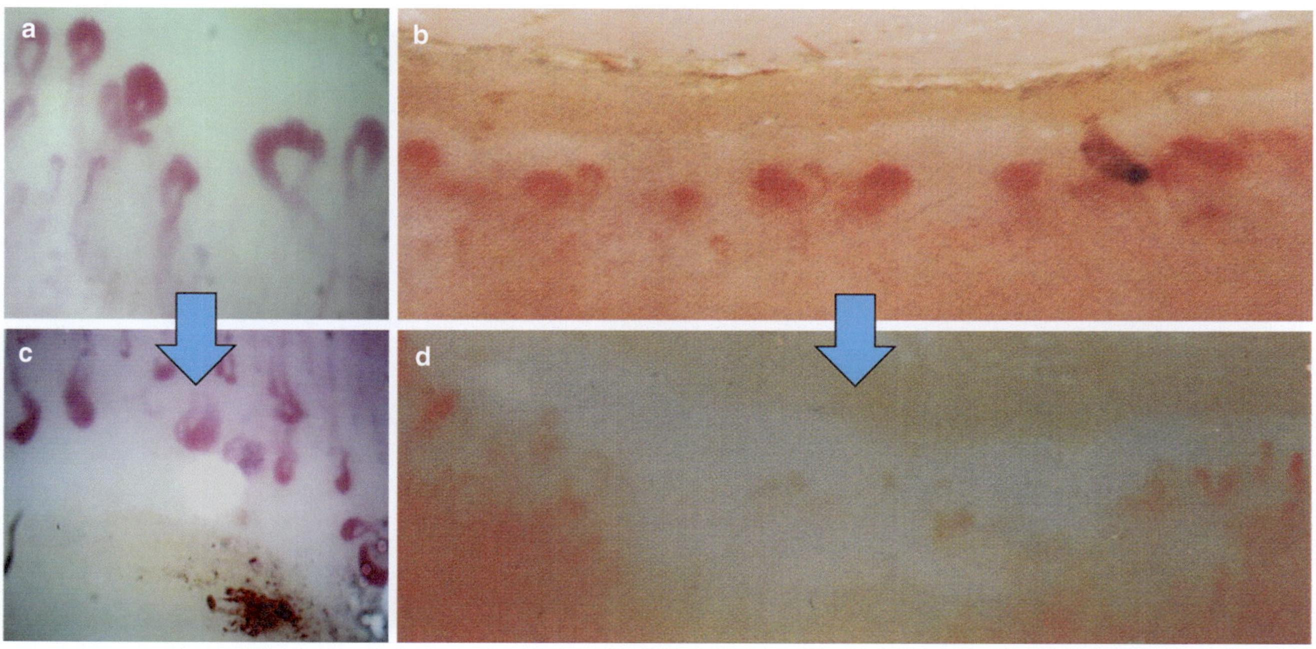

Fig. 20.2 Nailfold capillaroscopy. Early pattern with megacapillaries ('giant' capillaries) (**a**) which have evolved to microhaemorrhages (**c**). Active (**b**) and late (**d**) patterns

typically limited to specialist centres, including due to the high cost of the equipment. There is also a need to standardise the marked international variation in the thermographic protocols. Large-vessel involvement can be assessed by non-invasive arterial Doppler ultrasound including ankle–brachial pressure index, abnormalities of which indicate lower limb ischaemia. Anatomy of vascular lesions can be undertaken by CT, MRI and digital subtraction angiography. However, unlike the latter, CT and MRI provide poor visualisation of the distal vessels, and endovascular procedures cannot be undertaken.

Digital Ulcers in Systemic Sclerosis

Aetiopathogenesis

In general, SSc-DUs (Fig. 20.3) are believed to be driven by ischaemia, in particular, those that develop on the fingertips, although other aetiopathogenic drivers are likely important for ulcers occurring at different locations [41, 42]. Mechanical factors including recurrent trauma at vulnerable sites of the hands (e.g. overlying the small joints) and increased skin tension from tissue fibrosis will predispose to ulceration over the extensor (dorsal) aspects of the hands. Ulcers can also develop from underlying subcutaneous calcinosis deposition. The role of inflammation in the aetiopathogenesis of DUs is little understood to date. Increased peri-ulcer blood flow (e.g. as assessed by laser-based techniques) could theoretically promote healing (e.g. through neoangiogenesis) [43–45]. However, if excessive, this could potentially be tissue damaging through reperfusion injury [33]. Nailfold capillaroscopic abnormalities (e.g. reduced density) have been predictive of future DUs [46–49]. Furthermore, SSc-DUs have been reported to be associated with microangiopathic abnormalities of perilesional skin as assessed by capillaroscopy [50].

Clinical Features

DUs are common in patients with SSc, affecting around half of patients throughout the course of their disease, and with a point prevalence of approximately 10% [41, 51, 52]. The majority of patients will develop their first DU within the first 5 years of their disease and are often recurrent [41]. Any of the digits including the thumb can be affected and ulcers can also occur on the feet including the toes [53]. Ulcers often affect multiple fingers and both hands [53, 54]. DUs are often exceptionally painful and impact on all the physical and social activities including occupation [55, 56]. Ulcers in patients with SSc are associated with an enormous economic burden to society including through the need for hospitalisation and ambulatory care therapies [57]. DUs are often slow to heal, in particular, in the presence of complications (e.g. presence of infection or gangrene) [53].

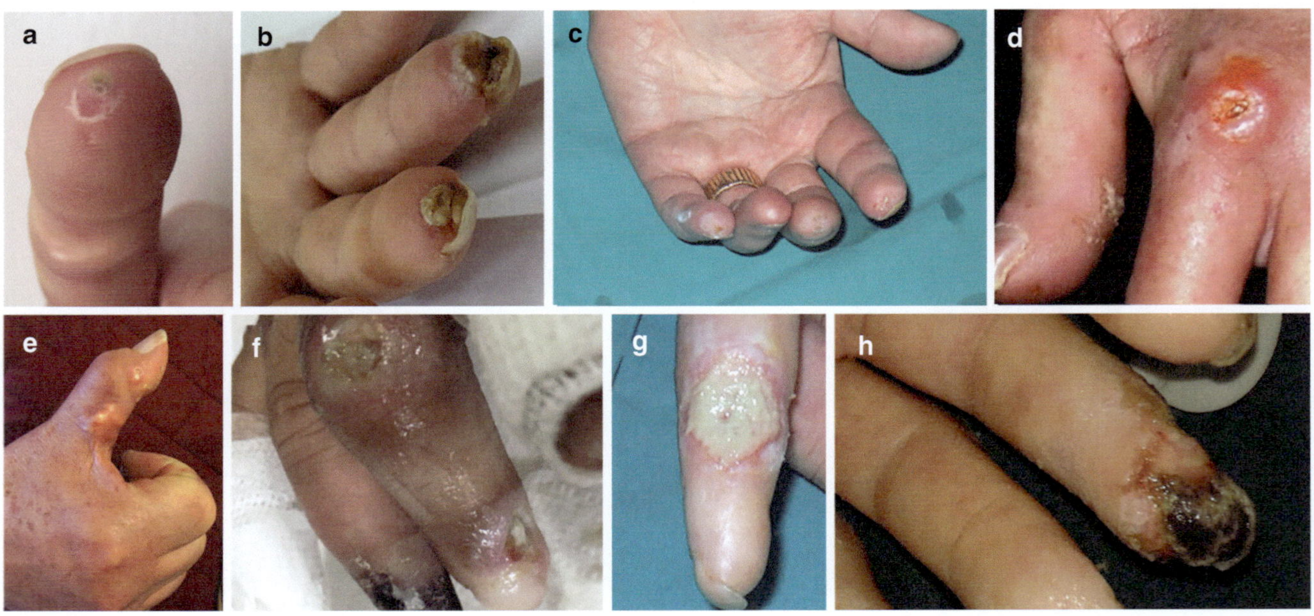

Fig. 20.3 Digital ulcers in systemic sclerosis. Fingertip DUs (**a–c**) including significant hyperkeratosis (**b**) and the presence of digital pitting scars (**c**). Ulcer occurring on the extensor (dorsal) aspect of the hand overlying the MCP joint (**d**). Ulceration related to underlying calcinosis (**e**). DU complications: infection (**f, g**) and digital ischaemia and gangrene (**h**)

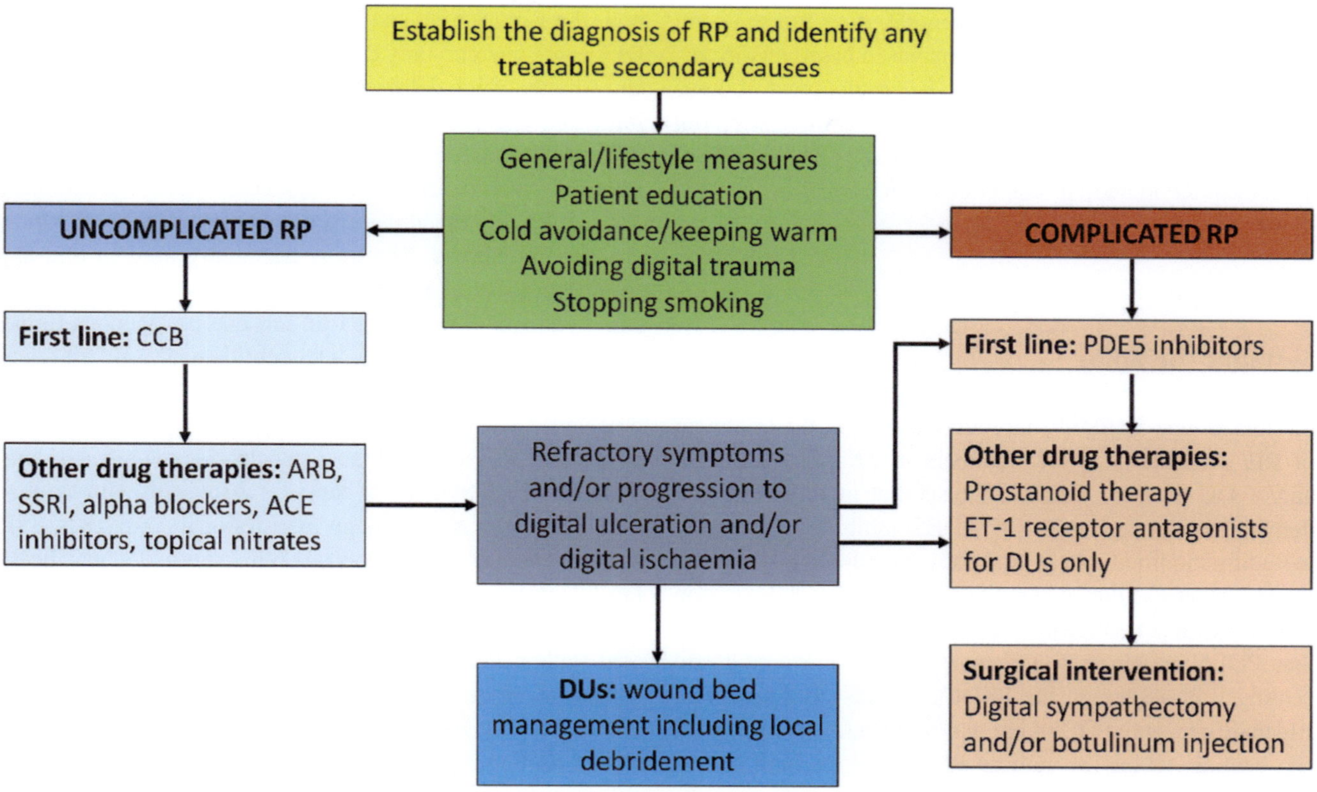

Fig. 20.4 Management of RP and DUs (adapted from expert guidance provided by the UK Scleroderma Study Group and the Scleroderma Clinical Trials Consortium/Canadian Scleroderma Research Group [29, 63]). *ACE* angiotensin-converting enzyme, *ARB* angiotensin receptor blocker, *CCB* calcium channel blocker, *ET* endothelin, *PDE5* phosphodiesterase type 5, *SSRI* selective serotonin receptor inhibitor

Management of RP and DUs

A key feature of management is to establish the diagnosis of RP and identify treatable secondary causes. Patients with SSc (and potentially other causes of SRP) are at risk of developing irreversible ischaemic digital lesions including DUs. We propose a practical approach to management (Fig. 20.4) based on the arbitrary division into 'uncomplicated RP' (e.g. PRP) and 'complicated RP' (e.g. patients with CTD-associated RP including complicated by DUs).

Uncomplicated RP

General/Lifestyle Measures

General/lifestyle measures are indicated in *all* patients with RP and should be delivered by a multidisciplinary team including rheumatology specialist nursing with prompt access to ulcer clinics [58]. Patients require appropriate, high-quality information throughout the course of the disease and can be signposted to national and international patient-led organisations [59, 60]. Key measures include keeping warm (e.g. by wearing multiple layers of clothing and gloves) and avoiding the cold. Patients should be strongly advised about the importance of smoking cessation which promotes vasoconstriction. All efforts must be made to avoid trauma to the digits to prevent the development of DU.

Pharmacological Therapy

Pharmacological therapy is indicated when patient's RP is refractory to the above-described general and lifestyle interventions. Calcium channel blockers (e.g. nifedipine) are generally considered the first-line drug treatment for uncomplicated RP [29, 61–63]. A recent meta-analysis that included 38 studies found low-to-moderate evidence for the benefit of CCBs in reducing the frequency, duration, severity, pain and disability associated with RP [64]. There was evidence that higher (compared to lower) doses are more effective and that patients with PRP derived greater benefit than those with SRP [64]. Other drug therapies that are used (usually after failure of CCB) by clinicians include drugs targeting the renin–angiotensin system (e.g. losartan and ACE inhibitors), alpha blockers (e.g. prazosin) and selective serotonin receptor antagonists (e.g. fluoxetine), the latter of which are useful in patients prone to systemic vasodilatory side effects [29, 63, 65–67]. In general, drug therapies are started at low dose and gradually increased based on the perceived benefit of treatment against the development of dose-limiting adverse side effects [29]. Clinicians often use drug therapies in combination, particularly in the context of SSc-associated RP including 'complicated' RP.

Complicated RP

Systemic Therapies

Internationally, clinicians are increasingly utilising phosphodiesterase type-5 (PDE5) inhibitors earlier in the treatment of RP, particularly in the treatment of SSc-associated RP and/or DU disease. A meta-analysis that included six randomised controlled trials of PDE5 inhibitors (sildenafil including modified release, tadalafil and vardenafil) showed moderate yet significant benefit (e.g. frequency and duration of attacks) in patients with SRP [68]. There is also evidence that PDE5 inhibition is effective for DU prevention and healing [69]. Although the SEDUCE study confirmed that sildenafil prevented DU, there was no benefit observed with DU healing, which the authors attribute to the high rate of ulcer healing in the placebo arm [70]. Prostanoids are indicated in the context of severe and/or refractory RP and digital ischaemic complications including ulcers and gangrene [29]. Such agents (e.g. iloprost and epoprostenol) are typically administered intravenously. Prostanoids are associated with an improvement in RP and also in DU healing and formation [71–74]. Differing intravenous-based regimens are used internationally [75]. However, treatment with prostanoids can be poorly tolerated due to systemic side effects (e.g. vasodilatory headache and myalgia) and patients often require hospitalisation for administration. Temporary discontinuation of oral vasodilatory agents can improve patient tolerability [76]. Previous studies of oral prostanoids have been largely disappointing due to patient tolerability. Data from two large randomised, double-blind, placebo-controlled trials demonstrated the efficacy of bosentan (an endothelin receptor antagonist) for DU prevention but not healing [77, 78]. However, this treatment effect was not reproduced in the DUAL-1 and DUAL-2 trials of macitentan (another endothelin receptor antagonist), which could in part be due to a more milder treated population in the contemporary era compared to the earlier RAPIDs studies [79].

Digital Ulcer Wound Bed Management

Optimal local wound bed management is essential for DUs and requires a systemic approach and should be delivered by a specialist multidisciplinary team [80]. The acronym 'TIME' is a useful approach, which can be used to identify and manage the key components involved in optimal wound healing [81]. ***Tissue management*** involves assessment of both the wound base and peri-lesional skin. The surface of DUs is not uncommonly covered by eschar/necrotic material and slough, which delays ulcer healing and is a reservoir for infection, and therefore requires removal by debridement [82]. Ulcer debridement is used to remove non-viable and infected tissue, debris and foreign bodies, and haematomas, and can be performed using a number of techniques, which are often combined. The most commonly used in SSc are 'sharp' (e.g. using a scalpel or curette) and 'autolytic' (i.e. using endogenous dressings to enhance endogenous tissue lysis) debridement [82, 83]. DU debridement can be exceptionally painful, and therefore, this requires adequate peri-procedural analgesia (topical and systemic) [84]. The choice of dressing is essential for autolytic debridement, and hydrocolloids are rarely used as they are associated with significant pain and can damage peri-lesional skin [82, 85]. ***Inflammation*** plays an important role in normal wound healing. Ulcers are often infected, in particular, by *Staphylococcus aureus* and also enteric organisms, and ***infection*** is associated with delayed wound healing [53, 86, 87]. ***Moisture*** stimulates wound healing, and an ulcer should never be allowed to dry out. However, excessive moisture inhibits wound healing. Again, the choice of dressing is essential, for example, hydrogels help to absorb/control excess wound exudate. The ***wound edge*** and epidermal advancement should be assessed. Normal wound edges appear pink from granulation tissue, whereas chronic wounds develop hyperproliferation and/or rolling of the wound edge.

Surgery

Surgical intervention should be considered as a last resort and is indicated for refractory RP and DU. Cervical sympathectomy is no longer performed due to subsequent recurrence of RP and the severe adverse side effect profile (e.g. Horner's syndrome) associated with the procedure [88]. There is increasing international experience with the use of digital (peri-arterial sympathectomy) and botulinum injection in the context of SSc-associated vasculopathy including DUs [89–93]. Digital amputation for extensive digital necrosis should be considered as a final resort. Natural autoamputation is usually better tolerated by patients and is associated with quite surprisingly minimal tissue loss. Indications for 'deep' surgical DU debridement include severe (and often worse nocturnal) uncontrollable pain, which could indicate the development of underlying digital necrosis (gangrene) or severe local infection complicated by septicaemia, including abscess formation.

Adjunctive Therapies

Clinicians sometimes consider a number of adjunctive therapies for severe RP and/or refractory DUs, although the evidence base to support these interventions is limited. Statins have a wide range of potentially beneficial effects on the endothelium (e.g. increased nitric oxide bioavailability) [94]. Improvement in both RP and DU disease has been reported with statins [95]. Antiplatelet and anticoagulant therapies are only usually considered in the context of acute digital ischaemia, which is refractory to the previously described interventions and/or suspected contributory thrombosis (e.g. of the proximal large vessels). However, to date the studies of such agents have been disappointing (e.g. in terms of DU prevention) [96, 97]. In addition, patients with SSc often have a tendency for gastrointestinal bleeding (e.g. from gastric antral vascular ectasia) and therefore the use of such agents must always be made on an individual patient risk vs. benefit basis. Oxidative stress has been implicated in the pathogenesis of both PRP and SSc-associated RP; however, to date, the evidence to support therapeutic intervention to restore this imbalance is limited, in particular in SSc [98–100].

Unmet Needs

There are a number of unmet needs relating to RP and DUs. Despite a wide therapeutic armoury, treatments are seldom fully effective and often poorly tolerated by patients. In an international survey that included responses from 443 individuals with RP (both PRP and SRP), only 16% reported that one or more of their current medications were considered 'effective' [22]. Similarly, in a study from the Digital Ulcers Outcome (DUO) Registry that included 1459 patients, over the course of ≥2 years of observation, 11.2% were identified to have 'chronic' DUs [101]. Patients have a limited ability to predict both the occurrence and impact of attacks of RP, and therefore, current treatment regimens can be considered as a 'preventative' and administered on a regular basis (as opposed to as required) [22].

A 'treat-to-target' approach has been proposed towards the drug initiation and escalation of oral vasodilator therapies for RP [102] akin to the treatment of many common rheumatological conditions (e.g. rheumatoid arthritis). However, this requires further research including to define the 'target/s' of such a treatment strategy for RP and whether this would differ between patient groups. For example, a recent study that included the responses from 1345 respondents from 15 countries identified that those with PRP more frequently defined their RP in terms of its impact on function/quality and pain compared to those with SRP [103], whereas those with SRP more frequently included specific body parts, colour change, management of attacks and other digital vascular complications, in their RP definition [103]. Akin to the modern pharmacological management of pulmonary hypertension, the benefit of sequential monotherapy vs. initial combination therapy should be explored. Furthermore, broader consensus is also required to determine whether such an approach should also seek to potentially modify other digital (e.g. ulcers) and visceral (e.g. cardiac) vasculopathic complications [102].

For DUs, a locally based approach to treatment could be very advantageous, in particular, from the likely absence of systemically mediated side effects. A range of different local approaches to treatment have been explored including (but not limited to) topical nitrates, platelet and vitamin E gels, phototherapy-based approaches, hyperbaric oxygen, amniotic membrane dressings and drugs which stimulate endothelial progenitor mobilisation (e.g. erythropoietin and GM CSF) [45, 104–111]. There is also some limited clinical experience with tissue/cell therapies, e.g. autologous fat grafting and variously administered mesenchymal stem cell transplantation to be effective for DU healing [112–116]. However, further rigorous investigation, including confirmatory trials, and the delineation of the timing of such investigations are currently required.

Patients report that they can predict and have explanations for DU development; such a pre-ulcer stage could provide an important 'window of opportunity' to intervene before the onset of irreversible tissue loss and ulceration [117]. Experts in SSc and RP have raised concerns about our current methods to assess treatment efficacy in RP and that this could impede drug development programmes for RP [118]. Important work has been undertaken to understand the patient experience of RP and SSc-DUs, which should hopefully result in the development of novel patient-reported outcome measures to capture the multi-faceted impact of these manifestations [23, 119–121]. Non-invasive imaging, in particular, nailfold capillaroscopy has been proposed as a putative biomarker and even potentially an outcome measure for clinical trials of SSc-associated vasculopathy [122–125]. The reliability of experts grading ulcers in SSc has been reported to be poor to moderate at best, which has major implications for DU clinical trials [126, 127]. Fortunately, significant work has been undertaken under the auspices of the World Scleroderma Foundation and the UK Scleroderma Study Group, which have developed and tested new DU definitions [128, 129]. Early validation of the composite DU Clinical Assessment Score (DUCAS) has demonstrated face, content and criterion validity and warrants further investigation [130]. Ultrasound has been successfully applied to measure a range of types of DUs in patients with SSc and could also provide novel insights into ulcer pathogenesis and complications (e.g. infection) [131–133, 135].

Conclusion

RP is common and associated with significant morbidity and is a key 'red flag' for SSc that provides a possible 'window of opportunity' for diagnosis and early intervention strategies. Key investigations are the detection of SSc microangiopathy by capillaroscopy and SSc-associated autoantibodies. DUs are associated with significant pain and disability in SSc and are often difficult to treat. Both RP and DU require a multidisciplinary team approach to management. Non-pharmacological management is required in all patients; however, patients with SRP almost always require treatment with drug therapies, including when complicated by digital ischaemia (e.g. ulcers). Surgical intervention, including digital debridement, should be considered as a final resort for intractable pain and complications (e.g. gangrene). Despite a wide therapeutic arsenal, RP and DUs are often very challenging to treat and our work is far from complete. Robust outcome measures are needed to facilitate clinical trials of new effective treatments for RP and DUs, including early phase studies of promising therapies, and to ensure that these are meaningful to the lived patient experience.

References

1. Maundrell A, Proudman SM. Epidemiology of Raynaud's phenomenon. In: Wigley FM, Herrick AL, Flavahan NA, editors. Raynaud's phenomenon, vol. 2. New York: Springer Science+Business Media; 2015. p. 21–35.
2. LeRoy EC, Medsger TA. Raynaud's phenomenon: a proposal for classification. Clin Exp Rheumatol. 1992;10(5):485–8.
3. Brennan P, Silman A, Black C, Bernstein R, Coppock J, Maddison P, et al. Validity and reliability of three methods used in the diagnosis of Raynaud's phenomenon. The UK Scleroderma Study Group. Br J Rheumatol. 1993;32(5):357–61.
4. Maricq HR, Weinrich MC. Diagnosis of Raynaud's phenomenon assisted by color charts. J Rheumatol. 1988;15(3):454–9.
5. Wigley FM. Raynaud's phenomenon. N Engl J Med. 2002;347(13):1001–8.
6. Maverakis E, Patel F, Kronenberg DG, Chung L, Fiorentino D, Allanore Y, et al. International consensus criteria for the diagnosis of Raynaud's phenomenon. J Autoimmun. 2014;48–49:60–5.
7. Garner R, Kumari R, Lanyon P, Doherty M, Zhang W. Prevalence, risk factors and associations of primary Raynaud's phenomenon: systematic review and meta-analysis of observational studies. BMJ Open. 2015;5(3):e006389.
8. Planchon B, Pistorius MA, Beurrier P, De Faucal P. Primary Raynaud's phenomenon. Age of onset and pathogenesis in a prospective study of 424 patients. Angiology. 1994;45(8):677–86.
9. Spencer-Green G. Outcomes in primary Raynaud phenomenon: a meta-analysis of the frequency, rates, and predictors of transition to secondary diseases. Arch Intern Med. 1998;158(6):595–600.
10. Koenig M, Joyal F, Fritzler MJ, Roussin A, Abrahamowicz M, Boire G, et al. Autoantibodies and microvascular damage are independent predictive factors for the progression of Raynaud's phenomenon to systemic sclerosis: a twenty-year prospective study of 586 patients, with validation of proposed criteria for early systemic sclerosis. Arthritis Rheum. 2008;58(12):3902–12.
11. Palmer KT, Griffin MJ, Syddall H, Cooper C, Coggon D. The clinical grading of Raynaud's phenomenon and vibration-induced white finger: relationship between finger blanching and difficulties in using the upper limb. Int Arch Occup Environ Health. 2002;75(1–2):29–36.
12. Nietert P, Shaftman S, Silver R, Wolf B, Egan B, Hunt K, et al. Raynaud phenomenon and mortality: 20+ years of follow-up of the Charleston Heart Study cohort. Clin Epidemiol. 2015;7:161–8.
13. Mueller M, Gschwandtner ME, Gamper J, Giurgea G-A, Charwat-Resl S, Kiener HP, et al. Relation of nailfold capillaries and autoantibodies to mortality in patients with Raynaud phenomenon. Circulation. 2016;133(5):509–17.
14. Herrick AL. Pathogenesis of Raynaud's phenomenon. Rheumatology (Oxford). 2005;44(5):587–96.
15. Herrick AL. The pathogenesis, diagnosis and treatment of Raynaud phenomenon. Nat Rev Rheumatol. 2012;8(8):469–79.
16. Flavahan NA. Pathophysiological regulation of the cutaneous vascular system in Raynaud's phenomenon. In: Wigley FM, Herrick AL, Flavahan NA, editors. Raynaud's phenomenon: a guide to pathogenesis and treatment. New York: Springer Science+Business Media; 2015. p. 57–79.
17. Meier FMP, Frommer KW, Dinser R, Walker UA, Czirjak L, Denton CP, et al. Update on the profile of the EUSTAR cohort: an analysis of the EULAR Scleroderma Trials and Research Group database. Ann Rheum Dis. 2012;71(8):1355–60.
18. van den Hoogen F, Khanna D, Fransen J, Johnson SR, Baron M, Tyndall A, et al. 2013 classification criteria for systemic sclerosis: an American College of Rheumatology/European League against Rheumatism collaborative initiative. Arthritis Rheum. 2013;65(11):2737–47.
19. LeRoy EC, Black C, Fleischmajer R, Jablonska S, Krieg T, Medsger TA, et al. Scleroderma (systemic sclerosis): classification, subsets and pathogenesis. J Rheumatol. 1988;15(2):202–5.
20. Wollersheim H, Thien T. The diagnostic value of clinical signs and symptoms in patients with Raynaud's phenomenon. A cross-sectional study. Neth J Med. 1990;37(5–6):171–82.
21. Merkel PA, Herlyn K, Martin RW, Anderson JJ, Mayes MD, Bell P, et al. Measuring disease activity and functional status in patients with scleroderma and Raynaud's phenomenon. Arthritis Rheum. 2002;46(9):2410–20.
22. Hughes M, Snapir A, Wilkinson J, Snapir D, Wigley FMFM, Herrick ALAL. Prediction and impact of attacks of Raynaud's phenomenon, as judged by patient perception. Rheumatology (Oxford). 2015;54(8):1443–7.
23. Pauling JD, Domsic RT, Saketkoo LA, Almeida C, Withey J, Jay H, et al. Multinational qualitative research study exploring the patient experience of Raynaud's phenomenon in systemic sclerosis. Arthritis Care Res (Hoboken). 2018;70(9):1373–84.
24. Bassel M, Hudson M, Taillefer SS, Schieir O, Baron M, Thombs BD. Frequency and impact of symptoms experienced by patients with systemic sclerosis: results from a Canadian National Survey. Rheumatology (Oxford). 2011;50(4):762–7.
25. Kwakkenbos L, Sanchez TA, Turner KA, Mouthon L, Carrier ME, Hudson M, et al. The association of sociodemographic and disease variables with hand function: a scleroderma patient-centered intervention network cohort study. Clin Exp Rheumatol. 2018;36:S88–94.
26. Avouac J, Fransen J, Walker UA, Riccieri V, Smith V, Muller C, et al. Preliminary criteria for the very early diagnosis of systemic sclerosis: results of a Delphi Consensus Study from EULAR Scleroderma Trials and Research Group. Ann Rheum Dis. 2011;70(3):476–81.
27. Bellando-Randone S, Matucci-Cerinic M. From Raynaud's phenomenon to very early diagnosis of systemic sclerosis—the VEDOSS approach. Curr Rheumatol Rev. 2013;9(4):245–8.
28. Chikura B, Moore T, Manning J, Vail A, Herrick AL. Thumb involvement in Raynaud's phenomenon as an indicator of underlying connective tissue disease. J Rheumatol. 2010;37(4):783–6.

29. Hughes M, Ong VHVHH, Anderson MEMEE, Hall F, Moinzadeh P, Griffiths B, et al. Consensus best practice pathway of the UK Scleroderma Study Group: digital vasculopathy in systemic sclerosis. Rheumatology (Oxford). 2015;54(11):2015–24.
30. Nihtyanova SI, Sari A, Harvey JC, Leslie A, Derrett-Smith EC, Fonseca C, et al. Using autoantibodies and cutaneous subset to develop outcome-based disease classification in systemic sclerosis. Arthritis Rheumatol (Hoboken, NJ). 2020;72(3):465–76.
31. Kayser C, Fritzler MJ. Autoantibodies in systemic sclerosis: unanswered questions. Front Immunol. 2015;6:167.
32. Hudson M, Pope J, Mahler M, Tatibouet S, Steele R, Baron M, et al. Clinical significance of antibodies to Ro52/TRIM21 in systemic sclerosis. Arthritis Res Ther. 2012;14(2):R50.
33. Hughes M, Allanore Y, Chung L, Pauling JD, Denton CP, Matucci-Cerinic M. Raynaud phenomenon and digital ulcers in systemic sclerosis. Nat Rev Rheumatol. 2020;16(4):208–21.
34. Bhakuni DS, Vasdev V, Garg MK, Narayanan K, Jain R, Mullick G. Nailfold capillaroscopy by digital microscope in an Indian population with systemic sclerosis. Int J Rheum Dis. 2012;15(1):95–101.
35. Berks M, Dinsdale G, Marjanovic E, Murray A, Taylor C, Herrick AL. Comparison between low cost USB nailfold capillaroscopy and videocapillaroscopy: a pilot study. Rheumatology (Oxford). 2020;60:3862 [Online ahead of print]. https://doi.org/10.1093/rheumatology/keaa72.
36. Cutolo M, Sulli A, Pizzorni C, Accardo S. Nailfold videocapillaroscopy assessment of microvascular damage in systemic sclerosis. J Rheumatol. 2000;27(1):155–60.
37. Smith V, Vanhaecke A, Herrick AL, Distler O, Guerra MG, Denton CP, et al. Fast track algorithm: how to differentiate a "scleroderma pattern" from a "non-scleroderma pattern". Autoimmun Rev. 2019;18(11):102394.
38. Ingegnoli F, Herrick AL, Schioppo T, Bartoli F, Ughi N, Pauling JD, et al. Reporting items for capillaroscopy in clinical research on musculoskeletal diseases: a systematic review and international Delphi consensus. Rheumatology (Oxford). 2020;60:keaa457 [Online ahead of print]. https://doi.org/10.1093/rheumatology/keaa457.
39. Ong YY, Nikoloutsopoulos T, Bond CP, Smith MD, Ahern MJ, Roberts-Thomson PJ. Decreased nailfold capillary density in limited scleroderma with pulmonary hypertension. Asian Pacific J Allergy Immunol. 1998;16(2–3):81–6.
40. Hofstee HMA, Vonk Noordegraaf A, Voskuyl AE, Dijkmans BAC, Postmus PE, Smulders YM, et al. Nailfold capillary density is associated with the presence and severity of pulmonary arterial hypertension in systemic sclerosis. Ann Rheum Dis. 2009;68(2):191–5.
41. Hachulla E, Clerson P, Launay D, Lambert M, Morell-Dubois S, Queyrel V, et al. Natural history of ischemic digital ulcers in systemic sclerosis: single-center retrospective longitudinal study. J Rheumatol. 2007;34(12):2423–30.
42. Hughes M, Murray A, Denton CP, Herrick AL. Should all digital ulcers be included in future clinical trials of systemic sclerosis-related digital vasculopathy? Med Hypotheses. 2018;116:101–4.
43. Ruaro B, Sulli A, Smith V, Paolino S, Pizzorni C, Cutolo M. Short-term follow-up of digital ulcers by laser speckle contrast analysis in systemic sclerosis patients. Microvasc Res. 2015;101:82–5.
44. Murray AK, Moore TL, Wragg E, Ennis H, Vail A, Dinsdale G, et al. Pilot study assessing pathophysiology and healing of digital ulcers in patients with systemic sclerosis using laser Doppler imaging and thermography. Clin Exp Rheumatol. 2016;5:100–5.
45. Hughes M, Moore T, Manning J, Wilkinson J, Dinsdale G, Roberts C, et al. Reduced perfusion in systemic sclerosis digital ulcers (both fingertip and extensor) can be increased by topical application of glyceryl trinitrate. Microvasc Res. 2017;111:32–6.
46. Smith V, Decuman S, Sulli A, Bonroy C, Piettte Y, Deschepper E, et al. Do worsening scleroderma capillaroscopic patterns predict future severe organ involvement? A pilot study. Ann Rheum Dis. 2012;71(10):1636–9.
47. Sebastiani M, Manfredi A, Vukatana G, Moscatelli S, Riato L, Bocci M, et al. Predictive role of capillaroscopic skin ulcer risk index in systemic sclerosis: a multicentre validation study. Ann Rheum Dis. 2012;71(1):67–70.
48. Smith V, Cutolo M, Herrick AL, Distler O, Becker M, Beltran E, et al. A multicenter, prospective cohort study using nailfold videocapillaroscopy and other clinical characteristics to determine the risk of developing new digital ulcers in patients with systemic sclerosis. Arthritis Rheumatol (Hoboken, NJ). 2014;66(10):S848–9.
49. Friedrich S, Friedrich S, Lüders S, Lüders S, Klotsche J, Klotsche J, et al. The first composite score predicting digital ulcers in systemic sclerosis patients using clinical data, imaging and patient history—CIP-DUS. Arthritis Res Ther. 2020;22(1):144.
50. Hughes M, Moore T, Manning J, Dinsdale G, Murray A, Herrick AL. Digital ulcers in systemic sclerosis are associated with microangiopathic abnormalities of peri-lesional skin as assessed by capillaroscopy. Scand J Rheumatol. 2017;46(1):81–2.
51. Tiev KP, Diot E, Clerson P, Dupuis-Siméon F, Hachulla E, Hatron PY, et al. Clinical features of scleroderma patients with or without prior or current ischemic digital ulcers: post-hoc analysis of a nationwide multicenter cohort (ItinérAIR-Sclérodermie). J Rheumatol. 2009;36(7):1470–6.
52. Ennis H, Vail A, Wragg E, Taylor A, Moore T, Murray A, et al. A prospective study of systemic sclerosis-related digital ulcers: prevalence, location, and functional impact. Scand J Rheumatol. 2013;42(6):483–6.
53. Amanzi L, Braschi F, Fiori G, Galluccio F, Miniati I, Guiducci S, et al. Digital ulcers in scleroderma: staging, characteristics and sub-setting through observation of 1614 digital lesions. Rheumatology (Oxford). 2010;49(7):1374–82.
54. Mouthon L, Carpentier PH, Lok C, Clerson P, Gressin V, Hachulla E, et al. Ischemic digital ulcers affect hand disability and pain in systemic sclerosis. J Rheumatol. 2014;41(7):1317–23.
55. Bérezné A, Seror R, Morell-Dubois S, de Menthon M, Fois E, Dzeing-Ella A, et al. Impact of systemic sclerosis on occupational and professional activity with attention to patients with digital ulcers. Arthritis Care Res. 2011;63(2):277–85.
56. Mouthon L, Carpentier PH, Lok C, Clerson P, Gressin V, Hachulla E, et al. Controlling the digital ulcerative disease in systemic sclerosis is associated with improved hand function. Semin Arthritis Rheum. 2017;46(6):759–66.
57. Morrisroe K, Stevens W, Sahhar J, Ngian G-S, Ferdowsi N, Hill CL, et al. Digital ulcers in systemic sclerosis: their epidemiology, clinical characteristics, and associated clinical and economic burden. Arthritis Res Ther. 2019;21(1):299.
58. Ngcozana T, Ong VH, Denton CP. Improving access to digital ulcer care through nurse-led clinic: a service evaluation. Musculoskeletal Care. 2020;18(1):92–7.
59. Hughes M, Baker A, Farrington S, Pauling JD. Patient organisation-led initiatives can play an important role in raising awareness about Raynaud's phenomenon and encourage earlier healthcare utilisation for high-risk groups. Ann Rheum Dis. 2019;78(3):439–41.
60. Devgire V, Martin AF, McKenzie L, Sandler RD, Hughes M. A systematic review of internet-based information for individuals with Raynaud's phenomenon and patients with systemic sclerosis. Clin Rheumatol. 2020;39(8):2363–7.
61. Kowal-Bielecka O, Fransen J, Avouac J, Becker M, Kulak A, Allanore Y, et al. Update of EULAR recommendations for the treatment of systemic sclerosis. Ann Rheum Dis. 2017;76(8):1327–39.
62. Denton C, Hughes M, Gak N, Vila J, Buch MH, Chakravarty K, et al. BSR and BHPR guideline for the treatment of systemic sclerosis. Rheumatology (Oxford). 2016;55(10):1906–10.

63. Fernández-Codina A, Walker KM, Pope JE, Scleroderma Algorithm Group. Treatment algorithms for systemic sclerosis according to experts. Arthritis Rheumatol. 2018;70(11):1820–8.
64. Rirash F, Tingey PC, Harding SE, Maxwell LJ, Tanjong Ghogomu E, Wells GA, et al. Calcium channel blockers for primary and secondary Raynaud's phenomenon. Cochrane Database Syst Rev. 2017;12(12):CD000467.
65. Harding SE, Tingey PC, Pope J, Fenlon D, Furst D, Shea B, et al. Prazosin for Raynaud's phenomenon in progressive systemic sclerosis. Cochrane Database Syst Rev. 2000;1998(2):CD000956.
66. Dziadzio M, Denton CP, Smith R, Howell K, Blann A, Bowers E, et al. Losartan therapy for Raynaud's phenomenon and scleroderma: clinical and biochemical findings in a fifteen-week, randomized, parallel-group, controlled trial. Arthritis Rheum. 1999;42(12):2646–55.
67. Coleiro B, Marshall SE, Denton CP, Howell K, Blann A, Welsh KI, et al. Treatment of Raynaud's phenomenon with the selective serotonin reuptake inhibitor fluoxetine. Rheumatology (Oxford). 2001;40(9):1038–43.
68. Roustit M, Blaise S, Allanore Y, Carpentier PH, Caglayan E, Cracowski J-L. Phosphodiesterase-5 inhibitors for the treatment of secondary Raynaud's phenomenon: systematic review and meta-analysis of randomised trials. Ann Rheum Dis. 2013;72(10):1696–9.
69. Tingey T, Shu J, Smuczek J, Pope J. Meta-analysis of healing and prevention of digital ulcers in systemic sclerosis. Arthritis Care Res (Hoboken). 2013;65(9):1460–71.
70. Hachulla E, Hatron PY, Carpentier P, Agard C, Chatelus E, Jego P, et al. Efficacy of sildenafil on ischaemic digital ulcer healing in systemic sclerosis: the placebo-controlled SEDUCE study. Ann Rheum Dis. 2016;75(6):1009–15.
71. Wigley FM, Seibold JR, Wise RA, McCloskey DA, Dole WP. Intravenous iloprost treatment of Raynaud's phenomenon and ischemic ulcers secondary to systemic sclerosis. J Rheumatol. 1992;19(9):1407–14.
72. Wigley FM, Wise RA, Seibold JR, McCloskey DA, Kujala G, Medsger TA, et al. Intravenous iloprost infusion in patients with Raynaud phenomenon secondary to systemic sclerosis. A multicenter, placebo-controlled, double-blind study. Ann Intern Med. 1994;120(3):199–206.
73. Cruz JE, Ward A, Anthony S, Chang S, Bae HB, Hermes-DeSantis ER. Evidence for the use of epoprostenol to treat Raynaud's phenomenon with or without digital ulcers. Ann Pharmacother. 2016;50(12):1060–7.
74. Law ST, Farber HW, Simms RW. Use of intravenous epoprostenol as a treatment for the digital vasculopathy associated with the scleroderma spectrum of diseases. J Scleroderma Relat Disord. 2017;2(3):208–12.
75. Negrini S, Magnani O, Matucci-Cerinic M, Carignola R, Data V, Montabone E, et al. Iloprost use and medical management of systemic sclerosis-related vasculopathy in Italian tertiary referral centers: results from the PROSIT study. Clin Exp Med. 2019;19(3):357–66.
76. Bellando-Randone S, Bruni C, Lepri G, Fiori G, Bartoli F, Conforti ML, et al. The safety of iloprost in systemic sclerosis in a real-life experience. Clin Rheumatol. 2018;37(5):1249–55.
77. Korn JH, Mayes M, Matucci Cerinic M, Rainisio M, Pope J, Hachulla E, et al. Digital ulcers in systemic sclerosis: prevention by treatment with bosentan, an oral endothelin receptor antagonist. Arthritis Rheum. 2004;50(12):3985–93.
78. Matucci-Cerinic M, Denton CP, Furst DE, Mayes MD, Hsu VM, Carpentier P, et al. Bosentan treatment of digital ulcers related to systemic sclerosis: results from the RAPIDS-2 randomised, double-blind, placebo-controlled trial. Ann Rheum Dis. 2011;70(1):32–8.
79. Khanna D, Denton CP, Merkel PA, Krieg T, Le Brun F-O, Marr A, et al. Effect of macitentan on the development of new ischemic digital ulcers in patients with systemic sclerosis: DUAL-1 and DUAL-2 randomized clinical trials. JAMA. 2016;315(18):1975–88.
80. Lebedoff N, Frech TM, Shanmugam VK, Fischer A, Erhardt D, Kolfenbach J, et al. Review of local wound management for scleroderma-associated digital ulcers. J Scleroderma Relat Disord. 2017;3(1):66–70.
81. Halim AS, Khoo TL, Saad AZM. Wound bed preparation from a clinical perspective. Indian J Plast Surg. 2012;45(2):193–202.
82. Hughes M, Alcacer-Pitarch B, Gheorghiu AM, Praino E, Sandler RD, Tavor Y, et al. Digital ulcer debridement in systemic sclerosis: a systematic literature review. Clin Rheumatol. 2020;39(3):805–11.
83. Hughes M, Alcacer-Pitarch B, Allanore Y, Baron M, Boin F, Bruni C, et al. Digital ulcers: should debridement be a standard of care in systemic sclerosis? Lancet Rheumatol. 2020;2(5):e302–7.
84. Braschi F, Bartoli F, Bruni C, Fiori G, Fantauzzo C, Paganelli L, et al. Lidocaine controls pain and allows safe wound bed preparation and debridement of digital ulcers in systemic sclerosis: a retrospective study. Clin Rheumatol. 2017;36(1):209–12. 7
85. Gualdi G, Monari P, Cammalleri D, Pelizzari L, Pinton PC. Hyaluronic acid-based products are strictly contraindicated in scleroderma-related skin ulcers. Wounds. 2019;31(3):81–4.
86. Giuggioli D, Manfredi A, Colaci M, Lumetti F, Ferri C. Scleroderma digital ulcers complicated by infection with fecal pathogens. Arthritis Care Res (Hoboken). 2012;64(2):295–7.
87. Haque A, Wyman M, Dargan D, Hughes M, Musson R, Cadick J, et al. Hand osteomyelitis in patients with secondary Raynaud phenomenon. J Clin Rheumatol. 2020;27:S342 [Online ahead of print]. https://doi.org/10.1097/RHU.0000000000001621.
88. Lowell RC, Gloviczki P, Cherry KJJ, Bower TC, Hallett JWJ, Schirger A, et al. Cervicothoracic sympathectomy for Raynaud's syndrome. Int Angiol. 1993;12(2):168–72.
89. Neumeister MW. Botulinum toxin type A in the treatment of Raynaud's phenomenon. J Hand Surg Am. 2010;35(12):2085–92.
90. Momeni A, Sorice SC, Valenzuela A, Fiorentino DF, Chung L, Chang J. Surgical treatment of systemic sclerosis-is it justified to offer peripheral sympathectomy earlier in the disease process? Microsurgery. 2015;35(6):441–6.
91. Bello RJ, Cooney CM, Melamed E, Follmar K, Yenokyan G, Leatherman G, et al. The therapeutic efficacy of botulinum toxin in treating scleroderma-associated Raynaud's phenomenon: a randomized, double-blind, placebo-controlled clinical trial. Arthritis Rheumatol. 2017;69(8):1661–9.
92. Satteson ES, Chung MP, Chung LS, Chang J. Microvascular hand surgery for digital ischemia in scleroderma. J Scleroderma Relat Disord. 2020;5(2):130–6.
93. Guerra MG, da Fonseca DG, Samões B, Videira T, Pinto P. Is botulinum toxin useful in systemic sclerosis related peripheral vasculopathy? A literature review. Reumatol Clin. 2020. pii: S1699-258X(20)30083-8.
94. Ladak K, Pope JE. A review of the effects of statins in systemic sclerosis. Semin Arthritis Rheum. 2016;45(6):698–705.
95. Abou-Raya A, Abou-Raya S, Helmii M. Statins: potentially useful in therapy of systemic sclerosis-related Raynaud's phenomenon and digital ulcers. J Rheumatol. 2008;35(9):1801–8.
96. Beckett VL, Conn DL, Fuster V, Osmundson PJ, Strong CG, Chao EY, et al. Trial of platelet-inhibiting drug in scleroderma. Double-blind study with dipyridamole and aspirin. Arthritis Rheum. 1984;27(10):1137–43.

97. Denton CP, Howell K, Stratton RJ, Black CM. Long-term low molecular weight heparin therapy for severe Raynaud's phenomenon: a pilot study. Clin Exp Rheumatol. 2000;18(4):499–502.
98. Herrick AL, Hollis S, Schofield D, Rieley F, Blann A, Griffin K, et al. A double-blind placebo-controlled trial of antioxidant therapy in limited cutaneous systemic sclerosis. Clin Exp Rheumatol. 2000;18(3):349–56.
99. Correa MJU, Mariz HA, Andrade LEC, Kayser C. [Oral N-acetylcysteine in the treatment of Raynaud's phenomenon secondary to systemic sclerosis: a randomized, double-blind, placebo-controlled clinical trial]. Rev Bras Reumatol. 2014;54(6):452–8.
100. Bruni C, Lepri G, Peruzzi F, Bellando-Randone S, Radicati A, Matucci-Cerinic M, et al. Antioxidant agents help primary Raynaud's phenomenon. Int Angiol. 2015;34(1):94–5.
101. Matucci-Cerinic M, Krieg T, Guillevin L, Schwierin B, Rosenberg D, Cornelisse P, et al. Elucidating the burden of recurrent and chronic digital ulcers in systemic sclerosis: long-term results from the DUO Registry. Ann Rheum Dis. 2016;75(10):1770–6.
102. Hughes M, Khanna DK, Pauling JD. Drug initiation and escalation strategies of vasodilator therapies for Raynaud's phenomenon: can we treat to target? Rheumatology (Oxford). 2020;59(3):464–6.
103. Murphy SL, Lescoat A, Alore M, Hughes M, Pauling JD, Sabbagh M, et al. How do patients define Raynaud's phenomenon? Differences between Primary and secondary disease. Clin Rheumatol. 2021;40:1611 [Online ahead of print]. https://doi.org/10.1007/s10067-021-05598-7.
104. Fiori G, Galluccio F, Braschi F, Amanzi L, Miniati I, Conforti ML, et al. Vitamin E gel reduces time of healing of digital ulcers in systemic sclerosis. Clin Exp Rheumatol. 2009;27(3 Suppl 54):51–4.
105. Inoue T, Yamaoka T, Murota H, Yokomi A, Tanemura A, Igawa K, et al. Effective oral psoralen plus ultraviolet a therapy for digital ulcers with revascularization in systemic sclerosis. Acta Derm Venereol. 2014;94(2):250–1.
106. Hughes M, Moore T, Manning J, Wilkinson J, Watson S, Samraj P, et al. A feasibility study of a novel low level light therapy for digital ulcers in systemic sclerosis. J Dermatolog Treat. 2019;30(3):251–7.
107. Frech TM, McNeill C, Lebiedz-Odrobina D, Lewis G. Amniotic membrane dressings: an effective therapy for SSc-related wounds. Rheumatology (Oxford). 2019;58(4):734–6.
108. Giuggioli D, Magistro R, Colaci M, Franciosi U, Caruso A, Ferri C. The treatment of skin ulcers in systemic sclerosis: use of granulocyte-colony stimulating factor (G-CSF) in 26 patients. Reumatismo. 2006;58(1):26–30.
109. Ferri C, Giuggioli D, Sebastiani M, Colaci M. Treatment of severe scleroderma skin ulcers with recombinant human erythropoietin. Clin Exp Dermatol. 2007;32(3):287–90.
110. Giuggioli D, Colaci M, Manfredi A, Mariano M, Ferri C. Platelet gel in the treatment of severe scleroderma skin ulcers. Rheumatol Int. 2012;32(9):2929–32.
111. Mirasoglu B, Bagli BS, Aktas S. Hyperbaric oxygen therapy for chronic ulcers in systemic sclerosis—case series. Int J Dermatol. 2017;56(6):636–40.
112. Del Papa N, Di Luca G, Sambataro D, Zaccara E, Maglione W, Gabrielli A, et al. Regional implantation of autologous adipose tissue-derived cells induces a prompt healing of long-lasting indolent digital ulcers in patients with systemic sclerosis. Cell Transplant. 2015;24(11):2297–305.
113. Del Papa N, Di Luca G, Andracco R, Zaccara E, Maglione W, Pignataro F, et al. Regional grafting of autologous adipose tissue is effective in inducing prompt healing of indolent digital ulcers in patients with systemic sclerosis: results of a monocentric randomized controlled study. Arthritis Res Ther. 2019;21(1):1–11.
114. Nevskaya T, Ananieva L, Bykovskaia S, Eremin I, Karandashov E, Khrennikov J, et al. Autologous progenitor cell implantation as a novel therapeutic intervention for ischaemic digits in systemic sclerosis. Rheumatology (Oxford). 2009;48(1):61–4.
115. Ishigatsubo Y, Ihata A, Kobayashi H, Hama M, Kirino Y, Ueda A, et al. Therapeutic angiogenesis in patients with systemic sclerosis by autologous transplantation of bone-marrow-derived cells. Mod Rheumatol. 2010;20(3):263–72.
116. Daumas A, Magalon J, Jouve E, Truillet R, Casanova D, Giraudo L, et al. Long-term follow-up after autologous adipose-derived stromal vascular fraction injection into fingers in systemic sclerosis patients. Curr Res Transl Med. 2017;65(1):40–3.
117. Hughes M, Pauling JD, Jones J, Denton CP, Domsic RT, Frech TM, et al. Patient experiences of digital ulcer development and evolution in systemic sclerosis. Rheumatology (Oxford). 2020;59(8):2156–8.
118. Pauling JD, Frech TM, Hughes M, Gordon JK, Domsic RT, Anderson ME, et al. Patient-reported outcome instruments for assessing Raynaud's phenomenon in systemic sclerosis: a SCTC vascular working group report. J Scleroderma Relat Disord. 2018;3(3):249–52.
119. Pauling JD, Saketkoo LA, Matucci-Cerinic M, Ingegnoli F, Khanna D. The patient experience of Raynaud's phenomenon in systemic sclerosis. Rheumatology (Oxford). 2019;58(1):18–26.
120. Hughes M, Pauling JD. Exploring the patient experience of digital ulcers in systemic sclerosis. Semin Arthritis Rheum. 2019;48(5):888–94.
121. Hughes M, Pauling JD, Jones J, Denton CP, Domsic RT, Frech TM, et al. A multi-centre qualitative study exploring the patient experience of digital ulcers in systemic sclerosis. Arthritis Care Res (Hoboken). 2020;72(5):723–33.
122. Cutolo M, Sulli A, Pizzorni C, Smith V. Capillaroscopy as an outcome measure for clinical trials on the peripheral vasculopathy in SSc—is it useful? Int J Rheumatol. 2010;2010:784947.
123. Dinsdale G, Moore T, O'Leary N, Berks M, Roberts C, Manning J, et al. Quantitative outcome measures for systemic sclerosis-related microangiopathy? Reliability of image acquisition in Nailfold Capillaroscopy. Microvasc Res. 2017;113:56–9.
124. Mihai C, Smith V, Dobrota R, Gheorghiu AM, Cutolo M, Distler O. The emerging application of semi-quantitative and quantitative capillaroscopy in systemic sclerosis. Microvasc Res. 2018;118:113–20.
125. Gheorghiu A, Oneata R, Ancuta I, Enuica A, Linte O, Macovei L, et al. Capillary loss reflects disease activity and prognosis in patients with systemic sclerosis. Exp Ther Med. 2020;20(4):3438–43.
126. Hughes M, Roberts C, Tracey A, Dinsdale G, Murray A, Herrick AL. Does the clinical context improve the reliability of rheumatologists grading digital ulcers in systemic sclerosis? Arthritis Care Res (Hoboken). 2016;68(9):1340–5.
127. Li W, Frech TM. The critical need for accurately defining digital ulcers in scleroderma. J Scleroderma Relat Disord. 2017;2(2):69–71.
128. Suliman YA, Bruni C, Johnson SR, Praino E, Alemam M, Borazan N, et al. Defining skin ulcers in systemic sclerosis: systematic literature review and proposed World Scleroderma Foundation (WSF) definition. J Scleroderma Relat Disord. 2017;2(2):115–20.
129. Hughes M, Tracey A, Bhushan M, Chakravarty K, Denton CP, Dubey S, et al. Reliability of digital ulcer definitions as proposed by the UK Scleroderma Study Group: a challenge for clinical trial design. J Scleroderma Relat Disord. 2018;3(2):170–4.

130. Bruni C, Ngcozana T, Braschi F, Pucci T, Piemonte G, Benelli L, et al. Preliminary validation of the digital ulcer clinical assessment score in systemic sclerosis. J Rheumatol. 2019;46(6):603–8.
131. Suliman YA, Kafaja S, Fitzgerald J, Wortsman X, Grotts J, Matucci-Cerrinic M, et al. Ultrasound characterization of cutaneous ulcers in systemic sclerosis. Clin Rheumatol. 2018;37(6):1555–61.
132. Hughes M, Moore T, Manning J, Dinsdale G, Herrick AL, Murray A. A pilot study using high-frequency ultrasound to measure digital ulcers: a possible outcome measure in systemic sclerosis clinical trials? Clin Exp Rheumatol. 2017;35 Suppl 1(4):218–9.
133. Hughes M, Bruni C, Cuomo G, Delle Sedie A, Gargani L, Gutierrez M, et al. The role of ultrasound in systemic sclerosis: on the cutting edge to foster clinical and research advancement. J Scleroderma Relat Disord. 2020;6:123 [Online ahead of print]. https://doi.org/10.1177/2397198320970394.
134. Pauling JD, Hughes M, Pope JE. Raynaud's phenomenon—an update on diagnosis, classification and management. Clin Rheumatol. 2019;38(12):3317–30.
135. Suliman YA, Bruni C, Hughes M, Matucci-Cerinic M, Furst DE. Ultrasonographic imaging of systemic sclerosis digital ulcers: A systematic literature review and validation steps. Semin Arthritis Rheum. 2021;51(2):425–9. https://doi.org/10.1016/j.semarthrit.2021.02.008. Epub 2021 Feb 19. PMID: 33677309.

Renal Crisis and Other Renal Manifestations

21

Christopher P. Denton and Marie Hudson

Introduction

Renal complications are an important clinical manifestation of systemic sclerosis. In particular, scleroderma renal crisis (SRC) is a hallmark internal organ complication and historically was the predominant cause of scleroderma-related death. Outcomes of SRC have improved but it remains a critical manifestation of the disease that must be diagnosed early and managed appropriately in collaboration with renal specialists. It is also now appreciated that other renal complications occur in SSc [1]. In many cases, there is co-occurrence of these different manifestations and this may account for the particular severity of SSc. Other causes of renal pathology should, however, always be considered in SSc and, with better treatment for SRC, are becoming more relevant to the management of the disease [2].

There have been clear improvements in survival after SRC over time [3, 4]. Several factors are probably responsible for this but undoubtedly, the routine use of ACE inhibitors to treat SRC, together with other advances in renal replacement therapy, has transformed outcome, thereby representing one of the most significant advances in scleroderma therapeutics [5]. There is clear improvement in early mortality from renal crisis, but this better outcome has highlighted the poor long-term outcome for scleroderma patients through complications of long-term dialysis or from other scleroderma complications.

C. P. Denton (✉)
Centre for Rheumatology, UCL Division of Medicine, Royal Free Hospital, London, UK
e-mail: c.denton@ucl.ac.uk

M. Hudson
Division of Rheumatology, Lady Davis Institute for Medical Research, Jewish General Hospital, Montréal, QC, Canada

Faculty of Medicine, McGill University, Montréal, QC, Canada
e-mail: marie.hudson@mcgill.ca

Renal Disease in SSc: The Spectrum of Involvement

Although SRC is the most important renal complication, manifested as accelerated phase hypertension accompanied by acute kidney injury (AKI), other processes that need to be considered in scleroderma include interstitial nephritis, glomerulonephritis, and renal vasculitis [6]. In addition, there is chronic renal vasculopathy and renal parenchymal fibrosis [7]. There is a high frequency of microscopic glomerular or tubular proteinuria for which the long-term significance is uncertain. These different complications will be discussed below.

Historical Aspects of SSc Renal Disease

Renal failure was first described in scleroderma in 1863 [8]. There was initial controversy concerning the specificity of this complication to scleroderma, but the link was established over the next 80 years and numerous case reports linked scleroderma with renal disease and increased mortality [9]. Microvascular changes showing the classic vascular changes were described even in patients who died of non-renal causes [10]. It was not until 1952, however, that Moore and Sheehan [11] identified a specific renal lesion as a major syndrome. They reported three scleroderma patients who developed acute hypertension and renal failure and died 6–8 weeks later. Concentric thickening of the intralobular arteries was found in all three cases and led to the term scleroderma renal crisis. Although bearing similarities to other forms of thrombotic microangiopathy associated AKI, there appear to be specific features of SRC that reflect the background autoimmune rheumatic disease, which impact on severity and outcome [12].

Y. Allanore et al. (eds.), *Scleroderma*, https://doi.org/10.1007/978-3-031-40658-4_21

Scleroderma Renal Crisis

Definition

Scleroderma renal crisis (SRC) is characterized by new onset of accelerated arterial hypertension and/or rapidly progressive oliguric renal failure during the course of SSc. One should not assume that non-malignant hypertension alone without uremia or other renal abnormalities is renal crisis. Likewise, urine abnormalities and/or mild uremia in a scleroderma patient are likely to have other explanations and should not be considered SRC [1]. The issue of specificity is also important, as other forms of thrombotic micro-angiopathy (TMA) may have striking similarity to SRC, and so, the presence of SSc becomes a critical aspect to diagnosis.

The absence of a gold standard and classification criteria for SRC are important challenges for research in this area. In an effort to overcome these challenges, the Scleroderma Clinical Trials Consortium (SCTC) Working Group on SRC has undertaken to develop and validate classification criteria for SRC. This international, multi-disciplinary group of experts was created in November 2015. A scoping review [13] and consensus study to develop a core set of items to define SRC identified 13 items in 5 domains, namely blood pressure, acute kidney injury, microangiopathic hemolytic anemia and thrombocytopenia, target organ dysfunction, and histopathology [13, 14]. Consensus was achieved on blood pressure cutoffs, and the Kidney Disease Improving Global Outcomes (KDIGO) definitions of acute kidney injury [15] were retained (Table 21.1). The Working Group has now ini-

Table 21.1 Core set of items to develop classification criteria for SRC [14]

Domain	Item	
Blood pressure	Acute rise in blood pressure defined as any of the following:	Systolic blood pressure ≥140 mmHg
		Diastolic blood pressure ≥90 mmHg
		A rise in systolic blood pressure ≥30 mmHg above normal
		A rise in diastolic blood pressure ≥20 mmHg above normal
	Blood pressure measurement should be taken twice separated by at least 5 min. If blood pressure readings are discordant, repeat readings should be obtained until two consistent readings are obtained.	
Kidney injury[a]	Acute kidney injury defined as any of the following:	Increase in serum creatinine by ≥26.5 µmol/L (≥0.3 mg/dL) within 48 h
		Increase in serum creatinine to ≥1.5 times baseline, which is known or presumed to have occurred within the prior 7 days
		Urine volume <0.5 mL/kg/h for 6 h
Microangiopathic hemolytic anemia and thrombocytopenia	New or worsening anemia not due to other causes.	
	Schistocytes or other red blood cell fragments on blood smear.	
	Thrombocytopenia ≤100,000, confirmed by manual smear.	
	Laboratory evidence of hemolysis, including elevated lactate dehydrogenase, reticulocytosis, and/or low/absent haptoglobin.	
	A negative direct anti-globulin test.	
Target organ dysfunction	*Hypertensive retinopathy* (hemorrhages, hard and soft (cotton wool) exudates, and/or disk edema, not attributable to other causes), confirmed by an ophthalmologist.	
	Hypertensive encephalopathy, characterized by headache, altered mental status, seizures, visual disturbances, and/or other focal or diffuse neurologic signs not attributable to other causes.	
	Acute heart failure, characterized by typical symptoms (e.g., breathlessness, ankle swelling, and fatigue) that may be accompanied by signs (e.g., elevated jugular venous pressure, pulmonary crackles, and peripheral edema).	
	Acute pericarditis, diagnosed with at least two of the four following criteria: (1) pericarditis chest pain; (2) pericardial rub; (3) new widespread ST elevation or PR depression on electrocardiogram; and (4) pericardial effusion (new or worsening) on cardiac echocardiography.	
Renal histopathology	Histopathological findings on kidney biopsy consistent with scleroderma renal crisis which may include the following: Small vessel (arcuate and interlobular arteries) changes that predominate over glomerular alterations. Glomerular changes of thrombotic microangiopathy may be present, with acute changes including fibrin thrombi and endothelial swelling, red blood cell fragments, and mesangiolysis, and chronic changes including double contours of the glomerular basement membrane. Nonspecific ischemic changes with corrugation of the glomerular basement membrane, and even segmental or global sclerosis of glomeruli may occur. Early vascular abnormalities include intimal accumulation of myxoid material, thrombosis, fibrinoid necrosis, and fragmented red blood cells, sometimes resulting in cortical necrosis. Narrowing and obliteration of the vascular lumen lead to glomerular ischemia. Juxtaglomerular apparatus hyperplasia, while relatively rare (10%), can be observed. Late changes are manifested by intimal thickening and proliferation (which lead to characteristic vascular "onion-skin" lesions), glomerulosclerosis, and interstitial fibrosis. Nonspecific tubular changes may also occur, including acute tubular injury in the early stage of injury, and later interstitial fibrosis and tubular atrophy. Since none of these findings are specific for SRC, the pathological diagnosis must be supported by appropriate clinical and serological data.	

[a] This is the definition of acute kidney injury from the Kidney Disease Improving Global Outcomes (KDIGO) guidelines [15]

tiated the *International Scleroderma Renal Crisis Survey II (ISRCS II)* to collect an inception SRC cohort and validate the core set using real-world clinical data. Importantly, data on patients with new-onset TMA are also being collected prospectively to determine the specificity of the core set variables. This project will generate the first validated classification criteria for SRC, which are expected to be used in future randomized trials and epidemiologic research of SSc.

Recently, it has been suggested that two groups of SRC might be considered, the tightly defined classical SRC and a less typical form that reflects TMA occurring in the context of SSc [16]. This is a potentially useful distinction, but it is likely that there will be substantial clinical and pathogenetic overlap between these groups.

Epidemiology

SRC was previously reported to affect up to 25% of SSc patients with early diffuse disease, but contemporary series seem to suggest that this may have fallen to as low as 5% [17–19]. A limitation is that previous data were generated in largely prevalent cohorts. In addition, it seems likely that frequency is strongly influenced by the population structure (genetic background and prevalence of autoantibodies). In the US Prospective Registry in Systemic Sclerosis (PRESS) cohort, the frequency of SRC in diffuse SSc was approximately 10% [17]. A UK cohort study also suggested a frequency in diffuse SSc of 14% compared with 3% in limited SSc [20]. On the other hand, a German study reported an overall frequency of SRC of 2.4% (1.4% in diffuse and 1% in limited SSc) [21] and the frequencies in Asian populations are among the lowest reported [22–24]. A meta-analysis reported in 2016 showed that the highest rates in SRC were reported in the United States, UK, and Australia and confirmed a strong association with anti-RNA polymerase III autoantibodies [25].

Experts have nonetheless perceived a decrease in the incidence of SRC over time. In the above-mentioned meta-analysis, although the overall rates appeared constant, there was a trend toward falling rates in dcSSc over time ($p = 0.16$) [25]. However, again, the studies driving that trend were an earlier US study with a higher rate [26] and a later European study with a lower rate [27]. Other possible explanations for falling rates over time include change in practice patterns, including less frequent use of corticosteroids and cyclosporine, and more frequent use of calcium channel blockers [28].

Interestingly, the incidence of renal crisis appears to have decreased since ACE inhibitors (ACEi) have been available, although there is no evidence that ACEi prevent renal crisis. Indeed, prior use of ACEi has been associated with worse long-term outcome and a higher frequency of long-term dialysis after SRC, as suggested by two independent cohort studies [20, 26] and confirmed by the first International Scleroderma Renal Crisis Survey [29]. The mechanism for this is unknown but it is possible that the low dose used in non-hypertensive patients is inadequate to handle the surge of renin when SRC is triggered but masks the acute manifestations which normally bring the patient to the attention of physicians early in the episode, turning the event into a less reversible, more chronic process.

Renal crisis is most often encountered early in the course of the disease, with 75% of SRC cases occurring less than 4 years after the first symptom attributable to scleroderma, and males are proportionately more frequently affected than females [18, 21, 25, 28–31]. However, late occurrences, even 20 years after disease onset also occur, and the impact of other treatment for SSc skin or organ-based disease might further change the timing and frequency of SRC. A higher risk of SRC has also been reported for African American patients within a recent large multicenter US cohort study with studies suggesting that African American patients are 3 times as likely as Caucasians to develop SRC [31]. In one series, it was reported that 22% of SRC may have this as the presenting feature of the disease, or at least not have a preexisting diagnosis of SSc even if attributable clinical features are present [20].

Historically, SRC was the leading cause of death in SSc. However, with the advent of angiotensin-converting enzyme (ACE) inhibitors, mortality rates have decreased considerably [18, 19]. Nevertheless, 5-year outcomes remain poor, 41% mortality, and 33% of patients remaining dialysis-dependent [20]. A recent systematic review of the literature showed that there is no convincing evidence of further improvement in the morbidity and mortality of SRC in the post-ACE inhibitor era [4].

Factors Predicting SRC

The characteristics of a typical SRC patient are well-recognized from several cohort studies. Many of these features or laboratory characteristics can be identified before the development of a renal crisis, and therefore, careful baseline assessment of all scleroderma cases for risk of crisis is essential. Patients with a greatly increased risk to develop this complication must be followed extremely closely for any hints of renal crisis. Patients with diffuse cutaneous scleroderma with skin thickening on the proximal extremities and/or the trunk are at greatest risk for SRC [31–33]. Far fewer patients with limited cutaneous scleroderma (previously termed the CREST syndrome) who have long-standing skin changes restricted to distal extremities ever develop renal crisis. There are even fewer cases of renal crisis documented in limited scleroderma patients with anti-centromere antibody [30, 34]. Thus, the vast majority of SRC cases (75–80%) occur in patients with diffuse skin involvement and rapid progression of skin thickening has been shown to be associated with development of SRC [35].

Some SRC cases occur in patients with less severe skin involvement but who are destined to develop typical diffuse scleroderma, although they only have minimal or even no skin changes at the time of the diagnosis of renal crisis. It is not infrequent for this type of patient with such minimal cutaneous and systemic findings to have the diagnosis of renal crisis made only at the time of kidney biopsy [36, 37]. There are several distinguishing features that are helpful to identify those patients who are likely to evolve to diffuse cutaneous disease. These patients almost always have a short duration of symptoms, often less than 1 year. Polyarthritis/arthralgias, puffy or swollen hands and legs, and carpal tunnel syndrome are a common complex of symptoms in patients with early diffuse scleroderma [38]. Although Raynaud's phenomenon eventually is almost universally found in scleroderma, its absence in early diffuse scleroderma is not uncommon. The presence of palpable tendon friction rubs, which occur in 65% of diffuse scleroderma patients, is an extremely helpful and predictive sign of diffuse scleroderma even prior to the development of diffuse cutaneous skin involvement [39]. Less than 5% of limited scleroderma patients ever have tendon rubs. Tendon friction rubs have been confirmed to be independent predictors of SRC (HR 2.33, 95% CI 1.03, 6.19) in a prospective EUSTAR cohort study that included 1301 SSc patients with disease duration ≤3 years and follow-up of at least 2 years [38].

Patients without known scleroderma who present with new isolated malignant hypertension should be carefully assessed for the presence of the other relevant risk factors. Autoantibodies may be helpful in predicting SRC. Antinuclear antibodies are seen in 95% of scleroderma; so, their presence may be helpful in determining whether a malignant hypertension patient could possibly have scleroderma. Anti-RNA polymerase III is a scleroderma-specific antibody that is seen almost exclusively in diffuse scleroderma, and up to 50% of patients with this antibody develop SRC [40–46]. In contrast, renal crisis occurs in only 10% of patients with anti-topoisomerase antibodies, which are also associated with diffuse skin disease [40].

Anti-RNA polymerase III antibodies have now been established as a robust risk factor for SRC, being present in more than 50% of SSc patients who develop SRC in some series [20] and associated with a significant increase in the odds of SRC (odds ratio [OR] 6.4, 95% confidence interval [CI] 3.4–12.2, $p < 0.001$) [43]. In a study from the European Scleroderma Trials and Research (EUSTAR) registry involving over 2800 SSc subjects, anti-RNA polymerase antibodies were independently associated with SRC (odds ratio 5.86, 95% confidence interval 2.6, 13.2) [21]. Of note, the prevalence of anti-RNA polymerase III antibodies in various studies is highly variable ranging from 0% to 41% [44]. Part of the variability is explained by geography with North American studies having overall higher rates (14%) than European studies (9%) [44]. Rates in the diffuse subset in the Pittsburgh cohort have been reported to be as high as 56% [45]. Interestingly, a recent report from The Royal Free cohort compared outcomes of SRC in anti-RNA polymerase III antibody-positive and anti-RNA polymerase III antibody-negative subjects [46]. Of the 150 cases with confirmed SRC, 61 (41%) were positive for anti-RNA polymerase III antibodies. The anti-RNA polymerase III antibody-positive cases were more likely to require dialysis compared to the anti-RNA polymerase III antibody-negative patients (51% vs 29%, $p = 0.07$) but they were also more likely to discontinue dialysis (53% vs 26%, $p = 0.01$) and had better survival (log rank $p = 0.003$). Whether this reflects differences in presentation and diagnosis, or in the underlying pathology remains unclear.

Most SSc sera that react with anti-RNA polymerases recognize more than one class of RNA polymerases. Anti-RNA polymerase I and III almost always co-exist, and among those, some sera also contain anti-RNA polymerase II [41, 47]. A group of Japanese investigators published a study of 583 SSc subjects, among whom 37 (6%) were positive for anti-RNA polymerase III by a commercially available ELISA and 17 (2.9%) developed SRC. There was a significantly higher frequency of SRC in anti-RNA polymerase III antibody-positive compared to anti-RNA polymerase III antibody-negative SSc patients (9 of 37 [24%] positive versus 8 of 546 [1%] negative, OR 21.6, 95% CI 7.8–60.3, $p < 0.00001$) [48]. The investigators further characterized the profiles of the 37 anti-RNA polymerase III antibody-positive subjects by immunoprecipitation and defined 2 groups, according to the presence or absence of anti-RNA polymerase II: 17 had anti-RNA polymerase I/II/III and 20 had anti-RNA polymerase I/III or III alone. In multivariate Cox proportional analysis, both anti-RNA polymerase I/II/III positivity (OR 11.0, 95% CI 1.6–222.8, $p = 0.0118$) and an ELISA index for anti-RNA polymerase III of ≥157 (OR 2.4 × 109, 95% CI 2.1-uncalculated, $p = 0.0093$) were independent factors associated with the development of SRC. These results were validated in an independent cohort [49]. Although the clinical usefulness of anti-RNA polymerase II may be limited by the fact that detection requires complex immunoprecipitation assays that are conducted in a limited number of laboratories, the higher ELISA index for anti-RNA polymerase III has better potential utility as a biomarker for SRC.

Antecedent hypertension is not usually present prior to SRC. Most often, there is a very acute onset of markedly elevated blood pressure. Normal blood pressures have been documented within 24 h prior to the onset of SRC hypertension [32]. Nonetheless, experts recommend that patients with early diffuse scleroderma should monitor their own blood pressure regularly and notify their physicians immediately when their blood pressure is persistently increased.

Systemic arterial hypertension, proteinuria, and chronic kidney disease have also recently been reported as risk factors for SRC [21, 50, 51]. However, earlier studies did not show that hypertension or renal abnormalities predicted SRC (insert Refs. [7, 35, 52–54]) and it remains possible that these "new" risk factors represent missed SRC.

Several non-renal abnormalities may precede SRC, including asymptomatic pericardial effusion, congestive heart failure, and/or arrhythmias and use of ACE inhibitors, although data for this are mixed regarding impact of susceptibility [20, 28, 29] as opposed to effect on long-term outcome [5]. New anemia, an uncommon manifestation of scleroderma, can be an early clue to renal crisis, particularly when microangiopathic hemolysis and thrombocytopenia are present in addition to the presence of high-risk autoantibodies such as anti-RNA polymerase III [16, 35, 54]. There have been further robust cohort studies that support the risk factors for SRC, confirming that ARA is strongly associated and also highlighting that outcomes are worse in those on ACEi [51]. This is important as they remain the cornerstone of management. It may be that future discrimination of distinct pathogenetic mechanisms may help to resolve the paradox that prior use of ACEi is associated with poor outcome but is an essential part of management [29].

Pericarditis has been associated with development of SRC [55], and cases of normotensive renal crisis can be especially challenging to diagnose and have poor outcome [56, 57]. Prior use of high-dose glucocorticoid frequently precedes the development of SRC [57, 58]. A case–control study matched 106 patients with renal crisis to other scleroderma patients based on features that would be associated with increased risks for renal crisis or the use of steroids [59]. Sex, disease subset, disease duration, extent of skin thickening, the presence of tendon friction rubs, and inflammatory myopathy were similar in both groups. Patients who received high-dose prednisone (>15 mg/day) were three times more likely to develop renal crisis in the next 6 months. High-dose steroids should be used with great caution and very close monitoring in patients with early diffuse scleroderma. In a cohort study from France, Guillevin et al. [3] found that the majority of SRC cases had been exposed to glucocorticoids prior to SRC and that this was significantly greater than control cases of SSc without SRC. However, this study has all of the well-appreciated limitations of a retrospective cohort design in a multicenter heterogeneous population of SSc, including confounding by indication. Glucocorticoid exposure prior to SRC has also been associated with worse outcomes. In the International Scleroderma Renal Crisis Survey, for every milligram of prednisone, the risk of death increased by 4% (hazard ratio [HR] 1.04, 95% CI 1.02, 1.07, $p < 0.01$) [29].

Clinical Presentation

Patients may complain of severe headache, blurred vision, or other encephalopathic symptoms with the onset of accelerated hypertension. Seizures may occur, although earlier diagnosis and better management of SRC should reduce the frequency of these events. Otherwise, the symptoms of renal crisis are nonspecific: increased fatigue, headache, dyspnea, or malaise. High-risk patients must be taught to take these symptoms seriously and should check their own blood pressure if these symptoms occur.

Most patients have striking elevations of blood pressure at the onset of SRC. Ninety percent have blood pressure levels greater than 150/90 mmHg, and 30% have diastolic recordings greater than 120 mmHg. Up to 10% of cases have been reported to have a normal blood pressure, although "normal" has to be interpreted case by case. Indeed, an increase of 20–30 mmHg or more in blood pressure in a patient with usually low normal pressures (e.g., increase from 95/60 to 140/85) can represent renal crisis. Thus, any change in blood pressure should lead to further testing and close monitoring. Normotensive renal crisis requires the presence of other features, primarily rapidly progressive unexplained azotemia and/or microangiopathic hemolytic anemia with thrombocytopenia. Pulmonary hemorrhage is a rare life-threatening problem, which has occurred in several of these patients [60]. It complicates the diagnosis and is a poor prognostic sign. Paradoxically, it appears that higher systolic or diastolic blood pressure at presentation may be associated with better long-term outcome in hypertensive SRC [20].

Patients with SRC often present with congestive heart failure (dyspnea, paroxysmal nocturnal dyspnea, or even pulmonary edema), serious ventricular arrhythmias (even cardiac arrest), pericarditis, and/or large pericardial effusions [55]. This is primarily from the stress of the hypertension on the heart, effects of hyperreninemia, and from fluid overload secondary to oliguric renal failure, although some patients with very severe disease also have primary scleroderma myocardial involvement contributing to these problems. Severe pulmonary hypertension secondary to the malignant systemic hypertension has also been seen but has a different course than the more frequent chronic pulmonary hypertension seen in limited scleroderma patients. Prompt control of the blood pressure usually improves these cardiac problems.

In some situations, SRC may be confused with other illnesses. Several cases of thrombotic thrombocytopenic purpura (TTP) have been reported in scleroderma patients, but it is unclear whether it was an isolated coexistent disease or just a different interpretation of SRC [61, 62]. A review of the 8 cases of TTP and scleroderma in the literature found that there were few differences between the patient subsets. Although a few "responded" to plasmapheresis, most were also treated with ACE inhibitors [63]. Fever and hemorrhagic manifestations were the only findings that distinguished the two conditions. A pilot study did not find abnormalities of the vWF-cleaving protease activity in 10 SRC patients [64]. If a diagnosis of TTP is made in a scleroderma patient, an ACE inhibitor should be used in conjunction with TTP treatment [65].

Rather than always representing a differential diagnosis, recently it has been appreciated that some cases of SRC have greater similarity with TTP and HUS including aHUS and this has implications for management. These cases need to be managed appropriately, and it is also likely that some cases represent an overlap with TTP. This is discussed in detail in a recent case series [16]. This also has therapeutic implications such as the possible use of complement-directed therapy. Clinical and laboratory features of other forms of TMA have been compared and contrasted with SRC [66, 67].

Laboratory Findings

Laboratory investigation of AKI in SRC is the main focus of initial investigations [68]. Serum creatinine is typically at least 150% of baseline value at presentation. This represents Stage 1 AKI in the most recent international consensus guidelines for AKI care [69]. Again, "normal" renal function needs to be interpreted cautiously since the creatinine value can reach this relative increase without rising above the normal absolute range in scleroderma patients with low muscle mass. Creatinine can rise rapidly in the first few days following onset of renal crisis and will usually continue to rise even once blood pressure has been adequately controlled. Although a slower increase of serum creatinine can occur over days to weeks, it is much more likely to increase by 0.5–1.0 mg/dL creatinine/day. It is important to recognize that even after antihypertensive therapy has effectively controlled blood pressure, the serum creatinine may continue to rise. The issue of whether the ACE inhibitor itself contributes to such increases is often raised, but in that setting we have not had any patient who has had significant improvement in serum creatinine after stopping the ACE inhibitor. Unfortunately, there are still situations where the serum creatinine continues to rise, and the patient develops renal failure in spite of adequate control of the blood pressure with ACE inhibitors. In these circumstances, alternative pathology or additional treatment measures should be considered including potential experimental interventions discussed later in the chapter.

There is usually both proteinuria and microscopic hematuria on dipstick urinalysis. Proteinuria is mild or moderate (generally <2 g/day) and microscopy can show microscopic hematuria (5–100 rbc/hpf) and granular casts [20]. These abnormalities are nonspecific in SSc and malignant hypertension.

Microangiopathic hemolytic anemia, which is characterized by normochromic, fragmented red blood cells, reticulocytosis, and thrombocytopenia, occurs in almost half of patients with SRC. The platelet count is rarely lower than 20,000/mm^3, and its improvement is often the first sign of adequate response to therapy even though the serum creatinine is continuing to increase. Patients are not usually symptomatic from this process although anemia may contribute to congestive heart failure. One series found a reduced platelet count in 50% of SRC patients and red cell fragments in 52% [20]. Other evidence of hemolysis, including a reduced serum haptoglobin level and/or a raised lactate dehydrogenase, should be sought. Given the remaining diagnostic uncertainty in this field, if a diagnosis of TTP or HUS is suspected in a scleroderma patient, we recommend that an ACE inhibitor be used in conjunction with plasmapheresis.

Potential biomarkers of SRC have been suggested. Circulating adhesion molecules in serum have shown association, and levels of NT-proBNP associate with poor renal outcome and need for long-term dialysis after SRC [70].

Recent studies have highlighted the potential of urinary protein analysis. This has focused on CKD but two markers that seem to associate with SSc-CKD include urinary ICAM-1 and urinary MCP-1. The latter has also proven informative in other renal complications of CTD such as SLE. The ability to correct urinary analytes for creatinine provides a powerful approach for studying candidate markers of local renal pathology that may be further explored in the future [71].

Physiological measurements have also been used to aid management. This includes assessment of the renal resistive index as a potential marker of risk or measurement of response to treatment. There are a number of promising reports, and studies are underway to assess the reliability and clinical utility of this measure outside the research setting [72–75].

Pathogenesis

Although the pathology of SSc focuses on an interplay between the innate and adaptive immune system, connective tissue and extracellular matrix metabolism, and vasculopathy in the microcirculation and microvasculature, SRC is principally an impairment of arterial blood flow in the kidney. First suggested by Steen et al. [35], a plausible model that explains clinical heterogeneity and the time course of the disease is that specific organ-based injury or damage occurs in susceptible individuals within the context of a unifying background of vasculopathy, fibrosis, and autoimmunity [1]. It is noteworthy that there is evidence of all of these different processes in the kidney in SSc [71]. It is particularly important to observe that these abnormalities are present even in the absence of SRC. Thus, they may reflect a background pathological state upon which a superimposed positive feedback loop driven by increased activity of the renin–angiotensin axis results in SRC.

The triggering event or events may include vascular injury. There are reports of confirmed viral infection triggering SRC [76], and this may explain the anecdotal observation that SRC is more frequent in the winter months when respiratory tract viral infections are most prevalent. There is an intriguing and potentially relevant link emerging between skin pathology, the renin–angiotensin system, and blood pressure control which could explain how skin activity in dcSSc might trigger the SRC process [77]. The dramatic response to therapeutic inhibition of the renin–angiotensin system in SRC (and historically improvement after nephrectomy) implicates renin overproduction as a central part of the pathogenesis of SRC. However, hyperreninemia is uncommon before the acute onset of SRC and if present does not predict future events [78]. Although anti-RNA polymerase III antibodies are strongly associated with SRC occurrence, there is no evidence for direct pathogenicity [79]. Thus, the initial trigger of SRC remains largely unknown.

The pathogenic mechanisms that lead to SRC have been defined through studies examining biopsy material and circulating molecular markers (Fig. 21.1). An acute event, probably vascular, appears to initiate a self-perpetuating cascade that leads to glomerular hypoperfusion and increased renin release. These events lead to release or activation of cytokines and growth factors that result in the typical proliferative vascular lesion of SRC. Hypertensive changes add to this constellation of events. Consistent with this model is the link between histopathological features and outcome that has been established in several studies. Thus, acute vascular injury is associated with worse outcome based on studies that have linked biopsy appearance to long-term outcome, such as the need for permanent dialysis [20, 80]. Of note, though, in the acute setting, the main diagnostic benefit of renal biopsy is to exclude other pathologies. In the longer term, it may help to inform renal prognosis (see below). Biopsy needs to be delayed until the patient is clinically stable with good blood pressure control and stable platelet count.

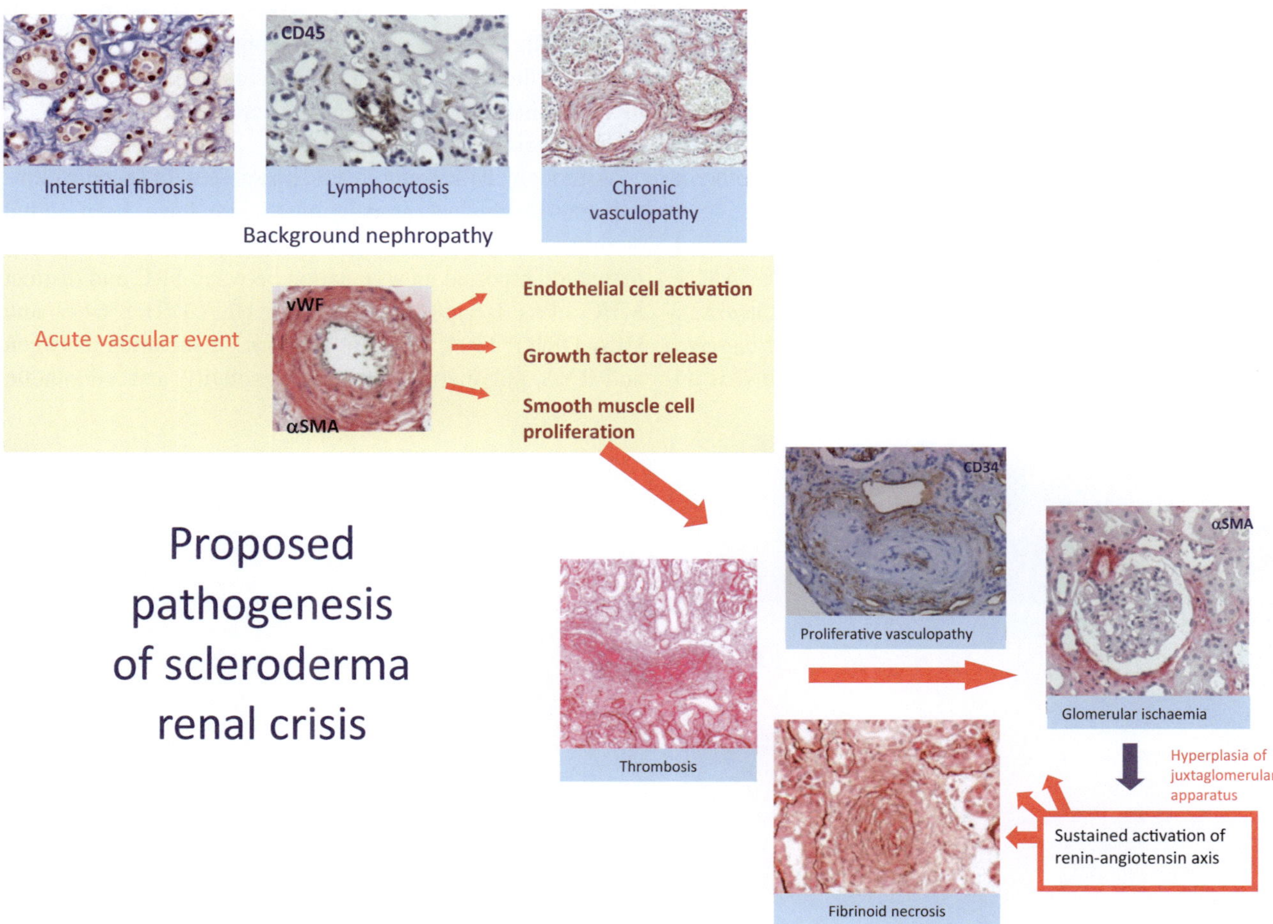

Fig. 21.1 Pathogenic processes underlying scleroderma renal crisis. Model of events that underlie development of SRC. It appears that background changes occur in many individuals but susceptibility and an acute triggering event result in SRC. Autopsy specimens confirm that inflammation, fibrosis, and chronic proliferative vasculopathy are often present in scleroderma but it is believed that an acute vascular injury or event that triggers hypertension results in other events that lead to glomerular ischemia and increased renin–angiotensin axis activity. This results in severe proliferative vasculopathy

The renal pathological findings in SRC are broadly the same as those seen in other causes of accelerated hypertension [20]. Fibrinoid necrosis is seen either in arterial walls or in the subintima in small arteries and arterioles (characteristically the interlobular and arcuate arteries). The resulting intimal thickening leads to narrowing or total obliteration of the lumen and a typical "onion skin" appearance (Fig. 21.2). Adventitial and peri-adventitial fibrosis, an indication of chronic vasculopathy seen in patients with SRC, is rarely seen in accelerated hypertension without scleroderma.

In particular, the renal pathological changes in SRC resemble those of the thrombotic microangiopathy (TMA) syndromes, in which dysregulation of the complement system is increasingly recognized and peritubular capillary complement 4d deposits have been associated with an increased risk of prolonged renal failure [67]. Complement is now implicated in SRC pathogenesis in a number of studies and also by the potential benefits of complement-targeting therapy including eculizumab [81]. Analysis of complement proteins indicates potential as biomarkers in some cases of SRC and suggests a role in a subset of patients [82].

Autoantibodies against vascular structures and receptors have also been implicated in SRC pathogenesis. These are markers of disease severity and associate with several outcomes. It is not clear yet whether they are drivers or markers of pathology, but they target relevant endothelial and cell surface receptors including angiotensin and endothelin receptors [83, 84].

Markers of renal injury have been reported to be increased prior to SRC. Studies examining serum levels of sVCAM-1 or vWF have shown that these may be increased at the onset, or preceding SRC [85]. Studies of other markers of damage such as adipokines and SSc are emerging. Lipocalin-2 is an adipokine that has been reported elevated in acute kidney injury and immunity. Its role in SSc was therefore explored in 50 SSc subjects with relatively early disease (mean duration of 3 years) who had not been previously treated with glucocorticoids or immunosuppressants [86]. Although the investigators reported that the prevalence of SRC was significantly higher in those with elevated serum lipocalin-2 levels compared to those with normal levels, the actual numbers were very small, with only 2 cases of SRC in the cohort. In addition, serum lipocalin-2 levels were inversely correlated with eGFR in SSc patients with eGFR <60 mL/min/1.73 m^2 ($r = -0.68$, $p = 0.035$) but not in those with eGFR >60 mL/min/1.73 m^2 ($r = 0.04$, $p = 0.79$). Along with these preliminary findings, the investigators also reported interesting associations between serum lipocalin-2 and skin scores (positive correlation) and right ventricular systolic pressures in subjects with normal eGFR (negative correlation), between lipocalin-2 expression in dermal fibroblasts and endothelial cells of lesional skin, and in dermal fibroblasts, but not endothelial cells, of bleomycin-treated mice. Finally, deficiency of transcription factor Fli1, which is implicated in SSc vasculopathy, induced lipocalin-2 expression in cultured endothelial cells. Further studies to confirm these results, in particular the role of lipocalin-1 as a biomarker for SRC, and to determine whether lipocalin-1 has a causal role in the pathogenesis SSc are required.

Although challenging in a rare disease with specific clinical and serological associations, there have been initial attempts to try to define genetic susceptibility for SRC. A first study reported an association between SRC and distinct MHC class I haplotypes, namely HLA-DRB1*0407 and HLA-DRB1*1304 [87]. In addition, association between anti-RNA polymerase antibody reactivity and endothelin

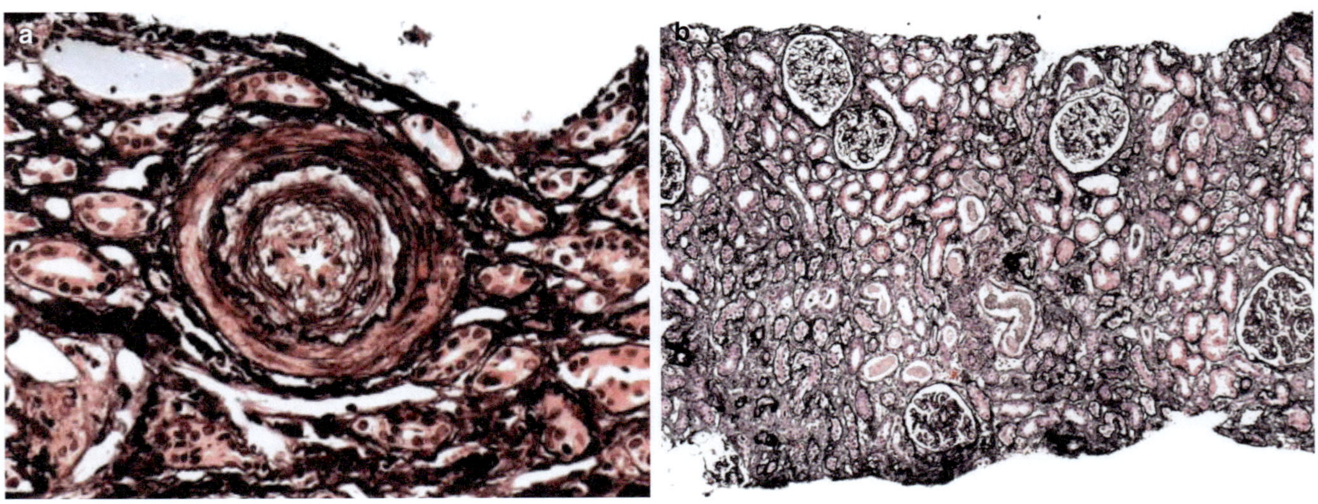

Fig. 21.2 Pathological predictors of outcome in scleroderma renal crisis. The hallmark features of scleroderma renal crisis include acute vascular injury (**a**) and interstitial fibrosis (**b**). Formal scoring suggests that the presence of severe acute vascular injury is associated with a poor prognosis and increased likelihood of permanent need for dialysis. Conversely, the extent of fibrotic scarring does not appear to reflect long-term renal outcome. Discussed further in Ref. [17]

receptor polymorphism has been suggested in another study [88]. More recently, a study focused on patients with anti-RNA polymerase antibody-positive disease and attempted to define differences between those cases with SRC and a cohort of anti-RNA polymerase antibody-positive cases followed for at least 5 years without developing SRC [89]. Interestingly, a SNP linked to GPATCH2L, a locus that is confirmed as a susceptibility factor for essential diastolic hypertension, was replicated in two SRC cohorts. In the same study, CTNND2, a gene associated with PAH in earlier work and operating as a negative regulator of Wnt signaling, was also identified in the discovery cohort. This is notable because overexpression of both proteins was seen in SRC biopsies compared with control renal tissue [89].

To date, there are no robust animal models that replicate the features of SRC. Attempts to induce hypertensive renal injury in transgenic strains that manifest features of SSc have been undertaken. So far, these studies support the concept that attenuated renal inflammation may be important in the uncontrolled proliferative vascular changes of SSc but have not provided fundamental insight into specific mechanisms of SRC [90].

Management

The most important aspect of management of renal crisis is early detection and blood pressure control. It is essential that high-risk patients are identified and that there is clear patient education and blood pressure monitoring. There should also be regular assessment of urine and biochemical indices of renal function.

In general, all SSc patients should receive education about the importance of having blood pressure monitoring, both regularly and at any time if symptoms such as headache, breathlessness, dizziness, or syncope develop. This is especially important in cases of dcSSc within 4 years of onset. We usually recommend home blood pressure monitoring twice weekly with instructions about individualized levels that should prompt medical review. Specialist nurses and patient "warning cards" can provide invaluable patient support in this context [91]. If new-onset hypertension or other relevant symptoms develop or if there is incidental finding of hypertension, urinalysis abnormality, or renal impairment, it is essential to obtain urgent specialist medical advice [92]. In this way, appropriate tests can be performed, and treatment initiated. Consensus best practice recommendations for management of scleroderma renal crisis have been published, and these provide an important opportunity to standardize approaches and share experience with physicians that may be less familiar with managing this complication [93].

Renal biopsy is particularly important in patients where there is any uncertainty about the diagnosis. If anything is atypical in the presentation, including normal blood pressure, active urinary sediment, or overlap features, it is important to confirm diagnosis and rule out other etiologies of kidney pathology, particularly glomerulonephritis. Renal biopsy for SRC can also provide valuable prognostic information, and scores have been developed. Interestingly, the chronic damage index that predicts long-term outcome in many renal pathologies does not appear to do so in SRC [20]. This underscores the concept that SRC is an acute event often superimposed upon background nephropathy. We perform renal biopsy as soon as clotting and blood pressure permit this to be safely undertaken, and this often provides useful prognostic information (see Fig. 21.2).

Once SRC is diagnosed, patients should be aggressively managed, preferably with hospitalization and careful blood pressure monitoring. Reflecting evidence-based recommendations [93], hypertension in SSc should prompt initiation of an ACE inhibitor or dose increased if already being taken. A short-acting ACE inhibitor may be preferable in hemodynamically unstable cases. However, ACE inhibition resistance is frequent, and our practice is to initiate a long-acting drug as soon as possible and escalate the dose daily to maximum. There is close monitoring with daily blood tests and aim for reduction of blood pressure to target as soon as possible, although in established SRC, this often takes some days. Renal function may continue to deteriorate during that time. It is important to increase the ACE inhibition dose to maximum—our practice is to double this every 24 h. Renal function may continue to deteriorate even after the initiation of ACE inhibition. This is an important point and should not lead to inappropriate reduction or discontinuation of ACE inhibition. We usually introduce other antihypertensives including calcium channel blockers, doxazocin, and clonidine if blood pressure remains unacceptably high. The goal is to rapidly achieve normal pre-SRC blood pressure.

Although angiotensin receptor blockers (ARB) are used, they should not replace ACE inhibitors because, unlike ACE inhibitors, they do not inhibit the degradation of bradykinin, which are potent vasodilators. Moreover, there are reports suggesting that ARB alone are less effective that ACEi in treating SRC [94]. Also, studies in other diseases have suggested that patients treated with both an ACE inhibitor and ARB are at higher risk for adverse events compared with those treated with only one agent. Beta-blocking drugs are contraindicated due to effects on peripheral circulation, and parenteral antihypertensives are usually not needed, although nitrate infusion is sometimes beneficial when pulmonary edema complicates SRC. There have been reports of using endothelin receptor antagonists in SRC [95], and this may be logical based on the high circulating levels of ET-1 reported in patients at the time of SRC [96] and studies demonstrating that endothelin ligand and receptor expression may be increased in SRC [97–99]. In addition, polymorphism in the endothelin ligand receptor axis [88] but not the ACE axis

[100] has been associated with scleroderma. The similarity of the pathology of SRC and precapillary PAH in SSc makes it plausible that an ERA might be beneficial for vascular repair post-SRC. However, results with bosentan, a non-selective endothelin-1 receptor antagonist, in an open-label trial have so far been disappointing [101]. The place of endothelin axis blockade is unclear at the present time and requires additional investigation.

In cases where renal replacement is required, this is generally by hemofiltration or hemodialysis, the choice of method being determined by hemodynamic stability and local facilities. Occasionally in more indolent cases, it may be possible to move to peritoneal dialysis as the first form of renal replacement.

Since SRC can be associated with a thrombotic microangiopathy and in view of recent evidence of the potential role of complement activation in other thrombotic microangiopathies such as atypical hemolytic uremic syndrome, the complement inhibitor eculizumab has been used in some cases of SRC [102]; however, the proper role of anti-complement therapy in the treatment of SRC remains to be established although it should presumably be considered only in SRC patients with evidence of microangiopathic hemolytic anemia. Similarly, the place for plasma exchange in SRC is uncertain as it has not been shown to be of benefit in SRC but is a central part of the management of some related conditions such as thrombotic thrombocytopenic purpura. It may be considered in cases that have severe MAHA and consumptive coagulopathy. However, there are no controlled clinical trial data available and case reports provide a mixed message concerning the benefits of this approach [63]. In any case, ACE inhibition must be used in conjunction with complement inhibitors or plasma exchange in the setting of SRC.

Organ-based complications are managed supportively, and this may include management of pulmonary edema or encephalopathy using standard approaches such as supplementary oxygen, ventilatory support, sedation, and/or anti-seizure medications according to clinical circumstances.

It is important to emphasize patient education and vigilance among patient and health professionals since it is critical to diagnose SRC as soon as possible. The unique challenges of managing renal crisis during pregnancy are discussed elsewhere in this textbook. Of note, though, the recent 2020 American College of Rheumatology Guideline for the Management of Reproductive Health in Rheumatic and Musculoskeletal Diseases recommends ACE inhibitors (or ARBs) in pregnant women who develop SRC [103].

Prevention

Patient education is critical together with risk stratification and vigilant monitoring of BP, urine, and renal function. There is no clear evidence that ACE inhibitors have prophylactic benefit. Earlier data from UK and French cohorts point to a worse long-term outcome in patients taking ACEi or ARB at time of SRC diagnosis. The basis for this is unclear and may relate to delays in diagnosis by masking hypertension or else aldosterone breakthrough in patients on chronic ACE inhibitors [104]. A large, controlled study of an ACE inhibitor, quinapril, did not show any preventative effect on vascular complications of SSc [105]. In that study, though, only subjects with either lcSSc or Raynaud's phenomenon were included, both groups at low risk of SRC. The International Scleroderma Renal Crisis Study was undertaken to investigate the prophylactic role of ACE inhibitors [29]. We found that exposure to ACE inhibitors prior to the onset of SRC was associated with a greater than two-fold increase in the risk of mortality (hazard ratio 2.42, 95% CI 1.0–5.75, $p = 0.046$). Of note, though, is that all the 16 subjects on ACE inhibitors prior to the onset of their SRC had some indication for this, including systemic hypertension ($n = 12$), Raynaud's phenomenon ($n = 2$), prophylaxis because of concurrent corticosteroid exposure ($n = 2$), and chronic renal insufficiency ($n = 1$). None of the subjects exposed to ACE inhibitors prior to SRC were on it as simple prophylaxis from SRC. Thus, it is possible that confounding by indication may have contributed to the poor outcomes. Two recent papers provide conflicting results on the effect of ACE inhibition prior to the onset of SRC, with one suggesting that it was a risk factor for SRC [51] while the other not [21]. Thus, at this time, the question of a prophylactic role of ACE inhibitors to prevent SRC remains largely unresolved. The updated EULAR guidelines for the treatment of SSc highlight the fact that published evidence does not support the preventative use of ACE inhibitors to decrease the risk of development or improve outcome of SRC [88].

Many groups performing autologous hematopoietic stem cell transplant (AHSCT) start full-dose ACE inhibition routinely a few weeks prior to the procedure [106, 107]. There is a strong belief that this may mitigate the risk of SRC which is considerable given the inherent fluid and glucocorticoid exposure associated with mobilization and conditioning in AHSCT. However, although AHSCT might be a possible risk factor for SRC, the role of prophylactic ACE inhibitors in this setting remains uncertain.

Long-term Outcomes

A systematic review of the literature on the mortality and morbidity associated with SRC was recently published [4]. Twenty studies with 14,059 SSc subjects, of which 854 had SRC and 4095 had SSc-associated end-stage renal disease (SSc-ESRD), met inclusion criteria. Cumulative mortality in the post-ACE inhibitor era was approximately 20% at 6 months, 30–36% at 1 year, 19–40% at 3 years, and almost 50% at 10 years from SRC onset. Although the introduction of ACE inhibitors resulted in a 50% improvement in SRC mortality, there was no further improvement thereafter. SRC mortality rates were proportionally higher than mortality rates associated with other SSc organ involvement. The rate of permanent dialysis after SRC in the post-ACE inhibitor era ranged from 19% to 40%.

Renal recovery after SRC is reported to occur in up to a quarter of patients up to 18 months after SRC [4]. Thus, in practice, decisions to proceed to renal transplant are often deferred for up to 2 years.

The use of ACE inhibitors should be indefinite as recurrence years after the initial event have occurred when these drugs were discontinued. Recurrence of SRC post-renal transplant has also been reported ranging from 2% to 9% [4]. In practice, though, it can be very difficult to distinguish recurrence from rejection and other etiologies of graft failure (e.g., nephrotoxic drugs and infections). In one report, recurrence of SRC in transplanted kidneys occurred after discontinuation of ACE inhibition [108].

Thus, SRC mortality and morbidity remain high and, while outcomes with ACE inhibitors have improved, earlier, more accurate diagnosis and treatment and novel treatments are required to improve outcomes of SRC.

Three to 17% of SRC patients undergo renal transplant [4]. Survival was better in SSc patients post-renal transplant (54–91%) compared to those on dialysis (31–56%). Graft survival has also improved over time and appears similar to that of patients with other types of ESRD.

Interstitial Renal Disease

Postmortem studies have confirmed that expression of fibrillar collagens is increased in SSc even in the absence of any clinical evidence of renal abnormality. However, there are some cases in which interstitial renal disease occurs as a consequence of drugs or other stimuli. It is unclear whether SSc cases are more susceptible to this, but interstitial nephritis remains an important differential diagnosis in any case of SSc with renal insufficiency.

Glomerulonephritis

Glomerulonephritis occurs in the context of overlap connective tissue disease, and there are often clinical or serological clues. In our cohort, all cases of glomerulonephritis had some serological features of lupus or positive ANCA. This is consistent with other reported cases [109]. Glomerulonephritis may occur as an isolated pathology, and clues are often present in the autoantibody profile of cases. On occasion, there may have been a scleroderma renal crisis before development of glomerulonephritis. Representative biopsies from cases of GN in SSc are shown in Fig. 21.3.

The significance of ANCA in SSc is important [110]. Series suggest that typical ANCA may be associated with glomerulonephritis [111] or small vessel vasculitis [112]. Typical and atypical ANCA are reported—the most frequent being MPO [113]. This provides strong justification for early renal biopsy as treatment for the vasculitis is paramount and

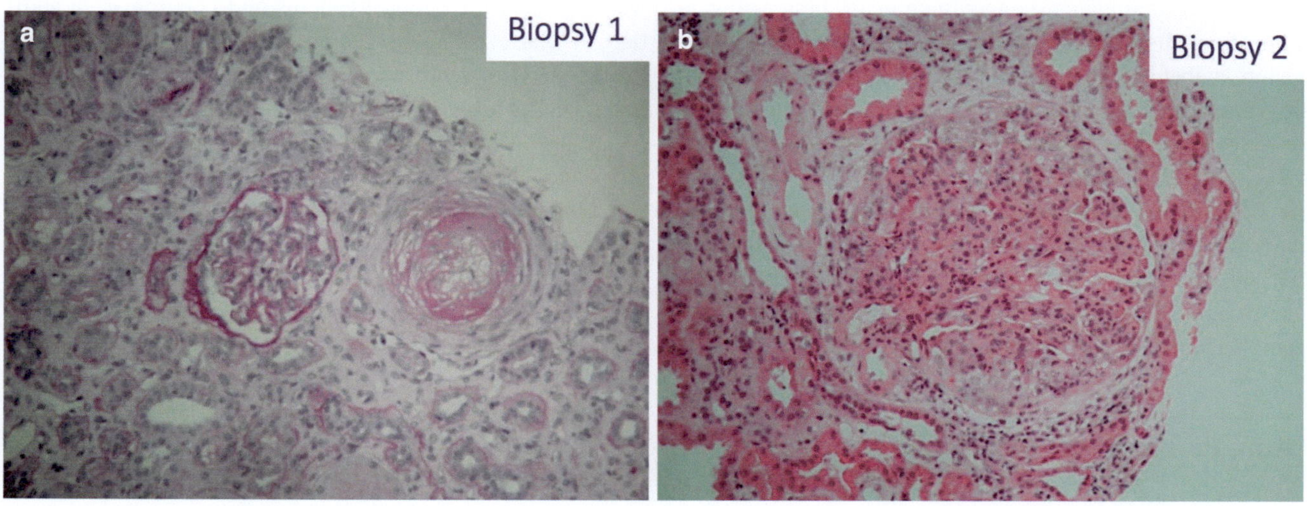

Fig. 21.3 Inflammatory renal pathology in scleroderma biopsy specimens. It is important to perform renal biopsy in cases of suspected glomerulonephritis. Clues for this include increased proteinuria, active urinary sediment, and/or serology. (**a**) In the upper case, this patient had previously demonstrated typical SRC on biopsy (**a**) with good outcome. There was later deterioration in renal function, increased proteinuria, and high titer anti-dsDNA antibodies. Repeat renal biopsy showed membranoproliferative glomerulonephritis (**b**). The lower case had early dcSSc and high titer ANCA and hematuria with normal renal function. The renal biopsy demonstrated vasculitis (**c**) and early crescentic glomerulonephritis (**d**)

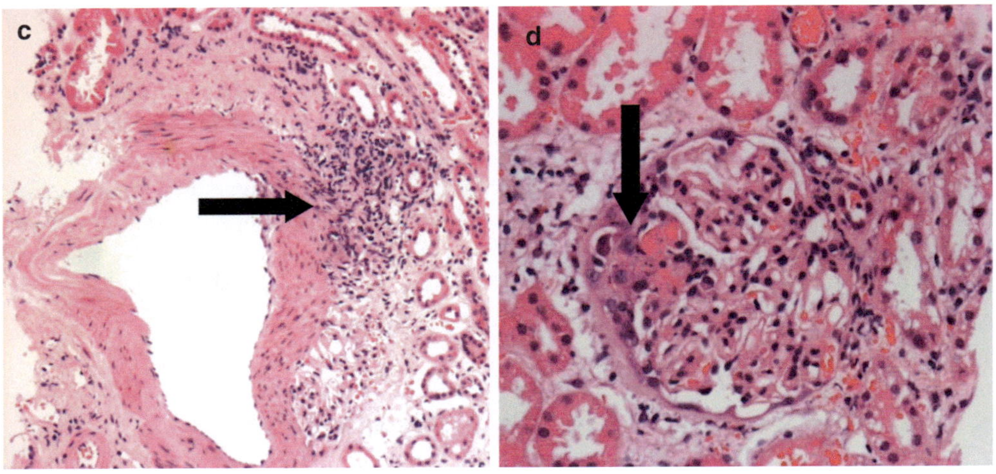

Fig. 21.3 (continued)

will involve high-dose glucocorticoids (and immunosuppression) that would otherwise be contraindicated in SSc. The association of ANCA vasculitis with SSc has recently been reviewed. Interestingly, MHC associations have been identified that may fit with this association for both conditions and also it is suggested that the distribution of vasculitic lesions is different for SSc-associated disease that could reflect concurrence of two distinct vasculopathic processes [113].

Chronic Kidney Disease (CKD) in Systemic Sclerosis

Other than SvRC and the entities mentioned above, renal disease in SSc has been reported to be common (up to 20% of subjects) and to result from a variety of causes, including both scleroderma-related (concomitant heart, lung, and gastrointestinal disease) and non-scleroderma-related (hypertension, diabetes, infection, and drugs such as non-steroidal anti-inflammatory drugs, penicillamine, and angiotensin-converting enzyme (ACE) inhibitors) [7, 53, 114]. However, in these situations, renal abnormalities tend to be mild (e.g., low GFR, proteinuria), renal function does not appear to deteriorate meaningfully over time, and prognosis of the renal disease tends to be generally favorable. Points to consider in clinical trials exploring CKD in SSc have been proposed [115].

Future Perspectives

Despite the marked improvement in outcome for the majority of patients with SRC since the introduction of ACE inhibitors, there is a significant subgroup for whom mortality remains high [116]. The poor long-term outcomes of SRC justify a continued search for novel treatment strategies. Some of the most exciting data emerging on the pathophysiology of SRC relate to endothelin-1, mostly because this is an actionable target. Endothelin-1 is known to contribute to other vascular manifestations of SSc including digital ulcers and pulmonary arterial hypertension. Elevated serum levels of endothelin-1 have now been reported in a small series of 27 SRC subjects and increased endothelin-1, and both endothelin-A and endothelin-B receptor expression were increased in SRC biopsies [97, 98]. In 2013, the Bosentan in Renal Disease-1 (BIRD-1) study reported the safety of bosentan, a non-selective endothelin-1 receptor antagonist, in addition to ACE inhibition in an open-label study of 6 SRC patients [99]. Unfortunately, the results of the *Effect of Bosentan in Scleroderma Renal Crisis (ScS-REINBO)* study, an open-label safety and efficacy study of bosentan, a non-selective endothelin-1 receptor antagonist, for new-onset SRC patients were disappointing [101], although the study was too small for a robust conclusion to be drawn. In addition, a phase II, single-center, randomized, placebo-controlled study of zibotentan, a novel selective endothelin-A, has recently been completed (ClinicalTrials.gov identifier: NCT02047708). The primary outcome measure, soluble vascular cell adhesion molecule 1 (sVCAM 1), was not informative but there was a significant change in the exploratory urinary marker MCP-1 and, notably, a statistically significant stabilization of eGFR in SSc-CKD patients receiving zibotentan compared with placebo. The final results are not yet fully published [117]. It is notable that a much larger recent study in diabetic CKD suggested renal function benefits in patients receiving atrasentan, a selective endothelin receptor blocker [118], in line with the benefits observed in the small trial of zibotentan in SSc-CKD. A number of other actionable targets of SRC, including direct renin inhibition and inhibitors of the complement cascade, remain to be studied [119]. The role of immunosuppression during the acute context of SRC or for the management of other renal manifestations of SSc needs to be delineated. In conclusion, outcomes and early mortality have improved dramatically but more needs to be achieved. Our ability to identify a subset of patients at high risk of developing the condition—those with early diffuse cutaneous systemic sclerosis and anti-RNA polymerase III antibodies in particular—offers hope that early diagnosis will improve this serious manifestation of SSc.

References

1. Denton CP, Lapadula G, Mouthon L, Muller-Ladner U. Renal complications and scleroderma renal crisis. Rheumatology (Oxford). 2009;48(Suppl 3):iii32–5.
2. Steen VD, Mayes MD, Merkel PA. Assessment of kidney involvement. Clin Exp Rheumatol. 2003;21(3 Suppl 29):S29–31.
3. Guillevin L, Bérezné A, Seror R, Teixeira L, Pourrat J, Mahr A, et al. Scleroderma renal crisis: a retrospective multicentre study on 91 patients and 427 controls. Rheumatology (Oxford). 2012;51(3):460–7.
4. Kim H, Lefebvre F, Hoa S, Hudson M. The changing mortality and morbidity of systemic sclerosis: 1970–2016. J Scleroderma Relat Disord. 2020 (online first).
5. Steen VD, Costantino JP, Shapiro AP, Medsger TA Jr. Outcome of renal crisis in systemic sclerosis: relation to availability of angiotensin converting enzyme (ACE) inhibitors [see comments]. Ann Intern Med. 1990;113(5):352–7.
6. Arnaud L, Huart A, Plaisier E, Francois H, Mougenot B, Tiev K, et al. ANCA-related crescentic glomerulonephritis in systemic sclerosis: revisiting the "normotensive scleroderma renal crisis". Clin Nephrol. 2007;68(3):165–70.
7. Steen VD, Syzd A, Johnson JP, Greenberg A, Medsger TA Jr. Kidney disease other than renal crisis in patients with diffuse scleroderma. J Rheumatol. 2005;32(4):649–55.
8. Auspitz H. Ein beit zur lehre vom haute-sklerem der erwachsenen. Wrin Med Wschr. 1863;13:739–55.
9. Osler W. The principles and practice of medicine. New York: Appleton; 1892. p. 993–8.
10. Goetz RH. The pathology of progressive systemic sclerosis (generalized scleroderma) with special reference to changes in the viscera. Clin Proc Grad Med Assoc. 1945;4:337–92.
11. Moore HC, Sheehan HL. The kidney of scleroderma. Lancet. 1952;1:68.
12. Keeler E, Fioravanti G, Samuel B, Longo S. Scleroderma renal crisis or thrombotic thrombocytopenic purpura: seeing through the masquerade. Lab Med. 2015;46(2):e39–44. https://doi.org/10.1309/LM72AM5XFHZYOQCB.
13. Hoa S, Stern EP, Denton CP, Hudson M, Scleroderma Clinical Trials Consortium Scleroderma Renal Crisis Working Group Investigators of the Scleroderma Clinical Trials Consortium Scleroderma Renal Crisis Working Group. Towards developing criteria for scleroderma renal crisis: a scoping review. Autoimmun Rev. 2017;16(4):407–15.
14. Butler EA, Baron M, Fogo AB, Frech T, Ghossein C, Hachulla E, et al. Generation of a core set of items to develop classification criteria for scleroderma renal crisis using consensus methodology. Arthritis Rheumatol. 2019;71(6):964–71.
15. Kellum J, Lameire N, Aspelin P, Barsoum R, Burdmann E, Goldstein S. Kidney Disease: Improving Global Outcomes (KDIGO) Acute Kidney Injury Work Group. KDIGO clinical practice guideline for acute kidney injury. Kidney Int. 2012;2(1):1–138.
16. Yamashita H, Kamei R, Kaneko H. Classifications of scleroderma renal crisis and reconsideration of its pathophysiology. Rheumatology (Oxford). 2019;58:2099–106. https://doi.org/10.1093/rheumatology/kez435.
17. Frech TM, Shanmugam VK, Shah AA, Assassi S, Gordon JK, Hant FN, Hinchcliff ME, Steen V, Khanna D, Kayser C, Domsic RT. Treatment of early diffuse systemic sclerosis skin disease. Clin Exp Rheumatol. 2013;31(2 Suppl 76):166–71. Epub 2013 Jul 23.
18. Steen VD, Medsger TA. Changes in causes of death in systemic sclerosis, 1972–2002. Ann Rheum Dis. 2007;66(7):940–4. https://doi.org/10.1136/ard.2006.066068. Epub 2007 Feb 28.
19. Rubio-Rivas M, Simeón-Aznar CP, Velasco C, Marí-Alfonso B, Espinosa G, Corbella X, Colunga-Argüelles D, Egurbide-Arberas MV, Ortego-Centeno N, Vargas-Hitos JA, Freire M, Ríos-Blanco JJ, Trapiella-Martínez L, Rodríguez-Carballeira M, Fonollosa-Pla V. Changes in the pattern of death of 987 patients with systemic sclerosis from 1990 to 2009 from the nationwide Spanish Scleroderma Registry (RESCLE). Clin Exp Rheumatol. 2017;35(Suppl 106):40–7.
20. Penn H, Howie AJ, Kingdon EJ, Bunn CC, Stratton RJ, Black CM, et al. Scleroderma renal crisis: patient characteristics and long-term outcomes. QJM. 2007;100(8):485–94.
21. Moinzadeh P, Kuhr K, Siegert E, Blank N, Sunderkoetter C, Henes J, Krusche M, Schmalzing M, Worm M, Schmeiser T, Günther C, Aberer E, Susok L, Riemekasten G, Kreuter A, Zeidler G, Juche A, Hadjiski D, Müller-Ladner U, Gaebelein-Wissing N, Distler JHW, Sárdy M, Krieg T, Hunzelmann N. Scleroderma renal crisis: risk factors for an increasingly rare organ complication. J Rheumatol. 2020;47:241–8. https://doi.org/10.3899/jrheum.180582.
22. Nishimagi E, Tochimoto A, Kawaguchi Y, Satoh T, Kuwana M, Takagi K, et al. Characteristics of patients with early systemic sclerosis and severe gastrointestinal tract involvement. J Rheumatol. 2007;34:2050–5.
23. Hashimoto A, Tejima S, Tono T, Suzuki M, Tanaka S, Matsui T, et al. Predictors of survival and causes of death in Japanese patients with systemic sclerosis. J Rheumatol. 2011;38:1931–9.
24. Foocharoen C, Mahakkanukrauh A, Suwannaroj S, Nanagara R. Spontaneous skin regression and predictors of skin regression in Thai scleroderma patients. Clin Rheumatol. 2011;30:1235–40.
25. Turk M, Pope JE. The frequency of scleroderma renal crisis over time: a meta-analysis. J Rheumatol. 2016;43:1350–5. https://doi.org/10.3899/jrheum.151353.
26. Steen VD, Medsger TA Jr. Severe organ involvement in systemic sclerosis with diffuse scleroderma. Arthritis Rheum. 2000;43:2437–44.
27. Walker UA, Tyndall A, Czirják L, Denton C, Farge-Bancel D, Kowal-Bielecka O, et al. Clinical risk assessment of organ manifestations in systemic sclerosis: a report from the EULAR Scleroderma Trials and Research Group database. Ann Rheum Dis. 2007;66:754–63.
28. Montanelli G, Beretta L, Santaniello A, Scorza R. Effect of dihydropyridine calcium channel blockers and glucocorticoids on the prevention and development of scleroderma renal crisis in an Italian case series. Clin Exp Rheumatol. 2013;31(2 Suppl 76):135–9.
29. Hudson M, Baron M, Tatibouet S, Furst DE, Khanna D, International Scleroderma Renal Crisis Study Investigators. Exposure to ACE inhibitors prior to the onset of scleroderma renal crisis-results from the International Scleroderma Renal Crisis Survey. Semin Arthritis Rheum. 2014;43(5):666–72.
30. Nihtyanova SI, Sari A, Harvey JC, Leslie A, Derrett-Smith EC, Fonseca C, Ong VH, Denton CP. Using autoantibodies and cutaneous subset to develop outcome-based disease classification in systemic sclerosis. Arthritis Rheumatol. 2020;72:465–76. https://doi.org/10.1002/art.41153.
31. Morgan ND, Shah AA, Mayes MD, Domsic RT, Medsger TAJ, Steen VD, Varga J, Carns M, Ramos PS, Silver RM, Schiopu E,

Khanna D, Hsu V, Gordon JK, Gladue H, Saketkoo LA, Criswell LA, Derk CT, Trojanowski MA, Shanmugam VK, Chung L, Valenzuela A, Jan R, Goldberg A, Remmers EF, Kastner DL, Wigley FM, Gourh P, Boin F. Clinical and serological features of systemic sclerosis in a multicenter African American cohort: analysis of the genome research in African American scleroderma patients clinical database. Medicine (Baltimore). 2017;96:e8980. https://doi.org/10.1097/MD.0000000000008980.
32. Traub YM, Shapiro AP, Rodnan GP, Medsger TA, McDonald RH Jr, Steen VD, et al. Hypertension and renal failure (scleroderma renal crisis) in progressive systemic sclerosis. Review of a 25-year experience with 68 cases. Medicine (Baltimore). 1983;62(6):335–52.
33. Steen VD, Medsger TA Jr. Epidemiology and natural history of systemic sclerosis. Rheum Dis Clin N Am. 1990;16(1):1–10.
34. Steen VD, Ziegler GL, Rodnan GP, Medsger TA Jr. Clinical and laboratory associations of anticentromere antibody in patients with progressive systemic sclerosis. Arthritis Rheum. 1984;27(2):125–31.
35. Steen VD, Medsger TA Jr, Osial TA Jr, Ziegler GL, Shapiro AP, Rodnan GP. Factors predicting development of renal involvement in progressive systemic sclerosis. Am J Med. 1984;76(5):779–86.
36. Korzets Z, Schneider M, Savin H, Ben Chetrit S, Bernheim J, Shitrit P, et al. Intriguing presentation of scleroderma renal crisis (scleroderma renal crisis sine scleroderma sine hypertension). Nephrol Dial Transplant. 1998;13(11):2953–6.
37. Molina JF, Anaya JM, Cabrera GE, Hoffman E, Espinoza LR. Systemic sclerosis sine scleroderma: an unusual presentation in scleroderma renal crisis. J Rheumatol. 1995;22(3):557–60.
38. Avouac J, Walker UA, Hachulla E, Riemekasten G, Cuomo G, Carreira PE, Caramaschi P, Ananieva LP, Matucci-Cerinic M, Czirjak L, Denton C, Ladner UM, Allanore Y, EUSTAR Collaborators. Joint and tendon involvement predict disease progression in systemic sclerosis: a EUSTAR prospective study. Ann Rheum Dis. 2016;75(1):103–9. https://doi.org/10.1136/annrheumdis-2014-205295. Epub 2014 Aug 27.
39. Steen VD, Medsger TA Jr. The palpable tendon friction rub: an important physical examination finding in patients with systemic sclerosis [see comments]. Arthritis Rheum. 1997;40(6):1146–51.
40. Bunn CC, Denton CP, Shi-wen X, Knight C, Black CM. Anti-RNA polymerases and other autoantibody specificities in systemic sclerosis. Br J Rheumatol. 1998;37(1):15–20.
41. Okano Y, Steen VD, Medsger TA Jr. Autoantibody reactive with RNA polymerase III in systemic sclerosis. Ann Intern Med. 1993;119(10):1005–13.
42. Rivolta R, Mascagni B, Berruti V, Di Palo FQ, Elli A, Scorza R, et al. Renal vascular damage in systemic sclerosis patients without clinical evidence of nephropathy. Arthritis Rheum. 1996;39(6):1030–4.
43. Nguyen B, et al. Association of RNA polymerase III antibodies with scleroderma renal crisis. J Rheumatol. 2010;37(5):1068; author reply 1069.
44. Sobanski V, Dauchet L, Lefevre G, Lambert M, Morell-Dubois S, Sy T, et al. Prevalence of anti-RNA polymerase III antibodies in systemic sclerosis: new data from a French cohort and a systematic review and meta-analysis. Arthritis Rheumatol. 2014;66(2):407–17.
45. Domsic RT, Nihtyanova SI, Wisniewski SR, Fine MJ, Lucas M, Kwoh CK, et al. Derivation and external validation of a prediction rule for five-year mortality in patients with early diffuse cutaneous systemic sclerosis. Arthritis Rheumatol. 2016;68(4):993–1003.
46. Lynch B, et al. The prognosis of scleroderma renal crisis in RNA-polymerase III antibody-positive compared to RNA-polymerase III antibody-negative patients. Rheumatology. 2014;53(Suppl 1):i179.
47. Kuwana M, et al. Autoantibody reactive with three classes of RNA polymerases in sera from patients with systemic sclerosis. J Clin Invest. 1993;91(4):1399–404.
48. Hamaguchi Y, et al. Clinical and immunologic predictors of scleroderma renal crisis in Japanese systemic sclerosis patients with anti-RNA polymerase III autoantibodies. Arthritis Rheumatol. 2015;67(4):1045–52.
49. Patel V, et al. Anti-RNA polymerase II antibodies in a US cohort of systemic sclerosis patients: comment on the article by Hamaguchi et al. Arthritis Rheumatol. 2015;67:2547.
50. Gordon SM, Stitt RS, Nee R, Bailey WT, Little DJ, Knight KR, et al. Risk factors for future scleroderma renal crisis at systemic sclerosis diagnosis. J Rheumatol. 2019;46(1):85–92.
51. Butikofer L, Varisco PA, Distler O, Kowal-Bielecka O, Allanore Y, Riemekasten G, et al. ACE inhibitors in SSc patients display a risk factor for scleroderma renal crisis-a EUSTAR analysis. Arthritis Res Ther. 2020;22(1):59.
52. Jaeger VK, Wirz EG, Allanore Y, Rossbach P, Riemekasten G, Hachulla E, Distler O, Airò P, Carreira PE, Balbir Gurman A, Tikly M, Vettori S, Damjanov N, Müller-Ladner U, Distler JHW, Li M, Walker UA. Incidences and risk factors of organ manifestations in the early course of systemic sclerosis: a longitudinal EUSTAR study. PLoS One. 2016;11:e0163894. https://doi.org/10.1371/journal.pone.0163894.
53. Caron M, Hudson M, Baron M, Nessim S, Steele R, Canadian Scleroderma Research Group. Longitudinal study of renal function in systemic sclerosis. J Rheumatol. 2012;39(9):1829–34.
54. Kingdon EJ, Knight CJ, Dustan K, Irwin AG, Thomas M, Powis SH, et al. Calculated glomerular filtration rate is a useful screening tool to identify scleroderma patients with renal impairment. Rheumatology (Oxford). 2003;42(1):26–33.
55. McWhorter JE, Leroy EC. Pericardial disease in scleroderma (systemic sclerosis). Am J Med. 1974;57(4):566–75.
56. Helfrich DJ, Banner B, Steen VD, Medsger TA Jr. Normotensive renal failure in systemic sclerosis. Arthritis Rheum. 1989;32(9):1128–34.
57. Kohno K, Katayama T, Majima K, Fujisawa M, Iida S, Fukami K, et al. A case of normotensive scleroderma renal crisis after high-dose methylprednisolone treatment [in process citation]. Clin Nephrol. 2000;53(6):479–82.
58. Yamanishi Y, Yamana S, Ishioka S, Yamakido M. Development of ischemic colitis and scleroderma renal crisis following methylprednisolone pulse therapy for progressive systemic sclerosis. Intern Med. 1996;35(7):583–6.
59. Steen VD, Medsger TA Jr. Case-control study of glucocorticoids and other drugs that either precipitate or protect from the development of scleroderma renal crisis. Arthritis Rheum. 1998;41(9):1613–9.
60. Bar J, Ehrenfeld M, Rozenman J, Perelman M, Sidi Y, Gur H. Pulmonary-renal syndrome in systemic sclerosis. Semin Arthritis Rheum. 2001;30(6):403–10.
61. Kapur A, Ballou SP, Renston JP, Luna E, Chung-Park M. Recurrent acute scleroderma renal crisis complicated by thrombotic thrombocytopenic purpura. J Rheumatol. 1997;24(12):2469–72.
62. Manadan AM, Harris C, Block JA. Thrombotic thrombocytopenic purpura in the setting of systemic sclerosis. Semin Arthritis Rheum. 2005;34(4):683–8.
63. Kfoury Baz EM, Mahfouz RA, Masri AF, Jamaleddine GW. Thrombotic thrombocytopenic purpura in a case of scleroderma renal crisis treated with twice-daily therapeutic plasma exchange. Ren Fail. 2001;23(5):737–42.
64. Torok KS, Cortese Hassett A, Kiss JE, Lucas M, Medsger TA. Scleroderma renal crisis and thrombotic thrombocytopenic purpura—are they related? ACR presentation 2008.

65. Lian EC. Pathogenesis of thrombotic thrombocytopenic purpura: ADAMTS13 deficiency and beyond. Semin Thromb Hemost. 2005;31(6):625–32.
66. Uriarte MH, Larrarte C, Rey LB. Scleroderma renal crisis debute with thrombotic microangiopathy: a successful case treated with eculizumab. Case Rep Nephrol. 2018;2018:6051083. https://doi.org/10.1155/2018/6051083.
67. Zuckerman JE, Chang A. Complement and renal thrombotic microangiopathy associated with hypertension and scleroderma. Adv Chronic Kidney Dis. 2020;27:149–54. https://doi.org/10.1053/j.ackd.2019.11.002.
68. Penn H, Denton CP. Diagnosis, management and prevention of scleroderma renal disease. Curr Opin Rheumatol. 2008;20(6):692–6.
69. KDIGO. Clinical practice guideline for acute kidney injury (AKI). Kidney Int Suppl. 2012;2(1):4.
70. Chighizola CB, Pregnolato F, Meroni PL, Denton CP, Ong VH. N-terminal pro brain natriuretic peptide as predictor of outcome in scleroderma renal crisis. Clin Exp Rheumatol. 2016;34(Suppl 100):122–8.
71. Stern EP, Unwin R, Burns A, Ong VH, Denton CP. Exploring molecular pathology of chronic kidney disease in systemic sclerosis by analysis of urinary and serum proteins. Rheumatol Adv Pract. 2021;5:rkaa083. https://doi.org/10.1093/rap/rkaa083.
72. Geraci G, Sorce A, Mulè G. The "Renocentric Theory" of renal resistive index: is it time for a copernican revolution? J Rheumatol. 2020;47:486–9. https://doi.org/10.3899/jrheum.190930.
73. Bruni C, Rosato E, Maestripieri V, Gigante A, Tesei G, Bellando-Randone S, Guiducci S, Chiostri M, El Aoufy K, Blagojevic J, Moggi-Pignone A, De Paulis A, Furst DE, Boddi M, Matucci-Cerinic M. The renal resistive index in systemic sclerosis: determinants, prognostic implication and proposal for specific age-adjusted cut-offs. Eur J Intern Med. 2019;70:43–9. https://doi.org/10.1016/j.ejim.2019.09.001.
74. Gigante A, Bruni C, Lepri G, Tesei G, Maestripieri V, Guiducci S, Moggi-Pignone A, Melchiorre D, Boddi M, Bellando-Randone S, Rosato E, Matucci-Cerinic M. The renal resistive index: a new biomarker for the follow-up of vascular modifications in systemic sclerosis. J Rheumatol. 2021;48:241–6. https://doi.org/10.3899/jrheum.191101.
75. Cianci R, Gigante A, Bagordo D, Pintus G, Giovannetti A, Lai S, Mazzaferro S, Rosato E. Renal resistive index in IgA nephropathy and renal scleroderma vasculopathy. Microvasc Res. 2021;133:104095. https://doi.org/10.1016/j.mvr.2020.104095.
76. Shimizu T, Iwamoto N, Okamoto M, Endo Y, Tsuji S, Takatani A, Igawa T, Umeda M, Fukui S, Sumiyoshi R, Kitamura M, Koga T, Kawashiri S-Y, Ichinose K, Tamai M, Nakamura H, Origuchi T, Nishino T, Kawakami A. Scleroderma renal crisis complicated with thrombotic microangiopathy triggered by influenza B virus infection. Intern Med. 2019;58:441–5. https://doi.org/10.2169/internalmedicine.1441-18.
77. Silva IMS, Assersen KB, Willadsen NN, Jepsen J, Artuc M, Steckelings UM. The role of the renin-angiotensin system in skin physiology and pathophysiology. Exp Dermatol. 2020;29:891–901.
78. Clements PJ, Lachenbruch PA, Furst DE, Maxwell M, Danovitch G, Paulus HE. Abnormalities of renal physiology in systemic sclerosis. A prospective study with 10-year followup. Arthritis Rheum. 1994;37(1):67–74.
79. Nihtyanova SI, Parker JC, Black CM, Bunn CC, Denton CP. A longitudinal study of anti-RNA polymerase III antibody levels in systemic sclerosis. Rheumatology (Oxford). 2009;48(10):1218–21. https://doi.org/10.1111/exd.14159.
80. Batal I, Domsic RT, Medsger TA, Bastacky S. Scleroderma renal crisis: a pathology perspective. Int J Rheumatol. 2010;54:3704.
81. Devresse A, Aydin S, Le Quintrec M, Demoulin N, Stordeur P, Lambert C, Gastoldi S, Pirson Y, Jadoul M, Morelle J. Complement activation and effect of eculizumab in scleroderma renal crisis. Medicine (Baltimore). 2016;95:e4459. https://doi.org/10.1097/MD.0000000000004459.
82. Okrój M, Johansson M, Saxne T, Blom AM, Hesselstrand R. Analysis of complement biomarkers in systemic sclerosis indicates a distinct pattern in scleroderma renal crisis. Arthritis Res Ther. 2016;18:267. https://doi.org/10.1186/s13075-016-1168-x.
83. Berger M, Steen VD. Role of anti-receptor autoantibodies in pathophysiology of scleroderma. Autoimmun Rev. 2017;16:1029–35. https://doi.org/10.1016/j.autrev.2017.07.019.
84. Riemekasten G, Philippe A, Näther M, Slowinski T, Müller DN, Heidecke H, Matucci-Cerinic M, Czirják L, Lukitsch I, Becker M, Kill A, van Laar JM, Catar R, Luft FC, Burmester GR, Hegner B, Dragun D. Involvement of functional autoantibodies against vascular receptors in systemic sclerosis. Ann Rheum Dis. 2011;70(3):530–6. https://doi.org/10.1136/ard.2010.135772. Epub 2010 Nov 15.
85. Denton CP, Bickerstaff MC, Shiwen X, Carulli MT, Haskard DO, Dubois RM, Black CM. Serial circulating adhesion molecule levels reflect disease severity in systemic sclerosis. Br J Rheumatol. 1995;34(11):1048–54.
86. Takahashi T, et al. A possible contribution of lipocalin-2 to the development of dermal fibrosis, pulmonary vascular involvement, and renal dysfunction in systemic sclerosis. Br J Dermatol. 2015;173:681.
87. Nguyen B, et al. HLA-DRB1*0407 and *1304 are risk factors for scleroderma renal crisis. Arthritis Rheum. 2011;63:530–4.
88. Fonseca C, Renzoni E, Sestini P, Pantelidis P, Lagan A, Bunn C, McHugh N, Welsh KI, Du Bois RM, Denton CP, Black C, Abraham D. Endothelin axis polymorphisms in patients with scleroderma. Arthritis Rheum. 2006;54:3034–42.
89. Stern EP, Guerra SG, Chinque H, Acquaah V, González-Serna D, Ponticos M, Martin J, Ong VH, Khan K, Nihtyanova SI, Harber M, Burns A, Mayes MD, Assassi S, Fonseca C, Denton CP. Analysis of anti-RNA polymerase III antibody-positive systemic sclerosis and altered GPATCH2L and CTNND2 expression in scleroderma renal crisis. J Rheumatol. 2020;47:1668–77. https://doi.org/10.3899/jrheum.190945.
90. Derrett-Smith E, et al. Perturbed response to experimental renal injury in a mouse model of systemic sclerosis. Rheumatology. 2014;53(Suppl 1):i176.
91. Shapiro L, et al. Development of a "renal crisis prevention card" as an educational tool aimed at improving outcomes in high-risk patients with systemic sclerosis. Arthritis Rheumatol. 2014;66:abstract 2716.
92. Kowal-Bielecka O, Landewe R, Avouac J, Chwiesko S, Miniati I, Czirjak L, et al. EULAR recommendations for the treatment of systemic sclerosis: a report from the EULAR Scleroderma Trials and Research group (EUSTAR). Ann Rheum Dis. 2009;68(5):620–8.
93. Lynch BM, Stern EP, Ong V, Harber M, Burns A, Denton CP. UK Scleroderma Study Group (UKSSG) guidelines on the diagnosis and management of scleroderma renal crisis. Clin Exp Rheumatol. 2016;34(Suppl 100):106–9.
94. Cheung WY, Gibson IW, Rush D, Jeffery J, Karpinski M. Late recurrence of scleroderma renal crisis in a renal transplant recipient despite angiotensin II blockade. Am J Kidney Dis. 2005;45(5):930–4.
95. Dhaun N, Macintyre IM, Bellamy CO, Kluth DC. Endothelin receptor antagonism and renin inhibition as treatment options for scleroderma kidney. Am J Kidney Dis. 2009;54(4):726–31.
96. Vancheeswaran R, Magoulas T, Efrat G, Wheeler-Jones C, Olsen I, Penny R, et al. Circulating endothelin-1 levels in systemic scle-

rosis subsets—a marker of fibrosis or vascular dysfunction? [see comments]. J Rheumatol. 1994;21(10):1838–44.
97. Kobayashi H, Nishimaki T, Kaise S, Suzuki T, Watanabe K, Kasukawa R, et al. Immunohistological study endothelin-1 and endothelin-A and B receptors in two patients with scleroderma renal crisis. Clin Rheumatol. 1999;18(5):425–7.
98. Mouthon L, Mehrenberger M, Teixeira L, Fakhouri F, Berezne A, Guillevin L, et al. Endothelin-1 expression in scleroderma renal crisis. Hum Pathol. 2011;42(1):95–102.
99. Penn H, et al. Targeting the endothelin axis in scleroderma renal crisis: rationale and feasibility. QJM. 2013;106(9):839–48.
100. Wipff J, Gallier G, Dieude P, Avouac J, Tiev K, Hachulla E, et al. Angiotensin-converting enzyme gene does not contribute to genetic susceptibility to systemic sclerosis in European Caucasians. J Rheumatol. 2009;36(2):337–40.
101. Bérezné A, Abdoul H, Karras A, Marie I, Huart A, Ficheux M, Queyrel V, Imbert B, Puéchal X, Hot A, Bienvenu B, Diot E, Moulin B, Quémeneur T, Kahn JE, Mouthon L, Guillevin for the French Vasculitis Study Group L. Bosentan in scleroderma renal crisis: a national open label prospective study [abstract]. Arthritis Rheumatol. 2017;69(Suppl 10). https://acrabstracts.org/abstract/bosentan-in-scleroderma-renal-crisis-a-national-open-label-prospective-study/. Accessed 26 Feb 2021.
102. Thomas CP, Nester CM, Phan AC, Sharma M, Steele AL, Lenert PS. Eculizumab for rescue of thrombotic microangiopathy in PM-Scl antibody-positive autoimmune overlap syndrome. Clin Kidney J. 2015;8(6):698–701.
103. Sammaritano LR, Bermas BL, Chakravarty EE, Chambers C, Clowse MEB, Lockshin MD, et al. 2020 American College of Rheumatology guideline for the management of reproductive health in rheumatic and musculoskeletal diseases. Arthritis Rheumatol. 2020;72(4):529–56.
104. Schrier RW. Aldosterone 'escape' vs 'breakthrough'. Nat Rev Nephrol. 2010;6(2):61.
105. Gliddon AE, Doré CJ, Black CM, McHugh N, Moots R, Denton CP, Herrick A, Barnes T, Camilleri J, Chakravarty K, Emery P, Griffiths B, Hopkinson ND, Hickling P, Lanyon P, Laversuch C, Lawson T, Mallya R, Nisar M, Rhys-Dillon C, Sheeran T, Maddison PJ. Prevention of vascular damage in scleroderma and autoimmune Raynaud's phenomenon: a multicenter, randomized, double-blind, placebo-controlled trial of the angiotensin-converting enzyme inhibitor quinapril. Arthritis Rheum. 2007;56:3837–46.
106. Sullivan KM, Goldmuntz EA, Keyes-Elstein L, McSweeney PA, Pinckney A, Welch B, Mayes MD, Nash RA, Crofford LJ, Eggleston B, Castina S, Griffith LM, Goldstein JS, Wallace D, Craciunescu O, Khanna D, Folz RJ, Goldin J, St Clair EW, Seibold JR, Phillips K, Mineishi S, Simms RW, Ballen K, Wener MH, Georges GE, Heimfeld S, Hosing C, Forman S, Kafaja S, Silver RM, Griffing L, Storek J, LeClercq S, Brasington R, Csuka ME, Bredeson C, Keever-Taylor C, Domsic RT, Kahaleh MB, Medsger T, Furst DE. Myeloablative autologous stem-cell transplantation for severe scleroderma. N Engl J Med. 2018;378:35–47. https://doi.org/10.1056/nejmoa1703327.
107. van Laar J, Spierings J. Upfront autologous HSCT versus immunosuppression in early diffuse cutaneous systemic sclerosis (UPSIDE). https://clinicaltrials.gov/ct2/show/NCT04464434.
108. Wierzbicki O, Khalidi N, Hudson M. Recurrence of scleroderma renal crisis in transplanted kidney leading to graft failure. J Rheumatol. 2016;43(6):1198 (abstract 122).
109. Herrera-Esparza R, Aguilar JL, Saucedo A, Gonzalez I, Lopez-Robles E, Avalos-Diaz E. Scleroderma with type III glomerulonephritis and MPO-ANCA antibodies in the serum. J Eur Acad Dermatol Venereol. 2005;19(5):617–20.
110. Casari S, Haeney M, Farrand S, Herrick A. Antineutrophil cytoplasmic antibodies a "Red Flag" in patients with systemic sclerosis. J Rheumatol. 2002;29(12):2666–7.
111. Mimura I, Hori Y, Matsukawa T, Uozaki H, Tojo A, Fujita T. Noncrescentic ANCA-associated renal crisis in systemic sclerosis. Clin Nephrol. 2008;70(2):183–5.
112. Anders HJ, Wiebecke B, Haedecke C, Sanden S, Combe C, Schlondorff D. MPO-ANCA-positive crescentic glomerulonephritis: a distinct entity of scleroderma renal disease? Am J Kidney Dis. 1999;33:e3.1.
113. Derrett-Smith EC, Nihtyanova SI, Harvey J, Salama AD, Denton CP. Revisiting ANCA-associated vasculitis in systemic sclerosis: clinical, serological and immunogenetic factors. Rheumatology (Oxford). 2013;52(10):1824–31.
114. Shanmugam VK, Steen VD. Renal manifestations in scleroderma: evidence for subclinical renal disease as a marker of vasculopathy. Int J Rheumatol. 2010;2010:538589.
115. Galluccio F, Müller-Ladner U, Furst DE, Khanna D, Matucci-Cerinic M. Points to consider in renal involvement in systemic sclerosis. Rheumatology (Oxford). 2017;56:v49–52. https://doi.org/10.1093/rheumatology/kex20122.
116. Steen VD. Scleroderma renal crisis. Rheum Dis Clin N Am. 2003;29(2):315–33.
117. Stern E, Host L, Escott K, Gilmour P, Wanjiku I, Ochiel R, Burns A, Unwin R, Ong V, Denton C. Evaluation of the highly selective endothelin a receptor antagonist zibotentan in systemic sclerosis associated chronic kidney disease [abstract]. Arthritis Rheumatol. 2019;71(Suppl 10). https://acrabstracts.org/abstract/evaluation-of-the-highly-selective-endothelin-a-receptor-antagonist-zibotentan-in-systemic-sclerosis-associated-chronic-kidney-disease/. Accessed 26 Feb 2021.
118. Heerspink HJL, Parving HH, Andress DL, Bakris G, Correa-Rotter R, Hou FF, Kitzman DW, Kohan D, Makino H, McMurray JJV, Melnick JZ, Miller MG, Pergola PE, Perkovic V, Tobe S, Yi T, Wigderson M, de Zeeuw D, SONAR Committees and Investigators. Atrasentan and renal events in patients with type 2 diabetes and chronic kidney disease (SONAR): a double-blind, randomised, placebo-controlled trial. Lancet. 2019;393(10184):1937–47. https://doi.org/10.1016/S0140-6736(19)30772-X. Epub 2019 Apr 14.
119. Gavriilaki E, Anagnostopoulos A, Mastellos DC. Complement in thrombotic microangiopathies: unraveling ariadne's thread into the labyrinth of complement therapeutics. Front Immunol. 2019;10:337. https://doi.org/10.3389/fimmu.2019.00337.

22 Cardiac Involvement: Evaluation and Management

Luna Gargani, Matteo Mazzola, and Sanjiv J. Shah

Introduction

Cardiac involvement in systemic sclerosis (SSc) is common, can present with protean manifestations, and when symptomatic portends a poor prognosis [1–6]. SSc can affect virtually any cardiac structure, thereby causing myocardial abnormalities (including myocardial fibrosis, left ventricular [LV] systolic dysfunction, and LV diastolic dysfunction), coronary microvascular ischemia, pericardial disease, conduction abnormalities (including brady- and tachyarrhythmias), and less commonly valvular disease [1–5]. Furthermore, cardiac manifestations of SSc can be primary (i.e., direct cardiac involvement due to the SSc disease process) or secondary to pulmonary arterial hypertension, interstitial lung disease, or significant kidney disease, all of which are common in patients with SSc [1, 6]. The purpose of this chapter was to focus on primary, direct cardiac involvement in SSc, with discussion of (1) epidemiology of cardiac involvement in SSc; (2) screening for cardiac involvement in SSc; (3) characterization of the pathophysiology, diagnosis, and management of specific cardiac lesions in SSc; (4) noninvasive and invasive tools for the detection and monitoring of cardiac involvement; and (5) areas of uncertainty in the study of cardiac involvement in SSc.

The successful evaluation and management of cardiac involvement in patients with SSc requires careful screening, a high index of suspicion given the broad and nonspecific symptoms associated with cardiac manifestations, and a multidisciplinary approach involving rheumatologists, cardiologists, and imaging specialists [6]. With the advent of novel non-invasive tests such as new biomarkers, tissue Doppler imaging, speckle-tracking echocardiography, and diffuse fibrosis imaging using cardiac magnetic resonance imaging (MRI), the screening, diagnosis, and research of cardiac manifestations of SSc should expand rapidly in the near future.

L. Gargani · M. Mazzola
Department of Surgical, Medical and Molecular Pathology and Critical Care Medicine, University of Pisa, Pisa, Italy
e-mail: luna.gargani@unipi.it

S. J. Shah (✉)
Northwestern University Feinberg School of Medicine, Chicago, IL, USA
e-mail: sanjiv.shah@northwestern.edu

Epidemiology of Cardiac Involvement in Systemic Sclerosis

Defining the epidemiology of cardiac involvement in SSc has proven to be difficult because of the wide variety of possible cardiac manifestations and variability in the types of diagnostic techniques used to diagnose SSc heart disease. Clinical symptoms can be considered as "late" events in a significant number of patients. Electrocardiography and chest radiography are insensitive techniques, whereas echocardiography (especially tissue Doppler imaging and speckle-tracking techniques), single photon emission computerized tomography (SPECT), radionuclide ventriculography, and magnetic resonance imaging (MRI) allow the detection of structural and functional cardiac lesions at a much earlier stage. From published studies, it appears that cardiac manifestations are quite common in SSc but the exact prevalence depends greatly on the patient population, definition of cardiac manifestations, and tests used to diagnose cardiac involvement. For example, rates of cardiac involvement in SSc for reduced LV ejection fraction [7], clinical cardiac involvement (defined as pericarditis, heart failure, severe arrhythmias, or conduction abnormalities) [8], abnormal tissue Doppler systolic or diastolic function [4, 9–11], and abnormal results on thallium scanning [12] have been found to be 5.4%, 30–35%, 40–60%, and >60–70%, respectively.

Y. Allanore et al. (eds.), *Scleroderma*, https://doi.org/10.1007/978-3-031-40658-4_22

Besides difficulties in estimating prevalence of cardiac manifestations, there is some controversy regarding the frequency of cardiac involvement in limited cutaneous versus diffuse cutaneous forms of SSc. Whereas some studies have found that both types of SSc have similar rates of cardiac involvement, others have found increased prevalence of cardiac manifestations in diffuse cutaneous SSc [1, 4, 8]. In a study of 1012 Italian patients with SSc, cardiac involvement was present in 32% of diffuse cutaneous SSc versus 23% in limited cutaneous SSc [8]. This finding was replicated in a large study of LV systolic dysfunction in SSc. Of 7073 patients with SSc, 383 had LV systolic dysfunction (defined as LV ejection fraction <55%), whereas 6690 had normal LV systolic function. SSc patients with LV systolic dysfunction were more likely to have diffuse cutaneous SSc compared to patients with normal LV systolic function (48% vs. 32%, respectively; $p = 0.001$) [7]. A recent study also found that patients with diffuse cutaneous SSc develop cardiac involvement sooner after diagnosis than limited cutaneous SSc patients [13]. Additional studies have found that the prevalence of cardiac involvement is especially high in the subset of patients with rapidly evolving skin involvement [14], anti-U3RNP antibodies [15], and/or skeletal myopathy [16]. From these studies, we can conclude that cardiac involvement occurs frequently in both limited and diffuse cutaneous forms of SSc but appears to be more common in the latter, and SSc patients at highest risk are those who have rapidly progressive skin disease, anti-U3RNP antibodies, and/or concomitant skeletal myopathy.

Several studies have examined the influence of cardiac involvement on death in SSc. In large series of SSc patients, when cardiac involvement appeared to be clinically evident, it has been found to be a poor prognostic factor [17]. In a study of patients with the diffuse cutaneous form of SSc, cardiac symptoms were observed in 15% of patients; at 10-year follow-up, cardiac involvement explained 20% of disease attributed deaths [18]. In a large cohort of Italian patients, 35% had cardiac symptoms or arrhythmia, with cardiac involvement alone accounting for 36% of deaths [8]. In French Canadian patients, 11.4% of deaths involved the heart [19]. An international meta-analysis of pooled cohorts of 11,526 person-years of follow-up [20] found that clinical cardiac involvement was present in 10% of patients. A multivariate analysis in this study demonstrated an increased hazard ratio for mortality of 2.8 (95% confidence interval 2.1–3.8) if cardiac involvement was present, and presence of cardiac involvement was the strongest predictor of mortality in this study [20]. These findings have been affirmed by more recent studies, the largest of which was a European study involving 5860 patients [21–24]. In this study, 55% of deaths were due to SSc, while 45% of deaths were thought to be unrelated to SSc. Of the SSc-related deaths, 26% were cardiac (predominantly heart failure and arrhythmias), whereas 29% of non-SSc-related deaths were due to cardiac causes. Thus, in patients with SSc, death due to cardiac disease is common and presence of cardiac involvement is an independent risk factor for death.

Screening and Diagnosis of Cardiac Involvement in Systemic Sclerosis

Given the poor prognosis associated with cardiac involvement in SSc, screening for the detection of subclinical cardiac disease (in addition to thorough evaluation of cardiac symptoms) is essential. Often times, details from the clinical history and physical examination provide important clues for the presence of cardiac involvement. Exertional lightheadedness, dizziness, or syncope can be a sign of pulmonary arterial hypertension, RV dysfunction, or arrhythmias. Chronic pericardial disease (both constrictive pericarditis and chronic pericardial effusion) often presents with symptoms of right-sided heart failure (lethargy, abdominal fullness, early satiety, and leg swelling). Myocardial disease and microvascular ischemia often do not cause specific symptoms until severe, at which point chest pain, shortness of breath, and overt left heart failure can occur. The sudden worsening of Raynaud's phenomenon (e.g., digital necrosis) may be an ominous sign of severe cardiac microvascular dysfunction and/or myocardial dysfunction leading to reduced cardiac output and reflexive systemic vasoconstriction. In these cases, urgent evaluation is often necessary so that therapies can be instituted to improve cardiac function.

Unlike interstitial lung disease and pulmonary arterial hypertension, optimal screening for direct cardiac involvement in SSc is unknown. Patients with SSc undergo routine Doppler echocardiography for pulmonary hypertension screening, so evaluation of possible direct cardiac involvement can and should be performed simultaneously. Given the ability of tissue Doppler imaging to detect subclinical systolic and diastolic dysfunction, this widely available technique should be performed on all patients with SSc.

Along with Doppler and tissue Doppler echocardiography, cardiac biomarker testing (with natriuretic peptides) is the other cornerstone in screening for cardiac involvement in SSc. In patients with symptoms or signs of cardiac involvement, and in patients with abnormal results on screening tests, detailed evaluation of possible forms of cardiac involvement should be undertaken as outlined in Table 22.1.

Table 22.1 Recommendations for evaluation of abnormal cardiac symptoms, signs, or screening studies in systemic sclerosis

Abnormal cardiac symptom, sign, or screening study	Recommendation for further evaluation specific to systemic sclerosis
Chest pain	Evaluate for myocardial microvascular ischemia with perfusion imaging (either nuclear or cardiac MRI); evaluate for pericarditis or pericardial effusion with ECG, echo, and cardiac MRI
Shortness of breath and exercise intolerance	If alternative causes (interstitial lung disease, pulmonary arterial hypertension) have been excluded, evaluate with natriuretic peptides (BNP or NT-proBNP); consider exercise testing to objectively document dyspnea and exercise intolerance (cardiopulmonary exercise testing can distinguish cardiac from pulmonary causes). If cardiac involvement suspected, evaluate further with echocardiography and cardiac MRI
Left heart failure (pulmonary edema or pulmonary vascular congestion)	Echocardiography, cardiac MRI with perfusion; consider constrictive pericarditis
Right heart failure (elevated jugular venous pressure, pleural effusion, hepatomegaly, ascites, and/or leg swelling)	echocardiography, cardiac MRI to look for constrictive pericarditis; if strong suspicion for constrictive pericarditis, evaluate further with simultaneous right and left heart catheterization
Palpitations	48-hour Holter monitor; if symptoms are infrequent, may need 30-day event monitor
Lightheadedness, dizziness, or syncope	48-hour Holter monitor; if symptoms are infrequent, may need 30-day event monitor; echocardiography to evaluate for structural heart disease and to exclude pulmonary arterial hypertension which can cause exertional lightheadedness or syncope
RV systolic dysfunction • TAPSE <1.6 cm [131]. • RV tissue Doppler *S'* <10 cm/s [131]. • RV fractional area change <0.35 [131]. • Septal flattening in systole or diastole ("D-shaped" LV in short axis).	Consider right heart catheterization to differentiate primary RV involvement (low or normal RV and PA systolic pressures) vs. secondary RV involvement due to pulmonary hypertension (high RV and PA systolic pressures)
LV systolic dysfunction • LV ejection fraction <55% [7, 133, 194].	Perfusion study (nuclear or cardiac MRI) to evaluate for microvascular (or macrovascular) ischemia; check for signs and symptoms of heart failure; consider coronary angiography to exclude epicardial coronary disease, especially in patients with EF <40–45% or if angina or atherosclerotic coronary artery disease risk factors are present
LV diastolic dysfunction • Impaired relaxation and/or evidence of elevated LV filling pressures [125, 127].	Evaluate for coronary artery disease, systemic hypertension, or microvascular ischemia; check for signs and symptoms of heart failure
Reduced LV tissue Doppler velocities • Lateral *S'* <10 cm/s [126]. • Lateral *e'* <10 cm/s if age <54 years; lateral *e'* <9 if age 55–65 years; or lateral *e'* <8 cm/s if age >65 years [126, 195].	More data are needed to determine optimal evaluation of systemic sclerosis patients with subclinical reduction in tissue Doppler velocities
Elevated natriuretic peptide levels • BNP >60 pg/mL [120]. • NT-proBNP >125 pg/mL [110].	If DLCO is decreased and/or RV dysfunction is present on echocardiography, proceed to right heart catheterization to evaluate for pulmonary hypertension; evaluate for LV systolic or diastolic dysfunction; check for signs and symptoms of heart failure

MRI magnetic resonance imaging, *RV* right ventricle, *LV* left ventricle, *S* systolic longitudinal tissue Doppler velocity, *e'* early diastolic longitudinal tissue Doppler velocity, *BNP* B-type natriuretic peptide, *NT-proBNP* N-terminal pro-B-type natriuretic peptide, *DLCO* diffusing capacity of carbon monoxide

Specific Cardiac Manifestations of Systemic Sclerosis

Given the diverse cardiac manifestations of SSc, understanding pathophysiology, clinical manifestations, diagnosis, and management of the various possibilities of cardiac involvement is essential. Figure 22.1 displays a schematic of the possible primary cardiac manifestations of SSc. In the following section, we review each of these specific forms of cardiac involvement in SSc in further detail. Primary cardiac involvement in SSc must be differentiated from secondary involvement, which can occur in the setting of pulmonary arterial hypertension, interstitial lung disease, systemic hypertension, and significant renal disease.

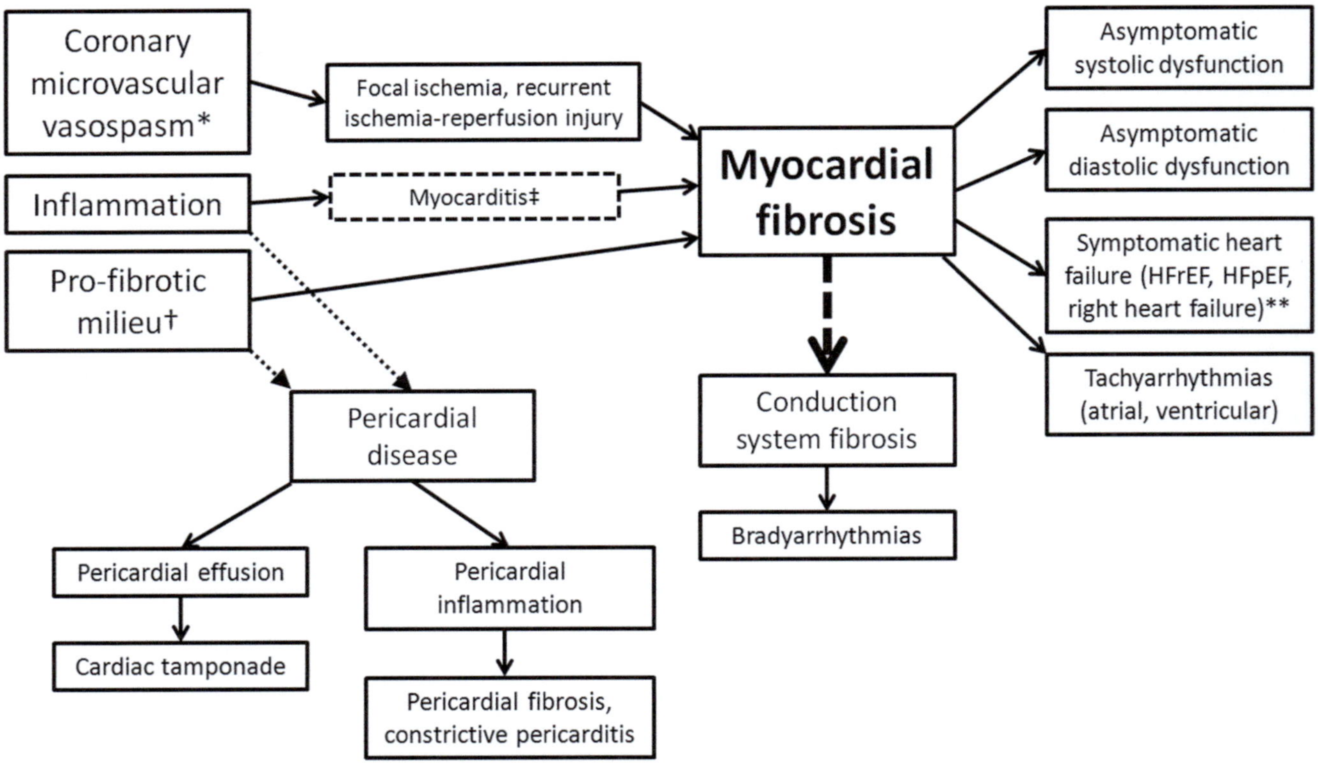

Fig. 22.1 Schematic diagram of primary cardiac manifestations of systemic sclerosis. *Coronary microvascular vasospasm may directly induce asymptomatic (or symptomatic) systolic and diastolic dysfunction and tachyarrhythmias. †Factors such as TGF-β1 and reactive oxygen species [191, 192]; ‡clinically active myocarditis can occur but is uncommon and typically associated with myositis; anecdotal reports of common "low-grade" cardiac inflammation have been reported [3] but there are no systematic studies which corroborate this observation; ***HFrEF* heart failure with reduced LV ejection fraction, *HFpEF* heart failure with preserved LV ejection fraction

Intrinsic Myocardial Disease: Myocardial Fibrosis and Microvascular Ischemia

Direct myocardial involvement in SSc often involves a combination of myocardial ischemia and fibrosis. As in other organs involved in SSc, there is a complex interplay between microvascular disease, possible low-grade inflammation, and the ultimate development of fibrosis, which is the hallmark of SSc-related myocardial disease.

Pathophysiology

In patients with SSc, the primary problem which ultimately leads to cardiac fibrosis and ventricular dysfunction is an abnormality of the coronary microcirculation, including vasospasm and recurrent ischemia–reperfusion injury [1, 4, 9]. There are several lines of evidence which support the conclusion that the microcirculation, and not traditional atherosclerotic coronary disease, is the site of abnormal myocardial blood flow in SSc. Histological examinations have revealed diffuse patchy fibrosis, with contraction band necrosis unrelated to epicardial coronary artery stenosis [25, 26] and concentric intimal hypertrophy associated with fibrinoid necrosis of intramural coronary arteries [27]. SSc cardiac fibrosis can be distinguished from atherosclerotic coronary artery disease because SSc involves the immediate subendocardium, which is usually spared in atherosclerotic heart disease. In addition, hemosiderin deposits are not typically seen in SSc but are found in atherosclerosis [3]. Furthermore, angina pectoris and myocardial infarction have been observed in SSc patients whose epicardial coronary arteries were normal. These findings suggest that extensive microvascular disease can occur in patients with SSc via mechanisms that are independent from atherosclerosis.

Vasospasm of the small coronary arteries and arterioles plays a major role in the early myocardial abnormalities in patients with SSc. These functional and reversible abnormalities were first demonstrated using thallium-201 SPECT; these studies, allowing the assessment of myocardial perfusion, provided evidence of early reversible ischemia. Myocardial perfusion defects in SSc patients were demonstrated either at rest, after exercise, or after cold stimulation [28–32]. Exercise-induced perfusion defects observed by scintigraphy were predictive of developing subsequent cardiac disease or death [33]. As these vasospastic lesions progress, they often lead to recurrent ischemia and reperfusion which leads to myocyte apoptosis and leads to replacement with fibroblasts and collagen deposits as fibrosis ensues.

Besides coronary vasospasm, there is also evidence to implicate impaired coronary vasodilator reserve in patients with SSc. Coronary vasodilator reserve at cardiac catheterization has been investigated in clinically symptomatic SSc patients with the diffuse cutaneous form of the disease [34]: At rest, the mean coronary sinus blood flow was not significantly different compared to control subjects; in contrast, after maximal coronary artery vasodilation with intravenous dipyridamole, the coronary vasodilator reserve was strikingly reduced. All the SSc patients had evidence of established myocardial involvement, confirmed using non-invasive procedures. Their coronary arteriograms were normal; endomyocardial biopsies showed fibrotic tissue and a typical SSc vascular lesion with concentric intimal hypertrophy. These results demonstrated that, despite normal epicardial coronary arteries, structural abnormalities of small coronary arteries or arterioles explained the strikingly reduced coronary reserve. Subsequent studies using contrast enhanced transthoracic Doppler before and after adenosine infusion confirmed the impaired coronary flow reserve in SSc patients without clinical evidence of cardiac involvement [35, 36].

Finally, direct myocardial inflammation can also occur and may cause acute myocarditis with resultant myocardial fibrosis. Myocardial inflammation may be acute or subacute and can result in rapid decline in cardiac function; whether low-grade chronic inflammation is present in SSc and contributes to the generalized fibrotic process and the slow decline of cardiac function in SSc is unknown and has only been reported anecdotally [3]. When severe myocarditis is present, it is often associated with skeletal muscle myositis [3, 37, 38], a finding which may represent a specific subset of SSc patient with an overlap syndrome of SSc and polymyositis.

Clinical Manifestations and Diagnosis

Recurrent vasospasm, poor vasodilator reserve, focal ischemia, and recurrent ischemia–reperfusion injury, and inflammation (when present) all culminate in the same end result: myocardial fibrosis. All of these pathologic insults can lead to the varied clinical manifestations of myocardial disease in SSc, which include asymptomatic LV systolic or diastolic dysfunction (which can occur several years prior to becoming clinically evident) and clinically overt heart failure (Fig. 22.2). Overt heart failure, in turn, can present as acute myocarditis or myopericarditis with a rapid decline in LV ejection fraction; chronic heart failure with reduced ejection fraction (systolic heart failure); or chronic heart failure with preserved ejection fraction (diastolic heart failure). In addi-

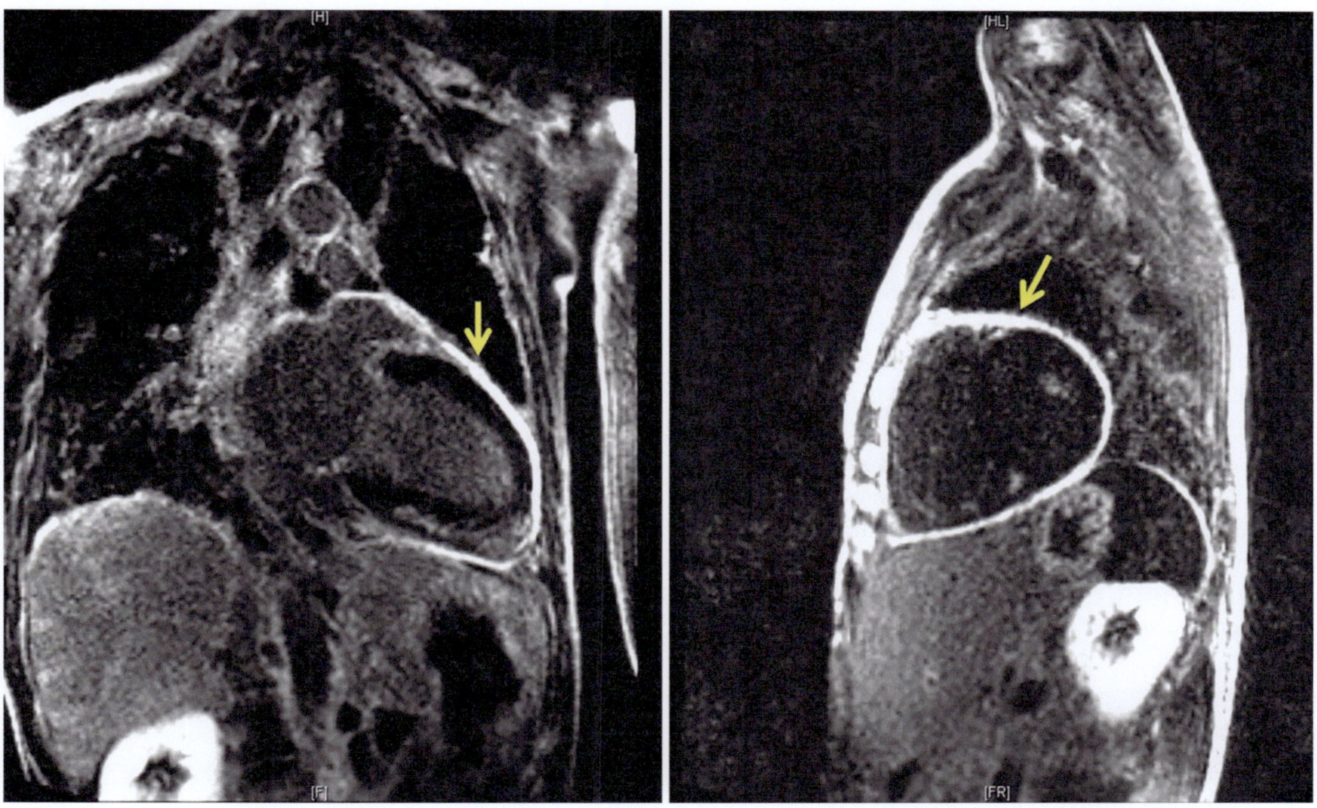

Fig. 22.2 Pericardial enhancement in a patient with diffuse cutaneous systemic sclerosis and constrictive pericarditis. Cardiac magnetic resonance imaging demonstrates intense signal uptake in the pericardium along with pericardial thickening in a 39-year-old man with severe, long-standing diffuse cutaneous systemic sclerosis and right heart failure due to constrictive pericarditis

tion, patients with SSc occasionally develop acute vasospastic crisis, which manifests as severe peripheral and cardiac Raynaud's phenomenon. These patients develop a rapid decline in cardiac output due to ischemia and reduced LV systolic function. This in turn leads to poor perfusion of the extremities, which exacerbates the severe Raynaud's phenomenon and can rapidly lead to digital necrosis if left untreated.

LV Systolic and Diastolic Dysfunction

Several studies, using radionuclide ventriculography, have demonstrated a decreased global LV ejection fraction (LVEF) in a minority of patients, although segmental dysfunction and exercise-induced LV dysfunction are more prevalent [39]. Studies of LV regional wall motion in SSc have shown that 29% of patients have one or more areas of hypokinesis [40]. In SSc patients with diffuse cutaneous disease, the group with thallium defect scores above the median had a significantly lower mean LVEF than the other group and all patients with abnormal resting LVEF had thallium scores above the median [12]. The link between myocardial perfusion abnormalities and dysfunction suggests a similar underlying mechanism for myocardial involvement in SSc. On transthoracic echocardiography, the presence of LVEF <50% has proven to be one of the most powerful predictors of mortality in SSc and has been included in the SCleroderma mOrtality Eustar (SCOpE) score, a tool to predict the risk of death at 3 years in patients with SSc [41].

Several studies have reported on the prevalence of diastolic dysfunction in SSc [42–46] and have shown that diastolic dysfunction is more common in SSc compared to controls [11]. Such abnormalities have been correlated with disease duration [47, 48] and have suggested that impaired diastolic relaxation of the left ventricle together is associated with a defective cardiac functional reserve [42]. Whether LV diastolic dysfunction in SSc is primary or secondary to other cardiac abnormalities is a subject of debate [43, 44]. Importantly, when diastolic dysfunction is present in SSc, it is associated with worse survival [48, 49], underscoring its importance as a marker of cardiac involvement in SSc. In a population study including 275 SSc patients in Norway, the presence of diastolic dysfunction was a strong predictor of death, with a higher hazard ratio than pulmonary hypertension (HR 3.7 [95% CI 1.69–8.14] vs. HR 2.0 [95% CI 1.1–3.9]) [50].

RV Dysfunction

Several studies have demonstrated a primary abnormality of RV function in SSc, independent of pulmonary hypertension [51–59]. A study by Meune et al. focused on cardiac function in 42 SSc patients with normal pulmonary arterial pressure and less than 5 years of disease duration compared to matched controls; radionuclide ventriculography showed that 16 SSc patients had reduced RVEF, three had reduced LVEF, and 10 had reduced peak filling rate, highlighting early RV systolic and left diastolic dysfunction [59]. Moreover, RVEF was correlated with both LVEF and peak filling rate, whereas no correlation was found with either pulmonary function impairment or pulmonary arterial pressure, strongly suggesting intrinsic myocardial involvement in these patients [59]. Others have found abnormalities in RV diastolic function using tissue Doppler imaging [58, 60] and tricuspid annular plane systolic excursion (TAPSE) [57].

Approach to the Patient with Clinical Symptoms or Signs of Possible Myocardial Involvement

In patients with shortness of breath, chest pain, heart failure symptoms, or frequent palpitations or arrhythmias, investigation of direct myocardial involvement is warranted. In these cases, echocardiography with tissue Doppler imaging and natriuretic peptides (BNP or NT-proBNP) can be very helpful as a first step. If microvascular ischemia is suspected, either SPECT or adenosine perfusion cardiac MRI can be performed. If available, we prefer cardiac MRI because of its increased sensitivity, higher spatial resolution, and ability to simultaneously evaluate the RV and pericardium along with LV structure and perfusion. In select cases, coronary angiography, invasive hemodynamic testing, or endomyocardial biopsy can be performed to assist in diagnosis and therapeutic decision-making. Patients who are found to have reduced LV ejection fraction (even if mildly reduced) should be monitored very closely for the possibility of acute vasospastic crisis or acute myocarditis since these can be life-threatening conditions.

Management

In SSc, treatment of direct myocardial involvement varies by clinical manifestation. The most well-studied has been treatment of microvascular ischemia, although it should be noted that there is a general lack of randomized controlled trials of therapies for cardiac involvement in SSc. Nevertheless, in single-arm, non-blinded studies, several vasodilators have been found to improve perfusion in SSc, further emphasizing the potential role of reversible vasospasm of the small coronary arteries. After intravenous administration of dipyridamole [61], as well as after treatment with nifedipine [62], nicardipine [63], or captopril [64], improved myocardial perfusion has been demonstrated in SSc patients using thallium-201 SPECT. Some myocardial perfusion defects were reversible, whereas others remained fixed, suggesting the co-existence of ischemic (functional) lesions accessible to reperfusion after relief of small coronary artery vasospasm and irreversible (fixed) lesions due to organic vessel disease or myocardial fibrosis [65]. The beneficial effect of nifedipine on myocardial perfusion and metabolism in SSc patients was also demonstrated using positron emission tomography

[66]; nifedipine caused a significant increase in 38K myocardial uptake, a significant decrease in 18FDG myocardial uptake, and a significant increase in the myocardial 38K/18FDG ratio, indicating improvement in both myocardial perfusion and myocardial metabolism. Nifedipine-induced improvement was confirmed using cardiac MRI, with a mean 38% increase of the global perfusion index and a significant decrease in the number of SSc patients with more than one segmental perfusion defect [67]. Similar results were observed using cardiac MRI for the assessment of the beneficial effect of bosentan, an oral dual endothelin receptor antagonist, on myocardial perfusion in SSc patients [68]. These findings suggest a major role for vasodilators in treating and preventing progression of microvascular disease in SSc.

The beneficial effect of vasodilators on ventricular dysfunction has also been demonstrated. Nicardipine was shown to acutely improve global LVEF and segmental abnormalities [69]. Improvements in both LVEF and RVEF after oral treatment with nicardipine and a correlation between improvement in LVEF and RVEF were demonstrated [59]. These results provide further evidence for the same pathogenic pathway, with reversible vasospastic small coronary artery disease inducing segmental and global cardiac dysfunction. Nifedipine significantly increased segmental (posterior wall) systolic and diastolic strain rates [67]. As peak systolic and early diastolic strain rates are respective markers of regional contractility and diastolic function, this study strongly suggested that nifedipine improved intrinsic myocardial properties; strain rate determined by tissue Doppler echocardiography is less load-dependent than other methods [70], and the afterload estimated by the systolic blood pressure heart rate product did not change significantly after nifedipine [67]. These results, together with the increased perfusion shown by MRI, suggested that an increase in myocardial perfusion might be the main determinant in the observed increased contractility, highlighting the global intrinsic beneficial effects of vasodilators such as nifedipine.

Thus, the beneficial effects of vasodilators, such as calcium channel blockers mostly of dihydropyridine type, angiotensin-converting enzyme inhibitors, and endothelin receptor antagonist, have been demonstrated in SSc patients, inducing a striking improvement in the early vasospastic reversible component of the "primary" SSc myocardial disease. The possibility of long-term beneficial effects of calcium channel blockers was demonstrated in a large series of 7073 SSc patients: Age, male gender, digital ulcerations, myositis, and lung involvement were independently associated with increased prevalence of LV dysfunction; in contrast, calcium channel blocker use appeared to be protective (odds ratio 0.41; 95% confidence interval 0.22–0.74) [7]. Although these data are highly promising, it should be noted that the aforementioned study was observational and therefore cannot prove a cause-and-effect relationship between calcium channel blocker use and reduction in incidence of LV dysfunction. Currently, vasodilators such as calcium channel blockers remain the best studied and validated for established myocardial disease in SSc, and given the aforementioned data can be considered for preventive therapy as well. It is unknown whether immunosuppressive therapy for myocardial disease is beneficial outside the realm of myocarditis (discussed below) or whether anti-fibrotic therapies will be beneficial based on available data. Dihydropyridine calcium channel blockers (e.g., amlodipine, nifedipine) have minimal negative inotropic effect and are generally well tolerated except for reflex tachycardia and lower extremity edema in some patients. All systemic vasodilators, including calcium channel blockers, should be used with caution in patients with severe pulmonary arterial hypertension because they can lead to severe systemic hypotension.

In SSc patients with overt LV systolic dysfunction (i.e., LVEF <40%), we advocate treatment with neurohormonal blockade given the beneficial effects of this therapeutic strategy in other forms of LV systolic dysfunction. ACE inhibitors or angiotensin receptor blockers are first-line treatments for SSc-associated LV systolic dysfunction given their utility in other manifestations of SSc (e.g., Raynaud's phenomenon, scleroderma renal disease). Beta-blockers can also be used, but we recommend the use of carvedilol given its combined beta- and alpha-blocking effects, which may help prevent exacerbation of Raynaud's phenomenon with other, more selective beta-blockers such as metoprolol. Mineralocorticoid receptor antagonists, such as spironolactone or eplerenone, can also be used in these patients.

In patients with acute myocarditis or myopericarditis, administration of immunosuppressive medications has been reported to improve LV ejection fraction and reduction in clinical symptoms [37, 71, 72]. Intravenous cyclophosphamide and corticosteroids have been used in this scenario, and a recent case series of myocarditis in SSc highlighted the importance of early diagnosis for successful treatment [72]. In patients with acute vasospastic crisis with myocardial involvement, urgent hospitalization (typically in an intensive care unit setting) and evaluation should be undertaken. These patients can have reduced LV ejection fraction and frequent arrhythmias along with worsening peripheral vasoconstriction. Unfortunately, there are little data on optimal treatment for this rare but life-threatening clinical scenario. Intravenous vasodilators, such as nitroprusside, may be useful to treat both LV systolic dysfunction and vasospasm; calcium channel blockers and ACE inhibitors can also be helpful in this situation. Intravenous prostacyclin has been used for acute worsening of peripheral vasoconstriction to prevent digital necrosis [73]; however, prostacyclins should be used with caution in patients with symptomatic heart failure due to LV systolic dysfunction because of their association with increased mortality in this patient population [74].

Coronary Artery Disease

Although coronary microvascular disease, and not epicardial coronary artery disease, has been thought to be the primary coronary manifestation of SSc, a prior study found that coronary artery calcium scores were higher in SSc compared to controls [75]. Subsequent studies, including a national cross-sectional cohort study and a systematic review with meta-analysis, found that coronary heart disease is more prevalent in SSc despite a lower number of cardiovascular risk factors in SSc compared to non-SSc controls [76, 77]. More recently, data from Danish administrative registries, including 2778 SSc patients, demonstrated an association between SSc diagnosis and a higher risk of developing myocardial infarction (HR 2.08 [95% CI 1.65–2.64]), ischemic stroke (HR 1.28 [95% CI 1.04–1.58]), and peripheral vascular disease (HR 5.73 [95% CI 4.63–7.09]). In this study, there was a higher prevalence of hypertension, treated dyslipidemia, and diabetes mellitus in patients with SSc compared to controls [78]. Given the findings of these studies, the mechanistic relationships between atherosclerosis, epicardial coronary artery disease, and coronary microvascular dysfunction in SSc require further investigation and exploration. Nevertheless, clinicians should have a low threshold to screen for atherosclerotic cardiovascular disease when caring for SSc patients.

Pericardial Disease

Patients with SSc can develop a range of complications due to pericardial disease, including pericardial inflammation, fibrinous pericarditis, fibrous pericarditis, pericardial effusion, pericardial adhesions, cardiac tamponade, and constrictive pericarditis [3]. Although rarely symptomatic, when significant pericardial disease is present, it can cause considerable morbidity in patients with SSc. The pathophysiology of pericardial disease in SSc is not well known.

Pericardial effusion is common in SSc and often asymptomatic. At autopsy, the prevalence of pericardial involvement has been reported to be as high as 78%; however, clinically symptomatic pericardial disease is only present in 5–16% [3, 79, 80]. Although pericardial abnormalities can often be detected in SSc, the presence of pericardial effusion should not be ignored because it can be a clue to impending scleroderma renal crisis and it can be seen in patients with pulmonary arterial hypertension. In patients with idiopathic pulmonary arterial hypertension, the presence of a pericardial effusion has been associated with poor prognosis [81–83], the mechanism thought to be one of impaired lymphatic drainage of pericardial fluid due to elevated right atrial pressure. In SSc patients with pulmonary arterial hypertension who have pericardial effusion, the etiology could be SSc, pulmonary arterial hypertension, or both. Regardless of the etiology, drainage of the pericardial effusion should be avoided in patients with pulmonary arterial hypertension [3]. In patients with SSc but no pulmonary arterial hypertension, the decision to drain the effusion should be made on a case-by-case basis but is generally reserved for patients who have developed life-threatening cardiac tamponade [84]. If symptoms of heart failure are present and can be attributed to the pericardial effusion, gentle diuresis is warranted.

Constrictive pericarditis is a syndrome that often presents as right-side heart failure, shortness of breath, fatigue, anorexia, and wasting. It can be difficult to diagnose in patients with SSc who are susceptible to both constriction (due to pericardial involvement) and restriction (due to myocardial involvement with fibrosis) [85, 86]. Thus, differentiation typically requires a multi-modality approach, including echocardiography, simultaneous RV and LV invasive hemodynamics, and cardiac MRI or CT [86]. Factors which increase the likelihood of constrictive pericarditis in SSc include diastolic septal bounce with increased respiratory variation in mitral inflow and preserved (or increased) tissue Doppler e' velocity, on echocardiography [87]; discordance of peak LV and RV pressures at peak inspiration on invasive hemodynamic testing [85], normal (or near-normal) BNP or NT-proBNP [88], and enhanced and/or thickened pericardium on cardiac MRI (see example, Fig. 22.2) or cardiac CT. Some patients with SSc will simultaneously have both constrictive and restrictive physiology, which can be very difficult to manage since pericardial stripping will not be beneficial and could result in severe morbidity or death in this situation. In these cases (and in patients in whom comorbidities preclude the possibility of pericardial stripping), intensive management with diuretics and sodium/fluid restriction will be essential in limiting symptoms and preserving quality of life.

Conduction Disease and Arrhythmias

Arrhythmias are frequent in SSc and have been reviewed in detail recently by Vacca et al. [89] Fibrosis of the conduction system disease can occur in SSc, and its relationship to myocardial fibrosis is variable [90]. When conduction system fibrosis occurs, it most commonly involves the sinoatrial node [91], though conduction system abnormalities in SSc are rarely symptomatic [92]. However, patients with SSc can develop palpitations, syncope, and even sudden death. Thus, recognition and identification of brady- and tachyarrhythmias is essential. Several ECG abnormalities have been reported in SSc, including P-wave notching, nonspecific ST-T wave abnormalities, right or left ventricular hypertrophy, and low voltage QRS, along with other abnormalities such as increased QT dispersion and decreased heart rate variability (a marker of autonomic dysfunction) summarized in detail by Lubitz et al. [92] A recent study found that abnormal spatial QRS-T angle, a marker of ventricular repolarization, predicts life-threatening ventricular arrhythmias in SSc [93]. Electrocardiographic abnormalities are also predictive of survival, although it is unclear whether these changes reflect overall disease burden or contribute to morbidity and mortality.

As opposed to the relatively low incidence of symptomatic conduction system disease and bradyarrhythmias, ventricular and supraventricular arrhythmias are common [3, 92, 94]. Up to two-thirds of patients have documented premature ventricular contractions (PVCs), and the prevalence of non-sustained ventricular tachycardia ranges from 7% to 30% [95]. Advanced age and SSc disease burden, and possibly extent of lung involvement, have been associated with arrhythmic burden. Unfortunately, there are very limited data on the use of SSc-specific therapies, vasodilators, anti-arrhythmics, or devices such as pacemakers or defibrillators in patients with SSc, which makes determining the best course of treatment difficult [92].

Based on available data for cardiac electrophysiologic abnormalities in SSc, we recommend screening for arrhythmias using ambulatory Holter or event monitoring in patients with symptoms of palpitations, lightheadedness, dizziness, or syncope. Exercise treadmill ECG testing can help identify arrhythmias that are exertional in nature. If arrhythmias are identified, they should be correlated to cardiac imaging (echocardiography) and given the lack of SSc-specific studies for treatment of arrhythmias, therapy should follow current treatment guidelines such as those available from the American Heart Association and European Society of Cardiology.

Cardiac Complications of Systemic Sclerosis Therapies

Some drugs used in the treatment of SSc have adverse cardiovascular effects which should be considered when treating patients with SSc. Of the drugs used to treat SSc, the ones with the best studied and most often reported adverse cardiac effects include cyclophosphamide [96] and hydroxychloroquine [97]. Cyclophosphamide-induced cardiac toxicity is uncommon when used at non-myeloablative doses for the treatment of SSc. However, cyclophosphamide can be associated with LV or RV systolic dysfunction at high doses, which are used prior to stem cell transplantation (which has been used to treat patients with SSc [98, 99]). Older age and an abnormal LV or RV ejection fraction prior to high-dose cyclophosphamide are known risk factors for the development of ventricular dysfunction and subsequent symptomatic heart failure. In rare cases, cyclophosphamide has been associated with the development of hemorrhagic myopericarditis [100], which can be variably associated with pericardial effusion and cardiac tamponade, and typically occurs early on after administration of the drug.

Although there are little data to support the use of hydroxychloroquine in SSc, some patients with SSc are nonetheless prescribed hydroxychloroquine as a treatment for symptomatic control of joint pain and arthritis. Despite a lack of studies for its use in SSc, there has been a report in the literature of restrictive cardiomyopathy associated with hydroxychloroquine in a patient with SSc [101], a complication which has been well-described in the literature in patients with other rheumatologic diseases such as rheumatoid arthritis and systemic lupus erythematosus who are often prescribed the drug. Hydroxychloroquine cardiotoxicity typically presents as symptomatic heart failure; however, it can also be associated with conduction system disease. If suspected, hydroxychloroquine toxicity can be diagnosed by endomyocardial biopsy, which shows vacuolization of myocytes on light microscopy and myelin figures and megamitochondria on electron microscopy [97, 101].

Aside from cyclophosphamide and hydroxychloroquine, imatinib mesylate and autologous stem cell transplantation are experimental therapies for SSc that can adversely affect the heart. Cardiotoxicity and severe heart failure have been reported in cancer patients treated with imatinib mesylate [102, 103]. Cardiotoxicity may be enhanced or more common in SSc patients treated with imatinib and related compounds given their anti-angiogenic effects. Although stem cell transplantation itself most likely does not cause cardiotoxicity, myeloablative doses of cyclophosphamide used prior to stem cell transplantation can result in cardiac toxicity (as described above), and patients with pre-existing cardiac dysfunction are at increased risk for morbidity and mortality with stem cell transplantation [98, 104]. Thus, prior to stem cell transplantation, careful screening is mandatory (typically with echocardiography, cardiac MRI, and cardiac catheterization) to exclude LV or RV dysfunction, pulmonary arterial hypertension, or significant pericardial disease [98, 105].

Tools for the Assessment of Cardiac Dysfunction in Systemic Sclerosis

Serum Biomarkers

Several biomarkers have been studied in SSc to determine their utility in diagnosing cardiac involvement and assisting with the management of SSc patients. Of these, natriuretic peptide and troponin tests have been the most frequently studied in SSc and appear to provide the most diagnostic information.

There are several types of natriuretic peptides, but the two most widely studied types are atrial natriuretic peptide (ANP) and B-type natriuretic peptide (BNP). ANP is primarily secreted by the atria, whereas BNP is primarily secreted by both the left and right ventricles [106]. Both ANP and BNP act to enhance systemic vasodilation, natriuresis, and diuresis via membrane-bound natriuretic peptide receptors, which are coupled to a cyclic GMP-dependent signaling cascade. As opposed to ANP, which is stored in pre-formed granules and can be released with minimal stimuli, BNP is synthesized and requires BNP gene expression. Therefore, BNP is more likely to be elevated after sustained elevation in ventricular wall stress and therefore has become the preferred natriuretic peptide for diagnostic use in the clinical setting. BNP originates from a precursor protein, pre-proBNP, which is cleaved into proBNP_{1-108} and then further cleaved into the biologically active BNP_{1-32} and the biologically inert amino-terminal (NT)-proBNP. Current commercial BNP assays measure both BNP_{1-108} and BNP_{1-32}, whereas NT-proBNP assays measure only NT-proBNP [107, 108].

BNP and NT-proBNP were initially studied as biomarkers for the identification of pulmonary hypertension in SSc patients. However, it is well known that BNP and NT-proBNP can increase not only in the setting of RV dysfunction (e.g., in pulmonary hypertension) but also in LV systolic dysfunction, LV diastolic dysfunction, and myocardial ischemia [107, 108]. Thus, natriuretic peptides may be better utilized as a screen for overall cardiac involvement in SSc as opposed to simply screening for pulmonary hypertension [109]. Indeed, in a study of 69 consecutive patients, Allanore and colleagues found that NT-proBNP diagnosed overall cardiac involvement (either LV systolic dysfunction, RV systolic dysfunction, or elevated pulmonary artery pressure) with an excellent area under the curve of 0.94 (95% CI 0.87–0.99) on receiver operator characteristic (ROC) analysis [110]. These authors additionally found that an NT-proBNP cutoff of 125 pg/mL (well within the "normal" range in non-SSc patients [107]) was optimal for the detection of cardiac involvement in SSc.

BNP vs. NT-proBNP in SSc

Most studies to date in SSc have examined NT-proBNP [109–119]. The main theoretical advantage to NT-proBNP is its longer half-life and increased stability [107]. However, since NT-proBNP is not cleared by the natriuretic peptide clearance receptor and is primarily excreted by the kidneys, renal dysfunction is more likely to cause higher NT-proBNP levels with less of an effect on BNP. In a single-center study, Cavagna and colleagues compared the utility of BNP and NT-proBNP for the diagnosis of pulmonary arterial hypertension in SSc and found that although pulmonary artery pressure correlated with both BNP and NT-proBNP, the former was slightly superior to the latter with higher area under the ROC curve (0.74 vs. 0.63, respectively) [120]. Furthermore, only BNP (and not NT-proBNP) was independently associated with pulmonary arterial hypertension diagnosis. Nonetheless, at the present time, there is insufficient data to determine whether one type of natriuretic peptide is superior to another in the diagnosis of cardiovascular disease in SSc. Given the importance of early identification of cardiovascular disease in SSc, either BNP or NT-proBNP should be used routinely in patients with SSc, as outlined below.

Practical Use of Natriuretic Peptides in Patients with SSc

Based on available studies, it appears that either BNP or NT-proBNP can be used in SSc for screening, diagnosis, and prognosis. As compared to the general population, it is also apparent that lower thresholds for BNP and NT-proBNP should be used to signify possible cardiovascular involvement in the patient with SSc. Levels of BNP >60 pg/mL or NT-proBNP >125 pg/mL should alert the clinician that there is potential for cardiovascular involvement in SSc. However, it should be noted that both cardiac and non-cardiac conditions can influence natriuretic peptide levels (Table 22.2), and these should be taken into consideration when interpreting results of BNP

Table 22.2 Factors which can influence natriuretic peptide levels

Factors associated with increased NP levels
LV systolic or diastolic dysfunction
RV systolic or diastolic dysfunction
Acute coronary syndrome
Valvular heart disease
Atrial arrhythmias (atrial fibrillation)
Pulmonary arterial hypertension and pulmonary venous hypertension
Interstitial lung disease if associated pulmonary hypertension
Pulmonary embolism
Older age
Female gender
Weight loss and cachexia
Renal insufficiency
Sepsis/critical illness
Anemia
High-output state (e.g., cirrhosis)
Glucocorticoids and excess cortisol levels
Hyperthyroidism
Malignancies
CNS injury (e.g., stroke and subarachnoid hemorrhage)
Factors associated with normal or decreased NP levels
Obesity
Constrictive pericarditis
Flash pulmonary edema
Cardiac medications (ACE inhibitors, ARBs, beta-blockers, diuretics, and spironolactone)

NP natriuretic peptides (i.e., BNP or NT-proBNP), *LV* left ventricle, *RV* right ventricle, *ACE* angiotensin-converting enzyme, *ARB* angiotensin receptor blocker. Data presented in table derived from literature on natriuretic peptides [106, 108, 196–198]

(or NT-proBNP) testing in SSc. Finally, when screening or diagnosing pulmonary hypertension in SSc, natriuretic peptides will likely perform best when coupled with other non-invasive data such as pulmonary artery systolic pressure and right ventricular function on echocardiography, and carbon monoxide diffusing capacity on pulmonary function testing.

Cardiac troponins have been studied extensively in the setting of coronary and non-coronary causes of myocyte necrosis. An initial small study found that cardiac troponin T was not elevated in patients with SSc [121]. However, a larger study (n = 161 SSc patients, n = 213 controls) that measured high-sensitivity troponin T (hsTnT) found that hsTnT levels were higher in SSc compared to controls and were associated with diffuse cutaneous SSc and pulmonary arterial hypertension [122]. If troponin is elevated in a patient with SSc, other potential causes include myopericarditis or non-SSc cardiovascular disease such as acute coronary syndrome or pulmonary embolism.

Echocardiography

Echocardiography, including Doppler and tissue Doppler imaging, serves a critical role in the assessment of cardiac involvement in SSc by providing information on cardiac structure, systolic dysfunction, diastolic dysfunction, pericardial disease, valvular disease, right ventricular function, and pulmonary hypertension. Many patients with SSc undergo routine annual screening with echocardiography. Routine echocardiographic measurements in SSc include left ventricular dimensions and volumes (including ejection fraction) and wall thickness (for assessment of hypertrophy); Doppler echocardiography for the evaluation of stenotic and regurgitant valvular lesions; identification of pericardial effusion; and estimation of pulmonary artery systolic pressure. Although these routine assessments are important, several newer echocardiographic techniques such as tissue Doppler imaging and right ventricular quantification are available and should be utilized in all patients with SSc.

Tissue Doppler Imaging

The assessment of myocardial tissue velocities using the Doppler technique has provided immense insight into longitudinal function of the heart. Since the heart is composed of longitudinal, circumferential, and radial fibers, global indices (such as ejection fraction) do not capture the full extent of myocardial dysfunction, especially in patients who have subclinical cardiac involvement. Because subendocardial fibers, which are mostly longitudinal in orientation, are most susceptible to microvascular ischemia, longitudinal systolic and diastolic dysfunction are often the earliest signs of cardiac impairment in SSc. By using a modified Doppler technique to identify low-velocity, high-amplitude signals found in myocardial tissue (as opposed to high-velocity, low-amplitude signals generated by red blood cells during traditional Doppler evaluation of blood flow), tissue Doppler imaging is able to measure longitudinal tissue velocities. Typically, velocities are measured at the septal and lateral mitral annulus. Waves generated include isovolumic contraction, systolic longitudinal velocity (S'), isovolumic relaxation, early diastolic longitudinal velocity (e'), and late (atrial) diastolic longitudinal velocity (a') (Fig. 22.3) [123]. Of these, S' can be used to identify early, subclinical LV systolic dysfunction in patients with SSc, whereas e' is critically important as a marker of LV diastolic dysfunction, particularly impaired relaxation. In addition, in patients with undifferentiated connective tissue disease at risk for SSc, tissue Doppler imaging has been able to reveal a mild impairment of LV and RV diastolic and systolic function [124]. The advent of tissue Doppler imaging has revolutionized the assessment of diastolic dysfunction because of the difficulties encountered with traditional Doppler mitral inflow imaging. Virtually, all traditional Doppler imaging indices, including transmitral E and A waves, E/A ratio, pulmonary venous flow, and early mitral deceleration time, suffer from a bimodal distribution during the progression from normal to abnormal [125]. For example, in normals, E/A ratio is elevated. As diastolic dysfunction ensues, E/A ratio reversal occurs and decreases to below 0.8 due to impaired LV relaxation. However, as diastolic dysfunction worsens, left atrial pressure rises and E/A ratio normalizes. Thus, mitral inflow and pulmonary venous flow patterns in normal and moderate ("pseudonormal") diastolic dysfunction can appear similar. Tissue Doppler e' has the advantage of decreasing linearly with worsening diastolic function and therefore can be used to differentiate normal diastolic function from moderate or severe diastolic dysfunction. Tissue Doppler e' velocity does decrease with normal aging, so the age of the patient must be considered when interpreting e' velocity and diastolic function in general. Fortunately, age-specific cutoffs for abnormal e' velocity exist [125, 126]. Thus, by using age-appropriate cutoffs for tissue Doppler e', one can identify diastolic dysfunction early in the patient with SSc. The presence of clinically significant diastolic dysfunction can be further ascertained by using the 2016 recommendations for the evaluation of left ventricular diastolic function of the American Society of Echocardiography (ASE) and European Association of Cardiovascular Imaging (EACVI). In these guidelines, two separate algorithms were proposed. Algorithm A should be applied to patients with preserved left ventricular ejection fraction (LVEF) (>50%) and unknown diastolic function, primarily for separating patients with normal from those with abnormal diastolic function. The four recommended

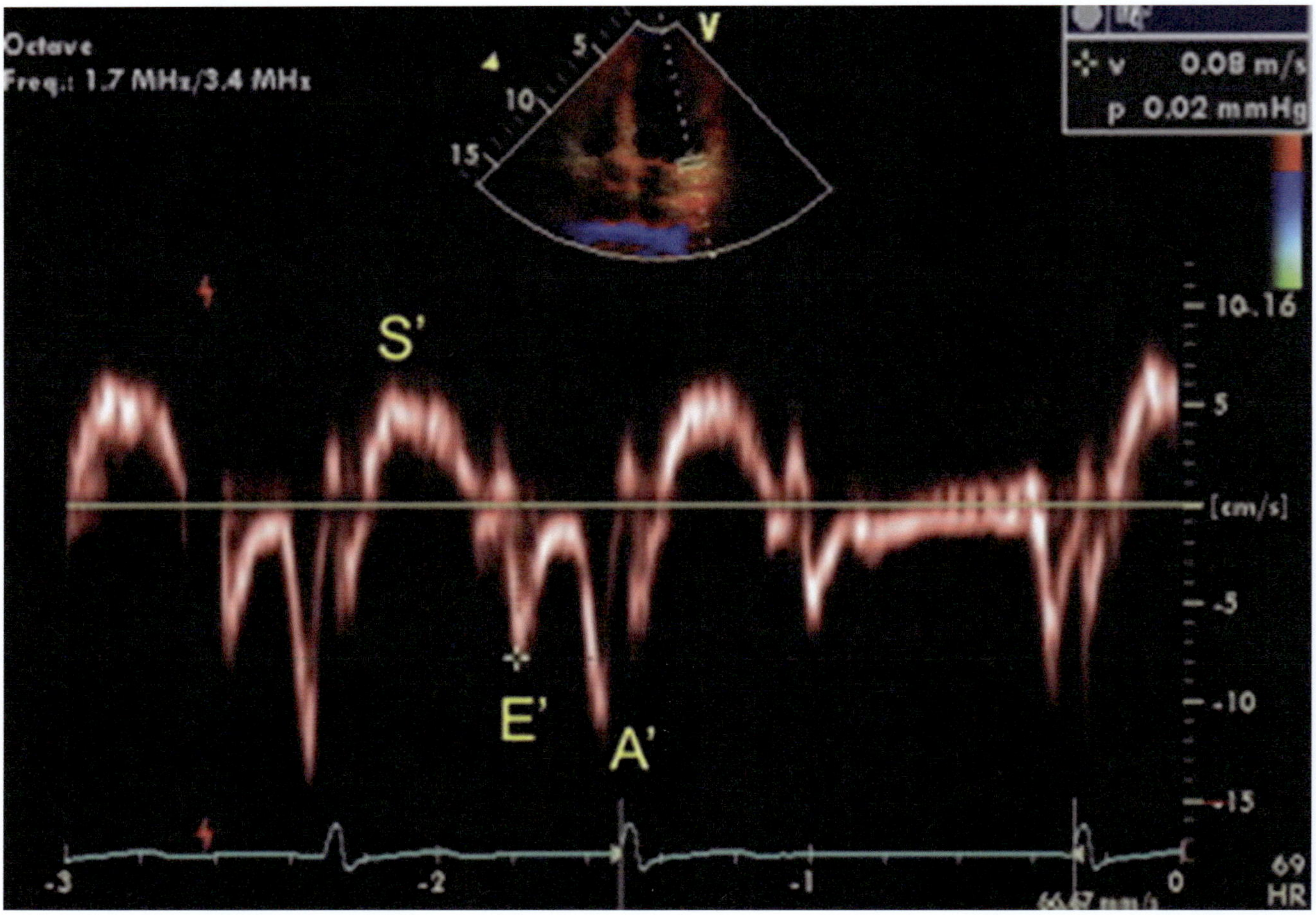

Fig. 22.3 Tissue Doppler imaging of the mitral annulus. *S′* systolic tissue velocity, *E′* early diastolic tissue velocity, *A′* late (atrial) diastolic tissue velocity, *IVC* isovolumic contraction, *IVR* isovolumic relaxation. Systolic and diastolic tissue velocities are decreased in this example of septal (medial) mitral annulus longitudinal tissue Doppler imaging from a 51-year-old woman with long-standing diffuse cutaneous systemic sclerosis

variables and their abnormal cutoff values are (1) *e′* velocity (septal *e′* <7 cm/s and/or lateral *e′* <10 cm/s); (2) *E*/*e′* ratio >14 (average of septal and lateral *E*/*e′* values); (3) left atrial (LA) maximum volume index >34 mL/m^2; and (4) peak tricuspid regurgitation (TR) velocity >2.8 m/s. In this context, LV diastolic function is normal if more than half of the available variables (at least 3) do not meet the cutoff values for identifying abnormal function. Algorithm B should be applied to patients with reduced LVEF (<50%) or with preserved LVEF and known or suspected diastolic dysfunction and is designed for estimating left ventricular (LV) filling pressure and grading diastolic function according to mitral flow velocities, mitral annular *e′* velocity, *E*/*e′* ratio, peak velocity of TR jet, LA maximum volume index, and other supplementary methods [127]. A more simplified approach, proposed by Oh et al., is shown in Fig. 22.4. According to this algorithm, it is possible to determine diastolic filling pressure based on the four parameters (septal *e′*, *E*/*e′*, LA maximum volume index, and TR velocity), regardless of LVEF and known diastolic dysfunction: When three or more are normal, filling pressure is normal, and when three or more are abnormal, filling pressure is elevated. After filling pressure assessment, diastolic grading can be assessed based on *E*/*A* ratio: Normal or grade 1 diastolic function is assigned to the subject with normal filling pressure with *E*/*A* >0.8 and ≤0.8, respectively, and grade 2 or 3 to the group with increased filling pressure with *E*/*A* <2 and ≥2, respectively [128].

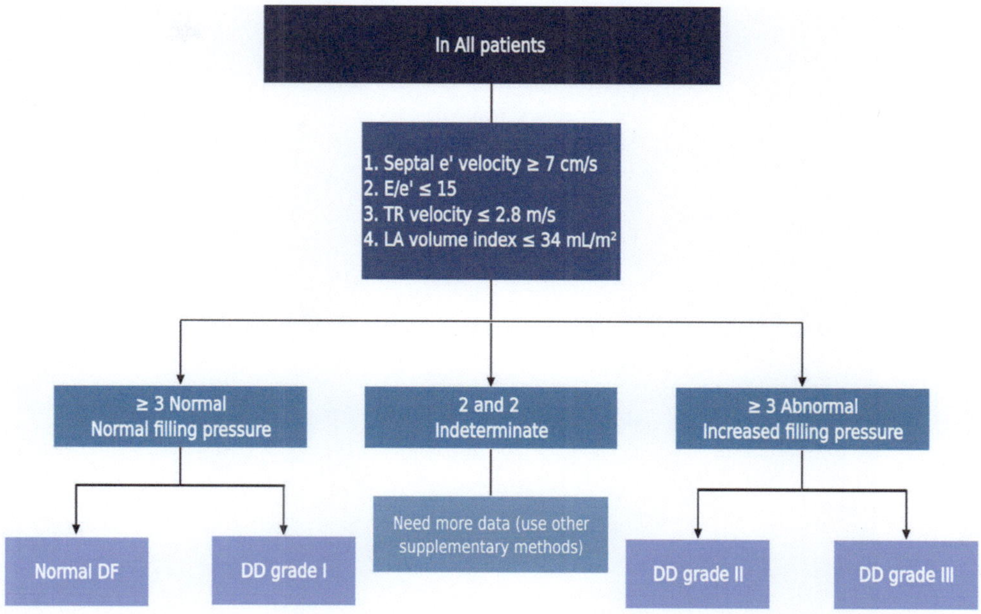

Fig. 22.4 Revised algorithm for assessment of diastolic filling pressure and diastolic function. *TR* tricuspid regurgitation, *LA* left atrium, *DF* diastolic function, *DD* diastolic dysfunction. Based on the four parameters (septal *e'*, *E*/*e'*, LA maximum volume index, and TR velocity), regardless of LVEF and known diastolic dysfunction, we can determine diastolic filling pressure. Diastolic grading can be assessed based on transmitral *E*/*A* ratio. (Revised from Oh et al. 2020 [128])

Right Ventricular Quantification

Although previously considered a passive conduit in the cardiopulmonary system, it is now well known that the right ventricle is extremely important in a wide variety of disease states, including SSc. In SSc, right ventricular dysfunction can be primary (due to direct myocardial involvement) or secondary (due to pulmonary hypertension from pulmonary vascular disease, left ventricular dysfunction, or interstitial lung disease). Thus, careful evaluation of the right ventricle can provide considerable insight into cardiovascular manifestations of SSc. Assessment of the right ventricle by echocardiography has been challenging due to its non-uniform, pyramidal shape [129]. However, advances in echocardiographic RV imaging [130], along with published guidelines for the quantification of the right ventricle [131], now allow for routine evaluation of the RV in SSc. Five parameters (RV fractional area change, TAPSE, tricuspid annular tissue Doppler *S*′, pulmonary artery systolic pressure, and the ratio of tricuspid regurgitant velocity to pulmonary artery velocity time integral [a non-invasive marker of pulmonary vascular resistance]) form the cornerstone of echocardiographic RV assessment in SSc (Figs. 22.5, 22.6, and 22.7). For the last two decades, three-dimensional echocardiography (3DE) has been improving and expanding the diagnostic capabilities of cardiac ultrasound. 3DE has identified relationships between RV volumes and EF to age and gender, which are very similar to those described by CMR [132]. Furthermore, assessment of RV volumes with 3DE overcomes the limitations of conventional two-dimensional echocardiography RV views with respect to orientation and reference point [133]. Accordingly, ASE/EACVI guidelines for cardiac chamber quantification by echocardiography in adults recommend 3DE assessment of RV volumes, in laboratories with experience in 3DE, when knowledge of RV volumes may be clinically important [133].

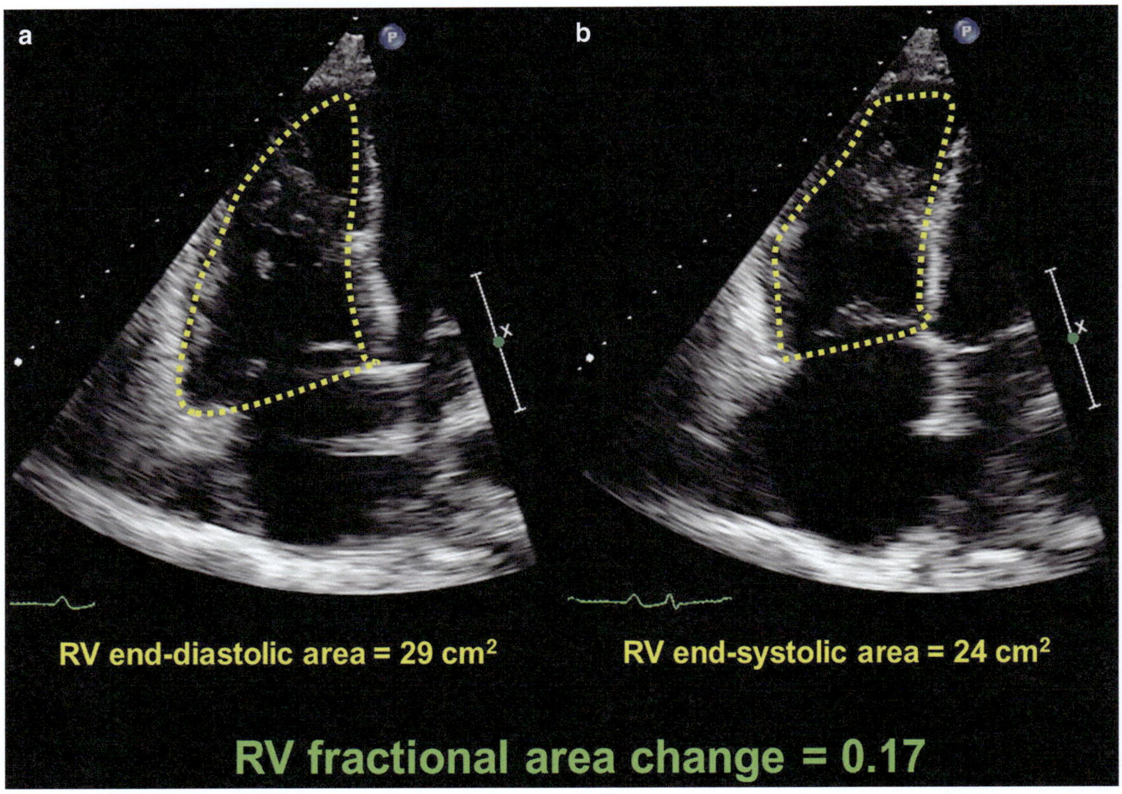

Fig. 22.5 Right ventricular fractional area change. *RV* right ventricle. Right ventricular fractional area change in a 63-year-old woman with limited cutaneous systemic sclerosis and pulmonary arterial hypertension. (**a**) RV end-diastolic area. (**b**) RV end-systolic area. RV fractional area change (= [RV end-diastolic area − RV end-systolic area]/RV end-diastolic area; normal [131] >0.35) is an echocardiographic marker of global RV systolic function

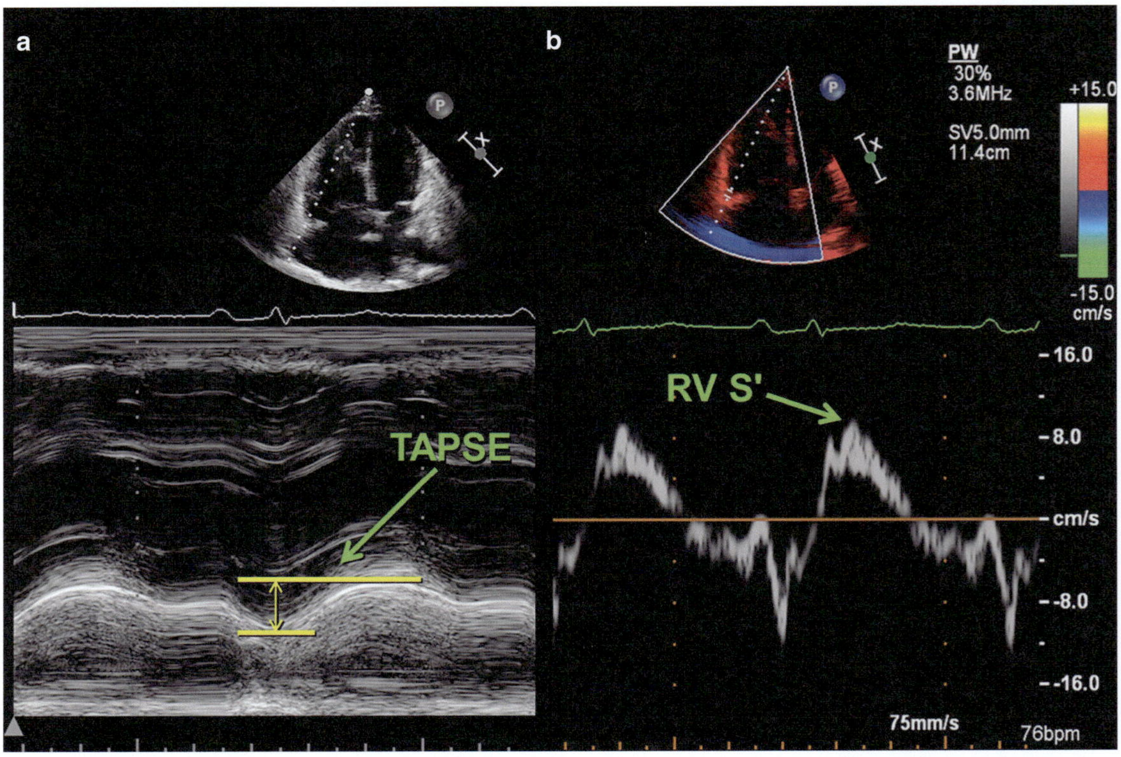

Fig. 22.6 Right ventricular longitudinal systolic function. *TAPSE* tricuspid annular plane systolic excursion (normal [131] >1.6 cm), *RV S′* right ventricular systolic longitudinal tissue Doppler velocity (normal [131] >10 cm/s). Images are from the same patient described in Fig. 22.2. Both TAPSE and RV *S′* are reduced, indicating a decrease in longitudinal RV systolic function. Both TAPSE and RV *S′* can be very useful if the RV is not well visualized or for the diagnosis of early RV dysfunction (prior to the reduction in global RV systolic function). (**a**) TAPSE. (**b**) Tricuspid annular tissue Doppler *S′*

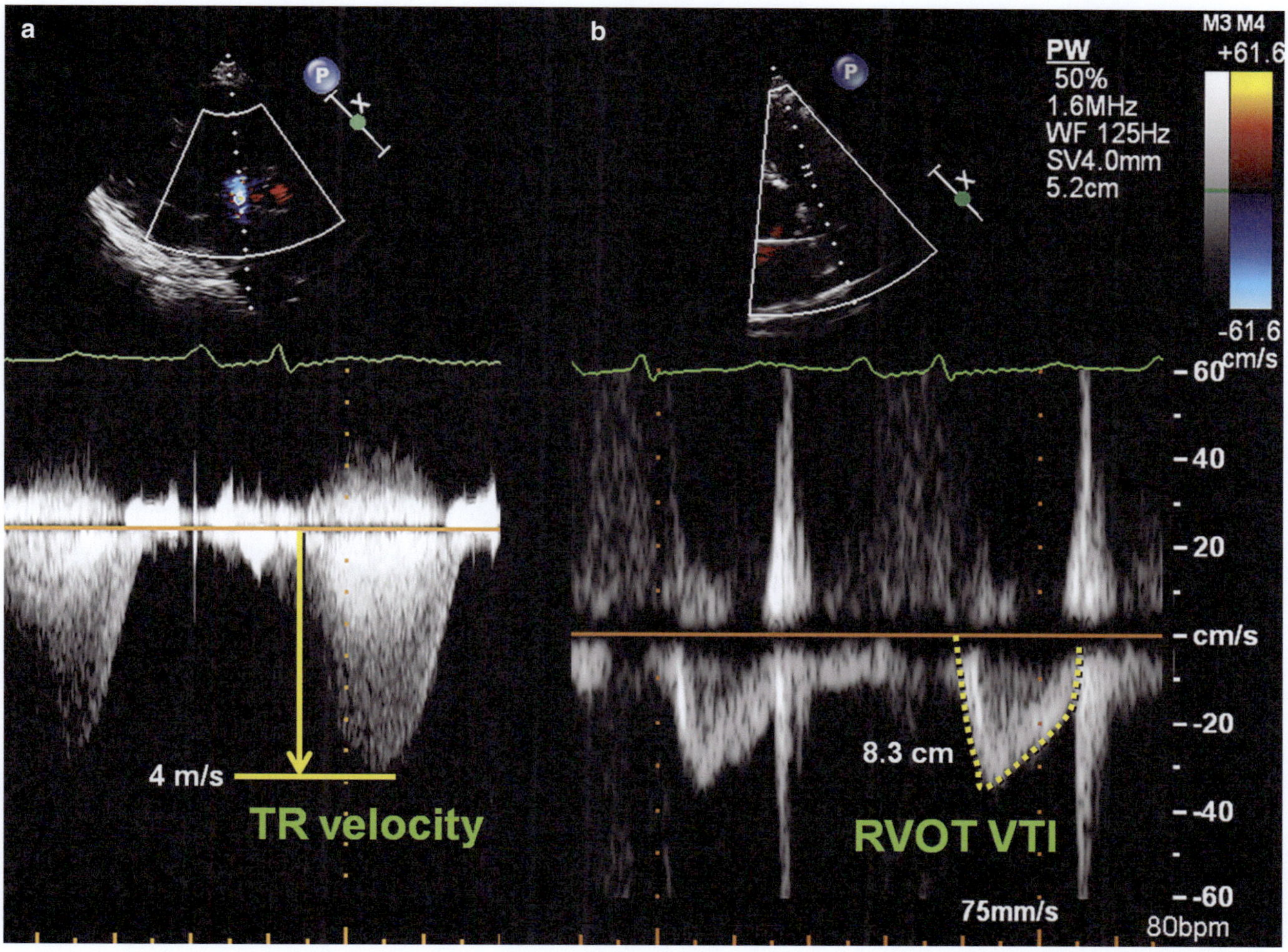

Fig. 22.7 Non-invasive estimation of pulmonary artery systolic pressure and pulmonary vascular resistance. *TR* tricuspid regurgitation, *RVOT VTI* right ventricular outflow tract velocity time integral (a measure of flow). Pulmonary vascular resistance can be estimated from the ratio of TR velocity (Panel **a**) to RVOT VTI (Panel **b**) which can help determine whether RV dysfunction is primary (due to intrinsic RV involvement) or secondary (due to pulmonary hypertension). If RV dysfunction is primary, TR velocity will be low and RVOT VTI will be low (with a normal or near-normal ratio [<0.18] [193]). If RV dysfunction is secondary to pulmonary hypertension, the ratio of TR velocity to RVOT VTI will be high (>0.18) [193]. In this example from the patient described in Figs. 22.2 and 22.3, ratio of TR velocity to RVOT VTI = 0.48; thus, estimated PVR is elevated and indicative of secondary RV dysfunction due to pulmonary hypertension

Nuclear Imaging, Cardiac MRI, and Cardiac Computed Tomography (CT)

Nuclear imaging techniques such as SPECT are currently the most commonly used method for the detection of abnormal myocardial perfusion. As described above, this technique, which relies on both a stressor (e.g., exercise, vasodilator, or cold stimuli in SSc) and an isotope (e.g., thallium-201), has been utilized to investigate myocardial ischemia in SSc [61]. Advances in nuclear imaging techniques, especially the use of positron emission tomography (PET) scanning, allow for enhanced resolution of the heart and may increase sensitivity for detection of microvascular ischemia in SSc [134]. However, detection of subendocardial ischemia by nuclear imaging is limited and inferior to perfusion imaging with cardiac MRI, which is discussed in detail below. Combined cardiac SPECT or PET and cardiac CT overcomes some of these limitations and can offer comprehensive assessment of the heart [135], though it remains to be seen if this type of study will be useful in SSc.

Both cardiac MRI and cardiac CT can provide valuable information on cardiac involvement in SSc. Either technique can be used to evaluation for pericardial disease and is invaluable for this purpose since echocardiography cannot reliably evaluate pericardial thickness and/or inflammation. However, given the frequent use of chest CT for evaluation of lung involvement in SSc, radiation exposure in these patients is not trivial. Therefore, cardiac MRI (which does not involve radiation exposure) may be preferable to cardiac CT.

Besides evaluation of pericardial disease, cardiac MRI is also the gold standard for assessment of cardiac structure given its high spatial resolution [2, 51, 79, 136]. Cardiac

MRI has been investigated in SSc and found to detect cardiac abnormalities with high sensitivity [137–140]. In one study of 52 patients with SSc, 75% had at least one detectable abnormality on cardiac MRI [79]. MRI is the reference standard for detection and quantification of myocardial fibrosis. The preferred imaging time for fibrosis detection is 15–20 min after gadolinium administration, when differences between scar, normal myocardium, and blood pool are maximal; therefore, it is referred to as late gadolinium enhancement (LGE) [141]. On gadolinium-enhanced cardiac MRI images in SSc, if diffuse enhancement is detected, the possibility of infiltrative disease is often entertained. Most often, however, severe diffuse fibrosis of the heart is the cause of the diffuse enhancement (thus the "infiltrative process" is infiltration by fibroblasts and collagen). In a population of 201 patients with SSc (90.5% women; 51 ± 14 years of age) without known SSc-related cardiac involvement, LGE with non-ischemic pattern was observed in 26.1% of patients and was linked to ventricular arrhythmias on ECG monitoring [142]. Furthermore, edema alters myocardial T2-relaxation and can therefore be detected by T2-weighted MRI (T2 ratio) [141]. In the Scleroderma Arrhythmia Clinical Utility Study (SAnCtUS), which enrolled 150 consecutive SSc patients from 8 European centers, %LGE and T2 ratio were significant predictors of ventricular rhythm disturbances, assessed using 24-h ECG monitoring [143]. Traditional vasodilator perfusion cardiac MRI can also reliably detect subendocardial ischemia (Fig. 22.8) by displaying a circumferential loss of perfusion in the subendocardium, a finding that is thought to be due to microvascular disease in SSc [136]. Finally, since evaluation of the RV is difficult using routine echocardiography, cardiac MRI is emerging as a vital technique for evaluation of RV structure and function [51] and may be useful in SSc for the differentiation of primary RV involvement from secondary RV involvement due to pulmonary arterial hypertension. In a cardiac MRI study of 50 SSc patients, Bezante and colleagues found that RV ejection fraction was decreased in SSc compared to controls (47 ± 7% vs. 58 ± 4%; $p < 0.0001$) and lower in diffuse cutaneous SSc when compared to limited cutaneous SSc (44 ± 6% vs. 48 ± 7%; $p = 0.03$) [51].

Cardiac Catheterization

Cardiac catheterization, the gold standard tool for assessment of hemodynamics and epicardial coronary anatomy, is necessary in patients with SSc when the diagnoses of pulmonary arterial hypertension, constrictive pericarditis, cardiac tamponade, or epicardial coronary artery disease are entertained. Cardiac catheterization also offers the opportunity for endomyocardial biopsy which may be necessary in SSc if there is suspicion of infiltrative cardiac disease, side effects of medications (e.g., hydroxychloroquine cardiomyopathy [101]), or active myocarditis [144]. Recent studies have also highlighted the utility of exercise testing at the time of right heart catheterization to determine the cause of unexplained dyspnea in SSc [145, 146]. Using a systematic strategy of identifying SSc patients with exercise-induced elevation in PA systolic pressure on echocardiography,

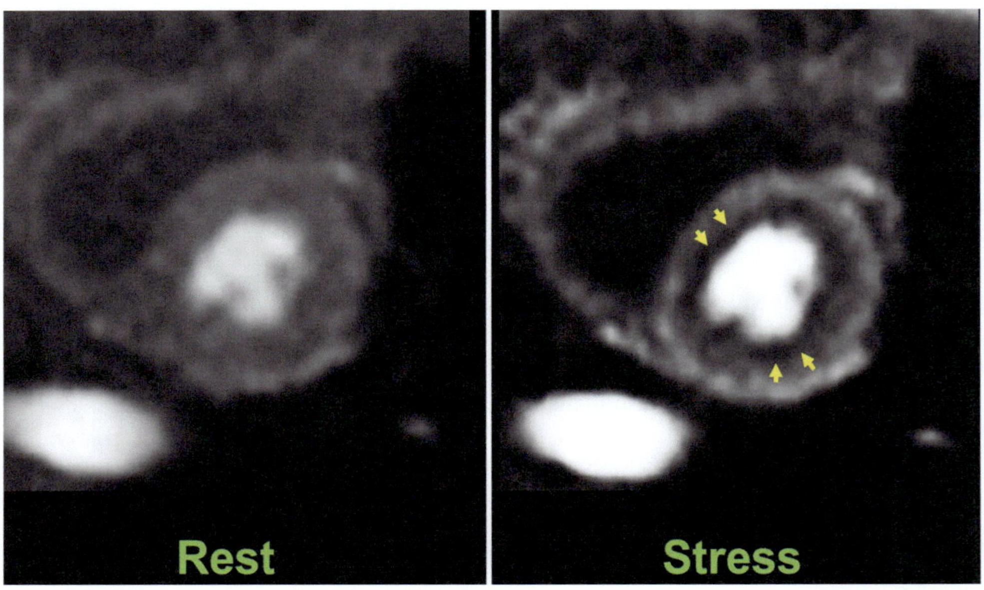

Fig. 22.8 Cardiac magnetic resonance imaging in systemic sclerosis: subendocardial ischemia. Short axis slice through the left ventricle showing subendocardial ischemia (arrows) due to microvascular disease. At rest, there is homogeneous uptake of contrast in the myocardium. At peak stress, the subendocardium is dark circumferentially (arrows), indicating that there is decreased perfusion in this territory (indicative of microvascular ischemia). (MRI images courtesy of Daniel C. Lee, M.D., Northwestern University Feinberg School of Medicine)

Hager et al. were able to demonstrate the ability of exercise invasive hemodynamic testing to differentiate exercise-induced pulmonary arterial hypertension from the much more common exercise-induced pulmonary venous hypertension [elevated pulmonary capillary wedge pressure (PCWP)] due to LV diastolic dysfunction [145]. Accordingly, current recommendations from the Sixth World Symposium on Pulmonary Hypertension (PH) suggest that in patients with PCWP 13–15 mmHg and high/intermediate probability of PH due to heart failure with preserved ejection fraction (HFpEF), provocative testing should be considered to uncover PH due to diastolic dysfunction [147]. However, for technical reasons and reliability of pressure recording, a fluid challenge can be preferred over exercise [147]. In a population including 25 SSc patients without PAH and 25 controls, after volume loading with saline infusion of 7 mL/kg over 5–10 min, increases in right atrial pressure (3 ± 1 vs. 2 ± 1 mmHg, $p = 0.03$), mean pulmonary artery pressure (5 ± 1 vs. 3 ± 1 mmHg, $p < 0.001$), and pulmonary capillary wedge pressure (PCWP; 5 ± 2 vs. 3 ± 1 mmHg, $p < 0.001$) were higher in SSc patients than in controls as a result of subclinical left ventricle diastolic dysfunction [148].

Although cardiac catheterization is an invasive procedure, it is minimally invasive and can be performed with minimal risks by experienced operators. Therefore, although it should be used judiciously, cardiac catheterization should not be avoided since it can provide a definitive diagnosis.

Arrhythmia Monitoring

Arrhythmias are common in SSc and can cause significant morbidity [3, 24, 149–151]. Several options are available for monitoring of arrhythmias. In SSc patients with frequent palpitations, 24- or 48-h Holter monitoring is likely to detect the cause of symptoms. However, in patients with less frequent symptoms or in patients with symptoms such as syncope, longer term (typically 30-day) event monitors are typically necessary. Newer devices for arrhythmia detection, such as the Zio patch (which collect electrocardiographic data for up to 14 days) and implantable loop recorders, which can detect arrhythmias indefinitely, are available and may extend the ability to detect arrhythmias in SSc.

Emerging Tools

Emerging tools likely to be included in a near future in the routine cardiac assessment of SSc heart disease include speckle-tracking echocardiography for the evaluation of myocardial strain [152–158], exercise echocardiography for the assessment of left and right ventricle systolic-diastolic reserve and pulmonary vascular reserve [159–162], cardiopulmonary exercise testing for quantification and characterization of exercise intolerance [164–166], MRI T1 mapping for the evaluation of diffuse cardiac fibrosis [167–169], and absolute perfusion cardiac MRI for the evaluation of microvascular coronary ischemia [170].

Speckle-Tracking Echocardiography for Measurement of Myocardial Strain

Although tissue Doppler imaging is widely available, this technique is used primarily for the measurement of tissue velocities. However, because different parts of the myocardium move at different velocities, the heart changes shape during its movement across the cardiac cycle and deformation occurs. Thus, tissue velocities do not tell the entire story of cardiac motion and cardiac mechanics. Myocardial strain is the fractional change in length of a segment of myocardium compared to its original length [152]. Strain is therefore a measure of cardiac deformation that differs from velocity. The fundamentals of strain imaging have been described in detail elsewhere [152, 171, 172]. Based on the association between cardiac fibrosis, circulating markers of fibrosis, and reduced myocardial strains in prior non-SSc studies [173, 174], measurement of strain in SSc may be a valuable tool for the assessment of preclinical myocardial involvement in SSc.

Myocardial strain, which occurs in the radial, circumferential, and longitudinal directions in the heart, is difficult to measure using tissue Doppler techniques because of this technique requires alignment of the Doppler ultrasound beam with the direction of myocardial motion [152, 153, 175]. Speckle-tracking echocardiography, which solves this problem by providing an angle-independent solution for measurement of myocardial deformation, uses a pattern-recognition type of software to follow naturally occurring acoustic markers (ultrasound speckles) throughout the cardiac cycle. Detection of spatial movement of this “fingerprint” (Fig. 22.9a) during the cardiac cycle allows direct calculation of strain (Fig. 22.9b, c). Speckle-tracking echocardiography is possible with commercially available echocardiography machines and thus can be applied to patients with SSc. Cardiac MRI also has the capability of measuring myocardial strain (e.g., MRI tagging technique [176]) and is considered the gold standard for non-invasive assessment of strain given the higher spatial resolution (albeit lower temporal resolution) of cardiac MRI compared with echocardiography. In the past 5 years, several speckle-tracking echocardiography studies in SSc have been published (Table 22.3) [157, 177–183]. These studies demonstrate the power of speckle-tracking echocardiography in detecting subclinical myocardial dysfunction in patients with SSc. This imaging technique has also been proposed as an alternative method of exploring atrial function as reservoir, conduit,

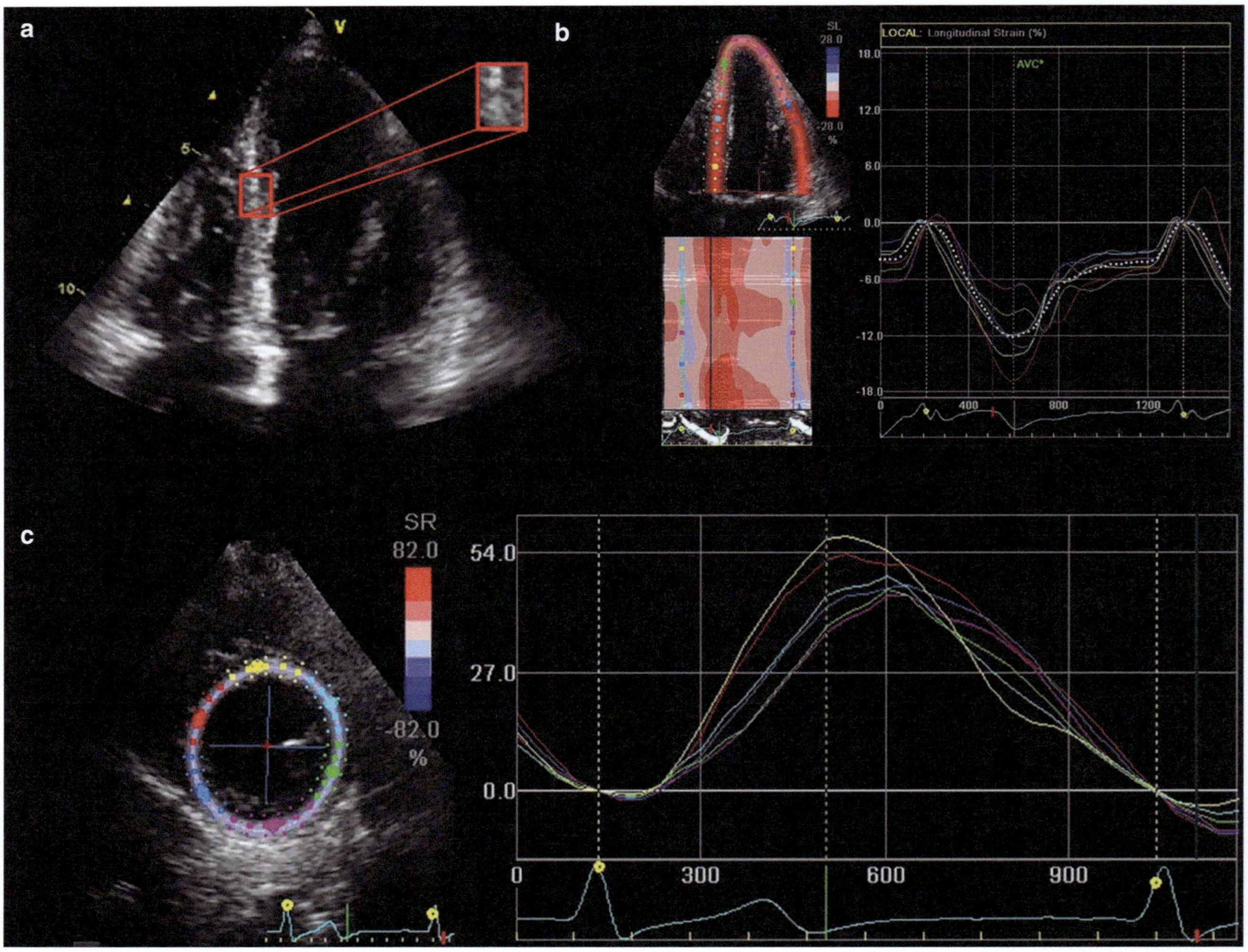

Fig. 22.9 Speckle-tracking echocardiography. (**a**) Speckle-tracking methodology showing "fingerprint" of ultrasound speckles which are tracked over the cardiac cycle. (**b**) Longitudinal and (**c**) radial strain curves from a patient with diffuse cutaneous systemic sclerosis. Note the reduction in peak global longitudinal strain (−12%) with preserved radial strain (+49%) suggestive of early subendocardial cardiac involvement

Table 22.3 Recent speckle-tracking echocardiography studies in systemic sclerosis

First author	Year	Sample size	Primary findings	Clinical implications
Agoston [157]	2014	42 SSc 42 controls	Despite similarly normal LVEF, pulmonary pressures, and left atrial (LA) volumes in SSc patients and controls, patients with SSc had significantly worse LA strain parameters.	Patients with SSc may have intrinsic left atrial dysfunction which can be an early sign of HFpEF
Atas [177]	2015	41 SSc 38 controls	Patients with SSc had had more frequent LV diastolic dysfunction, larger LA volumes, and worse LA strain parameters compared to controls.	
Cadeddu [178]	2015	45 SSc 20 controls	Compared to controls, SSc patients had higher *E*/*e*′ (a marker of LV filling pressures), larger LA volumes, and reduced LV contractile reserve, as assessed by exercise echocardiography with speckle-tracking (reduced global longitudinal strain at peak exercise).	Impaired LV contractile reserve may be reflective of underlying cardiac involvement in SSc and can be detected with speckle-tracking analysis of images obtained during exercise stress echocardiography
Cusma Piccione [179]	2013	29 SSc 30 controls	LV longitudinal and circumferential strains were lower (worse) in SSc compared to controls, and there was a significant correlation between anti-Scl-70 antibodies and longitudinal and circumferential strain parameters in SSc.	Patients with SSc have worse (more impaired) indices of cardiac mechanics compared to controls; these intrinsic abnormalities in myocardial function appear to be more prominent in patients with elevated anti-Scl-70 antibodies
Spethmann [180]	2012	22 SSc 22 controls	LV global longitudinal strain and strain rate were significantly worse in SSc compared to controls, particularly in the basal segments of the LV.	

Table 22.3 (contiuned)

First author	Year	Sample size	Primary findings	Clinical implications
Spethmann [181]	2014	19 SSc	In this pilot study, 19 SSc patients without pulmonary hypertension underwent speckle-tracking echocardiography at baseline and at 2 years of follow-up. LV ejection fraction and diastolic function remained unchanged, but LV global longitudinal strain decreased during follow-up.	LV global longitudinal strain, measured using speckle-tracking echocardiography, may be a sensitive marker of the longitudinal decline in LV function in SSc.
Tigen [182]	2014	53 SSc 26 controls	SSc patients had significantly lower longitudinal, circumferential, and radial LV strain compared to controls. Within the SSc group, 13/53 patients had a fragmented QRS on electrocardiography; SSc patients with a fragmented QRS had lower longitudinal strain values.	A fragmented QRS complex on routine 12-lead electrocardiography may be indicative of abnormal LV mechanics in SSc patients.
Yiu [183]	2011	104 SSc 37 controls	SSc patients had significantly worse LV longitudinal and circumferential strain compared to controls, despite similar LV ejection fraction between the two groups. Within the SSc groups, worse strain parameters correlated with (1) lower peak VO_2 on cardiopulmonary exercise testing and (2) more abnormal findings on 24-h electrocardiography (Holter monitoring).	Abnormal LV longitudinal and circumferential strain, detected by speckle-tracking echocardiography, is a marker of early LV systolic dysfunction in SSc and may underlie exercise intolerance and arrhythmias in these patients.

and pump and to detect early changes in atrial myocardial performance. In 42 SSc patients with normal LVEF and without any significant cardiac abnormalities, speckle-tracking imaging of left atrium demonstrated a reduced reservoir and conduit function compared to healthy controls [157]. Similarly, right atrial function assessed by speckle-tracking imaging was significantly impaired in SSc patients compared to control and presence of subtle right atrial dysfunction was associated with pulmonary fibrosis and with elevated pulmonary artery pressures or reduced left ventricular stroke volume during exercise [158].

Exercise Echocardiography

Exercise Doppler echocardiography can be used to investigate LV systolic and/or diastolic reserve and pulmonary vascular reserve during exertion [159–162]. In patients with SSc, several studies have reported with a high frequency of normal pulmonary arterial pressure at rest but abnormal hemodynamic response during stress, estimated by exercise Doppler echocardiography [160–162]. This high percentage of exercise-induced increase in systolic pulmonary arterial pressure clearly overestimates the subset of patients with SSc who will develop pulmonary arterial hypertension as pulmonary hemodynamic is dependent not only on pulmonary vascular resistance but also on left atrial pressure and cardiac output [160]. For these reasons, current guidelines discourage the clinical classification of exercise-induced pulmonary hypertension (ex-PH) [163]. Nevertheless, there is a growing body of evidence suggesting that ex-PH may represents an important group of high-risk patients requiring close serial monitoring for emerging RV failure and resting PAH [161]. Furthermore, exercise echocardiography represents an important non-invasive tool that allows for assessment of RV contractile reserve, an independent predictor of poor prognosis [161]. Future longitudinal studies are required to determine the utility of exercise echocardiography as a screening tool in patients with SSc at variable risk for PAH, and its prognostic relevance.

Cardiopulmonary Exercise Testing

Cardiopulmonary exercise testing (CPET) allows for a comprehensive analysis of the organ systems and pathways involved in the impaired physiological response to exercise, obtained by exercise gas exchange analysis, and enables the clinician to objectively quantify exercise intolerance and to investigate reasons for dyspnea and fatigue leading to precise differentiation between cardiac from pulmonary disorders [164]. In a study including 82 SSc patients, the application of a multiparametric CPET-modified algorithm categorized these patients into four distinct subgroups: (1) normal exercise capacity or subnormal but not limited by evident heart or lung disease; (2) respiratory limitation; (3) left ventricular dysfunction; and (4) pulmonary vasculopathy, thereby demonstrating the utility of CPET in the evaluation of the main cause of exercise limitation in SSc [165]. Moreover, peak oxygen uptake (peak VO_2) and the relationship between ventilation and carbon dioxide output (V_E/VCO_2 slope) have proven to be powerful prognosticators in SSc above and beyond established risk factors [166]. CPET coupled with exercise echocardiography can further combine exercise physiological data with non-invasive evaluations of cardiac function by measures of chamber volumes and geometry, valvular status, and systolic and diastolic function, including the evaluation of left atrial function and pulmonary vascular hemodynamics, and may be useful clinically [164].

Cardiac MRI T1 Mapping (Diffuse Fibrosis Imaging)

Cardiac MRI has emerged as the gold standard tool for the detection of myocardial scar (focal fibrosis), such as that

Table 22.4 Recent cardiac magnetic resonance imaging studies in systemic sclerosis

First author	Year	Sample size	Primary findings	Clinical implications
Barison [185]	2015	30 SSc 10 controls	On MRI T1 mapping, patients with SSc had increased extracellular volume (ECV) fraction in both the heart and the skeletal muscle, reflecting increased diffuse interstitial fibrosis in these tissues.	MRI T1 mapping ECV values appear to be useful in SSc for the detection of interstitial fibrosis. In SSc, the diffuse fibrosis that occurs in the heart may also occur in the skeletal muscle in parallel.
Di Cesare [137]	2013	58 SSc (all females)	Myocardial fibrosis (late gadolinium enhancement) was present in 25/58 (43%) of the SSc in a linear pattern (16 patients) and nodular pattern (9 patients).	In patients with SSc, cardiac MRI can detect focal scar (late gadolinium enhancement), diffuse interstitial fibrosis (T1 mapping), myocardial edema suggestive of myocarditis (T2 imaging), and subendocardial ischemia (perfusion imaging). These abnormalities have been correlated with biomarkers, NYHA functional class, and other imaging parameters indicative of cardiac dysfunction in SSc.
Mavrogeni [187]	2015	46 SSc (all dcSSc)	Of the 46 dcSSc patients, 2 had evidence of early myocarditis (myocardial edema on T2 imaging); the other 44 patients underwent a myocardial stress perfusion-fibrosis protocol and were found to have reduced myocardial perfusion reserve index (MPRI) compared to controls. Of the 11 SSc patients with 2-year follow-up MRI, all had deterioration in MPRI and 8/11 had diffuse subendocardial late gadolinium enhancement.	
Moroncini [138]	2014	26 SSc 13 controls	Of the 26 SSc patients, 54% had perfusion defects and 25% had late gadolinium enhancement.	
Rodriguez-Reyna [139]	2015	62 SSc	Of the 62 SSc patients, 79% had subendocardial perfusion detects, and 45% had late gadolinium enhancement, which was more common in dcSSc (59%) compared to lcSSc (33%) ($p = 0.04$). Patients with perfusion defects had higher values of high-sensitivity C-reactive protein.	
Sano [140]	2012	40 SSc	Of the 40 SSc patients, 17.5% had evidence of late gadolinium enhancement, the presence of which was associated with worse NYHA functional class.	
Thuny [186]	2014	33 SSc 16 controls	All 33 SSc patients studied had no significant echocardiographic abnormalities and no late gadolinium enhancement. SSc patients had higher ECV values on MRI T1 mapping compared to controls. ECV correlated with LA volume and grade of diastolic dysfunction.	

found in patients who have suffered a myocardial infarction and in some types of cardiomyopathies. This technique, which uses late gadolinium enhancement, relies on differential uptake of gadolinium in scarred (fibrotic) and adjacent non-scarred (non-fibrotic) myocardial tissue [184]. In patients with SSc, fibrosis is relatively diffuse and therefore cannot be detected readily using traditional late gadolinium enhancement. Fortunately, recent advances in cardiac MRI now allow determination of diffuse myocardial fibrosis using a T1 mapping technique [167–169]. Preliminary studies have now shown that the T1 mapping technique can be useful in SSc to detect diffuse interstitial fibrosis [185, 186]. In addition, T2 imaging, which detects myocardial edema, may be useful in the detection of early or overt myocarditis [187]. Table 22.4 summarizes recent studies published within the last 5 years that have investigated the utility of cardiac MRI in SSc.

Cardiac MRI Absolute Perfusion

Like the detection of myocardial scar, traditional methods for detecting abnormalities in myocardial perfusion (i.e., ischemia) also rely on relative differences between adjacent myocardial territories. Thus, currently available perfusion techniques are most helpful for focal epicardial coronary disease and less helpful for diffuse microvascular ischemia such as that seen in SSc. However, a novel technique of "absolute perfusion" has been developed using cardiac MRI and may solve the problem of detection of diffuse myocardial ischemia [6, 170]. By evaluating differences between enhancement of the myocardium and blood pool using mathematical techniques of deconvolution, absolute perfusion imaging with cardiac MRI may be a new way to diagnose and quantify myocardial ischemia in SSc and may provide insight on the effects of different classes of vasodilator therapy in SSc.

Summary: Recommendations and Unanswered Questions

Early diagnosis and treatment of direct cardiac involvement in SSc is essential given the considerable morbidity and mortality associated with cardiac manifestations. Based on available data, we recommend yearly screening with comprehensive echocardiography (including tissue Doppler imaging) and natriuretic peptide testing (either BNP or

NT-proBNP). If present, symptoms and signs of possible cardiac involvement should be thoroughly investigated, thereby ensuring timely intervention in the at-risk patient. For the most common type of cardiac involvement, intrinsic myocardial disease, treatment with vasodilators improves myocardial perfusion and may deter the development of overt LV systolic dysfunction by reducing progression to myocardial fibrosis. Nevertheless, despite considerable advances in our understanding of SSc cardiac involvement, several unanswered questions remain:

- Are there truly differences between diffuse and limited forms of SSc in terms of frequency of cardiac involvement? Although most studies have found that primary cardiac involvement is more common in diffuse cutaneous SSc, especially in patients with rapid progression of skin findings, gene expression data from skin biopsies in SSc patients [188] suggest that current classification of SSc is somewhat arbitrary. Therefore, it will be of interest to determine whether certain molecular subsets of patients will have more frequent cardiac involvement, while others do not.
- What are the best ways to screen for cardiac involvement? Current screening for cardiac involvement involves natriuretic peptides and echocardiography, including tissue Doppler imaging. However, the frequency of screening, and whether screening and early diagnosis of cardiac involvement changes clinical outcome, has yet to be determined. Furthermore, the utility of newer technologies such as speckle-tracking echocardiography, cardiac MRI diffuse fibrosis imaging, and absolute perfusion imaging is still unknown.
- Although vasodilator therapy with drugs such as calcium channel blockers and ACE inhibitors forms the cornerstone of treatment for myocardial involvement in SSc, randomized controlled trials are lacking, and the effect of these drugs on long-term outcomes is unknown. Furthermore, there are several novel medications currently in development (e.g., neprilysin inhibitors [189], soluble guanylate stimulators [190]) that may be particular beneficial for cardiac involvement in SSc given their mechanisms of action. However, the large number of patients required for adequately powered randomized clinical trials, coupled with the widespread use of vasodilators for Raynaud's phenomenon in SSc, will likely make the conduct of clinical studies challenging. Nevertheless, such studies must be performed, and the formation of large collaborative SSc research groups for multicenter clinical trials will assist in these endeavors.
- Can immunosuppressive therapy prevent progressive heart disease? Is cardiac fibrosis reversible? Current and newer drugs on the horizon for SSc may be able to address these questions, with the caveat that any improvement in cardiac function will have to be balanced with the potential for toxicity with these drugs.

Despite these unanswered questions, much has been learned about the cardiac manifestations of SSc, and it is hoped that ongoing investigations in this area will shed new light on prevention and treatment of cardiac disease in SSc.

Conclusions

Direct cardiac involvement is a frequent and early finding in SSc patients, both in the diffuse and limited cutaneous forms of the disease. There are several cardiac manifestations of SSc, each of which can cause considerable morbidity. The pathogenesis of direct cardiac involvement typically involves a general vasospastic mechanism that is thought to play a major role in SSc in general. Vasospasm of the small coronary arteries or arterioles initially impairs perfusion and function, which is reversible early but over time is followed by structural coronary arteriolar lesions leading to irreversible abnormalities. Therefore, early detection through screening is critical to prevent irreversible cardiac damage, especially since the presence of clinically overt cardiac involvement due to SSc is associated with adverse outcomes. Natriuretic peptides (either BNP or NT-proBNP) and tissue Doppler imaging have emerged as the most useful screening tools for cardiac involvement and form the cornerstone of cardiac assessment in SSc. Delayed enhancement cardiac MRI has also emerged as an extremely useful tool to evaluate abnormal cardiac structure, pericardial disease, perfusion, and diffuse fibrosis. Although the optimal strategies for combating cardiac manifestations of SSc have not been completely defined, there is accumulating evidence to suggest a major role of vasodilators early in the course of disease for the prevention of long-term cardiac morbidity and mortality. In the future, drugs that might prevent or treat structural vascular lesions (and fibrosis) might be extremely important. Therefore, more understanding of the molecular pathophysiology and optimal treatment of cardiac involvement in SSc is necessary, with the hope that novel treatments for cardiac disease can limit the morbidity and mortality of SSc overall.

Acknowledgements The authors would like to thank and acknowledge André Kahan MD, PhD, and J. Gerry Coghlan, M.D., for their important contributions as a co-author of the first and second editions of this chapter.

References

1. Kahan A, Coghlan G, McLaughlin V. Cardiac complications of systemic sclerosis. Rheumatology (Oxford). 2009;48 Suppl 3:iii45–8.
2. Allanore Y, Meune C, Kahan A. Systemic sclerosis and cardiac dysfunction: evolving concepts and diagnostic methodologies. Curr Opin Rheumatol. 2008;20:697–702.
3. Champion HC. The heart in scleroderma. Rheum Dis Clin N Am. 2008;34:181–90, viii.

4. Meune C, Vignaux O, Kahan A, Allanore Y. Heart involvement in systemic sclerosis: evolving concept and diagnostic methodologies. Arch Cardiovasc Dis. 2010;103:46–52.
5. Parks JL, Taylor MH, Parks LP, Silver RM. Systemic sclerosis and the heart. Rheum Dis Clin N Am. 2014;40:87–102.
6. Desai CS, Lee DC, Shah SJ. Systemic sclerosis and the heart: current diagnosis and management. Curr Opin Rheumatol. 2011;23:545–54.
7. Allanore Y, Meune C, Vonk MC, Airo P, Hachulla L, Caramaschi P, Riemekasten G, Cozzi F, Beretta L, Derk CT, Komocsi A, Farge D, Balbir A, Riccieri V, Distler O, Chiala A, Papa ND, Simic KP, Ghio M, Stamenkovic B, Rednic S, Host N, Pellerito R, Zegers E, Kahan A, Walker UA, Matucci-Cerinic M. Prevalence and factors associated with left ventricular dysfunction in the EULAR Scleroderma Trial and Research group (EUSTAR) database of patients with systemic sclerosis. Ann Rheum Dis. 2010;69:218–21.
8. Ferri C, Valentini G, Cozzi F, Sebastiani M, Michelassi C, La Montagna G, Bullo A, Cazzato M, Tirri E, Storino F, Giuggioli D, Cuomo G, Rosada M, Bombardieri S, Todesco S, Tirri G. Systemic sclerosis: demographic, clinical, and serologic features and survival in 1,012 Italian patients. Medicine (Baltimore). 2002;81:139–53.
9. Kahan A, Allanore Y. Primary myocardial involvement in systemic sclerosis. Rheumatology (Oxford). 2006;45 Suppl 4:iv14–7.
10. Meune C, Avouac J, Wahbi K, Cabanes L, Wipff J, Mouthon L, Guillevin L, Kahan A, Allanore Y. Cardiac involvement in systemic sclerosis assessed by tissue-doppler echocardiography during routine care: a controlled study of 100 consecutive patients. Arthritis Rheum. 2008;58:1803–9.
11. Plazak W, Zabinska-Plazak E, Wojas-Pelc A, Podolec P, Olszowska M, Tracz W, Bogdaszewska-Czabanowska J. Heart structure and function in systemic sclerosis. Eur J Dermatol. 2002;12:257–62.
12. Follansbee WP, Curtiss EI, Medsger TA, Steen VD, Uretsky BF, Owens GR, Rodnan GP. Physiologic abnormalities of cardiac function in progressive systemic sclerosis with diffuse scleroderma. N Engl J Med. 1984;310:142–8.
13. Fernandez-Codina A, Simeon-Aznar CP, Pinal-Fernandez I, Rodriguez-Palomares J, Pizzi MN, Hidalgo CE, Del Castillo AG, Prado-Galbarro FJ, Sarria-Santamera A, Fonollosa-Pla V, Vilardell-Tarres M. Cardiac involvement in systemic sclerosis: differences between clinical subsets and influence on survival. Rheumatol Int. 2017;37:75.
14. Perera A, Fertig N, Lucas M, Rodriguez-Reyna TS, Hu P, Steen VD, Medsger TA Jr. Clinical subsets, skin thickness progression rate, and serum antibody levels in systemic sclerosis patients with anti-topoisomerase I antibody. Arthritis Rheum. 2007;56:2740–6.
15. Steen VD. Autoantibodies in systemic sclerosis. Semin Arthritis Rheum. 2005;35:35–42.
16. Ranque B, Authier FJ, Berezne A, Guillevin L, Mouthon L. Systemic sclerosis-associated myopathy. Ann N Y Acad Sci. 2007;1108:268–82.
17. Clements PJ, Lachenbruch PA, Furst DE, Paulus HE, Sterz MG, Cardiac score. A semiquantitative measure of cardiac involvement that improves prediction of prognosis in systemic sclerosis. Arthritis Rheum. 1991;34:1371–80.
18. Steen VD, Medsger TA Jr. Severe organ involvement in systemic sclerosis with diffuse scleroderma. Arthritis Rheum. 2000;43:2437–44.
19. Scussel-Lonzetti L, Joyal F, Raynauld J-P, Roussin A, Rich E, Goulet J-R, Raymond Y, Senecal J-L. Predicting mortality in systemic sclerosis: analysis of a cohort of 309 French Canadian patients with emphasis on features at diagnosis as predictive factors for survival. Medicine (Baltimore). 2002;81:154–67.
20. Ioannidis JP, Vlachoyiannopoulos PG, Haidich AB, Medsger TA Jr, Lucas M, Michet CJ, Kuwana M, Yasuoka H, van den Hoogen F, Te Boome L, van Laar JM, Verbeet NL, Matucci-Cerinic M, Georgountzos A, Moutsopoulos HM. Mortality in systemic sclerosis: an international meta-analysis of individual patient data. Am J Med. 2005;118:2–10.
21. Al-Dhaher FF, Pope JE, Ouimet JM. Determinants of morbidity and mortality of systemic sclerosis in Canada. Semin Arthritis Rheum. 2010;39:269–77.
22. Czirjak L, Kumanovics G, Varju C, Nagy Z, Pakozdi A, Szekanecz Z, Szucs G. Survival and causes of death in 366 Hungarian patients with systemic sclerosis. Ann Rheum Dis. 2008;67:59–63.
23. Joven BE, Almodovar R, Carmona L, Carreira PE. Survival, causes of death, and risk factors associated with mortality in Spanish systemic sclerosis patients: results from a single university hospital. Semin Arthritis Rheum. 2010;39:285–93.
24. Tyndall AJ, Bannert B, Vonk M, Airo P, Cozzi F, Carreira PE, Bancel DF, Allanore Y, Muller-Ladner U, Distler O, Iannone F, Pellerito R, Pileckyte M, Miniati I, Ananieva L, Gurman AB, Damjanov N, Mueller A, Valentini G, Riemekasten G, Tikly M, Hummers L, Henriques MJ, Caramaschi P, Scheja A, Rozman B, Ton E, Kumanovics G, Coleiro B, Feierl E, Szucs G, Von Muhlen CA, Riccieri V, Novak S, Chizzolini C, Kotulska A, Denton C, Coelho PC, Kotter I, Simsek I, de la Pena Lefebvre PG, Hachulla E, Seibold JR, Rednic S, Stork J, Morovic-Vergles J, Walker UA. Causes and risk factors for death in systemic sclerosis: a study from the EULAR Scleroderma Trials and Research (EUSTAR) database. Ann Rheum Dis. 2010;69:1809–15.
25. Follansbee WP, Miller TR, Curtiss EI, Orie JE, Bernstein RL, Kiernan JM, Medsger TA. A controlled clinicopathologic study of myocardial fibrosis in systemic sclerosis (scleroderma). J Rheumatol. 1990;17:656–62.
26. Bulkley BH, Ridolfi RL, Salyer WR, Hutchins GM. Myocardial lesions of progressive systemic sclerosis. A cause of cardiac dysfunction. Circulation. 1976;53:483–90.
27. James TN. De subitaneis mortibus. VIII. Coronary arteries and conduction system in scleroderma heart disease. Circulation. 1974;50:844–56.
28. Alexander EL, Firestein GS, Weiss JL, Heuser RR, Leitl G, Wagner HN, Brinker JA, Ciuffo AA, Becker LC. Reversible cold-induced abnormalities in myocardial perfusion and function in systemic sclerosis. Ann Intern Med. 1986;105:661–8.
29. Gustafsson R, Mannting F, Kazzam E, Waldenstrom A, Hallgren R. Cold-induced reversible myocardial ischaemia in systemic sclerosis. Lancet. 1989;2:475–9.
30. Lekakis J, Mavrikakis M, Emmanuel M, Prassopoulos V, Papazoglou S, Papamichael C, Moulopoulou D, Kostamis P, Stamatelopoulos S, Moulopoulos S. Cold-induced coronary Raynaud's phenomenon in patients with systemic sclerosis. Clin Exp Rheumatol. 1998;16:135–40.
31. Long A, Duffy G, Bresnihan B. Reversible myocardial perfusion defects during cold challenge in scleroderma. Br J Rheumatol. 1986;25:158–61.
32. Mizuno R, Fujimoto S, Saito Y, Nakamura S. Cardiac Raynaud's phenomenon induced by cold provocation as a predictor of long-term left ventricular dysfunction and remodelling in systemic sclerosis: 7-year follow-up study. Eur J Heart Fail. 2010;12:268–75.
33. Steen VD, Follansbee WP, Conte CG, Medsger TA Jr. Thallium perfusion defects predict subsequent cardiac dysfunction in patients with systemic sclerosis. Arthritis Rheum. 1996;39:677–81.
34. Kahan A, Nitenberg A, Foult JM, Amor B, Menkes CJ, Devaux JY, Blanchet F, Perennec J, Lutfalla G, Roucayrol JC. Decreased coronary reserve in primary scleroderma myocardial disease. Arthritis Rheum. 1985;28:637–46.
35. Montisci R, Vacca A, Garau P, Colonna P, Ruscazio M, Passiu G, Iliceto S, Mathieu A. Detection of early impairment of coronary

flow reserve in patients with systemic sclerosis. Ann Rheum Dis. 2003;62:890–3.
36. Sulli A, Ghio M, Bezante GP, Deferrari L, Craviotto C, Sebastiani V, Setti M, Filaci G, Puppo F, Barsotti A, Cutolo M, Indiveri F. Blunted coronary flow reserve in systemic sclerosis: a sign of cardiac involvement in asymptomatic patients. Ann Rheum Dis. 2004;63:210–1.
37. Kerr LD, Spiera H. Myocarditis as a complication in scleroderma patients with myositis. Clin Cardiol. 1993;16:895–9.
38. West SG, Killian PJ, Lawless OJ. Association of myositis and myocarditis in progressive systemic sclerosis. Arthritis Rheum. 1981;24:662–8.
39. Follansbee WP, Zerbe TR, Medsger TA Jr. Cardiac and skeletal muscle disease in systemic sclerosis (scleroderma): a high risk association. Am Heart J. 1993;125:194–203.
40. Hegedus I, Czirjak L. Left ventricular wall motion abnormalities in 80 patients with systemic sclerosis. Clin Rheumatol. 1995;14:161–4.
41. Elhai M, Meune C, Boubaya M, Avouac J, Hachulla E, Balbir-Gurman A, Riemekasten G, Airò P, Joven B, Vettori S, Cozzi F, Ullman S, Czirják L, Tikly M, Müller-Ladner U, Caramaschi P, Distler O, Iannone F, Ananieva LP, Hesselstrand R, Becvar R, Gabrielli A, Damjanov N, Salvador MJ, Riccieri V, Mihai C, Szücs G, Walker UA, Hunzelmann N, Martinovic D, Smith V, Müller CS, Montecucco CM, Opris D, Ingegnoli F, Vlachoyiannopoulos PG, Stamenkovic B, Rosato E, Heitmann S, Distler JHW, Zenone T, Seidel M, Vacca A, Langhe E, Novak S, Cutolo M, Mouthon L, Henes J, Chizzolini C, Mühlen CAV, Solanki K, Rednic S, Stamp L, Anic B, Santamaria VO, De Santis M, Yavuz S, Sifuentes-Giraldo WA, Chatelus E, Stork J, Laar JV, Loyo E, de la Peña G, Lefebvre P, Eyerich K, Cosentino V, Alegre-Sancho JJ, Kowal-Bielecka O, Rey G, Matucci-Cerinic M, Allanore Y, EUSTAR Group. Mapping and predicting mortality from systemic sclerosis. Ann Rheum Dis. 2017;76(11):1897–905. https://doi.org/10.1136/annrheumdis-2017-211448. Epub 2017 Aug 23.
42. Valentini G, Vitale DF, Giunta A, Maione S, Gerundo G, Arnese M, Tirri E, Pelaggi N, Giacummo A, Tirri G, Condorelli M. Diastolic abnormalities in systemic sclerosis: evidence for associated defective cardiac functional reserve. Ann Rheum Dis. 1996;55:455–60.
43. Aguglia G, Sgreccia A, Bernardo ML, Carmenini E, Giusti De Marle M, Reali A, Morelli S. Left ventricular diastolic function in systemic sclerosis. J Rheumatol. 2001;28:1563–7.
44. Nakajima K, Taki J, Kawano M, Higuchi T, Sato S, Nishijima C, Takehara K, Tonami N. Diastolic dysfunction in patients with systemic sclerosis detected by gated myocardial perfusion SPECT: an early sign of cardiac involvement. J Nucl Med. 2001;42:183–8.
45. Rosato E, Maione S, Vitarelli A, Giunta A, Fontanella L, de Horatio LT, Cacciatore F, Proietti M, Pisarri S, Salsano F. Regional diastolic function by tissue Doppler echocardiography in systemic sclerosis: correlation with clinical variables. Rheumatol Int. 2009;29:913–9.
46. Kazzam E, Waldenstrom A, Landelius J, Hallgren R, Arvidsson A, Caidahl K. Non-invasive assessment of left ventricular diastolic function in patients with systemic sclerosis. J Intern Med. 1990;228:183–92.
47. Armstrong GP, Whalley GA, Doughty RN, Gamble GD, Flett SM, Tan PL, Sharpe DN. Left ventricular function in scleroderma. Br J Rheumatol. 1996;35:983–8.
48. Hinchcliff M, Desai CS, Varga J, Shah SJ. Prevalence, prognosis, and factors associated with left ventricular diastolic dysfunction in systemic sclerosis. Clin Exp Rheumatol. 2012;30:S30–7.
49. Faludi R, Kolto G, Bartos B, Csima G, Czirjak L, Komocsi A. Five-year follow-up of left ventricular diastolic function in systemic sclerosis patients: determinants of mortality and disease progression. Semin Arthritis Rheum. 2014;44:220–7.
50. Tennøe AH, Murbræch K, Andreassen JC, Fretheim H, Garen T, Gude E, Andreassen A, Aakhus S, Molberg Ø, Hoffmann-Vold AM. Left ventricular diastolic dysfunction predicts mortality in patients with systemic sclerosis. J Am Coll Cardiol. 2018;72(15):1804–13. https://doi.org/10.1016/j.jacc.2018.07.068.
51. Bezante GP, Rollando D, Sessarego M, Panico N, Setti M, Filaci G, Molinari G, Balbi M, Cutolo M, Barsotti A, Indiveri F, Ghio M. Cardiac magnetic resonance imaging detects subclinical right ventricular impairment in systemic sclerosis. J Rheumatol. 2007;34:2431–7.
52. George BJ, Kwan MD, Morris MJ. Isolated right ventricular failure in scleroderma heart disease. Cardiol Rev. 2004;12:279–81.
53. Giunta A, Tirri E, Maione S, Cangianiello S, Mele A, De Luca A, Valentini G. Right ventricular diastolic abnormalities in systemic sclerosis. Relation to left ventricular involvement and pulmonary hypertension. Ann Rheum Dis. 2000;59:94–8.
54. Gonzalez A, Seres L, Ferrer E, Valle V. Isolated right ventricular systolic dysfunction in scleroderma. Rev Esp Cardiol. 2008;61:990–1.
55. Hsiao SH, Lee CY, Chang SM, Lin SK, Liu CP. Right heart function in scleroderma: insights from myocardial Doppler tissue imaging. J Am Soc Echocardiogr. 2006;19:507–14.
56. Huez S, Roufosse F, Vachiery JL, Pavelescu A, Derumeaux G, Wautrecht JC, Cogan E, Naeije R. Isolated right ventricular dysfunction in systemic sclerosis: latent pulmonary hypertension? Eur Respir J. 2007;30:928–36.
57. Lee CY, Chang SM, Hsiao SH, Tseng JC, Lin SK, Liu CP. Right heart function and scleroderma: insights from tricuspid annular plane systolic excursion. Echocardiography. 2007;24:118–25.
58. Lindqvist P, Caidahl K, Neuman-Andersen G, Ozolins C, Rantapaa-Dahlqvist S, Waldenstrom A, Kazzam E. Disturbed right ventricular diastolic function in patients with systemic sclerosis: a Doppler tissue imaging study. Chest. 2005;128:755–63.
59. Meune C, Allanore Y, Devaux JY, Dessault O, Duboc D, Weber S, Kahan A. High prevalence of right ventricular systolic dysfunction in early systemic sclerosis. J Rheumatol. 2004;31:1941–5.
60. Meune C, Khanna D, Aboulhosn J, Avouac J, Kahan A, Furst DE, Allanore Y. A right ventricular diastolic impairment is common in systemic sclerosis and is associated with other target-organ damage. Semin Arthritis Rheum. 2016;45:439.
61. Kahan A, Devaux JY, Amor B, Menkes CJ, Weber S, Foult JM, Venot A, Guerin F, Degeorges M, Roucayrol JC. Pharmacodynamic effect of dipyridamole on thallium-201 myocardial perfusion in progressive systemic sclerosis with diffuse scleroderma. Ann Rheum Dis. 1986;45:718–25.
62. Kahan A, Devaux JY, Amor B, Menkes CJ, Weber S, Nitenberg A, Venot A, Guerin F, Degeorges M, Roucayrol JC. Nifedipine and thallium-201 myocardial perfusion in progressive systemic sclerosis. N Engl J Med. 1986;314:1397–402.
63. Kahan A, Devaux JY, Amor B, Menkes CJ, Weber S, Venot A, Guerin F, Degeorges M, Roucayrol JC. Nicardipine improves myocardial perfusion in systemic sclerosis. J Rheumatol. 1988;15:1395–400.
64. Kahan A, Devaux JY, Amor B, Menkes CJ, Weber S, Venot A, Strauch G. The effect of captopril on thallium 201 myocardial perfusion in systemic sclerosis. Clin Pharmacol Ther. 1990;47:483–9.
65. Ishida R, Murata Y, Sawada Y, Nishioka K, Shibuya H. Thallium-201 myocardial SPET in patients with collagen disease. Nucl Med Commun. 2000;21:729–34.
66. Duboc D, Kahan A, Maziere B, Loc'h C, Crouzel C, Menkes CJ, Amor B, Strauch G, Guerin F, Syrota A. The effect of nifedipine on myocardial perfusion and metabolism in systemic sclerosis. A positron emission tomographic study. Arthritis Rheum. 1991;34:198–203.
67. Vignaux O, Allanore Y, Meune C, Pascal O, Duboc D, Weber S, Legmann P, Kahan A. Evaluation of the effect of nifedipine upon

myocardial perfusion and contractility using cardiac magnetic resonance imaging and tissue Doppler echocardiography in systemic sclerosis. Ann Rheum Dis. 2005;64:1268–73.

68. Allanore Y, Meune C, Vignaux O, Weber S, Legmann P, Kahan A. Bosentan increases myocardial perfusion and function in systemic sclerosis: a magnetic resonance imaging and tissue-Doppler echography study. J Rheumatol. 2006;33:2464–9.
69. Kahan A, Devaux JY, Amor B, Menkes CJ, Weber S, Guerin F, Venot A, Strauch G. Pharmacodynamic effect of nicardipine on left ventricular function in systemic sclerosis. J Cardiovasc Pharmacol. 1990;15:249–53.
70. Smiseth OA, Ihlen H. Strain rate imaging: why do we need it? J Am Coll Cardiol. 2003;42:1584–6.
71. Stack J, McLaughlin P, Sinnot C, Henry M, MacEneaney P, Eltahir A, Harney S. Successful control of scleroderma myocarditis using a combination of cyclophosphamide and methylprednisolone. Scand J Rheumatol. 2010;39:349–50.
72. Pieroni M, De Santis M, Zizzo G, Bosello S, Smaldone C, Campioni M, De Luca G, Laria A, Meduri A, Bellocci F, Bonomo L, Crea F, Ferraccioli G. Recognizing and treating myocarditis in recent-onset systemic sclerosis heart disease: potential utility of immunosuppressive therapy in cardiac damage progression. Semin Arthritis Rheum. 2014;43:526–35.
73. Chung L, Fiorentino D. Digital ulcers in patients with systemic sclerosis. Autoimmun Rev. 2006;5:125–8.
74. Califf RM, Adams KF, McKenna WJ, Gheorghiade M, Uretsky BF, McNulty SE, Darius H, Schulman K, Zannad F, Handberg-Thurmond E, Harrell FE Jr, Wheeler W, Soler-Soler J, Swedberg K. A randomized controlled trial of epoprostenol therapy for severe congestive heart failure: the Flolan International Randomized Survival Trial (FIRST). Am Heart J. 1997;134:44–54.
75. Mok MY, Lau CS, Chiu SS, Tso AW, Lo Y, Law LS, Mak KF, Wong WS, Khong PL, Lam KS. Systemic sclerosis is an independent risk factor for increased coronary artery calcium deposition. Arthritis Rheum. 2011;63:1387–95.
76. Ngian GS, Sahhar J, Proudman SM, Stevens W, Wicks IP, Van Doornum S. Prevalence of coronary heart disease and cardiovascular risk factors in a national cross-sectional cohort study of systemic sclerosis. Ann Rheum Dis. 2012;71:1980–3.
77. Ungprasert P, Charoenpong P, Ratanasrimetha P, Thongprayoon C, Cheungpasitporn W, Suksaranjit P. Risk of coronary artery disease in patients with systemic sclerosis: a systematic review and meta-analysis. Clin Rheumatol. 2014;33:1099–104.
78. Butt SA, Jeppesen JL, Torp-Pedersen C, Sam F, Gislason GH, Jacobsen S, Andersson C. Cardiovascular manifestations of systemic sclerosis: a danish nationwide cohort study. J Am Heart Assoc. 2019;8(17):e013405. https://doi.org/10.1161/JAHA.119.013405. Epub 2019 Aug 24.
79. Hachulla AL, Launay D, Gaxotte V, de Groote P, Lamblin N, Devos P, Hatron PY, Beregi JP, Hachulla E. Cardiac magnetic resonance imaging in systemic sclerosis: a cross-sectional observational study of 52 patients. Ann Rheum Dis. 2009;68:1878–84.
80. Byers RJ, Marshall DA, Freemont AJ. Pericardial involvement in systemic sclerosis. Ann Rheum Dis. 1997;56:393–4.
81. Hinderliter AL, Willis PW 4th, Long W, Clarke WR, Ralph D, Caldwell EJ, Williams W, Ettinger NA, Hill NS, Summer WR, de Biosblanc B, Koch G, Li S, Clayton LM, Jobsis MM, Crow JW. Frequency and prognostic significance of pericardial effusion in primary pulmonary hypertension. PPH Study Group. Primary pulmonary hypertension. Am J Cardiol. 1999;84(481–484):A410.
82. Park B, Dittrich HC, Polikar R, Olson L, Nicod P. Echocardiographic evidence of pericardial effusion in severe chronic pulmonary hypertension. Am J Cardiol. 1989;63:143–5.
83. Habib G, Torbicki A. The role of echocardiography in the diagnosis and management of patients with pulmonary hypertension. Eur Respir Rev. 2010;19:288–99.
84. Wooten MD, Reddy GV, Johnson RD. Cardiac tamponade in systemic sclerosis: a case report and review of 18 reported cases. J Clin Rheumatol. 2000;6:35–40.
85. Nishimura RA. Constrictive pericarditis in the modern era: a diagnostic dilemma. Heart. 2001;86:619–23.
86. Hancock EW. Differential diagnosis of restrictive cardiomyopathy and constrictive pericarditis. Heart. 2001;86:343–9.
87. Dal-Bianco JP, Sengupta PP, Mookadam F, Chandrasekaran K, Tajik AJ, Khandheria BK. Role of echocardiography in the diagnosis of constrictive pericarditis. J Am Soc Echocardiogr. 2009;22:24–33; quiz 103–4.
88. Leya FS, Arab D, Joyal D, Shioura KM, Lewis BE, Steen LH, Cho L. The efficacy of brain natriuretic peptide levels in differentiating constrictive pericarditis from restrictive cardiomyopathy. J Am Coll Cardiol. 2005;45:1900–2.
89. Vacca A, Meune C, Gordon J, Chung L, Proudman S, Assassi S, Nikpour M, Rodriguez-Reyna TS, Khanna D, Lafyatis R, Matucci-Cerinic M, Distler O, Allanore Y. Cardiac arrhythmias and conduction defects in systemic sclerosis. Rheumatology (Oxford). 2014;53:1172–7.
90. D'Angelo WA, Fries JF, Masi AT, Shulman LE. Pathologic observations in systemic sclerosis (scleroderma). A study of fifty-eight autopsy cases and fifty-eight matched controls. Am J Med. 1969;46:428–40.
91. Ridolfi RL, Bulkley BH, Hutchins GM. The cardiac conduction system in progressive systemic sclerosis. Clinical and pathologic features of 35 patients. Am J Med. 1976;61:361–6.
92. Lubitz SA, Goldbarg SH, Mehta D. Sudden cardiac death in infiltrative cardiomyopathies: sarcoidosis, scleroderma, amyloidosis, hemachromatosis. Prog Cardiovasc Dis. 2008;51:58–73.
93. Gialafos E, Konstantopoulou P, Voulgari C, Giavri I, Panopoulos S, Vaiopoulos G, Mavrikakis M, Moyssakis I, Sfikakis PP. Abnormal spatial QRS-T angle, a marker of ventricular repolarisation, predicts serious ventricular arrhythmia in systemic sclerosis. Clin Exp Rheumatol. 2012;30:327–31.
94. Wozniak J, Dabrowski R, Luczak D, Kwiatkowska M, Musiej-Nowakowska E, Kowalik I, Szwed H. Evaluation of heart rhythm variability and arrhythmia in children with systemic and localized scleroderma. J Rheumatol. 2009;36:191–6.
95. Kostis JB, Seibold JR, Turkevich D, Masi AT, Grau RG, Medsger TA Jr, Steen VD, Clements PJ, Szydlo L, D'Angelo WA. Prognostic importance of cardiac arrhythmias in systemic sclerosis. Am J Med. 1988;84:1007–15.
96. Fraiser LH, Kanekal S, Kehrer JP. Cyclophosphamide toxicity. Characterising and avoiding the problem. Drugs. 1991;42:781–95.
97. Cotroneo J, Sleik KM, Rene Rodriguez E, Klein AL. Hydroxychloroquine-induced restrictive cardiomyopathy. Eur J Echocardiogr. 2007;8:247–51.
98. Burt RK, Oliveira MC, Shah SJ, Moraes DA, Simoes B, Gheorghiade M, Schroeder J, Ruderman E, Farge D, Chai ZJ, Marjanovic Z, Jain S, Morgan A, Milanetti F, Han X, Jovanovic B, Helenowski IB, Voltarelli J. Cardiac involvement and treatment-related mortality after non-myeloablative haemopoietic stem-cell transplantation with unselected autologous peripheral blood for patients with systemic sclerosis: a retrospective analysis. Lancet. 2013;381:1116–24.
99. Burt RK, Shah SJ, Dill K, Grant T, Gheorghiade M, Schroeder J, Craig R, Hirano I, Marshall K, Ruderman E, Jovanovic B, Milanetti F, Jain S, Boyce K, Morgan A, Carr J, Barr W. Autologous non-myeloablative haemopoietic stem-cell transplantation compared with pulse cyclophosphamide once per month for systemic sclerosis (ASSIST): an open-label, randomised phase 2 trial. Lancet. 2011;378:498–506.
100. Yamamoto R, Kanda Y, Matsuyama T, Oshima K, Nannya Y, Suguro M, Chizuka A, Hamaki T, Takezako N, Miwa A, Kami M, Mori S, Kojima T, Saito K, Itaoka Y, Kashida M. Myopericarditis

caused by cyclophosphamide used to mobilize peripheral blood stem cells in a myeloma patient with renal failure. Bone Marrow Transplant. 2000;26:685–8.
101. Soong TR, Barouch LA, Champion HC, Wigley FM, Halushka MK. New clinical and ultrastructural findings in hydroxychloroquine-induced cardiomyopathy—a report of 2 cases. Hum Pathol. 2007;38:1858–63.
102. Distler JH, Distler O. Cardiotoxicity of imatinib mesylate: an extremely rare phenomenon or a major side effect? Ann Rheum Dis. 2007;66:836.
103. Kerkela R, Grazette L, Yacobi R, Iliescu C, Patten R, Beahm C, Walters B, Shevtsov S, Pesant S, Clubb FJ, Rosenzweig A, Salomon RN, Van Etten RA, Alroy J, Durand JB, Force T. Cardiotoxicity of the cancer therapeutic agent imatinib mesylate. Nat Med. 2006;12:908–16.
104. Fujimaki K, Maruta A, Yoshida M, Sakai R, Tanabe J, Koharazawa H, Kodama F, Asahina S, Minamizawa M, Matsuzaki M, Fujisawa S, Kanamori H, Ishigatsubo Y. Severe cardiac toxicity in hematological stem cell transplantation: predictive value of reduced left ventricular ejection fraction. Bone Marrow Transplant. 2001;27:307–10.
105. Burt RK, Oliveira MC, Shah SJ. Cardiac assessment before stem cell transplantation for systemic sclerosis. JAMA. 2014;312:1803.
106. Daniels LB, Maisel AS. Natriuretic peptides. J Am Coll Cardiol. 2007;50:2357–68.
107. Maisel A, Mueller C, Adams K Jr, Anker SD, Aspromonte N, Cleland JG, Cohen-Solal A, Dahlstrom U, DeMaria A, Di Somma S, Filippatos GS, Fonarow GC, Jourdain P, Komajda M, Liu PP, McDonagh T, McDonald K, Mebazaa A, Nieminen MS, Peacock WF, Tubaro M, Valle R, Vanderhyden M, Yancy CW, Zannad F, Braunwald E. State of the art: using natriuretic peptide levels in clinical practice. Eur J Heart Fail. 2008;10:824–39.
108. Weber M, Hamm C. Role of B-type natriuretic peptide (BNP) and NT-proBNP in clinical routine. Heart. 2006;92:843–9.
109. Allanore Y, Meune C. N-terminal pro brain natriuretic peptide: the new cornerstone of cardiovascular assessment in systemic sclerosis. Clin Exp Rheumatol. 2009;27:59–63.
110. Allanore Y, Wahbi K, Borderie D, Weber S, Kahan A, Meune C. N-terminal pro-brain natriuretic peptide in systemic sclerosis: a new cornerstone of cardiovascular assessment? Ann Rheum Dis. 2009;68:1885–9.
111. Allanore Y, Borderie D, Meune C, Cabanes L, Weber S, Ekindjian OG, Kahan A. N-terminal pro-brain natriuretic peptide as a diagnostic marker of early pulmonary artery hypertension in patients with systemic sclerosis and effects of calcium-channel blockers. Arthritis Rheum. 2003;48:3503–8.
112. Mukerjee D, Yap LB, Holmes AM, Nair D, Ayrton P, Black CM, Coghlan JG. Significance of plasma N-terminal pro-brain natriuretic peptide in patients with systemic sclerosis-related pulmonary arterial hypertension. Respir Med. 2003;97:1230–6.
113. Williams MH, Handler CE, Akram R, Smith CJ, Das C, Smee J, Nair D, Denton CP, Black CM, Coghlan JG. Role of N-terminal brain natriuretic peptide (N-TproBNP) in scleroderma-associated pulmonary arterial hypertension. Eur Heart J. 2006;27:1485–94.
114. Mathai SC, Hassoun PM. N-terminal brain natriuretic peptide in scleroderma-associated pulmonary arterial hypertension. Eur Heart J. 2007;28:140–1; author reply 141.
115. Allanore Y, Borderie D, Avouac J, Zerkak D, Meune C, Hachulla E, Mouthon L, Guillevin L, Meyer O, Ekindjian OG, Weber S, Kahan A. High N-terminal pro-brain natriuretic peptide levels and low diffusing capacity for carbon monoxide as independent predictors of the occurrence of precapillary pulmonary arterial hypertension in patients with systemic sclerosis. Arthritis Rheum. 2008;58:284–91.
116. Choi HJ, Shin YK, Lee HJ, Kee JY, Shin DW, Lee EY, Lee YJ, Lee EB, Song YW. The clinical significance of serum N-terminal pro-brain natriuretic peptide in systemic sclerosis patients. Clin Rheumatol. 2008;27:437–42.
117. Dimitroulas T, Giannakoulas G, Karvounis H, Settas L. Limitations of the findings regarding the relationship between N-terminal pro-brain natriuretic peptide and systemic sclerosis-related pulmonary arterial hypertension: comment on the article by Allanore et al. Arthritis Rheum. 2008;58:2215–6; author reply 2216.
118. Carlo-Stella N, Belloli L, Biondi ML, Marasini B. Serum N-terminal pro-brain natriuretic peptide, a marker of skin thickness in systemic sclerosis? Clin Rheumatol. 2009;28:241–2.
119. Mathai SC, Bueso M, Hummers LK, Boyce D, Lechtzin N, Le Pavec J, Campo A, Champion HC, Housten T, Forfia PR, Zaiman AL, Wigley FM, Girgis RE, Hassoun PM. Disproportionate elevation of N-terminal pro-brain natriuretic peptide in scleroderma-related pulmonary hypertension. Eur Respir J. 2010;35:95–104.
120. Cavagna L, Caporali R, Klersy C, Ghio S, Albertini R, Scelsi L, Moratti R, Bonino C, Montecucco C. Comparison of brain natriuretic peptide (BNP) and NT-proBNP in screening for pulmonary arterial hypertension in patients with systemic sclerosis. J Rheumatol. 2010;37:2064–70.
121. Montagnana M, Lippi G, Volpe A, Salvagno GL, Biasi D, Caramaschi P, Guidi GC. Evaluation of cardiac laboratory markers in patients with systemic sclerosis. Clin Biochem. 2006;39:913–7.
122. Avouac J, Meune C, Chenevier-Gobeaux C, Borderie D, Lefevre G, Kahan A, Allanore Y. Cardiac biomarkers in systemic sclerosis: contribution of high-sensitivity cardiac troponin in addition to N-terminal pro-brain natriuretic peptide. Arthritis Care Res (Hoboken). 2015;67:1022–30.
123. Ho CY, Solomon SD. A clinician's guide to tissue Doppler imaging. Circulation. 2006;113:e396–8.
124. D'Alto M, Riccardi A, Argiento P, Di Stefano I, Romeo E, Iacono AM, D'Andrea A, Fasano S, Sanduzzi A, Bocchino M, Docimo L, Tolone S, Russo MG, Valentini G. Cardiac involvement in undifferentiated connective tissue disease at risk for systemic sclerosis (otherwise referred to as very early-early systemic sclerosis): a TDI study. Clin Exp Med. 2018;18(2):237–43. https://doi.org/10.1007/s10238-017-0477-y. Epub 2017 Oct 9.
125. Nagueh SF, Appleton CP, Gillebert TC, Marino PN, Oh JK, Smiseth OA, Waggoner AD, Flachskampf FA, Pellikka PA, Evangelista A. Recommendations for the evaluation of left ventricular diastolic function by echocardiography. J Am Soc Echocardiogr. 2009;22:107–33.
126. Henein M, Lindqvist P, Francis D, Morner S, Waldenstrom A, Kazzam E. Tissue doppler analysis of age-dependency in diastolic ventricular behaviour and filling: a cross-sectional study of healthy hearts (the Umea general population heart study). Eur Heart J. 2002;23:162–71.
127. Nagueh SF, Smiseth OA, Appleton CP, Byrd BF 3rd, Dokainish H, Edvardsen T, Flachskampf FA, Gillebert TC, Klein AL, Lancellotti P, Marino P, Oh JK, Popescu BA, Waggoner AD. Recommendations for the evaluation of left ventricular diastolic function by echocardiography: an update from the American Society of Echocardiography and the European Association of Cardiovascular Imaging. J Am Soc Echocardiogr. 2016;29(4):277–314. https://doi.org/10.1016/j.echo.2016.01.011.
128. Oh JK, Miranda WR, Bird JG, Kane GC, Nagueh SF. The 2016 diastolic function guideline: is it already time to revisit or revise them? JACC Cardiovasc Imaging. 2020;13(1 Pt 2):327–35. https://doi.org/10.1016/j.jcmg.2019.12.004.
129. Ho SY, Nihoyannopoulos P. Anatomy, echocardiography, and normal right ventricular dimensions. Heart. 2006;92(Suppl 1):i2–13.
130. Horton KD, Meece RW, Hill JC. Assessment of the right ventricle by echocardiography: a primer for cardiac sonographers. J Am Soc Echocardiogr. 2009;22:776–92; quiz 861–2.

131. Rudski LG, Lai WW, Afilalo J, Hua L, Handschumacher MD, Chandrasekaran K, Solomon SD, Louie EK, Schiller NB. Guidelines for the echocardiographic assessment of the right heart in adults: a report from the American Society of Echocardiography endorsed by the European Association of Echocardiography, a registered branch of the European Society of Cardiology, and the Canadian Society of Echocardiography. J Am Soc Echocardiogr. 2010;23:685–713; quiz 786–8.
132. Kawut SM, Lima JA, Barr RG, Chahal H, Jain A, Tandri H, Praestgaard A, Bagiella E, Kizer JR, Johnson WC, Kronmal RA, Bluemke DA. Sex and race differences in right ventricular structure and function: the multi-ethnic study of atherosclerosis-right ventricle study. Circulation. 2011;123(22):2542–51. https://doi.org/10.1161/CIRCULATIONAHA.110.985515.
133. Lang RM, Badano LP, Mor-Avi V, Afilalo J, Armstrong A, Ernande L, Flachskampf FA, Foster E, Goldstein SA, Kuznetsova T, Lancellotti P, Muraru D, Picard MH, Rietzschel ER, Rudski L, Spencer KT, Tsang W, Voigt JU. Recommendations for cardiac chamber quantification by echocardiography in adults: an update from the American Society of Echocardiography and the European Association of Cardiovascular Imaging. J Am Soc Echocardiogr. 2015;28(1):1–39.e14. https://doi.org/10.1016/j.echo.2014.10.003.
134. Schindler TH, Schelbert HR, Quercioli A, Dilsizian V. Cardiac PET imaging for the detection and monitoring of coronary artery disease and microvascular health. JACC Cardiovasc Imaging. 2010;3:623–40.
135. Kaufmann PA, Di Carli MF. Hybrid SPECT/CT and PET/CT imaging: the next step in noninvasive cardiac imaging. Semin Nucl Med. 2009;39:341–7.
136. Kobayashi H, Yokoe I, Hirano M, Nakamura T, Nakajima Y, Fontaine KR, Giles JT, Kobayashi Y. Cardiac magnetic resonance imaging with pharmacological stress perfusion and delayed enhancement in asymptomatic patients with systemic sclerosis. J Rheumatol. 2009;36:106–12.
137. Di Cesare E, Battisti S, Di Sibio A, Cipriani P, Giacomelli R, Liakouli V, Ruscitti P, Masciocchi C. Early assessment of subclinical cardiac involvement in systemic sclerosis (SSc) using delayed enhancement cardiac magnetic resonance (CE-MRI). Eur J Radiol. 2013;82:e268–73.
138. Moroncini G, Schicchi N, Pomponio G, Dziadzio M, della Costanza OP, Pierfederici A, Ferretti L, Pupita G, Valeri G, Agliata G, Salvolini L, Giovagnoni A, Gabrielli A. Myocardial perfusion defects in scleroderma detected by contrast-enhanced cardiovascular magnetic resonance. Radiol Med. 2014;119:885–94.
139. Rodriguez-Reyna TS, Morelos-Guzman M, Hernandez-Reyes P, Montero-Duarte K, Martinez-Reyes C, Reyes-Utrera C, Vazquez-La Madrid J, Morales-Blanhir J, Nunez-Alvarez C, Cabiedes-Contreras J. Assessment of myocardial fibrosis and microvascular damage in systemic sclerosis by magnetic resonance imaging and coronary angiotomography. Rheumatology (Oxford). 2015;54:647–54.
140. Sano M, Satoh H, Suwa K, Nobuhara M, Saitoh T, Saotome M, Urushida T, Katoh H, Shimoyama K, Suzuki D, Ogawa N, Takehara Y, Sakahara H, Hayashi H. Characteristics and clinical relevance of late gadolinium enhancement in cardiac magnetic resonance in patients with systemic sclerosis. Heart Vessel. 2015;30:779–88.
141. Mavrogeni SI, Kitas GD, Dimitroulas T, Sfikakis PP, Seo P, Gabriel S, Patel AR, Gargani L, Bombardieri S, Matucci-Cerinic M, Lombardi M, Pepe A, Aletras AH, Kolovou G, Miszalski T, van Riel P, Semb A, Gonzalez-Gay MA, Dessein P, Karpouzas G, Puntmann V, Nagel E, Bratis K, Karabela G, Stavropoulos E, Katsifis G, Koutsogeorgopoulou L, van Rossum A, Rademakers F, Pohost G, Lima JA. Cardiovascular magnetic resonance in rheumatology: current status and recommendations for use. Int J Cardiol. 2016;217:135–48. https://doi.org/10.1016/j.ijcard.2016.04.158. Epub 2016 Apr 27.
142. Gargani L, Todiere G, Guiducci S, Bruni C, Pingitore A, De Marchi D, Bellando Randone S, Aquaro GD, Bazzichi L, Mosca M, Lombardi M, Pepe A, Matucci-Cerinic M, Picano E. Early detection of Cardiac involvement in systemic sclerosis: the added value of magnetic resonance imaging. JACC Cardiovasc Imaging. 2019;12(5):927–8. https://doi.org/10.1016/j.jcmg.2018.09.025. Epub 2018 Dec 12.
143. Mavrogeni S, Gargani L, Pepe A, Monti L, Markousis-Mavrogenis G, De Santis M, De Marchi D, Koutsogeorgopoulou L, Karabela G, Stavropoulos E, Katsifis G, Bratis K, Bellando-Randone S, Guiducci S, Bruni C, Moggi-Pignone A, Dimitroulas T, Kolovou G, Bournia VK, Sfikakis PP, Matucci-Cerinic M. Cardiac magnetic resonance predicts ventricular arrhythmias in scleroderma: the Scleroderma Arrhythmia Clinical Utility Study (SAnCtUS). Rheumatology (Oxford). 2020;59(8):1938–48. https://doi.org/10.1093/rheumatology/kez494.
144. Cooper LT, Baughman KL, Feldman AM, Frustaci A, Jessup M, Kuhl U, Levine GN, Narula J, Starling RC, Towbin J, Virmani R. The role of endomyocardial biopsy in the management of cardiovascular disease: a scientific statement from the American Heart Association, the American College of Cardiology, and the European Society of Cardiology. Circulation. 2007;116:2216–33.
145. Hager WD, Collins I, Tate JP, Azrin M, Foley R, Lakshminarayanan S, Rothfield NF. Exercise during cardiac catheterization distinguishes between pulmonary and left ventricular causes of dyspnea in systemic sclerosis patients. Clin Respir J. 2013;7:227–36.
146. Ciurzynski M, Bienias P, Irzyk K, Kostrubiec M, Bartoszewicz Z, Siwicka M, Kurzyna M, Demkow U, Pruszczyk P. Exaggerated increase of exercise-induced pulmonary artery pressure in systemic sclerosis patients predominantly results from left ventricular diastolic dysfunction. Clin Res Cardiol. 2013;102:813–20.
147. Vachiéry JL, Tedford RJ, Rosenkranz S, Palazzini M, Lang I, Guazzi M, Coghlan G, Chazova I, De Marco T. Pulmonary hypertension due to left heart disease. Eur Respir J. 2019;53(1):1801897. https://doi.org/10.1183/13993003.01897-2018.
148. D'Alto M, Romeo E, Argiento P, Mattera Iacono A, Vettori S, Riccardi A, Allanore Y, D'Andrea A, Rea G, Bossone E, Valentini G, Naeije R, Golino P. Hemodynamic changes after acute fluid loading in patients with systemic sclerosis without pulmonary hypertension. Pulm Circ. 2019;9(1):2045894018816089. https://doi.org/10.1177/2045894018816089. Epub 2018 Nov 13.
149. Ciftci O, Onat AM, Yavuz B, Akdogan A, Aytemir K, Tokgozoglu L, Sahiner L, Deniz A, Ureten K, Kizilca G, Calguneri M, Oto A. Cardiac repolarization abnormalities and increased sympathetic activity in scleroderma. J Natl Med Assoc. 2007;99:232–7.
150. Can I, Onat AM, Aytemir K, Akdogan A, Ureten K, Kiraz S, Ertenli I, Ozer N, Tokgozoglu L, Oto A. Assessment of atrial conduction in patients with scleroderma by tissue doppler echocardiography and P wave dispersion. Cardiology. 2007;108:317–21.
151. Sergiacomi G, De Nardo D, Capria A, Manenti G, Fabiano S, Borzi M, De Sanctis G, Konda D, Sperandio M, Schillaci O, Masala S, Simonetti G, Fontana L. Non-invasive diagnostic and functional evaluation of cardiac and pulmonary involvement in systemic sclerosis. In Vivo. 2004;18:229–35.
152. Geyer H, Caracciolo G, Abe H, Wilansky S, Carerj S, Gentile F, Nesser HJ, Khandheria B, Narula J, Sengupta PP. Assessment of myocardial mechanics using speckle tracking echocardiography: fundamentals and clinical applications. J Am Soc Echocardiogr. 2010;23:351–69; quiz 453–5.
153. Blessberger H, Binder T. Non-invasive imaging: two dimensional speckle tracking echocardiography: basic principles. Heart. 2010;96:716–22.

154. Pavlopoulos H, Nihoyannopoulos P. Strain and strain rate deformation parameters: from tissue Doppler to 2D speckle tracking. Int J Cardiovasc Imaging. 2008;24:479–91.
155. Teske AJ, De Boeck BW, Melman PG, Sieswerda GT, Doevendans PA, Cramer MJ. Echocardiographic quantification of myocardial function using tissue deformation imaging, a guide to image acquisition and analysis using tissue Doppler and speckle tracking. Cardiovasc Ultrasound. 2007;5:27.
156. Haji K, Wong C, Wright L, Ramkumar S, Marwick TH. Left atrial strain performance and its application in clinical practice. JACC Cardiovasc Imaging. 2019;12(6):1093–101. https://doi.org/10.1016/j.jcmg.2018.11.009. Epub 2019 Jan 16.
157. Agoston G, Gargani L, Miglioranza MH, Caputo M, Badano LP, Moreo A, Muraru D, Mondillo S, Moggi Pignone A, Matucci Cerinic M, Sicari R, Picano E, Varga A. Left atrial dysfunction detected by speckle tracking in patients with systemic sclerosis. Cardiovasc Ultrasound. 2014;12:30. https://doi.org/10.1186/1476-7120-12-30.
158. D'Andrea A, D'Alto M, Di Maio M, Vettori S, Benjamin N, Cocchia R, Argiento P, Romeo E, Di Marco G, Russo MG, Valentini G, Calabrò R, Bossone E, Grünig E. Right atrial morphology and function in patients with systemic sclerosis compared to healthy controls: a two-dimensional strain study. Clin Rheumatol. 2016;35(7):1733–42. https://doi.org/10.1007/s10067-016-3279-9. Epub 2016 Apr 27.
159. Lancellotti P, Pellikka PA, Budts W, Chaudhry FA, Donal E, Dulgheru R, Edvardsen T, Garbi M, Ha JW, Kane GC, Kreeger J, Mertens L, Pibarot P, Picano E, Ryan T, Tsutsui JM, Varga A. The clinical use of stress echocardiography in non-ischaemic heart disease: recommendations from the European Association of Cardiovascular Imaging and the American Society of Echocardiography. Eur Heart J Cardiovasc Imaging. 2016;17(11):1191–229. https://doi.org/10.1093/ehjci/jew190. Erratum in: Eur Heart J Cardiovasc Imaging. 2017 May 1;18(8):832.
160. Gargani L, Pignone A, Agoston G, Moreo A, Capati E, Badano LP, Doveri M, Bazzichi L, Costantino MF, Pavellini A, Pieri F, Musca F, Muraru D, Epis O, Bruschi E, De Chiara B, Perfetto F, Mori F, Parodi O, Sicari R, Bombardieri S, Varga A, Cerinic MM, Bossone E, Picano E. Clinical and echocardiographic correlations of exercise-induced pulmonary hypertension in systemic sclerosis: a multicenter study. Am Heart J. 2013;165(2):200–7. https://doi.org/10.1016/j.ahj.2012.10.020. Epub 2012 Nov 28.
161. Kovacs G, Avian A, Wutte N, Hafner F, Moazedi-Fürst F, Kielhauser S, Aberer E, Brodmann M, Graninger W, Foris V, Olschewski A, Olschewski H. Changes in pulmonary exercise haemodynamics in scleroderma: a 4-year prospective study. Eur Respir J. 2017;50(1):1601708. https://doi.org/10.1183/13993003.01708-2016.
162. Madonna R, Morganti R, Radico F, Vitulli P, Mascellanti M, Amerio P, De Caterina R. Isolated exercise-induced pulmonary hypertension associates with higher cardiovascular risk in scleroderma patients. J Clin Med. 2020;9(6):1910. https://doi.org/10.3390/jcm9061910.
163. Galiè N, Humbert M, Vachiery JL, Gibbs S, Lang I, Torbicki A, Simonneau G, Peacock A, Vonk Noordegraaf A, Beghetti M, Ghofrani A, Gomez Sanchez MA, Hansmann G, Klepetko W, Lancellotti P, Matucci M, McDonagh T, Pierard LA, Trindade PT, Zompatori M, Hoeper M, ESC Scientific Document Group. 2015 ESC/ERS guidelines for the diagnosis and treatment of pulmonary hypertension: the Joint Task Force for the Diagnosis and Treatment of Pulmonary Hypertension of the European Society of Cardiology (ESC) and the European Respiratory Society (ERS): Endorsed by: Association for European Paediatric and Congenital Cardiology (AEPC), International Society for Heart and Lung Transplantation (ISHLT). Eur Heart J. 2016;37(1):67–119. https://doi.org/10.1093/eurheartj/ehv317. Epub 2015 Aug 29.
164. Guazzi M, Bandera F, Ozemek C, Systrom D, Arena R. Cardiopulmonary exercise testing: what is its value? J Am Coll Cardiol. 2017;70(13):1618–36. https://doi.org/10.1016/j.jacc.2017.08.012.
165. Boutou AK, Pitsiou GG, Siakka P, Dimitroulas T, Paspala A, Sourla E, Chavouzis N, Garyfallos A, Argyropoulou P, Stanopoulos I. Phenotyping exercise limitation in systemic sclerosis: the use of cardiopulmonary exercise testing. Respiration. 2016;91(2):115–23. https://doi.org/10.1159/000442888. Epub 2016 Jan 6.
166. Ewert R, Ittermann T, Habedank D, Held M, Lange TJ, Halank M, Winkler J, Gläser S, Olschewski H, Kovacs G. Prognostic value of cardiopulmonary exercise testing in patients with systemic sclerosis. BMC Pulm Med. 2019;19(1):230. https://doi.org/10.1186/s12890-019-1003-7.
167. Iles L, Pfluger H, Phrommintikul A, Cherayath J, Aksit P, Gupta SN, Kaye DM, Taylor AJ. Evaluation of diffuse myocardial fibrosis in heart failure with cardiac magnetic resonance contrast-enhanced T1 mapping. J Am Coll Cardiol. 2008;52:1574–80.
168. Messroghli DR, Greiser A, Frohlich M, Dietz R, Schulz-Menger J. Optimization and validation of a fully-integrated pulse sequence for modified look-locker inversion-recovery (MOLLI) T1 mapping of the heart. J Magn Reson Imaging. 2007;26:1081–6.
169. Messroghli DR, Radjenovic A, Kozerke S, Higgins DM, Sivananthan MU, Ridgway JP. Modified Look-Locker inversion recovery (MOLLI) for high-resolution T1 mapping of the heart. Magn Reson Med. 2004;52:141–6.
170. Lee DC, Johnson NP. Quantification of absolute myocardial blood flow by magnetic resonance perfusion imaging. JACC Cardiovasc Imaging. 2009;2:761–70.
171. Abraham TP, Dimaano VL, Liang HY. Role of tissue Doppler and strain echocardiography in current clinical practice. Circulation. 2007;116:2597–609.
172. Marwick TH. Measurement of strain and strain rate by echocardiography: ready for prime time? J Am Coll Cardiol. 2006;47:1313–27.
173. Plaksej R, Kosmala W, Frantz S, Herrmann S, Niemann M, Stork S, Wachter R, Angermann CE, Ertl G, Bijnens B, Weidemann F. Relation of circulating markers of fibrosis and progression of left and right ventricular dysfunction in hypertensive patients with heart failure. J Hypertens. 2009;27:2483–91.
174. Popovic ZB, Kwon DH, Mishra M, Buakhamsri A, Greenberg NL, Thamilarasan M, Flamm SD, Thomas JD, Lever HM, Desai MY. Association between regional ventricular function and myocardial fibrosis in hypertrophic cardiomyopathy assessed by speckle tracking echocardiography and delayed hyperenhancement magnetic resonance imaging. J Am Soc Echocardiogr. 2008;21:1299–305.
175. Mondillo S, Galderisi M, Mele D, Cameli M, Lomoriello VS, Zaca V, Ballo P, D'Andrea A, Muraru D, Losi M, Agricola E, D'Errico A, Buralli S, Sciomer S, Nistri S, Badano L. Speckle-tracking echocardiography: A new technique for assessing myocardial function. J Ultrasound Med. 2011;30:71–83.
176. Shehata ML, Cheng S, Osman NF, Bluemke DA, Lima JA. Myocardial tissue tagging with cardiovascular magnetic resonance. J Cardiovasc Magn Reson. 2009;11:55.
177. Atas H, Kepez A, Tigen K, Samadov F, Ozen G, Cincin A, Sunbul M, Bozbay M, Direskeneli H, Basaran Y. Evaluation of left atrial volume and function in systemic sclerosis patients using speckle tracking and real-time three-dimensional echocardiography. Anatol J Cardiol. 2016;16:316.
178. Cadeddu C, Deidda M, Giau G, Lilliu M, Cadeddu F, Binaghi G, Mura MN, Farci M, Del Giacco S, Manconi PE, Mercuro G. Contractile reserve in systemic sclerosis patients as a major

predictor of global cardiac impairment and exercise tolerance. Int J Cardiovasc Imaging. 2015;31:529–36.
179. Cusma Piccione M, Zito C, Bagnato G, Oreto G, Di Bella G, Carerj S. Role of 2D strain in the early identification of left ventricular dysfunction and in the risk stratification of systemic sclerosis patients. Cardiovasc Ultrasound. 2013;11:6.
180. Spethmann S, Dreger H, Schattke S, Riemekasten G, Borges AC, Baumann G, Knebel F. Two-dimensional speckle tracking of the left ventricle in patients with systemic sclerosis for an early detection of myocardial involvement. Eur Heart J Cardiovasc Imaging. 2012;13:863–70.
181. Spethmann S, Rieper K, Riemekasten G, Borges AC, Schattke S, Burmester GR, Hewing B, Baumann G, Dreger H, Knebel F. Echocardiographic follow-up of patients with systemic sclerosis by 2D speckle tracking echocardiography of the left ventricle. Cardiovasc Ultrasound. 2014;12:13.
182. Tigen K, Sunbul M, Ozen G, Durmus E, Kivrak T, Cincin A, Ozben B, Atas H, Direskeneli H, Basaran Y. Regional myocardial dysfunction assessed by two-dimensional speckle tracking echocardiography in systemic sclerosis patients with fragmented QRS complexes. J Electrocardiol. 2014;47:677–83.
183. Yiu KH, Schouffoer AA, Marsan NA, Ninaber MK, Stolk J, Vlieland TV, Scherptong RW, Delgado V, Holman ER, Tse HF, Huizinga TW, Bax JJ, Schuerwegh AJ. Left ventricular dysfunction assessed by speckle-tracking strain analysis in patients with systemic sclerosis: relationship to functional capacity and ventricular arrhythmias. Arthritis Rheum. 2011;63:3969–78.
184. Vohringer M, Mahrholdt H, Yilmaz A, Sechtem U. Significance of late gadolinium enhancement in cardiovascular magnetic resonance imaging (CMR). Herz. 2007;32:129–37.
185. Barison A, Gargani L, De Marchi D, Aquaro GD, Guiducci S, Picano E, Cerinic MM, Pingitore A. Early myocardial and skeletal muscle interstitial remodelling in systemic sclerosis: insights from extracellular volume quantification using cardiovascular magnetic resonance. Eur Heart J Cardiovasc Imaging. 2015;16:74–80.
186. Thuny F, Lovric D, Schnell F, Bergerot C, Ernande L, Cottin V, Derumeaux G, Croisille P. Quantification of myocardial extracellular volume fraction with cardiac MR imaging for early detection of left ventricle involvement in systemic sclerosis. Radiology. 2014;271:373–80.
187. Mavrogeni S, Bratis K, Karabela G, Spiliotis G, van Wijk K, Hautemann D, Reiber JH, Koutsogeorgopoulou L, Markousis-Mavrogenis G, Kolovou G, Stavropoulos E. Cardiovascular magnetic resonance imaging clarifies cardiac pathophysiology in early, asymptomatic diffuse systemic sclerosis. Inflamm Allergy Drug Targets. 2015;14:29.
188. Milano A, Pendergrass SA, Sargent JL, George LK, McCalmont TH, Connolly MK, Whitfield ML. Molecular subsets in the gene expression signatures of scleroderma skin. PLoS One. 2008;3:e2696.
189. Solomon SD, Zile M, Pieske B, Voors A, Shah A, Kraigher-Krainer E, Shi V, Bransford T, Takeuchi M, Gong J, Lefkowitz M, Packer M, McMurray JJ. The angiotensin receptor neprilysin inhibitor LCZ696 in heart failure with preserved ejection fraction: a phase 2 double-blind randomised controlled trial. Lancet. 2012;380:1387–95.
190. Pieske B, Butler J, Filippatos G, Lam C, Maggioni AP, Ponikowski P, Shah S, Solomon S, Kraigher-Krainer E, Samano ET, Scalise AV, Muller K, Roessig L, Gheorghiade M. Rationale and design of the SOluble guanylate Cyclase stimulatoR in heArT failurE Studies (SOCRATES). Eur J Heart Fail. 2014;16:1026–38.
191. Kapur NK. Transforming growth factor-{beta}: governing the transition from inflammation to fibrosis in heart failure with preserved left ventricular function. Circ Heart Fail. 2011;4:5–7.
192. Gabrielli A, Avvedimento EV, Krieg T. Scleroderma. N Engl J Med. 2009;360:1989–2003.
193. Abbas AE, Fortuin FD, Schiller NB, Appleton CP, Moreno CA, Lester SJ. A simple method for noninvasive estimation of pulmonary vascular resistance. J Am Coll Cardiol. 2003;41:1021–7.
194. Lang RM, Bierig M, Devereux RB, Flachskampf FA, Foster E, Pellikka PA, Picard MH, Roman MJ, Seward J, Shanewise JS, Solomon SD, Spencer KT, Sutton MS, Stewart WJ. Recommendations for chamber quantification: a report from the American Society of Echocardiography's Guidelines and Standards Committee and the Chamber Quantification Writing Group, developed in conjunction with the European Association of Echocardiography, a branch of the European Society of Cardiology. J Am Soc Echocardiogr. 2005;18:1440–63.
195. Solomon SD, Janardhanan R, Verma A, Bourgoun M, Daley WL, Purkayastha D, Lacourciere Y, Hippler SE, Fields H, Naqvi TZ, Mulvagh SL, Arnold JM, Thomas JD, Zile MR, Aurigemma GP. Effect of angiotensin receptor blockade and antihypertensive drugs on diastolic function in patients with hypertension and diastolic dysfunction: a randomised trial. Lancet. 2007;369:2079–87.
196. Baggish AL, van Kimmenade RR, Januzzi JL Jr. The differential diagnosis of an elevated amino-terminal pro-B-type natriuretic peptide level. Am J Cardiol. 2008;101:43–8.
197. Bettencourt PM. Clinical usefulness of B-type natriuretic peptide measurement: present and future perspectives. Heart. 2005;91:1489–94.
198. Rehman SU, Januzzi JL Jr. Natriuretic peptide testing in clinical medicine. Cardiol Rev. 2008;16:240–9.

Part V

Pulmonary Manifestations and Management

Yannick Allanore

Overview of Lung Involvement

23

Athol U. Wells

Introduction

In systemic sclerosis (SSc), interstitial lung disease (SSc-ILD) is a major source of morbidity. SSc-ILD is a frequent cause of death in SSc and, when severe, is often complicated by pulmonary hypertension (SSc-PH). With growing awareness of the high prevalence of ILD in SSc, there has been an increasing focus on the early identification of lung involvement. Other than the various interstitial pneumonias, interstitial lung disease processes are exceedingly rare in SSc with a handful of case reports of obliterative bronchiolitis, diffuse alveolar haemorrhage and significant pleural involvement and occasional cases of drug-induced lung disease. In this chapter, the approach to lung disease in SSc is discussed, including epidemiological implications, clinical features at presentation, prognostic evaluation and the management of SSc-ILD.

Epidemiological Considerations

SSc-ILD is a rare disease but has been widely studied as cohorts have been accumulated at expert centres, and in addition, the EUSTAR initiative has greatly expanded knowledge of the disease. In 46 pooled studies, the prevalence of SSc was 17.6/100,000 [1]. The estimated prevalence of SSc-ILD in SSc patients has varied greatly depending upon cohort inclusion characteristics, ranging from sub-clinical lung abnormalities ('pre-clinical disease'), detected from screening by CT or pulmonary function tests (PFT), to clinically significant disease. Overall, SSc-ILD is evident in approximately half of SSc-ILD patients with considerable variation depending upon the timing of evaluation after the initial onset of SSc. Thus, based on the prevalence of SSc [1], the prevalence of SSc-ILD is less than 10/100,000.

However, although SSc-ILD might be dismissed as a very rare disease in the general community, a very different picture emerges when interstitial lung disease (ILD) cohorts and patients presenting to rheumatologists are considered. In ILD populations at referral centres, ILD associated with connective tissue disease (CTD) consistently makes up 20–25% of patients, with SSc-ILD a significant minority of this sub-group. In rheumatological practice, ILD is more frequent in SSc than in other CTD. Rheumatoid arthritis is much more prevalent than SSc but much less frequently complicated by ILD: thus, rheumatoid lung and SSc-ILD are similar in prevalence. Thus, SSc-ILD is an important and significantly prevalent disease in respiratory and rheumatologic practice and, in those contexts, should not be viewed as rare disease.

The spectrum of SSc-ILD has been elucidated in large international collaborative databases, in which nomenclature [2] and diagnostic criteria are standardized and the problems of characterizing a rare disease have been overcome. The EUSTAR database, for example, includes more than 5800 SSc patients [3]. In that very large cohort, SSc mortality was most commonly due to SSc-ILD (35% of deaths related to SSc), followed by pulmonary hypertension (SSc-PH, 26% of deaths). Renal disease, the most frequent cause of SSc-related deaths before the millennium, has been mostly controlled by rigorous treatment of hypertension and now accounts for less than 5% of deaths [3]. SSc occurs more commonly in women (female:male ratio 5:1 in pooled studies) aged 30–50 years [1]. This profile broadly applies to SSc-ILD, and in US series, SSc-ILD risk is associated with African American ethnicity. Risk factors for the onset of SSc-ILD in SSc patients, discussed later, include diffuse cutaneous SSc, the presence of anti-topoisomerase antibodies (Scl70), older age at disease onset and a short duration of systemic disease [4–8].

A. U. Wells (✉)
Royal Brompton Hospital, London, UK
e-mail: rbhild@rbht.nhs.uk

Y. Allanore et al. (eds.), *Scleroderma*, https://doi.org/10.1007/978-3-031-40658-4_23

Histologic Features of SSc-ILD

In historical autopsy studies, interstitial fibrosis has been present histologically in a large majority of SSc patients, although often not evident prior to death [9]. In SSc-ILD, the spectrum of histological patterns mirrors that in the idiopathic interstitial pneumonias [10]. However, the prevalence and prognostic importance of individual histologic patterns differs substantially between SSc-ILD and idiopathic ILD. In the idiopathic interstitial pneumonias, usual interstitial pneumonia (UIP), corresponding to idiopathic pulmonary fibrosis (IPF), is the most frequent pattern, associated with a much worse outcome than other patterns. By contrast, nonspecific interstitial pneumonia (NSIP) is the most prevalent histologic pattern in SSc-ILD. In the largest series (n = 80) of SSc-ILD patients undergoing surgical biopsy [11], cellular or fibrotic NSIP was present in 78%. Less than a quarter of patients had potentially reversible histologic abnormalities; thus, in clinical practice, treatment of SSc-ILD may achieve stabilization but results in partial disease regression in only a minority of cases. Importantly, the distinction between UIP and NSIP had no prognostic significance. These observations were mirrored in smaller series, although a non-significant trend towards shorter survival in association with a UIP pattern was documented in one report [12].

The Detection of SSc-ILD

It is now universally recognized that SSc-ILD identification is by means of high-resolution computed tomography (HRCT) [13, 14]. HRCT appearances typically consist of prominent ground-glass evaluation with admixed reticulation and traction bronchiectasis in most cases but a low prevalence of honeycombing [15]. The high sensitivity of HRCT is advantageous but also creates difficulties in ascribing clinical significance when, as is often the case, abnormalities are very limited. Thus, the selection of patients for treatment, discussed later, requires the integration of symptoms, PFT and HRCT findings. The importance of baseline ILD severity in determining outcome has been underlined in a number of landmark historical studies [16–19].

Key Risk Factors for SSc-ILD in SSc Patients

SSc-ILD has been associated with both autoantibody findings and the presence of diffuse cutaneous disease in many series, with stronger linkage to autoantibody status [20, 21]. Anti-topoisomerase I (anti Scl-70) antibody positivity, present in more than 20% of SSc patients, is characterized by the development of pulmonary fibrosis in up to of cases [22]. However, anti-Scl70 positivity occurs in only 40% of SSc-ILD patients [23] and, thus, ILD is associated with many other autoantibody profiles. Anti-Scl70 levels have correlated with SSc-ILD severity [24, 25] but not with sufficient consistency to provide clinical utility. Anti-centromere antibody (ACA) positivity is seldom associated with clinically significant SSc-ILD but is associated with a greatly increased risk of SSc-PH [4, 26].

In summary, the nature of skin involvement and autoantibody status should be taken into account in anticipating the future development of SSc-ILD but the associations are insufficiently robust to serve as a basis for selective monitoring algorithms in routine practice.

Genetic and Pathogenetic Implications

Genetic predispositions to SSc [27, 28] do not have a direct bearing on the clinical approach to SSc-ILD as the overall familial linkage to SSc is weak, although it is believed that many gene variants may influence susceptibility, clinical phenotype and disease progression [29]. Similarly, although genetic linkages to Scl70 positivity [23, 30] and to SSc-ILD [31, 32] have been reported, these observations do not provide clinical useful information. Pathogenetic studies are explored in detail elsewhere in this volume but in terms of management, pathogenetic pathways believed to drive SSc-ILD have broadly include immune dysregulation in its various forms and pro-fibrotic pathways that are common to progressive fibrotic ILD.

Current Clinical Practice: Is Lung Disease Clinically Significant?

The overall approach to SSc-ILD is influenced by disease severity, the duration of systemic disease (as judged by SSc symptoms and not by Raynaud's phenomenon) and the presence of occupational exposures that might contribute to progression of SSc or SSc-ILD. Aspiration due to gastroesophageal regurgitation may contribute to the initiation or progression of SSc-ILD (this has yet to be validated) but should, in any case, be recognized as a cause of troublesome cough (due to a vagally mediated cough reflex).

Based on the prognostic significance of lung involvement, a pro-active approach in patients with SSc is increasingly taken with screening for ILD using PFT and HRCT. However, the presence of abnormalities is not synonymous with clinically significant disease. Perhaps, the greatest initial difficulty encountered by clinicians is the distinction between sub-clinical and clinically overt disease. The severity of exertional dyspnoea is often misleading as respiratory symptoms are notoriously nonspecific, not correlating well with pulmonary disease severity, as judged by PFT and HRCT. Exercise intolerance arises from many causes other than lung disease, including cardiac involvement, musculoskeletal disease and loss of fitness due to general debility. As a general guide, the absence of oxygen desaturation during a 6-minute walk test when the patient experiences exertional dyspnoea suggests that it largely results from extra-pulmonic limitation. Physical examination adds little to symptoms, PFT and CT in assigning clinical significance.

PFTs, used historically to define severity and to monitor SSc-ILD, play a key role in designating clinical significance. However, their limitations need to be understood. The 'normal' PFT range, varying from 80% to 120% of values predicted by age, height and gender [33], is a major confounder. An FVC value of 85% of predicted may equally represent absence of decline or a major reduction of 35% from a premorbid value of 120%. Severe reductions in PFT are reliably indicative of severe pulmonary disease. However, their high prevalence in historical cohorts [4] is less applicable to SSc patients evaluated at presentation with a view to early intervention. It is sometimes obvious that disease extent on HRCT is indicative of clinical significance but in many cases, abnormalities are limited.

In the case of SSc-PH, intervention is mostly confined to established PH but the early identification of those at higher risk allows monitoring to be targeted appropriately. In this regard, patterns of PFT impairment often allow the distinction between restrictive lung disease and predominant pulmonary vasculopathy. A disproportionate reduction in carbon monoxide diffusing capacity [DLco] (quantified as the gas transfer coefficient [Kco] or the FEV1/DLco ratio) is a helpful finding meriting the exclusion of PH and careful subsequent monitoring. An important caveat is that an apparently 'vasculopathic' profile can arise from the coexistence of emphysema and lung fibrosis, well documented in idiopathic interstitial pneumonia [34] but also encountered in SSc-ILD, including in lifelong smokers [35]. However, this scenario can be excluded by HRCT evaluation. Elevation of the FVC/DLco ratio has been validated as a marker of pulmonary vascular limitation in recent series [36, 37]. However, Kco reduction may be more robust as it is a highly reproducible measure. The FVC/DLco ratio is a composite of measured FVC, Kco and alveolar volume, with the latter two variables used to compute DLco [38].

HRCT has displaced chest radiography in the morphologic evaluation of ILD, with the chest radiograph insensitive in SSc-ILD detection [39]. An additional advantage enjoyed by HRCT is the confident identification of fibrotic disease, based on the admixture of ground glass and reticulation and, especially, the presence of traction bronchiectasis [13, 40, 41]. Precise measurement of disease extent is too arduous to be routinely applicable although this is likely to change when quantitative techniques eventually become widely available. However, rapid evaluation of disease extent on HRCT does at least allow the clinician to deal with the confounding effect of the PFT normal range, discussed earlier.

In summary, the identification of clinically significant lung disease requiring more frequent monitoring or, more often, immediate treatment is a multidisciplinary exercise requiring the reconciliation of symptoms, PFT severity, patterns of PFT impairment, HRCT and echocardiography.

Monitoring of Lung Disease in SSc

Serial PFTs are central to routine monitoring. However, as in interstitial lung disease in general, measurement variation creates difficulties. PFT trends reliably indicate change, as opposed to measurement variability, only when thresholds for 'significant change' are exceeded (e.g. a change in FVC exceeding 10% of baseline values). DLco trends are also helpful when FVC change is marginal but do not, in isolation, distinguish between SSc-ILD progression and worsening pulmonary vasculopathy. Alternative causes PFT decline must be considered, especially infection. Furthermore, PFT measurement variation can result in the under-statement of change, with a 5–10% serial reduction in FVC indicative of SSc-ILD progression. Thus, PFT trends most be reconciled with symptomatic change and, when appropriate, serial HRCT evaluation.

Serial HRCT should ideally be reserved for those patients in whom progression is suspected, based on PFT and symptomatic trends. HRCT is, in some cases, <u>too</u> sensitive in the identification of ILD progression. In the absence of a validated definition of 'significant' HRCT change, minor HRCT change is difficult to interpret in patients with stable PFT. The long-term risk of malignancy with excessive exposure to radiation should be kept in mind. Thus, serial HRCT should be performed case by case when important clinical questions are unanswered. In practice, this amounts to discordance between symptomatic change and pulmonary function trends, decline in DLco equally ascribable equally SSc-ILD progression and worsening pulmonary vasculopathy, and when alternative disease processes, such as opportunistic infection or drug-induced lung disease, are suspected.

In summary, the identification of progression of lung disease, the distinction between worsening SSc-ILD and worsening pulmonary vasculopathy and the exclusion of alternative disease processes are a multidisciplinary exercise, requiring the integration of symptoms and PFT trends and the judicious use of serial HRCT. It is usual to repeat PFT 3–6 monthly with less frequent monitoring when disease has been stable for at least 2 years.

Prognostic Evaluation of SSc-ILD: When Should Treatment Be Instituted?

The distinction between immediate treatment and meticulous monitoring is sometimes a close call, even when lung disease is clinically significant, with patient wishes often determining immediate management decisions. Thus, prognostic evaluation identifying a higher risk of subsequent progression plays a pivotal role in patient–doctor discussions. Based on accumulated clinical experience, risk stratification can be broadly defined from the severity of lung disease, duration of systemic disease and evidence of ongoing disease progression.

Severe lung disease is a consequence of previous repeated disease progression and is, in itself, indicative of a higher likelihood of future progression that is likely to be associated with major reduction in exercise tolerance and quality of life. The distinction between lower and higher risk SSc-ILD was quantified in a widely used staging system based on FVC and rapid semi-quantitative HRCT extent thresholds [19], validated in US and Australian cohorts [42, 43]. SSc-ILD is classified as 'extensive', when HRCT disease extent exceeds 20%, or, in cases with an 'indeterminate' disease extent, percentage predicted FVC of <70%. Extensive SSc-ILD is associated with a marked increased mortality and a shorter time to decline in PFT variables [19]. The risk of SSc-ILD progression is greater early after the onset of systemic disease and especially when lung disease precedes the cutaneous manifestations of SSc [4]. For practical purposes, SSc-ILD detected shortly after the onset of systemic disease is more likely to be intrinsically progressive, with a reduced threshold for therapeutic intervention. However, in SSc-ILD patients with minor PFT impairment and limited disease on HRCT after more than 5 years of systemic disease, evolution to severe fibrotic lung disease is less likely but must be closely monitored.

Recent disease progression of disease is, in itself, an additional indication for therapy. In SSc-ILD, decline in pulmonary function indices over 1–2 years, including serial FVC, DLco or Kco reduction, is associated with mortality, independently of baseline disease severity [44, 45].

No validated algorithm currently exists to integrate these considerations into a rigorous management algorithm: the decision to introduce therapy and the intensity of treatment decided case by case. Ancillary features of lung involvement have not provided rigorous guidance. The presence of pleuroparenchymal fibroelastosis (PPFE), affecting the visceral pleura and the sub-pleural parenchyma in up to 20% of SSc patients [46], is associated with increased mortality, but with only a marginal increase in serial FVC decline. There is an unmet need for biomarkers that accurately predict disease progression. Serum biomarkers investigated in SSc-ILD include MMP-7, surfactant protein-D [SP-D], Krebs von den Lungen-6 [KL-6] and C-C motif chemokine ligand 18 [CCL18] [47], with increased serum KL6 and CCL18 levels associated with progression in a large cohort [48]. Increased serum interleukin 6 levels are predictive of lung function decline and mortality in SSc-ILD patients, but only in limited disease, suggesting that this biomarker may be more relevant to earlier inflammatory disease [49]. However, serum biomarkers have not been validated as accurate in individual patients, as opposed to average sub-cohort change, and are not currently recommended in clinical practice. Finally, bronchoalveolar lavage (BAL) cellularity is no longer regarded as providing useful ancillary information guiding treatment decision, with no prognostic utility independently of disease severity [50, 51].

Management Considerations

SSc-ILD treatment studies and their application to clinical practice are covered in detail elsewhere in this volume. In brief, until recently, the unifying management approach has been the suppression of inflammation, based on a pathogenetic model in which inflammation precedes and leads to fibrosis (the inflammatory fibrotic model). Pivotal data justifying this approach have come from placebo-controlled trials of oral cyclophosphamide [18], intravenous cyclophosphamide [52], tocilizumab [53], a comparison between oral cyclophosphamide and mycophenolate mofetil [54], and a recent placebo-controlled trial of rituximab [55]. Other definitely studied treatments not based primarily on an inflammatory–fibrotic model, have consisted of bosentan [56], a failed therapy, and nintedanib [57], an anti-fibrotic agent that is likely to have a major future role in routine practice.

In the landmark SLS-1 trial, active treatment with oral cyclophosphamide was associated with statistically significant treatment benefits at 1 year on FVC levels, dyspnoea, skin thickening and quality of life [19]. A subsequent underpowered placebo-controlled trial of intravenous cyclophosphamide provided supportive but only marginally significant beneficial trends [52]. These studies prompted EULAR to recommend cyclophosphamide in SSc-ILD [58]. However, it was clear from the outset that cyclophosphamide is only partially efficacious and is also associated with significant toxicity. After completion of the SLS-1 study, less than 15% of participants were prescribed ongoing cyclophosphamide therapy by their primary physicians [59]. The benefits of treatment in the SLS-1 trial were mostly confined to patients with extensive fibrotic disease on HRCT, with a striking FVC benefit against placebo (>10%) in this patient subgroup [18].

The SLS1 and UK cyclophosphamide trials provided no guidance on optimal longer term management. In the SLS-1 cohort, therapeutic gains had been lost a year after treatment cessation [59]. Azathioprine, methotrexate and, more recently, mycophenolate mofetil (MMF) were widely used in the longer term in clinical practice without controlled data, although support for MMF usage came from a meta-analysis of safety and efficacy drawn from six observational studies [60]. Eventually, in the SLS-2 study, the efficacy and tolerability of mycophenolate and cyclophosphamide in SSc-ILD were compared [56]. The two agents were similarly efficacious, with MMF better tolerated and less toxic. Until very recently, no other therapies were validated in SSc-ILD. Corticosteroid therapy (doses in excess of prednisolone 15 mg daily) is contraindicated in SSc-ILD, due to an association with fatal renal crisis [61, 62].

However, the therapeutic landscape has now changed in SSc-ILD with the recent trials of tocilizumab [54], rituximab [55] and, especially, nintedanib [57]. The focuSSced trial of tocilizumab [54], in common with an earlier phase II trial of tocilizumab in SSc [63], with neither trial confined to SSc-ILD patients, demonstrated treatment benefits in attenuating FVC decline, in patients with mild PFT impairment and diffuse cutaneous SSc. Based on supportive trends in observational and underpowered controlled evaluations in SSc-ILD and ILD associated with inflammatory myopathy [64–68], a placebo-controlled trial of rituximab was recently undertaken. Although skin disease was the primary focus of the trial, a significant benefit in SSc-ILD was strongly suggested based on a key secondary end point [55].

Nintedanib, a tyrosine kinase inhibitor with anti-fibrotic effects evaluated in the SENSCIS nintedanib SSc-ILD trial [57], was found to reduce FVC decline against placebo by approximately 45% and was well tolerated. Importantly, the combination of mycophenolate and nintedanib in a large patient sub-group was with a suggestion of additive benefits [69]. The INBUILD trial of nintedanib in non-IPF fibrotic lung disease, progressing despite management, included a patient sub-group with SSc-ILD [70]. The treatment effect, uniform across ILD diagnostic sub-groups, was a proportional reduction in decline of over 50% associated with active treatment. Taken together, these trials validate nintedanib therapy in SSc-ILD, both as initial treatment and in lung disease progressing despite immunosuppressive therapy.

Other interventions are less studied in SSc-ILD. Bone marrow transplantation, evaluated in randomized studies, including patients with severe SSc-ILD [71, 72], is superior to conventional treatment in SSc, resulting in longer overall survival, longer disease-free survival and higher quality of life, when compared to conventional SSc treatment [71–73]. However, despite significant improvements in pulmonary function tests, this expensive and onerous treatment approach has not been adopted as standard therapy in severe SSc-ILD.

Taken together, pivotal trials in SSc-ILD have validated the use of cyclophosphamide, mycophenolate, nintedanib and tocilizumab in patients at risk of ILD progression. Immunosuppressive therapy is likely to remain first-line treatment in the majority of SSc-ILD patients as neither tocilizumab nor nintedanib has had benefits in extra-pulmonic disease. The optimal selection of patients to receive initial combination therapy with mycophenolate and nintedanib has yet to be defined.

It appears that SSc-ILD management has reached a crossroads with a recent expansion of treatment options. In the years to come, a period of consolidation will be needed with careful consideration of the best balance of treatments addressing immune dysregulation and those centred on pro-fibrotic pathways. In some patients, combination therapies will be necessary but at present there is no guidance on this opportunity. It is likely that treatment stratagems will be subdivided according to the severity of lung involvement. In limited SSc-ILD, mycophenolate is likely to remain the treatment of first choice and is, in any case, likely to be required in the management of systemic disease. Tocilizumab also appears to be more suited to limited disease, with the optimal role of rituximab yet to be ascertained.

However, as extensive SSc-ILD is associated with increased mortality, despite standard treatment, anti-fibrotic therapy (currently nintedanib) is likely to have a particularly important role in this major patient sub-group and is also validated as second-line treatment in patients progressing despite management. It appears likely that combination regimens will be increasingly used empirically. The urgent need for reliable biomarkers must be stressed, with the specific goal of distinguishing between upregulation of pro-inflammatory and pro-fibrotic pathways. Only with this information will it be possible to move towards precision medicine in this rapidly evolving field.

References

1. Bairkdar M, Rossides M, Westerlind H, et al. Incidence and prevalence of systemic sclerosis globally: a comprehensive systematic review and meta-analysis. Rheumatology (Oxford). 2021;60:3121–33.
2. American Thoracic Society/European Respiratory Society international multidisciplinary consensus classification of the idiopathic interstitial pneumonias. Am J Respir Crit Care Med. 2002;165:277–304.
3. Tyndal AJ, Banert B, Vonk M, et al. Causes and risk factors for death in systemic sclerosis: a study from the EULAR Scleroderma Trials and Research (EUSTAR) database. Ann Rheum Dis. 2010;69:1809–15.
4. Steen VD, Conte C, Owens GR, Medsger TA Jr. Severe restrictive lung disease in systemic sclerosis. Arthritis Rheum. 1994;37:1283–9.
5. Elhai M, Meune C, Boubaya M, et al. Mapping and predicting mortality from systemic sclerosis. Ann Rheum Dis. 2017;76:1897–905.

6. Li X, Qian Y-Q, Liu N, et al. Survival rate, causes of death, and risk factors in systemic sclerosis: a large cohort study. Clin Rheumatol. 2018;37:3051–6.
7. Mayes MD, Lacey JV Jr, Beebe-Dimmer J, et al. Prevalence, incidence, survival, and disease characteristics of systemic sclerosis in a large US population. Arthritis Rheum. 2003;48:2246–55.
8. Reveille JD. Ethnicity and race and systemic sclerosis: how it affects susceptibility, severity, antibody genetics, and clinical manifestations. Curr Rheumatol Rep. 2003;5:160–7.
9. D'Angelo WA, Fries JF, Masi AT, Shulman LE. Pathologic observations in systemic sclerosis (scleroderma). A study of fifty-eight autopsy cases and fifty-eight matched controls. Am J Med. 1969;46:428–40.
10. Tansey D, Wells AU, Colby TV, et al. Variations in histological patterns of interstitial pneumonia between connective tissue disorders and their relationship to prognosis. Histopathology. 2004;44:585–96.
11. Bouros D, Wells AU, Nicholson AG, et al. Histopathologic subsets of fibrosing alveolitis in patients with systemic sclerosis and their relationship to outcome. Am J Respir Crit Care Med. 2002;165:1581–6.
12. Fischer A, Swigris JJ, Groshong SD, et al. Clinically significant interstitial lung disease in limited scleroderma: histopathology, clinical features, and survival. Chest. 2008;134:601–5.
13. Launay D, Remy-Jardin M, Michon-Pasturel U, et al. High resolution computed tomography in fibrosing alveolitis associated with systemic sclerosis. J Rheumatol. 2006;33:1789–801.
14. Fischer A, Strek ME, Cottin V, et al. Proceedings of the American College of Rheumatology/Association of Physicians of Great Britain and Ireland Connective Tissue Disease–Associated Interstitial Lung Disease Summit: a multidisciplinary approach to address challenges and opportunities. Arthritis Rheumatol. 2019;71:182–95.
15. Desai SR, Veeraraghavan S, Hansell DM, et al. CT features of lung disease in patients with systemic sclerosis: comparison with idiopathic pulmonary fibrosis and nonspecific interstitial pneumonia. Radiology. 2004;232:560–7.
16. Wells AU, Cullinan P, Hansell DM, et al. Fibrosing alveolitis associated with systemic sclerosis has a better prognosis than lone cryptogenic fibrosing alveolitis. Am J Respir Crit Care Med. 1994;149:1583–90.
17. Kocheril SV, Appleton BE, Somers EC, et al. Comparison of disease progression and mortality of connective tissue disease-related interstitial lung disease and idiopathic interstitial pneumonia. Arthritis Rheum. 2005;53:549–57.
18. Tashkin DP, Elashoff R, Clements PJ, et al., Scleroderma Lung Study Research Group. Cyclophosphamide versus placebo in scleroderma lung disease N Engl J Med. 2006;354:2655–66.
19. Goh NS, Desai SR, Veeraraghavan S, et al. Interstitial lung disease in systemic sclerosis: a simple staging system. Am J Respir Crit Care Med. 2008;177:1248–54.
20. Nihtyanova SI, Sari A, Harvey JC, et al. Using autoantibodies and cutaneous subset to develop outcome-based disease classification in systemic sclerosis. Arthritis Rheumatol. 2020;72:465–76.
21. Walker UA, Tyndall A, Czirják L, et al. Clinical risk assessment of organ manifestations in systemic sclerosis: a report from the EULAR Scleroderma Trials And Research group database. Ann Rheum Dis. 2007;66:754–63.
22. Briggs DC, Vaughan RW, Welsh KI, et al. Immunogenetic prediction of pulmonary fibrosis in systemic sclerosis. Lancet. 1991;338:661–2.
23. Gilchrist FC, Bunn C, Foley PJ, et al. Class II HLA associations with autoantibodies in scleroderma: a highly significant role for HLA-DP. Genes Immun. 2001;2:76–81.
24. Kuwana M, Kaburaki J, Mimori T, Kawakami Y, Tojo T. Longitudinal analysis of autoantibody response to topoisomerase I in systemic sclerosis. Arthritis Rheum. 2000;43:1074–84.
25. Hu PQ, Fertig N, Medsger TA Jr, Wright TM. Correlation of serum anti-DNA topoisomerase I antibody levels with disease severity and activity in systemic sclerosis. Arthritis Rheum. 2003;48:1363–73.
26. Reveille JD, Solomon DH, American College of Rheumatology Ad Hoc Committee of Immunologic Testing Guidelines. Evidence-based guidelines for the use of immunologic tests: anticentromere, Scl-70, and nucleolar antibodies. Arthritis Rheum. 2003;49:399–412.
27. Feghali-Bostwick C, Medsger TA Jr, Wright TM. Analysis of systemic sclerosis in twins reveals low concordance for disease and high concordance for the presence of antinuclear antibodies. Arthritis Rheum. 2003;48:1956–63.
28. Zhou X, Tan FK, Wang N, et al. Genome-wide association study for regions of systemic sclerosis susceptibility in a Choctaw Indian population with high disease prevalence. Arthritis Rheum. 2003;48:2585–92.
29. Makino T, Jinnin M. Genetic and epigenetic abnormalities in systemic sclerosis. J Dermatol. 2016;43:10–8.
30. Allanore Y, Dieude P, Boileau C. Genetic background of systemic sclerosis: autoimmune genes take centre stage. Rheumatology (Oxford). 2010;49:203–10.
31. Stock CJW, Renzoni EA. Genetic predictors of systemic sclerosis-associated interstitial lung disease: a review of recent literature. Eur J Hum Genet. 2018;26:765–77.
32. Sumita Y, Sugiura T, Kawaguchi Y, et al. Genetic polymorphisms in the surfactant proteins in systemic sclerosis in Japanese: T/T genotype at 1580 C/T (Thr131Ile) in the SP-B gene reduces the risk of interstitial lung disease. Rheumatology (Oxford). 2008;47:289–91.
33. Standardized lung function testing. Official statement of the European Respiratory Society. Eur Respir J Suppl. 1993;16:1–100.
34. Wells AU, King AD, Rubens MB, Cramer D, du Bois RM, Hansell DM. Lone CFA: a functional-morphological correlation based on extent of disease on thin-section computed tomography. Am J Respir Crit Care Med. 1997;155:1367–75.
35. Cottin V, Nunes H, Mouthon L, Gamondes D, Lazor R, Hachulla E, et al. Combined pulmonary fibrosis and emphysema syndrome in connective tissue disease. Arthritis Rheum. 2011;63:295–304.
36. Nathan SD, Shlobin OA, Ahmad S, Urbanek S, Barnett SD. Pulmonary hypertension and pulmonary function testing in idiopathic pulmonary fibrosis. Chest. 2007;131:657–63.
37. Steen VD, Graham G, Conte C, Owens G, Medsger TA Jr. Isolated diffusing capacity reduction in systemic sclerosis. Arthritis Rheum. 1992;35:765–70.
38. Hughes JMB, Pride NB. Examination of the carbon monoxide diffusing capacity (DLCO) in relation to its KCO and VA components. Am J Respir Crit Care Med. 2012;186:132–9.
39. Schurawitzki H, Stiglbauer R, Graninger W, et al. Interstitial lung disease in progressive systemic sclerosis: high resolution CT versus radiography. Radiology. 1990;176:755–9.
40. Wells AU, Rubens MB, du Bois HDM. Serial CT in fibrosing alveolitis: prognostic significance of the initial pattern. Am J Roentgenol. 1993;161:1159–65.
41. Shah RM, Jimenez S, Wechsler R. Significance of ground-glass opacity on HRCT in long-term follow-up of patients with systemic sclerosis. J Thorac Imaging. 2007;22:120–4.
42. Khanna D, Nagaraja V, Tseng CH, et al. Predictors of lung function decline in scleroderma-related interstitial lung disease based on high-resolution computed tomography: implications for cohort enrichment in systemic sclerosis-associated interstitial lung disease trials. Arthritis Res Ther. 2015;17:372 (Online publication).
43. Moore OA, Goh N, Corte T, et al. Extent of disease on high-resolution computed tomography lung is a predictor of decline and mortality in systemic sclerosis-related interstitial lung disease. Rheumatology (Oxford). 2013;52:155–60.
44. Goh NS, Hoyles RK, Denton CP, et al. Short-term pulmonary function trends are predictive of mortality in interstitial lung dis-

ease associated with systemic sclerosis. Arthritis Rheumatol. 2017;69:1670–8.
45. Moore OA, Proudman SM, Goh N, et al. Quantifying change in pulmonary function as a prognostic marker in systemic sclerosis-related interstitial lung disease. Clin Exp Rheumatol. 2015;33(4 Suppl 91):S111–6.
46. Bonifazi M, Sverzellati N, Negri E, et al. Pleuroparenchymal fibroelastosis in systemic sclerosis: prevalence and prognostic impact. Eur Respir J. 2020;56:1902135.
47. DeMizio DJ, Bernstein EJ. Detection and classification of systemic sclerosis-related interstitial lung disease: a review. Curr Opin Rheumatol. 2019;31:553–60.
48. Elhai M, Hoffmann-Vold AM, Avouac J, et al. Performance of candidate serum biomarkers for systemic sclerosis-interstitial lung disease. Arthritis Rheumatol. 2019;71:672–82.
49. De Lauretis A, Sestini P, Pantelidis P, et al. Serum interleukin 6 is predictive of early functional decline and mortality in interstitial lung disease associated with systemic sclerosis. J Rheumatol. 2013;40:435–46.
50. Goh NS, Veeraraghavan S, Desai SR, et al. Bronchoalveolar lavage cellular profiles in patients with systemic sclerosis-associated interstitial lung disease are not predictive of disease progression. Arthritis Rheum. 2007;56:2005–12.
51. Strange C, Bolster MB, Roth MD, et al., Scleroderma Lung Study Research Group. Bronchoalveolar lavage and response to cyclophosphamide in scleroderma interstitial lung disease Am J Respir Crit Care Med. 2008;177:91–8.
52. Hoyles RK, Ellis RW, Wellsbury J, et al. A multicenter, prospective, randomized, double-blind, placebo-controlled trial of corticosteroids and intravenous cyclophosphamide followed by oral azathioprine for the treatment of pulmonary fibrosis in scleroderma. Arthritis Rheum. 2006; 54:3962–70.
53. Khanna D, Lin CJF, Furst DE, et al. Tocilizumab in systemic sclerosis: a randomised, double-blind, placebo-controlled, phase 3 trial. Lancet Respir Med. 2020;8:963–74.
54. Tashkin DP, Roth MD, Clements PJ, et al. Mycophenolate mofetil versus oral cyclophosphamide in scleroderma-related interstitial lung disease (SLS II): a randomised controlled, double-blind, parallel group trial. Lancet Respir Med. 2016;4:708–19.
55. Ebata S, Yoshizaki A, Oba K, et al. Safety and efficacy of rituximab in systemic sclerosis (DESIRES): a double-blind, investigator-initiated, randomised, placebo-controlled trial. Lancet Rheumatol. 2021;3:e489–97.
56. Seibold JR, Denton CP, Furst DE, et al. Randomized, prospective, placebo-controlled trial of bosentan in interstitial lung disease secondary to systemic sclerosis. Arthritis Rheum. 2010;62:2101–8.
57. Distler O, Highland KB, Gahlemann M, et al. Nintedanib for systemic sclerosis-associated interstitial lung disease. N Engl J Med. 2019;380:2518–28.
58. Kowal-Bielecka O, Landewe R, Avouac J, et al. EULAR recommendations for the treatment of systemic sclerosis: a report from the EULAR Scleroderma Trials And Research group (EUSTAR). Ann Rheum Dis. 2009;68:620–8.
59. Tashkin DP, Elashoff R, Clements PJ, et al. Effects of 1-year treatment with cyclophosphamide on outcomes at 2 years in scleroderma lung disease. Am J Respir Crit Care Med. 2007;176:1026–34.
60. Tzouvelekis A, Galanopoulos N, Bouros E, et al. Effect and safety of mycophenolate mofetil or sodium in systemic sclerosis-associated interstitial lung disease: a meta-analysis. Pulm Med. 2012;2012:143637.
61. Steen VD, Medsger TA Jr. Case-control study of corticosteroids and other drugs that could precipitate or protect from the development of scleroderma renal crisis. Arthritis Rheum. 1998;41:1613–9.
62. DeMarco PJ, Weisman MH, Seibold JR, et al. Predictors and outcomes of scleroderma renal crisis: the high-dose versus low-dose D-penicillamine in early diffuse systemic sclerosis trial. Arthritis Rheum. 2002;46:2983–9.
63. Khanna D, et al. Safety and efficacy of subcutaneous tocilizumab in systemic sclerosis: results from the open-label period of a phase II randomised controlled trial (faSScinate). Ann Rheum Dis. 2018;77:212–20.
64. Daoussis D, Liossis SN, Tsamandas AC, et al. Experience with rituximab in scleroderma: results from a 1-year, proof-of-principle study. Rheumatology. 2010;49:271–80.
65. Daoussis D, Liossis SN, Tsamandas AC, et al. Effect of long-term treatment with rituximab on pulmonary function and skin fibrosis in patients with diffuse systemic sclerosis. Clin Exp Rheumatol. 2012;30:S17–22.
66. Sem M, Molberg O, Lund MB, Gran JT. Rituximab treatment of the anti-synthetase syndrome: a retrospective case series. Rheumatology. 2009;48:968–71.
67. Keir GJ, Maher TM, Hansell DM, et al. Severe interstitial lung disease in connective tissue disease: rituximab as rescue therapy. Eur Respir J. 2012;40:641–8.
68. Daoussis D, Liossis SN, Tsamandas AC, et al. Experience with rituximab in scleroderma: results from a 1-year, proof-of-principle study. Rheumatology (Oxford). 2010;49:271–80.
69. Highland KB, Distler O, Kuwana M, et al. Efficacy and safety of nintedanib in patients with systemic sclerosis-associated interstitial lung disease treated with mycophenolate: a subgroup analysis of the SENSCIS trial. Lancet Respir Med. 2021;9:96–106.
70. Flaherty KR, Wells AU, Cottin V, et al. Nintedanib in progressive fibrosing interstitial lung diseases. N Engl J Med. 2019;381:1718–27.
71. Nash RA, McSweeney PA, Crofford LJ, et al. High-dose immunosuppressive therapy and autologous hematopoietic cell transplantation for severe systemic sclerosis: long-term follow-up of the US multicenter pilot study. Blood. 2007;110:1388–96.
72. van Laar JM, Farge D, Sont JK, et al. Autologous hematopoietic stem cell transplantation vs intravenous pulse cyclophosphamide in diffuse cutaneous systemic sclerosis: a randomized clinical trial. JAMA. 2014;311:2490–8.
73. Sullivan KM, Goldmuntz EA, Keyes-Elstein L, et al. Myeloablative autologous stem-cell transplantation for severe scleroderma. N Engl J Med. 2018;378:35–47.

Clinical Assessment of ILD

24

Anna-Maria Hoffmann-Vold, Kristin B. Highland, and Elisabeth Bendstrup

Key Points

- ILD is highly prevalent in systemic sclerosis and associated with high mortality.
- All SSc patients need screening for ILD.
- ILD is diagnosed by HRCT.
- Risk stratification for severe and progressive disease at diagnosis is important using multiple methods including HRCT and lung function test.
- ILD progression is frequent and monitoring of all SSc patients with ILD is necessary.

Epidemiology and Survival

ILD is Highly Prevalent in SSc

Interstitial lung disease (ILD) is highly prevalent in SSc but reported prevalence rates in the available literature are variable and likely reflect different design and populations in the underlying studies. Further complicating estimate is that the severity of ILD varies in SSc patients from minor findings to severe disease, and it is not known if all ILD findings will progress to clinical and/or symptomatic ILD. For example, ILD was found in 74% of all SSc patients who were referred to autopsy [1]. In the European Scleroderma Trial and Research (EUSTAR) cohort, 53% of all dcSSc and 35% of all lcSSc patients had ILD assessed by X-ray.

High-resolution computed tomography (HRCT) is the current gold standard for ILD diagnosis, and therefore, studies assessing the prevalence of ILD in unselected systemic sclerosis (SSc) cohorts using HRCT as a diagnostic tool for ILD provide the best estimates [2]. In the nationwide Norwegian SSc cohort, 80% of all SSc patients underwent HRCT for ILD screening [3]. ILD was reported to be prevalent in 50% of all SSc patients at time of their first HRCT assessment, with a prevalence of 75% in diffuse cutaneous SSc (dcSSc) and of 45% in limited cutaneous SSc (lcSSc) (Fig. 24.1). Significantly, the prevalence of severe ILD at time of diagnosis was 24%. This observation highlights that SSc-ILD presents early in the disease course, which has important clinical and management implications. These prevalence numbers are further supported by findings from the Dutch SSc cohort, where ILD on HRCT was found in 47% of all SSc patients [4]. Due to disease progression over the disease course, this number is increasing over time [3].

A.-M. Hoffmann-Vold (✉)
Department of Rheumatology, Oslo University Hospital, Oslo, Norway
e-mail: a.m.hoffmann-vold@medisin.uio.no

K. B. Highland
Department of Pulmonary Medicine, Cleveland Clinic, Cleveland, OH, USA
e-mail: HIGHLAK@ccf.org

E. Bendstrup
Department of Respiratory Diseases and Allergy, Aarhus University, Aarhus, Denmark
e-mail: kabend@rm.dk

Y. Allanore et al. (eds.), *Scleroderma*, https://doi.org/10.1007/978-3-031-40658-4_24

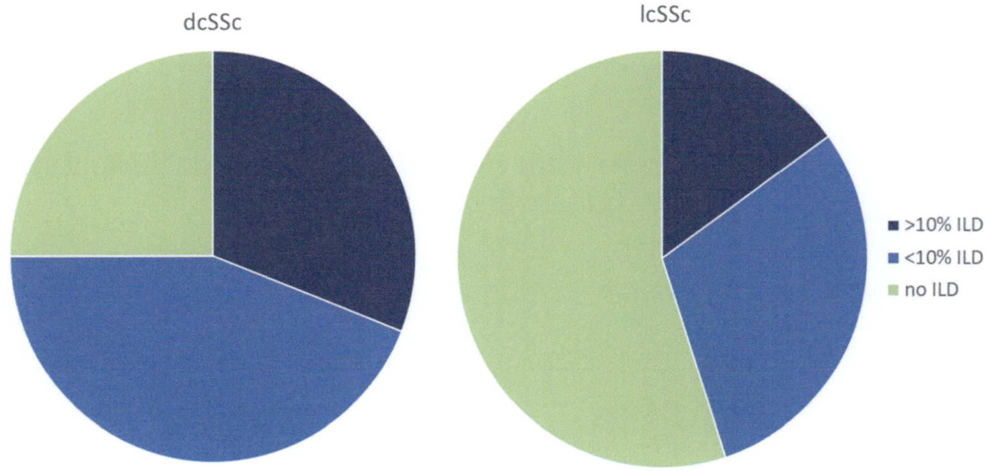

Fig. 24.1 Prevalence of no, limited and severe ILD in SSc in the nationwide Norwegian SSc cohort. (Hoffmann-Vold AM et al. Am J Respir Crit Care Med 2019;200:1258–66)

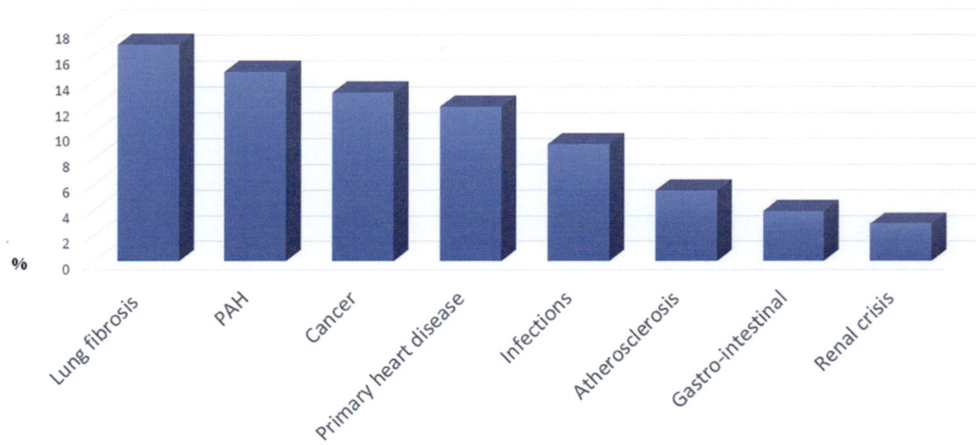

Fig. 24.2 Main causes of deaths in systemic sclerosis patients. (Modified figure based on Elhai M et al. Ann Rheum Dis 2017;76:1897–905)

ILD in SSc Is Associated with High Mortality

SSc-ILD is a leading cause of morbidity and mortality across all subtypes of SSc (Fig. 24.2). Even in patients with lcSSc, it is the third most common cause of death highlighting the impact of ILD regardless of skin subtype. Up to 18% of SSc-related deaths can be directly attributed to respiratory causes in all SSc-ILD patients. In SSc patients with severe ILD, it has been shown that 38% of deaths can be directly attributed to the ILD. Data from the Danish National Registry showed the hazard ratio (HR) for death in the overall SSc patient cohort was 2.8 (95% CI 2.4–3.3) compared with the general population and was increased in non-ILD SSc (HR 2.6, 95% CI 2.2–3.0) as well as in SSc-ILD (HR 4.2, 95% CI 3.2–5.4) [5]. In this study, younger age groups and males had the highest risk of death compared to a 1:4 matched control group [5].

The Risk of Death Is Directly Associated with the Extent of ILD on HRCT, with Impaired Lung Function, and with ILD Progression

Analyses performed in several independent cohorts have demonstrated that the risk of death in SSc patients is directly associated with the extent of lung involvement on HRCT [3, 6].

In 2008, Goh and colleagues showed that the degree of fibrosis by visual scoring on HRCT is associated with mortality [6]. Using these data, they developed an algorithm to classify patients with SSc-ILD into extensive and limited disease, which can be used in clinical practice. SSc patients with extensive ILD (>20% of fibrosis on HRCT) had a dramatically increased risk for mortality as compared to SSc patients with limited pulmonary involvement defined as <20% extent of ILD on HRCT [6]. For those patients with an

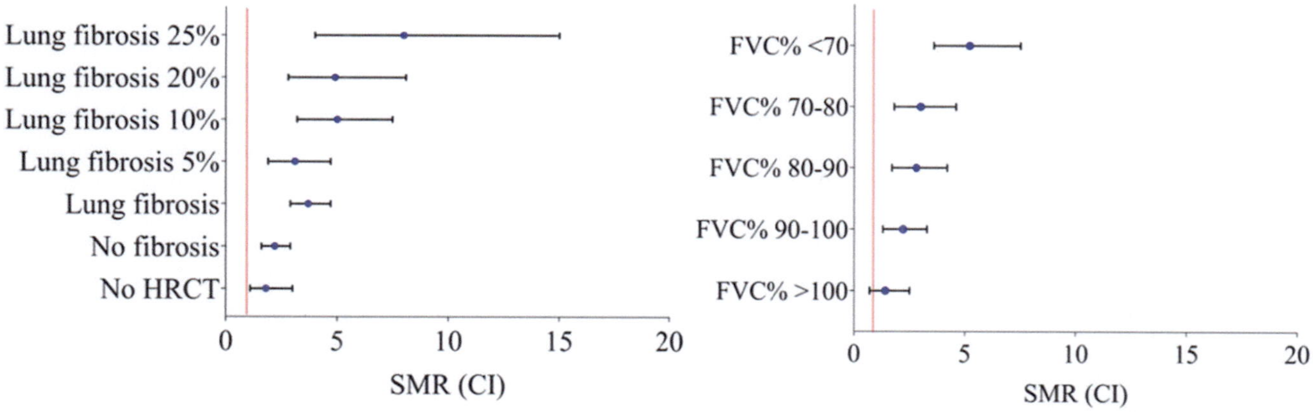

Fig. 24.3 Standard mortality rates (SMR) in SSc patients segregated by the extent of ILD on HRCT (**a**) and by FVC thresholds (**b**). (Hoffmann-Vold AM et al. Am J Respir Crit Care Med 2019;200:1258–66)

estimated involvement of 10–30% by HRCT, a forced vital capacity cut-off of 70% predicted further assisted in this dichotomous classification of limited (≥70% predicted) or extensive (<70% predicted) SSc-ILD.

In the large nationwide Norwegian SSc cohort, the standardized mortality ratio (SMR) was 2.2 for SSc patients with no lung fibrosis on HRCT and increased up to 8.0 for patients with >25% fibrosis on HRCT compared to a gender- and age-matched background population (Fig. 24.3) [3]. Similarly, mortality risk increased with a reduction in FVC, even when FVC remained in "normal" ranges for percent predicted (FVC ≥80% predicted) [1]. The impact of lung fibrosis on mortality was further confirmed in this study by the observation that cumulative survival is lower in patients with normal range FVC and evidence of ILD on HRCT as compared to patients with normal range FVC and no fibrosis on HRCT. ILD progression as defined by FVC decline has also shown to be associated with increased mortality and to be an even stronger predictor for mortality and then baseline FVC in post hoc analyses of the scleroderma lung studies (SLS) [7].

Screening SSc Patients for ILD

Given the high prevalence and its association with worse prognosis across all SSc subtypes as described above, all SSc patients need to be screened for ILD at time of SSc diagnosis and on a regular basis over the disease course if initially negative, as included in the consensus recommendations for SSc-ILD [8]. The frequency of screening over time in SSc patients with no initial signs of ILD on HRCT should be guided by risk factors of developing ILD combined with new respiratory symptoms and signs of ILD development [8].

The expert consensus recommendations for SSc-ILD state that all SSc patients should be screened with the following tools.

Respiratory Symptoms

Respiratory symptoms including dyspnea assessed by the Medical Research Council (MRC) score or the New York Heart Association (NYHA) functional class and the presence of cough should be assessed for screening of ILD. However, they are not mandatory nor specific for the presence of ILD [9]. The absence should be interpreted carefully as many patients even in the presence of obvious ILD on HRCT may be asymptomatic. This is especially true in early disease and/or when mobility is limited by non-pulmonary manifestations of SSc. Therefore, despite the absence of respiratory symptoms, screening for ILD is recommended for all SSc patients [8]. In the SENSCIS trial, where all patients needed to have an extent of ILD >10% on HRCT, around 30% did not have dyspnea and 20% no cough [10]. The clinical profiles of these patients about lung function and extent of HRCT did not significantly differ from patients with dyspnea and/or cough. Patient-related outcome measures assessing, for example, symptoms and quality of life, are used in research but not routinely in clinical practice.

It is important to note that patients with SSc may have respiratory symptoms related to other cardiopulmonary manifestations that can be seen in SSc, for example, chronic aspiration, infection related to immunosuppressant treatment, diaphragmatic muscle weakness, extrinsic restriction from severe thoracic skin involvement, pulmonary hypertension, diastolic dysfunction, other cardiac causes, and myositis. The contribution from deconditioning and other comorbidities such as chronic obstructive pulmonary disease (COPD) and coronary arteries disease should also be evaluated.

Auscultation and Physical Examination

Every patient with SSc should receive an auscultation as part of their physical examination. The lung examination of patients with ILD is frequently abnormal although findings may be nonspecific [9, 11]. Inspiratory velcro-like crackles can be present, typically at the lung bases, and are associated with a fibrotic NSIP or UIP pattern on HRCT [12]. Crackles are present early in the course of ILD, appearing first in the basal areas of the lung where the disease process initiates, with further progression to the upper zones. The presence of crackles, together with dyspnea or gas exchange abnormalities, may indicate ILD even if the chest radiograph is normal. Clubbing of the fingers in SSc-ILD is uncommon and when associated with SSc-ILD is typically a late manifestation of long-standing hypoxia and suggests advanced lung fibrosis. Clubbing can also be a harbinger of lung cancer.

Pulmonary Function Testing (PFT)

Pulmonary function testing (PFT) including FVC, total lung capacity (TLC), and diffusion capacity for carbon monoxide (DLCO) should be conducted in every patient with SSc to provide baseline parameters and should be repeated regularly in all patients with SSc [13]. Despite the established utility of PFTs, PFTs should not be used in isolation to screen for SSc-ILD and should be combined with other tools [14] due to their poor sensitivity. In the focuSSced trial, which evaluated tocilizumab in patients with early dcSSc, 64.1% of patients had evidence of ILD on HRCT despite a mean FVC greater than 80% predicted [15]. This study provided further evidence that not only can ILD occur early in the disease course, but patients with normal pulmonary function testing may already have clinically significant ILD [3, 14].

Of note, restrictive physiology may be of extrapulmonary origin such as diffuse skin involvement resulting in tightening of the chest, but the functional residual capacity should be preserved. Although an isolated reduced DLCO reduction may be seen in mild ILD or COPD, the presence of pulmonary vascular disease should be explored [16]. Furthermore, a reduction in DLCO out of proportion to FVC in patients with SSc-ILD (ratio of FVC% predicted to DLCO% predicted >1.6) is highly suspicious for the comorbid presence of pulmonary vascular disease [17].

HRCT

All patients with SSc should be screened at baseline with HRCT. The use of repeated HRCT over the disease course in patients with an initially normal HRCT should be guided by risk factors for developing ILD combined with respiratory symptoms and concerning changes in PFTs [18]. HRCT is the current gold standard for screening for ILD and is far superior to PFTs in detecting SSc-ILD. For example, in one study of patients with more than 20% extent of ILD on HRCT, only 37.5% had an FVC <80% predicted, which is in clinical practice often used as a threshold for ILD [14]. For screening in clinical practice, this means that two-thirds of all patients would not have been identified with ILD if only FVC would have been used as a screening tool, despite having extensive ILD on HRCT. Based on this observation, a baseline HRCT of the lungs is justified in all SSc patients, as new techniques have minimized radiation exposure [19]. The HRCT has the additional advantages of detecting other lung pathologies, but the high sensitivity for ILD is tempered by the yet unknown clinical significance of minor interstitial lung abnormalities (ILAs). [20].

Chest X-Rays

Chest X-ray has low sensitivity for the identification of ILD but a high specificity [21]. Importantly, a normal chest X-ray does not exclude the presence of SSc-ILD. It is not recommended to use chest X-ray as a screening tool for ILD in SSc.

Lung Ultrasound (LUS)

LUS is an attractive potential future tool for ILD screening as there is no risk of radiation exposure and it appears to be highly sensitive in detecting SSc-ILD; identification of more than 10 B-lines is associated with ILD [22]. As there are only a few studies showing its usefulness as a screening modality, it is not yet known if LUS can completely replace HRCT as a screening tool [23].

Screening Algorithm

Although the 2013 ACR/EULAR classification criteria for SSc include the presence of ILD as part of the diagnostic criteria, there are no evidence-based recommendations or guideline for screening of SSc-ILD, other than the expert consensus recommendations for SSc-ILD [8, 24]. The current local and national screening algorithms differ between expert centers and countries, and several different algorithms have been suggested [25].

Despite these differences, SSc patients are screened for ILD based on a combination of assessments of respiratory symptoms, PFTs, and HRCT. Follow-up PFT testing is often conducted for screening every 3–6 months for the next 3–5 years, and thereafter at least once a year [25]. The consensus on repeating HRCT for screening purpose is less clear. HRCT is often repeated when there is a clinically

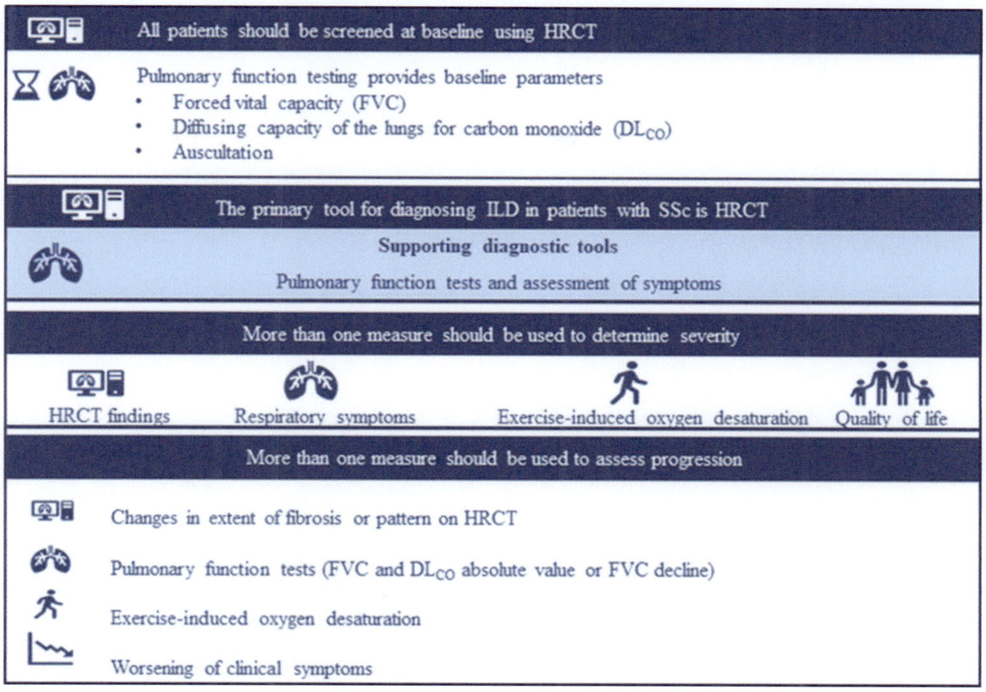

Fig. 24.4 Management algorithm of ILD in SSc based on a review of recent literature and a robust methodology including screening, diagnosis, treatment initiation, monitoring, and treatment escalation. [8]

meaningful decline in pulmonary function or development of respiratory symptoms, which could be attributed to SSc-ILD. In patients with SSc without lung changes on baseline HRCT, annual PFTs might be sufficient unless respiratory symptoms develop, but studies are lacking at this time point. Recently, worldwide experts joined together and defined guidelines for follow-up of SSc patients [26]. The lung was defined as one of the 10 items that needs annual follow-up, using clinical assessment (dyspnea, basal lung crackles), functional assessment using the NYHA functional classification, and PFT, but repeated imaging was not included [27] (Fig. 24.4).

ILD Diagnosis

Lung Physiology

Pulmonary function testing performed at baseline includes spirometry with measurement of dynamic lung volumes (forced expiratory volume in 1 second, FEV1, and FVC). In restrictive lung disease, both will typically be equally reduced with a normal or high FEV1/FVC ratio [28]. To confirm a restrictive ventilatory defect, body plethysmography with measurement of a reduced TLC and residual volume (RV) is relevant. DLCO will also typically be reduced (Fig. 24.5). FVC is the variable most widely used to show the level of restriction, and decline is closely related to a worse outcome. DLCO represents gas exchange and may be abnormal in interstitial lung disease as well as other parenchymal abnormalities including emphysema. It also may be reduced in the setting of pulmonary vascular disease. It must be corrected for hemoglobin as it is influenced by anemia and polycythemia and for lung volume if there is a history of resection. A six-minute walk test (6MWT) is a standardized, validated physiologic test often performed [29]. Oxygen desaturation on 6MWT is a marker of diffusion impairment, and reduced 6MWT distance and desaturation are associated with a worse prognosis [30]. Oxygen desaturation during 6MWT generally is not accurate with a finger oximeter in SSc patients with Raynaud phenomenon, and a forehead probe should be used. Distance should be cautiously interpreted in the correct clinical context as other cardiopulmonary (arthritis and myopathy/myositis) may also affect the results.

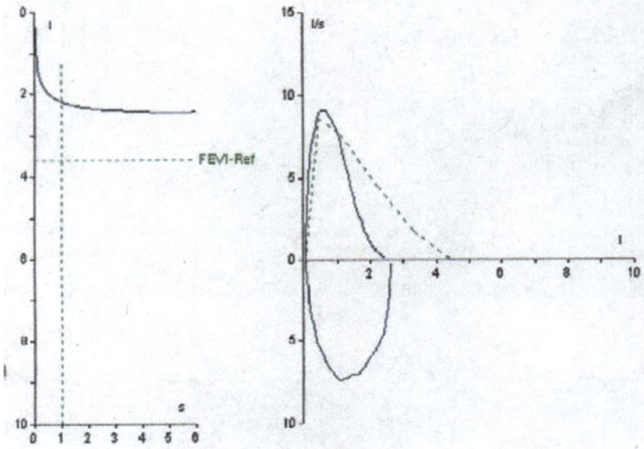

Spirometry and Flow-Volume :

parameter	unit	pred	act.	%pred
FVCex	l	4.46	2.61	59
FEV1	l	3.61	2.33	65
PEF	l/s	8.63	9.13	106
FEV1/FVC	%	77	89	115
FEV1/IVC	%	77	82	105
MEF25	l/s	1.73	1.24	71
MEF50	l/s	4.52	5.35	118
MEF75	l/s	7.57	9.05	120
MEF25-75	l/s	3.71	3.91	105
FVCin	l	4.46	2.64	59
PIF	l/s		7.40	
VC	l	4.46	2.85	64
IC	l	3.85	2.01	52
ERV	l	0.89	0.85	95

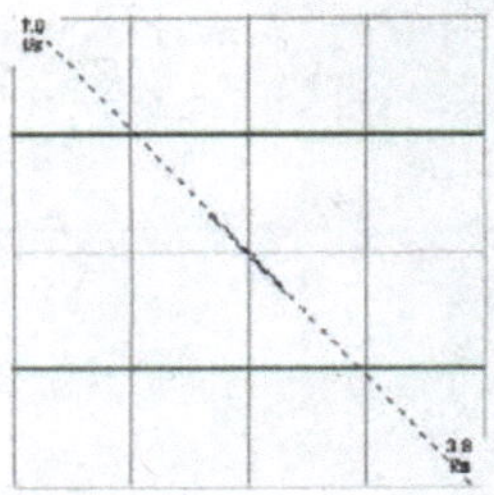

Volumes :

TGV	l	3.06	2.00	66
TLC	l	6.91	4.01	58
VC	l		2.85	
RV	l	2.17	1.16	53
TGV/TLC	%	55	50	91
RV/TLC	%	35	29	82

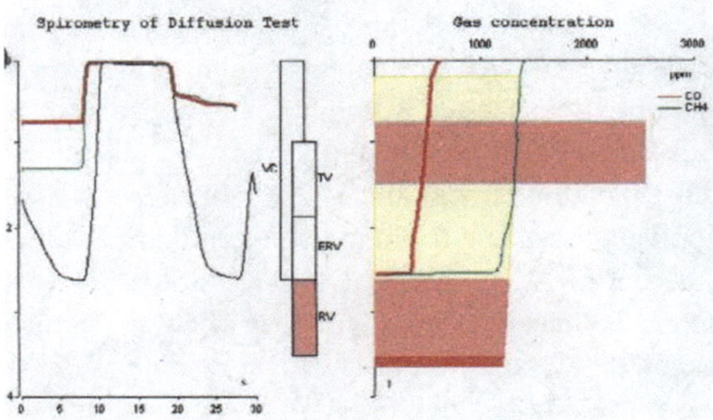

CO Diffusion (single breath):

parameter	unit	pred	act.	%pred
IVC CH4	l		2.63	
RV	l	2.26	0.90	40
TLC	l	6.98	3.53	51
RV/TLC	%	35	25	73
TLco	mmol/kPa/min	9.97	3.32	33
Kco	mmol/kPa/min/l	1.43	0.99	69
HB	mmol/l		10.70	
TLco(Hb)	mmol/kPa/min	9.97	3.08	31
Kco(Hb)	mmol/kPa/min/l	1.43	0.92	64
t diff.	s		11.63	
Vdiscard	ml		750	
Vsample	ml		750	

Fig. 24.5 Pulmonary function test in a patient with severe SSC-ILD showing reduced FVC, FEV1, TLC, RV, and DLCO

HRCT and Chest X-Ray

HRCT is the most important radiologic imaging technique as chest X-rays are not sufficiently sensitive to reliably show mild ILD or specific patterns of ILD.

Diagnostic HRCT should be performed using recommended scanning parameters, including inspiratory and expiratory images [31]. Prone positioning may also allow differentiation of dependent atelectasis and early interstitial lung disease. The typical ILD pattern in SSc-ILD is a non-specific interstitial pneumonia (NSIP) pattern followed by a usual interstitial pneumonia (UIP) pattern (Fig. 24.6), but other ILD patterns including organizing pneumonia (OP) can also be seen [32].

Fig. 24.6 HRCT images of different ILD patterns in SSc-ILD

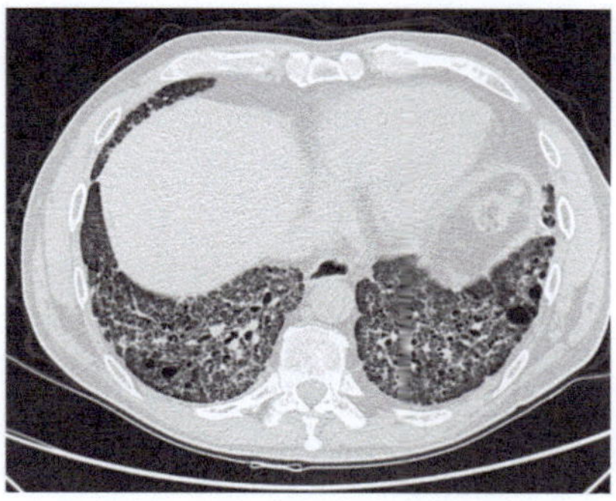	**Non-specific interstitial pneumonia (NSIP)** A typical NSIP pattern will show basal predominance with reticulation, ground glass opacities and traction bronchiectasis and bronchiectasis. Subpleural sparing is seen in approximately 30%.
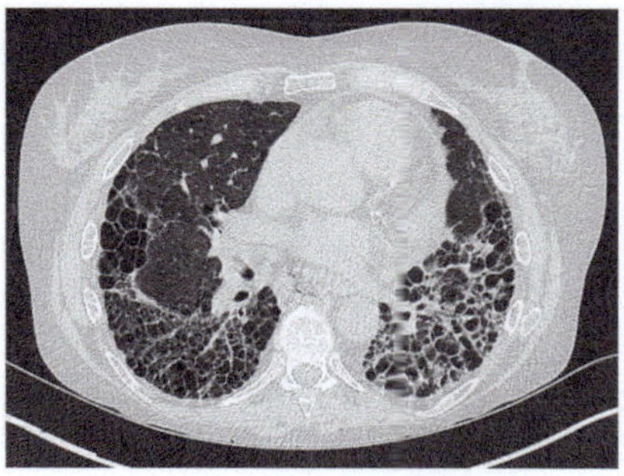	**Usual Interstitial pneumonia (UIP)** A typical UIP pattern will show a basal, peripheral localization with reticulation, traction bronchiectasis and honeycombing. Ground glass opacities, air trapping and nodules are absent.

BAL and Lung Biopsy

Bronchoalveolar lavage (BAL), and bronchoscopic or surgical lung biopsies are rarely needed as cyto-histopathology rarely adds further information for the diagnosis of SSc-ILD, treatment decisions, or prognosis [2, 33, 34]. Bronchoscopic techniques may be relevant in the acute setting for the diagnosis of lung infections, including opportunistic infections such as *pneumocystis jirovecii* emerging during immunomodulatory treatment, and when there is a suspicion of a potential malignancy. Currently, research is exploring the use of bronchoscopic techniques in a precision-based medicine approach to guide treatment decisions of either mono- or combination therapy of immunomodulatory or antifibrotic therapy.

Disease Course of ILD

The natural history of ILD in SSc is highly variable from mild and stable disease to rapidly progressive resulting in respiratory failure and death [35]. Historical observational studies have demonstrated that the greatest decline in lung function in SSc occurs early in the course of the disease [36]. Lately, it has also become clear that SSc-ILD patients may also show ILD progression later on in the disease course [37]. It has been shown that regardless of treatment, approximately 30% of patients with SSc-ILD show FVC decline in the following 12 months, 50% are stable, and the remaining patients show slight improvements in their lung function [37]. Among patients who do experience a decline in lung function, the rate of decline can be heterogeneous. Rapid progressors are a small subgroup of SSc-ILD patients that are critical to identify early [35, 37]. These patients will experience rapidly increasing lung parenchymal inflammatory and/or fibrotic changes leading to a substantial loss of lung function resulting in permanent lung damage and increased mortality. These patients should receive early and aggressive treatment (discussed in Chap. 27) and should be monitored very closely for response to therapy and for further ILD progression. Several factors have been described to be predictive for ILD progression or ILD-related mortality and are described below.

ILD Progression, Definitions, and Risk Factors for Progression

Paramount to defining ILD progression and characterizing clinical phenotypes of progressive SSc-ILD is reaching a consensus on how to define progression of ILD in SSc. While no valid definition of SSc-ILD disease progression has been established, a decline in FVC relative of ≥10% or a FVC decline of 5–9% in association with a DLCO decline of ≥15% over 12 months has been accepted widely to represent progression [37], and this definition is often used for research

Table 24.1 Risk factors for SSc-ILD progression

Clinical risk factors
• Short disease duration since onset of first non-Raynaud's symptom
• African American ethnicity
• Gastroesophageal reflux disease (GERD)
• Elevated C-reactive protein (CRP) and erythrocyte sedimentation rate (ESR)
• Clinical inflammatory manifestations (arthritis)
SSc subtype and skin changes
• Diffuse cutaneous SSc
• Extent of skin involvement measured by the mRSS
• Progressive skin fibrosis within 1 year
Autoantibody profile
• Anti-topoisomerase I antibody (ATA)
Pulmonary function and functional capacity
• FCV and DLCO at diagnosis
• Desaturation <94% at 6MWT
Imaging
• HRCT *without* fibrotic features is a *good* prognostic sign
Promising future prediction tools
• Circulating biomarkers: Krebs von den Lungen-6 (KL-6) and chemokine ligand 18 (CCl-18)
• New imaging tools: 18F-FDG-PET/CT, ultrasonography, MRI

purposes. A continuous FVC decline over time is also considered evidence of ILD progression as well as increasing extent of ILD on HRCT, increasing respiratory symptoms, and/or declining distance or desaturation on the 6-minute walking test [30, 38]. However, trained chest radiologists are essential to assess evolving extent of ILD over time [39, 40]. The evaluation should include change of extent of fibrosis and change of pattern [40]. Extrapulmonary factors are less likely to influence the results of HRCT imaging than of PFTs, which are influenced by biological and technical variations [29]. However, different scanners and scanning protocols may complicate valid comparison. Lastly, the need to escalate treatment, the initiation of supplemental oxygen therapy for ILD, and the need for lung transplantation should all be considered as signs of progressive ILD.

To enable timely treatment, it is of utmost importance to adequately identify the patients at risk for progression of ILD in the near future [41]. The following variables have been described to be predictive or prognostic for ILD progression in SSc-ILD patients (Table 24.1).

SSc Subtype and Skin Changes

Skin involvement is the hallmark of SSc. Skin assessment by the modified Rodnan skin score (mRSS) should be conducted at time of SSc diagnosis and on a regular basis at follow-up visits and can be used for prognostication of internal organ involvement including the lung [26]. The extent of skin involvement measured by the mRSS has been shown to be prognostic for progressive ILD defined by an FVC predicted decline >10% over 12 months [42]. Additionally, progressive skin fibrosis within 1 year is associated with decline in lung function and worse survival in dcSSc during follow-up [42]. Also, the presence of dcSSc is prognostic for ILD progression, especially in combination with other risk factors, such as early disease and increased inflammatory signs [15, 43]. Nevertheless, ILD can also occur and progress in patients with the limited cutaneous or sine scleroderma variants of SSc.

Autoantibody Profile

Autoantibody profiling is important for all patients with SSc at the time of diagnosis and has a high prognostic value for organ involvement in SSc [43–45]. The most frequent antibodies in SSc are anti-centromere antibody (ACA), anti-topoisomerase I antibody (ATA/Scl-70), and anti-RNA polymerase III antibody (RNAP-3) [46]. ATA is a prognostic marker for lung function decline and the development of severe ILD, especially in patients with short disease duration [43]. Some reports have shown that RNAP-3 is prognostic for ILD progression, which may also be correlated with rapid skin progression and short disease duration [47]. The knowledge about the prognostic value of other and less frequent SSc-related antibodies is limited.

Respiratory Symptoms and Functional Capacity

Respiratory symptoms should be recorded at every follow-up visit but it has not been shown that symptoms can be used for prognostication of ILD progression [9, 26]. 6MWT should also be conducted on a regular basis in all SSc-ILD patients. In patients with limited ILD, desaturation to <94% on 6-minute walk test and a history of arthritis as a sign of inflammation have been found to be prognostic for ILD progression after 1 year in the SPAR model [30].

Clinical Findings

Clinical findings and patient characteristics are also valuable prognostic factors, often in combination with each of the aforementioned factors or with each other. Short disease duration since onset of non-Raynaud's symptoms has been shown to be a strong risk factor for ILD progression in both observational and randomized clinical trials [15, 37, 45]. African American ethnicity is associated with an increased risk of progressive ILD [48]. For several years, there has been an ongoing debate regarding the role of gastroesophageal reflux disease (GERD) in SSc-related ILD [49]. GERD has recently been found in an analysis of SSc-ILD patients from the EUSTAR database to be a prognostic factor for ILD progression [37]. Signs of inflammation, such as increased C-reactive protein (CRP) or erythrocyte sedimentation rate (ESR) or clinical inflammatory manifestations (arthritis), have been shown to be a strong predictor for ILD progression, especially in combination with other risk factors such as disease duration [15, 42]. These risk factor combinations have also been used as successful enrichment strategies for clinical trials [15].

Pulmonary Function Tests

Reduced FVC in SSc-ILD patients has been reported to be an independent prognostic for ILD progression [50], whereas other studies have shown that preserved lung function is a risk factor for ILD progression [37]. A decreased DLCO at time of diagnosis of SSc-ILD has been associated with an increased risk for the development of severe ILD. Importantly, in patients with SSc, it is shown that there is reduced survival in patients with fibrotic changes on HRCT despite preserved pulmonary function FVC (80–100%) [3].

HRCT

A HRCT without evidence of lung fibrosis is a good prognostic factor since only a few patients with normal findings will develop ILD later during the disease course [18]. A significant change in extent of fibrosis on serial HRCT helps to identify patients with rapid ILD progression [39] consistent with the hypothesis that fibrosis begets fibrosis.

Circulating Biomarkers

There is an intense ongoing search for new circulating biomarkers to improve the ability to predict ILD progression [51]. To date, the only clinically useful biomarker is CRP, which has been shown to be a prognostic marker of progressive ILD. Krebs von den Lungen-6 (KL-6) and chemokine ligand 18 (CCL-18) are two promising biomarkers predictive of FVC decline but are currently not in clinical use [52].

New Imaging Techniques

In addition to the ongoing search for circulating biomarkers, several imaging techniques might prove to be useful. Currently, these techniques are applied in clinical research settings. Some studies have proposed that 18-F fluoro-deoxy-D-glucose positron-emission tomography/CT (18F-FDG-PET/CT) might be helpful to discriminate against active inflammatory lesions (ground glass) from pure fibrotic tissue [53, 54]. Ultrasound has been used to assess ILD in several studies. Recently, an OMERACT group evaluated the contribution of lung ultrasound for assessment of SSc-ILD [23]. Lung ultrasound is feasible and has shown content and face validity, but reliability and sensitivity to change still need to be demonstrated, making this tool not applicable for risk stratification in clinical practice.

Magnetic resonance imaging (MRI) could provide additive information compared to CT as on top of structural information, functional information is provided. Functional MRI might contribute to detect regional areas in the lung where fibrosis causes deformation during breathing [55]. However, up until now, only small studies have been performed and additional studies are needed to determine the sensitivity to change.

Also, several groups have analyzed the additive value of quantitative measurements of HRCT images to identify patients at risk [39, 40]. Although cross-sectional association between PFT and quantitative HRCT scores is demonstrated, additional predictive value still needs to be confirmed [56].

Monitoring

Because of the progressive nature of SSc-ILD, it is important that all patients with SSc-ILD are monitored over time. An individual monitoring plan should include monitoring of PFT, HRCT, 6MWD, clinical assessment, and respiratory symptoms (Fig. 24.7). Follow-up PFT testing after diagnosis

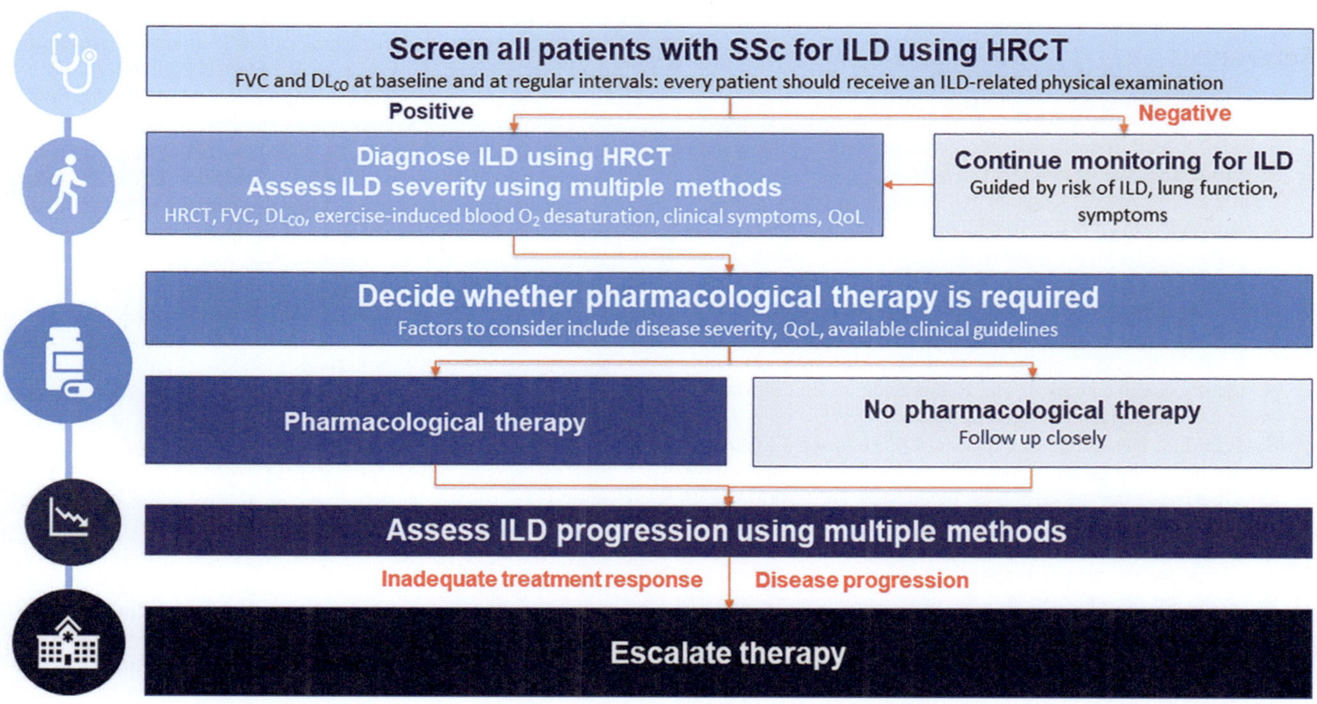

Fig. 24.7 Management algorithm of ILD in SSc based on a review of recent literature and a robust methodology including screening, diagnosis, treatment initiation, monitoring, and treatment escalation. (Hoffmann-Vold AM et al. Am J Respir Crit Care Med 2019;200:1258–66)

of ILD is often conducted every 3–6 months for the first 3–5 years and, thereafter at least once a year. It is recommended to perform simultaneously clinical assessment, mapping of respiratory symptoms, and 6MWD with assessment of oxygen saturation.

HRCT is often repeated when there is a clinically meaningful decline in pulmonary function or new onset or a change in respiratory symptoms.

Conclusion and Future Perspectives

ILD is a major contributor to SSc morbidity and mortality. Early diagnosis, facilitated by screening at baseline and during disease course, is crucial to allow for timely treatment, which can in turn improve outcomes. Screening and monitoring demand a repertoire of tools including symptom monitoring, clinical findings, PFT, HRCT, and exercise capacity. Imaging tools such as low-dose CT, ultrasonography, PET, and MRI are exciting developments but still need to be validation. Home monitoring with spirometry has shown to be promising in other forms of ILD including idiopathic pulmonary fibrosis and sarcoidosis. A telemedicine approach incorporating home spirometry with patient-related outcome measures such as dyspnea and cough questionnaires may allow us to intervene at the first hint of progression, but also needs to be validated [57, 58]. Finally, circulating biomarkers, specific for the development, and even more importantly for predicting disease progression, could help identify the group of patients in need of more comprehensive investigation and aggressive treatment.

References

1. Suzuki 1 A, Ohosone Y, Obana M, Mita S, Matsuoka Y, Irimajiri S, Fukuda J. Cause of death in 81 autopsied patients with rheumatoid arthritis. J Rheumatol. 1994;21(1):33–6.
2. Denton CP, Wells AU, Coghlan JG. Major lung complications of systemic sclerosis. Nat Rev Rheumatol. 2018;14(9):511–27.
3. Hoffmann-Vold AM, Fretheim H, Halse AK, et al. Tracking impact of interstitial lung disease in systemic sclerosis in a complete nationwide cohort. Am J Respir Crit Care Med. 2019;200:1258. Epub ahead of print.
4. Vonk MC, Broers B, Heijdra YF, et al. Systemic sclerosis and its pulmonary complications in The Netherlands: an epidemiological study. Ann Rheum Dis. 2009;68(6):961–5.
5. Hyldgaard C, Bendstrup E, Pedersen AB, Pedersen L, Ellingsen T. Interstitial lung disease in connective tissue diseases: survival patterns in a population-based cohort. J Clin Med. 2021;10(21):4830.
6. Goh NS, Desai SR, Veeraraghavan S, et al. Interstitial lung disease in systemic sclerosis: a simple staging system. Am J Respir Crit Care Med. 2008;177(11):1248–54.
7. Volkmann ER, Tashkin DP, Sim M, et al. Short-term progression of interstitial lung disease in systemic sclerosis predicts long-term survival in two independent clinical trial cohorts. Ann Rheum Dis. 2019;78(1):122–30.
8. Hoffmann-Vold A-M, Maher TM, Philpot EE, et al. The identification and management of interstitial lung disease in systemic sclerosis: evidence-based European consensus statements. Lancet Rheumatol. 2020;2(2):e71–83.
9. Tashkin DP, Volkmann ER, Tseng C-H, et al. Improved cough and cough-specific quality of life in patients treated for scleroderma-related interstitial lung disease. Chest. 2017;151(4):813–20.
10. Distler O, Highland KB, Gahlemann M, et al. Nintedanib for systemic sclerosis-associated interstitial lung disease. N Engl J Med. 2019;380:2518.
11. Cottin V, Cordier J-F. Velcro crackles: the key for early diagnosis of idiopathic pulmonary fibrosis? Eur Respir J. 2012;40(3):519–21.
12. Sellares J, Hernandez-Gonzalez F, Lucena CM, et al. Auscultation of Velcro crackles is associated with usual interstitial pneumonia. Medicine (Baltimore). 2016;95(5):e2573.
13. Bernstein EJ, Jaafar S, Assassi S, et al. Performance characteristics of pulmonary function tests for the detection of interstitial lung disease in adults with early diffuse cutaneous systemic sclerosis. Arthritis Rheumatol. 2020;72(11):1892–6.
14. Suliman YA, Dobrota R, Huscher D, et al. Brief report: pulmonary function tests: high rate of false-negative results in the early detection and screening of scleroderma-related interstitial lung disease. Arthritis Rheumatol. 2015;67(12):3256–61.
15. Khanna D, Lin CJF, Furst DE, et al. Tocilizumab in systemic sclerosis: a randomised, double-blind, placebo-controlled, phase 3 trial. Lancet Respir Med. 2020;8(10):963–74.
16. Galiè N, Humbert M, Vachiery J-L, et al. 2015 ESC/ERS Guidelines for the diagnosis and treatment of pulmonary hypertension. Eur Heart J. 2016;37(1):67–119.
17. Weatherald J, Montani D, Jevnikar M, Jaïs X, Savale L, Humbert M. Screening for pulmonary arterial hypertension in systemic sclerosis. Eur Respir Rev. 2019;28(153):190023.
18. Hoffmann-Vold AM, Aalokken TM, Lund MB, et al. Predictive value of serial high-resolution computed tomography analyses and concurrent lung function tests in systemic sclerosis. Arthritis Rheumatol. 2015;67(8):2205–12.
19. Frauenfelder T, Winklehner A, Nguyen TDL, et al. Screening for interstitial lung disease in systemic sclerosis: performance of high-resolution CT with limited number of slices: a prospective study. Ann Rheum Dis. 2014;73(12):2069–73.
20. Hatabu H, Hunninghake GM, Richeldi L, et al. Interstitial lung abnormalities detected incidentally on CT: a position paper from the Fleischner Society. Lancet Respir Med. 2020;8(7):726–37.
21. Epler GR, McLoud TC, Gaensler EA, Mikus JP, Carrington CB. Normal chest roentgenograms in chronic diffuse infiltrative lung disease. N Engl J Med. 1978;298(17):934–9.
22. Fairchild R, Chung M, Yang D, Sharpless L, Li S, Chung L. Development and assessment of a novel lung ultrasound interpretation criteria for the detection of interstitial lung disease in systemic sclerosis. Arthritis Care Res. 2020;73:1338.
23. Gutierrez M, Soto-Fajardo C, Pineda C, et al. Ultrasound in the assessment of interstitial lung disease in systemic sclerosis: a systematic literature review by the OMERACT ultrasound group. J Rheumatol. 2020;47(7):991–1000.
24. van den Hoogen F, Khanna D, Fransen J, et al. 2013 classification criteria for systemic sclerosis: an American college of rheumatology/European league against rheumatism collaborative initiative. Ann Rheum Dis. 2013;72(11):1747–55.
25. Roofeh D, Khanna D. Management of systemic sclerosis. Curr Opin Rheumatol. 2020;32(3):228–37.
26. Hoffmann-Vold AM, Distler O, Murray B, et al. Setting the international standard for longitudinal follow-up of patients with systemic sclerosis: a Delphi-based expert consensus on core clinical features. RMD Open. 2019;5(1):e000826.
27. Hoffmann-Vold AM, Maher TM, Philpot EE, et al. The identification and management of interstitial lung disease in systemic

sclerosis: evidence-based European consensus statements. Lancet Rheumatol. 2020. https://doi.org/10.1016/S2665-9913(19)30144-4.
28. Pellegrino R. Interpretative strategies for lung function tests. Eur Respir J. 2005;26(5):948–68.
29. ATS statement: guidelines for the six-minute walk test. Am J Respir Crit Care Med. 2002;166(1):111–7.
30. Wu W, Jordan S, Becker MO, et al. Prediction of progression of interstitial lung disease in patients with systemic sclerosis: the SPAR model. Ann Rheum Dis. 2018;77(9):1326–32.
31. Raghu G, Remy-Jardin M, Myers JL, et al. Diagnosis of idiopathic pulmonary fibrosis. An official ATS/ERS/JRS/ALAT clinical practice guideline. Am J Respir Crit Care Med. 2018;198(5):e44–68.
32. Shao T, Shi X, Yang S, et al. Interstitial lung disease in connective tissue disease: a common lesion with heterogeneous mechanisms and treatment considerations. Front Immunol. 2021;12(2092):684699.
33. Strange C, Bolster MB, Roth MD, et al. Bronchoalveolar lavage and response to cyclophosphamide in scleroderma interstitial lung disease. Am J Respir Crit Care Med. 2008;177(1):91–8.
34. Goh NSL, Veeraraghavan S, Desai SR, et al. Bronchoalveolar lavage cellular profiles in patients with systemic sclerosis–associated interstitial lung disease are not predictive of disease progression. Arthritis Rheum. 2007;56(6):2005–12.
35. Volkmann ER. Natural history of systemic sclerosis–related interstitial lung disease: how to identify a progressive fibrosing phenotype. J Scleroderma Relat Disord. 2020;5(2_Suppl):31–40.
36. Steen VMTJ. Severe organ involvement in systemic sclerosis with diffuse scleroderma. Arthritis Rheum. 2000;43(11):2437–44.
37. Hoffmann-Vold A-M, Allanore Y, Alves M, et al. Progressive interstitial lung disease in patients with systemic sclerosis-associated interstitial lung disease in the EUSTAR database. Ann Rheum Dis. 2021;80:219.
38. Flaherty KR, Wells AU, Cottin V, et al. Nintedanib in progressive fibrosing interstitial lung diseases. N Engl J Med. 2019;381(18):1718–27.
39. Goldin JG, Kim GHJ, Tseng CH, et al. Longitudinal changes in quantitative interstitial lung disease on computed tomography after immunosuppression in the scleroderma lung study II. Ann Am Thorac Soc. 2018;15(11):1286–95.
40. Kim HJ, Tashkin DP, Gjertson DW, et al. Transitions to different patterns of interstitial lung disease in scleroderma with and without treatment. Ann Rheum Dis. 2016;75(7):1367–71.
41. Distler O, Assassi S, Cottin V, et al. Predictors of progression in systemic sclerosis patients with interstitial lung disease. Eur Respir J. 2020;55(5):1902026.
42. Wu W, Jordan S, Graf N, et al. Progressive skin fibrosis is associated with a decline in lung function and worse survival in patients with diffuse cutaneous systemic sclerosis in the European Scleroderma Trials and Research (EUSTAR) cohort. Ann Rheum Dis. 2019;78:648.
43. Nihtyanova S, Schreiber B, Ong V, et al. Prediction of pulmonary complications and long-term survival in systemic sclerosis. Arthritis Rheumatol. 2014;66(6):1625–35.
44. Khanna D, Tashkin DP, Denton CP, Renzoni EA, Desai SR, Varga J. Aetiology, risk factors, and biomarkers in systemic sclerosis with interstitial lung disease. Am J Respir Crit Care Med. 2019;201:650.
45. Jaeger VK, Wirz EG, Allanore Y, et al. Incidences and risk factors of organ manifestations in the early course of systemic sclerosis: a longitudinal EUSTAR study. PLoS One. 2016;11(10):e0163894.
46. Fretheim H, Halse AK, Seip M, et al. Multidimensional tracking of phenotypes and organ involvement in a complete nationwide systemic sclerosis cohort. Rheumatology (Oxford). 2020;59:2920.
47. Hoffmann-Vold A, Midtvedt Ø, Tennøe A, et al. Cardiopulmonary disease development in anti-RNA polymerase III-positive patient cohort systemic sclerosis: comparative analyses from an unselected, prospective. J Rheumatol. 2017;44:459–65.
48. Assassi S, Sharif R, Lasky RE, et al. Predictors of interstitial lung disease in early systemic sclerosis: a prospective longitudinal study of the GENISOS cohort. Arthritis Res Ther. 2010;12(5):R166.
49. Gilson M, Zerkak D, Wipff J, et al. Prognostic factors for lung function in systemic sclerosis: prospective study of 105 cases. Eur Respir J. 2010;35(1):112–7.
50. Goh NS, Hoyles RK, Denton CP, et al. Short-term pulmonary function trends are predictive of mortality in interstitial lung disease associated with systemic sclerosis. Arthritis Rheumatol. 2017;69(8):1670–8.
51. Hoffmann-Vold A-M, Fretheim H, Meier C, Maurer B. Circulating biomarkers of systemic sclerosis—interstitial lung disease. J Scleroderma Relat Disord. 2020;5:239719831989485.
52. Elhai M, Hoffmann-Vold AM, Avouac J, et al. Performance of candidate serum biomarkers for systemic sclerosis-associated interstitial lung disease. Arthritis Rheumatol. 2019;71(6):972–82.
53. Röhrich M, Leitz D, Glatting FM, et al. Fibroblast activation protein–specific PET/CT imaging in fibrotic interstitial lung diseases and lung cancer: a translational exploratory study. J Nucl Med. 2022;63(1):127–33.
54. Bergmann C, Distler JHW, Treutlein C, et al. 68Ga-FAPI-04 PET-CT for molecular assessment of fibroblast activation and risk evaluation in systemic sclerosis-associated interstitial lung disease: a single-centre, pilot study. Lancet Rheumatol. 2021;3(3):e185–e94.
55. Chassagnon G, Martin C, Marini R, et al. Use of elastic registration in pulmonary MRI for the assessment of pulmonary fibrosis in patients with systemic sclerosis. Radiology. 2019;291(2):487–92.
56. Saldana DC, Hague CJ, Murphy D, et al. Association of computed tomography densitometry with disease severity, functional decline, and survival in systemic sclerosis-associated interstitial lung disease. Ann Am Thorac Soc. 2020;17(7):813–20.
57. Wijsenbeek MS, Holland AE, Swigris JJ, Renzoni EA. Comprehensive supportive care for patients with fibrosing interstitial lung disease. Am J Respir Crit Care Med. 2019;200(2):152–9.
58. Moor CC, Mostard RLM, Grutters JC, et al. Home monitoring in patients with idiopathic pulmonary fibrosis. A randomized controlled trial. Am J Respir Crit Care Med. 2020;202(3):393–401.

Lung Imaging Perspective in Scleroderma

25

Jonathan G. Goldin

Lung Imaging Perspective in Scleroderma

Introduction

The development of interstitial lung disease is common in patients with systemic sclerosis and is a major cause of their morbidity and mortality [1, 2]. Scleroderma-related interstitial lung disease (SSc-ILD) could precede the onset of both clinical symptoms and pulmonary function impairment [3, 4]. High-resolution CT (HRCT) has emerged as the most sensitive and specific diagnostic tool for both the early and accurate diagnosis of SSc-ILD [5, 6]. Beyond diagnosis, the extent of disease on HRCT has increasingly been found to be useful in predicting prognosis and for assessing disease progressions as part of the routine management of these patients [7]. Other imaging modalities, including Magnetic Resonance Imaging (MRI), Ultrasound, Positron Emission Tomography with Computed Tomography (PET-CT), and Optical Coherence Tomography (OCT) have also been found to have potential usefulness in the diagnosis and evaluation of SSc-ILD. In this chapter, we will review primarily the role of HRCT and introduce emerging technologies in the diagnosis and management of lung involvement in SSc-ILD.

J. G. Goldin (✉)
Radiology, Medicine and Biomedical Physics, David Geffen School of Medicine at UCLA, Los Angeles, CA, USA

Computer Vision and Imaging Biomarker Program, David Geffen School of Medicine at UCLA, Los Angeles, CA, USA

Departemt of Radiology, David Geffen School of Medcine, Los Angeles, CA, USA
e-mail: JGoldin@mednet.ucla.edu

HRCT in Scleroderma Lung Disease

Technique

It is important to acquire good quality images to optimize the evaluation of the lung parenchyma. It is generally accepted that a volumetric non-contrast enhanced, thin section (<2 mm) CT be acquired of the entire chest in the supine position. Images should be reconstructed with a smooth or moderate edge-enhancing algorithm [8–10]. All studies should be acquired at least at suspended breath hold, at total lung capacity after a maximum inspiration [9]. Radiation dose should be reduced to the lowest possible level that still allows sufficient image quality to evaluate the subtle parenchymal abnormalities that occur in SSc-ILD [11]. Advances in CT technology hardware and software have reduced the radiation dose of a CT study considerably without loss in image quality [12]. The average dose of HRCT studies used in the setting of patients with scleroderma is currently 2–4 mSv, which is similar to average background annual radiation risk which globally is between 2.5 and 3.9 mSv [11]. The radiation risks are considered small but are higher in young women, because of the increased sensitivity of breast tissue, who make up the majority of patients being diagnosed with systemic sclerosis [11, 13, 14]. The doses will likely reduce further with the development of novel dose-reducing algorithms and new generation detectors [15]. With the increased use of CT in monitoring change, it is important that whenever possible, the follow-up CT study be acquired on the same CT platform as the baseline study using the same acquisition parameters and standardized breath hold volume [9]. It is important that communication is clear between the referring physician and imaging technologist that the reason for the study is to specifically evaluate for SSc-LD. This clear communication is often the difference between a diagnostic and nondiagnostic CT examination.

Diagnosis of SSc-ILD on HRCT

HRCT is now recommended by several expert panels to be used along with pulmonary function tests to screen for ILD in patients with systemic sclerosis [16–18]. SSc-ILD is iden-

Y. Allanore et al. (eds.), *Scleroderma*, https://doi.org/10.1007/978-3-031-40658-4_25

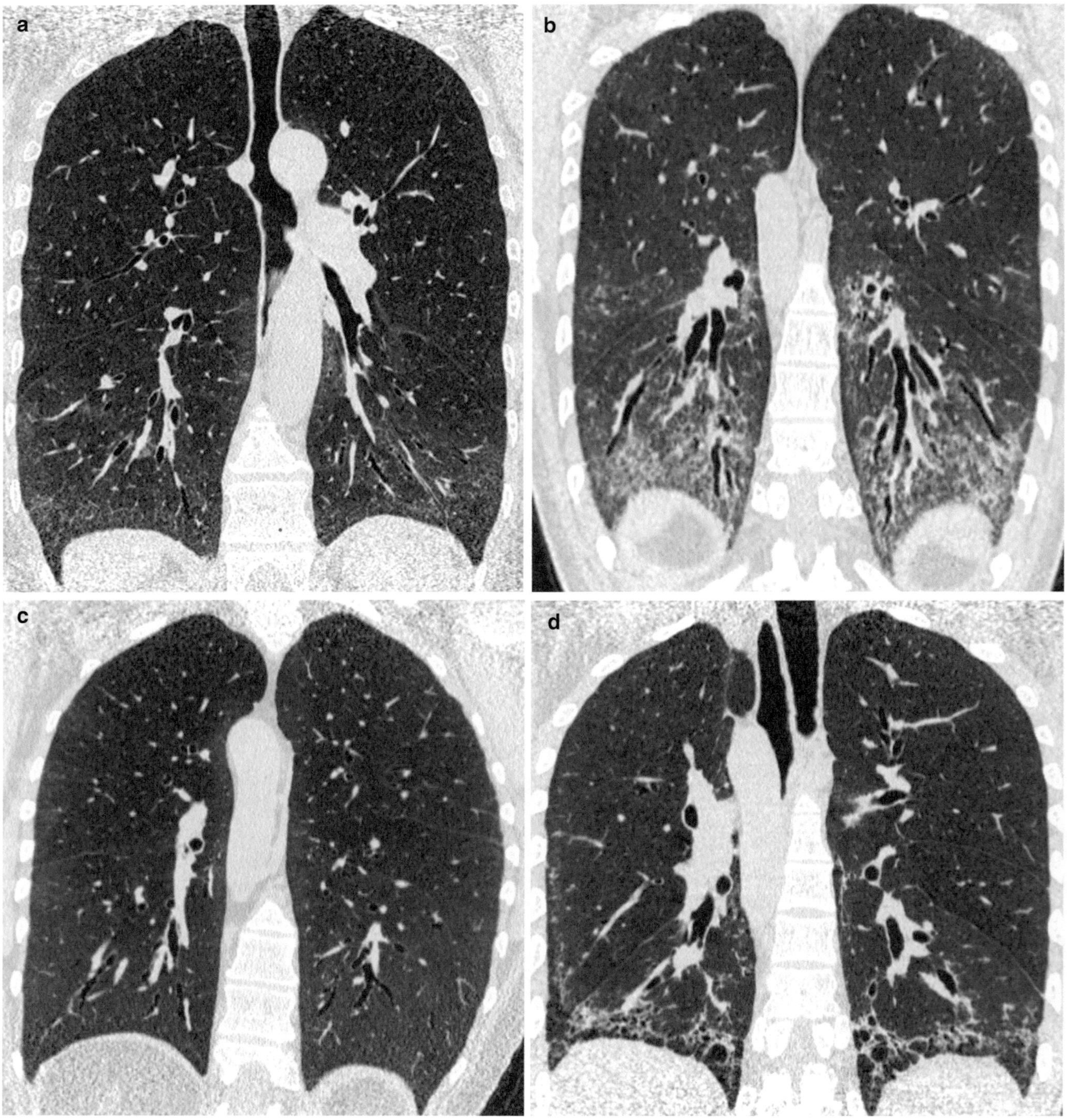

Fig. 25.1 The patterns of SSc-ILD. The most common pattern is that of nonspecific interstitial pneumonia (NSIPAQ3) characterized by a peribronchovascular, central more than peripheral predominant distribution of ground glass opacity (**a**) with varying extent of reticulation with architectural distortion sand-associated traction bronchiectasis (**b**). In some patients, diffuse subtle lower lobe predominant ground glass opacities are seen without any reticulation or architectural distortion (**c**). A pattern of usual interstitial pneumonia (UIP) Usual interstitial pneumonia (UIP) (as defined as sub-pleural lower lobe predominate pattern with reticular opacities with architectural distortion and associate honeycomb cysts reported can also be seen in a subset of patients

tified in up to 60% of patients with systemic sclerosis [19–21]. The most common abnormalities observed on HRCT include ground-glass opacities (defined as increased opacity through which normal anatomy can still be discerned), increased reticular and linear markings that may progress to pulmonary fibrosis (evidenced by associated architectural distortion with or without traction bronchiectasis and bronchiolectasis), and honeycomb cyst formation (defined as at least 3 hexagonal adjacent shaped cysts located in a subpleural location) (Fig. 25.1). The most common pattern is

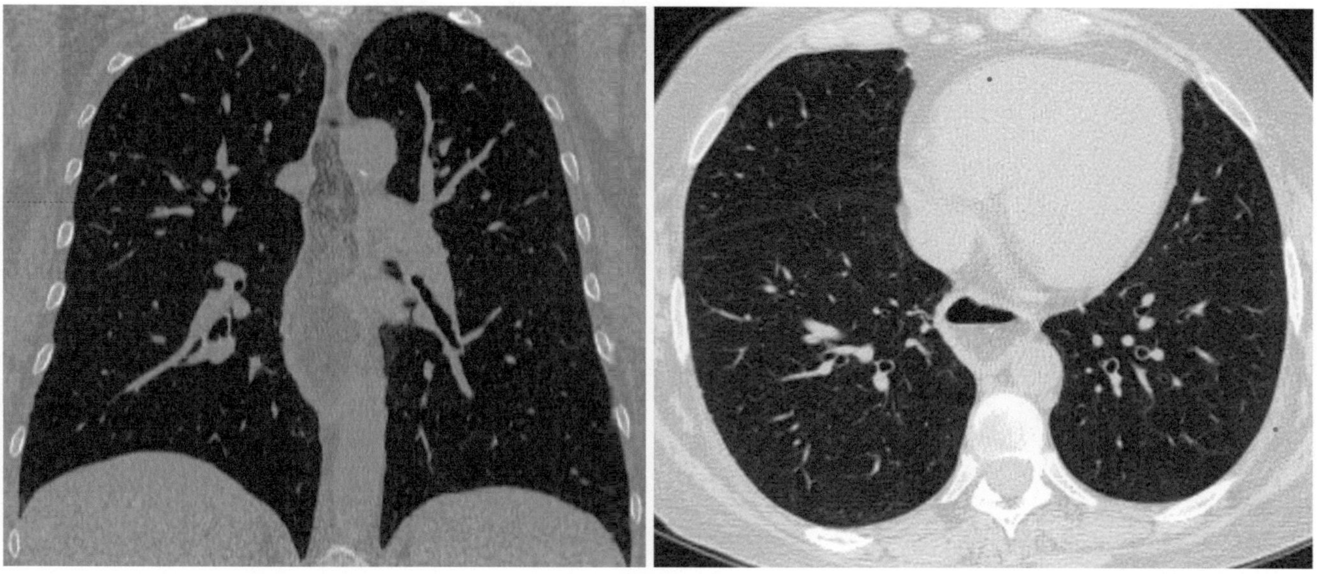

Fig. 25.2 Esophagus dilatation normal lungs. The presence of a dilated esophagus with air alone or on occasion with air and food/fluid is common finding in patients with Scleroderma. The relationship of a dilated esophagus to the development of SSc-ILD remains a topic of research. While some have suggested a relationship of a dilated esophagus with reflux as a putative cause of SSc-ILD, others have not found such a relationship. In this patient, there is clearly a markedly dilated esophagus with extensive food residue, yet no evidence for SSc-ILD or other process is currently seen in the lungs

that of nonspecific interstitial pneumonia (NSIP) characterized by a peribronchovascular, central more than peripheral predominant distribution [19]. A pattern of usual interstitial pneumonia (UIP) (as defined as sub-pleural lower lobe predominate pattern with associate honeycomb cysts reported in 11–36%) can also be seen [22–24]. In a very small number of cases, honeycombing is a predominate finding involving more than 70% of the lungs [25]. These findings suggest that patients with SSc-ILD may have either an NSIP or UIP predominant pattern or even a combination of both patterns [25–27]. This is consistent with the histopathologic findings of SSc-ILD, which include marked pulmonary fibrosis (PF) and honeycomb cystic change. The UIP findings in SSc-ILD tend to not extend along the lateral surfaces on a coronal view, as they tend to do in idiopathic pulmonary fibrosis (IPF), but have a straight margin from side to side [25, 26]. Multifocal coarse fibrosis of the visceral pleura and adjacent parenchyma in the upper lobes akin to pleuroparenchymal fibroelastosis (PPFE) has been reported in up to 18% of patients with SSC-ILD [28]. In asymptomatic patients with normal pulmonary function tests, the usual pattern is that of diffuse lower lobe predominate subtle ground glass opacities.

There are other features noted on HRCT that can be useful in supporting the diagnosis of SSc-ILD, when seen in association with the parenchymal abnormalities [27]. The most frequent and suggestive of these is the presence of a dilated esophagus with air alone or on occasion with air and food/fluid [29–31] (Fig. 25.2). The relationship of a dilated esophagus to the development of SSc-ILD remains a topic of research. While some have suggested a relationship of a dilated esophagus with reflux, a putative cause of SSc-ILD, others have not found such a relationship [27, 31, 32]. The presence of mildly enlarged mediastinal lymphadenopathy is likely reactive, and is also often observed in patients with SSc-ILD [31, 32]. The main pulmonary artery maybe enlarged due to comorbid pulmonary artery hypertension in patients with systemic sclerosis with or without evidence for SSc-ILD [33, 34].

Focal consolidation or ground glass opacities are not a feature of SSc-ILD and its presence raises the possibility of undercurrent infection, aspiration, or hemorrhage. It is important to review carefully for asymmetric focal ground glass opacities or incidental pulmonary nodules as patients with SSc-ILD have an increased risk of developing adenocarcinoma and other lung cancers [35] (Fig. 25.3).

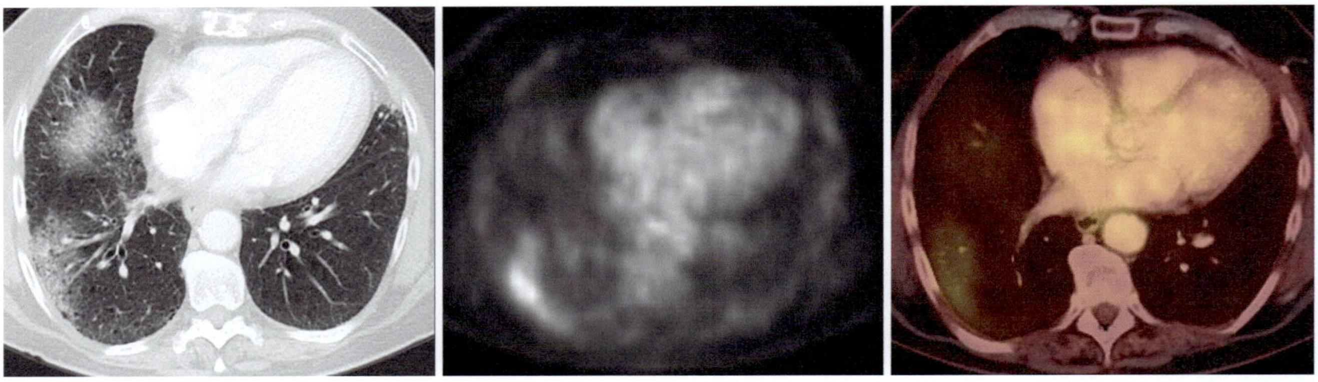

Fig. 25.3 Adenocarcinoma in SLS. Focal consolidation is not a feature of SSc-ILD and its presence raises the possibility of undercurrent infection, aspiration, or hemorrhage. Patients with SSc-ILD have an increased risk of developing adenocarcinoma, as seen in this case, where asymmetric focal ground glass opacity is identified in the right lower lobe, which is atypical for SSC-ILD that is more diffuse and symmetric. In addition, PET confirms the marked uptake in the same area in keeping with a diagnosis of cancer, which was confirmed on biopsy

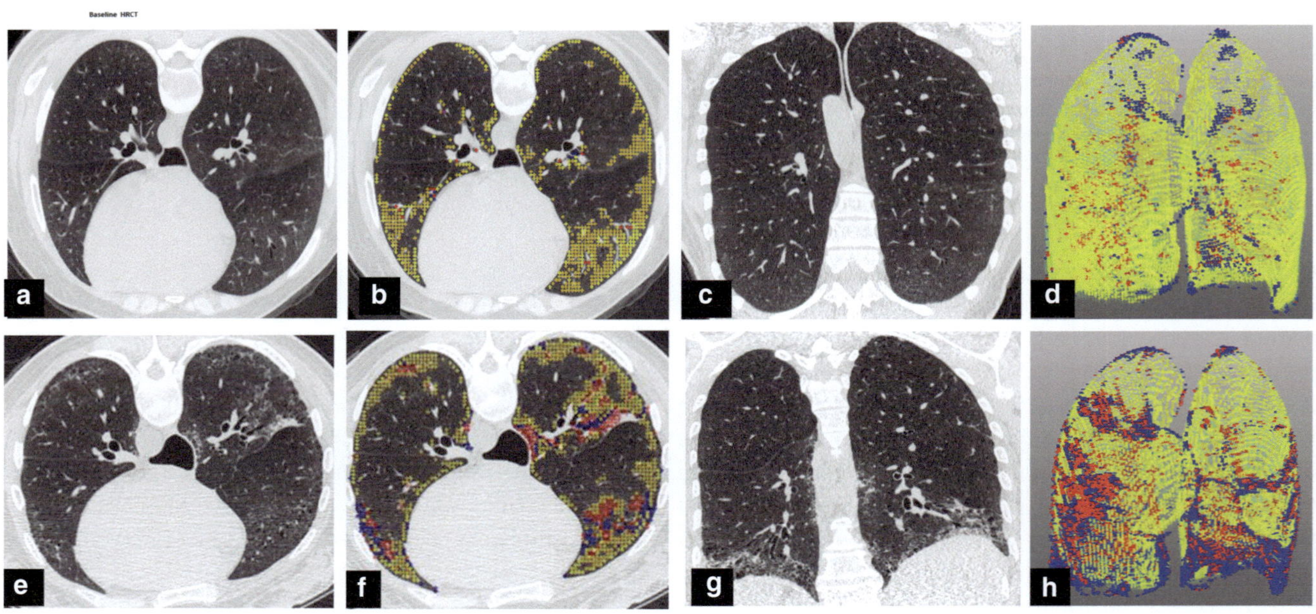

Fig. 25.4 Quantitative CT in SSc-ILD. Quantitative CT is emerging as method to detect and measure the presence extent and change over time of SSc-ILD disease in an example of 29 years old female whose percent predicted FVC was 83% and percent predicted DLCO 44% at baseline with HRCT images and the overlaid colors of QILD: In the first row, (**a**) axial HRCT at baseline, (**b**) overlaid image where the red and blue dots indicate QLF classification and yellow dots indicate the ground glass opacity. The sum of all colored dots is QILD classification, (**c**) coronal image, and (**d**) 3D rendering 1% QLF and 22% QILD score in whole lung; the second row, 5 year of follow-up (**e**) axial HRCT, (**f**) overlaid, (**g**) coronal, (**h**) 3D

Quantitative CT in SSc-ILD

Assessing Disease Extent

Volumetric thin section CT allows for the quantification of the extent of SSc-ILD as well as comorbid disease, in particular emphysema, by either visual estimation or direct measurement using computer vision algorithms. A useful simple visual approach estimates if the total extent of SSc-ILD parenchymal abnormality is clearly greater than 20% or less than 10% irrespective of the nature of the abnormality. If not clearly above or below these thresholds, then the extent is recorded as uncertain, and a secondary criterion is applied by dichotomizing the FVC as above or below 75% [36]. In other visual approaches, the lung is divided into upper-mid and lower zones or lobes and the individual amount of ground glass, reticulation, and honeycomb cysts are estimated within a range of percentages, usually a 4-point modified Likert scale or estimated to nearest 5% [37, 38]. However, all these methods are limited by being reader dependent, time consuming, and having significant inter- and intra-observer variation [39–42].

Quantitative measurement of lung involvement on CT can be assessed using automated post processing software (Fig. 25.4). This includes density measures of each voxel and applying defined threshold cut points for normal and abnormal lung. The area (or volume) occupied by voxels with attenuation values greater than those of normal lung parenchyma (e.g., above −400 HU threshold) represents the amount of interstitial lung tissue [43, 44]. An alternative to using defined density thresholds, parametric measures (kurtosis, skewness, and mean HU density) that describe the frequency distribution plot of lung densities in in the lung or lobe can be used to determine the presence and extent of SSc-ILD [43, 44]. Beyond density thresholds and parametric measures, machine-learned texture feature algorithms have been shown to be powerful in distinguishing between normal parenchyma and abnormal parenchymal abnormalities of SSc-ILD including fibrosis, ground glass, honeycomb cysts, and comorbid emphysema [45, 46]. Deep learning techniques have been shown to classify the pattern of ILD with essentially equivalent performance to subspecialist radiologists [47].

The precision, sensitivity, and absence of interobserver variability associated with QCT measures have made it an increasingly attractive substitute for visual CT analysis. QCT requires standardization of the CT acquisition and analysis akin to the standardization of spirometry, as the measures are heavily influenced by acquisition parameters and lung volume. Rapid and reproducible QCT analysis will likely become increasingly important in following patients. In addition, interrogation of 3D datasets by advanced computer vision and deep learning algorithm techniques may also permit identification of novel biomarkers of disease and prognostic CT features. By measuring the change in extent of SSc-ILD on follow-up CT, the progression of disease can be measured and can assess parenchymal disease progression even that may not always be reflected by changes in spirometry.

QCT as a Biomarker

The extent of SSc-ILD on CT assessed visually or with QCT has been shown to correlate with clinical and physiologic measures of disease severity [48–53]. Visual-based scores have been shown to correlate with both pulmonary function tests and skin involvement [54–57]. Density measures have also been shown to correlate diffusing capacity of lung for carbon monoxide (DLCO) and forced vital capacity (FVC) percentage predicted [43, 58]. Parametric measures of the extent of SSc-ILD correlate with pulmonary function tests and exercise oxygen desaturation [51, 59–65]. Patients with evidence of SSc-ILD on HRCT may however have a preserved FVC, although the single-breath DLCO, in such cases, is often modestly reduced. Consequently, HRCT is a more sensitive and specific diagnostic measure for the detection of SSc-ILD than pulmonary function tests (PFTs). Among PFTs, abnormalities in DLCO correlate best with the extent of ILD on HRCT [66].

The natural history of SSc-ILD is not well understood and although it tends to be progressive, the rate of progression varies. This has been seen in placebo arms in clinical trials where after 12 months, about a third of the subjects show stable disease and the remaining two-thirds varying degrees of progression. The extent of disease at baseline has been shown to be prognostic with respect to a greater rate of decline in FVC and early mortality using visual, density, parametric, and texture derived QCT measures [62, 67, 68]. The amount of interstitial lung disease abnormality has been shown in some studies to independently predict mortality in SSc-ILD when estimated by visual quantitation or directly measured by computer algorithms. Chest CT is not yet integrated in most mortality risk prediction models, which are otherwise predominantly based on spirometry and 6 minute walk tests (6MWT) [63, 69–74]. However, the measures used vary and the relationships are not seen in all studies [62, 75]. Identifying patients at risk of progression is important and so treatment can be initiated early in the course of the disease, especially in a context of recent positive data with antifibrotic drugs. Short-term changes in QCT measures over 6-month interval is associated with increased rate of deterioration of spirometry measures of pulmonary function.

For QCT to become routinely implemented into clinical practice, several challenges have to be overcome. Firstly, there is currently a reluctance to get CT scans due in part to the concern for radiation risk and lack of clear guidelines as to when and how often CT scans should be obtained in patients with SSc-ILD. Currently, the use of CT is guided by clinician preference and most often done due to worsening symptoms and discordance between symptoms and pulmonary function tests. The QIA algorithms have to be clinically validated, widely available, and cost effective. Although, currently being evaluated to date, no QCT method has been evaluated using the OMERACT (Outcome Measures in Rheumatology; https://omeract.org) criteria. Another challenge is socializing clinicians to become comfortable with the interpretation of QCT measures and understanding their additive value to understanding the disease extent and its implication for understanding their prognosis and making appropriate treatment decisions in clinical setting.

QCT as Measure of Drug Rx and Disease Progression

Several clinical trials have shown an impact on the progression on SSc-ILD (Fig. 25.5). The first was the Scleroderma Lung Study I, in which cyclophosphamide treatment led to slower progression of fibrosis compared with placebo [76]. This was followed by the Scleroderma Lung Study II, which reported similar efficacy and improved tolerability with mycophenolate mofetil in comparison with cyclophosphamide [77]. The SENSCIS® trial results [78] showed a positive impact of nintedanib on progression of SSC-ILD and

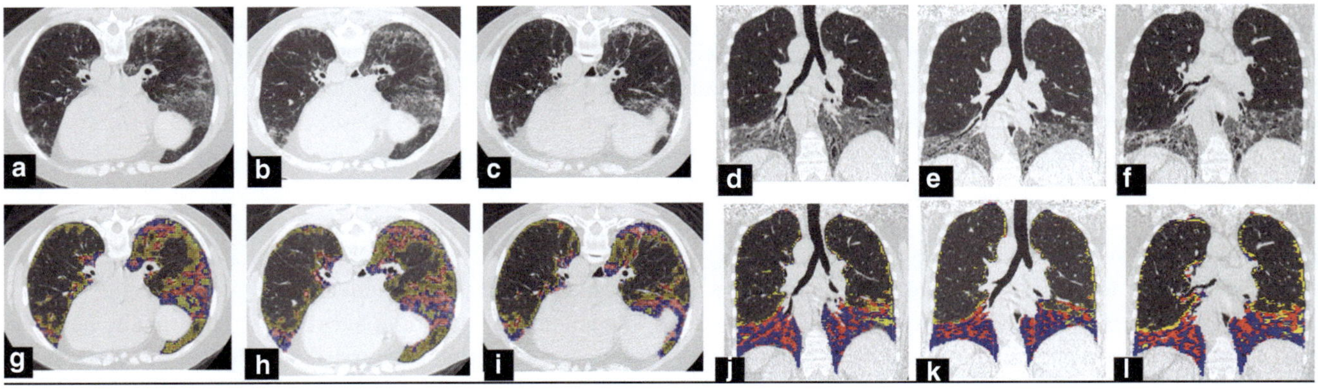

Fig. 25.5 Change overtime SSC-ILD. An example of 61 years old female whose percent predicted FVC was 79% and percent predicted DLCO 42% at baseline with HRCT images and the overlaid colors of QILD: (**a**) axial HRCT at baseline, (**b**) axial HRCT of 1 year of follow-up, (**c**) axial HRCT of approximate 3 years of follow-up, (**d–f**) coronal HRCT images of baseline, 1 year and 3 year follow-up HRCT scans; (**g**) overlaid 31% QILD score and 17% QLF score in whole lung at baseline where the red and blue dots indicate QLF classification and yellow dots indicate the ground glass opacity. The sum of all colored dots is QILD score. (**h**) Overlaid 28% QILD score and 18% QLF score in whole lung at 1 year, (**i**) overlaid 27% QILD score and 11% QLF score in whole lung approximately in 3 years; (**j–l**) are overlaid images of QLF and QILD classification of (**d–f**), respectively

became the first US Food and Drug Administration-approved treatment in patients with SSc-ILD. More recently, tocilizumab was shown to preserve lung function in people with early SSc-ILD and elevated acute-phase reactants.

In several of these trials, QCT was performed as an exploratory endpoint to assess treatment efficacy. In the SLS I Study QLF scores decreased by 2.6% in the cyclophosphamide group, whereas they increased by 9.1% in the placebo group, leading to ~12% difference ($P = 0.0027$). Significant associations were observed between changes in QLF and FVC, patient reported dyspnea score [79]. In the SLS II Study, treatment of SSc-ILD with either cyclophosphamide for 1 year, followed by placebo for a second year, or mycophenolate for 2 years was associated with a significant reduction (improvement) in the extent of SSC-ILD as measured by QILD score, of 2.51% in the pooled groups ($P = 0.001$). There was no significant difference in the QILD score improvement between the cyclophosphamide (−2.66%) and mycophenolate (−2.38%) groups when assessed separately ($P = 0.88$). For the pooled group, the 24-month changes in QILD scores in the whole lung correlated significantly with other outcomes, including 24-month changes in forced vital capacity), single-breath diffusing capacity of the lung for carbon monoxide and breathlessness as measured by the Transition Dyspnea Index ($\rho = -0.26$) [80]. In both the SLS I and SLS II trials, significantly favorable transitions from both ground-glass and lung fibrosis ILD patterns to a normal lung pattern as assessed by QCT were observed in patients undergoing immunosuppressive treatment for SSc-ILD, suggesting the usefulness of examining these transitions for insights into the underlying pathobiology of treatment response [81]. In the tocilizumab trial, it showed evidence of efficacy in SSc-ILD in patients with QCT evidence of lung disease [80, 81]. In the phase 3 tocilizumab randomized, double blind, placebo-controlled, QLF and QILD showed numeric improvements in lung fibrosis in participants treated with tocilizumab, supporting FVC results in the subgroup of participants with SSc-ILD at baseline [3].

To use QCT as a surrogate biomarker as a primary endpoint to establish drug efficacy, the minimal clinical important difference (MCID) must be established. These differences must not just be different between treatment groups, but must be shown to confer mortality benefit in the long term. To evaluate the relationship between changes, QILD and long-term survival in patients who participated in the Scleroderma Lung Study (SLS) 1 and 2 were studied. Progression of the radiographic extent of ILD of ≥2% was associated with worse long-term survival in the two independent SSc cohorts with extensive long-term follow up. The findings provide compelling evidence that using a MCID ≥2% changes in the radiographic extent of ILD may serve as a surrogate endpoint for mortality in patients with SSc [82].

Emerging Technologies

Ultrasound

Lung ultrasound has long been evaluated as a potential screening modality for the detection of ILD. The potential advantages include the absence of ionizing radiation, lower cost than CT or MRI, and ease of performing the study at the bedside. The presence of ILD is sensitively and accurately revealed by hyperechoic linear reverberations parallel to the pleura and that move with the lung called B Lines [83]. The number of B lines has been shown to correlate with the severity of interstitial lung disease [84–86]. The sensitivity and specificity of ultrasound for the detection of SSc-ILD is well below that of CT [85, 86]. Ultrasound is also limited to providing information about disease adjacent to the pleura and cannot give insight into the distribution or morphology of the lung disease. Thus, currently there is no consensus as to the usefulness of ultrasound in the routine screening of patients with scleroderma and its ability to detect change over time has not been established. Whether or not lung ultrasound is sensitive, enough to detect changes in the extent of ILD over time remains to be determined..

Magnetic Resonance Imaging (MRI)

Magnetic resonance imaging (MRI), utilizing ultrashort time-to-echo (UTE) sequences is emerging as a promising alternative to CT as it can provide both structure and function information without exposure to ionizing radiation [87, 88]. In the setting of IPF, MRI has been shown to be excellent in the detection of ILD, but to underestimate its extent. MRI may be useful to detect inflammatory versus fibrotic changes, not always discernable on CT. This has also been shown for patients with SSc-ILD who have more than 5% parenchymal involvement with a very high sensitivity (93%) and perfect specificity (100%). The degree of MRI-detected ILD correlated with the pulmonary function testing parameters, forced vital capacity (FVC) and diffusion capacity of the lung for carbon monoxide (DLCO) and the amount of ILD on HRCT. Using functional MRI images are acquired at both full inspiration and at end expiration, and then analyzed using algorithms that map voxels from the same region to assess lung dispensability as surrogate of compliance. Patients with SSc-ILD have reduced deformation of voxel location [89].

Hyperpolarized gas MRI can also be performed to enable detailed regional functional information as to ventilation and gas transfer across the interstitial space and into red blood cells [90]. This allows for the assessment of alveolar microstructure by measuring barrier thickness [91]. In SSc-ILD, like in those with IPF have an increased alveolar septal thickness compared to healthy volunteers. Hyperpolarized MRI has been demonstrated to detect changes in gas diffusion overtime in patients with IPF [92]. While ^{129}Xe MRI studies have predominately focused on IPF, its application to SSc-ILD may elucidate important functional.

MRI allows for molecular imaging by labeling standard MRI contrast agents with molecules or compounds that are indicative of the pathobiology of a disease process. In setting of patients with scleroderma, it has been suggested that endothelial injury that results in increased vascular permeability is central to the pathogenesis of SSc-ILD [93–99]. Increased vascular permeability resulting in leakage into the interstitium has been shown to contribute to the development of pulmonary fibrosis. By labeling gadolinium with albumin, the degree of extravasation can be measured and has shown that the rate of leakage is greatest in patients with fibrosis in both lung regions with and without fibrosis in patients with IPF and SSc-ILD [98, 99].*

Nuclear Medicine Imaging

Positron emission tomography (PET) CT is an imaging modality that enables noninvasive characterization of molecular processes in vivo. ^{18}F-fluorodeoxyglucose (FDG) is a commonly used PET radiotracer and has been observed in macrophages, neutrophils, and eosinophils and may detect cellular inflammation through the glycolysis of immune cells, as an indirect means to monitor fibrosis. The most readily available PET probe is fluorodeoxyglucose (^{18}F-FDG) which is utilized to quantify glucose uptake in tissues. Increased ^{18}F-FDG was demonstrated in patients with diffuse parenchymal lung disease, some of whom had connective tissue disease-associated ILD with higher uptake associating with mortality in IPF. Pulmonary FDG uptakes were higher in SSc patients than in controls, especially in those with ILD compared with those without ILD. Pulmonary FDG uptakes were positively correlated with the ILD severity (fibrosis extent, %FVC, and %DLCO) [100]. Semiquantitative assessment of ^{18}F-FDG PET/CT is able to distinguish ILD from non-affected lung tissue in SSc-ILD, suggesting that it may be used as a new biomarker for SSc-ILD inflammatory disease activity and treatment repose assessment in the future [101]. This is because potentially PET can stratify patients with predominantly ground glass opacities on HRCT into those due to inflammation vs fibrotic tissue, which is not possible on CT alone. The combination of PET and CT scan may provide synergistic metabolic and structural information about the SSc-ILD notwithstanding the challenges of cost and radiation dose that are limiting its current use. Another nuclear medicine test that has offered insights into the role of increased vascular permeability and leakage in the development of SSc-ILD is the measurements of clearance rate of the inhaled technetium-labeled diethylenediamine pentaacetate (^{99}Tc-DTPA). Patients with SSc-ILD demonstrated increased ^{99}Tc-DTPA clearance rates indicative of increased vascular leak and is associated with progression of FVC deterioration [96].

Optical Coherence Tomography (OCT)

Optical coherence tomography (OCT) is the only technique to provide very high resolution (<5 μm) in vivo insight into structure [102]. In the setting of scleroderma intravascular,

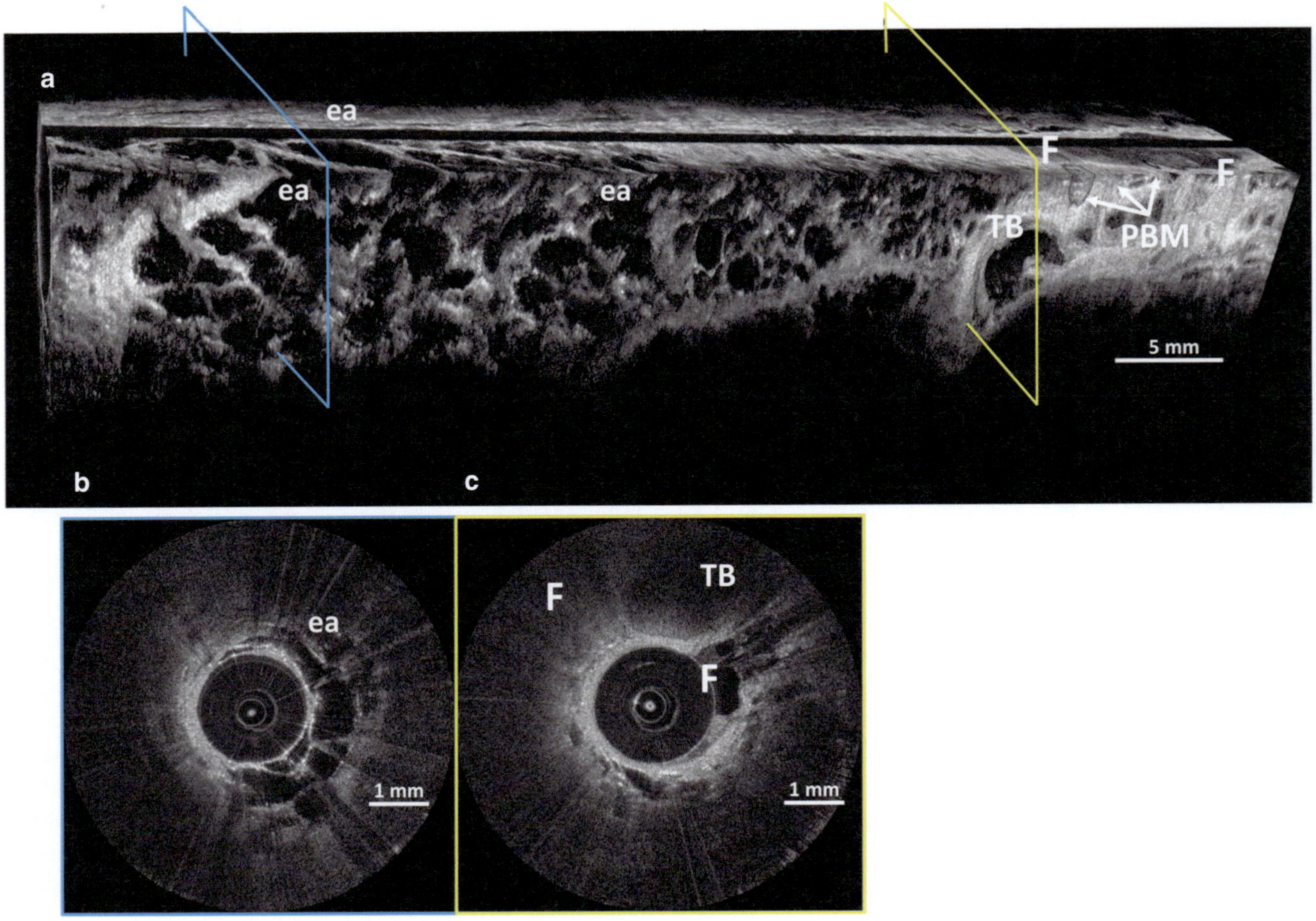

Fig. 25.6 OCT in a patient with SSC-ILD demonstrates airway-centered fibrosis. (**a**) In vivo volumetric and (**b**, **c**) cross-sectional EB-OCT imaging shows dense, signal-intense (light grey) fibrosis surrounding the proximal end of the airway (right side). Traction bronchiectasis within the fibrotic region appears as a cystically dilated, irregular airway branch point. Adjacent, smaller, irregular cystic structures are indicative of peribronchiolar metaplasia, often associated with traction bronchiectasis in airway-centered fibrosis. Distal to the airway-centered fibrosis, there is a transition to alveolated parenchyma with enlarged, rounded airspaces and intact alveolar walls (left side), indicative of hyperinflation. The EB-OCT cross-sections in B and C are taken from the locations on the volumetric image (**a**) indicated by the blue and yellow squares, respectively. *EB-OCT* endobronchial optical coherence tomography, *Ea* enlarged, rounded airspaces, *F* fibrosis, *PBM* peribronchiolar metaplasia, *TB* traction bronchiectasis. (Courtesy Dr. Lida Hariri)

OCT has provided insights into the morphology of peripheral small pulmonary arteries [103]. Endobronchial OCT is able to detect traction bronchiectasis and honeycombing in patients with ILD below the resolution of HRCT [104]. Beyond structure, OCT when integrated with fibrosis-specific molecular probes has the potential to evaluate fibrosis on a microscopic level (Fig. 25.6).

Conclusion

HRCT is currently the gold standard for early detection and accurate diagnosis of ILD in patients with SSc-ILD, and should be performed in all patients at the time of initial SSc diagnosis. Quantitative HRCT can also be used for prognosis and to monitor for disease progression in addition to serial lung function tests and other measures. Several emerging imaging technologies that should also be increasingly used to offer further insights into the pathobiology and nature of SSc-ILD. It is likely that these technologies will also have future role in the assessment of disease progression and evaluation of novel treatment therapies.

References

1. Giacomelli R, et al. Interstitial lung disease in systemic sclerosis: current and future treatment. Rheumatol Int. 2017;37(6):853–63.
2. Tyndall AJ, et al. Causes and risk factors for death in systemic sclerosis: a study from the EULAR Scleroderma Trials and Research (EUSTAR) database. Ann Rheum Dis. 2010;69(10):1809–15.
3. Khanna D, Lin C, Furst D, Wagner B, Zucchetto M, Raghu G, Martinez F, Goldin J, Siegel J, Denton C. Long-term

safety and efficacy of tocilizumab in early systemic sclerosis-interstitial lung disease: open-label extension of a phase 3 randomized controlled trial. Am J Respir Crit Care Med. 2022;205(6):674–84.
4. Doyle TJ, Hunninghake GM, Rosas IO. Subclinical interstitial lung disease: why you should care. Am J Respir Crit Care Med. 2012;185(11):1147–53.
5. Hax V, et al. Clinical algorithms for the diagnosis and prognosis of interstitial lung disease in systemic sclerosis. Semin Arthritis Rheum. 2017;47(2):228–34.
6. Molberg O, Hoffmann-Vold AM. Interstitial lung disease in systemic sclerosis: progress in screening and early diagnosis. Curr Opin Rheumatol. 2016;28(6):613–8.
7. Winstone TA, et al. Predictors of mortality and progression in scleroderma-associated interstitial lung disease: a systematic review. Chest. 2014;146(2):422–36.
8. Raghu G, et al. Diagnosis of idiopathic pulmonary fibrosis. An official ATS/ERS/JRS/ALAT clinical practice guideline. Am J Respir Crit Care Med. 2018;198(5):44–68.
9. Exam: CT thorax for interstitial lung disease. 2019. Available from: https://www.pulmonaryfibrosis.org/docs/default-source/medical-community-documents/ct-chest-for-ild-protocol.pdf?sfvrsn=0.
10. Lynch DA, et al. Diagnostic criteria for idiopathic pulmonary fibrosis: a Fleischner Society White Paper. Lancet Respir Med. 2018;6(2):138–53.
11. Goldin J, Beckett K. Risks of thoracic CT. Eur Respir Monogr. 2015;70:253–62.
12. Katsura M, Sato J, Akahane M, et al. Effects of pure and hybrid iterative reconstruction algorithms on high-resolution computed tomography in the evaluation of interstitial lung disease. Eur J Radiol. 2017;93:243–51.
13. National Research Council. Health risks from exposure to low levels of ionizing radiation: BEIR VII phase 2. Washington, DC: The National Academies Press; 2006. p. 422.
14. Silman AJ. Epidemiology of scleroderma. Ann Rheum Dis. 1991;50(Suppl 4):846–53.
15. Joycea S, O'Connor OJ, Maher MM, McEnteec MF. Strategies for dose reduction with specific clinical indications during computed tomography. Radiography. 2020;26(Suppl 2):S62–8.
16. Denton CP, Hughes M, Gak N, et al. BSR and BHPR guideline for the treatment of systemic sclerosis. Rheumatology. 2016;55(10):1906–10.
17. Kowal-Bielecka O, Fransen J, Avouac J, et al. Update of EULAR recommendations for the treatment of systemic sclerosis. Ann Rheum Dis. 2017;76(8):1327–39.
18. Hoffmann-Vold A-M, Maher TM, Philpot EE, et al. The identification and management of interstitial lung disease in systemic sclerosis: evidence-based European consensus statements. Lancet Rheumatol. 2020;2:e71–83.
19. Chung J, Walker CM, Hobbs S. Imaging features of systemic sclerosis-associated interstitial lung disease. J Vis Exp. 2020; https://doi.org/10.3791/60300. Epub ahead of print.
20. Suliman YA, Dobrota R, Huscher D, et al. Brief report: pulmonary function tests: high rate of false-negative results in the early detection and screening of scleroderma-related interstitial lung disease. Arthritis Rheumatol. 2015;67(12):3256–61.
21. Hoffmann-Vold AM, Fretheim H, Halse AK, et al. Tracking impact of interstitial lung disease in systemic sclerosis in a complete nationwide cohort. Am J Respir Crit Care Med. 2019;200:1258–66.
22. Branley HM. Pulmonary fibrosis in systemic sclerosis: diagnosis and management. Respir Med CME. 2010;3:10–4.
23. Engeler CE, Tashjian JH, Trenkner SW, Walsh JW. Ground-glass opacity of the lung parenchyma: a guide to analysis with high-resolution CT. Am J Roentgenol. 1993;160(2):249–51.
24. Goldin JG, et al. High-resolution CT scan findings in patients with symptomatic scleroderma-related interstitial lung disease. Chest. 2008;134(2):358–67.
25. Chung JH, et al. CT Features of the usual interstitial pneumonia pattern: differentiating connective tissue disease-associated interstitial lung disease from idiopathic pulmonary fibrosis. Am J Roentgenol. 2018;210(2):307–13.
26. Zhan X, et al. Differentiating usual interstitial pneumonia from nonspecific interstitial pneumonia using high-resolution computed tomography: the "Straight-edge Sign". J Thorac Imaging. 2018;33(4):266–70.
27. Farrokh D, Abbasi B, Fallah-Rastegar Y, Mirfeizi Z. The extrapulmonary manifestations of systemic sclerosis on chest high resolution computed tomography. Tanaffos. 2015;14(3):193–200.
28. Bonifazi M, Sverzellati N, Negri E, Jacob J, Egashira R, Moser J, Piciucchi S, Mei F, De Lauretis A, Visca D, Goh N, Bonini M, Cirilli L, LaVecchia C, Chua F, Kouranos V, Margaritopoulos G, Kokosi M, Maher TM, Gasparini S, Gabrielli A, Wells AU, Renzoni EA. Pleuroparenchymal fibroelastosis in systemic sclerosis: prevalence and prognostic impact. Eur Respir J. 2020;56:1902135. https://doi.org/10.1183/13993003.02135-2019.
29. Salaffi F, et al. Relationship between interstitial lung disease and oesophageal dilatation on chest high-resolution computed tomography in patients with systemic sclerosis: a cross-sectional study. Radiol Med. 2018;123(9):655–63.
30. Vonk MC, et al. Oesophageal dilatation on high-resolution computed tomography scan of the lungs as a sign of scleroderma. Ann Rheum Dis. 2008;67(9):1317–21.
31. Bhalla M, Silver RM, Shepard JA, McLoud TC. Chest CT in patients with scleroderma: prevalence of asymptomatic esophageal dilatation and mediastinal lymphadenopathy. AJR Am J Roentgenol. 1993;161(2):269.
32. Chowaniec M, Skoczynska M, Sokolik R, Wiland P. Interstitial lung disease in systemic sclerosis: challenges in early diagnosis and management. Reumatologia. 2018;56(4):249–54.
33. McCall RK, Ravenel JG, Nietert PJ, Granath A, Silver RM. Relationship of main pulmonary artery diameter to pulmonary arterial pressure in scleroderma patients with and without interstitial fibrosis. J Comput Assist Tomogr. 2014;38(2):163–8.
34. Pandey AK, et al. Predictors of pulmonary hypertension on high-resolution computed tomography of the chest in systemic sclerosis: a retrospective analysis. Can Assoc Radiol J. 2010;61(5):291–6.
35. Colaci M, et al. Lung cancer in scleroderma: results from an Italian rheumatologic center and review of the literature. Autoimmun Rev. 2013;12(3):374–9.
36. Goh NS, Desai SR, Veeraraghavan S, Hansell DM, Copley SJ, Maher TM, et al. Interstitial lung disease in systemic sclerosis: a simple staging system. Am J Respir Crit Care Med. 2008;177:1248–54. https://doi.org/10.1164/rccm.200706-877OC.
37. Warrick JH, Bhalla M, Schabel SI, et al. High resolution computed tomography in early scleroderma lung disease. J Rheumatol. 1991;18:1520–8.
38. Kazerooni EA, Martinez FJ, Flint A, et al. Thin-section CT obtained at 10-mm increments versus limited three-level thin-section CT for idiopathic pulmonary fibrosis: correlation with pathologic scoring. AJR Am J Roentgenol. 1997;169:977–83.
39. Ng CS, Desai SR, Rubens MB, et al. Visual quantitation and observer variation of signs of small airways disease at inspiratory and expiratory CT. J Thorac Imaging. 1999;14:279–85.
40. Aziz ZA, Wells AU, Hansell DM, et al. HRCT diagnosis of diffuse parenchymal lung disease: inter-observer variation. Thorax. 2004;59:506–11.
41. Sundaram B, Gross BH, Martinez FJ, et al. Accuracy of high-resolution CT in the diagnosis of diffuse lung disease: effect of predominance and distribution of findings. AJR Am J Roentgenol. 2008;191:1032–9.

42. Watadani T, Sakai F, Johkoh T, et al. Interobserver variability in the CT assessment of honeycombing in the lungs. Radiology. 2013;266:936–44.
43. Ninaber MK, Stolk J, Smit J, et al. Lung structure and function relation in systemic sclerosis: application of lung densitometry. Eur J Radiol. 2015;84:975–9.
44. Do K-H, Lee JS, Colby TV, et al. Nonspecific interstitial pneumonia versus usual interstitial pneumonia: differences in the density histogram of high-resolution CT. J Comput Assist Tomogr. 2005;29:544–8.
45. Kim HG, Tashkin DP, Clements PJ, et al. A computer-aided diagnosis system for quantitative scoring of extent of lung fibrosis in scleroderma patients. Clin Exp Rheumatol. 2010;28(5 Suppl 62):S26–35.
46. Zavaletta VA, Bartholmai BJ, Robb RA. High resolution multidetector CT-aided tissue analysis and quantification of lung fibrosis. Acad Radiol. 2007;14(7):772–87.
47. Walsh SLF, Calandriello L, Silva M, et al. Deep learning for classifying fibrotic lung disease on high-resolution computed tomography: a case-cohort study. Lancet Respir Med. 2018;6(11):837–45.
48. Roth MD, Tseng C-H, Clements PJ, et al. Predicting treatment outcomes and responder subsets in scleroderma related interstitial lung disease. Arthritis Rheum. 2011;63(9):2797–808.
49. Patiwetwitoon S, Wangkaew S, Euathrongchit J, et al. High-resolution computed tomographic findings in systemic sclerosis-associated interstitial lung disease: comparison between diffuse and limited systemic sclerosis. J Clin Rheumatol. 2012;18(5):229–33.
50. Le Gouellec N, Duhamel A, Perez T, et al. Predictors of lung function test severity and outcome in systemic sclerosis-associated interstitial lung disease. PLoS One. 2017;12(8):e0181692.
51. Khanna D, Nagaraja V, Tseng CH, et al. Predictors of lung function decline in scleroderma-related interstitial lung disease based on high-resolution computed tomography: implications for cohort enrichment in systemic sclerosis associated interstitial lung disease trials. Arthritis Res Ther. 2015;17:372.
52. Launay D, Remy-Jardin M, Michon-Pasturel U, et al. High resolution computed tomography in fibrosing alveolitis associated with systemic sclerosis. J Rheumatol. 2006;33(9):1789–801.
53. Tashkin DP, Volkmann ER, Tseng C-H. Relationship between quantitative radiographic assessments of interstitial lung disease and physiologic and clinical features of systemic sclerosis. Ann Rheum Dis. 2016;75(2):373–81.
54. Diot E, Boissinot E, Asquier E, et al. Relationship between abnormalities on high-resolution CT and pulmonary function in systemic sclerosis. Chest. 1998;114:1623–9.
55. Zompatori M, Leone MB, Giannotta M, et al. Pulmonary hypertension and systemic sclerosis: the role of high-resolution computed tomography. Radiol Med. 2013;118:1360–72.
56. Goldin JG, Lynch DA, Strollo DC, et al. High-resolution CT scan findings in patients with symptomatic scleroderma-related interstitial lung disease. Chest. 2008;134:358–67.
57. Hafez EA, Hamza SH, Morad CS, et al. Pulmonary manifestations in Egyptian patients with systemic sclerosis. Egypt Rheumatol. 2017;40:39–44.
58. Camiciottoli G, Orlandi I, Bartolucci M, et al. Lung CT densitometry in systemic sclerosis: correlation with lung function, exercise testing, and quality of life. Chest. 2007;131:672–81.
59. Ariani A, Silva M, Bravi E, et al. Operator-independent quantitative chest computed tomography versus standard assessment of interstitial lung disease related to systemic sclerosis: a multi-centric study. Mod Rheumatol. 2015;25:724–30.
60. Ariani A, Aiello M, Silva M, et al. Quantitative CT indexes are significantly associated with exercise oxygen desaturation in interstitial lung disease related to systemic sclerosis. Clin Respir J. 2017;11:983.
61. Ariani A, Silva M, Seletti V, et al. Quantitative chest computed tomography is associated with two prediction models of mortality in interstitial lung disease related to systemic sclerosis. Rheumatology (Oxford). 2017;56:922–7.
62. Saldana DC, Hague CJ, Murphy D, et al. Association of computed tomography densitometry with disease severity, functional decline, and survival in systemic sclerosis-associated interstitial lung disease. Ann Am Thorac Soc. 2020;17:813–20.
63. Goh NS, Hoyles RK, Denton CP, Hansell DM, Renzoni EA, Maher TM, et al. Short-term pulmonary function trends are predictive of mortality in interstitial lung disease associated with systemic sclerosis. Arthritis Rheumatol. 2017;69:1670–8. https://doi.org/10.1002/art.40130.
64. Takei R, et al. Radiographic fibrosis score predicts survival in systemic sclerosis-associated interstitial lung disease. Respirology. 2018;23(4):385–91.
65. Bakker ME, et al. Lung density and pulmonary artery diameter are predictors of pulmonary hypertension in systemic sclerosis. J Thorac Imaging. 2017;32(6):391–7.
66. Showalter K, et al. Performance of forced vital capacity and lung diffusion cutpoints for associated radiographic interstitial lung disease in systemic sclerosis. J Rheumatol. 2018;45(11):1572–6.
67. Ferrazza AM, Gigante A, Gasperini ML, et al. Assessment of interstitial lung disease in systemic sclerosis using the quantitative CT algorithm CALIPER. Clin Rheumatol. 2020;20:6–17.
68. Jacob J, Bartholmai BJ, Rajagopalan S, et al. Evaluation of computer-based computer tomography stratification against outcome models in connective tissue disease-related interstitial lung disease: a patient outcome study. BMC Med. 2016;14:190.
69. Ryerson CJ, O'Connor D, Dunne JV, et al. Predicting mortality in systemic sclerosis-associated interstitial lung disease using risk prediction models derived from idiopathic pulmonary fibrosis. Chest. 2015;148:1268–75.
70. Mango RL, Matteson EL, Crowson CS, et al. Assessing mortality models in systemic sclerosis-related interstitial lung disease. Lung. 2018;196:409–16.
71. Forestier A, Le Gouellec N, Béhal H, Kramer G, Perez T, Sobanski V, et al. Evolution of high-resolution CT-scan in systemic sclerosis-associated interstitial lung disease: description and prognosis factors. Semin Arthritis Rheum. 2020;50:1406–13. https://doi.org/10.1016/j.semarthrit.2020.02.015.
72. Kim EA, Johkoh T, Lee KS, Ichikado K, Koh EM, Kim TS, et al. Interstitial pneumonia in progressive systemic sclerosis: serial high-resolution CT findings with functional correlation. J Comput Assist Tomogr. 2001;25:757–63. https://doi.org/10.1097/00004728-200109000-00015.
73. Le Gouellec N, Duhamel A, Perez T, Hachulla AL, Sobanski V, Faivre JB, et al. Predictors of lung function test severity and outcome in systemic sclerosis-associated interstitial lung disease. PLoS One. 2017;12:e0181692. https://doi.org/10.1371/journal.pone.0181692.
74. Moore OA, Goh N, Corte T, Rouse H, Hennessy O, Thakkar V, et al. Extent of disease on high-resolution computed tomography lung is a predictor of decline and mortality in systemic sclerosis-related interstitial lung disease. Rheumatology. 2013;52:155–60. https://doi.org/10.1093/rheumatology/kes289.
75. Vanaken L, Landini N, Lenaerts J, Claeys E, Lenaerts J, Wuyts WA, et al. Progressive lung fibrosis and mortality can occur in early systemic sclerosis patients without pulmonary abnormalities at baseline assessment. Clin Rheumatol. 2020;39:3393–400. https://doi.org/10.1007/s10067-020-05105-4.
76. Tashkin D, Elashoff R, Clements P, Goldin J, Roth M, Furst D, et al. Cyclophosphamide versus placebo in scleroderma lung disease. N Engl J Med. 2006;354(25):2655–66.
77. Tashkin DP, et al. Mycophenolate mofetil versus oral cyclophosphamide in scleroderma-related interstitial lung disease (SLS II):

a randomised controlled, double-blind, parallel group trial. Lancet Respir Med. 2016;4(9):708–19.
78. Distler O, et al. Nintedanib for systemic sclerosis associated interstitial lung disease. N Engl J Med. 2019;380:2518–28.
79. Kim HJ, Brown MS, Elashoff R, Li G, Gjertson DW, Lynch DA, Strollo DC, Kleerup E, Chong D, Shah SK, Ahmad S, Abtin F, Tashkin DP, Goldin JG. Quantitative texture-based assessment of one-year changes in fibrotic reticular patterns on HRCT in scleroderma lung disease treated with oral cyclophosphamide. Eur Radiol. 2011;21(12):2455–65. https://doi.org/10.1007/s00330-011-2223-2. Epub 2011 Sep 17.
80. Goldin JG, Kim GHJ, Tseng CH, Volkmann E, Furst D, Clements P, Brown M, Roth M, Khanna D, Tashkin DP. Longitudinal changes in quantitative interstitial lung disease on computed tomography after immunosuppression in the scleroderma lung study II. Ann Am Thorac Soc. 2018;15(11):1286–95. https://doi.org/10.1513/AnnalsATS.201802-079OC.
81. Kim GHJ, Tashkin DP, Lo P, Brown MS, Volkmann ER, Gjertson DW, Khanna D, Elashoff RM, Tseng CH, Roth MD, Goldin JG. Using transitional changes on high-resolution computed tomography to monitor the impact of cyclophosphamide or mycophenolate mofetil on systemic sclerosis-related interstitial lung disease. Arthritis Rheumatol. 2020;72(2):316–25. https://doi.org/10.1002/art.41085. Epub 2019 Dec 26.
82. Volkman E, Tashkin D, Roth M, Goldin J, Kim G. Short-term changes in the radiographic extent of interstitial lung disease predict long-term mortality in systemic sclerosis. Ann Rheum Dis. 2021;80(Suppl 1):162–3.
83. Song GG, Bae S-C, Lee YH. Diagnostic accuracy of lung ultrasound for interstitial lung disease in patients with connective tissue diseases: a meta-analysis. Clin Exp Rheumatol. 2016;34:11–6.
84. Gargani L, Doveri M, D'Errico L, Frassi F, Bazzichi ML, Delle Sedie A, et al. Ultrasound lung comets in systemic sclerosis: a chest sonography hallmark of pulmonary interstitial fibrosis. Rheumatology (Oxford). 2009;48:1382–7.
85. Barskova T, Gargani L, Guiducci S, Randone SB, Bruni C, Carnesecchi G, et al. Lung ultrasound for the screening of interstitial lung disease in very early systemic sclerosis. Ann Rheum Dis. 2013;72:390–5.
86. Çakir Edis E, Hatipoğlu ON, Pamuk ÖN, Eraslan RM, Aktöz M, Tuncel SA. Effectiveness of thoracic ultrasonography in the evaluation of the severity of pulmonary involvement in patients with systemic sclerosis. Arch Rheumatol. 2016;31:364–70.
87. Lavelle LP, Brady D, McEvoy S, et al. Pulmonary fibrosis: tissue characterization using late-enhanced MRI compared with unenhanced anatomic high-resolution CT. Diagn Interv Radiol. 2017;23(2):106–11.
88. Mirsadraee S, Tse M, Kershaw L, et al. T1 characteristics of interstitial pulmonary fibrosis on 3T MRI-a predictor of early interstitial change? Quant Imaging Med Surg. 2016;6(1):42–9.
89. Chassagnon G, Martin C, Marini R, Vakalopolou M, Régent A, Mouthon L, et al. Use of elastic registration in pulmonary MRI for the assessment of pulmonary fibrosis in patients with systemic sclerosis. Radiology. 2019;182099:487.
90. Mammarappallil JG, Rankine L, Wild JM, Driehuys B. New developments in imaging idiopathic pulmonary fibrosis with hyperpolarized xenon magnetic resonance imaging. J Thorac Imaging. 2019;34:136–50.
91. Stewart NJ, Leung G, Norquay G, Marshall H, Parra-Robles J, Murphy PS, et al. Experimental validation of the hyperpolarized 129 Xe chemical shift saturation recovery technique in healthy volunteers and subjects with interstitial lung disease. Magn Reson Med. 2015;74:196–207.
92. Weatherley ND, Stewart NJ, Chan H-F, Austin M, Smith LJ, Collier G, et al. Hyperpolarised xenon magnetic resonance spectroscopy for the longitudinal assessment of changes in gas diffusion in IPF. Thorax. 2018;74:500.
93. Pearson JD. The endothelium: its role in scleroderma. Ann Rheum Dis. 1991;50(Suppl 4):866–71.
94. Dvorak HF. Tumors: wounds that do not heal: similarities between tumor stroma generation and wound healing. N Engl J Med. 1986;315(26):1650–9.
95. Shea BS, Brooks SF, Fontaine BA, Chun J, Luster AD, Tager AM. Prolonged exposure to sphingosine 1-phosphate receptor-1 agonists exacerbates vascular leak, fibrosis, and mortality after lung injury. Am J Respir Cell Mol Biol. 2010;43:662.
96. Fanti S, De Fabritiis A, Aloisi D, Dondi M, Marengo M, Compagnone G, et al. Early pulmonary involvement in systemic sclerosis assessed by technetium-99m-DTPA clearance rate. J Nucl Med. 1994;35:1933.
97. Wells AU, Hansell DM, Harrison NK, Lawrence R, Black CM, Bois du RM. Clearance of inhaled 99mTc-DTPA predicts the clinical course of fibrosing alveolitis. Eur Respir J. 1993;6:797–802.
98. Goh NSL, Desai SR, Anagnostopoulos C, Hansell DM, Hoyles RK, Sato H, et al. Increased epithelial permeability in pulmonary fibrosis in relation to disease progression. Eur Respir J. 2011;38:184–90.
99. Montesi SB, Rao R, Liang LL, Goulart HE, Sharma A, Digumarthy SR, et al. Gadofosveset-enhanced lung MRI to detect ongoing vascular leak in pulmonary fibrosis. Eur Respir J. 2018;51:1800171.
100. Ledoult E, Morelle M, Soussan M, Mékinian A, Béhal H, Sobanski V, Hachulla E, Huglo D, Le Gouellec N, Remy-Jardin M, Baillet C, Launay D. ^{18}F-FDG position emission tomography scanning in systemic sclerosis-associated interstitial lung disease: a pilot study. Arthritis Res Ther. 2021;23:76.
101. Peelen DM, Zwezerijnen BGJC, Nossent EJ, Meijboom LJ, Hoekstra OS, Van der Laken CJ, Voskuyl AE. The quantitative assessment of interstitial lung disease with positron emission tomography scanning in systemic sclerosis patients. Rheumatology (Oxford). 2020;59(6):1407–15. https://doi.org/10.1093/rheumatology/kez483.
102. Yonetsu T, Bouma BE, Kato K, Fujimoto JG, Jang IK. Optical coherence tomography—15 years in cardiology. Circ J. 2013;77:1933–40.
103. Schwaiger JP, et al. Optical coherence tomography evaluation of pulmonary arterial vasculopathy in systemic sclerosis. Sci Rep. 2017;7:43304. https://doi.org/10.1038/srep43304.
104. Hariri LP, Adams DC, Wain JC, Lanuti M, Muniappan A, Sharma A, et al. Endobronchial optical coherence tomography for low-risk microscopic assessment and diagnosis of idiopathic pulmonary fibrosis in vivo. Am J Respir Crit Care Med. 2018;197:949–52.

Treatment of Interstitial Lung Disease in Systemic Sclerosis

26

Muriel Elhai, Bruno Crestani,
Maria-Sinziana Muraru-Carbrune, and Yannick Allanore

Over the past 20 years, interstitial lung disease has emerged as the leading cause of morbidity and mortality in systemic sclerosis (SSc), accounting for 17% of SSc-related deaths in the last report from EUSTAR network [1–3]. This chapter will discuss the management of interstitial lung disease (ILD) in SSc with a focus on treatment strategy and drugs to use, relying on evidence-based data. Previous chapters in this textbook have discussed the pathogenesis of SSc-ILD in detail.

Natural History of ILD in SSc

ILD is common in SSc and typically occurs within the first 5 years of disease onset [4]. ILD can also be inaugural in about 4% of the patients [5] and is included in the classification criteria for SSc [6]. In autopsy studies, 74–100% of patients have lung involvement [7, 8]. Depending upon the cohort studied and on modalities used, ILD affects between 19% and 90% of SSc patients [9–12]. HRCT-defined pulmonary fibrosis was identified in 47% SSc patients in a British cohort [13] and 50% SSc patients in a national Norwegian cohort [11]. The mere detection of pulmonary fibrosis on HRCT, whatever its extension, was associated with a reduced survival in the Norwegian cohort, with the worst prognosis being observed in patients with >25% extension of opacities [11]. Physiologically, severe disease at baseline is associated with decreased survival, but increased mortality was evident in the group having FVC 90–100% at baseline in the national Norwegian cohort [11]. During follow-up, 40–75% will have changes in pulmonary function tests (PFTs) [12, 14, 15]. Progressive disease on HRCT or in PFTs during follow-up is associated with decreased survival [16–18].

Previous reports suggested that a majority of patients with normal baseline FVC remained stable during follow-up [19, 20]. Indeed, in analyzing 78 Greek patients with SSc, Plastiras and colleagues showed that almost 90% of the patients with normal FVC at initial assessment remained stable and were at low risk to develop decline in their FVC during subsequent follow-up [19]. Consistently, in an American cohort of 254 patients with SSc (with or without ILD), the majority of the cohort (85%) had slowly improving or stable trajectories, with a ≤1% increase in FVC per year. A smaller proportion of the cohort (15%) had declining trajectories, with rates of 2–3% decrease in FVC per year, all of them having low baseline FVC [20].

In a recent report from EUSTAR database including 826 SSc patients with ILD, almost 27% experienced lung progression over 1 year, of them 12% had significant progression (defined by a decline in forced vital capacity predicted (FVC% pred) >10%) and 15% a moderate progression (decline in FVC% pred >5%) [21]. Using a composite definition of progression based on FVC and diffusing capacity of the lung for

M. Elhai · M.-S. Muraru-Carbrune
Department of Rheumatology, University Hospital Zurich, University of Zurich, Zurich, Switzerland
e-mail: Muriel.Elhai@usz.ch; Maria-Sinziana.Muraru-Carbune@usz.ch

B. Crestani
APHP, Service de Pneumologie A, Constitutive Reference Center for Rare Pulmonary Diseases—OrphaLung, FHU APOLLO, Hôpital Bichat, Paris, France
e-mail: bruno.crestani@aphp.fr

Y. Allanore (✉)
Cochin Hospital, AP-HP, INSERM U1016, Paris University, Paris, France
e-mail: yannick.allanore@aphp.fr

Y. Allanore et al. (eds.), *Scleroderma*, https://doi.org/10.1007/978-3-031-40658-4_26

carbon monoxide (DLco), 14% of SSc patients with ILD had significant progression (decline in FVC% pred of >10%, or decline in FVC% pred ≥5–10% plus a decline in DLco% predicted (DLco% pred) ≥15%) while 13% had a moderate progression (decline in FVC% pred ≥5–10% without a decline in DLco% pred ≥15%). Among 535 patients with multiple FVC measurements over a 5-year period, FVC was stable in 39% and improved in 24%, with 37% experiencing FVC decline. When analyzing FVC changes from 1 year to the next, 67% experienced at least one episode of FVC decline. Of these, only a minority (8%) showed a rapid and continuous pattern of decline in FVC, while the majority was characterized by alternating periods of progression and stability [21].

Although baseline FVC was an independent predictor of subsequent decline, a moderate or significant progression also occurred in patients with normal baseline FVC. In a UK cohort of 215 patients with SSc-associated ILD, after 1 year, 21% had a significant progression defined by a change in FVC% pred >10%, while this rate rose to 32% if significant progression was defined by FVC and DLco [17]. Emphasizing the variability in ILD course in SSc patients, seven distinct trajectories of FVC were identified over a 12-year follow-up in the US cohort [20].

However, analysis of lung function decline in cohorts of SSc patients is subject to survival bias. This occurs when patients with a rapid rate of worsening have higher short-term mortality and thus do not contribute further measurements that would have continued to demonstrate this ongoing rapid progression. The absence of follow-up measurements from patients with rapid progression biases the total cohort's rate of change toward a less steep initial decline followed by a plateau that can mimic stabilization. This is what was observed in a Canadian cohort where the authors stratified their population by duration of survival and observed that patients with SSc-ILD could be categorized into subgroups with relatively consistent rates of progression over time. Despite long follow-up duration, they were unable to identify a plateau in the rate of progression for any subgroup, arguing against a stabilization of disease activity at any point in the disease course [22]. This observation goes against the common impression that disease progression occurs early in disease course, in the first 4–6 years after SSc onset [23]. A recent analysis of the EUSTAR database highlights that progression can occur even in the late stages of the disease [24]. Decline in FVC% pred >10% was observed in 41/347 (11.8%) and 32/228 (14%) SSc-ILD patients with disease duration 7–15 years and >15 years compared to 38/244 (15.6%) and 33/273 (15.6%) for disease duration <3 years and 3–7 years. Consistently, in the Scleroderma Lung Study, the rates of progression of lung disease were similar irrespective of disease duration [19]. However, when extensive radiographic disease was present, the rate of decline of FVC was highest in those with early disease (0–2 years). Despite an association with diffuse cutaneous SSc (dcSSc), a substantial proportion of limited cutaneous SSc (lcSSc) develop ILD with in some patients a rate of progression similar to dcSSc [25].

Altogether, these data show the high heterogeneity of ILD course in SSc, that progression can occur also in patients with a long disease duration, and especially that ILD can be slowly progressive over several years. This emphasizes the need of regular monitoring of SSc patients for progression of ILD, regardless of the disease duration and of comparing the PFTs and HRCT over several years (not only on the last two visits) to detect a slowly progressive disease.

Who Should Be Screened?

In a recent report of 6004 patients from EUSTAR cohort, 38% of patients had evidence of lung fibrosis on HRCT, highlighting that the probability to diagnose of ILD in any one SSc patient is high [21]. A considerable proportion of patients with SSc-ILD are asymptomatic, especially in the initial stages of disease [26]. It was also shown that cough is less frequent, less severe, and less often productive in SSc-ILD as compared to idiopathic pulmonary fibrosis [27]. Even if present, respiratory symptoms such as dyspnea upon exertion and cough are unspecific and can be related to ILD but also to pulmonary arterial hypertension (PAH), deconditioning, chronic anemia, and cardiac involvement [26]. Risk factors for the development of ILD in SSc include the pattern of skin disease with higher risk for diffuse cutaneous forms (dcSSc) and the antibody status with higher risk for anti-topoisomerase I, whereas anti-centromere are protective [21, 26, 28, 29]. Other risk factors include older age, male sex, African–American ethnicity, gastroesophageal reflux, low FVC, and DLco, although FVC and DLco changes can be secondary to ILD [21, 28–34]. Similarly, in a recent EUSTAR report including 826 SSc patients with ILD, half of the patients had lcSSc [21]. The probability of developing ILD is more strongly associated with the autoantibody profile than with the clinical classification of SSc. In the EUSTAR registry, 60.2% of patients with anti-topoisomerase 1 antibodies had ILD as compared to 21.3% of those with anticentromere antibodies [14], and stratification according to antibodies status predicted more accurately the presence of lung fibrosis and restrictive lung fibrosis during a median follow-up of 56 months than a classification according to the cutaneous subtype [35]. However, neither the clinical presentation of SSc nor the autoantibody profile is sufficient to select patients at high risk of ILD. Therefore, all patients with SSc should undergo evaluation to screen for ILD with chest HRCT and PFTs at diagnosis, and repeated during follow-up even in patients with normal FVC at baseline. PFTs should be repeated regularly in all patients (every 6 months in patients with ILD without indication to therapy, otherwise every 6–12 months according to patients) [36]. The frequency of screening and use of HRCT should be determined by the clinician, guided by the individual risk of ILD development/progression [36]. For this purpose, the ILD-RISC score was recently developed to help physicians to decide when to order HRCTs during the follow-up [37].

Who Is at Increased Risk of Progressive ILD?

ILD is characterized by great variability in disease course between patients, with rapid or slow progression, periods of stability alternating with periods of worsening, and progression that can occur in both early and late stages of the disease [21, 34]. This highlights the need of close monitoring of SSc patients especially with risk factors for ILD or ILD progression.

No parameter alone has been shown to be robust enough to accurately delineate the prognosis of ILD. Therefore, severity should be assessed using multiple parameters. In an analysis of 215 SSc patients followed for 10 years, both baseline PFTs and chest HRCTs were predictive of mortality risk. An extent of disease on HRCT >20% (as defined by the extent and coarseness of reticulation [fibrosis] and proportion of ground-glass opacity) was associated with increased mortality (hazard ratio [HR] 2.48, $p < 0.0005$). In this same cohort, subjects with a baseline FVC <70% also had increased mortality risk (HR 2.11, $p = 0.001$). When the two modalities were combined, patients with both an HRCT extent of ≥20% and an FVC% pred <70% had the highest mortality risk (HR 3.46, $p < 0.0005$) [16]. The prognostic value of FVC and extent of lung fibrosis at baseline was recently confirmed in a Norwegian cohort study [11].

Although severity at baseline is a major prognostic factor, a progressive disease more accurately predicted mortality than baseline parameters [38]. Using 12 months of data from the Scleroderma Lung Study (SLS) I and II, one post-hoc analysis defined a change (±) in FVC% pred of 3.0% as the minimum clinically important difference for progression according to patient-reported outcomes [39]. Consistently using data from SENSCIS trial investigating the efficacy and safety of nintedanib in SSc-ILD, a decrease of 3% in FVC% pred increased the risk of hospitalization and death [40]. Goh et al. showed that the most accurate predictor of mortality was an FVC% pred decline from baseline of ≥10% or an FVC% pred decline of 5–9% in association with a DLco% pred decline of ≥15% [17]. In the SPAR model, oxygen desaturation at the 6 min walk test (≤94%) and a history of arthritis predicted ILD progression (defined as a relative decrease in FVC% pred ≥15%, or FVC% pred ≥10% combined with DLco% pred ≥15%) at 1 year in patients with mild ILD (extent of lung fibrosis <20% on HRCT) [41]. The derived SPAR model combining both predictors (SPO2 and ARthritis) increased the prediction rate from 25.5% to 91.7% with an area under the curve (95% CI) of 0.83 (0.73–0.93). In the EUSTAR cohort, the strongest predictive factors for FVC decline over 5 years were male sex, higher modified Rodnan skin score, and reflux/dysphagia symptoms [21]. Circulating biomarkers have been studied with the aim of better identifying SSc-ILD patients at risk for progressive disease. Until now the most accurate biomarkers to predict disease progression (defined as a decline in FVC and/or mortality) are KL-6 and CCL18 [42]. However, they deserve further validation in routine practice and in prospective studies. Although bronchoalveolar lavage has often been used to assess ILD activity, its utility and clinical significance in SSc is in doubt. Analysis from both the SLS-1 [43] and another real-life cohort [44] showed that bronchoalveolar lavage was unable to predict either disease progression or response to cyclophosphamide.

A recent definition of ILD progression, which combines the increase in symptoms, the decline of FVC >5% pred or DLCO>10% pred, and the progression of lung fibrosis on HRCT, over the past 12 months, was proposed by an official ATS/ERS/JRS/ALAT clinical practice guideline committee [45]. The impact of this official definition of progression for SSc-ILD is still to be fully appreciated. This definition is different from the definition of ILD progression developed by Goh et al. (FVC% pred decline from baseline of ≥10% or an FVC% pred decline of 5–9% in association with a DLco% pred decline of ≥15%) [17], which is also the most commonly used in SSc-ILD patients and has been validated by an expert panel [36]. Regarding the time-period to define progression, decline over 1 year is usually used. However, slow lung function decline over longer time-periods seem to be common [21] and should also be considered as a progressive disease.

In Whom Should Treatment Be Considered?

European consensus guidelines consider that some patients with mild disease might not need pharmacological treatment [36]. The heterogeneity of SSc-ILD and the lack of robust predictive markers make it difficult to identify patients likely to progress and to determine the optimal time to initiate treatment.

It is well established that baseline lung function and its changes over time are highly predictive of survival. Although it is not yet known whether early treatment could be associated with the prevention of irreversible lung damage, one can hypothesize, that early treatment could contribute to preserving or slowing the decline in lung function in SSc-ILD. Waiting for patients to meet the severity criteria or for

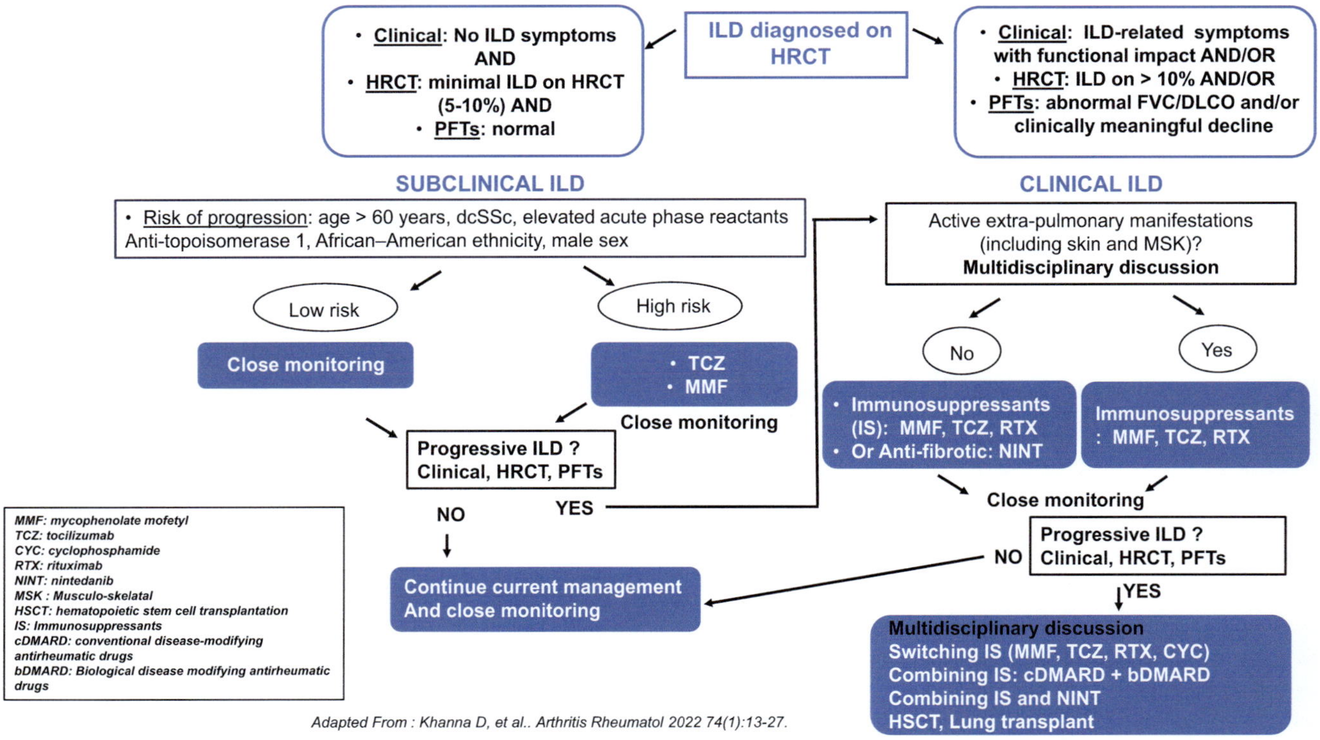

Fig. 26.1 Treatment algorithm for systemic sclerosis-interstitial lung disease based on evidence-based recommendations and clinical experiences. *The frequency of the screening should be guided by risk of ILD development/progression, in combination with symptoms. The frequency of HRCT should be guided by risk of ILD development/progression, in combination with PFTs and symptoms. **Disease progression can be defined by decline in FVC levels of more than 10% from baseline or decline in FVC greater than 5% to less than 10% and more than 15% relative decline in DLco or by increase in extent of ILD on HRCT. *DLco* diffusion capacity of carbon monoxide percentage predicted, *FVC* forced vital capacity percentage predicted, *HRCT* high-resolution chest computerized tomography, *PFT* pulmonary function testing, *dcSSc* diffuse cutaneous systemic sclerosis, *ILD* interstitial lung disease, *CRP* C-reactive protein. (Adapted from Roofeh D, et al. J Scleroderma Relat Disord. 2020. PMID: 35382226)

their lung function to deteriorate could instead lead to late initiation of treatment, missing a "window of opportunity" with the risk of irreversible lung damage.

Based on this assumption and the development of proven treatments with an acceptable safety profile, we suggest considering treatment for all patients with SSc who have clinical ILD (Fig. 26.1) defined by ILD symptoms with functional impact and/or more than minimal ILD (at least 10%) on HRCT and/or abnormal PFTs and/or sign of progression of PFTs according to Goh et al. [17] and/or evidence of progression on HRCT [4, 36]. Moreover, a treatment should be considered in patients at high-risk of progression (age > 60 years, African–American ethnicity, male sex, diffuse cutaneous subtype, anti-topoisomerase 1 antibodies, and systemic inflammation).

For untreated and treated patients, close monitoring (every 6 months) is required. Treated and untreated patients should be assessed using clinical symptoms, HRCT, pulmonary function tests, and exercise-induced oxygen desaturation to decide to initiate or escalate therapy [4, 36].

What Should Be Used When Treatment Is Indicated?

Although several agents have been proposed for improving or slowing the rate of progression of SSc-ILD, few have been subjected to a rigorous randomized controlled trial (RCT). We will focus our attention on treatments for with RCT-based evidence (Table 26.1).

Table 26.1 Summary of the randomized-controlled trials

Author, Year	*N*	Treatments groups	Population	Primary outcome	Results for ILD
Hoyles R, 2006 FAST	45 −22 CYC −23 PBO	PO Steroids low dose and IV CYC (600 mg/m²/month) (6 months) → PO AZA (2.5 mg/kg/day) vs. PBO	Lung fibrosis diagnosed on HRCT or lung biopsy	Change in % predicted FVC and corrected DLCO	ΔFVC: 2.4% (CYC) vs. −3 (PBO) ($p = 0.08$) ΔDLCO: −3.3% (CYC) vs. −3.2 (PBO) ($p = 0.64$)
Nadashkevich O, 2006	60 −30 CYC −30 AZA	PO CYC (2 mg/kg/day (1 year) → 1 mg/kg/day) vs. PO AZA (2.5 mg/kg/day (1 year) → 2 mg/kg/day)	Early dcSSc (<1 year)	mRSS; RP attack frequency; ESR; FVC; DLCO	ΔFVC: 3.3 ± 0.7% (CYC) vs. −1.1 ± 1.0% (AZA) ($p < 0.001$) ΔDLCO: 0 ± 1.6% (CYC) vs. −11.6 ± 1.3% (AZA) ($p < 0.001$)
Tashkin D, 2006 SLS I	145 −73 CYC −72 PBO	PO CYC 2 mg/kg/day vs. PBO	Active alveolitis on BAL or ground-glass opacity on HRCT Disease duration ≤7 years FVC: 45–85% Grad 2 exertional Dyspnoe (Mahler Dyspnoe Index)	FVC at 1 year (adjusted on baseline FVC)	ΔFVC: 2.53% [95% CI: 0.28–4.79] favoring CYC ($p < 0.03$)
Tashkin D, 2016 SLS II	126 −63 MMF −63 CYC	MMF (3 g) (2 year) vs. PO CYC (2 mg/kg/day) (1 year) → PBO (1 year)	18–75 years Ground-glass opacity on HRCT Disease duration ≤7 years FVC: 45–85% Grad 2 exertional Dyspnoe (Mahler Dyspnoe Index)	ΔFVC % over 24 months	ΔFVC % 2.19 (95% CI, 0.53–3.84) (MMF) vs. 2.88 (1.19–4.58) in CYC ($p = 0.24$)
Daoussis D, 2010	14 −8 RTX −6 CTRL	RTX (4 IV 375 mg/m² at baseline and 24 weeks) and standard therapy vs. standard therapy	Anti-topoisomerase 1 ILD (HRCT and/or PFT)	PFT at 1 year mRSS	ΔFVC: 10.25% (95% CI, 6.19–18.65) (RTX) vs. −5.04% (4.11–11.6) (CTRL), $p = 0.002$ ΔDLCO: 19.46% (3.7–30.8) (RTX) vs. −7.5% (1.4–26.57) (CTRL) $p = 0.023$
Sircar G, 2018	60 −30 RTX −30 CYC	RTX 1 g × 2 (D1 und D15) vs. IV CYC 500 mg/m²/month for 24 weeks	18–60 years; dcSSc; anti-topoisomerase 1 ILD on HRCT; FVC 45–85%	FVC% at 24-weeks	FVC: 61.30 (11.28) to 67.52 (13.59); $p = 0.002$ (RTX) vs. 59.25 (12.96) to 58.06 (11.23); $p = 0.496$ (CYC) ΔFVC: 9.46 (95% CI: 3.01–15.90), $p = 0.003$ (in favor of RTX)
Ebata S, 2021 DESIRES	49 −27 RTX −22 placebo	RTX 375 mg/m²/week for 4 weeks vs. PBO	20–79 years mRSS ≥10	Difference in mRSS from baseline to 24 weeks	ΔFVC% 0.09% (0.96) (RTX) vs. −2.87% (1.05) (PBO), difference: 2.96% (0.08–5.84), $p = 0.044$ ΔDLCO%: −1.32% (1.58) (RTX) vs. −3.56% (1.72) (PBO); difference: 2.24% (−2.47–6.94); $p = 0.34$; ΔILD extent:−0.32% (5.79) (RTX) vs. 2.39% (4.73) (PBO), difference:−2.71% (0.48–7.52), $p = 0.034$
Khanna D, 2018 faSScinate	87 −43 TCZ −44 PBO	TCZ 162 mg s.c./week vs. PBO for 48 weeks (double-blind), 96 weeks (open-label extension)	dcSSc Disease duration <5 years mRSS 15–40 Active disease (pre-specified mRSS/biomarker criteria)	Difference in mean change in mRSS from baseline to 24 weeks	Treatment difference: ΔFVC: 136 mL (9–264) ($p = 0.0368$) (week 24) and 120 mL (−23 to 262) ($p = 0.0990$) (week 48). ΔFVC% pred: −0.7 (95% CI:−3.2, 1.8) (TCZ) versus −4.5 (95% CI: −7.0, −1.9) (PBO) (week 24) and −2.6 (95% CI:−5.2, −0.1) (TCZ) versus −6.3 (95% CI:−8.9, −3.8) (PBO) (week 48)

(continued)

Table 26.1 (continued)

Author, Year	*N*	Treatments groups	Population	Primary outcome	Results for ILD
Khanna D, 2020 focuSSced	210 −104 TCZ −106 placebo	TCZ 162 mg s.c./week vs. PBO for 48 weeks	Active dcSSc Disease duration <5 years mRSS 15–35 CRP ≥6 mg/L or ESR ≥28 mm/h, or platelet ≥330 × 10^9/L	Difference in change in mRSS from baseline to week 48	LSM FVC% pred: −4.6 (PBO) vs. −0.4 (TCZ) (difference 4.2 [95% CI 2.0–6.4]; $p = 0.0002$) ΔFVC: −190 (PBO) vs. −24 (TCZ) (difference 167 [95% CI 83–250]; $p = 0.0001$). Δ extent lung fibrosis: 0.1 (0.0–0.3) (PBO) vs. 0.0 (−0.2 to 0.1) (TCZ) (difference: −0.1 [−0.3 to 0.05] ($p = 0.005$)). In SSc-ILD patients: LSM FVC% pred: −6.4 (PBO) vs. 0.1 (TCZ) (difference 6.5 [95% CI 3.4–9.5]; $p < 0.0001$), ΔFVC: −255 (PBO) vs. −14 (TCZ) (difference 241 [95% CI 124–358]; $p < 0.0001$) (Δ extent lung fibrosis: 0.4 (0.1–0.9) (PBO) vs. −0.2 (−0.8 to 0.1) (difference: −0.6 [−1.2 to 0.3] ($p = 0.0008$))
Distler O, 2019 SENSCIS	576 −288 NINT −288 PBO	PO nintedanib 150 mg × 2/day, vs. PBO	Disease duration ≤7 years Extent ILD ≥ 10% FVC ≥ 40% 30 ≤ DLCO ≤ 89%	Annual rate of decline in FVC (mL per year)	−52.4 mL/year (Nintedanib) vs. −93.3 mL/year (PBO) difference, 41.0 mL/year (95% CI: 2.9–79.0); $p = 0.04$
Burt RK, 2011 ASSIST	19 −10 HSCT −9 CYC	HSCT vs. IV CYC, 1000 mg/m²/month for 6 months	<60 years dcSSc (mRSS > 14) organ involvement (DLCO < 80% or ↓FVC ≥ 10% in the previous 12 months; ILD on HRCT; abnormal ECG; or gastrointestinal track involvement)	>25% decrease in mRSS or >10% increase in FVC at 12 months	ΔFVC 34% vs. −10% at 6 months ($p = 0.002$); ΔFVC 15% vs. −9% at 12 months ($p = 0.006$); ↓ extent of ILD in patients with HSCT ($p = 0.003$)
van Laar JM, 2014 ASTIS	156 −79 HSCT −77 CYC	HSCT vs. IV CYC 750 mg/m²/month × 12	dcSSc, 18–65 years old Disease duration ≤4 years mRSS >15 Involvement of heart, lungs, or kidney	Event-free survival	FVC: 6.3% (HSCT) vs. −2.8%; difference −9.1 (−14.7 to −2.5); ($p = 0.004$) TLC: 5.1% (HSCT) vs. −1.3%; difference −6.4 (−11.9 to −0.9); ($p = 0.02$)
Sullivan KM, 2018 SCOT	75 36 HSCT 39 CYC	HSCT vs. IV CYC 500 mg/m² → 750 mg/m²/month × 11	18–69 year old Disease duration ≤5 years Active ILD (BAL or HRCT) and FVC or DLCO < 70% or renal involvement	Composite Score at 54 months (death, event-free survival, FVC, HAQ, mRSS) at 54 months	Superiority HSCT for composite score: 20 (−58 to 55) vs. −8 (−58 to 55) ($p = 0.008$), 36% of patients in the HSCT group vs. 23% in the control group had a relative increase of FVC% pred by ≥10%,

CYC cyclophosphamide, *MMF* mycophenolate mofetil, *PBO* placebo, *AZA* azathioprine, *RTX* rituximab, *TCZ* tocilizumab, *NINT* nintedanib, *HSCT* autologous hematopoietic stem cell transplantation, *FVC* forced vital capacity% pred, *DLCO* diffusing capacity for carbon monoxide % pred, *SSc* Systemic sclerosis, *mRSS* modified Rodnan Skin score, *RP* Raynaud phenomenon, *ESR* erythrocyte sedimentation rate, *PFT* pulmonary function test, *HRCT* high resolution computed tomography, *BAL* bronchoalveolar lavage, *ILD* interstitial lung disease, *dcSSc* diffuse cutaneous systemic sclerosis, *HAQ* health assessment questionnaire

Cytotoxic Therapies

Cyclophosphamide

A variety of immunosuppressive agents has been considered as disease-modifying agents in SSc-ILD with cyclophosphamide being shown to be effective in an RCT.

Previous uncontrolled trials have suggested efficacy of oral or pulse cyclophosphamide in SSc-ILD [46, 47] and this led to a large randomized controlled trial, the Scleroderma Lung Study (SLS) [48]. The SLS was designed as a multicenter, double-blind RCT against placebo to evaluate the effectiveness and safety of oral cyclophosphamide administered for 1 year in 158 patients with symptomatic SSc-ILD who had evidence of active ILD by bronchoalveolar lavage (≥3% neutrophils and/or ≥2% eosinophils) and/or thoracic HRCT (any ground-glass opacity). After 1 year, therapy was stopped without maintenance treatment. The SLS was the first RCT to demonstrate the effectiveness of a compound in improving lung function (FVC and TLC) relative to placebo after a 1-year treatment period. Although the physiologic benefits of cyclophosphamide compared to placebo were quite modest (2.53% and 4.09% improvements in FVC%

pred and TLC% pred at 12 months, respectively; $p < 0.03$) [48], these results were supported by improvement in some patient-reported outcomes including transitional dyspnea index score and quality of life measures [49]. The benefit seemed to be larger in patients with more extensive lung disease with a greater decline in FVC over time among those who had more severe fibrosis at baseline in the placebo group, which was not observed in the cyclophosphamide group. In addition, follow-up HRCT scans revealed that the change in extent of fibrosis from baseline to 12 months was significantly worse in the placebo group ($p = 0.012$), and this difference was correlated with the favorable effect of cyclophosphamide on FVC, TLC, and dyspnea [50].

A retrospective analysis of the SLS data identified the severity of reticular infiltrates on baseline HRCT and the baseline modified Rodnan skin score as patient features that might be predictive of responsiveness to cyclophosphamide [51], suggesting that a greater extent in fibrosis is more likely to be responsive to anti-inflammatory/immunosuppressive therapy.

One of the hypotheses of the SLS was that 1 year of treatment with cyclophosphamide would be sufficient to prevent further disease progression without the need for ongoing immunosuppressive therapy, thereby obviating the risk of toxicity from ongoing treatment with cyclophosphamide [52]. However, despite the benefits observed up to 18 months after stopping the drug, they then dissipated and there was no difference with the placebo group at 2 years [53].

The Scleroderma Lung Study II (SLS II) was conducted, hypothesizing that mycophenolate mofetil for 2 years would be safer, better tolerated, and produce longer lasting improvements than cyclophosphamide for 12 months [54]. The adjusted FVC% pred (primary endpoint) improved from baseline to 24 months in both groups with no significant between-treatment difference ($p = 0.24$). In post-hoc analyses, improvements were also noticed for both treatments in dyspnea, cough [55], extent of HRCT ILD [56], and health-related quality of life [57]. After adjusting for baseline disease severity, there was no difference in the course of the FVC% pred nor the DLco% pred between the SLS I and II cyclophosphamide arms [58].

Consistently, in a randomized unblinded trial on early diffuse SSc, cyclophosphamide was associated with statistically significant improvement in the modified Rodnan skin score, FVC, and DLco as compared to azathioprine [59].

Despite some efficacy, the use of cyclophosphamide is limited by its significant toxicity. In-depth analysis of adverse events in SLS I showed a higher frequency of treatment-related adverse events in cyclophosphamide-treated patients during the first year (154 vs. 60; $p = 0.002$), and especially for mild to moderate leukopenia (19 vs. 0; $p < 0.0001$) [60]. There was no difference for serious related adverse events, or deaths [60]. Daily oral cyclophosphamide is associated with an increased risk of both hemorrhagic cystitis and bladder cancer, in a dose-dependent and/or duration-dependent manner. Moreover, hemorrhagic cystitis increases the risk of bladder cancer years later [61]. In SLS I, there were no differences in the occurrence of cancer (4 in cyclophosphamide vs. 2 in placebo) with only one carcinoma in-situ and hematuria was present in ten patients. In SLS II, only two patients had hematuria. IV cyclophosphamide is also used by some centers as it carries a lower risk of cystitis and probably also of bladder cancer (due to a lower cumulative dosage and prophylaxis with Mesna and fluids) [61]. Bruni et al. aimed to compare the relative efficacy and safety of PO- versus IV-cyclophosphamide using data from the EUSTAR centers and the Scleroderma Lung Studies I and II [62]. They enrolled 149 patients given PO-cyclophosphamide and 153 receiving IV-cyclophosphamide. ILD progressors rate was similar in both groups at the end of the treatment (11.4% in the PO group vs. 17.8% in the IV group) ($p = 0.146$) and at follow-up (14.8% vs. 11.5% ($p = 0.402$)). Interestingly, the median total dose of IV-cyclophosphamide was lower as PO-cyclophosphamide (39.5 g vs. 9.2 g). PO patients had more leukopenia ($p < 0.001$), hemorrhagic cystitis ($p = 0.011$), and alopecia ($p < 0.001$) at the end of treatment visit.

Azathioprine could have a role as a maintenance therapy. In a small observational study, 15 SSc patients with ILD received 18-months oral azathioprine as a maintenance therapy after 6-month intravenous cyclophosphamide [63]. Azathioprine was associated with stable or improved lung function in 70% and 51.8% of SSc patients at 6 months and 2 years. In another study, 45 consecutive SSc patients were treated with weekly pulses of 500 mg of cyclophosphamide up to 10-g cumulative dose followed by azathioprine in responders [64]. During follow-up, lung function parameters improved or remained stable in 87.5% of the 24 responders' patients. In another randomized controlled trial, 45 patients were randomized to receive low-dose prednisolone and 6 monthly infusions of cyclophosphamide (600 mg/m^2) followed by daily oral azathioprine or to placebo infusions followed by oral placebo [65]. Only 62% of the patients completed the first year of the study. Significantly, 9 patients (3 in the active treatment group, 6 in the placebo group) were withdrawn due to a significant decline in FVC or corrected DLco. At 12 months, a trend in improvement in FVC% pred was seen in the actively treated group, ($p = 0.08$), suggesting that IV cyclophosphamide followed by azathioprine could stabilize lung function in a subset of patients with the disease.

Mycophenolate Mofetil

Mycophenolate mofetil has emerged as a less toxic alternative to cyclophosphamide for treating SSc-ILD. Mycophenolate mofetil inhibits inosine monophosphate dehydrogenase and has been shown to deplete guanosine nucleotides, thereby suppressing T- and B-cell proliferation and promoting apoptosis of monocytes and other inflammatory cells, resulting in inhibition of cell-mediated immunity and antibody formation [66–68]. It also inhibits proliferation of smooth muscle cells and fibroblasts. Small open retrospective studies first showed a stabilization or an improvement of lung function in SSc-ILD [69–76]. In the SLS II, treatment of SSc-ILD with mycophenolate mofetil for 2 years or cyclophosphamide for 1 year both resulted in significant improvements in lung function over the 2-year course of the study without difference between both treatments [54]. Similarly, both mycophenolate mofetil and cyclophosphamide resulted in improvements in dyspnea index and Rodnan skin score with no significant difference between both groups. Fewer patients on mycophenolate mofetil than on cyclophosphamide prematurely withdrew from study drug (20 vs. 32) and the time to stopping treatment was shorter in the cyclophosphamide group ($p = 0.019$). A post-hoc analysis of SLS I and II compared the patients from the mycophenolate mofetil arm of SLS II with those from the placebo arm of SLS I. After adjustment for baseline disease severity, treatment with mycophenolate mofetil was associated with improved FVC% pred ($p < 0.0001$), DLco% pred ($p < 0.0001$), modified Rodnan skin score ($p < 0.0001$), and dyspnea ($p = 0.0112$) over 2 years as compared to placebo. At 12-months, 64.4% of the mycophenolate mofetil-treated patients and 28.8% of the placebo-treated patients had any improvement in FVC% pred. At 24 months, 71.7% of mycophenolate mofetil-treated patients and 37.5% of the placebo-treated patients had any improvement in FVC% pred. Interestingly, DLco and the DLco/alveolar volume ratio did not change in the mycophenolate mofetil group and worsened in the cyclophosphamide group [54], suggesting a positive effect of mycophenolate mofetil on pulmonary vascular remodeling.

Biological

Rituximab

Some case reports and open-labeled uncontrolled studies suggested an effect of rituximab as a rescue therapy in patients with progressive ILD [77–83]. In 2017, a EUSTAR study identified 146 SSc patients receiving rituximab for ILD [84]. After a median follow-up of 2 years, there was no significant change in FVC% pred or DLco% pred as compared to 9575 propensity-score matched patients. However, patients treated concomitantly with mycophenolate mofetil had a trend for better outcomes as compared with patients receiving rituximab alone. A meta-analysis has suggested some improvement in FVC and DLco under rituximab [85]. The first RCT compared rituximab and standard treatment in 14 SSc with anti-topoisomerase 1 antibodies and evidence of ILD [86]. After 1 year, there was an improvement in lung function in the rituximab group, whereas the control group experienced deterioration in the PFTs. This success was prolonged in an open 2-year observation of 33 patients receiving rituximab compared with patients treated with conventional treatments (methotrexate or azathioprine or mycophenolate mofetil) [87]. Among the 33 patients, 10 were also treated with mycophenolate mofetil. Direct comparison between the rituximab and the control group at the 2-year time point showed an upward trend for improvement in FVC and DLco in the rituximab group. The therapeutic benefit was sustained after 7 years for the five patients still followed. A randomized controlled trial compared the efficacy and safety of rituximab with cyclophosphamide in 60 patients with dcSSc [88]. At 6 months, FVC% pred had increased from 61.3 ± 11.3% to 67.5 ± 13.6% in the patients treated with rituximab ($p = 0.002$) vs. a nonsignificant decrease in patients receiving cyclophosphamide with a mean difference in FVC% pred of 9.5 ($p = 0.003$). Furthermore, a significantly higher percentage of patients experienced an improvement of more than 10% of FVC% pred in the rituximab group vs. in the cyclophosphamide group (27% vs. 7%, $p = 0.038$). There was also a significant improvement at 6 months in the 6-min walking test. The safety profile was also in favor of rituximab therapy, with a lower frequency of adverse events. Apart from its effect on lung function, in most of the studies, rituximab showed a positive effect on skin fibrosis [84, 88–90]. The DESIRES trial was the first randomized placebo-controlled trial to demonstrate an efficacy of rituximab against placebo on skin fibrosis [91]. Among the 56 patients, 25 patients in the rituximab group and 23 in the placebo group had ILD. The absolute change in mRSS 24 weeks after initiation of study treatment was lower in the rituximab group than in the placebo group (difference −8.44 [95% CI −11.00 to −5.88]; $p < 0.0001$). The change in FVC% pred at 24 weeks from baseline was significantly improved in the rituximab group compared with the placebo group (0.09% vs. −2.87%; difference 2.96% [95% CI 0.08–5.84]; $p = 0.044$). Moreover, after 24 weeks of follow-up, the extent of ILD was higher in the placebo group than in the rituximab group ($p = 0.034$). In the whole cohort, in a post-hoc analysis, patients with higher CRP levels tended to have a greater effect of rituximab. One serious adverse event leading to treatment discontinuation occurred in one patient in each group. The most common adverse event was upper respiratory infection, which occurred in 11 patients (39%) in the rituximab group and 10 patients (38%) in the placebo group. There were no deaths during follow-up. The results of RECITAL trial (NCT02990286) comparing rituximab (1000 mg given intravenously, twice at an interval of 2 weeks), with intravenously administered cyclophosphamide given monthly at a dose of 600 mg/m^2 for the treatment of connective tissue disease-associated ILD have been published [92, 93]. Of the 101 randomized to receive rituximab (n = 51) or cyclophosphamide (n = 50), 37 had SSc ILD (18 treated with rituximab and 19 with cyclophosphamide). At 24 weeks, both rituximab and cyclophosphamide improved FVC (97 ± 234 mL in the rituximab group and 99 ± 329 mL in the cyclophosphamide group) [93]. Rituximab caused fewer adverse events (445 vs. 646) and was associated with a reduction in corticosteroid exposure as compared to cyclophosphamide.

Tocilizumab

Previous data have shown elevated serum levels of IL-6 in patients with early diffuse SSc, correlating with the extent of skin fibrosis [94–96] and being predictive of early functional decline and of mortality in SSc-related ILD [97]. This evidence led to the hypothesis, that blocking IL-6 could halt disease progression, mainly regarding skin and lung involvement. Recently, two large randomized clinical trials have been published (faSScinate [98] and focuSSced [99]). Both trials were enriched for patients with evidence of systemic inflammation. The faSScinate trial [98] is a phase 2 multicenter RCT including 87 patients with early diffuse SSc, randomized to be treated with 162 mg tocilizumab weekly or placebo. In these patients, the average baseline FVC% pred was 80% vs. 82% in the control group. The primary endpoint, focused on improvements in mRSS was not met. Analysis of secondary lung outcomes demonstrated a smaller decrease in FVC from baseline for tocilizumab than for placebo at weeks 24 (difference: 136 mL [95% CI: 9, 264]; $p = 0.0368$) and 48 (difference: 120 mL [95% CI: −23, 262]; $p = 0.0990$). Fewer tocilizumab than placebo patients experienced worsening of FVC% pred ($p = 0.009$ at week 24 and $p = 0.0373$ at week 48). At weeks 24 and 48, respectively, 3% and 10% of tocilizumab-treated patients compared with 19% and 23% of placebo-treated patients experienced >10% decrease in FVC% pred from baseline. Changes in FVC% pred from baseline for tocilizumab versus placebo at weeks 24 and 48, respectively, were −0.7 (95% CI: −3.2, 1.8) versus −4.5 (95% CI: −7.0, −1.9) and −2.6 (95% CI: −5.2, −0.1) versus −6.3 (95% CI: −8.9, −3.8). HAQ-DI, clinician global VAS, and other patient-reported outcomes favored tocilizumab over placebo, though they did not reach statistical significance. In the larger and most recent phase 3 trial focuSSced [99], the primary endpoint on mRSS was not met, although participants treated with tocilizumab had a numerically greater reduction in skin sclerosis after 48 weeks ($p = 0.10$). Secondary analyses on lung function showed a significant difference in FVC% pred decline in favor of tocilizumab (−4.6 in the placebo group vs. −0.4 in the tocilizumab group (difference 4.2 [95% CI 2.0–6.4]; nominal $p = 0{\cdot}0002$)). Fifteen (17%) of 91 participants in the placebo group and 5 (5%) of 93 in the tocilizumab group had an absolute decline in FVC% pred of at least 10%. In the subgroup of SSc patients with ILD, least square mean changes in FVC% pred were −6.4 in the placebo group ($n = 66$) vs. 0.1 in the tocilizumab group ($n = 68$) (difference 6.5 [95% CI 3.4–9.5]; nominal $p < 0.0001$). Moreover, 9% of SSc ILD patients treated with tocilizumab vs. 25% of patients in the control population had a decline in FVC% pred ≥10%. The treatment led also to a stabilization in the extent of lung disease, whereas the placebo arm showed worsening of lung fibrosis on HRCT at 48 weeks. There was no difference between placebo and tocilizumab for DLco, patient-reported or physician-reported outcomes or HAQ-DI at week 48 [100]. In a small retrospective real-life study on 47 patients, 31 with serial lung function data available and 14 with lung fibrosis, the average decline in FVC was lower in tocilizumab-treated patients as compared to the control group [101]. However, the difference was statistically significant only for patients with anti-Scl70 antibodies ($p = 0.0058$), suggesting that tocilizumab may have greater benefit in this subgroup.

In an open extension study of focuSSced, patients from the tocilizumab (n = 92) and placebo groups (n = 89) transitioned to open-label tocilizumab injections from week 48 to week 96 [102]. Among them, 54 in the placebo-tocilizumab group and 60 in the continuous-tocilizumab group had SSc-ILD. Continued improvement in the modified Rodnan skin score were observed in both groups during the open-label period. Mean change in modified Rodnan skin score from baseline to week 96 was −8.4 (−10.0 to −6.8) for placebo-tocilizumab and −9.6 (−10.9 to −8.4) for continuous-tocilizumab. The benefits on ILD were sustained at 96 weeks with changes in FVC% pred from baseline to week 96 of −3.3 (−5.1 to −1.5) in the placebo-tocilizumab group and of −0.5 (−2.4 to 1.3) in the continuous-tocilizumab group. In a post hoc analysis among patients with ILD, mean change in FVC% pred from baseline to week 96 were −4.1 (−6.7 to −1.6) and −0.6 (−3.1 to 2.0), respectively [102]. The safety profile was similar to other tocilizumab trials, the main concern remaining a higher risk for infections. Based on these results, tocilizumab was recently approved by the FDA for prevention of lung function decline in patients with SSc-ILD, thus becoming the first biologic treatment acknowledged for this indication.

Antifibrotic

Nintedanib

Nintedanib is a tyrosine-kinase inhibitor inhibiting the proliferation, migration, and differentiation of fibroblasts, which demonstrated antifibrotic, anti-inflammatory, and vascular remodeling effects in animal models of ILD and of SSc-ILD [103, 104]. It was first approved for the treatment of patients with idiopathic pulmonary fibrosis before being assessed in ILD associated with SSc [105]. A phase 3 randomized, double-blind, placebo-controlled trial was conducted to investigate the efficacy and safety of nintedanib in patients with SSc-ILD (SENSCIS trial) [106]. Patients receiving low-dose prednisone and/or stable background therapy with mycophenolate mofetil or methotrexate were allowed to participate. Patients with clinically significant pulmonary hypertension and >3 digital ulcers or history of severe digital necrosis requiring hospitalization were excluded. Among the 576 included patients, 51.9% were of dcSSc and 60% were positive for anti-topoisomerase antibodies. The mean (±SD) FVC% pred at baseline was 72.5 ± 16.7% and the mean extent of fibrosis on HRCT was 36.0 ± 21.3%. Almost half of the patients (48.4%) were receiving mycophenolate mofetil at baseline. Patients were stratified according to the presence of anti-topoisomerase 1 antibodies. The difference in annual rate of change in FVC was 41.0 mL per year ($p = 0.04$) favoring nintedanib. At 52 weeks, 20.6% of SSc-patients in the nintedanib group and 28.5% in the placebo group had a decline in FVC% pred >5% (odds ratio, 0.65; 95% CI, 0.44–0.96). The effect was observed irrespective of the presence of cough or dyspnea at baseline [107]. The change in the modified Rodnan skin score was not different between both groups (−2.17 in the nintedanib group vs. −1.96 in the placebo group) (difference: −0.21 95% CI [−0.94, 0.53]). There was no significant difference in both groups regarding disability assessed by health assessment questionnaire disability index (HAQ-DI) [106].

The percentages of patients with any adverse event (283/288 vs. 276/288) and any serious adverse event (69/288 (24%) vs. 62/288 (21.5%)) were similar in both groups. Moreover, mortality was similar between the two groups with 10 deaths (3.5%) and 9 deaths (3.1%) in nintedanib and placebo groups, respectively. However, there were more events leading to the discontinuation of the treatment in the nintedanib group as compared to the placebo (46/288 (16.0%) vs. 25/288 (8.7%)). Consistently with what was observed in idiopathic pulmonary fibrosis [105], the most common adverse event was diarrhea, which was reported in 218 (75.7%) of the patients in the nintedanib group and in 91 (31.6%) of the patients in the placebo group. Although it is difficult to compare different trials, the proportion of patients with diarrhea was higher in the SENSCIS trial (75.7%) as compared to TOMORROW [108] (55.3%) and INPULSIS [109] trials (61.5% and 63.2%) including patients with idiopathic pulmonary fibrosis. One may hypothesize a higher digestive susceptibility in SSc patients. The diarrhea was classified as mild in 49.5% of the patients and moderate in 45% of them. Diarrhea was managed by reduction of nintedanib to 100 mg twice daily. Interestingly, the dose adjustments had no influence on rate of decline in FVC [110]. Other adverse events included nausea in 31.6% of the patients treated with nintedanib vs. 13.5% of the patients receiving placebo, vomiting and weight decrease (in 11.8% of the patients treated with nintedanib vs. 4.2% of the placebo-treated-patients). Elevations in liver enzymes at least three times the upper limit of the normal range were reported in 4.9% of the patients in the nintedanib group and in 0.7% of the patients treated with placebo [106]. For the management of nintedanib-related side effects, we recommend following the algorithms used in INPULSIS trials [109, 111]: (1) in cases of 4–8 extra-stools without effect on daily living, treatment with loperamide should be used without stopping the treatment, otherwise the treatment should be interrupted. If diarrhea persists more than 8 days despite optimal care, a dose reduction to 100 mg × 2/day is recommended with a secondary dose-reescalation; (2) in case of elevations in liver enzymes <5 times, the upper limit of the normal range, a dose reduction to 100 mg × 2/day is recommended until recovery, otherwise the treatment should be stopped.

The positive effect of nintedanib was confirmed in the INBUILD trial assessing efficacy and safety of nintedanib in 663 patients with progressive fibrosing ILDs including 39 SSc patients (23 of them received nintedanib) [112]. Progression in the 2 years preceding inclusion was defined by (1) relative decline of FVC% pred ≥10% or (2) relative decline of 5% ≤ FVC%pred < 10% and worsening of respiratory symptoms or increased extent of lung fibrosis on HRCT or (3) worsening of respiratory symptoms and increased extent of lung fibrosis on HRCT. Background immunosuppressants at inclusion were not allowed. In the overall population, the adjusted rate of decline in the FVC was −80.8 mL per year with nintedanib and −187.8 mL per year with placebo, for a between-group difference of 107.0 mL per year ($p < 0.001$). Subgroup analysis showed that the effect was consistent across type of ILDs including autoimmune ILDs (difference 104.0 [21.1–186.9]) [113]. In the specific subgroup of ILD associated with SSc, there was a trend to better improvement with nintedanib. The difference was more pronounced in patients with usual interstitial pneumonia (UIP) like pattern.

Interestingly, a post-hoc analysis of SENSCIS trial was performed on the subgroup of the patients receiving mycophenolate mofetil at baseline for at least 6 months [114]. In all, 139 (48%) of the nintedanib group and 140 (49%) of the patients in the placebo group were taking mycophenolate mofetil at baseline. In patients treated with nintedanib, the effect was observed irrespective of mycophenolate mofetil use. However, the annual rate of decline in FVC% pred was −40.2 mL per year with mycophenolate mofetil versus −63.9 mL in patients non-treated with mycophenolate mofetil, suggesting that the combination of mycophenolate mofetil and nintedanib is effective for SSc patients with ILD. The safety profile was acceptable. These results highlight that treatment regimens consisting of sequential add-on treatments might be favorable. Data about upfront combinations are still lacking.

An ongoing continuation trial, SENSCIS(R)-on (EudraCT 2016-003403-66), follows most of the SENSCIS study population and will provide data about treatment effect and stability measures. In 2020, the positive results of the SENSCIS trial have led to the approval by the United States Food and Drug Administration (FDA) and the European Medicines Agency (EMA) of the first drug for SSc-ILD. However, in some countries, nintedanib is only approved for progressive forms of SSc-ILD.

Transplantation

High-Dose Immunosuppressive Therapy and Hematopoietic Stem Cell Transplantation

The use of autologous hematopoietic stem cell transplantation (HSCT) as a treatment for hematologic malignancies dates back to the late 1960s. Among the treated patients, case reports were published describing remission of a coincidental autoimmune disease (connective tissue disease, rheumatoid arthritis) [115]. This led to the hypothesis that HSCT could be a salvage treatment option for patients with severe refractory autoimmune diseases and meanwhile, over 3000 patients with these conditions were undergoing HSCT [116].

SSc is the only rheumatologic condition in which RCT are not only available, but even showed superiority in long-term survival and organ manifestations compared to intravenous cyclophosphamide [117–119]. The goal of HSCT is to achieve clinical remission of the autoimmune disease through eradication of self-reactive B- and T-lymphocytes and regeneration of new self-tolerant cell populations [116].

The ASSIST [117] was the first randomized trial performed, being a single-center randomized phase II study and including 19 patients with diffuse SSc.

The HSCT regimen was lymphoablative and was compared to cyclophosphamide. All patients in the HSCT arm (10 patients) demonstrated a relevant improvement regarding the skin primary outcome. There was a significant improvement in FVC at 6 and 12 months as well as decrease in the extent of ILD after the HSCT as compared to controls. No deaths were reported. After a few years ASTIS [118] and SCOT [119] trials comparing HSCT to cyclophosphamide followed, being multicenter randomized phase III survival studies. There were 156 patients included in ASTIS, 87% having lung involvement. The mean change from baseline after 2 years follow-up was modestly better in the HSCT group. Event-free survival was significantly greater with HSCT compared with cyclophosphamide at year 1 (HR 0.52 [95% CI 0.28, 0.96]), year 2 (HR 0.35 [95% CI 0.16, 0 74]) and year 4 (HR 0.34 [95% CI 0.16, 0.74]). The mortality was higher in this trial than previously reported: after 5.8 years there were 19 deaths reported in the HSCT group (11 in the first year (10.1%) and additionally 3 cases of irreversible organ failure), while in the control group 23 deaths and 8 irreversible organ failures (7 of these patients died later) were documented. In the SCOT trial, 97% of the patients had pulmonary involvement (mean baseline FVC% pred 74% and DLCO% pred 53%) [119]. The primary end point was a global rank composite score (GRCS), consisting of relevant hierarchical outcomes: mortality, event-free survival (without organ failure), lung function, scleroderma HAQ, and modified Rodnan skin score. Superiority of HSCT compared to cyclophosphamide was shown on the primary outcome at 54 months. Moreover, 36% of patients in the HSCT group vs. 23% in the control group had a relative increase of FVC% pred by ≥10%, showing a relevant improvement. Regarding mortality, there were 3/36 deaths reported in the HSCT arm (1 treatment-related) and 11/39 deaths in the control group (none treatment-related).

Therefore, procedural risks, as well as long-term safety remain a concern—among the expected complications are viral, bacterial, or opportunistic infections secondary to the aggressive immunosuppression, including neutropenic fever [120], cardiac toxicity, infertility [121], alopecia. Long-term complications include a higher risk for hematologic (acute leukemia) and solid malignancies [120]. Based on the results of these trials and considering the treatment-related morbidity and mortality, HSCT should only be considered in carefully selected patients with rapidly progressive SSc and at high risk of organ failure [122].

Lung Transplantation

To date, there are no controlled clinical trials assessing the outcomes of patients undergoing lung transplantation for SSc-ILD in comparison to other treatment options. The 2009 EULAR recommendations for treatment of SSc [123], updated in 2017 [122], did not specifically address the role of lung transplantation. Historically, SSc-ILD was considered a contraindication for lung transplantation, because of concerns regarding the extrapulmonary manifestations, mainly renal disease [124]. The indication for lung transplantation in SSc-ILD was recently broadened based on data reported in ILD of other causes, but it is still performed rarely, in selected cases, accounting for only 1.1% of lung transplants of all-cause (2016 international registry report [125]).

A recent retrospective multicenter study [124] reported data about 90 patients with SSc-ILD and/or PAH, who underwent lung transplantation between 1993 and 2016 in 14 European centers, among these 40 patients having ILD and PAH, 30 patients ILD alone and 20 patients only PAH. The mean baseline FVC% pred in all patients was 54%, DLco% pred 25%, whereas in the group having ILD alone the mean FVC% pred was 47% and DLco% pred 27%.

The survival after 1, 3, and 5 years was 81%, 68%, and 61%, respectively, similar to those documented after lung transplantation for other reasons. Worse prognosis was associated with female gender and PAH as primary indication for the transplantation.

Previous studies examining the survival outcomes in lung transplantation for SSc-ILD showed similar results: a retrospective study comparing 72 patients with SSc-ILD to 311 patients with ILD of other causes and found similar 1- and 5-year survival rates: 81% SSc-ILD vs. 79% pulmonary fibrosis ($p = 0.743$) after 1 year, 66% vs. 58% ($p = 0.249$) after 5 years, respectively [126].

Based on the current data, lung transplantation can be considered in cases of severe, treatment-refractory ILD in patients with no- or mild extrapulmonary manifestations [127] and after a careful screening for coexisting PAH.

Future Therapies

Pirfenidone

Pirfenidone is approved for the treatment of idiopathic lung fibrosis [128]. A double-blind, randomized, placebo-controlled, pilot study assessed the efficacy and safety of pirfenidone in ILD associated with SSc [129]. Inclusion criteria were FVC% pred between 50% and 80%, DLco% pred >30%, and a disease duration of less than 7 years. In all, 34 SSc patients were randomized in 1:1 ratio to receive either pirfenidone (2403 mg/day) or placebo for 6 months. Primary outcome was the proportion of subjects with either stabilization or improvement in FVC% pred at 6 months. Stabilization/improvement in FVC% pred was seen in 16 (94.1%) and 13 (76.5%) subjects in the pirfenidone and placebo groups, respectively ($p = 0.33$). A multicenter phase-2 randomized controlled trial (Scleroderma Lung study III (NCT03221257)) assessing the efficacy and additive effects of a combination of mycophenolate mofetil and pirfenidone has been conducted but was prematurely stopped before the complete enrollment of the patients because of the sponsor decision.

Pirfenidone was tested in patients with progressive pulmonary fibrosis, defined as an annual decline of FVC of at least 5% predicted despite conventional therapy, based on at least three measurements within 6–24 months before enrolment, in the randomized placebo-controlled RELIEF study which included 8 patients with SSc-ILD out of 127 patients randomized [130]. Patients who received pirfenidone had a slower decline of FVC% pred from baseline to 48 weeks than those who received placebo. However, the findings need to be interpreted carefully in the context of the early termination of the trial. In patients with SSc-ILD who present with progressive fibrosis and who do not tolerate nintedanib, pirfenidone may be used as an alternative antifibrotic molecule.

Other Potential Therapies

Many drugs with antifibrotic properties are being tested in IPF patients and in progressive pulmonary fibrosis, that could prove of interest in SSc-ILD in the future, including inhibitors of the autotaxin pathway, NOX4 inhibitors, and integrin inhibitors [131–133]. Four molecules are entering phase 3 trials and might prove of interest in the near future.

Connective tissue growth factor (CTGF), also known as CCN2, is a matricellular protein, which constitutes a hub for the coordination of cell signaling and communication, with potent profibrotic properties. CTGF has been shown to be overexpressed in SSc [134]. CCN2 gene deletion in fibroblast has been shown to prevent bleomycin-induced lung fibrosis, and to limit the development of experimentally induced pulmonary hypertension in mice [134]. Pamvrelumab is a fully recombinant human monoclonal antibody targeting CTGF which gave interesting results in the phase 2 randomized, double-blind, placebo-controlled PRAISE trial which involved 103 patients (50 assigned to pamrevlumab and 53 to placebo) [135]. Pamrevlumab was given intravenously every 3 weeks over 48 weeks. Pamrevlumab reduced the decline of predicted FVC at week 48 (mean change from baseline −2.9% with pamrevlumab vs. −7.2% with placebo; between-group difference 4.3% [95% CI 0.4–8.3]). The proportion of patients with disease progression was lower in the pamrevlumab group than in the placebo group at week 48 (10.0% vs. 31.4%). Pamrevlumab was well tolerated, with a safety profile similar to that of placebo [135]. A phase 3 trial investigating the effect of pamrevlumab in IPF patients not receiving nintedanib or pirfenidone is ongoing (NCT03955146).

Pentraxin 2 (also known as serum amyloid P, SAP) is a naturally circulating serum protein and one of two short pentraxin protein family members, the other being C-reactive protein. SAP is produced in the liver and circulates as a highly stable pentamer. Each protomer of SAP contains two unique binding sites: a Ca^{2+}-dependent ligand binding site (ligands recognized by SAP include both pathogen-associated molecular patterns and danger- or damage-associated molecular patterns) and a receptor-binding site for recognition of specific Fcγ-receptors (FcγR). Pentraxin 2 has been shown to reduce experimentally induced lung fibrosis in mice, through monocyte-macrophage regulation in vivo [136–138]. Plasma levels of pentraxin 2 are reduced in IPF patients [137]. Recombinant pentraxin 2 was shown to reduce decline of FVC and decline of 6-min walk distance in a phase 2, randomized, double-blind, placebo-controlled trial in patients with IPF (78 patients received pentraxin 10 mg/kg intravenous every 4 weeks, and 39 received placebo) [139]. The least-squares mean change in FVC% pred from baseline to week 28 in patients treated with recombinant human pentraxin 2 was −2.5 vs. −4.8 for those in the placebo group (difference, +2.3 [90% CI, 1.1–3.5]; $p = 0.001$). The change in 6-min walk distance was −0.5 m for patients treated with recombinant human pentraxin 2 vs. −31.8 m for those in the placebo group (difference, +31.3 m [90% CI, 17.4–45.1]; $p < 0.001$) [139]. Cough and fatigue were more common in the recombinant human pentraxin 2 vs. placebo group. Long-term effects were confirmed in an open label extension study [140]. A phase 3 trial is ongoing in patients with IPF, with or without baseline antifibrotic treatment (NCT04552899).

Inhaled treprostinil, an analog of prostaglandin I2, is an established treatment in pulmonary hypertension. A recent study demonstrated that inhaled treprostinil improved the 6-min walk distance over 16 weeks in the INCREASE randomized controlled trial versus placebo in patients with lung fibrosis and pulmonary hypertension [141]. At week 16, the least-squares mean difference between the treprostinil group and the placebo group in the change from baseline in the 6-min walk distance was 31.12 m (95% confidence interval [CI], 16.85–45.39; $p < 0.001$). There was a reduction of 15% in NT-proBNP levels from baseline with inhaled treprostinil as compared with an increase of 46% with placebo. The positive results of the INCREASE trial have led to the approval by the FDA for pulmonary hypertension associated with interstitial lung disease (PH-ILD; WHO Group 3). Interestingly, a post-hoc analysis of the INCREASE trial [142] showed that inhaled treprostinil was associated with a placebo-corrected least squares mean improvement in FVC% pred of 1.8% (0.8; 0.2–3.4; $p = 0.028$) after 16 weeks, with a similar trend in patients with idiopathic interstitial pneumonia and patients with idiopathic pulmonary fibrosis in subgroup analysis. Interestingly, there was a reduced number of progression events in patients receiving inhaled treprostinil as compared to those receiving placebo (including lung disease exacerbation, FVC decline, cardiopulmonary hospitalization, and death). This is the basis for an ongoing phase 3 trial in patients with IPF (NCT04708782).

Phosphodiesterases are a class of enzymes, which degrade intracellular cyclic nucleotides, such as cyclic AMP and cyclic GMP, which are important mediators for fibroblast activation. BI 1015550, an oral preferential inhibitor of phosphodiesterase 4B, was shown to reduce FVC decline over 12 weeks in patients with IPF, with or without antifibrotics, in a placebo-controlled randomized clinical trial [143]. The most frequent adverse event was diarrhea. Two phase 3 trials are being initiated, in IPF patients (NCT05321069) and in patients with progressive pulmonary fibrosis (NCT05321082).

Supportive Care

Supportive care is an integral part of the management of patients with SSc-ILD [34]. Although, pulmonary rehabilitation has been shown to be safe and to improve functional exercise capacity, dyspnea, and quality of life in patients with ILD [144, 145], more disease specific studies are needed to prove its beneficial effect also for SSc-ILD. Regarding supplemental oxygen, a first prospective RCT with ambulatory oxygen showed a positive effect on quality of life and dyspnea [146]. Ten percent of the patients in this study had a diagnosis of CTD-ILD. This suggests that supplemental oxygen should be offered to patients with an oxygen desaturation on a 6 min walking test. Besides supportive measures, preventive advice is given in line with recommendations to all ILD patients. In the case of smoking, vaping, or other substance abuse, patients should strongly be encouraged to stop. In addition to these measures, an aggressive treatment for reflux is recommended in all SSc patients with ILD, as reflux has been associated with idiopathic pulmonary fibrosis, SSc ILD, and worsening of SSc ILD [21, 147].

Influenza and pneumococcal vaccinations are offered to all patients to prevent infections that may trigger an exacerbation or worsening of disease [34]. Patients treated with immunosuppressive drugs and/or with severe ILD might be considered at risk for a more severe disease course and higher mortality following the development of Severe Acute Respiratory Syndrome-Coronavirus-2 (SARS-CoV-2) virus infection [148]. In particular, rituximab therapy is associated with more severe SARS-CoV-2 infection [149]. A systematic review identified 25 cases of SARS-CoV-2 infection in SSc patients [150]. Information on disease course was available in nine cases. SARS-CoV-2 infection was severe in seven of nine, with three recorded deaths. Among the three patients with ILD, one developed a mild disease, one required intensive care unit level care and one died. Therefore, vaccination against SARS-CoV-2 is recommended in SSc patients. Increased prevalence of nonresponse to vaccine was observed in different auto-immune diseases including SSc, particularly in patients with ILD and in patients treated with glucocorticoids, mycophenolate mofetil, or rituximab [151]. Early determination of serum neutralizing antibody should be performed in SSc ILD patients to identify patients with suboptimal response, who could benefit from a booster-dose of vaccine.

Which Treatment to Which Patient?

The Eular recommendations for the treatment of SSc were published before the results of SLS-2, the SENSCIS study, and the focuSSced trials. In 2017, Canadian experts published new algorithms for treatment-decision in SSc [152]. Regarding ILD in SSc, 69% of experts agreed for induction therapy, mycophenolate mofetil as first-line, intravenous cyclophosphamide as second line and rituximab, whereas for maintenance, first-line treatment was mycophenolate mofetil and then azathioprine and cyclophosphamide as third-line.

The recent European consensus agreed that nintedanib (as monotherapy or in combination with mycophenolate mofetil) might be an effective option for treatment initiation or escalation, whereas mycophenolate mofetil or cyclophosphamide were considered in cases in which nintedanib was not an appropriate choice for patients. Consistently two recent expert reports proposed mycophenolate mofetil as the first-line choice for the treatment of diffuse SSc and ILD [153, 154]. Based on the available evidenced data, on our clinical experience, and recent recommendations [155, 156], we propose an algorithm to guide treatment-decision (Fig. 26.1). The algorithm relies on individual patient stratification based on clinical manifestations (extra-pulmonary involvement), disease severity, and risk of progression. As recently emphasized [34], the treatment for ILD strongly depends on the presence of other organ manifestations.

The first step is to screen SSc patients for other organ complications. The treatment should be decided in a multidisciplinary discussion involving also pneumologists.

In the subgroup of SSc-patients with extra-pulmonary manifestations including systemic inflammation, progressive skin, and musculoskeletal disease, mycophenolate mofetil, tocilizumab, or rituximab can be considered. Mycophenolate mofetil or rituximab will be preferred in cases of active skin disease, whereas tocilizumab will be the treatment of choice in cases of early disease with anti-topoisomerase 1 antibodies and evidence of systemic inflammation. Although there is no randomized controlled trial, for patients with concomitant active arthritis, rituximab and tocilizumab will be preferred, in regard to positive observational small-size studies [157, 158]. If the lung is the primary treatment indication and especially in the few patients with a predominant UIP pattern, nintedanib can be considered as a first-line therapy.

The treatment effect should be assessed after 3–6 months with clinical symptoms, PFTs, and 6-min walking test.

In nonresponders to a first-line therapy, we recommend a switch in immunosuppressants (mycophenolate, tocilizumab, or rituximab) or a combination of immunosuppressants (mycophenolate + rituximab or mycophenolate + tocilizumab). In patients with high-risk profile (extensive disease, exercise-induced blood oxygen desaturation), a step-up combined treatment (nintedanib + mycophenolate mofetil or tocilizumab + nintedanib) targeting both the immune system and the fibrotic component of the disease can be considered. In patients with progressive fibrosis who do not tolerate nintedanib, pirfenidone may be used as an alternative antifibrotic molecule.

In cases of progressive disease despite the second-line therapy, an escalation therapy is indicated (new switch, combination of immunosuppressants with anti-fibrotic, cyclophosphamide, autologous stem cell transplantation, or lung transplantation).

Autologous stem cell transplantation should be reserved to selected patients with progressive, severe, and multisystem disease despite previous mentioned treatments. Lung transplantation can be considered in case of severe isolated refractory lung involvement.

Pulmonary rehabilitation should be offered to every patient with exercise limitation due to SSc-ILD.

Conclusion

SSc-ILD is common and associated with significant morbidity and early mortality.

The high interindividual variability of SSc-ILD, both at baseline and during the course of the disease, complicates patient follow-up and treatment decisions.

While it was generally admitted that disease progression occurs early in the disease course, recent data highlights that it can also occur at late stages, warranting close monitoring using PFTs and HRCT throughout the course of the disease.

In recent years, insightful clinical trials have been published and great advances have been made in developing effective treatment options for SSc-ILD. Positive results from the SENSCIS trial led to the approval by drug agencies of the first drug for ILD in SSc, while tocilizumab was the first biologic therapy to be recognized in this indication based on the results of the faSScinate and focuSSced studies. Due to the positive results of the DESIRES study, rituximab has been approved in Japan for treatment of SSc.

Based on current available data, we recommend treatment for all patients with clinical ILD and/or high-risk patients and closely monitoring in untreated patients with clinical examination, PFTs and HRCT.

Although significant progress has been made in recent years in the development of effective therapies for SSc-ILD, several questions remain unanswered: the published clinical trials have primarily focused on immunosuppressive or antifibrotic therapies as monotherapy, but the benefit of an initial combination of treatments remains unknown. Moreover, the delay after which the treatment must be reevaluated and a switch or a combination of treatment considered remains unknown. From the perspective of a personalized approach to SSc, identifying subsets of patients more likely to benefit from immunosuppressive or antifibrotic therapy or a combination of both treatments should be a priority in the research agenda. This improved stratification could be based on the identification of new biomarkers (surrogate markers of inflammatory, fibrotic, or mixed disease stage), which deserve further study in the coming years. Moreover, the duration of the treatment remains unclear and there are currently no trials evaluating the possibility of stopping or reducing treatment during follow-up.

References

1. Elhai M, Meune C, Boubaya M, Avouac J, Hachulla E, Balbir-Gurman A, et al. Mapping and predicting mortality from systemic sclerosis. Ann Rheum Dis. 2017;76(11):1897–905.
2. Tyndall AJ, Bannert B, Vonk M, Airò P, Cozzi F, Carreira PE, et al. Causes and risk factors for death in systemic sclerosis: a study from the EULAR Scleroderma Trials and Research (EUSTAR) database. Ann Rheum Dis. 2010;69(10):1809–15.
3. Steen VD, Medsger TA. Changes in causes of death in systemic sclerosis, 1972–2002. Ann Rheum Dis. 2007;66(7):940–4.
4. Vonk MC, Walker UA, Volkmann ER, Kreuter M, Johnson SR, Allanore Y. Natural variability in the disease course of SSc-ILD: implications for treatment. Eur Respir Rev. 2021;30(159):200340.
5. Rubio-Rivas M, Corbella X, Pestaña-Fernández M, Tolosa-Vilella C, Guillen-Del Castillo A, Colunga-Argüelles D, et al. First clinical symptom as a prognostic factor in systemic sclerosis: results of a retrospective nationwide cohort study. Clin Rheumatol. 2018;37(4):999–1009.
6. van den Hoogen F, Khanna D, Fransen J, Johnson SR, Baron M, Tyndall A, et al. 2013 classification criteria for systemic sclerosis: an American College of Rheumatology/European League Against Rheumatism Collaborative Initiative. Ann Rheum Dis. 2013;72(11):1747–55.
7. Weaver AL, Divertie MB, Titus JL. Pulmonary scleroderma. Dis Chest. 1968;54(6):490–8.
8. D'Angelo WA, Fries JF, Masi AT, Shulman LE. Pathologic observations in systemic sclerosis (scleroderma). A study of fifty-eight autopsy cases and fifty-eight matched controls. Am J Med. 1969;46(3):428–40.
9. Schurawitzki H, Stiglbauer R, Graninger W, Herold C, Pölzleitner D, Burghuber OC, et al. Interstitial lung disease in progressive systemic sclerosis: high-resolution CT versus radiography. Radiology. 1990;176(3):755–9.
10. Vonk MC, Broers B, Heijdra YF, Ton E, Snijder R, van Dijk AP, et al. Systemic sclerosis and its pulmonary complications in The Netherlands: an epidemiological study. Ann Rheum Dis. 2009;68(6):961–5.
11. Hoffmann-Vold AM, Fretheim H, Halse AK, Seip M, Bitter H, Wallenius M, et al. Tracking impact of interstitial lung disease in systemic sclerosis in a complete nationwide cohort. Am J Respir Crit Care Med. 2019;200(10):1258–66.
12. Solomon JJ, Olson AL, Fischer A, Bull T, Brown KK, Raghu G. Scleroderma lung disease. Eur Respir Rev. 2013;22(127):6–19.
13. Nihtyanova SI, Sari A, Harvey JC, Leslie A, Derrett-Smith EC, Fonseca C, et al. Using autoantibodies and cutaneous subset to develop outcome-based disease classification in systemic sclerosis. Arthritis Rheumatol. 2020;72(3):465–76.
14. Walker UA, Tyndall A, Czirják L, Denton C, Farge-Bancel D, Kowal-Bielecka O, et al. Clinical risk assessment of organ manifestations in systemic sclerosis: a report from the EULAR Scleroderma Trials and Research group database. Ann Rheum Dis. 2007;66(6):754–63.
15. Clements PJ, Roth MD, Elashoff R, Tashkin DP, Goldin J, Silver RM, et al. Scleroderma lung study (SLS): differences in the presentation and course of patients with limited versus diffuse systemic sclerosis. Ann Rheum Dis. 2007;66(12):1641–7.
16. Goh NS, Desai SR, Veeraraghavan S, Hansell DM, Copley SJ, Maher TM, et al. Interstitial lung disease in systemic sclerosis: a simple staging system. Am J Respir Crit Care Med. 2008;177(11):1248–54.
17. Goh NS, Hoyles RK, Denton CP, Hansell DM, Renzoni EA, Maher TM, et al. Short-term pulmonary function trends are predictive of mortality in interstitial lung disease associated with systemic sclerosis. Arthritis Rheumatol. 2017;69(8):1670–8.
18. Volkmann ER, Tashkin DP, Roth MD, Goldin J, Kim GHJ. Early radiographic progression of scleroderma: lung disease predicts long-term mortality. Chest. 2021;161:1310.
19. Plastiras SC, Karadimitrakis SP, Ziakas PD, Vlachoyiannopoulos PG, Moutsopoulos HM, Tzelepis GE. Scleroderma lung: initial forced vital capacity as predictor of pulmonary function decline. Arthritis Rheum. 2006;55(4):598–602.
20. Man A, Davidyock T, Ferguson LT, Ieong M, Zhang Y, Simms RW. Changes in forced vital capacity over time in systemic sclerosis: application of group-based trajectory modelling. Rheumatology (Oxford). 2015;54(8):1464–71.
21. Hoffmann-Vold AM, Allanore Y, Alves M, Brunborg C, Airó P, Ananieva LP, et al. Progressive interstitial lung disease in patients with systemic sclerosis-associated interstitial lung disease in the EUSTAR database. Ann Rheum Dis. 2021;80(2):219–27.
22. Guler SA, Winstone TA, Murphy D, Hague C, Soon J, Sulaiman N, et al. Does systemic sclerosis-associated interstitial lung disease burn out? Specific phenotypes of disease progression. Ann Am Thorac Soc. 2018;15(12):1427–33.
23. Steen VD, Medsger TA Jr. Severe organ involvement in systemic sclerosis with diffuse scleroderma. Arthritis Rheum. 2000;43(11):2437–44.
24. Hoffmann-Vold AM, Brunborg C, Airò P, Ananyeva LP, Czirják L, Guiducci S, et al. POS0063 progressive interstitial lung disease is frequent also in late disease stages in systemic sclerosis patients from EUSTAR. Ann Rheum Dis. 2022;81(Suppl 1):248.
25. Frantz C, Huscher D, Avouac J, Hachulla E, Balbir-Gurman A, Riemekasten G, et al. Outcomes of limited cutaneous systemic sclerosis patients: results on more than 12,000 patients from the EUSTAR database. Autoimmun Rev. 2020;19(2):102452.
26. Perelas A, Silver RM, Arrossi AV, Highland KB. Systemic sclerosis-associated interstitial lung disease. Lancet Respir Med. 2020;8(3):304–20.
27. Cheng JZ, Wilcox PG, Glaspole I, Corte TJ, Murphy D, Hague CJ, et al. Cough is less common and less severe in systemic sclerosis-associated interstitial lung disease compared to other fibrotic interstitial lung diseases. Respirology. 2017;22(8):1592–7.
28. Sánchez-Cano D, Ortego-Centeno N, Callejas JL, Fonollosa Plá V, Ríos-Fernández R, Tolosa-Vilella C, et al. Interstitial lung disease in systemic sclerosis: data from the Spanish Scleroderma Study Group. Rheumatol Int. 2018;38(3):363–74.
29. Wangkaew S, Euathrongchit J, Wattanawittawas P, Kasitanon N, Louthrenoo W. Incidence and predictors of interstitial lung disease (ILD) in Thai patients with early systemic sclerosis: inception cohort study. Mod Rheumatol. 2016;26(4):588–93.
30. Le Gouellec N, Duhamel A, Perez T, Hachulla AL, Sobanski V, Faivre JB, et al. Predictors of lung function test severity and outcome in systemic sclerosis-associated interstitial lung disease. PLoS One. 2017;12(8):e0181692.
31. Tashkin DP, Volkmann ER, Tseng CH, Kim HJ, Goldin J, Clements P, et al. Relationship between quantitative radiographic assessments of interstitial lung disease and physiological and clinical features of systemic sclerosis. Ann Rheum Dis. 2016;75(2):374–81.
32. Al-Sheikh H, Ahmad Z, Johnson SR. Ethnic variations in systemic sclerosis disease manifestations, internal organ involvement, and mortality. J Rheumatol. 2019;46(9):1103–8.
33. Anna-Maria Hoffmann-Vold TMM, Philpot EE, Ashrafzadeh A, Barake R, Barsotti S, Bruni C, Carducci P, Carreira PE, Castellví I, Del Galdo F, Distler JHW, Foeldvari I, Fraticelli P, George PM, Griffiths B, Guillén-Del-Castillo A, Hamid AM, Horváth R, Hughes M, Kreuter M, Moazedi-Fuerst F, Olas J, Paul S, Rotondo C, Rubio-Rivas M, Seferian A, Tomčík M, Uzunhan Y, Walker UA, Więsik-Szewczyk E, Distler O. The identification and management of interstitial lung disease in systemic scle-

rosis: evidence-based European consensus statements. Lancet Rheumatol. 2020;2(2):e71–83.
34. Hoffmann-Vold AM, Allanore Y, Bendstrup E, Bruni C, Distler O, Maher TM, et al. The need for a holistic approach for SSc-ILD—achievements and ambiguity in a devastating disease. Respir Res. 2020;21(1):197.
35. Elhai M, Sritharan N, Boubaya M, Balbir-Gurman A, Siegert E, Hachulla E, et al. Stratification in systemic sclerosis according to autoantibody status versus skin involvment: a study of the prospective EUSTAR cohort. The Lancet Rheumatology. 2022;4(11):e785–94.
36. Hoffmann-Vold A-M, Maher TM, Philpot EE, Ashrafzadeh A, Barake R, Barsotti S, et al. The identification and management of interstitial lung disease in systemic sclerosis: evidence-based European consensus statements. Lancet Rheumatol. 2020;2(2):e71–83.
37. Bruni C, Tofani L, Fretheim H, Liem S, Velauthapillai A, Bjørkekjær HJ, et al. POS0388 developing a screening tool for the detection of interstitial lung disease in systemic sclerosis: the ILD-RISC risk score. Ann Rheum Dis. 2022;81(Suppl 1):449–50.
38. Volkmann ER, Tashkin DP, Sim M, Li N, Goldmuntz E, Keyes-Elstein L, et al. Short-term progression of interstitial lung disease in systemic sclerosis predicts long-term survival in two independent clinical trial cohorts. Ann Rheum Dis. 2019;78(1):122–30.
39. Kafaja S, Clements PJ, Wilhalme H, Tseng CH, Furst DE, Kim GH, et al. Reliability and minimal clinically important differences of forced vital capacity: results from the Scleroderma Lung Studies (SLS-I and SLS-II). Am J Respir Crit Care Med. 2018;197(5):644–52.
40. Kreuter M, Del Galdo F, Miede C, Khanna D, Wuyts WA, Hummers LK, et al. Impact of lung function decline on time to hospitalisation events in systemic sclerosis-associated interstitial lung disease (SSc-ILD): a joint model analysis. Arthritis Res Ther. 2022;24(1):19.
41. Wu W, Jordan S, Becker MO, Dobrota R, Maurer B, Fretheim H, et al. Prediction of progression of interstitial lung disease in patients with systemic sclerosis: the SPAR model. Ann Rheum Dis. 2018;77(9):1326–32.
42. Elhai M, Avouac J, Allanore Y. Circulating lung biomarkers in idiopathic lung fibrosis and interstitial lung diseases associated with connective tissue diseases: where do we stand? Semin Arthritis Rheum. 2020;50(3):480–91.
43. Strange C, Bolster MB, Roth MD, Silver RM, Theodore A, Goldin J, et al. Bronchoalveolar lavage and response to cyclophosphamide in scleroderma interstitial lung disease. Am J Respir Crit Care Med. 2008;177(1):91–8.
44. Goh NS, Veeraraghavan S, Desai SR, Cramer D, Hansell DM, Denton CP, et al. Bronchoalveolar lavage cellular profiles in patients with systemic sclerosis-associated interstitial lung disease are not predictive of disease progression. Arthritis Rheum. 2007;56(6):2005–12.
45. Raghu G, Remy-Jardin M, Richeldi L, Thomson CC, Inoue Y, Johkoh T, et al. Idiopathic pulmonary fibrosis (an update) and progressive pulmonary fibrosis in adults: an official ATS/ERS/JRS/ALAT clinical practice guideline. Am J Respir Crit Care Med. 2022;205(9):e18–47.
46. White B, Moore WC, Wigley FM, Xiao HQ, Wise RA. Cyclophosphamide is associated with pulmonary function and survival benefit in patients with scleroderma and alveolitis. Ann Intern Med. 2000;132(12):947–54.
47. Silver RM, Warrick JH, Kinsella MB, Staudt LS, Baumann MH, Strange C. Cyclophosphamide and low-dose prednisone therapy in patients with systemic sclerosis (scleroderma) with interstitial lung disease. J Rheumatol. 1993;20(5):838–44.
48. Tashkin DP, Elashoff R, Clements PJ, Goldin J, Roth MD, Furst DE, et al. Cyclophosphamide versus placebo in scleroderma lung disease. N Engl J Med. 2006;354(25):2655–66.
49. Khanna D, Yan X, Tashkin DP, Furst DE, Elashoff R, Roth MD, et al. Impact of oral cyclophosphamide on health-related quality of life in patients with active scleroderma lung disease: results from the scleroderma lung study. Arthritis Rheum. 2007;56(5):1676–84.
50. Goldin J, Elashoff R, Kim HJ, Yan X, Lynch D, Strollo D, et al. Treatment of scleroderma-interstitial lung disease with cyclophosphamide is associated with less progressive fibrosis on serial thoracic high-resolution CT scan than placebo: findings from the scleroderma lung study. Chest. 2009;136(5):1333–40.
51. Roth MD, Tseng CH, Clements PJ, Furst DE, Tashkin DP, Goldin JG, et al. Predicting treatment outcomes and responder subsets in scleroderma-related interstitial lung disease. Arthritis Rheum. 2011;63(9):2797–808.
52. Martinez FJ, McCune WJ. Cyclophosphamide for scleroderma lung disease. N Engl J Med. 2006;354(25):2707–9.
53. Tashkin DP, Elashoff R, Clements PJ, Roth MD, Furst DE, Silver RM, et al. Effects of 1-year treatment with cyclophosphamide on outcomes at 2 years in scleroderma lung disease. Am J Respir Crit Care Med. 2007;176(10):1026–34.
54. Tashkin DP, Roth MD, Clements PJ, Furst DE, Khanna D, Kleerup EC, et al. Mycophenolate mofetil versus oral cyclophosphamide in scleroderma-related interstitial lung disease (SLS II): a randomised controlled, double-blind, parallel group trial. Lancet Respir Med. 2016;4(9):708–19.
55. Tashkin DP, Volkmann ER, Tseng CH, Roth MD, Khanna D, Furst DE, et al. Improved cough and cough-specific quality of life in patients treated for scleroderma-related interstitial lung disease: results of Scleroderma Lung Study II. Chest. 2017;151(4):813–20.
56. Goldin JG, Kim GHJ, Tseng CH, Volkmann E, Furst D, Clements P, et al. Longitudinal changes in quantitative interstitial lung disease on computed tomography after immunosuppression in the Scleroderma Lung Study II. Ann Am Thorac Soc. 2018;15(11):1286–95.
57. Volkmann ER, Tashkin DP, LeClair H, Roth MD, Kim G, Goldin J, et al. Treatment with mycophenolate and cyclophosphamide leads to clinically meaningful improvements in patient-reported outcomes in scleroderma lung disease: results of Scleroderma Lung Study II. ACR Open Rheumatol. 2020;2(6):362–70.
58. Volkmann ER, Tashkin DP, Sim M, Li N, Khanna D, Roth MD, et al. Cyclophosphamide for systemic sclerosis-related interstitial lung disease: a comparison of Scleroderma Lung Study I and II. J Rheumatol. 2019;46(10):1316–25.
59. Nadashkevich O, Davis P, Fritzler M, Kovalenko W. A randomized unblinded trial of cyclophosphamide versus azathioprine in the treatment of systemic sclerosis. Clin Rheumatol. 2006;25(2):205–12.
60. Furst DE, Tseng CH, Clements PJ, Strange C, Tashkin DP, Roth MD, et al. Adverse events during the Scleroderma Lung Study. Am J Med. 2011;124(5):459–67.
61. Monach PA, Arnold LM, Merkel PA. Incidence and prevention of bladder toxicity from cyclophosphamide in the treatment of rheumatic diseases: a data-driven review. Arthritis Rheum. 2010;62(1):9–21.
62. Bruni C, Tashkin DP, Steen V, Allanore Y, Distler O, Grotts J, et al. Intravenous versus oral cyclophosphamide for lung and/or skin fibrosis in systemic sclerosis: an indirect comparison from EUSTAR and randomised controlled trials. Clin Exp Rheumatol. 2020;38 Suppl 125(3):161–8.
63. Bérezné A, Ranque B, Valeyre D, Brauner M, Allanore Y, Launay D, et al. Therapeutic strategy combining intravenous cyclophosphamide followed by oral azathioprine to treat worsening interstitial lung disease associated with systemic sclerosis: a retrospective multicenter open-label study. J Rheumatol. 2008;35(6):1064–72.

64. Iudici M, Cuomo G, Vettori S, Bocchino M, Sanduzzi Zamparelli A, Cappabianca S, et al. Low-dose pulse cyclophosphamide in interstitial lung disease associated with systemic sclerosis (SSc-ILD): efficacy of maintenance immunosuppression in responders and non-responders. Semin Arthritis Rheum. 2015;44(4):437–44.
65. Hoyles RK, Ellis RW, Wellsbury J, Lees B, Newlands P, Goh NS, et al. A multicenter, prospective, randomized, double-blind, placebo-controlled trial of corticosteroids and intravenous cyclophosphamide followed by oral azathioprine for the treatment of pulmonary fibrosis in scleroderma. Arthritis Rheum. 2006;54(12):3962–70.
66. Takebe N, Cheng X, Fandy TE, Srivastava RK, Wu S, Shankar S, et al. IMP dehydrogenase inhibitor mycophenolate mofetil induces caspase-dependent apoptosis and cell cycle inhibition in multiple myeloma cells. Mol Cancer Ther. 2006;5(2):457–66.
67. Colic M, Stojic-Vukanic Z, Pavlovic B, Jandric D, Stefanoska I. Mycophenolate mofetil inhibits differentiation, maturation and allostimulatory function of human monocyte-derived dendritic cells. Clin Exp Immunol. 2003;134(1):63–9.
68. Andrikos E, Yavuz A, Bordoni V, Ratanarat R, De Cal M, Bonello M, et al. Effect of cyclosporine, mycophenolate mofetil, and their combination with steroids on apoptosis in a human cultured monocytic U937 cell line. Transplant Proc. 2005;37(7):3226–9.
69. Swigris JJ, Olson AL, Fischer A, Lynch DA, Cosgrove GP, Frankel SK, et al. Mycophenolate mofetil is safe, well tolerated, and preserves lung function in patients with connective tissue disease-related interstitial lung disease. Chest. 2006;130(1):30–6.
70. Zamora AC, Wolters PJ, Collard HR, Connolly MK, Elicker BM, Webb WR, et al. Use of mycophenolate mofetil to treat scleroderma-associated interstitial lung disease. Respir Med. 2008;102(1):150–5.
71. Gerbino AJ, Goss CH, Molitor JA. Effect of mycophenolate mofetil on pulmonary function in scleroderma-associated interstitial lung disease. Chest. 2008;133(2):455–60.
72. Koutroumpas A, Ziogas A, Alexiou I, Barouta G, Sakkas LI. Mycophenolate mofetil in systemic sclerosis-associated interstitial lung disease. Clin Rheumatol. 2010;29(10):1167–8.
73. Owen C, Ngian GS, Elford K, Moore O, Stevens W, Nikpour M, et al. Mycophenolate mofetil is an effective and safe option for the management of systemic sclerosis-associated interstitial lung disease: results from the Australian Scleroderma Cohort Study. Clin Exp Rheumatol. 2016;34 Suppl 100(5):170–6.
74. Nihtyanova SI, Brough GM, Black CM, Denton CP. Mycophenolate mofetil in diffuse cutaneous systemic sclerosis—a retrospective analysis. Rheumatology (Oxford). 2007;46(3):442–5.
75. Liossis SN, Bounas A, Andonopoulos AP. Mycophenolate mofetil as first-line treatment improves clinically evident early scleroderma lung disease. Rheumatology (Oxford). 2006;45(8):1005–8.
76. Fischer A, Brown KK, Du Bois RM, Frankel SK, Cosgrove GP, Fernandez-Perez ER, et al. Mycophenolate mofetil improves lung function in connective tissue disease-associated interstitial lung disease. J Rheumatol. 2013;40(5):640–6.
77. McGonagle D, Tan AL, Madden J, Rawstron AC, Rehman A, Emery P, et al. Successful treatment of resistant scleroderma-associated interstitial lung disease with rituximab. Rheumatology (Oxford). 2008;47(4):552–3.
78. Yoo WH. Successful treatment of steroid and cyclophosphamide-resistant diffuse scleroderma-associated interstitial lung disease with rituximab. Rheumatol Int. 2012;32(3):795–8.
79. Smith V, Piette Y, van Praet JT, Decuman S, Deschepper E, Elewaut D, et al. Two-year results of an open pilot study of a 2-treatment course with rituximab in patients with early systemic sclerosis with diffuse skin involvement. J Rheumatol. 2013;40(1):52–7.
80. Moazedi-Fuerst FC, Kielhauser SM, Brickmann K, Hermann J, Lutfi A, Meilinger M, et al. Rituximab for systemic sclerosis: arrest of pulmonary disease progression in five cases. Results of a lower dosage and shorter interval regimen. Scand J Rheumatol. 2014;43(3):257–8.
81. Ebata S, Yoshizaki A, Fukasawa T, Miura S, Takahashi T, Sumida H, et al. Rituximab therapy is more effective than cyclophosphamide therapy for Japanese patients with anti-topoisomerase I-positive systemic sclerosis-associated interstitial lung disease. J Dermatol. 2019;46(11):1006–13.
82. Sari A, Guven D, Armagan B, Erden A, Kalyoncu U, Karadag O, et al. Rituximab experience in patients with long-standing systemic sclerosis-associated interstitial lung disease: a series of 14 patients. J Clin Rheumatol. 2017;23(8):411–5.
83. Lepri G, Avouac J, Airò P, Anguita Santos F, Bellando-Randone S, Blagojevic J, et al. Effects of rituximab in connective tissue disorders related interstitial lung disease. Clin Exp Rheumatol. 2016;34 Suppl 100(5):181–5.
84. Elhai M, Boubaya M, Distler O, Smith V, Matucci-Cerinic M, Alegre Sancho JJ, et al. Outcomes of patients with systemic sclerosis treated with rituximab in contemporary practice: a prospective cohort study. Ann Rheum Dis. 2019;78(7):979–87.
85. Goswami RP, Ray A, Chatterjee M, Mukherjee A, Sircar G, Ghosh P. Rituximab in the treatment of systemic sclerosis-related interstitial lung disease: a systematic review and meta-analysis. Rheumatology (Oxford). 2021;60(2):557–67.
86. Daoussis D, Liossis SN, Tsamandas AC, Kalogeropoulou C, Kazantzi A, Sirinian C, et al. Experience with rituximab in scleroderma: results from a 1-year, proof-of-principle study. Rheumatology (Oxford). 2010;49(2):271–80.
87. Daoussis D, Melissaropoulos K, Sakellaropoulos G, Antonopoulos I, Markatseli TE, Simopoulou T, et al. A multicenter, open-label, comparative study of B-cell depletion therapy with Rituximab for systemic sclerosis-associated interstitial lung disease. Semin Arthritis Rheum. 2017;46(5):625–31.
88. Sircar G, Goswami RP, Sircar D, Ghosh A, Ghosh P. Intravenous cyclophosphamide vs rituximab for the treatment of early diffuse scleroderma lung disease: open label, randomized, controlled trial. Rheumatology (Oxford). 2018;57(12):2106–13.
89. Jordan S, Distler JH, Maurer B, Huscher D, van Laar JM, Allanore Y, et al. Effects and safety of rituximab in systemic sclerosis: an analysis from the European Scleroderma Trial and Research (EUSTAR) group. Ann Rheum Dis. 2015;74(6):1188–94.
90. Daoussis D, Liossis SN, Tsamandas AC, Kalogeropoulou C, Paliogianni F, Sirinian C, et al. Effect of long-term treatment with rituximab on pulmonary function and skin fibrosis in patients with diffuse systemic sclerosis. Clin Exp Rheumatol. 2012;30(2 Suppl 71):S17–22.
91. Ebata S, Yoshizaki A, Oba K, Kashiwabara K, Ueda K, Uemura Y, et al. Safety and efficacy of rituximab in systemic sclerosis (DESIRES): a double-blind, investigator-initiated, randomised, placebo-controlled trial. Lancet Rheumatol. 2021;3:e489.
92. Saunders P, Tsipouri V, Keir GJ, Ashby D, Flather MD, Parfrey H, et al. Rituximab versus cyclophosphamide for the treatment of connective tissue disease-associated interstitial lung disease (RECITAL): study protocol for a randomised controlled trial. Trials. 2017;18(1):275.
93. Maher TM, Tudor VA, Saunders P, Gibbons GA, Fletcher SV, Denton CP, et al., RECITAL Investigators. Rituximab versus intravenous cyclophosphamide in patients with connective tissue disease-associated interstitial lung disease in the UK (RECITAL): a double-blind, double-dummy, randomised, controlled, phase 2b trial. Lancet Respir Med. 2023;11(1):45–54. https://doi.org/10.1016/S2213-2600(22)00359-9.
94. Hasegawa M, Sato S, Fujimoto M, Ihn H, Kikuchi K, Takehara K. Serum levels of interleukin 6 (IL-6), oncostatin M, soluble IL-6 receptor, and soluble gp130 in patients with systemic sclerosis. J Rheumatol. 1998;25(2):308–13.

95. Sato S, Hasegawa M, Takehara K. Serum levels of interleukin-6 and interleukin-10 correlate with total skin thickness score in patients with systemic sclerosis. J Dermatol Sci. 2001;27(2):140–6.
96. Scala E, Pallotta S, Frezzolini A, Abeni D, Barbieri C, Sampogna F, et al. Cytokine and chemokine levels in systemic sclerosis: relationship with cutaneous and internal organ involvement. Clin Exp Immunol. 2004;138(3):540–6.
97. De Lauretis A, Sestini P, Pantelidis P, Hoyles R, Hansell DM, Goh NS, et al. Serum interleukin 6 is predictive of early functional decline and mortality in interstitial lung disease associated with systemic sclerosis. J Rheumatol. 2013;40(4):435–46.
98. Khanna D, Denton CP, Jahreis A, van Laar JM, Frech TM, Anderson ME, et al. Safety and efficacy of subcutaneous tocilizumab in adults with systemic sclerosis (faSScinate): a phase 2, randomised, controlled trial. Lancet (London, England). 2016;387(10038):2630–40.
99. Khanna D, Lin CJF, Furst DE, Goldin J, Kim G, Kuwana M, et al. Tocilizumab in systemic sclerosis: a randomised, double-blind, placebo-controlled, phase 3 trial. Lancet Respir Med. 2020;8(10):963–74.
100. Roofeh D, Lin CJF, Goldin J, Kim GH, Furst DE, Denton CP, et al. Tocilizumab prevents progression of early systemic sclerosis associated interstitial lung disease. Arthritis Rheumatol (Hoboken, NJ). 2021;73(7):1301–10.
101. Suleman Y, Clark KEN, Cole AR, Ong VH, Denton CP. Real-world experience of tocilizumab in systemic sclerosis: potential benefit on lung function for anti-topoisomerase-positive patients. Rheumatology (Oxford). 2021;60(8):3945–6.
102. Khanna D, Lin CJF, Furst DE, Wagner B, Zucchetto M, Raghu G, et al. Long-term safety and efficacy of tocilizumab in early systemic sclerosis-interstitial lung disease: open-label extension of a phase 3 randomized controlled trial. Am J Respir Crit Care Med. 2022;205(6):674–84.
103. Huang J, Beyer C, Palumbo-Zerr K, Zhang Y, Ramming A, Distler A, et al. Nintedanib inhibits fibroblast activation and ameliorates fibrosis in preclinical models of systemic sclerosis. Ann Rheum Dis. 2016;75(5):883–90.
104. Huang J, Maier C, Zhang Y, Soare A, Dees C, Beyer C, et al. Nintedanib inhibits macrophage activation and ameliorates vascular and fibrotic manifestations in the Fra2 mouse model of systemic sclerosis. Ann Rheum Dis. 2017;76(11):1941–8.
105. Richeldi L, Cottin V, du Bois RM, Selman M, Kimura T, Bailes Z, et al. Nintedanib in patients with idiopathic pulmonary fibrosis: combined evidence from the TOMORROW and INPULSIS(®) trials. Respir Med. 2016;113:74–9.
106. Distler O, Highland KB, Gahlemann M, Azuma A, Fischer A, Mayes MD, et al. Nintedanib for systemic sclerosis-associated interstitial lung disease. N Engl J Med. 2019;380(26):2518–28.
107. Volkmann ER, Kreuter M, Hoffmann-Vold AM, Wijsenbeek M, Smith V, Khanna D, et al. Dyspnoea and cough in patients with systemic sclerosis-associated interstitial lung disease in the SENSCIS trial. Rheumatology (Oxford). 2022;61:4397.
108. Richeldi L, Costabel U, Selman M, Kim DS, Hansell DM, Nicholson AG, et al. Efficacy of a tyrosine kinase inhibitor in idiopathic pulmonary fibrosis. N Engl J Med. 2011;365(12):1079–87.
109. Richeldi L, du Bois RM, Raghu G, Azuma A, Brown KK, Costabel U, et al. Efficacy and safety of nintedanib in idiopathic pulmonary fibrosis. N Engl J Med. 2014;370(22):2071–82.
110. Seibold JR, Maher TM, Highland KB, Assassi S, Azuma A, Hummers LK, et al. Safety and tolerability of nintedanib in patients with systemic sclerosis-associated interstitial lung disease: data from the SENSCIS trial. Ann Rheum Dis. 2020;79(11):1478–84.
111. Corte T, Bonella F, Crestani B, Demedts MG, Richeldi L, Coeck C, et al. Safety, tolerability and appropriate use of nintedanib in idiopathic pulmonary fibrosis. Respir Res. 2015;16:116.
112. Flaherty KR, Wells AU, Cottin V, Devaraj A, Walsh SLF, Inoue Y, et al. Nintedanib in progressive fibrosing interstitial lung diseases. N Engl J Med. 2019;381(18):1718–27.
113. Wells AU, Flaherty KR, Brown KK, Inoue Y, Devaraj A, Richeldi L, et al. Nintedanib in patients with progressive fibrosing interstitial lung diseases-subgroup analyses by interstitial lung disease diagnosis in the INBUILD trial: a randomised, double-blind, placebo-controlled, parallel-group trial. Lancet Respir Med. 2020;8(5):453–60.
114. Highland KB, Distler O, Kuwana M, Allanore Y, Assassi S, Azuma A, et al. Efficacy and safety of nintedanib in patients with systemic sclerosis-associated interstitial lung disease treated with mycophenolate: a subgroup analysis of the SENSCIS trial. Lancet Respir Med. 2021;9(1):96–106.
115. Gratwohl A, Passweg J, Gerber I, Tyndall A, International Stem Cell Project for Autoimmune Diseases. Stem cell transplantation for autoimmune diseases. Best Pract Res Clin Haematol. 2001;14(4):755–76.
116. Swart JF, Delemarre EM, van Wijk F, Boelens JJ, Kuball J, van Laar JM, et al. Haematopoietic stem cell transplantation for autoimmune diseases. Nat Rev Rheumatol. 2017;13(4):244–56.
117. Burt RK, Shah SJ, Dill K, Grant T, Gheorghiade M, Schroeder J, et al. Autologous non-myeloablative haemopoietic stem-cell transplantation compared with pulse cyclophosphamide once per month for systemic sclerosis (ASSIST): an open-label, randomised phase 2 trial. Lancet (London, England). 2011;378(9790):498–506.
118. van Laar JM, Farge D, Sont JK, Naraghi K, Marjanovic Z, Larghero J, et al. Autologous hematopoietic stem cell transplantation vs intravenous pulse cyclophosphamide in diffuse cutaneous systemic sclerosis: a randomized clinical trial. JAMA. 2014;311(24):2490–8.
119. Sullivan KM, Goldmuntz EA, Keyes-Elstein L, McSweeney PA, Pinckney A, Welch B, et al. Myeloablative autologous stem-cell transplantation for severe scleroderma. N Engl J Med. 2018;378(1):35–47.
120. Daikeler T, Tichelli A, Passweg J. Complications of autologous hematopoietic stem cell transplantation for patients with autoimmune diseases. Pediatr Res. 2012;71(4 Pt 2):439–44.
121. Maciejewska M, Snarski E, Wiktor-Jedrzejczak W. A preliminary online study on menstruation recovery in women after autologous hematopoietic stem cell transplant for autoimmune diseases. Exp Clin Transplant. 2016;14(6):665–9.
122. Kowal-Bielecka O, Fransen J, Avouac J, Becker M, Kulak A, Allanore Y, et al. Update of EULAR recommendations for the treatment of systemic sclerosis. Ann Rheum Dis. 2017;76(8):1327–39.
123. Kowal-Bielecka O, Landewe R, Avouac J, Chwiesko S, Miniati I, Czirjak L, et al. EULAR recommendations for the treatment of systemic sclerosis: a report from the EULAR Scleroderma Trials and Research group (EUSTAR). Ann Rheum Dis. 2009;68(5):620–8.
124. Pradere P, Tudorache I, Magnusson J, Savale L, Brugiere O, Douvry B, et al. Lung transplantation for scleroderma lung disease: an international, multicenter, observational cohort study. J Heart Lung Transplant. 2018;37(7):903–11.
125. Yusen RD, Edwards LB, Dipchand AI, Goldfarb SB, Kucheryavaya AY, Levvey BJ, et al. The Registry of the International Society for Heart and Lung Transplantation: thirty-third adult lung and heart-lung transplant Report-2016; focus theme: primary diagnostic indications for transplant. J Heart Lung Transplant. 2016;35(10):1170–84.
126. Crespo MM, Bermudez CA, Dew MA, Johnson BA, George MP, Bhama J, et al. Lung transplant in patients with scleroderma compared with pulmonary fibrosis. Short- and long-term outcomes. Ann Am Thorac Soc. 2016;13(6):784–92.

127. Roofeh D, Lescoat A, Khanna D. Treatment for systemic sclerosis-associated interstitial lung disease. Curr Opin Rheumatol. 2021;33(3):240–8.
128. King TE Jr, Bradford WZ, Castro-Bernardini S, Fagan EA, Glaspole I, Glassberg MK, et al. A phase 3 trial of pirfenidone in patients with idiopathic pulmonary fibrosis. N Engl J Med. 2014;370(22):2083–92.
129. Acharya N, Sharma SK, Mishra D, Dhooria S, Dhir V, Jain S. Efficacy and safety of pirfenidone in systemic sclerosis-related interstitial lung disease-a randomised controlled trial. Rheumatol Int. 2020;40(5):703–10.
130. Behr J, Prasse A, Kreuter M, Johow J, Rabe KF, Bonella F, et al. Pirfenidone in patients with progressive fibrotic interstitial lung diseases other than idiopathic pulmonary fibrosis (RELIEF): a double-blind, randomised, placebo-controlled, phase 2b trial. Lancet Respir Med. 2021;9(5):476–86.
131. Slack RJ, Macdonald SJF, Roper JA, Jenkins RG, Hatley RJD. Emerging therapeutic opportunities for integrin inhibitors. Nat Rev Drug Discov. 2022;21(1):60–78.
132. Hecker L, Cheng J, Thannickal VJ. Targeting NOX enzymes in pulmonary fibrosis. Cell Mol Life Sci. 2012;69(14):2365–71.
133. Maher TM, van der Aar EM, Van de Steen O, Allamassey L, Desrivot J, Dupont S, et al. Safety, tolerability, pharmacokinetics, and pharmacodynamics of GLPG1690, a novel autotaxin inhibitor, to treat idiopathic pulmonary fibrosis (FLORA): a phase 2a randomised placebo-controlled trial. Lancet Respir Med. 2018;6(8):627–35.
134. Tam AYY, Horwell AL, Trinder SL, Khan K, Xu S, Ong V, et al. Selective deletion of connective tissue growth factor attenuates experimentally-induced pulmonary fibrosis and pulmonary arterial hypertension. Int J Biochem Cell Biol. 2021;134:105961.
135. Richeldi L, Fernández Pérez ER, Costabel U, Albera C, Lederer DJ, Flaherty KR, et al. Pamrevlumab, an anti-connective tissue growth factor therapy, for idiopathic pulmonary fibrosis (PRAISE): a phase 2, randomised, double-blind, placebo-controlled trial. Lancet Respir Med. 2020;8(1):25–33.
136. Murray LA, Rosada R, Moreira AP, Joshi A, Kramer MS, Hesson DP, et al. Serum amyloid P therapeutically attenuates murine bleomycin-induced pulmonary fibrosis via its effects on macrophages. PLoS One. 2010;5(3):e9683.
137. Murray LA, Chen Q, Kramer MS, Hesson DP, Argentieri RL, Peng X, et al. TGF-beta driven lung fibrosis is macrophage dependent and blocked by Serum amyloid P. Int J Biochem Cell Biol. 2011;43(1):154–62.
138. Castaño AP, Lin SL, Surowy T, Nowlin BT, Turlapati SA, Patel T, et al. Serum amyloid P inhibits fibrosis through Fc gamma R-dependent monocyte-macrophage regulation in vivo. Sci Transl Med. 2009;1(5):5ra13.
139. Raghu G, van den Blink B, Hamblin MJ, Brown AW, Golden JA, Ho LA, et al. Effect of recombinant human pentraxin 2 vs placebo on change in forced vital capacity in patients with idiopathic pulmonary fibrosis: a randomized clinical trial. JAMA. 2018;319(22):2299–307.
140. Raghu G, van den Blink B, Hamblin MJ, Brown AW, Golden JA, Ho LA, et al. Long-term treatment with recombinant human pentraxin 2 protein in patients with idiopathic pulmonary fibrosis: an open-label extension study. Lancet Respir Med. 2019;7(8):657–64.
141. Waxman A, Restrepo-Jaramillo R, Thenappan T, Ravichandran A, Engel P, Bajwa A, et al. Inhaled treprostinil in pulmonary hypertension due to interstitial lung disease. N Engl J Med. 2021;384(4):325–34.
142. Nathan SD, Waxman A, Rajagopal S, Case A, Johri S, DuBrock H, et al. Inhaled treprostinil and forced vital capacity in patients with interstitial lung disease and associated pulmonary hypertension: a post-hoc analysis of the INCREASE study. Lancet Respir Med. 2021;9(11):1266–74.
143. Richeldi L, Azuma A, Cottin V, Hesslinger C, Stowasser S, Valenzuela C, et al. Trial of a preferential phosphodiesterase 4B inhibitor for idiopathic pulmonary fibrosis. N Engl J Med. 2022;386(23):2178–87.
144. Garvey C. Interstitial lung disease and pulmonary rehabilitation. J Cardiopulm Rehabil Prev. 2010;30(3):141–6.
145. Dowman L, Hill CJ, May A, Holland AE. Pulmonary rehabilitation for interstitial lung disease. Cochrane Database Syst Rev. 2021;2(2):Cd006322.
146. Visca D, Mori L, Tsipouri V, Fleming S, Firouzi A, Bonini M, et al. Effect of ambulatory oxygen on quality of life for patients with fibrotic lung disease (AmbOx): a prospective, open-label, mixed-method, crossover randomised controlled trial. Lancet Respir Med. 2018;6(10):759–70.
147. Christmann RB, Wells AU, Capelozzi VL, Silver RM. Gastroesophageal reflux incites interstitial lung disease in systemic sclerosis: clinical, radiologic, histopathologic, and treatment evidence. Semin Arthritis Rheum. 2010;40(3):241–9.
148. Matucci-Cerinic M, Bruni C, Allanore Y, Clementi M, Dagna L, Damjanov NS, et al. Systemic sclerosis and the COVID-19 pandemic: World Scleroderma Foundation preliminary advice for patient management. Ann Rheum Dis. 2020;79(6):724–6.
149. Avouac J, Drumez E, Hachulla E, Seror R, Georgin-Lavialle S, El Mahou S, et al. COVID-19 outcomes in patients with inflammatory rheumatic and musculoskeletal diseases treated with rituximab: a cohort study. Lancet Rheumatol. 2021;3(6):e419–e26.
150. Russo B, Ben Shimol J, Matucci-Cerinic M, Bruni C. Systemic sclerosis and COVID-19: what's new in the literature. Clin Exp Rheumatol. 2021;39 Suppl 131(4):157–8.
151. Ferri C, Ursini F, Gragnani L, Raimondo V, Giuggioli D, Foti R, et al. Impaired immunogenicity to COVID-19 vaccines in autoimmune systemic diseases. High prevalence of non-response in different patients' subgroups. J Autoimmun. 2021;125:102744.
152. Fernández-Codina A, Walker KM, Pope JE. Treatment algorithms for systemic sclerosis according to experts. Arthritis Rheumatol. 2018;70(11):1820–8.
153. Bruni C, Furst DE. The burning question: to use or not to use cyclophosphamide in systemic sclerosis. Eur J Rheumatol. 2020;7(Suppl 3):S237–s41.
154. Volkmann ER, Chung A, Tashkin DP. Managing systemic sclerosis-related interstitial lung disease in the modern treatment era. J Scleroderma Relat Disord. 2017;2(2):72–83.
155. Khanna D, Lescoat A, Roofeh D, Bernstein EJ, Kazerooni EA, Roth MD, et al. Systemic sclerosis-associated interstitial lung disease: how to incorporate two food and drug administration-approved therapies in clinical practice. Arthritis Rheumatol. 2022;74(1):13–27.
156. Roofeh D, Distler O, Allanore Y, Denton CP, Khanna D. Treatment of systemic sclerosis-associated interstitial lung disease: Lessons from clinical trials. J Scleroderma Relat Disord. 2020;5(2 Suppl):61–71. PMID: 35382226
157. Giuggioli D, Lumetti F, Colaci M, Fallahi P, Antonelli A, Ferri C. Rituximab in the treatment of patients with systemic sclerosis. Our experience and review of the literature. Autoimmun Rev. 2015;14(11):1072–8.
158. Elhai M, Meunier M, Matucci-Cerinic M, Maurer B, Riemekasten G, Leturcq T, et al. Outcomes of patients with systemic sclerosis-associated polyarthritis and myopathy treated with tocilizumab or abatacept: a EUSTAR observational study. Ann Rheum Dis. 2013;72(7):1217–20.

Pathogenesis of Pulmonary Arterial Hypertension

27

Markella Ponticos, Michael H. Lee, Alan M. Holmes, and Rubin M. Tuder

Pulmonary arterial hypertension (PAH) is a progressive, incurable pulmonary vascular disease characterized by structural remodeling of the small pulmonary arteries and increased blood pressure in the pulmonary circulation, culminating in right ventricular failure. With an estimated prevalence of up to approximately 50 per million population [1, 2], PAH represents a form of precapillary pulmonary hypertension (PH), also categorized as group I Pulmonary Hypertension by the World Health Organization classification system [3].

Our understanding of PAH has been rapidly expanding in recent years. Since the first edition of this chapter, there have been several gains in new knowledge of cellular and molecular insights in the mechanism of the disease, based on technological breakthroughs in omics and next generation sequencing to characterize the disease, with a significant translation of much of this knowledge for therapeutic advantage of PAH patients.

The field of PAH has continued to evolve, marking the past decade with notable advancements [4]. The establishment of bone morphogenetic protein (BMP) type 2 receptor (BMPRII) and transforming growth factor-β (TGF-β) superfamily signaling as promising therapeutic targets is an example, one that particularly underscores the importance of a close interplay between clinical and fundamental research scientists. Not very long after the recognition of BMPRII mutations in PAH patients [5–8], benefit of restoring BMP9-BMPRII signaling was shown in animal studies [9–11] and the promising role of sotatercept, a ligand trap with affinity for activin and growth and differentiation factor (GDF), has now been demonstrated in a phase 2 clinical trial [12]. Tacrolimus, which acts on the same pathway, is now emerging as another potential therapeutic option [13, 14]. Although optimal ways to rebalance TGF-β superfamily signaling pathways are still being elucidated [15–17], BMP9-BMPRII augmentation represents a novel, anti-remodeling approach to managing PAH patients, beyond the paradigms of pulmonary vasodilation.

The past few years have also been marked by attempts to reevaluate diagnostic and therapeutic strategies in PAH management. At the Sixth World Symposium in Pulmonary Hypertension, held in 2018 (Nice, France), revising the hemodynamic definitions of PH was suggested, specifically lowering the mean pulmonary artery pressure (mPAP) cutoff from ≥25 to >20 mmHg, without a corresponding change in the cutoffs for pulmonary artery wedge pressure (≤15 mmHg) or pulmonary vascular resistance (≥3 Wood units) [3, 18]. This new diagnostic recommendation more accurately reflects physiologic mPAP values in healthy individuals [19], and it considers the prognostic importance of borderline elevated mPAP [20–22] and early treatment initiation in PAH

M. Ponticos (✉) · A. M. Holmes
Centre for Rheumatology, Division of Medicine, University College London, Royal Free Hospital, London, UK
e-mail: m.ponticos@ucl.ac.uk; alan.holmes@ucl.ac.uk

M. H. Lee
Division of Pulmonary and Critical Care Medicine, Department of Medicine, University of California San Francisco, San Francisco, CA, USA
e-mail: Michael.Lee8@ucsf.edu

R. M. Tuder
Division of Pulmonary Sciences and Critical Care Medicine, Department of Medicine, University of Colorado, Aurora, CO, USA
e-mail: rubin.tuder@cuanschutz.edu

Y. Allanore et al. (eds.), *Scleroderma*, https://doi.org/10.1007/978-3-031-40658-4_27

[23–26]. Although criticized for limited clinical impact and the paucity of data guiding treatment [27–29], the newly suggested mPAP cutoff of >20 mmHg, together with studies examining the inclusion of prostacyclin analogues as an initial therapy [30–32], represents collective effort to improve PAH outcomes by intervening at an early stage of disease, with upfront aggressive treatments.

The recent efforts to refine management of PAH patients is particularly fitting for PAH associated with SSc (SSc-PAH), which carries a particularly grim prognosis, with a shorter expected survival than other causes of PAH and even other subtypes of connective tissue disease-associated PAH (CTD-PAH) [33–36]. While SSc-PAH might also benefit from early, intensive therapy [37–42], SSc-PAH remains a major cause of death in SSc patients [43–47]. The currently incurable nature of PAH and the particularly poor outcome of SSc-PAH patients indicate the need for a deeper understanding of the PAH pathobiology, and an appreciation for its pathologic heterogeneity, which we further discuss in the following text. The development of pulmonary arterial hypertension (PAH) represents a serious comorbidity in collagen vascular diseases (CVD). This complication is commonly observed in SSc patients where the risk of developing PAH persists throughout the disease. Affecting up to 10% of patients, SSc appears to act as a susceptibility factor in the development of PAH [2, 3]. While significant progress has been made in understanding the pathological mechanisms that contribute to the development and progression of heritable and idiopathic forms of PAH, the relative pathogenic mechanisms that contribute to the development of PAH in SSc patients remain less appreciated. Indeed, SSc-PAH patients have a significantly poorer prognosis compared to other forms [4]. Here, we discuss the key pathological findings in PAH and fundamental pathobiological mechanisms implicated in the development and progression of PAH, particularly in SSc patients.

Although a few therapeutic candidates, such as anti-IL-6 tocilizumab [48, 49] and B lymphocyte-depleting rituximab [50], recently showed absent or inconclusive clinical benefits, the PAH field continues to explore novel treatments [4] (Table 27.1). These include serotonin synthesis inhibition with rodatristat (NCT04712669), anti-estrogen therapies with anastrozole [51] and tamoxifen (NCT03528902), and progenitor cells [52] (NCT03001414). While once associated with subdural hematomas and other safety concerns [53–55], imatinib mesylate is being reconsidered for PAH management (NCT04416750), particularly as an inhaled therapy (NCT05036135, NCT04903730). Seralutinib is another tyrosine kinase inhibitor being trialed (NCT04456998/NCT04816604). It is important to note that each of these treatment modalities represents the ongoing endeavor by the PAH field to uncover molecular and pathobiological underpinnings of the disease that underly individual pulmonary vascular lesions. Amid exciting clinical trials, appreciation of the pathobiological complexity and the pathologic heterogeneity of PAH will remain the cornerstone of novel therapies and improved outcomes.

Group 1 PAH contains, in addition to IPAH (and its closely related familial/genetic counterpart), related but also disparate diseases, including collagen vascular disease, HIV infection, anorectic and addiction-related drugs, and schistosomiasis [3]. While all of the forms of PAH have some shared pathology, there are structural differences in the scope of pulmonary vascular remodeling, which may underlie different pathogenetic processes. For instance, while pulmonary media and intima remodeling can occur in IPAH and collagen vascular disease-associated PAH (CVD-PAH) such scleroderma (SSc) associated PAH, an association with interstitial lung disease is predominantly seen in the latter. All forms of PAH have significant inflammation; however, the specific type of inflammatory cells and cytokines and how they affect pathogenesis may differ, such as between portopulmonary hypertension vs. schistosomiasis-associated PAH. It is becoming apparent that a TH1/M1-driven inflammation (characterized by activation of interferon-γ, TNF-α, IL12/IL18) or TH2/M2 inflammation (characterized by IL4/IL13, TGF-β, among others) may ultimately affect how a particular cause of PAH ultimately results in pulmonary vascular disease.

In studying PAH, we have to rely on the knowledge derived from shared and distinct insights gained from the conglomerate investigations in each subtype of disease. Indeed, despite the significant insights into PAH pathogenesis [56–59], we have still a lot to learn especially about which disease features are shared and which are unique. In addition, many key pathogenetic processes that are based mostly on investigations centered around IPAH may also appear to be shared, and it is imperative that we recognize the heterogeneity of the conditions in Group 1. In the present review, the authors chose to focus on key pathological features of PAH and then relate these alterations with key pathogenetic process. These include the role of growth factors, metabolic reprogramming, and inflammation.

In the current edition, we use the term "associated PAH," or APAH, to designate PAH arising secondary to systemic rheumatic diseases. APAH is also commonly referred to as connective tissue disease-associated PAH (CTD-PAH) and collagen vascular disease-associated PAH (CVD-PAH), all of which are synonymous with each other. In addition to the routinely used and widely established clinical subgroups of PAH (e.g., IPAH, FPAH, APAH, SSc-PAH, drug-induced PAH…etc.), in our discussion of disease heterogeneity, we introduce an additional categorization of pathology-based PAH patterns into four distinctive types: PAH-like pattern, FPAH-like pattern, APAH-like pattern, and VOD-like pattern.

Table 27.1 Pathways targeted for clinical intervention in PAH. This is an abridged list with only approved treatments (blue), trials with positive endpoints or ongoing trials included

Pathway	Drug	Target	Status	Reference or Clinicaltrials.gov ID
Endothelin-1 (ET-1)	Bosentan	ETA and ETB receptor	Approved	[217]
	Macitentan	ETA and ETB receptor	Approved	[218]
	Ambrisentan	ETA receptor	Approved	[219]
Prostacyclin (PGI_2)	Epoprostenol	PGI_2 receptor	Approved	[220]
	Treprostinil	PGI_2 receptor	Approved	[221, 222]
	Iloprost	PGI_2 receptor	Approved	[220]
	Selexipag	PGI_2 receptor	Approved	[71]
Nitric Oxide (NO)	Riociguat	soluble Guanylate Cyclase	Approved	[223]
	Sildenafil	Phosphodiesterase type 5	Approved	[224]
	Tadalafil	Phosphodiesterase type 5	Approved	[225]
Bone morphogenic protein (BMP)/Activin	Sotatercept	Activin (ligand trap)	Phase 2	[12]
BMP Receptor 2 signalling	Tacrolimus (FK506)	Calcineurin/BMPR2	Phase 2a	[14]
Tyrosine kinase /PDGF signalling	Imatinib (inhaled)	Tyrosine Kinase receptors, PDGFR	Phase 2b/3	NCT05036135
Tyrosine kinase/PDGF signaling	Seralutinib	Tyrosine Kinase receptors, PDGFR	Phase 2	NCT04456998 NCT04816604
Serotonin	Rodatristat Ethyl	Tryptophan Hydroxylase 1	Phase 2b	NCT04712669 [226]
Inflammation	Rituximab	B-lymphocyte antigen CD20	Phase 2	[50]
Inflammation	Elafin	Elastase-specific protease	Phase 1	[227]
Inflammation	Sulfasalazine	Cystine transporter subunit (xCT)	Phase 1	NCT04528056
Metabolism	Metformin	AMP-activated Protein kinase	Phase 2	[228]
Metabolism	Bardoxolone	Nrf2, NFkB	Phase 2	NCT02657356
Oestrogen signalling	Anastrozole	Aromatase	Phase 2	NCT03229499
Oestrogen signalling	Tamoxifen	Oestrogen receptor	Phase 2	NCT03528902
Angiotensin	Recombinant ACE2	Angiotensin-converting enzyme (ACE)	Phase 2	NCT01884051
Aldosterone	Spironolactone	Aldosterone receptor blocker	Phase 2	[229]
DNA repair	Olaparib	Poly(ADP-ribosyl)transferase	Phase 1b	NCT03782818
Epigenetic regulation	Apabetalone	Bromodomain-Containing Protein 4	Phase 1	NCT04915300
Dopamine	Zamicastat	Dopamine Beta-Hydroxylase	Phase 2	NCT04316143
Vasoactive Intestinal Peptide	Pemziviptadil	Vasoactive intestinal polypeptide receptor 1 and 2	Phase 2	NCT03795428

Pathology of Scleroderma-Associated Pulmonary Arterial Hypertension

In the prior edition of this chapter, we have described in detail the spectrum of the pulmonary vascular pathology of SSc-PAH [60]. Central to considering the pathological spectrum of pulmonary vascular lesions in SSc-PAH is the understanding of the structure of the pulmonary circulation. We strongly recommend that the reader refers to a more detailed description of this unique vascular architecture as it relates to pulmonary vascular physiology [61, 62]. In summary, a handful of three-dimensional casting-reconstruction studies demonstrated that a single pulmonary artery branch successively forms a fractal structure with 17 orders of vascular segments. The smallest identifiable segments by this approach are in the order of 25 μm diameter small arteries, which amount to approximately 25 million segments (the more distal segments down to the capillaries cannot be evaluated because of limitations of the casting method).

In 2012, we summarized our experience with 12 cases of CTD-PAH, including SSc-PAH [63]. In contrast to our initial impression that SSc-PAH has a more distinct pathology, with less or no plexiform lesions, the pathologic spectrum and frequency of the lesions were overall similar to the 48 cases of IPAH [64] in this cohort of the Pulmonary Hypertension Breakthrough Initiative (PHBI) (Fig. 27.1). Remarkably, we did not observe pulmonary venous disease as previously reported [65].

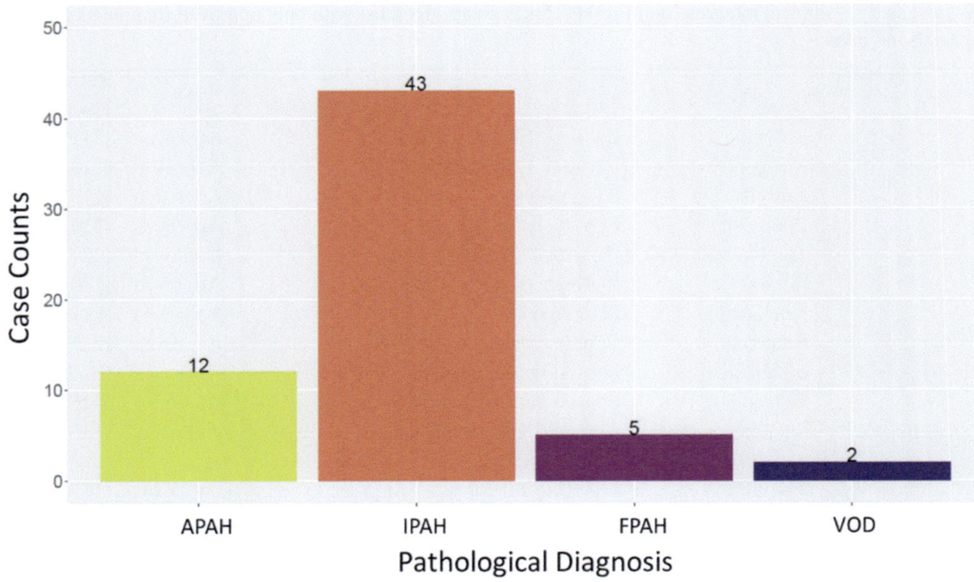

Fig. 27.1 Overall frequency of histopathological PAH patterns in the cohort. The IPAH pattern includes lungs with idiopathic PAH, PAH with congenital heart malformations ($n = 9$), drug and -associated. The familial or hereditary cases are included separately, though also with an IPAH morphology (FPAH). VOD (venocclusive disease). (Based and adapted on [63] with permission of the American Thoracic Society. Copyright © 2022 American Thoracic Society. All rights reserved. The American Journal of Respiratory and Critical Care Medicine is an official journal of the American Thoracic Society. Readers are encouraged to read the entire article for the correct context at [63]. The authors, editors, and The American Thoracic Society are not responsible for errors or omissions in adaptations)

Comparative Pathology of CTD-PAH vs. Other Forms of PAH

We have recently highlighted that a critical challenge in the field of PAH is the fact that the pathology of pulmonary vascular lesions is highly heterogeneous [66], both among lungs with similar underlying pathological patterns and among different regions of the same PAH lung. In this section, it is our goal to further underscore this heterogeneity, which involves a reassessment of the clinical vs. pathological characteristics found in the study of 2012. To achieve this goal, the published dataset was reevaluated using Principal Component Analyses using the R package. These data are best interpreted in the context of the original data [63].

The PHBI cohort was assembled with multiple clinical parameters pertinent to pulmonary hemodynamics, laboratory data, and patient demographics, ultimately leading to a tentative clinical diagnosis, such as idiopathic IPAH, associated PAH (APAH), and PAH-associated with congenital heart malformations, familial or hereditary PAH, and drug-induced PAH.

Based on our experience of the spectrum of the pathology of pulmonary vascular disease [61, 67, 68], we opted in the original publication for reporting the final diagnosis based on the pathological pattern rather than the underlying clinical diagnosis in Stacher et al. [63] (Fig. 27.2). The various clinical subtypes of PAH were pathologically categorized into the following three patterns: IPAH-like pattern, APAH-like pattern, and venoocclusive disease-like pattern.

The study on the modern pathology of PAH involved: characterization of the pulmonary vascular remodeling based on measurements of the intima, media, combined intima + media, and adventitia thickening in circular profiles of pulmonary arteries; assessment of the number of profiles of plexiform lesions; and a semiquantitative assessment of perivascular inflammation [63] (Fig. 27.3). Controls consisted of donor lungs that were rejected from the option of lung transplantation. We noted that these control lungs were segregated into two groups, one younger (22 lungs) and an older one, above 50 years of age, with more marked pulmonary vascular remodeling (6 lungs) (Fig. 27.4a, b, d). As it is apparent from the principal component analysis (PCA) of the control lungs, despite some superposition of the clustering of younger (CTL) and older groups, four older lungs (CTL2) separated from the younger control cluster (Fig. 27.5). It is of interest that the variance of the intima is the largest when the variance of the media is the lowest, while the variance of the adventitia thickening is intermediate between the intima and media. The variance of the intima tracks closely with that of the sum of the thickness of the intima and media. The implications of the increased remodeling, including aspects related to pulmonary vascular adaptation to age and decreased pulmonary vascular reserve, are discussed in more detail in the prior edition of this chapter [60].

The PAH cases had more marked intima, media, and combined intima + media thickening (Figs. 27.3 and 27.4a–d). The degree of these parameters of pulmonary vascular

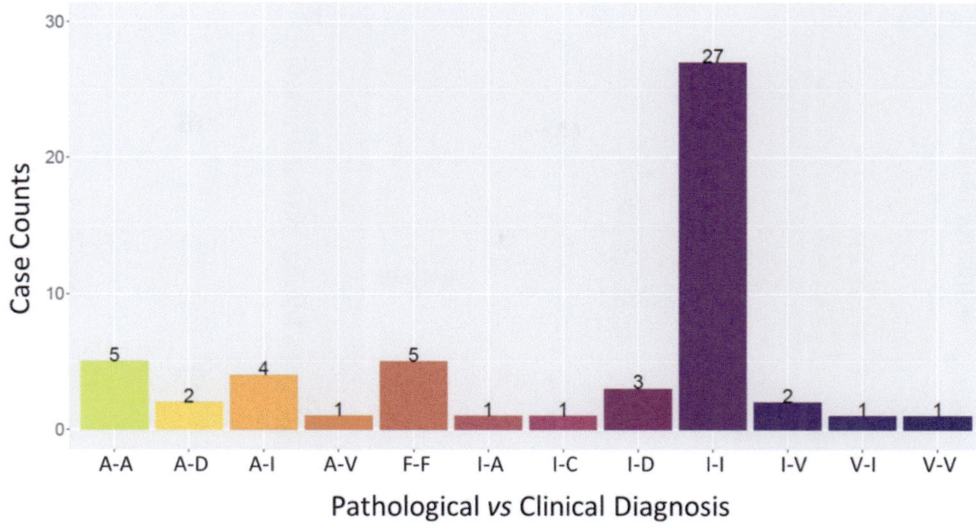

Fig. 27.2 Distribution of lungs based on the status of the concordance or discordance between the pathological pattern (First Letter = A: APAH, F: FPAH, I: IPAH, V: venocclusive disease) and the clinical diagnosis (second letter = A: APAH, D: drug induced PH, I: idiopathic PAH, C: Chronic Thromboembolic Disease, F: FPAH, V: venocclusive disease)

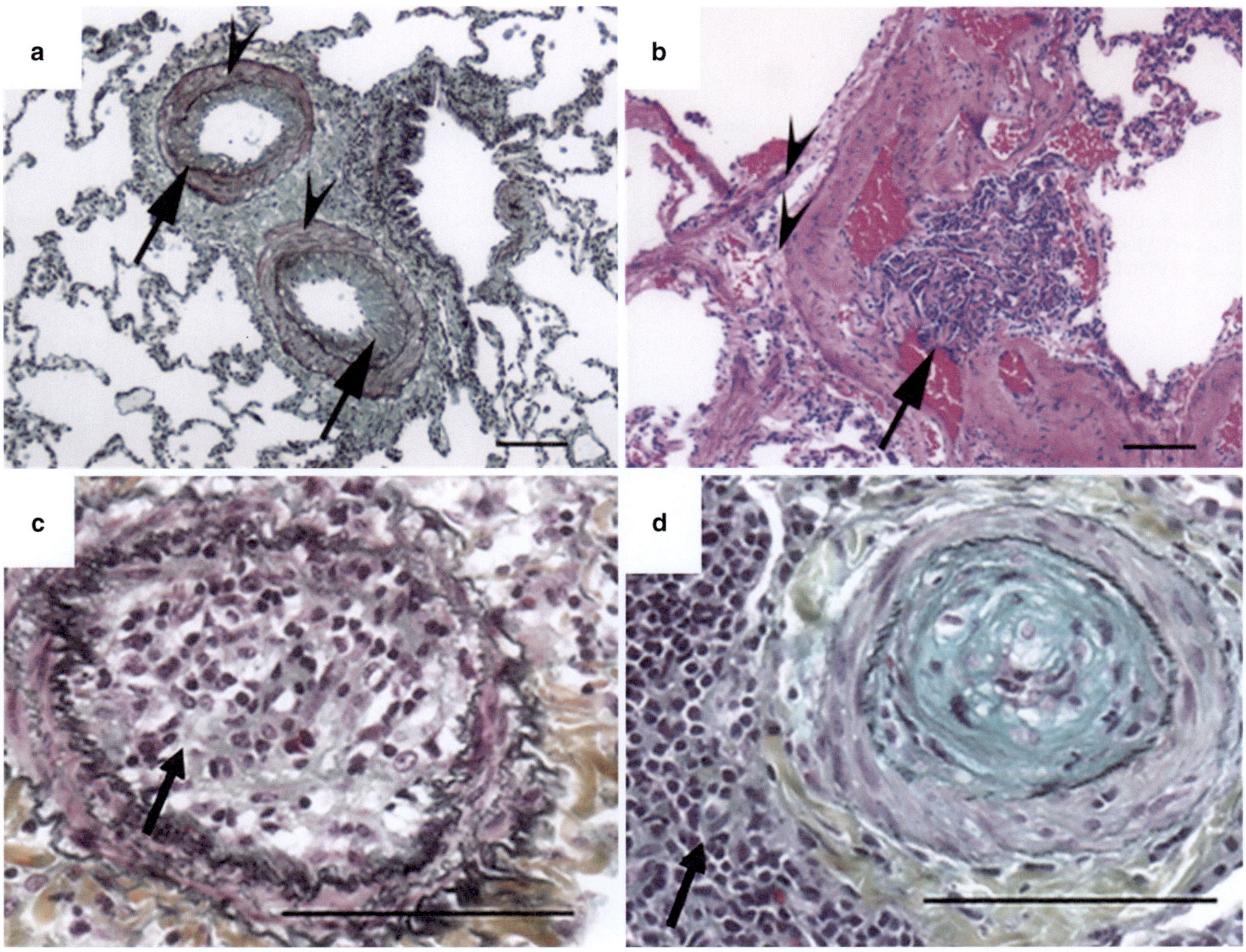

Fig. 27.3 Histopathological parameters indicative of pulmonary vascular remodeling in pulmonary arterial hypertension. (**a**) Intima thickening, media thickening (long arrows), and adventitia. The quantification of these parameters in control and PAH lungs is described in [63]. (**b**) Plexiform lesion (arrows), characteristic lesion in PAH. (**c**) Obliterative lesion with intravascular and perivascular inflammation (arrow). (**d**) Concentric lesion with lymphoid aggregate in the adventitia (arrow). (Based on [63] and reproduced with permission of the American Thoracic Society. Copyright © 2022 American Thoracic Society. All rights reserved. The American Journal of Respiratory and Critical Care Medicine is an official journal of the American Thoracic Society. Readers are encouraged to read the entire article for the correct context at [63]. The authors, editors, and The American Thoracic Society are not responsible for errors or omissions in adaptations)

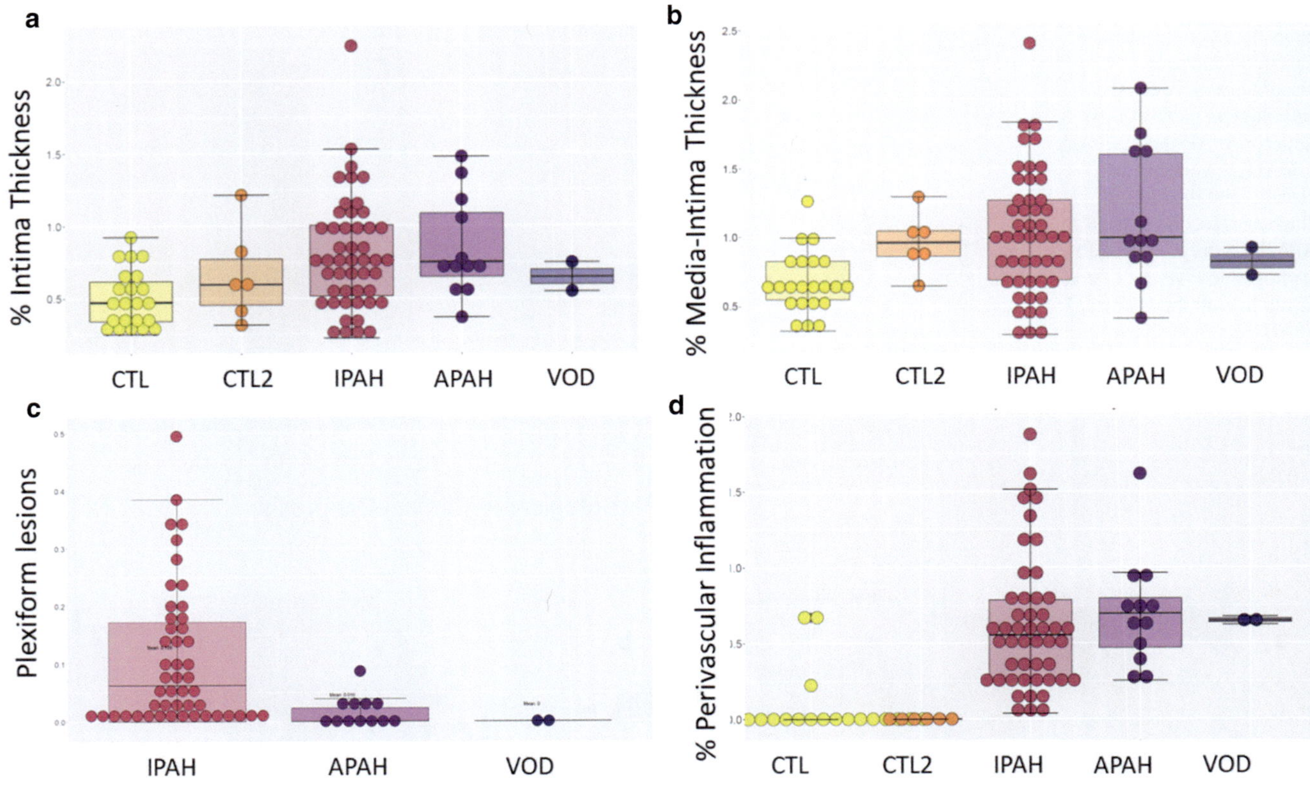

Fig. 27.4 Pulmonary vascular remodeling. (**a**) Intima thickness in control (CTL), aged controls (CTL2), IPAH, APAH, and venocclusive disease (VOD). (**b**) Media + intima thickening. (**c**) Number of profiles of plexifom lesion (note that control cases do not have plexiform lesion and were not included in the graph). (**d**) Perivascular inflammation score. (Based in [63])

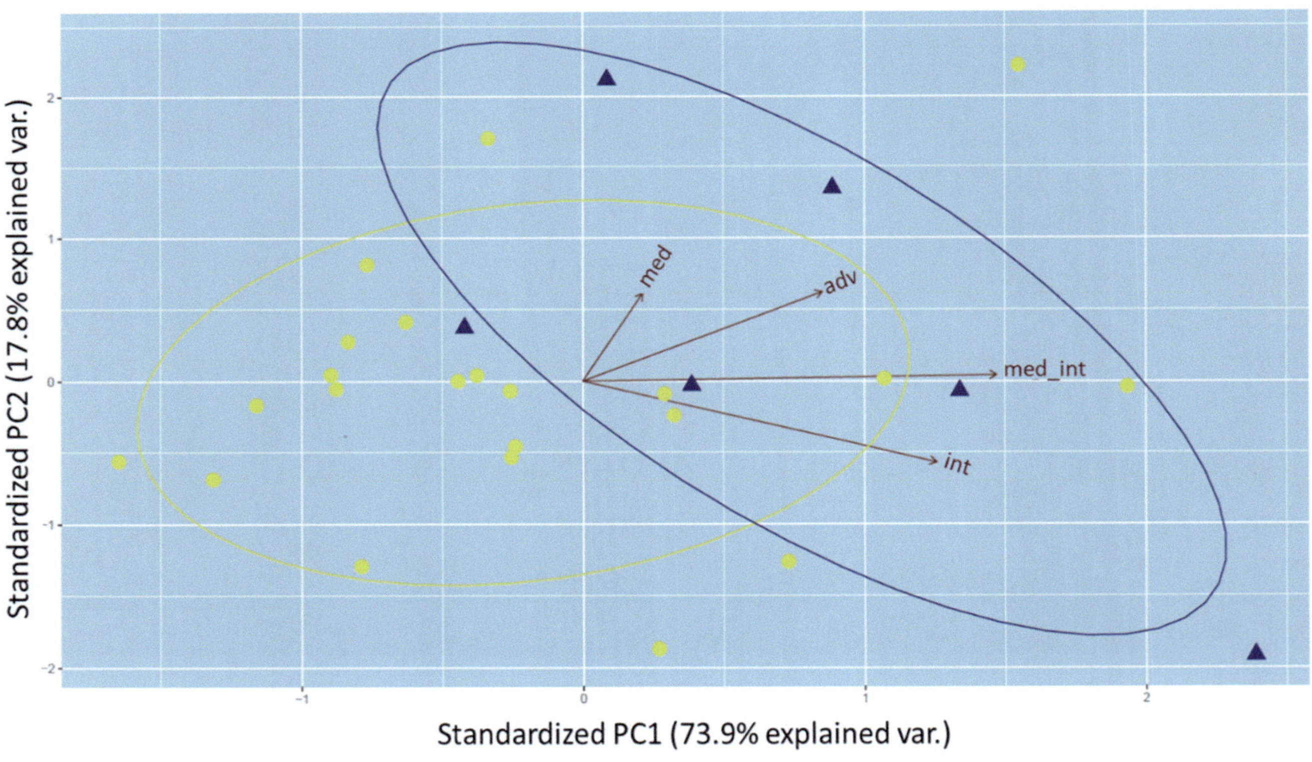

Fig. 27.5 Principal component analyses (PCA) of control (CTL, yellow) and aged controls (CTL2, blue) (based in [63]). Vectors indicate measure of variance along PC1 and PC2, involving intima thickness (int), media thickness (med), intima + media thickness (int_med), adventitia thickness (adv), number of profiles of plexiform lesions (plx) and perivascular inflammation score (inf). Each point represents the values of single lungs. (Based in [63])

remodeling is overall similar between pathologically diagnosed APAH vs. IPAH.

Plexiform lesions were detected in both pathological IPAH and APAH patterns (Fig. 27.4c). As a group, IPAH had a mean of tenfold higher number of plexiform lesion profiles per area sampled than the APAH pattern ($p < 0.001$). This supports our impression that plexiform lesions are not as frequently observed in APAH as in IPAH [7]. Notably, both IPAH and APAH demonstrated significant heterogeneity in the number of profiles of the plexiform lesion (as illustrated in Fig. E10 in Stacher et al. [63]).

The important association of perivascular inflammation with pulmonary vascular remodeling and pulmonary hemodynamics was underscored by the previous analyses of the PHBI cohort [63]. However, there were no significant differences between the IPAH- vs. APAH-pathological patterns (Fig. 27.4d). Again, as formerly underscored [63], there is significant heterogeneity in the inflammation score among the cases in the PAH group.

Examination of the pulmonary vascular remodeling data and a more detailed pathological analysis based on concordance vs. discordance between the pathological patterns and clinical diagnoses provide interesting insights into pathologic heterogeneity in PAH. The concordance between the pathological pattern and clinical diagnosis was observed in 5(12) APAH, all 5 familial/hereditary cases (as the IPAH morphology is like sporadic vs. hereditary PAH), and 27(34) sporadic PAH (Fig. 27.2). The discordance between the pathological vs. clinical diagnosis was more evident in cases of APAH, which was clinically interpreted as IPAH (4/12), drug-induced (amphetamine use) (2/12), or venocclusive disease (VOD) (1/12). Of the cases clinically diagnosed as APAH, three were due to scleroderma, one due to Lupus, and one due to rheumatoid arthritis. Interestingly, 2/4 of clinically diagnosed VODs had an APAH and an IPAH pattern (Fig. 27.2).

The discordant cases of APAH pathological patterns with a clinical diagnosis of drug-induced PH ($n = 2$) fell within the range of intima thickness seen in the concordant APAH cases (Fig. 27.2). A similar overall pattern was observed with media thickness as well (Fig. 27.6); it is noteworthy that the most prominent media remodeling was found in a case of IPAH pattern with the clinical diagnosis of chronic thromboembolic disease (I-C in Fig. 27.6) and IPAH pattern with the clinical diagnosis of VOD (I-V in Fig. 27.6).

Notwithstanding the novel findings related to perivascular inflammation in the PHBI study and its correlation with remodeling and hemodynamics, there were no significant differences based on concordance vs. discordance of pathological vs. clinical diagnosis (Fig. 27.7).

The PCA provided further interesting insights into the overall characteristics of the control vs. PAH cases. The PCA of control vs. PAH lungs (irrespective of the specific pathological pattern, i.e., all cases of APAH, IPAH, and VOD were considered as PAH) reveal some degree of shared clustering between the controls, and aged controls (labeled as CTL2), and the PAH lungs. There is a significant degree of heterogeneity in PAH cases as illustrated by the eight lungs that are plotted beyond the 0.68 ellipse probability. The variability is accounted mostly by the morphological parameters of the intima, media, intima + media, and adventitia thickness. Three of these eight lungs were APAH, while the remaining were IPAH patterns. Interestingly, two of the five IPAH patterns had a clinical diagnosis of APAH.

The PCA for the pathological patterns of APAH and IPAH reveals a marked sharing of the main clusters (Fig. 27.8). Ten APAH lungs (10/12) were also included in the 0.68 probability ellipse for IPAH, underscoring the marked shared pathological parameters between both pathological parameters. On the other hand, 14 of 48 IPAH pathological cases did not fall within the IPAH probability ellipse, highlighting the angle of heterogeneity of IPAH pathology. It is of interest that 7/12 APAH lungs were included in the IPAH probability ellipse, underscoring their shared variability with the morphological parameters. Intima, media, intima + media, and adventitia contributed most to the variability accounted in principal component or dimension 1 (dim1), while plexiform lesions and perivascular inflammation accounted for most of the variability in principal components or dimensions 2 and 3 (dim2 and dim3) (Fig. 27.9).

Eleven 11(53) cases fell outside the APAH and IPAH probability ellipses, i.e., those lungs with the highest levels of loading scores and therefore variability along with principal components 1 and 2. Only one of 11 had a discrepant APAH pathological vs. IPAH clinical diagnosis (with one that was APAH concordant). Interestingly, three of five FPAH fell outside the probability ellipses. In our original report, we documented the more marked remodeling in FPAH cases when compared with the sporadic IPAH pattern [63].

In conclusion, it is apparent from the original reporting and this reassessment that there is significant pathological heterogeneity in PAH, most notably in IPAH pathology. Moreover, there is a significant number of cases of APAH and IPAH pathology with a discrepant clinical diagnosis.

As we have outlined in our perspective on the cancer hypothesis of PAH [66], this pathological heterogeneity requires the incorporation of molecular tools to elucidate if the lesions in PAH have a similar molecular signature or their variability among different patients in both IPAH and APAH. Novel approaches reliant on digital special profiling are now available to answer these pressing questions.

Fig. 27.6 (**a**) Intima thickening, (**b**) Media thickening, (**c**) Perivascular inflammation in concordant vs. discordant cases. (First Letter = A: APAH, F: FPAH, I: IPAH, V: venocclusive disease) and the clinical diagnosis (second letter = A: APAH, D: drug induced PH, I: idiopathic PAH, C: Chronic Thromboembolic Disease, F: FPAH, V: venocclusive disease)

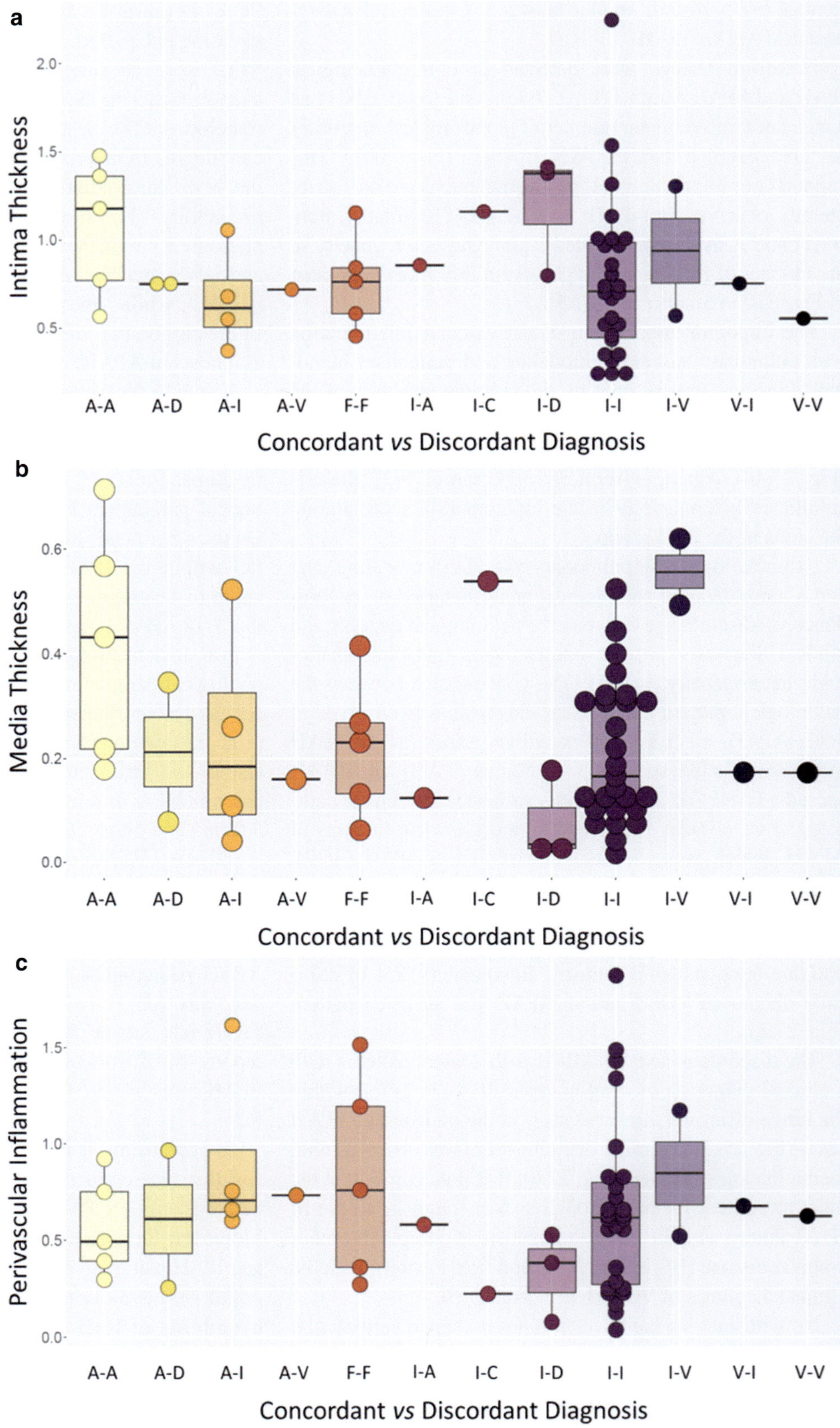

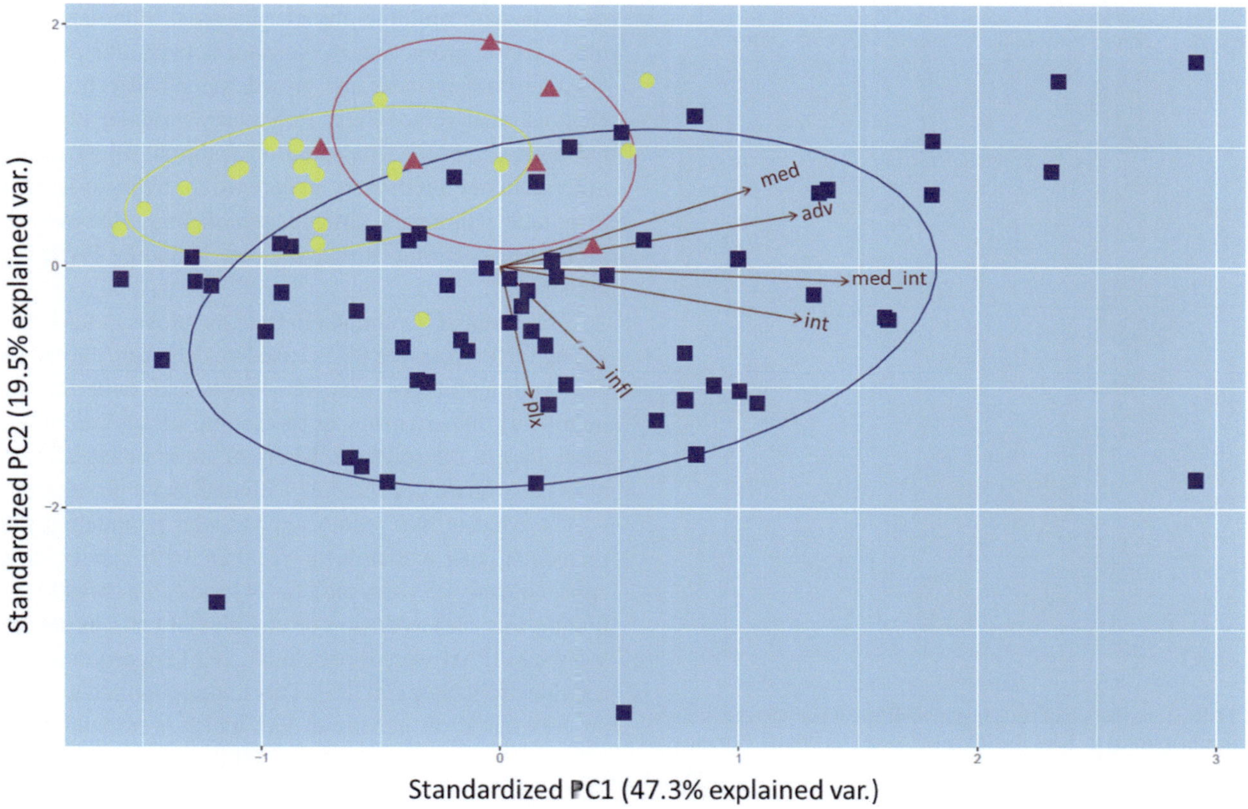

Fig. 27.7 PCA for PAH and control lungs (CTL, yellow) and aged controls (CTL2, blue) (based in [63]). Vectors indicate measure of variance along PC1 and PC2, involving intima thickness (int), media thickness (med), intima + media thickness (int_med), adventitia thickness (adv), number of profiles of plexiform lesions (plx) and perivascular inflammation score (inf) (based in [63]). Each point represents the values of single lungs

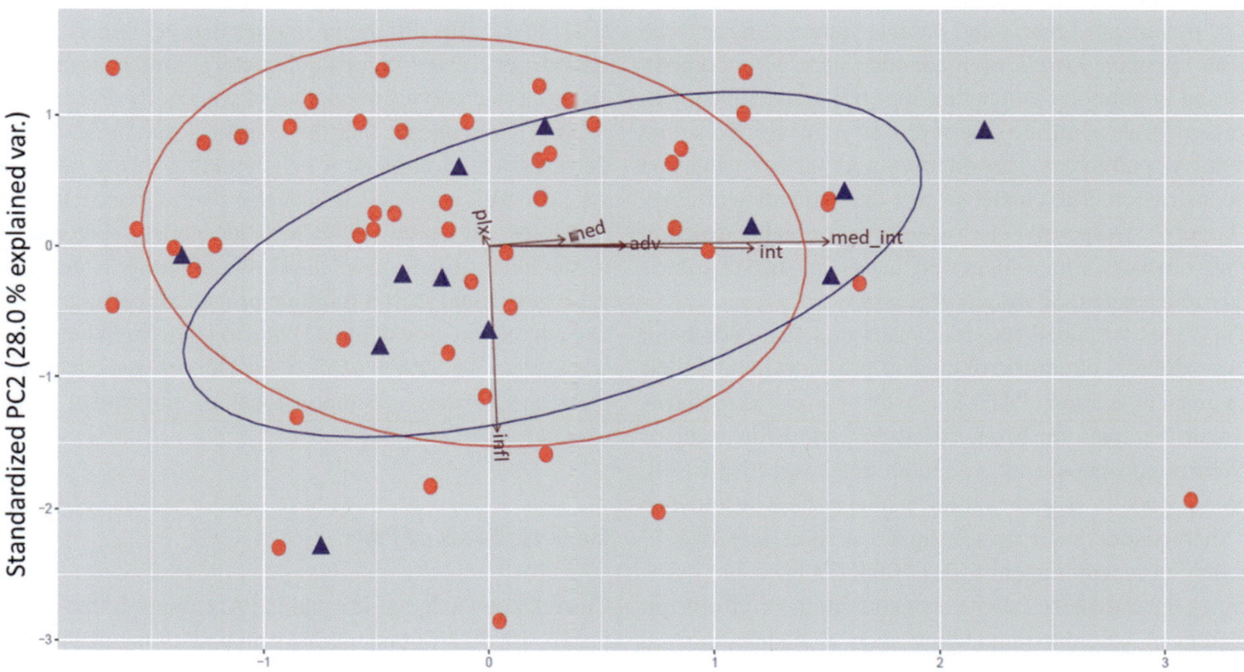

Fig. 27.8 PCA for APAH and IPAH morphological patterns. Principal component analyses (PCA) of APAH (Blue) and IPAH (red) (based in [63]). Vectors indicate measure of variance along PC1 and PC2, involving intima thickness (int), media thickness (med), intima + media thickness (int_med), adventitia thickness (adv), number of profiles of plexiform lesions (plx), and perivascular inflammation score (inf) (based in [63]). Each point represents the values of single lungs

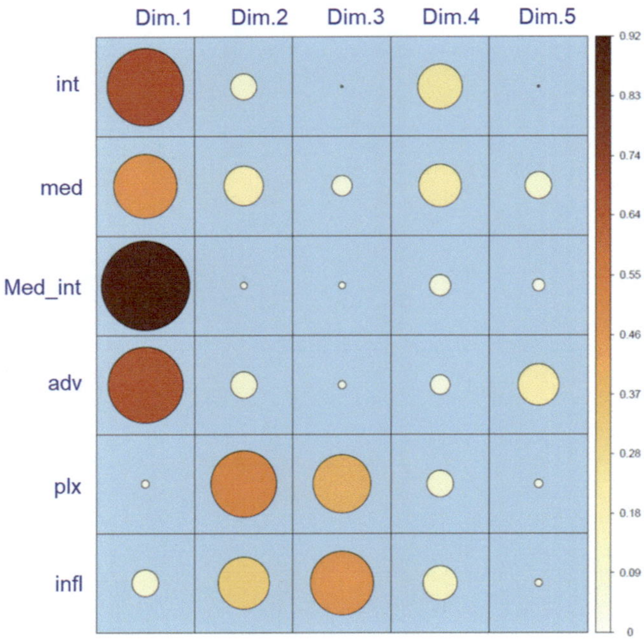

Fig. 27.9 Contribution of each histopathological parameter to components (dimensions) 1–5 of the PCA of APAH vs. IPAH pathological pattern. The relative size is a quantitative measure of the contribution. (Based in [63])

Pathogenetic Insights of PAH

For many decades, the main concepts underlying the pathogenesis of pulmonary hypertension involved vasoconstriction of pulmonary vessels and vascular remodeling and the role of hypoxia. Levels of mediators such as endothelin increased in pulmonary hypertension [69] and coupled with decreased levels of nitric oxide or prostacyclin which resulted in reduced pulmonary vasodilation, and further enhanced vasoconstriction. The challenge was that patients with PAH are largely unresponsive to vasodilators, notably calcium channel blockers, which suggested that established disease is largely independent of vasoconstriction.

The focus remained on vasoconstrictors like endothelin and vasodilators like nitric oxide and prostacyclin and their mechanism of action in PAH. The body of work led to two of the main therapies for PAH, based on endothelin receptor blockers or phosphodiesterase 5 inhibitors, respectively [70]. Ongoing work in targeting these pathways has resulted in new therapeutics such as selexipag, an oral selective IP prostacyclin-receptor agonist [71] (Table 27.1).

Other investigators have concentrated their efforts on mediators of vascular remodeling such as platelet-derived growth factor (PDGF) and TGFβ, among others. More recently, insights into the interplay of metabolism and gene mutations have expanded considerably the scope of key pathogenetic mechanisms involved in pulmonary hypertension. As with multiple chronic diseases, inflammation is a likely factor, promoting an interface between the pulmonary vascular compartment and growth signals affecting pulmonary vascular remodeling. Pulmonary vascular remodeling has been considered the result of abnormal injury/repair. In mild/moderate pulmonary hypertension, hypoxia is thought to initiate pulmonary vascular remodeling. However, what initiates remodeling in severe cases, including PAH, is still unclear.

The potential for endothelial cell apoptosis as the key triggering factor in severe PH is based on data from animal models. Auto-antibodies may be causal and underlie severe pulmonary hypertension in the setting of autoimmune diseases like in scleroderma. Many of these potential mechanisms also share key features with malignant processes.

The concept that pulmonary vascular remodeling shares molecular and pathological features with cancer is now approximately 25 years old [72–74] and came about from the finding that the expansion of endothelial cells in plexiform lesions in IPAH were monoclonal, i.e., they originated from a single progenitor cell [75]. This finding implied a selection process based on genetic events which were subsequently validated with the findings of BMPR2 mutations [6, 7] and TGFβ receptor 2 somatic instability [76]. Additional evidence of somatic genetic loss became evident when comparing primary cultures of pulmonary vascular cells from IPAH lungs with explanted lungs [77].

It is however worth mentioning that these events are restricted to IPAH; there is no current evidence that similar genetic processes affected other forms of PAH, including CVD-PAH. This difference implies that pulmonary vascular remodeling, involving pathologically similar lesions (see above), is stereotypic regardless of potentially diverse trigger factors. The concept that these lesions may arise from the derepression of progenitor cells residing in the pulmonary vascular wall may well fit into this overall concept; genetic events would occur within a single cell, giving rise to a monoclonal expansion in IPAH. On the other hand, nongenetic hits would recruit multiple progenitor cells, giving rise to a polyclonal growth in PAH due to left to right heart shunt; whether in SSc-PAH or Schistosomiasis-associated PAH, plexiform lesions are monoclonal or polyclonal remains unclear.

Genetic Basis of PAH

Current knowledge of idiopathic PAH assumes that approximately 25–30% of patients have an underlying genetic cause for the disease and are classified as heritable PAH (HPAH) [57]. Genetic studies on heritable PAH have identified a significant number of genes associated with susceptibility to developing the disease, which was first heralded by the identification of bone morphogenetic protein receptor type II (BMPR2) mutations, a member of the TGFβ superfamily, in PAH patients in the early 2000s [78]. Next-generation sequencing has more recently expanded the genetic landscape by broadening the mutation spectrum in known genes and identifying novel genetic risk alleles [56].

BMPR2 loss-of-function mutations account for the majority of heritable cases (82%) and 17% of IPAH cases and were the first mutations to be associated with PAH [79–81]. BMPR2 mutations exhibit incomplete penetrance and are inherited in an autosomal dominant fashion. Only 24% of carriers develop PAH [82] suggesting that other, as yet unknown genetic, epigenetic, and/or environmental factors may be required before the disease can manifest in carriers of BMPR2 mutations. More than 300 mutations have been described throughout the BMPR2 gene to date, including several frame-shifts, missense and nonsense mutations in critical regions, causing loss-of-function and resulting in PAH. Collectively, these mutations result in reduced expression of functional BMPR2 on the cell surface, and consequently in reduced signaling downstream of the receptor [83]. BMPR2 signaling inhibits the proliferation of vascular smooth muscle cells, while promoting the survival of pulmonary arterial endothelial cells, thereby protecting the pulmonary artery from damage and adverse inflammatory responses [84].

Other members of the TGFβ superfamily, including activin receptor-like kinase 1 (*ALK1 or ACVRL1*), endoglin (*ENG*), *SMAD1*, *SMAD4*, *SMAD8*, and *BMP9*, have been reported to contain mutations. Although these mutations are less frequent, they further establish the BMP signaling pathway in PAH pathogenesis [57]. Like BMPR2 mutations, these less common mutations exhibit incomplete penetrance and are also inherited in an autosomal dominant fashion. *ALK1* complexes with BMPR2 to form a functional receptor. Mutations in *ALK1* were more prevalent in 10% of pediatric PAH cases compared to adults PAH. In addition, mutations in the developmental *TBX4* gene are among the most common genetic causes of pediatric PAH suggesting an underlying developmental lung disease component [85]. Two new candidate genes with known functions in vasculogenesis and remodeling, *FBLN2* and *PDGFD* were also identified using rare variant analysis of a large international consortium [86].

Signal transducers and transcriptional modulators such as SMAD1 and SMAD8 act downstream of BMPR2 [87]. Once activated, BMPR2 phosphorylates SMAD1 and SMAD8, which translocate to the cell nucleus. SMAD1 and SMAD8, along with SMAD4 transcriptionally regulate many genes, including those that encode inhibitor of DNA binding (ID) proteins [87]. In pulmonary arterial smooth muscle cells, ID proteins mediate the antiproliferative effects of BMPs and BMPR2 signaling [88]. BMPR2 complexed with ALK1 can be preferentially activated by BMP9 in the pulmonary endothelium to maintain pulmonary vascular homeostasis and quiescence. Loss of BMP9 is thought to cause endothelial dysfunction and result in pulmonary vascular remodeling [10].

Rare variants have been identified in potassium (K^+) channels or accessory K^+ channel subunits are also associated with PAH. In 2013, novel mutations in KCNK3, the gene encoding the two-pore domain potassium channel TASK-1, were identified in patients with IPAH and HPAH, describing the first channelopathy in PAH. These heterozygous autosomal dominant KCNK3 mutations have a higher penetrance than BMPR2 mutations. Carriers of KCNK3 mutations develop a severe form of PAH, with raised mean pulmonary arterial pressures at right heart catheterization which failed to respond to acute vasodilator challenge [89]. Rare variants in ABCC8, which encodes sulfonylurea receptor 1 (SUR1), a regulatory subunit of the ATP-sensitive potassium channel associated with PAH, have also been identified resulting in decreased ATP-sensitive potassium channel function, which was pharmacologically recovered [90].

The advent of whole genome sequencing (WGS) and whole exome sequencing (WES) has increased our understanding of genes associated with predisposition and progression of PAH. To identify the missing heritability, WES was carried out on a collaborative European cohort of adult patients with IPAH and familial PAH. The study identified rare variants in *ATP13A3*, *AQP1*, and *SOX17*, a potential role of *GDF2*, which encodes a BMPR2 ligand, and a familial segregation of mutations in *AQP1* and *SOX17* in PAH [91]. In 2019, Rhodes et al. also reported in a large genome-wide association study that common genetic variation at loci in an enhancer near *SOX17* and in *HLA-DPA1/DPB1* is associated with PAH and propose that impairment of *SOX17* function maybe more prevalent in PAH than suggested by rare mutations in *SOX17* [92].

In the last 15 years, genetic and genomics studies of SSc patients have identified a number of genes associated with vascular complications, including the development of PAH. These genes include *IL23R* [93], *TNIP1* and *TNFAIP3* [94], *uPAR* [95], *TLR2* [96], *CAV* [97], *PPARγ* [98], *ATP8B4* [99], *MIF* [100], and *NKX2-5* [101]. Variants can broadly be classified in those affecting immune or inflammatory pathways and mechanisms and those which affect vascular structure and function.

Reported Interleukin 23 receptor gene (IL23R) polymorphisms identified susceptibility which is associated with anti-topoisomerase (ATA)-positive scleroderma and is protective against the development of pulmonary hypertension suggesting complex immunopathogenesis of SSc pulmonary hypertension [93]. Furthermore, polymorphisms in ubiquitin-modifying enzyme TNFAIP3, a key regulator of the NF-κB inflammatory signaling pathway, are associated with the development of diffuse cutaneous SSc (dcSSc), fibrosing alveolitis, and PAH [94]. More recently, studies of the Toll-like receptor genes (TLR) in scleroderma identified a rare functional polymorphism in the TLR2 gene associated with (ATA)-positive SSc patients and with the development of SSc-PAH. This polymorphism resulted in increased activation of IL-6 and TNFα by monocytes in response to TLR agonists [96]. More recently, whole-exome sequencing identified *ATP8B4*, which codes for ATPase phospholipid transporting 8B4 protein in immune cells, to be associated with a significant increase in the risk of SSc pulmonary complications and SSc-PAH. It catalyzes the hydrolysis of ATP coupled to the transport of aminophospholipids [99]. Macrophage migration inhibitory factor (MIF) gene encodes a constitutively expressed protein with an important role in autoimmune and inflammatory processes. A polymorphism in the promoter region of MIF is associated SSc-PAH resulting in increased MIF protein levels and is linked to several immune-mediated diseases [100].

Genetic variation in the promoter region of the Urokinase-type plasminogen activator receptor (uPAR) is associated with SSc vascular complications including digital ulceration and SSc-PAH has been identified. UPAR encodes a pleiotropic receptor, which is involved in fibrosis, immunity, angiogenesis, as well as vascular remodeling [95].

Caveolin-1 (CAV1) is essential for the formation of caveolae and is an inhibitor of tissue fibrosis. A protective polymorphism was associated with increased CAV1 protein expression in tissues of SSc patients [97]. Mutations in CAV1 that lead to a reduction in protein expression have also been identified in heritable PAH patients. CAV1 appears to modify TGFβ signaling, including the reduction in BMP signaling [97].

The multifunctional nuclear receptor peroxisome proliferator-activated receptor gamma (PPAR-γ) has potent anti-fibrotic effects, and its expression and activity are impaired in SSc patients. A case-control and meta-analysis study provided evidence of a polymorphism found in a con-coding region, which associates with pulmonary hypertension in a French cohort. The role of PPAR-γ dysfunction has been implicated in diverse cardiovascular pathologies [98].

NKX2-5 is a homeobox transcription factor that is required for the formation of the heart and vessels during development, with significant postnatal downregulation and reactivation in disease states, characterized by vascular remodeling. Disease-associated polymorphisms located in noncoding regions of *NKX2-5*, increase *NKX2-5* transcriptional activity and are associated with SSc-PAH [101].

Multiple genetic association studies in scleroderma have identified potential risk alleles, that play a role in adaptive and innate immune responses as well as fibrosis. It is noteworthy that currently the genetic/genomic landscape of SSc-associated PAH consists of genes regulating inflammation and vascular function which are markedly different from the genes observed in heritable and IPAH which are mainly associated with a reduction in BMPR2/SMAD activity. To date, no association to members of the TGFβ superfamily of receptors, including BMPR2 and ALK1, has been detected in SSc-PAH patients [102]. More research is required in assessing the relationship between genetic determinants, vascular phenotype, and the severity of SSc-PAH. At the dawn of the era of 'Big data' technologies, activities are likely to focus on integrating clinical data, imaging and multi-omic data in advancing our understanding in this area [103].

Pathogenic Factors and Signaling Pathways Implicated in the Development of PAH

Multiple proteins, lipids, and gases have been implicated in the various molecular mechanisms that result in PAH. Over the last two decades, the role of mediators such as endothelin, nitric oxide, and prostacyclin have been established and detailed mechanisms of their action in PAH have been delineated (Table 27.1). More recently, as our knowledge of the pathogenesis of PAH expanded, our understanding of mediators such as BMPs, Activin, PDGF, serotonin, and epigenetic components such as microRNAs (miRNAs) has also increased and has led to novel factors and emerging pathways that can be targeted for therapeutic advantage. Furthermore, new areas of study in PAH, such as inflammation and metabolism, are now providing mechanistic insights into the intricate and complex cross-talk between different cell types, factors, and pathways that drive disease pathology. We direct readers to several excellent reviews [61, 81, 87, 104] and shall focus on some well-established and some key emerging mediators.

The TGF-β/BMP Axis

The transforming growth factor (TGF-β) superfamily comprises more than 35 structurally related genes, which include bone morphogenetic proteins (BMP), and growth/differentiation factors and activins [87, 105–107]. The role of TGF-β, which in itself promotes the pro-fibrotic effects in numerous pathologies including SSc [108], is well described. In general terms, vascular remodeling is caused by the imbalance between various TGF-β family members resulting dysregulated signaling that results in vascular cell proliferation. The equilibrium is disturbed by overactive pro-proliferative SMAD2/3 signaling as well as deficient antiproliferative SMAD1/5/, ultimately resulting in the unrestricted proliferation of vascular endothelial and smooth muscle cells [109]. TGF-β has been implicated in promoting several of the cellular changes associated with vascular remodeling, including

SMC proliferation matrix deposition, and alterations in cell growth, particularly of endothelial cells whilst BMPs maintain vascular homeostasis [104, 110–117].

BMPR2 is a transmembrane serine/threonine kinase, which serves as a receptor for bone morphogenetic proteins (BMPs) [87]. BMPR2 is expressed on the surface of a wide range of cell types, including pulmonary arterial endothelial cells (PAECs) and Pulmonary arterial smooth muscle cells (PASMCs) [87]. In association with a co-receptor, BMPR2 can signal through multiple pathways, including the canonical SMAD1/5/8-dependent pathway [82, 87]. In normal PASMCs, ligation and subsequent activation of BMPR2 inhibits proliferation and promotes apoptosis [118]. PAH PASMCs harboring BMPR2 mutations are resistant to the growth-suppressive effects of BMPs, namely BMP2 and BMP4. Loss of responsiveness to the growth-suppressive effects of BMPs has also been reported in PASMCs derived from PAH patients lacking BMPR2 mutations, primarily as a consequence of downregulated BMPR2 expression or post-translational BMPR2 cleavage [9]. In PAECs, the BMPR2/ALK1 receptor complex signals selectively in response to the circulating ligands BMP9 and BMP10. BMP9 has been demonstrated to attenuate apoptosis in PAECs and strengthen the barrier function of the pulmonary endothelial monolayer. These effects are lost in PAECs isolated from PAH patients with BMPR2 mutations [10].

Although mutations in BMPR2 have not been identified in SSc patients, many proteins with a biased activity in favor of TGFβ or impaired BMP actions have been reported [119, 120]. Accumulative evidence in support is provided by TGF-β-driven preclinical models of SSc which spontaneously develop PAH and exhibit endothelial cell damage and a pulmonary vasculopathy [121]. Furthermore, there is a decrease of BMPR2 levels in SSc patients, associated with enhanced activity in downstream signaling components of the TGFβ pathways including Smad2 and MAPK [122]. The accumulation of evidence of decreased BMP signaling in SSc-PAH, albeit not from mutations in BMPR2, and increased TGFβ activity may still provide the underlying mechanism underpinning SSc-PAH although further mechanistic research is required in this area.

Much research has been caried out to address and restore the balance between BMPs and TGFβ activity. For example, the treatment of animals with BMP9 has been shown to reverse established PAH in preclinical models [10]. Although the role of BMP9 in PAH is becoming evident, its significance in SSc-PAH as yet remains unknown [10, 123–126]. GDF-15 may be a useful biomarker in PAH associated with SSc. GDP-15 may have a role in regulating inflammatory pathways by regulating apoptosis, cell repair, and cell growth, which are biological processes observed in cardiovascular and neoplastic disorders. Its presence in lung tissue may suggest a role in the pathology of the disease [127].

Other studies have used targeted gene delivery of BMPR2 to attenuate PAH [128] and inhibition of the TGF-β receptor ALK5 also prevents the development and progression of PAH [129]. As TGF-β signaling is crucial for many physiological functions, prolonged inhibition might lead to harmful side effects, although it has proved beneficial in persisting with more refined strategies to normalize TGF-β activity in PAH and other diseases [130, 131].

Recent studies have attempted to overcome the significant challenges in targeting the TGF-β/BMP axis, by focusing on a proposed mechanism that involves rebalancing pro-proliferative and antiproliferative signaling. The BMPR2-Smad1/5/8 pathway is downregulated in PAH leading to increased production of activin ligands, such as activin A, growth differentiation factor 8 (GDF8), and GDF11. As a result, the activin receptor type IIA (ActRIIA)–Smad2/3 pathway is upregulated. Increased phosphorylated Smad (pSmad)2/3 activity promotes expression of the endogenous BMP antagonists gremlin-1 and noggin. Gremlin-1 and noggin further reduce BMP–Smad1/5/8 signaling. The overall result is that antiproliferative signaling is reduced, shifting the balance toward pro-proliferative activin–Smad2/3 signaling, which leads to pulmonary vascular remodeling [11].

Sotatercept (Table 27.1), a fusion protein, sequesters excess activin ligands and growth differentiation factors, thereby reducing ActRIIA–Smad2/3 signaling and restoring balance between growth-promoting and growth-inhibiting signaling pathways [12]. Furthermore, Joshi et al. demonstrated that activin-class ligands are key mediators of inflammatory and immune responses in a model with severe experimental PAH. These authors clearly demonstrated that activin ligands may be important regulators of macrophage activation and perivascular infiltration in PAH lungs [132], suggesting the importance of these ligands in PAH inflammation (see section "Inflammation in PAH" below).

Serotonin (5-HT)

The 'serotonin hypothesis of PAH' arose over 40 years ago when patients taking the anorexigen aminorex fumarate were associated with an increased risk of developing PAH [133]. In the 1990s, it was reported that there was increased plasma serotonin in some patients with primary PH associated with platelet storage pool defect [134]. In PAH, platelet-driven and locally produced serotonin from lung tissue and arterial endothelial cells is thought to promote both vasoconstriction and remodeling of the pulmonary vasculature by inducing proliferation of pulmonary arterial fibroblasts and SMC [135, 136]. One way that serotonin promotes pulmonary smooth muscle cell proliferation and contraction is through receptor-mediated (5HT1B) vasoconstriction and receptor-independent uptake via the serotonin transporter (SERT) [135, 137]. SERT has been implicated in both clinical and experimental PAH, functionally activating the PDGFβ receptor to induce SMC proliferation [138]. Recently, SERT has been implicated in the pathogenesis of pulmonary hypertension in patients with chronic-obstructive pulmonary disease (Group 3) [139]. 5HT1B receptor expression is upregulated in PASMCs from female PAH patients potentially exacerbating the impact of increased serotonin levels [140]. A substantial upregulation of 5-HT(2B) receptor expression was noted in the pulmonary arteries in both animal models and IPAH patients [141, 142]. Serotonin has also been shown to induce ECM synthesis in interstitial fibroblasts from SSc patients via the 5-HT(2B) receptors in a TGFβ-dependent manner [143]. Although some studies have highlighted the dysregulation of components of the serotonin pathway in SSc and the links between vascular disease and tissue fibrosis [138], mechanistic details remain of the serotonin pathway unclear in the vasculature of SSc-PAH remains unclear. Several studies aimed to target the serotonin pathway including targeting receptor antagonists (e.g., ketanserin and terguride), receptor agonists (e.g., sumatriptan), or transporter reuptake inhibitors (e.g., fluoxetine) with disappointing results [144–147].

The rate-limiting step is serotonin biosynthesis production of 5-hydroxytryptophan from tryptophan by isoforms of tryptophan hydroxylase (TPH). TPH1 is associated with the production of serotonin in the periphery (outside the brain) and is overexpressed in the lungs and pulmonary arterial endothelial cells of patients with PAH and leads to excess local serotonin production [148]. Targeting TPH1 presents a logical strategy to improve vascular remodeling and treat PAH. Currently, a promising Phase 2b, double-blind, clinical trial (ELEVATE 2, NCT04712669) using rodatristat ethyl, a potent inhibitor of TPH1 is underway. Rodatristat efficacy has been demonstrated in monocrotaline and SUGEN hypoxia nonclinical models of PAH and robust dose-dependent reductions of 5-hydroxyindoleacetic acid, the major metabolite of serotonin in plasma and urine of healthy human subjects [136].

Platelet-Derived Growth Factor

In the last 25 years, many studies have highlighted the platelet-derived growth factor (PDGF) pathway as a major regulator of pulmonary vascular remodeling and PAH development [149–151]. PDGF is composed of two polypeptide chains A, B, C, and D leading to the formation of a dimeric protein (PDGF-AA, PDGF-BB, PDGF-CC, PDGF-DD, and PDGF-AB) [152], the best-studied being PDGF-AA and BB. Initially identified in platelets, PDGF isoforms are secreted from several cell types including macrophages, endothelial cells, vascular smooth muscle cells, and fibroblasts. PDGF is a potent mitogen and chemoattractant for fibroblasts, vascular smooth muscle cells, and endothelial cells [152]. It has often been implicated in PAH with increased circulating levels of PDGF-BB are elevated in IPAH patients [151] but not in SSc-PAH [153]. Conversely, PDGF receptor β (PDGFRβ) expression in SSc-PAH is broader and more intense in small- and post-capillary vessels compared to IPAH [154]. Furthermore, Baroni et al. reported that stimulatory autoantibodies against PDGFR may have a causal role in the pathogenesis of SSc [155]. In contrast, it remains unclear whether PDGFRα, which is a marker of mesenchymal stem cells and vascular progenitor cells, has a role in PAH [156].

Inhibition of the PDGF pathway is an attractive therapeutic strategy for the treatment of PAH. In animal studies, the PDGFR-β tyrosine kinase inhibitor Imatinib can reverse vascular remodeling via reduction in serotonin through inhibition of tryptophan hydroxylase 1 expression [157]. Other animal studies have demonstrated that imatinib reverses vascular remodeling in severe experimental pulmonary hypertension regardless of the initiating stimulus [158].

Administration of imatinib to PAH patients in two clinical trials showed a significant decrease in pulmonary vascular resistance (PVR) compared to a placebo and reported a significant improvement at 24 weeks in functional capacity [53, 159]. However, severe adverse events in the Imatinib group raised concern over safety. Currently, a new study (Clinicaltrials.gov id: NCT05036135) in IPAH and CTD-PAH is evaluating the safety and efficacy of AV-101 (a dry powder inhaled imatinib).

Inflammation in PAH

In the last decade, inflammation has emerged as a driving factor of the development of PAH. Extensive infiltration of T and B lymphocytes, monocytes, dendritic, and mast cells in the remodeled arteries and elevated levels of pro-inflammatory (e.g. interleukin-1β (IL-1β), IL-6, tumor necrosis factor α (TNFα)) and chemotactic (e.g. monocyte chemotactic protein-1 (MCP-1), IL-8) cytokines in the sera of PAH patients provides a growing body of evidence that early and persistent inflammation and altered immune responses underlie PAH pathophysiology [160, 161].

It is generally accepted that endothelial injury and concomitant upregulation of adhesion molecules are thought to promote the transmigration of these inflammatory cells into the vascular wall—the so-called 'inside-out' theory [162]. This is being increasingly contested, however, by the 'outside-in' hypothesis, which proposes that inflammation is initiated in the adventitial and perivascular layers and progresses inward toward the intima. Activated fibroblasts are thought to create a microenvironment permissive for the recruitment of circulating leukocytes through the production and retention of soluble factors, such as chemokines, cytokines, and growth factors in the adventitia of injured arteries [163]. Perivascular and adventitial accumulation of monocytes and macrophages as well as increased expression of proinflammatory cytokines and chemokines (GM-CSF, CCL2, CX3CL1, CXCL12, and IL6), have been consistently reported in patients with PAH and animal models. Frid et al. demonstrated recently a mechanism where immunoglobulin-driven dysregulated complement activation regulates proinflammatory and pro-proliferative processes in animal models of PAH and demonstrated that signaling of complement is a critical determinant of clinical outcome in PAH [164].

Among ongoing debate, the field has moved ahead with attempting to target inflammation clinically. One example of more selective targeting of pathological inflammation is the ongoing study of rituximab in scleroderma-associated PAH (ClinicalTrials.gov identifier: NCT01086540). Another example is anti-IL-6 therapy using tocilizumab [48, 49]. In SSc patients, tocilizumab reversed activation of TGF-β in dermal fibroblasts [165] and preserved lung function of patients with SSc interstitial lung disease [166]. However, a clinical trial on a group of IPAH and CTD-PAH patients, treatment with tocilizumab showed no significant effects on hemodynamic parameters of IPAH patients. A potential improvement was noted in the small subgroup of patients with CTD-associated PAH which requires further investigation [49].

BMPR2 has an anti-inflammatory role in pulmonary endothelial cells and therefore with reduced levels of BMPR2 would potentially lead to an increase of inflammation. Tian et al. found that an acute inflammatory insult caused endothelial-mesenchymal transdifferentiation (EndMT) of endothelial cells via canonical SMAD2/3 signaling. This can be reversed in by ALK5 or Smad3 knockdown or by ALK5 inhibition in Bmpr2 mutant rats [167]. This implies that targeting ALK5 or SMAD3 could potentially inhibit activin/GDF8/GDF11 signaling and implicate activin-driven inflammation in pulmonary vascular remodeling in PAH [132]. Joshi et al. also showed that Sotatercept reverses pulmonary vascular remodeling in severe experimental PAH by acting on perivascular macrophages which are activated by activin A. PAH patients have been shown to produce high levels of Activin A. Sotatercept also normalized IL6 levels induced by activin A, activin B, and GDF11 [132].

In the future, it may be useful to target inhibition of inflammation of at-risk individuals (such as those with SSc-PAH) to prevent the development of pulmonary vascular disease. Overall, blocking inflammation remains an attractive target in pulmonary hypertension.

Epigenetics of PAH

Since our last update and the emergence of nongenetic mechanisms which contribute to the cellular changes and the development of PAH, the pathological relevance in the context of SSc-PAH is also being explored.

Germ line pathological mutations have been identified in 17 genes thus far in PAH patients, the most prevalent occurring in ~25% of idiopathic PAH patients is in the BMPR2 gene [7]. In contrast genetic association in PAH patients with connective tissue diseases such as SSc is far from clear cut. Studies have highlighted the apparent phenocopying of SSc-PAH to disease-causing mutations identified in PAH. For example, we have previously shown the BMPRII protein in patients with SSc-PAH to be reduced [168]. More recently, mutations in the TET methyl-cytosine dioxygenase 2 (TET2) an important enzyme in DNA methylation were identified in PAH patients, and expression in PBMCs of TET2 was shown to be decreased in 86% of SSc-PAH patients relative to healthy subjects [169]. Interesting extensive CpG sites methylation in the BMPRII promoter region has been noted in SSc microvascular endothelial cells (SSc-MVECs), and these cells were more sensitive to apoptotic triggers than are control-MVECs [170]. It awaits future studies to assess if this is true for the pulmonary vasculature.

Histone acetylation is a key mechanism by which cell proliferation and survival is regulated. Zhao et al. demonstrated elevated protein levels of histone deacetylase (HDAC) 1 and 5 in PAH lungs. Administration of HDAC inhibitors reduced proliferation of PAH vascular fibroblasts and PDGF-stimulated growth of SMCs [171]. HDAC5 is also significantly increased in dermal ECs and fibroblasts from patients with SSc compared and leads to a reduction in expression of many genes including CYR61 resulting in dysregulated angiogenesis by ECs. In SSc fibroblasts, overexpression of CYR61 exhibits an antifibrotic effect, reducing the expression of profibrotic genes, including COL1A1 [172]. The pulmonary relevance of HDAC5 in SSc remains to be determined.

Micro RNAs (miRs) have been proposed as secreted biomarkers and mediators in the development of PAH [173, 174]. The growing relevance of miRNAs in modulating the pathogenic processes that contribute to the development of PAH is becoming more apparent in recent years. However, the relevance of these miRNAs in the development and progression of SSc-PAH lags. Within the context of FPAH and IPAH, a number of differentially expressed miRNAs have been identified that have relevance to PAH. Expression miR-96 is reduced in PASMCs from female patients with PAH, and negatively regulates the expression of the serotonin receptor 5-HT1BR. Restoration of miR-96 expression reduces the development of hypoxia-induced PH in mice [140]. Hypoxia can promote broader changes in miR expression impacting cellular functions. For example, hypoxia leads to the upregulation of miR-210 in SMC inhibiting apoptosis. Whereas miR-98 reduced in PAECs from PAH patients is repressed by hypoxia and regulates ET-1 expression and PAEC proliferation [173, 175].

More recently, Sindi et al. demonstrated that reduced KLF2 signaling is a common feature of human PAH and that KLF2-induced exosomal microRNAs; miR-181a-5p and miR-324-5p act together to attenuate pulmonary vascular remodeling [176]. Further epigenetic studies by the same group showed that endothelium-targeted miR-150 delivery prevented the disease in Sugen/hypoxia mice, while endothelial knockdown of miR-150 had adverse effects, miR-150 target genes revealed significant associations with PAH pathways, including proliferation, inflammation, and phospholipid signaling [177].

The utility of long noncoding RNAs (lncRNAs) in SSc as novel candidate biomarkers to support diagnosis and discriminate disease subtypes has recently been explored and ANCR and SPRY4-IT1 were found to positively correlate with SSc-PAH [178].

A deeper understanding of the epigenetic contribution to susceptibility and progression of PAH in SSc patients is needed.

Metabolism in PAH

Another area of pathogenetic significance in PAH is dysregulated metabolism. A large body of literature on PAH in humans and pulmonary hypertension (PH) in animal models have underscored an important role of altered pulmonary vascular cell metabolism in disease pathogenesis [179–181]. The significance of metabolic pathways as key promoters of cell proliferation and disease pathogenesis was first described in studies on cancer, a group of diseases that shares many other pathobiological similarities with PAH [73, 74, 182]. For example, cancer and PAH demonstrate upregulation of the transcription factor hypoxia inducible factor-1 (HIF-1), which activates genes involved in glycolysis as well as cell proliferation [183–185]. This connection between cell proliferation and metabolism has long been recognized in the cancer field, in which various metabolism-altering therapies are clinically approved [186].

Based on the similarities between cancer and the proliferative pulmonary vascular lesions in PAH [63], there have been growing efforts to understand the potential contribution of metabolic pathways to the PAH pathobiology and their therapeutic targetability [179–181]. Most heavily investigated is pulmonary vascular glucose metabolism, specifically a shift toward glycolysis coupled with suppressed glucose carbon oxidation via the mitochondrial tricarboxylic acid (TCA) cycle in PAH [187–189], a phenomenon known as the Warburg effect [72, 190, 191]. One potential mechanism of glycolysis-induced cell proliferation is NADPH generation from glucose carbons via the pentose phosphate pathway, thereby facilitating glutathione production, and nucleotide and lipid membrane synthesis [192, 193].

While its exact relevance specifically to SSc-PAH remains unclear, recent studies strongly suggest a link between glycolysis and pulmonary vascular cell proliferation. The presence of upregulated HIF-1 signaling, and increased glycolysis has been established in the whole lungs (e.g., increased ^{18}F-FDG uptake) [187–189] and pulmonary arterial cells of human PAH [184, 185, 187, 189], largely in idiopathic PAH. Systemic induction of mitochondrial glucose oxidation and suppression of glycolytic lactate production, achieved with the pharmacologic agent dichloroacetate, protected animals from pulmonary hypertension [194–196], and the same therapeutic strategy benefited a small number of carefully selected susceptible IPAH patients [197]. Other interventions to reduce glycolysis specifically in the vascular wall constituents, the endothelium and the smooth muscle cells, protected mice from hypoxia-induced pulmonary hypertension, which notably is distinct from PAH [198, 199]. Recent data indicate that HIF-1-dependent glycolysis in myeloid cells may also contribute to PH pathobiology, at least in the specific context of hypoxia-induced pulmonary hypertension [200, 201].

Metabolic substrates and pathways other than glucose metabolism likely promote PAH pathobiology. TCA cycle metabolites have been shown to promote cell proliferation [202–205] with numerous studies demonstrating mitochondrial dysregulation in diseased pulmonary arteries of PAH patients and animals with experimental pulmonary hypertension [61, 65, 82–85, 184, 187, 206–208]. Fatty acids represent an alternative carbon source for the mitochondrial TCA cycle, termed anaplerosis, the pathogenetic significance of which has long been recognized in cancer [209]. Fatty acid catabolism may be both a source of energy as well as carbons for macromolecule biosynthesis. For instance, fatty acid oxidation is necessary for endothelial cell proliferation [210] and likely contributes to the excessive endothelial growth seen in PAH [63, 73, 211]. Pulmonary vascular metabolism of amino acids, such as glutamine, represents another key pathogenetic process [212–214]. The aggregate of these observations underscores the individual and combine significance of the various metabolic pathways in promoting pulmonary vascular proliferation.

There are shortcomings however, applicable to the field of PAH in general in addition to SSc-PAH, which require further clarification before metabolism-altering therapies can be considered as a reliable therapeutic strategy. One largely unexamined area of critical importance regards how the various coexisting metabolic pathways interact with each other and affect the mitochondria to cause pulmonary vascular diseases. For instance, inhibition of fatty acid oxidation reciprocally induces glucose oxidation in the mitochondria, a phenomenon known as the Randle cycle [215], which in turn secondarily suppresses glycolysis. The combined and relative contributions of fatty acid oxidation and glycolysis to pulmonary vascular diseases remain unknown. Similarly, differential effects of the multiple carbon sources of TCA cycle intermediates (glucose, fatty acids, and glutamine) remain undefined.

Another area for future research is interrogation of metabolic pathways in a disease-specific and lesion-specific manner. Despite the cumulative data, evidence supporting a pathogenetic role of dysregulated pulmonary vascular metabolism specifically in SSc-PAH is lacking and merits future studies [185]. As discussed above, the varying frequency of plexiform lesions in SSc-PAH lungs compared to IPAH lungs suggests that, although similar in morphology, metabolic dysregulation might play a disease-specific, and even a patient or lesion-specific role in promoting pulmonary vascular proliferation. High-throughput quantification of metabolic targets in a spatially resolved manner with intact pulmonary vascular anatomy (e.g., in individual plexiform lesions), now enabled by new commercially available tools, is anticipated to provide key insights into how metabolic pathways contribute to SSc-PAH. Using omic strategies to determine metabolic profiles most informative to diagnosis or risk stratification is potentially another way to progress in this area [72, 216].

Concluding Remarks

In conclusion, the field of PAH has seen major recent advancements, adding to our understanding of the disease pathogenesis and identifying new avenues of therapeutic approaches. These insights stem from the discovery of genetic variants, various cell-signaling pathways, and epigenetic factors, collectively contributing to pulmonary vascular proliferation and clinically evident PAH.

Moving forward, addressing the following areas of uncertainty will be critical in enabling clinical applications of the new findings. The relevance of the abovementioned biologic pathways needs to be defined over the time course of disease development and in each subgroup of PAH. For instance, understanding the role of BMPR2 and TGF-β signaling at the onset of PAH as opposed during later stages of the disease will help determine when they can be optimally targeted to improve outcome. One challenge in studying PAH is the scarcity of human lung tissues in the early stages of the disease; methods allowing indirect assessment of the pulmonary arteries, for example using blood samples or imaging studies, will prove invaluable tools. Considering the pathobiologic and pathologic heterogeneities of PAH, significance of the molecular and genetic discoveries in IPAH will require validation in other cohorts, including SSc-PAH patients. Interactions and the collective impact of the various biologic pathways, for instance whether metabolic dysregulation affect inflammation, remain to be clarified. As the PAH field accrues multi-omic data, researchers and clinicians will benefit from establishing optimal ways to integrate various omics data with clinical data.

Acknowledgments We acknowledge support from grants awarded to R. M. Tuder: R24HL123767 and the Pulmonary Hypertension Breakthrough Initiative.

References

1. Badesch DB, Raskob GE, Elliott CG, et al. Pulmonary arterial hypertension: baseline characteristics from the REVEAL Registry. Chest. 2010;137(2):376–87. https://doi.org/10.1378/CHEST.09-1140.
2. Peacock AJ, Murphy NF, McMurrey JJV, Caballero L, Stewart S. An epidemiological study of pulmonary arterial hypertension. Eur Respir J. 2007;30(1):104–9. https://doi.org/10.1183/09031936.00092306.
3. Simonneau G. Haemodynamic definitions and updated clinical classification of pulmonary hypertension. Eur Respir J. 2019;53:1801913.
4. Condon DF, Agarwal S, Chakraborty A, et al. Novel mechanisms targeted by drug trials in pulmonary arterial hypertension. Chest. 2022;161(4):1060–72. https://doi.org/10.1016/J.CHEST.2021.10.010.
5. Deng Z, Haghighi F, Helleby L, et al. Fine mapping of PPH1, a gene for familial primary pulmonary hypertension, to a 3-CM region on chromosome 2q33. Am J Respir Crit Care Med. 1999;160(3 Pt 1):1055–9.
6. Deng Z, Morse JH, Slager SL, et al. Familial primary pulmonary hypertension (gene PPH1) is caused by mutations in the bone morphogenetic protein receptor-II gene. Am J Hum Genet. 2000;67(3):737–44. https://doi.org/10.1086/303059.
7. Lane KB, Machado RD, Pauciulo MW, et al. Heterozygous germline mutations in BMPR2, encoding a TGF-beta receptor, cause familial primary pulmonary hypertension. Nat Genet. 2000;26(1):81–4. https://doi.org/10.1038/79226.
8. Atkinson C, Stewart S, Upton PD, et al. Primary pulmonary hypertension is associated with reduced pulmonary vascular expression of type II bone morphogenetic protein receptor. Circulation. 2002;105(14):1672–8. https://doi.org/10.1161/01.CIR.0000012754.72951.3D.
9. Hurst LA, Dunmore BJ, Long L, et al. TNFα drives pulmonary arterial hypertension by suppressing the BMP type-II receptor and altering NOTCH signalling. Nat Commun. 2017;8:14079. https://doi.org/10.1038/ncomms14079.
10. Long L, Ormiston ML, Yang X, et al. Selective enhancement of endothelial BMPR-II with BMP9 reverses pulmonary arterial hypertension. Nat Med. 2015;21(7):777–85. https://doi.org/10.1038/nm.3877.
11. Yung LM, Yang P, Joshi S, et al. ACTRIIA-Fc rebalances activin/GDF versus BMP signaling in pulmonary hypertension. Sci Transl Med. 2020;12(543):eaaz5660. https://doi.org/10.1126/SCITRANSLMED.AAZ5660/SUPPL_FILE/AAZ5660_SM.PDF.
12. Humbert M, McLaughlin V, Gibbs JSR, et al. Sotatercept for the treatment of pulmonary arterial hypertension. N Engl J Med. 2021;384(13):1204–15. https://doi.org/10.1056/NEJMOA2024277.
13. Spiekerkoetter E, Tian X, Cai J, et al. FK506 activates BMPR2, rescues endothelial dysfunction, and reverses pulmonary hypertension. J Clin Invest. 2013;123:3600–13. https://doi.org/10.1172/JCI65592.

14. Spiekerkoetter E, Sung YK, Sudheendra D, et al. Randomised placebo-controlled safety and tolerability trial of FK506 (tacrolimus) for pulmonary arterial hypertension. Eur Respir J. 2017;50(3):1602449. https://doi.org/10.1183/13993003.02449-2016.
15. Zaiman AL, Podowski M, Medicherla S, et al. Role of the TGF-b/Alk5 signaling pathway in monocrotaline-induced pulmonary hypertension. Am J Respir Crit Care Med. 2008;177:896–905. https://doi.org/10.1164/rccm.200707-1083OC.
16. Yung LM, Nikolic I, Paskin-Flerlage SD, Scott Pearsall R, Kumar R, Yu PB. A selective transforming growth factor-β ligand trap attenuates pulmonary hypertension. Am J Respir Crit Care Med. 2016;194(9):1140–51. https://doi.org/10.1164/RCCM.201510-1955OC/SUPPL_FILE/DISCLOSURES.PDF.
17. Tu L, Desroches-Castan A, Mallet C, et al. Selective BMP-9 inhibition partially protects against experimental pulmonary hypertension. Circ Res. 2019;124(6):846–55. https://doi.org/10.1161/CIRCRESAHA.118.313356.
18. Galiè N, McLaughlin VV, Rubin LJ, Simonneau G. An overview of the 6th World Symposium on Pulmonary Hypertension. Eur Respir J. 2019;53(1):1802148. https://doi.org/10.1183/13993003.02148-2018.
19. Kovacs G, Berghold A, Scheidl S, Olschewski H. Pulmonary arterial pressure during rest and exercise in healthy subjects: a systematic review. Eur Respir J. 2009;34(4):888–94. https://doi.org/10.1183/09031936.00145608.
20. Maron BA, Hess E, Maddox TM, et al. Association of borderline pulmonary hypertension with mortality and hospitalization in a large patient cohort: insights from the veterans affairs clinical assessment, reporting, and tracking program. Circulation. 2016;133(13):1240–8. https://doi.org/10.1161/CIRCULATIONAHA.115.020207.
21. Kolte D, Lakshmanan S, Jankowich MD, Brittain EL, Maron BA, Choudhary G. Mild pulmonary hypertension is associated with increased mortality: a systematic review and meta-analysis. J Am Heart Assoc. 2018;7(18):e009729. https://doi.org/10.1161/JAHA.118.009729.
22. Douschan P, Kovacs G, Avian A, et al. Mild elevation of pulmonary arterial pressure as a predictor of mortality. Am J Respir Crit Care Med. 2018; https://doi.org/10.1164/rccm.201706-1215OC.
23. Humbert M, Sitbon O, Yaïci A, et al. Survival in incident and prevalent cohorts of patients with pulmonary arterial hypertension. Eur Respir J. 2010;36(3):549–55. https://doi.org/10.1183/09031936.00057010.
24. McLaughlin VV, Hoeper MM, Channick RN, et al. Pulmonary arterial hypertension-related morbidity is prognostic for mortality. J Am Coll Cardiol. 2018;71(7):752–63. https://doi.org/10.1016/J.JACC.2017.12.010.
25. Vizza CD, Badagliacca R, Messick CR, Rao Y, Nelsen AC, Benza RL. The impact of delayed treatment on 6-minute walk distance test in patients with pulmonary arterial hypertension: a meta-analysis. Int J Cardiol. 2018;254:299–301. https://doi.org/10.1016/J.IJCARD.2017.12.016.
26. Gaine S, Sitbon O, Channick RN, et al. Relationship between time from diagnosis and morbidity/mortality in pulmonary arterial hypertension: results from the phase III GRIPHON Study. Chest. 2021;160(1):277–86. https://doi.org/10.1016/j.chest.2021.01.066.
27. Kovacs G, Olschewski H. Debating the new haemodynamic definition of pulmonary hypertension: much ado about nothing? Eur Respir J. 2019;54(2):1901278. https://doi.org/10.1183/13993003.01278-2019.
28. Jaafar S, Visovatti S, Young A, et al. Impact of the revised haemodynamic definition on the diagnosis of pulmonary hypertension in patients with systemic sclerosis. Eur Respir J. 2019;54(2):1900586. https://doi.org/10.1183/13993003.00586-2019.
29. Simon J, Gibbs R, Torbicki A. Proposed new pulmonary hypertension definition: is 4 mm(Hg) worth re-writing medical textbooks? Eur Respir J. 2019;53(3):1900197. https://doi.org/10.1183/13993003.00197-2019.
30. D'Alto M, Badagliacca R, Argiento P, et al. Risk reduction and right heart reverse remodeling by upfront triple combination therapy in pulmonary arterial hypertension. Chest. 2020;157(2):376–83. https://doi.org/10.1016/J.CHEST.2019.09.009.
31. Chin KM, Sitbon O, Doelberg M, et al. Three- versus two-drug therapy for patients with newly diagnosed pulmonary arterial hypertension. J Am Coll Cardiol. 2021;78(14):1393–403. https://doi.org/10.1016/J.JACC.2021.07.057.
32. Boucly A, Savale L, Jaïs X, Humbert M, Sitbon O, Montani D. Sequential combination therapy with parenteral prostacyclin in BMPR2 mutations carriers. Pulm Circ. 2022;12(1):e12023. https://doi.org/10.1002/PUL2.12023.
33. Bull TM, Lee MH. The role of pulmonary arterial hypertension-targeted therapy in systemic sclerosis. F1000Res. 2019;8:F1000 Faculty Rev-2124. https://doi.org/10.12688/F1000RESEARCH.20313.1/DOI.
34. Condliffe R, Kiely DG, Peacock AJ, et al. Connective tissue disease-associated pulmonary arterial hypertension in the modern treatment era. Am J Respir Crit Care Med. 2009; https://doi.org/10.1164/rccm.200806-953OC.
35. Chung L, Farber HW, Benza R, et al. Unique predictors of mortality in patients with pulmonary arterial hypertension associated with systemic sclerosis in the REVEAL Registry. Chest. 2014;146(6):1494. https://doi.org/10.1378/CHEST.13-3014.
36. Chung L, Liu J, Parsons L, et al. Characterization of connective tissue disease-associated pulmonary arterial hypertension from REVEAL: identifying systemic sclerosis as a unique phenotype. Chest. 2010;138(6):1383. https://doi.org/10.1378/CHEST.10-0260.
37. Kovacs G, Maier R, Aberer E, et al. Borderline pulmonary arterial pressure is associated with decreased exercise capacity in scleroderma. Am J Respir Crit Care Med. 2009; https://doi.org/10.1164/rccm.200904-0563OC.
38. Bae S, Saggar R, Bolster MB, et al. Baseline characteristics and follow-up in patients with normal haemodynamics versus borderline mean pulmonary arterial pressure in systemic sclerosis: results from the PHAROS registry. Ann Rheum Dis. 2012;71(8):1335–42. https://doi.org/10.1136/ANNRHEUMDIS-2011-200546.
39. Gerry Coghlan J, Wolf M, Distler O, et al. Incidence of pulmonary hypertension and determining factors in patients with systemic sclerosis. Eur Respir J. 2018;51(4):1701197. https://doi.org/10.1183/13993003.01197-2017.
40. Valerio CJ, Schreiber BE, Handler CE, Denton CP, Coghlan JG. Borderline mean pulmonary artery pressure in patients with systemic sclerosis: transpulmonary gradient predicts risk of developing pulmonary hypertension. Arthritis Rheum. 2013;65(4):1074–84. https://doi.org/10.1002/art.37838.
41. Kolstad KD, Li S, Steen V, Chung L. Long-term outcomes in systemic sclerosis-associated pulmonary arterial hypertension from the Pulmonary Hypertension Assessment and Recognition of Outcomes in Scleroderma Registry (PHAROS). Chest. 2018;154(4):862–71. https://doi.org/10.1016/J.CHEST.2018.05.002.
42. Pan J, Lei L, Zhao C. Comparison between the efficacy of combination therapy and monotherapy in connective tissue disease associated pulmonary arterial hypertension: a systematic review and meta-analysis. Clin Exp Rheumatol. 2018;36(6):1095–102.
43. Denton CP, Khanna D. Systemic sclerosis. Lancet. 2017;390(10103):1685–99. https://doi.org/10.1016/S0140-6736(17)30933-9.
44. Tyndall AJ, Bannert B, Vonk M, et al. Causes and risk factors for death in systemic sclerosis: a study from the EULAR

Scleroderma Trials and Research (EUSTAR) database. Ann Rheum Dis. 2010;69(10):1809–15. https://doi.org/10.1136/ARD.2009.114264.
45. Steen VD, Medsger TA. Changes in causes of death in systemic sclerosis, 1972–2002. Ann Rheum Dis. 2007;66(7):940. https://doi.org/10.1136/ARD.2006.066068.
46. Morrisroe K, Stevens W, Huq M, et al. Survival and quality of life in incident systemic sclerosis-related pulmonary arterial hypertension. Arthritis Res Ther. 2017;19(1):122. https://doi.org/10.1186/S13075-017-1341-X.
47. Hao Y, Hudson M, Baron M, et al. Early mortality in a multinational systemic sclerosis inception cohort. Arthrit Rheumatol. 2017;69(5):1067–77. https://doi.org/10.1002/ART.40027.
48. Hashimoto-Kataoka T, Hosen N, Sonobe T, et al. Interleukin-6/interleukin-21 signaling axis is critical in the pathogenesis of pulmonary arterial hypertension. Proc Natl Acad Sci U S A. 2015;112(20):E2677–86. https://doi.org/10.1073/pnas.1424774112.
49. Toshner M, Church C, Harbaum L, et al. Mendelian randomisation and experimental medicine approaches to interleukin-6 as a drug target in pulmonary arterial hypertension. Eur Respir J. 2022;59(3):2002463. https://doi.org/10.1183/13993003.02463-2020.
50. Zamanian RT, Badesch D, Chung L, et al. Safety and efficacy of B-cell depletion with rituximab for the treatment of systemic sclerosis–associated pulmonary arterial hypertension: a multicenter, double-blind, randomized, placebo-controlled trial. Am J Respir Crit Care Med. 2021;204(2):209–21. https://doi.org/10.1164/RCCM.202009-3481OC/SUPPL_FILE/DISCLOSURES.PDF.
51. Kawut SM, Archer-Chicko CL, Demichele A, et al. Anastrozole in pulmonary arterial hypertension a randomized, double-blind, placebo-controlled trial. Am J Respir Crit Care Med. 2017;195:360–8. https://doi.org/10.1164/rccm.201605-1024OC.
52. Granton J, Langleben D, Kutryk MB, et al. Endothelial NO-synthase gene-enhanced progenitor cell therapy for pulmonary arterial hypertension: the PHACeT trial. Circ Res. 2015;117(7):645–54. https://doi.org/10.1161/CIRCRESAHA.114.305951.
53. Hoeper MM, Barst RJ, Bourge RC, et al. Imatinib mesylate as add-on therapy for pulmonary arterial hypertension: results of the randomized IMPRES study. Circulation. 2013;127(10):1128–38. https://doi.org/10.1161/CIRCULATIONAHA.112.000765.
54. Shah AM, Campbell P, Rocha GQ, et al. Effect of imatinib as add-on therapy on echocardiographic measures of right ventricular function in patients with significant pulmonary arterial hypertension. Eur Heart J. 2015; https://doi.org/10.1093/eurheartj/ehu035.
55. Frost AE, Barst RJ, Hoeper MM, et al. Long-term safety and efficacy of imatinib in pulmonary arterial hypertension. J Heart Lung Transplant. 2015;34(11):1366–75. https://doi.org/10.1016/J.HEALUN.2015.05.025.
56. Southgate L, Machado RD, Gräf S, Morrell NW. Molecular genetic framework underlying pulmonary arterial hypertension. Nat Rev Cardiol. 2020;17(2):85–95. https://doi.org/10.1038/S41569-019-0242-X.
57. Morrell NW, Aldred MA, Chung WK, et al. Genetics and genomics of pulmonary arterial hypertension. Eur Respir J. 2019;53(1):1801899.
58. Bourgeois A, Omura J, Habbout K, Bonnet S, Boucherat O. Pulmonary arterial hypertension: new pathophysiological insights and emerging therapeutic targets. Int J Biochem Cell Biol. 2018;104:9–13.
59. Thomas CA, Anderson RJ, Condon DF, de Jesus Perez VA. Diagnosis and management of pulmonary hypertension in the modern era: insights from the 6th World Symposium. Pulm Ther. 2020;6:9–22.
60. Tuder RM, Ponticos M, Holmes A. Pathogenesis of pulmonary arterial hypertension. In: Scleroderma: from pathogenesis to comprehensive management. Springer; 2016. p. 385–401. https://doi.org/10.1007/978-3-319-31407-5_26/COVER/.
61. Tuder RM. Pulmonary vascular remodeling in pulmonary hypertension. Cell Tissue Res. 2017;367(3):643–9. https://doi.org/10.1007/S00441-016-2539-Y.
62. Tuder RM, Stacher E, Robinson J, Kumar R, Graham BB. Pathology of pulmonary hypertension. Clin Chest Med. 2013;34(4):639–50. https://doi.org/10.1016/J.CCM.2013.08.009.
63. Stacher E, Graham BB, Hunt JM, et al. Modern age pathology of pulmonary arterial hypertension. Am J Respir Crit Care Med. 2012; https://doi.org/10.1164/rccm.201201-0164OC.
64. Tuder RM, Ponticos M, Holmes A. Pathogenesis of pulmonary arterial hypertension. Springer; 2016. https://doi.org/10.1007/978-3-319-31407-5_26.
65. Dorfmüller P, Montani D, Humbert M. Beyond arterial remodelling: pulmonary venous and cardiac involvement in patients with systemic sclerosis-associated pulmonary arterial hypertension. Eur Respir J. 2010;35(1):6–8. https://doi.org/10.1183/09031936.00081009.
66. Tuder RM, Stenmark KR. Perspective: pathobiological paradigms in pulmonary hypertension, time for reappraisal. Am J Physiol Lung Cell Mol Physiol. 2020;318(6):L1131. https://doi.org/10.1152/AJPLUNG.00067.2020.
67. Tuder RM, Zaiman AL. Pathology of pulmonary vascular disease. In: Peacock A, Rubin LJ, editors. Pulmonary circulation. 2nd ed. Arnold; 2004. p. 25–32.
68. Tuder RM, Marecki JC, Richter A, Fijalkowska I, Flores S. Pathology of pulmonary hypertension. Clin Chest Med. 2007;28(1):23. https://doi.org/10.1016/J.CCM.2006.11.010.
69. Giaid A, Yanagisawa M, Langleben D, et al. Expression of endothelin-1 in the lungs of patients with pulmonary hypertension. N Engl J Med. 1993;328(24):1732–9. https://doi.org/10.1056/NEJM199306173282402.
70. Humbert M, Sitbon O, Simonneau G. Treatment of pulmonary arterial hypertension. N Engl J Med. 2004;351(14):1425–36. https://doi.org/10.1056/NEJMra040291.
71. Sitbon O, Channick R, Chin KM, et al. Selexipag for the treatment of pulmonary arterial hypertension. N Engl J Med. 2015;373(26):2522–33. https://doi.org/10.1056/NEJMOA1503184/SUPPL_FILE/NEJMOA1503184_DISCLOSURES.PDF.
72. Rhodes CJ. The cancer hypothesis of pulmonary arterial hypertension: are polyamines the new Warburg? Eur Respir J. 2020;56(5):2002350. https://doi.org/10.1183/13993003.02350-2020.
73. Voelkel NF, Cool C, Lee SD, Wright L, Geraci MW, Tuder RM. Primary pulmonary hypertension between inflammation and cancer. Chest. 1998;114(3):225S–30S. https://doi.org/10.1378/CHEST.114.3_SUPPLEMENT.225S.
74. Rai PR, Cool CD, King JAC, et al. The cancer paradigm of severe pulmonary arterial hypertension. Am J Respir Crit Care Med. 2008;178(6):558–64. https://doi.org/10.1164/rccm.200709-1369PP.
75. Tuder RM, Radisavljevic Z, Shroyer KR, Polak JM, Voelkel NF. Monoclonal endothelial cells in appetite suppressant-associated pulmonary hypertension. Am J Respir Crit Care Med. 1999;158(6):1999–2001.
76. Yeager ME, Halley GR, Golpon HA, Voelkel NF, Tuder RM. Microsatellite instability of endothelial cell growth and apoptosis genes within plexiform lesions in primary pulmonary hypertension. Circ Res. 2001;88(1):E2–E11. https://doi.org/10.1161/01.RES.88.1.E2.
77. Aldred MA, Comhair SA, Varella-Garcia M, et al. Somatic chromosome abnormalities in the lungs of patients with pulmonary arterial hypertension. Am J Respir Crit Care Med. 2010; https://doi.org/10.1164/rccm.201003-0491OC.

78. Deng Z. Familial primary pulmonary hypertension (gene PPH1) is caused by mutations in the bone morphogenetic protein receptor-II gene. Am J Hum Genet. 2000;67:737–44.
79. Trembath RC, Thomson JR, Machado RD, et al. Clinical and molecular genetic features of pulmonary hypertension in patients with hereditary hemorrhagic telangiectasia. N Engl J Med. 2001;345(5):325–34. https://doi.org/10.1056/nejm200108023450503.
80. Ghataorhe P, Rhodes CJ, Harbaum L, Attard M, Wharton J, Wilkins MR. Pulmonary arterial hypertension—progress in understanding the disease and prioritizing strategies for drug development. J Intern Med. 2017;282(2):129–41. https://doi.org/10.1111/JOIM.12623.
81. Girerd B, Weatherald J, Montani D, Humbert M. Heritable pulmonary hypertension: from bench to bedside. Eur Respir Rev. 2017;26(145):170037. https://doi.org/10.1183/16000617.0037-2017.
82. Rabinovitch M. Molecular pathogenesis of pulmonary arterial hypertension. J Clin Invest. 2012;122(12):4306. https://doi.org/10.1172/JCI60658.
83. Evans JDW, Girerd B, Montani D, et al. BMPR2 mutations and survival in pulmonary arterial hypertension: an individual participant data meta-analysis. Lancet Respir Med. 2016;4(2):129–37. https://doi.org/10.1016/S2213-2600(15)00544-5.
84. Austin ED, Loyd JE. The genetics of pulmonary arterial hypertension. Circ Res. 2014;115(1):189–200. https://doi.org/10.1161/CIRCRESAHA.115.303404.
85. Zhu N. Exome sequencing in children with pulmonary arterial hypertension demonstrates differences compared with adults. Circ Genom Precis Med. 2018;11:e001887.
86. Zhu N, Swietlik EM, Welch CL, et al. Rare variant analysis of 4241 pulmonary arterial hypertension cases from an international consortium implicates FBLN2, PDGFD, and rare de novo variants in PAH. Genome Med. 2021;13(1):80. https://doi.org/10.1186/S13073-021-00891-1.
87. Morrell NW, Bloch DB, ten Dijke P, et al. Targeting BMP signalling in cardiovascular disease and anaemia. Nat Rev Cardiol. 2016; https://doi.org/10.1038/nrcardio.2015.156.
88. Yang J, Li X, Morrell NW. Id proteins in the vasculature: from molecular biology to cardiopulmonary medicine. Cardiovasc Res. 2014;104(3):388–98. https://doi.org/10.1093/CVR/CVU215.
89. Ma L, Roman-Campos D, Austin ED, et al. A novel channelopathy in pulmonary arterial hypertension abstract. N Engl J Med. 2013;369:351–61. https://doi.org/10.1056/NEJMoa1211097.
90. Bohnen MS, Ma L, Zhu N, et al. Loss of function ABCC8 mutations in pulmonary arterial hypertension. Circ Genom Precis Med. 2018;11(10):e002087. https://doi.org/10.1161/CIRCGEN.118.002087.
91. Gräf S. Identification of rare sequence variation underlying heritable pulmonary arterial hypertension. Nat Commun. 2018;9(1):1416.
92. Rhodes CJ, Kaakinen M, Ulrich A, et al. Genetic determinants of risk in pulmonary arterial hypertension: international genome; wide association studies and meta-analysis. Lancet Respir. 2019;7:227–38. https://doi.org/10.1016/S2213-2600(18)30409-0.
93. Agarwal SK, Gourh P, Shete S, et al. Association of interleukin 23 receptor polymorphisms with anti-topoisomerase-i positivity and pulmonary hypertension in systemic sclerosis. J Rheumatol. 2009;36(12):2715. https://doi.org/10.3899/JRHEUM.090421.
94. Dieudé P, Guedj M, Wipff J, et al. Association of the TNFAIP3 rs5029939 variant with systemic sclerosis in the European Caucasian population. Ann Rheum Dis. 2010;69(11):1958–64. https://doi.org/10.1136/ARD.2009.127928.
95. Manetti M, Allanore Y, Revillod L, et al. A genetic variation located in the promoter region of the UPAR (CD87) gene is associated with the vascular complications of systemic sclerosis. Arthritis Rheum. 2011;63(1):247–56. https://doi.org/10.1002/ART.30101.
96. Broen JCA, Bossini-Castillo L, van Bon L, et al. A rare polymorphism in the gene for Toll-like receptor 2 is associated with systemic sclerosis phenotype and increases the production of inflammatory mediators. Arthritis Rheum. 2012;64(1):264–71. https://doi.org/10.1002/art.33325.
97. Austin E. Whole exome sequencing to identify a novel gene (caveolin-1) associated with human pulmonary arterial hypertension. Circ Cardiovasc Genet. 2012;5:336–43.
98. Goncalves Marangoni R, Korman BD, Allanore Y, et al. A candidate gene study reveals association between a variant of the Peroxisome Proliferator-Activated Receptor Gamma (PPAR-γ) gene and systemic sclerosis. Arthritis Res Ther. 2011; https://doi.org/10.1186/s13075-015-0641-2.
99. Gao L, Emond MJ, Louie T, et al. Identification of rare variants in ATP8B4 as a risk factor for systemic sclerosis by Whole-Exome Sequencing and Blood Institute GO Exome Sequencing Project. Arthritis Rheum. 2016;68(1):191–200. https://doi.org/10.1002/art.39449.
100. Lara Bossini-Castillo A, Campillo-Davó D, López-Isac E, et al. A MIF promoter polymorphism is associated with the susceptibility to pulmonary arterial hypertension in diffuse cutaneous systemic sclerosis patients. J Rheumatol. 2017;44(10):1453–7.
101. Dritsoula A, Papaioannou I, Guerra SG, et al. Molecular basis for dysregulated activation of NKX2-5 in the vascular remodeling of systemic sclerosis. Arthritis Rheumatol. 2018;70(6):920–31. https://doi.org/10.1002/art.40419.
102. Koumakis E, Wipff J, Dieudé P, et al. TGFβ receptor gene variants in systemic sclerosis-related pulmonary arterial hypertension: results from a multicentre EUSTAR study of European Caucasian patients. Ann Rheum Dis. 2012;71(11):1900–3. https://doi.org/10.1136/ANNRHEUMDIS-2012-201755.
103. Rhodes CJ, Sweatt AJ, Maron BA. Harnessing big data to advance treatment and understanding of pulmonary hypertension. Circ Res. 2022;130(9):1423–44. https://doi.org/10.1161/CIRCRESAHA.121.319969.
104. Pardali E, Sanchez-Duffhues G, Gomez-Puerto MC, ten Dijke P. TGF-β-induced endothelial-mesenchymal transition in fibrotic diseases. Int J Mol Sci. 2017;18(10):2157. https://doi.org/10.3390/ijms18102157.
105. Derynck R, Budi EH. Specificity, versatility, and control of TGF-b family signaling. Sci Signal. 2019;12(570):eaav5183. https://doi.org/10.1126/SCISIGNAL.AAV5183.
106. Goumans MJ, Zwijsen A, ten Dijke P, Bailly S. Bone morphogenetic proteins in vascular homeostasis and disease. Cold Spring Harb Perspect Biol. 2018;10(2):a031989. https://doi.org/10.1101/CSHPERSPECT.A031989.
107. Tielemans B, Delcroix M, Belge C, Quarck R. TGFβ and BMPRII signalling pathways in the pathogenesis of pulmonary arterial hypertension. Drug Discov Today. 2019;24(3):703–16. https://doi.org/10.1016/J.DRUDIS.2018.12.001.
108. Ayers NB, Sun C, Chen SY. Transforming growth factor-β signaling in systemic sclerosis. J Biomed Res. 2018;32(1):3–12. https://doi.org/10.7555/JBR.31.20170034.
109. Andre P, Joshi SR, Briscoe SD, Alexander MJ, Li G, Kumar R. Therapeutic approaches for treating pulmonary arterial hypertension by correcting imbalanced TGF-β superfamily signaling. Front Med. 2022;8:2901. https://doi.org/10.3389/FMED.2021.814222/BIBTEX.
110. Gong H, Lyu X, Wang Q, Hu M, Zhang X. Endothelial to mesenchymal transition in the cardiovascular system. Life Sci. 2017;184:95–102. https://doi.org/10.1016/j.lfs.2017.07.014.
111. Reyes-Palomares A, Gu M, Grubert F, et al. Remodeling of active endothelial enhancers is associated with aberrant gene-regulatory networks in pulmonary arterial hypertension. Nat Commun. 2020;11(1):1673. https://doi.org/10.1038/S41467-020-15463-X.

112. Kim DJ, Dunleavey JM, Xiao L, et al. Suppression of TGFβ-mediated conversion of endothelial cells and fibroblasts into cancer associated (myo)fibroblasts via HDAC inhibition. Br J Cancer. 2018;118(10):1359–68. https://doi.org/10.1038/s41416-018-0072-3.
113. Teichert-Kuliszewska K. Bone morphogenetic protein receptor-2 signaling promotes pulmonary arterial endothelial cell survival: implications for loss-of-function mutations in the pathogenesis of pulmonary hypertension. Circ Res. 2006;98:209–17.
114. Good RB, Gilbane AJ, Trinder SL, et al. Endothelial to mesenchymal transition contributes to endothelial dysfunction in pulmonary arterial hypertension. Am J Pathol. 2015;185(7):1850–8. https://doi.org/10.1016/J.AJPATH.2015.03.019.
115. Zabini D, Granton E, Hu Y, et al. Loss of SMAD3 promotes vascular remodeling in pulmonary arterial hypertension via MRTF disinhibition. Am J Respir Crit Care Med. 2018;197(2):244–60. https://doi.org/10.1164/RCCM.201702-0386OC.
116. Mickael C, Kumar R, Hernandez-Saavedra D, et al. IL-6Ra in smooth muscle cells protects against schistosoma- and hypoxia-induced pulmonary hypertension. Am J Respir Cell Mol Biol. 2019;61(1):123–6. https://doi.org/10.1165/RCMB.2018-0277LE.
117. Calvier L, Chouvarine P, Legchenko E, Kokeny G, Mozes MM, Hansmann G. Chronic TGF-b1 signaling in pulmonary arterial hypertension induces sustained canonical Smad3 pathways in vascular smooth muscle cells. Am J Respir Cell Mol Biol. 2019;61(1):121–3. https://doi.org/10.1165/RCMB.2018-0275LE/SUPPL_FILE/DISCLOSURES.PDF.
118. Upton PD, Morrell NW. The transforming growth factor-β–bone morphogenetic protein type signalling pathway in pulmonary vascular homeostasis and disease. Exp Physiol. 2013;98(8):1262–6. https://doi.org/10.1113/EXPPHYSIOL.2012.069104.
119. Cahill E, Costello CM, Rowan SC, et al. Gremlin plays a key role in the pathogenesis of pulmonary hypertension. Circulation. 2012;125(7):920–30. https://doi.org/10.1161/CIRCULATIONAHA.111.038125.
120. Wellbrock J, Harbaum L, Stamm H, et al. Intrinsic BMP antagonist Gremlin-1 as a novel circulating marker in pulmonary arterial hypertension. Lung. 2015;193(4):567–70. https://doi.org/10.1007/S00408-015-9735-5/FIGURES/2.
121. Derrett-Smith EC, Dooley A, Gilbane AJ, et al. Endothelial injury in a transforming growth factor-dependent mouse model of scleroderma induces pulmonary arterial hypertension. Arthritis Rheum. 2013;65(11):2928–39. https://doi.org/10.1002/art.38078.
122. Gilbane AJ, Derrett-Smith E, Trinder SL, et al. Impaired bone morphogenetic protein receptor II signaling in a transforming growth factor-β-dependent mouse model of pulmonary hypertension and in systemic sclerosis. Am J Respir Crit Care Med. 2015;191(6):665–77. https://doi.org/10.1164/RCCM.201408--1464OC/SUPPL_FILE/DISCLOSURES.PDF.
123. Wang XJ. Germline BMP9 mutation causes idiopathic pulmonary arterial hypertension. Eur Respir J. 2019;53:1801609.
124. Wang G. Novel homozygous BMP9 nonsense mutation causes pulmonary arterial hypertension: a case report. BMC Pulm Med. 2016;16:17.
125. Hodgson J, Swietlik EM, Salmon RM, et al. Characterization of GDF2 mutations and levels of BMP9 and BMP10 in pulmonary arterial hypertension. Am J Respir Crit Care Med. 2020;201(5):575–85. https://doi.org/10.1164/RCCM.201906-1141OC.
126. Saito T, Bokhove M, Croci R, et al. Structural basis of the human endoglin-BMP9 interaction: insights into BMP signaling and HHT1. Cell Rep. 2017;19(9):1917–28. https://doi.org/10.1016/J.CELREP.2017.05.011.
127. Meadows CA, Risbano MG, Zhang L, et al. Increased expression of growth differentiation factor-15 in systemic sclerosis-associated pulmonary arterial hypertension. Chest. 2011;139(5):994. https://doi.org/10.1378/CHEST.10-0302.
128. Reynolds AM, Holmes MD, Danilov SM, Reynolds PN. Targeted gene delivery of BMPR2 attenuates pulmonary hypertension. Eur Respir J. 2012;39(2):329–43. https://doi.org/10.1183/09031936.00187310.
129. Long L, Crosby A, Yang X, et al. Altered bone morphogenetic protein and transforming growth factor-signaling in rat models of pulmonary hypertension potential for activin receptor-like kinase-5 inhibition in prevention and progression of disease. Circulation. 2009; https://doi.org/10.1161/CIRCULATIONAHA.108.821504.
130. Rol N, Kurakula KB, Happé C, Bogaard HJ, Goumans MJ. TGF-β and BMPR2 signaling in PAH: two black sheep in one family. Int J Mol Sci. 2018;19(9):2585. https://doi.org/10.3390/IJMS19092585.
131. Shi N, Wang Z, Zhu H, et al. Research progress on drugs targeting the TGF-β signaling pathway in fibrotic diseases. Immunol Res. 2022;70(3):276–88. https://doi.org/10.1007/S12026-022-09267-Y.
132. Joshi SR, Liu J, Bloom T, et al. Sotatercept analog suppresses inflammation to reverse experimental pulmonary arterial hypertension. Sci Rep. 2022;12(1):7803. https://doi.org/10.1038/s41598-022-11435-x.
133. Rothman RB, Ayestas MA, Dersch CM, Baumann MH. Aminorex, fenfluramine, and chlorphentermine are serotonin transporter substrates. Circulation. 1999;100(8):869–75. https://doi.org/10.1161/01.CIR.100.8.869.
134. Hervé P, Launay JM, Scrobohaci ML, et al. Increased plasma serotonin in primary pulmonary hypertension. Am J Med. 1995;99(3):249–54. https://doi.org/10.1016/S0002-9343(99)80156-9.
135. MacLean MMR. The serotonin hypothesis in pulmonary hypertension revisited: targets for novel therapies (2017 Grover Conference Series). Pulm Circ. 2018;8(2):2045894018759125. https://doi.org/10.1177/2045894018759125.
136. Lazarus HM, Denning J, Wring S, et al. A trial design to maximize knowledge of the effects of rodatristat ethyl in the treatment of pulmonary arterial hypertension (ELEVATE 2). Pulm Circ. 2022;12(2):e12088. https://doi.org/10.1002/PUL2.12088.
137. Penumatsa K, Abualkhair S, Wei L, et al. Tissue transglutaminase promotes serotonin-induced AKT signaling and mitogenesis in pulmonary vascular smooth muscle cells. Cell Signal. 2014;26(12):2818. https://doi.org/10.1016/J.CELLSIG.2014.09.002.
138. Dees C, Akhmetshina A, Zerr P, et al. Platelet-derived serotonin links vascular disease and tissue fibrosis. J Exp Med. 2011;208(5):961. https://doi.org/10.1084/JEM.20101629.
139. Frille A, Rullmann M, Becker GA, et al. Increased pulmonary serotonin transporter in patients with chronic obstructive pulmonary disease who developed pulmonary hypertension. Eur J Nucl Med Mol Imaging. 2021;48(4):1081–92. https://doi.org/10.1007/S00259-020-05056-7/TABLES/2.
140. Wallace E, Morrell NW, Yang XD, et al. A sex-specific microRNA-96/5-hydroxytryptamine 1B axis influences development of pulmonary hypertension. Am J Respir Crit Care Med. 2015;191:1432–42. https://doi.org/10.1164/rccm.201412-2148OC.
141. Long L, MacLean MR, Jeffery TK, et al. Serotonin increases susceptibility to pulmonary hypertension in BMPR2-deficient mice. Circ Res. 2006;98(6):818–27. https://doi.org/10.1161/01.RES.0000215809.47923.FD.
142. Launay JM, Hervé P, Peoc'h K, et al. Function of the serotonin 5-hydroxytryptamine 2B receptor in pulmonary hypertension. Nat Med. 2002;8(10):1129–35. https://doi.org/10.1038/NM764.
143. Chaturvedi S, Misra DP, Prasad N, et al. 5-HT2 and 5-HT2B antagonists attenuate pro-fibrotic phenotype in human adult dermal fibroblasts by blocking TGF-β1 induced non-canonical signaling pathways including STAT3: implications for fibrotic dis-

eases like scleroderma. Int J Rheum Dis. 2018;21(12):2128–38. https://doi.org/10.1111/1756-185X.13386.
144. McGoon MD, Vlietstra RE. Acute hemodynamic response to the S2-serotonergic receptor antagonist, ketanserin, in patients with primary pulmonary hypertension. Int J Cardiol. 1987;14(3):303–9. https://doi.org/10.1016/0167-5273(87)90200-2.
145. Dumitrascu R, Kulcke C, Konigshoff M, et al. Terguride ameliorates monocrotaline-induced pulmonary hypertension in rats. Eur Respir J. 2011;37(5):1104–18. https://doi.org/10.1517/14728222.2011.600692.
146. Macintyre PD, Bhargava B, Hogg KJ, Gemmill JD, Hillis WS. Brief rapid communication effect of subcutaneous sumatriptan, a selective 5HT1 agonist, on the systemic, pulmonary, and coronary circulation. Circulation. 1993;87(2):401–5.
147. Sodimu A, Bartolome S, Igenoza OP, Chin KM. Hemodynamic effects of fluoxetine in pulmonary arterial hypertension: an open label pilot study. Pulm Circ. 2020;10(4):2045894020971954. https://doi.org/10.1177/2045894020971954.
148. Humbert M, Labrune P, Sitbon O, et al. Pulmonary arterial hypertension and type-I glycogen-storage disease: the serotonin hypothesis. Eur Respir J. 2002;20(1):59–65. https://doi.org/10.1183/09031936.02.00258702.
149. Humbert M, Monti G, Fartoukh M, et al. Platelet-derived growth factor expression in primary pulmonary hypertension: comparison of HIV seropositive and HIV seronegative patients. Eur Respir J. 1998;11:554–9.
150. Humbert M, Guignabert C, Bonnet S, et al. Pathology and pathobiology of pulmonary hypertension: state of the art and research perspectives. Eur Respir J. 2019;53:1801887.
151. Perros F, Montani D, Dorfmüller P, et al. Platelet-derived growth factor expression and function in idiopathic pulmonary arterial. Hypertension. 2012;178(1):81–8. https://doi.org/10.1164/RCCM.200707-1037OC.
152. Antoniu SA. Targeting PDGF pathway in pulmonary arterial hypertension. Expert Opin Ther Targets. 2012;16(11):1055–63. https://doi.org/10.1517/14728222.2012.719500.
153. Riccieri V, Stefanantoni K, Vasile M, et al. Abnormal plasma levels of different angiogenic molecules are associated with different clinical manifestations in patients with systemic sclerosis. Clin Exp Rheumatol. 2011;29(2 SUPPL. 65):S46–52.
154. Overbeek MJ, Boonstra A, Voskuyl AE, et al. Platelet-derived growth factor receptor-β and epidermal growth factor receptor in pulmonary vasculature of systemic sclerosis-associated pulmonary arterial hypertension versus idiopathic pulmonary arterial hypertension and pulmonary veno-occlusive disease: a case-control study. Arthritis Res Ther. 2011;13(2):R61. https://doi.org/10.1186/AR3315.
155. Svegliati Baroni S, Santillo M, Bevilacqua F, et al. Stimulatory autoantibodies to the PDGF receptor in systemic sclerosis. N Engl J Med. 2006;354(25):2667–76. https://doi.org/10.1056/NEJMOA052955/SUPPL_FILE/NEJM_SVEGLIATIBARONI_2667SA1.PDF.
156. Dierick F, Héry T, Hoareau-Coudert B, et al. Resident PW1+ progenitor cells participate in vascular remodeling during pulmonary arterial hypertension. Circ Res. 2016;118(5):822–33. https://doi.org/10.1161/CIRCRESAHA.115.307035.
157. Ciuclan L, Hussey MJ, Burton V, et al. Imatinib attenuates hypoxia-induced pulmonary arterial hypertension pathology via reduction in 5-hydroxytryptamine through inhibition of tryptophan hydroxylase 1 expression. Am J Respir Crit Care Med. 2013;187(1):78–89. https://doi.org/10.1164/rccm.201206-1028OC.
158. Schermuly RT, Dony E, Ghofrani HA, et al. Reversal of experimental pulmonary hypertension by PDGF inhibition. J Clin Investig. 2005;115(10):2811. https://doi.org/10.1172/JCI24838.
159. Ghofrani HA, Morrell NW, Hoeper MM, et al. Imatinib in pulmonary arterial hypertension patients with inadequate response to established therapy. Am J Respir Crit Care Med. 2010;182(9):1171–7. https://doi.org/10.1164/rccm.201001-0123OC.
160. Rabinovitch M, Guignabert C, Humbert M, Nicolls MR. Inflammation and immunity in the pathogenesis of pulmonary arterial hypertension. Circ Res. 2014;115(1):165–75. https://doi.org/10.1161/CIRCRESAHA.113.301141.
161. Kumar R, Graham B. How does inflammation contribute to pulmonary hypertension? Eur Respir J. 2018;51(1):1702403. https://doi.org/10.1183/13993003.02403-2017.
162. Clapp LH, Gurung R. The mechanistic basis of prostacyclin and its stable analogues in pulmonary arterial hypertension: role of membrane versus nuclear receptors. Prostaglandins Other Lipid Mediat. 2015;120:56–71. https://doi.org/10.1016/J.PROSTAGLANDINS.2015.04.007.
163. Stenmark KR, Frid MG, Yeager M, et al. Targeting the adventitial microenvironment in pulmonary hypertension: a potential approach to therapy that considers epigenetic change. Pulm Circ. 2012;2(1):3–14. https://doi.org/10.4103/2045-8932.94817.
164. Frid MG, Alexandre McKeon B, Thurman JM, et al. Immunoglobulin-driven complement activation regulates proinflammatory remodeling in pulmonary hypertension. Am J Respir Crit Care Med. 2020;201(2):224–39. https://doi.org/10.1164/RCCM.201903-0591OC/SUPPL_FILE/DISCLOSURES.PDF.
165. Denton CP, Ong VH, Xu S, et al. Therapeutic interleukin-6 blockade reverses transforming growth factor-beta pathway activation in dermal fibroblasts: insights from the faSScinate clinical trial in systemic sclerosis. Ann Rheum Dis. 2018;77:1362–71. https://doi.org/10.1136/annrheumdis-2018-213031.
166. Khanna D, Lin CJF, Furst DE, et al. Tocilizumab in systemic sclerosis: a randomised, double-blind, placebo-controlled, phase 3 trial. Lancet Respir Med. 2020;8(10):963–74. https://doi.org/10.1016/S2213-2600(20)30318-0.
167. Tian W, Jiang X, Sung YK, et al. Phenotypically silent bone morphogenetic protein receptor 2 mutations predispose rats to inflammation-induced pulmonary arterial hypertension by enhancing the risk for neointimal transformation. Circulation. 2019;140(17):1409–25. https://doi.org/10.1161/CIRCULATIONAHA.119.040629.
168. Gilbane AJ, Derrett-Smith E, Trinder SL, Good RB, Pearce A, Denton CP, Holmes AM. Impaired bone morphogenetic protein receptor II signaling in a transforming growth factor-β-dependent mouse model of pulmonary hypertension and in systemic sclerosis. Am J Respir Crit Care Med. 2015;191:665–77.
169. Potus F, Pauciulo MW, Cook EK, et al. Novel mutations and decreased expression of the epigenetic regulator TET2 in pulmonary arterial hypertension. Circulation. 2020;141(24):1986. https://doi.org/10.1161/CIRCULATIONAHA.119.044320.
170. Wang Y, Kahaleh B. Epigenetic repression of bone morphogenetic protein receptor II expression in scleroderma. J Cell Mol Med. 2013;17(10):1291–9. https://doi.org/10.1111/JCMM.12105.
171. Zhao L, Chen CN, Hajji N, et al. Histone deacetylation inhibition in pulmonary hypertension: therapeutic potential of valproic acid and suberoylanilide hydroxamic acid. Circulation. 2012;126(4):455–67. https://doi.org/10.1161/CIRCULATIONAHA.112.103176.
172. Tsou PS, Khanna D, Sawalha AH. Identifying CYR61 as a potential anti-fibrotic and pro-angiogenic mediator in scleroderma. Arthritis Rheumatol. 2019;71(8):1350. https://doi.org/10.1002/ART.40890.
173. Zhou G, Chen T, Raj JU. MicroRNAs in pulmonary arterial hypertension. Am J Respir Cell Mol Biol. 2015; https://doi.org/10.1165/rcmb.2014-0166TR.
174. Meloche J, Pflieger A, Vaillancourt M, Graydon C, Provencher S, Bonnet S. miRNAs in PAH: biomarker, therapeutic target or both? Drug Discov Today. 2014;19(8):1264–9. https://doi.org/10.1016/J.DRUDIS.2014.05.015.

175. Kang BY, Park KK, Kleinhenz JM, et al. Peroxisome proliferator-activated receptor γ and microRNA 98 in hypoxia-induced endothelin-1 signaling. Am J Respir Cell Mol Biol. 2016;54(1):136–46. https://doi.org/10.1165/RCMB.2014-0337OC.
176. Sindi HA, Russomanno G, Satta S, et al. Therapeutic potential of KLF2-induced exosomal microRNAs in pulmonary hypertension. Nat Commun. 2020; https://doi.org/10.1038/s41467-020-14966-x.
177. Russomanno G, Jo KB, Abdul-Salam VB, et al. miR-150-PTPMT1-cardiolipin signaling in pulmonary arterial hypertension. Mol Ther Nucleic Acids. 2021;23:142–53. https://doi.org/10.1016/J.OMTN.2020.10.042.
178. Abd-Elmawla MA, Hassan M, Elsabagh YA, Alnaggar ARLR, Senousy MA. Deregulation of long noncoding RNAs ANCR, TINCR, HOTTIP and SPRY4-IT1 in plasma of systemic sclerosis patients: SPRY4-IT1 as a novel biomarker of scleroderma and its subtypes. Cytokine. 2020;133:155124. https://doi.org/10.1016/J.CYTO.2020.155124.
179. Tuder RM, Davis LA, Graham BB. Targeting energetic metabolism: a new frontier in the pathogenesis and treatment of pulmonary hypertension. Am J Respir Crit Care Med. 2012;185(3):260–6. https://doi.org/10.1164/RCCM.201108-1536PP.
180. Sutendra G, Michelakis ED. The metabolic basis of pulmonary arterial hypertension. Cell Metab. 2014;19(4):558–73. https://doi.org/10.1016/J.CMET.2014.01.004.
181. Cottrill KA, Chan SY. Metabolic dysfunction in pulmonary hypertension: the expanding relevance of the Warburg effect. Eur J Clin Investig. 2013;43(8):855–65. https://doi.org/10.1111/ECI.12104.
182. do Lee S, Shroyer KR, Markham NE, Cool CD, Voelkel NF, Tuder RM. Monoclonal endothelial cell proliferation is present in primary but not secondary pulmonary hypertension. J Clin Investig. 1998;101(5):927. https://doi.org/10.1172/JCI1910.
183. Semenza GL. Targeting HIF-1 for cancer therapy. Nat Rev Cancer. 2003;3(10):721–32. https://doi.org/10.1038/nrc1187.
184. Fijalkowska I, Xu W, Comhair SAA, et al. Hypoxia inducible-factor1α regulates the metabolic shift of pulmonary hypertensive endothelial cells. Am J Pathol. 2010;176(3):1130–8. https://doi.org/10.2353/AJPATH.2010.090832.
185. Tuder RM, Chacon M, Alger L, et al. Expression of angiogenesis-related molecules in plexiform lesions in severe pulmonary hypertension: evidence for a process of disordered angiogenesis. J Pathol. 2001;195(3):367–74. https://doi.org/10.1002/PATH.953.
186. Luengo A, Gui DY, van der Heiden MG. Targeting metabolism for cancer therapy. Cell Chem Biol. 2017;24(9):1161. https://doi.org/10.1016/J.CHEMBIOL.2017.08.028.
187. Xu W, Koeck T, Lara AR, et al. Alterations of cellular bioenergetics in pulmonary artery endothelial cells. Proc Natl Acad Sci U S A. 2007;104(4):1342. https://doi.org/10.1073/PNAS.0605080104.
188. Hagan G, Southwood M, Treacy C, et al. 18FDG PET imaging can quantify increased cellular metabolism in pulmonary arterial hypertension: a proof-of-principle study. Pulm Circ. 2011;1(4):448. https://doi.org/10.4103/2045-8932.93543.
189. Zhao L, Ashek A, Wang L, et al. Heterogeneity in lung 18FDG uptake in pulmonary arterial hypertension: potential of dynamic 18FDG positron emission tomography with kinetic analysis as a bridging biomarker for pulmonary vascular remodeling targeted treatments. Circulation. 2013;128(11):1214–24. https://doi.org/10.1161/CIRCULATIONAHA.113.004136.
190. Koppenol WH, Bounds PL, Dang CV. Otto Warburg's contributions to current concepts of cancer metabolism. Nat Rev Cancer. 2011;11(5):325–37. https://doi.org/10.1038/nrc3038.
191. Wunderlich V. Wegbereiter der modernen Krebsforschung: Theodor Boveri und Otto Warburg. BioSpektrum. 2020;26(6):687–90. https://doi.org/10.1007/S12268-020-1470-7.
192. van der Heiden MG, Cantley LC, Thompson CB. Understanding the Warburg effect: the metabolic requirements of cell proliferation NIH Public Access. Science (1979). 2009;324(5930):1029–33. https://doi.org/10.1126/science.1160809.
193. Lunt SY, van der Heiden MG. Aerobic glycolysis: meeting the metabolic requirements of cell proliferation. Annu Rev Cell Dev Biol. 2011;27:441–64. https://doi.org/10.1146/ANNUREV-CELLBIO-092910-154237.
194. Mcmurtry MS, Bonnet S, Wu X, et al. Dichloroacetate prevents and reverses pulmonary hypertension by inducing pulmonary artery smooth muscle cell apoptosis. Circ Res. 2004; https://doi.org/10.1161/01.RES.0000145360.16770.9f.
195. Michelakis ED, McMurtry MS, Wu XC, et al. Dichloroacetate, a metabolic modulator, prevents and reverses chronic hypoxic pulmonary hypertension in rats role of increased expression and activity of voltage-gated potassium channels. Circulation. 2002;105(2):244–50.
196. Guignabert C, Tu L, Izikki M, et al. Dichloroacetate treatment partially regresses established pulmonary hypertension in mice with SM22-targeted overexpression of the serotonin transporter. FASEB J. 2009; https://doi.org/10.1096/fj.09-131664.
197. Michelakis ED, Gurtu V, Webster L, et al. Inhibition of pyruvate dehydrogenase kinase improves pulmonary arterial hypertension in genetically susceptible patients. Sci Transl Med. 2017;9(413):eaao4583. https://doi.org/10.1126/SCITRANSLMED.AAO4583.
198. Cao Y, Zhang X, Wang L, et al. PFKFB3-mediated endothelial glycolysis promotes pulmonary hypertension. Proc Natl Acad Sci U S A. 2019;116(27):13394–403. https://doi.org/10.1073/PNAS.1821401116/SUPPL_FILE/PNAS.1821401116.SAPP.PDF.
199. Ball MK, Waypa GB, Mungai PT, et al. Regulation of hypoxia-induced pulmonary hypertension by vascular smooth muscle hypoxia-inducible Factor-1a. Am J Respir Crit Care Med. 2014;189:314–24. https://doi.org/10.1164/rccm.201302-0302OC.
200. Kojima H, Tokunou T, Takahara Y, et al. Hypoxia-inducible factor-1 α deletion in myeloid lineage attenuates hypoxia-induced pulmonary hypertension. Physiol Rep. 2019;7(7):e14025. https://doi.org/10.14814/PHY2.14025.
201. Wang L, Zhang X, Cao Y, et al. Mice with a specific deficiency of Pfkfb3 in myeloid cells are protected from hypoxia-induced pulmonary hypertension. Br J Pharmacol. 2021;178(5):1055–72. https://doi.org/10.1111/BPH.15339.
202. Martínez-Reyes I, Chandel NS. Mitochondrial TCA cycle metabolites control physiology and disease. Nat Commun. 2020;11(1):1–11. https://doi.org/10.1038/s41467-019-13668-3.
203. Selak MA, Armour SM, MacKenzie ED, et al. Succinate links TCA cycle dysfunction to oncogenesis by inhibiting HIF-prolylhydroxylase. Cancer Cell. 2005;7(1):77–85. https://doi.org/10.1016/J.CCR.2004.11.022.
204. Weinberg F, Hamanaka R, Wheaton WW, et al. Mitochondrial metabolism and ROS generation are essential for Kras-mediated tumorigenicity. Proc Natl Acad Sci U S A. 2010;107(19):8788–93. https://doi.org/10.1073/PNAS.1003428107/-/DCSUPPLEMENTAL.
205. Vasan K, Werner M, Chandel NS. Mitochondrial metabolism as a target for cancer therapy. Cell Metab. 2020;32(3):341–52. https://doi.org/10.1016/J.CMET.2020.06.019.
206. Paulin R, Dromparis P, Sutendra G, et al. Sirtuin 3 deficiency is associated with inhibited mitochondrial function and pulmonary arterial hypertension in rodents and humans. Cell Metab. 2014;20(5):827–39. https://doi.org/10.1016/J.CMET.2014.08.011.
207. Bonnet S, Michelakis ED, Porter CJ, et al. An abnormal mitochondrial-hypoxia inducible factor-1alpha-Kv channel pathway disrupts oxygen sensing and triggers pulmonary arterial hypertension in fawn hooded rats: similarities to human pulmo-

nary arterial hypertension. Circulation. 2006;113(22):2630–41. https://doi.org/10.1161/CIRCULATIONAHA.105.609008.
208. Sutendra G, Dromparis P, Wright P, et al. The role of Nogo and the mitochondria-endoplasmic reticulum unit in pulmonary hypertension. Sci Transl Med. 2011;3(88):88ra55. https://doi.org/10.1126/scitranslmed.3002194.
209. Carracedo A, Cantley LC, Paolo Pandolfi P. The process of cellular transformation and cancer progression involves genetic. Nat Rev Cancer. 2013;13:227–32. https://doi.org/10.1038/nrc3483.
210. Schoors S, Bruning U, Missiaen R, et al. Fatty acid carbon is essential for dNTP synthesis in endothelial cells. Nature. 2015;520(7546):192. https://doi.org/10.1038/NATURE14362.
211. Sutendra G, Bonnet S, Rochefort G, et al. Fatty acid oxidation and malonyl-CoA decarboxylase in the vascular remodeling of pulmonary hypertension. Sci Transl Med. 2010;2(44):44ra58. https://doi.org/10.1126/SCITRANSLMED.3001327/SUPPL_FILE/2-44RA58_SM.PDF.
212. Bertero T, Oldham WM, Cottrill KA, et al. Vascular stiffness mechanoactivates YAP/TAZ-dependent glutaminolysis to drive pulmonary hypertension. J Clin Invest. 2016;126(9):3313. https://doi.org/10.1172/JCI86387.
213. Bertero T, Perk D, Chan SY. The molecular rationale for therapeutic targeting of glutamine metabolism in pulmonary hypertension. Expert Opin Ther Targets. 2019;23(6):511. https://doi.org/10.1080/14728222.2019.1615438.
214. Chan SY, Rubin LJ. Metabolic dysfunction in pulmonary hypertension: from basic science to clinical practice. Eur Respir Rev. 2017;26(146):170094. https://doi.org/10.1183/16000617.0094-2017.
215. Randle PJ. Regulatory interactions between lipids and carbohydrates: the glucose fatty acid cycle after 35 years. Diabetes Metab Rev. 1998;14:263–83. https://doi.org/10.1002/(SICI)1099-0895(199812)14:4.
216. Long T, Hicks M, Yu HC, et al. Whole-genome sequencing identifies common-to-rare variants associated with human blood metabolites. Nat Genet. 2017;49(4):568–78. https://doi.org/10.1038/ng.3809.
217. Orst H, Lschewski O, Erald G, et al. Inhaled iloprost for severe pulmonary hypertension. Abstract. N Engl J Med. 2002;347:322–9.
218. Pulido T, Adzerikho I, Channick RN, et al. Macitentan and morbidity and mortality in pulmonary arterial hypertension. N Engl J Med. 2013;369(9):809–18. https://doi.org/10.1056/NEJMOA1213917/SUPPL_FILE/NEJMOA1213917_DISCLOSURES.PDF.
219. Galiè N, Olschewski H, Oudiz RJ, et al. Ambrisentan for the treatment of pulmonary arterial hypertension: results of the ambrisentan in pulmonary arterial hypertension, randomized, double-blind, placebo-controlled, multicenter, efficacy (ARIES) study 1 and 2. Circulation. 2008;117(23):3010–9. https://doi.org/10.1161/CIRCULATIONAHA.107.742510.
220. Obyn B, Arst RJ, Ewis R, Ubin LJ, Alker L, Ong WA, et al. A comparison of continuous intravenous epoprostenol (prostacyclin) with conventional therapy for primary pulmonary hypertension. N Engl J Med. 1996;334(5):296–301.
221. McLaughlin VV, Benza RL, Rubin LJ, et al. Addition of inhaled treprostinil to oral therapy for pulmonary arterial hypertension: a randomized controlled clinical trial. J Am Coll Cardiol. 2010;55(18):1915–22. https://doi.org/10.1016/J.JACC.2010.01.027.
222. Simonneau G, Barst RJ, Galie N, et al. Continuous subcutaneous infusion of treprostinil, a prostacyclin analogue, in patients with pulmonary arterial hypertension. Am J Respir Crit Care Med. 2012;165(6):800–4. https://doi.org/10.1164/AJRCCM.165.6.2106079.
223. Ghofrani HA, Galiè N, Grimminger F, et al. Riociguat for the treatment of pulmonary arterial hypertension. N Engl J Med. 2013;369(4):330–40. https://doi.org/10.1056/nejmoa1209655.
224. Galiè N, Ghofrani HA, Torbicki A, et al. Sildenafil citrate therapy for pulmonary arterial hypertension. N Engl J Med. 2005;353(20):2148–57. https://doi.org/10.1056/NEJMOA050010.
225. Galiè N, Brundage BH, Ghofrani HA, et al. Tadalafil therapy for pulmonary arterial hypertension. Circulation. 2009;119(22):2894–903. https://doi.org/10.1161/CIRCULATIONAHA.108.839274.
226. Lazarus H, Denning J, Kamau-Kelley W, Wring S, Palacios M, Humbert M. ELEVATE 2: a multicenter study of rodatristat ethyl in patients with WHO Group 1 pulmonary arterial hypertension (PAH). Eur Respir J. 2021;58(Suppl 65):PA1919. https://doi.org/10.1183/13993003.CONGRESS-2021.PA1919.
227. Sweatt AJ, Miyagawa K, Rhodes CJ, et al. Severe pulmonary arterial hypertension is characterized by increased neutrophil elastase and relative elafin deficiency. Chest. 2021;160(4):1442. https://doi.org/10.1016/J.CHEST.2021.06.028.
228. Brittain EL, Niswender K, Agrawal V, et al. Mechanistic phase II clinical trial of metformin in pulmonary arterial hypertension. J Am Heart Assoc. 2020;9(22):18349. https://doi.org/10.1161/JAHA.120.018349.
229. Safdar Z, Frost A, Basant A, Deswal A, O'Brian Smith E, Entman M. Spironolactone in pulmonary arterial hypertension: results of a cross-over study. Pulm Circ. 2020;10(2):1–8. https://doi.org/10.1177/2045894019898030.

Clinical Assessment of Pulmonary Hypertension

28

Stephanie M. Hon, Benoit Lechartier, Marc Humbert, and Harrison W. Farber

Introduction

Pulmonary arterial hypertension (PAH) is primarily a disease due to pulmonary vascular remodeling predominating on pulmonary arteries of less than 500 μm of diameter. PAH is a frequent complication of systemic sclerosis (SSc) observed with a prevalence of 8–12% [1–5]. In order to diagnose PAH, it is necessary to establish the appropriate cardiopulmonary hemodynamics as defined according to the sixth World Symposium on PH: mean pulmonary artery pressure (mPAP) ≥20 mmHg, pulmonary capillary wedge pressure (PCWP) or left ventricular end-diastolic pressure ≤15 mmHg, and a pulmonary vascular resistance (PVR) >3 Wood units. Currently, the only available method for detecting and assessing these and other important cardiopulmonary hemodynamic parameters (i.e., cardiac output) is right heart catheterization (RHC). Thus, RHC should be performed in all cases in which PAH is suspected. RHC will confirm the presence of pulmonary hypertension (PH) and its pre- and/or postcapillary mechanisms. RHC enables the establishment of a specific diagnosis of PAH, rules out other cardiac etiologies such as left ventricular failure, and assesses the degree of right heart dysfunction [6].

Within the last few decades, pulmonary fibrosis and PAH have become the leading causes of morbidity and mortality in SSc patients [7]. Despite advances and progresses in PAH therapy, prognosis of SSc-PAH is worse than other forms of PAH with a 1-year mortality reaching up to 30% [8]. The estimated 3-year survival among patients with PAH associated with SSc (SSc-PAH) is approximately 50% [9]. The development of PAH in SSc must be differentiated from PH due to chronic lung disease (pulmonary fibrosis) and/or hypoxia. Distinguishing PAH from PH due to pulmonary fibrosis is often difficult, especially since some patients can have both pulmonary fibrosis and a true pulmonary vasculopathy. However, if lung volumes (forced vital capacity (FVC) and/or total lung capacity (TLC)) are <60% of the predicted value and mPAP <35 mmHg at rest, PH is deemed more likely related to pulmonary fibrosis [10]. When lung volumes (TLC and/or FVC) are >70% of the predicted value, the PH is considered more likely to be PAH. When lung volumes (TLC and/or FVC) are between 60% and 70% of the predicted value, the diagnosis becomes more difficult; however, if mPAP is >35 mmHg, the PH is considered severe and most probably reflects a true pulmonary artery microangiopathy. Nevertheless, as noted, PH due to hypoxia/lung fibrosis and PAH may coexist in SSc patients. In this chapter, we will mainly focus on PAH.

Epidemiology

PAH is a frequent complication of SSc [1–5]. A meta-analysis of more than 3500 SSc patients showed that PAH prevalence in SSc, based on gold standard RHC definition, is slightly less than 10% [5]. In high-risk SSc patients, such as patients with a DLCO <60%, as in the DETECT study [11], PAH prevalence reaches 19%, while group 2 and group 3 PH in this study was 6%.

S. M. Hon · H. W. Farber
Pulmonary Hypertension Center, Tufts Medical Center, Boston, MA, USA
e-mail: shon@tuftsmedicalcenter.org; hfarber@tuftsmedicalcenter.org

B. Lechartier
Department of Respiratory Medicine, Hôpital Bicêtre, Paris, France

Department of Respiratory Medicine, Lausanne University Hospital, Lausanne, Switzerland
e-mail: benoit.lechartier@chuv.ch

M. Humbert (✉)
Department of Respiratory Medicine, Hôpital Bicêtre, Paris, France
e-mail: marc.humbert@bct.aphp.fr

Y. Allanore et al. (eds.), *Scleroderma*, https://doi.org/10.1007/978-3-031-40658-4_28

The incidence of SSc-PAH has been estimated in a large, multicenter cohort study of SSc patients using a revised screening algorithm for PAH diagnosis based on dyspnea and Doppler echocardiographic evaluation of tricuspid regurgitant jet velocity (TRJ) for referral of patients to RHC [12]. The overall incidence of PH was 1.37 cases per 100 patient-years [95% confidence interval 0.74–2.00] corresponding to PAH in 0.61 cases per 100 patient-years. Postcapillary PH had a similar incidence of 0.61 cases per 100 patient-years emphasizing the importance of a complete workup to rule out left heart disease in SSc patients presenting with PH [12]. Lastly, PH due to pulmonary fibrosis had an incidence of 0.15 cases per 100 patient-years. In all cases, it should be emphasized that RHC is mandatory for PAH diagnosis, as well as excluding a diagnosis of postcapillary PH. More recently, in a selected cohort of SSc patients with a DLCO <60% predicted, mPAP appeared to rise progressively during a 3-year follow-up and almost one-fourth of patients developed mPAP >25 mmHg using prospective RHC during follow-up [13].

PAH is generally considered a late complication of SSc [14] and represents a leading cause of morbidity and mortality, exceeding ILD in some registries [15]. Previous reports of the duration between diagnosis of SSc and onset of PAH vary according to study, ranging from 9.1 ± 6.6 years [16] to 14 ± 5 years [2]. Another study showed that PAH diagnosis occurred 6.3 ± 6.6 years after the first non-Raynaud's phenomenon symptom of SSc and that PAH can occur at any time following the diagnosis of SSc (in about half of cases within the first 5 years following the first non-Raynaud's symptom) [17]. In this study, patients with early-onset PAH (within the first 5 years following the first non-Raynaud's symptom) were older at the time of SSc diagnosis, with more severe pulmonary vascular disease and with a lower cardiac index and higher PVR than in patients with late-onset PAH.

Patients with limited cutaneous SSc are generally considered at greater risk of PAH than patients with diffuse cutaneous SSc [18–20]. However, diagnosis of PAH is often not based on RHC in these studies, and therefore, false-positive diagnosis of PAH or existence of postcapillary PH cannot be excluded in a significant proportion of cases. The frequency of diffuse cutaneous SSc observed in several registries is around 25% [2, 19], indicating that PAH should not be considered a specific vascular complication of limited cutaneous SSc alone.

Risk Factors

All subsets of SSc are at risk for development of PAH. However, several PAH risk factors have been shown in SSc, including the number of telangiectasias [21–23], reduced capillary nail fold density [21, 24], anticentromere antibodies, anti-topoisomerase antibodies, male gender, underlying pulmonary fibrosis, and Raynaud's phenomenon of greater than 3 years duration. SSc duration as a risk factor is more controversial, as indicated above [14, 16, 17, 21]. Other manifestations of SSc vasculopathy, such as digital ulcers, scleroderma renal crisis, and digital ischemia, have also been regarded as potential risk factors for development of PAH; however, studies have found no association between digital ulcers or digital ischemia and development of PAH [25, 26]. The strong association of PAH with >10 telangiectasias and the lack of clear association with digital ulcers, renal crisis, and digital ischemia suggest a shared pathogenesis with microvascular rather than macrovascular manifestations of SSc.

Screening: Why Is PAH Screening Needed in Scleroderma Patients?

PAH is a progressive disease with a poor prognosis, and SSc-PAH is particularly aggressive, accounting for 30% of deaths among SSc patients [8, 27]. If left untreated, SSc-PAH is associated with a median survival time of 1 year following diagnosis [28, 29]. Recent advances in diagnostic techniques and the emergence of evidence-based therapies for PAH facilitate earlier detection of the disease and, thus, earlier initiation of effective treatment [30]. Early detection of PAH and prompt initiation of effective therapy are considered an essential component of disease management, as patients diagnosed earlier in the course of the disease have a more pronounced benefit from therapy [30–32].

The predisposition of SSc patients to develop PAH as a complication means that with regular screening, the early diagnosis of PAH may be a realistic possibility in this patient population. Without screening, data from the French National Registry have shown that most patients are diagnosed in New York Heart Association (NYHA) functional class (FC) III or IV and, as such, are already severely compromised [4, 33]. Diagnosis of PAH in NYHA FC I or II is challenging, and even when patients become symptomatic, symptoms such as dyspnea and fatigue are nonspecific, and patients remain difficult to identify. Therefore, despite the potential for earlier diagnosis, SSc-PAH is still frequently identified late, with more than two-thirds of patients in NYHA FC III or IV at the time of diagnosis [12, 34, 35]. Of note, data from the French Registry have showed that, compared with patients in routine clinical practice, PAH detection programs in SSc are able to identify patients with milder forms of the disease, allowing earlier management and better outcomes: the 1-, 3-, 5-, and 8-year survival rates were 75%, 31%, 25%, and 17%, respectively, in the routine practice cohort, compared with 100%, 81%, 73%, and 64%, respectively, in the detection cohort ($p = 0.0037$) [36].

How Should PAH Screening Be Accomplished in Scleroderma Patients?

Screening is the systematic application of a test to identify individuals at sufficient risk of a specific disorder to warrant further investigation or direct preventive action, among persons who have not sought medical attention on account of symptoms of that disorder [36, 37]. Therefore, screening for PH/PAH applies to asymptomatic individuals belonging to groups in which PH/PAH is highly prevalent, such as SSc.

Echocardiography is currently the most effective screening tool to suspect PAH in SSc with the highest level of evidence of current tests used to screen for PAH [6]. For example, the 2015 ESC/ERS diagnostic algorithm in SSc patients with suspected PAH is based on the maximal TRJ velocity [6]:

1. A patient with a TRJ of ≤2.8 m/s or systolic PAP (sPAP) of ≤36 mmHg is unlikely to have PH, and RHC based on these measurements is not justified.
2. A patient with a TRJ of >3.4 m/s or sPAP of >50 mmHg is likely to have PH, and RHC is indicated to confirm the diagnosis.
3. In patients with a TRJ between these extremes (i.e., 2.9–3.4 m/s), other additional indicators of PH should be considered, and clinical judgment is required as to whether RHC is warranted [38].

This algorithm is relatively easy to follow, and using a slight adaptation of this, it has been possible to detect PAH in SSc patients following RHC dependent upon both echocardiographic readings and the presence or absence of dyspnea. Importantly, by using this adapted algorithm, 56.3% of patients were diagnosed in NYHA FC II [1, 12] (Fig. 28.1a).

There are other structural and functional echocardiographic features that could be used to indicate the need for diagnostic RHC in addition to criteria based on TRJ velocity. These signs provide assessment of the RV size and pressure overload, pattern of blood flow velocity out of the right ventricle, diameter of the pulmonary artery, and an estimate of right atrial pressure [6]. Resting echocardiography is recommended as a screening test in asymptomatic SSc patients, followed by annual screening with echocardiography, DLCO, and biomarkers [40, 41]. Importantly, exercise echocardiography has technical and methodological limitations and is not recommended for PH/PAH screening [6].

Additional clinical information that may be indicative of PH is a diffusing capacity for carbon monoxide (DLCO) of <60% of the predicted value in the absence of extensive interstitial lung disease (i.e., disease extent on High Resolution Computed Tomography (HRCT) >20% and/or FVC <70% of the predicted value) [6, 37, 42]. The **Australian Scleroderma Interest Group (ASIG)** algorithm correlates an FVC/DLCO ratio (both expressed as percentage of predicted values) ≥1.8, representative of a more pronounced reduction of gas transfer when compared to lung volume, to an increasing likelihood of pulmonary vascular disease [39]. As reported by Steen and Medsger [27], DLCO may be significantly decreased <60% of normal for many years prior to the occurrence of PAH. In contrast, although one-sixth of PAH-SSc patients have a DLCO >60% at PAH diagnosis, a DLCO >80% of the predicted value may exclude the diagnosis of PAH [12].

N-terminal pro-brain natriuretic peptide (NT-proBNP) levels are markers of myocardial wall stress and are also significantly correlated with RHC results [2, 43]. Even with a normal echocardiogram, NT-proBNP levels >3× the upper limit of normal is highly suggestive of PH. Elevated NT-proBNP levels may be predictive of PAH development in SSc patients [44], and as NT-proBNP detection is simple and noninvasive, it may be an attractive screening tool used alongside other parameters [37]. However, increased NT-proBNP levels are not specific of PAH, and elevated BNP or NT-proBNP levels do not differentiate left from right heart disease and cannot differentiate pre- from postcapillary PH. Moreover, normal NT-proBNP levels do not exclude PAH [45].

The **DETECT study** attempted to refine the screening process in SSc patients at increased risk of PAH (defined as SSc patients known for >3 years and DLCO <60% of the predicted value) [11]. These patients underwent a broad panel of noninvasive assessments followed by RHC. Of 466 SSc patients at increased risk of PAH, 87 (19%) had RHC-confirmed PAH. PAH was NYHA FC I/II in 64% of cases. A two-step composite score has been proposed in the DETECT study to select patients who should have a RHC [11]: six simple assessments in step 1 of the algorithm determined referral to echocardiography; then, in step 2, the step 1 prediction score and two echocardiographic variables determined referral to RHC. Studies evaluating performance of screening algorithms have demonstrated a sensitivity of 96–100%, specificity of only 35.3–48% and positive predictive value (PPV) of 35–68.6%, and negative predictive value (NPV) of 98–100% for the DETECT algorithm [11, 46, 47]. In comparison, the ASIG algorithm has a similar sensitivity of 94.1–100%, but a higher specificity at 54.5%, better PPV at 60–61.5% and similar NPV at 92.3–100% [39, 46]. In these studies, applying ESC/ERS guidelines to these patients had the lowest sensitivity at 91.4–96.3%, specificity at 31.8–32.3%, PPV at 51.6–55.3%, and NPV at 87.5–90.9% [39, 46, 47]. In other words, the DETECT algorithm recommended RHC in 62% of patients (referral rate) and missed 4% of PAH patients (false negatives). By comparison, applying ESC/ERS 2009 guidelines to these patients [40], 29% of diagnoses were missed while requiring a RHC referral rate of 40% [11].

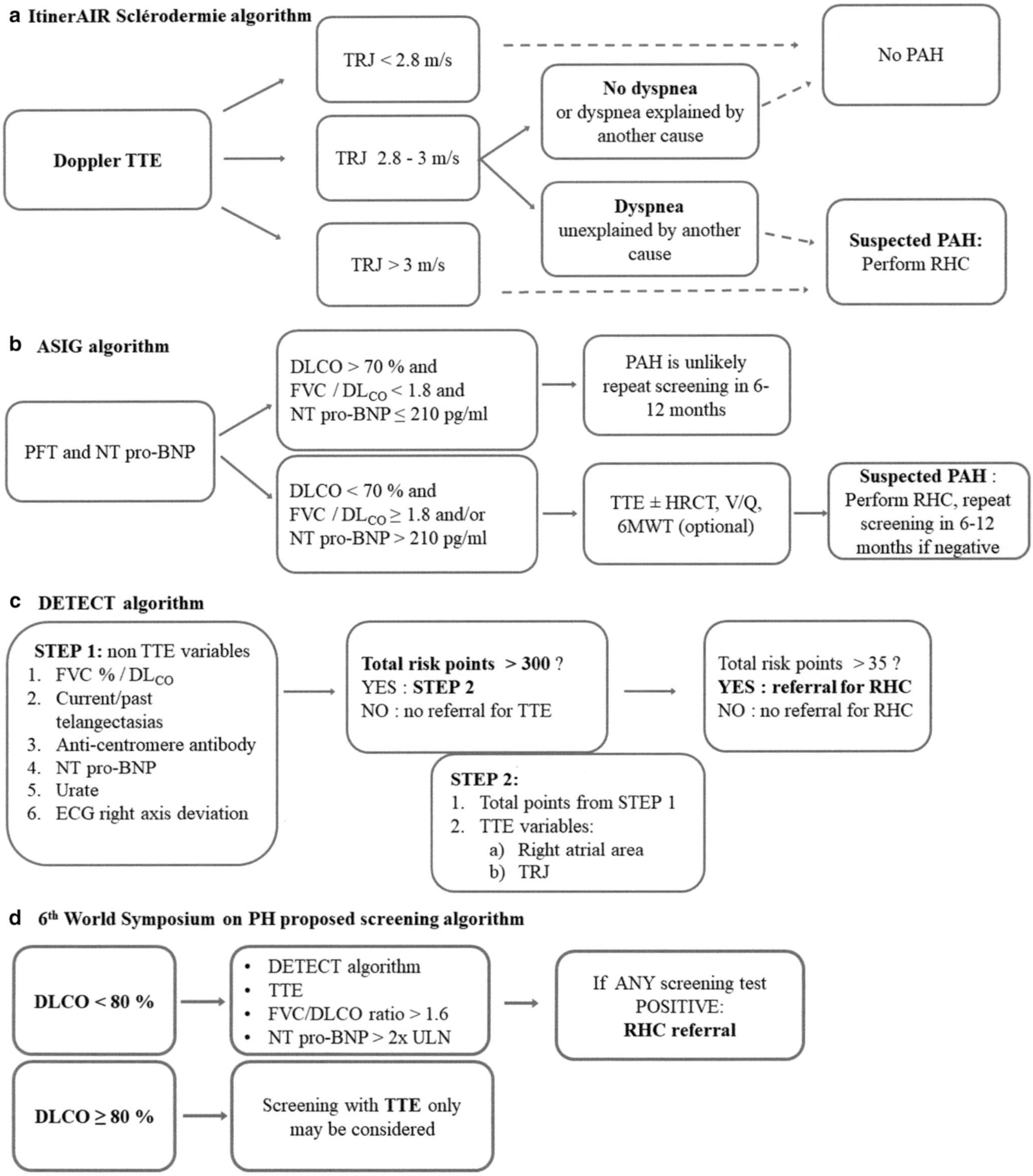

Fig. 28.1 Screening protocols proposed for SSc patients. (**a**) The ItinerAIR Sclérodermie algorithm. (**b**) The algorithm of the Australian Scleroderma Interest Group (ASIG). (**c**) The DETECT study. (**d**) The proposed screening algorithm from the 6th Wold Symposium on PH. *TRJ* tricuspid regurgitant jet, *sPAP* systolic pulmonary arterial pressure, *PAH* pulmonary arterial hypertension, *PH* pulmonary hypertension, *RHC* right heart catheterization. (Adapted from Hachulla et al. [12], Thakkar et al. [39], Coghlan et al. [11] and Galie et al. [6])

However, the following limitations should be noted with the use of DETECT algorithm: the online DETECT algorithm calculator is currently not accessible to US residents, it has not been validated for use in SSc patients with DLCO ≥60% predicted, and it does not provide further recommendations if the initial screening or echocardiographic results are low risk.

RHC in SSc patients may show borderline elevations in mPAP (ranging from 21 to 24 mmHg), relevant with the recent recommendations of the World Symposium [48]. In 2013, a study attempted to determine whether these patients are more likely to develop PH than those in whom mPAP is in the normal range [41]. Follow-up of a large single center cohort of SSc patients including 86 with borderline mPAP at baseline demonstrated that 29 of these patients later developed PH (of whom two cases were related to left heart disease). Patients with borderline mPAP were more likely to develop PH than patients with mPAP ≤20 mmHg (hazard ratio 3.7). A transpulmonary gradient (mPAP–PCWP) ≥11 mmHg at baseline also predicted progression to PH (hazard ratio 7.9). Of note, incident development of PAH was not benign, with a mortality of 18% within 3 years. Thus, SSc patients with borderline mPAP and an elevated transpulmonary gradient are more likely to progress to PH. Since then, the sixth World Symposium on PH has redefined precapillary PH with mPAP >20 mmHg from mPAP >25 mmHg with PVR >3 WU, in the presence of PCWP <15 mmHg [6]. Updated diagnostic work-up for SSc-PAH for patients with uncorrected DLCO ≥80% includes annual screening with TTE alone whereas patients with DLCO <80% should be screened with DETECT algorithm, TTE, FVC/DLCO ratio >1.6, and NT pro-BNP 2× upper limit of normal (ULN) and referred for RHC for any positive screening test [49].

Diagnosis and Evaluation

Patients with SSc-PAH tend to be asymptomatic early in the disease or only have symptoms related to involvement of other organs by SSc. Clinical symptoms are nonspecific, including progressive dyspnea with exertion and fatigue which are the most common initial presentation. However, functional impairment may be confounded by overall dysfunction from SSc, concomitant musculoskeletal disease, and lack of fitness. Physical examination findings may be absent early in the disease. Clinical findings include loud pulmonic component of the second heart sound and pulmonic/tricuspid regurgitant murmur.

Signs of right ventricular dysfunction become more evident as the disease progresses. Syncope, dyspnea at rest, chest pain, jugular vein extension, peripheral edema, and ascites generally indicate the development of right heart failure (Table 28.1) [50].

Diagnosis of PAH is suggested, in part, through the exclusion of other diseases. Pulmonary function testing, including measurement of DLCO, chest X-ray, ventilation/perfusion lung scintigraphy (and CT pulmonary angiography if needed), high-resolution computed tomography (HRCT) of the chest, echocardiography, laboratory testing for underlying diseases, and ECG are all employed for further signs of PAH or to diagnose a separate underlying cause.

Table 28.1 Clinical manifestations of PAH—primary symptom is dyspnea [50]

Preclinical	Symptomatic	Declining
Few symptoms manifest or are mistaken for lack of fitness	Increasing dyspnea on exertion	Dyspnea at rest
	Decreasing exercise tolerance	Severe impairment of exercise tolerance
	Fatigue	Hypoxemia
		Syncope
		Chest pain
		Edema
		Right heart failure
NYHA functional class I	NYHA functional class II–III	NYHA functional class IV

As indicated above, RHC is the gold standard for diagnosis of PAH, as well as providing prognostic parameters, such as cardiac index/output and right atrial pressure. Direct cardiac involvement can occur in SSc, affecting the myocardium, pericardium, and/or small intramyocardial vessels by vascular, fibrotic, and inflammatory changes. There is thus a higher prevalence of systolic or diastolic left ventricular dysfunction compared with idiopathic PAH [12, 48]. Patients with left heart disease may present with postcapillary PH (elevated PCWP). If PCWP is normal at baseline and left heart disease remains suspected, a fluid-loading test (or RHC at exercise) may be performed to identify diastolic left ventricle dysfunction which is common in patients with SSc [6, 51]. Studies have gathered data supporting the upper limit of normal of PCWP immediately after rapid infusion of 500 mL or 7 mL/kg saline does not exceed 18 mmHg [52]. A fluid challenge impacts the classification of PH in 20% of cases (most often by identifying occult left-sided heart failure) [53]. If appropriate, a left heart catheterization will allow better evaluation of an underlying left heart disease [51]. SSc-PAH patients more commonly present with pericardial effusion compared to idiopathic PAH, although it remains unknown whether the effusions are related to progressive right ventricular dysfunction or to the underlying inflammatory processes.

Pulmonary veno-occlusive disease (PVOD) is a less commonly recognized cause of precapillary PH in SSc but is not rare in SSc [54, 55]. When PVOD exists in SSc, it may lead to hydrostatic pulmonary edema without left ventricle dysfunction, frequently after treatment with pulmonary vasodilators [55]. Compared with isolated PAH, patients with PVOD often present with more severe hypoxemia and a more pronounced decrease of DLCO [55]. HRCT of the chest demonstrating centrilobular ground-glass opacities, increased septal lines, and lymph node enlargement is suggestive of PVOD in the setting of PH [55]. Similarly, occult alveolar hemorrhage on bronchoalveolar lavage in patients with PH is suggestive of PVOD. The diagnosis of PVOD is important, since pulmonary vasodilators are usually contraindicated in this form of PAH, and lung transplantation is the treatment of choice.

Natural History

The natural history of SSc-PAH is subclinical progression of pulmonary vascular injury and its consequences on the right side of the heart until dyspnea results. Once PAH has been recognized, the median survival before pulmonary vasodilator therapy was available was as low as 1–3 years [28, 29]. The eventual cause of death in SSc-PAH is usually the result of right heart failure [56]. As such, the combination of interstitial lung disease and SSc-PAH portends a much worse prognosis than isolated SSc-PAH; indeed, two large studies have shown <50% survival at 2 years in patients with both entities [2, 56].

Prognosis

Before specific PAH treatment era, the 3-year survival rate for patients with SSc-PAH was less than 35% [27]. Survival in two groups of matched patients with SSc-PAH has been reported: those treated with conventional medical therapy and prostanoids if needed (historical control group) and those treated with oral first-line treatment (current treatment era) [57]. Survival at 1 year was 68% in the historical control group, compared with 81% in the current treatment era group; the 2-year survival rates were 47% and 71%, respectively. Following the 2015 ESC/ERS PH guidelines [6], treatment of patients with SSc-PAH should follow the same algorithm as in idiopathic PAH as we now have a robust experience with oral and parenteral vasodilators use in SSc-PAH. Despite advances and progresses in PAH therapy, prognosis of SSc-PAH is worse than other forms of PAH with a 1-year mortality reaching up to 30% [8].

Mukerjee et al. reported that the prognosis of SSc-PAH is better if mPAP is mildly elevated at diagnosis. In patients with mPAP <32 mmHg, survival rates were 93% and 78% at 1 and 2 years, respectively [2]. Although one cannot rule out lead-time bias, these observations, as well as those reported above from the French Registry [4, 36], indicate that early detection of PAH may improve prognosis. Earlier diagnosis of PAH is a sine qua non condition for earlier management; however, whether earlier diagnosis is associated with increased life expectancy in SSc patients is not yet known. In a recent French report over the period of 2006–2017, survival improved over time in patients aged ≤70 years but not in older SSc-PAH [58].

Table 28.2 indicates signs and symptoms associated with prognosis and may guide clinical management.

Table 28.2 Prognosis factors according to recommendations [36]

Better prognosis	Determinants of prognosis	Worse prognosis
No	Clinical signs of right ventricular failure	Yes
Slow	Progression	Fast
No	Syncope	Yes
I, II	NYHA functional class	IV
>500 m	Walk test 6 min	<300 m
VO_2 max >15 mL/min/kg	Cardiopulmonary function	VO_2 max <12 mL/min/kg
Normal or quasi-normal	BNP/NT-proBNP (plasma rate)	Very high and increasing
No pericardial effusion	Echocardiography	Pericardial effusion
TAPSE >2.0 cm		TAPSE <1.5 cm
RAP <8 mmHg and CI ≥2.5 L/min/m^2	Hemodynamics	RAP >15 mmHg or CI ≤2.0 L/min/m^2

BNP brain natriuretic peptide, *CI* cardiac index, *6MWT* 6-min walk test, *RAP* right atrial pressure, *TAPSE* tricuspid annular plane systolic excursion, *NYHA* New York Heart Association

However, these prognosis factors have been extrapolated from patients with idiopathic PAH and may not be pertinent or achievable in patients with SSc-PAH (i.e., 6-min walk test >500 m) because of associated comorbidities, muscular involvement, and lower limb ischemia [59]. Moreover, there are multiple causes of dyspnea in SSc that may mask the intensity of dyspnea due to PAH [60]. It appears therefore necessary to identify specific SSc-PAH goals. However, if a patient with SSc-PAH remains in NYHA FC I/II after 4 months of treatment, prognosis is relatively good compared with patients who have deteriorated to NYHA FC III/IV during this period ($p = 0.007$). A cardiac index >2.71 L/min/m^2 is also associated with a better prognosis than a cardiac index of <2.71 L/min/m^2 ($p = 0.03$) [61]. Therefore, monitoring RHC 4 months after initiation of PAH therapy is recommended. If dyspnea or functional class status is not improved to appropriate levels and/or if cardiac index remains low, more aggressive therapy should be considered.

Prognosis in SSc-PAH Is Worse Than in Idiopathic PAH

Although the manifestations of PAH in SSc are similar to those in patients with PAH due to other etiologies, several independent studies have demonstrated increased morbidity and mortality in patients with SSc-PAH compared to patients with idiopathic PAH [9, 28]. Data from the REVEAL registry have showed that compared to patients with idiopathic PAH and other forms of PAH, connective tissue disease-associated PAH patients had more favorable hemodynamics at right heart catheterization yet had worse 6MWD, higher

BNP levels, increased likelihood of pericardial effusion, and worse 1-year survival [62]. Of the connective tissue disease-associated PAH, SSc-PAH had the worst prognosis and was associated with increased BNP levels, decreased DLCO, and increased mortality. These observations could be explained, in part, by the 50–80% incidence of concomitant interstitial lung disease in the SSc-PAH patients. Patients with SSc are also more likely to be chronically ill, have nutritional deficiencies from gastrointestinal involvement, and often have subclinical cardiac involvement with an increased propensity to arrhythmias. Therefore, increased mortality observed in SSc-PAH is most likely a result of a combination of factors: the presence of comorbidities in SSc-PAH and/or differences in the pathogenesis of PAH leading to a more severe phenotype in SSc-PAH. Supporting the latter possibility are observations of unique gene expression profiles in patients with IPAH and SSc-PAH in both lung tissue [4, 63] and peripheral blood cells [64, 65].

Increased mortality observed in SSc-PAH may also reflect the myocardium involvement in SSc that causes fibrosis and impaired microcirculatory function [66]. Eighty percent of necropsy case studies have demonstrated myocardial fibrosis as the pathological hallmark of this complication which likely contributes to inadequate compensation of the right ventricle to elevated afterload. Failure of the right ventricle to adapt to increased pulmonary afterload due to PAH lends itself to worse SSc-PAH morbidity, mortality, and decreased response to vasodilator therapy. Even in mild PAH (21–24 mmHg) in SSc patients, Nagel et al. found decreased 6MWD and reduced augmentation of RV output during exercise [67].

References

1. Hachulla E, Gressin V, Guillevin L, et al. Early detection of pulmonary arterial hypertension in systemic sclerosis: a French nationwide prospective multicenter study. Arthritis Rheum. 2005;52(12):3792–800.
2. Mukerjee D, St George D, Coleiro B, et al. Prevalence and outcome in systemic sclerosis associated pulmonary arterial hypertension: application of a registry approach. Ann Rheum Dis. 2003;62(11):1088–93.
3. Phung S, Strange G, Chung LP, et al. Prevalence of pulmonary arterial hypertension in an Australian scleroderma population: screening allows for earlier diagnosis. Intern Med J. 2009;39(10):682–91.
4. Humbert M, Sitbon O, Chaouat A, et al. Pulmonary arterial hypertension in France: results from a national registry. Am J Respir Crit Care Med. 2006;173(9):1023–30.
5. Avouac J, Airo P, Meune C, et al. Prevalence of pulmonary hypertension in systemic sclerosis in European Caucasians and metaanalysis of 5 studies. J Rheumatol. 2010;37(11):2290–8.
6. Galie N, Humbert M, Vachiery JL, et al. 2015 ESC/ERS Guidelines for the diagnosis and treatment of pulmonary hypertension: The Joint Task Force for the Diagnosis and Treatment of Pulmonary Hypertension of the European Society of Cardiology (ESC) and the European Respiratory Society (ERS): Endorsed by: Association for European Paediatric and Congenital Cardiology (AEPC), International Society for Heart and Lung Transplantation (ISHLT). Eur Respir J. 2015;46(4):903–75.
7. Steen VD, Medsger TA. Changes in causes of death in systemic sclerosis, 1972–2002. Ann Rheum Dis. 2007;66(7):940–4.
8. Chung L, Domsic RT, Lingala B, et al. Survival and predictors of mortality in systemic sclerosis-associated pulmonary arterial hypertension: outcomes from the pulmonary hypertension assessment and recognition of outcomes in scleroderma registry. Arthritis Care Res. 2014;66(3):489–95.
9. Fisher MR, Mathai SC, Champion HC, et al. Clinical differences between idiopathic and scleroderma-related pulmonary hypertension. Arthritis Rheum. 2006;54(9):3043–50.
10. Simonneau G, Gatzoulis MA, Adatia I, et al. Updated clinical classification of pulmonary hypertension. J Am Coll Cardiol. 2013;62(25 Suppl):D34–41.
11. Coghlan JG, Denton CP, Grunig E, et al. Evidence-based detection of pulmonary arterial hypertension in systemic sclerosis: the DETECT study. Ann Rheum Dis. 2014;73(7):1340–9.
12. Hachulla E, de Groote P, Gressin V, et al. The three-year incidence of pulmonary arterial hypertension associated with systemic sclerosis in a multicenter nationwide longitudinal study in France. Arthritis Rheum. 2009;60(6):1831–9.
13. Coghlan JG, Wolf M, Distler O, et al. Incidence of pulmonary hypertension and determining factors in patients with systemic sclerosis. Eur Respir J. 2018;51(4):1701197.
14. Medsger TA Jr. Natural history of systemic sclerosis and the assessment of disease activity, severity, functional status, and psychologic well-being. Rheum Dis Clin N Am. 2003;29(2):255–273, vi.
15. Simeon-Aznar CP, Fonollosa-Pla V, Tolosa-Vilella C, et al. Registry of the Spanish Network for Systemic Sclerosis: survival, prognostic factors, and causes of death. Medicine (Baltimore). 2015;94(43):e1728.
16. Coral-Alvarado P, Rojas-Villarraga A, Latorre MC, et al. Risk factors associated with pulmonary arterial hypertension in Colombian patients with systemic sclerosis: review of the literature. J Rheumatol. 2008;35(2):244–50.
17. Hachulla E, Launay D, Mouthon L, et al. Is pulmonary arterial hypertension really a late complication of systemic sclerosis? Chest. 2009;136(5):1211–9.
18. Chang B, Schachna L, White B, Wigley FM, Wise RA. Natural history of mild-moderate pulmonary hypertension and the risk factors for severe pulmonary hypertension in scleroderma. J Rheumatol. 2006;33(2):269–74.
19. MacGregor AJ, Canavan R, Knight C, et al. Pulmonary hypertension in systemic sclerosis: risk factors for progression and consequences for survival. Rheumatology (Oxford). 2001;40(4):453–9.
20. Scorza R, Caronni M, Bazzi S, et al. Post-menopause is the main risk factor for developing isolated pulmonary hypertension in systemic sclerosis. Ann N Y Acad Sci. 2002;966:238–46.
21. Cox SR, Walker JG, Coleman M, et al. Isolated pulmonary hypertension in scleroderma. Intern Med J. 2005;35(1):28–33.
22. Robert-Thomson PJ, Mould TL, Walker JG, Smith MD, Ahern MJ. Clinical utility of telangiectasia of hands in scleroderma and other rheumatic disorders. Asian Pac J Allergy Immunol. 2002;20(1):7–12.
23. Shah AA, Wigley FM, Hummers LK. Telangiectases in scleroderma: a potential clinical marker of pulmonary arterial hypertension. J Rheumatol. 2010;37(1):98–104.
24. Ong YY, Nikoloutsopoulos T, Bond CP, Smith MD, Ahern MJ, Roberts-Thomson PJ. Decreased nailfold capillary density in limited scleroderma with pulmonary hypertension. Asian Pac J Allergy Immunol. 1998;16(2–3):81–6.
25. Khimdas S, Harding S, Bonner A, et al. Associations with digital ulcers in a large cohort of systemic sclerosis: results from the Canadian Scleroderma Research Group registry. Arthritis Care Res. 2011;63(1):142–9.

26. Tiev KP, Diot E, Clerson P, et al. Clinical features of scleroderma patients with or without prior or current ischemic digital ulcers: post-hoc analysis of a nationwide multicenter cohort (ItinerAIR-Sclerodermie). J Rheumatol. 2009;36(7):1470–6.
27. Steen V, Medsger TA Jr. Predictors of isolated pulmonary hypertension in patients with systemic sclerosis and limited cutaneous involvement. Arthritis Rheum. 2003;48(2):516–22.
28. Kawut SM, Taichman DB, Archer-Chicko CL, Palevsky HI, Kimmel SE. Hemodynamics and survival in patients with pulmonary arterial hypertension related to systemic sclerosis. Chest. 2003;123(2):344–50.
29. Koh ET, Lee P, Gladman DD, Abu-Shakra M. Pulmonary hypertension in systemic sclerosis: an analysis of 17 patients. Br J Rheumatol. 1996;35(10):989–93.
30. Kiely DG, Lawrie A, Humbert M. Screening strategies for pulmonary arterial hypertension. Eur Heart J Suppl. 2019;21(Suppl K):K9–K20.
31. McLaughlin VV, Shillington A, Rich S. Survival in primary pulmonary hypertension: the impact of epoprostenol therapy. Circulation. 2002;106(12):1477–82.
32. Sitbon O, Humbert M, Nunes H, et al. Long-term intravenous epoprostenol infusion in primary pulmonary hypertension: prognostic factors and survival. J Am Coll Cardiol. 2002;40(4):780–8.
33. Weatherald J, Boucly A, Launay D, et al. Haemodynamics and serial risk assessment in systemic sclerosis associated pulmonary arterial hypertension. Eur Respir J. 2018;52(4):1800678.
34. Condliffe R, Kiely DG, Peacock AJ, et al. Connective tissue disease-associated pulmonary arterial hypertension in the modern treatment era. Am J Respir Crit Care Med. 2009;179(2):151–7.
35. Hachulla E, Carpentier P, Gressin V, et al. Risk factors for death and the 3-year survival of patients with systemic sclerosis: the French ItinerAIR-Sclerodermie study. Rheumatology (Oxford). 2009;48(3):304–8.
36. Humbert M, Yaici A, de Groote P, et al. Screening for pulmonary arterial hypertension in patients with systemic sclerosis: clinical characteristics at diagnosis and long-term survival. Arthritis Rheum. 2011;63(11):3522–30.
37. Khanna D, Gladue H, Channick R, et al. Recommendations for screening and detection of connective tissue disease-associated pulmonary arterial hypertension. Arthritis Rheum. 2013;65(12):3194–201.
38. D'Alto M, Romeo E, Argiento P, et al. Accuracy and precision of echocardiography versus right heart catheterization for the assessment of pulmonary hypertension. Int J Cardiol. 2013;168(4):4058–62.
39. Thakkar V, Stevens W, Prior D, et al. The inclusion of N-terminal pro-brain natriuretic peptide in a sensitive screening strategy for systemic sclerosis-related pulmonary arterial hypertension: a cohort study. Arthritis Res Ther. 2013;15(6):R193.
40. Galie N, Hoeper MM, Humbert M, et al. Guidelines for the diagnosis and treatment of pulmonary hypertension: the Task Force for the Diagnosis and Treatment of Pulmonary Hypertension of the European Society of Cardiology (ESC) and the European Respiratory Society (ERS), endorsed by the International Society of Heart and Lung Transplantation (ISHLT). Eur Heart J. 2009;30(20):2493–537.
41. Valerio CJ, Schreiber BE, Handler CE, Denton CP, Coghlan JG. Borderline mean pulmonary artery pressure in patients with systemic sclerosis: transpulmonary gradient predicts risk of developing pulmonary hypertension. Arthritis Rheum. 2013;65(4):1074–84.
42. Goh NS, Desai SR, Veeraraghavan S, et al. Interstitial lung disease in systemic sclerosis: a simple staging system. Am J Respir Crit Care Med. 2008;177(11):1248–54.
43. Blyth KG, Groenning BA, Mark PB, et al. NT-proBNP can be used to detect right ventricular systolic dysfunction in pulmonary hypertension. Eur Respir J. 2007;29(4):737–44.
44. Allanore Y, Borderie D, Avouac J, et al. High N-terminal pro-brain natriuretic peptide levels and low diffusing capacity for carbon monoxide as independent predictors of the occurrence of precapillary pulmonary arterial hypertension in patients with systemic sclerosis. Arthritis Rheum. 2008;58(1):284–91.
45. Cavagna L, Caporali R, Klersy C, et al. Comparison of brain natriuretic peptide (BNP) and NT-proBNP in screening for pulmonary arterial hypertension in patients with systemic sclerosis. J Rheumatol. 2010;37(10):2064–70.
46. Hao Y, Thakkar V, Stevens W, et al. A comparison of the predictive accuracy of three screening models for pulmonary arterial hypertension in systemic sclerosis. Arthritis Res Ther. 2015;17:7.
47. Guillen-Del Castillo A, Callejas-Moraga EL, Garcia G, et al. High sensitivity and negative predictive value of the DETECT algorithm for an early diagnosis of pulmonary arterial hypertension in systemic sclerosis: application in a single center. Arthritis Res Ther. 2017;19(1):135.
48. Simonneau G, Montani D, Celermajer DS, et al. Haemodynamic definitions and updated clinical classification of pulmonary hypertension. Eur Respir J. 2019;53(1):1801913.
49. Frost A, Badesch D, Gibbs JSR, et al. Diagnosis of pulmonary hypertension. Eur Respir J. 2019;53(1):1801904.
50. Rich S. Primary pulmonary hypertension. Prog Cardiovasc Dis. 1988;31(3):205–38.
51. Fox BD, Shimony A, Langleben D, et al. High prevalence of occult left heart disease in scleroderma-pulmonary hypertension. Eur Respir J. 2013;42(4):1083–91.
52. Borlaug BA. Invasive assessment of pulmonary hypertension: time for a more fluid approach? Circ Heart Fail. 2014;7(1):2–4.
53. D'Alto M, Romeo E, Argiento P, et al. Clinical relevance of fluid challenge in patients evaluated for pulmonary hypertension. Chest. 2017;151(1):119–26.
54. Dorfmuller P, Humbert M, Perros F, et al. Fibrous remodeling of the pulmonary venous system in pulmonary arterial hypertension associated with connective tissue diseases. Hum Pathol. 2007;38(6):893–902.
55. Gunther S, Jais X, Maitre S, et al. Computed tomography findings of pulmonary venoocclusive disease in scleroderma patients presenting with precapillary pulmonary hypertension. Arthritis Rheum. 2012;64(9):2995–3005.
56. Mathai SC, Hummers LK, Champion HC, et al. Survival in pulmonary hypertension associated with the scleroderma spectrum of diseases: impact of interstitial lung disease. Arthritis Rheum. 2009;60(2):569–77.
57. Williams MH, Das C, Handler CE, et al. Systemic sclerosis associated pulmonary hypertension: improved survival in the current era. Heart. 2006;92(7):926–32.
58. Hachulla E, Launay D, Boucly A, et al. Survival improved in patients aged ≤70 years with systemic sclerosis-associated pulmonary arterial hypertension during the period 2006 to 2017 in France. Chest. 2020;157(4):945–54.
59. Impens AJ, Wangkaew S, Seibold JR. The 6-minute walk test in scleroderma—how measuring everything measures nothing. Rheumatology (Oxford). 2008;47(Suppl 5):v68–9.
60. Hachulla E, Bervar JF, Launay D, et al. Dyspnea upon exertion in systemic scleroderma: from symptom to etiological diagnosis. Presse Med. 2009;38(6):911–26.
61. Launay D, Sitbon O, Le Pavec J, et al. Long-term outcome of systemic sclerosis-associated pulmonary arterial hypertension treated with bosentan as first-line monotherapy followed or not by the addition of prostanoids or sildenafil. Rheumatology (Oxford). 2010;49(3):490–500.
62. Chung L, Liu J, Parsons L, et al. Characterization of connective tissue disease-associated pulmonary arterial hypertension from REVEAL: identifying systemic sclerosis as a unique phenotype. Chest. 2010;138(6):1383–94.

63. Hsu E, Shi H, Jordan RM, Lyons-Weiler J, Pilewski JM, Feghali-Bostwick CA. Lung tissues in patients with systemic sclerosis have gene expression patterns unique to pulmonary fibrosis and pulmonary hypertension. Arthritis Rheum. 2011;63(3):783–94.
64. Christmann RB, Hayes E, Pendergrass S, et al. Interferon and alternative activation of monocyte/macrophages in systemic sclerosis-associated pulmonary arterial hypertension. Arthritis Rheum. 2011;63(6):1718–28.
65. Pendergrass SA, Hayes E, Farina G, et al. Limited systemic sclerosis patients with pulmonary arterial hypertension show biomarkers of inflammation and vascular injury. PLoS One. 2010;5(8):e12106.
66. Rangarajan V, Matiasz R, Freed BH. Cardiac complications of systemic sclerosis and management: recent progress. Curr Opin Rheumatol. 2017;29(6):574–84.
67. Nagel C, Marra AM, Benjamin N, et al. Reduced right ventricular output reserve in patients with systemic sclerosis and mildly elevated pulmonary artery pressure. Arthritis Rheumatol. 2019;71(5):805–16.

The Management of Pulmonary Arterial Hypertension in the Setting of Systemic Sclerosis

29

Stephen C. Mathai and Olivier Sitbon

Pulmonary hypertension (PH) commonly complicates systemic sclerosis (SSc). PH related to SSc can develop in multiple ways and thus be classified in any of the five groups of PH as defined by the current European guidelines [1, 2]. PH significantly impacts morbidity and mortality in SSc and along with interstitial lung disease (ILD), is currently the leading cause of death in this population. While advances in therapeutics have led to improvements in symptoms, functional capacity, and outcomes in patients with pulmonary arterial hypertension (PAH), the response to therapy in PAH related to SSc (PAH-SSc) is, in general, less robust than other forms of PAH. Unfortunately, there are few randomized clinical trials of these therapies in other forms of PH, and thus, treatment in these populations is challenging. However, newer therapeutic strategies, such as simultaneously targeting multiple pathways involved in the putative pathogenesis of the disease or utilizing inhaled therapies, suggest improved outcomes for SSc-PAH and have led to randomized trials in SSc-PH related to ILD. Focusing on supportive therapy, such as pulmonary rehabilitation, may also be important in the management of this complex disease.

S. C. Mathai (✉)
Division of Pulmonary and Critical Care Medicine, Department of Medicine, Johns Hopkins University School of Medicine, Baltimore, MD, USA
e-mail: smathai4@jhmi.edu

O. Sitbon
School of Medicine, Université Paris-Saclay, Le Kremlin-Bicêtre, France

Department of Respiratory and Intensive Care Medicine, AP-HP, Hôpital Bicêtre, Le Kremlin-Bicêtre, France

INSERM UMR_S 999, Hôpital Marie Lannelongue, Le Plessis-Robinson, France

Definition and Classification of Pulmonary Hypertension in Systemic Sclerosis

Pulmonary hypertension is a chronic disease of the pulmonary vasculature characterized by pulmonary vascular injury and remodeling that leads to increased pulmonary vascular resistance, right ventricular failure, and ultimately, death [1]. PH can develop in association with many different diseases, including connective tissue diseases (CTD) such as SSc, systemic lupus erythematosus, and mixed connective tissue disease, and can result from processes that primarily effect organ systems distinct from the pulmonary vasculature, such as the heart, lung parenchyma, liver, skin, and kidneys [2]. Direct pulmonary vascular involvement can occur from pulmonary embolism and from pulmonary vascular remodeling in response to endothelial damage without overt venous thromboembolism, known as pulmonary arterial hypertension (PAH).

At the Sixth World Symposium on Pulmonary Hypertension, the hemodynamic definition of PH was modified by lowering the diagnostic threshold of mean pulmonary artery pressure (mPAP) from ≥25 to >20 mmHg [3]. This change was based upon studies demonstrating the normal range of pulmonary pressures in healthy subjects (mPAP 14 ± 3 mmHg) and poor outcomes for patients with mPAP >20 mmHg [4–6]. Because the definition of PH is based on mPAP, it can only be diagnosed by right heart catheterization (RHC). PH is currently classified into one of five groups based upon associated diseases and risk factors [1, 2] (Fig. 29.1). SSc can affect multiple organ systems and thus, PH related to CTD can be associated with any of the five groups of PH. Most commonly, PH in CTD is either Group 1 (PAH) or Group 3 (PH related to lung disease). It can also be Group 2 (PH related to left heart disease), particularly in patients with SSc who frequently have diastolic dysfunction. PAH can occur in the absence of associated diseases or risk factors (idiopathic PAH or IPAH) or can complicate CTD

Y. Allanore et al. (eds.), *Scleroderma*, https://doi.org/10.1007/978-3-031-40658-4_29

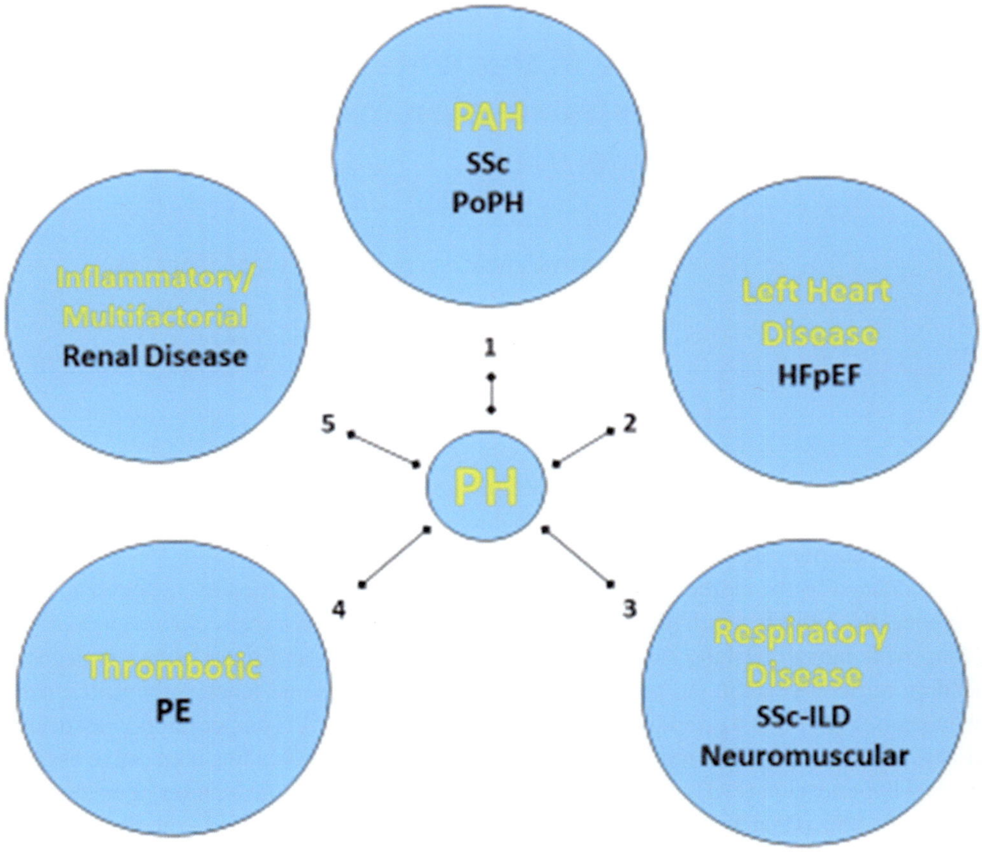

Fig. 29.1 Types of pulmonary hypertension in scleroderma. *PH* pulmonary hypertension, *PAH* pulmonary arterial hypertension, *PoPH* portopulmonary hypertension (related to primary biliary cirrhosis), *HFpEF* heart failure with preserved ejection fraction, *SSc-ILD* scleroderma-related interstitial lung disease, *PE* pulmonary embolism

(CTD-PAH), particularly SSc. Importantly, PAH refers to pulmonary vasculopathy with elevated mPAP in the absence of underlying heart or lung disease and underlying pulmonary embolism. This is an important distinction because most of the current targeted therapies are only approved for PAH; one recently has been approved for use in chronic thromboembolic PH (CTEPH) and in the US, for PH in the setting of interstitial lung disease (PH-ILD) [7]. Regardless of the cause, however, the presence of PH in any form is associated with an increased risk of morbidity and mortality [8–11].

Epidemiology of PH and Impact on Outcomes

PAH occurs in about 8–14% of patients with SSc when the diagnosis is properly established by RHC; higher estimates of PAH (up to 45% in certain series) have overestimated the prevalence due to use of echocardiography which has significant limitations in accuracy [12–15]. Risk factors for development of PAH within SSc populations include female sex, older age at diagnosis of SSc, longer duration of SSc, and limited disease (formerly known as the "CREST" syndrome) [16]. Because of the high risk of development of PAH in SSc, screening for PAH is recommended; an algorithm such as the one developed in the DETECT study that includes serum markers, physiologic data, and echocardiographic parameters may be employed [17]. However, whether early detection improves outcomes is unknown. Overall, outcomes in SSc-PAH are poor with worse survival than other forms of PAH such as IPAH and other forms of CTD-PAH [11, 18–21].

SSc patients can also develop PH related to interstitial lung disease (SSc-ILD), however, there are few data describing the incidence and prevalence of PH in SSc-ILD. While the presence of ILD in SSc in the absence of PH portends a poor prognosis, survival is even worse in SSc patients with combined ILD and PH [9, 10, 22–24]. In a cohort of 59 SSc-PH patients, 20 of whom had significant ILD (defined as a TLC <60% predicted or TLC between 60% and 70% predicted combined with moderate to severe fibrosis on high resolution CT of the chest), presence of ILD portended a fivefold increased risk of death compared to PAH [10]. A recent larger cohort study found survival remained poor in SSc patients with PH-ILD, but the risk of death for PH-ILD compared to PAH was attenuated [24]. Importantly, a recent randomized clinical trial of inhaled treprostinil included patients with PH-ILD demonstrated potential benefit and has been recently approved for treatment of this condition [7]. Whether this therapy impacts survival in SSc-related PH-ILD remains to be determined.

Exercise-Induced Pulmonary Hypertension

Recognition and diagnosis of early pulmonary vascular disease in SSc is challenging even when applying early detection strategies as noted above. An abnormal pulmonary vascular response to exercise has been postulated to represent early pulmonary vascular disease in patients without resting PH (mPAP ≤20 mmHg). While there remains controversy regarding the mode of exercise challenge and hemodynamic criteria, most experts agree that a pulmonary artery pressure to cardiac output slope of >3 mmHg/L/min with exercise identifies exercise-induced PH (Ex-PH) [25].

The impact of Ex-PH is particularly notable in SSc patients. In a cohort study of SSc patients, those with Ex-PH not only had worse outcomes than SSc patients without Ex-PH, but also had similar outcomes to those with PAH [26]. In SSc patients without resting PH (defined as a mPAP ≥25 mmHg), those patients with Ex-PH had significantly worse outcomes than those who did not demonstrate Ex-PH [27]. Despite these observations of the clinical relevance of Ex-PH in SSc, there are limited data to support treatment with PAH-specific therapies. One recent randomized clinical trial using ambrisentan in a cohort of patients with SSc and either Ex-PH or mild PH (defined as a mPAP between 21 and 24 mmHg) did not demonstrate significant changes in the primary outcome of mPAP [28].

SSc with Mildly Elevated Pulmonary Pressures

Prior cohort studies of SSc patients have demonstrated an increased risk for progression of pulmonary vascular disease and poor outcomes in patients with mildly elevated pulmonary pressures [9, 29]. The Sixth World Symposium on Pulmonary Hypertension recommended lowering the mPAP threshold for the diagnosis of PH, there were no specific recommendations offered regarding therapy for such patients. All currently approved therapies for PAH were evaluated in patients with mPAP ≥25 mmHg. Further, aside from the data from study referenced above, there are no studies examining the role of PAH-specific therapies in early PH. A small randomized clinical trial of sildenafil in SSc patients with mPAP between 21 and 24 mmHg is currently enrolling. (NCT04797286).

Risk Assessment in CTD-PAH

Assessment of risk at the time of diagnosis then regularly during the course of the disease is recommended by the current European guidelines [1, 2]. Risk assessment should be performed using a multidimensional approach including selected clinical, exercise, biochemical, imaging-derived, and hemodynamic variables [1, 2]. The main treatment goal is to achieve a low-risk status, which is associated with a low mortality risk. Several methods have been developed to assess the risk status (low-, intermediate, or high-risk) in patients with PAH, such as REVEAL scores and methods derived from the European guidelines risk stratification table [30–33]. All methods and scores can determine patient risk status. The study from the French PAH registry demonstrated that the number of noninvasive low-risk criteria achieved was a simple and valid method to determine a low-risk status in PAH [31]. The use of the REVEAL Lite 2 score, an abridged version of the REVEAL 2.0 Risk Score, resulted in similar findings [30]. Recent data from COMPERA and French Registries have shown that a 4-strata risk assessment method refined risk prediction, especially within the intermediate risk category of patients [34, 35]. The validity of this approach to risk assessment has also been studied specifically in SSc-PAH, using ESC/ERS prediction models and the REVEAL Risk Score Calculator [36–38].

Therapy for CTD-PAH: Overview

Historically, CTD-PAH patients, and in particular those with SSc-PAH, have less robust response to PAH-specific therapies when compared to other PAH populations. An older age, the presence of comorbidities, left heart involvement, interstitial lung disease, and pulmonary vein involvement are usually evoked to explain this finding. Using patient-level data from PAH registration trials, Rhee and colleagues found a higher rate of adverse events overall in CTD-PAH and an attenuated effect on quality of life [39]. Using the same data, the authors also report that CTD-PAH patients had minimal improvement in functional capacity in response to PAH therapies [40]. In contrast, a more recent meta-analysis of modern treatment strategies in CTD-PAH demonstrated improved outcomes overall for the CTD-PAH population [41]. However, while specific therapies for PAH have been studied in randomized clinical trials that have included patients with SSc-PAH, there have been only two study conducted exclusively in patients with SSc-PAH. Further, the classification of the specific CTD associated with PAH is often not reported in these clinical trials (Table 29.1). When reported, response to therapy in short-term studies seems to vary between types of CTD-PAH, with patients with SSc-PAH demonstrating the poorest response among the CTD population [42, 43]. However, since specific CTD diagnosis are not adjudicated, it is possible that misclassification of CTD exists and may influence observed associations between CTD type and response to therapy. Still, observational cohort studies have consistently demonstrated poorer survival for patients with SSc-PAH compared to other forms of CTD-PAH, suggesting poorer response to therapy in this population [9, 20].

Table 29.1 Inclusion of SSc patients in pivotal trials of PAH therapy

	CTD-PAH (*n*, overall %)	Type of CTD (*n*, % CTD)
Epoprostenol	111 (100%)	lcSSc: 77 (69%) dcSSc: 14 (13%) Others: 20 (18%)
Oral Treprostinil	110 (19%)	NR
Oral Treprostinil add-on	92 (26%)	NR
SC Treprostinil	90 (19%)	lcSSc: 20 (22%) dcSSc: 25 (28%) SLE: 25 (28%) MCTD: 17 (19%) Overlap: 3 (3%)
Inhaled Treprostinil	77 (33%)	NR
Inhaled Iloprost (AIR)	35 (17%)	NR
Inhaled Iloprost + Bosentan	NR	NR
Beraprost	13 (10%)	NR
Vardenafil (EVOLUTION)	20 (30%)	NR
Tadalafil (PHIRST)	95 (29%)	NR
Sildenafil + Epoprostenol (PACES)	55 (21%)	SSc: 31 (56%) SLE: 14 (25%) Other: 10 (18%)
Sildenafil (SUPER)	84 (30%)	SSc: 50 (60%) SLE: 19 (23%) MCTD: 8 (10%) SjS: 4 (5%) RA: 1 (1%)
Bosentan (EARLY)	33 (18%)	SSc: 15 (46%) SLE: 11 (6%) MCTD: 3 (9%) SjS: 1 (3%) Other: 1 (3%)
Bosentan (Study 351 + BREATHE)	66 (27%)	SSc: 52 (78%) SLE: 8 (12%) Overlap: 4 (6%) UCTD: 2 (3%)
Bosentan + Epoprostenol (BREATHE-2)	6 (18%)	SSc: 5 (83%) SLE: 1 (17%)
Ambrisentan (ARIES 1 + ARIES 2)	136 (35%)	NR
Sitaxsentan (STRIDE-1)	42 (24%)	SSc: 19 (45%) SLE: 15 (36%) MCTD: 7 (17%)
Macitentan (SERAPHIN)	224 (30.5%)	NR
Selexipag (GRIPHON)	334 (28.9%)	SSc: 170 (50.9%) SLE: 82 (24.5%) MCTD: 37 (11.1%) UCTD: 45 (13.4%)
Orenitram (FREEDOM-EV)	178 (25.8%)	NR
Rituximab	57 (100%)	SSc: 57 (100%)

General Measures

Despite a lack of specific data for SSc-PAH, consensus guidelines recommend the use of supplemental oxygen and diuretics [1, 2]. While anticoagulation could be considered in patients with IPAH based upon a high prevalence of in-situ thrombosis in histopathologic evaluation of lung tissue from patients with IPAH, use of this medication is not routinely recommended in SSc-PAH [44]. A recent large retrospective study regarding the utility of anticoagulation in SSc-PAH reported a strong trend toward worse outcomes in SSc-PAH patients treated with anticoagulation compared to those not treated (HR 1.82; 95% CI 0.94–3.54, $p = 0.08$) [45]. Some experts tend not to anticoagulate SSc-PAH patients based upon concerns about increased risk of gastrointestinal bleeding from vascular ectasias that may be common in SSc [16, 45, 46]. Furthermore, although the prevalence of in-situ thrombosis in IPAH patients may be high, these lesions may be less frequent in SSc-PAH patients [47]. There is an evolving evidence base to support pulmonary rehabilitation in PAH and based upon these studies, current guidelines recommend participation in such programs [1, 2, 48].

Anti-inflammatory Agents

Inflammation is a key mediator in the pathogenesis of SSc and accumulating evidence support the inflammatory nature of PAH [49]. Histologically, perivascular inflammatory infiltrates are observed around plexiform lesions in PAH [50]. In SSc-PAH, inflammatory infiltrates have been described around plexiform lesions, but not around uninvolved pulmonary vessels, implicating active inflammation as a key contributor to disease pathogenesis [51]. SSc-PAH has been described as a prototypical inflammatory disease, characterized by autoantibody-mediated endothelial cell injury, increased cytokine release, and increased expression of genes involved in the inflammatory response. In patients with other forms of connective tissue disease-associated PAH (systemic lupus erythematosus, mixed connective tissue disease), modest numbers have responded to anti-inflammatory treatment with cyclophosphamide and prednisone, demonstrating improvement in functional class, hemodynamic indices, and survival [52].

Unfortunately, a similar response to immunosuppressive therapy has not been observed in patients with SSc-PAH. Given the lack of demonstrated benefit and potential adverse effects of high-dose or long-term immunosuppressive therapies, these are generally not used for patients with SSc-PAH. In particular, the risk of scleroderma renal crisis with high-dose steroids dampens enthusiasm for its use in this patient population [53, 54]. A recently completed randomized controlled clinical trial of rituximab, a monoclonal antibody targeting CD20 on B cells, did not meet its primary endpoint of change in 6 min walk distance (6MWD) although there was a trend toward improvement [55]. Interestingly, in a post-hoc analysis, the authors found a panel of cytokines (rheumatoid factor, IL-2, and IL-17) that predicted response to rituximab. Thus, there remain no randomized trial data supporting the use of immunosuppression in the treatment of PAH in the setting of SSc.

Calcium Channel Blockers

Oral calcium channel blockers (nifedipine, diltiazem) given at high doses have proven to be an effective long-term therapy in a minority of IPAH patients (<7%) who demonstrate acute vasodilatation in response to nitric oxide, epoprostenol, or adenosine during hemodynamic testing [56, 57]. Unfortunately, the vast majority of patients with PAH related to connective tissue disease (>97%) fail to respond to acute vasodilators during hemodynamic testing [58]. Further, less than 1% of patients with PAH related to connective tissue disease treated with CCB have sustained response at 1 year [59]. In addition, there is a frequent pulmonary vein involvement in patients with SSc-PAH. In those patients, a positive acute response to vasodilator testing can be seen. However, initiation of CCB therapy in such patients with an acute vasodilator response always led to serious adverse event (severe pulmonary edema) and clinical deterioration [60]. Thus, although many SSc patients receive low-dose calcium channel blockers for Raynaud symptoms, high-dose calcium channel blocker therapy is not routinely prescribed for patients with SSc-PAH.

Prostaglandins

Prostacyclin, produced by endothelial cells, is a potent vasodilator, inhibits platelet aggregation, and effectively prevents the release of growth factors from endothelial cells, platelets, and macrophages [61]. As such, prostacyclin has the capacity to inhibit many of the fundamental abnormalities in PAH. In the United States, prostacyclin analogs are available for delivery via intravenous (epoprostenol, treprostinil), subcutaneous (treprostinil), inhaled (iloprost, treprostinil), and oral (treprostinil) routes. Continuous intravenous infusion of epoprostenol has been shown to provide sustained improvements in exercise capacity, pulmonary vascular resistance, mean pulmonary artery pressure, and quality of life in patients with PAH [62–64]. In one study of IPAH patients, epoprostenol was associated with improved survival over a 12-week period when compared to controls. Although no studies have demonstrated improved long-term survival in PAH patients with epoprostenol in randomized, controlled trials, IPAH patients with World Health Organization Functional Class 3 or 4 symptoms have demonstrated improved survival when compared to historical controls [65, 66].

In patients with SSc-PAH, a 12-week trial of IV epoprostenol was associated with increased exercise capacity, reduced symptoms, and improved functional class when compared to controls [67]. However, no short-term mortality benefit was seen. A prospective, non-controlled, open-label study of IV epoprostenol in SSc-PAH patients demonstrated a 1-year survival of 71% and 3-year survival of 48% [68]. These estimates were similar to those described in SSc-PAH patients taking various oral therapies. Further, when compared to patients with IPAH on epoprostenol, survival for SSc-PAH patients on epoprostenol also appeared worse [69]. Unfortunately, the therapy is cumbersome due to the short half-life of epoprostenol and instability at ambient temperatures. Requirements for frequent mixing and changing ice packs may be especially challenging for patients with sclerodactyly and Raynaud phenomena. Furthermore, IV epoprostenol requires continuous infusion through a dedicated indwelling central-venous catheter, resulting in increased risk of thromboembolic complications and catheter-associated infections. Finally, abrupt withdrawal of the therapy can lead to immediate rebound pulmonary vasoconstriction, a potentially fatal adverse effect.

To mitigate some of these complications, treprostinil, a tricyclic benzidine analog of epoprostenol, has been developed. Treprostinil is stable at ambient temperatures and has a longer half-life than epoprostenol. Treprostinil, delivered as a continuous, subcutaneous infusion (obviating the need for an indwelling catheter), resulted in reduced dyspnea, increased exercise capacity, and improved hemodynamics during a 12-week trial [70]. Unfortunately, injection site pain proved limiting for routine clinical practice. When delivered as a continuous intravenous infusion, treprostinil improved exercise capacity, symptoms, and World Health Organization functional status in a small, open-label study in PAH patients [71]. Although a central venous catheter is required, several benefits (including stability at ambient temperature and less frequent mixing) are appealing for treatment of SSc-PAH patients.

There are several other formulations of prostacyclin analogs that are currently available for use in the treatment of PAH and have been studied in CTD-PAH. Iloprost is formulated in both intravenous and inhaled versions, though only the inhaled form is approved for therapy of PAH in the US. IV iloprost has been studied in CTD patients without

PAH for treatment of peripheral vascular complications and shown to improve exercise capacity and hemodynamics compared to baseline values; however, no specific data exist in patients with CTD-PAH [72, 73]. Studies of inhaled iloprost in various forms of PAH, including CTD-PAH, have demonstrated significant improvements in functional class, exercise capacity, and hemodynamics compared to placebo. However, no disaggregated data for CTD-PAH are available [74].

Treprostinil is another prostacyclin analog that is chemically stable at room temperature and is available in IV, subcutaneous (SC) and inhaled forms; trials with an oral form of treprostinil are currently underway. Similar to IV epoprostenol, IV treprostinil must be delivered via a central catheter and continuous infusion pump. The SC formulation is also delivered via continuous infusion, but through a needle placed in the subcutaneous space. Ninety patients with various types of CTD associated PAH were included in the large randomized clinical trial of SC treprostinil (Table 29.1). The response in this subset, as reported by Oudiz and colleagues, suggested clinical efficacy, with improvements in dyspnea scores, functional capacity, and hemodynamics, though the change in 6MWD between treatment and placebo groups was of marginal statistical significance (25 m, $p = 0.055$) [75]. Although patients with CTD-PAH were included in the TRIUMPH study investigating the addition of inhaled treprostinil to bosentan or sildenafil and significant improvement in functional capacity was found, no subgroup analyses on CTD-PAH patients were reported [76].

The oral formulation of treprostinil was recently approved for use in patients with PAH based upon the results of several randomized clinical trials [77–79]. However, overall, the impact on functional capacity seemed marginal and less robust than other prostacyclin formulations. A more recent study, FREEDOM-EV, showed a statistically significant improvement in time to clinical worsening (TTCW) in patients on background PAH therapy who received oral treprostinil compared to placebo [80]. The impact on patients with CTD-PAH or SSc-PAH has not been reported.

A clinical trial examining the effect of selexipag, a novel therapy targeting the prostacyclin pathway via agonism of the prostacyclin receptor, on morbidity and mortality in PAH recently presented subgroup analyses of the CTD-PAH population included in the study [81]. This study was a randomized controlled of selexipag vs. placebo in patients with PAH; the majority of whom were prevalent patients on PAH therapy upon enrollment. Three hundred thirty-four (29%) of the 1156 PAH patients enrolled had CTD; 170 (51%) of these CTD patients had SSc. The primary outcome was TTCW, defined as disease progression or worsening that resulted in hospitalization, initiation of parenteral prostanoid therapy or long-term oxygen therapy, the need for lung transplantation or balloon atrial septostomy, or death from any cause. The reduction in TTCW for the CTD cohort was 41%, similar in magnitude to that observed in the other PAH populations in the study. When examining the SSc-PAH population alone, the reduction in risk was similar (44%, HR 0.56, 95% CI 0.34–0.91). Importantly, the side-effect profile in CTD-PAH patients was comparable to other PAH populations in the study. Since other formulations of prostaglandin therapies (parenteral in particular) may be less practical or feasible for SSc-PAH, oral formulations are important therapeutic options.

Prostaglandins, via their acute vasodilatory effects, have the potential to precipitate acute pulmonary edema in patients with pulmonary veno-occlusive disease. As the prevalence of pulmonary vein involvement in patients with SSc-PAH appears to be high, special consideration is required when initiating or titrating prostaglandins in this group [47, 82]. Overall, prostaglandins provide effective symptomatic relief and improve functional capacity in patients with SSc-PAH. However, no survival benefit has been detected to date, and other manifestations of SSc may limit the number of patients who will benefit from prostacyclin therapy. Nevertheless, IV epoprostenol is considered first-line therapy in severe PAH (WHO functional class 4) and in some patients as a bridge or alternative to lung transplantation [1, 2].

Endothelin Receptor Antagonists

Endothelin 1 is produced by endothelial cells and has direct vasoconstrictor and mitogenic effects on vascular smooth muscle cells. Endothelin's vasoconstrictive effects are mediated by two receptors (ERA, ERB) on pulmonary arterial smooth muscle cells. Conversely, ERB is also functional on endothelial cells, and stimulation mediates nitric oxide production and prostacyclin release, resulting in endothelial-mediated vasodilatation. Currently available endothelin receptor antagonists target both receptors (bosentan, macitentan), or selectively target ERA receptor A (ambrisentan).

The dual endothelin receptor antagonist bosentan has been shown to improve exercise capacity, functional class, hemodynamics, and dyspnea score after 12 weeks in a small, randomized controlled trial of patients with Class III PAH [83]. A subsequent larger randomized, controlled trial included a significant number of patients with SSc-PAH (22%), and demonstrated similar improvements in exercise capacity (measured by 6 min walk distance, 6MWD) and functional class [84]. However, post hoc analysis showed no increase in 6MWD in the SSc-PAH patients. Similarly, a retrospective review of IPAH and SSc-PAH patients treated with bosentan monotherapy at a single center showed improvements in functional status only in patients with IPAH [85].

No studies have demonstrated a survival benefit of bosentan in patients with any form of PAH. Post hoc subgroup analysis of a large randomized, controlled trial showed that patients with PAH related to connective tissue disease had improved 1- and 2-year survival when compared to historical controls [86]. However, Girgis et al. showed that SSc-PAH patients treated with bosentan monotherapy demonstrated a nonsignificant trend toward increased mortality when compared to IPAH patients [85].

Macitentan, a compound with increased receptor binding kinetics and enhanced tissue penetration, was recently studied in a large cohort of patients with PAH, including CTD associated disease. In the Study with an Endothelin Receptor Antagonist in Pulmonary Arterial Hypertension to Improve Clinical Outcome (SERAPHIN) trial, the impact of macitentan on the novel primary outcome of morbidity and mortality was tested in 742 patients with PAH [87]. Treatment with 10 mg daily of macitentan reduced the incidence of the composite end point of death, atrial septostomy, lung transplantation, initiation of treatment with intravenous or subcutaneous prostanoids, or worsening of PAH by 45% (HR = 0.55, 97.5% CI 0.39–0.76; $p < 0.001$). Approximately 30% of the cohort had CTD-PAH; and the dose of 10 mg exerted the same risk reduction for the primary endpoint also in this subgroup as compared to the overall group [87].

In an effort to selectively limit endothelin-mediated vasoconstriction while allowing vasodilatory effects, selective ERA antagonists have been developed. Ambrisentan has been associated with improved exercise capacity in patients with PAH in a randomized, controlled trial [88]. However, improvements in 6MWD were more pronounced in patients with IPAH (50–66 m) than in patients with SSc-PAH (15–23 m). While selective inhibitors appear to hold promise for symptomatic relief in patients with SSc-PAH, when used as a single agent, they appear to be more effective for patients with IPAH.

Phosphodiesterase Inhibitors/Soluble Guanylate Cyclase Stimulators

Sildenafil enhances the effects of nitric oxide on pulmonary vascular smooth muscle cells and causes pulmonary vasodilatation by inhibiting the enzyme phosphodiesterase-5 (PDE5). PDE5 is the predominant phosphodiesterase isoform in lung tissue and is responsible for catabolism of the nitric oxide second messenger cyclic guanosine monophosphate (cGMP). By inhibiting PDE5, sildenafil promotes accumulation of cGMP following nitric oxide stimulation, leading to smooth muscle cell relaxation and growth inhibition.

In patients with PAH, sildenafil has been shown to increase 6MWD after 12 weeks of therapy, with responses sustained after 1 year [89]. Additionally, sildenafil was associated with improved functional class and hemodynamic indices (including cardiac output), though there was no delay in the time to clinical worsening when compared to placebo. Approximately 20% of the subjects enrolled in this trial had SSc-PAH, most with class II or III disease. A post hoc, subgroup analysis of the 84 patients enrolled with connective tissue disease-associated PAH (45% of these with SSc-PAH) demonstrated improved 6MWD, improved hemodynamics, and a mild safety profile [90].

Tadalafil, a long-acting PDE5 inhibitor, is approved for once-daily administration for PAH in the United States. Recently, a large, randomized, controlled trial (including 23% of subjects with CTD-associated PAH) showed that daily administration of tadalafil improved 6MWD on average 20–33 m [91]. At the highest dose, tadalafil therapy was also associated with a reduced risk of clinical worsening after 16 weeks of therapy. Like sildenafil and side effects were mild. Disaggregated data for CTD-PAH population demonstrated improvement in functional capacity and improvements in TTCW with an increased risk of adverse events when compared to other PAH subgroups in the study [92].

Riociguat, a soluble guanylate cyclase stimulator that increases NO availability in pulmonary vasculature, is an approved therapy for PAH and for CTEPH. In a subgroup analysis of the Pulmonary Arterial Hypertension Soluble Guanylate Cyclase Stimulator Trial-1 (PATENT-1), CTD-PAH patients ($n = 111$) demonstrated an attenuated response in 6MWD (28 m vs. 36 m in the overall population) [93]. SSc-PAH patients ($n = 43$) in particular had less improvement in 6MWD (4 ± 43 m mean increase). A more recent study examining the impact of switching PAH patients with progressive clinical worsening while on established therapy with a PDE5i to riociguat (REPLACE study) showed that patients can benefit from switching to riociguat compared with PDE5i maintenance therapy in terms of clinical improvement and risk status [94]. The effect was consistent across predefined subgroups, including etiology of PAH [94]. As only 43 patients with CTD-PAH were included in the study, the role for riociguat in the management of CTD-PAH remains unclear.

Combination Therapy

As many of the agents described above work by affecting unique signaling pathways to promote pulmonary vasodilatation or inhibit pulmonary vasoconstriction, there may be additive or synergistic benefit to combining various agents in the treatment of PAH. So far, the results have been rather disappointing. Two studies have compared the addition of inhaled iloprost to placebo in patients taking bosentan monotherapy. While one study demonstrated a 30-m improvement in 6MWD, improved NYHA functional class, improved hemodynamics, and delayed time to worsening in patients receiving added iloprost, the other was stopped early due to futility, with no improvement in exercise capacity, functional class, or time to clinical worsening [95, 96]. In the multicenter PACES trial, PAH patients (11.6% with SSc-PAH) on long-term IV epoprostenol were randomized to receive added sildenafil versus placebo for 16 weeks [97]. Those randomized to the sildenafil arm demonstrated improved exercise capacity, hemodynamics (including cardiac output), and delayed time to clinical worsening when compared to those randomized to receive placebo.

Therapy with dual oral agents appears to be a rational approach, though the current data are limited. Two small, prospective, non-controlled studies showed improved 6MWD in IPAH patients when sildenafil was added to bosentan for clinical worsening [98, 99]. In one report, 12 patients with SSc-PAH showed no improvement in 6MWD after sildenafil was added to bosentan, and increased frequency of hepatotoxicity with combination therapy [99]. Careful consideration should be given to this combination, as bosentan is a CYP3A4 inducer and sildenafil is a CYP3A4 substrate. The combination may lead to reduced levels of sildenafil and increased levels of bosentan, though the clinical significance of this interaction remains unclear [100]. A recently published randomized, controlled trial examining the impact of adding bosentan to sildenafil in over 300 PAH patients did not demonstrate reduction in the incidence of achieving a composite endpoint of death, hospitalization for PAH, need for IV PAH therapy, atrial septostomy, lung transplantation, or worsening PAH. Subgroup analysis did not suggest response in the CTD-PAH patients who comprised about 25% of the study cohort [101]. However, in an open label real world experience, sequential combination of sildenafil with bosentan has shown favorable functional and hemodynamic results also in the PAH-CTD subgroup [102]. Data from the AMBITION study, in which treatment-naïve PAH patients were randomized to receive initial therapy with both tadalafil and ambrisentan or either drug alone suggests efficacy of this combination of PDE5I and ERA in reducing time to clinical failure, both in the overall PAH group and in the CTD-PAH group alone [103]. A subsequent subgroup analysis demonstrated improvements in TTCW not only in the CTD-PAH subgroup, but also in the SSc-PAH subgroup that were comparable to the overall cohort [104].

In a 36-week open-label study of treatment-naïve SSc-PAH patients with combination of ambrisentan and tadalafil, the investigators found significant improvement in symptoms, 6MWD, RV function as assessed by echocardiography and cardiac magnetic resonance imaging (CMR), and hemodynamics [105]. The improvement in right ventricular ejection fraction (RVEF) on CMR was particularly notable since the increase found was 2–3 times greater than the previously reported minimal clinically important difference for change in RVEF (Fig. 29.2).

The recently completed TRITON Study (The Efficacy and Safety of Initial Triple Versus Initial Dual Oral Combination Therapy in Patients with Newly Diagnosed Pulmonary Arterial Hypertension) examined the impact of initial treatment strategy of three oral agents (macitentan, tadalafil, and selexipag) versus two oral agents (macitentan and tadalafil) [106]. The primary endpoint of the study, dif-

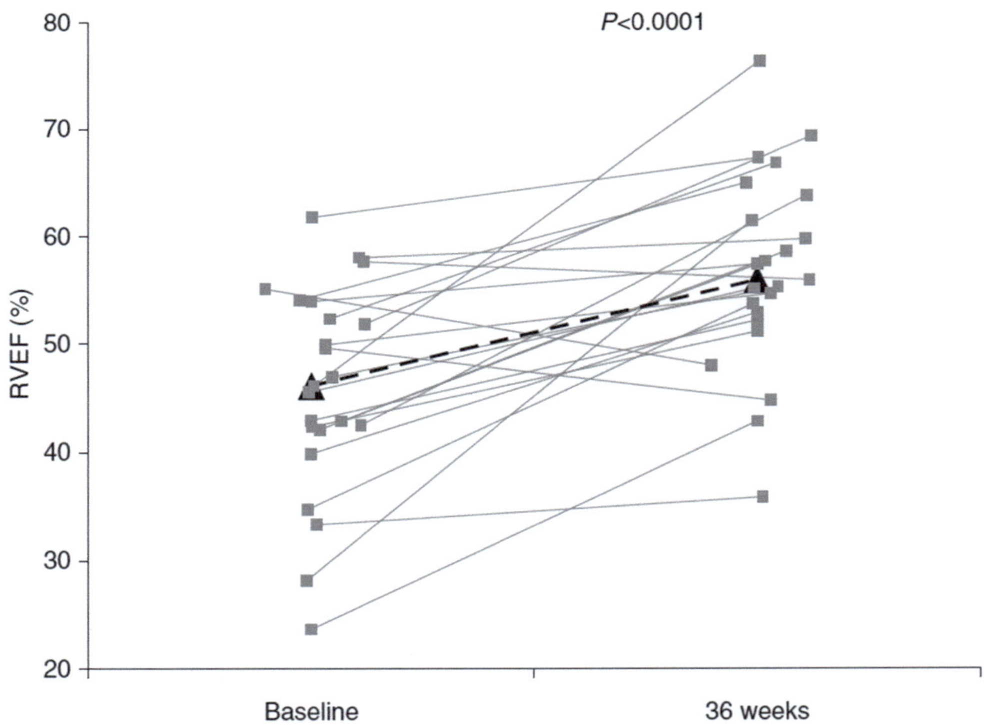

Fig. 29.2 Change in right ventricular ejection fraction assessed by cardiac magnetic resonance imaging in SSc-PAH patients treated with ambrisentan and tadalafil. Effect of combination therapy with ambrisentan and tadalafil on right ventricular ejection fraction (RVEF) from baseline to 36 weeks

ference in change in pulmonary vascular resistance between treatment arms, was not met. Subgroup analyses for the CTD-PAH population have not yet been reported.

Lung Transplantation

Although disease-specific therapy for severe PAH has reduced the referral of patients with PAH for lung transplantation, transplant remains a therapeutic option for select patients failing medical therapy [107]. Classically, the diagnosis of SSc has discouraged providers from proceeding with transplant, as frequent gastrointestinal involvement (namely esophageal dysmotility associated with reflux) raises concern for aspiration and damage to the allograft. However, international consensus recommendations do not preclude lung transplant for patients with SSc or other connective tissue diseases, as long as additional systemic manifestations are controlled [108]. Accordingly, 2-year survival was shown to be comparable (64%) among patients receiving lung transplant for SSc, interstitial lung disease, or IPAH [109]. An additional report from a single center recently showed that 1-year mortality, chronic rejection, infections, and pulmonary function were similar between 14 patients transplanted for pulmonary complications of SSc when compared to 38 patients with idiopathic pulmonary fibrosis [110]. Interestingly, more episodes of acute rejection were observed in SSc patients receiving transplant. A recent study using the United Network for Organ Sharing database found that while patients with SSc-ILD had a nearly 50% increased risk of death at 1 year post-transplant compared to patient with other forms of ILD, there was no difference in 1 year survival in patients with SSc-PAH compared to those with other forms of PAH [111]. These data suggest lung transplantation remains a viable option in carefully selected patients with SSc-PAH that proves refractory to medical management.

Summary and Future Directions

Despite the high prevalence of pulmonary involvement in SSc, including SSc-PAH and SSc-ILD-PH, and its major contribution to morbidity and mortality, treatment strategies for SSc-associated PH remain limited. Numerous clinical trials of currently available PAH-specific therapies have shown an inferior response in patients with SSc-PAH when compared to IPAH, but newer strategies, including initial combination therapy offer some hope for improved response in SSc-PAH. However, despite these advances, survival continues to lag behind patients with IPAH. The relative lack of efficacy in SSc-PAH when compared to IPAH may be related to fundamental differences in the pulmonary vasculopathy or in the greater incidence of intrinsic RV dysfunction observed in patients with SSc. Future investigational drug trials must continue to evaluate efficacy separately in patients with SSc-PAH.

References

1. Galiè N, Humbert M, Vachiery JL, Gibbs S, Lang I, Torbicki A, Simonneau G, Peacock A, Vonk Noordegraaf A, Beghetti M, Ghofrani A, Gomez Sanchez MA, Hansmann G, Klepetko W, Lancellotti P, Matucci M, McDonagh T, Pierard LA, Trindade PT, Zompatori M, Hoeper M. 2015 ESC/ERS Guidelines for the diagnosis and treatment of pulmonary hypertension: The Joint Task Force for the Diagnosis and Treatment of Pulmonary Hypertension of the European Society of Cardiology (ESC) and the European Respiratory Society (ERS): Endorsed by: Association for European Paediatric and Congenital Cardiology (AEPC), International Society for Heart and Lung Transplantation (ISHLT). Eur Heart J. 2016;37:67–119.
2. Galiè N, Humbert M, Vachiery JL, Gibbs S, Lang I, Torbicki A, Simonneau G, Peacock A, Vonk Noordegraaf A, Beghetti M, Ghofrani A, Gomez Sanchez MA, Hansmann G, Klepetko W, Lancellotti P, Matucci M, McDonagh T, Pierard LA, Trindade PT, Zompatori M, Hoeper M. 2015 ESC/ERS Guidelines for the diagnosis and treatment of pulmonary hypertension: The Joint Task Force for the Diagnosis and Treatment of Pulmonary Hypertension of the European Society of Cardiology (ESC) and the European Respiratory Society (ERS): Endorsed by: Association for European Paediatric and Congenital Cardiology (AEPC), International Society for Heart and Lung Transplantation (ISHLT). Eur Respir J. 2015;46:903–75.
3. Simonneau G, Montani D, Celermajer DS, Denton CP, Gatzoulis MA, Krowka M, Williams PG, Souza R. Haemodynamic definitions and updated clinical classification of pulmonary hypertension. Eur Respir J. 2019;53:1801913.
4. Kovacs G, Berghold A, Scheidl S, Olschewski H. Pulmonary arterial pressure during rest and exercise in healthy subject: a systematic review. Eur Respir J. 2009;34:888–94.
5. Maron BA, Hess E, Maddox TM, Opotowsky AR, Tedford RJ, Lahm T, Joynt KE, Kass DJ, Stephens T, Stanislawski MA, Swenson ER, Goldstein RH, Leopold JA, Zamanian RT, Elwing JM, Plomondon ME, Grunwald GK, Barón AE, Rumsfeld JS, Choudhary G. Association of borderline pulmonary hypertension with mortality and hospitalization in a large patient cohort: insights from the Veterans Affairs Clinical Assessment, Reporting and Tracking Program. Circulation. 2016;133:1240–8.
6. Assad TR, Maron BA, Robbins IM, Xu M, Huang S, Harrell FE, Farber-Eger EH, Wells QS, Choudhary G, Hemnes AR, Brittain EL. Prognostic effects and longitudinal hemodynamic assessment of borderline pulmonary hypertension. JAMA Cardiol. 2017;2:1361–8.
7. Waxman A, Restrepo-Jaramillo R, Thenappan T, Ravichandran A, Engel P, Bajwa A, Allen R, Feldman J, Argula R, Smith P, Rollins K, Deng C, Peterson L, Bell H, Tapson V, Nathan SD. Inhaled treprostinil in pulmonary hypertension due to interstitial lung disease. N Engl J Med. 2021;384:325–34.
8. Steen VD, Medsger TA. Changes in causes of death in systemic sclerosis, 1972–2002. Ann Rheum Dis. 2007;66:940–4.
9. Condliffe R, Kiely DG, Peacock AJ, Corris PA, Gibbs JS, Vrapi F, Das C, Elliot CA, Johnson M, DeSoyza J, Torpy C, Goldsmith K, Hodgkins D, Hughes RJ, Pepke-Zaba J, Coghlan JG. Connective tissue disease-associated pulmonary arterial hypertension in the modern treatment era. Am J Respir Crit Care Med. 2009;179:151–7.

10. Mathai SC, Hummers LK, Champion HC, Wigley FM, Zaiman A, Hassoun PM, Girgis RE. Survival in pulmonary hypertension associated with the scleroderma spectrum of diseases: impact of interstitial lung disease. Arthritis Rheum. 2009;60:569–977.
11. Chung L, Farber HW, Benza R, Miller DP, Parsons L, Hassoun PM, McGoon M, Nicolls MR, Zamanian RT. Unique predictors of mortality in patients with pulmonary arterial hypertension associated with systemic sclerosis in the REVEAL registry. Chest. 2014;146:1494–504.
12. Hachulla E, Gressin V, Guillevin L, Carpentier P, Diot E, Sibilia J, Kahan A, Cabane J, Francès C, Launay D, Mouthon L, Allanore Y, Phong Tiev K, Clerson P, de Groote P, Humbert M. Early detection of pulmonary arterial hypertension in systemic sclerosis: a French nationwide prospective multicenter study. Arthritis Rheum. 2005;52:3792–800.
13. Mukerjee D, St George D, Coleiro B, Knight C, Denton CP, Davar J, Black CM, Coghlan JG. Prevalence and outcome in systemic sclerosis associated pulmonary arterial hypertension: application of a registry approach. Ann Rheum Dis. 2003;62:1088–93.
14. Fisher MR, Forfia PR, Chamera E, Housten-Harris T, Champion HC, Girgis RE, Corretti MC, Hassoun PM. Accuracy of Doppler echocardiography in the hemodynamic assessment of pulmonary hypertension. Am J Respir Crit Care Med. 2009;179:615–21.
15. Rich JD, Shah SJ, Swamy RS, Kamp A, Rich S. Inaccuracy of Doppler echocardiographic estimates of pulmonary artery pressures in patients with pulmonary hypertension: implications for clinical practice. Chest. 2011;139:988–93.
16. Mathai SC. Pulmonary hypertension associated with connective tissue disease. Cardiol Clin. 2022;40:29–43.
17. Coghlan JG, Denton CP, Grunig E, Bonderman D, Distler O, Khanna D, Müller-Ladner U, Pope JE, Vonk MC, Doelberg M, Chadha-Boreham H, Heinzl H, Rosenberg DM, McLaughlin VV, Seibold JR, on behalf of the DETECT Study Group. Evidence-based detection of pulmonary arterial hypertension in systemic sclerosis: the DETECT study. Ann Rheum Dis. 2014;73:1340–9.
18. Fisher MR, Mathai SC, Champion HC, Girgis RE, Housten-Harris T, Hummers L, Krishnan JA, Wigley F, Hassoun PM. Clinical differences between idiopathic and scleroderma-related pulmonary hypertension. Arthritis Rheum. 2006;54:3043–50.
19. Kawut SM, Taichman DB, Archer-Chicko CL, Palevsky HI, Kimmel SE. Hemodynamics and survival in patients with pulmonary arterial hypertension related to systemic sclerosis. Chest. 2003;123:344–50.
20. Chung L, Liu J, Parsons L, Hassoun PM, McGoon M, Badesch DB, Miller DP, Nicolls MR, Zamanian RT. Characterization of connective tissue disease-associated pulmonary arterial hypertension from REVEAL: identifying systemic sclerosis as a unique phenotype. Chest. 2010;138:1383–94.
21. Kolstad KD, Li S, Steen V, Chung L, PHAROS Investigators. Long-term outcomes in systemic sclerosis-associated pulmonary arterial hypertension from the pulmonary hypertension assessment and recognition of outcomes in scleroderma registry (PHAROS). Chest. 2018;154:862–71.
22. Le Pavec J, Launay D, Mathai SC, Hassoun PM, Humbert M. Scleroderma lung disease. Clin Rev Allergy Immunol. 2011;40:104–16.
23. Launay D, Humbert M, Berezne A, Cottin V, Allanore Y, Couderc LJ, Bletry O, Yaici A, Hatron P-Y, Mouthon L, Le Pavec J, Clerson P, Hachulla E. Clinical characteristics and survival in systemic sclerosis-related pulmonary hypertension associated with interstitial lung disease. Chest. 2011;140:1016–24.
24. Chauvelot L, Gamondes D, Berthiller J, Nieves A, Renard S, Catella-Chatron J, Ahmad K, Bertoletti L, Camara B, Gomez E, Launay D, Montani D, Mornex JF, Prévot G, Sanchez O, Schott AM, Subtil F, Traclet J, Turquier S, Zeghmar S, Habib G, Reynaud-Gaubert M, Humbert M, Cottin V. Hemodynamic response to treatment and outcomes in pulmonary hypertension associated with interstitial lung disease versus pulmonary arterial hypertension in systemic sclerosis: data from a study identifying prognostic factors in pulmonary hypertension associated with interstitial lung disease. Arthritis Rheum. 2021;73:295–304.
25. Kovacs G, Herve P, Barbera JA, Chaouat A, Chemla D, Condliffe R, Garcia G, Grünig E, Howard L, Humbert M, Lau E, Laveneziana P, Lewis GD, Naeije R, Peacock A, Rosenkranz S, Saggar R, Ulrich S, Vizza D, Vonk Noordegraaf A, Olschewski H. An official European Respiratory Society statement: pulmonary haemodynamics during exercise. Eur Respir J. 2017;50:1700578.
26. Stamm A, Saxer S, Lichtblau M, Hasler ED, Jordan S, Huber LC, Bloch KE, Distler O, Ulrich S. Exercise pulmonary haemodynamics predict outcome in patients with systemic sclerosis. Eur Respir J. 2016;48:1658–67.
27. Zeder K, Avian A, Bachmaier G, Douschan P, Foris V, Sassmann T, Moazedi-Fuerst FC, Graninger WB, Hafner F, Brodmann M, Salmhofer W, Olschewski H, Kovacs G. Exercise pulmonary resistances predict long-term survival in systemic sclerosis. Chest. 2021;159:781–90.
28. Pan Z, Marra AM, Benjamin N, Eichstaedt CA, Blank N, Bossone E, Cittadini A, Coghlan G, Denton CP, Distler O, Egenlauf B, Fischer C, Harutyunova S, Xanthouli P, Lorenz HM, Grünig E. Early treatment with ambrisentan of mildly elevated mean pulmonary arterial pressure associated with systemic sclerosis: a randomized, controlled, double-blind, parallel group study (EDITA study). Arthritis Res Ther. 2019;21:217.
29. Valerio CJ, Schreiber BE, Handler CE, Denton CP, Coghlan JG. Borderline mean pulmonary artery pressure in patients with systemic sclerosis: transpulmonary gradient predicts risk of developing pulmonary hypertension. Arthritis Rheum. 2013;65:1074–84.
30. Benza RL, Kanwar MK, Raina A, Scott JV, Zhao CL, Selej M, Elliott CG, Farber HW. Development and validation of an abridged version of the REVEAL 2.0 risk score calculator, REVEAL Lite 2, for use in patients with pulmonary arterial hypertension. Chest. 2021;159:337–46.
31. Boucly A, Weatherald J, Savale L, Jaïs X, Cottin V, Prevot G, Picard F, de Groote P, Jevnikar M, Bergot E, Chaouat A, Chabanne C, Bourdin A, Parent F, Montani D, Simonneau G, Humbert M, Sitbon O. Risk assessment, prognosis and guideline implementation in pulmonary arterial hypertension. Eur Respir J. 2017;50:1700889.
32. Hoeper MM, Kramer T, Pan Z, Eichstaedt CA, Spiesshoefer J, Benjamin N, Olsson KM, Meyer K, Vizza CD, Vonk-Noordegraaf A, Distler O, Opitz C, Gibbs JSR, Delcroix M, Ghofrani HA, Huscher D, Pittrow D, Rosenkranz S, Grünig E. Mortality in pulmonary arterial hypertension: prediction by the 2015 European pulmonary hypertension guidelines risk stratification model. Eur Respir J. 2017;50:1700740.
33. Kylhammar D, Kjellström B, Hjalmarsson C, Jansson K, Nisell M, Söderberg S, Wikström G, Rådegran G. A comprehensive risk stratification at early follow-up determines prognosis in pulmonary arterial hypertension. Eur Heart J. 2018;39:4175–81.
34. Hoeper MM, Pausch C, Olsson KM, Huscher D, Pittrow D, Grünig E, Staehler G, Vizza CD, Gall H, Distler O, Opitz C, Gibbs JSR, Delcroix M, Ghofrani HA, Park D-H, Ewert R, Kaemmerer H, Kabitz HJ, Skowasch D, Behr J, Milger K, Halank M, Wilkens H, Seyfarth HJ, Held M, Dumitrescu D, Tsangaris I, Vonk-Noordegraaf A, Ulrich S, Klose H, Claussen M, Lange TJ, Rosenkranz S. COMPERA 2.0: a refined 4-strata risk assessment model for pulmonary arterial hypertension. Eur Respir J. 2022;60(1):2102311.
35. Boucly A, Weatherald J, Savale L, de Groote P, Cottin V, Prévot G, Chaouat A, Picard F, Horeau-Langlard D, Bourdin A, Jutant E-M, Beurnier A, Jevnikar M, Jaïs X, Simonneau G, Montani D,

Sitbon O, Humbert M. External validation of a refined 4-strata risk assessment score from the French pulmonary hypertension Registry. Eur Respir J. 2022;59(6):2102419.

36. Weatherald J, Boucly A, Launay D, Cottin V, Prévot G, Bourlier D, Dauphin C, Chaouat A, Savale L, Jaïs X, Jevnikar M, Traclet J, De Groote P, Simonneau G, Hachulla E, Mouthon L, Montani D, Humbert M, Sitbon O. Haemodynamics and serial risk assessment in systemic sclerosis associated pulmonary arterial hypertension. Eur Respir J. 2018;52:1800678.
37. Mercurio V, Diab N, Peloquin G, Housten-Harris T, Damico R, Kolb TM, Mathai SC, Hassoun PM. Risk assessment in scleroderma patients with newly diagnosed pulmonary arterial hypertension: application of the ESC/ERS risk prediction model. Eur Respir J. 2018;52:1800497.
38. Mullin CJ, Khair RM, Damico RL, Kolb TM, Hummers LK, Hassoun PM, Steen VD, Mathai SC, on behalf of the PHAROS Investigators. Validation of the REVEAL prognostic equation and risk score calculator in incident systemic sclerosis–associated pulmonary arterial hypertension. Arthritis Rheum. 2019;71:1691–700.
39. Rhee RL, Gabler NB, Praestgaard A, Merkel PA, Kawut SM. Adverse events in connective tissue disease-associated pulmonary arterial hypertension. Arthritis Rheum. 2015;67:2457–65.
40. Rhee RL, Gabler NB, Sangani S, Praestgaard A, Merkel PA, Kawut SM. Comparison of treatment response in idiopathic and connective tissue disease-associated pulmonary arterial hypertension. Am J Respir Crit Care Med. 2015;192:1111–7.
41. McLaughlin V, Zhao C, Coghlan JG, Chung LS, Mathai SC, Saggar R, Shah M, Hartney J, Khanna D. Long-term outcomes in patients with connective tissue disease–associated pulmonary arterial hypertension in the modern treatment era: meta-analyses of randomized, controlled trials and observational registries. Arthritis Rheum. 2021;73:837–47.
42. Galie N, Manes A, Negro L, Palazzini M, Bacchi-Reggiani ML, Branzi A. A meta-analysis of randomized controlled trials in pulmonary arterial hypertension. Eur Heart J. 2009;30:394–403.
43. Avouac J, Wipff J, Kahan A, Allanore Y. Effects of oral treatments on exercise capacity in systemic sclerosis related pulmonary arterial hypertension: a meta-analysis of randomised controlled trials. Ann Rheum Dis. 2008;67:808–14.
44. Pietra GG, Edwards WD, Kay JM, Rich S, Kernis J, Schloo B Ayres SM, Bergofsky EH, Brundage BH, Detre KM. Histopathology of primary pulmonary hypertension. A qualitative and quantitative study of pulmonary blood vessels from 58 patients in the National Heart, Lung, and Blood Institute, Primary Pulmonary Hypertension Registry. Circulation. 1989;80:1198–206.
45. Olsson KM, Delcroix M, Ghofrani HA, Tiede H, Huscher D, Speich R, Grünig E, Staehler G, Rosenkranz S, Halank M, Held M, Lange TJ, Behr J, Klose H, Claussen M, Ewert R, Opitz CF, Vizza CD, Scelsi L, Vonk-Noordegraaf A, Kaemmerer H Gibbs JSR, Coghlan G, Pepke-Zaba J, Schulz U, Gorenflo M, Pittrow D, Hoeper MM. Anticoagulation and survival in pulmonary arterial hypertension: results from the Comparative, Prospective Registry of Newly Initiated Therapies for Pulmonary Hypertension (COMPERA). Circulation. 2014;129:57–65.
46. Duchini A, Sessoms SL. Gastrointestinal hemorrhage in patients with systemic sclerosis and CREST syndrome. Am J Gastroenterol. 1998;93:1453–6.
47. Overbeek MJ, Vonk MC, Boonstra A, Voskuyl AE Vonk-Noordegraaf A, Smit EF, Dijkmans BA, Postmus PE, Mooi WJ, Heijdra Y, Grünberg K. Pulmonary arterial hypertension in limited cutaneous systemic sclerosis: a distinctive vasculopathy. Eur Respir J. 2009;34:371–9.
48. Mereles D, Ehlken N, Kreuscher S, Ghofrani S, Hoeper MM, Halank M, Meyer FJ, Karger G, Buss J, Juenger J, Holzapfel N, Opitz C, Winkler J, Herth FFJ, Wilkens H, Katus HA, Olschewski H, Grünig E. Exercise and respiratory training improve exercise capacity and quality of life in patients with severe chronic pulmonary hypertension. Circulation. 2006;114:1482–9.
49. Perros F, Humbert M, Dorfmüller P. Smouldering fire or conflagration? An illustrated update on the concept of inflammation in pulmonary arterial hypertension. Eur Respir Rev. 2021;30:210161.
50. Tuder RM, Archer SL, Dorfmuller P, Erzurum SC, Guignabert C, Michelakis E, Rabinovitch M, Schermuly R, Stenmark KR, Morrell NW. Relevant issues in the pathology and pathobiology of pulmonary hypertension. J Am Coll Cardiol. 2013;62:D4–D12.
51. Cool CD, Kennedy D, Voelkel NF, Tuder RM. Pathogenesis and evolution of plexiform lesions in pulmonary hypertension associated with scleroderma and human immunodeficiency virus infection. Hum Pathol. 1997;28:434–42.
52. Sanchez O, Sitbon O, Jais X, Simonneau G, Humbert M. Immunosuppressive therapy in connective tissue diseases-associated pulmonary arterial hypertension. Chest. 2006;130:182–9.
53. Guillevin L, Berezne A, Seror R, Teixeira L, Pourrat J, Mahr A, Hachulla E, Agard C, Cabane J, Vanhille P, Harle J-R, Deleveaux I, Mouthon L. Scleroderma renal crisis: a retrospective multicentre study on 91 patients and 427 controls. Rheumatology (Oxford). 2012;51:460–7.
54. Montanelli G, Beretta L, Santaniello A, Scorza R. Effect of dihydropyridine calcium channel blockers and glucocorticoids on the prevention and development of scleroderma renal crisis in an Italian case series. Clin Exp Rheumatol. 2013;31:135–9.
55. Zamanian RT, Badesch D, Chung L, Domsic RT, Medsger T, Pinckney A, Keyes-Elstein L, D'Aveta C, Spychala M, White RJ, Hassoun PM, Torres F, Sweatt AJ, Molitor JA, Khanna D, Maecker H, Welch B, Goldmuntz E, Nicolls MR. Safety and efficacy of B-cell depletion with rituximab for the treatment of systemic sclerosis-associated pulmonary arterial hypertension: a multicenter, double-blind, randomized, placebo-controlled trial. Am J Respir Crit Care Med. 2021;204:209–21.
56. Rich S, Kaufmann E, Levy PS. The effect of high doses of calcium-channel blockers on survival in primary pulmonary hypertension. N Engl J Med. 1992;327:76–81.
57. Sitbon O, Humbert M, Jaïs X, Ioos V, Hamid AM, Provencher S, Garcia G, Parent F, Hervé P, Simonneau G. Long-term response to calcium channel blockers in idiopathic pulmonary arterial hypertension. Circulation. 2005;111:3105–11.
58. Humbert M, Sitbon O, Chaouat A, Bertocchi M, Habib G, Gressin V, Yaici A, Weitzenblum E, Cordier J-F, Chabot F, Dromer C, Pison C, Reynaud-Gaubert M, Haloun A, Laurent M, Hachulla E, Simonneau G. Pulmonary arterial hypertension in France: results from a national registry. Am J Respir Crit Care Med. 2006;173:1023–30.
59. Montani D, Savale L, Natali D, Jaïs X, Herve P, Garcia G, Humbert M, Simonneau G, Sitbon O. Long-term response to calcium-channel blockers in non-idiopathic pulmonary arterial hypertension. Eur Heart J. 2010;31:1898–907.
60. Montani D, Lau EM, Dorfmüller P, Girerd B, Jaïs X, Savale L, Perros F, Nossent E, Garcia G, Parent F, Fadel E, Soubrier F, Sitbon O, Simonneau G, Humbert M. Pulmonary veno-occlusive disease. Eur Respir J. 2016;47:1518–34.
61. Vane JR, Anggard EE, Botting RM. Regulatory functions of the vascular endothelium. N Engl J Med. 1990;323:27–36.
62. Barst RJ, Rubin LJ, Long WA, McGoon MD, Rich S, Badesch DB, Groves BM, Tapson VF, Bourge RC, Brundage BH, Koerner SK, Langleben D, Keller CA, Murali S, Uretsky BF, Clayton LM, Jöbsis MM, Blackburn SD, Shortino D, Crow JW, Primary Pulmonary Hypertension Study Group. A comparison of continuous intravenous epoprostenol (prostacyclin) with conventional therapy for primary pulmonary hypertension. N Engl J Med. 1996;334:296–301.

63. McLaughlin VV, Genthner DE, Panella MM, Rich S. Reduction in pulmonary vascular resistance with long-term epoprostenol (prostacyclin) therapy in primary pulmonary hypertension. N Engl J Med. 1998;338:273–7.
64. Rubin LJ, Mendoza J, Hood M, McGoon M, Barst R, Williams WB, Diehl JH, Crow J, Long W. Treatment of primary pulmonary hypertension with continuous intravenous prostacyclin (epoprostenol) results of a randomized trial. Ann Intern Med. 1990;112:485–91.
65. Sitbon O, Humbert M, Nunes H, Parent F, Garcia G, Hervé P, Rainisio M, Simonneau G. Long-term intravenous epoprostenol infusion in primary pulmonary hypertension: prognostic factors and survival. J Am Coll Cardiol. 2002;40:780–8.
66. McLaughlin VV, Shillington A, Rich S. Survival in primary pulmonary hypertension: the impact of epoprostenol therapy. Circulation. 2002;106:1477–82.
67. Badesch DB, Tapson VF, McGoon MD, Brundage BH, Rubin LJ, Wigley FM, Rich S, Barst RJ, Barrett PS, Kral KM, Jöbsis MM, Loyd JE, Murali S, Frost A, Girgis R, Bourge RC, Ralph DD, Elliott CG, Hill NS, Langleben D, Schilz RJ, McLaughlin VV, Robbins IM, Groves BM, Shapiro S, Medsger TA. Continuous intravenous epoprostenol for pulmonary hypertension due to the scleroderma spectrum of disease. A randomized, controlled trial. Ann Intern Med. 2000;132:425–34.
68. Badesch DB, McGoon MD, Barst RJ, Tapson VF, Rubin LJ, Wigley FM, Kral KM, Raphiou IH, Crater GD. Longterm survival among patients with scleroderma-associated pulmonary arterial hypertension treated with intravenous epoprostenol. J Rheumatol. 2009;36:2244–9.
69. Fagan KA, Badesch DB. Pulmonary hypertension associated with connective tissue disease. Prog Cardiovasc Dis. 2002;45:225–34.
70. Simonneau G, Barst RJ, Galie N, Naeije R, Rich S, Bourge RC, Keogh A, Oudiz R, Frost A, Blackburn SD, Crow JW, Rubin LJ, Treprostinil Study Group. Continuous subcutaneous infusion of treprostinil, a prostacyclin analogue, in patients with pulmonary arterial hypertension: a double-blind, randomized, placebo-controlled trial. Am J Respir Crit Care Med. 2002;165:800–4.
71. Tapson VF, Gomberg-Maitland M, McLaughlin VV, Benza RL, Widlitz AC, Krichman A, Barst RJ. Safety and efficacy of IV treprostinil for pulmonary arterial hypertension: a prospective, multicenter, open-label, 12-week trial. Chest. 2006;129:683–8.
72. Caravita S, Wu SC, Secchi MB, Dadone V, Bencini C, Pierini S. Long-term effects of intermittent Iloprost infusion on pulmonary arterial pressure in connective tissue disease. Eur J Intern Med. 2011;22:518–21.
73. Hoeper MM, Gall H, Seyfarth HJ, Halank M, Ghofrani HA, Winkler J, Golpon H, Olsson KM, Nickel N, Opitz C, Ewert R. Long-term outcome with intravenous iloprost in pulmonary arterial hypertension. Eur Respir J. 2009;34:132–7.
74. Olschewski H, Simonneau G, Galiè N, Higenbottam T, Naeije R, Rubin LJ, Nikkho S, Speich R, Hoeper MM, Behr J, Winkler J, Sitbon O, Popov W, Ghofrani HA, Manes A, Kiely DG, Ewert R, Meyer A, Corris PA, Delcroix M, Gomez-Sanchez M, Siedentop H, Seeger W, Aerosolized Iloprost Randomized Study Group. Inhaled iloprost for severe pulmonary hypertension. N Engl J Med. 2002;347:322–9.
75. Oudiz RJ, Schilz RJ, Barst RJ, Galié N, Rich S, Rubin LJ, Simonneau G, Treprostinil Study Group. Treprostinil, a prostacyclin analogue, in pulmonary arterial hypertension associated with connective tissue disease. Chest. 2004;126:420–7.
76. McLaughlin VV, Benza RL, Rubin LJ, Channick RN, Voswinckel R, Tapson VF, Robbins IM, Olschewski H, Rubenfire M, Seeger W. Addition of inhaled treprostinil to oral therapy for pulmonary arterial hypertension: a randomized controlled clinical trial. J Am Coll Cardiol. 2010;55:1915–22.
77. Tapson VF, Torres F, Kermeen F, Keogh AM, Allen RP, Frantz RP, Badesch DB, Frost AE, Shapiro SM, Laliberte K, Sigman J, Arneson C, Galiè N. Oral treprostinil for the treatment of pulmonary arterial hypertension in patients on background endothelin receptor antagonist and/or phosphodiesterase type 5 inhibitor therapy (the FREEDOM-C study): a randomized controlled trial. Chest. 2012;142:1383–90.
78. Tapson VF, Jing Z-C, Xu K-F, Pan L, Feldman J, Kiely DG, Kotlyar E, McSwain CS, Laliberte K, Arneson C, Rubin LJ, FREEDOM-C2 Study Team. Oral treprostinil for the treatment of pulmonary arterial hypertension in patients receiving background endothelin receptor antagonist and phosphodiesterase type 5 inhibitor therapy (the FREEDOM-C2 study): a randomized controlled trial. Chest. 2013;144:952–8.
79. Jing Z-C, Parikh K, Pulido T, Jerjes-Sanchez C, White RJ, Allen R, Torbicki A, Xu K-F, Yehle D, Laliberte K, Arneson C, Rubin LJ. Efficacy and safety of oral treprostinil monotherapy for the treatment of pulmonary arterial hypertension: a randomized, controlled trial. Circulation. 2013;127:624–33.
80. White RJ, Jerjes-Sanchez C, Bohns Meyer GM, Pulido T, Sepulveda P, Wang KY, Grünig E, Hiremath S, Yu Z, Gangcheng Z, Yip WLJ, Zhang S, Khan A, Deng CQ, Grover R, Tapson VF, FREEDOM-EV Investigators. Combination therapy with oral treprostinil for pulmonary arterial hypertension. A double-blind placebo-controlled clinical trial. Am J Respir Crit Care Med. 2020;201:707–17.
81. Gaine S, Chin K, Coghlan G, Channick R, Di Scala L, Galiè N, Ghofrani HA, Lang IM, McLaughlin V, Preiss R, Rubin LJ, Simonneau G, Sitbon O, Tapson VF, Hoeper MM. Selexipag for the treatment of connective tissue disease-associated pulmonary arterial hypertension. Eur Respir J. 2017;50:1602493.
82. Dorfmuller P, Humbert M, Perros F, Sanchez O, Simonneau G, Muller KM, Capron F. Fibrous remodeling of the pulmonary venous system in pulmonary arterial hypertension associated with connective tissue diseases. Hum Pathol. 2007;38:893–902.
83. Channick RN, Simonneau G, Sitbon O, Robbins IM, Frost A, Tapson VF, Badesch DB, Roux S, Rainisio M, Bodin F, Rubin LJ. Effects of the dual endothelin-receptor antagonist bosentan in patients with pulmonary hypertension: a randomised placebo-controlled study. Lancet. 2001;358:1119–23.
84. Rubin LJ, Badesch DB, Barst RJ, Galie N, Black CM, Keogh A, Pulido T, Frost A, Roux S, Leconte I, Landzberg M, Simonneau G. Bosentan therapy for pulmonary arterial hypertension. N Engl J Med. 2002;346:896–903.
85. Girgis RE, Mathai SC, Krishnan JA, Wigley FM, Hassoun PM. Long-term outcome of bosentan treatment in idiopathic pulmonary arterial hypertension and pulmonary arterial hypertension associated with the scleroderma spectrum of diseases. J Heart Lung Transplant. 2005;24:1626–31.
86. Denton CP, Humbert M, Rubin L, Black CM. Bosentan treatment for pulmonary arterial hypertension related to connective tissue disease: a subgroup analysis of the pivotal clinical trials and their open-label extensions. Ann Rheum Dis. 2006;65:1336–40.
87. Pulido T, Adzerikho I, Channick RN, Delcroix M, Galiè N, Ghofrani H-A, Jansa P, Jing Z-C, Le Brun F-O, Mehta S, Mittelholzer CM, Perchenet L, Sastry BKS, Sitbon O, Souza R, Torbicki A, Zeng X, Rubin LJ, Simonneau G, SERAPHIN Investigators. Macitentan and morbidity and mortality in pulmonary arterial hypertension. N Engl J Med. 2013;369:809–18.
88. Galiè N, Olschewski H, Oudiz RJ, Torres F, Frost A, Ghofrani HA, Badesch DB, McGoon MD, McLaughlin VV, Roecker EB, Gerber MJ, Dufton C, Wiens BL, Rubin LJ. Ambrisentan for the treatment of pulmonary arterial hypertension results of the ambrisentan in pulmonary arterial hypertension, randomized, double-blind, placebo-controlled, multicenter, efficacy (ARIES) study 1 and 2. Circulation. 2008;117:3010–9.

89. Galiè N, Ghofrani HA, Torbicki A, Barst RJ, Rubin LJ, Badesch D, Fleming T, Parpia T, Burgess G, Branzi A, et al. Sildenafil citrate therapy for pulmonary arterial hypertension. N Engl J Med. 2005;353:2148–57.
90. Badesch DB, Hill NS, Burgess G, Rubin LJ, Barst RJ, Galiè N, Simonneau G, SUPER Study Group. Sildenafil for pulmonary arterial hypertension associated with connective tissue disease. J Rheumatol. 2007;34:2417–22.
91. Galiè N, Brundage BH, Ghofrani HA, Oudiz RJ, Simonneau G, Safdar Z, Shapiro S, White RJ, Chan M, Beardsworth A, Frumkin L, Barst RJ. Tadalafil therapy for pulmonary arterial hypertension. Circulation. 2009;119:2894–903.
92. Galiè N, Denton CP, Dardi F, Manes A, Mazzanti G, Li B, Varanese L, Esler A, Harmon C, Palazzini M. Tadalafil in idiopathic or heritable pulmonary arterial hypertension (PAH) compared to PAH associated with connective tissue disease. Int J Cardiol. 2017;235:67–72.
93. Humbert M, Coghlan JG, Ghofrani H-A, Grimminger F, He J-G, Riemekasten G, Vizza CD, Boeckenhoff A, Meier C, de Oliveira Pena J, Denton CP. Riociguat for the treatment of pulmonary arterial hypertension associated with connective tissue disease: results from PATENT-1 and PATENT-2. Ann Rheum Dis. 2017;76:422–6.
94. Hoeper MM, Al-Hiti H, Benza RL, Chang S-A, Corris PA, Gibbs JSR, Grünig E, Jansa P, Klinger JR, Langleben D, McLaughlin VV, Meyer GMB, Ota-Arakaki J, Peacock AJ, Pulido T, Rosenkranz S, Vizza CD, Vonk-Noordegraaf A, White RJ, Chang M, Kleinjung F, Meier C, Paraschin K, Ghofrani HA, Simonneau G, on behalf of the REPLACE investigators. Switching to riociguat versus maintenance therapy with phosphodiesterase-5 inhibitors in patients with pulmonary arterial hypertension (REPLACE): a multicentre, open-label, randomised controlled trial. Lancet Respir Med. 2021;9:573–84.
95. McLaughlin VV, Oudiz RJ, Frost A, Tapson VF, Murali S, Channick RN, Badesch DB, Barst RJ, Hsu HH, Rubin LJ. Randomized study of adding inhaled iloprost to existing bosentan in pulmonary arterial hypertension. Am J Respir Crit Care Med. 2006;174:1257–63.
96. Hoeper MM, Leuchte H, Halank M, Wilkens H, Meyer FJ, Seyfarth HJ, Wensel R, Ripken F, Bremer H, Kluge S, Hoeffken G, Behr J. Combining inhaled iloprost with bosentan in patients with idiopathic pulmonary arterial hypertension. Eur Respir J. 2006;28:691–4.
97. Simonneau G, Rubin LJ, Galiè N, Barst RJ, Fleming TR, Frost AE, Engel PJ, Kramer MR, Burgess G, Collings L, Cossons N, Sitbon O, Badesch DB, PACES Study Group. Addition of sildenafil to long-term intravenous epoprostenol therapy in patients with pulmonary arterial hypertension: a randomized trial. Ann Intern Med. 2008;149:521–30.
98. Hoeper MM, Faulenbach C, Golpon H, Winkler J, Welte T, Niedermeyer J. Combination therapy with bosentan and sildenafil in idiopathic pulmonary arterial hypertension. Eur Respir J. 2004;24:1007–10.
99. Mathai SC, Girgis RE, Fisher MR, Champion HC, Housten-Harris T, Zaiman A, Hassoun PM. Addition of sildenafil to bosentan monotherapy in pulmonary arterial hypertension. Eur Respir J. 2007;29:469–75.
100. Paul GA, Gibbs JS, Boobis AR, Abbas A, Wilkins MR. Bosentan decreases the plasma concentration of sildenafil when coprescribed in pulmonary hypertension. Br J Clin Pharmacol. 2005;60:107–12.
101. McLaughlin V, Channick RN, Ghofrani H-A, Lemarié J-C, Naeije R, Packer M, Souza R, Tapson VF, Tolson J, Hiti HA, Meyer G, Hoeper MM. Bosentan added to sildenafil therapy in patients with pulmonary arterial hypertension. Eur Respir J. 2015;46:405–13.
102. Dardi F, Manes A, Palazzini M, Bachetti C, Mazzanti G, Rinaldi A, Albini A, Gotti E, Monti E, Reggiani MLB, Galiè N. Combining bosentan and sildenafil in pulmonary arterial hypertension patients failing monotherapy: real-world insights. Eur Respir J. 2015;46:414–21.
103. Galiè N, Barberà JA, Frost AE, Ghofrani H-A, Hoeper MM, McLaughlin VV, Peacock AJ, Simonneau G, Vachiery J-L, Grünig E, Oudiz RJ, Vonk-Noordegraaf A, White RJ, Blair C, Gillies H, Miller KL, Harris JHN, Langley J, Rubin LJ. Initial use of ambrisentan plus tadalafil in pulmonary arterial hypertension. N Engl J Med. 2015;373:834–44.
104. Coghlan JG, Galiè N, Barberà JA, Frost AE, Ghofrani HA, Hoeper MM, Kuwana M, McLaughlin VV, Peacock AJ, Simonneau G, Vachiéry JL, Blair C, Gillies H, Miller KL, Harris JHN, Langley J, Rubin LJ, AMBITION investigators. Initial combination therapy with ambrisentan and tadalafil in connective tissue disease-associated pulmonary arterial hypertension (CTD-PAH): subgroup analysis from the AMBITION trial. Ann Rheum Dis. 2017;76:1219–27.
105. Hassoun PM, Zamanian RT, Damico R, Lechtzin N, Khair R, Kolb TM, Tedford RJ, Hulme OL, Housten T, Pisanello C, Sato T, Pullins EH, Corona-Villalobos CP, Zimmerman SL, Gashouta MA, Minai OA, Torres F, Girgis RE, Chin K, Mathai SC. Ambrisentan and tadalafil up-front combination therapy in scleroderma-associated pulmonary arterial hypertension. Am J Respir Crit Care Med. 2015;192:1102–10.
106. Chin KM, Sitbon O, Doelberg M, Feldman J, Gibbs JSR, Grünig E, Hoeper MM, Martin N, Mathai SC, McLaughlin VV, Perchenet L, Poch D, Saggar R, Simonneau G, Galiè N. Three-versus two-drug therapy for patients with newly diagnosed pulmonary arterial hypertension. J Am Coll Cardiol. 2021;78:1393–403.
107. Keogh AM, Mayer E, Benza RL, Corris P, Dartevelle PG, Frost AE, Kim NH, Lang IM, Pepke-Zaba J, Sandoval J. Interventional and surgical modalities of treatment in pulmonary hypertension. J Am Coll Cardiol. 2009;54:S67–77.
108. Orens JB, Estenne M, Arcasoy S, Conte JV, Corris P, Egan JJ, Egan T, Keshavjee S, Knoop C, Kotloff R, Martinez FJ, Nathan S, Palmer S, Patterson A, Singer L, Snell G, Studer S, Vachiery JL, Glanville AR. International guidelines for the selection of lung transplant candidates: 2006 update—a consensus report from the Pulmonary Scientific Council of the International Society for Heart and Lung Transplantation. J Heart Lung Transplant. 2006;25:745–55.
109. Schachna L, Medsger TA Jr, Dauber JH, Wigley FM, Braunstein NA, White B, Steen VD, Conte JV, Yang SC, McCurry KR, Borja MC, Plaskon DE, Orens JB, Gelber AC. Lung transplantation in scleroderma compared with idiopathic pulmonary fibrosis and idiopathic pulmonary arterial hypertension. Arthritis Rheum. 2006;54:3954–61.
110. Saggar R, Khanna D, Furst DE, Belperio JA, Park GS, Weigt SS, Kubak B, Ardehali A, Derhovanessian A, Clements PJ, Shapiro S, Hunter C, Gregson A, Fishbein MC, Lynch JP III, Ross DJ, Saggar R. Systemic sclerosis and bilateral lung transplantation: a single centre experience. Eur Respir J. 2010;36:893–900.
111. Bernstein EJ, Peterson ER, Sell JL, D'Ovidio F, Arcasoy SM, Bathon JM, Lederer DJ. Survival of adults with systemic sclerosis following lung transplantation: a nationwide cohort study. Arthritis Rheum. 2015;67:1314–22.

Part VI

Gastrointestinal Manifestations and Management

Ami A. Shah

Overview of Gastrointestinal Tract Involvement

30

Christopher P. Denton

Introduction

Gastrointestinal manifestations are the commonest internal organ complications of systemic sclerosis (SSc) and are a major cause of morbidity [1]. The commonest features are gastro-oesophageal reflux and chronic constipation, both reflecting altered gut motility and contractility. However there are many other manifestations that span the entire gastrointestinal tract. These include sicca symptoms akin to those typically observed in Sjogren's syndrome, together with all of the predictable secondary consequences of defective salivation [2]. Pharyngeal weakness and oesophageal dysmotility may both contribute to dysphagia as well as reflux symptoms and this includes oesophagitis. Stomach involvement includes delayed emptying with post-prandial bloating and also vascular complications, most notably gastric astral vascular ectasia (watermelon stomach) [3]. Other vascular lesions reminiscent of cutaneous telangiectasia can occur throughout the gastrointestinal tract and may be complicated by bleeding and anaemia. Small bowel involvement also manifests as altered motility and this can lead to episodes of ileus or pseudo-obstruction. Similar processes occur in the large bowel and recurrent distention and pain are important clinical problems that may require hospital-based treatment. Other consequences of slow intestinal transit include small intestinal bacterial overgrowth that may lead to diarrhoea, bloating and malabsorption [4]. Malnutrition is a frequent problem in SSc. It results in part from poor nutritional intake but pancreatic or mucosal enzyme deficiency also contributes and altered motility and mucosal and intestinal vasculature also contribute [5]. In some cases, nutritional support is needed and some cases require parenteral supplementation. Finally, anorectal involvement is a very common problem leading to anorectal incontinence. There may be associated or contributory manifestations such as rectal prolapse. Taken together, this range of GI manifestations contributes to the enormous personal impact of SSc and represents one of the most unmet clinical needs for SSc patients. The development of a validated assessment tool for SSc bowel complications has permitted more systematic and standardised assessment of the disease in a patient relevant way that will hopefully help in clinical research to improve outcomes and better define and understand the disease [6]. The SCTC-UCLA Scleroderma GI Assessment tool was developed to assess burden of diseases in a relevant and measurable way and is freely available for academic and clinical use (see http://bit.ly/UCLASCTCGIT).

Pathogenesis

The fundamental mechanisms underlying gastrointestinal tract pathology in SSc are likely to reflect the basic disease processes of inflammation, autoimmunity, fibrosis and vasculopathy [7]. There is also compelling evidence that there are enteric neuropathic mechanisms operating. The end consequence of these processes is undoubtedly a fibrotic bowel wall with poor intestinal blood flow and altered contractility together with likely reduction in the functional microcirculation that is intrinsic to the absorptive function of the intestine [8]. Many of the manifestations of bowel involvement including bloating, pseudo-obstruction and intestinal bacterial overgrowth can be unified through these pathological processes. However the symptoms of GI scleroderma are not always well correlated with structural or histopathological severity. In one genetically determined mouse model of scleroderma that is triggered by altered TGFbeta activity, there is evidence of adventitial and mural fibrosis in the large intestine with altered smooth muscle contractility and use of animal models may help to dissect out the sequence of events underlying progression of GI features [9]. This suggests that cofactors such as diet, medications and other comorbidities are likely to be extremely relevant. Although traditionally thought to be one of the most irreversible aspects of the dis-

C. P. Denton (✉)
Centre for Rheumatology and Connective Tissue Diseases, UCL Division of Medicine, Royal Free Hospital, London, UK
e-mail: c.denton@ucl.ac.uk

Y. Allanore et al. (eds.), *Scleroderma*, https://doi.org/10.1007/978-3-031-40658-4_30

ease, there is very often a favourable clinical outcome when individual components of the disease are tackled, and medical approaches that are effective in similar clinical processes occurring outside the context of SSc can be helpful. Some of these processes are considered in more detail below. The potential importance of immunological, and especially humoral, autoimmune processes is suggested by some reports of benefit from immunosuppressive treatments and especially for treatment with long-term intravenous immunoglobulin therapy [10].

The role of autoantibodies has been highlighted in several recent studies and has drawn analogy with other gastrointestinal tract disorders in which functional antibodies have been described [11]. There is now a body of data supporting this as a contributing mechanism in SSc and may have relevance beyond the gastrointestinal tract and anti-vinculin antibodies have been suggested as a possible biomarker [12, 13].

Another important area of increased study is the gut microbiome. This has been described in molecular detail and descriptive studies suggest that loss of microbial diversity may associate with increased symptoms. This is important for pathogenesis but also raised therapeutic possibilities. Thus the concept of faecal transplant to normalise microbiome has been proposed and initial studies have been reported [14]. A less invasive approach to beneficial modification gut dysbiosis is the potential use of probiotics in SSc [15]. Further research in this area is needed but it seems likely that gut flora in SSc is relevant to pathogenesis and treatment, and this is likely to be an area of future exploration [16].

Upper GI Complications

At the time of diagnosis, almost all SSc patients describe some symptoms of heartburn or dysphagia. These may be relatively mild and not always associated by patients with the other disparate symptoms of Raynaud's and skin changes that are typical of early stage SSc. They may be treated effectively with antacid therapy and the availability of routine proton pump inhibitors including without prescription, and has made this a much less significant issue for many patients. Although evidence for long-term benefit is sparse, it is clear from routine practice that these agents are remarkably effective, and many patients find that even short-term discontinuation results in severe return of intolerable symptoms of oesophagitis [17]. However in later stages of SSc, there are often very severe and refractory symptoms, and this may require high doses and combination of different antacid classes. In addition, some specific complications of long-term high-dose treatment with proton pump inhibitors are suggested by studies linking this to more severe calcinosis [18]. It is important to treat reflux occurring in the context of lung fibrosis as it may lead to progression or worsening of lung disease or to important superadded complications such as aspiration and infection. Simple measures to reduce mechanical aspects of reflux should also be recommended, especially as this might also benefit non-acid reflux. Emerging new imaging approaches that correlate with symptoms offer the prospect of more systematic or objective assessment and monitoring of treatments [19]. The effect of prokinetics is variable, perhaps because often the oesophagus is aperistaltic, and benefit needs to be balanced against potential risk of cardiac arrhythmias for some available agents. However, in some patients these are an additional treatment approach to consider.

Of the stomach complications of SSc, the most important is GAVE. This is under recognised but can lead to recurrent severe anaemia or precipitous falls in haematocrit that may require regular transfusion. If oral iron supplementation is not sufficient or feasible, especially in the context of PPI therapy, then parenteral iron treatments may be beneficial. Photocoagulation, especially with argon plasma-based therapy can be transformative although recurrent treatment is usually needed, and the success of this can be monitored by repeat endoscopy and regular monitoring of full blood count [20]. Barrett's metaplasia is increasingly recognised in SSc and may be a consequence of chronic reflux. Management is in line with other cases of this disease with regular surveillance and individual assessment of risk and need for additional treatment [21].

Midgut Disease

Weight loss and malnutrition are common in SSc. The most frequent mechanism is inadequate oral intake and this must be explored carefully so that patients try to maximise energy and protein consumption. This can be a real challenge due to the dental and mouth problems, dysphagia and post-prandial bloating, and the problems with lower bowel symptoms that may be improved when less is eaten. However oral nutritional supplements may be possible. Parenteral supplementation can be used intermittently or long-term enteral strategies with percutaneous gastrostomy or jejunostomy [22]. The latter is usually more feasible due to the problems of volume reflux associated with gastric feeding with risk of severe complications such as aspiration from reflux. Pancreatic enzyme supplements may be useful and other comorbidities such as coeliac disease should be excluded. Interestingly many patients do report benefit from dietary modification, and restriction of wheat, dairy products or red meat have all been reported to be useful in some cases. Probiotics may be useful although small intestinal bacterial overgrowth is also a common exacerbating factor that can be treated; broad spectrum antibiotics are used and can be given intermittently or if necessary, in rotation with different classes of agent [23]. The most effective treatment usually is ciprofloxacin or a similar agent, although many drugs are used including rifaximin when available. This has the theoretical advantage of not being absorbed and so may cause fewer systemic side effects. All SSc cases should be routinely assessed for clinically significant malnutrition, and the MUST questionnaire (*Malnutrition Universal Screening Tool*) provides a simple method to assess this [24]. If there is significant malnutrition, then expert input is needed and sometimes cases need to be referred to intestinal failure specialist to be considered for parenteral nutrition. This can be given intermittently and may not be total parenteral nutrition. Sometimes patients improve after medium-term treatment and are able to discontinue this form of feeding although these cases represent a minority.

There have been new studies of nutrition and appreciation that there may be systemic disease mechanisms that also impact on muscle and connective tissue growth and regeneration. This is important because of the emerging studies showing that severe gastrointestinal tract involvement and poor nutritional status associate with worse outcome and survival in SSc [25].

Lower GI Complications

Up to half of patients with SSc experience lower GI complications of the disease but these may be intermittent. In the most severe cases, there is severe constipation, sometimes leading to secondary complications such as sigmoid volvulus, diarrhoea that more often reflects midgut disease or pancreatic insufficiency and incontinence. The latter is underreported by patients but can be very debilitating. Treatments have been ineffective in part due to poor understanding of the pathology. More systematic studies have started to define better the links between investigational abnormality and symptoms and this is central to progress. Modern imaging approaches and functional studies are shedding light on the structural pathology of anorectal SSc [26]. Interestingly, in light of the multiple pathogenetic mechanisms that may operate, there is better correlation between altered neural function in the anorectum than structural change and this may be important in treatment [27]. There have been limited successes using sacral neuromodulation and this is often a method used in severe late-stage disease. Recently very preliminary data support alternative neurological approaches such as posterior tibial nerve stimulation, and this is a potential avenue for future treatment and this may be superior to conventional sacral nerve stimulation [28]. Better engagement with other incontinence approaches can also be valuable, and some approaches such as sphincter augmentation with fillers as well as more simple approaches such as voluntary muscle strengthening exercises may be used, including pelvic floor physical therapy, which can represent an important and well-tolerated first-line approach to symptoms of incontinence.

Recommended Approach to Gastrointestinal Tract Complications in Systemic Sclerosis

Although it has been conventional to take an anatomical approach to evaluation and classification of the GI manifestations of SSc, this has clear limitations since there is likely to be cross over in mechanism and overlap in symptoms, and so it has recently been proposed that a more problem-orientated approach may be better. This emerged from a systematic exercise in defining best practice management for the key GI complications of SSc and involved close collaboration between scleroderma specialists, gastroenterologists and nutritional experts. Pathways for the key complications have been suggested that are relevant generally [29]. A focus is on investigation and treatment together with treatment of other complications and GI comorbidities. Identifying the pointers for referral to specialist centres for investigation and treatment provide important keys to better management. The need for close cross-speciality collaboration is highlighted and likely to become the expected standard for future treatment and better outcomes for GI scleroderma.

Concluding Remarks

Although some aspects of GI disease in SSc have been effectively related and the outcomes and complications such as stricture of the lower oesophagus and bolus obstruction are now much rarer, there remain real problems for patients related to some of the commonest aspects of SSc. Closer collaboration between specialists, a more problem-orientated approach and use of innovative treatment strategies together will hopefully lead to more progress and better outcomes for some of the most difficult manifestations of SSc.

References

1. Thoua NM, Bunce C, Brough G, Forbes A, Emmanuel AV, Denton CP. Assessment of gastrointestinal symptoms in patients with systemic sclerosis in a UK tertiary referral centre. Rheumatology (Oxford). 2010;49(9):1770–5. https://doi.org/10.1093/rheumatology/keq147. Epub 2010 Jun 8. PubMed PMID: 20530510.
2. Baron M, Hudson M, Tatibouet S, Steele R, Lo E, Gravel S, Gyger G, El Sayegh T, Pope J, Fontaine A, Masetto A, Matthews D, Sutton E, Thie N, Jones N, Copete M, Kolbinson D, Markland J, Nogueira G, Robinson D, Fritzler M, Gornitsky M. Relationship between disease characteristics and orofacial manifestations in systemic sclerosis: Canadian Systemic Sclerosis Oral Health Study III. Arthritis Care Res (Hoboken). 2015;67(5):681–90. https://doi.org/10.1002/

acr.22490. PubMed PMID: 25303223; PubMed Central PMCID: PMC4464822.
3. Ghrénassia E, Avouac J, Khanna D, Derk CT, Distler O, Suliman YA, Airo P, Carreira PE, Foti R, Granel B, Berezne A, Cabane J, Ingegnoli F, Rosato E, Caramaschi P, Hesselstrand R, Walker UA, Alegre-Sancho JJ, Zarrouk V, Agard C, Riccieri V, Schiopu E, Gladue H, Steen VD, Allanore Y. Prevalence, correlates and outcomes of gastric antral vascular ectasia in systemic sclerosis: a EUSTAR case-control study. J Rheumatol. 2014;41(1):99–105. https://doi.org/10.3899/jrheum.130386. Epub 2013 Dec 1. PubMed PMID: 24293584.
4. Tauber M, Avouac J, Benahmed A, Barbot L, Coustet B, Kahan A, Allanore Y. Prevalence and predictors of small intestinal bacterial overgrowth in systemic sclerosis patients with gastrointestinal symptoms. Clin Exp Rheumatol. 2014;32(6 Suppl 86):S82–7. Epub 2014 Nov 3. PubMed PMID: 25372792.
5. Chua C-G, Wansaicheong GK-L, Lim W-C, Thong BY-H. Superior mesenteric artery syndrome: a potentially fatal but reversible gastrointestinal manifestation of systemic sclerosis. Case Rep Rheumatol. 2020;2020:8831417. https://doi.org/10.1155/2020/8831417.
6. Khanna D, Hays RD, Maranian P, Seibold JR, Impens A, Mayes MD, Clements PJ, Getzug T, Fathi N, Bechtel A, Furst DE. Reliability and validity of the University of California, Los Angeles Scleroderma Clinical Trial Consortium Gastrointestinal Tract Instrument. Arthritis Rheum. 2009;61(9):1257–63.
7. Manetti M, Neumann E, Milia AF, Tarner IH, Bechi P, Matucci-Cerinic M, Ibba-Manneschi L, Müller-Ladner U. Severe fibrosis and increased expression of fibrogenic cytokines in the gastric wall of systemic sclerosis patients. Arthritis Rheum. 2007;56(10):3442–7. PubMed PMID: 17907149.
8. Malandrini A, Selvi E, Villanova M, Berti G, Sabadini L, Salvadori C, Gambelli S, De Stefano R, Vernillo R, Marcolongo R, Guazzi G. Autonomic nervous system and smooth muscle cell involvement in systemic sclerosis: ultrastructural study of 3 cases. J Rheumatol. 2000;27(5):1203–6. PubMed PMID: 10813288.
9. Thoua NM, Derrett-Smith EC, Khan K, Dooley A, Shi-Wen X, Denton CP. Gut fibrosis with altered colonic contractility in a mouse model of scleroderma. Rheumatology (Oxford). 2012;51(11):1989–98. https://doi.org/10.1093/rheumatology/kes191. Epub 2012 Aug 20. PubMed PMID: 22908328.
10. Raja J, Nihtyanova SI, Murray CD, Denton CP, Ong VH. Sustained benefit from intravenous immunoglobulin therapy for gastrointestinal involvement in systemic sclerosis. Rheumatology. 2016;55(1):115–9.
11. Nakane S, Umeda M, Kawashiri S-Y, Mukaino A, Ichinose K, Higuchi O, Maeda Y, Nakamura H, Matsuo H, Kawakami A. Detecting gastrointestinal manifestations in patients with systemic sclerosis using anti-gAChR antibodies. Arthritis Res Ther. 2020;22:32. https://doi.org/10.1186/s13075-020-2128-z.
12. Adler BL, McMahan Z. Anti-vinculin autoantibodies in systemic sclerosis: a step toward a novel biomarker? Clin Rheumatol. 2021;40:809–11. https://doi.org/10.1007/s10067-020-05533-2.
13. Suliman Y, Kafaja S, Oh SJ, Alemam M, Bagnato G, Abignano G, Singh RR, Barlow G, Liu X, Valera I, Morales W, Rezaie A, Pimentel M, Del Galdo F, Furst DE. Anti-vinculin antibodies in scleroderma (SSc): a potential link between autoimmunity and gastrointestinal system involvement in two SSc cohorts. Clin Rheumatol. 2020; https://doi.org/10.1007/s10067-020-05479-5.
14. Fretheim H, Chung BK, Didriksen H, Bækkevold ES, Midtvedt Ø, Brunborg C, Holm K, Valeur J, Tennøe AH, Garen T, Midtvedt T, Trøseid M, Zarè H, Lund MB, Hov JR, Lundin KEA, Molberg Ø, Hoffmann-Vold A-M. Fecal microbiota transplantation in systemic sclerosis: a double-blind, placebo-controlled randomized pilot trial. PLoS One. 2020;15:e0232739. https://doi.org/10.1371/journal.pone.0232739.
15. Low AHL, Teng GG, Pettersson S, de Sessions PF, Ho EXP, Fan Q, Chu CW, Law AHN, Santosa A, Lim AYN, Wang YT, Haaland B, Thumboo J. A double-blind randomized placebo-controlled trial of probiotics in systemic sclerosis associated gastrointestinal disease. Semin Arthritis Rheum. 2019;49:411–9. https://doi.org/10.1016/j.semarthrit.2019.05.006.
16. Natalello G, Bosello SL, Paroni Sterbini F, Posteraro B, De Lorenzis E, Canestrari GB, Gigante L, Verardi L, Ferraccioli G, Sanguinetti M, Gremese E. Gut microbiota analysis in systemic sclerosis according to disease characteristics and nutritional status. Clin Exp Rheumatol. 2020;38(Suppl 125):73–84.
17. Pakozdi A, Wilson H, Black CM, Denton CP. Does long-term therapy with lansoprazole slow progression of oesophageal involvement in systemic sclerosis? Clin Exp Rheumatol. 2009;27(3 Suppl 54):5–8. PubMed PMID: 19796554.
18. Host LV, Campochiaro C, Afonso A, Nihtyanova SI, Denton CP, Ong VH. High proton pump inhibitor exposure increases risk of calcinosis in systemic sclerosis. Rheumatology (Oxford). 2021;60(2):849–54. https://doi.org/10.1093/rheumatology/keaa332. PMID: 32829395.
19. Abignano G, Mennillo GA, Lettieri G, Temiz Karadag D, Carriero A, Padula AA, Del Galdo F, Khanna D, D'Angelo S. UCLA Scleroderma Clinical Trials Consortium Gastrointestinal Tract 2.0 Reflux Scale correlates with impaired esophageal scintigraphy findings in Systemic Sclerosis. J Rheumatol. 2021; https://doi.org/10.3899/jrheum.201283.
20. Kar P, Mitra S, Resnick JM, Torbey CF. Gastric antral vascular ectasia: case report and review of the literature. Clin Med Res. 2013;11(2):80–5. https://doi.org/10.3121/cmr.2012.1036. Epub 2012 Dec 21. Review. PubMed PMID: 23262190; PubMed Central PMCID: PMC3692392.
21. Wipff J, Coriat R, Masciocchi M, Caramaschi P, Derk CT, Hachulla E, Riccieri V, Mouthon L, Krasowska D, Ananyeva LP, Kahan A, Matucci-Cerinic M, Chaussade S, Allanore Y. Outcomes of Barrett's oesophagus related to systemic sclerosis: a 3-year EULAR Scleroderma Trials and Research prospective follow-up study. Rheumatology (Oxford). 2011;50(8):1440–4. https://doi.org/10.1093/rheumatology/ker110. Epub 2011 Mar 16. PubMed PMID: 21415021.
22. Bharadwaj S, Tandon P, Gohel T, Corrigan ML, Coughlin KL, Shatnawei A, Chatterjee S, Kirby DF. Gastrointestinal manifestations, malnutrition, and role of enteral and parenteral nutrition in patients with scleroderma. J Clin Gastroenterol. 2015;49(7):559–64. https://doi.org/10.1097/MCG.0000000000000334. PubMed PMID: 25992813.
23. Frech TM, Khanna D, Maranian P, Frech EJ, Sawitzke AD, Murtaugh MA. Probiotics for the treatment of systemic sclerosis-associated gastrointestinal bloating/distention. Clin Exp Rheumatol. 2011;29(2 Suppl 65):S22–5. Epub 2011 May 12. PubMed PMID: 21586214.
24. Cereda E, Codullo V, Klersy C, Breda S, Crippa A, Rava ML, Orlandi M, Bonardi C, Fiorentini ML, Caporali R, Caccialanza R. Disease-related nutritional risk and mortality in systemic sclerosis. Clin Nutr. 2014;33(3):558–61. https://doi.org/10.1016/j.clnu.2013.08.010. Epub 2013 Sep 3. PubMed PMID: 24054278.
25. Smith E, Pauling JD. The efficacy of dietary intervention on gastrointestinal involvement in systemic sclerosis: a systematic literature review. Semin Arthritis Rheum. 2019;49:112–8. https://doi.org/10.1016/j.semarthrit.2018.12.001.
26. Thoua NM, Schizas A, Forbes A, Denton CP, Emmanuel AV. Internal anal sphincter atrophy in patients with systemic sclerosis. Rheumatology (Oxford). 2011;50(9):1596–602. https://doi.org/10.1093/rheumatology/ker153. Epub 2011 Apr 18. PubMed PMID: 21504990.
27. Thoua NM, Abdel-Halim M, Forbes A, Denton CP, Emmanuel AV. Fecal incontinence in systemic sclerosis is secondary to neu-

ropathy. Am J Gastroenterol. 2012;107(4):597–603. https://doi.org/10.1038/ajg.2011.399. Epub 2011 Nov 15. PubMed PMID: 22085820.

28. Butt S, Alam A, Cohen R, Krogh K, Buntzen S, Emmanuel A. Lack of effect of sacral nerve stimulation for incontinence in patients with systemic sclerosis. Color Dis. 2015;17(10):903–7. https://doi.org/10.1111/codi.12969.

29. Hansi N, Thoua N, Carulli M, Chakravarty K, Lal S, Smyth A, Herrick A, Ogunbiyi O, Shaffer J, Mclaughlin J, Denton C, Ong V, Emmanuel AV, Murray CD. Consensus best practice pathway of the UK scleroderma study group: gastrointestinal manifestations of systemic sclerosis. Clin Exp Rheumatol. 2014;32(6 Suppl 86):S214–21. Epub 2014 Nov 5. PubMed PMID: 25372804.

Upper Gastrointestinal Tract: Manifestations of Systemic Sclerosis

31

John O. Clarke and Nitin K. Ahuja

Introduction

Systemic sclerosis (SSc) is a chronic connective tissue disorder with multisystem involvement. The gastrointestinal (GI) tract is affected in up to 90% of patients [1–3], and gut involvement is a leading cause of morbidity. Symptoms vary based on location of involvement and degree of impairment; however, dysphagia, reflux, nausea, vomiting, pain, diarrhea, constipation, fecal incontinence, and weight loss are all commonly reported. GI involvement severely impacts quality of life and is a major cause of mortality associated with SSc [4].

While the esophagus is the most widely described site of GI involvement, SSc can affect any site within the GI tract from the mouth to the anus. This chapter will focus on foregut manifestations of SSc, ranging from the mouth to stomach, with an emphasis on both motility and bleeding. Involvement of other regions of the GI tract will be detailed in other chapters.

Oropharyngeal Cavity

Oropharyngeal manifestations of scleroderma are not well studied, with estimates of involvement ranging from 20% to 80% [5–7]. Sclerosis of the oropharyngeal mucosa, muscles associated with mastication, and salivary glands can lead to difficulty in speaking, chewing, and swallowing. Reported symptoms include head and neck numbness; tongue, hard palate, and soft palate fibrosis; microstomia; oral mucosa damage; perioral skin injury; xerostomia; periodontal ligament fibrous thickening; bone resorption; oral telangiectasia; trigeminal neuropathy; and significant dental caries. In addition, sicca symptoms are reported in up to 20% of SSc patients, and the associated decreased salivary gland activity is typically associated with mild oropharyngeal dysphagia due to lack of effective food bolus lubrication that impairs oropharyngeal transfer and esophageal transit. Significant perioral skin involvement can limit the aperture of the mouth and restrict food intake. Patients with a scleroderma-myositis overlap may also have pharyngeal muscle weakness, which may be suggested on videofluoroscopy.

Therapeutic options are often limited to dietary modifications using small bolus size, soft foods, and increased use of liquid supplementation during meals. Close follow-up with a dentist or oral specialist is also recommended, as is optimal oral hygiene. To date, there are not good data to suggest that oropharyngeal manifestations of SSc respond to any specific medical therapy. In our practices, however, we will often use over-the-counter oral moisturizers and have seen some benefit with use of these agents. Dedicated swallow therapy may also be of benefit for those patients with pharyngeal involvement.

J. O. Clarke (✉)
Division of Gastroenterology & Hepatology, Stanford University School of Medicine, Palo Alto, CA, USA
e-mail: john.clarke@stanford.edu

N. K. Ahuja
Division of Gastroenterology & Hepatology, University of Pennsylvania School of Medicine, Philadelphia, PA, USA
e-mail: Nitin.Ahuja@pennmedicine.upenn.edu

Y. Allanore et al. (eds.), *Scleroderma*, https://doi.org/10.1007/978-3-031-40658-4_31

Esophagus

The esophagus is the most commonly affected organ in the GI tract in SSc, with involvement seen in over 90% of patients via both pathology [8] and symptom assessment [9]. Symptoms are related to dysmotility and commonly consist of dysphagia, heartburn, and regurgitation. The pathogenesis of this dysfunction is still not clear, and prior investigations have suggested several potential mechanisms. Sjogren proposed a progression of GI SSc involvement composed of three distinct steps: (1) vascular damage, (2) neurogenic impairment, and (3) replacement of normal smooth muscle by fibrosis and atrophy [10]. Under this model, there is loss of response to prokinetic therapy as fibrosis develops, leading to progressive GI symptoms. To a certain extent, this theory remains speculative, however, as causal progression has never been demonstrated, and other competing theories exist. Autoantibodies directed against enteric neurons have been identified in a subset of SSc patients [11] as have antimuscarinic antibodies [12]. Responsiveness of the lower esophageal sphincter to exogenously administered methacholine, but not pharmacologic administration of agents acting via cholinergic neurons, supports the concept of a neurologic defect in SSc [13]. Autonomic dysfunction has also been posited as a potential mechanism [14]. In addition, there are contradictory data as to whether esophageal fibrosis is even present in these patients. A study using endoscopic ultrasound in patients with SSc revealed significant esophageal thickening as compared to unaffected controls [15]; however, in contrast, an autopsy study evaluating the esophagi of 74 patients with SSc showed significant atrophy (94% of patients) but no evidence of abnormal fibrosis [8]. It is notable that the autopsy study did not demonstrate a correlation between histopathology findings and disease duration. Interestingly, although the neurons within the myenteric plexus were intact, a reduction was demonstrated in the interstitial cells of Cajal important in modulating nerve-muscle interactions. In addition, no animal model for scleroderma esophageal disease exists, although there is a mouse model for colonic fibrosis [16].

In a novel experiment, Taroni and colleagues recently evaluated esophageal biopsies among patients with and without scleroderma. They performed molecular characterization of gene expression combined with detailed histological analysis and identified distinct subgroups with either an inflammatory gene expression signature or a proliferative/noninflammatory signature. They showed that these signatures appeared to be independent of traditional clinical markers of disease progression. Similar gene expression signatures previously identified in SSc skin biopsies were recapitulated in SSc esophageal biopsies, implying that the underlying pathogenesis in individual patients may be similar in different organ systems. This study also suggested disease heterogeneity across SSc patients. Numbers evaluated in this study were small, and clinical significance remains to be elucidated. That said, the mechanistic implications of this work are fascinating and potentially could lead to the development of future tissue biomarkers and recognition of molecular phenotypes with clinical implications [17].

Clinical Presentation and Complications

Symptoms attributable to esophageal dysfunction occur in the vast majority of patients with SSc and include heartburn, regurgitation, and dysphagia [7, 18–21]. Gastroesophageal reflux is of particular concern due to multiple contributing mechanisms, including peristaltic dysfunction, decreased lower esophageal sphincter (LES) pressure, delayed gastric emptying, autonomic dysfunction, occasional sicca syndrome (seen in 20% of patients), and occasionally an associated hiatal hernia [19]. Just as important as the loss of the LES as an antireflux barrier is the loss of reflux clearance mechanisms that include secondary peristalsis and salivary bicarbonate secretion. Medications used to treat other manifestations of SSc including phosphodiesterase inhibitors and calcium channel antagonists further impair LES function and may worsen reflux. Dysphagia for solid food is related to decreased or absent esophageal peristalsis. Despite the degree of functional impairment of esophageal motility, dysphagia is generally mild and intermittent owing to the ability of gravity to facilitate bolus transit. Furthermore, many patients, up to 40% in some series, are asymptomatic despite well-documented esophageal dysmotility [22–25]. The clinical situation, however, can be complicated if a stricture is present due to reflux, pill-induced esophagitis, *Candida*, or other etiologies. Compensatory strategies include assuming an upright posture during meals and use of liquids between swallows of solid food.

Esophageal dysmotility and reflux in the context of SSc can be associated with significant complications. Stricture formation is particularly prevalent and believed to be related to multiple possible etiologies, including reflux, pill-induced injury, and candidal infection. Prevalence of esophageal strictures in patients with SSc has been estimated to be as high as 29% [26]. The frequent administration of proton pump inhibitors (PPI) in SSc has, however, almost certainly reduced the prevalence of peptic strictures over the past two decades. A case-control study involving over 100,000 subjects evaluating risk factors for erosive esophagitis or esophageal stricture formation reported that a concurrent diagnosis of scleroderma was associated with an odds ratio of 6.1 for erosive esophagitis and 12.3 for stricture formation [27]. While reflux is believed to be the classic precipitant, candidal esophagitis is also worth considering given that patients with SSc typically have multiple risk factors, including chronic acid suppression, antibiotic administration, impaired esophageal motility, and use of immunosuppressive agents. One study reported colonization/infection rates of 15% with strictures associated with all cases [28].

The prevalence of Barrett's esophagus has been reported to be as high as 37% [29]; however, other investigators have reported significantly lower findings [26, 28]. Very recently, investigators from the Mayo Clinic Scottsdale reported a prevalence of 12.8% in female SSc patients [30]. Due to this wide variation, it is not entirely clear whether the prevalence of Barrett's esophagus in SSc patients exceeds that of the general public, but it likely does given the known risk factors and the recent Mayo report. Likewise, it is not clear that the risk of esophageal carcinoma is higher than baseline for patients with SSc [31]. It is also worth noting that most of the literature evaluating concerns for Barrett's esophagus and cancer predates widespread PPI use.

Finally, the natural history of esophageal dysmotility in SSc is not well studied; however, one recent publication evaluated patients seen over a 13-year period who had multiple esophageal scintigraphy transit studies performed. In this publication, esophageal motility worsened in 96% of patients with diffuse SSc as compared to 59% of patients with limited SSc [32].

Relationship to Pulmonary Disease

The relationship between reflux and pulmonary disease is not well established; however, reflux may contribute to pulmonary disease through two mechanisms: (1) microaspiration leading to direct injury and (2) vagal stimulation leading to bronchoconstriction. In addition, pulmonary disease may lead to increased reflux through alteration of esophageal/gastric pressure dynamics related to enhanced inspiratory force and diminished intrathoracic pressure, use of medications that decrease lower esophageal sphincter pressure (in particular bronchodilators and sildenafil), and potentially hiatal hernia formation. Given the morbidity and mortality associated with SSc lung disease, this relationship has substantial clinical importance.

Several studies have suggested a correlation between esophageal reflux and SSc lung disease [33–37]. However, this finding has not been universal as one study did not show any association [38]. Recently, this relationship has been evaluated with pH/impedance monitoring and high-resolution computed tomography, and a strong correlation was noted between interstitial lung disease and esophageal acid exposure, acid reflux numbers, nonacid reflux numbers, and proximal reflux (all with p values <0.01) [39]. Another study from the Canadian Scleroderma Research Group with over 1000 patients also showed a strong correlation between symptoms of esophageal dysmotility and worsening pulmonary function (also with p values <0.01) [40]. A very recent study from Italy evaluating 52 SSc patients over a 4-year period found no relationship between pulmonary involvement and esophageal involvement, but did find a relationship between pulmonary involvement and lower esophageal sphincter pressure [41]. Finally, a recent study from Thailand reported a correlation between interstitial pulmonary disease and esophageal dilation [42]. Given this information, the relationship between the two entities appears consistent and likely genuine; however, causality has not been established, and there are no data at present to prove that treatment of reflux in patients with SSc has any effect upon long-term pulmonary function [43].

Diagnostic Evaluation

Multiple diagnostic modalities exist to evaluate esophageal function and disease in patients with SSc. If dysphagia is present, a barium esophagram is often the initial study of choice as it provides information related to both structure and function. Dysphagia in SSc, however, is most commonly the result of dysmotility and not a structural lesion that can be visualized radiographically. On the other hand, while manometry is often considered the gold standard for esophageal function in SSc, it does not provide structural information and would not detect an esophageal stricture. Typical radiographic features include esophageal dilatation, presence of intraesophageal air, poor barium clearance, and a widely patent lower esophageal sphincter (Fig. 31.1) [44, 45]. Some experts have recommended that a barium esophagram be the initial study for all patients with suspected scleroderma [43]; however, the sensitivity of barium studies for detection of SSc-related dysmotility has been shown to be less than manometry in several studies [46–49]. For this reason, most authorities would not recommend a barium study as the initial test for assessment of esophageal motility in the absence of significant dysphagia [19, 50].

Esophagogastroduodenoscopy (EGD) should be considered in patients presenting with esophageal symptoms related to SSc. Esophagitis has been reported in 32–77% of SSc patients undergoing endoscopy [21–23, 27, 28, 36, 46, 51–53]; however, multiple studies have shown that symptoms do not necessarily correlate with esophageal injury and that even SSc patients with no symptoms can have significant esophageal damage (Fig. 31.2) [28, 52–54]. As detailed

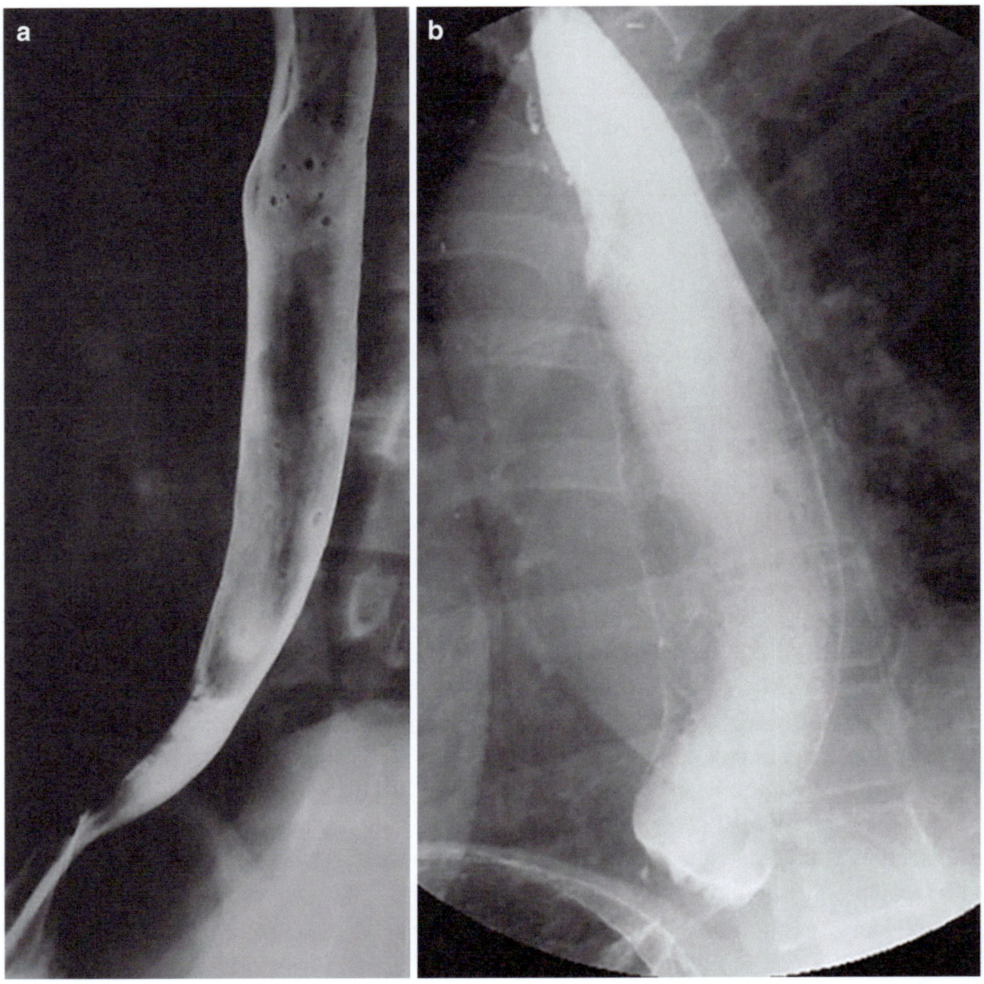

Fig. 31.1 Barium esophagram in scleroderma. Panel (**a**) depicts a normal esophagus with tapering at the esophagogastric junction. Panel (**b**) from a patient with scleroderma demonstrates pan esophageal dilatation

above, *Candida* and Barrett's esophagus are additional clinical concerns, neither of which can be reliably detected without endoscopy. For these reasons, some authorities recommend early endoscopy for all patients diagnosed with SSc [52]; there are no guidelines to support that position at present, however, and the decision to pursue endoscopy needs to be individualized given the relative risks and benefits of the procedure. Other potential benefits of endoscopy include tissue acquisition for Barrett's esophagus to exclude dysplasia, identification of sites of upper GI hemorrhage, and ability to perform dilation of esophageal strictures. In our practices, we usually pursue endoscopy specifically for symptoms refractory to medical intervention.

Esophageal manometry is considered the gold standard for assessment of esophageal motility in patients with SSc [19, 50, 55]. Abnormalities are detected in up to 90% of patients, even in the absence of symptoms [56]. Typical findings on manometry include low-contraction amplitudes in the distal esophagus and, in more advanced stages, esophageal aperistalsis with decreased lower esophageal sphincter pressure (Fig. 31.3). Classically, esophageal contractile forces are maintained in the proximal esophagus, and the upper esophageal sphincter is uninvolved [57]. Defects in proximal esophageal contractile function may indicate concomitant myositis (Fig. 31.3).

Recently, the Functional Lumen Imaging Probe (FLIP)—a Food and Drug Administration (FDA)-approved device that utilizes impedance planimetry to evaluate esophageal diameter, distensibility, and motility—has been used to characterize esophageal function in the context of SSc. Investigators have shown heterogeneity in primary and secondary peristalsis in SSc patients and wide discordance in esophageal distensibility [58]. These findings may have clinical relevance, but outcome studies are needed to determine whether this information affects clinical management.

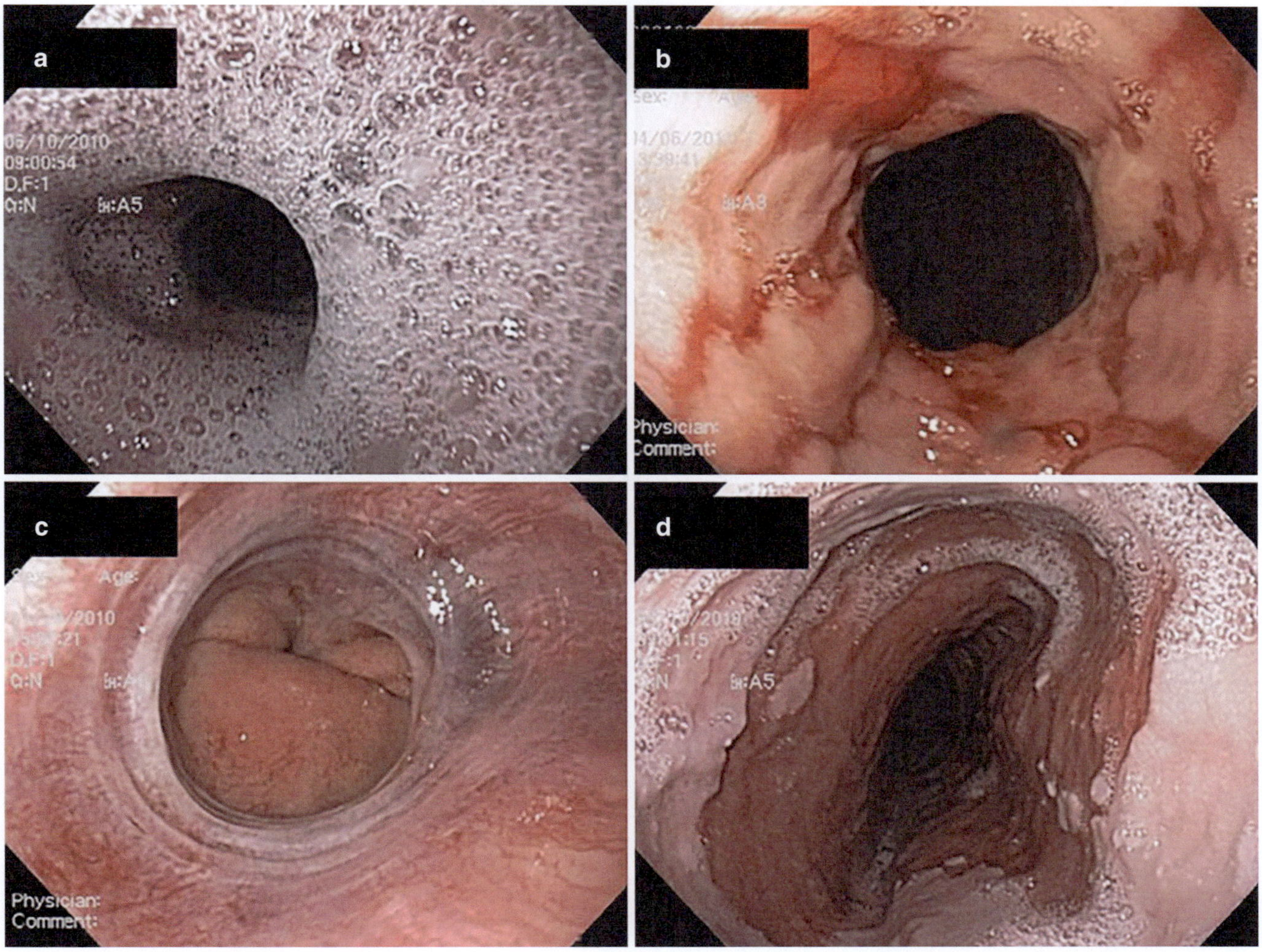

Fig. 31.2 Esophageal endoscopic findings in scleroderma. Panel (**a**) depicts retention of saliva within the esophagus. Panel (**b**) demonstrates reflux esophagitis with ulceration and stricture formation at the esophagogastric junction above a hiatal hernia. Panel (**c**) shows a peptic stricture. Panel (**d**) illustrates long segment Barrett's esophagus with small islands of squamous mucosa in a patient with scleroderma

Finally, for patients with suspected reflux or continued symptoms despite medical therapy, formal reflux testing is often employed [59]. Traditional reflux testing has consisted of a catheter-based pH study; however, two emerging technologies have been developed over the last two decades and have changed the landscape with regard to reflux testing. Wireless pH testing eliminates the need for a catheter and records esophageal pH over a 48–96 h span. It can be combined with endoscopy or can be placed without endoscopic guidance, if baseline endoscopic landmarks are known or a manometry is performed concurrently. Advantages of the wireless pH system include improved patient tolerability and prolonged recording periods that allow for increased detection of symptom-reflux correlation. The main limitation of wireless pH testing, though, is that it only looks at esophageal pH and does not allow assessment of weakly acidic or nonacidic reflux. The second emerging technology is combined pH-impedance, which allows simultaneous measurement of bolus flow and esophageal pH, thereby allowing separation of acidic, weakly acidic, and nonacidic reflux as well as assessment of the proximal extent of reflux. While PPI therapy effectively controls esophageal acid exposure, it does not eliminate nonacid reflux, which can be a major cause of morbidity in SSc patients owing to incompetency of the LES and delayed gastric emptying. Impedance technology has been studied in patients with SSc [39, 60] and does provide additional information; however, it requires an indwelling nasogastric tube for 24 h, which has its associated limitations. For clinical purposes, both modalities allow accurate assessment of reflux and can help guide clinical management in the context of ongoing reflux symptoms related to SSc [61].

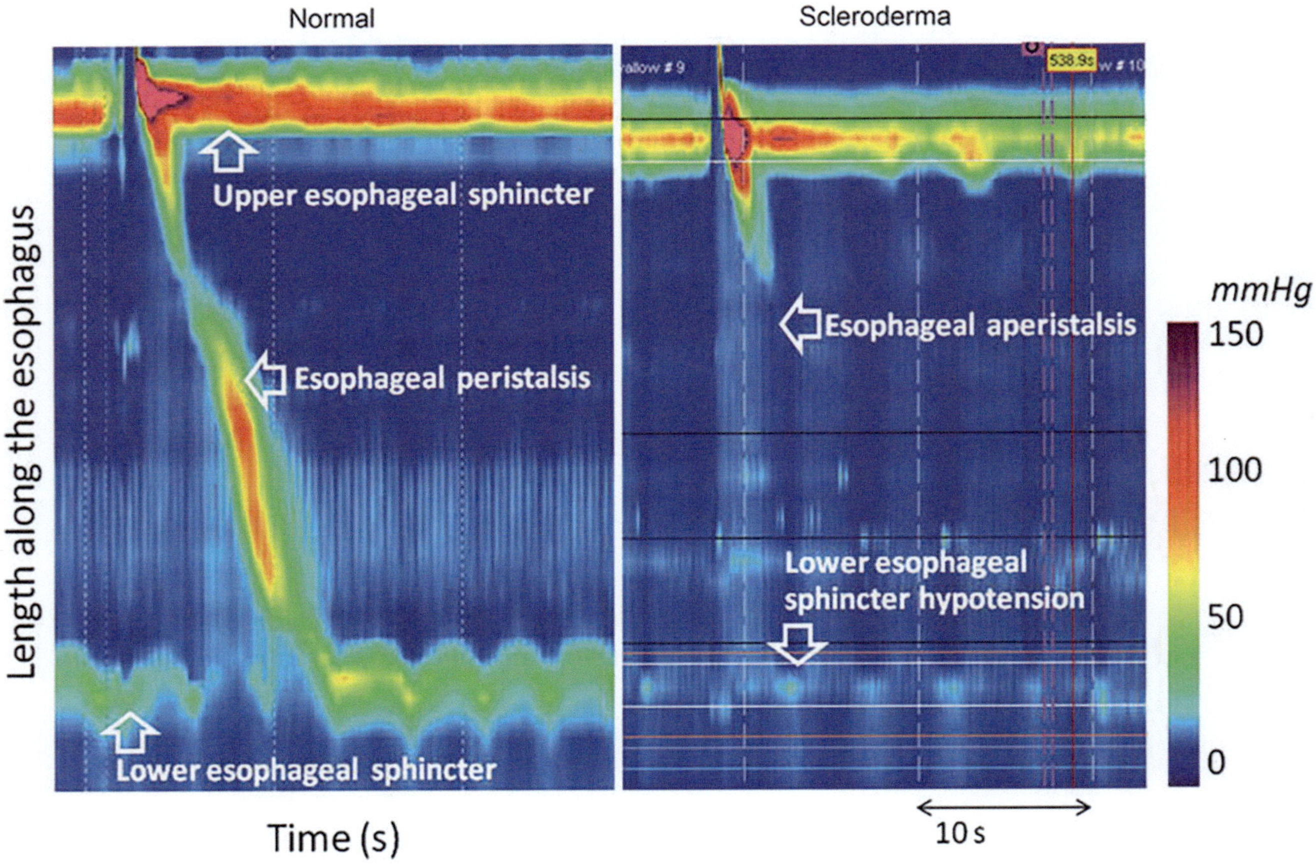

Fig. 31.3 High-resolution esophageal manometry contour plot in scleroderma. The left panel depicts a normal swallow with relaxation of the upper esophageal sphincter, sequential contractions in the esophageal body, and relaxation of the lower esophageal sphincter. The right panel from a patient with scleroderma demonstrates intact function of the upper esophageal sphincter and proximal esophagus but complete loss of contractile activity in the esophageal body and lower esophageal sphincter

Treatment

Treatment of esophageal disorders related to SSc can be challenging. Available therapies directed at slowing or reversing SSc progression including high-dose immunosuppression and stem cell transplantation have not demonstrated correction of the underlying GI dysmotility. Nevertheless, effective therapies exist for managing the consequences of esophageal dysfunction. For those with reflux, initial treatment often consists of lifestyle modifications, including elevation of the head of the bed; avoidance of meals within 3 or more hours of lying supine; and avoidance of alcohol, caffeine, nicotine, and other known reflux exacerbants (such as tomatoes, citrus, garlic, chocolate, peppermint, onions). Care should be taken to minimize medication use that could result in esophageal inflammation or altered esophageal motility. If therapy is required for Raynaud's syndrome, diltiazem may be considered over other smooth muscle relaxants as it may have less effect on lower esophageal sphincter pressure [62, 63].

Acid suppressive therapy with PPIs is the mainstay of therapy for reflux in patients with SSc. Specific randomized controlled trials showing efficacy of PPI use in patients with SSc are lacking; however, the efficacy of PPI use in the treatment of gastroesophageal reflux in the general population is well documented, and expert consensus (European League against Rheumatism Scleroderma Trials and Research group, UK Scleroderma Study Group) recommends PPI use for the prevention of SSc-related reflux disease, strictures, and esophageal ulcers [64, 65]. This recommendation is supported by several small studies showing improvement in either symptoms or esophagitis with prolonged PPI use [53, 66, 67]. Despite the above recommendation, it is not clear that PPI use changes the natural history of scleroderma, and there is still some debate as to whether treatment should be based on symptoms or objective measures of esophageal acid exposure [19]. There are also data to suggest that SSc patients may require higher PPI dosages than other patients with reflux symptoms [53, 68], which is not surprising given the impairment of multiple physiologic determinants of reflux in SSc. On the other hand, concerns exist regarding potential complications of long-term PPI therapy such as small intestinal bacterial overgrowth [69] and osteoporosis [70]. More recently, associations have been raised between

PPI use and a litany of concerns, including chronic kidney disease and dementia. However, it is important to note that these concerns are primarily based on weak and low-grade evidence and remain controversial [71, 72]. Histamine receptor blockers have also been employed with some efficacy, but the data behind their use are less robust than with PPI use [73, 74]. One study adding ranitidine to high-dose omeprazole in SSc patients showed no change in nocturnal acid breakthrough, reflux, or quality of life [75]. In our practice, we have not found histamine receptor blockers to work as well as PPI therapy in the SSc population and believe that the benefits of PPI use generally outweigh the risk given the frequency and severity of SSc esophageal involvement.

If symptoms progress despite high-dose acid suppressive therapy and lifestyle change, the next step in therapy is typically the addition of a prokinetic agent. This pharmacologic category has been shown to accelerate gastric emptying and increase lower esophageal sphincter pressure. Several small randomized controlled trials demonstrated efficacy of short-term cisapride [76–80]; however, cisapride has been withdrawn from the market in the United States due to fatal, albeit rare, arrhythmias associated with long QT syndrome and is available only in select countries or via Janssen Pharmaceuticals for compassionate use. Limited data support the use of metoclopramide in acute use [81–84]; however, long-term data demonstrating efficacy for metoclopramide are lacking, and safety concerns exist regarding long-term metoclopramide and tardive dyskinesia [85]. Limited data exist regarding erythromycin [86, 87]; however, this agent can be associated with tachyphylaxis and nausea in a substantial subset of patients and may not be ideal for long-term use. Domperidone has been suggested as a possible treatment [88] with fewer side effects than metoclopramide; however, there are limited data regarding domperidone in SSc patients, and this drug is not FDA-approved in the United States. In our practices, we tend to use either pyridostigmine or prucalopride. Pyridostigmine is an acetylcholinesterase inhibitor with a whole gut prokinetic effect. While it has a modest effect on gastric and esophageal motility, the safety profile is excellent, and there are data to support use in SSc [89, 90]. Similarly, prucalopride is a selective serotonin 5-HT4 agonist with a whole gut effect. While FDA-approved for constipation, it also has a foregut prokinetic effect, data to support use in SSc, and an excellent safety profile [91–93]. Overall, the clinical and physiologic benefits of available prokinetic agents in SSc are, at best, modest. Nevertheless, despite the limitations detailed above, a recent expert consensus recommends consideration of prokinetic drugs for the management of SSc-related symptomatic motility disturbances, including dysphagia and reflux [64].

A recent addition to the SSc dysmotility armamentarium has been buspirone, an oral 5-HT_{1A} receptor agonist which is believed to exert action on receptors in the esophagus and fundus. It was recently found to reduce symptom severity in patients with dyspepsia, presumably due to enhanced fundic accommodation [94]—and also to improve esophageal peristalsis and enhance lower esophageal sphincter pressure in healthy volunteers [95]. Investigators from Greece evaluated 20 SSc patients with manometry before and after buspirone administration and found that buspirone enhanced lower esophageal sphincter pressure and improved peristalsis [96]. The clinical implications of this work remain uncertain; buspirone may be an option for patients who remain symptomatic despite further therapy, but more data are required to confirm clinical efficacy and long-term safety.

In the event that gastroesophageal reflux cannot be controlled with medical therapy, surgical options do exist. Surgery is sometimes contemplated for relief of symptoms of heartburn or regurgitation that persist in spite of high-dose proton pump inhibition. The most common antireflux procedure performed today is the laparoscopic Nissen fundoplication; however, this can be associated with substantial dysphagia in SSc patients with severe dysmotility. The addition of even a minor degree of mechanical restriction at the esophagogastric junction in a SSc patient with absent esophageal peristalsis may result in the development of secondary achalasia. Early published series report postoperative dysphagia rates ranging from 31% to 71% [97–100]. Because of these reports, surgical intervention has typically been reserved for severe cases. A retrospective review of 23 SSc patients undergoing antireflux surgery revealed improved reflux and dysphagia postoperative rates with laparoscopic Roux-en-Y gastric bypass as compared to fundoplication [101]. Newer antireflux surgical procedures such as transoral incisionless fundoplication or magnetic sphincter augmentation do not have data to support use in SSc at present. Based on these studies, surgery is an option for select patients but is typically a last resort when medical therapy has been unsuccessful, and the risk of postoperative dysphagia needs to be considered. These data are reviewed in a recent systematic review [102].

Stomach

Gastric manifestations of SSc are highly variable and stem from both dysmotility and vascular ectasia. Symptoms of gastric dysmotility (including heartburn, regurgitation, nausea, bloating, epigastric pain, early satiety, and postprandial fullness) have been reported in approximately 50% of patients [7, 26, 55, 103, 104]. Bleeding related to gastric antral vascular ectasia is seen far less commonly and will be discussed later in this chapter [105, 106]. The pathogenesis of gastric dysmotility remains unclear but is believed to be related to both neuropathic and fibrotic changes as detailed above. Gastric involvement is associated with worsened morbidity and mortality [2, 3].

Clinical Presentation

Symptoms associated with gastric dysmotility are seen in approximately 50% of patients and include nausea, bloating, epigastric pain, early satiety, and postprandial fullness. In addition, gastric dysfunction also contributes to gastroesophageal reflux and may manifest only as traditional reflux symptoms, such as heartburn and regurgitation. Interestingly, the presence and severity of symptoms may not correlate with gastric dysfunction as measured by scintigraphy and electrogastrography (EGG) [104, 107, 108]; however, there are data to suggest that the presence of esophageal involvement corresponds with a higher rate of gastric involvement [7].

Multiple potential mechanisms have been hypothesized, and objective studies of gastric function have recorded widely divergent findings based on patient selection and study protocol. For example, gastric emptying has been recorded to be delayed in anywhere from 10% to 75% of SSc patients, based on studies using scintigraphy, radio-opaque markers, C^{13}-labeled breath tests, and ultrasonography [54, 55, 84, 107–114]. Hypothesized mechanisms whereby SSc impairs gastric motility include alterations in gastric accommodation, motility patterns, gastric myoelectrical activity, and gastric emptying [104]. The relative role of each of the aforementioned mechanisms is not clearly established at this time and may vary for individual patients.

Diagnostic Evaluation

There is no consensus regarding the appropriate initial study for the evaluation of gastric dysmotility in patients with SSc. Given the high prevalence of esophageal dysmotility and the nonspecific nature of the recorded symptoms, initial evaluation often consists of a barium contrast study and/or upper endoscopy. Barium contrast radiography allows a gross evaluation of gastric motility and exclusion of mechanical obstruction. Typical findings related to gastric involvement include a dilated stomach, hypomotility, and delayed transit, but barium contrast radiography is neither sensitive nor specific and is rarely if ever performed solely for assessment of gastric SSc involvement [45]. Similarly, upper endoscopy has utility in the evaluation of SSc and allows assessment of gastritis, peptic ulcer disease, esophagitis, and a gross assessment of pyloric contractions; however, the utility of endoscopy for SSc is primarily limited to assessment of inflammation and potential bleeding etiologies, whereas the role of endoscopy in assessment of gastric motility is limited. Retained food within the stomach during routine endoscopy can be suggestive of delayed gastric emptying, as patients are instructed to fast for approximately 8 h prior to the procedure. If identified in the setting of an accurate history of meal timing, retained food may obviate the need for additional testing for gastric transit.

Gastric emptying studies have been the traditional test of choice for evaluation of gastric motility. Studies employing a variety of techniques—including scintigraphy, radio-opaque markers, C^{13} breath tests, and ultrasonography—have reported abnormalities in gastric emptying in 10–75% of SSc patients, although the bulk of the studies appear to show impairment in approximately 50% of patients [26, 55, 84, 108, 111]. As these studies were performed in tertiary care facilities, these recorded values may overestimate the true prevalence of impaired gastric emptying in SSc. In the United States, the most commonly performed modality of gastric emptying study is scintigraphy, and normative values have been well established [115]. However, this study is not without controversy—it can be expensive, and symptoms do not always correlate with objective emptying abnormalities, both in SSc and other unrelated conditions [111, 116]. Recently, whole gut scintigraphy—extended to the entire GI tract—has also been pursued in SSc patients to assess for whole gut and regional dysmotility [117, 118]. Gastric emptying has also been assessed by other modalities, including radio-opaque marker transit [108], ultrasonography [114, 119], and breath testing [55, 120].

Gastric emptying has also been evaluated via a wireless capsule motility system (SmartPill) that provides prolonged recording of temperature, pH, and pressure. Whole transit is recorded over a several day period, and regional transit (gastric emptying, small intestinal transit, colonic transit) can be distinguished through analysis of the pH and pressure profiles. In theory, this technology offers the ability to measure whole gut and regional transit as well as segmental motility patterns without the need for radiation exposure or catheter-based monitoring; however, data are still emerging regarding appropriate normative values and subtleties of interpretation. In addition, to our knowledge there are no published data to date regarding the use of this technology in SSc patients. Finally, as the capsule is ingested, a theoretical risk of capsule retention does exist, and patients must be monitored to ensure the capsule has exited appropriately [121–123]. Of note, the data obtained with the transit of an indigestible capsule (wireless motility capsule) may not be the same as that of a digestible meal (scintigraphy); however, the two means of gastric investigation have been shown to have good correlation [122].

Gastric motility and myoelectrical activity can also be recorded using antroduodenal manometry (ADM) and electrogastrography (EGG). ADM consists of a manometry catheter which is passed transnasally and positioned so that pressure sensors are located in the duodenum and stomach. Prolonged pressure monitoring can be performed to allow assessment of migrating motor complex activity—in particular assessment of frequency, amplitude, and coordination of contractions. In patients with SSc, this technology can demonstrate decreased contractile amplitudes and disrupted patterns of motor activity [26, 124, 125]. EGG consists of multichannel surface recordings of gastric myoelectrical activity. The use of this technology has been largely experimental, and while abnormalities are frequently detected, it remains controversial whether EGG abnormalities correlate with either symptoms or delayed gastric emptying [111, 125, 126]. At present, both ADM and EGG are offered primarily in tertiary motility centers, and their role in routine clinical care of SSc patients remains unclear. In addition, the wireless capsule motility study has been compared directly to ADM with favorable correlation and may offer a less invasive means of obtaining similar data [121].

Treatment

Treatment of SSc-related gastric dysmotility can be challenging given a limited range of treatment options. Dietary modification is typically the first line of therapy, and a gastroparesis diet, consisting of multiple, small volume, low-fat meals, is often recommended. Liquid emptying may be preserved in certain cases, and liquid nutritional supplements and a soft diet that requires less emulsification may be of benefit, although the data behind this recommendation are limited. Enteral feeding and/or decompression via gastrostomy or jejunostomy is occasionally performed, although there are no data available regarding this approach. Similarly, limited data are available regarding the utilization of total parenteral nutrition, a strategy usually reserved for SSc patients with severe gastric and small bowel dysmotility. In our practices, we do our best to avoid enteral feeding, decompression, and parenteral nutrition and use them only as last-resort options.

Prokinetic agents have been the mainstay of therapy, although the data are relatively limited. Nevertheless, this approach is recommended by expert consensus panels [64, 65]. Metoclopramide is the only agent approved by the FDA in the United States for treatment of gastroparesis; however, it is associated with significant side effects including potentially irreversible tardive dyskinesia. Data regarding metoclopramide in SSc-related gastric dysmotility are limited to small studies evaluating short-term effects [82, 84, 124]. While short-term efficacy has been demonstrated, there are no data regarding long-term use or safety. In addition, there is a case report of one SSc patient who experienced bradycardia and cardiac arrest following metoclopramide administration [127].

Domperidone is a peripheral dopamine receptor antagonist that is believed to cross the blood-brain barrier less effectively than metoclopramide and may provide equal or superior efficacy with fewer side effects. There are limited data regarding usage of domperidone in SSc [128]; however, there are data to support the use of domperidone in other conditions associated with impaired gastric emptying [129, 130]. At present, this medication is not approved for use in the United States; however, it can be obtained via an FDA Investigational New Drug application and is also available in at least 50 other countries. Despite the lack of data in SSc, the use of this agent can be justified based on EULAR consensus recommendations [64], favorable side effect profile, and limited options available. There is concern for potential QT prolongation, and patients must be monitored closely if this agent is employed [131].

Erythromycin is a motilin agonist and has data to support usage in both scleroderma and unrelated conditions with impaired gastric emptying. Two short-term studies demonstrated improvement in gastric emptying with erythromycin administration; one of the studies also looked at symptom response and reported improvement in early satiety, nausea, vomiting, and abdominal pain [87, 109]. A single study looked at long-term use of erythromycin (up to 48 weeks in duration) and reported benefit; however, the patients in the study were also administered octreotide concurrently, and the relative merits of each agent were not clearly elucidated [132]. Of the available agents, erythromycin has been demonstrated to have the most potent gastric prokinetic function, but in practice it is often not as attractive as other options for several reasons. First, it is associated with tachyphylaxis. Second, side effects include cramps, nausea, diarrhea, ototoxicity, and QT interval prolongation, all of which may limit use [133]. Third, although erythromycin has potent prokinetic properties, a systematic review concluded that available studies do not establish efficacy of erythromycin in relieving symptoms of delayed gastric emptying [134]. For all of these reasons, erythromycin may be a less than ideal option for long-term use, although it does have the benefit of documented short-term improvement in SSc and availability in the United States.

Cisapride is a combined $5HT_4$ agonist/$5HT_3$ antagonist and is the most investigated prokinetic available for treatment of SSc-associated dysmotility. Small studies have demonstrated improvement in gastric emptying, antroduodenal motility, and symptoms with acute and chronic use [76, 104, 135]. However, cisapride was removed from the US market due to QT interval prolongation and numerous deaths related to cardiac arrhythmia. It is available on a limited basis for compassionate use; however, it should be used with caution, and close monitoring of the QT interval is required if this medication is initiated.

In our practices, we usually employ pyridostigmine or prucalopride as first-line prokinetic therapy for our SSc patients with gastric dysmotility due to the excellent safety profile of both agents. Pyridostigmine is an acetylcholinesterase inhibitor with a whole gut prokinetic effect that is FDA-approved for swallowing dysfunction in the context of myasthenia gravis. The main site of action is the small/large bowel, but there is some gastric effect and data to support use in SSc [89, 90]. Similarly, prucalopride is a selective serotonin 5-HT4 agonist with a whole gut effect that is FDA-approved for constipation. However, it has documented gastric effects and is similar mechanistically to cisapride with a much more favorable safety profile; it also has data to support use in SSc [91–93].

Alternative therapies have also been employed for SSc-associated gastric dysmotility and are worth considering given the drawbacks of more conventional options. Ginger has been shown to accelerate gastric emptying in normal individuals [136] and has been used to relieve pregnancy-associated nausea [137]. This agent has not been studied in SSc or gastroparesis, but given the innocuous side effect profile, it is worth considering as an adjunct therapy. Similarly, we have anecdotal benefit with STW-5 (Iberogast), a European herbal mixture with prokinetic effects, and will occasionally use this clinically due to benefit in other GI motility disorders and excellent safety profile.

Recently, there has also been research directed toward acupuncture and related entities as a potential remedy [138]. Acupressure to a specific GI-associated acupuncture site (PC6) was found to alter gastric myoelectrical activity (GMA) as assessed by EGG in patients with SSc in one small study. Interestingly, the alterations in GMA correlated with symptoms [139]. Based on this preliminary study, the same group evaluated the role of transcutaneous electrical nerve stimulation in symptomatic SSc patients for a 14-day trial. They reported improvement in heart rate variability, symptoms, and quality of life [140]. A further study by the same investigators showed improvement in GMA, decreased mean plasma VIP and motilin levels, increased IL-6 levels, and symptom improvement after a 14-day trial [141]. While further studies are needed, these preliminary investigations are encouraging.

Finally, endoscopic and surgical options have been posited. Botulinum toxin has been investigated in impaired gastric emptying. The proposed mechanism is that botulinum toxin injected into the pylorus may relieve gastric outlet obstruction and accelerate gastric emptying. Early anecdotal experience supported this assumption; however, more recent randomized controlled trials have not shown a benefit for botulinum toxin in idiopathic or diabetic gastroparesis, and for this reason, it has largely fallen out of favor unless there is documented pyloric spasm [142]. There are no data regarding the use of botulinum toxin in patients with SSc; however, as the physiology of SSc often results in impaired contractions and lower contractile amplitudes, one could argue that SSc-associated gastric dysmotility may be even more unlikely to respond to this therapy than patients with impaired gastric emptying related to other conditions [133]. Very recently, gastric per-oral endoscopic myotomy (G-POEM) has entered the therapeutic arena as a more controlled means to disrupt the pylorus and is gaining popularity for the treatment of gastroparesis. Data with regard to G-POEM and SSc are limited, but there is one case report detailing two SSc patients with gastric dysmotility refractory to medical therapy who derived benefit from this technique [143]. Other surgical options have also been proposed for impaired gastric emptying, including pyloric myotomy, subtotal gastrectomy, gastric bypass, and gastric electrical stimulation. At present, however, there are no data to support the use of any of these procedures in SSc-associated gastric dysmotility.

Gastric Antral Vascular Ectasia

GI hemorrhage is a known consequence of SSc and can be seen in up to 15% of SSc patients in a tertiary care facility [144]. Gastric antral vascular ectasia (GAVE), also known as watermelon stomach, is the major gastric manifestation which may lead to bleeding. This is an uncommon vascular condition that was first described in 1984 [145]. While classically associated with SSc, it is not specific to rheumatologic disorders and can also be seen in atrophic gastritis, diabetes mellitus, cirrhosis, chronic renal failure, heart disease, and autoimmune disorders. The true prevalence of GAVE in SSc is difficult to determine but appears to be relatively uncommon; the largest series to date to evaluate this issue reported a prevalence of 5.7% (15 cases in 274 SSc patients). This estimate may be low given that many patients may be asymptomatic in early stages, and the endoscopic findings of mild GAVE can be misinterpreted as antral gastritis by even experienced endoscopists [103]. A recent publication from the European League Against Rheumatism Scleroderma Trials and Research (EUSTAR) network estimated the prevalence of GAVE to be about 1% in SSc patients [146].

The pathogenesis of GAVE remains unclear. At the moment, there are two leading hypotheses. The first theory holds that antral mucosal prolapse and abnormal gastric motility may lead to submucosal ischemia and elongation/dilatation of mucosal vessels. This theory is supported by two lines of reasoning: (1) histological evidence of both fibromuscular hyperplasia and mucosal capillary dilatation and (2) documentation of select SSc patients with high-amplitude gastric antral contractions on antroduodenal manometry [105, 145, 147, 148]. The second theory suggests that GAVE may be related to SSc-associated cutaneous telangiectasia. This theory is supported by the fact that most patients with GAVE also have telangiectasia involving other regions of the body (in particular skin) and/or GI tract [105]. In either case, the predilection of this vascular abnormality for the gastric antrum may be related to the distinct motility patterns that characterize this region of the stomach in distinction to others.

Given the rarity of GAVE, its natural history is not well studied; however, available data suggest that the vast majority of SSc patients diagnosed with GAVE (81%) already have an established diagnosis of SSc at the time of their endoscopic GAVE diagnosis. In an additional 8% of patients, the diagnoses of SSc and GAVE were established concurrently, whereas in the remaining 11%, the diagnosis of GAVE preceded the diagnosis of SSc. In patients known to have a diagnosis of GAVE, the median time between SSc diagnosis and GAVE onset was 18 months. Given these data, GAVE appears to be an early manifestation of SSc and the majority of cases were diagnosed within 5 years of diagnosis. The prevalence of GAVE also appears to be similar in diffuse and limited SSc, although diagnosis may be earlier in diffuse SSc as opposed to limited. It is unclear whether GAVE activity is associated with SSc activity or a more aggressive SSc phenotype. One review reported that in the majority of patients, GAVE activity does not parallel SSc activity, and GAVE can occur or progress even when disease activity was not active on other fronts; however, another publication reported that in the majority of patients with diffuse SSc diagnosed with early GAVE, there was also a rapid progression of cutaneous disease [105, 106]. Finally, a EUSTAR case-control study of 49 patients with SSc and GAVE reported that patients with GAVE were associated with a vascular phenotype, including anti-RNA polymerase III antibodies and a high risk of renal crisis [146].

The classic clinical presentation of GAVE is iron-deficiency anemia related to occult GI bleeding. Available data suggest that this is the case in approximately 90% of patients with GAVE, and the mean hemoglobin at time of diagnosis has been reported to be 6.7 g/dL. Other clinical presentations include overt bleeding with melena or hematemesis, which occurs in only a minority of patients [105]. GAVE is sometimes confused with but is distinct from portal hypertensive gastropathy, with the latter entity involving the mucosa of the gastric fundus and body. The histopathology of GAVE demonstrates the presence of microvascular thrombi, vascular ectasia, spindle cell proliferation, and fibrohyalinosis.

The endoscopic appearance is classically described as erythematous streaks projecting from the pylorus in radial fashion throughout the antrum (Fig. 31.4). The term "watermelon stomach" was coined as these streaks appear similar to the outside of a watermelon [145]. Another endoscopic variant that has been described is referred to as "honeycomb stomach" and consists of diffuse angiodysplastic lesions that coalesce in the antrum [149]. Finally, a third variant has been described in which there are well-demarcated round or mushroom-shaped lesions formed by a tuft of ecstatic blood vessels [150]. In addition, involvement can extend proximal to the antrum in a subset of patients [105, 106].

Treatment for GAVE remains a challenge, and data are relatively limited. There are no randomized controlled trials for nonendoscopic treatments, and initial therapy is often supportive. Given that the majority of GAVE patients present with occult bleeding and iron-deficiency anemia, the first step is often iron replacement therapy, optimization of bleeding parameters (if necessary), and minimization or avoidance of medications that could either promote bleeding or injure the gastric mucosa [150, 151]. Proton pump inhibitors are also usually employed to decrease any further mucosal injury that may be potentiated by gastric acid [105]. Blood transfusions are often required given the low hemoglobin at diagnosis, other comorbidities, and slow response with the above measures. Despite conservative therapy, as many as 60–70% of patients remain transfusion dependent [150].

Endoscopic therapy has become the mainstay of treatment when supportive care is unsuccessful. Multiple endoscopic ablative modalities have been employed, including Nd:YAG (neodymium: yttrium aluminum garnet) laser, argon plasma coagulation (APC), bipolar electrocautery, heater probe, and argon laser. Traditionally, the mainstay of treatment was with the Nd:YAG laser system, and it has the largest literature to support use, with reported success rates of approximately 80% over multiple treatments; however, significant complications were reported, including hyperplastic polyps, multifocal gastric neoplasia, perforation, and death [105, 150]. APC is an electrocoagulation technique which induces superficial injury to the affected tissue through a high-frequency monopolar current conducted through ionized argon gas. As compared to Nd:YAG laser, APC offers the theoretical advantages of limited penetration depth and coagulation effect to the surrounding tissue, resulting in fewer complications. Published success rates for APC have been similar to those for Nd:YAG laser. Due to similar efficacy and less risk, APC has become the standard of care at present for endoscopic treatment of SSc-related GAVE [3, 105, 150].

Two new endoscopic techniques have entered the clinical arena and are worth considering: cryotherapy and radiofrequency ablation (RFA). Cryotherapy consists of the endoscopic application of either nitrous oxide or carbon dioxide (based on the system employed), resulting in a controlled thermal injury to the gastric mucosa. As opposed to Nd:YAG laser or APC, cryotherapy allows treatment of large mucosal areas relatively quickly and offers the potential for shorter procedure times and technical ease with perhaps equal efficacy. This modality may be especially beneficial for diffuse

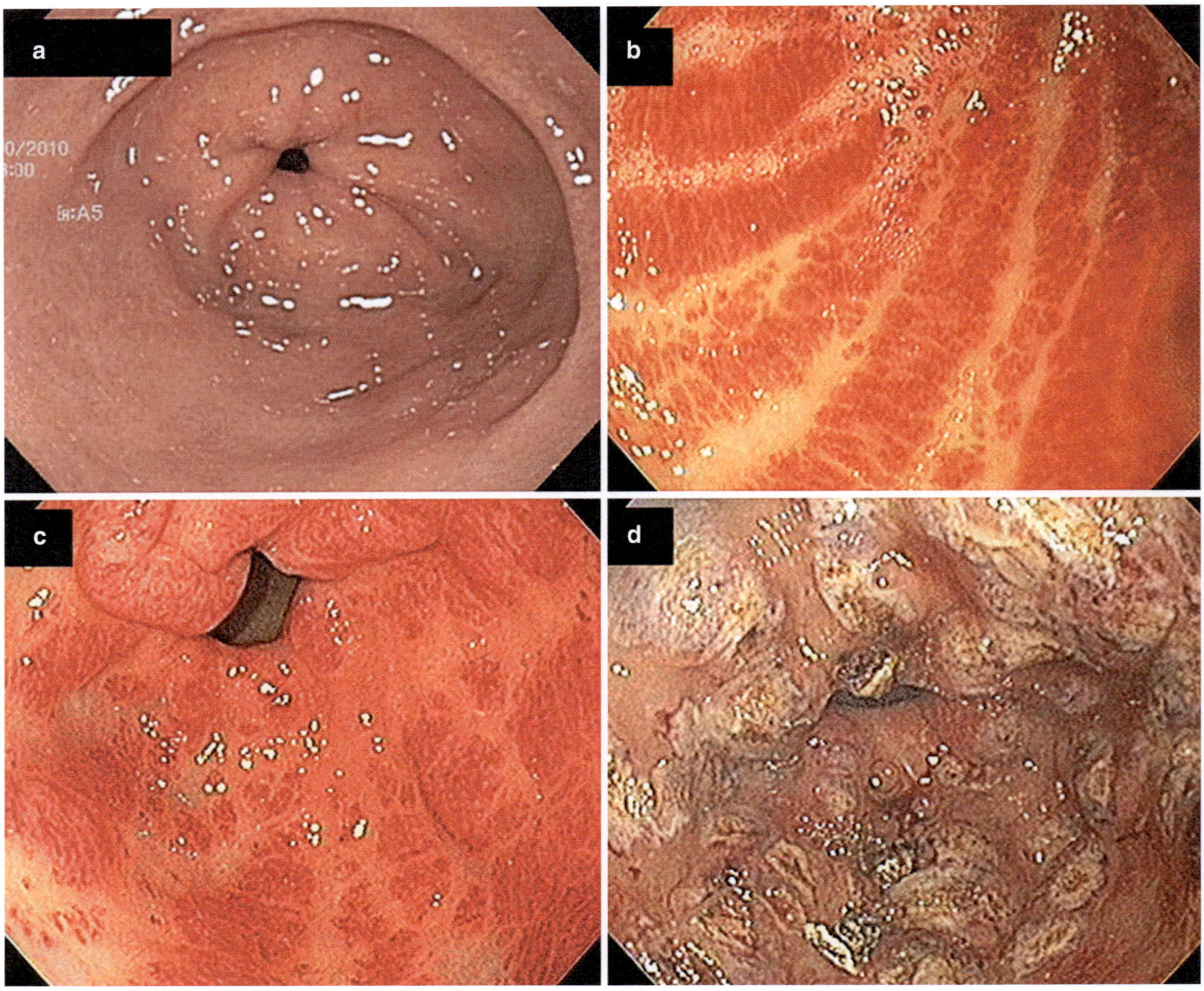

Fig. 31.4 Gastric endoscopic findings in scleroderma. Panel (**a**) shows the normal appearance to the gastric antrum. Panels (**b**, **c**) depict scleroderma patients with gastric antral vascular ectasia (GAVE) with erythematous, linear streaks along the long axis of the antrum. Panel (**d**) shows the appearance of GAVE immediately after therapy with argon plasma coagulation. The white patches represent superficial mucosal injury created by the therapy that rapidly heal and are replaced by normal gastric mucosa

GAVE with large areas of involvement. The first trial evaluating cryotherapy in the human GI tract was in 2003 and included seven patients with GAVE (71.4% response) [152]. A second study employing cryotherapy specifically for 12 patients with GAVE reported a 50% complete response rate and 50% partial response rate; however, it is worth noting that eight of the 12 patients enrolled in the study had previously been treated unsuccessfully with APC [153]. Of note, it is unclear from both studies whether any of the affected patients had SSc. Nevertheless, cryotherapy is worth considering in patients with disease refractory to APC, in particular in those patients with extensive involvement.

The second emerging endoscopic technology is RFA. This technology allows focused radio-frequency energy delivery to gastric tissue and results in a controlled superficial injury with uniform depth of ablation. There are recent extensive data regarding this technology in Barrett's esophagus, showing both efficacy and safety [154]. Recently, this technology was employed in six patients with GAVE with improvement in five of the six treated and no complications noted [155]. While the sample is small and it is unclear if any of the patients in the study had SSc, this technology may be used more frequently in the future given the growing usage of RFA in Barrett's esophagus and the increasing technical proficiency of endoscopists with this tool.

The number of medical therapies that have been attempted speaks to the inadequacies of current options. Steroids were attempted in several early reports with moderate success. Combining those reports, of 11 patients given steroids alone, 6 were reported to have complete resolution of bleeding;

however, another patient had hyperglycemia, and 4 patients had no response [150]. The potential benefits of steroids have to be weighed against the risks and potential caustic effect on GI mucosa. A separate case report detailed a single patient who received intravenous methylprednisolone and cyclophosphamide with complete resolution [156].

Cyclophosphamide is also an option for refractory GAVE. In addition to the single case report detailed above using cyclophosphamide in combination with steroids, there is a recent case series describing three patients with SSc-related GAVE treated with intravenous pulse cyclophosphamide, all of whom had improvement via both clinical and endoscopic parameters [157]. However, at present these data are limited to three patients, and additional confirmatory studies are needed.

Hormonal therapy was initially hypothesized as a treatment due to the observation that epistaxis associated with Osler-Weber-Rendu syndrome decreases during pregnancy and worsens postpartum. In an open pilot study looking at a combination of estrogen and progesterone for GAVE related to cirrhosis, four of six patients had complete cessation of bleeding. The endoscopic appearance was not altered, however, raising concern that bleeding would recur upon discontinuation. In addition, the long-term risks of hormonal therapy have to be considered, and it is worth mentioning that three of the six patients treated in this study developed gynecomastia and menorrhagia [158]. A few case reports support this approach, but data remain very limited, and this likely remains an option best suited for postmenopausal women or SSc patients judged to be too high risk for endoscopic approaches [150].

Octreotide is a third option that has been studied in cirrhotic patients with refractory vascular GI bleeding, some of whom had GAVE. Much of this benefit may have been from decreased portal pressure in the context of cirrhosis, and it is unclear if the same benefit would apply to patients with SSc. A case report describes a patient with SSc who received octreotide for GAVE without benefit [105]. Finally, there are additional case reports of other medical therapies for GAVE patients without SSc, including histamine receptor antagonists, calcitonin, tranexamic acid, interferon, serotonin antagonists, and thalidomide, although none of these have been reported for SSc-related GAVE [105, 150].

Surgical management has been reserved as the final option for those patients with GAVE who have failed endoscopic and medical treatment options. Antrectomy has been the most common procedure performed, but there is significant morbidity and mortality associated with this procedure, with one report suggesting a mortality rate of 7.4% (in all GAVE patients, not SSc-related GAVE specifically) [105, 150, 151]. Given this risk profile, antrectomy should be reserved as a last resort for SSc patients with GAVE; it is an option if all else fails.

References

1. LeRoy EC, Black C, Fleischmajer R, et al. Scleroderma (systemic sclerosis): classification, subsets and pathogenesis. J Rheumatol. 1988;15:202–5.
2. Clements PJ, Becvar R, Drosos AA, Ghattas L, Gabrielli A. Assessment of gastrointestinal involvement. Clin Exp Rheumatol. 2003;21:S15–8.
3. Forbes A, Marie I. Gastrointestinal complications: the most frequent internal complications of systemic sclerosis. Rheumatology (Oxford). 2009;48 Suppl 3:iii36–9.
4. Steen VD, Medsger TA. Changes in causes of death in systemic sclerosis, 1972–2002. Ann Rheum Dis. 2007;66:940–4.
5. Vitali C, Borghi E, Napoletano A, et al. Oropharyngolaryngeal disorders in scleroderma: development and validation of the SLS scale. Dysphagia. 2010;25:127–38.
6. Scardina GA, Mazzullo M, Messina P. Early diagnosis of progressive systemic sclerosis: the role of oro-facial phenomena. Minerva Stomatol. 2002;51:311–7.
7. Domsic R, Fasanella K, Bielefeldt K. Gastrointestinal manifestations of systemic sclerosis. Dig Dis Sci. 2008;53:1163–74.
8. Roberts CG, Hummers LK, Ravich WJ, Wigley FM, Hutchins GM. A case-control study of the pathology of oesophageal disease in systemic sclerosis (scleroderma). Gut. 2006;55:1697–703.
9. Thoua NM, Bunce C, Brough G, Forbes A, Emmanuel AV, Denton CP. Assessment of gastrointestinal symptoms in patients with systemic sclerosis in a UK tertiary referral centre. Rheumatology (Oxford). 2010;49:1770–5.
10. Sjogren RW. Gastrointestinal motility disorders in scleroderma. Arthritis Rheum. 1994;37:1265–82.
11. Howe S, Eaker EY, Sallustio JE, Peebles C, Tan EM, Williams RC Jr. Antimyenteric neuronal antibodies in scleroderma. J Clin Invest. 1994;94:761–70.
12. Goldblatt F, Gordon TP, Waterman SA. Antibody-mediated gastrointestinal dysmotility in scleroderma. Gastroenterology. 2002;123:1144–50.
13. Cohen S, Fisher R, Lipshutz W, Turner R, Myers A, Schumacher R. The pathogenesis of esophageal dysfunction in scleroderma and Raynaud's disease. J Clin Invest. 1972;51:2663–8.
14. Dessein PH, Joffe BI, Metz RM, Millar DL, Lawson M, Stanwix AE. Autonomic dysfunction in systemic sclerosis: sympathetic overactivity and instability. Am J Med. 1992;93:143–50.
15. Zuber-Jerger I, Muller A, Kullmann F, et al. Gastrointestinal manifestation of systemic sclerosis – thickening of the upper gastrointestinal wall detected by endoscopic ultrasound is a valid sign. Rheumatology (Oxford). 2010;49:368–72.
16. Thoua NM, Derrett-Smith EC, Khan K, Dooley A, Shi-Wen X, Denton CP. Gut fibrosis with altered colonic contractility in a mouse model of scleroderma. Rheumatology (Oxford). 2012;51:1989–98.
17. Taroni JN, Martyanov V, Huang CC, et al. Molecular characterization of systemic sclerosis esophageal pathology identifies inflammatory and proliferative signatures. Arthritis Res Ther. 2015;17:194.
18. Ostojic P, Damjanov N. Different clinical features in patients with limited and diffuse cutaneous systemic sclerosis. Clin Rheumatol. 2006;25:453–7.
19. Ebert EC. Esophageal disease in scleroderma. J Clin Gastroenterol. 2006;40:769–75.
20. Ebert EC. Esophageal disease in progressive systemic sclerosis. Curr Treat Options Gastroenterol. 2008;11:64–9.
21. Arif T, Masood Q, Singh J, Hassan I. Assessment of esophageal involvement in systemic sclerosis and morphea (localized scleroderma) by clinical, endoscopic, manometric and pH metric features: a prospective comparative hospital-based study. BMC Gastroenterol. 2015;15:24.

22. Abu-Shakra M, Guillemin F, Lee P. Gastrointestinal manifestations of systemic sclerosis. Semin Arthritis Rheum. 1994;24:29–39.
23. Ling TC, Johnston BT. Esophageal investigations in connective tissue disease: which tests are most appropriate? J Clin Gastroenterol. 2001;32:33–6.
24. Kaye SA, Siraj QH, Agnew J, Hilson A, Black CM. Detection of early asymptomatic esophageal dysfunction in systemic sclerosis using a new scintigraphic grading method. J Rheumatol. 1996;23:297–301.
25. Harper RA, Jackson DC. Progressive systemic sclerosis. Br J Radiol. 1965;38:825–34.
26. Weston S, Thumshirn M, Wiste J, Camilleri M. Clinical and upper gastrointestinal motility features in systemic sclerosis and related disorders. Am J Gastroenterol. 1998;93:1085–9.
27. El-Serag HB, Sonnenberg A. Association of esophagitis and esophageal strictures with diseases treated with nonsteroidal anti-inflammatory drugs. Am J Gastroenterol. 1997;92:52–6.
28. Zamost BJ, Hirschberg J, Ippoliti AF, Furst DE, Clements PJ, Weinstein WM. Esophagitis in scleroderma. Prevalence and risk factors. Gastroenterology. 1987;92:421–8.
29. Katzka DA, Reynolds JC, Saul SH, et al. Barrett's metaplasia and adenocarcinoma of the esophagus in scleroderma. Am J Med. 1987;82:46–52.
30. Snyder DL, Crowell MD, Kahn A, et al. Prevalence of Barrett's esophagus in female patients with scleroderma. Am J Gastroenterol. 2021;116:517–21.
31. Segel MC, Campbell WL, Medsger TA Jr, Roumm AD. Systemic sclerosis (scleroderma) and esophageal adenocarcinoma: is increased patient screening necessary? Gastroenterology. 1985;89:485–8.
32. Vischio J, Saeed F, Karimeddini M, et al. Progression of esophageal dysmotility in systemic sclerosis. J Rheumatol. 2012;39:986–91.
33. Denis P, Ducrotte P, Pasquis P, Lefrancois R. Esophageal motility and pulmonary function in progressive systemic sclerosis. Respiration. 1981;42:21–4.
34. Johnson DA, Drane WE, Curran J, et al. Pulmonary disease in progressive systemic sclerosis. A complication of gastroesophageal reflux and occult aspiration? Arch Intern Med. 1989;149:589–93.
35. Lock G, Pfeifer M, Straub RH, et al. Association of esophageal dysfunction and pulmonary function impairment in systemic sclerosis. Am J Gastroenterol. 1998;93:341–5.
36. Marie I, Dominique S, Levesque H, et al. Esophageal involvement and pulmonary manifestations in systemic sclerosis. Arthritis Rheum. 2001;45:346–54.
37. Kinuya K, Nakajima K, Kinuya S, Michigishi T, Tonami N, Takehara K. Esophageal hypomotility in systemic sclerosis: close relationship with pulmonary involvement. Ann Nucl Med. 2001;15:97–101.
38. Troshinsky MB, Kane GC, Varga J, et al. Pulmonary function and gastroesophageal reflux in systemic sclerosis. Ann Intern Med. 1994;121:6–10.
39. Savarino E, Bazzica M, Zentilin P, et al. Gastroesophageal reflux and pulmonary fibrosis in scleroderma: a study using pH-impedance monitoring. Am J Respir Crit Care Med. 2009;179:408–13.
40. Zhang XJ, Bonner A, Hudson M, Canadian Scleroderma Research Group, Baron M, Pope J. Association of gastroesophageal factors and worsening of forced vital capacity in systemic sclerosis. J Rheumatol. 2013;40:850–8.
41. Cozzani E, Muracchioli A, Murdaca M, et al. Correlation between skin and affected organs in 52 sclerodermic patients followed in a diseases management team: development of a risk prediction model of organi-specific complications. Front Immunol. 2021;12:588753.
42. Wangkaew S, Losuriya P, Euathrongchit J. Worsening of esophageal dilation is associated with increase in a high-resolution computed tomography score in early systemic sclerosis-associated interstitial lung disease. Clin Rheumatol. 2021;40:955–63.
43. Christmann RB, Wells AU, Capelozzi VL, Silver RM. Gastroesophageal reflux incites interstitial lung disease in systemic sclerosis: clinical, radiologic, histopathologic, and treatment evidence. Semin Arthritis Rheum. 2010;40:241–9.
44. Olive A, Juncosa S, Evison G, Maddison PJ. Air in the oesophagus: a sign of oesophageal involvement in systemic sclerosis. Clin Rheumatol. 1995;14:319–21.
45. Madani G, Katz RD, Haddock JA, Denton CP, Bell JR. The role of radiology in the management of systemic sclerosis. Clin Radiol. 2008;63:959–67.
46. Clements PJ, Kadell B, Ippoliti A, Ross M. Esophageal motility in progressive systemic sclerosis (PSS). Comparison of cine-radiographic and manometric evaluation. Dig Dis Sci. 1979;24:639–44.
47. Weihrauch TR, Korting GW. Manometric assessment of oesophageal involvement in progressive systemic sclerosis, morphea and Raynaud's disease. Br J Dermatol. 1982;107:325–32.
48. Jayanthi V, Srinivasan V, Nayak VM, Krishnamurthi V, Victor S. Comparative evaluation of cine-esophagogram with esophageal manometry in assessing esophageal motility in progressive systemic sclerosis. Indian J Gastroenterol. 1996;15:129–31.
49. Klein HA, Wald A, Graham TO, Campbell WL, Steen VD. Comparative studies of esophageal function in systemic sclerosis. Gastroenterology. 1992;102:1551–6.
50. Lock G, Zeuner M, Straub RH, et al. Esophageal manometry in systemic sclerosis: screening procedure or confined to symptomatic patients? Rheumatol Int. 1997;17:61–6.
51. Bassotti G, Battaglia E, Debernardi V, et al. Esophageal dysfunction in scleroderma: relationship with disease subsets. Arthritis Rheum. 1997;40:2252–9.
52. Thonhofer R, Siegel C, Trummer M, Graninger W. Early endoscopy in systemic sclerosis without gastrointestinal symptoms. Rheumatol Int. 2012;32(1):165–8.
53. Marie I, Ducrotte P, Denis P, Hellot MF, Levesque H. Oesophageal mucosal involvement in patients with systemic sclerosis receiving proton pump inhibitor therapy. Aliment Pharmacol Ther. 2006;24:1593–601.
54. Wegener M, Adamek RJ, Wedmann B, Jergas M, Altmeyer P. Gastrointestinal transit through esophagus, stomach, small and large intestine in patients with progressive systemic sclerosis. Dig Dis Sci. 1994;39:2209–15.
55. Savarino E, Mei F, Parodi A, et al. Gastrointestinal motility disorder assessment in systemic sclerosis. Rheumatology (Oxford). 2013;52:1095–100.
56. Rajapakse CN, Bancewicz J, Jones CJ, Jayson MI. Pharyngo-oesophageal dysphagia in systemic sclerosis. Ann Rheum Dis. 1981;40:612–4.
57. Mainie I, Tutuian R, Patel A, Castell DO. Regional esophageal dysfunction in scleroderma and achalasia using multichannel intraluminal impedance and manometry. Dig Dis Sci. 2008;53:210–6.
58. Carlson DA, Prescott JE, Germond E, et al. Heterogeneity of primary and secondary peristalsis in systemic sclerosis: a new model of "scleroderma esophagus". Neurogastroenterol Motil. 2021;34:e14284.
59. Hirano I, Richter JE. ACG practice guidelines: esophageal reflux testing. Am J Gastroenterol. 2007;102:668–85.
60. Carlo-Stella N, Belloli L, Barbera R, et al. Gastroesophageal reflux and lung disease in systemic sclerosis. Am J Respir Crit Care Med. 2009;179:1167; author reply 1168.
61. Carlson DA, Hinchcliff M, Pandolfino JE. Advances in the evaluation and management of esophageal disease of systemic sclerosis. Curr Rheumatol Rep. 2015;17:475.
62. Kahan A, Bour B, Couturier D, Amor B, Menkes CJ. Nifedipine and esophageal dysfunction in progressive systemic sclerosis. Arthritis Rheum. 1985;28:490–5.

63. Jean F, Aubert A, Bloch F, et al. Effects of diltiazem versus nifedipine on lower esophageal sphincter pressure in patients with progressive systemic sclerosis. Arthritis Rheum. 1986;29:1054–5.
64. Kowal-Bielecka O, Landewe R, Avouac J, et al. EULAR recommendations for the treatment of systemic sclerosis: a report from the EULAR Scleroderma Trials and Research group (EUSTAR). Ann Rheum Dis. 2009;68:620–8.
65. Hansi N, Thoua N, Carulli M, et al. Consensus best practice pathway of the UK scleroderma study group: gastrointestinal manifestations of systemic sclerosis. Clin Exp Rheumatol. 2014;32:S214–21.
66. Olive A, Maddison PJ, Davis M. Treatment of oesophagitis in scleroderma with omeprazole. Br J Rheumatol. 1989;28:553.
67. Hendel L. Hydroxyproline in the oesophageal mucosa of patients with progressive systemic sclerosis during omeprazole-induced healing of reflux oesophagitis. Aliment Pharmacol Ther. 1991;5:471–80.
68. Shoenut JP, Wieler JA, Micflikier AB. The extent and pattern of gastro-oesophageal reflux in patients with scleroderma oesophagus: the effect of low-dose omeprazole. Aliment Pharmacol Ther. 1993;7:509–13.
69. Gough A, Andrews D, Bacon PA, Emery P. Evidence of omeprazole-induced small bowel bacterial overgrowth in patients with scleroderma. Br J Rheumatol. 1995;34:976–7.
70. Reimer C. Safety of long-term PPI therapy. Best Pract Res Clin Gastroenterol. 2013;27:443–54.
71. Freedberg DE, Kim LS, Yang YX. The risks and benefits of long-term use of proton pump inhibitors: expert review and best practice advice from the American Gastroenterological Association. Gastroenterology. 2017;152:706–15.
72. Vaezi MF, Yang YX, Howden CW. Complications of proton pump inhibitor therapy. Gastroenterology. 2017;153:35–48.
73. Hendel L, Aggestrup S, Stentoft P. Long-term ranitidine in progressive systemic sclerosis (scleroderma) with gastroesophageal reflux. Scand J Gastroenterol. 1986;21:799–805.
74. Petrokubi RJ, Jeffries GH. Cimetidine versus antacid in scleroderma with reflux esophagitis. A randomized double-blind controlled study. Gastroenterology. 1979;77:691–5.
75. Janiak P, Thumshirn M, Menne D, et al. Clinical trial: the effects of adding ranitidine at night to twice daily omeprazole therapy on nocturnal acid breakthrough and acid reflux in patients with systemic sclerosis – a randomized controlled, cross-over trial. Aliment Pharmacol Ther. 2007;26:1259–65.
76. Horowitz M, Maddern GJ, Maddox A, Wishart J, Chatterton BE, Shearman DJ. Effects of cisapride on gastric and esophageal emptying in progressive systemic sclerosis. Gastroenterology. 1987;93:311–5.
77. Wehrmann T, Caspary WF. Effect of cisapride on esophageal motility in healthy probands and patients with progressive systemic scleroderma. Klin Wochenschr. 1990;68:602–7.
78. Kahan A, Chaussade S, Gaudric M, et al. The effect of cisapride on gastro-oesophageal dysfunction in systemic sclerosis: a controlled manometric study. Br J Clin Pharmacol. 1991;31:683–7.
79. Limburg AJ, Smit AJ, Kleibeuker JH. Effects of cisapride on the esophageal motor function of patients with progressive systemic sclerosis or mixed connective tissue disease. Digestion. 1991;49:156–60.
80. Wang SJ, La JL, Chen DY, Chen YH, Hsieh TY, Lin WY. Effects of cisapride on oesophageal transit of solids in patients with progressive systemic sclerosis. Clin Rheumatol. 2002;21:43–5.
81. Ramirez-Mata M, Ibanez G, Alarcon-Segovia D. Stimulatory effect of metoclopramide on the esophagus and lower esophageal sphincter of patients of patients with PSS. Arthritis Rheum. 1977;20:30–4.
82. Johnson DA, Drane WE, Curran J, et al. Metoclopramide response in patients with progressive systemic sclerosis. Effect on esophageal and gastric motility abnormalities. Arch Intern Med. 1987;147:1597–601.
83. Drane WE, Karvelis K, Johnson DA, Curran JJ, Silverman ED. Scintigraphic detection of metoclopramide esophageal stimulation in progressive systemic sclerosis. J Nucl Med. 1987;28:810–5.
84. Sridhar KR, Lange RC, Magyar L, Soykan I, McCallum RW. Prevalence of impaired gastric emptying of solids in systemic sclerosis: diagnostic and therapeutic implications. J Lab Clin Med. 1998;132:541–6.
85. Mercado U, Arroyo de Anda R, Avendano L, Araiza-Casillas R, Avendano-Reyes M. Metoclopramide response in patients with early diffuse systemic sclerosis. Effects on esophageal motility abnormalities. Clin Exp Rheumatol. 2005;23:685–8.
86. Fiorucci S, Distrutti E, Bassotti G, et al. Effect of erythromycin administration on upper gastrointestinal motility in scleroderma patients. Scand J Gastroenterol. 1994;29:807–13.
87. Folwaczny C, Laritz M, Meurer M, Endres SP, Konig A, Schindlbeck N. Effects of various prokinetic drugs on gastrointestinal transit times in patients with progressive systemic scleroderma. Z Gastroenterol. 1997;35:905–12.
88. Sjogren RW. Gastrointestinal features of scleroderma. Curr Opin Rheumatol. 1996;8:569–75.
89. Ahuja NK, Mische L, Clarke JO, et al. Pyridostigmine for the treatment of gastrointestinal symptoms in systemic sclerosis. Semin Arthritis Rheum. 2018;48:111–6.
90. McMahan ZH, Hummers LK. Gastrointestinal involvement in systemic sclerosis: diagnosis and management. Curr Opin Rheumatol. 2018;30:533–40.
91. Boeckxstaens GE, Bartelsman JF, Lauwers L, Tytgat GN. Treatment of GI dysmotility in scleroderma with the new enterokinetic agent prucalopride. Am J Gastroenterol. 2002;97:194–7.
92. Vigone B, Caronni M, Severino A, et al. Preliminary safety and efficacy profile of prucalopride in the treatment of systemic sclerosis-related intestinal involvement: results from the open label cross-over PROGASS study. Arthritis Res Ther. 2017;19:145.
93. Andrews CN, Woo M, Buresi M, et al. Prucalopride in diabetic and connective tissue disease-related gastroparesis: randomized placebo-controlled crossover pilot trial. Neurogastroenterol Motil. 2021;33:e13958.
94. Tack J, Janssen P, Masaoka T, Farre R, Van Oudenhove L. Efficacy of buspirone, a fundus-relaxing drug, in patients with functional dyspepsia. Clin Gastroenterol Hepatol. 2012;10:1239–45.
95. Di Stefano M, Papathanasopoulos A, Blondeau K, et al. Effect of buspirone, a 5-HT1A receptor agonist, on esophageal motility in healthy volunteers. Dis Esophagus. 2012;25:470–6.
96. Karamanolis GP, Panopoulos S, Karlaftis A, et al. Beneficial effect of the 5-HT1A receptor agonist buspirone on esophageal dysfunction associated with systemic sclerosis: a pilot study. United European Gastroenterol J. 2015;3:266–71.
97. Henderson RD, Pearson FG. Surgical management of esophageal scleroderma. J Thorac Cardiovasc Surg. 1973;66:686–92.
98. Orringer MB, Orringer JS, Dabich L, Zarafonetis CJ. Combined collis gastroplasty – fundoplication operations for scleroderma reflux esophagitis. Surgery. 1981;90:624–30.
99. Mansour KA. Surgery for scleroderma of the esophagus: a 12-year experience. Updated in 1995. Ann Thorac Surg. 1995;60:227.
100. Poirier NC, Taillefer R, Topart P, Duranceau A. Antireflux operations in patients with scleroderma. Ann Thorac Surg. 1994;58:66–72; discussion 73.
101. Kent MS, Luketich JD, Irshad K, et al. Comparison of surgical approaches to recalcitrant gastroesophageal reflux disease in the patient with scleroderma. Ann Thorac Surg. 2007;84:1710–5; discussion 75–6.
102. Aiolfi A, Nosotti M, Matushima K, et al. Surgical treatment of recalcitrant gastroesophageal reflux disease in patients with sys-

temic sclerosis: a systematic review. Langenbecks Arch Surg. 2021;406:1353–61.
103. Szamosi S, Szekanecz Z, Szucs G. Gastrointestinal manifestations in Hungarian scleroderma patients. Rheumatol Int. 2006;26:1120–4.
104. Sallam H, McNearney TA, Chen JD. Systematic review: pathophysiology and management of gastrointestinal dysmotility in systemic sclerosis (scleroderma). Aliment Pharmacol Ther. 2006;23:691–712.
105. Marie I, Ducrotte P, Antonietti M, Herve S, Levesque H. Watermelon stomach in systemic sclerosis: its incidence and management. Aliment Pharmacol Ther. 2008;28:412–21.
106. Ingraham KM, O'Brien MS, Shenin M, Derk CT, Steen VD. Gastric antral vascular ectasia in systemic sclerosis: demographics and disease predictors. J Rheumatol. 2010;37:603–7.
107. Maddern GJ, Horowitz M, Jamieson GG, Chatterton BE, Collins PJ, Roberts-Thomson P. Abnormalities of esophageal and gastric emptying in progressive systemic sclerosis. Gastroenterology. 1984;87:922–6.
108. Marie I, Levesque H, Ducrotte P, et al. Gastric involvement in systemic sclerosis: a prospective study. Am J Gastroenterol. 2001;96:77–83.
109. Fiorucci S, Distrutti E, Gerli R, Morelli A. Effect of erythromycin on gastric and gallbladder emptying and gastrointestinal symptoms in scleroderma patients is maintained medium term. Am J Gastroenterol. 1994;89:550–5.
110. Pfaffenbach B, Adamek RJ, Hagemann D, et al. Effect of progressive systemic sclerosis on antral myoelectrical activity and gastric emptying. Z Gastroenterol. 1996;34:517–21.
111. Franck-Larsson K, Hedenstrom H, Dahl R, Ronnblom A. Delayed gastric emptying in patients with diffuse versus limited systemic sclerosis, unrelated to gastrointestinal symptoms and myoelectric gastric activity. Scand J Rheumatol. 2003;32:348–55.
112. Marycz T, Muehldorfer SM, Gruschwitz MS, et al. Gastric involvement in progressive systemic sclerosis: electrogastrographic and sonographic findings. Eur J Gastroenterol Hepatol. 1999;11:1151–6.
113. Mittal BR, Wanchu A, Das BK, Ghosh PP, Sewatkar AB, Misra RN. Pattern of gastric emptying in patients with systemic sclerosis. Clin Nucl Med. 1996;21:379–82.
114. Wedmann B, Wegener M, Adamek RJ, el Gammal S. Gastrobiliary motility after liquid fatty meal in progressive systemic sclerosis. A sonographic study. Dig Dis Sci. 1994;39:565–70.
115. Abell TL, Camilleri M, Donohoe K, et al. Consensus recommendations for gastric emptying scintigraphy: a joint report of the American Neurogastroenterology and Motility Society and the Society of Nuclear Medicine. Am J Gastroenterol. 2008;103:753–63.
116. Talley NJ. Diabetic gastropathy and prokinetics. Am J Gastroenterol. 2003;98:264–71.
117. Adler B, Hummers LK, Pasricha PJ, McMahan ZH. Gastroparesis in systemic sclerosis: a detailed analysis using whole-gut scintigraphy. Rheumatology. 2022;61:4503.
118. McMahan ZH, Tucker AE, Perin J, et al. Relationship between gastrointestinal transit, Medsger gastrointestinal severity, and University of California – Los Angeles Scleroderma Clinical Trial Consortium Gastrointestinal Tract 2.0 symptoms in patients with systemic sclerosis. Arthritis Care Res. 2022;74:442–50.
119. Bortolotti M, Bolondi L, Santi V, Sarti P, Brunelli F, Barbara L. Patterns of gastric emptying in dysmotility-like dyspepsia. Scand J Gastroenterol. 1995;30:408–10.
120. Tang DM, Friedenberg FK. Gastroparesis: approach, diagnostic evaluation, and management. Dis Mon. 2011;57:74–101.
121. Cassilly D, Kantor S, Knight LC, et al. Gastric emptying of a nondigestible solid: assessment with simultaneous SmartPill pH and pressure capsule, antroduodenal manometry, gastric emptying scintigraphy. Neurogastroenterol Motil. 2008;20:311–9.
122. Kuo B, McCallum RW, Koch KL, et al. Comparison of gastric emptying of a nondigestible capsule to a radio-labelled meal in healthy and gastroparetic subjects. Aliment Pharmacol Ther. 2008;27:186–96.
123. Parkman HP. Assessment of gastric emptying and small-bowel motility: scintigraphy, breath tests, manometry, and SmartPill. Gastrointest Endosc Clin N Am. 2009;19:49–55, vi.
124. Rees WD, Leigh RJ, Christofides ND, Bloom SR, Turnberg LA. Interdigestive motor activity in patients with systemic sclerosis. Gastroenterology. 1982;83:575–80.
125. Marie I, Levesque H, Ducrotte P, et al. Manometry of the upper intestinal tract in patients with systemic sclerosis: a prospective study. Arthritis Rheum. 1998;41:1874–83.
126. McNearney TA, Sallam HS, Hunnicutt SE, et al. Gastric slow waves, gastrointestinal symptoms and peptides in systemic sclerosis patients. Neurogastroenterol Motil. 2009;21:1269–e120.
127. Tung A, Sweitzer B, Cutter T. Cardiac arrest after labetalol and metoclopramide administration in a patient with scleroderma. Anesth Analg. 2002;95:1667–8, table of contents.
128. Foocharoen C, Chunlertrith K, Mairiang P, et al. Effectiveness of add-on therapy with domperidone vs alginic acid in proton pump inhibitor partial response gastro-oesophageal reflux disease in systemic sclerosis: randomized placebo-controlled trial. Rheumatology. 2017;56:214–22.
129. Patterson D, Abell T, Rothstein R, Koch K, Barnett J. A double-blind multicenter comparison of domperidone and metoclopramide in the treatment of diabetic patients with symptoms of gastroparesis. Am J Gastroenterol. 1999;94:1230–4.
130. Parkman HP, Jacobs MR, Mishra A, et al. Domperidone treatment for gastroparesis: demographic and pharmacogenetic characterization of clinical efficacy and side-effects. Dig Dis Sci. 2011;56:115–24.
131. Buffery PJ, Strother RM. Domperidone safety: a mini-review of the science of QT prolongation and clinical implications of recent global regulatory recommendations. N Z Med J. 2015;128:66–74.
132. Verne GN, Eaker EY, Hardy E, Sninsky CA. Effect of octreotide and erythromycin on idiopathic and scleroderma-associated intestinal pseudoobstruction. Dig Dis Sci. 1995;40:1892–901.
133. Masaoka T, Tack J. Gastroparesis: current concepts and management. Gut Liver. 2009;3:166–73.
134. Maganti K, Onyemere K, Jones MP. Oral erythromycin and symptomatic relief of gastroparesis: a systematic review. Am J Gastroenterol. 2003;98:259–63.
135. Linke R, Meier M, Muenzing W, Folwaczny C, Schnell O, Tatsch K. Prokinetic therapy: what can be measured by gastric scintigraphy? Nucl Med Commun. 2005;26:527–33.
136. Wu KL, Rayner CK, Chuah SK, et al. Effects of ginger on gastric emptying and motility in healthy humans. Eur J Gastroenterol Hepatol. 2008;20:436–40.
137. Chaiyakunapruk N, Kitikannakorn N, Nathisuwan S, Leeprakobboon K, Leelasettagool C. The efficacy of ginger for the prevention of postoperative nausea and vomiting: a meta-analysis. Am J Obstet Gynecol. 2006;194:95–9.
138. Sallam HS, McNearney TA, Chen JD. Acupuncture-based modalities: novel alternative approaches in the treatment of gastrointestinal dysmotility in patients with systemic sclerosis. Explore (NY). 2014;10:44–52.
139. Wollaston DE, Xu X, Tokumaru O, Chen JD, McNearney TA. Patients with systemic sclerosis have unique and persistent alterations in gastric myoelectrical activity with acupressure to Neiguan point PC6. J Rheumatol. 2005;32:494–501.
140. Sallam H, McNearney TA, Doshi D, Chen JD. Transcutaneous electrical nerve stimulation (TENS) improves upper GI symptoms

and balances the sympathovagal activity in scleroderma patients. Dig Dis Sci. 2007;52:1329–37.
141. McNearney TA, Sallam HS, Hunnicutt SE, Doshi D, Chen JD. Prolonged treatment with transcutaneous electrical nerve stimulation (TENS) modulates neuro-gastric motility and plasma levels of vasoactive intestinal peptide (VIP), motilin and interleukin-6 (IL-6) in systemic sclerosis. Clin Exp Rheumatol. 2013;31:140–50.
142. Friedenberg FK, Palit A, Parkman HP, Hanlon A, Nelson DB. Botulinum toxin A for the treatment of delayed gastric emptying. Am J Gastroenterol. 2008;103:416–23.
143. Gonzalez JM, Granel B, Barthet M, Vitton V. G-POEM may be an optional treatment for refractory gastroparesis in systemic sclerosis. Scand J Gastroenterol. 2020;55:777–9.
144. Duchini A, Sessoms SL. Gastrointestinal hemorrhage in patients with systemic sclerosis and CREST syndrome. Am J Gastroenterol. 1998;93:1453–6.
145. Jabbari M, Cherry R, Lough JO, Daly DS, Kinnear DG, Goresky CA. Gastric antral vascular ectasia: the watermelon stomach. Gastroenterology. 1984;87:1165–70.
146. Ghrenassia E, Avouac J, Khanna D, et al. Prevalence, correlates and outcomes of gastric antral vascular ectasia in systemic sclerosis: a EUSTAR case-control study. J Rheumatol. 2014;41:99–105.
147. Gostout CJ, Viggiano TR, Ahlquist DA, Wang KK, Larson MV, Balm R. The clinical and endoscopic spectrum of the watermelon stomach. J Clin Gastroenterol. 1992;15:256–63.
148. Suit PF, Petras RE, Bauer TW, Petrini JL Jr. Gastric antral vascular ectasia. A histologic and morphometric study of "the watermelon stomach". Am J Surg Pathol. 1987;11:750–7.
149. Chawla SK, Ramani K, Lo Presti P. The honeycomb stomach: coalesced gastric angiodysplasia. Gastrointest Endosc. 1990;36:516–8.
150. Sebastian S, O'Morain CA, Buckley MJ. Review article: Current therapeutic options for gastric antral vascular ectasia. Aliment Pharmacol Ther. 2003;18:157–65.
151. Dulai GS, Jensen DM. Treatment of watermelon stomach. Curr Treat Options Gastroenterol. 2006;9:175–80.
152. Kantsevoy SV, Cruz-Correa MR, Vaughn CA, Jagannath SB, Pasricha PJ, Kalloo AN. Endoscopic cryotherapy for the treatment of bleeding mucosal vascular lesions of the GI tract: a pilot study. Gastrointest Endosc. 2003;57:403–6.
153. Cho S, Zanati S, Yong E, et al. Endoscopic cryotherapy for the management of gastric antral vascular ectasia. Gastrointest Endosc. 2008;68:895–902.
154. Shaheen NJ, Sharma P, Overholt BF, et al. Radiofrequency ablation in Barrett's esophagus with dysplasia. N Engl J Med. 2009;360:2277–88.
155. Gross SA, Al-Haddad M, Gill KR, Schore AN, Wallace MB. Endoscopic mucosal ablation for the treatment of gastric antral vascular ectasia with the HALO90 system: a pilot study. Gastrointest Endosc. 2008;67:324–7.
156. Lorenzi AR, Johnson AH, Davies G, Gough A. Gastric antral vascular ectasia in systemic sclerosis: complete resolution with methylprednisolone and cyclophosphamide. Ann Rheum Dis. 2001;60:796–8.
157. Schulz SW, O'Brien M, Maqsood M, Sandorfi N, Del Galdo F, Jimenez SA. Improvement of severe systemic sclerosis-associated gastric antral vascular ectasia following immunosuppressive treatment with intravenous cyclophosphamide. J Rheumatol. 2009;36:1653–6.
158. Tran A, Villeneuve JP, Bilodeau M, et al. Treatment of chronic bleeding from gastric antral vascular ectasia (GAVE) with estrogen-progesterone in cirrhotic patients: an open pilot study. Am J Gastroenterol. 1999;94:2909–11.

32 Lower Gastrointestinal Tract Involvement: Understanding the Interplay of Motility, the Microbiome, and Nutrition

Elizabeth R. Volkmann and Zsuzsanna McMahan

Introduction

Gastrointestinal (GI) tract dysfunction in systemic sclerosis (SSc) is common, affecting more than 90% of patients. Dysfunction of the small and/or large bowel is estimated to occur in up to 50% of patients with SSc and often results in significant morbidity and mortality [1–3]. Patients may experience marked GI distress, as manifested by distention, bloating, chronic diarrhea, recurrent pseudo-obstruction, severe refractory constipation, and fecal incontinence, and may ultimately require total parenteral nutrition (TPN) to sustain life [2, 4, 5]. Several studies have determined that GI distress is associated with a poor quality of life due to the development of depression, anxiety, disability, and social isolation [6–8]. The etiology of lower GI dysfunction in SSc is thought to be multifactorial and may result from an interplay between delayed GI transit, dysbiosis, dietary intolerances, and other environmental exposures (e.g., medication side effects) [1, 9–11]. Prokinetic therapies are available to treat dysmotility, though supportive data are largely related to extrapolations from the general GI motility literature. Such interventions are often most effective in specific regions of the gut (e.g., prucalopride for delayed colonic transit; metoclopramide for gastroparesis) [12, 13], and may produce distinct effects in different areas of the GI tract (e.g., mirtazapine may enhance gastric motility, but cause constipation) [14–16]. In addition, therapies targeting motility are not uniformly effective across all patients, especially when GI symptoms are also driven by dysbiosis or food intolerance. As a result, it is important for physicians to identify the etiology of symptoms and characterize the region(s) of GI dysfunction in symptomatic patients to optimally formulate therapeutic plans. In this chapter, we provide an overview of what is known about the prevalence, pathophysiology, clinical presentation, diagnosis, and treatment of patients with SSc who experience various complications of the small intestine, colon, and anorectum.

Anatomy and Histopathology of the Lower Bowel in SSc

In SSc, endothelial cell abnormalities lead to the release of reactive species (cytokines, chemokines, and growth factors) and fibrocyte recruitment in a genetically susceptible host [17]. Progressive smooth muscle atrophy, fibroproliferative vasculopathy, and/or tissue fibrosis develop and may negatively impact internal organ function. Interestingly, however, the response of the GI tissue to the SSc disease milieu may be somewhat distinct from that of other organ systems, as smooth muscle atrophy and neuropathy predominate over the extent of fibrosis and vasculopathy that are striking in other organ systems [18, 19].

E. R. Volkmann (✉)
Division of Rheumatology, Department of Medicine, University of California, Los Angeles, CA, USA
e-mail: evolkmann@mednet.ucla.edu

Z. McMahan
Division of Rheumatology, Department of Medicine, McGovern Medical School, Houston, TX, USA
e-mail: zsuzsanna.h.mcmahan@uth.tmc.edu

Y. Allanore et al. (eds.), *Scleroderma*, https://doi.org/10.1007/978-3-031-40658-4_32

The anatomy of the GI tract is comprised of four main layers that are conserved from the esophagus through the colon and include the mucosa which is the innermost luminal layer, submucosa, muscularis propria (externa), and the outermost adventitia (a.k.a. serosa). The inner mucosa is composed of three sublayers: (1) the epithelium, which includes glandular tissue; (2) lamina propria, which is a loose layer of connective tissue providing vascular support for the epithelium and often includes lymphoid follicles and plasma cells; and (3) the muscularis mucosa, which is a thin double layer of smooth muscle that supports local movement of the mucosa (see Fig. 32.1). The submucosa is the next layer, and it is also comprised of loose connective tissue and contains nerves, larger blood vessels, lymphatics, and may contain mucous secreting glands. The muscularis propria surrounds the submucosa and plays a significant role in peristalsis using its inner circular muscle layer and outer longitudinal muscle layer, to support the passage of food through the gut. The outer adventitia layer contains blood vessels, lymphatics, and nerves and is covered by the visceral peritoneum.

In SSc, the layer that is the most profoundly affected in the lower GI tract is the muscularis propria [18–20]. While the histopathological changes of the small bowel and colon in SSc are characterized in few studies, existing data demonstrates preservation of epithelial morphology and villous structures. Light microscopy demonstrates collagen deposition surrounding the Brunner's glands [21]. An increase in submucosal and serosal collagen and elastin as well as marked atrophy of the smooth muscle layers are seen on full-thickness biopsies. Autopsy data from 58 patients with SSc demonstrated dilation and atony of the duodenal loop in the majority of patients (72%) [18]. Nearly half of patients had evidence of muscle atrophy, dilation, and/or fibrosis, which was significantly higher than in controls (48% vs. 2%; $p < 0.001$). In the colon, muscle atrophy, dilation, or fibrosis of the large intestine was observed in SSc patients but not in controls [18]. The authors highlighted that atrophy was usually a more prominent finding than fibrosis, supporting the hypothesis that an enteric neuropathy or primary myopathy is likely an important driver of SSc GI pathogenesis. Findings in the external muscle layers demonstrate a reduced number of smooth muscle cells and junctions between smooth muscle cells [18]. Some perineuronal collagen cuffing, neuronal degeneration (in the absence of collagen cuffing), and perivascular fibrosis were also described. In the anorectum of patients with SSc, the histopathology of the rectum reveals axonal and smooth muscle cell degeneration. In both symptomatic and asymptomatic patients, there is evidence of thinning and atrophy of the internal anal sphincter, with sparing of the external anal sphincter [22, 23].

Dysmotility of the Small and Large Bowel in SSc

GI tract dysmotility is a major contributor to the clinical GI manifestations of SSc. Both the small intestine and colon may be affected, though colonic dysmotility is more frequently observed [1, 24]. The hypothesis that SSc-GI disease is at least partially attributed to neuropathic and myopathic mechanisms is supported by physiologic studies in SSc. Myopathic processes are generally associated with normal but low-amplitude contractions, while neuropathic disorders are usually associated with uncoordinated contractions. In SSc, migrating motor complexes (MMCs), or spontaneous peristaltic waves that occur during fasting, are absent and are instead replaced by irregular and/or low-amplitude contractile activity. Following a meal, this uncoordinated activity may continue, though the normal contractile response of the intestine to a meal may be absent. In addition, duodenal hyperactivity with uncoordinated activity, which is often observed in patients with diabetic neuropathy, is also seen in SSc [25].

Constipation is the most common manifestation of colonic involvement in SSc [24, 26]. Physiologic studies demon-

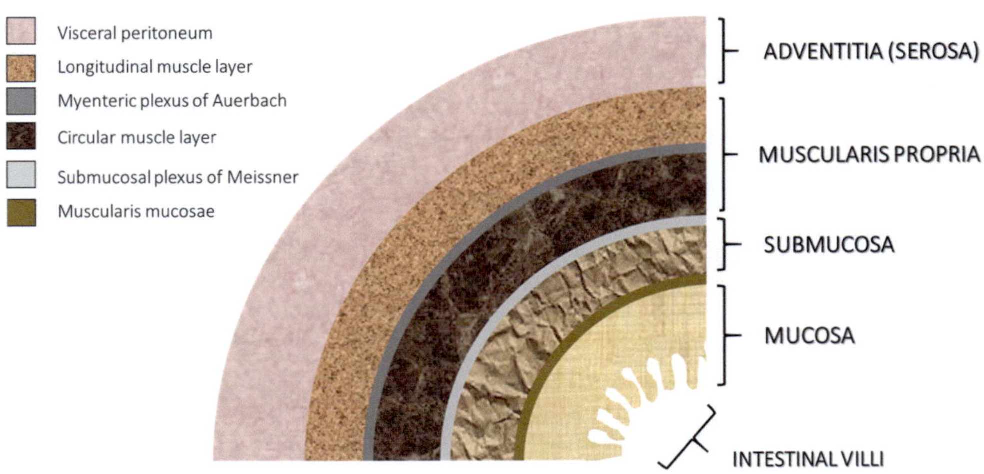

Fig. 32.1 Anatomy of the GI tract

strate an absent gastrocolic reflex in early SSc, suggesting that abnormalities in neural reflexes also play an important role in colonic dysfunction and lead to constipation primarily due to slow transit [1, 27–29]. Anorectal dysfunction is also common and usually manifests as fecal incontinence [26, 30]. Continence is normally controlled by the combined functioning of the pelvic floor, rectum, and anal sphincters (internal and external). Resting anal tone is maintained by the internal anal sphincter, which is composed of smooth muscle and more likely to be affected in SSc. Its dysfunction is associated with passive fecal incontinence [31]. Patients with fecal incontinence have reduced resting anal tone [32, 33]. In addition, the rectoanal inhibitory response, which helps to maintain continence, is impaired in symptomatic patients with SSc [23].

Hypotheses for the Etiology of Dysmotility in SSc

Intrinsic neurons in the myenteric plexus play a dominant role in the contractile activity of the GI tract [34]. Stimulatory neuromuscular communication is largely facilitated by acetylcholine, acting predominantly via the muscarinic-3 receptor (M3R) on smooth muscle. Importantly, disruption of this neuromuscular communication may result in progressive smooth muscle atrophy [35]. The identification of GI dysmotility early in the disease process is important, as there is a window of opportunity to intervene when the smooth muscle is still functional and responsive to prokinetic agents. As the smooth muscle begins to atrophy, GI tract-related symptoms progress and become less responsive to prokinetic agents. Ultimately, prokinetic agents become largely ineffective due to severe smooth muscle atrophy.

The concept of progressive smooth muscle atrophy was studied by Cohen in the 1970s when he examined functional denervation of the smooth muscle in the esophagus [36]. In the early stages of SSc, stimulation with edrophonium and gastrin-1 (compounds that act indirectly through stimulation of cholinergic nerves) failed to stimulate smooth muscle motility, while methacholine (a direct stimulator of smooth muscle) did stimulate motility. This observation suggests that in the early stages of SSc, the GI smooth muscle becomes hypomotile due to denervation, but that this denervated smooth muscle remains capable of responding to direct stimulation (i.e., methacholine in the initial experiments and potentially in clinical practice with promotility agents, such as prucalopride, cisapride, erythromycin, domperidone, metoclopramide, and octreotide). However, in patients with SSc of longer disease duration, the GI tract did not respond to direct stimulation, suggesting that the smooth muscle had atrophied [36]. In clinical practice, these patients often fail treatment with promotility agents.

Historically, the initial injury to the neural function of the GI tract was deemed a consequence of the progressive SSc-related vasculopathy affecting the vasa nervosum [25, 36]. Vascular changes include myointimal proliferation with narrowing and irregularity of the lumen and disruption of the internal elastic lamina of small arteries. Capillary basement membranes are thickened and laminated with relative sparing of the veins [25]. Interestingly, however, the areas of vascular change in the GI tract do not appear to correlate with areas of smooth muscle atrophy [19]. Increasing data suggest that autoantibodies to muscarinic 3 receptors (M3R) may play an important role in the development of GI dysmotility, specifically in a subset of SSc patients with early onset pseudo-obstruction or malabsorption. In one study, effects on intestinal motility were assessed after rats were immunized with purified immunoglobulin G (IgG) from the sera of patients with SSc who had antimyenteric neuronal antibodies [37]. Passive immunization led to the prolongation and disruption of rat intestinal myoelectrical activity, though there was no effect on the myoelectric activity when the rats were immunized with the IgG of normal healthy controls. In another study, the IgG from patients with SSc inhibited M3R activation in the smooth muscle cells of the internal anal sphincter of rats [38]. The removal of the antibodies reversed this effect. Subsequent studies of the effects of IgG from patients with SSc on healthy human smooth muscle tissue showed similar results [39].

Other autoantibodies associated with non-SSc GI dysmotility [e.g., GI dysmotility associated with autonomic dysfunction and irritable bowel syndrome (IBS)] are also described in SSc patients with GI symptoms. Anti-gAChR autoantibodies were identified in 14% (7/50) patients with SSc. The mean level of anti-gAChRα3 autoantibodies in SSc patients with gastrointestinal manifestations was significantly higher than that in SSc patients without gastrointestinal manifestations ($p = 0.001$) [40]. Antivinculin antibodies, which are associated primarily with inflammatory bowel disease (IBD) are described in SSc and associated with more significant GI symptoms [41]. Importantly, however, no objective outcome measures of GI motility were utilized in either study, and therefore, additional data are needed to determine whether: (1) these antibodies associate with GI dysmotility; and (2) these antibodies play a role in causing disease. Other autoantibodies are also associated with more severe GI symptoms and/or complications in patients with SSc (e.g., U1RNP, U3RNP, RNPC3, CENP), though no clear link determining causality has been identified [42–44].

Small Bowel Involvement in SSc and the Approach to Diagnosis and Management

Small Bowel Dysmotility

Small bowel dysmotility is estimated to affect between 40% and 88% of patients with SSc based on manometry studies, though many of these patients may be asymptomatic at the time of the study [45, 46]. Symptoms of small bowel involvement may include diarrhea, unintentional weight loss, distention, and bloating (Table 32.1) [11, 47]. Prior to attributing these symptoms to SSc, it is important to first exclude other causes of GI symptoms which are prevalent in the general population, such as infection, as well as inflammatory or infiltrative bowel diseases (e.g., sarcoidosis, amyloidosis), overlapping autoimmune bowel diseases, such as IBD and Celiac diseases, and malignancy. While these conditions may overlap in patients with SSc, they are not necessarily enriched among patients with SSc [48]. Once these considerations are excluded, several SSc-related GI complications should also be considered.

To diagnose small bowel dysmotility, various radiographic studies may be employed. An abdominal X-ray may identify dilated bowel loops with or without the classic "hide-bound" appearance indicative of tightly packed valvulae conniventes in the duodenum and jejunum [49]. Small intestinal manometry screens for low-amplitude contractions with either absent or prolonged migrating motor complexes, although it takes multiple hours to perform and is limited to the assessment of the proximal small bowel [11, 49]. Scintigraphy (see Fig. 32.2), wireless motility capsules, and CT/MRI enterography are also utilized; however, wireless motility capsules are contraindicated in patients with known, severe gastroparesis or GI strictures [49]. Data supporting the application of promotility agents in the manage-

Table 32.1 Clinical phenotype of SSc patients with lower GI dysfunction based on anatomic region of involvement

Anatomic region	Clinical phenotype
Small bowel	**Bloating/Excess Gas**: Commonly occurs after eating simple carbohydrates (e.g., monosaccharides, disaccharides) **Abdominal pain**: A less frequent symptom, but can occur after ingestion of large meals, especially if gastroparesis is present **Change in stool smell or diarrhea**: An indicator that malabsorption and/or SIBO may be present
Colon	**Constipation**: Often begins as a gradual decrease in bowel movements, but can progress to complete inability to evacuate without daily medical management **Diarrhea**: Less frequent phenotype, but when present can be severe leading to volume loss, electrolyte, and metabolic imbalances that require ongoing attention and evaluation **Alternating Constipation/Diarrhea**: The predominant symptom is generally constipation, but patients can have episodic diarrhea due to issues such as overflow and adverse effects of stimulant laxatives **Abdominal cramping**: Can occur immediately after eating and/or prior to evacuation
Anorectum	**Fecal incontinence**: Can range from occasional leakage of stool when passing gas to complete loss of bowel control **Urgency**: Patients have a sudden urge to evacuate bowels, and can occur in patients with both constipation- and diarrhea-predominant lower GI symptoms

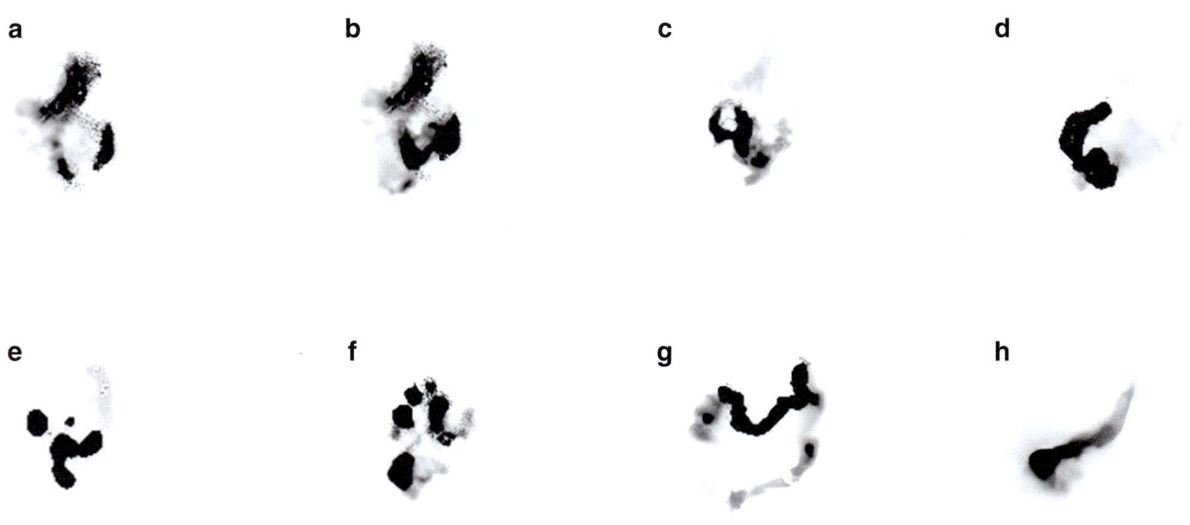

Fig. 32.2 Images of whole gut scintigraphy from patient with SSc with delayed colonic transit. The eight panels below demonstrate radionucleotide passing from the stomach (Panel **a**) through the small bowel (Panels **b–d**) and into the colon (Panels **e–g**) in a 72-h period. Radionucleotide was not fully evacuated from the colon at 72 h indicated delayed transit (Panel **h**)

ment of small intestinal dysmotility in SSc remain limited; however, octreotide and prucalopride have both demonstrated benefit (Table 32.2) [50–52]. For the management of diarrhea, dietary modifications to enhance stool consistency, empiric antibiotics for presumed SIBO (see below), and/or a trial of loperamide may be used [46]. It is important that agents that slow motility should be avoided until infectious causes of diarrhea are excluded, and their use should subsequently be minimized as such medications may increase risk of pseudo-obstruction in SSc [49].

Table 32.2 Promotility agents used in SSc: clinical indications and mechanism of action

Drug	Primary clinical indication(s)	Primary effects on the GI tract	Important considerations
Metoclopramide	Esophageal dysmotility, refractory GERD, and/or gastroparesis [53]	Increased frequency of esophageal contraction, increased LES pressures, improved gastric emptying	Risk of serious neurological adverse effects including tardive dyskinesia, dystonia, depression, Parkinsonism, and neuroleptic malignant syndrome
Bethanechol	Esophageal dysmotility, GERD [54–56]	Increased distal esophageal contraction amplitudes, increased LES pressures	Contraindicated in patients with hyperthyroidism, peptic ulcer disease, bronchial asthma, bradycardia or hypotension, vasomotor instability, coronary artery disease, epilepsy, and parkinsonism
Cisapride	Refractory GERD, esophageal dysmotility [57, 58], gastroparesis, chronic constipation	No significant improvement in esophageal emptying, but increased LES pressure; increased gastric emptying and fundic contractions	Cardiac adverse effects such as serious ventricular arrhythmias and sudden cardiac death; no longer FDA approved in the United States
Erythromycin	Esophageal dysmotility [59], gastroparesis [60]	Accelerated esophageal and gastric motility [61]	Tachyphylaxis; caution with prolonged QT/cardiac arrhythmia; avoid in patients with myasthenia gravis and skeletal muscle disorders
Buspirone	Refractory GERD, esophageal dysmotility [62, 63], early satiety [64]	Enhanced esophageal peristalsis and lower esophageal sphincter (LES) function; enhanced gastric accommodation [65]	Risk of serotonin syndrome; restlessness may appear shortly after initiation of treatment
Mirtazapine	Gastroparesis [66, 67], weight loss [16]	Enhanced gastric emptying; may decrease diarrhea	Common side effects include weight gain, increased appetite, increased sleep, bad dreams; caution in patients with constipation; avoid in patients with hyperlipidemia, mania, seizures, glaucoma, QT prolongation, muscle disease
Baclofen	GERD [68], gastroparesis	Inhibition of transient lower esophageal sphincter relaxation, improved GER [68], stimulation of gastric motility [68, 69]	Caution in patients with constipation; avoid in patients with psychosis, seizures, chronic kidney disease, functional bladder disorders
Pyridostigmine	Esophageal dysmotility [54], gastroparesis [70], chronic intestinal-pseudo-obstruction [71], delayed small bowel transit, chronic constipation [72–74]	Accelerated GI transit, especially colonic [73]	Contraindicated in mechanical intestinal or urinary obstruction, and particular caution should be used in its administration to patients with bronchial asthma
Domperidone	Esophageal dysmotility, GERD [53], gastroparesis [75], chronic constipation [76]	Accelerated overall gastrointestinal transit; reduction in nausea and vomiting	May cause cardiac arrhythmia, QT prolongation; no longer FDA approved in the United States; avoid in patients with electrolyte disturbances, cardiac, hepatic or renal problems, GI bleeding, and pregnancy
Prucalopride	Chronic constipation [77], ileus [78], intestinal pseudo-obstruction [79], gastroparesis [80]	Increased gastric, small bowel, and colonic transit	Avoid in patients with significant depression, intestinal perforation or obstruction due to structural or functional disorder of the gut wall; obstructive ileus; severe inflammatory conditions of the intestinal tract (e.g., IBD, toxic megacolon/megarectum)
Tegaserod	Esophageal dysmotility [81], small and large bowel delayed transit	Increased gastric emptying, and small bowel and colonic transit; induction of MMCs [82, 83]	Ischemic cardiovascular events; avoid in patients with a history of MI, stroke, angina, etc. FDA approved for IBS-C in women under age 65 in the United States
Linaclotide, plecanatide	Delayed colonic transit, constipation [84, 85]	Increased cecal pH; accelerated colonic motility [86, 87]	Generally well-tolerated, minimal systemic absorption; avoid in patients with GI obstruction and diarrhea

Small Intestinal Bacterial Overgrowth and Malabsorption

Small intestinal bacterial overgrowth (SIBO) is a common complication of the small bowel in patients with SSc. It may be a consequence of small bowel dysmotility, large bowel dysmotility in the context of a weakened ileocecal valve, or chronic gastric acid suppression [88]. The prevalence of SIBO in symptomatic patients is estimated to be between 30% and 62.5%; however, inconsistencies in outcome measures (i.e., diagnostic modalities, symptom presentation) likely contribute to this high variability in reported SIBO prevalence. Nausea, vomiting, early satiety, postprandial bloating, abdominal distention, diarrhea, excessive flatulence, fecal soilage, weight loss, and cachexia may all be observed in patients with SIBO [89]. A prospective study of 120 SSc patients exhibiting symptoms of SIBO demonstrated that both weight loss in the past 6 months, longer disease duration, as well as increased self-reported SSc-GI symptoms were associated with SIBO diagnosis [90]. Dysmotility of the smooth muscle in the small intestine, particularly the loss of MMC, leads to stasis and stagnation of intestinal contents, allowing the migration of colonic bacteria into the small intestine [25, 91]. Conjugated bile acids are necessary for the breakdown and absorption of fats within the small intestine. Some bacteria are able to deconjugate bile acids within the small intestine [89]. Deconjugated bile acids are less able to absorb fat, leading to a calorie deficit and deficiencies of fat-soluble vitamins. Clinically, this may result in steatorrhea. In addition, patients may experience problems related to increased bloating, abdominal pain and distention, and flatulence, as bacteria in the small intestine metabolize sugars and carbohydrates, which produce gas. SIBO may also result in villous atrophy, which reduces the absorptive surface area, thereby diminishing nutrient absorption [92]. If left untreated, this process can lead to chronic and severe malnutrition; therefore, the early identification of SIBO, malabsorption, and/or dysmotility is critical [25]. See below for additional information related to optimizing nutritional intake in SSc.

The jejunal culture is the gold standard for diagnosis of SIBO, where $>10^5$ organisms/mL is considered a positive result. The application of the jejunal culture for the diagnosis of SIBO is limited in the SSc patient population as it is invasive, and the use of anesthesia may be risky in SSc patients with cardiopulmonary involvement [93]. The hydrogen and methane breath tests after an oral glucose or lactulose bolus are the only diagnostic tests for SIBO that are specifically validated in SSc. While the specificity of breath testing is high (78–100%), sensitivities range from 62% to 93%, rendering this a suboptimal screening strategy [49]. Ultimately, a high clinical suspicion in the setting of a negative workup to exclude other causes (e.g., infection, inflammatory/infiltrative diseases, malignancy, as described further above) is the most common approach to diagnosing SIBO. Treatment for SIBO often involves the use of broad-spectrum antibiotics, though data supporting for this approach are mixed [94–98]. In our clinical practice, we most frequently use rifaximin as initial therapy. There is limited data to support one antibiotic regimen versus another, though rifaximin has the most robust data to support its use [98–100]. There is no consensus on the appropriate dosing of rifaximin for SIBO, and therefore the current AGA guidelines [97] suggest a regimen of dividing a total daily dose of 800–1200 mg. The length of antibiotic therapy also varies, with studies ranging 1–4 weeks of therapy. Several guidelines support repeated or rotating antibiotic courses as recurrence rates are high (e.g., 44% of cases by 9 months) [46, 97, 101]. Other antibiotics that have been evaluated in uncontrolled SSc-SIBO studies included ciprofloxacin, norfloxacin, amoxicillin, and metronidazole with varying success rates [97]. However, as described further below, the long-term consequences of repeated courses of antibiotics are unknown.

Pancreatic Insufficiency

A significant reduction in pancreatic secretions is necessary to cause malabsorption. Small studies ($n = 16$; $n = 20$) suggest that it is common for patients with SSc to have a reduction in their pancreatic exocrine function [102, 103]. However, this reduction is only large enough to be considered clinically significant in a few patients. A recent study confirmed this after no association between clinically significant pancreatic exocrine dysfunction and SSc was identified in a cohort of 112 patients with SSc compared to 52 controls [104]. In the few affected patients, it is important to be aware that malabsorption related to pancreatic insufficiency may result in numerous vitamin and mineral deficiencies. Fat-soluble vitamin (A, D, E, and K) malabsorption may be caused by bacterial bile acid deconjugation or pancreatic enzyme insufficiency. However, any reduction in vitamin K levels may be partially compensated by its production by intestinal bacteria. Absorption of water-soluble vitamins may also be impaired. A trial of pancreatic enzymes may be helpful in select patients in whom significant pancreatic insufficiency is suspected. A recent review focused on the practical assessment and management of exocrine pancreatic insufficiency is beyond the scope of this chapter but may be further explored here [105].

Colonic Involvement in SSc and the Approach to Diagnosis and Management

Colonic manifestations in SSc are estimated to affect up to 50% of all patients [1, 24]. Symptoms of colonic involvement in SSc may include abdominal pain, distention, constipation, and tenesmus, with less common manifestations including fecal impaction and recurrent intestinal pseudo-obstruction [11]. Slow transit constipation is the most common finding, though long-term complications may include pseudodiverticula, ulcerations, volvulus, and very rarely perforation or infarction are reported [106–108]. A recent study demonstrated that delayed colonic transit is positively associated with female sex, telangiectasia, anticentromere antibodies, past history of smoking, and a Medsger GI severity score of ≥3 [44].

Constipation

Constipation is defined by the AGA as a subjective symptom, which may include the traditional "definition" of less than 3 weekly bowel movements, but may also encompass symptoms of "hard stools, a feeling of incomplete evacuation, abdominal discomfort, bloating, and distention" [109]. A careful history and physical is important in characterizing symptoms and ruling out other systemic contributors (e.g., endocrine, metabolic) [46]. Colonoscopy is an appropriate first step for patients who are due for age-appropriate colon cancer screenings, or patients reporting "alarm symptoms," such as sudden-onset constipation, hematochezia, or unintentional weight loss [109].

An empiric trial of stool-bulking agents and/or laxatives is recommended for patients who have no endoscopic findings to explain constipation symptoms [109]. In patients with an infrequent urge to void and difficulty evacuating the colon, osmotic laxatives (e.g., polyethylene glycol or milk of magnesia) may improve symptoms; however, they may also exacerbate symptoms of bloating in patients with slow transit. Colonic secretory agents such as lubiprostone, linaclotide, and plecanatide are currently used to treat chronic idiopathic constipation [109–111]. As these agents are minimally absorbed, they should conceivably be safe to use in the SSc population, though studies on safety and efficacy in SSc are lacking.

When a laxative trial for constipation fails, patients are considered candidates for additional colonic transit studies, according to the AGA. Complications of colonic dysmotility, such as colonic dilation, perforation dysmotility, pseudo-obstruction, or fecal impaction, can be identified with radiographic imaging (e.g., abdominal radiographs, computed tomography) [27, 112]. Large bowel manometry is less frequently utilized for the diagnosis of colonic dysmotility given the length of procedure time and the cardiopulmonary limitations associated with anesthesia. Sitz markers enable the study of colonic transit over several days; however, concerns related to pellet retention and bowel perforation in patients with severely delayed transit exist [113]. It is important to note that identifying the presence of dysmotility does not consistently correlate with symptom severity, therefore the whole clinical picture should be considered prior to initiating therapy [1, 114]. Prokinetic therapies, such prucalopride, may be considered following a diagnosis of slow transit constipation in symptomatic patients [52, 114–116]. Collaboration with an experienced SSc gastroenterologist may lead to improved patient outcomes, particularly in patients who continue to have symptoms despite medical therapy.

Pseudo-Obstruction

Intestinal pseudo-obstruction is a rare complication of SSc, affecting less than 10% of patients [117]. It is characterized by the failure of the intestinal tract to propel its luminal contents in a forward direction, in the absence of any mechanical obstruction. Recurrent clinical episodes of pseudo-obstruction are defined as either acute or chronic (obstructive symptoms for >6 months). A recent study suggested that episodes of pseudo-obstruction and malabsorption in patients with SSc are most commonly associated with delayed colonic transit [1].

SSc patients with acute intestinal pseudo-obstruction most commonly present with symptoms of nausea (77%) and/or abdominal pain (50%) [1, 118, 119]. Other common symptoms include constipation, diarrhea, vomiting, and distention and postprandial bloating [118]. Patients may also report an inability to pass flatus and a progressively increasing abdominal girth (greater than that with SIBO). Older age, male sex, diffuse cutaneous disease, myopathy, and opioid use are associated with an increased risk of pseudo-obstruction [117]. The presence of autoantibodies to RNA polymerase-3 may be associated with a lower risk of pseudo-obstruction [117]. Bowel rest, decompression, and nutritional support, often in the setting of hospitalization, are the mainstay of therapy.

Pneumatosis (Cystoides) Intestinalis

Pneumatosis intestinalis is a very rare complication of SSc [120, 121]. It is characterized by the presence of multiple gas-filled cysts within the intestinal wall. The pathogenesis is unproven, despite several hypotheses being proposed. These include mucosal breaks from immunosuppressive agents (e.g., steroids) causing shrinkage of Peyer's patches, which disrupts mucosal integrity; bacterial carbohydrate fermentation leading to production of gaseous end products which are absorbed into the luminal wall; and SSc-related atrophy and fibrosis leading to increased wall permeability [122–125]. Most of the literature on pneumotosis cystoides intestinalis exists in the form of case reports with limited population level data [126–129]. A generalized review of a population with this diagnosis, not specific to SSc, found that the colon was the most commonly affected representing 46% of cases, followed by small bowel (27%) and simultaneous involvement of the small and large bowel (7%) [130]. Pneumoperitoneum is a frequent complication, with one case series of 37 patients demonstrating an incidence rate of 87% [128].

Intestinal Pseudodiverticula

In contrast to true diverticula, which contain all the layers of the parent structure, pseudodiverticula are composed solely of mucosa projecting through a muscular wall. In patients with SSc, they are thought to be due to intestinal smooth muscle loss and gaseous products inflating the intestines, which cause weak hypomotile areas on the antimesenteric side to dilate [131]. These outpouchings are visible on contrast studies, usually better demonstrated on postevacuation images [131–133].

The Anorectum

The anorectum is the second most affected region of the GI tract in patients with SSc. Up to 50–70% of patients report symptoms of anorectal dysfunction, with fecal incontinence (38%) being the most common symptom. Nearly 20% of patients also report a need for regular digital stimulation or evacuation [134]. An impaired rectoanal inhibitory response (RAIR) is correlated with fecal incontinence symptoms, and some studies also suggest that incontinence may correlate with a lower mean resting pressure of the internal anal sphincter [23, 135]. However, prior to RAIR assessment, the American College of Gastroenterology (ACG) guidelines and other groups recommend first addressing other conditions that predispose to fecal incontinence, such as diarrhea, pelvic floor trauma (particularly obstetric injury such as prolapse), and neuropathy [136].

A complete history and physical exam are central to the diagnosis of anorectal involvement. Fecal impaction and anal sphincter tone may easily be evaluated with a digital rectal exam, which is important in differentiating anorectal from colonic involvement [137]. Aside from the physical exam, anorectal manometry (ARM) will assess the resting tone of the internal and external anal sphincters [138]. In SSc, ARM will reveal that the internal anal sphincter is affected more often than the external sphincter [33, 139, 140].

For patients with confirmed anorectal dysfunction, the ACG strongly recommends pelvic floor rehabilitation therapy [140] and evidence from SSc studies supports this therapeutic approach [141]. The ACG guidelines outline several other alternative invasive options for the management of fecal incontinence in patients who do not respond to symptom-modifying therapies or pelvic exercises, including minimally invasive sphincter-bulking agents (weak recommendation), sacral nerve stimulation (strong recommendation), and surgical options (i.e., sphincteroplasty, artificial anal sphincters, and colostomy).

Gastrointestinal Bleeding

GI bleeding risk is significantly higher in SSc relative to patients without SSc [142, 143]. The most common causes of small intestinal bleeding by video capsule endoscopy in 50 patients with SSc were found to be small intestinal telangiectasia (26.9%) and small intestinal angiodysplasia (38.5%) [144, 145]. Patients with GI vascular lesions were more likely to have the limited cutaneous subtype of SSc (73.3% limited cutaneous subtype vs. 26.7% diffuse cutaneous subtype, $N = 15$) [144]. Many patients with GI bleeding are initially asymptomatic, and the presence of iron deficiency-related anemia may serve as the first sign of blood loss. As these vascular abnormalities, particularly those in the small bowel, can be difficult to diagnose and treat, they are frequently the culprit of recurrent bleeds [144, 146]. A standard GI bleeding workup should be pursued in all symptomatic patients or those with signs of iron deficiency anemia, starting with a bidirectional endoscopy, followed by consideration for capsule study, computed tomography or magnetic resonance enterography, and subsequently push or balloon endoscopy [147, 148]. Given the complexities of using general anesthesia in SSc, patients should be referred to an experienced center for these latter studies.

Malnutrition

Malnutrition is a serious complication of SSc that is often underdiagnosed, particularly among patients with multiorgan involvement. Studies have demonstrated that up to 18% of patients with SSc are at risk for malnutrition based on the Malnutrition Universal Screening Tool (MUST) criteria [149]. The causes of malnutrition are multifactorial and include malabsorption as well as decreased oral intake which may be attributable to a variety of causes (e.g., dysphagia, dysmotility, depression, disability, adverse effects of medications). Patients with end-stage lung disease may also be affected as patients with severe ILD may require higher caloric intake due to increased basal metabolic requirements (i.e., pulmonary cachexia). Prior studies identified increased GI complaints, decreased oral aperture, abdominal distension, and physician-assessed possible malabsorption as additional risk factors for malnutrition [149]. The treatment of malnutrition includes dietary supplementation of nutrient deficiencies and in severe cases, total parental nutrition (TPN). TPN is generally reserved for patients who cannot maintain a healthy body mass index (BMI) with oral intake alone or those who have signs of severe malnutrition.

Discovering biomarkers for predicting malnutrition in SSc in an evolving area of research as traditional biomarkers may not consistently predict outcomes in this disease state. For example, a recent meta-analysis of 111 studies of hospitalized non-SSc older adults demonstrated that low BMI and low concentrations of albumin, hemoglobin, total cholesterol, prealbumin, and total protein were associated with an increased risk of malnutrition [150]. In contrast, a study of 258 patients with SSc demonstrated that serum albumin level was not a useful marker of malnutrition [151]. Another study of 160 patients with SSc followed at a single center found that serum prealbumin was independently associated with malnutrition with an odds ratio of 8.6 [152]. Future, prospective and longitudinal studies are needed to identify and validate reliable biomarkers of malnutrition in patients with SSc.

Medication Adverse Effects

A number of the medications used to manage clinical complications of SSc may also elicit GI symptoms. Such symptoms may be indistinguishable from those directly related to SSc-GI dysfunction. For example, the initiation of mycophenolate mofetil (MMF) is often associated with GI symptoms in patients with SSc, although these symptoms often resolve following the cessation of the drug. In addition, treatment with nintedanib is associated with an increased risk of GI symptoms (e.g., diarrhea), and such symptoms appear to be a dose-dependent effect. Therefore, during the evaluation of any GI symptoms in patients with SSc, it is important to consider treatment-related adverse effects/toxicity in the differential diagnosis.

Alterations in the GI Microbiome in SSc

Dysbiosis in SSc

GI microbiota alteration (i.e., dysbiosis) may moderate the relationship between the SSc-related motility dysfunction described above and the clinical phenotype of SSc-GI disease [153, 154]. The GI microbiota is a metabolically active, homeostatic organ deemed to play a central role in immune function and host health [155]. Comprised of microorganisms [e.g., bacteria (predominantly), archaea, fungi, eukaryotes, and viruses] residing in the mucous membranes of the human intestine, the GI microbiota has emerged as a key environmental factor in diverse autoimmune diseases, including IBD [155], rheumatoid arthritis [155], as well as multiple sclerosis [156]. In IBD, in particular, dysbiosis is a recognized feature of the disease state [157], and restoration of GI microbiota composition represents a key therapeutic strategy [157].

In SSc, recent studies demonstrate that alteration of the commensal microbiota exists across various SSc patient populations (Table 32.3). In the first study to characterize the GI microbiome in SSc, Volkmann and colleagues demonstrated that patients with SSc had distinct microbial community dif-

Table 32.3 Select genus level differences in lower GI microbiota in SSc patients compared with unaffected controls

Genus	Abundance relative to controls	Cohort location	Potential clinical correlates
Lactobacillus	Increased	Los Angeles, CA, USA[a] Oslo, Norway Lund, Sweden Piacenza, Italy Rome, Italy	*Lactobacillus* may play a role in motility based on preclinical [173] and clinical studies [174]
Ruminococcus	Increased	Los Angeles, CA, USA[a] Rome, Italy	Increased *Ruminococcus gnavus* is associated with symptoms of Crohn's disease [175]
Clostridium	Decreased	Los Angeles, CA, USA (2016) Oslo, Norway Rome, Italy Lund, Sweden[b]	Commensal genus involved maintaining intestinal homeostasis across multiple studies [176]
Bacteroides	Decreased	Los Angeles, CA, USA (2017) Oslo, Norway	Commensal genus; decreased abundance of the species *B. fragilis* has been associated with increased SSc-GI symptoms in cross-sectional [158] and longitudinal studies [167]
Faecalibacterium	Decreased	Los Angeles, CA, USA (2017) Oslo, Norway Lund, Sweden[c] Piacenza, Italy[c]	Commensal genus; decreased abundance of the species *F. prausnitzii* has been associated with increased disease activity in Crohn's disease [177]

[a] Increased in both stool and colonic lavage samples from the same patients [158, 178]
[b] In the Swedish cohort, the family *Clostridiaceae* was decreased in SSc. The family contains the genus *Clostridium*
[c] In the Swedish and Italian cohorts, the species *Faecalibacterium prausnitzii* was decreased in SSc. It is the sole known species of the genus *Faecalibacterium*

ferences compared with unaffected, age- and sex-matched controls in an examination of colonic lavage specimens from the cecum and sigmoid areas [158]. In this study, SSc patients had decreased abundance of beneficial commensal genera (e.g., *Faecalibacterium* and *Clostridium*), as well as increased abundance of pathobiont genera (e.g., *Fusobacterium*, *Ruminococcus*, and *Akkermansia*). In a subsequent study of stool specimens from patients with SSc, the pathobionts, *Fusobacterium*, *Ruminococcus*, *Akkermansia*, were again enriched in patients with SSc compared with unaffected controls [157]. Additional studies have also found increased abundance of *Ruminococcus* [159] and *Akkermansia* [160]. While the exact pathogenic role of these genera in SSc is unclear, both *Ruminococcus* and *Akkermansia* have been implicated as mediators of specific complications of Crohn's disease, a condition that is similar to SSc, in both inflammatory and fibrosing pathological features [161]. For instance, in a large, multicenter study of patients with Crohn's disease in North America, increased *Ruminococcus* abundance was associated with increased stricturing complications [161].

Dysbiosis and SSc-GI Symptoms

In SSc, increased abundance of the pathobiont, *Fusobacterium*, was associated with increased severity of GI symptoms [158], as measured by the UCLA GIT 2.0 [162]. *Fusobacterium* is a candidate biomarker of disease activity [163] and a predictor of future disease severity [161] in IBD. In addition to *Fusobacterium*, increased abundance of *Desulfovibrio* was observed in SSc patients with GI involvement relative to SSc patients without GI involvement [164]. This sulfate-reducing bacteria has been found in higher abundance in patients with active IBD [165], and a recent study demonstrated that the relative abundance of *Desulfovibrio* was associated depression in patients with ulcerative colitis [166].

Depletions in commensal bacteria may also contribute to GI manifestations of SSc. For example, decreased abundance of *Bacteroides fragilis* was associated with increased GI symptoms (e.g., total GIT 2.0 scores, diarrhea domain score, and bloating/distension domain score) in SSc [158]. In addition, in the first longitudinal study of the GI microbiome in SSc, decreased abundance of *Bacteroides fragilis* at baseline was associated with increased SSc-GI symptoms over time, even after adjustment for potential confounders [167]. In this study, SSc patients underwent microbiome evaluation and symptom assessment every 3 months over a 12-month period. Notably, no significant changes in the abundance, nor the presence/absence of specific genera were observed within subjects over the study period. The findings suggest that if changes occur in the GI microbiota over the SSc disease course, these changes may evolve over a longer time period.

Dysbiosis and SSc Features

Specific SSc features may also be associated with unique alterations of the GI microbiota. In a study of two relatively large, independent SSc cohorts from Los Angeles, USA and Lund, Sweden, Andréasson and colleagues found that disease duration, the presence of interstitial lung disease (ILD), small intestine bacterial overgrowth (SIBO), and any immunosuppression use were independently associated with lower GI microbial composition in SSc [168]. In an earlier study of patients from Lund, dysbiosis was also more common among patients with ILD [169]. While the directionality of these reported associations is unknown, these findings suggest that specific SSc manifestations may result in and/or be moderated by changes in the GI microbiome.

The Relationship Between Nutrition and the SSc-GI Microbiome

Dietary Modifications and the GI Microbiome

Additional factors may also underlie GI microbial composition in SSc, including diet. In the aforementioned study of SSc patients from Los Angeles and Lund, significant genus level differences were observed between the two cohorts even after adjustment for disease duration, ILD, SIBO, and any immunosuppression use [168] (Table 32.3). Specifically, the SSc patients from Los Angeles had increased abundance of the pathobionts *Streptococcus* and *Ruminococcus* compared with the SSc patients from Lund. Nutritional intake patterns could conceivably account for some of these differences. A number of studies have demonstrated that alterations in diet can cause substantial changes in GI microbial composition. For instance, a longitudinal study of a multigenerational Asian American cohort demonstrated that emigration to the US was associated with a significant reduction in GI microbial diversity and function [170]. Studies have also demonstrated that changes in the GI microbiota can occur rapidly after a dietary intervention. One study, for example, found that assignment either to a plant-based diet or animal-based diet led to rapid shifts (within 5 days) in the GI microbiota [171]. Another study demonstrated that adherence to a low-gluten versus high-gluten diet was associated with moderate changes in the GI microbiota, as well as decreased self-reported bloating [172]. In this study, 60 healthy adults were randomly assigned to one of the two diets for 8 weeks, followed by an 8-week crossover period. The study also found a reduction in both fasting and postprandial hydrogen exhalation after a standardized test meal following the low-gluten diet compared with the high-gluten diet.

While no studies have directly assessed the effects of a dietary intervention on the GI microbiota in patients with SSc, our group recently demonstrated that restricted intake of short-chain fermentable oligosaccharides, disaccharides, monosaccharides, and polyols (low FODMAP) was not associated with alterations in the GI microbiota in patients with SSc [179]. In this small, observational study, SSc patients adhering to the low-FODMAP diet also had no difference in self-reported GI symptoms compared with patients consuming FODMAPs. The findings suggest that although the low-FODMAP diet is commonly recommended to alleviate GI symptoms in SSc, the evidence supporting this dietary recommendation is lacking. Furthermore, long-term adherence to a low-FODMAP diet is often problematic, as FODMAPs are prebiotics, which support the GI microbiota, and they are also a rich source of healthy plant foods.

Although no direct evidence exists to support the implementation of a specific diet in SSc, data from other disease states may guide future research and clinical practice in this area. Table 32.4 summarizes potential nutritional strategies to consider in patients with SSc. For example, in patients with SIBO and/or bloating, adherence to a diet low in refined grains, starch, and added sugars may be beneficial. A large Dutch study ($N = 1135$) found that total intake of carbohydrates was the strongest predictor of diminished GI bacterial diversity, followed by the consumption of beer, bread, and soda [172]. Moreover, increased consumption of carbohydrates is associated with increased abundance of *Methanobrevibacter*, a methane producer from by-products of bacterial fermentation [180]. Among specific carbohydrates, limiting fructose consumption may also help to curtail GI symptoms in SSc. In a single-center cohort study of 80 patients with SSc, 40% of patients exhibited fructose malabsorption based on a breath test [180]. The SSc patients with fructose malabsorption reported increased GI symptoms at baseline; however, when these patients adhered to a low-fructose diet for 1 month, their GI symptoms decreased.

Table 32.4 Summary of potential interventions to modify the GI microbiota

Modification	Microbiota effect	Potential clinical implications
Decrease carbohydrates	Increase microbial diversity [201]	Decrease in distension/bloating symptoms [9]
Increase omega-3 polyunsaturated fatty acids	Increase abundance of commensal genera [183]	Decrease in intestinal inflammation [184]
Increase consumption of foods naturally rich in probiotics	Increase abundance of commensal genera [202]	Improve GI motility [187]
Increase consumption of foods naturally rich in prebiotics	Increase abundance of commensal genera [188, 189]	Improve GI symptoms [191, 203]
Limit unnecessary use of antibiotics	Antibiotics promote dysbiosis [194]	Curtail progression of SSc-GI disease
Fecal microbial transplantation	Restore dysbiosis [200]	Improve GI symptoms [200]

Omega-3 Polyunsaturated Fatty Acids

Increased consumption of omega-3 polyunsaturated fatty acids may exert beneficial effects on the GI microbiota in SSc. Studies have demonstrated that a Western diet high in animal protein is associated with an increased ratio of omega-6 to omega-3 fatty acids and a reduction in the production of anti-inflammatory compounds, such as short-chain fatty acids [181]. A relatively large study of adult female twins found that even after adjusting for dietary fiber intake, increased consumption and circulating levels of omega-3 fatty acids were associated with increased alpha diversity, a measure of species richness of the GI microbiota [182]. Although no studies have assessed whether increased consumption of omega-3 fatty acids could improve GI symptoms in patients with SSc, one small randomized, open-label, crossover trial of omega-3 fatty acid supplementation in healthy adults found that supplementation of a mixture of eicosapentaenoic acid (EPA) and docosahexaenoic acid (DHA) led to reversible alterations in the abundance of several genera, including *Bifidobacterium* and *Lactobacillus* [183]. Interestingly, the supplement was given in two formulations (as a nutraceutical in the form of capsules and as functional drink that was EPA- and DHA-rich), and the study found that the functional drink had a greater impact on GI microbial composition compared with nutraceutical supplementation. This observation suggests that increasing the consumption of foods with naturally occurring omega-3 polyunsaturated fatty acids may be more impactful than taking a nutraceutical fatty acid supplement. In addition to modifying the GI microbiome, increased consumption of omega-3 fatty acids may lead to an increase in the production of resolvins. Resolvins are thought to play a key role in terminating inflammatory processes and could potentially help to mitigate the propagation of inflammation in SSc [184].

Probiotics

Increased consumption of foods naturally comprised of probiotics could represent another means of restoring balance in the GI microbiota in SSc. Probiotic-rich foods include fermented (e.g., sauerkraut, tempeh, Kombucha) and cultured (e.g., yogurt, kephir, cheese) food products. A few studies have assessed the impact of probiotic supplementation in

SSc with mixed results. One open-label study found a symptomatic benefit of probiotic supplementation in SSc [184], while two randomized controlled trials (RCTs) found that probiotic supplementation did not improve GI symptoms [185, 186]. Similar to omega-3 supplementation, consumption of food naturally rich in probiotics may prove more effective than the administration of a nutraceutical probiotic supplement. A small study found that consumption of yogurt enriched with *Bifidobacterium longum* led to an acceleration in mouth-to-cecum transit time [187]. Since many patients with SSc exhibit delayed GI transit [1], this approach could potentially help to alleviate bloating and constipation in affected SSc patients. Of note, certain probiotic-rich foods that are high in lactose (e.g., milks derived from animals) should be avoided in patients with SSc who are intolerant to lactose, and nondairy alternatives can be recommended instead (e.g., plant- or nut-based milk products).

Prebiotics

Prebiotics are nondigestible dietary substances that feed intestinal microbes, which in turn can modify the abundance of commensal bacteria [188]. For example, studies have demonstrated that ingestion of short-chain fructooligosaccharides, a common prebiotic, leads to increased abundance of fecal *Bifidobacteria* counts [188, 189]. After fermentation, the degradation products of prebiotics include short-chain fatty acids, which may protect against inflammation. In one preclinical study, mice fed a high-prebiotic diet had increased circulating levels of short-chain fatty acids and less allergic airway disease in the lung compared with mice fed a low-prebiotic diet [190]. Prebiotics include fructans, galactooligosaccharides, glucose-derived oligosaccharides, as well as noncarbohydrate oligosaccharides (e.g., cocoa-derived flavanols) and naturally occur in a plethora of healthy food sources, including Jerusalem artichoke, chicory, asparagus, sugar beet, garlic, soybeans, and seaweeds [190]. No studies have evaluated the impact of prebiotic ingestion on GI microbial composition or symptoms in SSc; however, some studies have found a therapeutic benefit in the treatment of irritable bowel syndrome [191] and Crohn's disease [191]. While some patients with SSc-GI dysfunction may not tolerate consumption of prebiotic-rich foods in their raw form, many patients can tolerate small amounts of these foods if they are cooked well in soups or purees.

Antibiotics

Rotating cycles of antibiotics are often used to treat SSc patients with SIBO as described above [192]. This intervention typically yields a transient and short-lived improvement in GI symptoms [193]. While no studies have assessed the long-term effects of repeated antibiotic use in SSc, studies in other disease states have demonstrated that antibiotic use actually promotes dysbiosis [194]. For example, a longitudinal study of children initiating treatment for Crohn's disease found that treatment with antibiotics in the previous 6 months was associated with increased microbial dysbiosis, as well as enrichment of certain fungi, such as *Candida* [194]. In addition, a large retrospective cohort study in the UK found that any exposure to a tetracycline antibiotic for the treatment of acne was associated with a significant increase in the development of IBD, particularly Crohn's disease [195]. Based on these studies, it is possible that repeated antibiotic exposure for the treatment of SIBO in SSc may actually cause more harm than good, and future studies are needed to assess the long-term effects of antibiotic use on progression of GI dysfunction in SSc.

Fecal Microbiota Transplantation

Fecal microbiota transplantation (FMT) may potentially help to improve GI dysbiosis in SSc. Highly effective for the treatment of recurrent *Clostridium difficle* infection [196], FMT has been studied in other disorders, including IBD [197] and metabolic syndrome [198]. However, a rigorous systematic review of the safety and efficacy of FMT in IBD demonstrated a lack of quality evidence supporting the use of this intervention, as well as a deficiency in reported data on long-term maintenance of remission [198].

A small FMT study in patients with SSc found that four out of five patients randomized to receive gastroduodenoscopy transfer of commercially available anaerobic cultivated human intestinal microbiota experienced an improvement in GI symptoms at 4 and/or 16 weeks compared with two out of four in the placebo arm [198]. While these preliminary results are promising, safety is an ongoing concern with this therapeutic approach. One patient experienced a duodenal perforation during gastroduodenoscopy in the study [199], and serious and fatal complications can occur when inadequate screening measures allow the transmission of microorganisms that can cause adverse infectious events [200]. This can be especially worrisome in an SSc patient receiving treatment with immunosuppressive therapies for their condition.

Conclusions

The GI tract is the most common internal organ system affected in SSc and has a major impact on patient-related quality of life and mortality [200]. Despite its high prevalence and clinical burden, SSc-related GI disease remains an area where diagnostic strategies are complex and limited treatment options exist. The present review highlighted the known clinical and pathophysiological features of lower GI dysfunction in SSc, focusing on the biological mechanisms underlying dysmotility and the emerging evidence that bacterial dysbiosis may be a feature of the SSc disease state. The interplay between motility and dysbiosis represents an evolving area of research that may potentially reveal new therapeutic targets. Understanding whether GI microbial balance contributes to progressive dysmotility in SSc (or vice versa) and how this may occur will provide opportunities to therapeutically modify the course of SSc-GI disease and potentially improve patient outcomes.

Importantly, the treatment options presented in this chapter are largely used to ameliorate symptoms of SSc-GI disease. Aside from the small studies mentioned above evaluating the efficacy of probiotics in SSc, few RCTs exist for this clinical dimension of SSc. There are a number of possibilities to explain the dearth of RCTs in this area. One likely explanation is the lack of objective outcome measures of SSc-GI disease. In contrast to the skin and lung disease of SSc, no valid SSc-GI study endpoints exist. In addition, the symptoms of GI involvement are heterogeneous and improved patient phenotyping may help to enrich trial cohorts to study specific GI manifestations of SSc (e.g., constipation, diarrhea, etc.). Finally, the symptoms of GI disease are not always addressed during patient visits to the same extent as other more obvious features of the disease are. Patients may be reluctant to discuss symptoms of fecal incontinence, for example, unless prompted in a sensitive and compassionate manner by their provider.

In summary, the GI tract represents an important clinical dimension of SSc. Numerous unanswered questions remain regarding the pathophysiology and treatment of SSc-GI disease, leaving an opening for future research and discovery in this area.

Acknowledgments We would like to thank the authors of the prior version of this chapter for their contributions in the second edition.

References

1. McMahan ZH, Tucker AE, Perin J, Volkmann ER, Kulkarni S, Ziessman HA, et al. The relationship between gastrointestinal transit, Medsger GI severity, and UCLA GIT 2.0 symptoms in patients with systemic sclerosis. Arthritis Care Res (Hoboken). 2020; https://doi.org/10.1002/acr.24488.
2. McMahan ZH, Paik JJ, Wigley FM, Hummers LK. Determining the risk factors and clinical features associated with severe gastrointestinal dysmotility in systemic sclerosis. Arthritis Care Res (Hoboken). 2018;70(9):1385–92. https://doi.org/10.1002/acr.23479.
3. Steen VD, Medsger TA. Severe organ involvement in systemic sclerosis with diffuse scleroderma. Arthritis Rheum. 2000;43(11):2437–44. https://doi.org/10.1002/1529-0131(200011)43:11<2437::AID-ANR10>3.0.CO;2-U.
4. Nagaraja V, McMahan ZH, Getzug T, Khanna D. Management of gastrointestinal involvement in scleroderma. Curr Treat Opt Rheumatol. 2015;1(1):82–105. https://doi.org/10.1007/s40674-014-0005-0.
5. Jaovisidha K, Csuka ME, Almagro UA, Soergel KH. Severe gastrointestinal involvement in systemic sclerosis: report of five cases and review of the literature. Semin Arthritis Rheum. 2005;34(4):689–702. https://doi.org/10.1016/j.semarthrit.2004.08.009.
6. Umar SB, Griffing L, Garcia H, Foxx-Orenstein AE, DiBaise JK, Crowell MD. The impact of pelvic floor and lower gastrointestinal symptoms on quality of life in women with systemic sclerosis. J Clin Gastroenterol. 2016;50(6):e55–9. https://doi.org/10.1097/MCG.0000000000000405.
7. Nietert PJ, Mitchell HC, Bolster MB, Curran MY, Tilley BC, Silver RM. Correlates of depression, including overall and gastrointestinal functional status, among patients with systemic sclerosis. J Rheumatol. 2005;32(1):51–7.
8. Omair MA, Lee P. Effect of gastrointestinal manifestations on quality of life in 87 consecutive patients with systemic sclerosis. J Rheumatol. 2012;39(5):992–6. https://doi.org/10.3899/jrheum.110826.
9. Marie I, Leroi AM, Gourcerol G, Levesque H, Ménard JF, Ducrotte P. Fructose malabsorption in systemic sclerosis. Medicine (Baltimore). 2015;94(39):e1601. https://doi.org/10.1097/MD.0000000000001601.
10. Volkmann ER, Hoffmann-Vold AM, Chang YL, Jacobs JP, Tillisch K, Mayer EA, et al. Systemic sclerosis is associated with specific alterations in gastrointestinal microbiota in two independent cohorts. BMJ Open Gastroenterol. 2017;4(1):e000134. https://doi.org/10.1136/bmjgast-2017-000134.
11. Kröner PT, Tolaymat OA, Bowman AW, Abril A, Lacy BE. Gastrointestinal manifestations of rheumatological diseases. Am J Gastroenterol. 2019;114(9):1441–54. https://doi.org/10.14309/ajg.0000000000000260.
12. Emmanuel A, Cools M, Vandeplassche L, Kerstens R. Prucalopride improves bowel function and colonic transit time in patients with chronic constipation: an integrated analysis. Am J Gastroenterol. 2014;109(6):887–94. https://doi.org/10.1038/ajg.2014.74.
13. Camilleri M, Parkman HP, Shafi MA, Abell TL, Gerson L, American College of Gastroenterology. Clinical guideline: management of gastroparesis. Am J Gastroenterol. 2013;108(1):18–37; quiz 8. https://doi.org/10.1038/ajg.2012.373.
14. Song HR, Bahk WM, Woo YS, Jeong JH, Kwon YJ, Seo JS, et al. Efficacy and tolerability of generic mirtazapine (mirtax) for major depressive disorder: multicenter, open-label, uncontrolled, prospective study. Clin Psychopharmacol Neurosci. 2015;13(2):144–9. https://doi.org/10.9758/cpn.2015.13.2.144.
15. Tack J, Ly HG, Carbone F, Vanheel H, Vanuytsel T, Holvoet L, et al. Efficacy of mirtazapine in patients with functional dyspepsia and weight loss. Clin Gastroenterol Hepatol. 2016;14(3):385–92.e4. https://doi.org/10.1016/j.cgh.2015.09.043.
16. Carbone F, Vanuytsel T, Tack J. The effect of mirtazapine on gastric accommodation, gastric sensitivity to distention, and nutrient tolerance in healthy subjects. Neurogastroenterol Motil. 2017;29(12) https://doi.org/10.1111/nmo.13146.
17. Cutolo M, Soldano S, Smith V. Pathophysiology of systemic sclerosis: current understanding and new insights. Expert Rev Clin Immunol. 2019;15(7):753–64. https://doi.org/10.1080/1744666X.2019.1614915.
18. D'Angelo WA, Fries JF, Masi AT, Shulman LE. Pathologic observations in systemic sclerosis (scleroderma). A study of fifty-eight autopsy cases and fifty-eight matched con-

trols. Am J Med. 1969;46(3):428–40. https://doi.org/10.1016/0002-9343(69)90044-8.
19. Roberts CG, Hummers LK, Ravich WJ, Wigley FM, Hutchins GM. A case-control study of the pathology of oesophageal disease in systemic sclerosis (scleroderma). Gut. 2006;55(12):1697–703. https://doi.org/10.1136/gut.2005.086074.
20. Stafford-Brady FJ, Kahn HJ, Ross TM, Russell ML. Advanced scleroderma bowel: complications and management. J Rheumatol. 1988;15(5):869–74.
21. Cohen S. The gastrointestinal manifestations of scleroderma: pathogenesis and management. Gastroenterology. 1980;79(1):155–66.
22. Thoua NM, Schizas A, Forbes A, Denton CP, Emmanuel AV. Internal anal sphincter atrophy in patients with systemic sclerosis. Rheumatology (Oxford). 2011;50(9):1596–602. https://doi.org/10.1093/rheumatology/ker153.
23. Thoua NM, Abdel-Halim M, Forbes A, Denton CP, Emmanuel AV. Fecal incontinence in systemic sclerosis is secondary to neuropathy. Am J Gastroenterol. 2012;107(4):597–603. https://doi.org/10.1038/ajg.2011.399.
24. Brandler JB, Sweetser S, Khoshbin K, Babameto M, Prokop LJ, Camilleri M. Colonic manifestations and complications are relatively under-reported in systemic sclerosis: a systematic review. Am J Gastroenterol. 2019;114(12):1847–56. https://doi.org/10.14309/ajg.0000000000000397.
25. Sjogren RW. Gastrointestinal motility disorders in scleroderma. Arthritis Rheum. 1994;37(9):1265–82. https://doi.org/10.1002/art.1780370902.
26. Sattar B, Chokshi RV. Colonic and anorectal manifestations of systemic sclerosis. Curr Gastroenterol Rep. 2019;21(7):33. https://doi.org/10.1007/s11894-019-0699-0.
27. Wang SJ, Lan JL, Chen DY, Chen YH, Hsieh TY, Lin WY. Colonic transit disorders in systemic sclerosis. Clin Rheumatol. 2001;20(4):251–4. https://doi.org/10.1007/s100670170038.
28. Battle WM, Snape WJ Jr, Wright S, Sullivan MA, Cohen S, Meyers A, et al. Abnormal colonic motility in progressive systemic sclerosis. Ann Intern Med. 1981;94(6):749–52. https://doi.org/10.7326/0003-4819-94-6-749.
29. Basilisco G, Barbera R, Vanoli M, Bianchi P. Anorectal dysfunction and delayed colonic transit in patients with progressive systemic sclerosis. Dig Dis Sci. 1993;38(8):1525–9. https://doi.org/10.1007/BF01308615.
30. Luciano L, Granel B, Bernit E, Harle JR, Baumstarck K, Grimaud JC, et al. Esophageal and anorectal involvement in systemic sclerosis: a systematic assessment with high resolution manometry. Clin Exp Rheumatol. 2016;34 Suppl 100(5):63–9.
31. Engel AF, Kamm MA, Talbot IC. Progressive systemic sclerosis of the internal anal sphincter leading to passive faecal incontinence. Gut. 1994;35(6):857–9. https://doi.org/10.1136/gut.35.6.857.
32. Sallam HS, McNearney TA, Chen JZ. Anorectal motility and sensation abnormalities and its correlation with anorectal symptoms in patients with systemic sclerosis: a preliminary study. ISRN Gastroenterol. 2011;2011:402583. https://doi.org/10.5402/2011/402583.
33. Fynne L, Worsøe J, Laurberg S, Krogh K. Faecal incontinence in patients with systemic sclerosis: is an impaired internal anal sphincter the only cause? Scand J Rheumatol. 2011;40(6):462–6. https://doi.org/10.3109/03009742.2011.579575.
34. Furness JB, Callaghan BP, Rivera LR, Cho HJ. The enteric nervous system and gastrointestinal innervation: integrated local and central control. Adv Exp Med Biol. 2014;817:39–71. https://doi.org/10.1007/978-1-4939-0897-4_3.
35. Keely SJ. Epithelial acetylcholine—a new paradigm for cholinergic regulation of intestinal fluid and electrolyte transport. J Physiol. 2011;589(Pt 4):771–2. https://doi.org/10.1113/jphysiol.2010.204263.
36. Cohen S, Fisher R, Lipshutz W, Turner R, Myers A, Schumacher R. The pathogenesis of esophageal dysfunction in scleroderma and Raynaud's disease. J Clin Invest. 1972;51(10):2663–8. https://doi.org/10.1172/JCI107084.
37. Eaker EY, Kuldau JG, Verne GN, Ross SO, Sallustio JE. Myenteric neuronal antibodies in scleroderma: passive transfer evokes alterations in intestinal myoelectric activity in a rat model. J Lab Clin Med. 1999;133(6):551–6. https://doi.org/10.1016/s0022-2143(99)90184-1.
38. Singh J, Mehendiratta V, Del Galdo F, Jimenez SA, Cohen S, DiMarino AJ, et al. Immunoglobulins from scleroderma patients inhibit the muscarinic receptor activation in internal anal sphincter smooth muscle cells. Am J Physiol Gastrointest Liver Physiol. 2009;297(6):G1206–13. https://doi.org/10.1152/ajpgi.00286.2009.
39. Singh J, Cohen S, Mehendiratta V, Mendoza F, Jimenez SA, Dimarino AJ, et al. Effects of scleroderma antibodies and pooled human immunoglobulin on anal sphincter and colonic smooth muscle function. Gastroenterology. 2012;143(5):1308–18. https://doi.org/10.1053/j.gastro.2012.07.109.
40. Nakane S, Umeda M, Kawashiri SY, Mukaino A, Ichinose K, Higuchi O, et al. Detecting gastrointestinal manifestations in patients with systemic sclerosis using anti-gAChR antibodies. Arthritis Res Ther. 2020;22(1):32. https://doi.org/10.1186/s13075-020-2128-z.
41. Suliman Y, Kafaja S, Oh SJ, Alemam M, Bagnato G, Abignano G, et al. Anti-vinculin antibodies in scleroderma (SSc): a potential link between autoimmunity and gastrointestinal system involvement in two SSc cohorts. Clin Rheumatol. 2020; https://doi.org/10.1007/s10067-020-05479-5.
42. McMahan ZH, Domsic RT, Zhu L, Medsger TA, Casciola-Rosen L, Shah AA. Anti-RNPC-3 (U11/U12) antibodies in systemic sclerosis in patients with moderate-to-severe gastrointestinal dysmotility. Arthritis Care Res (Hoboken). 2019;71(9):1164–70. https://doi.org/10.1002/acr.23763.
43. Steen VD. The many faces of scleroderma. Rheum Dis Clin N Am. 2008;34(1):1–15; v. https://doi.org/10.1016/j.rdc.2007.12.001.
44. Cheah J, Perin J, Volkmann ER, Hummers L, Wigley F, McMahan Z. A systematic assessment of demographics, clinical and serological features associated with colonic hypomotility in systemic sclerosis [abstract]. Arthritis Rheumatol. 2020;72(Suppl 10).
45. Sallam H, McNearney TA, Chen JD. Systematic review: pathophysiology and management of gastrointestinal dysmotility in systemic sclerosis (scleroderma). Aliment Pharmacol Ther. 2006;23(6):691–712. https://doi.org/10.1111/j.1365-2036.2006.02804.x.
46. Hansi N, Thoua N, Carulli M, Chakravarty K, Lal S, Smyth A, et al. Consensus best practice pathway of the UK Scleroderma Study Group: gastrointestinal manifestations of systemic sclerosis. Clin Exp Rheumatol. 2014;32(6 Suppl 86):S214–21.
47. McFarlane IM, Bhamra MS, Kreps A, Iqbal S, Al-Ani F, Saladini-Aponte C, et al. Gastrointestinal manifestations of systemic sclerosis. Rheumatology (Sunnyvale). 2018;8(1):235. https://doi.org/10.4172/2161-1149.1000235.
48. Nisihara R, Utiyama SR, Azevedo PM, Skare TL. Celiac disease screening in patients with scleroderma. Arq Gastroenterol. 2011;48(2):163–4. https://doi.org/10.1590/s0004-28032011000200014.
49. Sakkas LI, Simopoulou T, Daoussis D, Liossis SN, Potamianos S. Intestinal involvement in systemic sclerosis: a clinical review. Dig Dis Sci. 2018;63(4):834–44. https://doi.org/10.1007/s10620-018-4977-8.
50. Soudah HC, Hasler WL, Owyang C. Effect of octreotide on intestinal motility and bacterial overgrowth in scleroderma. N Engl J Med. 1991;325(21):1461–7. https://doi.org/10.1056/NEJM199111213252102.

51. Nikou GC, Toumpanakis C, Katsiari C, Charalambopoulos D, Sfikakis PP. Treatment of small intestinal disease in systemic sclerosis with octreotide: a prospective study in seven patients. J Clin Rheumatol. 2007;13(3):119–23. https://doi.org/10.1097/RHU.0b013e3180645d2a.
52. Vigone B, Caronni M, Severino A, Bellocchi C, Baldassarri AR, Fraquelli M, et al. Preliminary safety and efficacy profile of prucalopride in the treatment of systemic sclerosis (SSc)-related intestinal involvement: results from the open label cross-over PROGASS study. Arthritis Res Ther. 2017;19(1):145. https://doi.org/10.1186/s13075-017-1340-y.
53. Maddern GJ, Kiroff GK, Leppard PI, Jamieson GG. Domperidone, metoclopramide, and placebo. All give symptomatic improvement in gastroesophageal reflux. J Clin Gastroenterol. 1986;8(2):135–40.
54. Blonski W, Vela MF, Freeman J, Sharma N, Castell DO. The effect of oral buspirone, pyridostigmine, and bethanechol on esophageal function evaluated with combined multichannel esophageal impedance-manometry in healthy volunteers. J Clin Gastroenterol. 2009;43(3):253–60. https://doi.org/10.1097/MCG.0b013e318167b89d.
55. O'Rourke A, Weinberger P, Morrison M, Conklin J, Postma G. Topical bethanechol for the improvement of esophageal dysmotility: a pilot study. Ann Otol Rhinol Laryngol. 2013;122(8):481–6. https://doi.org/10.1177/000348941312200801.
56. Agrawal A, Hila A, Tutuian R, Mainie I, Castell DO. Bethanechol improves smooth muscle function in patients with severe ineffective esophageal motility. J Clin Gastroenterol. 2007;41(4):366–70. https://doi.org/10.1097/01.mcg.0000225542.03880.68.
57. Smout AJ, Bogaard JW, Grade AC, ten Thije OJ, Akkermans LM, Wittebol P. Effects of cisapride, a new gastrointestinal prokinetic substance, on interdigestive and postprandial motor activity of the distal oesophagus in man. Gut. 1985;26(3):246–51. https://doi.org/10.1136/gut.26.3.246.
58. Staiano A, Clouse RE. The effects of cisapride on the topography of oesophageal peristalsis. Aliment Pharmacol Ther. 1996;10(6):875–82. https://doi.org/10.1046/j.1365-2036.1996.94266000.x.
59. Chrysos E, Tzovaras G, Epanomeritakis E, Tsiaoussis J, Vrachasotakis N, Vassilakis JS, et al. Erythromycin enhances oesophageal motility in patients with gastro-oesophageal reflux. ANZ J Surg. 2001;71(2):98–102. https://doi.org/10.1046/j.1440-1622.2001.02005.x.
60. Arts J, Caenepeel P, Verbeke K, Tack J. Influence of erythromycin on gastric emptying and meal related symptoms in functional dyspepsia with delayed gastric emptying. Gut. 2005;54(4):455–60. https://doi.org/10.1136/gut.2003.035279.
61. Kao CH, Wang SJ, Pang DY. Effects of oral erythromycin on upper gastrointestinal motility in patients with non-insulin-dependent diabetes mellitus. Nucl Med Commun. 1995;16(9):790–3. https://doi.org/10.1097/00006231-199509000-00011.
62. Di Stefano M, Papathanasopoulos A, Blondeau K, Vos R, Boecxstaens V, Farré R, et al. Effect of buspirone, a 5-HT1A receptor agonist, on esophageal motility in healthy volunteers. Dis Esophagus. 2012;25(5):470–6. https://doi.org/10.1111/j.1442-2050.2011.01275.x.
63. Karamanolis GP, Panopoulos S, Denaxas K, Karlaftis A, Zorbala A, Kamberoglou D, et al. The 5-HT1A receptor agonist buspirone improves esophageal motor function and symptoms in systemic sclerosis: a 4-week, open-label trial. Arthritis Res Ther. 2016;18:195. https://doi.org/10.1186/s13075-016-1094-y.
64. Van Oudenhove L, Kindt S, Vos R, Coulie B, Tack J. Influence of buspirone on gastric sensorimotor function in man. Aliment Pharmacol Ther. 2008;28(11–12):1326–33. https://doi.org/10.1111/j.1365-2036.2008.03849.x.
65. Scheerens C, Tack J, Rommel N. Buspirone, a new drug for the management of patients with ineffective esophageal motility? United European Gastroenterol J. 2015;3(3):261–5. https://doi.org/10.1177/2050640615585688.
66. Kumar N, Barai S, Gambhir S, Rastogi N. Effect of mirtazapine on gastric emptying in patients with cancer-associated anorexia. Indian J Palliat Care. 2017;23(3):335–7. https://doi.org/10.4103/IJPC.IJPC_17_17.
67. Gooden JY, Takahashi PY. Mirtazapine treatment of diabetic gastroparesis as a novel method to reduce tube-feed residual: a case report. J Med Case Rep. 2013;7:38. https://doi.org/10.1186/1752-1947-7-38.
68. Omari TI, Benninga MA, Sansom L, Butler RN, Dent J, Davidson GP. Effect of baclofen on esophagogastric motility and gastroesophageal reflux in children with gastroesophageal reflux disease: a randomized controlled trial. J Pediatr. 2006;149(4):468–74. https://doi.org/10.1016/j.jpeds.2006.05.029.
69. Andrews PL, Wood KL. Systemic baclofen stimulates gastric motility and secretion via a central action in the rat. Br J Pharmacol. 1986;89(3):461–7. https://doi.org/10.1111/j.1476-5381.1986.tb11145.x.
70. Pasha SF, Lunsford TN, Lennon VA. Autoimmune gastrointestinal dysmotility treated successfully with pyridostigmine. Gastroenterology. 2006;131(5):1592–6. https://doi.org/10.1053/j.gastro.2006.06.018.
71. O'Dea CJ, Brookes JH, Wattchow DA. The efficacy of treatment of patients with severe constipation or recurrent pseudo-obstruction with pyridostigmine. Color Dis. 2010;12(6):540–8. https://doi.org/10.1111/j.1463-1318.2009.01838.x.
72. Manini ML, Camilleri M, Grothe R, Di Lorenzo C. Application of pyridostigmine in pediatric gastrointestinal motility disorders: a case series. Paediatr Drugs. 2018;20(2):173–80. https://doi.org/10.1007/s40272-017-0277-6.
73. Bharucha AE, Low PA, Camilleri M, Burton D, Gehrking TL, Zinsmeister AR. Pilot study of pyridostigmine in constipated patients with autonomic neuropathy. Clin Auton Res. 2008;18(4):194–202. https://doi.org/10.1007/s10286-008-0476-x.
74. Ahuja NK, Mische L, Clarke JO, Wigley FM, McMahan ZH. Pyridostigmine for the treatment of gastrointestinal symptoms in systemic sclerosis. Semin Arthritis Rheum. 2018;48(1):111–6. https://doi.org/10.1016/j.semarthrit.2017.12.007.
75. Schey R, Saadi M, Midani D, Roberts AC, Parupalli R, Parkman HP. Domperidone to treat symptoms of gastroparesis: benefits and side effects from a large single-center cohort. Dig Dis Sci. 2016;61(12):3545–51. https://doi.org/10.1007/s10620-016-4272-5.
76. Reddymasu SC, Soykan I, McCallum RW. Domperidone: review of pharmacology and clinical applications in gastroenterology. Am J Gastroenterol. 2007;102(9):2036–45. https://doi.org/10.1111/j.1572-0241.2007.01255.x.
77. Shin A. Patient considerations in the management of chronic constipation: focus on prucalopride. Patient Prefer Adherence. 2016;10:1373–84. https://doi.org/10.2147/PPA.S92550.
78. Smart CJ, Malik KI. Prucalopride for the treatment of ileus. Expert Opin Investig Drugs. 2017;26(4):489–93. https://doi.org/10.1080/13543784.2017.1301427.
79. Oustamanolakis P, Tack J. Prucalopride for chronic intestinal pseudo-obstruction. Aliment Pharmacol Ther. 2012;35(3):398–9. https://doi.org/10.1111/j.1365-2036.2011.04947.x.
80. Langworthy J, Parkman HP, Schey R. Emerging strategies for the treatment of gastroparesis. Expert Rev Gastroenterol Hepatol. 2016;10(7):817–25. https://doi.org/10.1586/17474124.2016.1150175.
81. Fox M, Menne D, Stutz B, Fried M, Schwizer W. The effects of tegaserod on oesophageal function and bolus

transport in healthy volunteers: studies using concurrent high-resolution manometry and videofluoroscopy. Aliment Pharmacol Ther. 2006;24(7):1017–27. https://doi.org/10.1111/j.1365-2036.2006.03090.x.
82. Nasr I, Rao SS, Attaluri A, Hashmi SM, Summers R. Effects of tegaserod and erythromycin in upper gut dysmotility: a comparative study. Indian J Gastroenterol. 2009;28(4):136–42. https://doi.org/10.1007/s12664-009-0048-6.
83. Degen L, Petrig C, Studer D, Schroller S, Beglinger C. Effect of tegaserod on gut transit in male and female subjects. Neurogastroenterol Motil. 2005;17(6):821–6. https://doi.org/10.1111/j.1365-2982.2005.00715.x.
84. Fukudo S, Miwa H, Nakajima A, Kinoshita Y, Kosako M, Hayashi K, et al. High-dose linaclotide is effective and safe in patients with chronic constipation: a phase III randomized, double-blind, placebo-controlled study with a long-term open-label extension study in Japan. Neurogastroenterol Motil. 2019;31(1):e13487. https://doi.org/10.1111/nmo.13487.
85. Bassotti G, Usai Satta P, Bellini M. Plecanatide for the treatment of chronic idiopathic constipation in adult patients. Expert Rev Clin Pharmacol. 2019;12(11):1019–26. https://doi.org/10.1080/17512433.2019.1670057.
86. Farmer AD, Ruffle JK, Hobson AR. Linaclotide increases cecal pH, accelerates colonic transit, and increases colonic motility in irritable bowel syndrome with constipation. Neurogastroenterol Motil. 2019;31(2):e13492. https://doi.org/10.1111/nmo.13492.
87. Andresen V, Camilleri M, Busciglio IA, Grudell A, Burton D, McKinzie S, et al. Effect of 5 days linaclotide on transit and bowel function in females with constipation-predominant irritable bowel syndrome. Gastroenterology. 2007;133(3):761–8. https://doi.org/10.1053/j.gastro.2007.06.067.
88. Chander Roland B, Mullin GE, Passi M, Zheng X, Salem A, Yolken R, et al. A prospective evaluation of ileocecal valve dysfunction and intestinal motility derangements in small intestinal bacterial overgrowth. Dig Dis Sci. 2017;62(12):3525–35. https://doi.org/10.1007/s10620-017-4726-4.
89. Marie I, Ducrotté P, Denis P, Menard JF, Levesque H. Small intestinal bacterial overgrowth in systemic sclerosis. Rheumatology (Oxford). 2009;48(10):1314–9. https://doi.org/10.1093/rheumatology/kep226.
90. Tauber M, Avouac J, Benahmed A, Barbot L, Coustet B, Kahan A, et al. Prevalence and predictors of small intestinal bacterial overgrowth in systemic sclerosis patients with gastrointestinal symptoms. Clin Exp Rheumatol. 2014;32(6 Suppl 86):S82–7.
91. Bures J, Cyrany J, Kohoutova D, Förstl M, Rejchrt S, Kvetina J, et al. Small intestinal bacterial overgrowth syndrome. World J Gastroenterol. 2010;16(24):2978–90. https://doi.org/10.3748/wjg.v16.i24.2978.
92. Jansson-Knodell CL, Hujoel IA, Rubio-Tapia A, Murray JA. Not all that flattens villi is celiac disease: a review of enteropathies. Mayo Clin Proc. 2018;93(4):509–17. https://doi.org/10.1016/j.mayocp.2017.10.025.
93. Sawadpanich K, Soison P, Chunlertrith K, Mairiang P, Sukeepaisarnjaroen W, Sangchan A, et al. Prevalence and associated factors of small intestinal bacterial overgrowth among systemic sclerosis patients. Int J Rheum Dis. 2019;22(4):695–9. https://doi.org/10.1111/1756-185X.13495.
94. Di Stefano M, Quigley EMM. The diagnosis of small intestinal bacterial overgrowth: two steps forward, one step backwards? Neurogastroenterol Motil. 2018;30(11):e13494. https://doi.org/10.1111/nmo.13494.
95. Quigley EM. Small intestinal bacterial overgrowth: what it is and what it is not. Curr Opin Gastroenterol. 2014;30(2):141–6. https://doi.org/10.1097/MOG.0000000000000040.
96. Shah SC, Day LW, Somsouk M, Sewell JL. Meta-analysis: antibiotic therapy for small intestinal bacterial overgrowth. Aliment Pharmacol Ther. 2013;38(8):925–34. https://doi.org/10.1111/apt.12479.
97. Quigley EMM, Murray JA, Pimentel M. AGA clinical practice update on small intestinal bacterial overgrowth: expert review. Gastroenterology. 2020;159(4):1526–32. https://doi.org/10.1053/j.gastro.2020.06.090.
98. Rezaie A, Pimentel M, Rao SS. How to test and treat small intestinal bacterial overgrowth: an evidence-based approach. Curr Gastroenterol Rep. 2016;18(2):8. https://doi.org/10.1007/s11894-015-0482-9.
99. Gatta L, Scarpignato C. Systematic review with meta-analysis: rifaximin is effective and safe for the treatment of small intestine bacterial overgrowth. Aliment Pharmacol Ther. 2017;45(5):604–16. https://doi.org/10.1111/apt.13928.
100. Parodi A, Sessarego M, Greco A, Bazzica M, Filaci G, Setti M, et al. Small intestinal bacterial overgrowth in patients suffering from scleroderma: clinical effectiveness of its eradication. Am J Gastroenterol. 2008;103(5):1257–62. https://doi.org/10.1111/j.1572-0241.2007.01758.x.
101. Kowal-Bielecka O, Fransen J, Avouac J, Becker M, Kulak A, Allanore Y, et al. Update of EULAR recommendations for the treatment of systemic sclerosis. Ann Rheum Dis. 2017;76(8):1327–39. https://doi.org/10.1136/annrheumdis-2016-209909.
102. Hendel L, Worning H. Exocrine pancreatic function in patients with progressive systemic sclerosis. Scand J Gastroenterol. 1989;24(4):461–6. https://doi.org/10.3109/00365528909093075.
103. Cobden I, Axon AT, Rowell NR. Pancreatic exocrine function in systemic sclerosis. Br J Dermatol. 1981;105(2):189–93. https://doi.org/10.1111/j.1365-2133.1981.tb01204.x.
104. Bozovic G, Pullerits R, Ståhl A, Ydström K, Wenger D, Marsal J, et al. Exocrine pancreatic function is preserved in systemic sclerosis. Arthritis Res Ther. 2019;21(1):52. https://doi.org/10.1186/s13075-019-1840-z.
105. Struyvenberg MR, Martin CR, Freedman SD. Practical guide to exocrine pancreatic insufficiency - breaking the myths. BMC Med. 2017;15(1):29. https://doi.org/10.1186/s12916-017-0783-y.
106. Stupalkowska W, Mahler-Araujo B, Bennett J, Gourgiotis S. Spontaneous bowel perforation in the setting of colonic involvement with scleroderma. BMJ Case Rep. 2020;13(1):e233220. https://doi.org/10.1136/bcr-2019-233220.
107. Koklu H, Kav T, Altan E, Tseveldorj N, Yekeduz E. A rare complication of systemic sclerosis in an elderly patient: spontaneous colonic perforation. Gastroenterol Nurs. 2018;41(4):352–4. https://doi.org/10.1097/SGA.0000000000000406.
108. Bloch F, Phat VN, Camilléri JP, Vayssairat M, Fiessinger JN, Mallet L, et al. Colonic involvement in systemic sclerosis: report of a case with perforation (author's transl). Gastroenterol Clin Biol. 1981;5(6–7):655–62.
109. Locke GR, Pemberton JH, Phillips SF. American Gastroenterological Association Medical Position Statement: guidelines on constipation. Gastroenterology. 2000;119(6):1761–6. https://doi.org/10.1053/gast.2000.20390.
110. Drossman DA, Chey WD, Johanson JF, Fass R, Scott C, Panas R, et al. Clinical trial: lubiprostone in patients with constipation-associated irritable bowel syndrome—results of two randomized, placebo-controlled studies. Aliment Pharmacol Ther. 2009;29(3):329–41. https://doi.org/10.1111/j.1365-2036.2008.03881.x.
111. Lembo AJ, Kurtz CB, Macdougall JE, Lavins BJ, Currie MG, Fitch DA, et al. Efficacy of linaclotide for patients with chronic constipation. Gastroenterology. 2010;138(3):886–95.e1. https://doi.org/10.1053/j.gastro.2009.12.050.
112. Vischio J, Matlyuk-Urman Z, Lakshminarayanan S. Benign spontaneous pneumoperitoneum in systemic sclerosis. J Clin

Rheumatol. 2010;16(8):379–81. https://doi.org/10.1097/RHU.0b013e3181ffeb49.
113. Rao SS, Rattanakovit K, Patcharatrakul T. Diagnosis and management of chronic constipation in adults. Nat Rev Gastroenterol Hepatol. 2016;13(5):295–305. https://doi.org/10.1038/nrgastro.2016.53.
114. Staller K, Barshop K, Ananthakrishnan AN, Kuo B. Number of retained radiopaque markers on a colonic transit study does not correlate with symptom severity or quality of life in chronic constipation. Neurogastroenterol Motil. 2018;30(5):e13269. https://doi.org/10.1111/nmo.13269.
115. Wang SJ, Lan JL, Chen DY, Chen YH, Hsieh TY, Lin WY. Effects of cisapride on colonic transit in patients with progressive systemic sclerosis. Clin Rheumatol. 2002;21(4):271–4. https://doi.org/10.1007/s100670200072.
116. Bassotti G, Usai Satta P, Bellini M. Prucalopride for the treatment of constipation: a view from 2015 and beyond. Expert Rev Gastroenterol Hepatol. 2019;13(3):257–62. https://doi.org/10.1080/17474124.2019.1568238.
117. Dein E, Kuo PL, Hong YS, Hummers LK, Mecoli CA, McMahan ZH. Evaluation of risk factors for pseudo-obstruction in systemic sclerosis. Semin Arthritis Rheum. 2019;49(3):405–10. https://doi.org/10.1016/j.semarthrit.2019.05.005.
118. Zapatier JA, Ukleja A. Intestinal obstruction and pseudo-obstruction in patients with systemic sclerosis. Acta Gastroenterol Latinoam. 2013;43(3):227–30.
119. Mecoli C, Purohit S, Sandorfi N, Derk CT. Mortality, recurrence, and hospital course of patients with systemic sclerosis-related acute intestinal pseudo-obstruction. J Rheumatol. 2014;41(10):2049–54. https://doi.org/10.3899/jrheum.131547.
120. Devgun P, Hassan H. Pneumatosis cystoides intestinalis: a rare benign cause of pneumoperitoneum. Case Rep Radiol. 2013;2013:353245. https://doi.org/10.1155/2013/353245.
121. Siddall JK, Hetherington JW, Cooper EH, Newling DW, Robinson MR, Richards B, et al. Biochemical monitoring of carcinoma of prostate treated with an LH-RH analogue (Zoladex). Br J Urol. 1986;58(6):676–82. https://doi.org/10.1111/j.1464-410x.1986.tb05911.x.
122. Cobden I, Rothwell J, Axon AT, Dixon MF, Lintott DJ, Rowell NR. Small intestinal structure and passive permeability in systemic sclerosis. Gut. 1980;21(4):293–8. https://doi.org/10.1136/gut.21.4.293.
123. Sequeira W. Pneumatosis cystoides intestinalis in systemic sclerosis and other diseases. Semin Arthritis Rheum. 1990;19(5):269–77. https://doi.org/10.1016/0049-0172(90)90049-l.
124. Keyting WS, McCarver RR, Kovarik JL, Daywitt AL. Pneumatosis intestinalis: a new concept. Radiology. 1961;76:733–41. https://doi.org/10.1148/76.5.733.
125. Yale CE, Balish E, Wu JP. The bacterial etiology of pneumatosis cystoides intestinalis. Arch Surg. 1974;109(1):89–94. https://doi.org/10.1001/archsurg.1974.01360010067017.
126. Mitsuyoshi Y, Takakura K, Kobayashi T, Ogawa N, Sakurai T, Nakano M, et al. Chronic intestinal pseudo-obstruction with pneumatosis cystoides intestinalis in a patient with systemic sclerosis: a case report. Medicine (Baltimore). 2019;98(18):e15480. https://doi.org/10.1097/MD.0000000000015480.
127. Singh G, Johnson C, Gill R, De Cruz P. Pneumatosis cystoides intestinalis (PCI) in a patient with undiagnosed systemic sclerosis. BMJ Case Rep. 2018; https://doi.org/10.1136/bcr-2018-225175.
128. Kaneko M, Sasaki S, Teruya S, Ozaki K, Ishimaru K, Terai E, et al. Pneumatosis cystoides intestinalis in patients with systemic sclerosis: a case report and review of 39 japanese cases. Case Rep Gastrointest Med. 2016;2016:2474515. https://doi.org/10.1155/2016/2474515.
129. Fujita M, Nakano Y, Yagita M. Successful treatment of prokinetic-resistant intestinal pseudo-obstruction and pneumatosis cystoides intestinalis in systemic sclerosis with metronidazole. Rheumatol Int. 2017;37(7):1213–5. https://doi.org/10.1007/s00296-017-3668-7.
130. Morris MS, Gee AC, Cho SD, Limbaugh K, Underwood S, Ham B, et al. Management and outcome of pneumatosis intestinalis. Am J Surg. 2008;195(5):679–82; discussion 82–3. https://doi.org/10.1016/j.amjsurg.2008.01.011.
131. Scutellari PN, Cinotti A, Orzincolo C, Cavallari L, Dovigo L, Menegale G, et al. Changes in the small and large intestines in systemic sclerosis. Radiol Med. 1990;80(6):876–81.
132. Bluestone R, Macmahon M, Dawson JM. Systemic sclerosis and small bowel involvement. Gut. 1969;10(3):185–93. https://doi.org/10.1136/gut.10.3.185.
133. Rohrmann CA, Ricci MT, Krishnamurthy S, Schuffler MD. Radiologic and histologic differentiation of neuromuscular disorders of the gastrointestinal tract: visceral myopathies, visceral neuropathies, and progressive systemic sclerosis. AJR Am J Roentgenol. 1984;143(5):933–41. https://doi.org/10.2214/ajr.143.5.933.
134. Trezza M, Krogh K, Egekvist H, Bjerring P, Laurberg S. Bowel problems in patients with systemic sclerosis. Scand J Gastroenterol. 1999;34(4):409–13. https://doi.org/10.1080/003655299750026434.
135. Heyt GJ, Oh MK, Alemzadeh N, Rivera S, Jimenez SA, Rattan S, et al. Impaired rectoanal inhibitory response in scleroderma (systemic sclerosis): an association with fecal incontinence. Dig Dis Sci. 2004;49(6):1040–5. https://doi.org/10.1023/b:ddas.0000034569.85066.69.
136. Wald A, Bharucha AE, Cosman BC, Whitehead WE. ACG clinical guideline: management of benign anorectal disorders. Am J Gastroenterol. 2014;109(8):1141–57; Quiz 58. https://doi.org/10.1038/ajg.2014.190.
137. Tantiphlachiva K, Rao P, Attaluri A, Rao SS. Digital rectal examination is a useful tool for identifying patients with dyssynergia. Clin Gastroenterol Hepatol. 2010;8(11):955–60. https://doi.org/10.1016/j.cgh.2010.06.031.
138. Massone C, Milone L, Parodi A, Pandolfo N, Rebora A. Anorectal involvement is frequent in limited systemic sclerosis. Acta Derm Venereol. 2002;82(6):446–8. https://doi.org/10.1080/000155502762064593.
139. Koh CE, Young CJ, Wright CM, Byrne CM, Young JM. The internal anal sphincter in systemic sclerosis. Dis Colon Rectum. 2009;52(2):315–8. https://doi.org/10.1007/DCR.0b013e31819a5d59.
140. Franck-Larsson K, Graf W, Eeg-Olofsson KE, Axelson HW, Rönnblom A. Physiological and structural anorectal abnormalities in patients with systemic sclerosis and fecal incontinence. Scand J Gastroenterol. 2014;49(9):1076–83. https://doi.org/10.3109/00365521.2014.913188.
141. Collins J, Mazor Y, Jones M, Kellow J, Malcolm A. Efficacy of anorectal biofeedback in scleroderma patients with fecal incontinence: a case-control study. Scand J Gastroenterol. 2016;51(12):1433–8. https://doi.org/10.1080/00365521.2016.1218537.
142. Lin YT, Chuang YS, Wang JW, Wu PH. High risk of gastrointestinal hemorrhage in patients with systemic sclerosis. Arthritis Res Ther. 2019;21(1):301. https://doi.org/10.1186/s13075-019-2078-5.
143. Michel A, González-Pérez A, Sáez ME, García Rodríguez LA. Risk of bleeding events among patients with systemic sclerosis and the general population in the UK: a large population-based cohort study. Clin Rheumatol. 2020;39(1):19–26. https://doi.org/10.1007/s10067-019-04588-0.

144. Marie I, Antonietti M, Houivet E, Hachulla E, Maunoury V, Bienvenu B, et al. Gastrointestinal mucosal abnormalities using videocapsule endoscopy in systemic sclerosis. Aliment Pharmacol Ther. 2014;40(2):189–99. https://doi.org/10.1111/apt.12818.
145. Duchini A, Sessoms SL. Gastrointestinal hemorrhage in patients with systemic sclerosis and CREST syndrome. Am J Gastroenterol. 1998;93(9):1453–6. https://doi.org/10.1111/j.1572-0241.1998.00462.x.
146. Khanlou H, Malhotra A, Friedenberg F, Rothstein K. Jejunal telangiectasias as a cause of massive bleeding in a patient with scleroderma. Rev Rhum Engl Ed. 1999;66(2):119–21.
147. Ko CW, Siddique SM, Patel A, Harris A, Sultan S, Altayar O, et al. AGA clinical practice guidelines on the gastrointestinal evaluation of iron deficiency anemia. Gastroenterology. 2020;159(3):1085–94. https://doi.org/10.1053/j.gastro.2020.06.046.
148. Otani K, Watanabe T, Shimada S, Hosomi S, Nagami Y, Tanaka F, et al. Clinical utility of capsule endoscopy and double-balloon enteroscopy in the management of obscure gastrointestinal bleeding. Digestion. 2018;97(1):52–8. https://doi.org/10.1159/000484218.
149. Baron M, Hudson M, Steele R, Canadian Scleroderma Research Group. Malnutrition is common in systemic sclerosis: results from the Canadian scleroderma research group database. J Rheumatol. 2009;36(12):2737–43. https://doi.org/10.3899/jrheum.090694.
150. Zhang Z, Pereira SL, Luo M, Matheson EM. Evaluation of blood biomarkers associated with risk of malnutrition in older adults: a systematic review and meta-analysis. Nutrients. 2017;9(8):829. https://doi.org/10.3390/nu9080829.
151. Baron M, Hudson M, Steele R, Canadian Scleroderma Research Group (CSRG). Is serum albumin a marker of malnutrition in chronic disease? The scleroderma paradigm. J Am Coll Nutr. 2010;29(2):144–51. https://doi.org/10.1080/07315724.2010.10719828.
152. Caporali R, Caccialanza R, Bonino C, Klersy C, Cereda E, Xoxi B, et al. Disease-related malnutrition in outpatients with systemic sclerosis. Clin Nutr. 2012;31(5):666–71. https://doi.org/10.1016/j.clnu.2012.02.010.
153. Bellocchi C, Volkmann ER. Update on the gastrointestinal microbiome in systemic sclerosis. Curr Rheumatol Rep. 2018;20(8):49. https://doi.org/10.1007/s11926-018-0758-9.
154. Volkmann ER, Hoffmann-Vold AM. Gastrointestinal tract microbiota modifications in systemic sclerosis. Eur J Rheumatol. 2020;7(Suppl 3):S228–36. https://doi.org/10.5152/eurjrheum.2019.19103.
155. Koboziev I, Reinoso Webb C, Furr KL, Grisham MB. Role of the enteric microbiota in intestinal homeostasis and inflammation. Free Radic Biol Med. 2014;68:122–33. https://doi.org/10.1016/j.freeradbiomed.2013.11.008.
156. Schepici G, Silvestro S, Bramanti P, Mazzon E. The gut microbiota in multiple sclerosis: an overview of clinical trials. Cell Transplant. 2019;28(12):1507–27. https://doi.org/10.1177/0963689719873890.
157. de Souza HS, Fiocchi C. Immunopathogenesis of IBD: current state of the art. Nat Rev Gastroenterol Hepatol. 2016;13(1):13–27. https://doi.org/10.1038/nrgastro.2015.186.
158. Volkmann ER, Chang YL, Barroso N, Furst DE, Clements PJ, Gorn AH, et al. Association of systemic sclerosis with a unique colonic microbial consortium. Arthritis Rheumatol. 2016;68(6):1483–92. https://doi.org/10.1002/art.39572.
159. Bosello S, Sterbini FP, Natalello G, Canestrari G, Parisi F, Sanguinetti M, et al. The intestinal involvement in systemic sclerosis is characterized by a peculiar gut microbiota [abstract]. Arthritis Rheumatol. 2016;68(Suppl 10).
160. Patrone V, Puglisi E, Cardinali M, Schnitzler TS, Svegliati S, Festa A, et al. Gut microbiota profile in systemic sclerosis patients with and without clinical evidence of gastrointestinal involvement. Sci Rep. 2017;7:14874. https://doi.org/10.1038/s41598-017-14889-6.
161. Kugathasan S, Denson LA, Walters TD, Kim MO, Marigorta UM, Schirmer M, et al. Prediction of complicated disease course for children newly diagnosed with Crohn's disease: a multicentre inception cohort study. Lancet. 2017;389(10080):1710–8. https://doi.org/10.1016/S0140-6736(17)30317-3.
162. Khanna D, Hays RD, Maranian P, Seibold JR, Impens A, Mayes MD, et al. Reliability and validity of the University of California, Los Angeles Scleroderma Clinical Trial Consortium Gastrointestinal Tract Instrument. Arthritis Rheum. 2009;61(9):1257–63. https://doi.org/10.1002/art.24730.
163. Strauss J, Kaplan GG, Beck PL, Rioux K, Panaccione R, Devinney R, et al. Invasive potential of gut mucosa-derived Fusobacterium nucleatum positively correlates with IBD status of the host. Inflamm Bowel Dis. 2011;17(9):1971–8. https://doi.org/10.1002/ibd.21606.
164. Bellocchi C, Fernández-Ochoa Á, Montanelli G, Vigone B, Santaniello A, Milani C, et al. Microbial and metabolic multi-omic correlations in systemic sclerosis patients. Ann N Y Acad Sci. 2018;1421(1):97–109. https://doi.org/10.1111/nyas.13736.
165. Rowan F, Docherty NG, Murphy M, Murphy B, Calvin Coffey J, O'Connell PR. Desulfovibrio bacterial species are increased in ulcerative colitis. Dis Colon Rectum. 2010;53(11):1530–6. https://doi.org/10.1007/DCR.0b013e3181f1e620.
166. Humbel F, Rieder JH, Franc Y, Juillerat P, Scharl M, Misselwitz B, et al. Association of alterations in intestinal microbiota with impaired psychological function in patients with inflammatory bowel diseases in remission. Clin Gastroenterol Hepatol. 2020;18(9):2019–29.e11. https://doi.org/10.1016/j.cgh.2019.09.022.
167. Volkmann ER, Hoffmann-Vold A-M, Chang Y-L, Lagishetty V, Clements PJ, Midtvedt Ø, et al. Longitudinal characterisation of the gastrointestinal tract microbiome in systemic sclerosis. Eur Med J. 2020;5:110–8.
168. Andréasson K, Lee SVL, Wu M, Howlett N, English J, Hesselstrand RJJ, Volkmann ER. Disease features of systemic sclerosis are associated with alterations in gastrointestinal microbial composition in two independent cohorts [abstract]. Arthritis Rheumatol 2020;72(Suppl 10).
169. Andréasson K, Alrawi Z, Persson A, Jönsson G, Marsal J. Intestinal dysbiosis is common in systemic sclerosis and associated with gastrointestinal and extraintestinal features of disease. Arthritis Res Ther. 2016;18(1):278. https://doi.org/10.1186/s13075-016-1182-z.
170. Vangay P, Johnson AJ, Ward TL, Al-Ghalith GA, Shields-Cutler RR, Hillmann BM, et al. US immigration westernizes the human gut microbiome. Cell. 2018;175(4):962–72.e10. https://doi.org/10.1016/j.cell.2018.10.029.
171. David LA, Maurice CF, Carmody RN, Gootenberg DB, Button JE, Wolfe BE, et al. Diet rapidly and reproducibly alters the human gut microbiome. Nature. 2014;505(7484):559–63. https://doi.org/10.1038/nature12820.
172. Hansen LBS, Roager HM, Søndertoft NB, Gøbel RJ, Kristensen M, Vallès-Colomer M, et al. A low-gluten diet induces changes in the intestinal microbiome of healthy Danish adults. Nat Commun. 2018;9(1):4630. https://doi.org/10.1038/s41467-018-07019-x.
173. Wang B, Mao YK, Diorio C, Wang L, Huizinga JD, Bienenstock J, et al. Lactobacillus reuteri ingestion and IK(Ca) channel blockade have similar effects on rat colon motility and myenteric neurones. Neurogastroenterol Motil. 2010;22(1):98–107, e33. https://doi.org/10.1111/j.1365-2982.2009.01384.x.
174. Dimidi E, Christodoulides S, Fragkos KC, Scott SM, Whelan K. The effect of probiotics on functional constipation in adults: a systematic review and meta-analysis of randomized controlled trials. Am J Clin Nutr. 2014;100(4):1075–84. https://doi.org/10.3945/ajcn.114.089151.

175. Hall AB, Yassour M, Sauk J, Garner A, Jiang X, Arthur T, et al. A novel Ruminococcus gnavus clade enriched in inflammatory bowel disease patients. Genome Med. 2017;9(1):103. https://doi.org/10.1186/s13073-017-0490-5.
176. Guo P, Zhang K, Ma X, He P. *Clostridium* species as probiotics: potentials and challenges. J Anim Sci Biotechnol. 2020;11:24. https://doi.org/10.1186/s40104-019-0402-1.
177. Prosberg M, Bendtsen F, Vind I, Petersen AM, Gluud LL. The association between the gut microbiota and the inflammatory bowel disease activity: a systematic review and meta-analysis. Scand J Gastroenterol. 2016;51(12):1407–15. https://doi.org/10.1080/00365521.2016.1216587.
178. Volkmann ER. Intestinal microbiome in scleroderma: recent progress. Curr Opin Rheumatol. 2017;29(6):553–60. https://doi.org/10.1097/BOR.0000000000000429.
179. Howlett N, Lee S, Lagishetty V, McMahan Z, Wu M, Jacobs J, Volkmann E, et al. Low FODMAP diet is not associated with decreased gi symptoms or changes in GI microbial composition in patients with systemic sclerosis [abstract]. Arthritis Rheumatol. 2020;72(Suppl 10).
180. Hoffmann C, Dollive S, Grunberg S, Chen J, Li H, Wu GD, et al. Archaea and fungi of the human gut microbiome: correlations with diet and bacterial residents. PLoS One. 2013;8(6):e66019. https://doi.org/10.1371/journal.pone.0066019.
181. Costantini L, Molinari R, Farinon B, Merendino N. Impact of omega-3 fatty acids on the gut microbiota. Int J Mol Sci. 2017;18(12):2645. https://doi.org/10.3390/ijms18122645.
182. Menni C, Zierer J, Pallister T, Jackson MA, Long T, Mohney RP, et al. Omega-3 fatty acids correlate with gut microbiome diversity and production of N-carbamylglutamate in middle aged and elderly women. Sci Rep. 2017;7(1):11079. https://doi.org/10.1038/s41598-017-10382-2.
183. Watson H, Mitra S, Croden FC, Taylor M, Wood HM, Perry SL, et al. A randomised trial of the effect of omega-3 polyunsaturated fatty acid supplements on the human intestinal microbiota. Gut. 2018;67(11):1974–83. https://doi.org/10.1136/gutjnl-2017-314968.
184. Avanoğlu Güler A, Rossi FW, Bellando-Randone S, Prevete N, Tufan A, Manetti M, et al. The role of endogenous eicosapentaenoic acid and docosahexaenoic acid-derived resolvins in systemic sclerosis. Front Immunol. 2020;11:1249. https://doi.org/10.3389/fimmu.2020.01249.
185. Low AHL, Teng GG, Pettersson S, de Sessions PF, Ho EXP, Fan Q, et al. A double-blind randomized placebo-controlled trial of probiotics in systemic sclerosis associated gastrointestinal disease. Semin Arthritis Rheum. 2019;49(3):411–9. https://doi.org/10.1016/j.semarthrit.2019.05.006.
186. Marighela TF, Arismendi MI, Marvulle V, Brunialti MKC, Salomão R, Kayser C. Effect of probiotics on gastrointestinal symptoms and immune parameters in systemic sclerosis: a randomized placebo-controlled trial. Rheumatology (Oxford). 2019;58(11):1985–90. https://doi.org/10.1093/rheumatology/kez160.
187. Bartram HP, Scheppach W, Gerlach S, Ruckdeschel G, Kelber E, Kasper H. Does yogurt enriched with Bifidobacterium longum affect colonic microbiology and fecal metabolites in health subjects? Am J Clin Nutr. 1994;59(2):428–32. https://doi.org/10.1093/ajcn/59.2.428.
188. Bouhnik Y, Raskine L, Simoneau G, Paineau D, Bornet F. The capacity of short-chain fructo-oligosaccharides to stimulate faecal bifidobacteria: a dose-response relationship study in healthy humans. Nutr J. 2006;5:8. https://doi.org/10.1186/1475-2891-5-8.
189. Bouhnik Y, Achour L, Paineau D, Riottot M, Attar A, Bornet F. Four-week short chain fructo-oligosaccharides ingestion leads to increasing fecal bifidobacteria and cholesterol excretion in healthy elderly volunteers. Nutr J. 2007;6:42. https://doi.org/10.1186/1475-2891-6-42.
190. Trompette A, Gollwitzer ES, Yadava K, Sichelstiel AK, Sprenger N, Ngom-Bru C, et al. Gut microbiota metabolism of dietary fiber influences allergic airway disease and hematopoiesis. Nat Med. 2014;20(2):159–66. https://doi.org/10.1038/nm.3444.
191. Silk DB, Davis A, Vulevic J, Tzortzis G, Gibson GR. Clinical trial: the effects of a trans-galactooligosaccharide prebiotic on faecal microbiota and symptoms in irritable bowel syndrome. Aliment Pharmacol Ther. 2009;29(5):508–18. https://doi.org/10.1111/j.1365-2036.2008.03911.x.
192. Miller JB, Gandhi N, Clarke J, McMahan Z. Gastrointestinal involvement in systemic sclerosis: an update. J Clin Rheumatol. 2018;24(6):328–37. https://doi.org/10.1097/RHU.0000000000000626.
193. Lauritano EC, Gabrielli M, Scarpellini E, Ojetti V, Roccarina D, Villita A, et al. Antibiotic therapy in small intestinal bacterial overgrowth: rifaximin versus metronidazole. Eur Rev Med Pharmacol Sci. 2009;13(2):111–6.
194. Lewis JD, Chen EZ, Baldassano RN, Otley AR, Griffiths AM, Lee D, et al. Inflammation, antibiotics, and diet as environmental stressors of the gut microbiome in pediatric Crohn's disease. Cell Host Microbe. 2015;18(4):489–500. https://doi.org/10.1016/j.chom.2015.09.008.
195. Margolis DJ, Fanelli M, Hoffstad O, Lewis JD. Potential association between the oral tetracycline class of antimicrobials used to treat acne and inflammatory bowel disease. Am J Gastroenterol. 2010;105(12):2610–6. https://doi.org/10.1038/ajg.2010.303.
196. van Nood E, Vrieze A, Nieuwdorp M, Fuentes S, Zoetendal EG, de Vos WM, et al. Duodenal infusion of donor feces for recurrent Clostridium difficile. N Engl J Med. 2013;368(5):407–15. https://doi.org/10.1056/NEJMoa1205037.
197. Rossen NG, Fuentes S, van der Spek MJ, Tijssen JG, Hartman JH, Duflou A, et al. Findings from a randomized controlled trial of fecal transplantation for patients with ulcerative colitis. Gastroenterology. 2015;149(1):110–8.e4. https://doi.org/10.1053/j.gastro.2015.03.045.
198. Vrieze A, Van Nood E, Holleman F, Salojärvi J, Kootte RS, Bartelsman JF, et al. Transfer of intestinal microbiota from lean donors increases insulin sensitivity in individuals with metabolic syndrome. Gastroenterology. 2012;143(4):913–6.e7. https://doi.org/10.1053/j.gastro.2012.06.031.
199. Fretheim H, Chung BK, Didriksen H, Bækkevold ES, Midtvedt Ø, Brunborg C, et al. Fecal microbiota transplantation in systemic sclerosis: a double-blind, placebo-controlled randomized pilot trial. PLoS One. 2020;15(5):e0232739. https://doi.org/10.1371/journal.pone.0232739.
200. DeFilipp Z, Bloom PP, Torres Soto M, Mansour MK, Sater MRA, Huntley MH, et al. Drug-resistant. N Engl J Med. 2019;381(21):2043–50. https://doi.org/10.1056/NEJMoa1910437.
201. Zhernakova A, Kurilshikov A, Bonder MJ, Tigchelaar EF, Schirmer M, Vatanen T, et al. Population-based metagenomics analysis reveals markers for gut microbiome composition and diversity. Science. 2016;352(6285):565–9. https://doi.org/10.1126/science.aad3369.
202. Singh RK, Chang HW, Yan D, Lee KM, Ucmak D, Wong K, et al. Influence of diet on the gut microbiome and implications for human health. J Transl Med. 2017;15(1):73. https://doi.org/10.1186/s12967-017-1175-y.
203. Lindsay JO, Whelan K, Stagg AJ, Gobin P, Al-Hassi HO, Rayment N, et al. Clinical, microbiological, and immunological effects of fructo-oligosaccharide in patients with Crohn's disease. Gut. 2006;55(3):348–55. https://doi.org/10.1136/gut.2005.074971.

Part VII

Skin, Musculoskeletal and Other Complications

Lorinda Chung

33 Evaluation and Management of Skin Disease

Nicolas Hunzelmann and Flavia V. Castelino

Phototherapy for Skin Fibrosis

Similar to SSc, in localized scleroderma activation of proinflammatory and profibrotic pathways leads to excessive collagen production and a decrease of matrix metalloproteinase (MMP) activity responsible for collagen degradation. Current options for treatment of the fibrotic process are limited and include immunosuppressive agents as well as phototherapy. It is well known, that UV-light exerts a multitude of effects on the skin including inhibition of T-cell activation, inflammatory cell apoptosis as well as the induction of collagen degradation and remodeling. Phototherapy and photochemotherapy are therefore often considered in the therapeutic ladder of treating skin fibrosis primarily in localized scleroderma.

UVB (290–320 nm) is considered to have too short of a wavelength to induce a significant change in scleroderma skin, even in targeted sources such as the 308-nm excimer laser. UVA wavelengths are longer (320–400 nm) and penetrate more deeply into the skin reaching the connective tissue. Mechanisms of action relate to modulation of cytokine synthesis, to enhanced remodeling of the connective tissue via upregulation of collagen-degrading matrix metalloproteinase, as well as increased apoptosis of T cells. For instance, a recent serologic study of nine patients who received PUVA (Psoralen + UVA) and three who received topical PUVA demonstrated a statistically significant increase in circulating TNF-alpha in 8/12 subjects that was accompanied by a clinically significant improvement in the modified Rodnan skin score in 11/12 subjects [1].

N. Hunzelmann (✉)
Department of Dermatology, University of Cologne, Cologne, Germany
e-mail: nico.hunzelmann@uni-koeln.de

F. V. Castelino
Division of Rheumatology, Massachusetts General Hospital/Harvard Medical School, Boston, MA, USA
e-mail: FCASTELINO@mgh.harvard.edu

Use of phototherapy for the treatment of skin sclerosis should be guided by the phase of the fibrotic process (early phase vs. late phase), the degree of disease activity, and whether there has been progression of the fibrosis. In the early phase with limited skin involvement, UVA1 or photochemotherapy (bath-PUVA, systemic PUVA) should be considered. In analogy to the successful treatment of localized scleroderma with UVA modalities, a number of uncontrolled studies indicate a beneficial effect on skin fibrosis in SSc [2, 3]. However, controlled studies are still lacking. The challenge in treating skin fibrosis with PUVA is that it is often difficult to define a treatment endpoint. The potential risk of skin cancers such as squamous cell carcinoma and melanoma limits its appropriateness for long-term treatment, particularly in patients with light constitutive pigmentation [4].

Phototherapy may lead to postinflammatory hyperpigmentation of skin areas which previously appeared unaffected by the disease, causing concern for the patient. This usually reflects low-grade inflammation of the skin, which after successful treatment, reacts with postinflammatory hyperpigmentation that usually persists at least for several months following the discontinuation of treatment and is most pronounced and persistent in patients with Fitzpatrick skin type III or greater. Those patients should be counseled that the hyperpigmentation will take approximately a year to resolve.

UVA-1 treatment (340–400 nm) has the advantage of generating high-irradiation levels that in contrast to PUVA therapy does not require a photosensitizing agent. However, UVA-1 light boxes are difficult for many patients to find close to home, as they are large lie-down units (as opposed to stand-up design for UVB or UVA) that are costly for providers to purchase and to maintain. UVA-1 also causes deep tanning, which can worsen postinflammatory hyperpigmentation. Reported treatment regimens have been highly variable. High-dose (~130 J/cm^2), medium-dose (~50–60 J/cm^2), and low-dose (~10–30 J/cm^2) UVA-1 regimens have all been reported to result in improvement in scleroderma skin.

Y. Allanore et al. (eds.), *Scleroderma*, https://doi.org/10.1007/978-3-031-40658-4_33

Clearly larger-scale randomized controlled trials are needed for further evaluation [5].

Photopheresis (extracorporeal photochemotherapy) has shown promise in several uncontrolled studies [6] but failed to demonstrate a favorable effect in a randomized crossover study [7]. It can be used as second line or adjuvant therapy in early progressive disease preferably of less than 2 years duration.

Lipodystrophy

Lipodystrophy overlying inflammatory lesions such as plaques of localized scleroderma is well described. The most frequently encountered cosmetically significant forms of this are generally linear scleroderma, especially when presenting in the en coup de sabre form affecting the face, and the Parry-Romberg variant of linear scleroderma in which there is associated progressive hemifacial atrophy. Additionally, there can be prominent fat loss on the limbs or trunk in association with cutaneous fibrosis in systemic sclerosis. Since the subcutaneous fat often recovers as skin softens, the adipocytes are likely compressed by the tight fibrotic dermis rather than destroyed.

Treatment

Injectable soft tissue fillers may improve atrophic changes in inactive lesions. Consultation with a plastic surgeon or a procedural dermatologist with experience in treating patients with morphea is essential. Noninvasive treatment of facial lipodystrophy is often preferred by patients when feasible, as opposed to surgical approaches such as microvascular-free tissue transfer. With 10 years of treatment efficacy established in HIV-associated lipoatrophy, and now being used widely for esthetic facial revolumization, poly-L-lactic acid (Sculptra®, PLLA) is a good option for these patients. Typically, a series of at least three treatments are needed, with each entailing topical anesthetic in addition to 1% lidocaine without epinephrine mixed into the injected material. The viscous suspension is injected into the areas of volume deficiency using a crosshatch linear threading technique in combination with depot injections where necessary. No active inflammation should be present at the time of treatment for an optimal result, as PLLA has the potential to produce inflammatory nodules. In a paper describing PLLA treatment of four patients with linear scleroderma of the face and two with Parry-Romberg syndrome, two developed subcutaneous nodules [8]. While this is a known potential complication of PLLA treatment, a more dilute preparation than used in those cases has improved outcomes. The other filler with FDA approval for the treatment of HIV-associated lipoatrophy is Radiesse®, which consists of calcium hydroxyapatite microspheres suspended in an aqueous gel carrier. Because the microspheres can be seen on X-rays or CT scans, it should not be injected in areas that may require monitoring with those modalities. Hyaluronic acid injectable dermal fillers such as Juvéderm may be suitable for revolumizing in scleroderma patients since they are used widely to treat age-related volume loss and do not carry as high a risk of nodule formation as does PLLA; they can also be dissolved with hyaluronidase if need be.

Surgical options such as autologous fat transfer can return symmetry and contour to lesions with substantial deep atrophy [9]. Before cosmetic enhancement may be considered, there should be substantial evidence of disease inactivity. The main advantage of autologous fat in comparison to other soft tissue fillers is the lack of risk for hypersensitivity or foreign body reactions.

Xerosis Cutis and Pruritus

Therapy of xerosis and itch is an important component of multimodal therapy in SSc patients. Since scleroderma skin thickening causes loss of periadnexal fat, the adnexa (hair follicles, sebaceous glands, eccrine glands) can be compressed resulting in frequent loss of skin appendages. This translates clinically to reduced sebum production and consequent xerosis and itch. This process is often accompanied by alopecia and hypohidrosis. As skin softens, the alopecia sometimes dramatically reverses with hypertrichosis (Fig. 33.1). Scleroderma skin is often rough and slightly erythematous, resembling an eczematous dermatitis. This dermatitis can produce varying degrees of pruritus. Small papules of prurigo nodularis can arise in areas of chronic

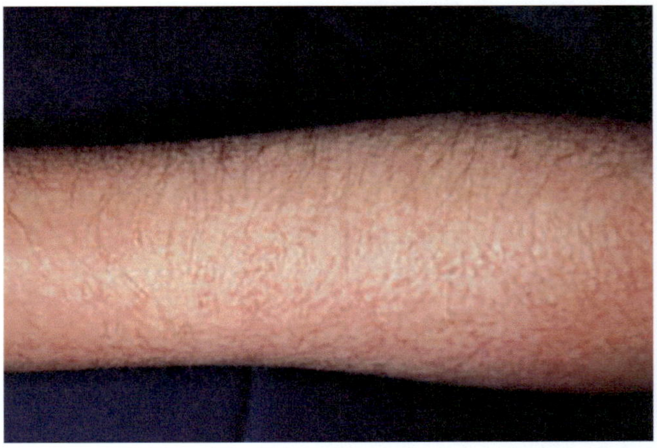

Fig. 33.1 Hypertrichosis in the setting of skin softening. (Courtesy of F.M. Wigley)

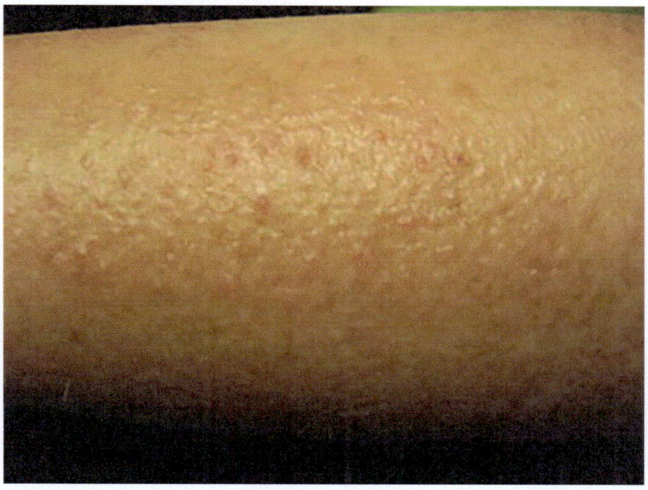

Fig. 33.2 Cobblestoning of the forearm in diffuse scleroderma. (Courtesy of F.M. Wigley)

rubbing or excoriation, giving the skin a "cobblestoned" appearance (Fig. 33.2).

In patients with SSc, itch may be present in up to 60% of cases and a correlation with disease severity has been described [10]. In addition, the presence of itch correlates independently with the severity of skin hardening and greater GI involvement, and remained predominantly stable in the course of the disease [11]. The exact causative mechanisms for itch in SSc still have yet to be elucidated. Inflammatory processes in the dermis, the subsequent loss of skin appendages by the fibrotic process, entrapping of sensory nerve fibers in combination with the loss of the ability to synthesize appropriate amounts of "endogenous lipids and emollients" are components of this symptom. As a result of other comorbidities, pruritus is often not taken sufficiently into consideration with patient well-being. It may significantly affect quality of life, contribute to sleep disturbances, and mood disorders. The differential diagnosis of pruritus encompasses a wide array of dermatological and nondermatological diseases [12]. Medical history (including onset, duration, location, quality, and severity of itch) and skin examination are the basis of an initial assessment. In chronic pruritus (i.e., persisting longer than 6 weeks), a complete dermatological examination is mandatory to exclude comorbidities and underlying systemic diseases. A number of drugs may additionally induce or maintain chronic pruritus.

Treatment

Topical therapy is the mainstay of initial treatment. For maintenance of the skin barrier to prevent dry skin, it is important that patients hydrate and moisturize their skin. Emollients with a high-water content favoring resorption can be effective but do not improve skin texture or pruritus. Hence, an emollient containing urea (3–10%), lactic acid (1–5%, increasing hydration), and a higher percentage of glycerol (up to 20%) should be recommended. Moisturizing lotions that are thin enough to be dispensed through a pump contain too much water to be sufficiently moisturizing for scleroderma skin. Instead, creams that are dispensed in a jar (as tubes can be difficult to use with sclerodactyly) are ideal. Also for patients with milder pruritus, a mid-potency topical steroid compounded 1:1 with a rich emollient (such as triamcinolone acetonide 0.1% cream 1:1 with Eucerin or CeraVe cream) is a first-line treatment. In patients with skin fragility in whom topical steroids would be inadvisable, topical calcineurin inhibitors such as tacrolimus or pimecrolimus ointment are an excellent alternative. Patients should be advised that these can cause a very warm or even burning sensation in the skin that subsides within 2–3 days into use. In patients in whom pruritus is pronounced, a short course of super potent topical steroids (such as clobetasol propionate 0.05% ointment, or cream if ointment cannot be tolerated) to decrease the inflammation and pruritus can be considered. Avoidance of frequent washing and bathing is strongly recommended.

For patients with a more pronounced eczematous dermatitis, narrowband UVB treatment (NBUVB, 311 nm) can be extraordinarily helpful as a steroid-sparing treatment strategy. Three times weekly treatment is needed to achieve optimal clearance, and then it should be tapered to twice-weekly treatment for 4 weeks, followed by weekly treatment for 4 weeks. NBUVB is not as effective for weekly maintenance therapy as PUVA, so if a patient is clear at that point, treatment can be discontinued with the understanding that it will be resumed should the dermatitis flare significantly. Usually, UV therapy is combined with topical treatment. Systemic therapy of the underlying disease by DMARDs as methotrexate, mycophenolate mofetil, biologics as rituximab or cyclophosphamide in severely affected patients with dcSSc leads to a reduction of the inflammation and can influence the extent of itching.

Systemic antipruritics can be helpful, but not uniformly so. Antihistamines are widely used as a treatment for chronic itch in systemic diseases. However, conventional doses of antihistamines, either sedating first-generation or nonsedating second-generation antihistamines have not yet proven effective in controlled studies. Fexofenadine 180 mg can be an effective first-line antihistamine. An antidepressant with H1/H2 antihistamine activity, doxepin, can be very helpful in some patients. It should be taken every 24 h and timed for several hours before bed so that the peak effect occurs during deep sleep. Gabapentin and pregabalin are antiepileptic and anxiolytic drugs which are also used in neuropathic pain and chronic severe pruritus [13].

Telangiectasias

Telangiectasias (also termed telangiectases) are a hallmark of scleroderma skin disease and are now included in the EULAR/ACR systemic sclerosis classification criteria [14]. They blanch on diascopy and represent dilated postcapillary venules without evidence of inflammation or neovascularization. They can be seen in both limited and diffuse forms of SSc and are more evident in patients with lighter skin. Interestingly, the number of telangiectasias increases with disease duration, even in cases when the skin and other manifestations of the disease seem clinically quiescent. The lesions are apparent first on the face, fingers, palms, and mucous membranes, and then later in the disease course appear on the arms and trunk (chest and back). Rarely, they are seen on the legs and feet. It is hypothesized that they may arise due to decreased oxygen tension in the skin and are a clinical biomarker of microvascular pathology as the extent of telangiectasias has been shown to correlate with a more severe vascular phenotype [15] with increased right ventricular systolic pressure and the development of pulmonary hypertension in scleroderma patients [16, 17].

Stellate telangiectasias, which are more linear, can be seen in any form of scleroderma. Geometric mat telangiectasias are most prominently seen in limited SSc, but are also a component of diffuse disease. They can also be seen concurrently, with mat telangiectasias against a background of less prominent stellate telangiectasias (Fig. 33.3). Mat telangiectasias are often evident on the lips (Fig. 33.4) and, as a presenting sign can be confused with Osler-Weber-Rendu disease (hereditary hemorrhagic telangiectasia, HHT). However, recurrent epistaxis is pathognomonic of HHT rather than scleroderma; HHT patients often have arteriovenous malformations in the lungs and other organs that are not seen in scleroderma, and HHT does not have associated skin fibrosis. Rarely, cutaneous telangiectasias can bleed, most commonly on thin mucous membranes such as the lip and nasal mucosa. Telangiectasias should not be confused with rosacea. Rosacea is a common disease and is characterized by a more diffuse spreading of telangiectatic vessels involving the nose and cheeks.

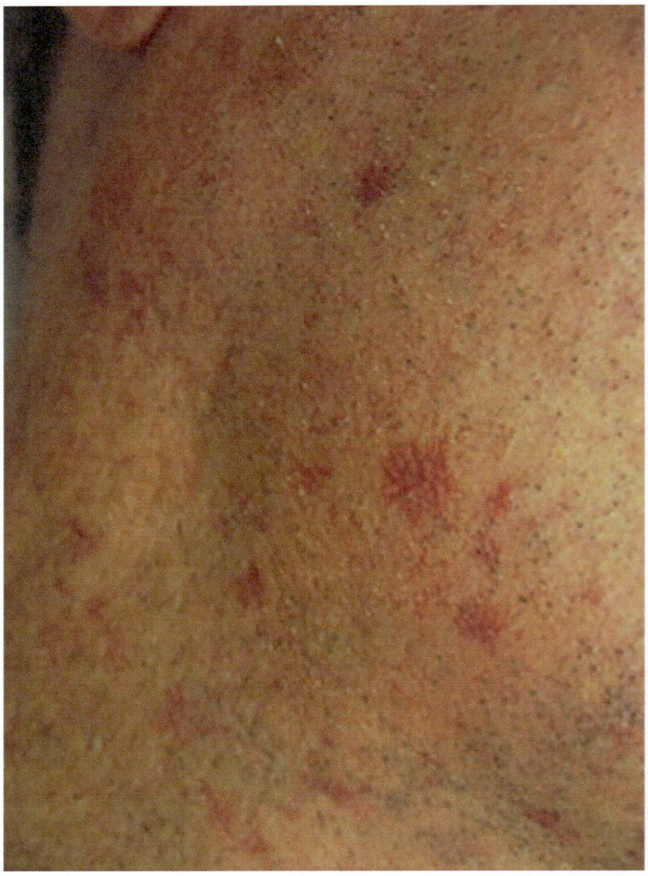

Fig. 33.3 Mat telangiectasias adjacent to stellate telangiectasias. (Courtesy of F.M. Wigley)

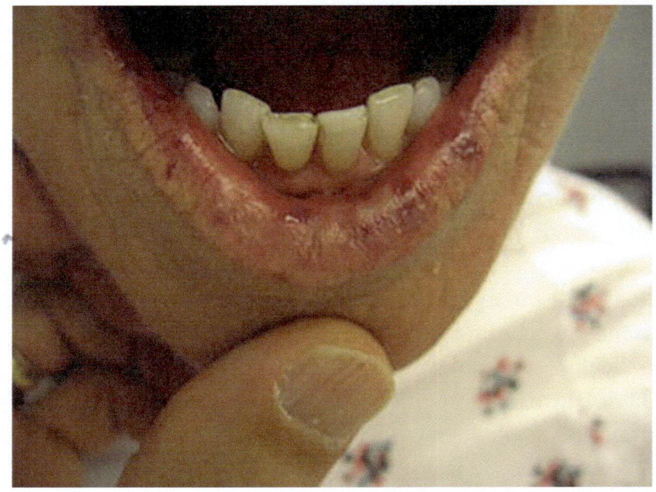

Fig. 33.4 Mat telangiectasias on the lips. (Courtesy of F.M. Wigley)

Treatment

Telangiectasias involving the face are perceived by many patients as a stigma of their disease and can significantly affect their quality of life. Telangiectasias can be treated safely and effectively with laser therapy. Either intense pulsed light (IPL) with a 560 nm or similar filter depending on the device, the 585-nm or 595-nm pulsed dye laser, or the 1064-nm Nd:YAG laser are effective modalities [18, 19]. Usually, several treatments are needed for optimal result. Since these laser treatments are nonablative (do not disrupt the integrity of the epidermis), there is no risk for infection or scarring unless blistering results from excessive energy delivered from the laser. With appropriate settings, this is a rare complication. Posttreatment purpura is common when a pulsed dye laser is used. The associated discomfort is brief and minimal. In general, a test spot should be performed before an entire area is treated. Laser treatment is often possible in darker skin types by decreasing the fluence and increasing the pulse width, with caution not to cause depigmentation. Telangiectasias tend to reaccumulate over time, generally making repeated treatments necessary; this may pose a cost issue for patients as insurance companies often deem treatment to be cosmetic and may not reimburse costs associated with laser therapy. Specialized cosmetics (camouflage) are also often used to cover the affected areas.

Dyspigmentation

The prevalence of skin pigmentation disorders in SSc patients has recently reported to reach more than 30% [20]. Three types have been described, i.e., salt and pepper dyspigmentation, diffuse hyperpigmentation, and combined hyper- and hypopigmentation.

Salt and pepper leukoderma is frequently seen in association with the diffuse form of systemic sclerosis, more commonly than in the limited or localized forms. It manifests as patches of depigmentation with preserved perifollicular pigmentation. This results in a speckled appearance resembling salt and pepper (Fig. 33.5a, b). By contrast, vitiligo is characterized by depigmented maculae without perifollicular sparing (Fig. 33.6), typically favoring the hands, genitalia, and peri-ocular, -oral skin. A Wood's lamp (320–400 nm) examination can demonstrate whether depigmentation (total loss of pigment) versus hypopigmentation (partial loss of pigment) has occurred, as depigmentation will fluoresce with a brighter blue-white than will hypopigmentation.

In some cases of systemic sclerosis, patients will develop a diffuse hyperpigmentation, also called melanoderma. Diffuse hyperpigmentation appears to be associated with a more severe disease course, e.g., digital ulcers and diffuse SSc [20]. Melanoderma in the context of SSc has to be differentiated from similar changes seen, e.g., in adrenal insufficiency.

The pathogenesis of salt and pepper leukoderma is unclear but probably relates to an autoimmune assault on melanocytes, with the perifollicular-sparing reflecting sites of comparative immune privilege. Vitiligo also remains idiopathic, but humoral and cellular immune activity against melanocytes is hypothesized.

Combined hyper- and hypopigmentation reflecting inflammatory or postinflammatory changes is seen commonly in scleroderma. After an inflammatory phase has resolved, hypopigmentation or hyperpigmentation may remain in that area for at least a year. Postinflammatory pigmentation changes are often more ill-defined than the pigmentary change seen in vitiligo or salt and pepper leukoderma.

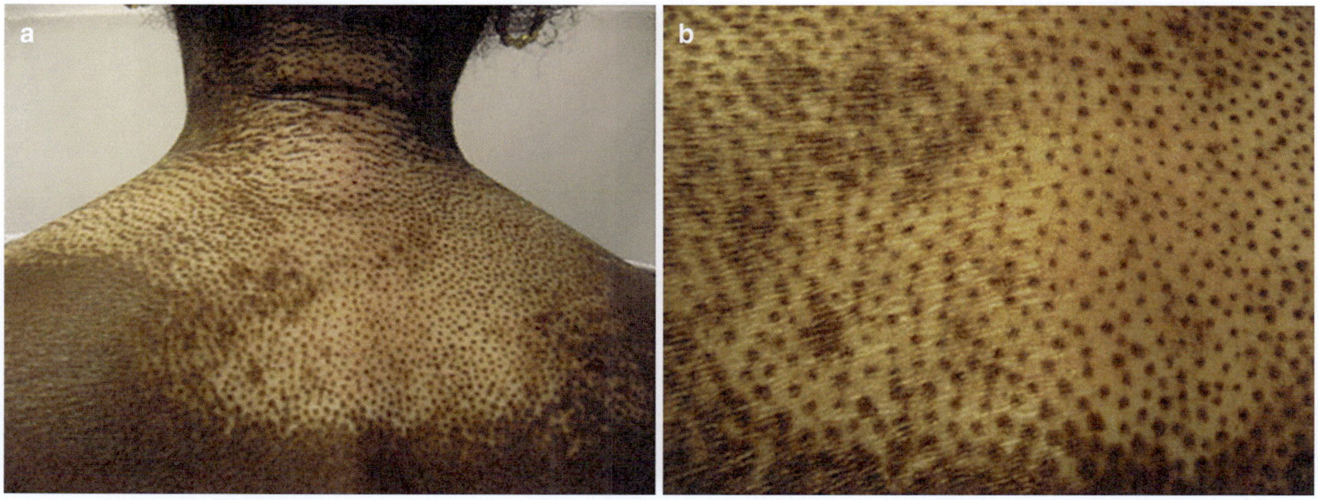

Fig. 33.5 (**a**) Salt and pepper leukoderma. (**b**) Preservation of perifollicular pigmentation in salt and pepper leukoderma. (Courtesy of F.M. Wigley)

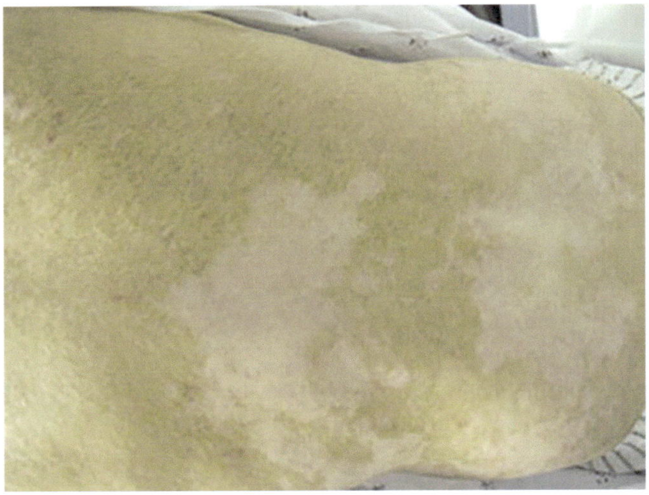

Fig. 33.6 Vitiligo in diffuse scleroderma. (Courtesy of F.M. Wigley)

Treatment

Salt and pepper leukoderma is notoriously difficult to treat. NBUVB would be the first-line phototherapy approach and may induce pigmentation in a minority of patients. Patients who have not improved could progress to PUVA photochemotherapy. The excimer laser (308 nm) offers targeted UVB treatment of vitiligo so that nonlesional skin does not get unnecessary UV exposure, and adjunct treatment with topical vitamin D derivatives may augment its efficacy per a left/right comparative single-blinded clinical trial [21].

Repigmentation in vitiligo occurs perifollicularly first, giving an appearance similar to salt and pepper leukoderma. For either condition, if no significant improvement is noted after 3 months of dose- and frequency-optimized phototherapy, it should be discontinued as perpetual intense UV exposure can increase the risk of skin cancer.

Since vitiligo and leukoderma are not a dangerous condition and more of a cosmetic concern, the long-term use of high-potency topical steroids is inadvisable, particularly in scleroderma, as it can cause significant epidermal atrophy with prominent telangiectasias.

Postinflammatory hyperpigmentation can be challenging to treat in scleroderma skin, as commonly prescribed hydroquinone compounds may provoke treatment-limiting inflammation. Hydroquinone, a tyrosinase inhibitor, needs to be compounded with a steroid, a retinoid, and an antioxidant for optimal pigment lightening effect; however, increasing the steroid level to prevent inflammation of scleroderma skin that can be easily sensitized from the hydroquinone and retinoid can lead to skin atrophy. Nonprescription skin brighteners that are very effective against postinflammatory hyperpigmentation have emerged, such as Elure Advanced Brightening Lotion which uses lignin peroxidase as an alternative to a tyrosinase inhibitor and does not cause treatment-related inflammation, thus making it suitable for sensitive or sensitized skin. In combination with mineral sunscreens applied rigorously in sun-exposed areas, these topical skin brighteners can improve postinflammatory hyperpigmentation significantly. Specialized cosmetics (camouflage) are often used to cover the affected, visible areas such as the face.

Nail Involvement in SSc

Nail involvement in SSc is often an under reported manifestation of SSc. Prolonged tissue ischemia can lead to fibrosis of the matrix that manifests with beaking as a form of pseudoclubbing of the nails (Fig. 33.7). This is also known as "parrot beak nails." Inflammation of the matrix can lead to pitting (Fig. 33.8) or beading—larger teardrop-shaped indentations in the nail plate. The periungual skin can become hyperkeratotic due to xerosis and inflammation, leading to ragged cuticles (Fig. 33.9). Pterygium inversum unguium, in which the distal nail groove is obliterated by an aberrant connection between the nail plate and the hyponychium, can result from ischemia [22]. Here the hyponychium attaches to the underside of the nail as it grows. Splinter hemorrhages may also be present. Typically distal splinter hemorrhages may appear secondary to trauma (Fig. 33.10), and proximal splinter hemorrhages often reflect vascular injury. In a single center study evaluating nail changes in SSc, patients had fre-

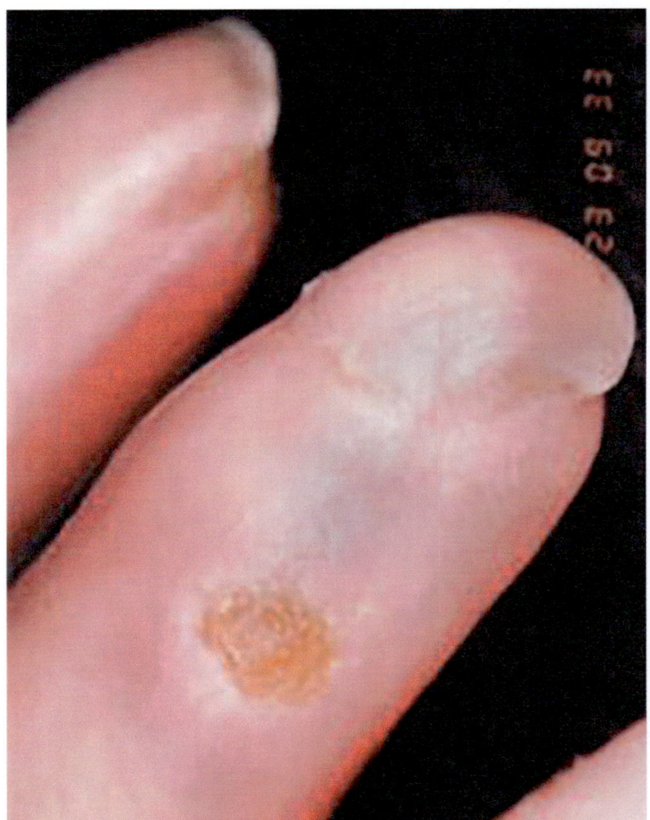

Fig. 33.7 Beaking of the nails. (Courtesy of F.M. Wigley)

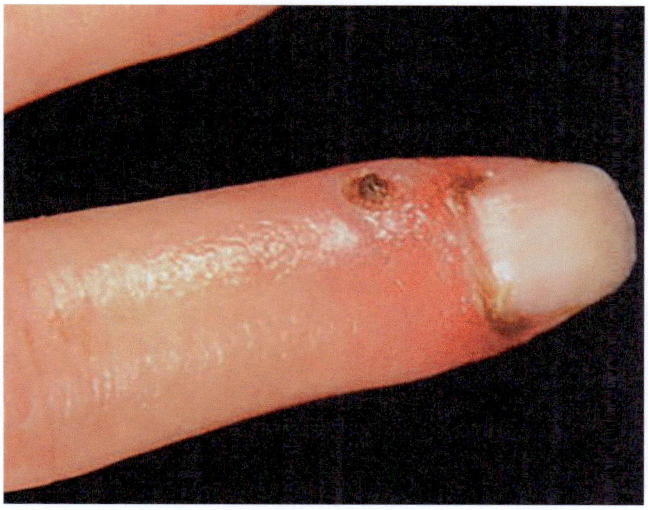

Fig. 33.8 Nail plate pitting. (Courtesy of F.M. Wigley)

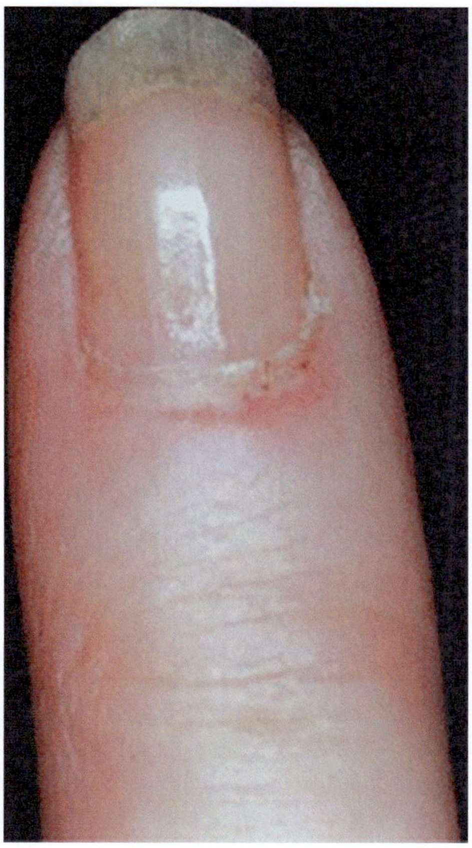

Fig. 33.9 Ragged cuticles. (Courtesy of F.M. Wigley)

quent surface abnormalities including longitudinal ridging (53.5%), thickened (41.1%) and irregular (40.3%) cuticles, scleronychia (thickening of nails) (41.1%), hyponychium hyperkeratosis (thickening of skin under the nail) (37.2%), pterygium inversum unguis (17.1%), and splinter hemorrhages (32.6%) [23].

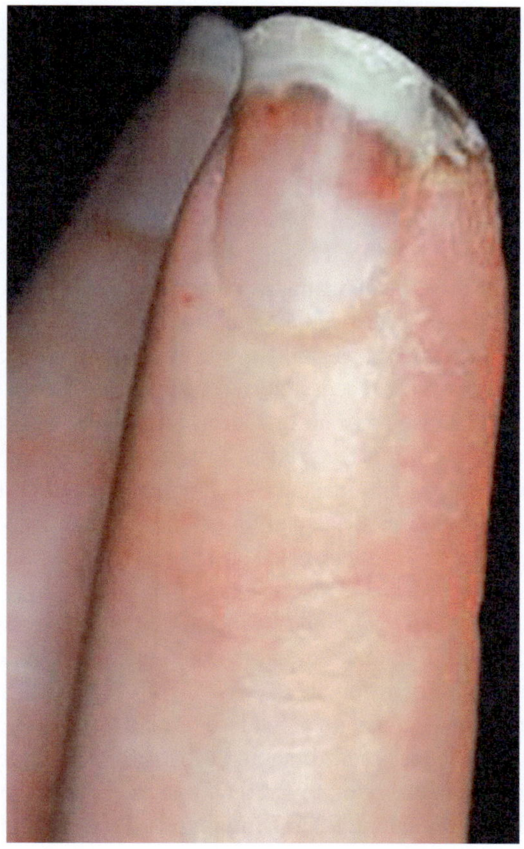

Fig. 33.10 Distal splinter hemorrhages secondary to trauma. (Courtesy of F.M. Wigley)

Treatment

Topical agents penetrate the nail plate poorly, so onychodystrophy is difficult to treat topically. For ragged cuticles, a steroid-containing nongreasy treatment such as Locoid Lipocream® (hydrocortisone butyrate 0.1% cream) is generally well tolerated at bedtime for flare-ups. For the daytime, barrier creams such as MimyX® can work very well to minimize xerosis of the skin of the hands and periungual area when used every morning. Additionally, over the counter cuticle creams work well to keep the area moisturized and can be reapplied throughout the day.

Orofacial Manifestations

Microstomia and mouth furrowing are the top orofacial concerns for adults with SSc [24]. Microstomia or limited mouth opening is a common and debilitating cutaneous manifestation of SSc. It is present in approximately 43–80% of adults with SSc [25, 26]. Microstomia is mainly caused by submucosal collagen deposits that contribute to fibrosis in the perioral tissue. This results in difficulty with eating, speaking, oral hygiene, and dental care.

Treatment

Historically oral aperture exercises have been used for the treatment of microstomia. Naylor and colleagues compared mouth-stretching and oral augmentation exercises to a set of traditional orofacial grimacing exercises in a randomized, controlled trial in nine patients with SSc (five in the experimental group, four in the comparison group). Both groups showed an increase in maximal oral aperture after 3 months of exercise, but no statistically significant difference was found between the two groups, perhaps due to insufficient statistical power [27]. A more recent study evaluated the effect of a home orofacial exercise program in which participants with an oral aperture of <40 mm received an orofacial exercise program which included daily manual mouth-stretching and oral augmentation exercises twice daily for 6 min for 6 months [28]. While the study did not meet the primary endpoint at 6 months, larger oral aperture was noted at 3 months.

More recently hyaluronidase injections have been reported as a possible treatment strategy to provide some relief for patients with microstomia [29]. As SSc fibrosis is associated with increased deposition of hyaluronic acid and collagen, the hyaluronidase treatment is thought to work by hydrolyzing these components to improve skin tightening. The use of adipose tissue as a natural filler to improve contours and enhance remodeling is increasingly being investigated and improvement of oral opening has been observed [30]. It is assumed that mesenchymal stem-like cells, endothelial progenitor cells present in the grafted fat, mediate this process [31].

Ulcerations

Ulcerations can be related to several etiologies in scleroderma. Ischemic skin ulcers are discussed in a separate section of this book. Traumatic ulcerations occur readily in the setting of sclerodactyly, particularly over the interphalangeal joints (Fig. 33.11), and often occur on the ears, elbows, and ankle areas. Ulcerations over the distal interphalangeal joints (DIP) and proximal interphalangeal joints (PIP) in particular relate to repetitive microtrauma over tightened skin with decreased blood flow resulting in poor wound healing. Ulcerations on the distal fingertips can be secondary to trauma, but often are primarily ischemic in origin (Fig. 33.12). A clue to this is surrounding pale cool skin. Shallow ulcers can also be seen in the setting of skin fragility. Ulcers that are monomorphic and linear are likely the result of excoriations, while those that are more ill-defined likely relate to associated xerosis and dermatitis. Other reported causes of skin ulcerations in scleroderma patients include complications of calcinosis cutis or paronychia, cutaneous vasculitis, and rarely, bullous pemphigoid or pyoderma gangrenosum.

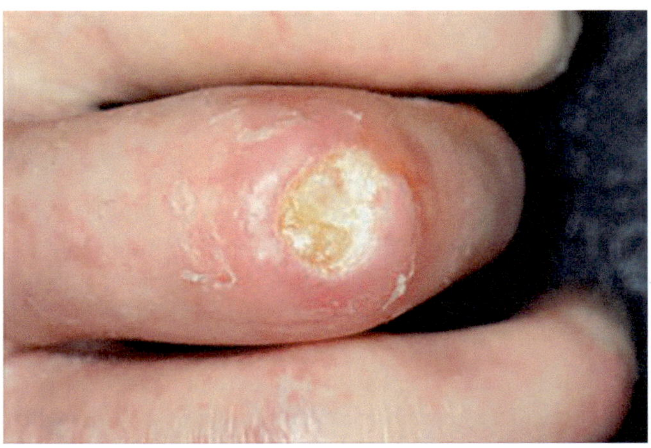

Fig. 33.11 Traumatic ulceration over interphalangeal joint

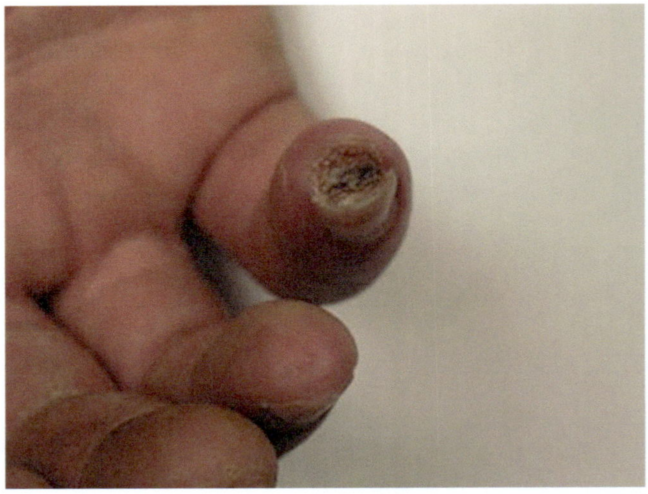

Fig. 33.12 Ischemic fingertip ulceration. (Courtesy of F.M. Wigley)

Treatment

Fingertip ulcers must be protected from trauma and infection. Keeping an ulcer moist significantly aids in wound healing. For ulcers with surrounding erythema, edema, warmth, or tenderness, a culture should be the first step to assess whether an ulcer is infected and whether systemic antibiotics are needed. For infected ulcers, silver-containing dressings are optimal for their antimicrobial benefits. Since the silver ions confer the antimicrobial effect, a moist wound bed is essential for those dressings to be effective. For infected ulcers with exudate, or for noninfected ulcers with exudate in which you want to prevent secondary infection, silver-containing hydrofiber dressings like Aquacel Ag (available over the counter) are an ideal choice as they absorb drainage, protect the skin, and prevent infection. For infected ulcers without exudate, mupirocin 2% ointment can be used to moisten the wound bed before application of the silver-containing dressing. Of note, many silver-containing dressings contain sulfa and should be used with caution in sulfa-allergic patients. For noninfected ulcers without exudate, the healing area should be kept moist with Vaseline or Aquaphor and should be protected from trauma with gel blister pads or similar cushioned bandage. Wet-to-dry dressings are not optimal as they tend to pull viable tissue away from the wound bed with each dressing change and therefore slow the healing process.

Pain can be a treatment challenge in the management of ulcers. Topical anesthetics such as ELMA or lidocaine ointment should be avoided as they commonly provoke skin irritation and contact dermatitis that can be difficult to distinguish from signs of infection and can slow wound healing. Appropriate wound dressings are a better solution for pain management and can reduce pain to a far greater degree than topical anesthetics are able. Additionally, wound dressings shield the healing skin from trauma. For a painful dry ulcer that is noninfected, a hydrogel dressing like Curagel keeps the wound moist and reduces pain significantly by decreasing nerve impulses that transmit the sensation of pain. Hydrogels donate moisture to the wound for an optimal healing environment, but must be applied under Adaptiq or other Vaseline-impregnated gauze as a secondary dressing to maintain moisture. Hydrogels should not be used on tunneled ulcers as they can form a gelatinous mass that is difficult to remove completely. Hydrogel dressings should be changed daily. If this is difficult for a particular patient due to sclerodactyly or other concerns, hydrocolloid dressings can be left in place for up to 7 days. To avoid skin tearing after prolonged wear of a hydrocolloid dressing, patients should be cautioned to lift a corner of the dressing and stretch it parallel to the skin before attempting to remove it, so that the adhesive bonds break for easier removal [32]. For painful noninfected ulcers with exudate, a silver-containing hydrofiber dressing reduces wound pain similar to a hydrogel or hydrocolloid does in dry wounds.

If an ulcer heals with excess granulation tissue, topical in-office application of silver nitrate is a very effective treatment. Several treatments may be needed, and patients should be advised that the treated tissue will look gray or black and that this is not a cause for alarm but rather the result of silver transferring onto the skin.

Topical antibiotics can be useful in preventing secondary infection or treating mild superficial infection, but over-the-counter options such as Neosporin and bacitracin frequently incite an allergic or irritant contact dermatitis when used on compromised skin such as the site of an ulcer. Even if a patient has used these topical antibiotics previously without a reaction, mupirocin 2% ointment (Bactroban) is a better choice for ulcer treatment since it very rarely causes dermatitis on wounds and protects against MRSA, which is increasingly common in wounds of patients with frequent hospital contact.

To clean the ulcerated area between dressing changes, a dilute vinegar solution is gentle and effective at treating bacterial and fungal colonization. This solution can be prepared at home by mixing one teaspoon of plain white vinegar with two cups of water. To use, patients should dip a clean, soft cloth into the vinegar solution, place the wet cloth against the affected area gently pressing to ensure that the vinegar solution wets the skin, and then rinse and repeat for 10–15 min. The antibiotic ointment or gelatinous residue from a hydrogel dressing should be readily removed through this soaking process without any rubbing of the skin needed. Bleach soaks are another good option for wound cleaning in between dressing changes, but should not exceed 0.025% in concentration.

Wound care can be discontinued when an ulcer reepithelializes completely. In general, it is not advisable to let ulcers develop an eschar as this will slow healing. However, for very small punctate ulcers that will heal quickly by secondary intention, this may be reasonable management.

Future Directions

The next steps forward in skin-directed therapy of scleroderma will capitalize on the progress in systemically applied drugs as well as drug delivery systems for topical therapies. For instance, mediators of type 2 inflammation are increasingly recognized as a potential treatment target to modulate inflammatory processes in the skin. Janus kinase (JAK) inhibitors affecting these pathways are currently in development for systemic and topical treatment. Encouraging results are already reported for the use of JAK inhibition in diffuse cutaneous systemic sclerosis and in other diseases, e.g., graft versus host disease, vitiligo, and pruritus [33, 34]. Additionally, advances in autologous tissue transfer are emerging as a means of inducing tissue remodeling in areas affected by atrophy and fibrosis. The ability to treat the cutaneous manifestations of scleroderma without systemic morbidities stemming from immunosuppression or immunomodulation will be a significant advance in the field and offers an exciting opportunity to mollify what has to date been one of the most problematic areas of scleroderma skin disease management.

References

1. Usmani N, Murphy A, Veale D, et al. Photochemotherapy for systemic sclerosis: effect on clinical and molecular markers. Clin Exp Dermatol. 2010;35:608–13.
2. Morita A, Kobayashi K, Isomura I, Tsuji T, Krutmann J. UVA1 phototherapy for scleroderma in systemic sclerosis. J Am Acad Dermatol. 2000;43(4):670–4.

3. Connolly KL, Griffith JL, McEvoy M, Lim HW. Ultraviolet A1 phototherapy beyond morphea: experience in 83 patients. Photodermatol Photoimmunol Photomed. 2015;31(6):289–95.
4. Patel RV, Clark LN, Lebwohl M, et al. Treatments for psoriasis and the risk of malignancy. J Am Acad Dermatol. 2009;60:1001–7.
5. Breuckmann F, Gambichler T, Altmeyer P, Kreuter A. UVA/UVA1 phototherapy and PUVA photochemotherapy in connective tissue diseases and related disorders: a research based review. BMC Dermatol. 2004;4(1):11.
6. Knobler RM, French LE, Kim Y, Bisaccia E, Graninger W, Nahavandi H, et al. A randomized, double-blind, placebo-controlled trial of photopheresis in systemic sclerosis. J Am Acad Dermatol. 2006;54(5):793–9.
7. Enomoto DN, Mekkes JR, Bossuyt PM, Yong SL, Out TA, Hoekzema R, et al. Treatment of patients with systemic sclerosis with extracorporeal photochemotherapy (photopheresis). J Am Acad Dermatol. 1999;41(6):915–22.
8. Onesti MG, Troccola A, Scuderi N. Volumetric correction using poly-L-lactic acid in facial asymmetry: Parry Romberg syndrome and scleroderma. Dermatol Surg. 2009;35:1368–75.
9. Barin EZ, Cinal H, Cakmak MA, Tan O. Treatment of linear scleroderma (en coup de sabre) with dermal fat grafting. J Cutan Med Surg. 2016;20(3):269–71.
10. Razykov I, Thombs BD, Hudson M, Bassel M, Baron M, Canadian Scleroderma Research Group. Prevalence and clinical correlates of pruritus in patients with systemic sclerosis. Arthritis Rheum. 2009;61(12):1765–70.
11. Razykov I, Levis B, Hudson M, Baron M, Thombs BD, Canadian Scleroderma Research Group. Prevalence and clinical correlates of pruritus in patients with systemic sclerosis: an updated analysis of 959 patients. Rheumatology (Oxford). 2013;52(11):2056–61.
12. Stander S, Weisshaar E, Mettang T, Szepietowski JC, Carstens E, Ikoma A, et al. Clinical classification of itch: a position paper of the International Forum for the Study of Itch. Acta Derm Venereol. 2007;87(4):291–4.
13. Kaur R, Sinha VR. Antidepressants as antipruritic agents: a review. Eur Neuropsychopharmacol. 2018;28(3):341–52.
14. van den Hoogen F, Khanna D, Fransen J, Johnson SR, Baron M, Tyndall A, et al. 2013 classification criteria for systemic sclerosis: an American College of Rheumatology/European League Against Rheumatism Collaborative Initiative. Ann Rheum Dis. 2013;72:1747–55.
15. Hurabielle C, Avouac J, Lepri G, de Risi T, Kahan A, Allanore Y. Skin teleangiectasia and the identification of a subset of systemic sclerosis patients with severe vascular disease. Arthritis Care Res (Hoboken). 2016;68:1021–7.
16. Shah AA, Wigley FM, Hummers LK. Telangiectases in scleroderma: a potential clinical marker of pulmonary arterial hypertension. J Rheumatol. 2010;37:98–104.
17. Jouvray M, Launay D, Dubucquoi S, Sobanski V, Podevin C, Lambert M, et al. Whole body distribution and clinical association of teleangiectases in systemic sclerosis. JAMA Dermatol. 2018;154(7):796–805.
18. Halachmi S, Gabari O, Cohen S, Koren R, Amitai DB, Lapidoth M. Telangiectasis in CREST syndrome and systemic sclerosis: correlation of clinical and pathological features with response to pulsed dye laser treatment. Lasers Med Sci. 2014;29:137–40.
19. Dinsdale G, Murray A, Moore T, Ferguson J, Wilkinson J, Richards H, Griffiths CE, Herrick AL. A comparison of intense pulsed light and laser treatment of telangiectases in patients with systemic sclerosis: a within-subject randomized trial. Rheumatology (Oxford). 2014;53:1422–30.
20. Leroy V, Henrot P, Barnetche T, Cario M, Darrigade AS, Manicki P, et al. Association of skin hyperpigmentation disorders with digital ulcers in systemic sclerosis: analysis of a cohort of 239 patients. J Am Acad Dermatol. 2019;80(2):478–84.
21. Goldinger SM, Dummer R, Schmid P, et al. Combination of 308-nm xenon chloride Excimer laser and topical calcipotriol in vitiligo. J Eur Acad Dermatol Venereol. 2007;21:504–8.
22. Sherber NS, Wigley FM, Scher RK. Autoimmune disorders: nail signs and therapeutic approaches. Dermatol Ther. 2007;20:17–30.
23. Marie I, Gremain V, Nassermadji K, Richard L, Joly P, Menard JF, Levesque H. Nail involvement in systemic sclerosis. J Am Acad Dermatol. 2017;76(6):1115–23. https://doi.org/10.1016/j.jaad.2016.11.024. Epub 2016 Dec 20. PMID: 28010889
24. Paquette DL, Falanga V. Cutaneous concerns of scleroderma patients. J Dermatol. 2003;30:438–43.
25. Eversole LR, Jacobsen PL, Stone CE. Oral and gingival changes in systemic sclerosis (scleroderma). J Periodontol. 1984;55:175–8.
26. Scardina GA, Messina P. Systemic sclerosis: description and diagnostic role of the oral phenomena. Gen Dent. 2004;52:42–7.
27. Naylor WP, Douglass CW, Mix E. The nonsurgical treatment of microstomia in scleroderma: a pilot study. Oral Surg Oral Med Oral Pathol. 1984;57:508–11.
28. Yuen HK, Marlow NM, Reed SG, Mahoney S, Summerlin LM, Leite R, et al. Effect of orofacial exercises on oral aperture in adults with systemic sclerosis. Disabil Rehabil. 2012;34(1):84–9.
29. Melvin OG, Hunt KM, Jacobson ES. Hyaluronidase treatment of scleroderma-induced microstomia. JAMA Dermatol. 2019;155(7):857–9.
30. Del Papa N, Caviggioli F, Sambataro D, Zaccara E, Vinci V, Di Luca G, et al. Autologous fat grafting in the treatment of fibrotic perioral changes in patients with systemic sclerosis. Cell Transplant. 2015;24(1):63–72.
31. Daumas A, Magalon J, Delaunay F, Abellan M, Philandrianos C, Sabatier F, et al. Fat grafting for treatment of facial scleroderma. Clin Plast Surg. 2020;47(1):155–63.
32. Lee JC, Kandula S, Sherber NS. Beyond wet-to-dry: a rational approach to treating chronic wounds. Eplasty. 2009;9:e14.
33. Solimani F, Meier K, Ghoreschi K. Emerging topical and systemic JAK inhibitors in dermatology. Front Immunol. 2019;10:2847.
34. Khanna D, Bush E, Nagaraja V, Koenig A, Khanna P, Young A, et al. Tofacitinib in early diffuse cutaneous systemic sclerosis—results of phase I/II investigator initiated, double-blind randomized placebo-controlled trial [abstract]. Arthritis Rheumatol. 2019;71(Suppl 10):1–3.

Calcinosis

34

Antonia Valenzuela and Lorinda Chung

Introduction

Calcinosis cutis is the deposition of insoluble calcium in the skin and subcutaneous tissues. It is a manifestation of several autoimmune connective tissue diseases (ACTDs) including systemic sclerosis (SSc). Calcinosis has a substantial impact on quality of life as it is often associated with pain, and functional impairment. Herein, we review the most current knowledge regarding associated clinical factors, pathogenesis, diagnostic approach, and treatment options.

Definition of Calcinosis

Calcinosis cutis is a disorder characterized by calcium deposition in the skin and subcutaneous tissues. It is associated with several autoimmune connective tissue diseases (ACTDs) including systemic sclerosis (SSc), dermatomyositis (DM), mixed connective tissue diseases (MCTDs), and, more rarely, systemic lupus erythematosus (SLE) [1]. There are five subtypes of calcinosis: dystrophic, metastatic, iatrogenic, idiopathic, and calciphylaxis [2]. Dystrophic calcinosis is the subtype associated with ACTD, and it is defined as the deposition of calcified material in damaged tissue in the setting of normal serum calcium and phosphate levels [3].

A. Valenzuela
Department of Clinical Immunology and Rheumatology, Pontificia Universidad Católica de Chile, Santiago, Chile
e-mail: antonia.valenzuela@uc.cl

L. Chung (✉)
Division of Immunology & Rheumatology, Stanford University School of Medicine and Palo Alto VA Health Care System, Palo Alto, CA, USA
e-mail: shauwei@stanford.edu

Epidemiology, Distribution, and Clinical Associations of Calcinosis in Systemic Sclerosis

Calcinosis is not uncommon in SSc, but the prevalence varies depending on racial backgroud. A large retrospective multicenter international cohort study led by the Scleroderma Clinical Trials Consortium (SCTC) of 5280 patients with SSc showed that 1290 patients (24.4%) had calcinosis, with similar prevalence estimates in Caucasians, African Americans, and Hispanic populations [4]. Moreover, a subsequent SCTC prospective study, which included 568 consecutive SSc patients, showed that 215 (38%) patients had calcinosis by imaging and/or physical examination [5]. However, in a multicenter study of 1009 African Americans patients with SSc, the prevalence of calcinosis was only 18% [6], while in Mexican and Malaysian cohorts, the estimated prevalence was 37% and 49% respectively [7, 8]. This large range is likely attributable to variable patient populations.

Calcinosis in SSc occurs most frequently in the hands [5, 7, 9], particularly the fingers, and within the fingers, most commonly in the thumbs or index of the dominant hand [10, 11]. Other locations are the arms/forearms (7–27%), knee/proximal lower extremity (10–22%), feet (18%), and hip (6.7%) [5, 12]. Calcinosis can also affect the trunk, chest, and buttocks, and more obscure locations such as the maxillary sinuses, breasts [13], and spinal and paraspinal tissues [14–18]. Interestingly, in a recent study of 77 SSc patients who had X-ray of the hands and thoracic or thoracoabdominal and pelvic CT scan or lumbar CT scan during the course of 1 year, 20 (26%) had calcinosis of the hands, and 64 (83%) exhibited at least one calcification of the spine, primarily the thoracic spine [19].

Calcinosis is known to be a long-term complication in SSc, presenting more than 10 years after the first non-Raynaud's symptom [4, 5]. Several clinical features have been found to be associated with calcinosis. One study of 103 consecutively recruited patients with SSc found that male gender and digital ulcers (DU) were significant inde-

Y. Allanore et al. (eds.), *Scleroderma*, https://doi.org/10.1007/978-3-031-40658-4_34

pendent predictive factors for radiological progression of calcinosis (HR 3.99, 95% CI 1.45–12.13, and HR 3.16, 95% CI 1.22–9.43, respectively) [20]. Several studies have confirmed the association between the presence of calcinosis and DU [4–6, 20–23], as well as with other microvascular disease manifestations of SSc, such as late nailfold capillary pattern [24, 25], and acroosteolysis [5, 26]. In addition, an association with macrovascular disease, specifically with ulnar artery occlusion, has also been described, even in the absence of DU [24, 27].

Traditionally, calcinosis has been linked to limited cutaneous SSc (lcSSc), in association with positive anticentromere antibody (ACA) [5, 28–30]. However, in Mexican, Canadian, and Malaysian cohorts, calcinosis was associated with diffuse cutaneous SSc (dcSSc) [7, 8, 23]. Similarly, antinucleolar and antitopoisomerase (Scl-70) antibodies were more prevalent in Mexican patients with calcinosis [7], and in a cohort of 1305 SSc patients from the Canadian Scleroderma Research Group (CSRG) registry, ACA but also RNA-polymerase-III antibody were predictors of calcinosis [23]. On the other hand, other studies have not found associations between calcinosis and cutaneous subtype, or a specific autoantibody profile [5, 6], suggesting that these may be influenced by ethnic background or geographic region. A more consistent association has been found between calcinosis and anti-PM/Scl (anti-PM-100 and anti-PM-75) autoantibody in SSc patients [4, 31–33], which has also been reported in DM patients [34]; however, since this autoantibody is only present in 2–11% of SSc patients [35], these results must be interpreted with caution.

Calcinosis has also been associated with an increased prevalence of vitamin D deficiency and secondary hyperparathyroidism, [36], osteoporosis [4, 37], and increased vertebral fracture [38] suggesting a potential role of bone metabolism in the pathogenesis of calcinosis. Another interesting study of a retrospective cohort of 199 SSc patients and a prospective cohort of 215 consecutive SSc patients found that the risk of calcinosis at any time was increased in those with more than 10 years of exposure to proton pump inhibitors (PPI) (OR = 1.04, $p < 0.001$). The authors hypothesized that PPI may promote tissue calcification via vascular endothelial cell injury [39].

Clinical Presentation and Complications of Calcinosis

Calcinosis usually presents as chalky-white to yellow papules, plaques or nodules of the dermis, panniculus or deeper subcutaneous structures (Fig. 34.1). More rarely, calcinosis may present as large calcified masses (pseudotumoral calcinosis) (Fig. 34.2). A recent study of 629 living and deceased SSc cases from two referrals centers in France and Italy showed that 19 (3%) living and 7 (1%) deceased patients were affected by pseudotumoral calcinosis, defined as calcinosis with a maximum diameter >2 cm, confirmed by imaging. Pseudotumoral calcinosis was commonly symmetrical, present in multiple sites, and often associated with a severe vascular phenotype [40]. Attempts to classify calcinosis according to their macroscopic and radiological features have been published. A study of 112 SSc patients (52 with calcinosis) divided 316 calcinotic lesions into visible/palpable (47.4%) and nonvisible/palpable (52.6%). Visible/palpable lesions were further clustered as mousse (31.8%) or stone (68.2%). All calcinotic lesions, both visible and nonvisible, were classified as stone (91.4%), net (3.8%), and plate (4.8%) based on X-ray appearance [9].

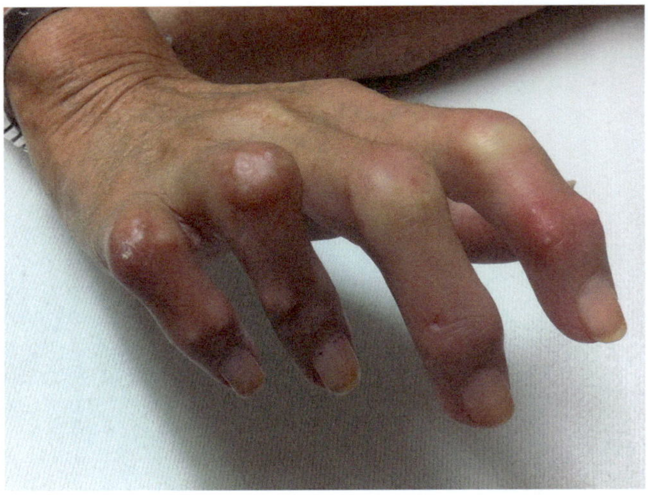

Fig. 34.1 Calcinosis of the fingers

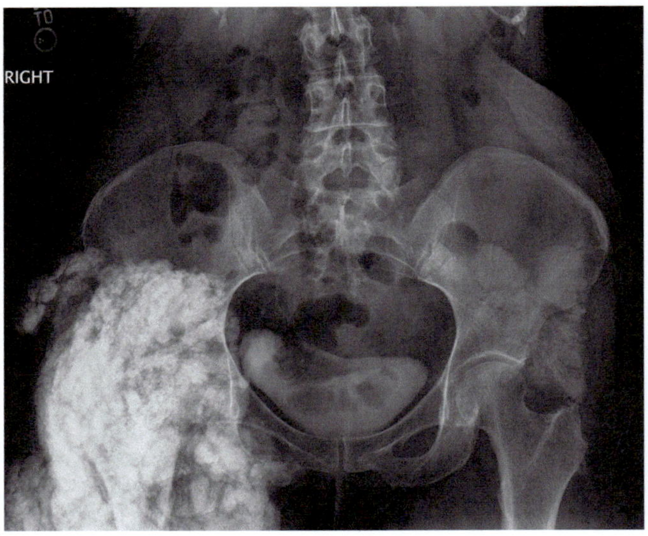

Fig. 34.2 Frontal radiograph of the right hip in a 57-year-old female with SSc demonstrates extensive pseudotumoral calcinosis around the hip, hemipelvis, and proximal thigh

SSc-related calcinosis tends to slowly progress over time. A single center study showed radiographic progression of calcinosis, defined as at least one new calcification or increase in the size of at least one calcification, in 27 patients (26%) of 103 consecutively recruited SSc patients [20]. A more recent prospective study of 39 SSc patients with calcinosis who had baseline and 1-year anteroposterior hand radiographs showed a median of progression of 12.8% as assessed by a radiologic scoring system specifically developed and validated for SSc-calcinosis (Scleroderma Clinical Trials Consortium (SCTC) radiologic scoring system) [41]. In this study, 16 patients (41%) experienced progression of calcinosis over 1 year; 18 (46%) remained stable; and 5 (13%) had improvement [42].

Common complications of calcinosis are pain/tenderness, impaired function, ulceration at the site of lesions, spontaneous extrusion of calcinosis through the skin, and infection [2, 5, 43]. Pain may be related to calcinosis over pressure areas or to associated inflammation. Importantly, calcinosis clearly worsens patients' disability, function, and symptoms, as demonstrated in the SCTC prospective study, where calcinosis was an independent predictor of dysfunction and pain as assessed by patient-reported outcomes, contributing as much as arthritis to the disability index [5]. Patients may also complain of a "toothpaste-like" material extruding from the skin, which can be a point of entry for infections. Spreading redness and thick green/yellow discharge from a lesion are signs of infection and warrant antibiotic therapy. When cultured, the most frequent organism identified has been *Staphylococcus aureus* [43, 44].

Composition of Calcinosis and Pathogenesis

The composition of SSc-related calcinosis resembles that of bone, with hydroxyapatite (HA) as the primary mineral component [45]. The analysis of spontaneously draining calcinosis material from ten SSc patients using X-ray diffraction, a tool for identifying precipitated crystallized phases, confirmed that HA—in variable proportions—was the only inorganic material. In addition, most drained samples contained >50% organic material as a minor component [46].

The detailed pathophysiology of calcinosis in SSc remains poorly understood. However, several mechanisms have been proposed, including vascular hypoxia, chronic tissue inflammation, recurrent trauma, and disruption in bone mineralization.

As mentioned above, several clinical studies suggest that vascular ischemia may contribute to calcinosis development [5, 6, 20, 23, 26, 47]. In addition, Davies et al. demonstrated increased expression of the hypoxia-associated glucose transporter molecule (GLUT-1) in skin biopsies of SSc patients with calcinosis [48]. Similarly, the same group evaluated the expression of recognized markers of oxidative stress, the advanced glycation/lipoperoxidation end products (AGEs), and their receptor (RAGE), and concluded that it was greater in the dermis of patients with SSc, especially in those with calcinosis, when compared to healthy controls [49]. Another study showed that upregulation of VEGF, a potent angiogenic factor induced by hypoxia, was associated with increased osteoclast activity in SSc patients with acroosteolysis, 73% of whom had calcinois [50]. This hypoxia-induced osteoclast activity in SSc may also be involved in the development of calcinosis, and we are currently evaluating this [6, 30, 37].

The role of chronic tissue inflammation in the subsequent development of calcinosis is unclear [1, 2, 51]. Inflammatory cell infiltration in and around calcinosis lesions has been described; however, inflammation may be a result rather than the actual cause of HA deposition [45]. Similar to vascular calcification, inflammation in association with premature cellular aging, and senescence promoted by persistent DNA damage by oxidative stress, may be a key pathway driving dystrophic calcification [52]. Particularly, interleukin-6 (IL-6), a procalcific inflammatory mediator in both vascular calcification and rheumatic calcinosis, has been proposed to be involved in driving these disorders [52].

The association between calcinosis and long disease duration indicates that cumulative disease damage may be important in the development of calcinosis. Likewise, the fact that the index finger and thumb are the two digits most affected by calcinosis raises the potential role for repetitive trauma in the pathogenesis of SSc-related calcinosis [10, 11]. As areas of recurrent trauma, they may be more susceptible to the development of calcinosis due to the impaired compensatory angiogenesis that characterizes the proliferative obliterative vasculopathy seen in the distal digits in SSc [53].

There is some evidence of systemic alterations in mineral metabolism in patients with SSc-associated calcinosis. Inorganic pyrophosphate (PPi) and inorganic phosphate (Pi) are important mediators of calcification, with PPi inhibiting and Pi promoting HA crystal growth [45]. Genetic mutations causing disruption of PPi/Pi metabolism pathways lead to various ectopic calcification phenotypes in humans, specifically pseudoxanthoma elasticum (PXE), generalized arterial calcification of infancy (GACI), and arterial calcification due to CD73 deficiency (ACDC), caused by mutations in ABCC6, ENPP1, and NT5E, respectively [54]. A study of 33 subjects (19 control and 14 SSc, 5 of whom had SSc-calcinosis) demonstrated the lowest mean PPi levels in the SSc-calcinosis group supporting the role of a systemic imbalance of mineralization inhibitors and promotors in SSc patients with calcinosis [55]. The development of mouse models that mimic heritable ectopic mineralization disorders, specifically PXE, GACI, and ACDC has helped in understanding the process leading to calcium deposition in the extracellular matrix [54, 56]. These conditions have phenotypic similarities with the "acquired" forms of dystrophic calcification. The ABCC6$^{-/-}$ mice develop mineral deposits in the extracellular matrix of connective tissues in a number of organs. These deposits have been found to consist of calcium and phosphate, forming HA crystals, similar to that in patients with SSc [57]. The ENPP1$^{-/-}$ mice lack nucleotide pyrophosphatase phosphodiesterase 1 (NPP1), which is involved in the formation of inorganic pyrophosphate (PPi) (inhibitor of hydroxyapatite crystal formation) [58]. These mice develop severe disruption to the architecture and mineralization of long bones, and dysregulation of calcium/phosphate homeostasis, confirming the critical role of PPi as an antimineralization factor [56]. NT5E$^{-/-}$ mice demonstrate periarticular and ligamentous calcification as well as increased Pi/PPi ratios [56]. This gene encodes CD73, which converts AMP to adenosine, supporting a role for this metabolic pathway in inhibiting ectopic tissue calcification [59].

Fetuin A, another known inhibitor of systemic calcification, was found to be significantly lower in serum of patients with calcinosis as compared to those without calcinosis in a study of 23 SSc patients (15 with calcinosis) [60]. Finally, circulating osteoprotegerin (OPG), the decoy receptor of the receptor activator of nuclear factor-κB ligand (RANKL), inhibits bone resorption and promotes mineralization. In one study, OPG levels were measured in 60 SSc patients, eight of whom had calcinosis, and found to be significantly higher in those with active DU and calcinosis. The authors hypothesize that this may be due to an inadequate compensatory response of OPG as an inhibitor of bone resorption [61]. Other regulators of calcification include osteonectine, a promoter of calcification, which has been found to be increased in endothelial cells and fibroblasts of SSc patients, particularly in those with calcinosis compared with those without calcinosis [62]. Poly(ADP-ribose) polymerase (PARP) enzymes are another proposed promoter of HA nucleation of mineralized deposits, and are overexpressed in response to DNA damage. Although not evaluated in SSc-related calcinosis, studies have demonstrated that overexpression of PARP-1 in rat aortas increased vascular calcification and osteogenic differentiation of vascular smooth muscle cells [63].

More studies are necessary to better define the roles of hypoxia, inflammation, and metabolic derangements in the pathogenesis of calcinosis and to identify other mechanisms that may be involved.

Diagnosis

While calcinosis is often clearly visible or palpable on physical exam, imaging can help confirm the diagnosis of subclinical deposits, and determine the extent and severity of calcinotic lesions. Plain radiography is the recommended initial imaging for calcinosis [64] given its low cost and comparable information to three-dimensional modalities [65] (Fig. 34.3). A radiographic scoring system for hand calcinosis was developed and validated to standardize the measurement of calcium deposits for clinical and research purposes [41]. This scoring system takes into account the hand area covered, density, number, and anatomic location of calcinosis lesions to provide an estimate of calcinosis burden, with excellent inter- and intra-rater reliability (ICC = 0.89, 95% CI 0.86–0.92, and ICC = 0.89, 95% CI 0.8–0.97, respectively). Another X-ray-based classification of calcinosis has also been proposed based on shapes and patterns of the lesions [9]. This approach divides clinically nonvisible but palpable cal-

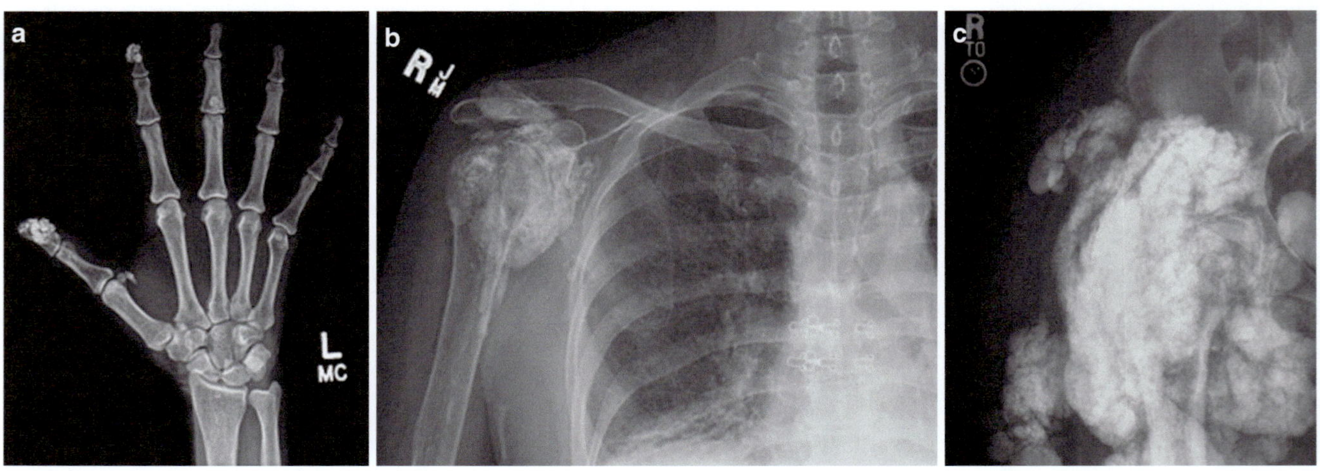

Fig. 34.3 (**a**) "Wet cotton-wool appearance" of calcinosis on radiography of the hands. (**b**) Anteroposterior radiograph of the right shoulder in a 58-year-old female with long-standing scleroderma demonstrates calcinosis around the glenohumeral and acromioclavicular joints, with calcification extending distally along the bicipital groove. Linear opacities are seen at the right lung base compatible with the underlying interstitial lung disease related to scleroderma. (**c**) Frontal radiograph of the right hip in a 57-year-old female with scleroderma demonstrates extensive calcinosis around the hip, hemipelvis, and proximal thigh

cinosis into three subtypes: stone, net, and plate. The authors showed that the net form took the longest time to heal (mean 140 ± 22 days), while stone calcinosis took the shortest (30 ± 12 days), suggesting that this categorization has clinical significance in the management and prognosis of calcinosis.

Calcinosis is also amenable to evaluation by ultrasound (US), which, although operator-dependent, has the benefits of being a noninvasive, nonionizing, point of care imaging modality (Fig. 34.4). Calcinosis in US can be identified as hyperechoic lesions with or without shadowing, located in the skin, soft tissue, tendons, peritendinous or periarticular areas. Freire et al. detected calcinosis in 17/44 (39%) SSc patients using US with a high sensitivity (89%) compared to radiographs [66]. In a more recent study of 43 SSc patients (19 diffuse, 24 limited), US identified 13 (30.2%) patients with calcinosis, while calcinosis was seen in 17 (39.5%) patients by radiographs. Sensitivity and specificity for US were 61% and 95% by zone, 78% and 98% by hand, and 76% and 100% by patient, respectively [27].

Various forms of computerized tomography (CT) imaging have been examined for evaluation of calcinosis. Dual-energy computed tomography (DECT), a modern technique used for assessing monosodium urate deposits in soft tissue from patients with gout, has recently been proposed as a useful modality to evaluate SSc-calcinosis of the hands (Fig. 34.5). A study of 16 SSc patients with clinically

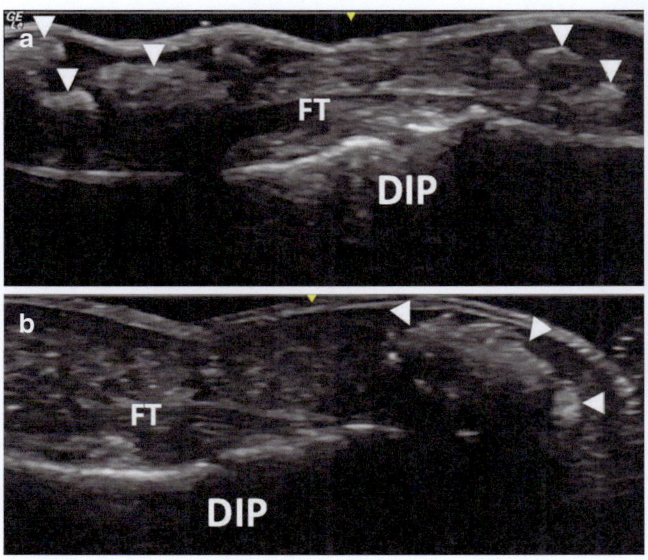

Fig. 34.4 Ultrasonography of the palmar aspect of two distal fingers with calcinosis. (**a**) Multiple calcinosis lesions (arrowheads) both proximal and distal to the DIP joint; increased density in these lesions to the left of the DIP (proximal) results in acoustic shadowing, unlike the less dense lesions to the right of the DIP (distal). (**b**) Ultrasound's submillimeter resolution can reveal fine structural detail as demonstrated in this fingertip calcinosis lesion (arrowheads). *FT* flexor tendon, *DIP* distal interphalangeal joint. (Courtesy of Dr. Robert Fairchild)

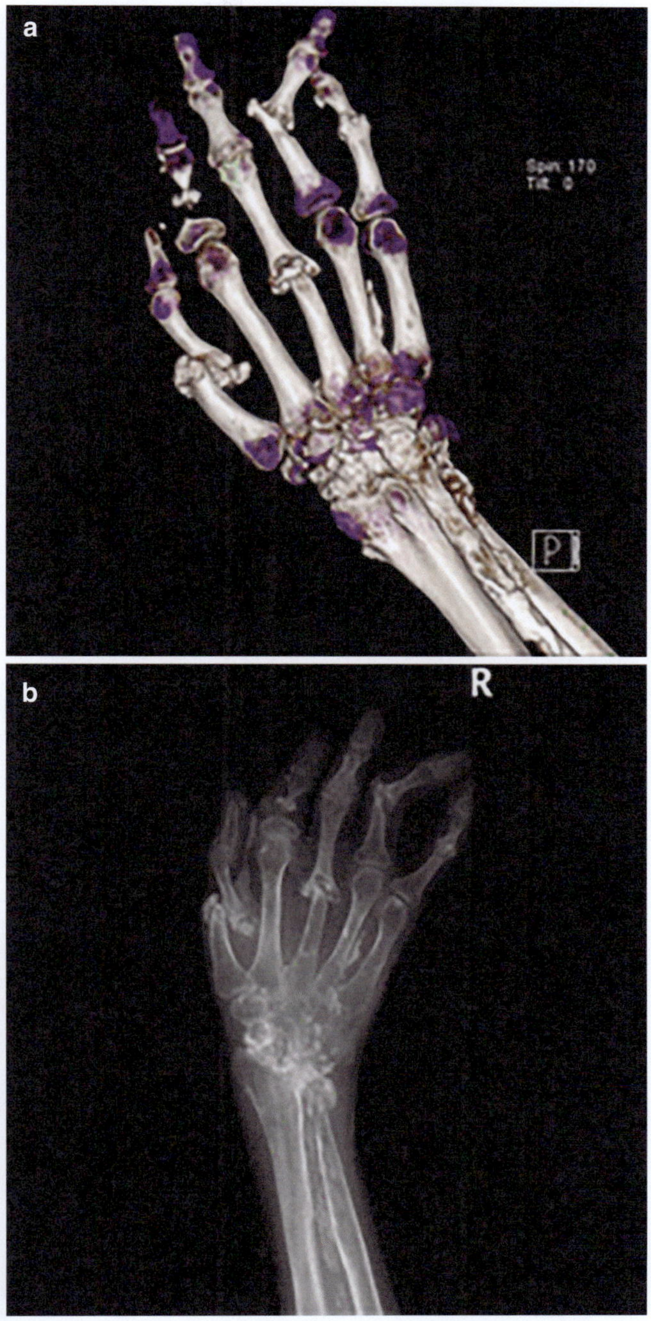

Fig. 34.5 Calcinosis in dual-energy computed tomography. Two views of the right hand with extensive calcinosis seen throughout the fingers and carpal bones and surrounding the remaining proximal second phalanx. (**a**) Dual-energy computed tomography. (**b**) Hand radiography. (Reprinted with permission from Hsu V et al. *J Rheumatol*. 2015;42(2))

apparent calcinosis demonstrated successful detection of calcinosis in the subcutaneous tissue, tendon sheaths, carpal tunnel, and adjacent to muscles with DECT, and with better details than radiography due to extensive finger contractures or osteopenia adjacent to large calcinosis deposits [67]. Computer vision algorithms, such as convolutional neural network (CNN) have been applied to DECT hand images of SSc patients for more precise measurement of calcinosis [68]. Cinematic rendering (CR) CT, a new 3-D photorealistic visualization technique was used in addition to traditional 3-D CT methods to evaluate calcinosis in one patient with DM/SSc overlap [69] (Fig. 34.6). Of note, multidetector computed tomography (MDCT) may better assess the extent of calcinotic lesions due to improved resolution and 3D capabilities compared to traditional CT [70] (Fig. 34.7).

Magnetic resonance imaging (MRI) can also detect calcinosis deposits, providing better visualization of edema or inflammation of surrounding tissue [71]. Interestingly, a study of 15 SSc patients with clinically apparent calcinosis compared X-ray, CT, and MRI for the detection of calcinosis showing that both the density (compared to radiography and MRI) and volume (compared to MRI) were significantly higher with CT [65] (Fig. 34.8).

Finally, a recent small pilot study of three DM and three SSc patients with new calcinosis deposits within the past 6 months who underwent ^{18}F-NaF PET/CT as well as a clinical examination for assessment of calcinosis showed that ^{18}F-NaF PET/CT detected heterogeneous uptake in calcinosis deposits that appeared homogeneous on CT (Fig. 34.9) The authors suggested that ^{18}F-NaF PET/CT identifies actively calcifying and subclinical deposits that are not apparent on CT [72]. Further studies are needed to determine whether US, CT, MRI or PET might be more useful in the assessment and measurement of calcinosis burden than plain radiography.

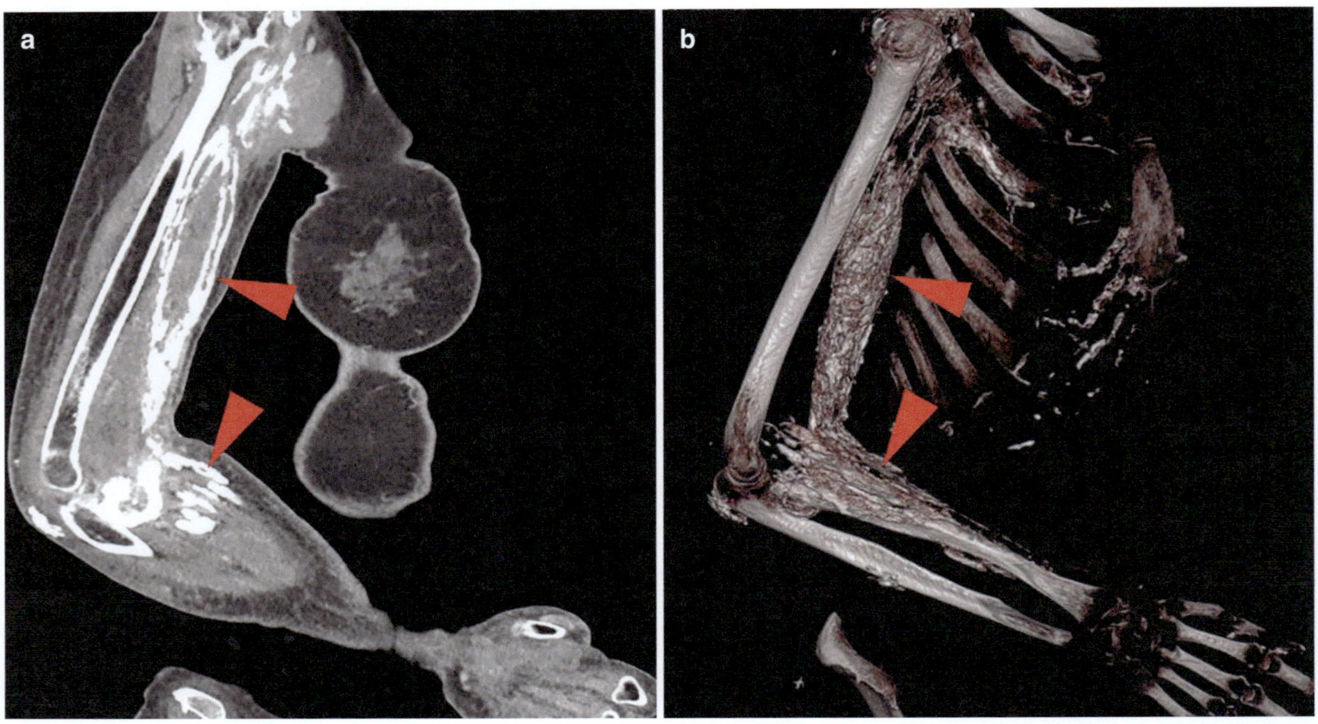

Fig. 34.6 (**a**) Sagittal, contrast-enhanced two-dimensional CT image, and (**b**) volume-rendered 3-D CT image of the patient demonstrating calcinosis (red arrowheads) of the biceps brachii and brachioradialis compartments and overlying subcutaneous soft tissues. *CT* computed tomography. (Reprinted with permission from Rowe et al. *J Rheumatol*. 2019;46(5):539–40)

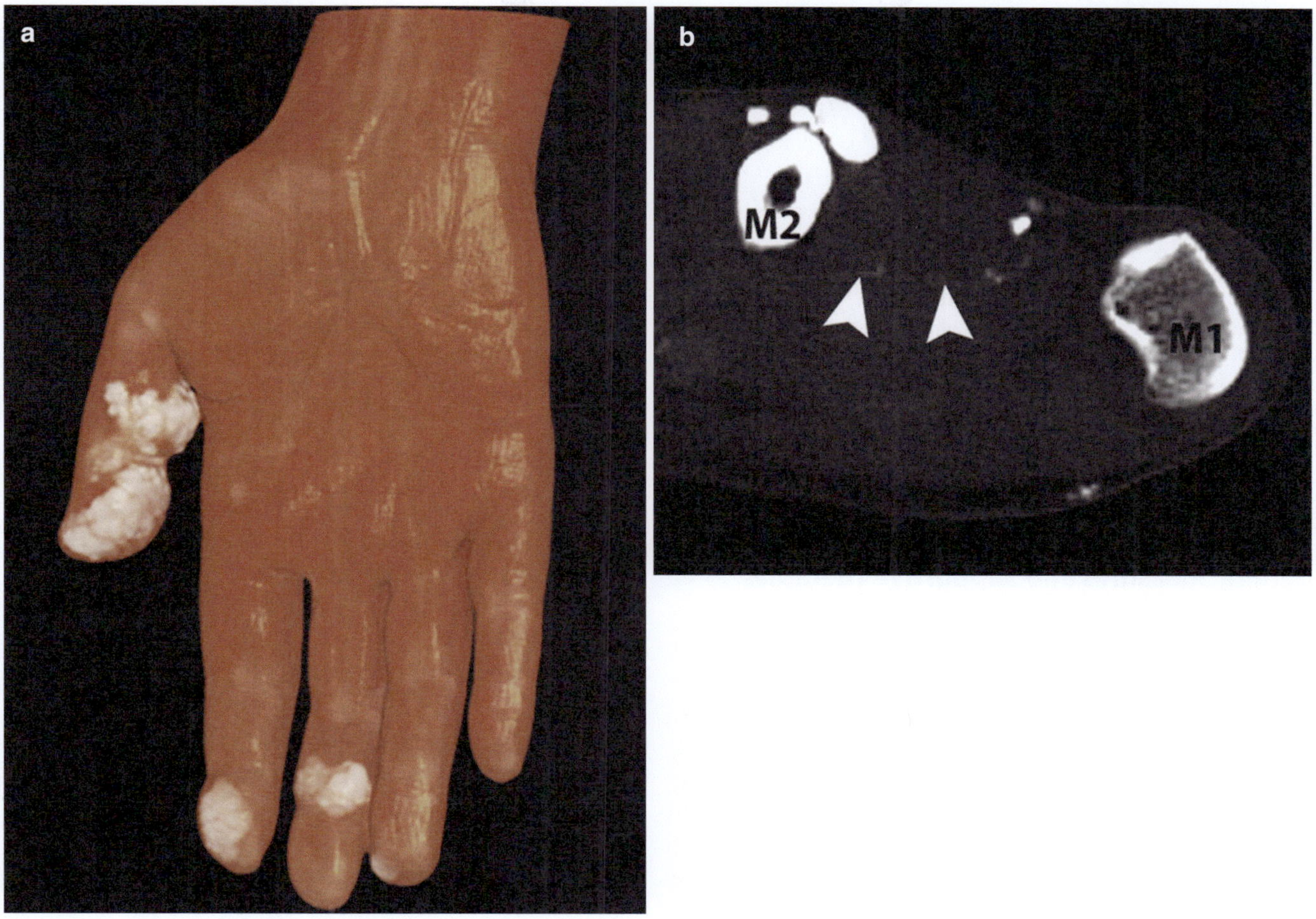

Fig. 34.7 (**a**) Volume-rendered MDCT image of the left hand displays calcinosis involving the thumb, the index, and the middle finger. (**b**) Axial-unenhanced MDCT image of the left hand depicts the thin linear distribution of calcinosis in the intermuscular plane of the first commissure (arrowheads). *M1* first metacarpal, *M2* second metacarpal. (Reprinted with permission from Freire V et al. *Radiology*. 2013;269(3))

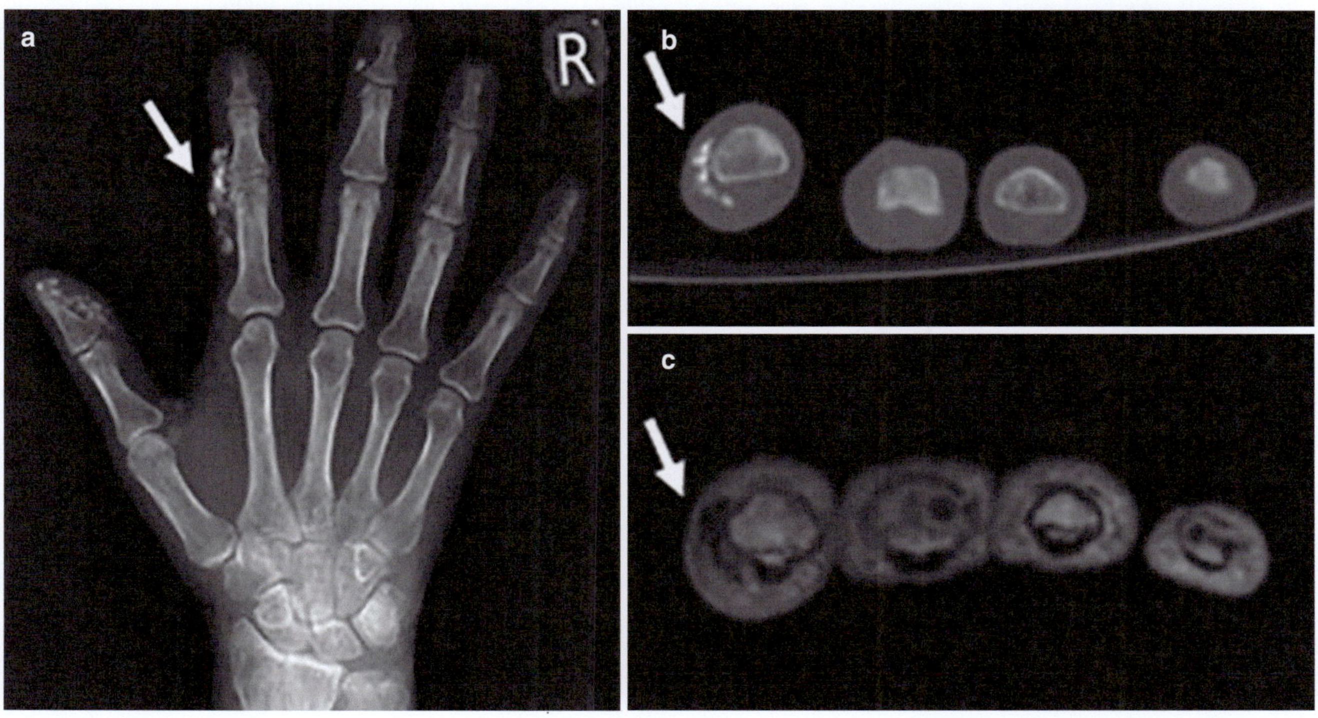

Fig. 34.8 The same calcinotic lesions (white arrows) can be seen by radiography (**a**), CT (**b**), and MRI (**c**). (Reprinted with permission from Hughes M et al. *Semin Arthritis Rheum*. 2019;49(2):279–82)

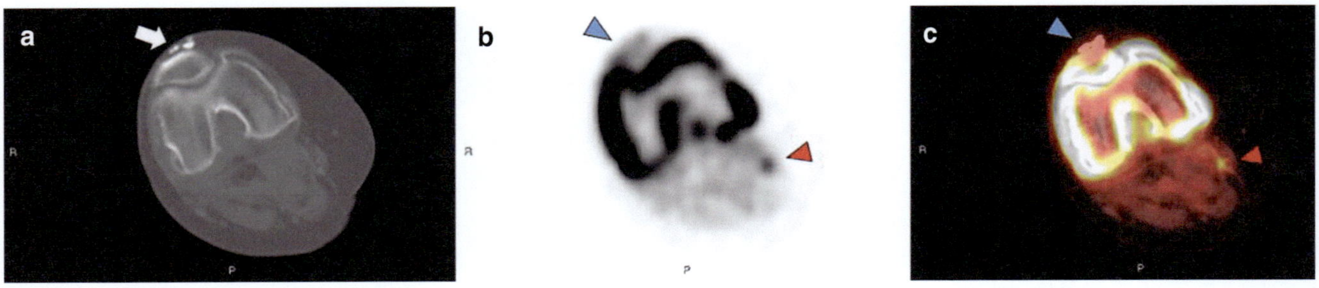

Fig. 34.9 Calcinosis involving the quadriceps and patellar tendon on axial CT bone window (**a**) and axial ^{18}F-NaF PET/CT (**b** and **c**). Blue arrowheads demonstrate mild activity along this calcified complex, red arrowheads demonstrate focal PET signal activity located along the semimembranosus muscle without associated calcification on CT, suggesting increased sensitivity of ^{18}F-NaF PET imaging in detecting pre-calcified disease involvement. (Reprinted with permission from authors, from Richardson et al. Arthritis Rheumatol. 2020; 72(suppl 10))

Treatment of Calcinosis

General Measures and Supportive Therapies

Treatment of calcinosis remains a major clinical challenge in patients with SSc. General measures include improving blood flow to the extremities by avoiding trauma, stress, smoking, and cold exposure. Supportive therapies such as antibiotics for infections, pain medications, and wound care are also key. If there is suspicion for superinfection of calcinotic lesions, antibiotics covering *Streptococci* and *Staphylococci*, such as cephalexin, dicloxacillin, or clindamycin, should be prescribed. If pain is present, acetaminophen, nonsteroidal anti-inflammatory agents, and even opioids can help [73]. If calcinosis becomes ulcerated, standard wound care with hydrocolloid membrane products, such as DuoDerm, may be useful [74]. A recent study compared the efficacy of Holoil®, a plant-based extract oil, for treating skin ulcers associated with calcinosis in 21 SSc patients versus 20 SSc patients who received standard local treatment. Complete healing of skin ulcers occurred in 15/33 (45%) of calcinosis lesions within a mean time of 40.1 ± 16.3 days, as compared with only 4/26 (15.4%) in the control group ($p = 0.0237$).

Medical Therapies

Several medications have been tried for the management of calcinosis, with variable results (Table 34.1). None have received regulatory approval since the supporting evidence mainly comes from small retrospective studies, case series, and case reports, and until recently, there have not been any validated outcome measures to study these agents in randomized clinical trials. In addition, the clinical impact of these interventions requires a prolonged observation period. A recent systematic review aimed to assess the efficacy and tolerance of available treatments for calcinosis cutis in patients with DM and SSc, and identified 11 therapeutic classes, surgery, and physical therapies among 30 studies (288 patients) as potential treatment options for calcinosis cutis [75].

Table 34.1 Pharmacological treatments of calcinosis in systemic sclerosis

Treatment	Proposed mechanism of action	Drug dosage	Number of responses/ numbers of patients treated	References
Vasodilators				
Diltiazem	Reduce intracellular calcium influx	240–480 mg/day for 1–12 years	4/4	Palmieri et al. [76]
		120 mg/day for 2 years	1/1	Dolan et al. [77]
		240 mg/day for 5 years	1/1	Farah et al. [78]
		<480 mg/day for unknown duration	9/17	Balin et al. [79]
		180 mg/day for 1–15 years	3/12	Vayssairat et al. [28]
Treprostinil	Causes direct vasodilation of pulmonary and systemic arterial vascular beds and inhibition of platelet aggregation	1 mg (0.25–7.625 mg) TID for 1 year	4/5	Chung et al. [81]
Anti-inflammatories				
Triamcinolone acetonide injection	Reduces secondary inflammation from calcinosis	Intralesional 20 mg/mL every 4–8 weeks for 6 months	1/1	Hazen et al. [82]
Minocycline	Anti-inflammatory and calcium-binding properties. Suppress PARP-1 and inhibit mineralization of human vascular smooth muscle cells in vitro	50–100 mg/day for 3.5 years	8/9	Robertson et al. [83]
		50–200 mg/day for 6–12 weeks	34/78	Fonseca et al. [84]
Colchicine	Inhibits microtubule polymerization, and disrupts leukocyte chemotaxis and phagocytosis	1 mg/day for 2 months	1/1	Fuchs et al. [87]
		1 mg/day for 4 months	1/1	Vereecken et al. [88]
		<1.2 mg/day for unknown duration	3/8	Balin et al. [79]
Intravenous immunoglobulin	Anti-inflammatory properties, possibly related to suppression of activated macrophages	2 g/day in a 4-day protocol once a month × 5 cycles	1/1	Schanz et al. [91]
Infliximab	Monoclonal antibody anti-TNF-α	3 mg/kg IV at 0, 2 and 6 weeks, and every 8 weeks × 7 months	1/1	Tosonidou et al. [92]
Rituximab	Humanized chimeric anti-CD20 monoclonal antibody	375 mg/m^2 IV weekly × 4	1/1	De Paula et al. [93]
		375 mg/m^2 IV weekly × 4	3/6	Giugglioli et al. [94]
		4 weekly infusions (375 mg/m^2) with repeated dose in 6 months	1/1	Daoussis et al. [95]
		1 or more cycles (1 g × 2 weeks)	4/8	Narvaez et al. [96]
		500 mg on day 0 and day 14, and then twice every 3 months	3/3	Moazedi-Fuerst et al. [97]
		1 gram IV × 2 at 2 week-interval and then every 6 months	0/1	Hurabielle et al. [98]
		2 infusions at 2-week intervals, 1 g each and 1 g 6 months later	0/1	Poormoghim et al. [99]

(continued)

Table 34.1 (continued)

Treatment	Proposed mechanism of action	Drug dosage	Number of responses/ numbers of patients treated	References
Interferes with calcium metabolism				
Sodium thiosulfate Topical	May dissolve calcium deposits and promote local vasodilation and wound healing	25% sodium metabisulfite BID	1/1	Barrio-Diaz et al. [100]
		25% STS compounded in zinc oxide ointment for mean duration of 3.9 months	11/15	Ma et al. [101]
		10% STS for at least 4 weeks	6/6	von Hodenberg [102]
		STS for 3–7 months	0/4	Pelrine et al. [103]
Intralesional		STS 1–3 g/week × 1 year	2/2	Goosens et al. [104]
		STS 12.5–150 mg × 1–4 times	5/5	Baumgartner-Nielsen et al. [105]
Intravenous		25 g two times weekly for 6 months	0/3	Song et al. [106]
		20 g/day, 5 days/month, at least 6 cycles	0/1	Mageau et al. [107]
Bisphosphonates	Inhibits macrophage proinflammatory cytokine production and reduces bone resorption	Risedronate × 6 months	1/1	Fujii et al. [110]
Warfarin	Prevents carboxylation of glutamic acid by reducing levels of MGP	1 mg/day	2/6	Traineau et al. [75]

BID twice a day, *TID* three times a day, *IV* intravenous, *PARP*-1 poly(ADP-ribose) polymerase-1, *TNF-α* tumor necrosis factor alpha, *STS* sodium thiosulfate, *MGP* matrix gamma-carboxyglutamic acid protein

Vasodilators

Calcium Channel Blockers

Calcium channel blockers (CCB) reduce intracellular calcium influx, altering the formation and crystallization of the calcium nidus in affected tissues. Diltiazem is the most well-studied CCB for treating calcinosis. Early case reports showed encouraging results with 240–480 mg/day of diltiazem for calcinosis in SSc patients [76–78]. These results were confirmed in a retrospective cohort of 78 patients with autoimmune connective tissue diseases showing that diltiazem was effective in 9 of 17 patients as first-line therapy [79]. However, a larger retrospective study did not show a beneficial effect on radiographs from 12 SSc patients treated with 180 mg/day of diltiazem for 1–15 years [28]. An observational study using 5-year follow-up data from the Canadian Scleroderma Research Group showed no significant associations between the use of CCBs and calcinosis (OR 0.9, 95% CI 0.73–1.05), except in patients with disease duration <5 years, in whom the use of CCB was associated with decreased risk of calcinosis (OR 0.62, 95% CI 0.45–0.86) [80].

Treprostinil

Treprostinil is a prostacyclin analog that causes direct vasodilation of pulmonary and systemic arterial vascular beds and inhibition of platelet aggregation, and is approved in the United States for the treatment of pulmonary arterial hypertension (PAH). A recent prospective, open-label pilot study of 12 SSc patients with radiologically confirmed calcinosis of the hands evaluated the utility of oral treprostinil in the prevention of radiographic progression of calcinosis over 1 year. Only five patients completed the study, with the remainder experiencing intolerable side effects, particularly headaches and gastrointestinal side effects. Four out of the five patients who completed the study had stability of calcinosis on hand radiographs at 1 year, with a median tolerated dosage of 1 mg TID, as assessed by the SCTC radiographic scoring system [81].

Anti-inflammatories

Triamcinolone Acetonide Injection

Corticosteroid injections are well tolerated and palliative and may be effective in reducing secondary inflammation from calcinosis. In one published case of a patient with SSc and calcinosis, injection of the margins of the lesion with 20 mg/mL of triamcinolone acetonide suspension at 4–8 week intervals resulted in healing at 12 months [82].

Minocycline

This tetracycline antibiotic has anti-inflammatory and calcium-binding properties. In a case series of nine lcSSc patients with calcinosis, 50 or 100 mg/day of minocycline for a mean of 3.5 years resulted in reduced ulceration and inflammation, with a modest decrease in the size of deposits in eight patients [83]. The largest series of 78 SSc patients with calcinosis treated with minocycline 50–200 mg/day for 6–12 weeks in repeated courses showed that 34 patients (43.6%) reported clinical improvement in calcinosis-related symptoms with acceptable tolerability [84]. Interestingly, minocycline has been shown to suppress PARP-1 and inhibit mineralization of human vascular smooth muscle cells in vitro [85].

Colchicine

Colchicine induces anti-inflammatory effects by inhibiting microtubule polymerization, and hence disrupting leukocyte chemotaxis and phagocytosis. Since inflammation often accompanies calcinosis and may be involved in resultant ulceration, colchicine has been used for the treatment of these lesions, but only a few reports in patients with SSc have been published [86]. One patient with SSc and prepatellar calcinosis received 1 mg/day of oral colchicine, and had regression of the associated local inflammation and healing of associated skin ulcers after 2 months of follow-up [87]. Another patient with linear scleroderma and ulcerated cutaneous calcinosis was treated with colchicine 1 mg/day, with healing of the ulcerations after 4 months [88]. Balin et al. reported that three out of eight patients with ACTD who received colchicine (<1.2 mg/day) responded favorably, with one patient having a complete response [79].

Intravenous Immunoglobulins

The use of intravenous immunoglobulins (IVIG) in the treatment of calcinosis is mostly restricted to DM patients, and with mixed results [89, 90]. There is one report of a patient with lcSSc and disabling calcinosis of the left index finger who was free of symptoms after 5 months of IVIG [91]. The authors hypothesize that this effect was based on its anti-inflammatory properties, possibly related to suppression of activated macrophages.

Biologic Agents

Although, tumor necrosis factor-alpha inhibitors might be useful for treating juvenile DM [75], there is not much data on SSc. A patient with SSc-myositis overlap and refractory calcinosis treated with infliximab 3 mg/kg infused at 0, 2, and 6 weeks, and every 8 weeks thereafter, experienced reduction in size of calcifications and no new deposits at 41 months in serial CT imaging [92].

Most literature on biologics for SSc-related calcinosis have focused on rituximab (RTX), with promising results [75]. One lcSSc patient with extensive, frequently ulcerating, and painful calcinotic lesions was treated with two courses of rituximab (four weekly infusions of 375 mg/m^2 each) 18 months apart. Twelve months after the therapy was initiated, she experienced reduction in size of multiple lesions as assessed by physical examination, and her pain improved substantially [93]. Additionally, a series of ten SSc patients treated with RTX for ILD, skin fibrosis, and/or arthritis, reported improvement in three of six patients who had calcinosis [94]. A beneficial effect on calcinosis of four weekly infusions of RTX (375 mg/m^2) with repeated dose in 6 months in a 53-year-old woman with lcSSc was reported, showing an improvement in the size and number of calcifications within 12 months [95]. A more recent single-center observational study of eight patients with refractory SSc-related calcinosis treated with one or more cycles of RTX (1 g × 2 weeks) showed that four (50%) had a significant sustained improvement in the visual analog scale for pain of at least 50% and no new episodes of local inflammation or skin ulceration. Additionally, two patients (25%) had complete resolution or significant reduction in the size of the calcifications on X-ray, according to the SCTC radiographical scoring system after at least 12 months of RTX treatment [96]. Finally, a study reported the outcomes of five SSc patients treated with RTX 500 mg on day 0 and day 14, with repeated courses every 3 months. Three patients had calcinosis cutis affecting the hands and the integument, which resolved in the first 6 months of rituximab treatment, with no relapse after 1–2 years of follow-up [97]. In contrast, Hurabielle et al. reported the case of a female SSc patient with calcinosis on her right wrist, who received two infusions of rituximab (1 g each) at a 2-week interval and then every 6 months, for interstitial lung disease and arthritis. This patient experienced remarkable worsening of the number and size of calcifications revealed by X-ray [98]. A similar case of a patient with lcSSc and widespread calcinosis cutis showed no response to two courses of RTX at 2-week intervals, at baseline, and 6 months later [99]. As summarized above, RTX in SSc-associated calcinosis has shown inconsistent efficacy, and randomized trials are necessary to further delineate whether there is a role for RTX for the treatment of calcinosis [75].

Interferes with Calcium Metabolism

Sodium Thiosulfate

Topical, intralesional and intravenous (IV) sodium thiosulfate (STS) have been studied as treatments for calcinosis.

Four patients with calcinosis (one with SSc, two with DM, and fourth one with radiodermatitis after breast cancer) showed significant decrease in size, erythema, and pain with topical 25% sodium metabisulfite (SM), a metabolite of STS. The authors hypothesized that topical SM may dissolve calcium deposits and promote local vasodilation and wound healing [100]. Similarly, a case series of 26 patients with ACTD treated with topical 25% STS compounded in zinc oxide ointment (incuding 15 with SSc) from the Mayo Clinic, reported that 19 (68%) experienced clinical improvement, defined as total resolution or regression of the lesion without recurrence, at a mean follow-up of 3.9 months [101]. A recent case series reported that all six lcSSc patients with small calcinosis lesions (<2 mm) at the fingertips who were treated with 10% STS formulation for at least 4 weeks, experienced a substantial reduction in the number and/or diameter of lesions [102]. However, in a small retrospective study that included four patients with SSc-related calcinosis, no significant change in calcinosis SCTC radiologic scores was seen at 6 months with topical STS, and one patient did not tolerate treatment due to erythema and inflammation of ulcerating calcinosis [103].

Goossens et al. reported two cases of weekly intralesional injections of 1–3 g STS leading to pain relief, functional improvement, and 59% size reduction after 12 months [104]. A larger series describes the treatment of eight lesions in six patients (five with SSc and one with nephrogenic systemic fibrosis) with injections of 12.5–275 mg STS 150 mg/mL for up to 4 weeks. By weeks 4 and 12, the lesions decreased in size by 67% and 90%, respectively, and all patients reported improved pain and disability [105].

A report of three patients with ACTD-associated calcinosis treated with IV STS, after failing multiple prior therapies, did not show any notable clinical improvement of calcinosis [106]. However, another series of four patients (lcSSc, DM, JDM, SLE) demonstrated improvement in calcinosis after six cycles of IV STS except in the patient with lcSSc [107]. A retrospective analysis of 80 calcinosis lesions treated with either topical, intralesional, and intravenous STS showed that topical STS completely resolved all lesions <0.2 cm, 78% of 0.2–0.3 cm, but only 20% of 0.3–0.5 cm calcinosis lesions. Intralesional STS injections were successful for all calcifications <2 cm, but failed to resolve lesions >2 cm. Intravenous STS failed to resolve the tumoral calcinosis lesions [108]. In summary, intralesional and topical STS may have some therpeutic utility for the treatment of small calcinotic lesions.

Bisphosphonates

Bisphosphonates may be useful in reversing the calcification process by inhibiting macrophage proinflammatory cytokine production and reducing bone resorption [109]. Bisphosphonates might be a useful treatment option for calcinosis in patients with DM [75]; however, few data are available for SSc patients. A case report describes resolution of calcinosis in a patient with lcSSc after 6 months of risedronate therapy for glucocorticoid-induced osteoporosis [110].

Warfarin

Low-dose warfarin has been used for treatment of ACTD-calcinosis, based on the rationale that it reduces the levels of matrix gamma-carboxyglutamic acid protein (MGP) by preventing carboxylation of glutamic acid [111]. A systematic review identified five studies investigating the role of warfarin for calcinosis (most commonly prescribed dose of 1 mg/day), with a total of 19 patients, including 6 with SSc. The partial response rate ranged from 0% to 66% with no complete response observed in all but one study [75]. On the basis of the results of these studies, they conclude that low-dose warfarin should not be used for calcinosis cutis.

Nonmedical Therapies

A prospective study of nine patients (three with SSc) with calcinosis found that three extracorporeal shock wave lithotripsy (ESWL) sessions at 3-week intervals reduced the size and pain from calcinosis at 6 months [112]. A recent 12-week study of three weekly sessions of ESWL on calcinosis lesions in four SSc patients found a reduction in lesion size in three patients and pain improvement in two patients [113]. In a case report of a SSc female with extensive leg ulcerations and calcifications, ESWL was well tolerated and reduced the size of ulcers and pain [114]. The carbon dioxide (CO) laser-tissue vaporization procedure allows excellent visualization and vaporization of calcium deposits and has been shown to improve pain and function in selected patients with SSc-calcinosis [115, 116]. Patients with large, localized, and symptomatic lesions especially located over tendons, blood vessels, and nerves should be referred for surgery [117, 118]. In the Mayo Clinic experience, all 11 patients who underwent surgical excision alone and 16 out of 17 patients who received medical and surgical therapy responded to treatment. In contrast, only 7 of 19 patients treated with medical therapy alone had any response [79]. Specific techniques such as curettage of calcinosis [119] or debulking with a high-speed microburr [120] effectively reduce pain and disability scores, but lesions can recur.

Conclusions

Calcinosis is a common problem in patients with SSc. It most frequently affects the hands, particularly the fingers. Although pathogenesis is unclear, there is evidence supporting chronic inflammation, vascular hypoxia, local trauma, and dysregulation of bone matrix proteins as potential mechanisms. There are no universally effective medical treatments for calcinosis in patients with SSc; however, limited data have been published supporting the use of several pharmacological therapies including minocycline, and STS. Surgical excision of calcinosis remains the mainstay for treatment. Clinical trials using novel outcome measures are necessary to determine the efficacy of current and emerging treatments.

References

1. Chander S, Gordon P. Soft tissue and subcutaneous calcification in connective tissue diseases. Curr Opin Rheumatol. 2012;24(2):158–64.
2. Boulman N, Slobodin G, Rozenbaum M, Rosner I. Calcinosis in rheumatic diseases. Semin Arthritis Rheum. 2005;34(6):805–12.
3. Reiter N, El-Shabrawi L, Leinweber B, Berghold A, Aberer E. Calcinosis cutis: Part I. Diagnostic pathway. J Am Acad Dermatol. 2011;65(1):1–12; quiz 13–4.
4. Valenzuela A, Baron M, Herrick AL, Proudman S, Stevens W, Rodriguez-Reyna TS, et al. Calcinosis is associated with digital ulcers and osteoporosis in patients with systemic sclerosis: a Scleroderma Clinical Trials Consortium study. Semin Arthritis Rheum. 2016;46(3):344–9.
5. Valenzuela A, Baron M, Rodriguez-Reyna TS, Proudman S, Khanna D, Young A, et al. Calcinosis is associated with ischemic manifestations and increased disability in patients with systemic sclerosis. Semin Arthritis Rheum. 2020;50(5):891–6.
6. Morgan ND, Shah AA, Mayes MD, Domsic RT, Medsger TA Jr, Steen VD, et al. Clinical and serological features of systemic sclerosis in a multicenter African American cohort: analysis of the genome research in African American scleroderma patients clinical database. Medicine (Baltimore). 2017;96(51):e8980.
7. Cruz-Domínguez MP, García-Collinot G, Saavedra MA, Medina G, Carranza-Muleiro RA, Vera-Lastra OL, et al. Clinical, biochemical, and radiological characterization of the calcinosis in a cohort of Mexican patients with systemic sclerosis. Clin Rheumatol. 2017;36(1):111–7.
8. Sujau I, Ng CT, Sthaneshwar P, Sockalingam S, Cheah TE, Yahya F, et al. Clinical and autoantibody profile in systemic sclerosis: baseline characteristics from a West Malaysian cohort. Int J Rheum Dis. 2015;18(4):459–65.
9. Bartoli F, Fiori G, Braschi F, Amanzi L, Bruni C, Blagojevic J, et al. Calcinosis in systemic sclerosis: subsets, distribution and complications. Rheumatology (Oxford). 2016;55(9):1610–4.
10. Gauhar R, Wilkinson J, Harris J, Manning J, Herrick AL. Calcinosis preferentially affects the thumb compared to other fingers in patients with systemic sclerosis. Scand J Rheumatol. 2016;45(4):317–20.
11. Hughes M, Hodgson R, Harris J, Porter N, Jackson S, Kirwadi A, et al. Further evidence that calcinosis is associated with repetitive trauma in systemic sclerosis. Semin Arthritis Rheum. 2020;50(1):E4–5.
12. Sari-Kouzel H, Hutchinson CE, Middleton A, Webb F, Moore T, Griffin K, et al. Foot problems in patients with systemic sclerosis. Rheumatology (Oxford). 2001;40(4):410–3.
13. Tang EY, Varughese S, Herrick AL. Systemic sclerosis-related calcinosis can affect the breast—but malignancy should always be excluded. Scand J Rheumatol. 2020;1-2:78.
14. Delvino P, Biglia A, Bellis E, Monti S, Bozzalla Cassione E, Zanframundo G, et al. Lumbar spondylolisthesis associated with systemic sclerosis-related spinal calcinosis: an unusual clinical case. Rheumatology (Oxford). 2020;59:3999.
15. Motegi SI, Sekiguchi A, Yonemoto Y, Mieda T, Chikuda H, Ishikawa O. Demographic and clinical characteristics of spinal calcinosis in systemic sclerosis: possible association with peripheral angiopathy. J Dermatol. 2019;46(1):33–6.
16. Gossner J, Krahlisch J. Intraspinal calcinosis in systemic sclerosis. Joint Bone Spine. 2019;86(5):644.
17. Maraković J, Marinović T, Jeleč V, Dlaka D, Muller D, Blažević A, et al. Intraspinal calcinosis mimicking intervertebral disc extrusion: a clinical and surgical case report. Surg Neurol Int. 2018;9:166.
18. Tan CK, Suresh E. Cervical and lumbar paraspinal calcinosis in systemic sclerosis. Reumatismo. 2016;68(4):203–5.
19. Bauer E, Fauny M, Tanguy M, Albuisson E, Mandry D, Huttin O, et al. Relationship between calcifications and structural lesions on hand radiography and axial calcifications on CT-scan: a retrospective study in systemic sclerosis. Medicine (Baltimore). 2020;99(43):e22443.
20. Avouac J, Mogavero G, Guerini H, Drapé JL, Mathieu A, Kahan A, et al. Predictive factors of hand radiographic lesions in systemic sclerosis: a prospective study. Ann Rheum Dis. 2011;70(4):630–3.
21. Sakata K, Kaneko Y, Yasuoka H, Takeuchi T. Association of radiographic findings in hand X-ray with clinical features and autoantibodies in patients with systemic sclerosis. Clin Rheumatol. 2020;39(1):113–8.
22. Tolosa-Vilella C, Morera-Morales ML, Simeón-Aznar CP, Marí-Alfonso B, Colunga-Arguelles D, Callejas Rubio JL, et al. Digital ulcers and cutaneous subsets of systemic sclerosis: clinical, immunological, nailfold capillaroscopy, and survival differences in the Spanish RESCLE Registry. Semin Arthritis Rheum. 2016;46(2):200–8.
23. Baron M, Pope J, Robinson D, Jones N, Khalidi N, Docherty P, et al. Calcinosis is associated with digital ischaemia in systemic sclerosis-a longitudinal study. Rheumatology (Oxford). 2016;55(12):2148–55.
24. Lescoat A, Coiffier G, de Carlan M, Droitcourt C, Ballerie A, Cazalets C, et al. Combination of capillaroscopic and ultrasonographic evaluations in systemic sclerosis: results of a cross-sectional study. Arthritis Care Res (Hoboken). 2018;70(6):938–43.

25. Walsh JS, Fairley JA. Calcifying disorders of the skin. J Am Acad Dermatol. 1995;33(5 Pt 1):693–706; quiz 7–10.
26. Johnstone EM, Hutchinson CE, Vail A, Chevance A, Herrick AL. Acro-osteolysis in systemic sclerosis is associated with digital ischaemia and severe calcinosis. Rheumatology (Oxford). 2012;51(12):2234–8.
27. Fairchild R, Chung M, Sharpless L, Li S, Chung L. Ultrasound detection of calcinosis and association with ulnar artery occlusion in patients with systemic sclerosis. Arthritis Care Res (Hoboken). 2020;73:1332.
28. Vayssairat M, Hidouche D, Abdoucheli-Baudot N, Gaitz JP. Clinical significance of subcutaneous calcinosis in patients with systemic sclerosis. Does diltiazem induce its regression? Ann Rheum Dis. 1998;57(4):252–4.
29. Mahmood M, Wilkinson J, Manning J, Herrick AL. History of surgical debridement, anticentromere antibody, and disease duration are associated with calcinosis in patients with systemic sclerosis. Scand J Rheumatol. 2016;45(2):114–7.
30. Pai S, Hsu V. Are there risk factors for scleroderma-related calcinosis? Mod Rheumatol. 2018;28(3):518–22.
31. Wodkowski M, Hudson M, Proudman S, Walker J, Stevens W, Nikpour M, et al. Clinical correlates of monospecific anti-PM75 and anti-PM100 antibodies in a tri-nation cohort of 1574 systemic sclerosis subjects. Autoimmunity. 2015;48(8):542–51.
32. D'Aoust J, Hudson M, Tatibouet S, Wick J, Mahler M, Baron M, et al. Clinical and serologic correlates of anti-PM/Scl antibodies in systemic sclerosis: a multicenter study of 763 patients. Arthritis Rheumatol. 2014;66(6):1608–15.
33. Richardson C, Perin J, Zeger S, Wigley F, Hummers L, Casciola-Rosen L, Rosen A, Shah A. A heavy burden of calcinosis reflects cumulative disease damage in scleroderma [abstract]. Arthritis Rheumatol. 2020;72(Suppl 10).
34. De Lorenzo R, Pinal-Fernandez I, Huang W, Albayda J, Tiniakou E, Johnson C, et al. Muscular and extramuscular clinical features of patients with anti-PM/Scl autoantibodies. Neurology. 2018;90(23):e2068–e76.
35. Tartar DM, Chung L, Fiorentino DF. Clinical significance of autoantibodies in dermatomyositis and systemic sclerosis. Clin Dermatol. 2018;36(4):508–24.
36. Braun-Moscovici Y, Furst DE, Markovits D, Rozin A, Clements PJ, Nahir AM, et al. Vitamin D, parathyroid hormone, and acroosteolysis in systemic sclerosis. J Rheumatol. 2008;35(11):2201–5.
37. Omair MA, Pagnoux C, McDonald-Blumer H, Johnson SR. Low bone density in systemic sclerosis. A systematic review. J Rheumatol. 2013;40(11):1881–90.
38. Fauny M, Bauer E, Albuisson E, Perrier-Cornet J, Deibener J, Chabot F, et al. Vertebral fracture prevalence and measurement of the scanographic bone attenuation coefficient on CT-scan in patients with systemic sclerosis. Rheumatol Int. 2018;38(10):1901–10.
39. Host LV, Campochiaro C, Afonso A, Nihtyanova SI, Denton CP, Ong VH. High proton pump inhibitor exposure increases risk of calcinosis in systemic sclerosis. Rheumatology (Oxford). 2020;60:849.
40. Zanatta E, Desportes M, Do HH, Avouac J, Doria A, Feydy A, et al. Pseudotumoral calcinosis in systemic sclerosis: data from systematic literature review and case series from two referral centres. Semin Arthritis Rheum. 2020;50:1339.
41. Chung L, Valenzuela A, Fiorentino D, Stevens K, Li S, Harris J, et al. Validation of a novel radiographic scoring system for calcinosis affecting the hands of patients with systemic sclerosis. Arthritis Care Res (Hoboken). 2015;67(3):425–30.
42. Valenzuela A, Chung M, Rodríguez-Reyna T, Proudman S, Baron M, Castelino F, Hsu V, Li S, Fiorentino D, Stevens K, Chung L. Change in calcinosis over 1 year using the SCTC Radiologic Scoring System for calcinosis of the hands in patients with systemic sclerosis [abstract]. Arthritis Rheumatol. 2019;71(Suppl 10).
43. Hughes M, Freemont TJ, Denton J, Herrick AL. Infected calcinosis of the knee in limited cutaneous systemic sclerosis. J Rheumatol. 2012;39(10):2043–4.
44. Bussone G, Berezné A, Mouthon L. Infectious complications of systemic sclerosis. Presse Med. 2009;38(2):291–302.
45. Richardson C, Plaas A, Varga J. Calcinosis in systemic sclerosis: updates in pathophysiology, evaluation, and treatment. Curr Rheumatol Rep. 2020;22(10):73.
46. Hsu VM, Emge T, Schlesinger N. X-ray diffraction analysis of spontaneously draining calcinosis in scleroderma patients. Scand J Rheumatol. 2017;46(2):118–21.
47. Koutaissoff S, Vanthuyne M, Smith V, De Langhe E, Depresseux G, Westhovens R, et al. Hand radiological damage in systemic sclerosis: comparison with a control group and clinical and functional correlations. Semin Arthritis Rheum. 2011;40(5):455–60.
48. Davies CA, Jeziorska M, Freemont AJ, Herrick AL. The differential expression of VEGF, VEGFR-2, and GLUT-1 proteins in disease subtypes of systemic sclerosis. Hum Pathol. 2006;37(2):190–7.
49. Davies CA, Herrick AL, Cordingley L, Freemont AJ, Jeziorska M. Expression of advanced glycation end products and their receptor in skin from patients with systemic sclerosis with and without calcinosis. Rheumatology (Oxford). 2009;48(8):876–82.
50. Park JK, Fava A, Carrino J, Del Grande F, Rosen A, Boin F. Association of acroosteolysis with enhanced osteoclastogenesis and higher blood levels of vascular endothelial growth factor in systemic sclerosis. Arthritis Rheumatol. 2016;68(1):201–9.
51. Nakamura T, Hirakawa K, Takaoka H, Iyama K. Dystrophic calcinosis with both a huge calcified mass in the cervical spine and calcification in the chest wall in a patient with rheumatoid overlap syndrome. Clin Rheumatol. 2016;35(5):1403–9.
52. Tsakali SS, Shanahan CM. Calcinosis: insights from other calcinoses. Curr Opin Rheumatol. 2020;32(6):472–8.
53. Cantatore FP, Maruotti N, Corrado A, Ribatti D. Angiogenesis dysregulation in the pathogenesis of systemic sclerosis. Biomed Res Int. 2017;2017:5345673.
54. Li Q, van de Wetering K, Uitto J. Pseudoxanthoma elasticum as a paradigm of heritable ectopic mineralization disorders: pathomechanisms and treatment development. Am J Pathol. 2019;189(2):216–25.
55. Hsu V, Schlesinger N, Li Q, Varga J. Reduced circulating levels of inorganic pyrophosphate are associated with ectopic calcification in scleroderma spectrum disorders [abstract]. Arthritis Rheumatol. 2019;71(Suppl 10).
56. Li Q, Jiang Q, Uitto J. Ectopic mineralization disorders of the extracellular matrix of connective tissue: molecular genetics and pathomechanisms of aberrant calcification. Matrix Biol. 2014;33:23–8.
57. Kavukcuoglu NB, Li Q, Pleshko N, Uitto J. Connective tissue mineralization in Abcc6−/− mice, a model for pseudoxanthoma elasticum. Matrix Biol. 2012;31(4):246–52.
58. Mackenzie NC, Zhu D, Milne EM, van't Hof R, Martin A, Darryl Quarles L, et al. Altered bone development and an increase in FGF-23 expression in Enpp1(−/−) mice. PLoS One. 2012;7(2):e32177.
59. St Hilaire C, Ziegler SG, Markello TC, Brusco A, Groden C, Gill F, et al. NT5E mutations and arterial calcifications. N Engl J Med. 2011;364(5):432–42.
60. Belloli L, Ughi N, Massarotti M, Marasini B, Biondi ML, Brambilla G. Role of fetuin-A in systemic sclerosis-associated calcinosis. J Rheumatol. 2010;37(12):2638–9.
61. Dovio A, Data V, Carignola R, Calzolari G, Vitetta R, Ventura M, et al. Circulating osteoprotegerin and soluble RANK ligand in systemic sclerosis. J Rheumatol. 2008;35(11):2206–13.

62. Davies CA, Jeziorska M, Freemont AJ, Herrick AL. Expression of osteonectin and matrix Gla protein in scleroderma patients with and without calcinosis. Rheumatology (Oxford). 2006;45(11):1349–55.
63. Wang C, Xu W, An J, Liang M, Li Y, Zhang F, et al. Poly(ADP-ribose) polymerase 1 accelerates vascular calcification by upregulating Runx2. Nat Commun. 2019;10(1):1203.
64. Shahi V, Wetter DA, Howe BM, Ringler MD, Davis MD. Plain radiography is effective for the detection of calcinosis cutis occurring in association with autoimmune connective tissue disease. Br J Dermatol. 2014;170(5):1073–9.
65. Hughes M, Hodgson R, Harris J, Porter N, Jackson S, Kirwadi A, et al. Imaging calcinosis in patients with systemic sclerosis by radiography, computerised tomography and magnetic resonance imaging. Semin Arthritis Rheum. 2019;49(2):279–82.
66. Freire V, Bazeli R, Elhai M, Campagna R, Pessis É, Avouac J, et al. Hand and wrist involvement in systemic sclerosis: US features. Radiology. 2013;269(3):824–30.
67. Hsu V, Bramwit M, Schlesinger N. Use of dual-energy computed tomography for the evaluation of calcinosis in patients with systemic sclerosis. Clin Rheumatol. 2015;34(9):1557–61.
68. Chandrasekaran AC, Fu Z, Kraniski R, Wilson FP, Teaw S, Cheng M, et al. Computer vision applied to dual-energy computed tomography images for precise calcinosis cutis quantification in patients with systemic sclerosis. Arthritis Res Ther. 2021;23(1):6.
69. Rowe SP, Fritz J, Fishman EK. Soft tissue calcinosis universalis visualized with novel 3-D computed tomography cinematic rendering. J Rheumatol. 2019;46(5):539–40.
70. Freire V, Becce F, Feydy A, Guérini H, Campagna R, Allanore Y, et al. MDCT imaging of calcinosis in systemic sclerosis. Clin Radiol. 2013;68(3):302–9.
71. Kimball AB, Summers RM, Turner M, Dugan EM, Hicks J, Miller FW, et al. Magnetic resonance imaging detection of occult skin and subcutaneous abnormalities in juvenile dermatomyositis. Implications for diagnosis and therapy. Arthritis Rheum. 2000;43(8):1866–73.
72. Richardson C, Javadi M, Shah A, Solnes L, Wigley F, Hummers L, Christopher-Stine L. 18F-NaF PET/CT identifies active calcium uptake in calcinosis due to dermatomyositis and scleroderma [abstract]. Arthritis Rheumatol. 2020;72(Suppl 10).
73. Ughi N, Crotti C, Ingegnoli F. Effectiveness and safety of oxycodone/naloxone in the management of chronic pain in patients with systemic sclerosis with recurrent digital ulcers: two case reports. Clin Interv Aging. 2016;11:307–11.
74. Netsch D. Calcinosis cutis: WOC nurse management. J Wound Ostomy Continence Nurs. 2018;45(1):83–6.
75. Traineau H, Aggarwal R, Monfort JB, Senet P, Oddis CV, Chizzolini C, et al. Treatment of calcinosis cutis in systemic sclerosis and dermatomyositis: a review of the literature. J Am Acad Dermatol. 2020;82(2):317–25.
76. Palmieri GM, Sebes JI, Aelion JA, Moinuddin M, Ray MW, Wood GC, et al. Treatment of calcinosis with diltiazem. Arthritis Rheum. 1995;38(11):1646–54.
77. Dolan AL, Kassimos D, Gibson T, Kingsley GH. Diltiazem induces remission of calcinosis in scleroderma. Br J Rheumatol. 1995;34(6):576–8.
78. Farah MJ, Palmieri GM, Sebes JI, Cremer MA, Massie JD, Pinals RS. The effect of diltiazem on calcinosis in a patient with the CREST syndrome. Arthritis Rheum. 1990;33(8):1287–93.
79. Balin SJ, Wetter DA, Andersen LK, Davis MD. Calcinosis cutis occurring in association with autoimmune connective tissue disease: the Mayo Clinic experience with 78 patients, 1996–2009. Arch Dermatol. 2012;148(4):455–62.
80. Li G, Adachi JD, Cheng J, Thabane L, Hudson M, Fritzler MJ, et al. Relationship between calcium channel blockers and skin fibrosis in patients with systemic sclerosis. Clin Exp Rheumatol. 2017;35 Suppl 106(4):56–60.
81. Chung M, Vergara AMV, Catanese B, Li S, Stevens K, Chung L. A pilot study to evaluate the safety and efficacy of Treprostinil in the treatment of calcinosis in patients with systemic sclerosis [abstract]. Arthritis Rheumatol. 2020;72(Suppl 10).
82. Hazen PG, Walker AE, Carney JF, Stewart JJ. Cutaneous calcinosis of scleroderma. Successful treatment with intralesional adrenal steroids. Arch Dermatol. 1982;118(5):366–7.
83. Robertson LP, Marshall RW, Hickling P. Treatment of cutaneous calcinosis in limited systemic sclerosis with minocycline. Ann Rheum Dis. 2003;62(3):267–9.
84. Fonseca C, Ong V, Denton C. Minocycline for refractory calcinosis in systemic sclerosis: a single-centre observational cohort study [abstract]. Arthritis Rheumatol. 2019;71(Suppl 10).
85. Müller KH, Hayward R, Rajan R, Whitehead M, Cobb AM, Ahmad S, et al. Poly(ADP-ribose) links the DNA damage response and biomineralization. Cell Rep. 2019;27(11):3124–38.e13.
86. Gutierrez A Jr, Wetter DA. Calcinosis cutis in autoimmune connective tissue diseases. Dermatol Ther. 2012;25(2):195–206.
87. Fuchs D, Fruchter L, Fishel B, Holtzman M, Yaron M. Colchicine suppression of local inflammation due to calcinosis in dermatomyositis and progressive systemic sclerosis. Clin Rheumatol. 1986;5(4):527–30.
88. Vereecken P, Stallenberg B, Tas S, de Dobbeleer G, Heenen M. Ulcerated dystrophic calcinosis cutis secondary to localised linear scleroderma. Int J Clin Pract. 1998;52(8):593–4.
89. Asano Y, Ihn H, Asashima N, Yazawa N, Mimura Y, Jinnin M, et al. A case of diffuse scleroderma successfully treated with high-dose intravenous immune globulin infusion. Rheumatology (Oxford). 2005;44(6):824–6.
90. Fredi M, Bartoli F, Cavazzana I, Ceribelli A, Carabellese N, Tincani A, et al. Calcinosis in poly-dermatomyositis: clinical and laboratory predictors and treatment options. Clin Exp Rheumatol. 2017;35(2):303–8.
91. Schanz S, Ulmer A, Fierlbeck G. Response of dystrophic calcification to intravenous immunoglobulin. Arch Dermatol. 2008;144(5):585–7.
92. Tosounidou S, MacDonald H, Situnayake D. Successful treatment of calcinosis with infliximab in a patient with systemic sclerosis/myositis overlap syndrome. Rheumatology (Oxford). 2014;53(5):960–1.
93. de Paula DR, Klem FB, Lorencetti PG, Muller C, Azevedo VF. Rituximab-induced regression of CREST-related calcinosis. Clin Rheumatol. 2013;32(2):281–3.
94. Giuggioli D, Lumetti F, Colaci M, Fallahi P, Antonelli A, Ferri C. Rituximab in the treatment of patients with systemic sclerosis. Our experience and review of the literature. Autoimmun Rev. 2015;14(11):1072–8.
95. Daoussis D, Antonopoulos I, Liossis SN, Yiannopoulos G, Andonopoulos AP. Treatment of systemic sclerosis-associated calcinosis: a case report of rituximab-induced regression of CREST-related calcinosis and review of the literature. Semin Arthritis Rheum. 2012;41(6):822–9.
96. Narváez J, Pirola JP, LLuch J, Juarez P, Nolla JM, Valenzuela A. Effectiveness and safety of rituximab for the treatment of refractory systemic sclerosis associated calcinosis: a case series and systematic review of the literature. Autoimmun Rev. 2019;18(3):262–9.
97. Moazedi-Fuerst FC, Kielhauser SM, Bodo K, Graninger WB. Dosage of rituximab in systemic sclerosis: 2-year results of five cases. Clin Exp Dermatol. 2015;40(2):211–2.
98. Hurabielle C, Allanore Y, Kahan A, Avouac J. Flare of calcinosis despite rituximab therapy. Semin Arthritis Rheum. 2014;44(2):e5–6.

99. Poormoghim H, Andalib E, Almasi AR, Hadibigi E. Systemic sclerosis and calcinosis cutis: response to rituximab. J Clin Pharm Ther. 2016;41(1):94–6.
100. Del Barrio-Díaz P, Moll-Manzur C, Álvarez-Veliz S, Vera-Kellet C. Topical sodium metabisulfite for the treatment of calcinosis cutis: a promising new therapy. Br J Dermatol. 2016;175(3):608–11.
101. Ma JE, Ernste FC, Davis MDP, Wetter DA. Topical sodium thiosulfate for calcinosis cutis associated with autoimmune connective tissue diseases: the Mayo Clinic experience, 2012–2017. Clin Exp Dermatol. 2019;44(5):e189–e92.
102. von Hodenberg C, Neufeld M, Wohlrab J, Meyer D, Ehrchen J, Sunderkötter C. Topical sodium thiosulfate: a reliable treatment for digital calcinosis cutis—a case series with six patients. J Dtsch Dermatol Ges. 2020;18:1181.
103. Pelrine E, Gordon JK, Baron M, Spiera RF. Sodium thiosulfate in calcinosis [abstract]. Arthritis Rheumatol. 2015;67(Suppl 10).
104. Goossens J, Courbebaisse M, Caudron E, Bahans C, Vacquerie V, Melchior J, et al. Efficacy of intralesional sodium thiosulfate injections for disabling tumoral calcinosis: two cases. Semin Arthritis Rheum. 2017;47(3):451–5.
105. Baumgartner-Nielsen J, Olesen AB. Treatment of skin calcifications with intra-lesional injection of sodium thiosulphate: a case series. Acta Derm Venereol. 2016;96(2):257–8.
106. Song P, Fett NM, Lin J, Merola JF, Costner M, Vleugels RA. Lack of response to intravenous sodium thiosulfate in three cases of extensive connective tissue disease-associated calcinosis cutis. Br J Dermatol. 2018;178(6):1412–5.
107. Mageau A, Guigonis V, Ratzimbasafy V, Bardin T, Richette P, Urena P, et al. Intravenous sodium thiosulfate for treating tumoral calcinosis associated with systemic disorders: report of four cases. Joint Bone Spine. 2017;84(3):341–4.
108. Howard RM, Smith GP. Treatment of calcinosis cutis with sodium thiosulfate therapy. J Am Acad Dermatol. 2020;83:1518.
109. Dima A, Balanescu P, Baicus C. Pharmacological treatment in calcinosis cutis associated with connective-tissue diseases. Rom J Intern Med. 2014;52(2):55–67.
110. Fujii N, Hamano T, Isaka Y, Ito T, Imai E. Risedronate: a possible treatment for extraosseous calcification. Clin Calcium. 2005;15(Suppl 1):75–8; discussion 8–9.
111. Herrick AL, Gallas A. Systemic sclerosis-related calcinosis. J Scleroderma Relat Disord. 2016;1(2):194–203.
112. Sultan-Bichat N, Menard J, Perceau G, Staerman F, Bernard P, Reguiaï Z. Treatment of calcinosis cutis by extracorporeal shock-wave lithotripsy. J Am Acad Dermatol. 2012;66(3):424–9.
113. Blumhardt S, Frey DP, Toniolo M, Alkadhi H, Held U, Distler O. Safety and efficacy of extracorporeal shock wave therapy (ESWT) in calcinosis cutis associated with systemic sclerosis. Clin Exp Rheumatol. 2016;34 Suppl 100(5):177–80.
114. Sparsa A, Lesaux N, Kessler E, Bonnetblanc JM, Blaise S, Lebrun-Ly V, et al. Treatment of cutaneous calcinosis in CREST syndrome by extracorporeal shock wave lithotripsy. J Am Acad Dermatol. 2005;53(5 Suppl 1):S263–5.
115. Bottomley WW, Goodfield MJ, Sheehan-Dare RA. Digital calcification in systemic sclerosis: effective treatment with good tissue preservation using the carbon dioxide laser. Br J Dermatol. 1996;135(2):302–4.
116. Chamberlain AJ, Walker NP. Successful palliation and significant remission of cutaneous calcinosis in CREST syndrome with carbon dioxide laser. Dermatol Surg. 2003;29(9):968–70.
117. Merlino G, Germano S, Carlucci S. Surgical management of digital calcinosis in CREST syndrome. Aesthet Plast Surg. 2013;37(6):1214–9.
118. Fujimoto M, Asano Y, Ishii T, Ogawa F, Kawakami T, Kodera M, et al. The wound/burn guidelines—4: guidelines for the management of skin ulcers associated with connective tissue disease/vasculitis. J Dermatol. 2016;43(7):729–57.
119. Saddic N, Miller JJ, Miller OF III, Clarke JT. Surgical debridement of painful fingertip calcinosis cutis in CREST syndrome. Arch Dermatol. 2009;145(2):212–3.
120. Lapner MA, Goetz TJ. High-speed burr debulking of digital calcinosis cutis in scleroderma patients. J Hand Surg Am. 2014;39(3):503–10.

Tendons, Joints, and Bone

35

Elisabetta Zanatta, Maya H. Buch, and Yannick Allanore

While tethering of the skin is the clinical hallmark of systemic sclerosis (SSc), many patients may develop musculoskeletal (MSK) symptoms as an early sign of the disease and/or during the course of their illness [1]. Up to 20% of patients with SSc report joint symptoms as early as 1 year or more prior to diagnosis and a third within the same year of diagnosis. Manifestations may be varied ranging from carpal tunnel syndrome and arthralgia to frank inflammatory arthritis and bony lesions. Joint symptoms have been reported to be present in 66% of patients with SSc and muscle symptoms in half of the patients, the latter with a predominance of muscle weakness and myalgia [2]. Musculoskeletal involvement has been shown to strongly contribute to disability and impaired quality of life in SSc, reducing the performance of everyday occupation [1, 3–6]. Indeed, several cross-sectional studies have been reported over the recent years, all highlighting the major impact of MSK involvement on the quality of life in SSc. One report examined patients' beliefs and investigated the relationship between these beliefs, symptom reports, and clinical/demographic variables. This study included a total of 49 patients who underwent clinical examination and completed the Revised Illness Perception Questionnaire. The symptoms most frequently associated with SSc were stiff joints (79%), pain (75%), and fatigue (75%). Over 96% of patients believed that their condition would be chronic and 78% believed that the condition had serious consequences on their lives. Patients with diffuse cutaneous SSc (dcSSc) reported more significant consequences of the condition and less personal control of their SSc compared with patients with limited cutaneous disease (lcSSc) [7].

Joint pain was found to be the most common type of pain in 42 consecutive patients with SSc (78.6% of patients) and was associated with a more severe disease, impaired quality of life, and significant symptoms of depression [8]. Furthermore, in a large international survey, patients ranked MSK involvement third behind Raynaud's syndrome and gastrointestinal involvement among key factors impairing their daily life [9]. Thus, unsurprisingly, a recent study involving 4252 patients from the German Network for SSc [10] found that physical therapy (e.g., lymphatic drainage, exercise and heat therapy) was more frequently prescribed in patients with MSK involvement (up to 69.8%) as compared to the overall SSc population (37.4%), with the maximum odds ratio (OR) for patients presenting arthritis (OR 3.83 (95% confidence interval, CI 2.89–5.08)).

The involvement of hand joints seems to have the greatest impact on daily activities and quality of life. In 1193 patients with SSc from the Scleroderma Patient-centered Intervention Network Cohort, the presence of moderate to severe small joint contractures, digital ulcers, and the severity of Raynaud's phenomenon were the factors more tightly associated with higher Cochin Hand Function Scale scores (i.e., more impaired hand function) [11]. A detailed analysis of hand function in 30 patients with SSc revealed that dexterity was on average reduced to 68–80% and grip force to 46–65% vs. healthy subjects. Finger flexion and extension were the most impaired aspects of hand function. Activities building on hand and arm function were harder to perform than activities depending on lower limb function. Stiffness, grip force, and dexterity had the highest strength of association with difficulties of daily living activities after Raynaud's phenomenon, which was the master symptom [12]. A recent report

E. Zanatta (✉)
Rheumatology Unit, Department of Medicine (DIMED), University Hospital of Padova, Padova, Italy
e-mail: elisabetta.zanatta@unipd.it

M. H. Buch
Department of Rheumatology, Centre for Musculoskeletal Research, School of Biological Sciences, Faculty of Biology, Medicine & Health, University of Manchester, Manchester, UK

NIHR Manchester Biomedical Research Centre, Manchester Academic Health Science Centre, Manchester University Foundation Trust, Manchester, UK
e-mail: maya.buch@manchester.ac.uk

Y. Allanore
Rheumatology Department, Cochin Hospital, APHP, Université Paris Cité, Paris, France
e-mail: yannick.allanore@aphp.fr

Y. Allanore et al. (eds.), *Scleroderma*, https://doi.org/10.1007/978-3-031-40658-4_35

also suggests that the modified Rodnan skin score (mRSS)—besides hand span and grip strength—has significant bearing on hand function in SSc [13]. Moreover, this study confirmed that the impairment of hand function evaluated by the Duruöz Hand Index (DHI) may be similar to that observed in rheumatoid arthritis (RA). In fact, even in the first study which demonstrated the reliability and validity of the DHI in SSc, the mean (SD) total score of 21.10 ± 19.25 (0–66) was higher than or similar to those reported in series of patients with RA or digital osteoarthritis (17 (SD) and 19 (SD), respectively) [4].

This chapter will provide an overview of the spectrum of tendon, joint, bone, and soft tissue involvement in SSc to further highlight the multisystem nature of this condition and will review the different therapeutic approaches that may be employed.

Articular and Tendon Involvement

Tendon Involvement

Clinical Presentations

Tendon abnormalities were first described in 1876 by Westphal, who noticed "coarse cracking and crepitus of finger and knees" in a 23-year-old woman with dcSSc. In 1961, Shulman et al. attributed these grating sensations to fibrinous deposits on the surface of tendon sheaths and overlying fascia. Rodnan and Medsger described this finding as "leathery crepitus" on palpation of the knees, wrists, fingers, and ankles during motion in 19 of 53 patients [14]. These are termed tendon friction rubs, and in the leg, are usually localized to the tibialis anterior, or less frequently, the peroneus muscles. In the forearm, they are usually localized to the flexor or extensor muscles, immediately proximal to the wrist. Median nerve compression with carpal tunnel syndrome may occur. In advanced disease, fibrous deposits within the tendon sheaths might be responsible for a cracking noise during joint movements. The bursae may also be affected especially at the trochanteric or olecranon regions, with sometimes recurrent bursitis with or without associated regional arthritis. An example of magnetic resonance imaging (MRI) illustrating trochanteric bursitis associated with hip synovitis in a patient with dcSSc is presented on Fig. 35.1. The inflammatory proliferative tenosynovitis may lead in rare cases to tendon rupture, which is illustrated in Fig. 35.2a–f [15]. Pathologic examination of biopsies and of tissue obtained at necropsy has revealed thickening of the tendon sheath and deposits of fibrin on the surface of the sheaths and tendons that are similar to those in the case of synovium of the suprapatellar bursa. There appears to be relatively little inflammatory reaction.

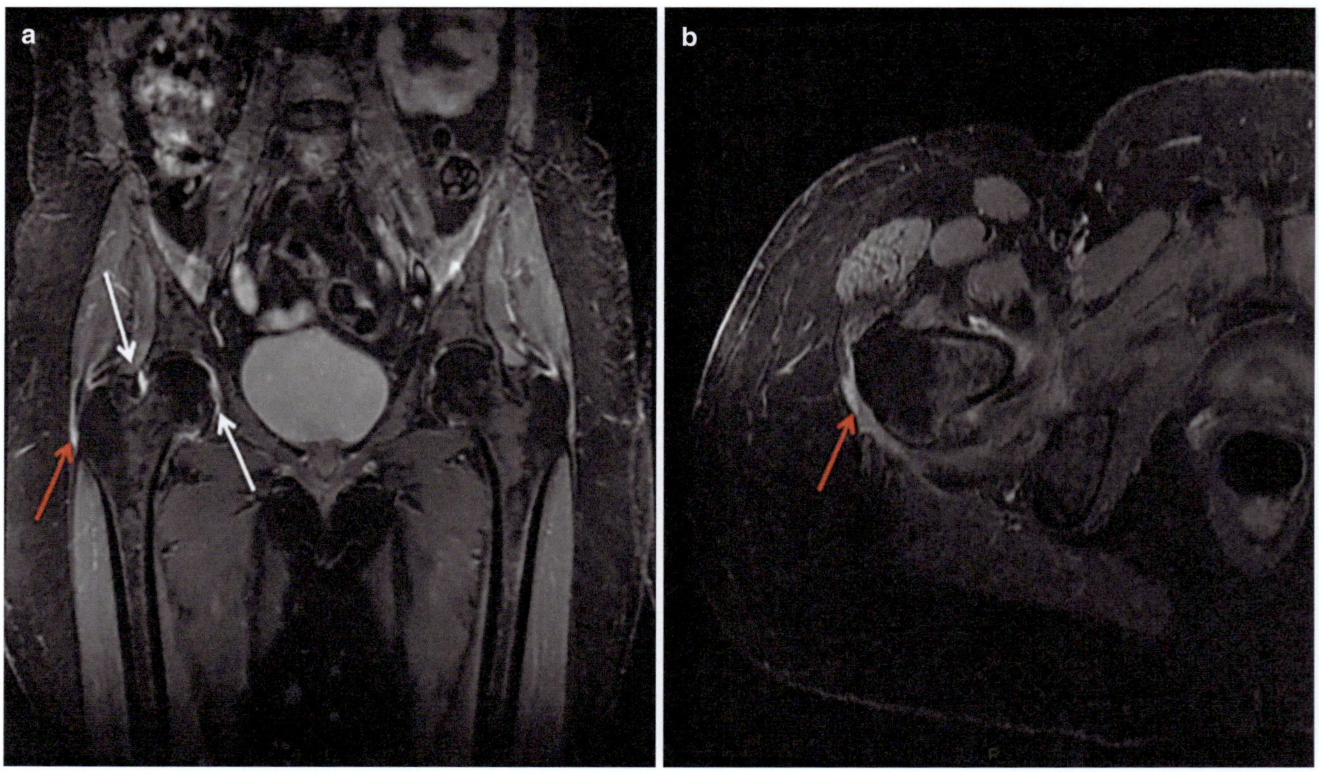

Fig. 35.1 (**a**, **b**) Magnetic resonance imaging (MRI) showing an association of trochanteric bursitis (red arrow) with hip synovitis (white arrow) in a patient with diffuse cutaneous systemic sclerosis

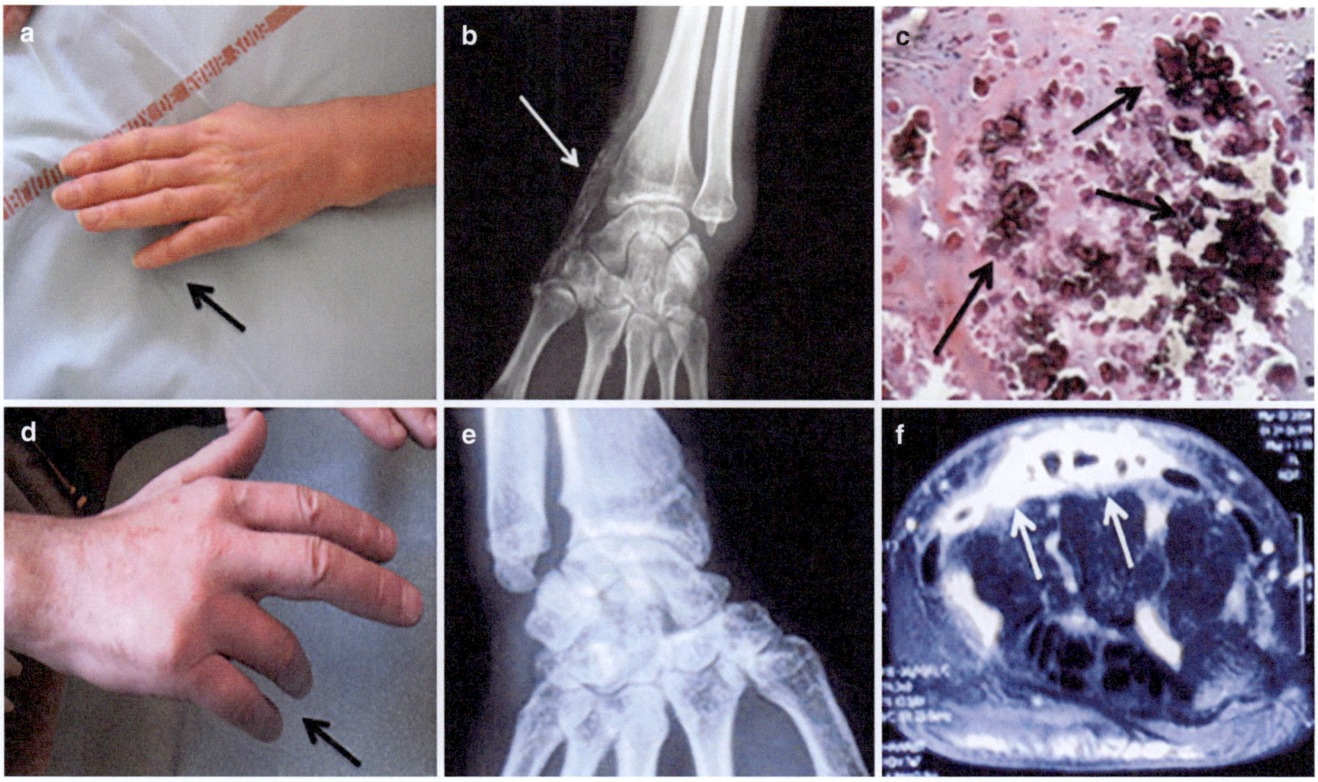

Fig. 35.2 (**a–f**) Tendon rupture in two patients with diffuse cutaneous systemic sclerosis. (**a–c**) Spontaneous rupture of the fifth extensor tendon (**a**). The X-ray did not show any cause of tendon rupture but revealed calcifications of the extensor carpi radialis longus tendon (**b**). Histology obtained after surgical reinsertion of the tendon showed large calcium and fibrin deposits (black arrow) on the surface of the sheaths (**c**). (**d–f**) Spontaneous rupture of the fourth and fifth extensor tendons (**d**). The X-ray showed radiocarpal joint space narrowing and radioulnar erosion (**e**). MRI revealed extensor tenosynovitis (white arrows) (**f**) and radioulnar joint synovitis.

Prevalence

Tendon involvement is not uncommon in SSc; in fact, it was reported in 10 of 98 patients in the leg and 23/98 in the forearm [16]. In the EUSTAR (EULAR Scleroderma Trials and Research) database, the point prevalence of tendon friction rubs was 11% (802/7286 patients) in 2010 [17] and 12.9% (2434/18871 patients) in December 2020 (*unpublished data*). At both time points, their prevalence was lower than previously reported in a large North American study including 1305 patients with SSc. In this study, rubs were observed in 28.2% (368/1305) of patients with SSc [18]. This different point prevalence could partly be explained by the higher proportion of patients with the diffuse cutaneous subset in the American study (49% vs. 33%). Furthermore, certain intrinsic racial differences may also partially explain the higher frequency of tendon friction rubs in North American cohorts. In a study that only included patients with early dcSSc, the point prevalence was considerably higher in the Pittsburgh cohort than in the London Royal Free cohort (59% vs. 22%, respectively) [19]. The prevalence of clinical tendon involvement in SSc is provided in Table 35.1.

The frequency of tendon involvement has been assessed by ultrasound (US) in two studies [23, 24], which found a point prevalence of 27% (14/52 patients and 12/44 patients, respectively). Tendon involvement in SSc is often characterized by evidence of low-grade inflammation (Fig. 35.3) or by its complete absence. In this regard, ultrasonography detected two types of tenosynovitis: an inflammatory type associated with power Doppler signal and a sclerosing type characterized by hyperechoic tendon sheath thickening [23]. Notably, no patients affected by RA exhibited sclerosing tenosynovitis. In another US study conducted in 103 patients with SSc, inflammatory and sclerosing tenosynovitis were recorded in 3.9% and 18.4% of patients, respectively [25]. MRI is more sensitive than US in detecting tenosynovitis in general, with a prevalence of 81.3% vs. 43.7%, respectively, in a study including 16 SSc patients with hand arthralgia [26]. Nevertheless, both ultrasound and MRI might be useful to discern tenosynovitis secondary to fibrous deposits on the surface of the tendon sheaths (Figs. 35.3a–c and 35.4a) from the changes of inflammatory tenosynovitis (Fig. 35.4b–e). Notably, a layered pattern (similar to the appearance of an artichoke heart) of tenosynovitis was common in SSc patients.

Table 35.1 Prevalence of clinical tendon involvement

	Khanna et al. [20] (n = 134 dcSSc)	Ostojic et al. [21] (n = 105)	Ostojic et al. [22] (n = 60)	Avouac et al. [17] (n = 7286)	Steen and Medsger [18] (n = 1305)	Elhai et al. [23] (n = 52)	Freire et al. [24] (n = 1122)
Frequency of tendon involvement, n (%)	49 (37%)	16 (15%)	9 (15%)	802 (11%)	368 (28%)	3 (6%)	63 (6%)

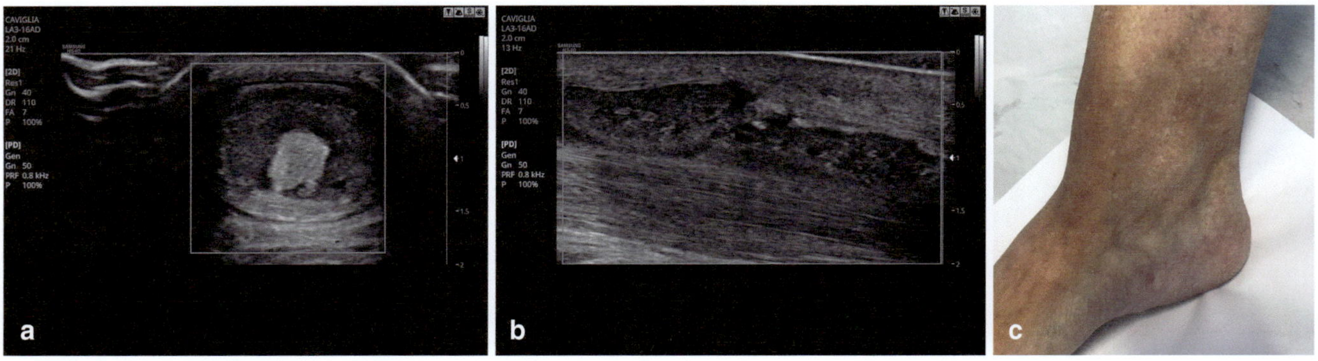

Fig. 35.3 (**a**–**c**) Sclerosing tenosynovitis: US-assessed transverse (**a**) and longitudinal (**b**) view of tibialis anterior tendon characterized by dishomogeneous sheath thickening with iso-hypoechoic effusion and hyperechoic spots. (**c**) Anterior swelling of the ankle due to tenosynovitis of the tibialis anterior tendon

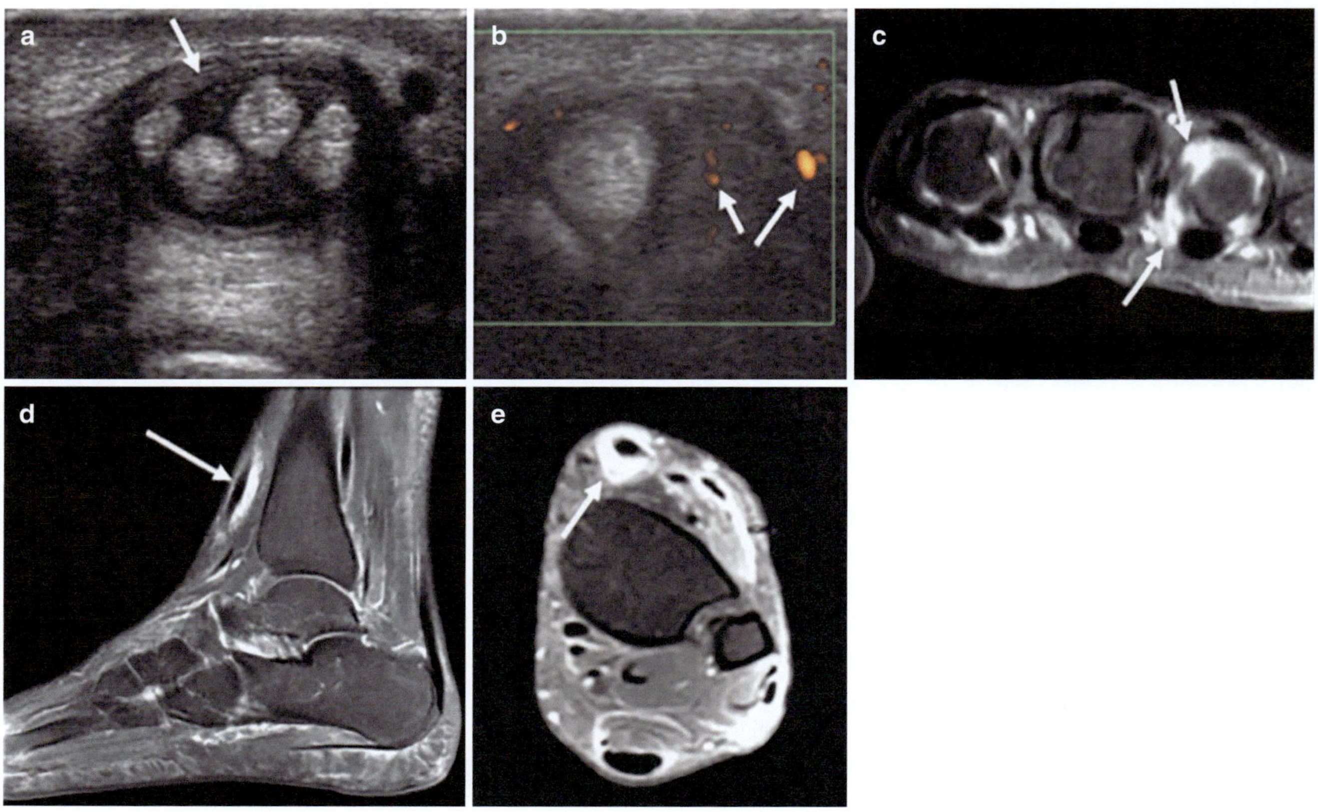

Fig. 35.4 (**a**, **b**) Fibrotic tenosynovitis of extensor digitorum communis (**a**) and inflammatory tenosynovitis of extensor carpi ulnaris (**b**), assessed by ultrasonography. (**c**–**e**) MRI showing hand flexor and extensor (**c**) and tibialis anterior (**d**, **e**) inflammatory tenosynovitis

Enthesitis and Synovio-Entheseal Complex Involvement

The enthesis is the site of attachment of tendons, ligaments, fascia, or joint capsule to bone. The inflammation of the enthesis—enthesitis—which is one of the most important and typical characteristics of spondyloarthritis (SpA), has been recently investigated in SSc. US has allowed rheumatologists to explore the enthesis in detail, finding different elemental lesions. Furthermore, it has been highlighted in recent years that the enthesis forms with the synovial lining an "entheseal organ" coined synovio-entheseal complex (SEC). The two main scores for assessing enthesitis by US are the Glasgow Ultrasound Enthesitis Scoring System (GUESS) [27], which evaluates in greyscale only four types of lesions in the enthesis of lower limbs (maximum score 36), and the more complex Madrid Sonographic Enthesitis Index (MASEI), which assesses six entheses (the bilateral triceps, the quadriceps, both proximal and distal patellar and Achilles tendons and the proximal insertion of the plantar aponeurosis) and six elementary lesions including power Doppler (maximum score 136) [28].

In one study, 52 patients with SSc and a total of 624 entheses were evaluated by US. Except for plantar aponeurosis, MASEI scores and all tendon and ligament thickness were higher in patients with SSc than in healthy controls [29]. Importantly, in patients with SSc, MASEI scores positively correlated with age, mRSS, and the grade of dyspnea, whereas a negative correlation was found with handgrip strength and 36-item short form (SF-36) physical component summary score. A subsequent study [30] in 100 patients with SSc recorded a higher GUESS score in patients (median 4, interquartile range, IQR 2.0–7.0) than in controls (median 1, IQR 0.0–3.0) ($p < 0.001$). Moreover, SEC involvement was evaluated on the entheses of the lateral epicondylar common extensor tendon, highlighting more frequent US-B mode alterations and power Doppler signal in patients than in controls. In this regard, it has been hypothesized that both skin thickening typical of scleroderma and the frequently low body fat mass of these patients may contribute to altering the distribution of mechanical forces on the underlying enthesis and SEC.

Correlation with SSc Features and Prognosis

Tendon involvement is more prevalent in patients with the diffuse cutaneous subset and early disease. It is also associated with signs of severe vascular, muscle, and renal involvement and decreased survival [17, 18]. In particular, the data from the EUSTAR database highlighted the independent association in multivariate analysis between tendon friction rubs and digital ulcerations (OR 1.21, 95% CI 1.01–1.44), muscle weakness (OR 1.42, 95% CI 1.18–1.70), pulmonary fibrosis on plain chest X-ray (OR 1.22, 95% CI 1.02–1.46), and proteinuria detected with a urinalysis dipstick (OR 1.38, 95% CI 1.02–1.87). Tendon friction rubs are associated with active disease [20] and must be taken into account in calculating the EUSTAR revised activity index: their presence contributes to the total score with 2.25 points [31]. Indeed, a prospective analysis of the EUSTAR database also confirmed that tendon friction rubs are an independent predictor of skin progression and the further occurrence of scleroderma renal crisis [32]. More recently, a Spanish multicenter study conducted in 1506 patients with SSc confirmed that tendon friction rubs were a predictive factor for 10-year mortality in both male and female patients [33] and their presence was also included in a 6-variable prediction rule for 5-year mortality in patients with early diffuse SSc [19].

Sclerosing tenosynovitis evaluated in a US study [25] was more frequently observed in men (OR 6.32, 95% CI 2.17–18.41), as well as in patients with anti-RNA polymerase III positivity (OR 10.93, 95% CI 1.84–65.12), dcSSc (OR 18.24, 95% CI 4.80–69.32), interstitial lung disease (OR 6.09, 95% CI 1.86–19.98), and inflammatory arthralgia as first non-Raynaud symptom (OR 14.64, 95% CI 2.58–83.10). Importantly, all patients with tendon friction rubs at clinical examination had tenosynovitis on US, and patients with sclerosing tenosynovitis on US were more likely to have tendon friction rubs [23].

These results highlight that tendon friction rubs are an important physical finding, as they often precede widespread skin thickening, are associated with more severe disease, and are a poor prognostic marker. In patients with recent onset of Raynaud's phenomenon and swollen fingers, the finding of palpable tendon friction rubs should lead to a suspicion of SSc. Searching for friction rubs should be a routine part of the physical examination to aid in early diagnosis and assessment of the disease. US evidence of sclerosing tenosynovitis may also been sought, as it is more frequent in patients with tendon friction rubs and seems highly specific for scleroderma.

Treatment

The treatment of tendon involvement is usually symptomatic, since its evolution is usually favorable after the first years of the disease course. For the most part, tenosynovitis will respond to nonsteroidal anti-inflammatory drugs (NSAIDs) and low-dose corticosteroids. Surgery may be required in rare cases of tendon rupture, as illustrated by the two cases presented who required surgical reinsertion of their extensor tendons (see Fig. 35.2). In some cases, and in particular the early stages of SSc, tendon friction rubs may also resolve following immunosuppressive treatment.

The evidence that enthesopathy and SEC involvement may share the same microanatomical localization in SSc and SpA, combined with the in vitro demonstration that interleukin (IL)-23 and IL-17 upregulate the collagen production in SSc fibroblasts [34, 35], seems to indicate that the IL-23/

IL-17 axis might play a role also in the pathogenesis of SSc enthesopathy. However, further studies are needed to help elucidate for a role of IL-23/IL-17 and therefore the use of IL-23/IL-17 targeted approach in the treatment of SSc-related refractory enthesopathy.

Carpal Tunnel Syndrome

Carpal tunnel syndrome is commonly observed in early dcSSc, although no large study has evaluated its prevalence accurately. One electrophysiological study investigated the characteristics of the canalicular passage nerve involvement in SSc comprising 34 patients of less than 5 years disease duration. Fourteen (44%) patients showed a decrement of the median nerve terminal latency index and seven (22%) of either the median or the ulnar nerve, without severe lesions. Indeed, carpal tunnel syndrome is often the basis for the presenting symptom to a physician. In particular, the co-occurrence of Raynaud's syndrome together with carpal tunnel syndrome should trigger further investigation for a potential connective tissue disorder.

In a controlled study that included 64 SSc patients asymptomatic for hand symptoms and 30 controls, median nerve was measured using high-resolution real-time US of the carpal tunnel. The median nerve cross-sectional area, the transverse (major axis), and the flattening ratio (defined as the ratio of the nerve's major to minor axis) diameters appeared to be increased in patients with SSc compared to controls, whereas the anteroposterior (minor axis) was similar. All SSc measures were higher than controls in all phases of disease and independently of duration of SSc, extent of skin involvement, cutaneous subset (limited or diffuse), and phase of skin involvement (edematous, atrophic, fibrotic) [36]. It is noteworthy that this study failed to identify any link between median nerve involvement and friction rubs, flexor tenosynovitis, or radiocarpal synovitis. And, despite thickening of the skin, subcutaneous deposits, and tenosynovitis, symptoms of numbness in the median nerve are much less frequent in SSc in comparison, for example, to RA. This suggests that carpal tunnel syndrome may not be a consequence of *ab extrinseco* compression and raises the hypothesis that ischemia of *vasa nervorum*, following vasospasm, may contribute to its pathogenesis. Another report of a smaller sample size also showed data that support this hypothesis of a vascular-dependent neuropathy in SSc rather than a compressive mechanism or an autoimmune-dependent neuropathy [37]. More recently, a study on 24 patients with SSc was able to demonstrate increased stiffness of the median nerve in SSc as compared to patients with idiopathic carpal tunnel syndrome and healthy subjects. In fact, the elastic ratio measured at pisiform level and at forearm level was significantly higher (i.e., a lower elasticity of the nerve) compared to the other two groups [38]. Interestingly, and in contrast to the aforementioned study [36], in patients with SSc the median nerve cross-sectional area was similar to controls and lower than in patients with idiopathic carpal tunnel syndrome. Although the concomitant involvement of joint and tendon was not assessed in this study, these findings suggest that—in addition to the possible ischemia of *vasa nervorum*, the involvement of the connective tissue of the nerve itself might play a role in the development of carpal tunnel syndrome.

The choice of treatment is typically determined by the severity of the symptoms. Initial treatment usually includes rest and immobilization of the wrist in a splint. Those whose occupations aggravate the symptoms may modify their daily activities. Ergonomic modification, for example adjustment of computer keyboards and chair height, may optimize comfort. Similarly, NSAIDs are sometimes offered for decreasing inflammation and reducing pain, but their side effects in SSc are a major concern. Thus, corticosteroids are frequently injected directly into the carpal tunnel. This usually brings rapid symptomatic relief of the symptoms with minimal side effects and can be repeated with any recurrence in symptoms. Most patients with carpal tunnel syndrome improve with such conservative measures. Corticosteroid-resistance and persistence symptoms, however, often warrant surgical decompression. Occasionally, chronic lesions of the median nerve may result in continued numbness and weakness; although surgical treatment may be considered, improvement at this stage is questionable. Nevertheless, surgical carpal tunnel release is usually very effective in symptomatic and even refractory patients [39].

Joint Involvement

Clinical Presentation

Arthralgia is quite frequent in SSc, occurring in up to 80% of patients, and is among the most frequent presenting symptoms of scleroderma [40]. At an early stage of the disease, confusion with RA is not uncommon but Raynaud's phenomenon and skin involvement are major signs indicating a connective tissue disorder and SSc. In very early dcSSc, arthralgia may be difficult to assess because of rapidly progressing skin involvement leading to skin tethering and pain. Nevertheless, clinical findings are often minimal at the onset, and generalized arthralgia with slight pain and stiffness is common, with the bowing of the fingers suggested as a useful early diagnostic sign [41]. Patients may exhibit localized joint tenderness or swelling and, albeit usually mild, joint effusion and inflammation may occur and be a source of initial diagnostic confusion. The onset may be acute or insidious, oligoarticular, or polyarticular in pattern. The same joints are generally affected repeatedly and arthralgia is not migratory. Virtually, all joints may be affected with the fingers (in particular the metacarpophalangeal (MCP) and proximal interphalangeal (PIP) joints), wrists, and ankles predominating.

There may be limitation in the range of motion or loss in all planes of wrist motion, MCP flexion, PIP extension, and thumb abduction, opposition, and flexion. The distal interphalangeal (DIP) joint may become fixed in midrange flexion. The result is a claw-type deformity with MCP extension, PIP flexion, thumb adduction, and the wrist in neutral position.

The course of the joint manifestations is either intermittent or chronic remittent. As the cutaneous involvement progresses, there is an inexorable tethering and contracture of the underlying joints with impairment of movement and function. Moreover, the co-occurrence of fibromyalgia must also be taken into account, since it has been observed in 20–30% of SSc depending on the diagnostic tool used [42].

The cross-sectional analysis of the EUSTAR database has revealed that the presence of synovitis is associated with increased levels of acute-phase reactants, markers of severe vascular disease, and muscle weakness. The presence of raised acute-phase reactants indicates systemic inflammation and has a strong association with synovitis [43]. Among 1545 patients enrolled in the Australian Scleroderma Cohort Study, increased C-Reactive Protein (CRP) levels but not Erythrocyte sedimentation rate (ESR) were significantly associated with the presence of synovitis and tendon friction rubs [44].

The presence of synovitis may be related to an overlap with RA or, more likely, to the existence of primary arthritis specific to SSc [45–48]. Several data support that overlap of SSc and RA is very unusual. The prevalence of SSc-RA overlap seems close to 1–5% and its incidence is 5% [43]. Moreover, one study from our group showed in a population of 120 SSc patients a point prevalence of radiographic erosive arthritis of 18%, whereas only two SSc patients (2%) with erosive arthritis fulfilled the ACR criteria for RA [49]. In a study with a larger sample size ($n = 7286$), much lower values for the prevalence of synovitis were reported with synovitis affecting only one in eight patients with SSc [17]. These data are supported by the low frequency of anti-cyclic citrullinated peptide (anti-CCP) antibodies in patients with SSc, which are highly specific for RA [50–52]. Another study that described the clinical and laboratory features of 15 patients with SSc-RA overlap suggested a distinct entity based on characteristic features: generalized skin fibrosis, severe seropositive erosive polyarthritis, pulmonary fibrosis, anti-topoisomerase-I antibodies, and HLA haplotype DR4. None of the reported patients had destructive DIP involvement [53]. A more recent meta-analysis confirmed this clinical phenotype in anti-CCP-positive SSc patients [54].

Multicenter interventional trials have measured the presence of synovitis as a "modified Ritchie index" whereby the presence of swelling and tenderness of the MCP joints, wrists, elbows, and knees have been recorded. The disease activity score (DAS)-28 has been recommended as a core assessment tool for inflammatory arthritis in patients with SSc [1]. However, a recent study conducted in patients with early dcSSc showed an excellent inter and intra-observer reliability in the assessment of tendon joint count (TJC), but not in swollen joint count (SJC) [55]. This difficulty in assessing SJC, as well as the poor association between physical examination and musculoskeletal findings, may be attributable to overlapping skin fibrosis. In this regard, it bears noting that among the seven core arthritis measures used in clinical practice to assess the response in RA [56], only three functional assessments have undergone validation in SSc using the OMERACT filter criteria: the Disability Index of the Health Assessment Questionnaire (HAQ-DI), the Cochin Hand Function Scale, and the Hand Mobility in Scleroderma (HAMIS). A modified HAMIS using four items is currently being evaluated [57].

Prevalence

Joint involvement has been described as an initial manifestation in 12–65% of patients with SSc and as a possible manifestation in up to 46–97% of patients [1, 58]. A systematic study on articular manifestations in 38 patients with SSc detected tenderness, stress pain, or effusions in approximately 61% of patients. Ten patients had small effusions confined to the knees, with the exception of one PIP joint. The pattern was symmetrical polyarticular in 61%, oligoarticular in 22%, and monoarticular in 17% of patients. A retrospective analysis of 100 patients investigating the clinical features of hand and foot involvement in SSc identified foot arthralgia and arthritis in 23% and 14% of patients, respectively, and hand arthralgia and arthritis in 9% and 11% of patients, respectively [16, 59]. In 2010, a systematic cross-sectional examination of the EUSTAR registry, which included more than 7000 patients, identified synovitis in 16% (1191/7286) of patients with SSc, indicating synovial involvement may be a common feature in scleroderma [17]. The point prevalence of joint contracture, resulting from joint destruction turning into ankylosis and fibrotic changes in the skin, was 31% (2264/7286). In December 2020, the point prevalence of joint synovitis and joint contractures in the EUSTAR database was 21.7% (4086/18,871) and 34.8% (6558/18,871), respectively (*unpublished data*). In particular, the increased diagnosis of synovitis compared to 2010 could be attributable to the widespread use of ultrasonography in addition to clinical examination.

Imaging Studies

We have learned from the management of RA that musculoskeletal US is very useful for detecting synovitis that is "subclinical." Sonography shows synovitis as abnormal hypoechoic (relative to subdermal fat) intra-articular tissue that is poorly compressible and that exhibits Doppler signal with color or power Doppler imaging (Fig. 35.5). In several patients, tendon and articular involvement may coexist (Fig. 35.5).

One can speculate that it may be even more useful in SSc in which swelling can be subtle, especially in the fingers and hands. Furthermore, since ultrasound can detect inflammatory activity, the monitoring of inflammatory activity with power Doppler ultrasonography could be very valuable.

An Italian study that included 45 consecutive patients with SSc assessed articular involvement using US [60]. Joint effusion and synovial proliferation were found in 22 (49%) and 19 (42%) of patients, respectively (Table 35.2); synovial proliferation was associated with increased intra-articular power Doppler signals in 11 patients. The prevalence of synovitis detected with US (i.e., effusion and/or synovial proliferation) was significantly higher than that found by clinical examination (i.e., tenderness and/or swelling) (26 vs. 15 of 45 cases; $p = 0.03$). Some correlation between synovitis and acute-phase reactants was also observed.

A second study [23] assessed ultrasonographic hand features in 52 patients with SSc (Table 35.2). This study confirmed the more frequent detection of synovitis with US than with clinical examination (46% vs. 15%; $p < 0.01$), although 57% of patients had borderline mildly inflammatory activity with mostly Doppler grade 1.

Another study performed on 44 patients with SSc also demonstrated the utility of ultrasonography in the assessment of hand and wrist involvement in SSc, particularly for the detection of synovitis, which was detected in 12 patients (27%) [24] (Table 35.2). Recently, the systematic power Doppler ultrasonography evaluation of the hands of 103 SSc patients revealed synovial involvement in 33/103 (32%) of patients, with synovitis in 21 (64% of them) and inflammation in 18 (55%) with more frequent power Doppler positivity in the wrist and MCP joints. Furthermore, inflammatory synovitis was associated with CRP levels >5 mg/L, pericarditis, and inflammatory arthralgia [25].

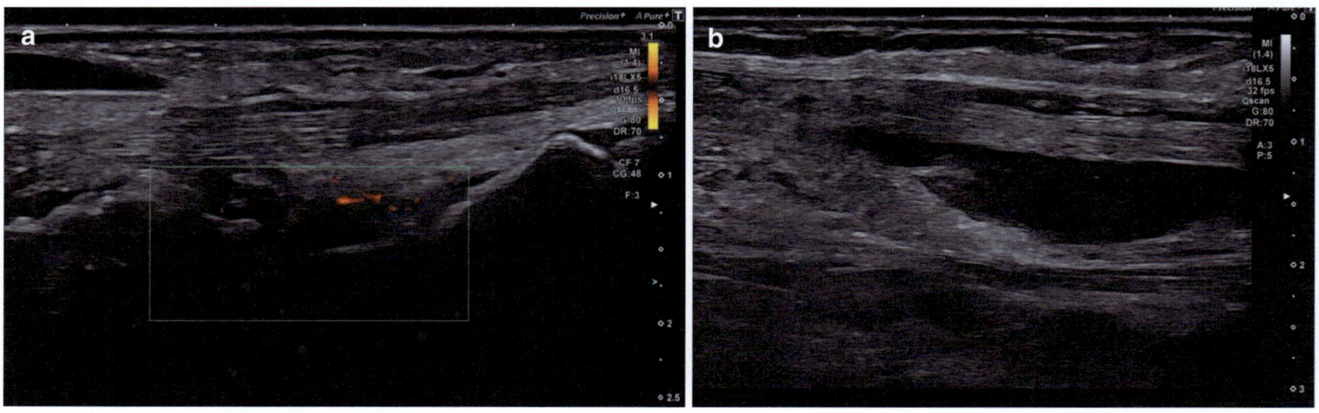

Fig. 35.5 (**a**) US-assessed synovial distension of the radiocarpal joint with low-grade power Doppler signal and hypoechoic effusion in the extensor tendon sheath (**b**) Tenosynovitis of the flexor tendons characterized by sheath thickening with iso-hypoechoic effusion

Table 35.2 Prevalence of joint involvement with ultrasonography and MRI

	Ultrasonography			MRI	
	Cuomo et al. [60] ($n = 45$)	Elhai et al. [23] ($n = 52$)	Freire et al. [24] ($n = 44$)	Low et al. [61] ($n = 17$)	Allanore et al. [62] ($n = 38$)
Frequency of synovitis, n (%)	22 (49%)	24 (46%)	17 (39%)	19 (50%)	8 (47%)
	19 (42%) with synovial proliferation	68 regions explored:	52 regions explored:		
		33 (48%) power Doppler grade 1	28/52 (54%) power Doppler grade 1		
		6 (9%) power Doppler grade 2 or 3	5/52 (10%) power Doppler grade 2 or 3		
Frequency of joint space narrowing, n (%)	8 (18%)	No data	No data	No data	No data
	MCP: 8 (100%)				
	PIP: 2 (25%)				
Frequency of erosions, n (%)	5 (11%)	No data	No data	7 (41%)	No data
	Wrist: 1 (20%)			Wrist: 2 (29%)	
	MCP: 4 (80%)			MCP: 5 (71%)	
				PIP: 2 (29%)	

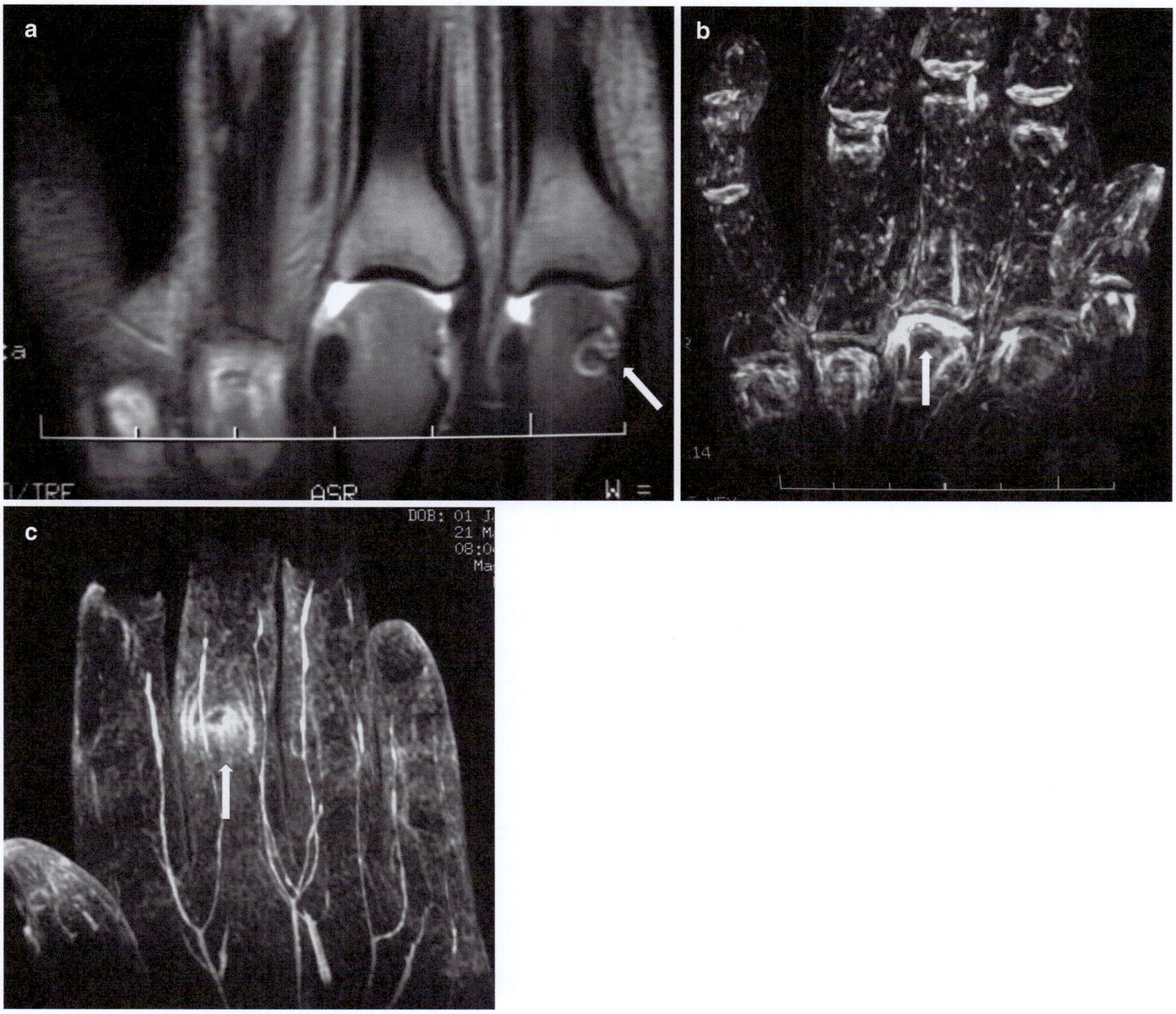

Fig. 35.6 (**a**) MRI showing synovitis, and erosion at fourth MCP joints (white arrow). Magnetic resonance angiography revealing synovitis, particularly at the third MCP joint (**b**) and third PIP joint (**c**) (white arrows)

Other than hand and wrist, ankle and foot synovitis was also evaluated in a recent French study which confirmed that US was more sensitive in detecting at least one joint with synovitis than physical examination (52% vs. 25%; $p = 0.025$) [63]. Notably, among the 55 SSc patients included, 29% had ankle and/or foot synovitis, mostly located at metatarsophalangeal joints (25.5%).

MRI is also a very promising research tool to detect synovitis (Table 35.2). MRI reveals proliferative synovitis as thickening of the synovial membrane that appears as rapid enhancement after the administration of gadolinium; it is also well shown on fat-suppressed gadolinium-enhanced T1-weighted image (Fig. 35.6a). Hand inflammatory joint disease has been assessed by MRI in 17 patients with history of joint pain or swelling [61]. Ten patients had inflammatory MRI findings with synovitis (n = 8), joint effusion (n = 7), or tenosynovitis (n = 8). In another series of 17 patients with SSc and arthralgia but no overt inflammatory arthritis, while both MRI and ultrasound were useful for characterizing synovial inflammation in SSc, MRI appeared clearly more sensitive than US in this setting [64]. Another study compared MRI and ultrasonography to detect inflammatory arthropathy in SSc patients with hand arthralgia [26]. MRI and ultrasonography were both shown to be useful to characterize synovial inflammation, but MRI was also found more sensitive in this setting.

With regard to the burden of the vasculopathy in SSc, magnetic resonance angiography (MRA) has appeared as an appealing technique to assess hand vascular involvement. MRA can indeed be used to identify and quantitatively characterize the vascular disease in SSc fingers. We have described in a cross-sectional study the major arterial and venous involvement that can be identified using MRA. In addition, micro-MRA has also been used to focus on fingers, and non-enhanced MR angiography has also been used to improve the evaluation of the hand vasculature in vasospastic disorders [65, 66]. MRA also enables detection of synovitis (Fig. 35.6b, c), and in our study evaluating hand MRA in 38 SSc patients, 19 patients had one or more joints with synovitis and 4 one or more areas with tenosynovitis [62].

Laboratory Findings

Rheumatoid factor (RF) positivity may occur in about 30% of SSc patients [49, 67]. This test appears to be nonspecific and does not serve to distinguish patients with SSc with MSK manifestations from those without [49]. In 100 Caucasian SSc patients, the presence of anti-CCP antibodies but not RF positivity was found to be associated with arthritis [68]. However, in a series of 34 patients with a current or past history of articular symptoms selected from 300 consecutive patients with SSc, a distinctive subset of 10 patients with deforming arthritis was characterized. These patients more frequently had limited cutaneous subtype, anti-centromere antibody, and also positive RF (80% vs. 13%; $p < 0.05$). Seven out of these ten fulfilled RA classification criteria, but anti-CCP status was not known at this time [69]. A recent study [70] found a higher prevalence of RF positivity in lcSSc and SSc sine scleroderma compared to dcSSc (15.7% and 20%, respectively in the former vs. 9% in the latter). Notably, RF may also be found in patients with SSc-associated secondary Sjögren's syndrome, which is common in SSc and occurs more frequently in patients with lcSSc and positive anti-centromere antibody [69, 71]. Unlike RF, the detection of anti-CCP antibodies might be of great help in identifying uncommon cases of SSc-RA overlap [50]. Several cross-sectional studies estimated that the point prevalence of anti-CCP antibodies in patients with SSc ranged from 1% to 15% (Table 35.3). In a recent meta-analysis including 1231 SSc patients from 13 observational studies, the mean prevalence of anti-CCP antibodies was 9.2% [54]. Some studies also suggested the potential diagnostic value of this test to identify patients with SSc also having RA, with a sensitivity ranging from 50% to 100% and a diagnostic specificity of about 95% [50–52, 72–74, 77]. However, the presence of RF or anti-CCP antibodies does not seem to directly correlate with the clinical or radiographic pattern of arthritis, including the subset of patients with erosions on X-ray, which supports the existence of a primary inflammatory and erosive arthropathy in SSc independent of RA [49].

Anti-Ku antibodies are found in a wide spectrum of connective tissue diseases, including overlap syndromes with SSc and myositis. Synovitis and joint contractures have been found to be associated with anti-Ku antibodies in patients with SSc. A strong association has also been identified between these antibodies and the presence of muscle weakness/atrophy and muscle enzyme elevation [78].

Analysis of the synovial fluid generally reveals normal or modestly increased leukocyte concentrations of less than 2000 cells/mm^3 and a predominantly mononuclear infiltrate [79]. Rarely, frankly inflamed synovial fluid with inclusion-containing cells indistinguishable from the ragocytes (leukocytes with peripheral cytoplasmic inclusions) of RA has been reported [80]. Immunocytologic studies have revealed that these inclusion bodies contain large amounts of fibrin and/or fibrin breakdown products as well as the immunoglobulins (Ig) G and IgM. Synovial biopsies from SSc joints have demonstrated histological evidence of inflammation in the synovial membrane, as well as inflammatory infiltrates in the subsynovium and perivascular tissues, with lymphocytic and plasma cell infiltration; these features are associated with superficial fibrin deposition and focal microvascular obliteration [79, 81]. In contrast to RA, however, the usual proliferation of synovial hyperplasia and pannus formation typical of RA does not occur in the SSc. Instead, fibrin accumulation in the synovial lining cells, with atrophy of the synovial cells leading to fibrosis, is observed, similar to that present in the dermis.

Joint Involvement as a Correlate of Prognosis in SSc

Analysis of the EUSTAR database revealed that synovitis was present in SSc patients at all disease stages. However, patients with synovitis and early disease (date of first non-Raynaud's symptom <5 years) were more likely to experience diffuse cutaneous thickening (Fig. 35.7).

Table 35.3 Point prevalence of anti-CCP antibodies in systemic sclerosis

	Avouac et al. [49] (*n* = 120)	Morita et al. [51] (*n* = 114)	Generini et al. [72] (*n* = 55)	Marrone et al. [52] (*n* = 60)	Ingegnoli et al. [73] (*n* = 75)	Ueda-Hayakawa et al. [74] (*n* = 146)	Payet et al. [75] (*n* = 44)	Farkas et al. [76] (*n* = 168)
Prevalence of anti-CCP, *n* (%)	2 (1.5%)	3 (2.6%)	4 (7%)	5 (8%)	8 (11%)	18 (12%)	7 (16%)	10 (6%)
Sensitivity of anti-CCP for the diagnosis of associated rheumatoid arthritis	100%	86%	50%	83%	75%	64%	No data	No data

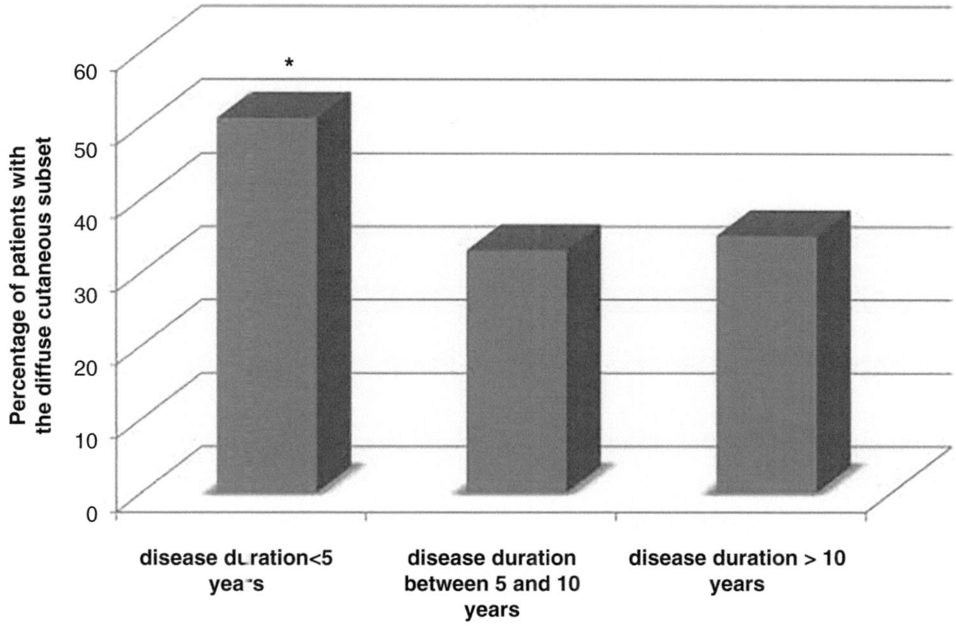

Fig. 35.7 Patients with synovitis and early disease (date of first non-Raynaud's symptom <5 years) are more likely to experience diffuse cutaneous thickening. *$P < 0.05$ vs. patients with disease duration >5 years

This observation raises the question of the prognostic value of synovitis in patients with early SSc to identify those with potential risk of developing the diffuse cutaneous subset, which has a more fulminant course.

Two prospective cohort studies including one from the EUSTAR database have identified joint synovitis as a predictor of overall disease progression. The first study included 1301 patients with SSc with disease duration ≤3 years at inclusion and with a follow-up of at least 2 years (mean follow-up: 4.5 ± 2.2 years) [32]. Joint synovitis, detected by clinical examination, was independently predictive of the worsening of the mRSS (≥30% and ≥5 points) and of the further occurrence of new ischemic digital ulcers and decreased left ventricular ejection fraction. The second study was performed on 637 SSc patients with the diffuse cutaneous subset [82]. Joint synovitis was also identified in univariate and multivariate analyses as a predictor for progressive skin fibrosis and confirmed in a second validation cohort (188 patients with dcSSc) as an independent predictor of progressive skin fibrosis within 1 year. The presence of arthritis ever was also found to be predictive of interstitial lung disease progression in two independent SSc cohorts. A prediction model for lung disease progression, combining the presence of both oxygen saturation $SpO_2 \leq 94\%$ after 6 min walking test and arthritis ever, was established in the derivation cohort and validated in the multinational validation cohort [83]. The fact that arthritis is one of the two main determinants of this robust evidence-based prediction model—the SPAR model—further highlights its important prognostic significance in SSc.

Another study conducted in the EUSTAR database aiming to predict mortality in SSc provides more evidence [84]. In fact, the presence of joint contractures was independently associated with mortality in multivariable analysis, and thus incorporated into a risk of mortality score, which has proven to accurately predict 3-year mortality in SSc patients.

The examination of the EUSTAR database also identified a strong association between synovitis and elevation of acute-phase reactants (ESR ≥28 mm and CRP ≥10 mg/L), reflecting systemic inflammation. This suggests that joint involvement has a close relationship with systemic inflammation in SSc [49]. This is supported by the infiltration of inflammatory cells in SSc synovial biopsies [79]. Further studies are warranted to determine if joint involvement is the main contributor to systemic inflammation in SSc, as is observed in RA.

Radiologic Features: Structural Osteoarticular Lesions

Many distinctive radiographic abnormalities have been recognized in patients with SSc. Articular lesions from juxta-articular osteoporosis and joint space narrowing to frank erosions have been reported throughout the MCP, PIP, and DIP joints, as well as the wrist. Selective involvement of the first carpometacarpal phalangeal joint might be a distinctive feature of SSc. The described abnormalities include bilateral resorption of the trapezium and adjacent metacarpal bone along with intra-articular calcification and erosions [85]. The detection of pencil-in-cup deformity in hands and feet, considered to be relatively specific for psoriasis arthropathy, has also been reported [59]. The frequency of hand radiographic erosions is estimated between 5% and 40% (Table 35.4) [1, 49, 59, 67, 87]. Joint space narrowing is not uncommon in SSc; its point prevalence on X-ray has been reported to be about 30%, with a predominant involvement of DIP joints (Table 35.4) [1, 49, 59, 67, 87]. Joint space narrowing has been found with ultrasonography in 8/45 (18%) SSc patients.

Table 35.4 Prevalence of hand radiographic lesions in systemic sclerosis

	Avouac et al. [49] (*n* = 120)	Baron et al. [1] (*n* = 38)	La Montagna et al. [16] (*n* = 51)	La Montagna et al. [59] (*n* = 76)	Brun et al. [86] (*n* = 41)	Koutaissoff et al. [87] (*n* = 167)	Blocka et al. [67] (*n* = 55)	Ingegnoli et al. [73] (*n* = 75)	Erre et al. [88] (*n* = 41)
Joint involvement, *n* (%):									
Erosion	25 (21)	15 (40)	10 (20)	8 (10.5)	9 (21)	30 (18)	12 (22)	11 (16)	8 (19)
Joint space narrowing	35 (28)	13 (34)	17 (33)	31 (41)	10 (24)	102 (61)	n.d.	n.d.	29 (71)
Bone involvement, *n* (%):									
Radiological demineralization	28 (23)	16 (42)	32 (63)	12 (16)	7 (17)	n.d.	n.d.	17 (23)	4 (10)
Acro-osteolysis	26 (22)	14 (37)	25 (55)	22 (29)	11 (27)	41 (25)	28 (51)	13 (17)	7 (17)
Soft tissue involvement, *n* (%):									
Flexion contracture	32 (27)	n.d.	n.d.	31 (41)	n.d.	n.d.	45 (82)	n.d.	11 (27)
Calcinosis	28 (23)	19 (50)	18 (35)	45 (59)	18 (44)	25 (15)	14 (25)	19 (25)	12 (29)

n.d. no data

Modern techniques such as US and MRI have also been used to describe structural articular lesions. Point prevalence of erosions assessed by ultrasonography on 45 SSc patients was 11% (5/45 patients) [60]. In the two studies using MRI, hand erosions were detected in 16% (6/38 patients) and 41% (7/17 patients) [61, 62]. It is noteworthy that the predictive value of erosions detected by MRI is not known and remains to be determined. The pathogenesis of erosions is still unknown, although several hypotheses have been raised on the mechanisms underlying their formation. Erosions might arise secondary to inflammatory synovitis, or they might represent focal resorptive changes resulting from the continuous traction of tendons underlying demineralized bone, or they might represent a localized manifestation of an unexplained, more widespread osseous resorptive phenomenon recognized to affect various regions of the skeleton. In this regard, the resorption and osteonecrosis of the lunate bone may sometimes be observed in SSc patients (Fig. 35.8a, b), and in our experience especially in those exhibiting a particularly severe vascular phenotype. In the feet, the presence of erosions in the MTP joints could be due to an increase in plantar foot pressures identified in patients with SSc, similar to the association of erosions and abnormal plantar pressures that has been reported in patients with RA [59, 89, 90].

In a recent controlled study involving 120 patients, erosive arthritis, as defined by the occurrence of both erosions and joint space narrowing, was found in 22 (18%) SSc patients [50] (Fig. 35.9a–d). The 5-year longitudinal follow-up of these patients, with a systematic examination of dual time-point X-ray, showed a total radiographic progression of erosive arthritis in 24 (23%) patients with SSc. Among these, 10 had developed incident erosive arthritis, defined by the occurrence on the second X-ray of at least 1 erosion and joint space narrowing, and 14 experienced worsening of their baseline lesions, defined by the occurrence on the second X-ray of at least 1 new erosion and/or joint space narrowing [91]. The presence of erosive arthritis was not associated at baseline with any SSc characteristics or with the presence of RF or anti-CCP antibodies. This is in accordance with previous studies that failed to show correlation between erosive arthritis and clinical or laboratory variables [48, 67].

Despite its high frequency, we did not identify any independent predictor of the progression of erosive arthritis in SSc [91]. This lack of predictive factor for erosive arthritis might be related to the multifactorial aspects of SSc arthropathy [92]. An overlap with RA should be considered, but was found only in two patients with erosive arthritis at baseline and in one patient with worsened erosive arthritis. The possibility of erosive osteoarthritis should also be considered, particularly in light of the nature of the erosions [89], the low frequency of persistent clinical synovitis in patients with development of erosive arthritis (5/24, 21%), the high frequency of DIP joint involvement, and the large proportion in our sample of postmenopausal women. Finally, erosive arthropathy could also be as a direct result of SSc and considered as an integral feature of this disease.

There is thus a need to clarify the precise nature of the arthropathy observed in SSc in order to further identify valid predictors of the progression of erosive arthritis directly related to SSc. As reliable predictors of the future course of erosive arthritis are still unknown, patients should be followed up regularly, with clinical examination and regular X-rays. Moreover, this lack of valid predictors may significantly limit the use of potentially effective drugs [93]. Recent developments of new imaging techniques in SSc should allow an early detection of erosive arthritis, before being detected on X-ray, and likely increase the chance of defining accurate predictors [60–62].

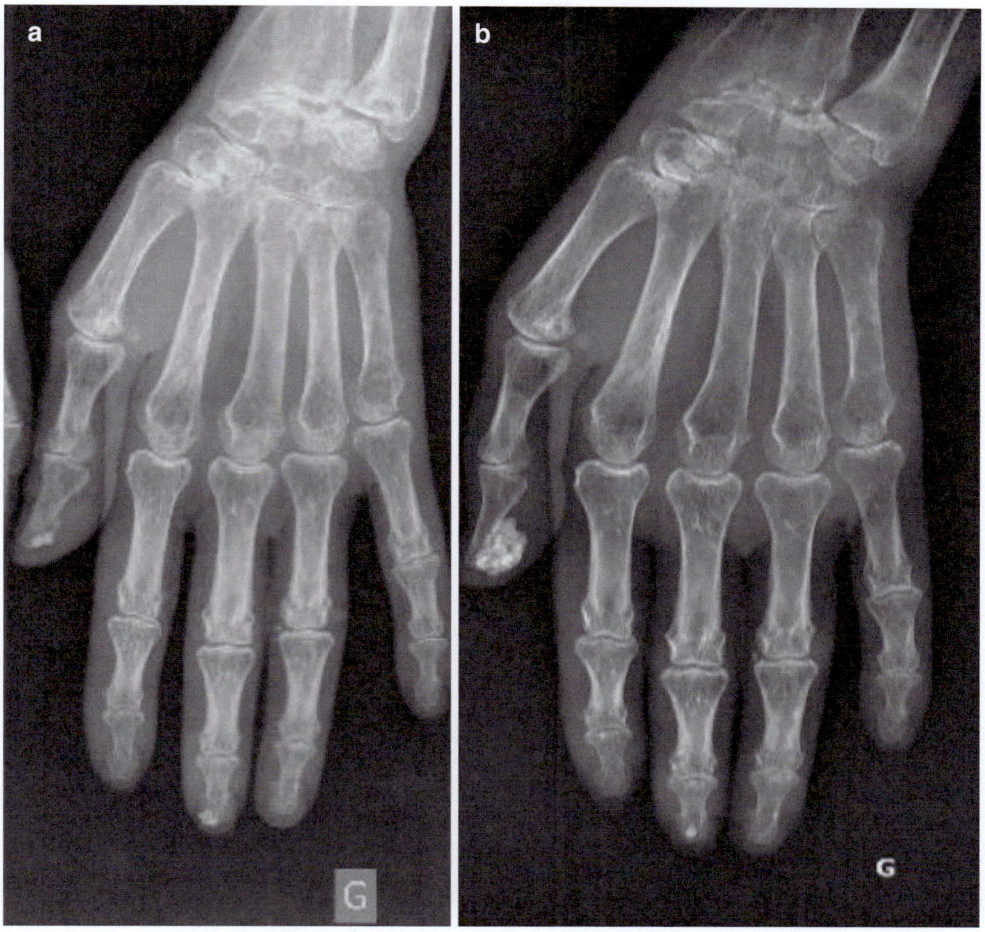

Fig. 35.8 (**a**, **b**) Sequential X-ray images of osteonecrosis of the left lunate in a patient with diffuse cutaneous systemic sclerosis in 2013 (**a**) and 2018 (**b**)

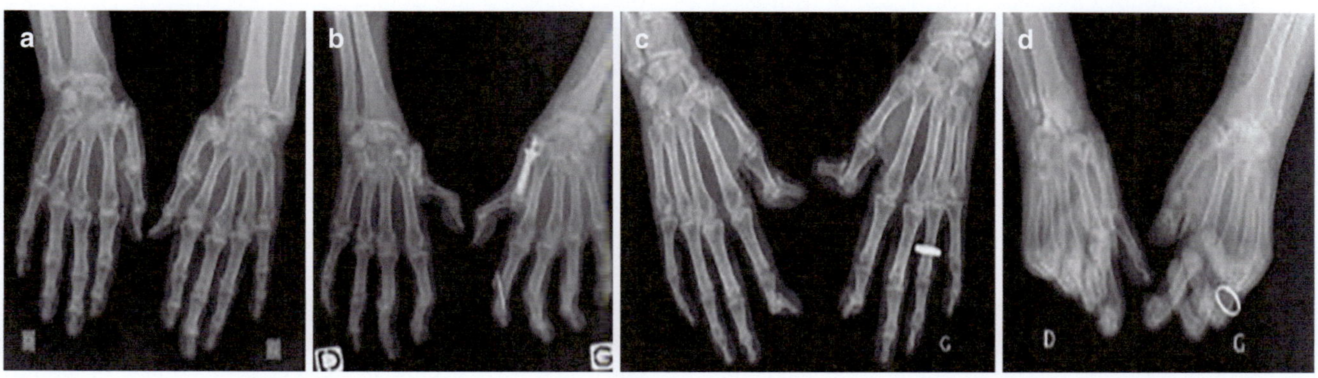

Fig. 35.9 (**a**–**d**) Four cases of erosive radiographic arthritis characterized by erosions and joint space narrowing involving the wrist, MCP, PIP, and/or DIP joints

Management

Pharmacological Treatments

The management of articular involvement is essentially symptomatic. Supportive therapies or disease-modifying antirheumatic drugs (DMARDs) have not yet been systematically evaluated for the treatment of articular involvement in SSc in randomized controlled trials (RCTs). Only two recent RCTs considered and analyzed joint involvement as a secondary outcome measure [94, 95]. However, the effect of these drugs (i.e., tocilizumab and abatacept) in reducing TJC was not significant, despite several observational studies showing promising results.

For the most part, the minor MSK symptoms of SSc, such as arthralgia, respond to simple NSAIDs treatment. Caution should be exercised, however, with this class of drugs because of the enhanced risk of gastroesophageal abnormalities or bleeding and impaired renal function in this group of patients. Low-dose corticosteroids (<10 mg/day) may also have some value for the symptomatic treatment of inflammatory arthritis or tenosynovitis. Employing a similar approach to RA, methotrexate (MTX) is typically used for the treatment of an inflammatory arthritis. Subcutaneous route may be used to mitigate against gastrointestinal symptoms and ensure effective bioavailability. Cyclophosphamide has also been considered, although secondary analyses of the scleroderma lung study did not show any significant effects on articular outcomes. Specifically, there were no significant differences between placebo and cyclophosphamide groups for joint swelling and joint tenderness at 12 and 24 months [96].

A small, pilot study of 6 months of intravenous immunoglobulin therapy in seven women with SSc and severe, refractory inflammatory joint involvement reported reduction in joint pain and tenderness, together with improvement of quality of life. Reliable conclusions from this small case series cannot be drawn; however, it use may be reserved in patients with severe and refractory articular involvement. The cost of immunoglobulin therapy is an additional factor that would limit their use [97]. The same group [98] also investigated ten SSc patients with joint involvement treated with hydroxychloroquine for at least 6 months and observed a trend for improvement in synovitis on US ($p = 0.008$) as compared to matched SSc patients with joint involvement. However, these findings gathered from a small retrospective series have not been confirmed on a larger scale and to date there is not a defined indication for the use of hydroxychloroquine in SSc patients with articular involvement.

The introduction of biologic DMARDs has led to a new era in the treatment of inflammatory rheumatic conditions and is of increasing interest in SSc-related arthritis. The efficacy of tumor necrosis factor (TNF) inhibitors on inflammatory joint symptoms was suggested in a retrospective study performed on 18 patients treated with etanercept over a period of 2–66 months [99]. Fifteen of these 18 patients had "positive responses" (not defined in the "letter to the editor" report), with apparent significant decrease in signs of inflammation or synovitis on follow-up examination and complete resolution of joint symptoms in some patients. Mean HAQ-DI scores also decreased with therapy, paralleling the improvement in joint disease. Despite these promising preliminary results, no other study has assessed the potential efficacy of TNF-inhibitors in SSc-related arthritis. This may be due to concerns about the safety of this therapeutic class in SSc. One case of fatal exacerbation of fibrosing alveolitis has been reported in a patient with SSc following adalimumab treatment [100] and very rare cases of fatal exacerbation of pulmonary fibrosis while on treatment with TNF-inhibitors described in patients with RA at the time of introduction of these therapies [101] have further deterred their use. Nevertheless, a 26-week open-label pilot study was performed on 16 patients that aimed to assess the safety of infliximab in dcSSc. One hundred twenty-seven adverse events (10 severe) occurred in 16 patients. Of these, 19 adverse events were directly related to infliximab treatment. Moreover, infusion reactions directly related to infliximab led to early treatment discontinuation in 8/16 patients [102]. Separately, infliximab did not show a clear overall benefit at week 26, although articular involvement was not included as an outcome measure. Thus, these data may limit the further evaluation of this class of drug in SSc-related arthritis in formal RCTs.

A three-round Delphi exercise was performed among EUSTAR centers to obtain expert consensus on the use of TNF-inhibitors in SSc [103]. Most EUSTAR experts recommended the use of TNF-inhibitors only as part of RCTs and discouraged off-label use in individual patients outside of clinical trials. Arthritis was considered a manifestation that might respond to TNF-inhibitors, and the group recommended that the response of SSc arthritis to TNF-inhibitors should be investigated in more detail. Robust, controlled trials demonstrating the safety and efficacy of TNF-inhibitors for joint involvement in patients with SSc are needed before employed in clinical practice.

Rituximab, a chimeric monoclonal antibody against the protein CD20 that is well-established in the management of RA, might also be beneficial for the treatment of SSc arthritis. However, no study has yet formally assessed rituximab for this specific indication. Open-label trials and one large observational study from the EUSTAR database [104] have indicated a good efficacy of rituximab in improving skin fibrosis and stabilizing lung function in SSc, although articular involvement was not evaluated in any of these studies [105, 106]. Further research assessing the efficacy of rituximab in SSc-related joint disease is now warranted before this treatment is recommended.

The EUSTAR group has recorded observations following treatment with tocilizumab, a chimeric monoclonal antibody against IL-6 receptor in refractory SSc. This study revealed a trend toward articular improvement in cases of polyarthritis, but with a weak decline in signs of dermatologic or pulmonary involvement [107]. A decrease in the DAS-28 was reported of 1.8 ± 1.5 (2.8 ± 0.6 before the last infusion administered at 6 months vs. 4.6 ± 1.0 at the beginning, $p = 0.02$) with a decrease in the TJCs of 5 (4.2 ± 4.3 vs. 9.2 ± 8.6) and in the SJCs of 0.5 (3.0 ± 4.4 vs. 3.5 ± 3). A good EULAR response was observed in three out of five patients.

FaSScinate was a phase II, double blind, placebo-controlled clinical trial with the purpose to evaluate the efficacy of tocilizumab on the cutaneous involvement in recent onset and evolving dcSSc [94]. Favorable trends in skin score for tocilizumab were detected, though the primary skin score endpoint was not met (difference in the least squares mean, LSM change of mRSS at 24 weeks −2.70, 95% CI –5.85 to 0.45; $p = 0.0915$). In addition, fewer patients in the tocilizumab group than in the placebo group had a decline in % Forced vital capacity (FVC) at 48 weeks ($p = 0.0373$). Of note, randomization in this study was stratified by joint involvement at baseline (<4 vs. ≥4 joints on the 28 tender joint count). In patients with joint involvement, change from baseline at 24 weeks and 48 weeks in 28 tender joint count (secondary endpoint) showed a favorable trend in the tocilizumab group vs. the placebo group, but data were not statistically significant.

A recent case series and literature review [108] including 16 patients treated with tocilizumab for a median duration of 18.5 months showed a significant reduction of the mRSS ($p < 0.001$) and an improvement of joint and MSK involvement in 80% and 75% of patients, respectively. Patients with early SSc responded better to tocilizumab ($p = 0.001$).

The EUSTAR group has also collected observations on the effects of abatacept on articular involvement in SSc [107, 109]. Like tocilizumab, favorable effects on inflammatory articular involvement were obtained after 11 months of treatment with abatacept with a good EULAR response in 6 out of 11 patients [107]. A subsequent retrospective observational EUSTAR study [109] confirmed that in 27 SSc patients treated with abatacept, the number of tender and swollen joints decreased at 12 months vs. baseline ($p < 0.03$ and $p < 0.02$, respectively). Moreover, abatacept also had a beneficial effect on HAQ-DI, morning stiffness, and mRSS.

In the phase II, randomized, double-blind, placebo-controlled trial of abatacept in dcSS, the primary endpoint (i.e., change in mRSS over 12 months) was not met, with an adjusted mean treatment difference of −1.75 units ($p = 0.28$) [95]. By contrast, HAQ-DI and a composite measure were significantly better with abatacept. A potential effect on articular involvement was evaluated as secondary outcome measure and no differences in the swollen joint count were found between the abatacept and placebo groups at 12 months (LSM ± SEM 0.75 ± 0.84, $p = 0.37$) and tender joint count (LSM ± SEM 0.76 ± 1.28, $p = 0.55$). Notably, among patients who needed escape therapy (26%), polyarthritis was the reason in three patients in the placebo group vs. 0 patient in the abatacept group.

Thus, the observational data reported from the EUSTAR group and recent case-series suggest that both tocilizumab and abatacept may be considered in SSc patients with inflammatory articular involvement refractory to conventional DMARDs (i.e., MTX, leflunomide). The discrepancy between these real-life data and results from recent RCTs suggest the need to better define SSc-specific MSK outcomes in RCTs, in order to obtain more robust conclusions.

Clements [110] suggested a treatment algorithm for SSc-arthritis according to the subclassification of patients as affected by erosive polyarthritis, RA, and psoriatic arthritis-like and nonerosive lupus-like polyarthritis. The absence of appropriately designed RCTs to specifically address MSK manifestations of SSc argues for such a pragmatic approach. Typically, glucocorticoids (mainly systemic and/or local in case of monoarthritis) may be a first-line approach in SSc patients with arthritis and with early consideration of MTX in patients with polyarticular involvement. The clinical response to hydroxychloroquine seems rather unsatisfactory in SSc patients with polyarthritis, although it may be considered in cases of mild polyarthralgia. A switch to leflunomide may be considered in SSc patients who do not respond to MTX, with rituximab, tocilizumab, and abatacept as subsequent treatments. TNF-inhibitors should be considered only in cases refractory to the aforementioned biologics.

Developing SSc-Specific MSK Outcome Measures for Future RCTs

A major unmet need in the management of (inflammatory) MSK manifestations of SSc is that accurate outcome measures are yet to be defined. Lack of standardized and validated outcome measures that represent and are sensitive to SSc-MSK manifestations has meant intervention trials either do not evaluate for these or utilize borrowed endpoints. This means trials have been limited in the extent to which they inform on the efficacy of treatments on MSK manifestations. As summarized earlier, studies in SSc have often employed the DAS28 outcome measure used in RA trials and selected individual components such as tender and swollen joint counts. The DAS28, however, is a surrogate for joint synovitis, the primary basis for DMARDs change in RA, but is not designed to capture the underlying MSK pathophysiological processes of SSc.

The development of an outcome measure requires the identification of core 'domain(s)' and at least one applicable measurement instrument. In the case of MSK manifestations of SSc, the domains should detect tendon and synovial joint involvement. In addition, there is arguably the need to be able to discriminate between inflammatory and fibrosing pathology when evaluating anti-inflammatory and immune modulating agents. In line with the principles of successful outcome measures [111], such an instrument must prove to be truthful (with construct, content, face, and criterion validity), discriminative, and feasible. The development of specific MSK outcome measures and their application in future appropriately designed clinical trials would improve the management and outcomes in people with SSc.

Non-pharmacological Management Strategies

Non-pharmacological interventions are an important adjunct to pharmacotherapy in reducing the burden of disease and enhancing quality of life.

The current literature on rehabilitation techniques in SSc consists of studies evaluating the effectiveness of paraffin wax treatment, hand and face stretching exercises, connective tissue massage and joint manipulation, splints, aerobic exercise, and resistance training. The data seem promising, except for splints, for the improvement in joint motion, hand function, and cardiopulmonary endurance. However, except for a few RCTs, the majority of studies involved small sample sizes and no control groups. Thus, larger randomized controlled studies are needed to fully determine the effectiveness of rehabilitation techniques for persons with SSc, in order to improve quality of life and work disability, which are major burdens in early SSc as well [112].

As previously mentioned, the joint involvement of the hand seems to have the greatest impact on daily activities and quality of life. In this regard, occupational therapy—especially if integrated with a self-administered stretching program—might have a role in improving hand function and activities of daily living, even through the use of devices such as modified handles on kitchen utensils, jar opening devices, button hooks, etc. [113, 114].

Surgery of the hand for SSc is generally considered for pain reduction, severe fixed deformities with functional limitations, ulceration, and calcinosis. The goals of surgery are limited and include pain relief, repositioning the digits, providing a functional position of fusion, and in some cases modest mobilization through resection arthroplasty, to marginally improve finger function for patients with marked preexisting limitations. Surgical reconstruction of severely flexed PIP joints by straightening and fusing them is quite successful if the MCP joints are mobile. This procedure may increase function and reduce the frequency of dorsal skin ulceration. Some rigid, deformed digits benefit from MCP joint resection to overcome contracture, reposition the digits, and introduce a small range of mobility. Surgical wounds generally heal well following fusion of the PIP or DIP joints [115]. Nevertheless, as the benefit of these surgical procedures can be minimal and complications can occur, surgery for hand contractures is generally not advised in SSc, but, if performed, it should be performed by an experienced hand surgeon [116].

Non-articular Musculoskeletal Manifestations

Calcinosis

Non-articular abnormalities are prominent in SSc and sometimes very specific. Indeed, subcutaneous calcifications may be seen as a hallmark of SSc in comparison to other connective tissue disorders (Fig. 35.10a, b). Several studies using

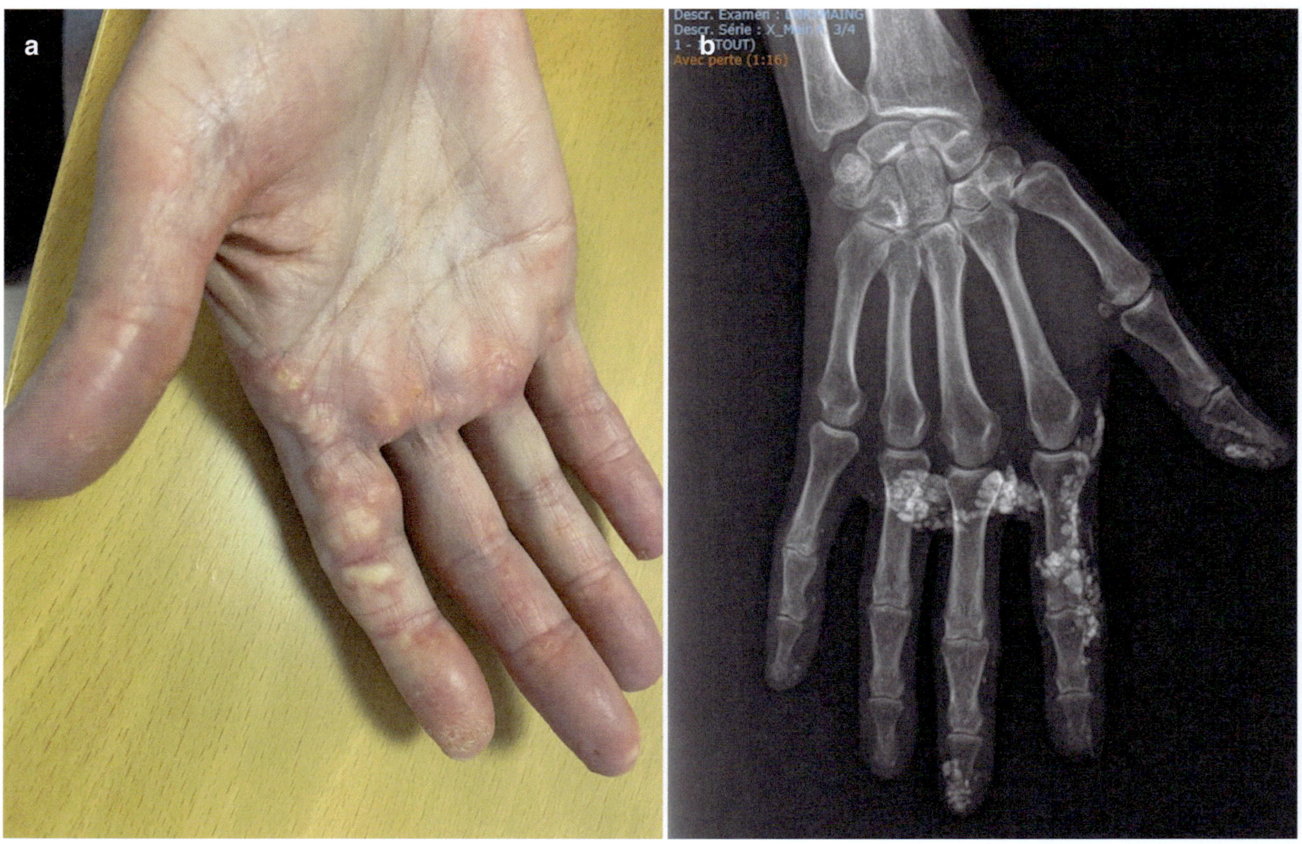

Fig. 35.10 (**a**, **b**) Severe calcinosis of the right hand, as it appears in photo (**a**) and conventional X-ray (**b**).

consecutive X-ray or ultrasonography of the hands have allowed clarification of its point prevalence, which is about 20–30% (Table 35.4) [49, 60, 87]. The incidence of radiographic calcinosis of the hands after a median duration of 5 years was 14% in a recent study from our group [91]. Calcinosis may also occur less frequently in other locations such as feet, knees, and legs. In a large retrospective cohort study conducted in 5218 SSc patients, the prevalence of calcinosis was 24.7% [117], whereas a recent literature review indicated that it may range from 18% to 49% [118].

A recent study evaluated more than 300 calcinosis lesions from 52 SSc patients and proposed to classify calcinosis in SSc as mousse, stone, net, and plate according to clinical and X-ray features [119]. The study also found an association between mousse calcinosis with pulmonary arterial hypertension and stone calcinosis with pulmonary involvement. It is noteworthy that calcinosis predominates at sites of repetitive stress or pressure, suggesting that trauma and/or ischemia may contribute to its pathogenesis as this is well known for shoulder calcifications. Indeed, recent evidence has shown that the index finger, and to a lesser extent, the thumb are the two digits most affected by calcinosis [120]. Furthermore, calcinosis has been found to be associated with digital ulcerations, teleangectasia, and with the late nailfold videocapillaroscopy pattern and especially with severe capillary loss, which strengthens the link between these radiographic lesions and digital destructive vasculopathy [49, 117, 121]. In addition, digital ulcers have recently been identified as independent predictors of radiographic progression of calcinosis (Hazard Ratio, HR 3.16, 95% CI 1.22–9.43) [91]. It bears noting that some SSc patients may also develop very large calcified masses (Figs. 35.11a, b and 35.12). In this regard, following a systematic review of the literature (SLR) and our cases, we have proposed that "pseudotumoral" should be the term used in SSc to define calcinosis larger than 2 cm, which tend to develop in multiple sites (especially the hands, shoulders, elbows, and hips) and more often are periarticular and symmetrically distributed [122]. Furthermore, pseudotumoral forms appear to mostly affect patients who exhibit a severe vascular phenotype, further corroborating the fact that ischemia may play a prominent role in the pathogenesis of calcinosis in SSc.

Despite many attempts, there is still a lack of efficient treatments for calcinosis [123–126]. The natural course and

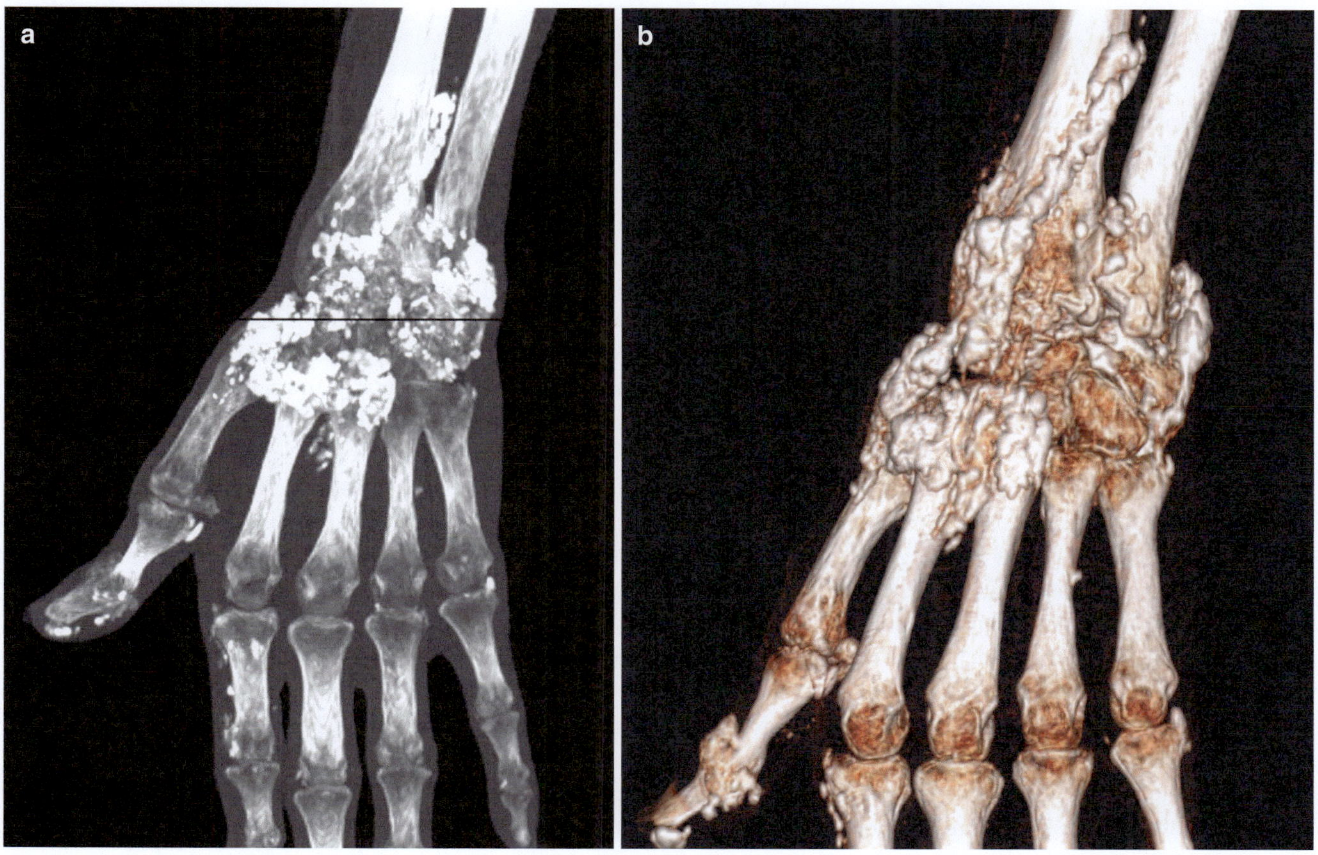

Fig. 35.11 (**a**, **b**) Pseudotumoral calcinosis of the left wrist assessed by CT-scan in coronal maximum intensity projection (MIP) image (**a**) and in 3D coronal volume-rendering image (**b**)

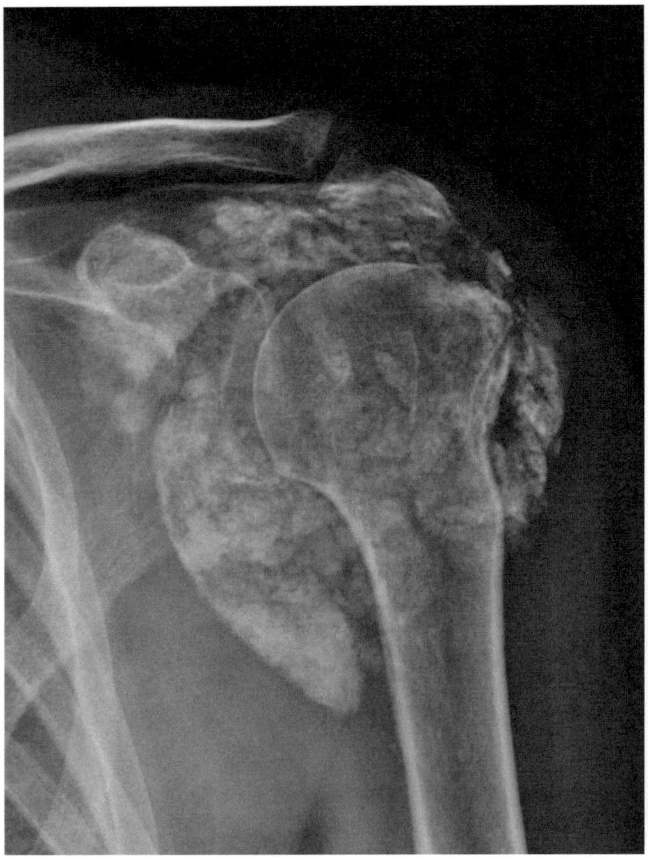

Fig. 35.12 Pseudotumoral calcinosis of the left shoulder assessed by conventional X-ray

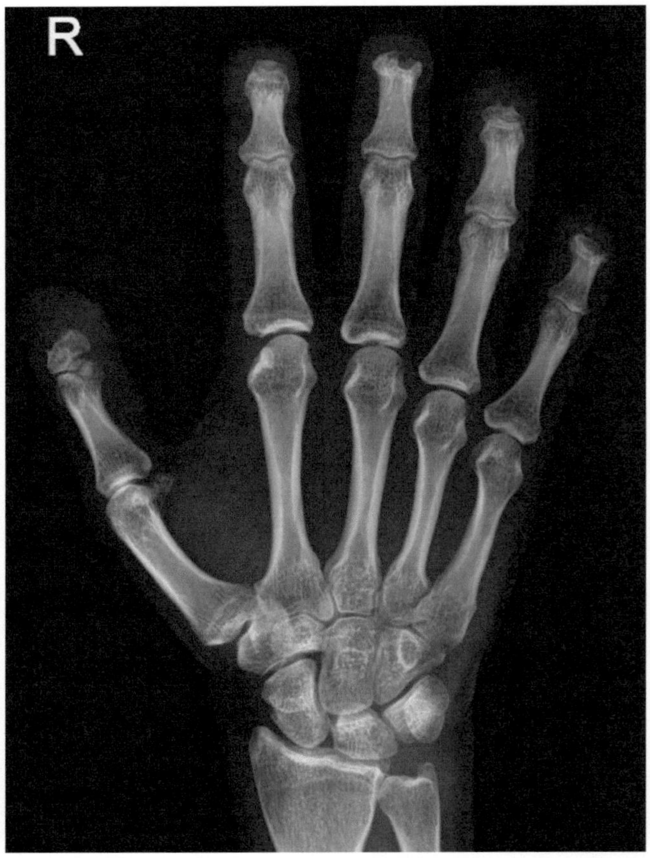

Fig. 35.13 Acro-osteolysis involving all the terminal phalanges of the right hand in a young female patient with dcSSc

strong heterogeneity of calcinosis are very challenging and have prevented clinical trials until now. The results of our prospective study suggest that the treatment of calcinosis should primarily target SSc vasculopathy [91]. This may be supported by data reported on shoulder tendinitis in which calcinosis usually appears close to tendon ischemic sites [127]. Nevertheless, no robust data confirmed that calcium channel blockers have a positive effect on calcinosis. The effects of other treatments, including bisphosphonates, warfarin, and minocycline, remain controversial and were obtained through small series [118, 128–130]. Considering pseudotumoral forms, our recent case series and SLR have highlighted the lack of effective medical treatment, with some reporting benefits with colchicine exclusively in reducing the inflammation around calcinosis, though no drug proved effective in reducing the size of calcinosis [122]. Surgical excision of calcinosis is the only measure that provided moderate results, also with respect to pain relief and function. However, the procedure requires extensive incisions and carries a risk of slower wound healing, and thus should be limited to selected cases (e.g., with recurrent pain and ulceration/overinfection or spinal forms with nerve compression) [115, 122].

Acro-Osteolysis

Osseous resorption is another common finding and hand acro-osteolysis occurs in about 20% of the patients [49, 59, 116] (Table 35.4 and Fig. 35.13). Furthermore, other locations may be involved such as the carpal bones, radius, ulna, ribs, mandible, clavicle, humerus, and cervical spine [131]. In a group of 134 Mediterranean patients, the incidence of vitamin D deficiency appeared to be 42%, and secondary hyperparathyroidism was surprisingly high at 22%. The authors observed some correlation between these abnormalities and the occurrence of acro-osteolysis and calcinosis [132]. In another study performed in two European countries, we also found that vitamin D insufficiency and deficiency rates were very high and comparable between the two populations: 74/90 (82%) vs. 57/66 (86%) for insufficiency and 29/90 (32%) vs. 15/66 (23%) for deficiency, in the French and Italian patient groups, respectively [133]. The cohorts were not influenced by vitamin D supplementation, which was not statistically different in the two groups. In the combined populations, a significant negative correlation was found between low vitamin D levels and European Disease Activity Score, and an even more significant correlation was found with acute-phase reactants. Low levels of vitamin D were associated with the systolic pulmonary artery pressure (sPAP) estimated by echocardiography. No association was observed with calcinosis or acro-osteolysis and hyperparathyroidism. In multivariate analysis, vitamin D deficiency was associated with sPAP ($p = 0.02$). This suggests that common vitamin D supplementation does not correct the deficiency in SSc patients and that a higher dose is probably needed, especially in those with high inflammatory activity or severe disease. In line with the above results, calcinosis (HR 6.17, 95% CI 1.16–47.23) and digital ulcers (HR 12.43, 95% CI 1.97–88.40) were identified as independent predictors of the radiographic progression of acro-osteolysis [91]. The current evidence supports hypoxia as the common pathophysiological denominator of digital vasculopathy and enhanced osteoclastic activity in SSc-associated acro-osteolysis [134]. In fact, the hypoxia-inducible transcription factor HIF-1α and higher levels of vascular endothelial grow factor (VEGF) play a critical role in increasing osteoclastogenesis and seem to contribute to acro-osteolysis [135].

These data suggest that patients with severe digital vasculopathy are at higher risk of sustaining radiographic progression of bone resorption and further support the role of vascular injury playing a critical role in such lesions, possibly due to repeated vasospasm, as previously suggested [136]. The association of acro-osteolysis and severe capillary loss observed with nailfold videocapillaroscopy also supports these findings. Severe acro-osteolysis is more likely to occur with neoangiogenesis (defined as irregular enlargement of the capillaries, disorganization of the normal capillary array, and ramified/bushy capillaries), which may suggest an attempt to compensate for bone resorption [121].

Unfortunately, no medical therapy has proven effective on acro-osteolysis. As there have been suggestions of a vascular pathogenesis, it could be speculated that an optimized control of Raynaud's phenomenon and more aggressive vasodilator therapy may help prevent or slow this complication. However, to date, there is no evidence from observational studies or clinical trials.

Bone Involvement

Many studies have established an increased risk of bone loss and fracture in individuals with chronic inflammatory conditions. These patients are at increased risk for osteoporosis for many reasons: the glucocorticoid medications often prescribed for the treatment can trigger significant bone loss. In addition, pain and loss of joint function caused by the disease can result in inactivity, further increasing osteoporosis risk. Studies also show that bone loss in RA may occur as a direct result of the inflammatory disease. By contrast, it is still unknown whether osteoporosis is truly increased in SSc or whether this association has been observed in some studies as a result of other confounding risk factors. Indeed, small sample size and clinical heterogeneity of SSc study samples have led to underpowered and imprecise estimates of the risk for the development of osteoporosis [137]. Currently, there are no recommendations for the systematic screening of osteoporosis in SSc and therefore, recommendations made for the general population should be applied.

In a series of 43 postmenopausal SSc patients and 47 healthy postmenopausal women, excluding severe SSc, a higher frequency of osteoporosis in the lumbar spine (32.5%) and femoral neck (51.1%) was observed in SSc patients when compared to controls (14.8% vs. 19.1%; $p < 0.01$). Multiple linear regression analysis revealed an association between the presence of SSc and low bone mineral density. Lean mass was an important factor related to osteoporosis [138]. In another cross-sectional study including 71 SSc, 139 RA, and 227 healthy women, the prevalence of osteoporosis and fracture was similar in SSc and RA and was for both higher than in healthy controls (osteoporosis: 30% in SSc, 32% in RA, and 11% in controls; fracture: 35% in SSc, 33% in RA, and 10% in controls) [139]. Multivariate analysis identified disease duration as a risk factor of osteoporosis in SSc. Age and low 25(OH)D levels were recognized as risk factors of fracture in SSc. In a recent study [140], Vitamin D deficiency was found in 60% of SSc patients vs. 39% of controls ($p = 0.003$). Thus, these results support the performance of BMD measurements together with vitamin D levels in patients with SSc. In another report, 27/61 SSc patients presented osteopenia and 14/61 osteoporosis. Bone mineral density results in fertility, and post-menopausal SSc patients were independent of the SSc clinical variants, race, and previous use of corticosteroids and cyclophosphamide. However, a low density was associated with a low body mass index [141, 142]. Some other series were less demonstrative and therefore there is no strong evidence in the literature for consistently lower bone mineral density scores in SSc [143]. Premature menopause, corticosteroid use, major disability, or other factors secondary to SSc (malabsorption, low weight, or sometimes systemic inflammation) may be causal factors or confounders in SSc. As regards potential associations with other clinical manifestations of SSc, bone loss has been more frequently found in patients with digital ulcers, calcinosis, and pulmonary involvement [117, 140, 142]. More work is needed to determine the precise risk or the lack of specific risk of osteoporosis in SSc patients and to define adapted management.

Conclusions and Perspectives

Musculoskeletal involvement is frequent in SSc and represents a heavy burden. It is multifaceted and injury of several structures, such as tendon, joint, bone, or soft tissue, can occur. Its clinical diagnosis and management in SSc may be particularly challenging owing to some peculiar features of the disease such as concomitant skin involvement, subcutaneous edema, and frequently a more subtle MSK inflammation. In this regard, clinical and radiographic studies with large sample size have allowed a better estimation of the frequency of joint involvement and identified subsets of SSc patients with higher risk of developing joint, bone, or soft tissue involvement. In addition, several prospective studies have identified joint and tendon involvement as predictors of skin, lung, and overall disease progression. Several pilot studies have underlined the potential interest of other imaging techniques, such as ultrasonography, MRI, or MRA, for the early detection of articular, tendon, or soft tissue involvement. Larger studies are needed to confirm these results and validate these tools in clinical practice and estimate their predictive value. Finally, although the understanding of osteoarticular pathogenesis has significantly increased in the last years, optimal treatments of inflammatory joint disease, tenosynovitis, bone resorption, and calcinosis remain to be determined. In particular for refractory SSc-arthritis, recent observational studies have reported interesting results with some biological therapies (i.e., tocilizumab and abatacept), but these findings have not been corroborated in RCTs. This highlights an urgent need to better define new MSK outcomes to be evaluated in RCTs, in order to significantly improve the management of these manifestations, resulting in less morbidity and better quality of life for SSc patients.

References

1. Baron M, Lee P, Keystone EC. The articular manifestations of progressive systemic sclerosis (scleroderma). Ann Rheum Dis. 1982;41:147–52.
2. Hietaharju A, Jaaskeläinen S, Kalimo H, Hietarinta M. Peripheral neuromuscular manifestations in systemic sclerosis (scleroderma). Muscle Nerve. 1993;16:1204–12.
3. Mau W, Listing J, Huscher D, Zeidler H, Zink A, Schneider M, et al. Employment across chronic inflammatory rheumatic diseases and comparison with the general population. J Rheumatol. 2005;32:721–8.
4. Brower LM, Poole JL. Reliability and validity of the Duruöz Hand Index in persons with systemic sclerosis (scleroderma). Arthritis Care Res. 2004;51:805–9.
5. Poole JL, Gallegos M, O'Linc S. Reliability and validity of the Arthritis Hand Function Test in adults with systemic sclerosis (scleroderma). Arthritis Care Res. 2000;13:69–73.
6. Poole JL, Steen VD. The use of the health assessment questionnaire (HAQ) to determine physical disability in systemic sclerosis. Arthritis Rheum. 1991;4:27–31.
7. Richards HL, Herrick AL, Griffin K, Gwilliam PDH, Loukes J, Fortune DG. Systemic sclerosis: patients' perceptions of their condition. Arthritis Care Res. 2003;49:689–96.
8. Ostojic P, Jankovic K, Djurovic N, Stojic B, Knezevic-Apostolski S, Bartolovic D. Common causes of pain in systemic sclerosis: frequency, severity, and relationship to disease status, depression, and quality of life. Pain Manag Nurs. 2019;20:331–6.
9. Frantz C, Avouac J, Distler O, Amrouche F, Godard D, Kennedy AT, et al. Impaired quality of life in systemic sclerosis and patient perception of the disease: a large international survey. Semin Arthritis Rheum. 2016;46:115–23.
10. Belz D, Moinzadeh P, Riemekasten G, Henes J, Müller-Ladner U, Blank N, et al. Large variability of frequency and type of physical therapy in patients in the German Network for Systemic Sclerosis. Arthritis Care Res. 2020;72:1041–8.
11. Kwakkenbos L, Sanchez TA, Turner KA, Mouthon L, Carrier ME, Hudson M, et al. The association of sociodemographic and disease variables with hand function: a Scleroderma Patient-centered Intervention Network cohort study. Clin Exp Rheumatol. 2018;36:S88–94.
12. Sandqvist G, Eklund M, Åkesson A, Nordenskiöld U. Daily activities and hand function in women with scleroderma. Scand J Rheumatol. 2004;33:102–7.
13. Erol K, Gok K, Cengiz G, Ozgocmen S. Hand functions in systemic sclerosis and rheumatoid arthritis and influence on clinical variables. Int J Rheum Dis. 2018;21:249–52.
14. Rodnan GP, Medsger TA. The rheumatic manifestations of progressive systemic sclerosis (scleroderma). Clin Orthop Relat Res. 1968;57:81–93.
15. Rosenbaum LH, Swartz WM, Rodnan GP, Medsger TA. Wrist drop in progressive systemic sclerosis (scleroderma): complete rupture of the extensor tendon mechanism. Arthritis Rheum. 1985;28:586–9.
16. La Montagna G, Baruffo A, Tirri R, Buono G, Valentini G. Foot involvement in systemic sclerosis: a longitudinal study of 100 patients. Semin Arthritis Rheum. 2002;31:248–55.
17. Avouac J, Walker U, Tyndall A, Kahan A, Matucci-Cerinic M, Allanore Y, et al. Characteristics of joint involvement and relationships with systemic inflammation in systemic sclerosis: results from the EULAR Scleroderma Trial and Research Group (EUSTAR) database. J Rheumatol. 2010;37:1488–501.
18. Steen VD, Medsger TA Jr. The palpable tendon friction rub: an important physical examination finding in patients with systemic sclerosis. Arthritis Rheum. 1997;40:1146–51.
19. Domsic RT, Nihtyanova SI, Wisniewski SR, Fine MJ, Lucas M, Kwoh CK, et al. Derivation and external validation of a prediction rule for five-year mortality in patients with early diffuse cutaneous systemic sclerosis. Arthritis Rheumatol. 2016;68:993–1003.
20. Khanna PP, Furst DE, Clements PJ, Maranian P, Indulkar L, Khanna D, et al. Tendon friction rubs in early diffuse systemic sclerosis: prevalence, characteristics and longitudinal changes in a randomized controlled trial. Rheumatology (Oxford). 2010;49:955–9.
21. Ostojic P, Damianov N. Different clinical features in patients with limited and diffuse cutaneous systemic sclerosis. Clin Rheumatol. 2006;25:453–7.
22. Ostojic P, Damianov N. Indices of the Scleroderma Assessment Questionnaire (SAQ) can be used to demonstrate change in patients with systemic sclerosis over time. Joint Bone Spine. 2008;75:286–90.
23. Elhai M, Guerini H, Bazeli R, Avouac J, Freire V, Drapé JL, et al. Ultrasonographic hand features in systemic sclerosis and correlates with clinical, biologic, and radiographic findings. Arthritis Care Res. 2012;64:1244–9.

24. Freire V, Bazeli R, Elhai M, Campagna R, Pessis É, Avouac J, et al. Hand and wrist involvement in systemic sclerosis: US features. Radiology. 2013;269:824–30.
25. Lescoat A, Ballerie A, Belhomme N, Cazalets C, de Carlan M, Droitcourt C, et al. Synovial involvement assessed by power Doppler ultra-sonography in systemic sclerosis: results of a cross-sectional study. Rheumatology (Oxford). 2018;57:2012–21.
26. Abdel-Magied RA, Lotfi A, Abdelgawad EA. Magnetic resonance imaging versus musculoskeletal ultrasonography in detecting inflammatory arthropathy in systemic sclerosis patients with hand arthralgia. Rheumatol Int. 2013;33:1961–6.
27. Balint PV, Kane D, Wilson H, McInnes IB, Sturrock RD. Ultrasonography of entheseal insertions in the lower limb in spondyloarthropathy. Ann Rheum Dis. 2002;61:905–10.
28. De Miguel E, Cobo T, Muñoz-Femández S, Naredo E, Usón J, Acebes JC, et al. Validity of enthesis ultrasound assessment in spondyloarthropathy. Ann Rheum Dis. 2009;68:169–74.
29. Kilic E, Kilic G, Akgul O, Ozgocmen S. Presence of enthesopathy demonstrated with ultrasonography in systemic sclerosis. Mod Rheumatol. 2015;25:731–6.
30. Terenzi R, Karalilova R, Lepri G, Bruni C, Bellando-Randone S, Manetti M, et al. Enthesopathy and involvement of synovio-entheseal complex in systemic sclerosis: an ultrasound pilot study. Rheumatology (Oxford). 2020;59:580–5.
31. Valentini G, Iudici M, Walker UA, Jaeger VK, Baron M, Carreira P, et al. The European Scleroderma Trials and Research group (EUSTAR) task force for the development of revised activity criteria for systemic sclerosis: derivation and validation of a preliminarily revised EUSTAR activity index. Ann Rheum Dis. 2017;76:270–6.
32. Avouac J, Walker UA, Hachulla E, Riemekasten G, Cuomo G, Carreira PE, et al. Joint and tendon involvement predict disease progression in systemic sclerosis: a EUSTAR prospective study. Ann Rheum Dis. 2016;75:103–9.
33. Dapena MF, Rivera A, Sopeña B, Vilella CT, Guillén-Del Castillo A, Argüelles DC, et al. Clinical and epidemiological differences between men and women with systemic sclerosis: a study in a Spanish systemic sclerosis cohort and literature review. Clin Exp Rheumatol. 2017;35:S89–97.
34. Nakayama W, Jinnin M, Tomizawa Y, Nakamura K, Kudo H, Inoue K, et al. Dysregulated interleukin-23 signalling contributes to the increased collagen production in scleroderma fibroblasts via balancing microRNA expression. Rheumatology (Oxford). 2017;56:145–55.
35. Yang X, Yang J, Xing X, Wan L, Li M. Increased frequency of Th17 cells in systemic sclerosis is related to disease activity and collagen overproduction. Arthritis Res Ther. 2014;16(1):R4.
36. Bandinelli F, Kaloudi O, Candelieri A, Conforti ML, Casale R, Cammarata S, et al. Early detection of median nerve syndrome at the carpal tunnel with high-resolution 18 MHz ultrasonography in systemic sclerosis patients. Clin Exp Rheumatol. 2010;28:S15–8.
37. Tagliafico A, Panico N, Resmini E, Derchi LE, Ghio M, Martinoli C. The role of ultrasound imaging in the evaluation of peripheral nerve in systemic sclerosis (scleroderma). Eur J Radiol. 2011;77:377–82.
38. Yagci I, Kenis-Coskun O, Ozsoy T, Ozen G, Direskeneli H. Increased stiffness of median nerve in systemic sclerosis. BMC Musculoskelet Disord. 2017;18:434.
39. Machet L, Vaillant L, Machet MC, Esteve E, Muller C, Khallouf R, et al. Carpal tunnel syndrome and systemic sclerosis. Dermatology. 1992;185:101–3.
40. Clements PJ, Allanore Y, Khanna D, Singh M, Furst DE. Arthritis in systemic sclerosis: systematic review of the literature and suggestions for the performance of future clinical trials in systemic sclerosis arthritis. Semin Arthritis Rheum. 2012;41:801–14.
41. Palmer DG, Hale GM, Grennan DM, Pollock M. Bowed fingers. A helpful sign in the early diagnosis of systemic sclerosis. J Rheumatol. 1981;8:266–72.
42. Perrot S, Peixoto M, Dieudé P, Hachulla E, Avouac J, Ottaviani S, et al. Patient phenotypes in fibromyalgia comorbid with systemic sclerosis or rheumatoid arthritis: influence of diagnostic and screening tests. Screening with the FiRST questionnaire, diagnosis with the ACR 1990 and revised ACR 2010 criteria. Clin Exp Rheumatol. 2017;35:35–42.
43. Avouac J, Airò P, Dieude P, Caramaschi P, Tiev K, Diot E, et al. Associated autoimmune diseases in systemic sclerosis define a subset of patients with milder disease: results from 2 large cohorts of European Caucasian patients. J Rheumatol. 2010;37:608–14.
44. Ross L, Stevens W, Rabusa C, Wilson M, Ferdowsi N, Walker J, et al. The role of inflammatory markers in assessment of disease activity in systemic sclerosis. Clin Exp Rheumatol. 2018;36 Suppl 113:126–34.
45. Fairley JL, Hansen D, Proudman S, Sahhar J, Ngian GS, Walker J, et al. Clinical characteristics and survival in systemic sclerosis-mixed connective tissue disease and systemic sclerosis-overlap syndrome. Arthritis Care Res. 2020;73:732. https://doi.org/10.1002/acr.24167. PMID: 32058672.
46. Cohen MJ, Persellin RH. Coexistence of rheumatoid arthritis and systemic sclerosis in four patients. Scand J Rheumatol. 1982;11:241–5.
47. Armstrong RD, Gibson T. Scleroderma and erosive polyarthritis: a disease entity? Ann Rheum Dis. 1982;41:141–6.
48. Baron M, Srolovitz H, Lander P, Kapusta M. The coexistence of rheumatoid arthritis and scleroderma: a case report and review of the literature. J Rheumatol. 1982;9:947–50.
49. Avouac J, Guerini H, Wipff J, Assous N, Chevrot A, Kahan A, et al. Radiological hand involvement in systemic sclerosis. Ann Rheum Dis. 2006;65:1088–92.
50. Avouac J, Gossec L, Dougados M. Diagnostic and predictive value of anti-cyclic citrullinated protein antibodies in rheumatoid arthritis: a systematic literature review. Ann Rheum Dis. 2006;65:845–51.
51. Morita Y, Muro Y, Sigiura K, Tomita Y. Anti-cyclic citrullinated peptide antibody in systematic sclerosis. Clin Exp Rheumatol. 2008;26:542–7.
52. Marrone M, Chialà A, Tampoia M, Iannone F, Raho L, Covelli M, et al. Prevalence of anti-CCP antibodies in systemic sclerosis. Reumatismo. 2011;59:20–4.
53. Horiki T, Moriuchi J, Takaya M, Uchiyama M, Hoshina Y, Inada K, et al. The coexistence of systemic sclerosis and rheumatoid arthritis in five patients. Arthritis Rheum. 1996;39:152–6.
54. Laustriat G, Ruyssen-Witrand A, Constantin A, Barnetche T, Adoue D, Cantagrel A, et al. Anti-citrullinated peptides antibodies in systemic sclerosis: meta-analysis of frequency and meaning. Joint Bone Spine. 2018;85:147–53.
55. Gordon JK, Girish G, Berrocal VJ, Zhang M, Hatzis C, Assassi S, et al. Reliability and validity of the tender and swollen joint counts and the modified Rodnan skin score in early diffuse cutaneous systemic sclerosis: analysis from the prospective registry of early systemic sclerosis cohort. J Rheumatol. 2017;44:791–4.
56. Felson DT, Anderson JJ, Boers M, Bombardier C, Chernoff M, Fried B, et al. The American College of Rheumatology preliminary core set of disease activity measures for rheumatoid arthritis clinical trials. Arthritis Rheum. 1993;36:729–40.
57. Sandqvist G, Nilsson JÅ, Wuttge DM, Hesselstrand R. Development of a modified hand mobility in Scleroderma (HAMIS) test and its potential as an outcome measure in systemic sclerosis. J Rheumatol. 2014;41:2186–92.
58. Winkelmann RK. Systemic scleroderma: a clinical study of 727 cases. Arch Dermatol. 1961;84:359–71.

59. La Montagna G, Sodano A, Capurro V, Malesci D, Valentini G. The arthropathy of systemic sclerosis: a 12 month prospective clinical and imaging study. Skelet Radiol. 2005;34:35–41.
60. Cuomo G, Zappia M, Abignano G, Iudici M, Rotondo A, Valentini G. Ultrasonographic features of the hand and wrist in systemic sclerosis. Rheumatology (Oxford). 2009;48:1414–7.
61. Low AHL, Lax M, Johnson SR, Lee P. Magnetic resonance imaging of the hand in systemic sclerosis. J Rheumatol. 2009;36:961–4.
62. Allanore Y, Seror R, Chevrot A, Kahan A, Drapé JL. Hand vascular involvement assessed by magnetic resonance angiography in systemic sclerosis. Arthritis Rheum. 2007;56:2747–54.
63. Hubac J, Gilson M, Gaudin P, Clay M, Imbert B, Carpentier P. Ultrasound prevalence of wrist, hand, ankle and foot synovitis and tenosynovitis in systemic sclerosis, and relationship with disease features and hand disability. Joint Bone Spine. 2020;87:229–33.
64. Chitale S, Ciapetti A, Hodgson R, Grainger A, O'connor P, Goodson NJ, et al. Magnetic resonance imaging and musculoskeletal ultrasonography detect and characterize covert inflammatory arthropathy in systemic sclerosis patients with arthralgia. Rheumatology (Oxford). 2010;49:2357–61.
65. Wang J, Yarnykh VL, Molitor JA, Nash RA, Chu B, Wilson GJ, et al. Micro magnetic resonance angiography of the finger in systemic sclerosis. Rheumatology (Oxford). 2008;47:1239–43.
66. Sheehan JJ, Fan Z, Davarpanah AH, Hodnett PA, Varga J, Carr JC, et al. Nonenhanced MR angiography of the hand with flow-sensitive dephasing-prepared balanced SSFP sequence: initial experience with systemic sclerosis. Radiology. 2011;259:248–56.
67. Blocka KLN, Bassett LW, Furst DE, Clements PJ, Paulus HE. The arthropathy of advanced progressive systemic sclerosis. Arthritis Rheum. 1981;24:874–84.
68. Wielosz E, Majdan M, Dryglewska M, Zwolak R. Anti-CCP antibodies and rheumatoid factor in systemic sclerosis: prevalence and relationships with joint manifestations. Adv Clin Exp Med. 2018;27:1253–7.
69. Misra R, Darton K, Jewkes RF, Black CM, Maini RN. Arthritis in scleroderma. Rheumatology (Oxford). 1995;34:831–7.
70. Kamalaksha S, White DHN, Solanki KK. Significance of combined anti-CCP antibodies and rheumatoid factor in a New Zealand cohort of patients with systemic sclerosis. Int J Rheum Dis. 2018;21:1430–5.
71. Avouac J, Sordet C, Depinay C, Ardizonne M, Vacher-Lavenu MC, Sibilia J, et al. Systemic sclerosis-associated Sjögren's syndrome and relationship to the limited cutaneous subtype: results of a prospective study of sicca syndrome in 133 consecutive patients. Arthritis Rheum. 2006;54:2243–9.
72. Generini S, Steiner G, Miniati I, Conforti ML, Guiducci S, Skriner K, et al. Anti-hnRNP and other autoantibodies in systemic sclerosis with joint involvement. Rheumatology (Oxford). 2009;48:920–5.
73. Ingegnoli F, Galbiati V, Zeni S, Meani L, Zahalkova L, Lubatti C, et al. Use of antibodies recognizing cyclic citrullinated peptide in the differential diagnosis of joint involvement in systemic sclerosis. Clin Rheumatol. 2007;26:510–4.
74. Ueda-Hayakawa I, Hasegawa M, Kumada S, Tanaka C, Komura K, Hamaguchi Y, et al. Usefulness of anti-cyclic citrullinated peptide antibody and rheumatoid factor to detect rheumatoid arthritis in patients with systemic sclerosis. Rheumatology (Oxford). 2010;49:2135–9.
75. Payet J, Goulvestre C, Bialé L, Avouac J, Wipff J, Job-Deslandre C, et al. Antyciclic citrullinated peptide antibodies in rheumatoid arthritis and nonrheumatoid disorders: experience with 1162 patients. J Rheumatol. 2014;41:2395–402.
76. Farkas N, Szabó A, Lóránd V, Péter Sarlós D, Minier T, Prohászka Z, et al. Clinical usefulness of measuring red blood cell distribution width in patients with systemic sclerosis. Rheumatology (Oxford). 2014;53:1439–45.
77. Santiago M, Baron M, Miyachi K, Fritzler MJ, Abu-Hakima M, Leclercq S, et al. A comparison of the frequency of antibodies to cyclic citrullinated peptides using a third generation anti-CCP assay (CCP3) in systemic sclerosis, primary biliary cirrhosis and rheumatoid arthritis. Clin Rheumatol. 2008;27:77–83.
78. Rozman B, Čučnik S, Sodin-Semrl S, Czirják L, Varjú C, Distler O, et al. Prevalence and clinical associations of anti-Ku antibodies in patients with systemic sclerosis: a European EUSTAR-initiated multi-centre case-control study. Ann Rheum Dis. 2008;67:1282–6.
79. Schumacher HR. Joint involvement in progressive systemic sclerosis (scleroderma): a light and electron microscopic study of synovial membrane and fluid. Am J Clin Pathol. 1973;60:593–600.
80. Hollander JL, McCarty DJ Jr, Astorga G, Castro-Murillo E. Studies on the pathogenesis of rheumatoid joint inflammation. I. the "R.A. Cell" and a working hypothesis. Ann Intern Med. 1965;62:271–80.
81. Barry M, Katz L, Cooney L. An unusual articular presentation of progressive systemic sclerosis. Arthritis Rheum. 1983;26:1041–3.
82. Maurer B, Graf N, Michel BA, Müller-Ladner U, Czirják L, Denton CP, et al. Prediction of worsening of skin fibrosis in patients with diffuse cutaneous systemic sclerosis using the EUSTAR database. Ann Rheum Dis. 2015;74:1124–31.
83. Wu W, Jordan S, Becker MO, Dobrota R, Maurer B, Fretheim H, et al. Prediction of progression of interstitial lung disease in patients with systemic sclerosis: the SPAR model. Ann Rheum Dis. 2018;77:1326–32.
84. Elhai M, Meune C, Boubaya M, Avouac J, Hachulla E, Balbir-Gurman A, et al. Mapping and predicting mortality from systemic sclerosis. Ann Rheum Dis. 2017;76:1897–905.
85. Resnick D, Greenway G, Vint VC, Robinson CA, Piper S. Selective involvement of the first carpometacarpal joint in scleroderma. Am J Roentgenol. 1978;131:283–6.
86. Brun B, Serup J, Hagdrup H. Radiological changes of the hands in systemic sclerosis. Acta Derm Venereol. 1983;63:349–52.
87. Koutaissoff S, Vanthuyne M, Smith V, De Langhe E, Depresseux G, Westhovens R, et al. Hand radiological damage in systemic sclerosis: comparison with a control group and clinical and functional correlations. Semin Arthritis Rheum. 2011;40:455–60.
88. Erre GL, Marongiu A, Fenu P, Faedda R, Masala A, Sanna M, et al. The "sclerodermic hand": a radiological and clinical study. Joint Bone Spine. 2008;75:426–31.
89. Allali F, Tahiri L, Senjari A, Abouqal R, Hajjaj-Hassouni N. Erosive arthropathy in systemic sclerosis. BMC Public Health. 2007;22(7):260.
90. van der Leeden M, Steultjens M, Dekker JHM, Prins APA, Dekker J. Forefoot joint damage, pain and disability in rheumatoid arthritis patients with foot complaints: the role of plantar pressure and gait characteristics. Rheumatology (Oxford). 2006;45:465–9.
91. Avouac J, Mogavero G, Guerini H, Drapé JL, Mathieu A, Kahan A, et al. Predictive factors of hand radiographic lesions in systemic sclerosis: a prospective study. Ann Rheum Dis. 2011;70:630–3.
92. Avouac J, Clements PJ, Khann D, Furst DE, Allanore Y. Articular involvement in systemic sclerosis. Rheumatology (Oxford). 2012;51:1347–56.
93. Clements P, Allanore Y, Furst DE, Khanna D. Points to consider for design clinical trials in systemic sclerosis patients with arthritic involvement. Rheumatology (Oxford). 2017;56(Suppl_5):v23–6.
94. Khanna D, Denton CP, Jahreis A, van Laar JM, Frech TM, Anderson ME, et al. Safety and efficacy of subcutaneous tocilizumab in adults with systemic sclerosis (faSScinate): a phase 2, randomised, controlled trial. Lancet. 2016;387(10038):2630–40.
95. Khanna D, Spino C, Johnson S, Chung L, Whitfield M, Denton CP, et al. Abatacept in early diffuse cutaneous systemic sclerosis—results of a phase 2 investigator-initiated, multicenter, double-

blind randomized placebo-controlled trial. Arthritis Rheumatol. 2019;72:125–36.
96. Au K, Mayes MD, Maranian P, Clements PJ, Khanna D, Steen VD, et al. Course of dermal ulcers and musculoskeletal involvement in systemic sclerosis patients in the scleroderma lung study. Arthritis Care Res (Hoboken). 2010;62:1772–8.
97. Nacci F, Righi A, Conforti ML, Miniati I, Fiori G, Martinovic D, et al. Intravenous immunoglobulins improve the function and ameliorate joint involvement in systemic sclerosis: a pilot study. Ann Rheum Dis. 2007;66:977–9.
98. Bruni C, Praino E, Guiducci S, Bellando-Randone S, Furst DE, Matucci-Cerinic M. Hydroxychloroquine and joint involvement in systemic sclerosis: preliminary beneficial results from a retrospective case-control series of an EUSTAR center. Joint Bone Spine. 2017;84:747–8.
99. Lam GK, Hummers LK, Woods A, Wigley FM. Efficacy and safety of etanercept in the treatment of scleroderma-associated joint disease. J Rheumatol. 2007;34:1636–7.
100. Allanore Y, Devos-François G, Caramella C, Boumier P, Jounieaux V, Kahan A. Fatal exacerbation of fibrosing alveolitis associated with systemic sclerosis in a patient treated with adalimumab. Ann Rheum Dis. 2006;65:834–5.
101. Ostor AJK, Crisp AJ, Somerville MF, Scott DGI. Fatal exacerbation of rheumatoid arthritis associated fibrosing alveolitis in patients given infliximab. Br Med J. 2004;329:1266.
102. Denton CP, Engelhart M, Tvede N, Wilson H, Khan K, Shiwen X, et al. An open-label pilot study of infliximab therapy in diffuse cutaneous systemic sclerosis. Ann Rheum Dis. 2009;68:1433–9.
103. Distler JH, Jordan S, Airo P, Alegre-Sancho J, Allanore Y, Balbir Gurman A, et al. Is there a role for TNFα antagonists in the treatment of SSc? EUSTAR expert consensus development using the Delphi technique. Clin Exp Rheumatol. 2011;29:S40–5.
104. Elhai M, Boubaya M, Distler O, Smith V, Matucci-Cerinic M, Alegre Sancho JJ, et al. Outcomes of patients with systemic sclerosis treated with rituximab in contemporary practice: a prospective cohort study. Ann Rheum Dis. 2019;78:979–87.
105. Lafyatis R, Kissin E, York M, Farina G, Viger K, Fritzler MJ, et al. B cell depletion with rituximab in patients with diffuse cutaneous systemic sclerosis. Arthritis Rheum. 2009;60:578–83.
106. Daoussis D, Liossis SNC, Tsamandas AC, Kalogeropoulou C, Kazantzi A, Sirinian C, et al. Experience with rituximab in scleroderma: results from a 1-year, proof-of-principle study. Rheumatology (Oxford). 2010;49:271–80.
107. Elhai M, Meunier M, Matucci-Cerinic M, Maurer B, Riemekasten G, Leturcq T, et al. Outcomes of patients with systemic sclerosis-associated polyarthritis and myopathy treated with tocilizumab or abatacept: a EUSTAR observational study. Ann Rheum Dis. 2013;72:1217–20.
108. Zacay G, Levy Y. Outcomes of patients with systemic sclerosis treated with tocilizumab: case series and review of the literature. Best Pract Res Clin Rheumatol. 2018;32:563–71.
109. Castellví I, Elhai M, Bruni C, Airò P, Jordan S, Beretta L, et al. Safety and effectiveness of abatacept in systemic sclerosis: the EUSTAR experience. Semin Arthritis Rheum. 2020;50:1489–93.
110. Clements P. Management of musculoskeletal involvement in systemic sclerosis. Curr Treat Options Rheumatol. 2016;2:61–8.
111. Beaton DE, Maxwell LJ, Shea BJ, Wells GA, Boers M, Grosskleg S, et al. Instrument selection using the OMERACT filter 2.1: the OMERACT methodology. J Rheumatol. 2019;46:1028–35.
112. Sandqvist G, Hesselstrand R, Petersson IF, Kristensen LE. Work disability in early systemic sclerosis: a longitudinal population-based cohort study. J Rheumatol. 2015;42:1794–800.
113. Stefanantoni K, Sciarra I, Iannace N, Vasile M, Caucci M, Sili Scavalli A, et al. Occupational therapy integrated with a self-administered stretching programme on systemic sclerosis patients with hand involvement. Clin Exp Rheumatol. 2016;34 Suppl 100:157–61.
114. Zanatta E, Rodeghiero F, Pigatto E, Galozzi P, Polito P, Favaro M, et al. Long-term improvement in activities of daily living in women with systemic sclerosis attending occupational therapy. Br J Occup Ther. 2017;80:417–22.
115. Bogoch ER, Gross DK. Surgery of the hand in patients with systemic sclerosis: outcomes and considerations. J Rheumatol. 2005;32:642–8.
116. Young A, Namas R, Dodge C, Khanna D. Hand impairment in systemic sclerosis: various manifestations and currently available treatment. Curr Treat Opt Rheumatol. 2016;2:252–69.
117. Valenzuela A, Baron M, Herrick AL, Proudman S, Stevens W, Rodriguez-Reyna TS, et al. Calcinosis is associated with digital ulcers and osteoporosis in patients with systemic sclerosis: a Scleroderma Clinical Trials Consortium study. Semin Arthritis Rheum. 2016;46:344–9.
118. Valenzuela A, Song P, Chung L. Calcinosis in scleroderma. Curr Opin Rheumatol. 2019;30:554–61.
119. Bartoli F, Fiori G, Braschi F, Amanzi L, Bruni C, Blagojevic J, et al. Calcinosis in systemic sclerosis: subsets, distribution and complications. Rheumatology. 2016;55:1610–4.
120. Hughes M, Hodgson R, Harris J, Porter N, Jackson S, Kirwadi A, et al. Further evidence that calcinosis is associated with repetitive trauma in systemic sclerosis. Semin Arthritis Rheum. 2020;50:E4–5.
121. Moradet L, Avouac J, Sammour M, Baron M, Kahan A, Feydy A, et al. Late nailfold videocapillaroscopy pattern associated with hand calcinosis and acro-osteolysis in systemic sclerosis. Arthritis Care Res. 2016;68:366–73.
122. Zanatta E, Desportes M, Do HH, Avouac J, Doria A, Feydy A, et al. Pseudotumoral calcinosis in systemic sclerosis: data from systematic literature review and case series from two referral centres. Semin Arthritis Rheum. 2020;50:1339–47.
123. Vayssairat M, Hidouche D, Abdoucheli-Baudot N, Gaitz JP. Clinical significance of subcutaneous calcinosis in patients with systemic sclerosis. Does diltiazem induce its regression? Ann Rheum Dis. 1998;57:252–4.
124. Farah MJ, Palmieri GMA, Sebes JI, Cremer MA, Massie JD, Pinals RS. The effect of diltiazem on calcinosis in a patient with the CREST syndrome. Arthritis Rheum. 1990;33:1287–93.
125. Narváez J, Pirola JP, LLuch J, Juarez P, Nolla JM, Valenzuela A. Effectiveness and safety of rituximab for the treatment of refractory systemic sclerosis associated calcinosis: a case series and systematic review of the literature. Autoimmun Rev. 2019;18:262–9.
126. Palmieri GMA, Sebes JI, Aelion JA, Moinuddin M, Ray MW, Wood GC, et al. Treatment of calcinosis with diltiazem. Arthritis Rheum. 1995;38:1646–54.
127. Matsumoto I, Ito Y, Tomo H, Nakao Y, Takaoka K. Ossified mass of the rotator cuff tendon in the subacromial bursa. Clin Orthop Relat Res. 2005;437:247–50.
128. Metzger AL, Singer FR, Bluestone R, Pearson CM. Failure of disodium etidronate in calcinosis due to dermatomyositis and scleroderma. N Engl J Med. 1974;291:1294–6.
129. Cukierman T, Elinav E, Korem M, Chajek-Shaul T. Low dose warfarin treatment for calcinosis in patients with systemic sclerosis. Ann Rheum Dis. 2004;63:1341–3.
130. Robertson LP, Marshall RW, Hickling P. Treatment of cutaneous calcinosis in limited systemic sclerosis with minocycline. Ann Rheum Dis. 2003;62:267–9.
131. Mugino H, Ikemura K. Progressive systemic sclerosis with spontaneous fracture due to resorption of the mandible: a case report. J Oral Maxillofac Surg. 2006;64:1137–9.
132. Braun-Moscovici Y, Furst DE, Markovits D, Rozin A, Clements PJ, Nahir AM, et al. Vitamin D, parathyroid hormone, and acroosteolysis in systemic sclerosis. J Rheumatol. 2008;35:2201–5.
133. Vacca A, Cormier C, Piras M, Mathieu A, Kahan A, Allanore Y. Vitamin D deficiency and insufficiency in 2 independent cohorts of patients with systemic sclerosis. J Rheumatol. 2009;36:1924–9.

134. Siao-Pin S, Damian LO, Muntean LM, Rednic S. Acroosteolysis in systemic sclerosis: an insight into hypoxia-related pathogenesis. Exp Ther Med. 2016;12:3459–63.
135. Park JK, Fava A, Carrino J, Del Grande F, Rosen A, Boin F. Association of acroosteolysis with enhanced osteoclastogenesis and higher blood levels of vascular endothelial growth factor in systemic sclerosis. Arthritis Rheumatol. 2016;68:201–9.
136. Scharer L, Smith DW, Rodan GP, Holling HE, Scharer L, Smith DW. Resorption of the terminal phalanges in scleroderma. Arthritis Rheum. 1969;12:51–63.
137. Loucks J, Pope JE. Osteoporosis in scleroderma. Semin Arthritis Rheum. 2005;34:678–82.
138. Souza RBC, Borges CTL, Takayama L, Aldrighi JM, Pereira RMR. Systemic sclerosis and bone loss: the role of the disease and body composition. Scand J Rheumatol. 2006;35:384–7.
139. Avouac J, Koumakis E, Toth E, Meunier M, Maury E, Kahan A, et al. Increased risk of osteoporosis and fracture in women with systemic sclerosis: a comparative study with rheumatoid arthritis. Arthritis Care Res. 2012;64:1871–8.
140. Horváth Á, Végh E, Pusztai A, Petho Z, Hamar A, Czókolyová M, et al. Complex assessment of bone mineral density, fracture risk, vitamin D status, and bone metabolism in Hungarian systemic sclerosis patients. Arthritis Res Ther. 2019;21:274.
141. Sampaio-Barros PD, Costa-Paiva L, Filardi S, Sachetto Z, Samara AM, Marques-Neto JF. Prognostic factors of low bone mineral density in systemic sclerosis. Clin Exp Rheumatol. 2005;23:180–4.
142. Caimmi C, Caramaschi P, Barausse G, Orsolini G, Idolazzi L, Gatti D, et al. Bone metabolism in a large cohort of patients with systemic sclerosis. Calcif Tissue Int. 2016;99:23–9.
143. Neumann K, Wallace DJ, Metzger AL. Osteoporosis—less than expected in patients with scleroderma? J Rheumatol. 2000;27:1822–3.

Skeletal Muscle Involvement

36

Julie J. Paik and Britta Maurer

Prevalence and Epidemiology

Skeletal myopathy is an underappreciated, yet important manifestation of systemic sclerosis (SSc). While it is associated with poor outcomes such as disability and death, skeletal muscle involvement has not been widely recognized as a distinct organ that can be affected in systemic sclerosis. In earlier studies, the prevalence of skeletal myopathy in scleroderma had a wide range from 14% to 96% [1–7] depending on the diagnostic criteria that were used to define muscle involvement. In more recent studies, the prevalence of muscle weakness in a United States (US) scleroderma cohort has been reported to be approximately 25% [8], whereas a meta-analysis in 2013 reported that the prevalence of proximal muscle weakness was 16% and myositis was 13% [9].

Risk Factors Associated with Skeletal Myopathy

Consistent risk factors associated with myopathy in systemic sclerosis have been reported in large international cohorts. In a large Canadian Scleroderma Cohort, patients with a myopathy were more likely to be male, younger, and have diffuse scleroderma when compared to those who did not have a skeletal myopathy [10]. Similarly, in a recently published Chinese cohort, patients with a myopathy were more likely to have diffuse scleroderma, interstitial lung disease, gastrointestinal involvement, pulmonary hypertension, and pericardial effusion when compared to those who did not have myopathy. In both studies, it is clear that those who have a myopathy had a more severe clinical phenotype and poor outcomes. In fact, survival was lower in those with a skeletal myopathy when compared to those without a myopathy with 10 year survival rates ranging from 81.4% to 84.0% in those with myopathy vs. 94% in those without a myopathy [10, 11].

Evaluation of Skeletal Muscle Involvement

Given that skeletal myopathy is associated with a worse prognosis, it is imperative that a careful evaluation of skeletal muscle involvement is conducted in patients with SSc. In this section, we will highlight useful diagnostic tools to assess for skeletal muscle involvement.

Muscle Strength Testing

We believe that the assessment of muscle strength in all patients should be used as a screening tool. Similar to patients with an inflammatory myopathy, it is common for scleroderma patients to present with symmetric proximal muscle weakness. Therefore, at minimum, assessment of proximal muscles (neck flexors, arm abductors, and hip flexors) should be done at regular intervals. Since SSc patients can have contractures of the hands/fingers due to the skin thickening, it may be difficult to isolate distal weakness. Nevertheless, since there are rare reports of overlap inclusion body myositis and heritable myopathies with SSc, assessment of the distal muscles should also be performed [12].

J. J. Paik (✉)
Division of Rheumatology, Johns Hopkins University School of Medicine, Baltimore, MD, USA
e-mail: jpaik1@jhmi.edu

B. Maurer
Department of Rheumatology and Immunology, University Hospital Bern, University of Bern, Bern, Switzerland

Y. Allanore et al. (eds.), *Scleroderma*, https://doi.org/10.1007/978-3-031-40658-4_36

Muscle Enzymes

Laboratory assessment of muscle involvement including creatine kinase (CK) and aldolase (aldolase) can give insight to ongoing muscle disease in SSc. However, it is important to note that muscle enzyme elevation may not be seen in all cases of myopathy in SSc. In fact, in the EUSTAR cohort, elevated CK levels were reported to be 4.4% in limited scleroderma and 11.3% in the those with diffuse scleroderma [13]. In those with clear overlap myositis, elevated muscle enzymes are classically seen in patients with SSc. In patients with overlap polymyositis or dermatomyositis, it has been reported that up to 50–96% of SSc patients have elevated muscle enzymes [6, 14]. Of note, very elevated CK levels can herald the onset of myositis such as a necrotizing myopathy and can be a useful method to detect muscle disease in SSc. Aldolase can also be an important laboratory test for muscle involvement. In fact, Toledano and colleagues demonstrated that an elevated serum aldolase level of 9 IU/L or higher had a 89% sensitivity and 67% specificity for predicting which patients would develop persistent muscle disease [15].

Other muscle enzymes such as AST and ALT have also been reported to be elevated in the Toledano study. However, the predictive power of plasma aldolase for identifying subsequent myopathy in SSc was significantly higher than those of CK or transaminase enzymes (AST, ALT). Elevated troponin has been reported in multiple studies in SSc patients with myopathy or overlap myositis. In one study of 195 SSc patients where 63 (32.3%) had an elevated troponin, those who had an elevated troponin also had an association with a history of skeletal myositis ($p < 0.01$) [16]. Another study of 8 patients with fibrosis alone on skeletal muscle biopsy, or a fibrosing myopathy, found that 5 of 6 (83.3%) who had a troponin checked had an elevated troponin [17]. Lastly, a more recent study of 35 patients with scleroderma-associated myopathy demonstrated that increased LDH (defined as LDH of >190 U/L) was seen in 62% (14 of 24) of patients with diffuse SSc, while it was only seen in 36% (4 of 11) of patients with limited SSc [18].

Electromyography (EMG) and Nerve Conduction Study (NCS)

Electromyography (EMG) and nerve conduction studies (NCS) are important diagnostic tools to determine the etiology of muscle weakness. A well characterized cohort of 35 French SSc patients with a myopathy demonstrated that of the 14 patients who had an EMG, 93% (13 of 14) of the patients had myopathic features and 4 (29%) had combined myopathic and neuropathic findings [19]. Similarly, in a well-characterized US cohort of 42 patients with muscle disease, 48.9% (19 of 39) had an irritable myopathy, while 16 of 39 (41.3%) had a non-irritable myopathy [20]. Therefore, an EMG/NCS can help establish whether a myopathic or neuropathic process (i.e., motor neuron disease or neuropathy) is contributing to the patient's weakness and it can also guide the decision of which muscle to biopsy. It is advisable to have the EMG performed only on one side so that it will not affect the results of the muscle biopsy.

Magnetic Resonance Imaging (MRI) of Muscles

Magnetic resonance imaging (MRI) of the muscles can be a very valuable tool in assessing for (1) active disease and (2) chronicity or damage. In inflammatory myopathies, MRI T2 STIR is routinely used to assess for muscle inflammation. However, there are only very limited studies in scleroderma muscle disease. Schanz and colleagues performed a study using whole body MRI in 18 scleroderma patients and demonstrated that muscle weakness is associated with fasciitis and muscle edema [21]. In another study of scleroderma-associated myopathy, muscle MRI demonstrated that there was more prominent fascial edema than intramuscular edema in those with a fibrosing myopathy compared to an inflammatory myopathy on muscle biopsy [22]. In our experience, similar to an EMG, MRI of the muscles can be a useful tool to guide a muscle biopsy, especially when working in conjunction with an experienced musculoskeletal radiologist.

Muscle Biopsy

Muscle biopsy should be considered in all scleroderma patients who are weak and/or have elevated muscle enzymes. The reason is that a muscle biopsy that demonstrates an inflammatory myopathy can change the immunosuppressive treatment in these patients. Furthermore, there is clear evidence that patients who have inflammation or necrosis on biopsy have a favorable response to treatment [19]. Since there may be concern for poor healing after biopsy in scleroderma patients with severe skin disease, risks and benefits should be carefully weighed. In our experience, however, most patients tolerate a muscle biopsy without any severe complications. Distinct muscle histopathologic features will be discussed in detail below.

Muscle Histopathology

Predominance of Muscle Fibrosis Without Inflammation or Necrosis Is a Unique Feature of Scleroderma Muscle Disease

In this section, we will highlight studies that demonstrate that muscle histopathology may guide not only treatment, but also give insight into prognosis of SSc patients with skeletal muscle involvement. The first study to rigorously characterize muscle pathology in SSc was done in 1968 by Medsger and colleagues [1]. In this study, muscle tissue was obtained in 36 cases with only 18 containing open muscle biopsies with 19 containing postmortem or autopsy specimens. While fibrosis was found in up to 13 (36%) of the muscle specimens, it was hard to discern the clinical relevance since some were from autopsy cases. Nevertheless, subsequent studies also reported that up to 58% of muscle biopsies had endomysial and perimysial fibrosis in scleroderma-associated myopathy [2, 23].

More recently, a study performed at the Johns Hopkins Scleroderma Center demonstrated that patients with predominant fibrosis on muscle biopsy, or a fibrosing myopathy, had a unique clinical phenotype [17]. Histopathology demonstrating a fibrosing myopathy is shown in Fig. 36.1.

This study was the first to describe the clinical phenotype of SSc patients with a fibrosing myopathy. It was observed that patients with a fibrosing myopathy tended to have diffuse cutaneous scleroderma, be more commonly African American, and have lower creatine kinase levels when compared to those with an inflammatory myopathy. It was also reported that these patients had a significantly higher rate of mortality (5 of 8 (62.5%) vs. 4 of 29 (14.3%), $p = 0.0005$). This study further corroborated the importance of obtaining a muscle biopsy in SSc patients, especially since those with a fibrosing myopathy tended to have lower CK levels but higher mortality rates.

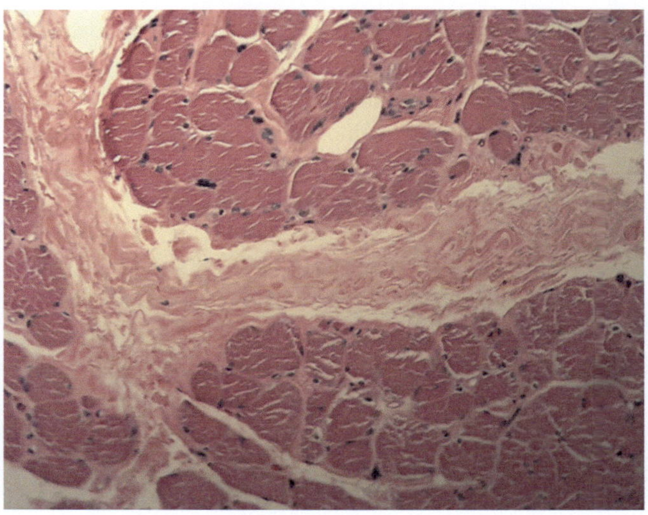

Fig. 36.1 Hematoxylin and eoxin stain of deltoid muscle 10× demonstrate perimysial and endomysial fibrosis in a patient with systemic sclerosis

At the University of Siena in Italy, muscle biopsies were performed in 35 SSc patients who presented with clinical or EMG findings of muscle involvement [18]. This study included a wealth of histopathologic data including ultrastructural analysis from electron microscopy. In addition, these patients had a muscle biopsy at the onset of muscle involvement, early in their scleroderma disease process. Multifocal endomysial fibrosis without prominent necrosis or regeneration was seen in 81% (28 of 35) of SSc patients compared to 32% (11 of 35) of patients with an idiopathic inflammatory myopathy (IIM) ($p < 0.05$). Vascular involvement, represented by VEGF-A staining, was also statistically much higher when compared to patients with inflammatory myopathy. Other studies have also reported vascular changes such as endothelial cell swelling, basement membrane lamination, intimal hypertrophy, and loss of capillary density in muscle biopsies from SSc patients [23, 24].

Inflammation and Necrosis Are Prevalent Findings in Scleroderma Muscle Disease

In 2009, Ranque and colleagues evaluated muscle biopsies of 35 patients with scleroderma-associated myopathy. Twenty-two of the 35 (63%) muscle biopsies demonstrated mononuclear inflammation. Myofiber necrosis was seen in 22 of 35 (63%) of the muscle biopsies and fibrosis was seen in 8 of 22 (24%). Muscle inflammation on biopsy was associated with good muscle prognosis (as defined as improvement in muscle grading and myalgia intensity, or if no muscle weakness or myalgia, normalization or greater than 50% decrease in CK levels) when compared to those without inflammation that was statistically significant [19, 25]. This study highlighted the importance of obtaining muscle biopsies and confirming the histopathologic findings since treatment of those with inflammation/necrosis had much better prognosis.

In 2015, a series of 42 weak patients with SSc who had muscle biopsies conducted for clinical evaluation were retrospectively assigned into histopathologic categories [20]. These categories were adapted from the European Neuro Muscular Centre criteria [26], and the muscle biopsies were grouped into the following categories: polymyositis, dermatomyositis, nonspecific myositis, necrotizing myopathy, acute denervation, and fibrosis only. Nonspecific myositis (36%) and necrotizing myopathy (21%) were the most common histopathologic categories in weak scleroderma patients. This also agreed with another study that demonstrated that in 25 patients with SSc-polymyositis (PM) overlap, 96% of this subset had necrotic muscle fibers [27].

Immunostaining of Muscle Biopsies

The characterization of cellular infiltrates in scleroderma-associated myopathy has not been well described. In the previously described study, immunostaining demonstrated that CD8 cells, CD4 cells, and CD20 cells were found in 18%, 15%, and 15% of the 39 muscle biopsies, respectively [20]. This is consistent with an earlier study of 11 scleroderma muscle biopsies demonstrating that perimysial exudates consisting mainly of CD8 T cells and macrophages were the most common type of cellular infiltrate [28]. Complement deposition on vascular walls has also been described [19, 29], and MHC 1 upregulation has been described in most studies [19, 20, 27]. A more robust characterization will be needed in the future in order to develop targeted therapies for scleroderma muscle disease.

Autoantibodies

Autoantibodies in scleroderma-associated muscle disease are primarily found in those with overlap myositis. One of the most widely recognized autoantibodies is anti-PM-Scl with most patients presenting some degree of both diseases (scleroderma and either polymyositis or dermatomyositis). First described in 1977, the clinical features of these patients have been appreciated in greater detail over the years [30, 31]. In a large US scleroderma cohort of 2425 patients, the prevalence of anti-PM-Scl was only 3% (76 of 2425). Of those, only 33 (1.4%) had an inflammatory myopathy [32]. When compared to those without anti-PM-Scl antibodies, antibody-positive patients had higher prevalence of muscle disease (51% vs. 14%, $p < 0.0001$). When anti-PM-Scl antibodies are detected in myositis cohorts, the range is much higher, up to 20–51% [6, 33, 34]. In a recent study performed in 41 myositis patients with anti-PM-Scl antibodies, only 30% of the patients met the 2013 ACR/EULAR criteria for systemic sclerosis, highlighting the heterogeneity of patients who are positive for anti-PM-Scl autoantibodies [35].

Anti-Ku autoantibodies have also been reported in patients who have both scleroderma and myositis. The prevalence in the EUSTAR SSc cohort has been reported to be quite low at 2.2% [36]. Using a case-control design, anti-Ku antibodies were found to be significantly associated with myositis, arthritis, and joint contractures in this cohort. Autoantibodies to RuvBL1 and RubL2 have also been found almost exclusively in SSc patients with diffuse disease and myositis. However, similar to anti-Ku and anti-PM-Scl, the prevalence of this autoantibody in a large US SSc cohort was quite low at 1.9% [37].

Anti-U3RNP has also been reported in patients with both scleroderma and myositis. The prevalence is variable ranging from 18% to 54% [38–40], but the phenotype has been more clearly appreciated as SSc patients with this autoantibody tend to be African American and have diffuse skin disease with GI dysmotility. Most recently, anti-SMN autoantibodies have been reported in a small subset of SSc patients with scleroderma and myositis or "scleromyositis" who tend to have calcinosis, but infrequent ILD and renal crisis [41].

Scleroderma-specific autoantibodies have also been detected in patients with scleroderma-associated myopathy. A negative association has been reported for anti-centromere antibodies [33, 42]. Of the 1330 patients who were positive for anti-Scl-70 in the EUSTAR cohort, muscle disease characteristics were as follows: 32% were found to have muscle weakness, 16% with muscle atrophy, and 8.7% with CK elevation [13]. The prevalence of ACA positivity in SSc patients with muscle inflammation has been reported to be 1%, similarly anti-RNA polymerase III is infrequent at 4%, and 9% in those with Scl-70 antibodies [42]. In contrast, it is reported to be more frequent in those with antibodies to PM-Scl (58%) and U3RNP (18%) [42].

Novel Imaging Modalities

Whole body MRI has been used to detect muscle disease in SSc as noted above. While there was no comparison to SSc patients without muscle involvement, this study by Schanz and colleagues demonstrated that muscle weakness correlated with fasciitis and muscle edema on imaging [21]. In a more recent study, blood oxygenation level-dependent (BOLD) magnetic resonance imaging (MRI) was conducted in 11 consecutive SSc patients and 12 healthy volunteers. Even though the vast majority of SSc patients lacked skeletal weakness or CK elevation, more intense oxygen desaturation during ischemia was observed compared to controls ($p = 0.02$). These findings led the investigators to conclude that this novel imaging technique, BOLD MRI, can detect significant impairment of skeletal muscle microcirculation in SSc [43]. Additional advanced MRI techniques such as T2 and T1 mapping and Diffusion Weighted Imaging were recently reported in a small number of SSc patients with skeletal muscle disease [44]. Seven patients who met the 2013 ACR/EULAR criteria for SSc and three healthy controls underwent research multiparametric MRI. The obturator muscles of the pelvis were preferentially affected by SSc compared to healthy controls ($p = 0.02$). Figure 36.2 demonstrates an example of a SSc patient with prominent muscle edema in the obturator externus muscles (blue) bilaterally and fasciitis (red).

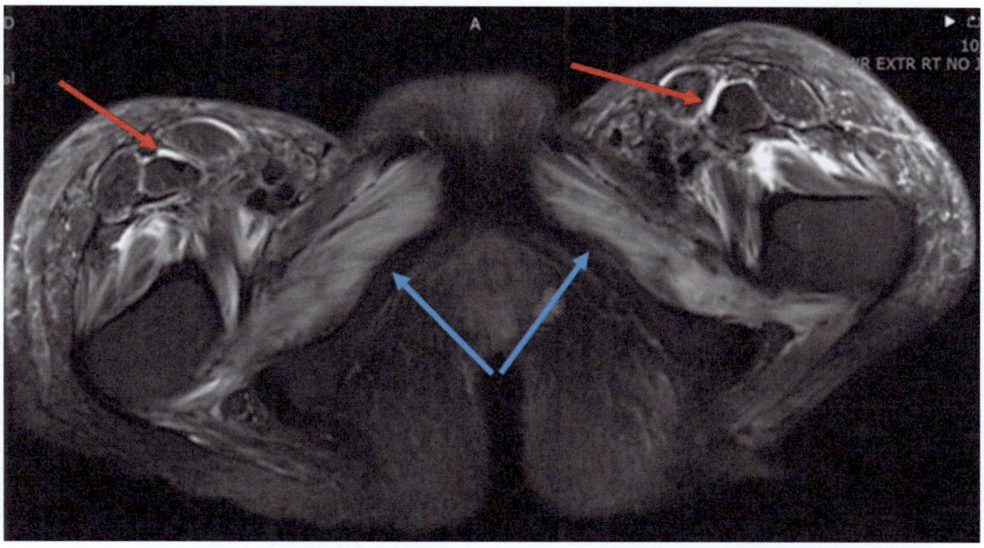

Fig. 36.2 MRI T2 STIR of the thighs. Red arrows demonstrate marked fasciitis of the anterior compartment. Blue arrows demonstrate bilateral muscle edema of the obturator muscles

Treatments and Prognosis

There are no prospective randomized clinical trials in the treatment of scleroderma-associated myopathy. A report of seven SSc patients receiving abatacept showed a trend for improvement in their muscle disease, but these results did not reach statistical significance [45]. While there is no evidence-based treatment algorithm, it is clear from multiple studies that SSc patients with muscle inflammation and necrosis have better outcomes than those who do not [25] As noted previously, SSc patients with a fibrosing myopathy tended to not improve with treatment and had a higher risk for mortality. Nonetheless, of the three patients with a fibrosing myopathy who were treated aggressively and early, the outcome of these patients was positive with improved muscle strength [17]. Further research is necessary to delineate the most efficacious treatments and timing for the various histopathologic subtypes of SSc muscle disease.

Based on our experience in treating skeletal muscle disease in SSc, we advise that treatment be aggressive and prompt once detected. A potential treatment algorithm based on histopathologic diagnoses is noted in Table 36.1. Based on the efficacy of mycophenolate mofetil in the treatment of skin and lung disease in SSc, the first-line therapy that is most appropriate for skeletal muscle involvement is mycophenolate mofetil (MMF) [46–49]. It is well known that MMF is very effective in the treatment of myositis [50, 51]. Second, intravenous immunoglobulin (IVIG) can be considered especially in those with overlap myositis [52]. Third, rituximab can also be considered given the efficacy of rituximab in myositis and also its reported effects in scleroderma skin disease [53–56]. Steroids should be used with caution particularly in those with early diffuse cutaneous SSc due to the high risk for renal crisis. Overall, since disability and death are higher in those with skeletal muscle involvement, and effective therapies are available, early diagnosis and treatment is imperative.

Table 36.1 Histopathologic diagnosis and potential treatment of SSc-associated myopathy

Histopathologic diagnoses in SSc-associated myopathy	SSc phenotype	Potential treatment
Inflammatory myopathy[a]	Diffuse or limited scleroderma	Can consider steroids first line if patient is very weak, but doses greater than 20 mg/daily should be avoided. First-line immunosuppressant: Mycophenolate mofetil. If no improvement after 3 months, consider IVIG ± Rituximab
Fibrosing myopathy	Diffuse > limited, higher prevalence of African American, high risk for cardiac involvement	Unknown, Mycophenolate mofetil first and after 3 months would consider IVIG ± rituximab

[a] Inflammatory myopathy includes the following: polymyositis, non-specific myositis, dermatomyositis, and necrotizing myopathy

Conclusion

Skeletal myopathy is an underappreciated manifestation of systemic sclerosis that deserves greater attention because of its impact on important outcomes such as disability and mortality. Evaluation of muscle disease should include at minimum muscle strength testing and muscle enzymes for screening. If a patient screens positive, further evaluation with EMG, muscle MRI, and in particular muscle biopsy should be strongly considered since patients with muscle inflammation are known to have a better prognosis when treated with immunosuppression. Novel muscle imaging modalities may eventually replace invasive studies or be an adjunctive tool in the assessment of muscle disease in scleroderma. Of the many organs that are already involved in scleroderma, such as skin, lung, and the gastrointestinal tract, muscle involvement is unique in that there are more therapeutic options, and if treated (in particular those with inflammation on biopsy), will demonstrate a clinically significant response. Therefore, it is important to screen and evaluate all patients with SSc for muscle disease.

References

1. Medsger TA, Rodnan GP, Moossy J, Vester JW. Skeletal muscle involvement in progressive systemic sclerosis (scleroderma). Arthritis Rheum. 1968;11:554–68.
2. Thompson JM, Bluestone R, Bywaters EGL, Dorling J, Johnson M. Skeletal muscle involvement in systemic sclerosis. Ann Rheum Dis. 1969;28:281.
3. Clements PJ, Furst DE, Campion DS, Bohan A, Harris R, Levy J, et al. Muscle disease in progressive systemic sclerosis: diagnostic and therapeutic considerations. Arthritis Rheum. 1978;21:62–71.
4. West SG, Killian PJ, Lawless OJ. Association of myositis and myocarditis in progressive systemic sclerosis. Arthritis Rheum. 1981;24:662–7.
5. Hausmanowa-Petrusewicz I, Jabłońska S, Błaszczyk M, Matz B. Electromyographic findings in various forms of progressive systemic sclerosis. Arthritis Rheum. 1982;25:61–5.
6. Mimori T. Scleroderma-polymyositis overlap syndrome. Clinical and serologic aspects. Int J Dermatol. 1987;26:419–25.
7. Follansbee WP, Zerbe TR, Medsger TA. Cardiac and skeletal muscle disease in systemic sclerosis (scleroderma): a high risk association. Am Heart J. 1993;125:194–203.
8. Paik JJ, Wigley FM, Mejia AF, Hummers LK. Severity of muscle weakness independently associates with disability as measured by the Health Assessment Questionnaire-Disability Index (HAQ-DI) in scleroderma. Arthritis Care Res (Hoboken). 2016;68:1695. https://doi.org/10.1002/acr.22870.
9. Muangchan C, Markland J, Robinson D, Jones N, Khalidi N, Docherty P, et al. The 15% rule in scleroderma: the frequency of severe organ complications in systemic sclerosis. A systematic review. J Rheumatol. 2013;40:1545–56.
10. Jung M, Bonner A, Hudson M, Baron M, Pope JE, Canadian Scleroderma Research Group (CSRG). Myopathy is a poor prognostic feature in systemic sclerosis: results from the Canadian Scleroderma Research Group (CSRG) cohort. Scand J Rheumatol. 2014;43:217–20. https://doi.org/10.3109/03009742.2013.868512.
11. Zhou M, Jiang L, Nie L, Chen T, Zhang T, Sun W, et al. Myopathy is a risk factor for poor prognosis of patients with systemic sclerosis: a retrospective cohort study. Medicine (Baltimore). 2020;99:e21734. https://doi.org/10.1097/MD.0000000000021734.
12. Kusaoi M, Fukazawa T, Hirashima M, Morita Y, Yamaji C, Takai S, et al. A case of inclusion body myositis with systemic sclerosis. Mod Rheumatol. 2003;13:87–9. https://doi.org/10.3109/s101650300014.
13. Walker UA, Tyndall A, Czirják L, Denton C, Farge-Bancel D, Kowal-Bielecka O, et al. Clinical risk assessment of organ manifestations in systemic sclerosis: a report from the EULAR Scleroderma Trials And Research group database. Ann Rheum Dis. 2007;66:754–63. https://doi.org/10.1136/ard.2006.062901.
14. Troyanov Y, Targoff IN, Tremblay J-L, Goulet J-R, Raymond Y, Senécal J-L. Novel classification of idiopathic inflammatory myopathies based on overlap syndrome features and autoantibodies: analysis of 100 French Canadian patients. Medicine (Baltimore). 2005;84:231–49.
15. Tolédano C, Gain M, Kettaneh A, Baudin B, Johanet C, Chérin P, et al. Aldolase predicts subsequent myopathy occurrence in systemic sclerosis. Arthritis Res Ther. 2012;14:R152. https://doi.org/10.1186/ar3888.
16. Bosello S, De Luca G, Berardi G, Canestrari G, de Waure C, Gabrielli FA, et al. Cardiac troponin T and NT-proBNP as diagnostic and prognostic biomarkers of primary cardiac involvement and disease severity in systemic sclerosis: a prospective study. Eur J Intern Med. 2019;60:46–53. https://doi.org/10.1016/j.ejim.2018.10.013.
17. Paik JJ, Wigley FM, Shah AA, Corse AM, Casciola-Rosen L, Hummers LK, et al. Association of fibrosing myopathy in systemic sclerosis and higher mortality. Arthritis Care Res (Hoboken). 2017;69:1764–70. https://doi.org/10.1002/acr.23291.
18. Corallo C, Cutolo M, Volpi N, Franci D, Aglianò M, Montella A, et al. Histopathological findings in systemic sclerosis-related myopathy: fibrosis and microangiopathy with lack of cellular inflammation. Ther Adv Musculoskelet Dis. 2017;9:3–10. https://doi.org/10.1177/1759720X16671928.
19. Ranque B, Authier F-J, Le-Guern V, Pagnoux C, Berezne A, Allanore Y, et al. A descriptive and prognostic study of systemic sclerosis-associated myopathies. Ann Rheum Dis. 2009;68:1474–7.
20. Paik JJ, Wigley FM, Lloyd TE, Corse AM, Casciola-Rosen L, Shah AA, et al. Spectrum of muscle histopathologic findings in forty-two scleroderma patients with weakness. Arthritis Care Res (Hoboken). 2015;67:1416–25. https://doi.org/10.1002/acr.22620.
21. Schanz S, Henes J, Ulmer A, Kötter I, Fierlbeck G, Claussen CD, et al. Magnetic resonance imaging findings in patients with systemic scleroderma and musculoskeletal symptoms. Eur Radiol. 2013;23:212–21. https://doi.org/10.1007/s00330-012-2584-1.
22. Paik JJ, Ahlawat S, DelGrande, F, Hummers LK, Wigley FM, Shah AA, et al. Predominant fasciitis and mild intramuscular edema on muscle magentic resonance imaging in scleroderma associated myopathy. Arthritis Rheumatol. 2018;70.
23. Ringel RA, Brick JE, Brick JF, Gutmann L, Riggs JE. Muscle involvement in the scleroderma syndromes. Arch Intern Med. 1990;150:2550–2.
24. Scarpelli M, Montironi R, Tulli D, Sisti S, Matera G, Magi Galluzzi C, et al. Quantitative analysis of quadriceps muscle biopsy in systemic sclerosis. Pathol Res Pract. 1992;188:603–6. https://doi.org/10.1016/S0344-0338(11)80064-6.
25. Ranque B, Bérezné A, Le-Guern V, Pagnoux C, Allanore Y, Launay D, et al. Myopathies related to systemic sclerosis: a case–control study of associated clinical and immunological features. Scand J Rheumatol. 2010;39:498–505. https://doi.org/10.3109/03009741003774626.
26. Hoogendijk JE, Amato AA, Lecky BR, Choy EH, Lundberg IE, Rose MR, et al. 119th ENMC International Workshop: trial design in adult idiopathic inflammatory myopathies, with the exception of inclusion body myositis, 10–12 October 2003, Naarden, The Netherlands. Neuromuscul Disord. 2004;14:337–45. https://doi.org/10.1016/j.nmd.2004.02.006.
27. Bhansing KJ, van Riel PLCM, van Engelen BGM, Fransen J, Vonk MC. Patients with systemic sclerosis/polymyositis overlap have a worse survival rate than patients without it. J Rheumatol. 2016;43:1838–43. https://doi.org/10.3899/jrheum.151425.
28. Arahata K, Engel AG. Monoclonal antibody analysis of mononuclear cells in myopathies. I: Quantitation of subsets according to diagnosis and sites of accumulation and demonstration and counts of muscle fibers invaded by T cells. Ann Neurol. 1984;16:193–208. https://doi.org/10.1002/ana.410160206.

29. Ranque B, Authier F-J, Berezne A, Guillevin L, Mouthon L. Systemic sclerosis-associated myopathy. Ann N Y Acad Sci. 2007;1108:268–82. https://doi.org/10.1196/annals.1422.029.
30. Wolfe JF, Adelstein E, Sharp GC. Antinuclear antibody with distinct specificity for polymyositis. J Clin Invest. 1977;59:176–8. https://doi.org/10.1172/JCI108616.
31. Treadwell EL, Alspaugh MA, Wolfe JF, Sharp GC. Clinical relevance of PM-1 antibody and physiochemical characterization of PM-1 antigen. J Rheumatol. 1984;11:658–62.
32. Koschik RW, Fertig N, Lucas MR, Domsic RT, Medsger TA. Anti-PM-Scl antibody in patients with systemic sclerosis. Clin Exp Rheumatol. 2012;30:S12–6.
33. Pakozdi A, Nihtyanova S, Moinzadeh P, Ong VH, Black CM, Denton CP. Clinical and serological hallmarks of systemic sclerosis overlap syndromes. J Rheumatol. 2011;38:2406–9. https://doi.org/10.3899/jrheum.101248.
34. Aguila LA, Lopes MRU, Pretti FZ, Sampaio-Barros PD, Carlos de Souza FH, Borba EF, et al. Clinical and laboratory features of overlap syndromes of idiopathic inflammatory myopathies associated with systemic lupus erythematosus, systemic sclerosis, or rheumatoid arthritis. Clin Rheumatol. 2014;33:1093–8. https://doi.org/10.1007/s10067-014-2730-z.
35. De Lorenzo R, Pinal-Fernandez I, Huang W, Albayda J, Tiniakou E, Johnson C, et al. Muscular and extramuscular clinical features of patients with anti-PM/Scl autoantibodies. Neurology. 2018;90:e2068–76. https://doi.org/10.1212/WNL.0000000000005638.
36. Rozman B, Cucnik S, Sodin-Semrl S, Czirják L, Varjú C, Distler O, et al. Prevalence and clinical associations of anti-Ku antibodies in patients with systemic sclerosis: a European EUSTAR-initiated multi-centre case-control study. Ann Rheum Dis. 2008;67:1282–6. https://doi.org/10.1136/ard.2007.073981.
37. Kaji K, Fertig N, Medsger TA, Satoh T, Hoshino K, Hamaguchi Y, et al. Autoantibodies to RuvBL1 and RuvBL2: a novel systemic sclerosis-related antibody associated with diffuse cutaneous and skeletal muscle involvement. Arthritis Care Res (Hoboken). 2014;66:575–84. https://doi.org/10.1002/acr.22163.
38. Tormey VJ, Bunn CC, Denton CP, Black CM. Anti-fibrillarin antibodies in systemic sclerosis. Rheumatology (Oxford). 2001;40:1157–62. https://doi.org/10.1093/rheumatology/40.10.1157.
39. Aggarwal R, Lucas M, Fertig N, Oddis CV, Medsger TA. Anti-U3 RNP autoantibodies in systemic sclerosis. Arthritis Rheum. 2009;60:1112–8. https://doi.org/10.1002/art.24409.
40. Okano Y, Steen VD, Medsger TA. Autoantibody to U3 nucleolar ribonucleoprotein (fibrillarin) in patients with systemic sclerosis. Arthritis Rheum. 1992;35:95–100. https://doi.org/10.1002/art.1780350114.
41. Landon-Cardinal O, Baril-Dionne A, Hoa S, Meyer A, Leclair V, Bourré-Tessier J, et al. Recognising the spectrum of scleromyositis: HEp-2 ANA patterns allow identification of a novel clinical subset with anti-SMN autoantibodies. RMD Open. 2020;6:e001357. https://doi.org/10.1136/rmdopen-2020-001357.
42. Steen VD. Autoantibodies in systemic sclerosis. Semin Arthritis Rheum. 2005;35:35–42. https://doi.org/10.1016/j.semarthrit.2005.03.005.
43. Partovi S, Schulte A-C, Aschwanden M, Staub D, Benz D, Imfeld S, et al. Impaired skeletal muscle microcirculation in systemic sclerosis. Arthritis Res Ther. 2012;14:R209. https://doi.org/10.1186/ar4047.
44. Paik JJ, Wigley FM, Hummers LK, Jacobs M. Advanced multiparametric magnetic resonance imaging of muscle for detection and quantification of muscle disease in systemic sclerosis [abstract]. Arthritis Rheumatol. 2020;70(Suppl 10).
45. Elhai M, Meunier M, Matucci-Cerinic M, Maurer B, Riemekasten G, Leturcq T, et al. Outcomes of patients with systemic sclerosis-associated polyarthritis and myopathy treated with tocilizumab or abatacept: a EUSTAR observational study. Ann Rheum Dis. 2013;72:1217–20. https://doi.org/10.1136/annrheumdis-2012-202657.
46. Boulos D, Ngian G-S, Rajadurai A, Elford K, Stevens W, Proudman S, et al. Long-term efficacy and tolerability of mycophenolate mofetil therapy in diffuse scleroderma skin disease. Int J Rheum Dis. 2017;20:481–8. https://doi.org/10.1111/1756-185X.13035.
47. Hinchcliff M, Toledo DM, Taroni JN, Wood TA, Franks JM, Ball MS, et al. Mycophenolate mofetil treatment of systemic sclerosis reduces myeloid cell numbers and attenuates the inflammatory gene signature in skin. J Invest Dermatol. 2018;138:1301–10. https://doi.org/10.1016/j.jid.2018.01.006.
48. Le EN, Wigley FM, Shah AA, Boin F, Hummers LK. Long-term experience of mycophenolate mofetil for treatment of diffuse cutaneous systemic sclerosis. Ann Rheum Dis. 2011;70:1104–7. https://doi.org/10.1136/ard.2010.142000.
49. Tashkin DP, Roth MD, Clements PJ, Furst DE, Khanna D, Kleerup EC, et al. Mycophenolate mofetil versus oral cyclophosphamide in scleroderma-related interstitial lung disease (SLS II): a randomised controlled, double-blind, parallel group trial. Lancet Respir Med. 2016;4:708–19. https://doi.org/10.1016/S2213-2600(16)30152-7.
50. Hervier B, Masseau A, Mussini J-M, Audrain M, Hamidou MA. Long-term efficacy of mycophenolate mofetil in a case of refractory antisynthetase syndrome. Joint Bone Spine. 2009;76:575–6. https://doi.org/10.1016/j.jbspin.2009.02.004.
51. Moghadam-Kia S, Aggarwal R, Oddis CV. Treatment of inflammatory myopathy: emerging therapies and therapeutic targets. Expert Rev Clin Immunol. 2015;11:1265–75. https://doi.org/10.1586/1744666X.2015.1082908.
52. Dalakas MC, Illa I, Dambrosia JM, Soueidan SA, Stein DP, Otero C, et al. A controlled trial of high-dose intravenous immune globulin infusions as treatment for dermatomyositis. N Engl J Med. 1993;329:1993–2000. https://doi.org/10.1056/NEJM199312303292704.
53. Aggarwal R, Bandos A, Reed AM, Ascherman DP, Barohn RJ, Feldman BM, et al. Predictors of clinical improvement in rituximab-treated refractory adult and juvenile dermatomyositis and adult polymyositis. Arthritis Rheumatol (Hoboken, NJ). 2014;66:740–9. https://doi.org/10.1002/art.38270.
54. Oddis CV, Reed AM, Aggarwal R, Rider LG, Ascherman DP, Levesque MC, et al. Rituximab in the treatment of refractory adult and juvenile dermatomyositis and adult polymyositis: a randomized, placebo-phase trial. Arthritis Rheum. 2013;65:314–24. https://doi.org/10.1002/art.37754.
55. Sem M, Molberg O, Lund MB, Gran JT. Rituximab treatment of the anti-synthetase syndrome: a retrospective case series. Rheumatology (Oxford). 2009;48:968–71. https://doi.org/10.1093/rheumatology/kep157.
56. Jordan S, Distler JHW, Maurer B, Huscher D, van Laar JM, Allanore Y, et al. Effects and safety of rituximab in systemic sclerosis: an analysis from the European Scleroderma Trial and Research (EUSTAR) group. Ann Rheum Dis. 2015;74:1188–94. https://doi.org/10.1136/annrheumdis-2013-204522.

Cancer in Systemic Sclerosis

37

Ami A. Shah and Masataka Kuwana

Epidemiology of Cancer in SSc

Most epidemiologic studies have demonstrated that patients with scleroderma have an increased age- and gender-adjusted risk of cancer compared to the general population (SIRs or RR ranging from 1.4 to 4.2), with only two studies reporting no increase in risk (Table 37.1) [1–16]. In two recent systematic reviews and meta-analyses, investigators summarized this risk increase and examined whether patients with scleroderma were at higher risk for particular tumor types. The first conducted by Bonifazi and colleagues [13] pooled 16 original studies with more than 7000 scleroderma patients. Patients with scleroderma had an increased cancer risk overall (summary RR 1.75, 95% CI 1.41, 2.18) and were noted to have a higher risk of lung cancer (summary RR 4.35, 95% CI 2.08, 9.09) and hematologic neoplasms (summary RR 2.24, 95% CI 1.53, 3.29) in particular. While there was insufficient data to perform a meta-analysis for liver and esophageal cancers, an increased risk of these tumor types was also noted in most of the original studies that examined these cancer sites.

Onishi and colleagues [14] performed another high quality systematic review and meta-analysis of cancer risk in scleroderma. They evaluated six studies with over 6600 scleroderma patients. In this review, the pooled SIR for all cancers was 1.41 (95% CI 1.18, 1.68), and they noted that there was an increased risk of lung (pooled SIR 3.18, 95% CI 2.09, 4.85), bladder (in women only, pooled SIR 2.80, 95% CI 1.36, 5.76), hematologic (pooled SIR 2.57, 95% CI 1.79, 3.68), liver (pooled SIR 4.36, 95% CI 2.0, 9.51), and nonmelanoma skin (in men only, pooled SIR 2.34, 95% CI 1.25, 4.59) cancers in scleroderma patients compared to the general population. Overall the risk of malignancy was higher in male patients with scleroderma (pooled SIR 1.85, 95% CI 1.49, 2.31), and the authors postulated that this may be related to more smoking among men compared to women. The risk of cancer was also higher in the 12 months following a scleroderma diagnosis (SIR 2.79) than >12 months after diagnosis (SIR 1.40, $p = 0.003$), suggesting that there may be a biological link between cancer and scleroderma or that there is a cancer detection bias among patients with new onset disease.

Other studies have also demonstrated that patients with scleroderma have an increased risk of head and neck [12, 18] cancers. In one US study, scleroderma patients had a 25-fold increased incidence of tongue cancer and a 9.6-fold increased risk of oropharyngeal carcinomas (all squamous cell carcinomas) [18], whereas in a Taiwanese population scleroderma patients had a 3.67-fold increased risk of cancers of the oral cavity and pharynx [12]. Numerous investigators have probed whether there is a higher risk of gender-specific tumor types, such as breast, cervical, ovarian, uterine, prostate, or testicular cancers. These studies have not consistently demonstrated that there is an increased risk of these cancer sites. However, breast and prostate cancer risk may be increased around the time of scleroderma onset, particularly in unique serologic subsets [16, 19–21]. Recent data also suggest that scleroderma patients may have an increased risk of both nonmelanoma and melanoma skin cancers [16, 21, 22].

In patients with SSc, malignancy is one of the most common non-SSc related causes of death [23, 24]. The presence of cancer increases the risk of death and health care costs in patients with SSc [16, 25, 26].

A. A. Shah (✉)
Johns Hopkins University School of Medicine, Baltimore, MD, USA
e-mail: Ami.Shah@jhmi.edu

M. Kuwana
Nippon Medical School Graduate School of Medicine, Tokyo, Japan
e-mail: kuwanam@nms.ac.jp

Y. Allanore et al. (eds.), *Scleroderma*, https://doi.org/10.1007/978-3-031-40658-4_37

Table 37.1 Risk of cancer in scleroderma from cohort studies, national registries, and systematic reviews and meta-analyses. Adapted with permission from [17]

Author (year)	SSc population	Comparator cancer registry	SSc *N*	SIR or RR (95% CI)	Types of cancer	Potential risk factors identified
Roumm (1985) [1]	Pittsburgh cohort living in Pittsburgh metro area (US)	Third National Cancer Survey of 1969–1971	262	1.81 (N/A)	Lung cancer	Pulmonary fibrosis
Abu-Shakra (1993) [2]	Scleroderma clinic at Wellesley Hospital (Canada)	Ontario population data from 1985 to 1986 National Cancer Incidence Reporting System	248	2.1 (1.52–2.91)	Lung, breast, cervix, oral cavity, melanoma, prostate, testicle, uterus	Older age at scleroderma onset
Rosenthal (1993) [3]	Inpatient registry (6 counties, Sweden)	Swedish National Cancer Registry	233	2.4 (1.5–3.6)	Lung, non-Hodgkin's lymphoma	
Rosenthal (1995) [4]	Inpatient registry (whole country, Sweden)	Swedish national	917	1.5 (1.2–1.9)	Lung, nonmelanoma skin, liver	
Hill (2003) [5]	South Australian scleroderma registry	South Australian	441	1.99 (1.46–2.65)	Lung	
Chatterjee (2005) [6]	Michigan scleroderma registry (US)	Metro Detroit (SEER)	538	0.91 (0.66–1.22)	Liver cancer	Limited scleroderma, black females (liver)
Derk (2006) [7]	Jefferson Scleroderma Center (US)	SEER registry	2040	1.55 (1.16–1.93)	Esophageal, oropharyngeal	Older age at scleroderma diagnosis, smoking, family history of cancer
Kang (2009) [8]	Korean SSc patients evaluated at Kangnam St Mary's Hospital	Korean National Cancer Centre database	112	4.2 (2.3–6.1)	Lung, stomach, esophagus, liver, pancreas	Male sex
Olesen (2010) [9]	Danish National Registry of Patients	Danish Cancer Registry	2040	1.5 (1.3–1.7)	Lung, hematologic, immune-related cancers (including nonmelanoma skin)	Male sex
Siau (2011) [10]	South West England (Bristol region, UK)	South West Cancer Intelligence Service Registry	68	3.15 (1.77–5.20)	Hematologic	
Hashimoto (2012) [11]	Kitasato University Hospital scleroderma cohort (Japan)	Research Group for the Population-based Cancer Registration	405	1.24 (0.77–1.71)	Lung	
Kuo (2012) [12]	Catastrophic illness registry of the Taiwan National Health Insurance Research Dataset	National Health Insurance dataset	2053	1.63 (1.31–2.01)	Lung, Oral cavity, and pharynx, hematologic	
Bonifazi (2013) [13]	Meta-analysis of observational studies			1.75 (1.41–2.18)	Lung, hematologic	
Onishi (2013) [14]	Meta-analysis of population-based cohort studies		6641	1.41 (1.18–1.68)	Lung, liver, hematologic, non-Hodgkin's, leukemia, bladder, nonmelanoma skin (men)	Male sex, first 12 months after diagnosis
Zhang (2013) [15]	Meta-analysis of observational studies		7183	N/A	Lung, non-Hodgkin's lymphoma, hematopoietic	
Morrisroe (2020) [16]	Australian Scleroderma Cohort Study (ASCS)	Australian state-based cancer registries	1727	2.15 (1.84–2.49)	Lung	Older age at scleroderma onset, ILD, PAH, extended use of calcium channel blockers

Potential Risk Factors and Mechanisms That May Explain the Increased Cancer Risk

It remains unclear whether particular scleroderma characteristics are risk factors for cancer in scleroderma. While the Onishi meta-analysis did not detect a difference in cancer risk by scleroderma cutaneous subtype [14], other studies have suggested that the risk of cancer may be higher in patients with diffuse scleroderma than those with limited scleroderma [5]. Patients who are older when they develop the first clinical signs of scleroderma are also at higher risk of cancer [2, 16, 27, 28].

Many investigations have suggested that chronic inflammation and damage from scleroderma itself may predispose patients to the development of malignancy. It has been hypothesized that lung cancers may develop in the context of pulmonary scar [29, 30], and patients with idiopathic pulmonary fibrosis have been shown to have an increased risk of lung cancer even after adjusting for smoking status [31]. Alternatively, fibrosis may develop in the lung as a host response to an underlying lung neoplasm. In scleroderma, the data are controversial with some studies suggesting a higher risk of lung cancer in patients with interstitial lung disease [2, 8, 16, 32] and others contradicting this [14, 33]. Similarly, the risk of esophageal cancer may be greater in patients with severe gastroesophageal reflux disease who develop Barrett's esophagus [34]. Patients with an overlap syndrome with primary biliary cirrhosis, particularly those with advanced histologic findings or biochemical nonresponse to ursodeoxycholic acid therapy, may have a higher risk of hepatocellular carcinoma [35, 36].

Another concern is that cytotoxic or immunosuppressive therapies employed to treat scleroderma may trigger the development of malignancy. This is a complicated issue as there is often a problem of confounding by indication; patients who are treated with cyclophosphamide for interstitial lung disease in scleroderma may have a higher risk of lung cancer, although whether this is related to the drug or damage from the disease itself is unclear. However, it is well established that patients treated with cyclophosphamide for other diseases have a higher risk of bladder and hematologic neoplasms, especially with exposure to higher cumulative doses or smoking [37, 38]. It remains controversial whether other immunosuppressive therapies employed to treat scleroderma are associated with an increased cancer risk. Mycophenolate mofetil is being employed more commonly in scleroderma to treat severe cutaneous disease, interstitial lung disease, and overlap syndromes with inflammatory myositis. While cancer risk with mycophenolate use has not been well studied in scleroderma, data from the transplant literature are conflicting as to whether or not there is an increased risk of lymphoma and nonmelanoma skin cancers with mycophenolate use [39–42]. Data from the transplant literature also suggest that there may be an elevated risk of primary CNS lymphoma in patients treated with mycophenolate [43], with new case reports of this diagnosis occurring in scleroderma also [44]. It is difficult to draw inferences from the transplant population as these patients are often on multiple concomitant immunosuppressive therapies, a practice that is less common in scleroderma. Lastly, recent data suggest that non-immunosuppressive therapies used to treat scleroderma, such as calcium channel blockers, may associate with increased cancer risk [16].

While immunosuppressive therapies employed to treat scleroderma and severe disease itself may be risk factors for the development of cancer, cancer therapies themselves may also increase the risk of developing scleroderma or scleroderma-like disease. For example, bleomycin, paclitaxel, gemcitabine, and carboplatin have been reported to trigger skin sclerosis and development or exacerbation of Raynaud's phenomenon and ischemic digits [45–50]. Immunotherapies that prime and amplify host immune responses to destroy neoplasms have also been reported to trigger new onset autoimmune disease or exacerbate previously quiescent rheumatic disease [51]. Scleroderma-like skin changes and critical digital ischemia have been described after immune checkpoint inhibitor therapy, although often these cases do not report the presence of other disease features or classical scleroderma autoantibodies [52–57]. The risk of scleroderma after immune checkpoint inhibitor therapy has been assessed in VigiBase, the World Health Organization global Individualized Case Safety Report database [55]. These data suggest that the risk of scleroderma may be increased with use of anti-PD-1 agents like nivolumab and pembrolizumab. Lastly, radiation therapy may trigger severe skin thickening in patients with preexisting scleroderma [58, 59] or development of localized scleroderma in patients without an antecedent history of a connective tissue disease [60].

Another potential mechanism that may explain the increased risk of cancer among scleroderma patients includes a shared genetic susceptibility for both cancer and autoimmunity. A common inciting environmental exposure, such as silica, could also trigger the development of scleroderma and cancer [61, 62].

Data Suggesting That a Subset of Systemic Sclerosis Is a Paraneoplastic Disease

While all of these mechanisms likely play a role in the cancer-scleroderma relationship, a recent accumulation of data strongly suggests that scleroderma may be a paraneoplastic disease in some patients. As in dermatomyositis, a subset of patients with scleroderma is diagnosed with cancer within a short interval of the first clinical signs of scleroderma [1, 2,

63–67]. This has been most striking in patients with breast cancer [64–66], where breast cancer diagnoses are often detected within 2 years of scleroderma onset. However, the temporal clustering of cancer diagnosis with the first clinical signs of scleroderma likely extends to multiple other tumor types. In a large US scleroderma cohort, it was detected that cancer diagnoses peaked around scleroderma onset with 22.7% of cancer diagnoses developing within 2 years of the first non-Raynaud's scleroderma symptom [28]. Anecdotal reports of cancer therapy halting the scleroderma disease process also raise the question of whether scleroderma is a paraneoplastic disease in some patients [68–70].

An initial investigation of 23 scleroderma patients with cancer was performed to examine whether unique clinical or serologic features are associated with a close temporal relationship between cancer diagnosis and scleroderma onset [67]. In this study, scleroderma patients with cancer and anti-RNA polymerase III autoantibodies (anti-POLR3) had a unique clustering of cancer with scleroderma onset that was not detected among patients with anti-topoisomerase I or anticentromere antibodies. Interestingly, these patients also had unique nucleolar RNA polymerase III expression in their cancerous tissues (Fig. 37.1), in spite of nucleoplasmic expression of RNA polymerase III in normal cells. This suggests that ectopic expression of scleroderma autoantigens in cancer cells may associate with scleroderma-specific immune responses.

The clustering of cancer with scleroderma onset among patients with anti-POLR3 antibodies has since been confirmed in multiple international investigations (Table 37.2). Interestingly, anti-POLR3 antibodies have never been detected in cancer patients without rheumatic disease, including women with breast cancer and patients with lung cancer [75, 76].

While the observation of a short cancer-scleroderma interval is most striking among patients with anti-POLR3 antibodies (Table 37.2), many of these cohorts had patients with a clustering of cancer with scleroderma onset among other autoantibody specificities. In the US investigation, this was most evident in patients who developed scleroderma at an older age, particularly among those with anti-topoisomerase I antibodies or those who were ANA-positive but negative for the three most common scleroderma antibodies (anti*c*entromere, anti-*t*opoisomerase I, and anti-RNA *p*olymerase III or CTP-negative) [28]. These data raise the question of whether cancer may be an important trigger of the immune response more broadly among scleroderma patients, especially since other scleroderma autoantigens, such as topoisomerase I, may play a key role in cancer fitness [77]. In one investigation, two patients with scleroderma and late lung cancer diagnoses had significant increases in anti-topoisomerase 1 antibody levels at the time of lung cancer diagnosis [78]. Furthermore, study of longitudinal serum samples revealed that these patients' sera reacted with new, previously unrecognized epitopes of the topoisomerase 1 molecule after lung cancer diagnosis [78]. Additional studies have identified that anti-RNPC3 (also known as anti-U11/U12) antibodies may also associate with an increased risk of cancer around the time of scleroderma onset [79, 80]. In one study, patients with anti-PM/Scl antibodies had an increased risk of cancer, though not cancer within a short interval of SSc onset [26]. In an intriguing case report, a patient with a pancreatic neoplasm had increased nuclear expression of PM/Scl-100 in her tumor tissue and had clinical remission of her SSc after resection of her malignancy [70]. These data further support the possibility that cancers may be an antigen source that drive rheumatic disease [67, 77, 78].

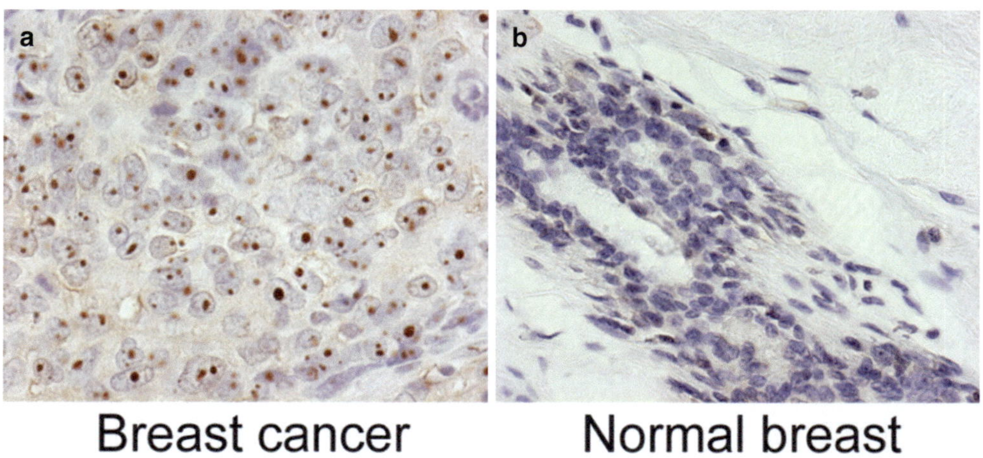

Fig. 37.1 Nucleolar RNA polymerase III expression is prominent in cancerous tissue from scleroderma patients with RNA polymerase III autoantibodies. Paraffin sections from cancerous breast tissue from a scleroderma patient with anti-RNA polymerase III antibodies (**a**) and from normal breast tissue (**b**). Tissue sections were stained with antibodies against RNA polymerase III. Brown color shows RNA polymerase III staining, and blue (Mayer's hematoxylin counterstain) shows nuclei. Original magnification ×40. (Reproduced with permission from [67])

Table 37.2 Risk of contemporaneous cancer in SSc patients with anti-POLR3 antibodies compared to SSc patients without anti-POLR3

Author	Year published	Cohort location	SSc *N*	Definition of short cancer-scleroderma interval[a]	OR (95% CI)[b] or prevalence (%, *p*-value)
Airo et al. [71]	2011	Italy	360	−6 months to +12 months	18.8% anti-POLR3 vs. 0% anti-topo vs. 0.4% anti-centromere, $p < 0.001$
Nikpour et al. [27]	2011	Australia	451	±5 years	4.2 (1.3–13.4)[c]
Moinzadeh et al. [20]	2014	United Kingdom	2177	±3 years	5.83 (3.21–10.92)[d]
Shah et al. [28]	2015	United States	1044	±2 years	5.08 (1.60–16.1)[e]
Saigusa et al. [72]	2015	Japan	261	−6 months to +12 months	13.6% anti-POLR3 vs. 0% anti-topo vs. 0.7% anti-centromere, $p < 0.01$
Lazzaroni et al. [73]	2017	Europe (EUSTAR)	357[f]	−6 months to +12 months	7.38 (1.61–33.8)
Callejas-Moraga et al. [74]	2019	Spain	221[f]	±5 years	7.7% anti-POLR3+ vs. 3.6% anti-POLR3−, $p = 0.28$
Morrisroe et al. [16]	2020	Australia	1727	Within 5 years	2.14 (1.03–4.45)[g]

POLR3 RNA polymerase III, *topo* topoisomerase-1
[a]Values are anchored to SSc onset where negative values precede SSc onset and + values denote time after SSc onset
[b]Comparing SSc patients with anti-POLR3 to SSc patients without anti-POLR3 unless otherwise noted
[c]Adjusted for age at SSc onset, smoking, subtype, immunosuppression
[d]Adjusted for age and sex
[e]Adjusted for age at SSc onset, race, sex, smoking, scleroderma subtype, anti-topoisomerase 1, and anti-centromere antibody status
[f]Case control study with univariable analysis reported. In Lazzaroni et al., cases consisted of 158 anti-POLR3+ patients and 199 anti-POLR3− SSc controls. In Callejas-Moraga et al., cases consisted of 26 anti-POLR3+ patients and 195 anti-POLR3− SSc controls
[g]Adjusted for age at SSc onset, sex, race, smoking, extended immunosuppressive therapy use, and digital ulceration

Genetic Alteration of Autoantigens in Malignancies May Be an Antigen Source That Triggers Scleroderma

The data demonstrating unique nucleolar RNA polymerase III expression in cancerous tissues from scleroderma patients with anti-POLR3 antibodies raised the question of whether autoimmunity may be triggered by structural alterations of RNA polymerase III in cancers from these patients, thereby resulting in recognition as a "foreign antigen" by the immune system [81]. To address this possibility, a group of investigators searched for missense mutations in the *POLR3A* gene, which encodes the largest subunit of RNA polymerase III (RPC155), in cancers from 16 scleroderma patients, 8 with anti-POLR3 antibodies, and 8 with anti-topoisomerase I or anticentromere antibodies [81]. Three of the eight patients with anti-POLR3 antibodies had evidence of somatic, missense variants in *POLR3A*. Each of these three patients had a different mutation resulting in a single amino acid change of RPC155, and two of these three patients exhibited mutation-specific T cell immune responses. There was evidence that the immune response that may have been initiated against the mutated subunit of RNA polymerase III spread to the wild-type version, as autoantibodies that cross-reacted with both wild-type and mutant RNA polymerase III were detected. In addition to somatic mutations in *POLR3A*, loss of heterozygosity at the *POLR3A* locus was also detected in five of the eight patients with anti-POLR3 antibodies (two of whom also had somatic mutations). In contrast, no genetic alterations were detected in the *POLR3A* locus in tumors from patients with anti-topoisomerase I or anticentromere antibodies [81].

These data provided further evidence to support a paraneoplastic model of disease pathogenesis, wherein mutated autoantigens result in the generation of T cell responses specific to mutant proteins and B cell responses cross-reactive with both mutant and wild-type proteins (Fig. 37.2) [77]. Due to subsequent antibody-mediated uptake of wild-type proteins by antigen-presenting cells, T cell responses may then be directed against the wild-type molecule [77]. These immune effector cells may cross-react with self-tissue, resulting in target tissue damage [77]. It has been shown that myositis autoantigens are detectable in immature, regenerating myoblasts in myositis muscle, and this antigen source may sustain and propagate the autoimmune response [82]. Data regarding a causal relationship between autoantibody responses and a pathogenic process are limited in scleroderma, although one study reported immunization of topoisomerase I in conjunction with adjuvant-induced scleroderma-like skin sclerosis and lung fibrosis in mice [83]. Alternatively, autoantibody production and scleroderma development may be independent consequences, both of which result from cancer development. In this regard, development of scleroderma-like skin lesions was reported in patients with cancer, which produces a large amount of fibrogenic factors, including TGF-β [84–86].

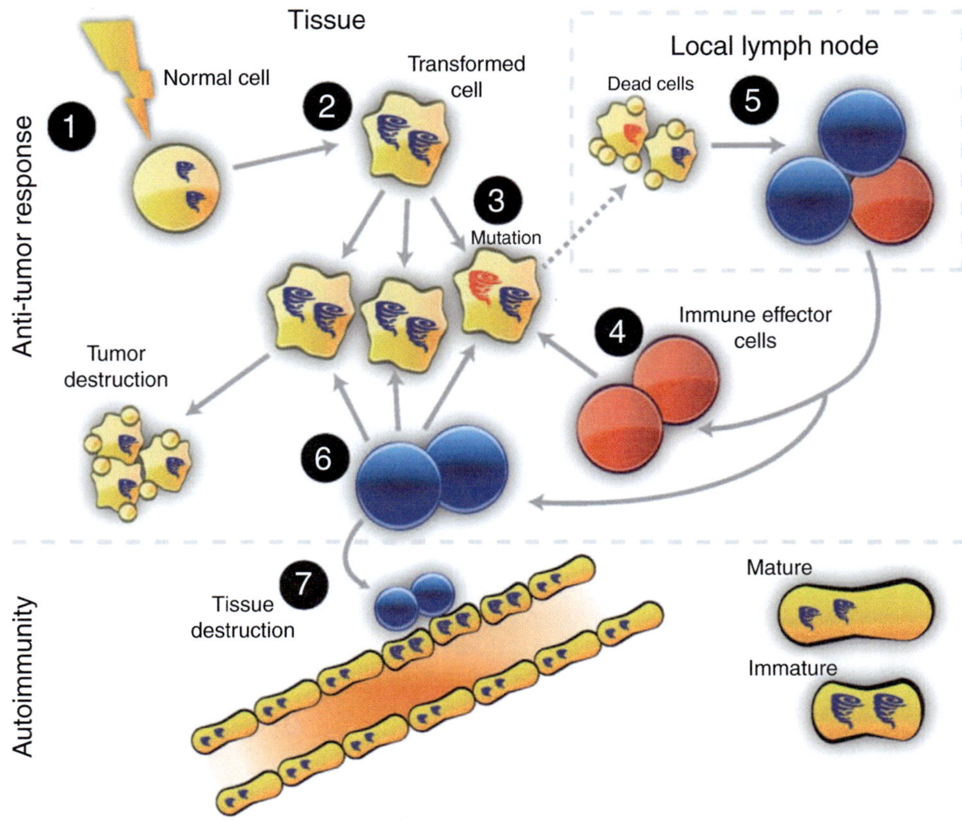

Fig. 37.2 Paraneoplastic model. Transformation of normal cells (**1**) may result in gene expression patterns that resemble immature cells involved in tissue healing (**2**). Occasionally, autoantigens become mutated (**3**); these are not driver mutations, and not all cancer cells have them. The first immune response is directed against the mutated form of the antigen (**4**) and may spread to the wild-type version (**5**). Immune effector cells directed against the mutant (depicted in red) delete exclusively cancer cells containing the mutation (**6**). Immune effector cells directed against the wild-type (depicted in blue) delete cancer cells without the mutation and also cross-react with the patient's own tissues (particularly immature cells expressing high levels of antigen, found in damaged/repairing tissue) (**7**). Once autoimmunity has been initiated, the disease is self-propagating. Immature cells (expressing high antigen levels) that repair the immune-mediated injury can themselves become the targets of the immune response, sustaining an ongoing cycle of damage/repair that provides the antigen source that fuels the autoimmune response. (Reproduced with permission from [77])

Autoantibodies and Clinical Phenotype May Define Tumor Risk, Type, and Timing

Epidemiologic and mechanistic data suggesting a model of cancer-induced autoimmunity raise the question of whether early cancer detection and treatment could improve both cancer and scleroderma outcomes. While published reports from many international scleroderma cohorts have demonstrated an increased risk of cancer around the time of scleroderma onset in patients with anti-POLR3 antibodies, a major limitation of these studies was that cancer risk was ascertained in scleroderma patients with an anti-POLR3 immune response compared to scleroderma patients without anti-POLR3 antibodies. An important question is whether this risk increase is greater than that expected in the general population, as this would suggest a role for enhanced cancer detection strategies in patients with anti-POLR3 antibodies. Igusa and colleagues investigated cancer risk in 2383 scleroderma patients compared to the US Surveillance, Epidemiology and End Results (SEER) registry [21]. Cancer incidence over time was examined in autoantibody and cutaneous subsets, as shown in Fig. 37.3. While cancer risk was not increased in scleroderma patients overall, those with anti-POLR3 antibodies and CTP-negative patients had an increased risk of cancer around the time of scleroderma onset. Within 3 years of scleroderma onset, patients with anti-POLR3 antibodies and diffuse scleroderma had an increased risk of breast cancer (SIR 5.14, 95% CI 2.66–8.98), prostate cancer (SIR 7.17, 95% CI 1.95–18.4), and tongue cancer (SIR 43.9, 95% CI 5.31–158.5), while those with anti-POLR3 and limited scleroderma had an increased risk of lung cancer (SIR 10.4, 95% CI 1.26–37.7). Within 3 years of scleroderma onset, CTP-negative patients with limited scleroderma had an increased risk of breast cancer (SIR 4.44, 95% CI 1.92–8.74) and melanoma (SIR 7.10, 95% CI 1.46–20.8), whereas CTP-negative patients with diffuse scleroderma had an increased risk of tongue cancer (SIR 40.5, 95% CI 1.02–225.5). These data demonstrate the importance of using biologically relevant filters, such as autoantibodies, cutaneous subtype, and timing, to risk stratify patients with scleroderma. Further work is needed to validate these findings and investigate the value of targeted cancer detection strategies in scleroderma patients with distinct immune responses.

Unique Scleroderma Immune Responses, Alone or in Combination, May Be Cancer-Protective

An important and unexpected finding from Igusa et al. was that patients with anti-centromere antibodies had a decreased risk of cancer compared to that expected in the general population after accounting for age, sex, race, ethnicity, and calendar-time (Fig. 37.3) [21]. Prior studies in small breast cancer cohorts have demonstrated the presence of anti-centromere antibodies associates with improved disease-free and overall survival [87–89]. Given data in SLE that suggest anti-DNA antibodies can have direct anticancer effects in cells with DNA repair defects [90], this raises the hypothesis that anti-centromere immune responses could exert an anticancer effect in scleroderma [21]. Further work is needed to validate these epidemiologic findings and study its mechanistic basis.

While compelling data support a model of cancer-induced autoimmunity in patients with anti-POLR3, it is important to note that ~80–85% of patients with this specificity do not

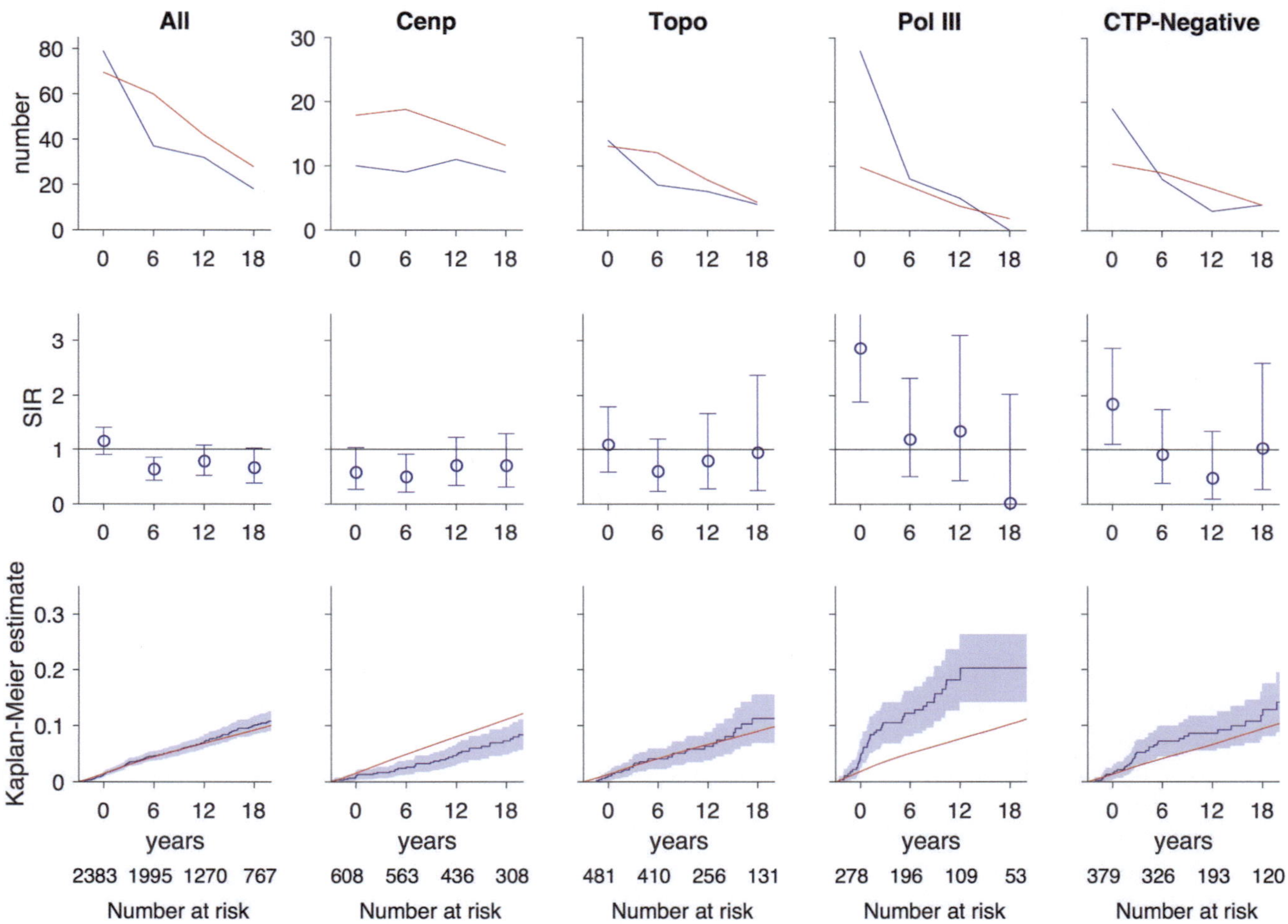

Fig. 37.3 Risk of all cancers over time. In each graph, the *x*-axis reflects time from scleroderma onset (defined as time zero). Top and middle rows, each time window represents a 6-year period (±3 years); for example, data plotted at time zero reflect cancer risk within ±3 years of scleroderma onset. The number at risk for each time window is denoted at the bottom of the graph. Top row, the observed number of cancer cases (blue) is presented in comparison with the number of cancer cases that are expected based on SEER data (red). Middle row, the ratio between the observed and expected cancer cases, is presented as a standardized incidence ratio (SIR) along with its 95% confidence interval. Values of 1 denote a cancer risk equivalent to that of the background population. Bottom row, the cumulative incidence of cancer among scleroderma patients (solid blue line) starting at 3 years before scleroderma onset is presented with 95% confidence intervals (shaded blue region). Red lines represent the expected cumulative incidence of cancer based on SEER data for the general population. Scleroderma patients with anti-centromere antibodies appear to have a decreased risk of cancer over time. Scleroderma patients with pol III antibodies and the CTP-Negative group have an increased risk of cancer that is prominent at scleroderma onset. The cumulative incidence of cancer is significantly higher than that observed in the general population among patients with pol III autoantibodies. (Adapted with permission [21])

have a cancer diagnosis over follow up. One hypothesis is that cancer is a trigger for the development of scleroderma in patients with anti-POLR3 antibodies, but the immune response is variably successful in eliminating cancer or maintaining it in equilibrium such that it does not clinically emerge [91]. This raises the important question of whether a broader immune response could have a more potent anticancer effect than an immune response directed against a narrower set of targets.

In a study of 168 scleroderma patients with anti-POLR3 antibodies (80 with a history of cancer, 88 without cancer after at least 5 years of follow up), it was found that antibodies targeting the large subunit of RNA polymerase I (RPA194) were enriched in patients without cancer [91]. This is intriguing in light of recent studies demonstrating that BMH21, a small molecule inhibitor of RNA polymerase I, has antitumor activity in multiple cancer cell lines in vitro and in animal models [92]. Functional studies are needed to define whether anti-RPA194 immune responses have similar anticancer properties.

Emerging data also suggest that anti-Th/To antibodies may also associate with a lower risk of a short cancer-scleroderma interval [93]. In a case control study of 804 scleroderma patients (403 with cancer, 401 without cancer after at least 5 years of follow up), patients with antibodies against components of the Th/To complex (hPOP1, RPP25, RPP30, and/or RPP40) were less likely to develop cancer within 3 years of scleroderma onset. Interestingly, anti-Th/To antibodies were detected in a small number of patients with anti-POLR3 also. Among patients with anti-POLR3 antibodies, none of the patients who also had anti-hPOP1 had cancer diagnosed within 3 years of scleroderma onset compared to 24% of patients with anti-POLR3 antibodies who did not have anti-Th/To antibodies.

While these findings require external validation and further study with respect to general population comparators, these data suggest that unique scleroderma immune responses, alone or in combination, may modify cancer risk. This is supported by a recent study showing that ANA positivity is an independent predictor of favorable prognosis in scleroderma patients with cancer, possibly suggesting potential role of scleroderma humoral autoimmunity in anticancer benefit [94]. In particular, for patients with anti-POLR3 antibodies, testing for the presence of additional autoantibodies could improve precision in cancer risk assessment. For instance, those with anti-POLR3 alone may warrant more intensive cancer detection strategies, whereas those with anti-POLR3 + anti-RPA194 or those with anti-POLR3 + anti-Th/To may only need age, sex, and risk factor appropriate cancer screening tests. This could be beneficial to minimize the harms (e.g., radiation exposure, false-positive tests) and costs of overscreening in patients with anti-POLR3 antibodies.

Implications for Cancer Screening and Scleroderma Therapeutics

The optimal approach for cancer screening in scleroderma remains unknown. The recent data supporting a model of cancer-induced autoimmunity among patients with anti-POLR3 autoantibodies suggest that aggressive malignancy screening may be warranted at the clinical onset of scleroderma [73, 95]. In particular, these data raise the question of whether early cancer diagnosis and treatment could play a significant role in achieving scleroderma remission.

The EUSTAR group conducted a Delphi exercise including 82 providers from EUSTAR centers [73]. For scleroderma patients with anti-POLR3 antibodies, there was a high level of agreement that cancer screening should be performed at the time of scleroderma diagnosis. Possible recommendations included: (1) screening for breast cancer in women, (2) performing other cancer screening tests based on age, sex, and clinical suspicion, and (3) continuing cancer surveillance in the first 2–5 years after SSc diagnosis.

It is the authors' practice to perform comprehensive, age- and gender-appropriate cancer screening in all new patients with scleroderma according to guidelines established in the United States [95]. In women, we recommend pelvic exams and Pap smears every 3 years starting at age 21 or every 5 years if HPV testing has been performed, with shorter intervals if there have been prior abnormal results [96]. While Pap smears are typically not recommended beyond the age of 65, we suggest that this be done once in older patients with new onset of scleroderma. While the current recommendations for mammography screening in the United States general population are controversial, it is our practice to follow a more aggressive screening protocol with annual mammography starting at age 40. For men younger than age 40, we recommend an annual testicular examination, and for older gentleman, we discuss the risks and benefits of digital rectal examination and prostate-specific antigen testing given the controversies of this test for prostate cancer screening. We initiate colonoscopy screening for colon cancer at the age of 45 with testing every 10 years if the baseline study is normal [97]. While it is not recommended that colonoscopies be performed in individuals above the age of 75 due to anticipated life expectancy, in older patients with new onset scleroderma, we recommend this test to ensure there is not an underlying colonic malignancy that may drive disease.

Further testing should be considered if particular risk factors are present. Patients who have refractory gastroesophageal reflux disease despite high-dose proton pump inhibitor therapy are referred for upper endoscopy, and sequential screenings are performed in those with (1) Barrett's esophagus at 1–3 year intervals depending on the presence of dysplasia or (2) severe erosive esophagitis at intervals suggested by the evaluating gastroenterologist

[98]. Low-dose chest computed tomography (CT) is now recommended for patients aged 55–74 with a 30+ pack year smoking history if they continue to smoke or have quit in the last 15 years [99]. Baseline high-resolution chest CT scan may have been performed already in scleroderma patients who are at high risk for interstitial lung disease, including African Americans, those with topoisomerase 1 antibodies or diffuse cutaneous disease, and those with a restrictive ventilatory defect or forced vital capacity decline greater than 10% of predicted. For patients with cirrhosis from primary biliary cirrhosis, the American Association for the Study of Liver Diseases recommends cross-sectional imaging (usually ultrasound) with or without alpha fetoprotein levels at 6–12 month intervals [100]. Patients with dysphagia that persists without an identifiable cause (such as severe xerostomia, pharyngeal muscle weakness, or esophageal stricture) may require further examination by an otolaryngologist for evaluation of head and neck cancers. Serum protein electrophoresis, serum immunofixation, and peripheral blood flow cytometry may be useful initial tests in the evaluation of new cytopenias not otherwise explained by immunosuppressive therapies, and consultation with a hematologist and bone marrow biopsy may be required. It is also important to carefully evaluate patients with current or antecedent immunosuppressive exposure to monitor for long-term cancer risks. Annual urinalysis and urine cytology are recommended in patients with prior cyclophosphamide exposure, and full skin examination is suggested in patients treated with mycophenolate mofetil.

Lastly, we consider more aggressive cancer surveillance in select patients who are considered to be at particularly elevated risk of cancer including patients with: (1) anti-POLR3 autoantibodies, (2) an older age of scleroderma onset, (3) atypical, aggressive, or treatment unresponsive disease, (4) profound weight loss or other constitutional features out of proportion with disease severity, or (5) patients with a personal or striking family history of cancer. While there are no established trials of cancer screening in these patients, further evaluation with CT of the chest, abdomen and pelvis, or whole body PET-CT and serum tumor markers may be warranted. In patients with anti-POLR3 antibodies in particular, there may be a role for breast MRI, chest CT, PSA testing, and ENT examination given the increased risk of breast, lung, prostate, and tongue cancer seen in these patients [21].

Complexity of Cancer Care in Patients with SSc

The occurrence of cancer in patients with systemic inflammatory rheumatic conditions like scleroderma significantly increases the complexity of medical decision making. Often there is reluctance to treat patients with scleroderma with conventional cancer therapies, such as radiation therapy, or use immune checkpoint inhibitors. In one study comparing patients with autoimmune rheumatic disease and lung cancer to those with lung cancer alone, only 69.5% of patients with autoimmune disease received standard of care compared to 97.3% of those with lung cancer alone [101]. Interestingly, there were no differences in survival observed despite these differences in care [101]. There has been debate whether SSc is a contraindication to radiation with the concern of exaggerated radiation-induced fibrosis in patients with SSc. In a two-center study examining radiation and SSc outcomes in SSc patients with breast cancer, ~50% of patients developed skin thickening in the radiation port, but there was no evidence of lung or generalized skin disease flare [102]. There were no differences in disease duration, SSc subtype, or autoantibody status between patients who developed localized skin thickening in the field of radiation and those who did not [102]. Further study is required to define the risks of radiation in patients with SSc, particularly across cancer sites and radiation modalities. The risk of severe radiation toxicities may be less with newer radiation therapy techniques, such as 3D conformal approaches, dose-fractionated radiotherapy, improved dose homogeneity, and brachytherapy [102, 103]. Further work is also needed to define the risks of immune checkpoint inhibitor therapy in patients with preexisting SSc. In the authors' experience to date, generalized disease flares have not been observed with careful patient selection (unpublished data). It is important to individualize decision making for patients with SSc and cancer. Close multidisciplinary discussion between rheumatologists, medical oncologists, radiation oncologists, surgeons, and patients can be beneficial to customize care. In particular, it is important to factor in a patient's SSc disease activity and severity, the tumor type and stage, potential cancer, and survival outcomes under the different treatment options under consideration, possible exacerbation of disease activity with cancer therapy, and the patient's preferences and tolerance for risk [102].

Summary

The relationship between scleroderma and malignancy is complex, with many potential explanations for the increased risk of cancer in patients with scleroderma. Emerging data suggest that subsets of scleroderma patients, identified by distinct immune responses, may have paraneoplastic disease. Careful malignancy screening should be considered in patients with new onset scleroderma, and further study is required to understand whether cancer therapy may be effective treatment for scleroderma.

References

1. Roumm AD, Medsger TA Jr. Cancer and systemic sclerosis. An epidemiologic study. Arthritis Rheum. 1985;28(12):1336–40.
2. Abu-Shakra M, Guillemin F, Lee P. Cancer in systemic sclerosis. Arthritis Rheum. 1993;36(4):460–4.
3. Rosenthal AK, McLaughlin JK, Linet MS, Persson I. Scleroderma and malignancy: an epidemiological study. Ann Rheum Dis. 1993;52(7):531–3.
4. Rosenthal AK, McLaughlin JK, Gridley G, Nyren O. Incidence of cancer among patients with systemic sclerosis. Cancer. 1995;76(5):910–4.
5. Hill CL, Nguyen AM, Roder D, Roberts-Thomson P. Risk of cancer in patients with scleroderma: a population based cohort study. Ann Rheum Dis. 2003;62(8):728–31.
6. Chatterjee S, Dombi GW, Severson RK, Mayes MD. Risk of malignancy in scleroderma: a population-based cohort study. Arthritis Rheum. 2005;52(8):2415–24.
7. Derk CT, Rasheed M, Artlett CM, Jimenez SA. A cohort study of cancer incidence in systemic sclerosis. J Rheumatol. 2006;33(6):1113–6.
8. Kang KY, Yim HW, Kim IJ, Yoon JU, Ju JH, Kim HY, Park SH. Incidence of cancer among patients with systemic sclerosis in Korea: results from a single centre. Scand J Rheumatol. 2009;38(4):299–303.
9. Olesen AB, Svaerke C, Farkas DK, Sorensen HT. Systemic sclerosis and the risk of cancer: a nationwide population-based cohort study. Br J Dermatol. 2010;163(4):800–6.
10. Siau K, Laversuch CJ, Creamer P, O'Rourke KP. Malignancy in scleroderma patients from south west England: a population-based cohort study. Rheumatol Int. 2011;31(5):641–5.
11. Hashimoto A, Arinuma Y, Nagai T, Tanaka S, Matsui T, Tohma S, Endo H, Hirohata S. Incidence and the risk factor of malignancy in Japanese patients with systemic sclerosis. Intern Med. 2012;51(13):1683–8.
12. Kuo CF, Luo SF, Yu KH, Chou IJ, Tseng WY, Chang HC, Fang YF, Chiou MJ, See LC. Cancer risk among patients with systemic sclerosis: a nationwide population study in Taiwan. Scand J Rheumatol. 2012;41(1):44–9.
13. Bonifazi M, Tramacere I, Pomponio G, Gabrielli B, Avvedimento EV, La Vecchia C, Negri E, Gabrielli A. Systemic sclerosis (scleroderma) and cancer risk: systematic review and meta-analysis of observational studies. Rheumatology. 2013;52(1):143–54.
14. Onishi A, Sugiyama D, Kumagai S, Morinobu A. Cancer incidence in systemic sclerosis: meta-analysis of population-based cohort studies. Arthritis Rheum. 2013;65(7):1913–21.
15. Zhang JQ, Wan YN, Peng WJ, Yan JW, Li BZ, Mei B, Chen B, Yao H, Yang GJ, Tao JH, et al. The risk of cancer development in systemic sclerosis: a meta-analysis. Cancer Epidemiol. 2013;37(5):523–7.
16. Morrisroe K, Hansen D, Huq M, Stevens W, Sahhar J, Ngian GS, Ferdowsi N, Hill C, Roddy J, Walker J, et al. Incidence, risk factors, and outcomes of cancer in systemic sclerosis. Arthritis Care Res (Hoboken). 2020;72(11):1625–35.
17. Mecoli CA, Rosen A, Casciola-Rosen L, Shah AA. Advances at the interface of cancer and systemic sclerosis. J Scleroderma Relat Disord. 2021;6(1):50–7.
18. Derk CT, Rasheed M, Spiegel JR, Jimenez SA. Increased incidence of carcinoma of the tongue in patients with systemic sclerosis. J Rheumatol. 2005;32(4):637–41.
19. Colaci M, Giuggioli D, Vacchi C, Lumetti F, Iachetta F, Marcheselli L, Federico M, Ferri C. Breast cancer in systemic sclerosis: results of a cross-linkage of an Italian Rheumatologic Center and a population-based Cancer Registry and review of the literature. Autoimmun Rev. 2014;13(2):132–7.
20. Moinzadeh P, Fonseca C, Hellmich M, Shah AA, Chighizola C, Denton CP, Ong VH. Association of anti-RNA polymerase III autoantibodies and cancer in scleroderma. Arthritis Res Ther. 2014;16(1):R53.
21. Igusa T, Hummers LK, Visvanathan K, Richardson C, Wigley FM, Casciola-Rosen L, Rosen A, Shah AA. Autoantibodies and scleroderma phenotype define subgroups at high-risk and low-risk for cancer. Ann Rheum Dis. 2018;77(8):1179–86.
22. Boozalis E, Shah AA, Wigley F, Kang S, Kwatra SG. Morphea and systemic sclerosis are associated with an increased risk for melanoma and nonmelanoma skin cancer. J Am Acad Dermatol. 2019;80(5):1449–51.
23. Hao Y, Hudson M, Baron M, Carreira P, Stevens W, Rabusa C, Tatibouet S, Carmona L, Joven BE, Huq M, et al. Early mortality in a multinational systemic sclerosis inception cohort. Arthritis Rheumatol. 2017;69(5):1067–77.
24. Butt SA, Jeppesen JL, Fuchs C, Mogensen M, Engelhart M, Torp-Pedersen C, Gislason GH, Jacobsen S, Andersson C. Trends in incidence, mortality, and causes of death associated with systemic sclerosis in Denmark between 1995 and 2015: a nationwide cohort study. BMC Rheumatol. 2018;2:36.
25. Rubio-Rivas M, Corbella X, Guillén-Del-Castillo A, Tolosa Vilella C, Colunga Argüelles D, Argibay A, Vargas Hitos JA, Todolí Parra JA, González-Echávarri C, Ortego-Centeno N, et al. Spanish scleroderma risk score (RESCLESCORE) to predict 15-year all-cause mortality in scleroderma patients at the time of diagnosis based on the RESCLE cohort: derivation and internal validation. Autoimmun Rev. 2020;19(5):102507.
26. Bernal-Bello D, de Tena JG, Guillén-Del Castillo A, Selva-O'Callaghan A, Callejas-Moraga EL, Marín-Sánchez AM, Fonollosa-Pla V, Simeón-Aznar CP. Novel risk factors related to cancer in scleroderma. Autoimmun Rev. 2017;16(5):461–8.
27. Nikpour M, Hissaria P, Byron J, Sahhar J, Micallef M, Paspaliaris W, Roddy J, Nash P, Sturgess A, Proudman S, et al. Prevalence, correlates and clinical usefulness of antibodies to RNA polymerase III in systemic sclerosis: a cross-sectional analysis of data from an Australian cohort. Arthritis Res Ther. 2011;13(6):R211.
28. Shah AA, Hummers LK, Casciola-Rosen L, Visvanathan K, Rosen A, Wigley FM. Examination of autoantibody status and clinical features associated with cancer risk and cancer-associated scleroderma. Arthritis Rheumatol. 2015;67(4):1053–61.
29. Bobba RK, Holly JS, Loy T, Perry MC. Scar carcinoma of the lung: a historical perspective. Clin Lung Cancer. 2011;12(3):148–54.
30. Yu YY, Pinsky PF, Caporaso NE, Chatterjee N, Baumgarten M, Langenberg P, Furuno JP, Lan Q, Engels EA. Lung cancer risk following detection of pulmonary scarring by chest radiography in the prostate, lung, colorectal, and ovarian cancer screening trial. Arch Intern Med. 2008;168(21):2326–2332; discussion 2332.
31. Hubbard R, Venn A, Lewis S, Britton J. Lung cancer and cryptogenic fibrosing alveolitis. A population-based cohort study. Am J Respir Crit Care Med. 2000;161(1):5–8.
32. Peters-Golden M, Wise RA, Hochberg M, Stevens MB, Wigley FM. Incidence of lung cancer in systemic sclerosis. J Rheumatol. 1985;12(6):1136–9.
33. Pontifex EK, Hill CL, Roberts-Thomson P. Risk factors for lung cancer in patients with scleroderma: a nested case-control study. Ann Rheum Dis. 2007;66(4):551–3.
34. Wipff J, Allanore Y, Soussi F, Terris B, Abitbol V, Raymond J, Chaussade S, Kahan A. Prevalence of Barrett's esophagus in systemic sclerosis. Arthritis Rheum. 2005;52(9):2882–8.
35. Trivedi PJ, Lammers WJ, van Buuren HR, Pares A, Floreani A, Janssen HL, Invernizzi P, Battezzati PM, Ponsioen CY, Corpechot C, et al. Stratification of hepatocellular carcinoma risk in primary biliary cirrhosis: a multicentre international study. Gut. 2015;65:321.

36. Cavazza A, Caballeria L, Floreani A, Farinati F, Bruguera M, Caroli D, Pares A. Incidence, risk factors, and survival of hepatocellular carcinoma in primary biliary cirrhosis: comparative analysis from two centers. Hepatology. 2009;50(4):1162–8.
37. Faurschou M, Sorensen IJ, Mellemkjaer L, Loft AG, Thomsen BS, Tvede N, Baslund B. Malignancies in Wegener's granulomatosis: incidence and relation to cyclophosphamide therapy in a cohort of 293 patients. J Rheumatol. 2008;35(1):100–5.
38. Monach PA, Arnold LM, Merkel PA. Incidence and prevention of bladder toxicity from cyclophosphamide in the treatment of rheumatic diseases: a data-driven review. Arthritis Rheum. 2010;62(1):9–21.
39. Brewer JD, Colegio OR, Phillips PK, Roenigk RK, Jacobs MA, Van de Beek D, Dierkhising RA, Kremers WK, McGregor CG, Otley CC. Incidence of and risk factors for skin cancer after heart transplant. Arch Dermatol. 2009;145(12):1391–6.
40. Marcen R, Galeano C, Fernandez-Rodriguez A, Jimenez-Alvaro S, Teruel JL, Rivera M, Burgos FJ, Quereda C. Effects of the new immunosuppressive agents on the occurrence of malignancies after renal transplantation. Transplant Proc. 2010;42(8):3055–7.
41. Bichari W, Bartiromo M, Mohey H, Afiani A, Burnot A, Maillard N, Sauron C, Thibaudin D, Mehdi M, Mariat C, et al. Significant risk factors for occurrence of cancer after renal transplantation: a single center cohort study of 1265 cases. Transplant Proc. 2009;41(2):672–3.
42. Robson R, Cecka JM, Opelz G, Budde M, Sacks S. Prospective registry-based observational cohort study of the long-term risk of malignancies in renal transplant patients treated with mycophenolate mofetil. Am J Transplant. 2005;5(12):2954–60.
43. Crane GM, Powell H, Kostadinov R, Rocafort PT, Rifkin DE, Burger PC, Ambinder RF, Swinnen LJ, Borowitz MJ, Duffield AS. Primary CNS lymphoproliferative disease, mycophenolate and calcineurin inhibitor usage. Oncotarget. 2015;6(32):33849–66.
44. Robinett DM, Hummers LK, Morris M, Duffield AS, Shah AA. Primary CNS lymphoma in scleroderma: a case series. J Scleroderma Relat Disord. 2021;6(2):214–9.
45. Berger CC, Bokemeyer C, Schneider M, Kuczyk MA, Schmoll HJ. Secondary Raynaud's phenomenon and other late vascular complications following chemotherapy for testicular cancer. Eur J Cancer. 1995;31A(13–14):2229–38.
46. Bessis D, Guillot B, Legouffe E, Guilhou JJ. Gemcitabine-associated scleroderma-like changes of the lower extremities. J Am Acad Dermatol. 2004;51(2 Suppl):S73–6.
47. Clowse ME, Wigley FM. Digital necrosis related to carboplatin and gemcitabine therapy in systemic sclerosis. J Rheumatol. 2003;30(6):1341–3.
48. Cohen IS, Mosher MB, O'Keefe EJ, Klaus SN, De Conti RC. Cutaneous toxicity of bleomycin therapy. Arch Dermatol. 1973;107(4):553–5.
49. Finch WR, Rodnan GP, Buckingham RB, Prince RK, Winkelstein A. Bleomycin-induced scleroderma. J Rheumatol. 1980;7(5):651–9.
50. De Angelis R, Bugatti L, Cerioni A, Del Medico P, Filosa G. Diffuse scleroderma occurring after the use of paclitaxel for ovarian cancer. Clin Rheumatol. 2003;22(1):49–52.
51. Ioannou Y, Isenberg DA. Current evidence for the induction of autoimmune rheumatic manifestations by cytokine therapy. Arthritis Rheum. 2000;43(7):1431–42.
52. Barbosa NS, Wetter DA, Wieland CN, Shenoy NK, Markovic SN, Thanarajasingam U. Scleroderma induced by pembrolizumab: a case series. Mayo Clin Proc. 2017;92(7):1158–63.
53. Shenoy N, Esplin B, Barbosa N, Wieland C, Thanarajasingam U, Markovic S. Pembrolizumab induced severe sclerodermoid reaction. Ann Oncol. 2017;28(2):432–3.
54. Cho M, Nonomura Y, Kaku Y, Nakabo S, Endo Y, Otsuka A, Kabashima K. Scleroderma-like syndrome associated with nivolumab treatment in malignant melanoma. J Dermatol. 2019;46(1):e43–4.
55. Terrier B, Humbert S, Preta LH, Delage L, Razanamahery J, Laurent-Roussel S, Mestiri R, Beaudeau L, Legendre P, Goupil F, et al. Risk of scleroderma according to the type of immune checkpoint inhibitors. Autoimmun Rev. 2020;19(8):102596.
56. Gambichler T, Strutzmann S, Tannapfel A, Susok L. Paraneoplastic acral vascular syndrome in a patient with metastatic melanoma under immune checkpoint blockade. BMC Cancer. 2017;17(1):327.
57. Khaddour K, Singh V, Shayuk M. Acral vascular necrosis associated with immune-check point inhibitors: case report with literature review. BMC Cancer. 2019;19(1):449.
58. Varga J, Haustein UF, Creech RH, Dwyer JP, Jimenez SA. Exaggerated radiation-induced fibrosis in patients with systemic sclerosis. JAMA. 1991;265(24):3292–5.
59. Abu-Shakra M, Lee P. Exaggerated fibrosis in patients with systemic sclerosis (scleroderma) following radiation therapy. J Rheumatol. 1993;20(9):1601–3.
60. Colver GB, Rodger A, Mortimer PS, Savin JA, Neill SM, Hunter JA. Post-irradiation morphoea. Br J Dermatol. 1989;120(6):831–5.
61. Lacasse Y, Martin S, Gagne D, Lakhal L. Dose-response meta-analysis of silica and lung cancer. Cancer Causes Control. 2009;20(6):925–33.
62. McCormic ZD, Khuder SS, Aryal BK, Ames AL, Khuder SA. Occupational silica exposure as a risk factor for scleroderma: a meta-analysis. Int Arch Occup Environ Health. 2010;83(7):763–9.
63. Duncan SC, Winkelmann RK. Cancer and scleroderma. Arch Dermatol. 1979;115(8):950–5.
64. Forbes AM, Woodrow JC, Verbov JL, Graham RM. Carcinoma of breast and scleroderma: four further cases and a literature review. Br J Rheumatol. 1989;28(1):65–9.
65. Launay D, Le Berre R, Hatron PY, Peyrat JP, Hachulla E, Devulder B, Hebbar M. Association between systemic sclerosis and breast cancer: eight new cases and review of the literature. Clin Rheumatol. 2004;23(6):516–22.
66. Lee P, Alderdice C, Wilkinson S, Keystone EC, Urowitz MB, Gladman DD. Malignancy in progressive systemic sclerosis—association with breast carcinoma. J Rheumatol. 1983;10(4):665–6.
67. Shah AA, Rosen A, Hummers L, Wigley F, Casciola-Rosen L. Close temporal relationship between onset of cancer and scleroderma in patients with RNA polymerase I/III antibodies. Arthritis Rheum. 2010;62(9):2787–95.
68. Hasegawa M, Sato S, Sakai H, Ohashi T, Takehara K. Systemic sclerosis revealing T-cell lymphoma. Dermatology. 1999;198(1):75–8.
69. Juarez M, Marshall R, Denton C, Evely R. Paraneoplastic scleroderma secondary to hairy cell leukaemia successfully treated with cladribine. Rheumatology. 2008;47(11):1734–5.
70. Bruni C, Lages A, Patel H, Nihtyanova SI, Green B, AbuHilal M, Harvey J, Ong VH, Matucci Cerinic M, Derrett-Smith E, et al. Resolution of paraneoplastic PM/Scl-positive systemic sclerosis after curative resection of a pancreatic tumour. Rheumatology (Oxford). 2017;56(2):317–8.
71. Airo P, Ceribelli A, Cavazzana I, Taraborelli M, Zingarelli S, Franceschini F. Malignancies in Italian patients with systemic sclerosis positive for anti-RNA polymerase III antibodies. J Rheumatol. 2011;38(7):1329–34.
72. Saigusa R, Asano Y, Nakamura K, Miura S, Ichimura Y, Takahashi T, Toyama T, Taniguchi T, Noda S, Aozasa N, et al. Association of anti-RNA polymerase III antibody and malignancy in Japanese patients with systemic sclerosis. J Dermatol. 2015;42(5):524–7.
73. Lazzaroni MG, Cavazzana I, Colombo E, Dobrota R, Hernandez J, Hesselstrand R, Varju C, Nagy G, Smith V, Caramaschi P, et al. Malignancies in patients with anti-RNA polymerase III antibodies and systemic sclerosis: analysis of the EULAR scleroderma trials

and research cohort and possible recommendations for screening. J Rheumatol. 2017;44(5):639–47.
74. Callejas-Moraga EL, Guillén-Del-Castillo A, Marín-Sánchez AM, Roca-Herrera M, Balada E, Tolosa-Vilella C, Fonollosa-Pla V, Simeón-Aznar CP. Clinical features of systemic sclerosis patients with anti-RNA polymerase III antibody in a single centre in Spain. Clin Exp Rheumatol. 2019;37 Suppl 119(4):41–8.
75. Shah AA, Rosen A, Hummers LK, May B, Kaushiva A, Roden RBS, Armstrong DK, Wigley FM, Casciola-Rosen L, Visvanathan K. Evaluation of cancer-associated myositis and scleroderma autoantibodies in breast cancer patients without rheumatic disease. Clin Exp Rheumatol. 2017;35 Suppl 106:71.
76. Betteridge ZE, Priest L, Cooper RG, McHugh NJ, Blackhall F, Lamb JA. Investigation of myositis and scleroderma specific autoantibodies in patients with lung cancer. Arthritis Res Ther. 2018;20(1):176.
77. Shah AA, Casciola-Rosen L, Rosen A. Review: Cancer-induced autoimmunity in the rheumatic diseases. Arthritis Rheumatol. 2015;67(2):317–26.
78. Kuwana M, Fujii T, Mimori T, Kaburaki J. Enhancement of anti-DNA topoisomerase I autoantibody response after lung cancer in patients with systemic sclerosis. A report of two cases. Arthritis Rheum. 1996;39(4):686–91.
79. Xu GJ, Shah AA, Li MZ, Xu Q, Rosen A, Casciola-Rosen L, Elledge SJ. Systematic autoantigen analysis identifies a distinct subtype of scleroderma with coincident cancer. Proc Natl Acad Sci U S A. 2016;113(47):E7526–34.
80. Shah AA, Xu G, Rosen A, Hummers LK, Wigley FM, Elledge SJ, Casciola-Rosen L. Brief report: Anti-RNPC-3 antibodies as a marker of cancer-associated scleroderma. Arthritis Rheumatol. 2017;69(6):1306–12.
81. Joseph CG, Darrah E, Shah AA, Skora AD, Casciola-Rosen LA, Wigley FM, Boin F, Fava A, Thoburn C, Kinde I, et al. Association of the autoimmune disease scleroderma with an immunologic response to cancer. Science. 2014;343(6167):152–7.
82. Casciola-Rosen L, Nagaraju K, Plotz P, Wang K, Levine S, Gabrielson E, Corse A, Rosen A. Enhanced autoantigen expression in regenerating muscle cells in idiopathic inflammatory myopathy. J Exp Med. 2005;201(4):591–601.
83. Yoshizaki A, Yanaba K, Ogawa A, Asano Y, Kadono T, Sato S. Immunization with DNA topoisomerase I and Freund's complete adjuvant induces skin and lung fibrosis and autoimmunity via interleukin-6 signaling. Arthritis Rheum. 2011;63(11):3575–85.
84. Bielefeld P. Systemic scleroderma and malignant diseases. A review of the literature. La Revue de medecine interne/ fondee par la Societe nationale francaise de medecine interne. 1991;12(5):350–4.
85. Fujii T, Mimori T, Kimura N, Satoh S, Hirakata M. Pseudoscleroderma associated with transforming growth factor beta1-producing advanced gastric carcinoma: comment on the article by Varga. Arthritis Rheum. 2003;48(6):1766–1767; author repy 1767–8.
86. Querfeld C, Sollberg S, Huerkamp C, Eckes B, Krieg T. Pseudoscleroderma associated with lung cancer: correlation of collagen type I and connective tissue growth factor gene expression. Br J Dermatol. 2000;142(6):1228–33.
87. Atalay C, Atalay G, Yilmaz KB, Altinok M. The role of anti-CENP-B and anti-SS-B antibodies in breast cancer. Neoplasma. 2005;52(1):32–5.
88. Atalay C, Dogan L, Atalay G. Anti-CENP-B antibodies are associated with prolonged survival in breast cancer. Future Oncol. 2010;6(3):471–7.
89. Fritzler MJ, Rattner JB, Luft LM, Edworthy SM, Casiano CA, Peebles C, Mahler M. Historical perspectives on the discovery and elucidation of autoantibodies to centromere proteins (CENP) and the emerging importance of antibodies to CENP-F. Autoimmun Rev. 2011;10(4):194–200.
90. Hansen JE, Chan G, Liu Y, Hegan DC, Dalal S, Dray E, Kwon Y, Xu Y, Xu X, Peterson-Roth E, et al. Targeting cancer with a lupus autoantibody. Sci Transl Med. 2012;4(157):157ra142.
91. Shah AA, Laiho M, Rosen A, Casciola-Rosen L. Protective effect against cancer of antibodies to the large subunits of both RNA polymerases I and III in scleroderma. Arthritis Rheumatol. 2019;71(9):1571–9.
92. Peltonen K, Colis L, Liu H, Trivedi R, Moubarek MS, Moore HM, Bai B, Rudek MA, Bieberich CJ, Laiho M. A targeting modality for destruction of RNA polymerase I that possesses anticancer activity. Cancer Cell. 2014;25(1):77–90.
93. Mecoli CA, Adler BL, Yang Q, Hummers LK, Rosen A, Casciola-Rosen L, Shah AA. Cancer in systemic sclerosis: analysis of antibodies against components of the Th/To complex. Arthritis Rheumatol. 2020;73:315.
94. Watad A, McGonagle D, Bragazzi NL, Tiosano S, Comaneshter D, Shoenfeld Y, Cohen AD, Amital H. Autoantibody status in systemic sclerosis patients defines both cancer risk and survival with ANA negativity in cases with concomitant cancer having a worse survival. Oncoimmunology. 2019;8(6):e1588084.
95. Shah AA, Casciola-Rosen L. Cancer and scleroderma: a paraneoplastic disease with implications for malignancy screening. Curr Opin Rheumatol. 2015;27(6):563–70.
96. Sawaya GF, Kulasingam S, Denberg T, Qaseem A. Cervical cancer screening in average-risk women: best practice advice from the clinical guidelines Committee of the American College of Physicians. Ann Intern Med. 2015;162:851.
97. Davidson KW, Barry MJ, Mangione CM, Cabana M, Caughey AB, Davis EM, Donahue KE, Doubeni CA, Krist AH, Kubik M, et al. Screening for colorectal cancer: US Preventive Services Task Force recommendation statement. JAMA. 2021;325(19):1965–77.
98. Shaheen NJ, Weinberg DS, Denberg TD, Chou R, Qaseem A, Shekelle P, Clinical Guidelines Committee of the American College of Physicians. Upper endoscopy for gastroesophageal reflux disease: best practice advice from the clinical guidelines committee of the American College of Physicians. Ann Intern Med. 2012;157(11):808–16.
99. National Lung Screening Trial Research Team, Aberle DR, Adams AM, Berg CD, Black WC, Clapp JD, Fagerstrom RM, Gareen IF, Gatsonis C, Marcus PM, et al. Reduced lung-cancer mortality with low-dose computed tomographic screening. N Engl J Med. 2011;365(5):395–409.
100. Lindor KD, Gershwin ME, Poupon R, Kaplan M, Bergasa NV, Heathcote EJ, American Association for Study of Liver Diseases. Primary biliary cirrhosis. Hepatology. 2009;50(1):291–308.
101. Jacob S, Rahbari K, Tegtmeyer K, Zhao J, Tran S, Helenowski I, Zhang H, Walunas T, Varga J, Dematte J, et al. Lung cancer survival in patients with autoimmune disease. JAMA Netw Open. 2020;3(12):e2029917.
102. Shah DJ, Hirpara R, Poelman CL, Woods A, Hummers LK, Wigley FM, Wright JL, Parekh A, Steen VD, Domsic RT, et al. Impact of radiation therapy on scleroderma and cancer outcomes in scleroderma patients with breast cancer. Arthritis Care Res (Hoboken). 2018;70(10):1517–24.
103. Yoon SM, Chu FI, Ruan D, Steinberg ML, Raldow A, Lee P. Assessment of toxic effects associated with dose-fractionated radiotherapy among patients with cancer and comorbid collagen vascular disease. JAMA Netw Open. 2021;4(2):e2034074.

Overlooked Manifestations

38

Ami A. Shah and Fredrick M. Wigley

Oral Manifestations

Oral involvement in scleroderma is associated with varying degrees of orofacial manifestations including rigidity of facial skin, thin and retracted lips, perioral wrinkling (rhytids), a reduced mouth opening (microstomia), mask-like facial appearance, telangiectasia, xerostomia, periodontitis, and resorption of structures of the mandible [1, 2]. In 2016, a review of 45 published articles found limitation of mouth opening (69.8%), widening of the periodontal ligament (67.3%), xerostomia (63.4%), telangiectasia (36.2%), and bone lesions (34.5%) among patients with scleroderma [3]. Oral complications have a major impact not only on mouth function, but also on facial appearance and patient quality of life and yet evaluating and managing these features are often overlooked [4]. A systematic review of the literature found a correlation between oropharyngeal features and quality of life of patients with scleroderma [5]. A questionnaire-based survey found there was a significant correlation between alexithymia and esthetic concerns, including dissatisfaction with self-appearance and mouth disability, suggesting that facial changes exerted a major impact on the psychological health of patients with scleroderma [6]. In addition to psychological distress from these cosmetic changes [7], alterations in facial architecture can impair dental care and contribute to malnutrition due to fatigue with chewing and reduced capacity to eat large boluses of solid food. A useful scale has been developed to measure disability [8]. The major factors accounting for disability are microstomia, periodontal disease, xerostomia, and cosmetic concerns [5, 8].

Microstomia has been reported in up to 80% of patients with scleroderma [9], and decreased oral mobility and strength significantly impairs quality of life [10]. The reduced oral aperture makes daily oral hygiene and dental treatment more complex and challenging, and at times, patients are denied dental care altogether because of restricted access to the oral cavity [11]. A narrowed oral aperture correlates with poorer oral hygiene and with increased numbers of dental caries [12]. Studies have demonstrated that simple oral exercise regimens may be effective treatments for microstomia. A 6-month clinical trial of nine patients with scleroderma compared two different exercise programs [13]. While the control group performed facial grimacing exercises, the experimental group did three mouth stretching exercises plus an oral augmentation exercise using tongue depressors. The mouth stretching exercises consisted of placing the right thumb in the corner of the left side of the mouth and stretching, placing the left thumb in the right side of the mouth and stretching, and then doing both sides simultaneously. Three sets of five stretches were performed. Patients then used tongue depressors placed diagonally across the posterior teeth to open the oral cavity by stretching the facial skin and musculature. After holding this pose for several minutes, repetitions were encouraged with brief rest periods. Patients were encouraged to gradually increase the number of tongue depressors used. The experimental group in this study achieved a 5.6 mm increase in vertical oral opening compared to a 3 mm increase in the control group. Pizzo and colleagues studied a similar but slightly modified exercise regimen over an 18-week period [14]. They noted a mean increase in oral opening of 10.7 mm. By the end of the study, all patients noted greater ease in eating, speaking, and maintaining oral hygiene; denture insertion was easier in edentulous patients. These simple exercises can easily be taught to scleroderma patients in both rheumatologists and dentists' offices and may improve oral function and quality of life (Fig. 38.1). In a third study, 28 participants, with a mean oral aperture of <40 mm at baseline, were randomized to orofacial exercise instructions (n = 13) or no exercises

A. A. Shah (✉)
Division of Rheumatology, Department of Medicine, Johns Hopkins University School of Medicine, Baltimore, MD, USA
e-mail: Ami.Shah@jhmi.edu

F. M. Wigley
Division of Rheumatology, Department of Medicine, The Johns Hopkins University School of Medicine, Baltimore, MD, USA
e-mail: fwig@jhmi.edu

Y. Allanore et al. (eds.), *Scleroderma*, https://doi.org/10.1007/978-3-031-40658-4_38

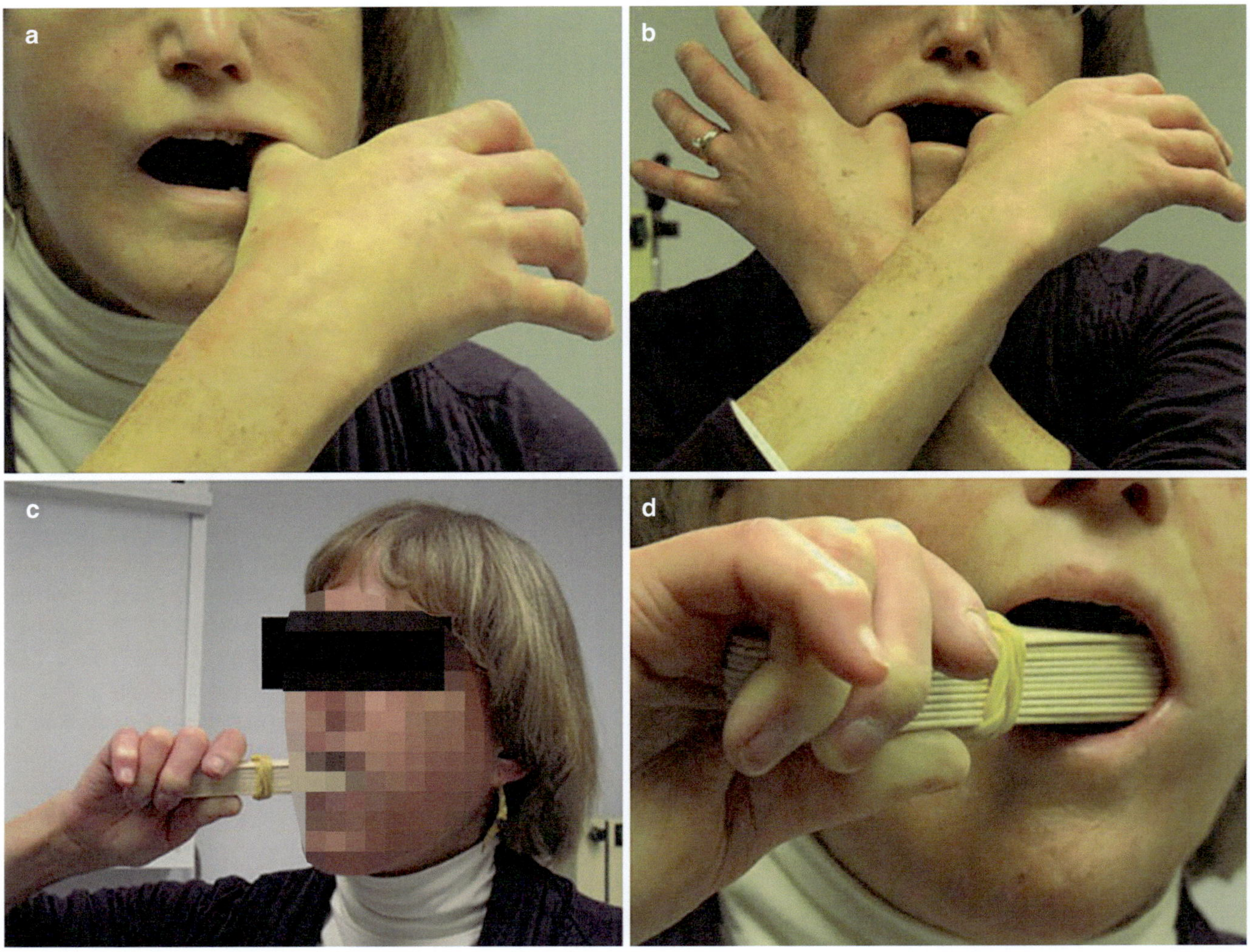

Fig. 38.1 Sample exercises to maximize oral opening. (**a**) The patient places the right thumb in the corner of the left side of the mouth and stretches for 10–15 s. Then, the patient places the left thumb in the corner of the right side of the mouth and stretches (not shown). (**b**) After doing each side, the patient stretches both sides simultaneously. Steps (**a**) and (**b**) should be repeated five to ten times. (**c**) A stack of tongue depressors bound by a rubber band is inserted into the mouth from the front middle teeth to the back molars on one side. The patient uses as many tongue depressors as necessary to stretch the facial skin and musculature. After holding the pose for several minutes, the contralateral side is stretched in the same manner (not shown). Repetitions and gradually increasing the number of tongue depressors used are encouraged. (**d**) A closer view of the angle of insertion

(n = 15) [15]. The patients demonstrated a significantly larger increase in oral aperture at 3 months for the intervention group compared with those receiving no exercise (2.81 vs. −0.61 mm, $p = 0.01$). However, this effect did not last at the 6-month evaluation (2.75 vs. 2.33 mm, $p = 0.19$) with adherence rates to the orofacial exercise of only 48.9% [15]. Rehabilitation focused on lip and tongue strength and mobility, which are essential for mouth function, was performed using orofacial exercises conducted by speech therapists [16]. After treatment, there was an improvement in lip and tongue mobility and strength and maximum mouth opening.

Fat grafting has been shown to improve skin quality and improve contour irregularities, may be helpful in the treatment of patients with scleroderma, and is now used for perioral therapy [17–19]. An uncontrolled study of 16 patients treated with autologous fat injection ranging from 15 to 40 mL found by clinical assessment a significantly improved mouth opening capacity and mouth handicap score [20]. In this study, the esthetic and/or functional results of fat injection were satisfying to 80% of the patients. Autologous stem cell-enriched lipotransfer significantly improved the effects of orofacial fibrosis in a cohort of 62 patients with scleroderma. Mouth function (MHISS) was significantly improved (6.85 ± 5.07) ($p < 0.0001$) after treatment. All psychological measures were significantly improved: DAS 24 (12.1 ± 9.5) ($p < 0.0001$); HADS-anxiety (2.8 ± 3.2) ($p < 0.0001$), HADS-depression (2.0 ± 3.1) ($p < 0.0001$); BFNE (2.9 ± 4.3) ($p < 0.0001$); VAS (3.56 ± 4.1) ($p < 0.0001$). Multiple treatments further improved mouth function ($p < 0.05$), DAS ($p < 0.0001$) and VAS ($p = 0.01$) scores [21]. These studies support the idea that stem cells in autologous fat may provide both functional and cosmetic improvements that are sustained, but long-term follow-up studies are needed. Commissurotomy is described in case reports, but is infrequently used to treat microstomia due to concerns about poor wound healing and lack of long-term benefit.

Xerostomia is a common problem in scleroderma, occurring in up to 70% of scleroderma patients [22–24], and concomitant Sjogren's syndrome may occur in 12–21% of patients depending on which Sjogren's diagnostic criteria are used [22, 25, 26]. A study using diagnostic criteria of the American-European Consensus Group (AECG) found grade 3 and/or grade 4 sialoadenitis in 33.9% of 74 patients with sicca symptoms suggesting that Sjogren's syndrome was common among patients with scleroderma [27]. Xerostomia may be secondary to salivary gland fibrosis involving capillary walls and excretory ducts [22, 26, 28, 29], a pathological finding that is distinct and more common than the lymphocytic infiltrates generally seen in Sjogren's syndrome. A study compared the lymphocyte focus score, plasma cell focus, fibrosis degree, and serum autoantibody positivity rate in 43 patients with primary Sjogren's (pSS) and 26 patients with scleroderma and Sjogren's. The plasma cell focus was statistically significantly higher in pSS cases ($p = 0.003$). No difference was seen between the subtypes in terms of lymphocyte focus score, fibrosis, and autoantibody positivity [30]. Unstimulated salivary flow rates correlate with glandular sclerosis [28]. One survey found that low saliva production was associated with specific Sjogren's autoantibodies (Ro52/TRIM21, SSA/Ro60, or SSB/La) [31]. Salivary flow contributes to dysphagia, which may also be limited in scleroderma due to tongue fibrosis and limited tongue mobility [11, 32]. Increased dental caries and *Candida* infections are also complications [32]. Treatment of xerostomia is challenging and requires a multifaceted approach including the use of sugarless candies and mints, lozenges, saliva substitutes, pharmacological agents to stimulate salivary flow, small sips of water throughout the day, and frequent oral hygiene visits [32]. Avoidance of aggravating medications, such as anticholinergic agents, that dry mucous membranes is critical.

A survey of the oral health of 163 patients with scleroderma compared to 231 healthy controls found that patients had more missing teeth, more periodontal disease, less saliva production, and overall poorer quality of oral health [33]. A second study by the same investigators found oral health measures associated with global quality of life but not with various measures of disease severity [34]. A third survey found that tooth loss was associated with poor upper extremity function, gastrointestinal reflux disease, and decreased saliva [31]. Periodontal disease has been reported in up to 95% of scleroderma patients, and the most common finding is periodontal ligament distension [9, 23, 24, 35, 36]. A case-control study of 54 patients and 55 non-disease controls found a significantly higher measure of periodontal disease defined by the clinical attachment loss: the distance from the cemento-enamel junction to the bottom of the sulcus or periodontal pocket (3.92 mm in scleroderma vs. 2.59 mm in controls, $p < 0.05$). Periodontal disease correlated with mRSS in the overall scleroderma group and with the mean duration of disease in patients with limited SSc ($p = 0.007$), even after adjusting this correlation for the presence of the major organ involvement [37].

A case-control study of 50 patients and 43 healthy controls reported that telangiectasia (42/50, 84%) and reduced mouth opening (35/50, 70%) were the most frequent orofacial findings among patients. The periodontitis frequency was much higher in patients than in healthy controls (90.7% versus 48.83%; $p < 0.001$). In addition, patients with scleroderma presented a distinctive pattern of periodontitis, with low probing pocket depth, higher gingival recession, higher periodontal attachment loss, and lower gingival bleeding index values [38]. The association between scleroderma and periodontitis was examined in 58 patients and 52 control patients, matched for age and sex. Adjusted for age and sex, patients with scleroderma had a 0.52 mm higher periodontal attachment loss (a measure of the elapsed periodontal disease process) compared with controls (95% CI 0.16–0.88; $p = 0.005$) [39]. This association remained significant independent of demographic and lifestyle characteristics, including age, sex, education, smoking status, and alcohol consumption. Increased periodontal disease may not be solely due to poor oral hygiene; in one study, patients with scleroderma had more periodontal disease but similar plaque and calculus scores compared to controls [24]. In the same study, the width of tooth roots was not increased as well, suggesting that a wide periodontal ligament (PDL) may occur at the expense of adjacent socket bone [24]. Tooth mobility may result, occurring in 62% of scleroderma patients in one study [9, 24]. In one survey, significant correlations between number of teeth with PDL widening and Medsger disease severity scale ($r = 0.702$, $p = 0.028$), modified Rodnan skin score ($r = 0.821$, $p = 0.01$), disease subset (diffuse vs. limited, $r = 0.782$, $p = 0.041$ vs. $r = 0.451$, $p = 0.05$, respectively), anti-topoisomerase I antibodies ($r = 0.568, p = 0.012$), age ($r = 0.872$, $p = 0.01$), and disease duration ($r = 0.811$, $p = 0.01$) were demonstrated [40]. A study investigated the prevalence of oral manifestations and temporomandibular disorders (TMD) in 80 patients with scleroderma compared with 80 sex- and age-matched healthy controls [41]. A higher prevalence of TMDs was observed in the scleroderma group (92.5%) compared to healthy patients (75.0%); more muscle pain on chewing, the sensation of a stuck or locked jaw, and arthralgia were commonly reported symptoms in the scleroderma group.

Bony resorption of the mandibular angle, coronoid process, condylar head, and digastric region [9, 24, 42] may contribute to reduced oral strength and mobility in scleroderma, and in one study, mandibular erosions were associated with the presence of periodontal membrane thickening [24]. A cross-sectional study in 43 patients with scleroderma and matching controls receiving systematic oral assessments (full mouth dental/periodontal) and imaging using tridimensional cone beam computed tomography confirmed widening of PDL and mandibular erosions as common dental findings in scleroderma. A study of 159 subjects systematically assessed the relationship between disease features and oral radiographic abnormalities in scleroderma [43]. Widening of the PDL involving at least 1 tooth was present in 38% of subjects, and 14.5% had at least 1 site in the mandible with an erosion. In analyses adjusting for age, disease duration, sex, smoking, and education, there was a significant association between the number of teeth with widening of the PDL and disease severity assessed by the physician global assessment (PGA) (relative risk [RR] 1.19, 95% CI 1.02–1.39, $p = 0.028$). Analyses replacing the PGA with the skin score, disease subset, or anti-topoisomerase I antibodies confirmed the relationship with indices of disease severity [43]. This study supported the idea that global measures of disease severity are associated with a wide PDL perhaps as a consequence of a generalized overproduction of collagen in scleroderma.

Because an obliterative vasculopathy of small blood vessels has been observed in a thickened periodontal ligament from a scleroderma patient [44], it has been suggested that poor perfusion in scleroderma may increase susceptibility to periodontal disease [24]. Oral microcirculation was lower in all regions of the mouth in a study of 20 patients with scleroderma compared to 20 age- and gender-matched controls using Sidestream Dark Field imaging [45].

Telangiectasia often develops on oral mucous membranes in patients with limited or diffuse disease, yet these lesions often go unnoticed. Telangiectasia may bleed following trauma, but generally do not present a significant clinical risk when found intra-orally. Extraoral lesions are often cosmetically unpleasant with challenges of finding adequate creams and makeup products to cover them. Light-based treatments such as pulsed dye laser can remove lesions, but recurrence is common.

A summary of scleroderma oral manifestations and management options is provided in Table 38.1. An excellent patient guide on basic oral hygiene is available through the Scleroderma Foundation [46] and can be found online at https://www.scleroderma.org/site/SPageServer/?pagename=body_mouth#.X-ERDGhKh9M. Limited hand dexterity and joint range of motion correlate with increased decayed surfaces and dental caries [12]. Worse gingival inflammation has been associated with poor hand dexterity and decreased flossing habits [47]. A low-cost solution to this problem may be to have the dentist mold a custom grip on the toothbrush handle with dental acrylic [46]. If this is ineffective, an electric toothbrush may need to be considered [46]. The use of assistive devices including power toothbrush and Reach Access Flosser along with oral-facial exercises improved gingival inflammation [48]. In addition to recommending child-sized toothbrushes with wide flat handles, it is suggested that patients with microstomia have a second toothbrush with all but the end two rows of bristles tweezed out to clean the cheek sides of the upper and lower teeth. Specific oral exercises, toothbrush brands, floss types, fluoride agents, and products to treat xerostomia are recommended in a concise format that is easy for patients to digest. It is notable that a survey found that depression and difficulty performing flossing decreased dental care [49].

Table 38.1 Summary of management options for oral manifestations and barriers to good oral hygiene

Clinical finding	Management options
1. Microstomia	Daily oral exercises (see Fig. 38.1) to maximize oral aperture
	Child-sized toothbrushes with only two rows of bristles to enhance cleaning of cheek sides of the teeth
	Education re: eating smaller parcels of food
2. Dental decay and caries	Early referral to an experienced dentist or dental specialist for preventive and regular dental and periodontal care
	Frequent fluoride treatments (every 3 months)
	Encourage flossing; specific floss brands for various clinical situations are provided in reference [46]
3. Xerostomia	Eliminate medications that dry mucous membranes
	Treat with stimulators of muscarinic cholinergic receptors (pilocarpine, cevimeline)
	Sugarless candies/mints
	Saliva substitutes
	Nonalcoholic mouth washes
	Frequent dental hygiene visits
4. Hand contractures	Referral to hand occupational therapy for assistive devices to aid in dental care
	Mold custom grip on toothbrush handle with dental acrylic
	Consider electric toothbrushes with soft brush filaments

In the setting of tooth loss, implants may be considered in those with adequate bone levels [32]. If dentures are required, frequent dental visits should be continued for denture adjustments and evaluation of the oral mucosa's ability to withstand pressure without atrophy [32]. In addition, collapsible dentures have been designed for patients with microstomia [50]. Recent new technology using digital methods with intraoral scanning and computer-aided manufacturing provides a better method to make a removable partial denture in patients with severe microstomia [51].

Audiovestibular Disease

Observational and case-controlled surveys show that unappreciated hearing loss and other auditory symptoms are prevalent among patients with scleroderma [52–64]. Sensorineural hearing loss (SNHL) involves the inner ear, cochlea, or the auditory nerve. In an initial report detailing cranial nerve involvement in ten patients with scleroderma, three patients were noted to have tinnitus and two patients had hearing loss [52]. Berrettini and colleagues studied 31 unselected scleroderma patients, 62% of whom reported audiovestibular symptoms [53]. Objective hearing loss was detected in 14 patients (10 with SNHL, 4 with mixed sensorineural and conductive hearing loss), and in all cases, the site of the lesion was cochlear. Four patients had abnormal vestibular function, and one patient had calcification of the tympanic membrane. A study of 20 unselected patients were compared to 26 healthy controls matched for age and sex [54]. This study found that patients with scleroderma had significantly poorer mean hearing thresholds than the control group for 0.5, 1, 6, and 8 kHz. In eight patients (40%), there was SNHL, mostly bilateral and symmetrical. Furthermore, no relation was seen between hearing level and duration, type, and severity of the scleroderma. Using a structured questionnaire focused on otological symptoms and risk factors for hearing loss, 26 patients with diffuse scleroderma (dcSSc) were age- and sex-matched with two individuals each [55]. The questionnaire revealed auditory complaints in 54% of the dcSSc patients (25% hearing loss, 21% tinnitus, and 21% dizziness); almost half (46%) of the dcSSc patients were diagnosed as having hearing loss on audiogram compared to only 19% in the control group ($p = 0.01$). All dcSSc patients with hearing loss had a sensorineural component. A study of 35 patients focused on cases with limited cutaneous scleroderma (lcSSc) and anti-centromere protein B antibodies and compared them to 59 age-, sex-, and ethnically matched controls [56]. While 54% of lcSSc patients reported subjective hearing loss compared to 0% of controls, objective hearing loss on audiogram was detected in 77% of lcSSc patients compared to 26% of controls ($p < 0.001$). Hearing loss was bilateral in most cases and was attributed to asymmetric SNHL in 11 patients and symmetric SNHL in 13 patients. The audiometric curve was flat in 13 patients with high-frequency hearing loss in 14 patients. Scleroderma subjects had a higher prevalence of abnormal tympanograms, absent stapedius reflexes, abnormal oculocephalic responses, head-shaking nystagmus, and abnormal caloric tests and clinical tests of sensory integration and balance compared to controls. Overall, these findings provided evidence of inner and middle ear compromise resulting in auditory and vestibular dysfunction. One of the few observational studies with longitudinal data reported audiological evaluations of 12 individuals revealing progression of hearing loss not explained by a new comorbid condition [57].

A complete ENT examination and audiological evaluation with pure tone, impedance, and speech audiometry were performed in 34 scleroderma patients and 45 age-matched healthy subjects [58]. Sensorineural hearing loss was detected in 20% of patients with scleroderma, and a quarter of patients had hearing loss affecting the middle and mainly high frequencies. Speech audiometry identified word recognition scores compatible with cochlear disease. There were no differences in age, systemic manifestations, disease duration, autoantibody profile, or drug therapy comparing patients with and without hearing loss. Interestingly, a patulous Eustachian tube was identified in three patients; the authors postulated that this finding could be secondary to an inflammatory myopathy affecting major muscles surrounding the Eustachian tube, microvascular abnormalities resulting in chronic ischemia, or fibrosis causing tendon dysfunction.

While high-frequency SNHL is reported in several surveys and in many reports, the etiology is still unclear. Pathology in one case suggests a middle and inner ear vasculopathy may be responsible [59]. Histologic findings have found enlarged and thickened blood vessels, perivascular fibrosis, and reduced numbers of outer hair cells. A case-control study showed that 33% of patients with scleroderma had vestibular impairment that significantly is associated with both nailfold capillary patterns and a vascular severity score ($p = 0.049$ and $p = 0.046$, respectively), suggesting that microvascular disease may account for the dysfunction [60]. However, another study of 54 patients and 60 controls found objective hearing loss, SNHL, abnormal pure tone audiometry, and speech recognition thresholds were significantly higher among patients compared to the control group; but they found no significant correlation with digital ulcers, digital pitting scars, interstitial lung disease, abnormal pulmonary artery pressure, gastrointestinal involvement, patterns of capillaroscopy, or any components of capillary changes with hearing loss [61].

A study of 42 patients with scleroderma (35 with limited skin disease and anti-centromere protein B antibodies, 7 with diffuse skin disease) and 74 age-, sex-, and ethnically matched controls performed Dix-Hallpike maneuvers, cephalic rotational tests, and clinical tests of sensory integration and balance [62]. Seven patients (17%) fulfilled criteria for benign paroxysmal positional vertigo (BPPV) compared to zero controls ($p < 0.001$). BPPV was related to the posterior semicircular canal in two patients with lcSSc and to the horizontal semicircular canal in five patients (three limited, two diffuse). Twenty patients with scleroderma (48%) had abnormal postural control, largely vestibular in origin, compared to 10% of controls ($p < 0.0001$). Because of the predominance of peripheral vestibular abnormalities, the authors postulated an ischemic etiology or an intralabyrinthine autoimmune process as potential trigger of disease.

A careful medical history probing for the use of ototoxic medications (e.g., sildenafil, high-dose nonsteroidal anti-inflammatory drugs or aspirin, loop diuretics, aminoglycoside antibiotics) is essential in patients with scleroderma who have audiovestibular symptoms. Patients with hearing loss should be referred for otolaryngology evaluation and audiometry, and tests of vestibular function should be considered in patients with dizziness, vertigo, and poor balance. If the onset of hearing loss, aural fullness, or tinnitus is sudden or rapid, this constitutes an otologic emergency until proven otherwise. Urgent referral to an otolaryngologist for audiometry and confirmation of SNHL is necessary, as prompt institution of intratympanic corticosteroids may improve or restore hearing [65]. In one case report of a patient who presented with bilateral SNHL as the first manifestation of scleroderma, hearing improved with high doses of methotrexate and intravenous immunoglobulin [63]. Similarly, Abou-Taleb and colleagues reported a woman with bilateral mixed hearing loss in the context of longstanding scleroderma who had improved hearing and speech discrimination after cyclophosphamide therapy [59]. Lastly, a cochlear implant was used to treat one woman with scleroderma, who had double-stranded DNA antibodies and an auditory neuropathy [64]. A well-designed approach is needed in that therapeutic options for SNHL and other audiovestibular manifestations in scleroderma are not studied in great depth. Further investigation of therapeutic options, including the use of immunosuppressive therapy, is warranted.

Thyroid Dysfunction

Thyroid dysfunction is prevalent in scleroderma and can mimic active disease as many symptoms of hypothyroidism and hyperthyroidism overlap with scleroderma features. Treatments for thyroid disease are readily available and effective [66]. Fatigue evaluated among patients with scleroderma with either clinical or subclinical hypothyroidism improved after appropriate thyroid therapy [67]. Thyroid fibrosis, autoimmune thyroiditis resulting in hypothyroidism, and hyperthyroidism from Graves' disease are frequent and often unsuspected findings in scleroderma. Autoimmune thyroid disease should especially be sought in patients with primary biliary cirrhosis, CREST features, and Sjogren's syndrome as there are reports of these autoimmune diseases clustering together [68, 69]. In autopsy studies, thyroid gland fibrosis is more prevalent in scleroderma patients than in matched controls [70, 71], and in one study, all hypothyroid scleroderma patients had glandular fibrosis [71]. A single-center, prospective, cross-sectional study carried out on 106 consecutive consenting patients (limited or diffuse) using ultrasound methods found a decrease in thyroid volume that correlated with thyroid dysfunction suggesting disease was due to thyroid fibrosis [72]. Lymphocytic infiltration characteristic of Hashimoto's thyroiditis was infrequent [71], despite a strong association between hypothyroidism and high serum titers of antithyroid antibodies. In one study of 719 scleroderma patients, 38% had autoimmune thyroid disease and 9% of patients had a first-degree relative with autoimmune thyroid disease [73].

In a Hungarian population, the prevalence of Hashimoto's thyroiditis and Graves' disease was 220-fold higher and 102-fold higher, respectively, in patients with scleroderma than in the general population [74]. Using a chronic diseases registry, a survey including 2431 patients with scleroderma and 12,710 age- and sex-matched controls found that age ($p < 0.0001$, OR 1.03 [95% CI 1.02–1.04]), female sex ($p = 0.0015$, OR 1.86 [95% CI 1.27–2.74]), and diagnosis of scleroderma ($p = 0.0011$, OR 1.81 [95% CI 1.27–2.58]) were all independently associated with hyperthyroidism [75]. Autoimmune-induced thyroid disease was identified in 14.3% of 210 Japanese patients with scleroderma; 29 with hypothyroidism (Hashimoto's disease) and one with hyperthyroidism (Graves' disease) [76]. This compared to 7.2% in the general Japanese population. Demographic and clinical features revealed that female sex, anti-centromere antibody positivity, the complication of Sjogren's syndrome, severe facial skin sclerosis, and atrophy of the thyroid gland were prevalent among the patients with thyroid disease [76].

Hashimoto thyroiditis is characterized by high serum concentrations of anti-thyroglobulin (anti-Tg) antibodies and antithyroid peroxidase (anti-TPO) antibodies. In particular, antithyroid peroxidase (TPO) antibodies are more commonly observed in scleroderma than in controls [77–80], and it has been suggested that anti-TPO antibodies may identify the subset of patients at risk for subsequent thyroid dysfunction [77]. Scleroderma patients with normal basal thyroid function often have an exaggerated thyroid-stimulating hormone (TSH) response to thyrotropin-releasing hormone consistent with subclinical hypothyroidism [81, 82]. Antonelli and colleagues assessed the prevalence of clinical and subclinical thyroid disorders in 202 scleroderma patients compared to 404 controls matched on age and gender [78]. The authors specifically assessed for thyroid disease in a population that had a similar iodine intake. Among females, there were significantly increased relative odds of thyroid disease among scleroderma patients compared to controls including subclinical hypothyroidism [OR 3.2 (95% CI 1.8–5.7)], clinical hypothyroidism [OR 14.5 (95% CI 2.3–90.9)], anti-TPO positivity [OR 2.7 (95% CI 1.8–4.1)], thyroid ultrasound hypoechoic pattern [OR 3.2 (95% CI 2.2–4.7)], thyroid autoimmunity [OR 3.7 (95% CI 2.6–5.4)], and small thyroid volumes <6 mL [1.8 (95% CI 2.2–52.4)]. The relative odds of having thyroid autoimmunity were also higher in male scleroderma patients compared to male controls. Mean TSH values were higher in scleroderma women and anti-TPO titers were higher in scleroderma patients in general than in controls. Three female scleroderma patients had Graves' disease compared to no female controls. Scleroderma patients with thyroid autoimmunity had a longer scleroderma disease duration than scleroderma patients without thyroid autoimmunity. A follow-up study by the same investigators showed a high incidence of thyroid disorders including hypothyroidism, thyroid dysfunction, anti-TPO antibody positivity, and appearance of a hypoechoic thyroid pattern [83]. A study in Japan found that 27.6% (58/210) of patients had either or both anti-Tg and anti-TPO antibodies compared to the reported 12.8% in healthy Japanese adults [76]. A survey in New Zealand found anti-Tg antibodies in 34.2% of limited scleroderma (lcSSc) and 33.3% of diffuse scleroderma (dcSSc) patients [84]. Anti-TPO antibodies were present in 34.2% of lcSSc and 33.3% of dcSSc patients. Thyroid dysfunction was found in 11.7% (10 of 85 patients). Another study found an increased prevalence of anti-TPO antibodies in patients with limited SSc compared to healthy controls but not diffuse scleroderma [85].

Patients with scleroderma and hyperthyroidism also are reported to have 1.54-fold increased mortality rate, emphasizing the importance of screening for thyroid disease in this population [74]. A survey ($n = 77$) to determine the impact of thyroid disease on pregnancy in scleroderma found that Hashimoto's thyroiditis increased the risk of pregnancy failure among women with scleroderma [86]. A controlled survey of 327 unselected patients showed that papillary thyroid cancer had a higher prevalence in patients with scleroderma than in age- and gender-matched iodine-deficient controls, and iodine-sufficient controls [87]. This study found that autoimmune thyroid involvement and hypothyroidism were more frequently observed in patients with scleroderma than in the comparison groups, in agreement with results from other studies, and emphasized the importance careful thyroid evaluation by ultrasound, FT4, TSH, and anti-TPO antibody measurements.

A review of the literature studying the association of thyroid disorders and scleroderma strongly recommends periodically monitoring for thyroid function in the routine clinical evaluations of patients with scleroderma [88]. Special attention should be given to females with a high risk (a borderline high though normal TSH value, the presence of anti-TPO antibodies, and a hypoechoic pattern showing a small thyroid) of developing thyroid dysfunction [88].

Liver Disease

While initial autopsy studies did not find more liver disease than expected in a comparison to a non-scleroderma group, the relative risk of chronic liver disease is reported to be 2.5–4.3 times higher in patients with scleroderma compared to the general population [70, 89, 90]. Abnormal liver function is common in clinical practice and often related to coexistent disorders including hepatic steatosis, coincidental viral infections, and drug toxicity. A survey of 44 patients with scleroderma suggested liver fibrosis was a common finding; 13.6% of cases had liver stiffness as measured using transient elastography to assess the degree of liver fibrosis [91]. A study using a registry including 2431 patients with scleroderma and 12,710 controls found that the rates for both hepatitis B viral (HBV) and hepatitis C viral (HCV) infection were higher in patients as compared to controls (1.56 vs. 0.5% and 1.23 vs. 0.65%, respectively) [92]. After adjusting for age, sex, socioeconomic status, smoking, alcohol abuse, and dialysis treatment, scleroderma was found to be independently associated with both HBV and HCV [OR 2.97 (1.92–4.53) and OR 1.73 (1.10–2.66), respectively] [92]. Primary biliary cholangitis (PBC, previously called primary biliary cirrhosis), autoimmune hepatitis (AIH), nodular regenerative hyperplasia (NRH), steatosis, primary sclerosing cholangitis (PSC), and idiopathic portal hypertension may develop in scleroderma in isolation or at times together [93, 94]. A cross-sectional analysis of 1572 patients with scleroderma recruited in a large Spanish multicenter cohort found hepatobiliary involvement (HBI) in 118 (7.5%) patients [95]. PBC was recorded in 67 (4.3%), autoimmune hepatitis in 19 (1.2%), and anti-mitochondrial negative PBC in 6 (0.4%). Other causes of HBI included secondary liver diseases ($n = 11$, 0.7%), scleroderma-related HBI ($n = 7$, 0.4%), nodular regenerative hyperplasia ($n = 3$, 0.2%), liver cirrhosis ($n = 3$, 0.2%), and HBI of unknown origin ($n = 2$, 0.1%). There is reported evidence for an autoimmune process targeting liver autoantigens in a cohort of 63 scleroderma patients compared to 100 healthy controls in scleroderma [96]. The prevalence of the liver autoantibodies anti-mitochondrial antibody (AMA), anti-smooth muscle antibodies (SMAs), and liver-kidney microsomal (LKM-1) autoantibody was increased among scleroderma patients [96].

Primary biliary cholangitis is a chronic and progressive inflammatory obliteration of intrahepatic biliary ducts leading to fibrosis and cholestatic symptoms of pruritis and jaundice [97]. In the early 1970s, an overlap of PBC with scleroderma was recognized [98]. The prevalence of PBC among patients with scleroderma is about 2–2.5% [99–101], and it has been estimated that 3.9–15% of patients with PBC have scleroderma [102–105]. A recent survey evaluating 100 patients with PBC found a total of 23% to have scleroderma using sensitive criteria for the diagnosis of scleroderma with Raynaud's phenomenon, nailfold capillary microscopy, and autoantibodies [106]. Primary biliary cholangitis may develop years before or after the diagnosis of scleroderma [101, 103], though concurrent onset has been reported. Prior epidemiological studies have demonstrated that although PBC may develop in patients with limited or diffuse scleroderma, it is much more common among the limited subset, particularly in patients with anti-centromere antibodies (ACAs) [99–101]. One study demonstrated that 93% of patients with PBC with scleroderma were of the limited subtype [107]. A survey of patients with localized scleroderma (morphea) found AMA positivity in 6.6% of patients and 4 (4.39%) had PBC [108].

Many investigators have compared patients with both PBC and scleroderma to either patients with PBC alone or patients with scleroderma alone. These studies have demonstrated that patients with a PBC-scleroderma overlap (a) are more likely to be ACA-positive than either of the other groups [109, 110], (b) are older and have a longer scleroderma disease duration than those with scleroderma alone [99], and (c) are more likely to have Sjogren's syndrome than those with limited scleroderma alone [110]. Indeed, in one study 91% of patients with a PBC-scleroderma overlap had keratoconjunctivitis sicca such that the authors suggested using the acronym PACK (**P**BC, **A**CA, **C**REST, **K**eratoconjunctivitis sicca) syndrome to remember the key features of the disease [103].

Anti-centromere antibodies occur in up to 30% of patients with PBC [111–113] and up to 90% of patients with PBC and scleroderma [114]. The anti-mitochondrial antibodies (AMAs), which are classically associated with PBC, may occur in up to 25% of patients with scleroderma [99, 115–117]. Anti-mitochondrial antibodies are highly correlated to the presence of ACA [100, 115] and increased pruritis in scleroderma [115]. Although there is a strong correlation between ACA and AMA, patients with PBC who are AMA-negative are more likely to have a secondary autoimmune disease, such as scleroderma or Sjogren's syndrome, than those who are AMA-positive [104, 118].

It is important to consider both assay methodology and the need for additional autoantibody testing when evaluating a patient suspected of having PBC. In a study of 817 patients with scleroderma, 16 patients (2%) had confirmed PBC [99]. Testing for AMA by indirect immunofluorescence had a sensitivity of only 43.8% with a specificity of 98.9%. Using an M2-enhanced (MIT3) ELISA assay, the sensitivity increased to 81.3% with only a slight decrease in specificity (94.6%). When the authors combined the testing for AMA by ELISA with another autoantibody that is highly specific for PBC (sp100), sensitivity increased to 100% with a specificity of 92.6%. The authors suggested performing sp100 autoantibody testing in patients who have a persistent cholestatic picture, but are AMA negative, to improve detection of PBC. Testing for this autoantibody also has prognostic value, because a sp100-positive patient may progress more rapidly from early- to late-stage PBC [119].

Liver biopsy is not routinely required to diagnose PBC in the appropriate clinical setting: including an elevated alkaline phosphatase level, positive anti-mitochondrial antibody, elevated IgM fraction, and exclusion of other causes of extrahepatic biliary obstruction. A biopsy should be considered in patients where the differential diagnosis is unclear in that there are many mimics of PBC. These include granulomatous liver disease, drug toxicity, steatosis in an obese subject, autoimmune hepatitis due to an atypical laboratory profile (positive ANA, elevated IgG fraction, transaminitis out of proportion to alkaline phosphatase elevation), or nodular regenerative hyperplasia due to the presence of non-cirrhotic portal hypertension or a hepatic vascular insult.

Early detection of PBC and institution of ursodeoxycholic acid (UDCA), a hydrophilic bile acid, may be helpful; UDCA was the first treatment for primary biliary cholangitis approved by the US Food and Drug Administration (FDA) in 1997. Therapy with UDCA improves hepatic biochemical parameters [120] and may reduce mortality [121, 122]. Initial therapy for all patients with PBC is UDCA at a total daily dose of 13–15 mg/kg, given orally and usually administered twice daily. Improvement in liver biochemical tests (alkaline phosphatase) is typically observed within three months of starting UDCA, although symptoms such as fatigue often do not improve with treatment. Therefore, it is imperative that rheumatologists consider PBC in the differential diagnosis of scleroderma patients with pruritis or abnormal liver function tests. Normalization of alkaline phosphatase values is associated with an improved prognosis, and liver function tests should continue to be monitored in these patients two to three times per year. Treatment with bile acid sequestrants such as cholestyramine or colestipol may be helpful for pruritis [123]. In patients with PBC and scleroderma, surveillance for metabolic bone disease is also essential.

About 40% percent of patients have an inadequate biochemical response after 1 year of UDCA. Alternative therapy should be considered in those patients if liver function is not improved after 1 year [124]. Obeticholic acid is derived from chenodeoxycholic acid and is an agonist of the farnesoid X receptor leading to inhibition of transcription of the gene encoding cholesterol 7α hydroxylase (CYP7A1), which catalyzes the synthesis of bile acids. Obeticholic acid can be used as monotherapy or in combination with UDCA; but there is a black box warning pointing out the need to monitor liver function periodically in patients taking obeticholic acid and to use a reduced dose in those patients who have Child-Pugh class B or C cirrhosis. Other therapy under study include fibrates (fenofibrate, a specific peroxisome proliferator-activated receptor [PPAR] alpha agonist, and bezafibrate, a pan-PPAR agonist), corticosteroids, B cell depletion (rituximab), and other farnesoid X receptor agonists [124]. Corticosteroids can be especially helpful in patients with overlap PBC and autoimmune hepatitis [124].

In a study from the United Kingdom, 43 patients with PBC and scleroderma were matched on serum bilirubin concentration at initial visit to 86 patients with PBC alone [101]. Overall survival was similar between the groups, but the risk of liver transplantation was significantly lower in the PBC-scleroderma group (16%) than in the PBC alone group (26%) due to less severe liver disease. The rate of bilirubin increase, a marker of severity, was less in the PBC-scleroderma group than those with PBC alone. Although there were fewer liver-related deaths in the scleroderma group, there was an increase in non-liver deaths due to scleroderma, and therefore overall survival did not differ between the two groups. Interestingly, hepatic complications were not different between the groups except the incidence of first occurrence of spontaneous bacterial peritonitis and septicemia, which were higher in PBC patients with scleroderma than in those without scleroderma.

In addition to PBC, autoimmune hepatitis may develop in limited scleroderma and can overlap with PBC in the same patient [94, 125–130]. Autoimmune hepatitis is characterized by liver inflammation on biopsy including interface hepatitis, hypergammaglobulinemia, and autoantibodies (ANA, anti-smooth muscle, anti-liver-kidney microsome type 1, anti-soluble liver antigen) [131, 132]. In one study, a review of 35 cases with biopsy-proven autoimmune hepatitis revealed that two patients developed scleroderma [133]. In our center's experience, affected patients have limited cutaneous disease and respond to immunosuppressive therapy [126]. Therefore, liver biopsy and evaluation of histology may be critical in identifying this subset of patients.

Nodular regenerative hyperplasia (NRH) of the liver is reported in varied rheumatic diseases and is also known as non-cirrhotic portal hypertension, diffuse nodular hyperplasia, or nodular transformation of the liver [132, 134]. This condition is characterized by transformation of hepatic parenchyma into nodules consisting of hyperplastic hepatocytes without significant fibrosis [132]. One theory is that hepatic ischemia either due to alterations in hepatic perfusion or direct hepatic vascular bed injury may contribute to the pathogenesis of this condition. Nodular regenerative hyperplasia may present incidentally during the evaluation of abnormal liver function tests, with chronic abdominal pain, or as portal hypertension with signs of hepatosplenomegaly, bleeding esophageal varices, or ascites [132]. Four out of 278 patients with established scleroderma had biopsy-proven NRH resulting in a prevalence of symptomatic NRH of 1.4% [135]. Nodular regenerative hyperplasia may also occur concurrent with PBC and scleroderma [93]. Diagnosis requires histologic examination, and it has been suggested that liver biopsy should be obtained in patients with rheumatic diseases who have persistently abnormal liver function tests, hepatosplenomegaly, or a risk factor for thrombosis (e.g., antiphospholipid antibodies) [132].

Other hepatic findings in scleroderma may include steatosis, where fatty liver may account for 20% of liver disturbance in scleroderma [125], primary sclerosing cholangitis [136], or idiopathic portal hypertension [125, 137, 138]. These liver diseases are reported primarily in case reports; however, and it is difficult to conclude whether these conditions are related to or associated with scleroderma.

Given the risk of these hepatic complications, the rheumatologist should screen all patients with scleroderma, particularly those with the limited subtype, with basic labs including transaminases and an alkaline phosphatase. If elevated transaminases are abnormal, then a search for hepatic and non-hepatic causes, including inflammatory myopathies, is essential. Although anti-mitochondrial antibodies can be present years before onset of PBC, routine screening with these antibodies is controversial, as many of these patients may never develop symptomatic or clinically relevant liver disease. In the scleroderma patient with a classic constellation of findings for PBC (elevated alkaline phosphatase, positive anti-mitochondrial antibody, elevated IgM fraction, and exclusion of extrahepatic biliary obstruction), liver biopsy may not be required. If the alkaline phosphatase does not normalize with UDCA treatment or if the differential diagnosis remains broad, liver biopsy should be performed given that these conditions may overlap with another liver disorder and therefore impact prognosis and therapy.

Lower Urinary Tract

Lower urinary tract symptoms (LUTS) such as urinary frequency, nocturia, hesitancy, decreased stream, suprapubic pain, urinary incontinence, and hematuria are now recognized as common among patients with scleroderma, yet they are unappreciated and not ideally managed. One survey noted that only 24% of patients with scleroderma who had urinary incontinence remembered being asked by a health provider about urinary symptoms [139]. Yet a recent uncontrolled survey involving 334 patients categorizing LUTS into issues of bladder storage, voiding, and post-micturition reported that only 4% of patients had no symptoms; the most frequent being nocturia, followed by urinary incontinence for women and terminal dribble for men [140]. These same investigators reported that the prevalence of urinary incontinence was 63% (95% CI 60–68%) [139]. Limited cutaneous scleroderma (lcSSc) and anti-centromere antibodies were both significantly associated with urinary incontinence even after adjusting for age, sex, disability, diabetes, BMI, caffeine consumption, dyspnea, fecal incontinence, abnormal bowel movement, or the presence of overlapping rheumatic disease [139].

A survey done in an ambulatory setting by questionnaire reported that among the 121 (87%) responders, frequent urination was reported by 79 (66.3%) patients, urge incontinence leaks occurred in 47 (39.4%) patients, urine leakage related to coughing, sneezing, or laughing was reported by 50 (42%) patients, and small amount of urine leakage (drops) by 28 (23.6%) patients [141]. Severe vesico-sphincter events or severe anal incontinence occurred in 3.4% and 12.4% of cases, respectively. Frequent urination (66.3%) and anal incontinence to gas (50.4%) were the most frequent severe symptoms. There were no correlations with age, sex, or scleroderma characteristics. In multivariate analysis, moderate or severe vesico-sphincter events were associated with higher anxiety and depression scores and lower SF-36 scores.

An investigation evaluated the frequency of LUTS and sexual dysfunction in patients with scleroderma attending a specialized clinic and associated these symptoms with clinical and functional parameters including disability and quality of life [142]. The most frequent LUTS among the 73 patients (13 males) were overactive bladder (n = 11, 84.6%) and dysuria (n = 8, 61.5%) for males and overactive bladder (n = 51, 85%) and incontinence (n = 29, 48.3%) for females. Sexual disorders were associated with short disease duration ($p = 0.01$) and high depression ($p = 0.04$) scores. For men, 7/8 (87.5%) had erectile dysfunction (mean IIEF-5 score 16 [5.3]).

A survey of 175 women with scleroderma found fecal incontinence in 62 (39%) patients, urinary incontinence in 55 (34%), dual incontinence in 37 (23%), and pelvic pain in 31 (19%) [141]. Pelvic floor symptoms reduced measures of quality of life compared to patients without those symptoms.

One of the few controlled studies compared LUTS in 42 patients with scleroderma to 50 age- and gender-matched healthy subjects [143]. They found that patients showed a significantly higher prevalence of urinary symptoms (69% vs. 40%, $p = 0.005$) and severity of urinary incontinence (52% vs. 18%, $p < 0.005$) and overactive bladder (45% vs. 20%, $p < 0.01$) than healthy controls.

A scleroderma disease process (e.g., fibrosis, microvascular disease, or secondary dysautonomia) and/or comorbid conditions (e.g., age, pelvic floor muscle weakness, fluid imbalance from cardiopulmonary disease, medications) can cause LUTS. One survey failed to find a direct or independent link between skin fibrosis, scleroderma vascular involvement (e.g., pulmonary hypertension, Raynaud's phenomenon, and ulceration), or cardiopulmonary symptoms and LUTS [140]. While one of the few case-controlled autopsy studies did not find an abnormal degree of bladder fibrosis among patients with scleroderma [70], there are several cases reported with bladder stiffness with dysfunction and pathological evidence consistent with excess connective tissue and bladder fibrosis [142, 144–148]. A study comparing 21 female scleroderma patients to 15 age- and gender-matched controls detected a large variation in premictional bladder volume and reduced bladder emptying in scleroderma patients (89.8 ± 13.1% bladder emptying in scleroderma patients vs. 97.4 ± 4.1% in controls) [142]. Twenty-nine percent of patients had bladder volumes more than two standard deviations (SDs) above the mean for controls and 33% of patients had bladder volumes more than two SDs below the mean for controls. Patients with long-standing scleroderma (>14 years) had higher bladder volumes, and the authors postulated that bladder fibrosis might result in decreased distensibility and contractility of the bladder. A study reported functional bladder alterations with failed detrusor activity in four of nine patients [147]. These abnormalities did correlate with histologic findings. Three patients with detrusor areflexia had collagen accumulation in the small arteries of the detrusor along with tortuous, enlarged capillary loops, and areas of capillary loss. Two patients with detrusor areflexia had fibrotic replacement of the bladder smooth muscle.

On occasion, scleroderma-related vascular anomalies such as A-V malformations seen in the bladder mucosa lead to micro- or macro-hematuria [149]. There are cases of severe gross hematuria from bladder telangiectasia requiring blood transfusions and one case was successfully treated with diathermocoagulation [149].

Sarcopenia can occur in patients with severe scleroderma and associate with functional disability [150–152]. In a survey comparing patients to normal healthy controls, overactive bladder positively correlated with sarcopenia ($p < 0.001$), and both overactive bladder and urinary incontinence significantly correlated with reduced BMD ($p < 0.05$, $p = 0.001$) [143].

Circulating autoantibodies directed against cholinergic muscarinic type-3 receptor (M_3-R) are present in the serum of patients with scleroderma, and there is evidence that they associate with bowel dysfunction [153]. There is speculation that these antibodies can target M3 muscarinic receptors, disrupting autonomic function, and lead to bladder dysfunction [154]. A report used urodynamic testing, assessment of autonomic nervous system, and bladder pathology in 23 female patients with scleroderma [146]. Five patients had frequent daytime urination, one had urge incontinence, and the remaining patients were asymptomatic. In only three patients, urodynamic alterations was detected, but signs of parasympathetic dysfunction were identified in 13 cases, 9 of whom also had sympathetic dysfunction. Two patients with autonomic dysfunction had urinary symptoms, and three had bladder dysfunction. Interestingly, abnormal bladder pathology was common: 78% of patients had increased connective tissue in the lamina propria and interstitial fibrosis separating smooth muscle bundles (12 patients with mild fibrosis, 4 moderate, 2 severe), and 7 patients had proliferative changes in small arteries. There was no correlation between urinary symptoms and urodynamic features with the severity of bladder fibrosis.

Attention to LUTS is important in every patient with scleroderma. There are no studies to provide guidance for scleroderma-specific treatment for LUTS, but a standard approach makes sense. For example, one should follow guidelines for evaluation and management of urinary incontinence used in the general population [155]. Scleroderma patients with urinary symptoms may require formal urological evaluation including urodynamic testing with clinical symptoms of bladder autonomic dysfunction and cystoscopy in patients with hematuria to evaluate for bladder telangiectasia and to exclude other causes including malignancy. Management of LUTS usually does not need surgical intervention, although surgery helped a patient with a thickened, poorly distensible bladder who suffered from dysuria, frequency, and urinary incontinence [148].

Erectile Dysfunction

Erectile dysfunction (ED) in scleroderma was first described in 1981 [156]. These authors described five male patients with scleroderma who presented with impotence as a significant initial feature of their disease. Endocrinologic, urological, and psychiatric evaluations failed to reveal an alternative cause for impotence. None of the patients took medications known to alter sexual function. All of these patients had preservation of libido throughout their illness, but absent or greatly diminished erectile function. None had evidence for large-vessel vascular disease. Subsequently, Nowlin and colleagues [157] performed a study of ten patients with scleroderma who were evaluated for sexual function. Five of these reported complete impotence and three partial impotence. Endocrinologic evaluation, including measurements of serum testosterone, prolactin, estradiol, follicle-stimulating hormone, and luteinizing hormones, was normal in all patients.

Since these early reports, several other descriptions of ED in male patients with scleroderma have been reported [158–160]. In most of these reports, comprehensive evaluations for other causes of impotence attributed the ED directly to scleroderma. The prevalence of ED in scleroderma has varied from 27% to 81% [157, 161].

More recently, ED was studied in 130 men with scleroderma by the European Scleroderma Trials and Research (EUSTAR) group [162]. Of the 130 men studied, only 17.7% had normal erectile function scores. ED in these patients occurred earlier in the disease and was associated with severe cutaneous, muscular or renal involvement of scleroderma, elevated pulmonary pressures, and restrictive lung disease. The authors concluded that severe ED is a common and early symptom in men with scleroderma.

In order to determine if ED is more common in scleroderma than in other chronic rheumatic diseases, Hong and colleagues [161], in a case-control study, evaluated men with scleroderma and rheumatoid arthritis (RA). The authors found that 81% of men with scleroderma had ED—three times more commonly than in RA. In both scleroderma and RA, ED was associated with the presence of Raynaud's phenomenon (80% of men with RP vs. 50% of men without RP). The authors report that ED frequently developed within the first 3 years of disease onset and was a prominent symptom in these involved patients. The association of ED with RP in both of these patient populations suggested to these authors that microvascular involvement of the penis was responsible for this symptom.

Rosato and colleagues [163] investigated ED in 20 patients with scleroderma using color Doppler ultrasound examination in the cavernous arteries and correlated these changes with disease severity and digital vascular damage. They further evaluated these patients using nailfold videocapillaroscopy, Sexual Health Inventory for Men (SHIM), and Medsger Disease Severity Scale (DSS). In all patients studied, a reduction in SHIM was present. Greater vascular damage correlated with low SHIM scores. The authors concluded that the degree of ED in the patients correlated with the severity of the vascular damage. Using more sophisticated methodologies for measuring genital blood flow, these authors confirmed their previous observation [164]. However, Keck and colleagues [165] studied 86 men with scleroderma with and without ED and performed nailfold capillaroscopy. Specific nailfold findings did not associate with the coexistence of ED in these patients. They also could not find a correlation based on the stage or duration of scleroderma.

Pathogenesis of ED in the general population is a neurovascular phenomenon, which depends on neural integrity, a functional vascular system, and healthy corporal tissues. Normal erectile function involves three synergistic and simultaneous processes: (1) neurologically mediated increase in penile arterial inflow, (2) relaxation of corporal smooth muscle, and (3) restriction of venous outflow from the penis. The corpus cavernosum of the penis is composed of a meshwork of interconnected smooth muscle cells lined by vascular endothelium. The small resistance helicine arteries that supply blood to the corpus cavernosum during penile tumescence are also lined by endothelial cells and underlying smooth muscle. Pathological alteration in the anatomy of the penile vasculature or impairment of any combination of neurovascular processes can result in ED [162]. The severity of ED is associated with vascular risk factors such as atherosclerosis, hypertension, hypercholesterolemia, diabetes mellitus, and cigarette smoking. Clinical and basic science investigations on aging, diabetes, hypercholesterolemia, and hypertension show that endothelial dysfunction is a major contributing factor to penile vascular pathology [166, 167]. Endothelial dysfunction can impair penile blood flow into the penis and thus cause ED. ED associated with scleroderma is thought to be due to underlying vasculopathic (endothelial and penile arterial dysfunction) and fibrotic changes in the penile vascular bed [168]. Pathological findings suggest penile arterial alterations such as increased collagen to smooth muscle density in the small helicine arteries of the penis as well as increased collagen deposition in the corporal sinusoids [168]. These pathological findings are associated with arteriogenic and veno-occlusive ED.

Since both fibrosis and microvasculopathy occur as prominent features of scleroderma, it is possible that either one of these, or both, contribute to the pathogenesis of ED. Microvascular disease in the circulation of the penis may impede the distending pressure required for penile erection. In addition, autonomic nervous system alterations may interfere with neurogenic control of penile vascular tone and contribute to ED. Autonomic dysfunction is described in scleroderma [169–171]. Penile fibrosis, although a late finding in scleroderma, could contribute to the inability to obtain sufficient distending pressure to achieve an erection. In order to investigate these various hypotheses, researchers have focused on noninvasive methods to evaluate penile blood flow. In a report by Nowlin et al. [157], penile blood flow, evaluated by Doppler, was normal in all five impotent and one partially potent patient. Of the age-matched controls with RA, none had impotence or reduced penile blood flow. Aversa and colleagues studied the penile vasculature in scleroderma using the duplex ultrasound technique in 15 male patients with scleroderma [172]. Nine of the 15 patients had moderate to severe ED. Severely impaired mean peak systolic velocities in the presence of mild venous leakage were found in these patients. Granchi and colleagues [173] reported that penile smooth muscle cells synthesized endothelin-1 (ET-1), one of the main regulators of microvascular contractility. In general, patients with scleroderma-associated ED have rapidly progressive decline in erectile function [172].

Reports of fibrosis of penile structures in the development of ED have emerged over the years. Pathologic examinations have shown greater than normal connective tissue infiltration of the testes and other genital organs in patients with scleroderma [174]. Rossman and Zorgniotti [160] described three male patients with scleroderma and impotence in whom the corpus cavernosum had been extensively replaced with connective tissue. These authors postulated that extensive fibrosis resulted in limited blood flow and the inability of the venous sinusoids to distend appropriately. In a clinicopathological study by Nehra and colleagues [168], hemodynamic testing on a patient who underwent a penile implant revealed diffuse corporeal veno-occlusive dysfunction. The excised corporeal tissue demonstrated severe fibrosis. Pro-fibrotic cytokines including transforming growth factor beta and platelet-derived growth factor are overexpressed in the corpora cavernosa under various hypoxic conditions [175, 176]. Under similar hypoxic conditions, penile smooth muscle cells release ET-1, which may stimulate fibroblast proliferation. It is likely that ED in scleroderma has a multifactorial etiology [177, 178] and develops due to both microvascular abnormalities and penile fibrosis.

Evaluation of patients with scleroderma and ED should systematically include attention to medications known to be associated with ED, symptoms of depression, and assessment of comorbidities including smoking, diabetes mellitus, hypertension, and peripheral vascular disease. An evaluation of an endocrine disorder should also be carried out including serum testosterone levels. Referral to a urologist should be initiated in order to perform a penile duplex Doppler ultrasound evaluation of the penis in order to determine the penile vascular status which can help manage both medical and surgical therapy [178]. If the duplex Doppler ultrasound of the penis shows severe penile fibrosis with poor arterial inflow to the corpora cavernosa of the penis after pharmacostimulation, then this may warrant placement of a penile prosthesis [168, 172, 178].

Treatment and pharmacologic management of ED in scleroderma have received little attention. In small series, there does not appear to be support for calcium channel blockers or other vasodilators in treating this condition. Certainly, PDE 5 inhibitors (PDE5Is) are the first-line ED therapy in scleroderma [178–180]. However, on demand PDE5Is generally have been ineffective in improving erectile function in most case series [177], but studies to guide management are needed. A trial of either sildenafil (50 mg qd) or tadalafil (10 mg qd) on a daily basis for a period of 2–3 weeks is recommended. Extrapolating from the experience in men without scleroderma, sildenafil can be increased to 100 mg or tadalafil to 20 mg daily. Inability to achieve satisfactory erections during this trial period suggests that the PDE 5 inhibitors will not be helpful. Patients who do not respond to medications should be referred to a urologist for duplex Doppler ultrasound of the penis and an evaluation for other treatments including intracavernous injection therapy with vasoactive agents, a vacuum constrictive device, or possible placement of an inflatable penile prosthesis. A vacuum constriction device is an external pump that a man with erectile dysfunction can use to get and maintain an erection. The pump helps the penis to become erect and a band attached to the pump helps to maintain the erection.

Duplex Doppler ultrasound of the penis shows that men with scleroderma often have severe penile fibrosis and impaired penile arterial smooth muscle relaxation [168, 178], making them a hard-to-treat ED population of patients. If the penile ultrasound shows an intact penile vascular bed with good response to pharmacostimulation with vasoactive agents such as prostaglandin E1, phentolamine, and papaverine, then local intracavernous injection therapy can be used.

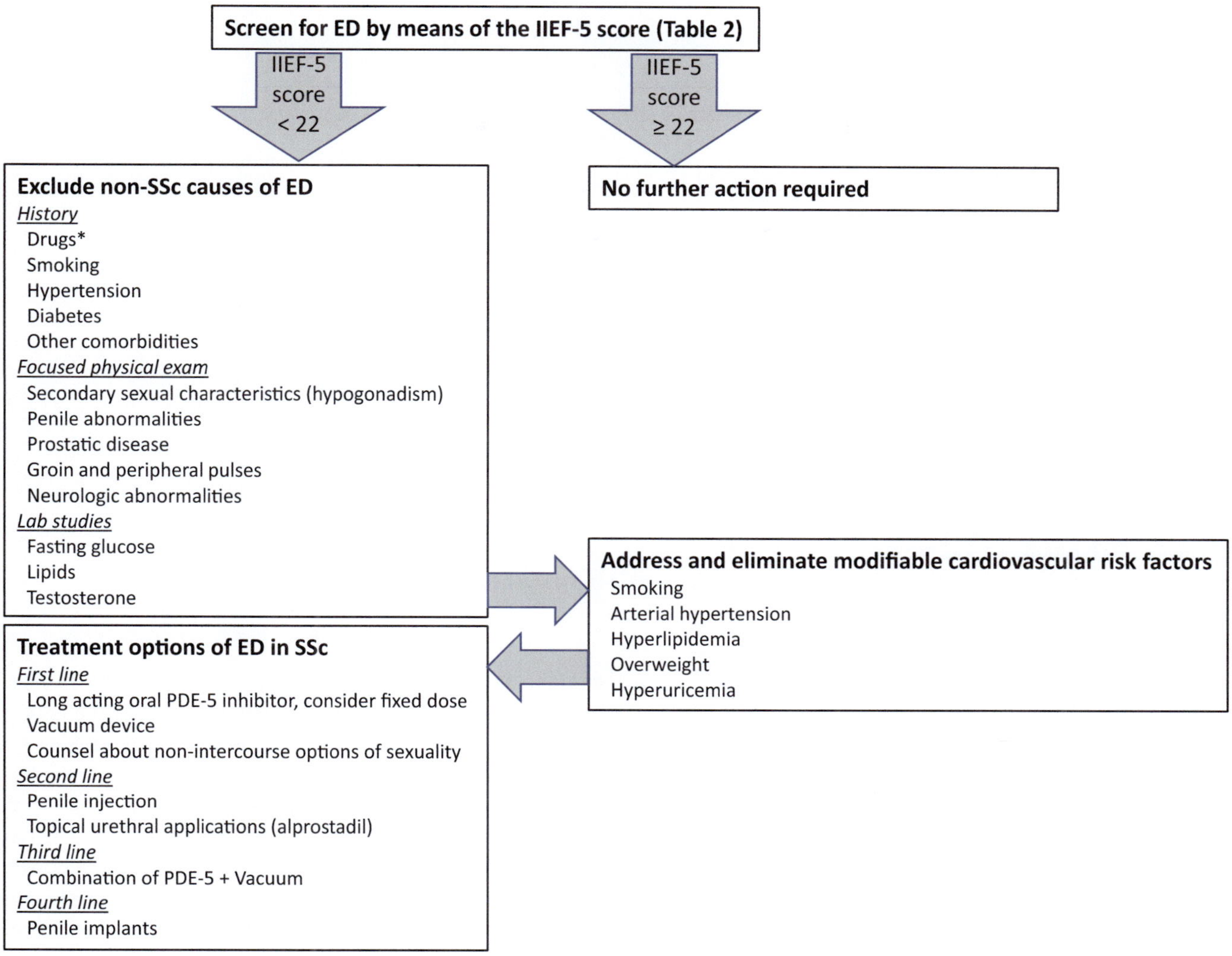

Fig. 38.2 Approach to evaluating ED in men with SSc (Adapted with permission from [181]). *Drugs include diuretics (thiazides, spironolactone), antihypertensive drugs (calcium-channel blockers, beta-blockers, methyldopa, clonidine, reserpine, guanethidine), cardiac or cholesterol drugs (digoxin, gemfibrozil, clofibrate), antidepressants (selective serotonin-reuptake inhibitors, tricyclic antidepressants, lithium, monoamine oxidase inhibitors), tranquilizers (butyrophenones, phenothiazines), H2 antagonists (ranitidine, cimetidine), hormones (progesterone, estrogens, corticosteroids, luteinizing hormone-releasing hormone antagonists, 5α-reductase inhibitors, cyproterone acetate), cytotoxic agents (methotrexate), immunomodulators (interferon-α), anticholinergic agents (disopyramide, anticonvulsants), recreational drugs (alcohol, cocaine)

However, if there is a poor response to pharmacostimulation, then a vacuum device with banding or a penile prosthesis can be used. During the time of prosthesis placement, Nehra and colleagues have shown that excision of severely fibrotic corporal tissue is necessary to place an inflatable penile prosthesis [168]. The published data suggest that experts can place inflatable penile prostheses in patients with scleroderma without undue complications such as infection or penile erosion [177, 178]. However, experience with the use of penile prostheses in scleroderma is limited and the duration of benefit and long-term safety are not well defined. A recent review outlined an approach to the evaluation and treatment of patients with ED (Fig. 38.2) using a validated 5 item questionnaire to screen patients (Table 38.2) [181, 182].

Table 38.2 Erectile dysfunction screening questionnaire

The IIEF-5 questionnaire[a]					
Over the past 6 months					
1. How do you rate your **confidence** that you could get and keep an erection?	Very low 1	Low 2	Moderate 3	High 4	Very high 5
2. When you had erections with sexual stimulation, how often were your erections hard enough for penetration?	Almost never/never 1	A few times (much less than half the time) 2	Sometimes (about half the time) 3	Most times (much more than half the time) 4	Almost always/always 5
3. During sexual intercourse, **how often** were you able to maintain your erection after you had penetrated (entered) your partner?	Almost never/never 1	A few times (much less than half the time) 2	Sometimes (about half the time) 3	Most times (much more than half the time) 4	Almost always/always 5
4. During sexual intercourse, **how difficult** was it to maintain your erection to completion of intercourse?	Extremely difficult 1	Very difficult 2	Difficult 3	Slightly difficult 4	Not difficult 5
5. When you attempted sexual intercourse, how often was it satisfactory for you?	Almost never/never 1	A few times (much less than half the time) 2	Sometimes (about half the time) 3	Most times (much more than half the time) 4	Almost always/always 5

Reproduced with permission from [182]

[a] The IIEF-5 score is the sum of the ordinal responses to the five items; thus, the score can range from 5 to 25

Avascular Necrosis of Bone

Avascular necrosis of the carpal scaphoid bone and lunate of the wrist is reported in patients with scleroderma [183–188]. This can occur in the absence of potential risk factors for avascular necrosis of bone including steroid use, specific trauma, antiphospholipid autoantibodies, or comorbid conditions such as diabetes or hyperlipidemia [187]. Patients present with wrist pain with minimal, if any, signs of inflammation and thus the presence of avascular necrosis may be underdiagnosed and mistaken for arthritis or tendonitis. Case series report that avascular necrosis of the lunate bone is most common and is associated with severe Raynaud's, suggesting that scleroderma vascular disease and bone ischemia are the causative factors [184, 187, 188]. Ulnar artery occlusion was reported in three of five cases, implicating underlying scleroderma related macrovascular disease [187]. Standard radiographs may miss avascular necrosis even in an advanced stage. A survey of 26 patients using magnetic resonance imaging found pathologic bone marrow edema in 18% of lunate bones, suggesting early stages of lunate osteonecrosis [189]. Treatment is often nonsurgical with conservative measures of wrist support, occupational therapy, and pain control. Surgical therapy includes attempts at placing a vascularized bone graft or removal of the damaged bone with stabilization of the wrist to reduce pain and disability.

Neurological Manifestations

Compared to the recognized visceral organ involvement in scleroderma, neurological manifestations are less common and often related to comorbid non-scleroderma conditions or complications of scleroderma-related organ failure. In fact, early studies of organ involvement in scleroderma rarely reported neurological disease. Leinwand and colleagues [190], in 1954, reported over 150 cases of scleroderma but did not include any mention of neurologic abnormalities. In 1955, Piper and Hellwig [191] reported foci of ischemic necrosis in 3 of 17 brains of scleroderma patients at autopsy, but no clinical correlations were reported. Tuffanelli and Winkler [192] reported a large series of 727 patients with scleroderma and described 2 patients with grand mal seizures and 4 with minimal seizure activity. In a comprehensive review of 130 patients with scleroderma by Gordon and Silverstein [193], 24 patients were found to have 28 neurological manifestations, but none were definitely related to the scleroderma disease process itself. In a study of 58 autopsy cases and 58 age-matched controls, D'Angelo and colleagues [70] did not report any pathologic cases of nervous system involvement in scleroderma.

However, recent surveys report several neurological manifestations that may be related to complications of the scleroderma disease process. Lee and colleagues [194] reported in a prospective survey of 125 patients with scleroderma that 7 (5.6%) were found to have defined neurologic lesions, 4 with carpal tunnel syndrome, and 1 each with trigeminal neuralgia, mononeuritis multiplex, and peripheral neuropathy. Amaral and colleagues [195] reported a variety of neurological manifestations including central nervous system (CNS) involvement (headache, seizures, and cognitive impairment), depression and anxiety, myopathy, trigeminal neuropathy, peripheral sensory motor polyneuropathy, and carpal tunnel syndrome. There is also evidence that autonomic neuropathy plays a key role in organ dysfunction. A systematic literature review of neurologic involvement in scleroderma [195] found autonomic nervous system (ANS) dysfunction to be common and typically involved cardiovascular and gastrointestinal systems.

Cranial nerve involvement in scleroderma with evidence of trigeminal neuropathy is compelling. It is postulated that microvascular disease with secondary deposition of fibrous tissue contributes to the nerve damage and compression. Beighton and colleagues [196] first reported trigeminal sensory neuropathy in a patient who later developed scleroderma. Ashworth and Tait [197] reported this sensory deficit in five patients classified as having scleroderma, but two of the five had features of systemic lupus erythematosus. Farrell and Medsger [198] noted trigeminal neuropathy in 16 of 442 consecutive patients (4%) with scleroderma evaluated at the University of Pittsburgh between 1972 and 1980. Teasdall and colleagues [52] described ten patients with scleroderma who developed cranial nerve involvement. Trigeminal neuropathy was a presenting feature in five patients; the glossopharyngeal nerve was involved in one patient. Taste was impaired in one patient and tongue fasciculations were present in another. Tinnitus was noted in three patients and facial weakness was present in five. The trigeminal lesions appeared to be peripheral since the sensory deficits occurred over those parts of the face innervated by distal branches of the trigeminal nerve. A case report described a patient with diffuse scleroderma whose trigeminal neuropathy responded to treatment with steroids and methotrexate [199].

Cerebrovascular abnormalities in patients with scleroderma may be more common than previously recognized. There have been isolated reports of CNS arteritis [200–202] and cerebritis [203]. Recent studies have suggested more specific vascular brain involvement [204–206]. These are noted as calcifications of cerebral arteries on computed tomography (CT) scans [203] and white matter lesions (WMLs) on magnetic resonance imaging (MRI) [206]. Subsequent to these studies, Terrier and colleagues [207] studied 63 patients with scleroderma and found severe cerebrovasculopathy on CT scan in 22 patients and on MRI in 38 patients. Those patients with severe cerebrovasculopathy were more likely to have pulmonary arterial hypertension and showed a tendency to have scleroderma renal crisis. In another MRI study, 30 female SSc patients and 30 age-matched controls underwent brain MRIs [208]. CNS involvement in the form of white matter hyperintense foci was more common in patients with scleroderma. CNS lesions in these patients correlated with clinical features including headaches, depression, and peripheral vascular disease. A study of 72 patients with scleroderma with no CNS symptoms and 42 healthy controls used a Doppler ultrasound to measure the carotid intima-media thickness (CIMT) [209]. Brain fluid-attenuated inversion recovery (FLAIR)-MRI and diffusion-weighted MRI (DWI) were done. Patients with scleroderma had more CIMT, higher CRP, and more brain MRI hyperintense lesions than controls ($p < 0.05$). The FLAIR-MRI showed multiple hyperintense lesions in 24 patients (33%), ranging 0–36 lesions. The MRI with positive FLAIR lesions likely represented some CNS small vessel disease, including increased atherosclerosis, since the lesions correlated with increased CIMT.

Vascular changes of hypertension and atherosclerosis may be the underlying cause of CNS lesions rather than direct involvement of cerebral vessels with scleroderma vascular disease. Evidence in other autoimmune diseases suggests an increased risk of atherosclerosis, but the development of accelerated atherosclerosis in scleroderma is less clear. A systematic search identified studies of atherosclerosis in scleroderma [210]. Compared to healthy controls, patients with scleroderma had a higher prevalence of coronary atherosclerosis, peripheral vascular disease, and cerebrovascular calcification. The meta-analysis showed that patients with scleroderma had increased CIMT (summary mean difference 0.11 mm, 95% CI 0.05–0.17 mm; $p = 0.0006$) and lower FMD% (summary mean difference − 3.07%, 95% CI −5.44% to −0.69%; $p = 0.01$) compared to controls [210]. A case-control study of 40 patients with scleroderma and 40 healthy age and sex matched controls used Doppler measures of CIMT [211]. They found the presence of premature atherosclerosis associated with traditional cardiovascular risk factors such as age, dyslipidemia, and obesity (BMI) as well as with the use of steroids and markers of inflammation such as CRP and ESR [211]. Forty-six female patients with scleroderma and 46 age- and ethnicity-matched controls underwent carotid US to assess the presence of plaque and CIMT [212]. Patients with scleroderma had more plaque (45.6% vs. 19.5%, $p = 0.01$) but similar CIMT compared with controls. Compared to rheumatoid arthritis (RA) patients, a systemic disease with well-defined high atherosclerotic burden, subclinical atherosclerosis is comparable between scleroderma and RA [213]. A total of 110 patients with scleroderma (102 females and 8 males, mean ± SD age 50.5 ± 11.9 years), 110 age- and sex-matched RA patients, and 51 healthy subjects without CV disease were examined with ultrasonography (US). Twenty-one (19.1%) patients with scleroderma, 24 (21.8%) RA patients, and 3 (5.9%) healthy subjects had subclinical atherosclerosis (scleroderma versus RA: $p = 0.62$, scleroderma versus healthy subjects: $p = 0.029$) [214]. While there is evidence of an increase in CIMT in scleroderma, there is controversial evidence for increased macro-vascular complications such as stroke or myocardial infarction. One survey of four retrospective cohort studies did find a statistically significant elevated ischemic stroke risk in patients with scleroderma with a pooled risk ratio of 1.68 (95% CI 1.26–2.24) [215].

There is evidence that the vascular disease seen in scleroderma may affect the eye. Postmortem studies show abnormalities of the choroidal vasculature as well as exudates in the retina [216, 217]. Grennan and Foster [218] investigated the choroidal and retinal vasculature in a group of patients with early as well as advanced scleroderma by using routine funduscopic examination, screening for keratoconjunctivitis sicca (KCS), and preforming fluorescein angiograms. Two of the ten patients with scleroderma had KCS, similar to the incidence found in other series [219]. Fluorescein angiography demonstrated abnormalities of perfusion affecting the choriocapillaris and small choroidal arterioles. All but one of the patients was normotensive. Retinopathy [220, 221] and central retinal vein occlusion [222] have also been described in scleroderma. A case-control study measured subfoveal thicknesses of the choroid as well as all three choroidal vascular sublayers and submacular perfusion in 12 patients with scleroderma and 12 matched controls using optical coherence tomography angiography (OCTA) [223]. Choroidal microcirculation was impaired in scleroderma, even in patients without ophthalmological symptoms [223]. A systematic literature review of eye involvement demonstrates limited proven associations between scleroderma and ocular abnormalities [224]. While dry eye symptoms may be more common and the choroidal vasculature appears affected to a greater extent than the retinal microcirculation, the authors concluded that the limited number of patients included in published studies renders it hazardous to draw overall conclusions [224].

Migraine headache is a frequent symptom in the general population and the coincidence noted in studies related to scleroderma could occur by chance. Goldberg and colleagues [225] found 16 cases with well-documented scleroderma and migraine phenomena. Pal and colleagues [226] noted migraines in 32% of patients with scleroderma. Headaches occurred in 23.7% of patients in a large systematic literature review of neurological manifestations in scleroderma [195].

The prevalence of involvement of the peripheral nervous system is unclear. Compression neuropathies including carpal tunnel syndrome, ulnar nerve, and tarsal tunnel syndrome occur in scleroderma, with carpal tunnel syndrome a common presenting symptom [227–230]. A survey of 120 patients found total pain frequency was 69% and neuropathic pain was 35.9% of the entire patient group [231]. The high frequency of neuropathic pain seen in these patients with scleroderma was associated with low quality or life [231]. Richter [232] reported a patient with quadriparesis and peripheral neuropathy who, at autopsy, had peripheral nerve histopathology that revealed epi- and perineural fibrosis with demyelination and axonal degeneration. In a study of the nerve network of the skin, Pawlowski and Warsaw [233] documented fragmentation of the nerve fibers of the skin in patients with scleroderma. Fleischmajer and colleagues [234] also found cellular infiltrates in the perineurium of patients with diffuse cutaneous scleroderma. In a review of 130 patients with scleroderma, Gordan and Silverstein [193] were unable to demonstrate any clinical manifestations of peripheral neuropathy. Very few studies have reported the use of electrodiagnostic testing as a means of delineating the existence of peripheral neurologic involvement in scleroderma. Christopher and Robinson [235] performed electrodiagnostic studies including determination of conduction velocities in motor and sensory nerves on 17 patients with scleroderma compared to a control group of 22 patients without peripheral neuropathy. There was a statistically significant reduction in values of mean conduction velocity in ulnar and median sensory nerves of the upper extremities in patients with scleroderma. Only the peroneal nerve of the lower extremity revealed decreased conduction velocity. Poncelet and Connolly [236] studied 14 patients with scleroderma who underwent a complete neurologic examination, nerve conduction studies (NCS), and quantitative sensory testing (QST). Neurologic examination revealed reduced vibrations or pinprick sensation in the upper extremity, focal muscle atrophy or proximal weakness, and decreased deep tendon reflexes. NCS showed reduced sensory nerve action potentials in one patient and carpal tunnel syndrome in another. QST of the upper and lower extremity revealed increased cold or vibration detection threshold in 8 of the 14 patients. The authors conclude that peripheral neuropathy occurs at a higher frequency in scleroderma than was previously appreciated. The prevalence of length-dependent peripheral neuropathy was studied using signs and symptoms of neuropathy derived from the Total Neuropathy Score (TNS) and standardized nerve conduction study (NCS) [237]. Seventeen of 60 (28%) patients had evidence of a peripheral neuropathy as defined by the presence of neuropathic symptoms on the TNS (12 of 60) and/or electrophysiologic evidence of neuropathy (5 subjects with neuropathic symptoms and 5 without neuropathic symptoms). Subjects with neuropathy were more likely to be male (60% versus 40%; $p = 0.02$), African American (41% versus 4.6%; $p = 0.001$), have diabetes mellitus (17.7% versus 0%; $p = 0.02$), have limited cutaneous scleroderma (82.3% versus 53.5%; $p = 0.04$), and have anti-U1 RNP antibodies (23.5% versus 0%; $p = 0.009$) than those without neuropathy. A potential non-scleroderma etiology for the peripheral neuropathy such as diabetes mellitus was found in 82.3% (14 of 17) of subjects with neuropathy.

Impaired vibratory perception is one of the early signs of peripheral neuropathy. A case-control study of 20 consecutive patients with scleroderma and 20 healthy controls evaluated for peripheral neuropathy in both feet using the 10-g Semmes-Weinstein monofilament examination [238]. Two controls and 12 of the scleroderma patients demonstrated abnormal vibratory sense (one-sided Fishers' exact, $p < 0.002$). The prevalence of sensory loss to monofilament in the scleroderma patients was identical to diabetic patients. The interpretation of defects in vibratory sense is complex because of the influence of the viscoelastic properties of the skin and subcutaneous tissue. This is particularly important in scleroderma in which thickened fibrotic skin may alter vibratory perception thresholds. Dahlgaard and colleagues [239] measured the vibratory perception threshold in patients with diffuse cutaneous scleroderma, but found no clinical evidence of peripheral neuropathy. The vibratory perception threshold was significantly elevated on sclerotic skin test loci, but remained normal on loci with normal skin suggesting that the scleroderma skin caused a dampening effect on external vibration. A study by Poncelet and Connolly [236] confirmed the impact of the skin texture on measuring the sense of vibration.

There is evidence that dysregulation of the autonomic nervous system (ANS) is playing a role in scleroderma resulting in abnormal vascular reactivity, gastrointestinal dysmotility, and alterations of heart rate and blood pressure. A survey of 104 patients with scleroderma using the Composite Autonomic Symptom Score (COMPASS)-31 questionnaire, a validated tool to assess symptoms of autonomic dysfunction, found that the mean COMPASS-31 score in this cohort was 24.9 ± 15.5, higher than COMPASS-31 scores from previously published healthy controls (8.9 ± 8.7) [240]. Some of the clinical manifestations of dysautonomia are common (e.g., Raynaud's phenomenon; gastrointestinal reflux), but others are more subtle (e.g., exercise intolerance, orthostatic changes, or secretory dysfunction). The underlying pathogenesis of dysregulation of the ANS focuses on the microvascular disease, secondary fibrosis, and direct autoimmune-mediated injury to the nervous system.

One argument is that scleroderma microvascular disease is the primary event leading to secondary nervous system injury. Another theory is that vascular neurogenic control is the putative mechanism that alters normal vascular reactivity and leads to progressive tissue disease or organ dysfunction. The sympathetic and parasympathetic nervous system play a major role in vasomotor integrity. Early studies focused on direct measurements of circulating catecholamines on the morphologic assessment of autonomic nerve endings or plexuses in the skin. Peacock [241] found elevated levels of epinephrine and norepinephrine in the plasma of patients with Raynaud's phenomenon before and after cold stimulation. However, the assays used for catecholamine determination were not reliable and these abnormal levels could not be reproduced [242]. In 1972, Sapira and colleague [243] reported on resting venous plasma catecholamine concentrations and urinary catecholamine excretion patterns in patients with Raynaud's and scleroderma and could find no evidence of catecholamine excess. Studies of the nerve network of the skin in scleroderma found characteristic morphologic changes (degeneration and regeneration) in the nerve ending in various stages of the disease [233]. However, it is not clear whether such changes are primary or a secondary phenomenon. Most now agree that abnormal vascular reactivity is due to a "local fault" of the vessel with evidence of endothelial injury and upregulation of adrenergic receptors with abnormal responses to catecholamine and other vasoactive mediators.

Abnormal autonomic nervous system function is implicated in scleroderma with diminished/absent peristalsis of the body of the esophagus, reduced lower esophageal sphincter pressure, delayed gastric emptying, abnormal colonic motility, and anal rectal sphincter incompetence [244–246]. Lock and colleagues [247] noted evidence of ANS dysfunction in 12 of 77 patients with scleroderma who also had manometric changes of esophageal dysmotility. The primary event in the pathogenesis of gastrointestinal involvement in scleroderma is likely a neural lesion followed by secondary smooth muscle atrophy and then clinical symptoms of dysmotility. The first study suggesting an early neuropathic phase in scleroderma- related gastrointestinal disease demonstrated that the esophageal smooth muscle responded to the direct acting agent methacholine, a muscarinic receptor agonist, but not to edrophonium, an agent that increases acetylcholine (Ach) [248]. Another study found abnormality in intestinal activation by mechanical and hormonal stimuli while duodenal myoelectric activity was intact [249]. These studies suggested dysregulation of ACh release from the myenteric cholinergic neurons as an early defect causing gastrointestinal dysmotility. A case-control survey of autopsy tissue from 74 patients with scleroderma and 74 age-, race-, and sex-matched controls investigated histological evidence of esophageal muscle atrophy, the degree of vascular changes, inflammatory infiltration, fibrosis, abnormalities of the myenteric plexus, and reduction of interstitial cells of Cajal (ICC) using a predesigned semiquantitative descriptive method [250]. The pathological findings of the esophagus were inconsistent with either an ischemic or an inflammatory process. Loss of circular and longitudinal smooth muscle in the distal scleroderma esophagus was associated with fewer ICC, suggesting a loss of normal neural function as a primary pathological process. Studies demonstrate that gastrointestinal dysmotility in scleroderma is associated with circulating autoantibodies against the muscarinic-3 receptor (M_3-R) [251, 252]. These autoantibodies inhibited the contraction of smooth muscle cells directly stimulated with a cholinergic agent, supporting the concept of immune-mediated neuron injury. Both scleroderma and diabetes (DM) manifest abnormalities to the microvascular circulation and characteristic gastrointestinal changes (delayed gastric emptying, colonic hypomotility, anal sphincter dysfunction) [253–257], and erectile dysfunction [257]. Autonomic neuropathy occurs frequently in DM [257–259] and may contribute to the gastrointestinal lesions as well as male erectile failure. The similar organ malfunction and microvascular disease present in scleroderma and DM supports the concept of ANS dysfunction playing a role in scleroderma.

There is evidence that abnormal autonomic nervous control of the heart is present and can identify subclinical cardiac involvement in patients with scleroderma [260]. Suarez-Almazor and colleagues [261] studied 16 consecutive patients with diffuse cutaneous scleroderma and performed standard noninvasive clinical and electrocardiographic procedures for the detection of cardiovascular autonomic insufficiency. Cardiovascular autonomic insufficiency did not appear to be a significant feature of scleroderma. Dessein and Gledhill [262] also studied cardiovascular autonomic function in eight patients with scleroderma compared with healthy volunteers matched by age, sex, and race. Six of the eight patients had abnormal values for one or more of the ANS tests performed; autonomic involvement was "severe" in four of the six patients. In 1992, Dessein and colleagues [169] further evaluated autonomic function in 34 patients with scleroderma using five noninvasive cardiovascular autonomic function tests as well as sequential plasma catecholamine estimations at rest during standing and during sustained handgrip. Autonomic testing in these patients revealed autonomic dysfunction in each patient, while neurologic symptoms were present in 33 of the 34 patients. They concluded that ANS dysfunction is extremely common in scleroderma, characterized by parasympathetic impairment and marked sympathetic overactivity. Heart rate variability (HRV) is a noninvasive test used to assess the cardiac autonomic system. A study compared autonomic HRV parameters at rest and during activity in a population of patients with scleroderma compared to normal controls [263]. They showed a reduced vagal and increased sympathetic modulation at rest and a blunted autonomic response to orthostatic responses in comparison to controls. Twenty patients with scleroderma and ten age-, sex- and body mass index-matched healthy controls underwent assessment of autonomic nervous activity by ambulatory HRV using time and frequency domains [264]. The high frequencies measured by HRV, modulated mainly by parasympathetic system, were lower ($p = 0.003$) in patients than healthy controls (normalized HZ units: 30 [16–42] vs. 36.5 [24–44]). This suggested that sympathetic hyperactivity was due to reduction of parasympathetic activity in patients with scleroderma. Cardiopulmonary exercise testing showed a relationship between autonomic dysfunction as measured by HRV and decreased exercise tolerance in patients with scleroderma [265]. An assessment using body mass index and HRV measures observed a correlation between autonomic dysfunction and nutritional status in scleroderma, suggesting that poor nutrition can influence cardiac function [266].

Overall, these data suggest that an insult to the nervous system may be fundamental to the secondary dysfunction of specific organ systems in patients with scleroderma.

Summary

Systemic sclerosis is a complex human disease resulting in tissue fibrosis likely triggered by an inflammatory autoimmune process. Although Raynaud's phenomenon, skin sclerosis, and dysfunction of gastrointestinal, cardiopulmonary, and musculoskeletal systems are widely recognized clinical manifestations, several important clinical problems of this multisystem disease are often overlooked and result in significant morbidity. Awareness of these neglected manifestations, including oral, audiovestibular, thyroid, liver, lower urinary tract, erectile, bone necrosis, and neurological features, will help in the design of appropriate management strategies and hopefully improve clinical outcomes.

Acknowledgments The authors would like to thank Dr. Edward Lally for his contributions to this chapter in the second edition.

References

1. Veale BJ, Jablonski RY, Frech TM, Pauling JD. Orofacial manifestations of systemic sclerosis. Br Dent J. 2016;221(6):305–10.
2. Jung S, Martin T, Schmittbuhl M, Huck O. The spectrum of orofacial manifestations in systemic sclerosis: a challenging management. Oral Dis. 2017;23(4):424–39.
3. Hadj Said M, Foletti JM, Graillon N, Guyot L, Chossegros C. Orofacial manifestations of scleroderma. A literature review. Rev Stomatol Chir Maxillofac Chir Orale. 2016;117(5):322–6.
4. Isola G, Migliorati M, Dalessandri D, Matarese G. Systemic sclerosis: small mouth, big burden? Autoimmun Rev. 2018;17(3):323–4.
5. Smirani R, Truchetet ME, Poursac N, Naveau A, Schaeverbeke T, Devillard R. Impact of systemic sclerosis oral manifestations on patients' health-related quality of life: a systematic review. J Oral Pathol Med. 2018;47(9):808–15.
6. Basta F, Margiotta DPE, Mazzuca C, Batani V, Dolcini G, Moras P, et al. Factors related to alexithymia in patients with systemic sclerosis: a tight relationship with facial image dissatisfaction. Rheumatol Int. 2019;39(3):461–7.
7. van Lankveld WG, Vonk MC, Teunissen H, van den Hoogen FH. Appearance self-esteem in systemic sclerosis—subjective experience of skin deformity and its relationship with physician-assessed skin involvement, disease status and psychological variables. Rheumatology (Oxford). 2007;46(5):872–6.
8. Mouthon L, Rannou F, Bérezné A, Pagnoux C, Arène JP, Foïs E, et al. Development and validation of a scale for mouth handicap in systemic sclerosis: the Mouth Handicap in Systemic Sclerosis scale. Ann Rheum Dis. 2007;66(12):1651–5.
9. Marmary Y, Glaiss R, Pisanty S. Scleroderma: oral manifestations. Oral Surg Oral Med Oral Pathol. 1981;52(1):32–7.
10. Vitali C, Borghi E, Napoletano A, Polini F, Caronni M, Ammenti P, et al. Oropharyngolaryngeal disorders in scleroderma: development and validation of the SLS scale. Dysphagia. 2010;25(2):127–38.
11. Eversole LR, Jacobsen PL, Stone CE. Oral and gingival changes in systemic sclerosis (scleroderma). J Periodontol. 1984;55(3):175–8.
12. Poole JL, Brewer C, Rossie K, Good CC, Conte C, Steen V. Factors related to oral hygiene in persons with scleroderma. Int J Dent Hyg. 2005;3(1):13–7.

13. Naylor WP, Douglass CW, Mix E. The nonsurgical treatment of microstomia in scleroderma: a pilot study. Oral Surg Oral Med Oral Pathol. 1984;57(5):508–11.
14. Pizzo G, Scardina GA, Messina P. Effects of a nonsurgical exercise program on the decreased mouth opening in patients with systemic scleroderma. Clin Oral Investig. 2003;7(3):175–8.
15. Yuen HK, Marlow NM, Reed SG, Mahoney S, Summerlin LM, Leite R, et al. Effect of orofacial exercises on oral aperture in adults with systemic sclerosis. Disabil Rehabil. 2012;34(1):84–9.
16. Vitali C, Baldanzi C, Crispiatico V, Polini F, Ammenti P, Montesano A, et al. Effect of impairment-oriented and function-oriented exercises on mouth function in subjects with systemic sclerosis. Folia Phoniatr Logop. 2020;72(5):389–401.
17. Strong AL, Rubin JP, Kozlow JH, Cederna PS. Fat grafting for the treatment of scleroderma. Plast Reconstr Surg. 2019;144(6):1498–507.
18. Daumas A, Magalon J, Delaunay F, Abellan M, Philandrianos C, Sabatier F, et al. Fat grafting for treatment of facial scleroderma. Clin Plast Surg. 2020;47(1):155–63.
19. Blezien O, D'Andrea F, Nicoletti GF, Ferraro GA. Effects of fat grafting containing stem cells in microstomia and microcheilia derived from systemic sclerosis. Aesthet Plast Surg. 2017;41(4):839–44.
20. Gheisari M, Ahmadzadeh A, Nobari N, Iranmanesh B, Mozafari N. Autologous fat grafting in the treatment of facial scleroderma. Dermatol Res Pract. 2018;2018:6568016.
21. Almadori A, Griffin M, Ryan CM, Hunt DF, Hansen E, Kumar R, et al. Stem cell enriched lipotransfer reverses the effects of fibrosis in systemic sclerosis. PLoS One. 2019;14(7):e0218068.
22. Avouac J, Sordet C, Depinay C, Ardizonne M, Vacher-Lavenu MC, Sibilia J, et al. Systemic sclerosis-associated Sjogren's syndrome and relationship to the limited cutaneous subtype: results of a prospective study of sicca syndrome in 133 consecutive patients. Arthritis Rheum. 2006;54(7):2243–9.
23. Rout PG, Hamburger J, Potts AJ. Orofacial radiological manifestations of systemic sclerosis. Dentomaxillofac Radiol. 1996;25(4):193–6.
24. Wood RE, Lee P. Analysis of the oral manifestations of systemic sclerosis (scleroderma). Oral Surg Oral Med Oral Pathol. 1988;65(2):172–8.
25. Avouac J, Airo P, Dieude P, Caramaschi P, Tiev K, Diot E, et al. Associated autoimmune diseases in systemic sclerosis define a subset of patients with milder disease: results from 2 large cohorts of European Caucasian patients. J Rheumatol. 2010;37(3):608–14.
26. Drosos AA, Andonopoulos AP, Costopoulos JS, Stavropoulos ED, Papadimitriou CS, Moutsopoulos HM. Sjogren's syndrome in progressive systemic sclerosis. J Rheumatol. 1988;15(6):965–8.
27. Kobak S, Oksel F, Aksu K, Kabasakal Y. The frequency of sicca symptoms and Sjogren's syndrome in patients with systemic sclerosis. Int J Rheum Dis. 2013;16(1):88–92.
28. Hebbar M, Janin A, Huglo D, Copin MC, Lafyatis R, Devulder B, et al. Xerostomia in systemic sclerosis: systematic evaluation by salivary scintigraphy and lip biopsy in thirty-four patients. Arthritis Rheum. 1994;37(3):439–41.
29. Janin A, Gosselin B, Gosset D, Hatron PY, Sauvezie B. Histological criteria of Sjogren's syndrome in scleroderma. Clin Exp Rheumatol. 1989;7(2):167–9.
30. Kucuk U, Sarioglu S, Cetin P, Sari I, Birlik M. Histopathological differences between primary Sjogren's syndrome and Sjogren's syndrome accompanied by scleroderma. Indian J Pathol Microbiol. 2018;61(3):319–22.
31. Baron M, Hudson M, Tatibouet S, Steele R, Lo E, Gravel S, et al. Relationship between disease characteristics and orofacial manifestations in systemic sclerosis: Canadian Systemic Sclerosis Oral Health Study III. Arthritis Care Res. 2015;67(5):681–90.
32. Fischer DJ, Patton LL. Scleroderma: oral manifestations and treatment challenges. Spec Care Dentist. 2000;20(6):240–4.
33. Baron M, Hudson M, Tatibouet S, Steele R, Lo E, Gravel S, et al. The Canadian systemic sclerosis oral health study: orofacial manifestations and oral health-related quality of life in systemic sclerosis compared with the general population. Rheumatology. 2014;53(8):1386–94.
34. Baron M, Hudson M, Tatibouet S, Steele R, Lo E, Gravel S, et al. The Canadian systemic sclerosis oral health study II: the relationship between oral and global health-related quality of life in systemic sclerosis. Rheumatology. 2015;54(4):692–6.
35. Rowell NR, Hopper FE. The periodontal membrane in systemic sclerosis. Br J Dermatol. 1977;96(1):15–20.
36. Alexandridis C, White SC. Periodontal ligament changes in patients with progressive systemic sclerosis. Oral Surg Oral Med Oral Pathol. 1984;58(1):113–8.
37. Isola G, Williams RC, Lo Gullo A, Ramaglia L, Matarese M, Iorio-Siciliano V, et al. Risk association between scleroderma disease characteristics, periodontitis, and tooth loss. Clin Rheumatol. 2017;36(12):2733–41.
38. Gomes da Silva GS, Maymone de Melo ML, Leao JC, Carvalho AT, Porter S, Duarte A, et al. Oral features of systemic sclerosis: a case-control study. Oral Dis. 2019;25(8):1995–2002.
39. Pischon N, Hoedke D, Kurth S, Lee P, Dommisch H, Steinbrecher A, et al. Increased periodontal attachment loss in patients with systemic sclerosis. J Periodontol. 2016;87(7):763–71.
40. Iordache C, Antohe ME, Chirieac R, Ancuta E, Tanculescu O, Ancuta C. Volumetric cone beam computed tomography for the assessment of oral manifestations in systemic sclerosis: data from an EUSTAR cohort. J Clin Med. 2019;8(10):1620.
41. Crincoli V, Fatone L, Fanelli M, Rotolo RP, Chiala A, Favia G, et al. Orofacial manifestations and temporomandibular disorders of systemic scleroderma: an observational study. Int J Mol Sci. 2016;17(7):1189.
42. Burchfield C, Vorrasi J. Maxillofacial implications of scleroderma and systemic sclerosis: a case report and literature review. J Oral Maxillofac Surg. 2019;77(6):1203–8.
43. Baron M, Hudson M, Dagenais M, Macdonald D, Gyger G, El Sayegh T, et al. Relationship between disease characteristics and oral radiologic findings in systemic sclerosis: results from a Canadian Oral Health Study. Arthritis Care Res. 2016;68(5):673–80.
44. Gores RJ. Dental characteristics associated with acrosclerosis and diffuse scleroderma. J Am Dent Assoc. 1957;54(6):755–9.
45. Sha M, Griffin M, Denton CP, Butler PE. Sidestream Dark Field (SDF) imaging of oral microcirculation in the assessment of systemic sclerosis. Microvasc Res. 2019;126:103890.
46. Foundation S. Oral, facial and dental problems. 2020. https://www.scleroderma.org/site/SPageServer/?pagename=body_mouth#.X-ERDGhKh9M.
47. Yuen HK, Weng Y, Reed SG, Summerlin LM, Silver RM. Factors associated with gingival inflammation among adults with systemic sclerosis. Int J Dent Hyg. 2014;12(1):55–61.
48. Yuen HK, Weng Y, Bandyopadhyay D, Reed SG, Leite RS, Silver RM. Effect of a multi-faceted intervention on gingival health among adults with systemic sclerosis. Clin Exp Rheumatol. 2011;29(2 Suppl 65):S26–32.
49. Yuen HK, Hant FN, Hatfield C, Summerlin LM, Smith EA, Silver RM. Factors associated with oral hygiene practices among adults with systemic sclerosis. Int J Dent Hyg. 2014;12(3):180–6.
50. Gozde Turk A, Ulusoy M. A collapsible partial denture for a patient with limited mouth opening induced by scleroderma: a clinical report. J Prosthodont. 2015;24(4):334–8.
51. Zhang Y, Luo J, Zhang Y, Wu J. Rehabilitation for a scleroderma patient with severe microstomia using digital and conventional methods. J Am Dent Assoc. 2020;151(9):684–90.

52. Teasdall RD, Frayha RA, Shulman LE. Cranial nerve involvement in systemic sclerosis (scleroderma): a report of 10 cases. Medicine (Baltimore). 1980;59(2):149–59.
53. Berrettini S, Ferri C, Pitaro N, Bruschini P, Latorraca A, Sellari-Franceschini S, et al. Audiovestibular involvement in systemic sclerosis. ORL J Otorhinolaryngol Relat Spec. 1994;56(4):195–8.
54. Maciaszczyk K, Waszczykowska E, Pajor A, Bartkowiak-Dziankowska B, Durko T. Hearing organ disorders in patients with systemic sclerosis. Rheumatol Int. 2011;31(11):1423–8.
55. Monteiro TA, Christmann RB, Bonfa E, Bento RF, Novalo-Goto ES, Vasconcelos LG. Hearing loss in diffuse cutaneous systemic scleroderma. Scand J Rheumatol. 2011;40(6):467–71.
56. Amor-Dorado JC, Arias-Nunez MC, Miranda-Filloy JA, Gonzalez-Juanatey C, Llorca J, Gonzalez-Gay MA. Audiovestibular manifestations in patients with limited systemic sclerosis and centromere protein-B (CENP-B) antibodies. Medicine (Baltimore). 2008;87(3):131–41.
57. Silva MM, Araujo RPC, Araujo F, Valente JS, Corona AP. Hearing alterations in systemic sclerosis. Codas. 2019;31(1):e20170119.
58. Kastanioudakis I, Ziavra N, Politi EN, Exarchakos G, Drosos AA, Skevas A. Hearing loss in progressive systemic sclerosis patients: a comparative study. Otolaryngol Head Neck Surg. 2001;124(5):522–5.
59. Abou-Taleb A, Linthicum FH Jr. Scleroderma and hearing loss: (histopathology of a case). J Laryngol Otol. 1987;101(7):656–62.
60. Bassyouni IH, Emad Y, Rafaat HA, Dabbous AO. Relationship between nailfold capillary abnormalities and vestibular dysfunction in systemic sclerosis. Joint Bone Spine. 2011;78(3):266–9.
61. Shenavandeh S, Hashemi SB, Masoudi M, Nazarinia MA, Zare A. Hearing loss in patients with scleroderma: associations with clinical manifestations and capillaroscopy. Clin Rheumatol. 2018;37(9):2439–46.
62. Amor-Dorado JC, Barreira-Fernandez MP, Arias-Nunez MC, Gomez-Acebo I, Llorca J, Gonzalez-Gay MA. Benign paroxysmal positional vertigo and clinical test of sensory interaction and balance in systemic sclerosis. Otol Neurotol. 2008;29(8):1155–61.
63. Deroee AF, Huang TC, Morita N, Hojjati M. Sudden hearing loss as the presenting symptom of systemic sclerosis. Otol Neurotol. 2009;30(3):277–9.
64. Santarelli R, Scimemi P, Dal Monte E, Genovese E, Arslan E. Auditory neuropathy in systemic sclerosis: a speech perception and evoked potential study before and after cochlear implantation. Eur Arch Otorhinolaryngol. 2006;263(9):809–15.
65. Singh A, Kumar Irugu DV. Sudden sensorineural hearing loss—a contemporary review of management issues. J Otol. 2020;15(2):67–73.
66. Nicholson D, White S, Lipson A, Jacobs RP, Borenstein DG. Progressive systemic sclerosis and Graves' disease. Report of three cases. Arch Intern Med. 1986;146(12):2350–2.
67. Antonelli A, Fallahi P, Di Bari F, Giuggioli D, Ferrari SM, Ferri C. Fatigue in patients with systemic sclerosis and hypothyroidism. A review of the literature and report of our experience. Clin Exp Rheumatol. 2017;35 Suppl 106(4):193–7.
68. Nakamura T, Higashi S, Tomoda K, Tsukano M, Sugi K. Primary biliary cirrhosis (PBC)-CREST overlap syndrome with coexistence of Sjogren's syndrome and thyroid dysfunction. Clin Rheumatol. 2007;26(4):596–600.
69. Horita M, Takahashi N, Seike M, Nasu S, Takaki R. A case of primary biliary cirrhosis associated with Hashimoto's thyroiditis, scleroderma and Sjogren's syndrome. Intern Med. 1992;31(3):418–21.
70. D'Angelo WA, Fries JF, Masi AT, Shulman LE. Pathologic observations in systemic sclerosis (scleroderma). A study of fifty-eight autopsy cases and fifty-eight matched controls. Am J Med. 1969;46(3):428–40.
71. Gordon MB, Klein I, Dekker A, Rodnan GP, Medsger TA Jr. Thyroid disease in progressive systemic sclerosis: increased frequency of glandular fibrosis and hypothyroidism. Ann Intern Med. 1981;95(4):431–5.
72. Singh PK, Sharma SK, Sinha A, Dutta P. Can thyroid volume predict thyroid dysfunction in patients with systemic sclerosis? A prospective cross-sectional study from a tertiary care center in North West India. Clin Rheumatol. 2016;35(3):765–9.
73. Hudson M, Rojas-Villarraga A, Coral-Alvarado P, Lopez-Guzman S, Mantilla RD, Chalem P, et al. Polyautoimmunity and familial autoimmunity in systemic sclerosis. J Autoimmun. 2008;31(2):156–9.
74. Biro E, Szekanecz Z, Czirjak L, Danko K, Kiss E, Szabo NA, et al. Association of systemic and thyroid autoimmune diseases. Clin Rheumatol. 2006;25(2):240–5.
75. Akuka A, Watad A, Comaneshter D, Cohen AD, Amital H, Bragazzi NL. Systemic sclerosis patients are at higher risk of hyperthyroidism and have a worse survival than those without hyperthyroidism: A nationwide population-based cohort study. Eur J Clin Investig. 2019;49(12):e13177.
76. Toki S, Motegi S, Yamada K, Uchiyama A, Ishikawa O. Demographic and clinical features of autoimmune thyroid disorder in Japanese patients with systemic sclerosis. J Dermatol. 2014;41(12):1053–7.
77. Marasini B, Ferrari PA, Solaro N, Selmi C. Thyroid dysfunction in women with systemic sclerosis. Ann N Y Acad Sci. 2007;1108:305–11.
78. Antonelli A, Ferri C, Fallahi P, Cazzato M, Ferrari SM, Sebastiani M, et al. Clinical and subclinical autoimmune thyroid disorders in systemic sclerosis. Eur J Endocrinol. 2007;156(4):431–7.
79. Lippi G, Caramaschi P, Montagnana M, Salvagno GL, Volpe A, Guidi GC. Thyroid status in patients with systemic sclerosis. J Clin Rheumatol. 2006;12(6):322–4.
80. Innocencio RM, Romaldini JH, Ward LS. Thyroid autoantibodies in autoimmune diseases. Medicina (B Aires). 2004;64(3):227–30.
81. Kahl LE, Medsger TA Jr, Klein I. Prospective evaluation of thyroid function in patients with systemic sclerosis (scleroderma). J Rheumatol. 1986;13(1):103–7.
82. De Keyser L, Narhi DC, Furst DE, Huberman AK, Ross R, Clements J, et al. Thyroid dysfunction in a prospectively followed series of patients with progressive systemic sclerosis. J Endocrinol Investig. 1990;13(2):161–9.
83. Antonelli A, Fallahi P, Ferrari SM, Mancusi C, Giuggioli D, Colaci M, et al. Incidence of thyroid disorders in systemic sclerosis: results from a longitudinal follow-up. J Clin Endocrinol Metab. 2013;98(7):E1198–202.
84. Solanki KK, Al-Majmuei M, White DHN. High prevalence of antithyroid antibodies in a New Zealand cohort of patients with systemic sclerosis. J Clin Rheumatol. 2018;24(5):264–71.
85. Danielides S, Mavragani CP, Katsakoulas I, Zintzaras E, Drosos AA, Vlachoyiannopoulos PG, et al. Increased prevalence of antithyroid antibodies in patients with limited scleroderma. Scand J Rheumatol. 2011;40(4):299–303.
86. Triggianese P, Conigliaro P, Chimenti MS, Barbato C, Greco E, Kroegler B, et al. Systemic sclerosis: exploring the potential interplay between thyroid disorders and pregnancy outcome in an Italian cohort. Isr Med Assoc J. 2017;19(8):473–7.
87. Antonelli A, Ferri C, Ferrari SM, Di Domenicantonio A, Giuggioli D, Galleri D, et al. Increased risk of papillary thyroid cancer in systemic sclerosis associated with autoimmune thyroiditis. Rheumatology. 2016;55(3):480–4.
88. Fallahi P, Ruffilli I, Giuggioli D, Colaci M, Ferrari SM, Antonelli A, et al. Associations between systemic sclerosis and thyroid diseases. Front Endocrinol (Lausanne). 2017;8:266.

89. Bartholomew LG, Cain JC, Winkelmann RK, Baggenstoss AH. Chronic disease of the liver associated with systemic scleroderma. Am J Dig Dis. 1964;9:43–55.
90. Robinson D Jr, Eisenberg D, Nietert PJ, Doyle M, Bala M, Paramore C, et al. Systemic sclerosis prevalence and comorbidities in the US, 2001–2002. Curr Med Res Opin. 2008;24(4):1157–66.
91. Lee SW, Kim BK, Park JY, Kim DY, Ahn SH, Song JJ, et al. Disease duration and Medsger's severity score are associated with significant liver fibrosis in patients with systemic sclerosis. Clin Exp Rheumatol. 2015;33(4 Suppl 91):S68–74.
92. Tiosano S, Cohen AD, Amital H. The association between hepatitis B, hepatitis C and systemic sclerosis: a cross-sectional study. Curr Opin Rheumatol. 2019;31(5):493–8.
93. McMahon RF, Babbs C, Warnes TW. Nodular regenerative hyperplasia of the liver, CREST syndrome and primary biliary cirrhosis: an overlap syndrome? Gut. 1989;30(10):1430–3.
94. Efe C, Ozaslan E, Nasiroglu N, Tunca H, Purnak T, Altiparmak E. The development of autoimmune hepatitis and primary biliary cirrhosis overlap syndrome during the course of connective tissue diseases: report of three cases and review of the literature. Dig Dis Sci. 2010;55(8):2417–21.
95. Mari-Alfonso B, Simeon-Aznar CP, Guillen-Del Castillo A, Rubio-Rivas M, Trapiella-Martinez L, Todoli-Parra JA, et al. Hepatobiliary involvement in systemic sclerosis and the cutaneous subsets: characteristics and survival of patients from the Spanish RESCLE Registry. Semin Arthritis Rheum. 2018;47(6):849–57.
96. Skare TL, Nisihara RM, Haider O, Azevedo PM, Utiyama SR. Liver autoantibodies in patients with scleroderma. Clin Rheumatol. 2011;30(1):129–32.
97. Lleo A, Leung PSC, Hirschfield GM, Gershwin EM. The pathogenesis of primary biliary cholangitis: a comprehensive review. Semin Liver Dis. 2020;40(1):34–48.
98. Reynolds TB, Denison EK, Frankl HD, Lieberman FL, Peters RL. Primary biliary cirrhosis with scleroderma, Raynaud's phenomenon and telangiectasia. New syndrome. Am J Med. 1971;50(3):302–12.
99. Assassi S, Fritzler MJ, Arnett FC, Norman GL, Shah KR, Gourh P, et al. Primary biliary cirrhosis (PBC), PBC autoantibodies, and hepatic parameter abnormalities in a large population of systemic sclerosis patients. J Rheumatol. 2009;36(10):2250–6.
100. Jacobsen S, Halberg P, Ullman S, Van Venrooij WJ, Hoier-Madsen M, Wiik A, et al. Clinical features and serum antinuclear antibodies in 230 Danish patients with systemic sclerosis. Br J Rheumatol. 1998;37(1):39–45.
101. Rigamonti C, Shand LM, Feudjo M, Bunn CC, Black CM, Denton CP, et al. Clinical features and prognosis of primary biliary cirrhosis associated with systemic sclerosis. Gut. 2006;55(3):388–94.
102. Floreani A, Franceschet I, Cazzagon N, Spinazze A, Buja A, Furlan P, et al. Extrahepatic autoimmune conditions associated with primary biliary cirrhosis. Clin Rev Allergy Immunol. 2015;48(2–3):192–7.
103. Powell FC, Schroeter AL, Dickson ER. Primary biliary cirrhosis and the CREST syndrome: a report of 22 cases. Q J Med. 1987;62(237):75–82.
104. Watt FE, James OF, Jones DE. Patterns of autoimmunity in primary biliary cirrhosis patients and their families: a population-based cohort study. QJM. 2004;97(7):397–406.
105. Abraham S, Begum S, Isenberg D. Hepatic manifestations of autoimmune rheumatic diseases. Ann Rheum Dis. 2004;63(2):123–9.
106. Zheng B, Vincent C, Fritzler MJ, Senecal JL, Koenig M, Joyal F. Prevalence of systemic sclerosis in primary biliary cholangitis using the new ACR/EULAR classification criteria. J Rheumatol. 2017;44(1):33–9.
107. Chalifoux SL, Konyn PG, Choi G, Saab S. Extrahepatic manifestations of primary biliary cholangitis. Gut Liver. 2017;11(6):771–80.
108. Bali G, Szilvasi A, Inotai D, Varga A, Sardy M, Karpati S, et al. Comorbidity of localized scleroderma and primary biliary cholangitis. J Dtsch Dermatol Ges. 2018;16(11):1323–7.
109. Akimoto S, Ishikawa O, Takagi H, Miyachi Y. Immunological features of patients with primary biliary cirrhosis (PBC) overlapping systemic sclerosis: a comparison with patients with PBC alone. J Gastroenterol Hepatol. 1998;13(9):897–901.
110. Akimoto S, Ishikawa O, Muro Y, Takagi H, Tamura T, Miyachi Y. Clinical and immunological characterization of patients with systemic sclerosis overlapping primary biliary cirrhosis: a comparison with patients with systemic sclerosis alone. J Dermatol. 1999;26(1):18–22.
111. Agmon-Levin N, Shapira Y, Selmi C, Barzilai O, Ram M, Szyper-Kravitz M, et al. A comprehensive evaluation of serum autoantibodies in primary biliary cirrhosis. J Autoimmun. 2010;34(1):55–8.
112. Nakamura M, Kondo H, Mori T, Komori A, Matsuyama M, Ito M, et al. Anti-gp210 and anti-centromere antibodies are different risk factors for the progression of primary biliary cirrhosis. Hepatology. 2007;45(1):118–27.
113. Gao L, Tian X, Liu B, Zhang F. The value of antinuclear antibodies in primary biliary cirrhosis. Clin Exp Med. 2008;8(1):9–15.
114. Liberal R, Grant CR, Sakkas L, Bizzaro N, Bogdanos DP. Diagnostic and clinical significance of anti-centromere antibodies in primary biliary cirrhosis. Clin Res Hepatol Gastroenterol. 2013;37(6):572–85.
115. Gupta RC, Seibold JR, Krishnan MR, Steigerwald JC. Precipitating autoantibodies to mitochondrial proteins in progressive systemic sclerosis. Clin Exp Immunol. 1984;58(1):68–76.
116. Norman GL, Bialek A, Encabo S, Butkiewicz B, Wiechowska-Kozlowska A, Brzosko M, et al. Is prevalence of PBC underestimated in patients with systemic sclerosis? Dig Liver Dis. 2009;41(10):762–4.
117. Pope JE, Thompson A. Antimitochondrial antibodies and their significance in diffuse and limited scleroderma. J Clin Rheumatol. 1999;5(4):206–9.
118. Sakauchi F, Mori M, Zeniya M, Toda G. Antimitochondrial antibody negative primary biliary cirrhosis in Japan: utilization of clinical data when patients applied to receive public financial aid. J Epidemiol. 2006;16(1):30–4.
119. Zuchner D, Sternsdorf T, Szostecki C, Heathcote EJ, Cauch-Dudek K, Will H. Prevalence, kinetics, and therapeutic modulation of autoantibodies against Sp100 and promyelocytic leukemia protein in a large cohort of patients with primary biliary cirrhosis. Hepatology. 1997;26(5):1123–30.
120. Goulis J, Leandro G, Burroughs AK. Randomised controlled trials of ursodeoxycholic-acid therapy for primary biliary cirrhosis: a meta-analysis. Lancet. 1999;354(9184):1053–60.
121. Floreani A, Caroli D, Variola A, Rizzotto ER, Antoniazzi S, Chiaramonte M, et al. A 35-year follow-up of a large cohort of patients with primary biliary cirrhosis seen at a single centre. Liver Int. 2011;31(3):361–8.
122. Jones DE, Al-Rifai A, Frith J, Patanwala I, Newton JL. The independent effects of fatigue and UDCA therapy on mortality in primary biliary cirrhosis: results of a 9 year follow-up. J Hepatol. 2010;53(5):911–7.
123. Nishio A, Neuberger J, Gershwin ME. Management of patients with primary biliary cirrhosis: a practical guide. BioDrugs. 1999;12(3):159–73.
124. Shah RA, Kowdley KV. Current and potential treatments for primary biliary cholangitis. Lancet Gastroenterol Hepatol. 2020;5(3):306–15.
125. Kojima H, Uemura M, Sakurai S, Ann T, Ishii Y, Imazu H, et al. Clinical features of liver disturbance in rheumatoid diseases: clinicopathological study with special reference to the cause of liver disturbance. J Gastroenterol. 2002;37(8):617–25.

126. Shah AA, Wigley FM. Often forgotten manifestations of systemic sclerosis. Rheum Dis Clin N Am. 2008;34(1):221–38; ix.
127. Ishikawa M, Okada J, Shibuya A, Kondo H. CRST syndrome (calcinosis cutis, Raynaud's phenomenon, sclerodactyly, and telangiectasia) associated with autoimmune hepatitis. Intern Med. 1995;34(1):6–9.
128. Marie I, Levesque H, Tranvouez JL, Francois A, Riachi G, Cailleux N, et al. Autoimmune hepatitis and systemic sclerosis: a new overlap syndrome? Rheumatology. 2001;40(1):102–6.
129. Yabe H, Noma K, Tada N, Mochizuki S, Nagano M. A case of CREST syndrome with rapidly progressive liver damage. Intern Med. 1992;31(1):69–73.
130. West M, Jasin HE, Medhekar S. The development of connective tissue diseases in patients with autoimmune hepatitis: a case series. Semin Arthritis Rheum. 2006;35(6):344–8.
131. Friedman LS, Gee MS, Misdraji J. Case records of the Massachusetts General Hospital. Case 39-2010. A 19-year-old woman with nausea, jaundice, and pruritus. N Engl J Med. 2010;363(26):2548–57.
132. Perez Ruiz F, Orte Martinez FJ, Zea Mendoza AC, Ruiz del Arbol L, Moreno Caparros A. Nodular regenerative hyperplasia of the liver in rheumatic diseases: report of seven cases and review of the literature. Semin Arthritis Rheum. 1991;21(1):47–54.
133. Assandri R, Monari M, Montanelli A. Development of systemic sclerosis in patients with autoimmune hepatitis: an emerging overlap syndrome. Gastroenterol Hepatol Bed Bench. 2016;9(3):211–9.
134. Kaburaki J, Kuramochi S, Fujii T, Kuwana M, Tojo T, Ikeda Y, et al. Nodular regenerative hyperplasia of the liver in a patient with systemic sclerosis. Clin Rheumatol. 1996;15(6):613–6.
135. Graf L, Dobrota R, Jordan S, Wildi LM, Distler O, Maurer B. Nodular regenerative hyperplasia of the liver: a rare vascular complication in systemic sclerosis. J Rheumatol. 2018;45(1):103–6.
136. Fraile G, Rodriguez-Garcia JL, Moreno A. Primary sclerosing cholangitis associated with systemic sclerosis. Postgrad Med J. 1991;67(784):189–92.
137. Moschos J, Leontiadis GI, Kelly C, Henry J, Kadis S. Idiopathic portal hypertension complicating systemic sclerosis: a case report. BMC Gastroenterol. 2005;5:16.
138. Kogawa H, Migita K, Ito M, Takii Y, Daikoku M, Nakao M, et al. Idiopathic portal hypertension associated with systemic sclerosis and Sjogren's syndrome. Clin Rheumatol. 2005;24(5):544–7.
139. John G, Allanore Y, Polito P, Piantoni S, Fredi M, Avouac J, et al. The limited cutaneous form of systemic sclerosis is associated with urinary incontinence: an international multicentre study. Rheumatology. 2017;56(11):1874–83.
140. John G, Avouac J, Piantoni S, Polito P, Fredi M, Cozzi F, et al. Prevalence and disease-specific risk factors for lower urinary tract symptoms in systemic sclerosis: an international multicenter study. Arthritis Care Res. 2018;70(8):1218–27.
141. Umar SB, Griffing L, Garcia H, Foxx-Orenstein AE, DiBaise JK, Crowell MD. The impact of pelvic floor and lower gastrointestinal symptoms on quality of life in women with systemic sclerosis. J Clin Gastroenterol. 2016;50(6):e55–9.
142. Kucharz EJ, Jonderko G, Rubisz-Brzezinska J, Konca A, Jarczyk R. Premictional volume and contractility of the urinary bladder in patients with systemic sclerosis. Clin Rheumatol. 1996;15(2):118–20.
143. Pacini G, Paolino S, C Trombetta A, Goegan F, Pizzorni C, Alessandri E, et al. Lower urinary tract symptoms in systemic sclerosis: a detailed investigation. Rheumatology. 2020;59(6):1315–24.
144. Raz S, Boxer R, Waisman J, Sukov RJ. Scleroderma of lower urinary tract. Urology. 1977;9(6):682–3.
145. Lally EV, Kaplan SR, Susset JG, Trebbin WM, Klutz WS, Cohen SI. Pathologic involvement of the urinary bladder in progressive systemic sclerosis. J Rheumatol. 1985;12(4):778–81.
146. Minervini R, Morelli G, Minervini A, Pampaloni S, Tognetti A, Fiorentini L, et al. Bladder involvement in systemic sclerosis: urodynamic and histological evaluation in 23 patients. Eur Urol. 1998;34(1):47–52.
147. Lazzeri M, Beneforti P, Benaim G, Corsi C, Ciambrone V, Marrapodi E, et al. Vesical dysfunction in systemic sclerosis (scleroderma). J Urol. 1995;153(4):1184–7.
148. La Civita L, Fiorentini L, Tognetti A, Pasero G, Ferri C. Severe urinary bladder involvement in systemic sclerosis. Case report and review of the literature. Clin Exp Rheumatol. 1998;16(5):591–3.
149. De Luca A, Terrone C, Tirri E, Rossetti SR, Valentini G. Vesical telangiectasias as a cause of macroscopic hematuria in systemic sclerosis. Clin Exp Rheumatol. 2001;19(1):93–4.
150. Siegert E, March C, Otten L, Makowka A, Preis E, Buttgereit F, et al. Prevalence of sarcopenia in systemic sclerosis: assessing body composition and functional disability in patients with systemic sclerosis. Nutrition. 2018;55–56:51–5.
151. Caimmi C, Caramaschi P, Venturini A, Bertoldo E, Vantaggiato E, Viapiana O, et al. Malnutrition and sarcopenia in a large cohort of patients with systemic sclerosis. Clin Rheumatol. 2018;37(4):987–97.
152. Corallo C, Fioravanti A, Tenti S, Pecetti G, Nuti R, Giordano N. Sarcopenia in systemic sclerosis: the impact of nutritional, clinical, and laboratory features. Rheumatol Int. 2019;39(10):1767–75.
153. Kumar S, Singh J, Kedika R, Mendoza F, Jimenez SA, Blomain ES, et al. Role of muscarinic-3 receptor antibody in systemic sclerosis: correlation with disease duration and effects of IVIG. Am J Physiol Gastrointest Liver Physiol. 2016;310(11):G1052–60.
154. John G. Systemic sclerosis and urinary symptoms: a complex pathophysiology. Clin Rheumatol. 2020;39(1):5–8.
155. Vaughan CP, Markland AD. Urinary incontinence in women. Ann Intern Med. 2020;172(3):ITC17–32.
156. Lally EV, Jimenez SA. Impotence in progressively systemic sclerosis. Ann Intern Med. 1981;95(2):150–3.
157. Nowlin NS, Brick JE, Weaver DJ, Wilson DA, Judd HL, Lu JK, et al. Impotence in scleroderma. Ann Intern Med. 1986;104(6):794–8.
158. Klein LE, Posner MS. Progressive systemic sclerosis and impotence. Ann Intern Med. 1981;95(5):658–9.
159. Sukenik S, Abarbanel JM, Buskila D, Potashnik G, Horowitz J. Impotence, carpal tunnel syndrome and peripheral neuropathy as presenting symptoms in progressive systemic sclerosis. J Rheumatol. 1987;14(3):641–3.
160. Rossman B, Zorgniotti AW. Progressive systemic sclerosis (scleroderma) and impotence. Urology. 1989;33(3):189–92.
161. Hong P, Pope JE, Ouimet JM, Rullan E, Seibold JR. Erectile dysfunction associated with scleroderma: a case-control study of men with scleroderma and rheumatoid arthritis. J Rheumatol. 2004;31(3):508–13.
162. Foocharoen C, Tyndall A, Hachulla E, Rosato E, Allanore Y, Farge-Bancel D, et al. Erectile dysfunction is frequent in systemic sclerosis and associated with severe disease: a study of the EULAR Scleroderma Trial and Research group. Arthritis Res Ther. 2012;14(1):R37.
163. Rosato E, Aversa A, Molinaro I, Pisarri S, Spera G, Salsano F. Erectile dysfunction of sclerodermic patients correlates with digital vascular damage. Eur J Intern Med. 2011;22(3):318–21.
164. Rosato E, Barbano B, Gigante A, Aversa A, Cianci R, Molinaro I, et al. Erectile dysfunction, endothelium dysfunction, and microvascular damage in patients with systemic sclerosis. J Sex Med. 2013;10(5):1380–8.
165. Keck AD, Foocharoen C, Rosato E, Smith V, Allanore Y, Distler O, et al. Nailfold capillary abnormalities in erectile dysfunction

of systemic sclerosis: a EUSTAR group analysis. Rheumatology. 2014;53(4):639–43.
166. Bivalacqua TJ, Usta MF, Champion HC, Kadowitz PJ, Hellstrom WJ. Endothelial dysfunction in erectile dysfunction: role of the endothelium in erectile physiology and disease. J Androl. 2003;24(6 Suppl):S17–37.
167. Burnett AL. Metabolic syndrome, endothelial dysfunction, and erectile dysfunction: association and management. Curr Urol Rep. 2005;6(6):470–5.
168. Nehra A, Hall SJ, Basile G, Bertero EB, Moreland R, Toselli P, et al. Systemic sclerosis and impotence: a clinicopathological correlation. J Urol. 1995;153(4):1140–6.
169. Dessein PH, Joffe BI, Metz RM, Millar DL, Lawson M, Stanwix AE. Autonomic dysfunction in systemic sclerosis: sympathetic overactivity and instability. Am J Med. 1992;93(2):143–50.
170. Morelli S, Piccirillo G, Fimognari F, Sgreccia A, Ferrante L, Morabito G, et al. Twenty-four hour heart period variability in systemic sclerosis. J Rheumatol. 1996;23(4):643–5.
171. Malandrini A, Selvi E, Villanova M, Berti G, Sabadini L, Salvadori C, et al. Autonomic nervous system and smooth muscle cell involvement in systemic sclerosis: ultrastructural study of 3 cases. J Rheumatol. 2000;27(5):1203–6.
172. Aversa A, Proietti M, Bruzziches R, Salsano F, Spera G. The penile vasculature in systemic sclerosis: a duplex ultrasound study. J Sex Med. 2006;3(3):554–8.
173. Granchi S, Vannelli GB, Vignozzi L, Crescioli C, Ferruzzi P, Mancina R, et al. Expression and regulation of endothelin-1 and its receptors in human penile smooth muscle cells. Mol Hum Reprod. 2002;8(12):1053–64.
174. Varga J, Lally E, Jimenez S. Endocrinopathy and other visceral organ involvement in progressive systemic sclerosis. Systemic sclerosis: scleroderma. New York: Wiley; 1988. p. 267–78.
175. Aversa A, Basciani S, Visca P, Arizzi M, Gnessi L, Frajese G, et al. Platelet-derived growth factor (PDGF) and PDGF receptors in rat corpus cavernosum: changes in expression after transient in vivo hypoxia. J Endocrinol. 2001;170(2):395–402.
176. Faller DV. Endothelial cell responses to hypoxic stress. Clin Exp Pharmacol Physiol. 1999;26(1):74–84.
177. Walker UA, Tyndall A, Ruszat R. Erectile dysfunction in systemic sclerosis. Ann Rheum Dis. 2009;68(7):1083–5.
178. Aversa A, Bruzziches R, Francomano D, Rosato E, Salsano F, Spera G. Penile involvement in systemic sclerosis: new diagnostic and therapeutic aspects. Int J Rheumatol. 2010;2010:708067.
179. Proietti M, Aversa A, Letizia C, Rossi C, Menghi G, Bruzziches R, et al. Erectile dysfunction in systemic sclerosis: effects of long-term inhibition of phosphodiesterase type-5 on erectile function and plasma endothelin-1 levels. J Rheumatol. 2007;34(8):1712–7.
180. Aversa A, Caprio M, Rosano GM, Spera G. Endothelial effects of drugs designed to treat erectile dysfunction. Curr Pharm Des. 2008;14(35):3768–78.
181. Jaeger VK, Walker UA. Erectile dysfunction in systemic sclerosis. Curr Rheumatol Rep. 2016;18(8):49.
182. Rosen RC, Cappelleri JC, Smith MD, Lipsky J, Pena BM. Development and evaluation of an abridged, 5-item version of the International Index of Erectile Function (IIEF-5) as a diagnostic tool for erectile dysfunction. Int J Impot Res. 1999;11(6):319–26.
183. Rennie C, Britton J, Prouse P. Bilateral avascular necrosis of the lunate in a patient with severe Raynaud's phenomenon and scleroderma. J Clin Rheumatol. 1999;5(3):165–8.
184. Matsumoto AK, Moore R, Alli P, Wigley FM. Three cases of osteonecrosis of the lunate bone of the wrist in scleroderma. Clin Exp Rheumatol. 1999;17(6):730–2.
185. Agus B. Bilateral aseptic necrosis of the lunate in systemic sclerosis. Clin Exp Rheumatol. 1987;5(2):155–7.
186. Kawai H, Tsuyuguchi Y, Yonenobu K, Inoue A, Tada K. Avascular necrosis of the carpal scaphoid associated with progressive systemic sclerosis. Hand. 1983;15(3):270–3.
187. Frerix M, Kroger K, Szalay G, Muller-Ladner U, Tarner IH. Is osteonecrosis of the lunate bone an underestimated feature of systemic sclerosis? A case series of nine patients and review of literature. Semin Arthritis Rheum. 2016;45(4):446–54.
188. Zegarra-Mondragon S, Llop-Vilaltella M, Sifuentes-Giraldo WA, de la Puente Bujidos C. Osteonecrosis of the lunate associated with systemic sclerosis: report of 4 cases. Reumatol Clin. 2019;15(5):e70–1.
189. Akbayrak E, Dinser R, Muller-Ladner U, Tarner IH. Low-field magnetic resonance imaging study on carpal arthritis in systemic sclerosis—low-grade erosive arthritis of carpal bones is an unexpected and frequent disease manifestation. Arthritis Res Ther. 2013;15(1):R2.
190. Leinwand I, Duryee AW, Richter MN. Scleroderma; based on a study of over 150 cases. Ann Intern Med. 1954;41(5):1003–41.
191. Piper WN, Helwig EB. Progressive systemic sclerosis; visceral manifestations in generalized scleroderma. AMA Arch Derm. 1955;72(6):535–46.
192. Tuffanelli DL, Winkelmann RK. Systemic scleroderma, A clinical study of 727 cases. Arch Dermatol. 1961;84:359–71.
193. Gordon RM, Silverstein A. Neurologic manifstations in progressive systemic sclerosis. Arch Neurol. 1970;22(2):126–34.
194. Lee P, Bruni J, Sukenik S. Neurological manifestations in systemic sclerosis (scleroderma). J Rheumatol. 1984;11(4):480–3.
195. Amaral TN, Peres FA, Lapa AT, Marques-Neto JF, Appenzeller S. Neurologic involvement in scleroderma: a systematic review. Semin Arthritis Rheum. 2013;43(3):335–47.
196. Beighton P, Gumpel JM, Cornes NG. Prodromal trigeminal sensory neuropathy in progressive systemic sclerosis. Ann Rheum Dis. 1968;27(4):367–9.
197. Ashworth B, Tait GB. Trigeminal neuropathy in connective tissue disease. Neurology. 1971;21(6):609–14.
198. Farrell DA, Medsger TA Jr. Trigeminal neuropathy in progressive systemic sclerosis. Am J Med. 1982;73(1):57–62.
199. Miguel D, Darr-Foit S, Tittelbach J, Elsner P. Trigeminal neuropathy responding to systemic corticosteroids and methotrexate in a patient with diffuse cutaneous systemic sclerosis. Eur J Dermatol. 2017;27(1):82–3.
200. Lee JE, Haynes JM. Carotid arteritis and cerebral infarction due to scleroderma. Neurology. 1967;17(1):18–22.
201. Estey E, Lieberman A, Pinto R, Meltzer M, Ransohoff J. Cerebral arteritis in scleroderma. Stroke. 1979;10(5):595–7.
202. Abers MS, Iluonakhamhe EK, Goldsmith CE, Kass JS. Central nervous system vasculitis secondary to systemic sclerosis. J Clin Neurosci. 2013;20(8):1168–70.
203. Wise TN, Ginzler EM. Scleroderma cerebritis, an unusual manifestation of progressive systemic sclerosis. Dis Nerv Syst. 1975;36(2):60–2.
204. Heron E, Fornes P, Rance A, Emmerich J, Bayle O, Fiessinger JN. Brain involvement in scleroderma: two autopsy cases. Stroke. 1998;29(3):719–21.
205. Heron E, Hernigou A, Chatellier G, Fornes P, Emmerich J, Fiessinger JN. Intracerebral calcification in systemic sclerosis. Stroke. 1999;30(10):2183–5.
206. Sardanelli F, Iozzelli A, Cotticelli B, Losacco C, Cutolo M, Sulli A, et al. White matter hyperintensities on brain magnetic resonance in systemic sclerosis. Ann Rheum Dis. 2005;64(5):777–9.
207. Terrier B, Charbonneau F, Touze E, Berezne A, Pagnoux C, Silvera S, et al. Cerebral vasculopathy is associated with severe vascular manifestations in systemic sclerosis. J Rheumatol. 2009;36(7):1486–94.
208. Mohammed RH, Sabry YY, Nasef AA. Brain MRI screening showing evidences of early central nervous system involve-

ment in patients with systemic sclerosis. Rheumatol Int. 2011;31(5):667–71.
209. Gamal RM, Abozaid HSM, Zidan M, Abdelmegid MAF, Abdel-Razek MR, Alsayed SA, et al. Study of MRI brain findings and carotid US features in systemic sclerosis patients, relationship with disease parameters. Arthritis Res Ther. 2019;21(1):95.
210. Au K, Singh MK, Bodukam V, Bae S, Maranian P, Ogawa R, et al. Atherosclerosis in systemic sclerosis: a systematic review and meta-analysis. Arthritis Rheum. 2011;63(7):2078–90.
211. Sedky Abdou MM, El Desouky SM, Helmy El Kaffas KM, Ahmed Hassan AM. Premature atherosclerosis in systemic sclerosis patients: its relation to disease parameters and to traditional risk factors. Int J Rheum Dis. 2017;20(3):383–9.
212. Schiopu E, Au KM, McMahon MA, Kaplan MJ, Divekar A, Singh RR, et al. Prevalence of subclinical atherosclerosis is increased in systemic sclerosis and is associated with serum proteins: a cross-sectional, controlled study of carotid ultrasound. Rheumatology. 2014;53(4):704–13.
213. Dimitroulas T, Baniotopoulos P, Pagkopoulou E, Soulaidopoulos S, Nightingale P, Sandoo A, et al. Subclinical atherosclerosis in systemic sclerosis and rheumatoid arthritis: a comparative matched-cohort study. Rheumatol Int. 2020;40(12):1997–2004.
214. Ozen G, Inanc N, Unal AU, Korkmaz F, Sunbul M, Ozmen M, et al. Subclinical atherosclerosis in systemic sclerosis: not less frequent than rheumatoid arthritis and not detected with cardiovascular risk indices. Arthritis Care Res. 2016;68(10):1538–46.
215. Ungprasert P, Sanguankeo A, Upala S. Risk of ischemic stroke in patients with systemic sclerosis: a systematic review and meta-analysis. Mod Rheumatol. 2016;26(1):128–31.
216. Maclean H, Guthrie W. Retinopathy in scleroderma. Trans Ophthalmol Soc U K. 1970;89:209–20.
217. Farkas TG, Sylvester V, Archer D. The choroidopathy of progressive systemic sclerosis (scleroderma). Am J Ophthalmol. 1972;74(5):875–86.
218. Grennan DM, Forrester J. Involvement of the eye in SLE and scleroderma. A study using fluorescein angiography in addition to clinical ophthalmic assessment. Ann Rheum Dis. 1977;36(2):152–6.
219. Alarcon-Segovia D, Ibanez G, Hernandez-Ortiz J, Velazquez-Forero F, Gonzalez-Jimenez Y. Sjogren's syndrome in progressive systemic sclerosis (scleroderma). Am J Med. 1974;57(1):78–85.
220. Ashton N, Coomes EN, Garner A, Oliver DO. Retinopathy due to progressive systemic sclerosis. J Pathol Bacteriol. 1968;96(2):259–68.
221. Kraus A, Guerra-Bautista G, Espinoza G, Barojas E, Quiroz-Mercado H, Sanchez-Echeverri G, et al. Defects of the retinal pigment epithelium in scleroderma. Br J Rheumatol. 1991;30(2):112–4.
222. Littlejohn GO, Urowitz MB, Pavlin CJ. Central retinal vein occlusion and scleroderma: implications for sclerodermatous vascular disease. Ann Rheum Dis. 1981;40(1):96–9.
223. Ranjbar M, Rothe M, Klapa S, Lange T, Prasuhn M, Grisanti S, et al. Evaluation of choroidal substructure perfusion in patients affected by systemic sclerosis: an optical coherence tomography angiography study. Scand J Rheumatol. 2020;49(2):141–5.
224. Kreps EO, Carton C, Cutolo M, Cutolo CA, Vanhaecke A, Leroy BP, et al. Ocular involvement in systemic sclerosis: a systematic literature review, it's not all scleroderma that meets the eye. Semin Arthritis Rheum. 2019;49(1):119–25.
225. Goldberg NC, Duncan SC, Winkelmann RK. Migraine and systemic scleroderma. Arch Dermatol. 1978;114(4):550–1.
226. Pal B, Gibson C, Passmore J, Griffiths ID, Dick WC. A study of headaches and migraine in Sjogren's syndrome and other rheumatic disorders. Ann Rheum Dis. 1989;48(4):312–6.
227. Alonso-Ruiz A, Leiva-Santana C. Carpal tunnel syndrome in scleroderma-like syndromes. J Rheumatol. 1985;12(5):1030.
228. Machet L, Vaillant L, Machet MC, Esteve E, Muller C, Khallouf R, et al. Carpal tunnel syndrome and systemic sclerosis. Dermatology. 1992;185(2):101–3.
229. Bandinelli F, Kaloudi O, Candelieri A, Conforti ML, Casale R, Cammarata S, et al. Early detection of median nerve syndrome at the carpal tunnel with high-resolution 18 MHz ultrasonography in systemic sclerosis patients. Clin Exp Rheumatol. 2010;28(5 Suppl 62):S15–8.
230. Mondelli M, Romano C, Della Porta PD, Rossi A. Electrophysiological evidence of "nerve entrapment syndromes" and subclinical peripheral neuropathy in progressive systemic sclerosis (scleroderma). J Neurol. 1995;242(4):185–94.
231. Cuzdan N, Turk I, Sarpel T, Erken E, Alparslan ZN. Neuropathic pain: is it an underestimated symptom in systemic sclerosis? Clin Rheumatol. 2018;37(7):1845–51.
232. Richter RB. Peripheral neuropathy and connective tissue disease. J Neuropathol Exp Neurol. 1954;13(1):168–80.
233. Pawlowski A. The nerve network of the skin in diffuse scleroderma and clinically similar conditions. Arch Dermatol. 1963;88:868–73.
234. Fleischmajer R, Perlish JS, Reeves JR. Cellular infiltrates in scleroderma skin. Arthritis Rheum. 1977;20(4):975–84.
235. Christopher RP, Robinson H. Studies of nerve conduction in patients with scleroderma. South Med J. 1972;65(6):668–72.
236. Poncelet AN, Connolly MK. Peripheral neuropathy in scleroderma. Muscle Nerve. 2003;28(3):330–5.
237. Paik JJ, Mammen AL, Wigley FM, Shah AA, Hummers LK, Polydefkis M. Symptomatic and electrodiagnostic features of peripheral neuropathy in scleroderma. Arthritis Care Res. 2016;68(8):1150–7.
238. Frech TM, Smith G, Reily M, Chamberlain J, Murtaugh MA, Penrod J, et al. Peripheral neuropathy: a complication of systemic sclerosis. Clin Rheumatol. 2013;32(6):885–8.
239. Dahlgaard T, Nielsen VK, Kristensen JK. Vibratory perception in patients with generalized scleroderma. Acta Derm Venereol. 1980;60(2):119–22.
240. Adler BL, Russell JW, Hummers LK, McMahan ZH. Symptoms of autonomic dysfunction in systemic sclerosis assessed by the COMPASS-31 questionnaire. J Rheumatol. 2018;45(8): 1145–52.
241. Peacock JH. Peripheral venous blood concentrations of epinephrine and norepinephrine in primary Raynaud's disease. Circ Res. 1959;7:821–7.
242. Kontos HA, Wasserman AJ. Effect of reserpine in Raynaud's phenomenon. Circulation. 1969;39(2):259–66.
243. Sapira JD, Rodnan GP, Scheib ET, Klaniecki T, Rizk M. Studies of endogenous catecholamines in patients with Raynaud's phenomenon secondary to progressive systemic sclerosis (scleroderma). Am J Med. 1972;52(3):330–7.
244. Gabrielli A, Avvedimento EV, Krieg T. Scleroderma. N Engl J Med. 2009;360(19):1989–2003.
245. Sjogren RW. Gastrointestinal motility disorders in scleroderma. Arthritis Rheum. 1994;37(9):1265–82.
246. Abu-Shakra M, Guillemin F, Lee P. Gastrointestinal manifestations of systemic sclerosis. Semin Arthritis Rheum. 1994;24(1): 29–39.
247. Lock G, Straub RH, Zeuner M, Antoniou E, Holstege A, Scholmerich J, et al. Association of autonomic nervous dysfunction and esophageal dysmotility in systemic sclerosis. J Rheumatol. 1998;25(7):1330–5.
248. Cohen S, Fisher R, Lipshutz W, Turner R, Myers A, Schumacher R. The pathogenesis of esophageal dysfunction in scleroderma and Raynaud's disease. J Clin Invest. 1972;51(10):2663–8.
249. DiMarino AJ, Carlson G, Myers A, Schumacher HR, Cohen S. Duodenal myoelectric activity in scleroderma. Abnormal responses to mechanical and hormonal stimuli. N Engl J Med. 1973;289(23):1220–3.

250. Roberts CG, Hummers LK, Ravich WJ, Wigley FM, Hutchins GM. A case-control study of the pathology of oesophageal disease in systemic sclerosis (scleroderma). Gut. 2006;55(12):1697–703.
251. Singh J, Cohen S, Mehendiratta V, Mendoza F, Jimenez SA, Dimarino AJ, et al. Effects of scleroderma antibodies and pooled human immunoglobulin on anal sphincter and colonic smooth muscle function. Gastroenterology. 2012;143(5):1308–18.
252. Singh J, Mehendiratta V, Del Galdo F, Jimenez SA, Cohen S, DiMarino AJ, et al. Immunoglobulins from scleroderma patients inhibit the muscarinic receptor activation in internal anal sphincter smooth muscle cells. Am J Physiol Gastrointest Liver Physiol. 2009;297(6):G1206–13.
253. Feldman M, Schiller LR. Disorders of gastrointestinal motility associated with diabetes mellitus. Ann Intern Med. 1983;98(3):378–84.
254. Yang R, Arem R, Chan L. Gastrointestinal tract complications of diabetes mellitus. Pathophysiology and management. Arch Intern Med. 1984;144(6):1251–6.
255. Schiller LR, Santa Ana CA, Schmulen AC, Hendler RS, Harford WV, Fordtran JS. Pathogenesis of fecal incontinence in diabetes mellitus: evidence for internal-anal-sphincter dysfunction. N Engl J Med. 1982;307(27):1666–71.
256. Camilleri M. Clinical practice. Diabetic gastroparesis. N Engl J Med. 2007;356(8):820–9.
257. Nathan DM. Long-term complications of diabetes mellitus N Engl J Med. 1993;328(23):1676–85.
258. O'Brien IA, O'Hare JP, Lewin IG, Corrall RJ. The prevalence of autonomic neuropathy in insulin-dependent diabetes mellitus: a controlled study based on heart rate variability. Q J Med. 1986;61(234):957–67.
259. Watkins PJ. Diabetic autonomic neuropathy. N Engl J Med. 1990;322(15):1078–9.
260. Di Franco M, Paradiso M, Riccieri V, Basili S, Mammarella A, Valesini G. Autonomic dysfunction and microvascular damage in systemic sclerosis. Clin Rheumatol. 2007;26(8):1278–83.
261. Suarez-Almazor ME, Bruera E, Russell AS. Normal cardiovascular autonomic function in patients with systemic sclerosis (CREST variant). Ann Rheum Dis. 1988;47(8):672–4.
262. Dessein PH, Gledhill RF. More on autonomic neuropathy in systemic sclerosis. Ann Rheum Dis. 1988;47(3):261–3.
263. Rodrigues GD, Tobaldini E, Bellocchi C, Santaniello A, Caronni M, Severino A, et al. Cardiac autonomic modulation at rest and during orthostatic stress among different systemic sclerosis subsets. Eur J Intern Med. 2019;66:75–80.
264. Gigante A, Galea N, Borrazzo C, Tubani L, Liberatori M, Ciolina F, et al. Role of autonomic dysfunction in the regulation of myocardial blood flow in systemic sclerosis evaluated by cardiac magnetic resonance. Int J Rheum Dis. 2019;22(6):1029–35.
265. Di Paolo M, Gigante A, Liberatori M, Sardo L, Marinelli P, Rossetti M, et al. Effects of autonomic dysfunction on exercise tolerance in systemic sclerosis patients without clinical and instrumental evidence of cardiac and pulmonary involvement. Clin Exp Rheumatol. 2018;36 Suppl 113(4):61–7.
266. Rosato E, Gigante A, Liberatori M, Gasperini ML, Barbano B, Amoroso A, et al. Altered diurnal cardiac sympathovagal balance correlates with nutritional status indexes in systemic sclerosis patients. J Biol Regul Homeost Agents. 2017;31(4):1133–8.

Pregnancy

39

Melody Chung and Lorinda Chung

Sexuality in Women with Systemic Sclerosis

As SSc can have a profound effect on a woman's life, a significant component of pregnancy is whether women feel well enough for sexual activity. Female sexual response is a complex and multifactorial process involving neurogenic, vasogenic, psychogenic, and hormonal factors. The impairment of the normal female sexual response leads to female sexual dysfunction, which is defined as the reduction in orgasm intensity, decreased desire, dyspareunia, recurring decrease in sexual arousal, and/or less satisfaction [1].

Female sexual dysfunction has been found to be significantly higher among SSc patients than in the general population [2, 3], with contributions from both physical and psychological factors. Physical changes due to SSc can have an unfavorable impact on sexual function in women, either by directly affecting reproductive organ systems or by causing functional derangements in other organs affected by the chronic disease. Direct effects of SSc on the genital tract include vaginal tightness and dryness (with low levels of lubrication from changes in vaginal mucosa leading to dyspareunia), constricted introitus, early menopause, and small-sized uterus which may adversely influence sexual relations [4]. Clinical manifestations of SSc such as skin tightening (including changes in skin around the face, oral aperture, breasts, and breast muscle), digital ulcers, joint contractures, gastrointestinal manifestations (including heartburn), and Raynaud's phenomenon also contribute to pain and discomfort [4–6]. Symptoms such as fatigue, chronic pain, arthralgias, muscle weakness, cough, dyspnea, and reduced exercise capacity may also interfere with sexual acts [3]. These symptoms can decrease sexual enjoyment in SSc patients and prevent their partners from engaging in sexual activity for the fear of causing discomfort or pain [3]. With regards to psychological aspects, the physical change in SSc patients related to disfiguring skin thickening affects body image and sexuality. Lower body esteem has been associated with more sexual dysfunction in SSc patients [7]. In contrast, another study reported that body image dissatisfaction did not correlate with reduced sexual function and was less important than pain in determining sexual function [8]. In SSc, emotional and psychological burden such as depressive symptoms, marital dissatisfaction, and fibromyalgia were associated with impaired sexual functioning and distress [2, 3, 9].

Women with SSc remain sexually active overall in spite of several disease-related physical and psychological difficulties, with approximately 40–60% of women still engaging in sexual activity [10, 11]. In an American study of 101 SSc women, of the 40% who were not sexually active, only 17% listed SSc as the primary reason for sexual inactivity, instead citing other reasons for inactivity such as lack of a partner, personal choice, and health status of partner [3]. However, of SSc women who are sexually active, the level of sexual impairment remains high, ranging from 44 to 61%. In one multicentric study from Canada and the UK, women with SSc were significantly less likely to be sexually active (OR = 0.34, 95% CI = 0.28–0.42) compared to women in the general population even after adjusting for age and marital status, and, among sexually active women, significantly more likely to be sexually impaired (OR = 1.88, 95% CI = 1.42–2.49) [10]. These women with SSc also showed significantly worse lubrication and higher pain scores compared to women in the general population with similar sexual impairment scores. In a study of 547 SSc women, sexual impairment was independently associated with older age, higher skin scores, and more severe breathing problems; in contrast, predictors of sexual activity were younger age, fewer gastrointestinal symptoms, and less severe Raynaud's

M. Chung
Division of Rheumatology, Mid-Atlantic Permanente Group, Gaithersburg, MD, USA
e-mail: melody.chung@kp.org

L. Chung (✉)
Division of Immunology & Rheumatology, Stanford University School of Medicine and Palo Alto VA Health Care System, Palo Alto, CA, USA
e-mail: shauwei@stanford.edu

Y. Allanore et al. (eds.), *Scleroderma*, https://doi.org/10.1007/978-3-031-40658-4_39

phenomenon [11]. This study also identified vaginal pain as the most prominent symptom which clearly distinguished women with and without sexual impairment.

Quality of life studies in SSc women has found stronger associations of sexual function with psychological rather than physical features. Sexual function was correlated with the SF-36 mental component score in female patients with SSc, but not with the physical component score [2, 3, 7]. In contrast, a Turkish study evaluating 30 SSc sexually active female patients found significantly lower SF-36 scores across all domains (including physical function) compared to controls [12]. These SSc patients also had significantly worse scores with respect to sexual desire, arousal, lubrication, orgasm, sexual satisfaction, and pain compared to controls. Reproductive organ and genital tract abnormalities in SSc females can cause reduced desire and decrease of the orgasmic response as well, and SSc females have been found to have a lower number and less intensity of orgasms compared to women with rheumatoid arthritis [4].

Dysregulation of the female sexual response in SSc women is thought to be due to microvascular impairment, similar to erectile dysfunction in males. One study investigated the clitoral blood flow in a small number of SSc female patients compared with healthy controls. Using color Doppler ultrasound, clitoral blood flow was found to be reduced in SSc females and associated with digital ulcer history and capillaroscopic modification [13]. While PDE-5 inhibitors are the mainstay of treatment for male erectile dysfunction, its use in the treatment of female sexual arousal problems is less efficacious in the general population [14] and has not been studied extensively in SSc.

Sexual dysfunction is a major issue for female SSc patients, with a high prevalence and great impact on quality of life. However, these issues are frequently not addressed by both clinicians and patients [15]. The topics related to sexual female problems are sensitive and patients often feel embarrassed or uncomfortable to talk about their problems with their health-care providers, who may also not feel adequately trained to initiate and address sexual issues. Rheumatologists and general practitioners should discuss sexual health with patients with SSc by paying attention to both psychological and physical problems (including depression), counseling them on strategies to adapt to a chronic disease, and referring them to specialists when appropriate [7]. Some steps that patients can take to improve comfort during sexual activity include use of vaginal lubricants to decrease vaginal dryness and dyspareunia, adjusting the room temperature to keep warm, avoiding meals and elevating the bed prior to sexual activity, and having open communication with partners about finding comfortable and pain-free positions. Patients can, in many situations, adapt to some of the problems and anticipate difficulties by being more prepared and educated on these issues.

Fertility

Fertility in women with SSc is a complex issue because many factors, both physical and psychological, affect the ability and desire to be sexually active and to consider pregnancy. Infertility is a heterogeneous condition that can be related to immunological mechanisms, pregnancy loss, disease burden, therapy, and personal choices regarding family size. It is difficult to draw clear conclusions concerning fertility in women with SSc due to limited studies and potential methodological biases. Studies have shown mixed results with respect to pregnancy rates and frequency of pregnancy difficulties among women with SSc, both prior to and after the diagnosis.

In early reports from the 1950s, women with SSc were thought to have diminished fertility because of the low incidence of pregnancy, but most women had completed all their pregnancies prior to SSc symptom onset and diagnosis. In one of the largest studies evaluating infertility in SSc women, Steen surveyed 214 women with SSc, 167 women with rheumatoid arthritis, and 105 healthy controls about their obstetric histories [16]. They found a statistically significant higher rate of nulliparity among women with an autoimmune rheumatic disease (21% SSc, 23% RA, 12% controls, $p < 0.05$), but this difference disappeared after adjusting for factors such as the number of women who had never married, who were sexually inactive, or who had chosen not to have children. Among the three groups, there were similar rates of infertility (2–5%), delays in conception more than 1 year (12–15%), and successful pregnancy in patients with a period of prior infertility (37–43%). During infertility evaluations, SSc patients were more likely to be counseled about possible causes of infertility such as fallopian tube obstruction or endometriosis. However, there were no unique findings causing infertility that could be attributed specifically to SSc, and some fertility problems were related to their partners instead.

Some studies have suggested that infertility may be present even before the onset of SSc disease [17, 18]. Englert found a higher incidence of infertility and a longer time to conceive in women prior to the diagnosis of SSc compared with healthy controls, but not compared with women with primary Raynaud's phenomenon [18].

Pathogenesis in SSC Pregnancies

Placental Pathology and Vasculopathy

Given the widespread vasculopathy present in SSc patients, there are concerns that the same pathophysiologic changes may also occur in the placental vasculature [19]. Histopathologic examinations of placentas from a limited number of SSc pregnancies are reported; all found normal placental weight for gestational age [20, 21]. Studies in SSc placentas have shown severe fibrosis and abnormal vascular remodeling. One study of three placentas from SSc patients (gestational age at delivery between 34 and 38 weeks) found evidence of decidual vasculopathy with stromal fibrosis and infarcts in chronic villi despite normal, healthy clinical outcomes [20]. In another case, an SSc patient with IUGR was found to have increased resistance in the umbilical artery by Doppler examination at 31 weeks of gestational age. Examination of the placenta after delivery at 37 weeks found numerous placental infarcts, placental mesenchymal dysplasia, decreased vascularity, and stromal fibrosis, all consistent with changes secondary to decidual vasculopathy [22]. In the largest study to date, 13 placentas from SSc patients were examined and correlated with perinatal outcomes [21]. Five of the 13 placentas demonstrated marked decidual vasculopathy, four of which were associated with intrauterine fetal demise between weeks 16 and 30. Chorioamnionitis and accelerated placental maturation complicated the majority of other placentas. These findings are similar to what is seen in pregnancies complicated by pregnancy-induced hypertension. Thus, placental abnormalities may be present in SSc pregnancies, even in the absence of clinical perinatal complications, and the more severe manifestations of placental vasculature may contribute to intrauterine growth restriction, preterm delivery, and death.

In a study of cord blood of neonates born to mothers with systemic autoimmune diseases (including SSc, systemic lupus erythematosus, mixed connective tissue disease, Sjogren's syndrome, and rheumatoid arthritis), elevated serum concentrations of multiple cytokines were found in the umbilical artery and vein in 11 of 17 neonates [23]. The disease was controlled in all mothers, and none had chorioamnionitis. Fetal growth restriction and non-reassuring fetal status of unknown cause were all found in the hypercytokinemia group. The authors hypothesized that the high level of cytokines in cord blood originates in neither the mother nor the placenta but in fetal immune tissues. Further work is needed to investigate the immunological mechanisms of hypercytokinemia in larger sample sizes of neonates and mothers with systemic autoimmune diseases.

Fetal Microchimerism

SSc has a strong predilection for women, a peak incidence in women following childbearing years, and clinical similarities to chronic graft-versus-host disease that occurs after allogeneic stem cell transplantation. Fetal microchimerism (the bidirectional transfer of cells between mother and fetus during gestation and delivery, followed by perpetuation of small amounts of foreign cells or DNA in the host for years or decades, potentially leading to a graft-versus-host-like effect) has been hypothesized to be implicated in the pathogenesis of SSc. Indirect support for this hypothesis is provided both by an increased frequency of persistent fetal cells among women with SSc and a history of pregnancy (as compared with normal women with a history of pregnancy) and by the presence of fetal cells in the involved skin of such patients [24, 25]. However, these associations do not prove causality and thus further research is needed in this area.

Pregnancy Outcomes

Miscarriage

Several studies (but not all) suggest that women with SSc have an increased risk of miscarriage after diagnosis, potentially related to the underlying vasculopathy associated with the disease [18, 26, 27]. Similar to other autoimmune diseases, antiphospholipid antibody positivity may also be associated with venous thrombosis and miscarriage in SSc patients [28]. In a meta-analysis including observational data published between 1950 and 2018, pregnancies in women with SSc had a higher risk of miscarriage compared with healthy controls (OR 1.6, 95% CI 1.22–2.22) [29]. The rate of spontaneous miscarriage has also been reported to be higher among women who became pregnant prior to disease diagnosis when compared with control individuals [26, 30]. It has been hypothesized that these blighted pregnancies could result in microchimerism, which has been discussed as a potential mechanism of disease pathogenesis in SSc [26].

In contrast to these findings, other studies suggest that the risk of miscarriage in SSc women can be comparable to the general healthy population when monitored as high-risk pregnancies [31–34] with the exception of patients with late diffuse SSc who may experience a higher risk for miscarriage [32]. Steen prospectively studied 59 women with SSc who had 91 pregnancies during a 10-year period and found no increase in the frequency of miscarriage after SSc onset except in those with long-standing diffuse cutaneous SSc greater than 4 years of symptoms (42% in SSc women vs. 13% in rheumatoid arthritis and control group) [32]. Taraborelli also found a low miscarriage rate (4% of SSc pregnancies), but defined miscarriage as <10 weeks [31].

Premature Delivery

Premature delivery is defined as delivery prior to 37 completed weeks of gestation. Preterm birth complications are estimated to be responsible for one-third of neonatal deaths and can have long-term effects on neurodevelopmental functioning as well as increased risk of chronic disease in adulthood.

Premature births appear to be higher in SSc than in the general population [35, 36], ranging from 11 to 40% of pregnancies in SSc women compared to 11% of all live births worldwide [37]. Steen's retrospective series found that premature births occurred slightly more frequently in both SSc patients and rheumatoid arthritis patients compared with neighborhood control subjects [16]. An expanded study by the same group of investigators retrospectively obtained reproductive histories. Women with SSc were more likely than those without SSc to have adverse outcomes of pregnancy after the onset of their rheumatic disease, particularly premature births (29% vs. 5% in historical controls) [32].

In an Australian population-based cohort, the frequency of preterm births was also significantly higher than in the general obstetric population (30% vs. 7%; unadjusted RR 4.80, 95% CI 3.03–7.61) [38]. This risk remained high even after adjusting for maternal age, country of birth, socioeconomic status, maternal residence, chronic hypertension, pregestational diabetes, smoking during pregnancy, parity, and multiple births (adjusted RR 4.19, 95% CI 2.56–6.86).

Similarly, in the prospective IMPRESS study (Italian Multicentric Study on Pregnancy in Systemic Sclerosis), SSc women ($n = 99$) were significantly more likely to have premature deliveries (25% vs. 12%, OR 2.53, 95% CI 1.55–4.10, $p < 001$) and severe preterm deliveries (<34 weeks of gestation) (10% vs. 5%, $p = 0.03$) compared to the general obstetric population [31]. Univariable analyses found that women with SSc who had preterm deliveries had a higher rate of corticosteroid use, intrauterine growth restriction, and very-low birth weights. Maternal age, disease duration, Medsger Severity Score for SSc, disease subtype, and presence of anti-centromere antibodies or antiphospholipid antibodies were not associated with prematurity. On multivariable analyses, corticosteroid use was the only variable associated with higher preterm deliveries, whereas use of folic acid and unexpectedly anti-topoisomerase positivity were protective factors. Most preterm deliveries (72%) were iatrogenic and ordered by the patient's obstetrician, suggesting that the prevention of fetal or maternal complications may be responsible for earlier deliveries.

Preeclampsia

Preeclampsia is a multisystem disorder characterized by new onset hypertension (systolic blood pressure ≥ 140 mmHg or diastolic blood pressure ≥ 90 mmHg) and proteinuria and/or organ dysfunction after 20 weeks of gestation. Eclampsia corresponds to the development of grand mal seizures in women with preeclampsia. The worldwide prevalence of preeclampsia and eclampsia has been estimated at 4.6% and 1.4% of all deliveries, respectively [39]. Prevalence of hypertensive disorders of pregnancy in SSc has been estimated between 2–23% [31, 38, 40]. Chakravarty reported that the proportion of hypertensive disorders (23%) in SSc patients was significantly higher than controls (8%) in a small study [40].

Although some studies have not found a significant increase in preeclampsia in SSc patients [32], a population-based study of pregnancy outcomes utilizing an administrative hospital discharge database found an increased risk of hypertensive disorders including preeclampsia [40]. In a meta-analysis, women with SSc were more prone to develop gestational hypertension and to undergo C-section [8]. Poor obstetric outcomes after a diagnosis of SSc may be related to the vasculopathy associated with the disease as well as immune system abnormalities [9, 10].

Interestingly, a few small studies have been performed on obstetric outcomes *prior* to a diagnosis of SSc. One case-control study found that women who later developed SSc had twice the odds of having had a pregnancy complicated by a hypertensive disorder compared to women who never developed SSc or an autoimmune disease [30]. A Danish population-based register study found a nonsignificant increased risk of subsequent SSc diagnosis among women with preeclampsia [30]. In a small matched case-control study, nonstatistically significant increased rates of obstetric complications (such as preeclampsia) were found prior to SSc diagnosis compared to the general obstetric population [41]. Some authors have hypothesized that altered fetal origin microchimerism seen in preeclampsia may contribute to subsequent development of autoimmune conditions postpartum such as SSc. Another possibility is that women who are later diagnosed with SSc could already have subclinical features of the disease during pregnancy leading to placental infarction, which then results in adverse pregnancy outcomes, particularly vascular complications such as intrauterine growth restriction (IUGR) and hypertension.

Intrauterine Growth Restriction and Small for Gestational Age Infants

IUGR refers to a fetus who does not achieve the expected in utero growth potential due to genetic or environmental factors. It is defined as an estimated fetal weight below the tenth percentile and ultrasonographic findings of fetal abdominal circumference below the fifth percentile for gestational age. Small for gestational age (SGA) infants are newborns whose birth weight is below the tenth percentile for gestational age. Women with SSc can have successful pregnancies, but they have a higher-than-normal risk of preterm delivery, IUGR, and SGA infants [16].

Chakravarty used the 2002–2004 U.S. Nationwide Inpatient Sample of the Healthcare Cost and Utilization Project to estimate the number of obstetric hospitalizations and deliveries among women with SSc and in the general population [40]. SSc was associated with an increased risk of IUGR (OR 3.74, 95% CI 1.51–9.28) and increased length of hospital stay. In the IMPRESS study, SSc patients had a significantly increased frequency of IUGR (6% vs. 1%) and babies with very-low birth weight (5% vs. 1%) compared to the general obstetric population [31]. Much higher rates of SGA infants (50%) were found in Chung's relatively small study of SSc patients [36]. Data suggest an increase in IUGR even among women who later develop SSc compared to healthy controls [30]; however, it is difficult to ascertain whether pregnancy complications may be very early manifestations of SSc in otherwise asymptomatic women or a risk factor for the future development of SSc [42]. These findings might represent epiphenomena of SSc vasculopathy affecting the placenta, as histopathologic studies from a limited number of cases showed decidual vascular abnormalities, placental mesenchymal dysplasia, and chronic villi infarcts [20, 21].

Neonatal Mortality

Infant deaths were quite common in individual case reports. In Chung's series of seven women with SSc with a total of 12 pregnancies, fetal loss complicated two pregnancies in women with severe diffuse cutaneous SSc and antiphospholipid syndrome [36]. Other cases were associated with the acute exacerbation of SSc complications in the mother. However, no large studies to date have found a statistically or clinically excessive number of neonatal deaths compared with controls.

Effects of Pregnancy on Systemic Sclerosis

In addition to understanding the effects of SSc on pregnancy, it is equally important to consider the effect that pregnancy may have upon the disease itself (Table 39.1). Evaluation of the potential effects of pregnancy on the SSc course is challenging, since many pregnancy symptoms are similar to SSc symptoms (e.g., edema, arthralgias, gastrointestinal reflux, and shortness of breath). Early small studies described cases of poor maternal outcomes due to renal crisis [19, 43], whereas subsequent larger studies by Steen and the IMPRESS centers found no significant changes in disease status during pregnancy [16, 31, 32]. In a prospective study by Steen, 61% of pregnant SSc women had overall stable disease status, 20% experienced some improvement, and 20% experienced some worsening [32]. There were no differences in 10-year survival between SSc women with or without a pregnancy. In general, progressive cutaneous disease during or after pregnancy is uncommon.

Table 39.1 Effects of pregnancy on systemic sclerosis

SSc involvement	Change during pregnancy
Overall	Disease generally stable
Raynaud's phenomenon	Improved during pregnancy, worse after or during complicated deliveries
Skin	Can have onset during pregnancy and some diffuse SSc have progression of skin postpartum
Joints	More arthralgias, similar to non-scleroderma pregnancy
Gastrointestinal	More reflex, similar to non-scleroderma pregnancy
Cardiopulmonary	Shortness of breath from scleroderma problems aggravated as in other diseases and managed as they would be in any pregnancy with compromised cardiopulmonary status. Women with pregestational pulmonary artery hypertension have a higher maternal mortality rate, particularly during delivery, and are strongly advised against pregnancy.
Kidney	Renal crisis occurs during early diffuse scleroderma with or without pregnancy. Management must be with ACE inhibitors in spite of risks to the baby.

Renal Disease

Renal crisis remains the most dreaded and life-threatening complication of SSc pregnancies and necessitates prompt institution of ACE inhibitor therapy despite its potential teratogenicity. ACE inhibitors are indicated at any stage of the pregnancy if renal crisis is suspected. Unlike blood pressure elevations due to preeclampsia or in non-SSc pregnancies, SSc pregnancies complicated by renal crisis must be treated aggressively with ACE inhibitors. In order to minimize the risk for renal crisis, pregnancies should be avoided in rapidly progressive diffuse disease as such patients are at a greater risk for developing serious cardiopulmonary and renal problems early in the disease.

Renal crisis can be difficult to distinguish from preeclampsia due to similar findings of hypertension and proteinuria. Some blood tests may help differentiate the two: elevated uric acid and liver function tests are more frequent in preeclampsia, while progressive daily increases in serum creatinine and microangiopathic hemolytic anemia are typical of renal crisis. Renal biopsy can be helpful, but it is not recommended during pregnancy due to high risk of pregnancy complications [20]. New and specific biomarkers for early preeclampsia have been proposed, such as the ratio of soluble fms-like tyrosine kinase-1 (sFlt-1) to placental growth factor (PlGF) [22], but their specificity remains to be evaluated in SSc pregnancies.

Recent studies of SSc pregnancies have found a lower incidence of renal crisis than reported in the early literature. In a prospective study by Steen, among 91 pregnancies from 59 women, there were 3 cases of renal crises during pregnancy, all in women with early diffuse cutaneous SSc [32].

In the IMPRESS study, there were no renal crises during the 109 pregnancies; however, a 30-year-old woman with diffuse cutaneous SSc suffered from renal crisis 1 month after delivering an SGA infant at 37 weeks. She started high-dose ACE-inhibitors and bosentan and stopped dialysis after 4 years, but developed chronic kidney disease [31].

Musculoskeletal and Gastrointestinal Disease

Other pregnancy symptoms are frequently seen in SSc patients. Musculoskeletal complaints in pregnancy in general are common, including carpal tunnel syndrome, muscle leg cramps, arthralgias, and back pain. SSc patients are not immune to any of these problems, and it is difficult to determine whether they occur more than expected in this population. Likewise, gastrointestinal symptoms, particularly esophageal reflux and constipation, occur with increased frequency in both SSc and during normal pregnancy [44]; it is not surprising that SSc patients during pregnancy complain of increased reflux, early satiety, or constipation. It is also likely that patients may not report mild-to-moderate increases in these symptoms as they may consider them to be changes related to pregnancy rather than the underlying disease. For example, during any normal pregnancy, the tone of the lower half of the esophagus becomes profoundly depressed during the last two trimesters contributing to increased reflux [45, 46], thus reflux may be related to physiologic changes from pregnancy rather than worsening SSc.

Raynaud's Phenomenon and Digital Ulceration

Of all vascular complications of SSc, Raynaud's phenomenon tends to improve during pregnancy, only to worsen postpartum [17]. Since Raynaud's is characterized by vascular hyperreactivity and vasospasm, pregnancy may potentially improve peripheral blood flow by increasing blood volume and decreasing systemic vascular resistance. Less is known about the development of or healing of digital ulcerations. Return to prepregnancy hemodynamics often leads to return of baseline peripheral circulatory complications. There have been only a few case reports of acute gangrenous changes developing late in pregnancy; these were associated with the use of beta-blockers or with other problems including complicated deliveries, sepsis, or increased systemic hypertension [36, 47, 48].

Cardiopulmonary Disease

Women with SSc do not seem to have greater adverse outcomes from cardiopulmonary problems than one would expect in other pregnant patients with similar underlying cardiopulmonary issues [49–51]. Other than increased shortness of breath (typical in most pregnant women due to increased basal oxygen consumption and alveolar ventilation), there is no evidence that pregnancy increases the severity of SSc pulmonary fibrosis. SSc patients may have undetected myocardial damage, and this could in theory cause cardiac dysfunction and compromise during the cardiovascular stress of pregnancy.

Pulmonary Arterial Hypertension

Pulmonary arterial hypertension (PAH) is a serious complication which usually occurs in anti-centromere positive, limited cutaneous SSc patients who have long-standing disease and who often have the onset of SSc at an older age. Pregnant women with pulmonary hypertension are at increased risk of complications and death for both mother and fetus. Maternal mortality rates in pregnant women with pulmonary hypertension have been reported to be as high as 30–56% [52]. Even with the advent of pulmonary vascular-targeted medications, maternal mortality remains very high. Any pregnant woman with pulmonary hypertension is at extremely high risk for severe hemodynamic complications because of the low reserve of the pulmonary arterioles to reduce vascular resistance to accommodate the increased blood volume and cardiac output that occurs during pregnancy. Delivery appears to be the most vulnerable period for cardiovascular collapse and maternal death in the pregnant pulmonary hypertension patient, because of the acute increase in cardiac output during the second stage of labor with the return of uterine blood back to the maternal systemic vascular beds [19, 53, 54]. Pregnant women with underlying PAH are at extremely high risk for acute hospitalization during pregnancy (OR 4.67, 95% CI 2.88–7.57), developing hypertensive disorders of pregnancy (OR 5.62, 95% CI 2.60–12.15) and increased length of hospital stay [40]. Women who carry a diagnosis of pulmonary hypertension should be strongly counseled to avoid pregnancy as it remains a condition associated with high risks for maternal and fetal morbidity and mortality.

Pregnancy Management

All pregnancies in women with SSc should be considered high risk for pregnancy morbidity (including premature and small full-term infants) as well as disease-related complications. In addition to a rheumatologist familiar with SSc, pregnant patients should be followed closely by an obstetrician experienced in high-risk pregnancies. At the onset of pregnancy, a SSc patient should be carefully evaluated to determine the disease subtype, duration of symptoms, as well as the extent and severity of visceral involvement. Women at greater risk of having more active, aggressive disease include those with less than 4 years of SSc symptoms,

Table 39.2 Management of scleroderma patients during pregnancy, labor, and delivery

Preterm
1. Early evaluation of extent of scleroderma organ involvement and autoantibody analysis, including echocardiogram and pulmonary function tests
2. Discontinue use of disease-remitting drugs with teratogenic potential (i.e., mycophenolate mofetil, methotrexate, etc.) before pregnancy
3. High-risk obstetric care
4. Minimal use of proton pump inhibitors, histamine blockers, or calcium channel blockers for gastrointestinal and vascular problems
5. Avoidance of corticosteroids
6. More frequent monitoring of fetal size and uterine activity
7. Frequent blood pressure monitoring
8. Aggressive treatment of any hypertension (preeclampsia or others)
9. Close observation and treatment for premature labor (avoid beta-adrenergic agonists)
Labor and delivery
1. Epidural anesthesia is preferred
2. Special warming of delivery room, intravenous fluids, patients themselves (e.g., extra blankets, thermal socks, gloves)
3. Venous access before delivery
4. Careful attention to the episiotomy and cesarean section incisions, which generally heal without difficulty
Postdelivery
1. Continued careful monitoring postpartum, with early reinstitution of medication and aggressive treatment of hypertension, if it is present (do not assume it will resolve following delivery)

diffuse cutaneous SSc, and anti-topoisomerase or RNA polymerase III antibodies when compared to those with long-standing disease with anti-centromere antibody [55]. When organs are severely damaged (i.e., severe cardiomyopathy with ejection fraction <30%, pulmonary hypertension, severe restrictive lung disease with forced vital capacity <50% of predicted, malabsorption, or renal insufficiency), the decision to terminate the pregnancy may have to be considered depending on the risks to the mother and the infant. Patient, partner, and all physicians involved in her care will need to make this difficult decision together. The high risk of preterm labor necessitates special management throughout the pregnancy as described in Table 39.2.

Management of Renal Crisis during Pregnancy

Renal crisis remains the most dreaded complication of a SSc pregnancy, since this may be life-threatening for both mother and child and is associated with high early mortality. Renal crisis usually occurs early in the course of the disease in patients with diffuse cutaneous skin involvement. Management of renal crisis during pregnancy in SSc is described in Table 39.3. Those with early, rapidly progressive, diffuse skin thickening should have their blood pressures monitored closely at least three to five times a week and avoid becoming pregnant since intrinsically they are at higher risk of developing renal crisis. The presence of even mild elevation in blood pressure compared with previous levels should be considered potentially very serious. A search for evidence of elevated serum creatinine levels, proteinuria, microangiopathic hemolytic anemia, and uric acid should be done promptly to differentiate this condition from preeclampsia. If the serum creatinine is increasing in this setting, particularly in the setting of microangiopathy and the absence of increased liver function tests (i.e., to differentiate from HELLP), a diagnosis of renal crisis must be assumed.

Table 39.3 Management of renal crisis during pregnancy in scleroderma

1. New-onset hypertension must be taken seriously
2. Search for evidence of increased creatinine, proteinuria, or microangiopathic hemolytic anemia, elevated liver function, and uric acid
3. Do not assume it is preeclampsia
4. Try to control blood pressure with other medications, but if not controlled or if creatinine increases, add small doses of an ACE inhibitor
5. Controlling blood pressure may be lifesaving to the mother and baby even with the risks of fetopathy from ACE inhibitor toxicity

Renal crisis necessitates prompt institution of ACE inhibitor therapy at any stage of the pregnancy, despite its potential teratogenicity. There are major difficulties in the decision to use ACE inhibitors during pregnancy, since ACE inhibitors are usually contraindicated in the second and third trimesters of pregnancy because they can cause significant fetal abnormalities such as oligohydramnios, anuria, renal failure, pulmonary hypoplasia, and fetal death [56]. Successful use of captopril or other ACE inhibitors during pregnancy has been documented in SSc [32, 57]. Captopril is perhaps the best choice in the setting of pregnancy as it can be easily and quickly titrated, and it appears to be associated with lower risk of fetopathy than other ACE inhibitors or ARBs.

It is possible to try non-ACE inhibitors to control blood pressure early on, but they may not successfully control the renal crisis process and ACE inhibitors may be necessary. If the blood pressure remains high, the risk to the mother may outweigh the risk of fetal toxicity as adequately controlled blood pressure could be lifesaving to the fetus as well. If elective C-section is planned, one should begin an ACE inhibitor and not assume the blood pressure will improve after delivery.

Management of Pregnancy in Mothers with Prior Renal Crisis

The management of SSc during pregnancy is challenging, particularly for pregnant women who have survived prior renal crisis. After an episode of renal crisis, ACE inhibitors are required to maintain blood pressure control and renal function indefinitely. Pregnancy in patients after renal crisis may be successful, but potential disastrous outcomes both to the mother and the infant are possible especially in patients with poor blood pressure control.

Steen described ten women from an SSc cohort who had 12 pregnancies after an episode of renal crisis [58]. Four of these women who remained on ACE inhibitors throughout pregnancy had five healthy babies. Two other women discontinued ACE inhibitors prior to or early in pregnancy, and their blood pressures were successfully managed with other medications including calcium channel blockers. None of these infants had any significant evidence of ACE inhibitor toxicity. In the small series, the worst outcomes occurred in patients who had very poor blood pressure control.

There are several possible approaches that a patient can take if she desires a pregnancy after renal crisis, but they each involve significant risk. If the patient discontinues the ACE inhibitor and the blood pressure is not controlled, then the ACE inhibitor must be reinstituted. Otherwise, she is likely to experience severe deterioration in renal function and potential harm to the fetus as well. Another strategy is to use a small dose of ACE inhibitor along with non-ACE inhibitor medication to control blood pressure along with close monitoring of oligohydramnios or other signs of fetal abnormalities. In any situation, the patient and her spouse must seriously consider a variety of options and potential outcomes before deciding whether to become pregnant or continue a pregnancy. Although SSc patients have had successful pregnancy outcomes while on ACE inhibitors, the use of these drugs during the third trimester of pregnancy is associated with an increased risk of serious kidney problems in the baby.

Management of Pulmonary Hypertension During Pregnancy

According to the 2015 European Society of Cardiology/European Respiratory Society (ESC/ERS) Guidelines for the diagnosis and treatment of pulmonary hypertension, PAH patients are advised to avoid pregnancy (class of recommendation I, level of evidence C) [59]. There are significant risks of right heart failure and maternal mortality particularly during the early postpartum period, but the outcome of pregnancy in PAH has improved in the modern management era when PAH is well controlled [60]. Pregnant patients with PAH should be informed of the high risk of pregnancy and termination of pregnancy may need to be discussed.

Patients who choose to continue pregnancy should be treated with advanced disease-targeted therapies, planned elective delivery, and effective close collaboration between obstetricians and the PAH team [59]. Careful monitoring of arterial oxygen saturation, cardiac rhythm, and blood pressure are recommended for PAH patients in the peripartum period. The use of pulmonary function studies with carbon monoxide to assess diffusion capacity is considered safe during pregnancy [19]. Advanced therapies (prostacyclin analogues, phosphodiesterase inhibitors, endothelin-receptor antagonists, and nitric oxide) have revolutionized PAH management and have been used in pregnancy [61]. Low-dose subcutaneous heparin prophylaxis is generally recommended in pregnant women with PAH, but some patients may require higher levels of anticoagulation (e.g., patients with a history of thromboembolic events or atrial fibrillation). The optimal mode of delivery (vaginal vs. C-section) in patients with PAH remains a matter of debate. Vaginal delivery is associated with smaller shifts in blood volume, fewer clotting or bleeding complications, and a lower risk of infection [61]. However, C-section may become necessary in cases of maternal hemodynamic deterioration or fetal distress requiring urgent delivery.

Management of Delivery

Pregnancy in SSc is an anesthetic challenge that needs to be carefully considered and discussed before delivery. A multidisciplinary approach should be used for delivery planning and anesthetic management with obstetricians, neonatologists, maternal-fetal medicine specialists, pulmonologists, cardiologists, critical care physicians, and obstetric anesthesiologists.

SSc presents several mechanical difficulties due to thickening skin, secondary tissue contractures, and vasoconstriction. This may make it difficult to obtain venous access, take accurate vital signs, or position the limbs for delivery. Venous access, even if it requires a central line and consideration of a Swan–Ganz catheter, may be necessary if cardiopulmonary compromise, hypertension, or renal dysfunction are present. Direct arterial line placement should be avoided as cannulation of peripheral arteries for invasive blood pressure monitoring may induce Raynaud's phenomenon, provoke vasospasm, and cause ischemia and subsequent distal necrosis, thus femoral arterial pressure monitoring may need to be used instead. Other measures that could prevent problems related to Raynaud's phenomenon during delivery should be routinely used, including warming the delivery room and using warm intravenous fluids, thermal socks, and warm external compresses.

Some pathophysiological aspects of SSc pose problems for anesthetic management, regardless of the anesthesia type and whether obstetric delivery is by the vaginal route or C-section. There are no specific contraindications to the use of any type of anesthesia, although the selection must be guided by identification of organ dysfunction. The anesthesiologist must be aware of the organs involved, severity of the disease, and associated anesthetic considerations and potential risks in order to safely manage the patient with SSc. Literature regarding anesthetic care of patients with SSc during labor and delivery is limited to case reports [62].

Regional anesthesia, particularly an epidural block, allows the most benefit during delivery. Not only does it provide adequate anesthesia, but it provides peripheral vasodilatation and increased skin perfusion of the lower extremities [50, 63]. Smaller-than-normal doses of regional anesthesia have been suggested because SSc patients may exhibit prolonged motor and sensory blockade after delivery [63]. Although cases of uncomplicated general anesthesia have been described in pregnant SSc patients, there are significant risks including difficulty with intubation due to reduced oral aperture as well as concerns about aspiration. Rapid-sequence induction or awake fiberoptic intubation (when a difficult airway is anticipated) should be considered due to aspiration risk secondary to SSc and pregnancy. There should be no hesitation to perform a C-section if medically necessary because even the tightest abdominal skin usually heals if care is taken in the surgical repair of the incision.

Postnatal care should include continued attentiveness to monitoring disease activity, particularly progressive skin changes, new signs of cardiopulmonary disease, or new hypertension, so therapeutic intervention can begin immediately. There are no data on postpartum depression being greater in SSc than in any pregnancy, but given the complexity of the situation, providers should be on the alert for emotional distress. Close observation for physical or emotional disease and early therapeutic intervention are indicated. Necessary medications that had been disrupted specifically because of the pregnancy should be reinstituted promptly, provided they are not contraindicated during breastfeeding, or the patient decides against breastfeeding.

Summary

Sexual dysfunction is a major issue for female SSc patients, with a high prevalence and great impact on quality of life that should be addressed by physicians. There have been some suggestions that infertility and miscarriages are increased in SSc patients. Although pregnancy in SSc may be uneventful with both good maternal and fetal outcomes, complications such as hypertensive disorders of pregnancy can occur and thus careful antenatal evaluations, discussion of potential problems, and participation in a high-risk obstetric monitoring program are very important to optimize the outcome. The high risk of premature and small infants may be minimized with specialized obstetric and neonatal care.

Women with diffuse cutaneous SSc are at a greater risk for developing serious cardiopulmonary and renal problems early in the disease, so they should be encouraged to delay pregnancy until the disease stabilizes. All patients who become pregnant during this high-risk time should be monitored extremely carefully particularly for renal crisis. Renal crisis remains one of the most serious and life-threatening complications of a SSc pregnancy and necessitates prompt institution of ACE inhibitors despite its potential teratogenicity, as it may be lifesaving to the mother. SSc women with PAH should be counseled to avoid pregnancy due to high rates of maternal and fetal morbidity and mortality. With the exception of these complications, careful planning, close monitoring, and aggressive management should allow women with SSc to have a high likelihood of a successful pregnancy.

References

1. Basson R, Berman J, Burnett A, Derogatis L, Ferguson D, Fourcroy J, et al. Report of the international consensus development conference on female sexual dysfunction: definitions and classifications. J Urol. 2000;163(3):888–93.
2. Schouffoer AA, van der Marel J, Ter Kuile MM, Weijenborg PT, Voskuyl A, Vliet Vlieland CW, et al. Impaired sexual function in women with systemic sclerosis: a cross-sectional study. Arthritis Rheum. 2009;61(11):1601–8.
3. Impens AJ, Rothman J, Schiopu E, Cole JC, Dang J, Gendrano N, et al. Sexual activity and functioning in female scleroderma patients. Clin Exp Rheumatol. 2009;27(3 Suppl 54):38–43.
4. Bhadauria S, Moser DK, Clements PJ, Singh RR, Lachenbruch PA, Pitkin RM, et al. Genital tract abnormalities and female sexual function impairment in systemic sclerosis. Am J Obstet Gynecol. 1995;172(2 Pt 1):580–7.
5. Bruni C, Raja J, Denton CP, Matucci-Cerinic M. The clinical relevance of sexual dysfunction in systemic sclerosis. Autoimmun Rev. 2015;14(12):1111–5.
6. Wilson D, Goerzen J, Fritzler MJ. Treatment of sexual dysfunction in a patient with systemic sclerosis. J Rheumatol. 1993;20(8):1446–7.
7. Maddali Bongi S, Del Rosso A, Mikhaylova S, Baccini M, Matucci CM. Sexual function in Italian women with systemic sclerosis is affected by disease-related and psychological concerns. J Rheumatol. 2013;40(10):1697–705.
8. Knafo R, Haythornthwaite JA, Heinberg L, Wigley FM, Thombs BD. The association of body image dissatisfaction and pain with reduced sexual function in women with systemic sclerosis. Rheumatology (Oxford). 2011;50(6):1125–30.
9. CeC F, da Mota LM, Oliveira AC, de Carvalho JF, Lima RA, Simaan CK, et al. Frequency of sexual dysfunction in women with rheumatic diseases. Rev Bras Reumatol. 2013;53(1):35–46.
10. Levis B, Burri A, Hudson M, Baron M, Thombs BD, (CSRG) CSRG. Sexual activity and impairment in women with systemic sclerosis compared to women from a general population sample. PLoS One. 2012;7(12):e52129.
11. Levis B, Hudson M, Knafo R, Baron M, Nielson WR, Hill M, et al. Rates and correlates of sexual activity and impairment among women with systemic sclerosis. Arthritis Care Res (Hoboken). 2012;64(3):340–50.
12. Uçar İ, Turgay B, Küçükşahin O, Özkan Uçar E, Turgay M. Sexual dysfunction in patients with systemic sclerosis. Turk J Med Sci. 2018;48(6):1104–8.
13. Rosato E, Gigante A, Barbano B, La Marra F, Molinaro I, Quarta S, et al. Clitoral blood flow in systemic sclerosis women: correlation with disease clinical variables and female sexual dysfunction. Rheumatology (Oxford). 2013;52(12):2238–42.

14. Chivers ML, Rosen RC. Phosphodiesterase type 5 inhibitors and female sexual response: faulty protocols or paradigms? J Sex Med. 2010;7(2 Pt 2):858–72.
15. Schmalzing M, Nau LF, Gernert M, Froehlich M, Schwaneck EC, Pecher AC, et al. Sexual function in German women with systemic sclerosis compared to women with systemic lupus erythematosus and evaluation of a screening test. Clin Exp Rheumatol. 2020;38(Suppl. 125):59–64.
16. Steen VD, Medsger TA. Fertility and pregnancy outcome in women with systemic sclerosis. Arthritis Rheum. 1999;42(4):763–8.
17. Silman AJ, Black C. Increased incidence of spontaneous abortion and infertility in women with scleroderma before disease onset: a controlled study. Ann Rheum Dis. 1988;47(6):441–4.
18. Englert H, Brennan P, McNeil D, Black C, Silman AJ. Reproductive function prior to disease onset in women with scleroderma. J Rheumatol. 1992;19(10):1575–9.
19. Chakravarty EF. Vascular complications of systemic sclerosis during pregnancy. Int J Rheumatol. 2010;2010:287248. https://doi.org/10.1155/2010/287248.
20. Ibba-Manneschi L, Manetti M, Milia AF, Miniati I, Benelli G, Guiducci S, et al. Severe fibrotic changes and altered expression of angiogenic factors in maternal scleroderma: placental findings. Ann Rheum Dis. 2010;69(2):458–61.
21. Doss BJ, Jacques SM, Mayes MD, Qureshi F. Maternal scleroderma: placental findings and perinatal outcome. Hum Pathol. 1998;29(12):1524–30.
22. Papakonstantinou K, Hasiakos D, Kondi-Paphiti A. Clinicopathology of maternal scleroderma. Int J Gynaecol Obstet. 2007;99(3):248–9.
23. Takahashi N, Nagamatsu T, Fujii T, Takahashi K, Tsuchida Y, Fujio K. Extremely high levels of multiple cytokines in the cord blood of neonates born to mothers with systemic autoimmune diseases. Cytokine. 2020;127:154926.
24. Artlett CM, Smith JB, Jimenez SA. Identification of fetal DNA and cells in skin lesions from women with systemic sclerosis. N Engl J Med. 1998;338(17):1186–91.
25. Nelson JL, Furst DE, Maloney S, Gooley T, Evans PC, Smith A, et al. Microchimerism and HLA-compatible relationships of pregnancy in scleroderma. Lancet. 1998;351(9102):559–62.
26. Giordano M, Valentini G, Lupoli S, Giordano A. Pregnancy and systemic sclerosis. Arthritis Rheum. 1985;28(2):237–8.
27. Slate WG, Graham AR. Scleroderma and pregnancy. Am J Obstet Gynecol. 1968;101(3):335–41.
28. Sobanski V, Lemaire-Olivier A, Giovannelli J, Dauchet L, Simon M, Lopez B, et al. Prevalence and clinical associations of antiphospholipid antibodies in systemic sclerosis: new data from a French cross-sectional study, systematic review, and meta-analysis. Front Immunol. 2018;9:2457.
29. Blagojevic J, AlOdhaibi KA, Aly AM, Bellando-Randone S, Lepri G, Bruni C, et al. Pregnancy in systemic sclerosis (SSc): results of systematic review and meta-analysis. J Rheumatol. 2020;47(6):881–7.
30. van Wyk L, van der Marel J, Schuerwegh AJ, Schouffoer AA, Voskuyl AE, Huizinga TW, et al. Increased incidence of pregnancy complications in women who later develop scleroderma: a case control study. Arthritis Res Ther. 2011;13(6):R183.
31. Taraborelli M, Ramoni V, Brucato A, Airò P, Bajocchi G, Bellisai F, et al. Brief report: successful pregnancies but a higher risk of preterm births in patients with systemic sclerosis: an Italian multicenter study. Arthritis Rheum. 2012;64(6):1970–7.
32. Steen VD. Pregnancy in women with systemic sclerosis. Obstet Gynecol. 1999;94(1):15–20.
33. Steen VD, Conte C, Day N, Ramsey-Goldman R, Medsger TA. Pregnancy in women with systemic sclerosis. Arthritis Rheum. 1989;32(2):151–7.
34. Siamopoulou-Mavridou A, Manoussakis MN, Mavridis AK, Moutsopoulos HM. Outcome of pregnancy in patients with autoimmune rheumatic disease before the disease onset. Ann Rheum Dis. 1988;47(12):982–7.
35. Kolstad KD, Mayo JA, Chung L, Chaichian Y, Kelly VM, Druzin M, et al. Preterm birth phenotypes in women with autoimmune rheumatic diseases: a population-based cohort study. BJOG. 2020;127(1):70–8.
36. Chung L, Flyckt RL, Colón I, Shah AA, Druzin M, Chakravarty EF. Outcome of pregnancies complicated by systemic sclerosis and mixed connective tissue disease. Lupus. 2006;15(9):595–9.
37. Sobanski V, Launay D, Depret S, Ducloy-Bouthors AS, Hachulla E. Special considerations in pregnant systemic sclerosis patients. Expert Rev Clin Immunol. 2016;12(11):1161–73.
38. Chen JS, Roberts CL, Simpson JM, March LM. Pregnancy outcomes in women with rare autoimmune diseases. Arthritis Rheumatol. 2015;67(12):3314–23.
39. Abalos E, Cuesta C, Grosso AL, Chou D, Say L. Global and regional estimates of preeclampsia and eclampsia: a systematic review. Eur J Obstet Gynecol Reprod Biol. 2013;170(1):1–7.
40. Chakravarty EF, Khanna D, Chung L. Pregnancy outcomes in systemic sclerosis, primary pulmonary hypertension, and sickle cell disease. Obstet Gynecol. 2008;111(4):927–34.
41. Chung MP, Kolstad KD, Dontsi M, Postlethwaite D, Manwani P, Zhao H, et al. Increased rates of obstetric complications prior to systemic sclerosis diagnosis. Arthritis Care Res (Hoboken). 2020;47(6):881–7.
42. Chakravarty E. Pre-disease pregnancy complications and systemic sclerosis: pathogenic or pre-clinical? Arthritis Res Ther. 2012;14(1):102.
43. Lidar M, Langevitz P. Pregnancy issues in scleroderma. Autoimmun Rev. 2012;11(6-7):A515–9.
44. Calhoun BC. Gastrointestinal disorders in pregnancy. Obstet Gynecol Clin N Am. 1992;19(4):733–44.
45. Ulmsten U, Sundström G. Esophageal manometry in pregnant and nonpregnant women. Am J Obstet Gynecol. 1978;132(3):260–4.
46. Van Thiel DH, Gavaler JS, Joshi SN, Sara RK, Stremple J. Heartburn of pregnancy. Gastroenterology. 1977;72(4 Pt 1):666–8.
47. Avrech OM, Golan A, Pansky M, Langer R, Caspi E. Raynaud's phenomenon and peripheral gangrene complicating scleroderma in pregnancy—diagnosis and management. Br J Obstet Gynaecol. 1992;99(10):850–1.
48. Smith CA, Pinals RS. Progressive systemic sclerosis and postpartum renal failure complicated by peripheral gangrene. J Rheumatol. 1982;9(3):455–8.
49. Raymond R, Underwood DA, Moodie DS. Cardiovascular problems in pregnancy. Cleve Clin J Med. 1987;54(2):95–104.
50. Thompson J, Conklin KA. Anesthetic management of a pregnant patient with scleroderma. Anesthesiology. 1983;59(1):69–71.
51. Sullivan JM, Ramanathan KB. Management of medical problems in pregnancy—severe cardiac disease. N Engl J Med. 1985;313(5):304–9.
52. Sun X, Feng J, Shi J. Pregnancy and pulmonary hypertension: an exploratory analysis of risk factors and outcomes. Medicine (Baltimore). 2018;97(44):e13035.
53. Madden BP. Pulmonary hypertension and pregnancy. Int J Obstet Anesth. 2009;18(2):156–64.
54. Huang S, DeSantis ER. Treatment of pulmonary arterial hypertension in pregnancy. Am J Health Syst Pharm. 2007;64(18):1922–6.
55. Steen VD. The many faces of scleroderma. Rheum Dis Clin N Am. 2008;34(1):1–15. v
56. Bullo M, Tschumi S, Bucher BS, Bianchetti MG, Simonetti GD. Pregnancy outcome following exposure to angiotensin-converting enzyme inhibitors or angiotensin receptor antagonists: a systematic review. Hypertension. 2012;60(2):444–50.

57. Baethge BA, Wolf RE. Successful pregnancy with scleroderma renal disease and pulmonary hypertension in a patient using angiotensin converting enzyme inhibitors. Ann Rheum Dis. 1989;48(9):776–8.
58. Steen VD. Management of pregnancy in SSc renal crisis. Arthritis Rheum. 2002;52:S45. Ref Type: Abstract
59. Galiè N, Humbert M, Vachiery JL, Gibbs S, Lang I, Torbicki A, et al. 2015 ESC/ERS guidelines for the diagnosis and treatment of pulmonary hypertension. Rev Esp Cardiol (Engl Ed). 2016;69(2):177.
60. Jaïs X, Olsson KM, Barbera JA, Blanco I, Torbicki A, Peacock A, et al. Pregnancy outcomes in pulmonary arterial hypertension in the modern management era. Eur Respir J. 2012;40(4):881–5.
61. Bédard E, Dimopoulos K, Gatzoulis MA. Has there been any progress made on pregnancy outcomes among women with pulmonary arterial hypertension? Eur Heart J. 2009;30(3):256–65.
62. Moaveni D, Cohn J, Brodt J, Hoctor K, Ranasinghe J. Scleroderma and pulmonary hypertension complicating two pregnancies: use of neuraxial anesthesia, general anesthesia, epoprostenol and a multidisciplinary approach for cesarean delivery. Int J Obstet Anesth. 2015;24(4):375–82.
63. Eisele JH, Reitan JA. Scleroderma, Raynaud's phenomenon, and local anesthetics. Anesthesiology. 1971;34(4):386–7.

Vaccinations in Patients with Systemic Sclerosis

40

Elana J. Bernstein and John D. Pauling

The Justification for Vaccination Programmes in ARDs

The autoimmune rheumatic diseases (ARDs) are associated with higher rates of serious infection caused by the dysregulated immune responses inherent within the diseases themselves and the widespread use of immunomodulatory treatments across this heterogenous group of diseases. Rheumatologists have an important role in advocating and encouraging vaccine uptake, although studies have indicated that advice from treating rheumatologists is sometimes responsible for poor uptake of vaccines among eligible patients [1, 2]. There have been reports of vaccination rates for influenza and pneumococcus of ~50% among eligible ARD populations, despite immunomodulatory drug use and a high prevalence of additional relevant co-morbidities that would further benefit from vaccination [2]. Reasons for this may include concerns regarding the clinical effectiveness of vaccinations in patients receiving immunomodulatory therapies, concerns regarding the potential risk of disease flare post-vaccination, and an under-estimation of the burden of infectious diseases such as influenza and pneumococcus within our patient populations [2].

E. J. Bernstein (✉)
Columbia University/New York-Presbyterian Hospital Scleroderma Center, Division of Rheumatology, Department of Medicine, Columbia University Vagelos College of Physicians and Surgeons, Columbia University Irving Medical Center, New York, NY, USA
e-mail: ejb2153@cumc.columbia.edu

J. D. Pauling
Department of Rheumatology, North Bristol NHS Trust, Bristol, UK

Musculoskeletal Research Unit, Bristol Medical School Translational Health Sciences, University of Bristol, Bristol, UK
e-mail: John.pauling@nbt.nhs.uk

Risk of Precipitating ARDs Following Vaccination

Infectious pathogens, and viruses in particular, have been implicated as key environmental triggers in the emergence of ARDs in genetically susceptible individuals. The loss of self-tolerance is thought to be precipitated by a range of factors including "molecular mimicry" (caused by the structural similarity between viruses and self-antigens), "bystander activation" (in which an exaggerated anti-viral immune response propagates a pro-inflammatory environment that enhances autoreactive T cell activation in response to sequestered self-antigens released from microbial cells), and "epitope spreading" (whereby autoreactive T cells – themselves sometimes immortalized by the virus itself – spread to target additional self-antigens) [3]. Viruses such as Dengue fever have been implicated in the emergence of ARDs in case reports and population-based cohort studies [4]. Indeed, seasonal variation in infectious pathogen transmission may contribute to seasonal variation in onset and flares of autoimmune diseases [5]. Unsurprisingly, this has raised concerns about the potential for vaccines to precipitate or worsen ARDs. A number of vaccines have been implicated in the occurrence of ARDs, including hepatitis B, Bacillus Calmette-Guerin (BCG), tetanus, typhoid, influenza, diphtheria, and measles, mumps, and rubella (MMR) [6]. Human leukocyte antigen (HLA) genes (mirroring those responsible for ARDs) and genetic variants of interleukin-4 and interferon regulatory factors have been proposed to be associated with vaccine-induced autoimmunity. While the epidemiological evidence for vaccine-induced autoimmunity is insufficient to attribute causality, the apparent association has led to proposals to consider carefully the potential adverse impact of vaccinations in patients with a history of allergies, those with genetic risk factors, and/or those with a family history of autoimmunity [6].

A large case-control study comprising nearly 2000 incident cases of RA did not identify any association between the administration of commonly used vaccines and the subsequent development of RA (including among potentially

Y. Allanore et al. (eds.), *Scleroderma*, https://doi.org/10.1007/978-3-031-40658-4_40

higher risk groups such as smokers and those carrying the HLA DRB1 shared epitope) [7]. Reviews of the literature and cases reported to the Vaccine Adverse Event Reporting System (VAERS) have identified numerous cases of potential ARDs with arthritis, myelitis, optic neuritis, and pancytopenias following vaccinations against influenza, hepatitis B, and others [8, 9]. Reports of positive re-challenge adverse events appear to provide further evidence of the potential for vaccines to trigger or worsen ARDs [9], although such reports are strongly susceptible to publication bias. Large epidemiological studies have indicated vaccines are not an important cause of ARDs, although investigators should remain vigilant for the possibility that specific high-risk subgroups of patients (e.g., those carrying certain genetic haplotypes) may be at higher risk of reacting adversely to vaccinations than others – signals that could be overlooked in large cohort studies [10].

The potential pathogenic role of infectious agents has also led to hopes that vaccines could be used to abrogate potentially pathogenic autoreactive immune responses while preserving host immune responses to infectious pathogens [11]. Putative vaccine types that could help prevent or arrest the progression of autoimmunity include DNA (enabling cells to transiently express the self-antigen encoded by DNA to induce Th2 immunity), peptides of naturally occurring epitopes to act as tolerogens, MHC-II peptides, tolerogenic vaccines (comprising cytokines fused to self-antigens to eliminate autoreactive T-cells), and T-cell receptor-based vaccines [11, 12]. The potential anti-inflammatory actions of existing vaccinations such as the live BCG vaccine have also been espoused across a number of immune-mediated diseases, at least in pre-clinical models [13].

Risk of Exacerbating ARDs Following Vaccination

There have also been concerns raised about the safety of vaccination in patients with existing ARDs, and the specific risk of precipitating flares of pre-existing ARDs. This is thought to be an important contributing factor to poor vaccine uptake among patients with ARDs. Influenza vaccination does not appear to be associated with flares of rheumatoid arthritis (RA) [14] or systemic lupus erythematosus (SLE) [15]. Similarly, hepatitis B vaccine is not associated with flares of SLE in patients who are not taking high-dose corticosteroids or other immunosuppressive medications [16]. Other studies have confirmed the safety and efficacy (albeit with blunted serological responses) of influenza vaccination among patients with a diverse range of ARDs [17, 18].

The American College of Rheumatology (ACR) has recommended that all killed (pneumococcal, influenza, and hepatitis B), recombinant (HPV), and live attenuated (herpes zoster) vaccinations be given to all patients with RA before starting a biologic or non-biologic DMARD [19, 20].

Risk of Sclerosing Skin Disease Following Vaccination

There have been several case reports about the development of morphea following immunizations. For example, Torrelo et al. reported two cases of morphea profunda in young children following vaccinations: the first was a case of an 8-month-old boy who developed morphea profunda at the site of intramuscular injection of his third dose of the diphtheria, tetanus, pertussis vaccination, 2–3 weeks following the vaccination; and the second was a case of a 2-year-old girl who developed morphea profunda at age 15 months at the site of injection of the measles, mumps, and rubella vaccine [21]. Khaled et al. reported a case of a 2-year-old girl who developed morphea profunda at the site of the third dose of the diphtheria-pertussis-tetanus vaccination, 3 months following the immunization [22]. Drago et al. reported a case of a 50-year-old female who developed generalized morphea 2 weeks after receiving the second dose of the adsorbed tetanus toxoid vaccination [23].

Benmously Mlika et al. reported a case of a 9-month-old boy who developed morphea profunda 2 weeks following the third dose of the hepatitis B vaccination [24], and Schmutz et al. reported cases of a 5-year-old girl and 36-year-old female who developed localized scleroderma at the sites of recent hepatitis B vaccinations [25]. Viladomiu et al. reported a case of a 12-month-old boy who developed morphea profunda at the age of 6 months, approximately 20 days following intramuscular injection of the second dose of the 13-valent pneumococcal conjugate vaccine [26]. Requena Lopez et al. reported a case of a 67-year-old female who developed morphea and generalized extragenital lichen sclerosis et atrophicus 10 days following intramuscular influenza vaccination [27]. Finally, Matsumoto and Yamamoto reported a case of an 8-year-old girl who developed generalized morphea and linear scleroderma that began at the site of a (BCG) vaccination she had received more than 7 years prior [28].

Impact of Immunomodulatory Treatments on Vaccine Efficacy

The use of immunosuppressive medications is one of the key reasons why vaccination in ARDs is desirable. Minimizing cumulative glucocorticoid exposure and cyclophosphamide dosing in high-risk groups such as people >65 years old with vasculitis is associated with lower rates of complications secondary to infections such as herpes zoster and pneumonia (compared to conventional treatment) [29]. It is generally accepted that immunosuppressed populations are at higher risk of complications of influenza and that humoral serological responses to vaccines are attenuated in these populations [30]. Nonetheless, seroconversion to non-adjuvanted influenza A/H1N1 vaccination in mixed connective tissue disease patients is comparable to healthy controls and is not influenced by disease manifestations such as lymphopenia or immunoglobulin levels, or by use of immunomodulatory therapy [31]. A prospective vaccination study of mixed populations of ARDs suggested that seroprotection following influenza vaccination was more readily achieved in connective tissue disease and spondyloarthropathy compared with RA and vasculitis [32]. In juvenile ARD, influenza vaccination is safe and, while serological responses are blunted, seroconversion is sufficient to confer protection [33]. The majority of patients with SLE mount a sufficient immune response to vaccines despite background immunosuppressive therapy, although serological responses to hepatitis B should be confirmed to ensure immunity [34]. Similarly, hepatitis B vaccination appears to be associated with an adequate serological response in patients with inactive SLE who are not taking high-dose corticosteroids or other immunosuppressive medications [16]. Conventional DMARDs do not appear to influence serological responses to influenza vaccine in SLE patients compared to healthy controls [15]. Glucocorticoids, meanwhile, appear to blunt serological responses to influenza type B antigen (but not type A antigens) in SLE patients [15]. Glucocorticoids were the major factors blunting serological response to influenza vaccination in children [33].

Among renal transplant recipients receiving cyclosporine and glucocorticoids, those who also received mycophenolate mofetil (MMF) had a blunted humoral immune response to influenza vaccination compared to those treated with azathioprine and controls (with ~80% failing to mount a >four-fold rise in titre to one of 3 antigens in those exposed to MMF, compared to only ~40% in the azathioprine group and ~ 20% in the control arm) [35]. Methotrexate, rituximab, and abatacept are also associated with reduced rates of seroprotection following influenza vaccination [32]. A linear decline in serological responses also occurs with age [32].

Given its role targeting B cell maturation, the potential impact of rituximab on immunity has been examined. Hypogammaglobulinemia following rituximab is associated with an increased frequency of serious infections, highlighting the importance of prior vaccination [36]. Humoral responses to specific vaccines have been tested in patients with hypogammaglobulinemia and/or infections, following rituximab therapy. Adequate response to tetanus occurred in 93% of subjects, but suboptimal responses to pneumococcus and haemophilus were identified in 59% and 72% of patients, respectively (which persisted at 6 weeks in over half of patients and sometimes necessitated the use of immunoglobulin replacement) [36]. Serological responses to influenza vaccination are also suppressed following rituximab therapy for RA, particularly within 6 months of administration, whereas humoral responses in patients with RA treated with methotrexate alone were comparable to controls [14]. Similarly, patients with RA treated with rituximab (alongside methotrexate) have been shown to have a reduced serological response to pneumococcal polysaccharide vaccine. For example, only 57% of patients treated with rituximab achieved a twofold rise in titre, compared with 82% of patients treated with methotrexate alone [37]. The effect of rituximab was not uniform across different vaccines, however. For example, responses to tetanus toxoid vaccine were similar in both groups with ~40% of both rituximab-treated and methotrexate monotherapy-treated RA patients achieving a fourfold increase in antibody titre following tetanus toxoid immunization [37]. Humoral responses to influenza vaccination are modestly restored to normal expected levels 6–10 months after rituximab administration [14]. Previous influenza vaccination is associated with higher pre- and post-vaccination titres in patients with RA treated with rituximab [14].

In patients with RA already receiving immunomodulatory treatments who have not previously been vaccinated, the ACR has recommended that all killed (pneumococcal, influenza, and hepatitis B) and recombinant (human papillomavirus [HPV]) vaccinations be administered [19, 20]. The ACR has recommended the use of live attenuated zoster vaccine in patients already receiving conventional synthetic (cs) DMARD therapies (including combination therapy), but *not* biologic therapies, due to theoretical concerns rather than data confirming a specific risk in patients receiving such treatment [19, 20].

Re-Vaccination Following Autologous Hematopoietic Stem Cell Transplantation

The most powerful form of immunomodulatory intervention for patients with SSc is myeloablative autologous hematopoietic stem cell transplant (HSCT). This therapy appears to result in loss of immunological memory in the majority of patients with prior neoantigen vaccination, but memory to recall antigen is preserved in many patients [38]. Other treatments that may occasionally be used in ARDs such as extracorporeal photopheresis do not appear to dampen primary responses to vaccinations [39].

Re-vaccination is an important part of the management of SSc patients who undergo autologous HSCT (Table 40.1) [40, 41]. Live vaccinations should not be administered until 24 months post-HSCT and then only if a patient is immunocompetent [41].

Table 40.1 Suggested vaccine schedule following autologous hematopoietic stem cell transplantation

	Time Post-HSCT			
Vaccine	6 months	9 months	12 months	18 months
13-valent Pneumococcal conjugate (PCV13)	✓	✓	✓	
23-valent Pneumococcal polysaccharide (PPSV23)				✓
Diphtheria, tetanus, and acellular pertussis (DTaP)	✓	✓	✓	
Haemophilus influenzae type b conjugate (Hib)	✓	✓	✓	
Seasonal inactivated influenza[a]	✓			
Inactivated polio (IPV)	✓	✓	✓	
Hepatitis B	✓	✓	✓	

[a]Annual vaccination

Safety of Live Vaccines in ARDs

Live vaccines have raised specific concerns in the context of ARDs. The lack of evidence has forced many manufacturers to advise against the use of live vaccinations in patients receiving immunomodulatory therapy. As previously discussed, the ACR does not recommend the use of live attenuated zoster vaccine in patients already receiving biologic therapies, due to theoretical concerns of serious adverse events [19, 20].

While live vaccines are generally contraindicated in persons receiving immunosuppressive medication, case series of patients inadvertently immunized with the yellow fever vaccine despite receiving immunosuppressive treatments suggest they are still able to mount a protective serological response with a low incidence of adverse effects, although caution is still warranted in such patients when considering use of live vaccines [42]. A recent study examined the routine use of yellow fever vaccine in patients with stable low disease activity who were able to discontinue existing immunomodulatory treatments for a pre-specified period prior to vaccination (ranging from 3 months for csDMARDs to >6 months following rituximab) [43]. The study identified a lower and delayed seroconversion rate in these patients compared to healthy controls, although the yellow fever vaccine was safe and immunogenic in the majority of patients [43].

The live attenuated vaccine against herpes zoster is contraindicated in immunocompromised people, in whom serious adverse events have been reported, although it has been noted that few of these reports concerned patients with ARDs receiving csDMARDs. A case control study examining autoimmune adverse events following administration of the zoster vaccine did identify a twofold increased risk of arthritis and alopecia, but no increased risk of SLE or any other defined ARDs [44]. The live attenuated varicella zoster vaccine appears to be safe and well tolerated among children with ARDs, although serological responses are lower than among their healthy counterparts [45]. Humoral and cellular responses to newer varicella zoster vaccination in patients with paediatric ARDs are comparable to that of healthy controls, despite background treatment with methotrexate (and for some corticosteroids and/or biologics) and does not appear to be associated with disease flares [46].

Uptake of Vaccination Programmes in Patients with ARDs

There appears to be a low uptake of vaccines among patients with ARDs. Allowing for marked geographic variation in uptake, an international cohort study of 3920 patients with RA identified 25.3% (95% confidence interval [CI] 23.8–26.5) coverage for influenza and ~17.2% (95% CI 16.0–18.4) for pneumococcus [47]. Similar coverage for influenza vaccination (~30%) has been observed in patients with vasculitis and SSc, compared with uptake of approximately 70% in eligible patients >65 years among the general population of France within the same period of study [48]. Reassuringly, older age and additional co-morbidities were associated with higher vaccination rates [47, 49], but non-smoking and higher educational status were also associated with higher uptake of vaccinations, indicating potential socioeconomic factors that favour more affluent patients which may influence vaccine uptake [47]. Negative stories circulated by anti-vaccination lobby groups may have had an impact on immunization coverage and may have contributed to geographic variation in vaccine provision among countries with similar socioeconomic profiles. The low rates of pneumococcal vaccine uptake are of particular concern, given higher risk rates of hospital admission for pneumococcal disease among patients with ARDs (with rate ratios as high as 4.2 for SSc and 5.0 for both polyarteritis nodosa and SLE, compared with 3.7 for diabetes mellitus) [50]. Complex interventions have been developed and tested in patients with ARDs to increase coverage of influenza, pneumococcus, and zoster vaccinations, with modest effects [51].

A handful of studies have evaluated the vaccination rate in patients with SSc. For example, Pope et al. compared self-reported vaccination history since age 18 years between 65 adults with SSc and 196 controls with non-inflammatory musculoskeletal disorders [52]. They found no difference between the two groups in rate of vaccinations – 49% of the SSc group recalled receiving vaccinations in adulthood, compared to 50% of the controls (p-value = 0.90). Mouthon et al. evaluated the influenza vaccination rate among adults with SSc [53]. Of the 177 SSc patients surveyed, 69 (39%) had received an influenza vaccination the previous year. Of these 69 vaccinated patients, 54% were immunized because of a general practitioner's recommendation and 20% because of a specialist's recommendation. Seventy-eight of the 108 (72.2%) unvaccinated patients had at least one indication for influenza vaccination: 22 (28.2%) were ≥ 65 years of age; 28 (35.9%) received corticosteroids; 28 (35.9%) received other immunosuppressants; 44 (56.4%) had ILD; and 12 (15.4%) had pulmonary arterial hypertension. The most common reasons cited for not receiving the influenza vaccination among the 108 SSc patients who were not immunized were: no physician had recommended it (36.1%); fear of side effects (23.1%); and fear of inefficacy (4%).

Another study evaluating seasonal influenza and pneumococcal vaccination rates in a cohort of 91 SSc patients reported that 63 (69.2%) were vaccinated against seasonal influenza and 68 (74.7%) against *Streptococcus pneumoniae*. Age > 65 years (odds ratio [OR] 31.68, 95% CI 4.89–205.29) and use of immunosuppressive therapy (OR 31.98, 95% CI 4.33–236.36) were both associated with influenza vaccination in a multivariable analysis. Age > 65 years (OR 6.10, 95% CI 1.43–25.99), use of immunosuppressive therapy (OR 11.24, 95% CI 42.38–52.97), and cardiovascular disease (OR 8.18, 95% CI 1.10–60.86) were associated with pneumococcal vaccination in a multivariable analysis [54].

Bizjak et al. performed a retrospective cohort study of children with ARDs and fibromyalgia at a single center in Slovenia to assess vaccination status and reasons for not vaccinating [1]. Two of the 187 included participants had juvenile SSc. Vaccination status was complete in both of these juvenile SSc patients.

Vaccination Immunogenicity and Safety in Patients with Systemic Sclerosis

Pneumococcal Vaccination

Some studies suggest that patients with SSc are at a greater risk for invasive pneumococcal disease. Wotton and Goldacre used the Oxford Record Linkage Study (ORLS)1 (1963–1998), ORLS2 (1999–2008), and English national linked Hospital Episode Statistics (HES) (1999–2008) databases to determine the risk of invasive pneumococcal disease (i.e., pneumococcal pneumonia, septicemia, or meningitis) in hospitalized patients with autoimmune diseases, including SSc [50]. The time periods of ORLS1 and ORLS2 correspond to time periods before and after the introduction of routine pneumococcal vaccination in England, respectively. ORLS1 contained 427 SSc patients, ORLS2 481, and HES 9308. Patients with SSc had a higher risk of invasive pneumococcal disease compared to a control cohort in all three databases, adjusted for age in 5-year bands, sex, calendar year, and district of residence in ORLS1 and ORLS2 and for age in 5-year bands, sex, calendar year, region of residence, and deprivation score associated with area of residence in HES (ORLS1: rate ratio [RR] 5.77, 95% CI 2.63–11.0; ORLS2: RR 4.97, 95% CI 3.07–7.62; HES: RR 4.26, 95% CI 3.84–4.72).

Mercado et al. evaluated the immunogenicity of the 23-valent pneumococcal polysaccharide vaccine (PPSV23) in 18 consecutive adults with SSc [55]. Antibody concentrations to the four most common antigens encountered in their region were measured pre-vaccination and 4 weeks post-vaccination. One-hundred percent of the patients achieved a ≥ two-fold increase in antibody titer to at least one of the four capsular antigens, while 83% experienced a ≥ two-fold increase in antibody titer to at least three of the four capsular antigens. Antibody levels were re-measured at 1-year post-vaccination in 10 of the 18 participants. The mean antibody level to each of the four capsular antigens was lower at 1 year than at 4 weeks post-vaccination.

In a prospective study, 44 SSc patients (12 of whom were taking DMARDs, 32 of whom were not) and 49 controls were immunized with either the 13-valent pneumococcal conjugate vaccine (PCV13) or PPSV23 vaccine [56]. Pre-vaccination antibody levels against the 6B and 23F serotypes were similar between SSc patients taking DMARDs, SSc patients not taking DMARDs, and controls. Four to six weeks following vaccination, antibody levels against both serotypes had statistically significantly increased from baseline among SSc patients not taking DMARDs and controls. However, among SSc patients taking DMARDs, only antibodies against serotype 6B had statistically significantly increased from baseline. The authors report that the PCV13 and PPSV23 vaccines were generally well tolerated.

Hepatitis B Vaccination

There have not been any large studies looking at hepatitis B vaccination in adult SSc. Patel et al. performed a retrospective chart review of 75 children (aged 3–18 years) with morphea, atopic dermatitis, or psoriasis who were prescribed methotrexate and had anti-Hepatitis B surface antibody titers [57]. All participants had completed the hepatitis B vaccination series. The authors characterized participants as non-responders to hepatitis B vaccination if their anti-Hepatitis B surface antibody titers were < 10 mIU/mL. Four patients with morphea were categorized as responders, and four patients with morphea were categorized as non-responders.

Influenza Vaccination

The Advisory Committee on Influenza Practices of the Centers for Disease Control recommends routine annual influenza vaccination for all people ≥6 months of age who do not have contraindications [58]. During the 2006–2007 influenza season, Setti et al. performed a single center, open label study of a virosomal influenza vaccine that contained 15 µg of hemagglutinin for each of the following strains of influenza virus: A/Wisconsin/67/2005 (H3N2) (A/Hiroshima/52/2005 IVR-142); A/New Caledonia/20/99 (H1N1) (A/New Caledonia/20/99 IVR-116); B/Malaysia/2506/2004 (B/Malaysia/2506/2004) [59]. Fifty adults with dcSSc and 20 age- and sex-matched healthy controls were included. Patients were excluded if they were receiving prednisone >1 mg/kg/day, cyclosporine-A >300 mg/day, mycophenolate mofetil >1000 mg/day, or methotrexate >15 mg/week for >1 month; if they were receiving any tumor necrosis factor-inhibitor at any dosage; or if they had received a blood transfusion or intravenous immunoglobulin within the prior 3 months. Of the 46 dcSSc patients who completed this study, and depending on the hemagglutination inhibition test used (i.e., guinea pig erythrocytes or human 0-type erythrocytes), 47% had protective titers of influenza antibodies against the A/H3N2 (Wisconsin, 67/2005) strain, 40–47% against the A/H1N1 (New Caledonia, 20/99) strain, and 20–50% against the B (Malaysia, 2506/2004) strain prior to vaccination. At 1 month following vaccination, and depending on the hemagglutination inhibition test used, 80–83% had a rise in antibody titers against the A/H3N2 (Wisconsin, 67/2005) strain, 76–88% had a rise in antibody titers against the A/H1N1 (New Caledonia, 20/99) strain, and 74–89% had a rise in antibody titers against the B (Malaysia, 2506/2004) strain. The authors defined seroprotection as an antibody titer of ≥1:40. At 1 month following vaccination, and depending on the hemagglutination inhibition test used, 67–73% of dcSSc patients were protected against the A/H3N2 (Wisconsin, 67/2005) strain, 73–80% against the A/H1N1 (New Caledonia, 20/99) strain, and 67–80% against the B (Malaysia, 2506/2004) strain. No flu-like episodes or serious vaccination-related adverse events were reported during the follow-up period.

Kostianovsky et al. performed a prospective, open label, single center study to evaluate the immunogenicity and safety of the seasonal and A/H1N1 influenza vaccines in adults with ARDs [17]. Participants received the seasonal influenza vaccine at baseline, the first dose of the A/H1N1 influenza vaccine 3–6 weeks later, and the second dose of the A/H1N1 influenza vaccine 3 weeks after the first. The seasonal influenza vaccine contained 15 µg of hemagglutinin for each of the following strains of influenza virus: A/Brisbane/59/2007/3/2006 (H1N1); A/Brisbane/10/2007 (H3N2); and B/Brisbane/60/2008. One-hundred ninety-nine patients were included, of whom 34 had SSc. Of the 33 SSc patients who received the seasonal influenza vaccine, 29 (87.9%) became seroprotected and 12 (41.4%) of them seroconverted. The geometric mean titer increased from 24.3 at baseline to 88.3 at week 3, which is a 3.63-fold increase. Of the 34 SSc patients who received the A/H1N1 influenza vaccine, 24 (70.6%) became seroprotected and 13 (54.2%) of them seroconverted. The geometric mean titer increased from 19.7 at baseline (which is 3–6 weeks following the seasonal influenza vaccine) to 60.3 at week 6, which is a 3.06-fold increase. Thirty-two of the 173 participants (18%) who received the seasonal influenza vaccine and 45 of the 197 participants (23%) who received at least one dose of the A/H1N1 influenza vaccine developed local injection site reactions. The percentage of participants who developed systemic reactions was even lower – 1% of those who received the seasonal influenza vaccine and 4% of those who received at least one dose of the A/H1N1 influenza vaccine. One participant with SSc developed a mild flare of myositis/arthritis and a calcinosis abscess.

Saad et al. performed a prospective, open label, single center study to assess the immunogenicity and safety of the non-adjuvanted influenza A H1N1/2009 vaccine in 1668 adults with ARDs compared to 234 healthy controls [18]. One-hundred twenty-seven (7.6%) of the patients had SSc. Prior to immunization, 18.1% of the SSc patients were seroprotected. Following immunization, 81.1% of SSc patients were seroprotected and 73.2% had seroconverted. In comparison, 11.5% of the controls were seroprotected prior to immunization, 82.9% were seroprotected following immunization, and 76.9% had seroconverted. The geometric mean titer pre- and post-vaccination in participants with SSc was 11.2 and 134.4, respectively, which is a 12-factor-increase. In comparison, the geometric mean titer pre- and post-vaccination in controls was 9.3 and 122.9, respectively, which is a 13.2-factor-increase. The vaccine was generally well tolerated. No severe adverse effects were reported. A smaller proportion of patients with ARDs than controls experienced local injection site reactions (8.3% vs. 14.1%, p-value = 0.007). The frequency of mild systemic reactions was similar between both groups (24.6% in patients with ARDs vs. 25.6% in controls, p-value = 0.75). A greater proportion of patients with ARDs than controls experienced arthralgia (9% vs. 3.8%, p-value = 0.005) and fever (3.9% vs. 1.2%, p-value = 0.04).

Sampaio-Barros et al. performed a prospective, open label, single center study to assess the immunogenicity and safety of the non-adjuvanted, monovalent A(H1N1)pdm09 influenza vaccine in 92 adults with SSc compared to 92 age- and sex-matched healthy controls [60]. The active substance in the A(H1N1)pdm09 influenza vaccine is a split, inactivated influenza virus containing antigens equivalent to the A/California/7/2009 (H1N1) virus-like strain. Prior to immunization, 20.7% of the SSc patients were seroprotected compared to 12.0% of the controls (p-value = 0.11). Following immunization, 83.7% of the SSc patients were seroprotected compared to 76.1% of the controls (p-value = 0.20), and 76.1% of the SSc patients had seroconverted compared to 72.8% of the controls (p-value = 0.61). The geometric mean titer pre- and post-vaccination in participants with SSc was 11.3 and 166.1, respectively, which is a 14.7-factor-increase. In comparison, the geometric mean titer pre- and post-vaccination in controls was 8.8 and 104.1, respectively, which is an 11.8-factor-increase. The difference in factor-increases in geometric mean titers between SSc patients and controls was not statistically significant (14.7 vs. 11.8, p-value = 0.34). Following immunization, there were no statistically significant differences in seroprotection rates, seroconversion rates, or geometric mean titer factor-increases between SSc patients with the diffuse vs. limited subtype, between those with an mRSS ≥14 vs. <14, or between those taking vs. not taking immunosuppressive medications. A similar proportion of SSc patients and controls reported local injection site reactions (7.6% vs. 10.9%, p-value = 0.45) and minor systemic reactions (25.0% vs. 31.5%, p-value = 0.33). There were no statistically significant differences in rates of local injection site reactions or minor systemic reactions between SSc patients with the diffuse vs. limited subtype, between those with an mRSS ≥14 vs. <14, or between those taking vs. not taking immunosuppressive medications.

Litinsky et al. performed a prospective, open label study at three medical centers to assess the efficacy and safety of a trivalent influenza subunit vaccine (H1N1 A/Brisbane/59/2007 [TGA 2008/81B] [H1N1], H3N2 A/Uruguay/716/2007 [A/Brisbane/10/2007-like, NIBSC 8/124] [H3N2] and B B/Brisbane/60/2008 [TGA 2009/82/B]) in 26 consecutive SSc patients compared to 16 age- and sex-matched healthy hospital personnel [61]. Compared to pre-vaccination, at 6 weeks post-vaccination, both the SSc patients and controls had increases in the geometric mean titers of haemagglutination inhibition (HI) antibodies against all 3 influenza antigens (H1N1, H3N2, and B). The increase in geometric mean titer at 6 weeks post-vaccination against the H3N2 antigen in SSc patients receiving immunosuppressive therapy ($n = 7$) was not statistically significant. However, the increase in geometric mean titer at 6 weeks post-vaccination against the H1N1 and B antigens in SSc patients receiving immunosuppressive therapy was statistically significant. None of the SSc patients or controls developed a local reaction following vaccination. Two of the SSc patients developed mild upper respiratory tract infections.

Aikawa et al. performed a prospective, open label study to assess the immunogenicity and safety of the non-adjuvanted influenza A H1N1/2009 in 237 children with ARDs and 91 age-matched healthy controls aged 9–21 years [33]. One dose of the H1N1 A/California/7/2009-like virus vaccine (A/California/7/2009/Butantan Institute/Sanofi Pasteur) was administered intramuscularly to all participants. Of the 11 participants with juvenile scleroderma (5 with SSc and 6 with localized scleroderma), 27.3% had a seroprotective antibody titer of ≥1:40 before vaccination. At 21 days following immunization, 90.9% had a seroprotective antibody titer. The geometric mean titer pre- and post-vaccination in the participants with juvenile scleroderma was 12.1 and 181.5, respectively, which was a 15-factor-increase. No reduced protective immunogenicity in the participants with juvenile scleroderma was observed.

Yellow Fever Vaccination

Valim et al. performed a prospective, open label, single center study to assess the safety and immunogenicity of the 17DD-Yellow Fever vaccine in 211 adults with ARDs and 38 healthy controls [43]. Seven patients had SSc. One (14%) of the SSc patients experienced a local adverse effect, compared to 8 (3%) of the healthy controls (p-value = 0.50). Four (57%) of the SSc patients experienced a systemic adverse effect compared to 8 (21%) of the healthy controls (p-value = 0.07). Seropositivity rates at day 28 were similar between SSc patients (5/6, 83%) and healthy controls (22/23, 96; p-value = 0.29), although the geometric mean titer was lower in SSc patients than in healthy controls (206 vs. 440, p-value = 0.09). Yellow fever viremia was undetectable in the 2 SSc patients in whom it was measured.

Oliveira, Mota, and Santos-Neto evaluated seroconversion in patients with ARDs who were treated with immunosuppressives or immunomodulators and were inadvertently revaccinated against yellow fever [42]. Thirty-one adult females were included, 27 (87.1%) of whom were seropositive for protection against yellow fever. Two of the 31 included patients had SSc, although the authors did not report seropositivity by disease. One of the SSc patients developed fever and rhinorrhea following the yellow fever vaccination.

In a case series of 70 adults with ARDs who were vaccinated against yellow fever within the prior 60 days, 2 (2.9%) of the patients had SSc [62]. Sixteen (22.9%) patients reported an adverse event, one of whom had SSc.

Measles Vaccination

In a study of the relationship between natural and infection-induced antibodies in patients with ARDs, Borocz et al. found that 144 of 157 (91.7%) SSc patients had IgG anti-measles antibodies [63].

Varicella Vaccination

Pileggi et al. performed a prospective, open label, single center study to assess the safety and immunogenicity of the live attenuated varicella virus vaccine in 25 children and adolescents (aged 2–19 years) with juvenile ARDs who were taking methotrexate compared to 18 healthy children and adolescent controls (ages 2–18 years) [45]. One out of the 3 juvenile scleroderma patients had equivocal pre-immunization anti-varicella zoster virus (VZV) IgG titers and was therefore excluded from the immunogenicity analysis. All 3 juvenile scleroderma patients were taking both methotrexate and prednisone. Of the 2 juvenile scleroderma patients who were negative for pre-immunization anti-VZV IgG titers, 1 (50%) developed anti-VZV IgG titers 4–6 weeks following immunization. This patient maintained anti-VZV IgG titers 1 year following the varicella virus vaccination. None of the juvenile scleroderma patients developed a vaccine-related rash.

Groot et al. performed a prospective, open label, single center study to assess the immunogenicity of the live attenuated varicella virus vaccine in 49 children (25 of whom were previously included in the aforementioned study by Pileggi et al.[45]) and adolescents (aged 2–17 years) with juvenile ARDs who were taking methotrexate ± other immunosuppressants compared to 18 healthy children and adolescent controls (ages 3–18 years) [46]. Varicella vaccination resulted in a statistically significant increase in VZV-specific antibodies in the 5 included patients with juvenile scleroderma. One of the juvenile scleroderma patients who was taking methotrexate and corticosteroids reported an elevated temperature (that remained <38 °C and lasted 1–3 days) and a mild vesicular rash within 2 weeks following vaccination. One juvenile scleroderma patient who was receiving methotrexate and corticosteroids and had low VZV-specific antibody concentration after vaccination developed chickenpox at least 1 year following immunization. The course of the episode of chickenpox was similar to that of healthy children, with fever and vesicular lesions.

Human Papillomavirus Vaccination

Recent work has demonstrated that women with ARDs have an increased risk of high- and low-grade cervical dysplasia, comparable to that of those with HIV infection [64, 65]. Risk factors for pre-malignant cervical lesions in ARDs include exposure to glucocorticoids and other immunomodulatory agents, particularly cyclophosphamide [65]. The HPV vaccines appear to be safe and immunogenic in females with ARDs and it is hoped that vaccination programmes will decrease the future risk of cervical dysplasia in women with ARDs [64, 65]. Preliminary data suggest there is no increased risk of autoimmune disorders, including connective tissue diseases, in women receiving the quadrivalent HPV vaccine [66]. Similarly, there are no data that indicate a relationship between HPV vaccination and worsening of ARDs [67]. HPV carriage is similar in SSc as in controls, but multi-HPV carriage may be higher in SSc and, when considered alongside the established increased risk of malignancy associated with SSc, HPV vaccination may be of particular importance in SSc patients [68].

Severe Acute Respiratory Syndrome Coronavirus 2 (SARS-CoV-2)

The recent emergence of SARS-CoV-2 has led to an accelerated vaccination programme to achieve population-based immunity to COVID-19, the disease that results from SARS-CoV-2. To date, there have been no studies reporting any specific issues around safety and seroprotection status within SSc patient populations. COVID-19 vaccination should be offered to patients with SSc, particularly those with pre-existing pulmonary complications and those receiving immunosuppressive therapy. There is no particular type of COVID-19 vaccine that is preferred for patients with SSc. Therefore, patients with SSc should receive whichever COVID-19 vaccine is available to them. The timing of vaccination (e.g., around rituximab administration) should be informed by approaches taken with other vaccines. Decisions around choice and timing of COVID-19 vaccinations should be based upon shared decision-making between patients and physicians, although there is guidance emerging from the American College of Rheumatology (currently under peer-review but the living document is available from: https://www.rheumatology.org/Portals/0/Files/COVID-19-Vaccine-Clinical-Guidance-Rheumatic-Diseases-Summary.pdf) and other groups to support such decision making.

Conclusions

Patients with ARDs, including SSc, have a higher risk of morbidity and mortality from vaccine-preventable infections than the general population, primarily due to the immunosuppressive medications used to treat these diseases. Thus, it is critical that patients with SSc be immunized against vaccine-preventable diseases, such as influenza and pneumococcus. Rheumatologists should encourage their patients with SSc and other ARDs to receive the necessary vaccinations, as this will likely help improve vaccine uptake among patients with ARDs.

References

1. Bizjak M, Blazina S, Zajc Avramovic M, Markelj G, Avcin T, Toplak N. Vaccination coverage in children with rheumatic diseases. Clin Exp Rheumatol. 2020;38(1):164–70.
2. Assala M, Groh M, Blanche P, Vinter C, Cohen P, Le Guern V, et al. Pneumococcal and influenza vaccination rates in patients treated with corticosteroids and/or immunosuppressive therapies for systemic autoimmune diseases: a cross-sectional study. Joint Bone Spine. 2017;84(3):365–6. https://doi.org/10.1016/j.jbspin.2016.03.013.
3. Smatti MK, Cyprian FS, Nasrallah GK, Al Thani AA, Almishal RO, Yassine HM. Viruses and autoimmunity: a review on the potential interaction and molecular mechanisms. Viruses. 2019;11(8) https://doi.org/10.3390/v11080762.
4. Li HM, Huang YK, Su YC, Kao CH. Increased risk of autoimmune diseases in dengue patients: a population-based cohort study. J Infect. 2018;77(3):212–9. https://doi.org/10.1016/j.jinf.2018.03.014.
5. Watad A, Azrielant S, Bragazzi NL, Sharif K, David P, Katz I, et al. Seasonality and autoimmune diseases: the contribution of the four seasons to the mosaic of autoimmunity. J Autoimmun. 2017;82:13–30. https://doi.org/10.1016/j.jaut.2017.06.001.
6. Vadala M, Poddighe D, Laurino C, Palmieri B. Vaccination and autoimmune diseases: is prevention of adverse health effects on the horizon? EPMA J. 2017;8(3):295–311. https://doi.org/10.1007/s13167-017-0101-y.
7. Bengtsson C, Kapetanovic MC, Kallberg H, Sverdrup B, Nordmark B, Klareskog L, et al. Common vaccinations among adults do not increase the risk of developing rheumatoid arthritis: results from the Swedish EIRA study. Ann Rheum Dis. 2010;69(10):1831–3. https://doi.org/10.1136/ard.2010.129908.
8. Mamarabadi M, Baisre A, Leitch M, Hsu V, Kanduri JS, Chen S. Case of anti-single recognition particle-mediated necrotizing myopathy after influenza vaccination. J Clin Neuromuscul Dis. 2018;19(4):211–6. https://doi.org/10.1097/CND.0000000000000208.
9. Geier MR, Geier DA. A case-series of adverse events, positive re-challenge of symptoms, and events in identical twins following hepatitis B vaccination: analysis of the vaccine adverse event reporting system (VAERS) database and literature review. Clin Exp Rheumatol. 2004;22(6):749–55.
10. Vial T, Descotes J. Autoimmune diseases and vaccinations. Eur J Dermatol. 2004;14(2):86–90.
11. Zhang N, Nandakumar KS. Recent advances in the development of vaccines for chronic inflammatory autoimmune diseases. Vaccine. 2018;36(23):3208–20. https://doi.org/10.1016/j.vaccine.2018.04.062.
12. Marciani DJ. Effects of immunomodulators on the response induced by vaccines against autoimmune diseases. Autoimmunity. 2017;50(7):393–402. https://doi.org/10.1080/08916934.2017.1373766.
13. Lagranderie M, Guyonvarc'h PM. The interplay between bacillus Calmette-Guerin and Treg cells and its role to prevent or cure inflammatory diseases. Expert Rev Clin Immunol. 2014;10(6):741–5. https://doi.org/10.1586/1744666X.2014.909286.
14. van Assen S, Holvast A, Benne CA, Posthumus MD, van Leeuwen MA, Voskuyl AE, et al. Humoral responses after influenza vaccination are severely reduced in patients with rheumatoid arthritis treated with rituximab. Arthritis Rheum. 2010;62(1):75–81. https://doi.org/10.1002/art.25033.
15. Wallin L, Quintilio W, Locatelli F, Cassel A, Silva MB, Skare TL. Safety and efficiency of influenza vaccination in systemic lupus erythematosus patients. Acta Reumatol Port. 2009;34(3):498–502.
16. Kuruma KA, Borba EF, Lopes MH, de Carvalho JF, Bonfa E. Safety and efficacy of hepatitis B vaccine in systemic lupus erythematosus. Lupus. 2007;16(5):350–4. https://doi.org/10.1177/0961203307078225.
17. Kostianovsky A, Charles P, Alves JF, Goulet M, Pagnoux C, Le Guern V, et al. Immunogenicity and safety of seasonal and 2009 pandemic a/H1N1 influenza vaccines for patients with autoimmune diseases: a prospective, monocentre trial on 199 patients. Clin Exp Rheumatol. 2012;30(1 Suppl 70):S83–9.
18. Saad CG, Borba EF, Aikawa NE, Silva CA, Pereira RM, Calich AL, et al. Immunogenicity and safety of the 2009 non-adjuvanted influenza a/H1N1 vaccine in a large cohort of autoimmune rheumatic diseases. Ann Rheum Dis. 2011;70(6):1068–73. https://doi.org/10.1136/ard.2011.150250.
19. Singh JA, Furst DE, Bharat A, Curtis JR, Kavanaugh AF, Kremer JM, et al. 2012 update of the 2008 American College of Rheumatology recommendations for the use of disease-modifying antirheumatic drugs and biologic agents in the treatment of rheumatoid arthritis. Arthritis Care Res (Hoboken). 2012;64(5):625–39. https://doi.org/10.1002/acr.21641.
20. Singh JA, Saag KG, Bridges SL Jr, Akl EA, Bannuru RR, Sullivan MC, et al. 2015 American College of Rheumatology Guideline for the treatment of rheumatoid arthritis. Arthritis Rheumatol. 2016;68(1):1–26. https://doi.org/10.1002/art.39480.
21. Torrelo A, Suarez J, Colmenero I, Azorin D, Perera A, Zambrano A. Deep morphea after vaccination in two young children. Pediatr Dermatol. 2006;23(5):484–7. https://doi.org/10.1111/j.1525-1470.2006.00289.x.
22. Khaled A, Kharfi M, Zaouek A, Rameh S, Zermani R, Fazaa B, et al. Postvaccination morphea profunda in a child. Pediatr Dermatol. 2012;29(4):525–7. https://doi.org/10.1111/j.1525-1470.2011.01548.x.
23. Drago F, Rampini P, Lugani C, Rebora A. Generalized morphoea after antitetanus vaccination. Clin Exp Dermatol. 1998;23(3):142. https://doi.org/10.1046/j.1365-2230.1998.00324.x.
24. Benmously Mlika R, Kenani N, Badri T, Hammami H, Hichri J, Haouet S, et al. Morphea profunda in a young infant after hepatitis B vaccination. J Am Acad Dermatol. 2010;63(6):1111–2. https://doi.org/10.1016/j.jaad.2009.02.047.
25. Schmutz JL, Posth M, Granel F, Trechot P, Barbaud A. Localized scleroderma after hepatitis B vaccination. Presse Med. 2000;29(19):1046.
26. Viladomiu Edel A, Valls AT, Zabaleta BA, Moreno AJ, Perez NO. Deep morphea in a child after pneumococcal vaccination. Indian J Dermatol Venereol Leprol. 2014;80(3):259–60. https://doi.org/10.4103/0378-6323.132259.
27. Requena Lopez S, Hidalgo Garcia Y, Gomez Diez S, Vivanco AB. Morphea and extragenital lichen Sclerosus et atrophicus after influenza vaccination. Actas Dermosifiliogr. 2018;109(1):86–8. https://doi.org/10.1016/j.ad.2017.05.016.
28. Matsumoto M, Yamamoto T. Pediatric generalized morphea that developed at a BCG vaccination site. Actas Dermosifiliogr. 2015;106(2):150–2. https://doi.org/10.1016/j.ad.2014.06.012.
29. Pagnoux C, Guillevin L. Reply to: importance of immunisation of elderly subjects before immunosuppressive treatment. Clin Exp Rheumatol. 2016;34(1 Suppl 95):S21.
30. Kunisaki KM, Janoff EN. Influenza in immunosuppressed populations: a review of infection frequency, morbidity, mortality, and vaccine responses. Lancet Infect Dis. 2009;9(8):493–504. https://doi.org/10.1016/S1473-3099(09)70175-6.
31. Miossi R, Fuller R, Moraes JC, Ribeiro AC, Saad CG, Aikawa NE, et al. Immunogenicity of influenza H1N1 vaccination in mixed connective tissue disease: effect of disease and therapy. Clinics (Sao Paulo). 2013;68(2):129–34. https://doi.org/10.6061/clinics/2013(02)oa02.

32. Adler S, Krivine A, Weix J, Rozenberg F, Launay O, Huesler J, et al. Protective effect of A/H1N1 vaccination in immune-mediated disease--a prospectively controlled vaccination study. Rheumatology (Oxford) 2012;51(4):695–700. doi: https://doi.org/10.1093/rheumatology/ker389.
33. Aikawa NE, Campos LM, Silva CA, Carvalho JF, Saad CG, Trudes G, et al. Glucocorticoid: major factor for reduced immunogenicity of 2009 influenza a (H1N1) vaccine in patients with juvenile autoimmune rheumatic disease. J Rheumatol. 2012;39(1):167–73. https://doi.org/10.3899/jrheum.110721.
34. O'Neill SG, Isenberg DA. Immunizing patients with systemic lupus erythematosus: a review of effectiveness and safety. Lupus. 2006;15(11):778–83. https://doi.org/10.1177/0961203306069355.
35. Smith KG, Isbel NM, Catton MG, Leydon JA, Becker GJ, Walker RG. Suppression of the humoral immune response by mycophenolate mofetil. Nephrol Dial Transplant. 1998;13(1):160–4. https://doi.org/10.1093/ndt/13.1.160.
36. Md Yusof MY, Vital EM, McElvenny DM, Hensor EMA, Das S, Dass S, et al. Predicting severe infection and effects of hypogammaglobulinemia during therapy with rituximab in rheumatic and musculoskeletal diseases. Arthritis Rheumatol. 2019;71(11):1812–23. https://doi.org/10.1002/art.40937.
37. Bingham CO 3rd, Looney RJ, Deodhar A, Halsey N, Greenwald M, Codding C, et al. Immunization responses in rheumatoid arthritis patients treated with rituximab: results from a controlled clinical trial. Arthritis Rheum. 2010;62(1):64–74. https://doi.org/10.1002/art.25034.
38. Brinkman DM, Jol-van der Zijde CM, ten Dam MM, te Boekhorst PA, ten Cate R, Wulffraat NM, et al. Resetting the adaptive immune system after autologous stem cell transplantation: lessons from responses to vaccines. J Clin Immunol. 2007;27(6):647–58. https://doi.org/10.1007/s10875-007-9120-0.
39. Suchin KR, Cassin M, Washko R, Nahass G, Berkson M, Stouch B, et al. Extracorporeal photochemotherapy does not suppress T- or B-cell responses to novel or recall antigens. J Am Acad Dermatol. 1999;41(6):980–6. https://doi.org/10.1016/s0190-9622(99)70257-4.
40. Rubin LG, Levin MJ, Ljungman P, Davies EG, Avery R, Tomblyn M, et al. 2013 IDSA clinical practice guideline for vaccination of the immunocompromised host. Clin Infect Dis. 2014;58(3):e44–100. https://doi.org/10.1093/cid/cit684.
41. Prevention CfDCa: General Best Practice Guidelines for Immunization: Best Practices Guidance of the Advisory Committee on Immunization Practices (ACIP). https://www.cdc.gov/vaccines/hcp/acip-recs/general-recs/immunocompetence.html (2020). Accessed December 23 2020.
42. Oliveira AC, Mota LM, Santos-Neto LL, Simoes M, Martins-Filho OA, Tauil PL. Seroconversion in patients with rheumatic diseases treated with immunomodulators or immunosuppressants, who were inadvertently revaccinated against yellow fever. Arthritis Rheumatol. 2015;67(2):582–3. https://doi.org/10.1002/art.38960.
43. Valim V, Machado K, Miyamoto ST, Pinto AD, Rocha PCM, Serrano EV, et al. Planned yellow fever primary vaccination is safe and immunogenic in patients with autoimmune diseases: a prospective non-interventional study. Front Immunol. 2020;11:1382. https://doi.org/10.3389/fimmu.2020.01382.
44. Lai YC, Yew YW. Severe autoimmune adverse events post herpes zoster vaccine: a case-control study of adverse events in a National Database. J Drugs Dermatol. 2015;14(7):681–4.
45. Pileggi GS, de Souza CB, Ferriani VP. Safety and immunogenicity of varicella vaccine in patients with juvenile rheumatic diseases receiving methotrexate and corticosteroids. Arthritis Care Res (Hoboken). 2010;62(7):1034–9. https://doi.org/10.1002/acr.20183.
46. Groot N, Pileggi G, Sandoval CB, Grein I, Berbers G, Ferriani VPL, et al. Varicella vaccination elicits a humoral and cellular response in children with rheumatic diseases using immune suppressive treatment. Vaccine. 2017;35(21):2818–22. https://doi.org/10.1016/j.vaccine.2017.04.015.
47. Hmamouchi I, Winthrop K, Launay O, Dougados M. Low rate of influenza and pneumococcal vaccine coverage in rheumatoid arthritis: data from the international COMORA cohort. Vaccine. 2015;33(12):1446–52. https://doi.org/10.1016/j.vaccine.2015.01.065.
48. Lanternier F, Henegar C, Mouthon L, Blanche P, Guillevin L, Launay O. Low influenza-vaccination rate among adults receiving immunosuppressive therapy for systemic inflammatory disease. Ann Rheum Dis. 2008;67(7):1047. https://doi.org/10.1136/ard.2007.081703.
49. Costello R, Winthrop KL, Pye SR, Brown B, Dixon WG. Influenza and pneumococcal vaccination uptake in patients with rheumatoid arthritis treated with immunosuppressive therapy in the UK: a retrospective cohort study using data from the clinical practice research datalink. PLoS One. 2016;11(4):e0153848. https://doi.org/10.1371/journal.pone.0153848.
50. Wotton CJ, Goldacre MJ. Risk of invasive pneumococcal disease in people admitted to hospital with selected immune-mediated diseases: record linkage cohort analyses. J Epidemiol Community Health. 2012;66(12):1177–81. https://doi.org/10.1136/jech-2011-200168.
51. Baker DW, Brown T, Lee JY, Ozanich A, Liss DT, Sandler DS, et al. A multifaceted intervention to improve influenza, pneumococcal, and herpes zoster vaccination among patients with rheumatoid arthritis. J Rheumatol. 2016;43(6):1030–7. https://doi.org/10.3899/jrheum.150984.
52. Pope JE, Goodwin JL, Ouimet JM, Krizova A, Laskin M. Infections are not increased in scleroderma compared to non-inflammatory musculoskeletal disorders prior to disease onset. Open Rheumatol J. 2007;1:12–7. https://doi.org/10.2174/1874312900701010012.
53. Mouthon L, Mestre C, Berezne A, Poiraudeau S, Marchand C, Guilpain P, et al. Low influenza vaccination rate among patients with systemic sclerosis. Rheumatology. 2010;49(3):600–6. https://doi.org/10.1093/rheumatology/kep440.
54. Murdaca G, Noberasco G, Battaglini A, Vassallo C, Giusti F, Greco M, et al. Systemic sclerosis and vaccinations: a register-based cohort study about seasonal influenza and Streptococcus pneumoniae vaccination rate and uptake from Liguria regional center, Northwest Italy. Vaccines (Basel). 2020;8(2) https://doi.org/10.3390/vaccines8020204.
55. Mercado U, Acosta H, Diaz-Molina R. Antibody response to pneumococcal polysaccharide vaccine in systemic sclerosis. J Rheumatol. 2009;36(7):1549–50. https://doi.org/10.3899/jrheum.081227.
56. Hesselstrand R, Nagel J, Saxne T, Geborek P, Skattum L, Kapetanovic MC. Immunogenicity and safety of pneumococcal vaccination in patients with systemic sclerosis. Rheumatology. 2018;57(4):625–30. https://doi.org/10.1093/rheumatology/kex471.
57. Patel DP, Treat JR, Castelo-Socio L. Decreased hepatitis B vaccine response in pediatric patients with atopic dermatitis, psoriasis, and morphea. Vaccine. 2017;35(35 Pt B):4499-500 https://doi.org/10.1016/j.vaccine.2017.07.025.
58. Grohskopf LA, Alyanak E, Broder KR, Blanton LH, Fry AM, Jernigan DB, et al. Prevention and control of seasonal influenza with vaccines: recommendations of the advisory committee on immunization practices — United States, 2020–21 influenza season. MMWR Recomm Rep 2020;69(No. RR-8):1-24. doi: http://dx.doi.org/10.15585/mmwr.rr6908a1.
59. Setti M, Fenoglio D, Ansaldi F, Filaci G, Bacilieri S, Sticchi L, et al. Flu vaccination with a virosomal vaccine does not affect clinical course and immunological parameters in scleroderma patients. Vaccine. 2009;27(25–26):3367–72. https://doi.org/10.1016/j.vaccine.2009.01.078.

60. Sampaio-Barros PD, Andrade DCO, Seguro LCP, Pasoto SG, Viana VST, Ribeiro ACM, et al. Pandemic non-adjuvanted influenza a H1N1 vaccine in a cohort of patients with systemic sclerosis. Rheumatology. 2018;57(10):1721–5. https://doi.org/10.1093/rheumatology/kex330.
61. Litinsky I, Balbir A, Zisman D, Mandelboim M, Mendelson E, Feld J, et al. Vaccination against influenza in patients with systemic sclerosis. Clin Exp Rheumatol. 2012;30(2 Suppl 71):S7–11.
62. Mota LM, Oliveira AC, Lima RA, Santos-Neto LL, Tauil PL. Vaccination against yellow fever among patients on immunosuppressors with diagnoses of rheumatic diseases. Rev Soc Bras Med Trop. 2009;42(1):23–7. https://doi.org/10.1590/s0037-86822009000100006.
63. Borocz K, Simon D, Erdo-Bonyar S, Kovacs KT, Tuba E, Czirjak L, et al. Relationship between natural and infection-induced antibodies in systemic autoimmune diseases (SAD): SLE, SSc and RA. Clin Exp Immunol. 2020; https://doi.org/10.1111/cei.13521.
64. Foster E, Malloy MJ, Jokubaitis VG, Wrede CDH, Butzkueven H, Sasadeusz J, et al. Increased risk of cervical dysplasia in females with autoimmune conditions-results from an Australia database linkage study. PLoS One. 2020;15(6):e0234813. https://doi.org/10.1371/journal.pone.0234813.
65. Raposo A, Tani C, Costa J, Mosca M. Human papillomavirus infection and cervical lesions in rheumatic diseases: a systematic review. Acta Reumatol Port. 2016;41(3):184–90.
66. Grimaldi-Bensouda L, Guillemot D, Godeau B, Benichou J, Lebrun-Frenay C, Papeix C, et al. Autoimmune disorders and quadrivalent human papillomavirus vaccination of young female subjects. J Intern Med. 2014;275(4):398–408. https://doi.org/10.1111/joim.12155.
67. Vichnin M, Bonanni P, Klein NP, Garland SM, Block SL, Kjaer SK, et al. An overview of quadrivalent human papillomavirus vaccine safety: 2006 to 2015. Pediatr Infect Dis J. 2015;34(9):983–91. https://doi.org/10.1097/INF.0000000000000793.
68. Martin M, Mougin C, Pretet JL, Gil H, Meaux-Ruault N, Puzenat E, et al. Screening of human papillomavirus infection in women with systemic sclerosis. Clin Exp Rheumatol. 2014;32(6 Suppl 86):S-145-8

Part VIII

Management and Outcome Assessment

Christopher P. Denton, Yannick Allanore, and Ami A. Shah

41 Overview of Management and Outcome Assessment in Systemic Sclerosis

Christopher P. Denton, Ami A. Shah, and Yannick Allanore

A cornerstone of good clinical practice and effective development of new treatments is the availability of feasible and validated clinical outcome measures that can be used in clinical trials. This chapter provides a brief overview and summarises the challenges and context of outcome development. As in other aspects of the disease, some of the progress has resulted from translating lessons from other areas of medicine and rheumatology into the arena of systemic sclerosis. Management principles are considered, and approaches to investigate and treat the major clinical manifestations of SSc are presented as well as providing an overview of current and emerging outcome measures.

Principles of Management

Early diagnosis and treatment of systemic sclerosis is critical and has been shown to increase ascertainment of organ-based disease [1]. Currently, more than half of SSc patients die as a direct result of disease complications and the frequency is now well established from the review of the EUSTAR database and other single-centre cohorts [2]. All patients should have systematic investigation early in the disease and at regular intervals during follow-up.

Improvements in managing scleroderma renal crisis, pulmonary arterial hypertension and interstitial lung disease have resulted in greater prominence and priority for the nonlethal burden of SSc including gut involvement, Raynaud's phenomenon, fatigue, calcinosis and impact on quality of life. The evaluation and assessment tools that are used in clinical practice and trials are summarised below.

Outcome Measure Development

Outcome measures are important to objectively assess disease and to demonstrate changes in activity and severity that may reflect natural history or response to treatment. Some generic assessment tools such as performance status or quality-of-life measures may be used in many different disease states. This has the advantage of comparability across diverse conditions but at a potential cost of disease-specific assessments. Other tools such as the Health Assessment Questionnaire Disability Index (HAQ-DI) may be adopted from other disease areas and used unmodified or adapted to be more relevant to systemic sclerosis [3]. Organ-based assessment tools such as renal function indices or lung function are transferable across diseases. In terms of disease-specific outcomes, there has been a particular focus on the use of skin assessment by the modified Rodnan skin score [4]. This is a semiquantitative assessment tool examining palpated skin thickness at 17 sites. It has been demonstrated to reflect outcome and clinical progression and has been used as primary end point in many trials. However, it is no longer considered the gold standard tool due to challenges of reliable assessment, the confounding effect of diversity between patients and a natural history that has led to major improvements in placebo-treated subjects, together with limited short-term sensitivity to change and poor correlation with more global patient-reported outcomes.

Role of OMERACT in Development and Testing of New Outcome Measures

The OMERACT organisation has been central to the development, validation and dissemination of outcome measures for rheumatic diseases. Although initially focused on

C. P. Denton (✉)
Division of Medicine, University College London, London, UK
e-mail: c.denton@medsch.ucl.ac.uk

A. A. Shah (✉)
Division of Rheumatology, Department of Medicine, Johns Hopkins University School of Medicine, Baltimore, MD, USA
e-mail: Ami.Shah@jhmi.edu

Y. Allanore
Paris University, Cochin Hospital, AP-HP, INSERM U1016, Paris, France

Y. Allanore et al. (eds.), *Scleroderma*, https://doi.org/10.1007/978-3-031-40658-4_41

rheumatoid arthritis, it has now broadened to include many rheumatic and musculoskeletal diseases and has been instrumental in elevating standards of assessment and practice in rheumatology. Central to the initiative is the conceptual framework of the OMERACT filter that has a broad view of validation and utility of potential outcome measures. The filter has been updated and is now based on the following three key principles or pillars: truth, discrimination and feasibility [5]. These are tested for any candidate outcome measure through a series of questions that first consider content and face validity, then ask if it is practical to use and finally move on to assess whether the numeric scores make sense and can discriminate groups of interest. Discrimination includes test–retest reliability, longitudinal construct validity, thresholds of meaning and sensitivity to change. To be fully validated, an outcome measure needs to satisfy the different domains. Some measures have attained this although not many that are relevant to systemic sclerosis. Regular meetings and greater inclusion have ensured that OMERACT remains relevant and central to outcome development in systemic sclerosis.

Defining and Quantifying Damage and Disease Activity

Different rheumatic diseases have allowed the concepts of damage, activity and severity to be developed. They are highly relevant to clinical impact and outcome evaluation. In simple terms, the severity of disease is reflected by the amount of damage that has occurred and impacts on how patients feel, function and survive and so has great relevance to health authorities and drug approval standards. Damage is likely to be irreversible [6]. Activity is a more dynamic process that reflects the driving factors that lead to damage and determine severity, but activity encompasses aspects of disease that are more variable and critically may diminish as part of natural history or in response to treatment [7]. Severity is a more nebulous concept that indicates aspects of damage and activity [8]. In a disease like systemic sclerosis, progression of damage can be regarded as activity. In other diseases such as vasculitis or rheumatoid arthritis, there are much more clear definitions of disease activity and so goals for treatment or low disease activity or remission are more achievable than in systemic sclerosis [9].

Systemic Sclerosis as a Multi-Compartment Disease

Systemic sclerosis is a particular challenge because of the multifaceted nature that impacts on patient quality of life and disease impact. Thus, patients may show different levels of activity or severity across different disease domains. This is also a particular challenge in developing and validating surrogate or biomarkers based upon blood analyte measurement since systemic levels of a marker might reflect the disease process at multiple sites. Thus, high levels could reflect relatively low levels of disease across many compartments such as skin, vasculature or lungs or particularly severe involvement of just one component of SSc. Sampling of lesional tissue or environment can be achieved in the research setting through biopsy of skin or internal organs, dermal blister fluid, broncho-alveolar lavage or urine [10], and this can provide insight into local disease biology and markers. There are attempts to use local sampling to deconvolute multiplex plasma analysis and develop single-compartment composite markers [11].

Composite Outcome Measures

The multifaceted nature of systemic sclerosis makes composite measures relevant and attractive because they can capture disease in ways that allow comparison of different patients. For overall disease in SSc, the CRISS was developed and secured provisional American College of Rheumatology (ACR) endorsement [12]. This is a tractable approach that incorporates two steps to reflect clinical practice. It is essentially a response index that designates a patient as improved or not improved based upon step 1 that reflects major organ-based disease. If this has progressed or occurred, then a patient has not improved. If no step 1 event has occurred, then step 2 is a weighted calculation of change in five domains that reflect usual assessment of SSc through HAQ, mRSS, physician and patient global and lung function (FVC). This has been developed and tested in early dcSSc and in studies with placebo has performed well. Unfortunately, a recent trial allowing background immunosuppression was negative because this treatment in both arms achieved a good response by CRISS. A revised CRISS is now being evaluated that uses unweighted integration of measures at step 2, and it is anticipated that this may prove more robust and useful in current clinical trials [13]. These approaches are discussed in more detail in subsequent chapters.

Patient-Reported Outcomes

Generic patient-reported measures are usually applied in trials and practice including EQ-5D and SF-36. These are limited by the major impact of SSc that means the measures often do not reflect improvement of single aspects of disease. More specific measures of quality of life have been developed and are being validated, including ScleroID [14]. Functional indices such as HAQ and hand function measures including the COCHIN questionnaire are routinely used. Organ-specific PROs include the skin assessment [15] and lung questionnaires, but these have not shown reproducible or meaningful effect of drugs that have been approved based on FVC change and so better PROs are needed. This is important to capture disease impact and how patients feel and function that are priorities for regulators in evaluating new potential treatments for SSc.

Biomarkers

There are no fully validated surrogates or biomarkers for SSc but several promising candidates as markers of fibrosis including the enhanced liver fibrosis (ELF) score [16]. As discussed above, it seems likely that single-compartment markers are more feasible and useful as they can augment other assessment tools and be incorporated into composite tools such as DETECT. Including candidate biomarker studies in clinical trials has helped to establish utility, and markers for lung fibrosis (e.g. KL6 [17]) and SSc renal disease have emerged from recent clinical trials. Biomarkers can be prognostic or predictive. In the future, pharmacodynamic markers may also emerge and be included as potential trial end points. This might be especially valuable in early-phase trials to select treatments for further study in trials that measure clinical impact and benefit.

Organ-Specific Treatment and Outcomes

The assessment of key organs and systems is the cornerstone of good management of SSc and has been shown to improve ascertainment of significant disease and be associated with improved outcome, plausibly through earlier diagnosis and treatment. There are measures that are transferable from other branches of medicine that are already established as well as SSc-specific assessment. Manifestations such as overlap arthritis or myositis may be assessed using outcomes developed for other musculoskeletal diseases. Other complications such as calcinosis remain very challenging for outcome assessment.

Skin Assessment and Treatment

Whilst the mRSS is considered a "gold standard" for assessment of skin severity and has been considered validated by applying the OMERACT filter, it has performed better in cohort studies as an outcome predictor than as an end point in clinical trials. Nevertheless, some studies have emerged with this as a positive primary end point. Other assessment tools include imaging modalities such as high-frequency ultrasound, OCT and the Raman spectroscopy. PROs include the SSPRO that is a measure of skin impact and holds promise as a useful end point in trials. The COVID-19 pandemic led to development of a remote self-assessment tool for skin severity (PASTUL) that is undergoing further evaluation for broader application in clinical practice [18]. Immunosuppression with methotrexate and mycophenolate mofetil is the cornerstone of management of skin in most patients with diffuse cutaneous SSc [19] although biological agents such as rituximab may be considered in some cases [20] and patients with severe refractory disease may be considered for autologous haematopoietic stem cell transplantation [21]. Other approaches are discussed further in the relevant chapters of this textbook.

Lung Fibrosis

There are now approved treatments for SSc-ILD based upon slowing of progression of FVC decline in clinical trials. Whilst tocilizumab has been shown to be effective in early-stage disease in dcSSc with evidence of disease activity, conventional immunosuppression with mycophenolate mofetil or cyclophosphamide is also frequently used. Nintedanib slows progression of SSc-ILD and has broad benefits in patients with progressive disease [22] and may show greater benefit in combination with immunosuppression. This is a major step forward for patients and for clinical investigators. However, FVC has been the only variable that has proved useful in trials. DLco is valuable as a prognostic marker but not in short-term trials. This may reflect the intrinsic variability of this important measure. Imaging outcomes are now being developed including quantitative evaluation of CT extent and pattern of fibrosis. Automated or computer-assisted algorithms have been applied successfully to trial data sets and may be applied to routine clinical practice in the future. Thus, it is likely that further progress in meaningful assessment of lung outcomes will emerge for future trials [23]. One limitation might be raised with regard to the measurement of clinical symptoms where improvement in dyspnoea could not be demonstrated to improve using available assessment tools despite efficient drugs, but functional consequences, through PFTs and walking test, and structural damages through HRCT offer a highly relevant platform to measure accurately ILD.

Pulmonary Hypertension

Pulmonary arterial hypertension (PAH) is an important complication of systemic sclerosis and is discussed in detail elsewhere in this volume. Tools for prediction of risk are applied in practice, including DETECT [24] to guide towards the performance of right heart catheterisation, which remains the gold standard for diagnosis of pulmonary hypertension. Moreover, composite risk scores that incorporate clinical and investigational threshold determinants of low, intermediate, or high risk or mortality are now central to drive optimal management of SSc-PAH. In trials, event-driven morbidity–mortality end points have replaced short-term evaluation of exercise capacity by SMWT. This has been important in establishing current standards of combination treatment for SSc-PAH that are now proven to improve long-term survival and outcome. There are multiple approved therapies for SSc-PAH, and other drugs are under evaluation. Regular and systematic screening is therefore important to permit referral to specialised pulmonary hypertension centres for diagnosis and treatment in line with expert recommendations [25].

Gut Disease

Gastrointestinal tract symptoms are frequent and a major burden in systemic sclerosis. The SSc-specific UCLA-SCTC-GIT 2.0 is a well-developed patient-reported outcome that documents and quantifies symptom burden related to key domains of gut involvement [26]. It has proven valuable for cohort observational research and seen to demonstrate change over time. This is a major burden for patients, and so assessment is vital as a first step towards more effective treatment and better outcomes. Treatment is generally symptomatic using acid-suppressive therapy such as proton-pump inhibitors and prokinetic agents, including prucalopride. Other specific complications include small intestinal bacterial overgrowth which can respond to antibiotics and gastric antral vascular ectasia that can be managed using argon plasma or radiofrequency endoscopic vascular ablation [27].

Raynaud's and Digital Vasculopathy

Vasodilator drugs such as calcium channel blockers are routinely used to treat Raynaud's. Refractory cases of digital ulceration may respond to selective phosphodiesterase antagonists including sildenafil or to bosentan, an endothelin receptor blocker [28]. The most established tool applied to Raynaud's assessment in clinical trials is the Raynaud Condition Score (RCS). Although the RCS is considered a valid measure, it has been challenging in trials to demonstrate differences between active treatment arms and placebo. This has led to the development of a measure more specific for SSc, the Assessment of Systemic sclerosis-associated RAynaud's Phenomenon (ASRAP) questionnaire [29]. ASRAP is likely to be used in future studies based upon good performance and validation. This tool is an excellent example for applying strict development methods and validation to achieve the goal of a feasible and useful outcome measure. Other assessment outcomes for vasculopathy include digital ulcer counts and burden. Although feasible and used to gain regulatory approval of drugs, there are still challenges in assessing ulcers due to variable local clinical practice and the complex natural history of ulcers. In addition, inter-observer differences in assessing and classifying ulcers have been a particular challenge. Vascular imaging can help in the management by looking at large vessels and potential impaired circulation. Moreover, microcirculation measures by laser Doppler or thermography are under development but are still missing validation to reach requirements to be used in clinical trials.

Cardiac Disease

Cardiac involvement in systemic sclerosis is common. It can present with protean manifestations, and when symptomatic, portends a poor prognosis with reduced survival [30]. SSc can affect virtually any cardiac structure, thereby causing myocardial inflammation or fibrosis, coronary microvascular ischemia, pericardial disease, arrhythmias, conduction abnormalities and less commonly valvular disease. Moreover, cardiac manifestations of SSc can be primary (direct cardiac involvement due to the SSc disease process) or secondary to lung or significant kidney disease [31]. Doppler echocardiography, resting ECG (and 24-h Holter) and cardiac biomarker testing are the cornerstone in screening for cardiac involvement. If damages are suspected, cardiac MRI has emerged as a key tool with high sensitivity, spatial resolution and ability to simultaneously evaluate the RV and pericardium along with LV structure and perfusion [32]. Further support for MRI as a stratification tool comes from a study using hierarchical clustering analysis of an unselected cohort of cases that identifies distinct cardiovascular phenotypes are associated with prognosis in systemic sclerosis [33]. In select cases, coronary angiography, invasive hemodynamic testing or endomyocardial biopsy can be performed to assist in diagnosis and therapeutic decision-making. In the dedicated chapter, emerging tools including speckle-tracking echocardiography, exercise echocardiography, cardiopulmonary exercise testing, MRI T1 mapping for the evaluation of diffuse cardiac fibrosis and absolute perfusion cardiac MRI are discussed.

Concluding Remarks

In conclusion, outcome measures are central to good management and evaluation of SSc and there has been substantial progress in this field based upon clinical trial data and observational cohort analysis. It is important that outcomes are developed using modern methodology and tested rigorously.

References

1. Nihtyanova SI, Tang EC, Coghlan JG, Wells AU, Black CM, Denton CP. Improved survival in systemic sclerosis is associated with better ascertainment of internal organ disease: a retrospective cohort study. QJM. 2010;103(2):109–15. https://doi.org/10.1093/qjmed/hcp174. Epub 2009 Dec 4.
2. Elhai M, Meune C, Boubaya M, Avouac J, Hachulla E, Balbir-Gurman A, Riemekasten G, Airò P, Joven B, Vettori S, Cozzi F, Ullman S, Czirják L, Tikly M, Müller-Ladner U, Caramaschi P, Distler O, Iannone F, Ananieva LP, Hesselstrand R, Becvar R, Gabrielli A, Damjanov N, Salvador MJ, Riccieri V, Mihai C, Szücs G, Walker UA, Hunzelmann N, Martinovic D, Smith V, Müller CS, Montecucco CM, Opris D, Ingegnoli F, Vlachoyiannopoulos PG, Stamenkovic B, Rosato E, Heitmann S, Distler JHW, Zenone T, Seidel M, Vacca A, Langhe E, Novak S, Cutolo M, Mouthon L, Henes J, Chizzolini C, Mühlen CAV, Solanki K, Rednic S, Stamp L, Anic B, Santamaria VO, De Santis M, Yavuz S, Sifuentes-Giraldo WA, Chatelus E, Stork J, Laar JV, Loyo E, de la Peña G, Lefebvre P, Eyerich K, Cosentino V, Alegre-Sancho JJ, Kowal-Bielecka O, Rey G, Matucci-Cerinic M, Allanore Y, EUSTAR Group. Mapping and predicting mortality from systemic sclerosis. Ann Rheum Dis. 2017;76(11):1897–905. https://doi.org/10.1136/annrheumdis-2017-211448. Epub 2017 Aug 23.
3. Allanore Y, Bozzi S, Terlinden A, Huscher D, Amand C, Soubrane C, Siegert E, Czirják L, Carreira PE, Hachulla E, Zanatta E, Li M, Airò P, Mendoza FA, Rosato E, Distler O, EUSTAR Collaborators. Health Assessment Questionnaire-Disability Index (HAQ-DI) use in modelling disease progression in diffuse cutaneous systemic sclerosis: an analysis from the EUSTAR database. Arthritis Res Ther. 2020;22(1):257. https://doi.org/10.1186/s13075-020-02329-2.
4. Herrick AL, Assassi S, Denton CP. Skin involvement in early diffuse cutaneous systemic sclerosis: an unmet clinical need. Nat Rev Rheumatol. 2022;18(5):276–85. https://doi.org/10.1038/s41584-022-00765-9. Epub 2022 Mar 15.
5. Maxwell LJ, Beaton DE, Boers M, D'Agostino MA, Conaghan PG, Grosskleg S, Shea BJ, Bingham CO III, Boonen A, Christensen R, Choy E, Doria AS, Hill CL, Hofstetter C, Kroon FP, Leung YY, Mackie S, Meara A, Touma Z, Tugwell P, Wells GA. The evolution of instrument selection for inclusion in core outcome sets at OMERACT: Filter 2.2. Semin Arthritis Rheum. 2021;51(6):1320–30. https://doi.org/10.1016/j.semarthrit.2021.08.011. Epub 2021 Aug 28.
6. Ferdowsi N, Huq M, Stevens W, Hudson M, Wang M, Tay T, Burchell JL, Mancuso S, Rabusa C, Sundararajan V, Prior D, Proudman SM, Baron M, Nikpour M, Scleroderma Clinical Trials Consortium Damage Index Working Group, The Australian Scleroderma Interest Group, Canadian Scleroderma Research Group, Scleroderma Clinical Trials Consortium Damage Index Working Group, The Australian Scleroderma Interest Group, Canadian Scleroderma Research Group. Development and validation of the Scleroderma Clinical Trials Consortium Damage Index (SCTC-DI): a novel instrument to quantify organ damage in systemic sclerosis. Ann Rheum Dis. 2019;78(6):807–16. https://doi.org/10.1136/annrheumdis-2018-214764. Epub 2019 Mar 30.
7. Valentini G, Iudici M, Walker UA, Jaeger VK, Baron M, Carreira P, Czirják L, Denton CP, Distler O, Hachulla E, Herrick AL, Kowal-Bielecka O, Pope J, Müller-Ladner U, Riemekasten G, Avouac J, Frerix M, Jordan S, Minier T, Siegert E, Ong VH, Vettori S, Allanore Y. The European Scleroderma Trials and Research group (EUSTAR) task force for the development of revised activity criteria for systemic sclerosis: derivation and validation of a preliminarily revised EUSTAR activity index. Ann Rheum Dis. 2017;76(1):270–6. https://doi.org/10.1136/annrheumdis-2016-209768. Epub 2016 Sep 12.
8. Medsger TA Jr, Silman AJ, Steen VD, Black CM, Akesson A, Bacon PA, Harris CA, Jablonska S, Jayson MI, Jimenez SA, Krieg T, Leroy EC, Maddison PJ, Russell ML, Schachter RK, Wollheim FA, Zacharaie H. A disease severity scale for systemic sclerosis: development and testing. J Rheumatol. 1999;26(10):2159–67.
9. Nagaraja V, Matucci-Cerinic M, Furst DE, Kuwana M, Allanore Y, Denton CP, Raghu G, Mclaughlin V, Rao PS, Seibold JR, Pauling JD, Whitfield ML, Khanna D. Current and future outlook on disease modification and defining low disease activity in systemic sclerosis. Arthritis Rheumatol. 2020;72(7):1049–58. https://doi.org/10.1002/art.41246. Epub 2020 May 18.
10. Stern EP, Unwin R, Burns A, Ong V, Denton CP. Exploring molecular pathology of chronic kidney disease in systemic sclerosis by analysis of urinary and serum proteins. Rheumatol Adv Pract. 2021;5(1):rkaa083. https://doi.org/10.1093/rap/rkaa083.
11. Clark KE, Csomor E, Campochiaro C, Galwey N, Nevin K, Morse MA, Teo YV, Freudenberg J, Ong VH, Derrett-Smith E, Wisniacki N, Flint S, Denton CP. Integrated analysis of dermal blister fluid proteomics and genome-wide skin gene expression in systemic sclerosis: an observational study. Lancet Rheumatol. 2022;4(7):e507–16.
12. Khanna D, Berrocal VJ, Giannini EH, Seibold JR, Merkel PA, Mayes MD, Baron M, Clements PJ, Steen V, Assassi S, Schiopu E, Phillips K, Simms RW, Allanore Y, Denton CP, Distler O, Johnson SR, Matucci-Cerinic M, Pope JE, Proudman SM, Siegel J, Wong WK, Wells AU, Furst DE. The American College of Rheumatology provisional composite response index for clinical trials in early diffuse cutaneous systemic sclerosis. Arthritis Rheumatol. 2016;68(2):299–311. https://doi.org/10.1002/art.39501.
13. Khanna D, Huang S, Lin CJF, Spino C. New composite endpoint in early diffuse cutaneous systemic sclerosis: revisiting the provisional American College of Rheumatology Composite Response Index in Systemic Sclerosis. Ann Rheum Dis. 2021;80(5):641–50. https://doi.org/10.1136/annrheumdis-2020-219100. Epub 2020 Nov 30.
14. Becker MO, Dobrota R, Garaiman A, Debelak R, Fligelstone K, Tyrrell Kennedy A, Roennow A, Allanore Y, Carreira PE, Czirják L, Denton CP, Hesselstrand R, Sandqvist G, Kowal-Bielecka O, Bruni C, Matucci-Cerinic M, Mihai C, Gheorghiu AM, Mueller-Ladner U, Sexton J, Kvien TK, Heiberg T, Distler O. Development and validation of a patient-reported outcome measure for systemic sclerosis: the EULAR Systemic Sclerosis Impact of Disease (ScleroID) questionnaire. Ann Rheum Dis. 2022;81(4):507–15. https://doi.org/10.1136/annrheumdis-2021-220702. Epub 2021 Nov 25.
15. Man A, Correa JK, Ziemek J, Simms RW, Felson DT, Lafyatis R. Development and validation of a patient-reported outcome instrument for skin involvement in patients with systemic sclerosis. Ann Rheum Dis. 2017;76(8):1374–80. https://doi.org/10.1136/annrheumdis-2016-210534. Epub 2017 Feb 17.
16. Abignano G, Cuomo G, Buch MH, Rosenberg WM, Valentini G, Emery P, Del Galdo F. The enhanced liver fibrosis test: a clinical grade, validated serum test, biomarker of overall fibrosis in systemic sclerosis. Ann Rheum Dis. 2014;73(2):420–7. https://doi.org/10.1136/annrheumdis-2012-202843. Epub 2013 Mar 19.
17. Stock CJW, Hoyles RK, Daccord C, Kokosi M, Visca D, De Lauretis A, Alfieri V, Kouranos V, Margaritopoulos G, George PM, Molyneaux PL, Chua F, Maher TM, Abraham DJ, Ong V, Donovan J, Sestini P, Denton CP, Wells AU, Renzoni EA. Serum markers of pulmonary epithelial damage in systemic sclerosis-associated interstitial lung disease and disease progression. Respirology. 2021;26(5):461–8. https://doi.org/10.1111/resp.13988. Epub 2020 Dec 17.
18. Spierings J, Ong V, Denton CP. PASTUL questionnaire: a tool for self-assessment of scleroderma skin during the COVID-19 pandemic. Ann Rheum Dis. 2021;80(6):819–20. https://doi.org/10.1136/annrheumdis-2020-219775. Epub 2021 Jan 29.
19. Khanna D, Furst DE, Maranian P, Seibold JR, Impens A, Mayes MD, Clements PJ, Getzug T, Hays RD. Minimally important dif-

ferences of the UCLA Scleroderma Clinical Trial Consortium Gastrointestinal Tract Instrument. J Rheumatol. 2011;38(9):1920–4. https://doi.org/10.3899/jrheum.110225. Epub 2011 Jul 1.
20. Herrick AL, Pan X, Peytrignet S, Lunt M, Hesselstrand R, Mouthon L, Silman A, Brown E, Czirják L, Distler JHW, Distler O, Fligelstone K, Gregory WJ, Ochiel R, Vonk M, Ancuţa C, Ong VH, Farge D, Hudson M, Matucci-Cerinic M, Balbir-Gurman A, Midtvedt Ø, Jordan AC, Jobanputra P, Stevens W, Moinzadeh P, Hall FC, Agard C, Anderson ME, Diot E, Madhok R, Akil M, Buch MH, Chung L, Damjanov N, Gunawardena H, Lanyon P, Ahmad Y, Chakravarty K, Jacobsen S, MacGregor AJ, McHugh N, Müller-Ladner U, Riemekasten G, Becker M, Roddy J, Carreira PE, Fauchais AL, Hachulla E, Hamilton J, İnanç M, McLaren JS, van Laar JM, Pathare S, Proudman S, Rudin A, Sahhar J, Coppere B, Serratrice C, Sheeran T, Veale DJ, Grange C, Trad GS, Denton CP. Treatment outcome in early diffuse cutaneous systemic sclerosis: the European Scleroderma Observational Study (ESOS). Ann Rheum Dis. 2017;76(7):1207–18. https://doi.org/10.1136/annrheumdis-2016-210503. Epub 2017 Feb 10.
21. Yarkan Tuğsal H, Zengin B, Kenar G, Önen F, Birlik M. Rituximab on lung, skin, and joint involvement in patients with systemic sclerosis: a case series study and review of the literature. Int J Rheum Dis. 2022; https://doi.org/10.1111/1756-185X.14333. Epub ahead of print.
22. Shah A, Spierings J, van Laar JM, Sullivan KM. Re-evaluating inclusion criteria for autologous hematopoietic stem cell transplantation in advanced systemic sclerosis: Three successful cases and review of the literature. J Scleroderma Relat Disord. 2021;6(2):199–205. https://doi.org/10.1177/2397198320985766. Epub 2021 Jan 14.
23. Roofeh D, Barratt SL, Wells AU, Kawano-Dourado L, Tashkin D, Strand V, Seibold J, Proudman S, Brown KK, Dellaripa PF, Doyle T, Leonard T, Matteson EL, Oddis CV, Solomon JJ, Sparks JA, Vassallo R, Maxwell L, Beaton D, Christensen R, Townsend W, Khanna D. Outcome measurement instrument selection for lung physiology in systemic sclerosis associated interstitial lung disease: a systematic review using the OMERACT filter 2.1 process. Semin Arthritis Rheum. 2021;51(6):1331–41. https://doi.org/10.1016/j.semarthrit.2021.08.001. Epub 2021 Aug 20.
24. Coghlan JG, Denton CP, Grünig E, Bonderman D, Distler O, Khanna D, Müller-Ladner U, Pope JE, Vonk MC, Doelberg M, Chadha-Boreham H, Heinzl H, Rosenberg DM, McLaughlin VV, Seibold JR, DETECT Study Group. Evidence-based detection of pulmonary arterial hypertension in systemic sclerosis: the DETECT study. Ann Rheum Dis. 2014;73(7):1340–9. https://doi.org/10.1136/annrheumdis-2013-203301. Epub 2013 May 18.
25. Galiè N, Channick RN, Frantz RP, Grünig E, Jing ZC, Moiseeva O, Preston IR, Pulido T, Safdar Z, Tamura Y, McLaughlin VV. Risk stratification and medical therapy of pulmonary arterial hypertension. Eur Respir J. 2019;53(1):1801889. https://doi.org/10.1183/13993003.01889-2018.
26. Khanna D, Lescoat A, Roofeh D, Bernstein EJ, Kazerooni EA, Roth MD, Martinez F, Flaherty KR, Denton CP. Systemic sclerosis-associated interstitial lung disease: how to incorporate two food and drug administration-approved therapies in clinical practice. Arthritis Rheumatol. 2022;74(1):13–27. https://doi.org/10.1002/art.41933. Epub 2021 Nov 10.
27. Cheah JX, Khanna D, McMahan ZH. Management of scleroderma gastrointestinal disease: Lights and shadows. J Scleroderma Relat Disord. 2022;7(2):85–97. https://doi.org/10.1177/23971983221086343. Epub 2022 Apr 19.
28. Hughes M, Allanore Y, El Aoufy K, Denton CP, Khanna D, Krieg T, Matucci-Cerinic M. A practical approach to the management of digital ulcers in patients with systemic sclerosis: a narrative review. JAMA Dermatol. 2021;157(7):851–8. https://doi.org/10.1001/jamadermatol.2021.1463.
29. Pauling JD, Frech TM, Hughes M, Gordon JK, Domsic RT, Anderson ME, Ingegnoli F, McHugh NJ, Johnson SR, Hudson M, Boin F, Ong VH, Matucci-Cerinic M, Altorok N, Scolnik M, Nikpour M, Shah A, Pope JE, Khanna D, Herrick AL. Patient-reported outcome instruments for assessing Raynaud's phenomenon in systemic sclerosis: a SCTC Vascular Working Group Report. J Scleroderma Relat Disord. 2018;3(3):249–52. https://doi.org/10.1177/2397198318774307. Epub 2018 May 24.
30. Sun G, Yafasova A, Andersson C, McMurray JJV, Jhund PS, Docherty KF, Faurschou M, Nielsen CT, Schou M, Gislason GH, Torp-Pedersen C, Fosbøl EL, Køber L, Butt JH. Gender- and age-specific rates of heart failure and other adverse cardiovascular outcomes in systemic sclerosis. Rheumatology (Oxford). 2022:keac072. https://doi.org/10.1093/rheumatology/keac072. Epub ahead of print.
31. Bruni C, Buch MH, Furst DE, De Luca G, Djokovic A, Dumitru RB, Giollo A, Polovina M, Steelandt A, Bratis K, Suliman YA, Milinkovic I, Baritussio A, Hasan G, Xintarakou A, Isomura Y, Markousis-Mavrogenis G, Tofani L, Mavrogeni S, Gargani L, Caforio AL, Tschöpe C, Ristic A, Klingel K, Plein S, Behr ER, Allanore Y, Kuwana M, Denton CP, Khanna D, Krieg T, Marcolongo R, Galetti I, Zanatta E, Tona F, Seferovic P, Matucci-Cerinic M. Primary systemic sclerosis heart involvement: a systematic literature review and preliminary data-driven, consensus-based WSF/HFA definition. J Scleroderma Relat Disord. 2022;7(1):24–32.
32. De Luca G, Palmisano A, Campochiaro C, Vignale D, Cavalli G, Bruno E, Sartorelli S, Ferlito A, Peretto G, Sala S, Matucci-Cerinic M, Dagna L, Esposito A. Cardiac magnetic resonance in systemic sclerosis myocarditis: the value of T2 mapping to detect myocardial inflammation. Rheumatology (Oxford). 2022:keac098. https://doi.org/10.1093/rheumatology/keac098. Online ahead of print.
33. Knight DS, Karia N, Cole AR, Maclean RH, Brown JT, Masi A, Patel RK, Razvi Y, Chacko L, Venneri L, Kotecha T, Martinez-Naharro A, Kellman P, Scott-Russell AM, Schreiber BE, Ong VH, Denton CP, Fontana M, Coghlan JG, Muthurangu V. Distinct cardiovascular phenotypes are associated with prognosis in systemic sclerosis: a cardiovascular magnetic resonance study. Eur Heart J Cardiovasc Imaging. 2022:jeac120. https://doi.org/10.1093/ehjci/jeac120. 2023;24(4):463–71.

Management of Progressive Skin Involvement in Diffuse Scleroderma

42

Eric Hachulla and Ariane L. Herrick

Introduction

Earlier chapters have described how there are two major subtypes of systemic sclerosis (SSc): limited cutaneous and diffuse cutaneous. This chapter deals solely with the rarer, diffuse cutaneous subtype (dcSSc). The diffuse subtype is defined by skin involvement commencing distally then extending, often rapidly, to involve proximal limb (proximal to elbows and/or knees) and/or the trunk.

It is well recognized that the degree of skin involvement and the speed of its progression provide a highly visible mirror of the overall disease process in patients with dcSSc. The modified Rodnan skin score (mRSS) [1], which is a measure of skin thickening, associates with the degree of internal organ involvement and with survival: patients with high skin scores have reduced survival [2–4]. Domsic et al. [5] reported that in patients with dcSSc, 'skin thickness progression rate' (the mRSS at first visit divided by patient reported duration of skin thickening) predicted early mortality and development of scleroderma renal crisis. Wu et al. [6], in an analysis of the European Scleroderma Trials and Research [EUSTAR] cohort, found that among 1021 patients with dcSSc, the 78 'skin progressors' had lower survival and deterioration in lung function, compared to 943 'non-progressors'. Conversely, reduction in skin thickening has been shown to be associated with improved survival [7] and reduced internal organ involvement [8].

E. Hachulla
Univ. Lille, Inserm, CHU Lille, Service de Médecine Interne et Immunologie Clinique, Centre de référence des maladies autoimmunes systémiques rares du Nord et Nord-Ouest de France (CeRAINO), U1286—INFINITE—Institute for Translational Research in Inflammation, Lille, France
e-mail: Eric.HACHULLA@CHRU-LILLE.FR

A. L. Herrick (✉)
Division of Musculoskeletal and Dermatological Sciences, The University of Manchester, Northern Care Alliance NHS Foundation Trust, Manchester Academic Health Science Centre, Manchester, UK
e-mail: ariane.herrick@manchester.ac.uk

However, what is less well recognized is that the skin thickening ('scleroderma' = hard skin) of early dcSSc is in itself a major source of pain, disability, and disfigurement. In this chapter we shall first give a brief description of the skin thickening in patients with dcSSc and of its associated morbidity. We shall then describe risk factors for progressive skin involvement and how to monitor disease progression/treatment response. Then we focus on treatment, starting with 'general measures' (including analgesia and physiotherapy), then discussing immunosuppressive therapies, recent clinical trials of targeted therapies, and autologous stem cell transplantation.

Clinical Features

In dcSSc, skin thickening commences distally and dcSSc could therefore initially be confused with limited cutaneous disease (lcSSc). 'Red flags' that the patient may have diffuse disease are a short duration of extremity skin thickening, a short as opposed to a long history of Raynaud's phenomenon (in dcSSc, Raynaud's phenomenon may develop *after* the onset of skin thickening), and finger/hand swelling, sometimes leading to an incorrect initial diagnosis of inflammatory arthritis. The oedema around the hand and wrist of early phase disease frequently leads to carpal tunnel syndrome, which resolves as the oedema evolves into fibrosis. The skin involvement then progresses proximally, becoming progressively tighter, often with contractures (Fig. 42.1). The skin is often itchy.

In dcSSc, the extremities (particularly the fingers) are always involved. If a patient with proximal and/or truncal skin thickening does not have finger involvement, then this is unlikely to be dcSSc and the diagnosis should therefore be questioned.

Y. Allanore et al. (eds.), *Scleroderma*, https://doi.org/10.1007/978-3-031-40658-4_42

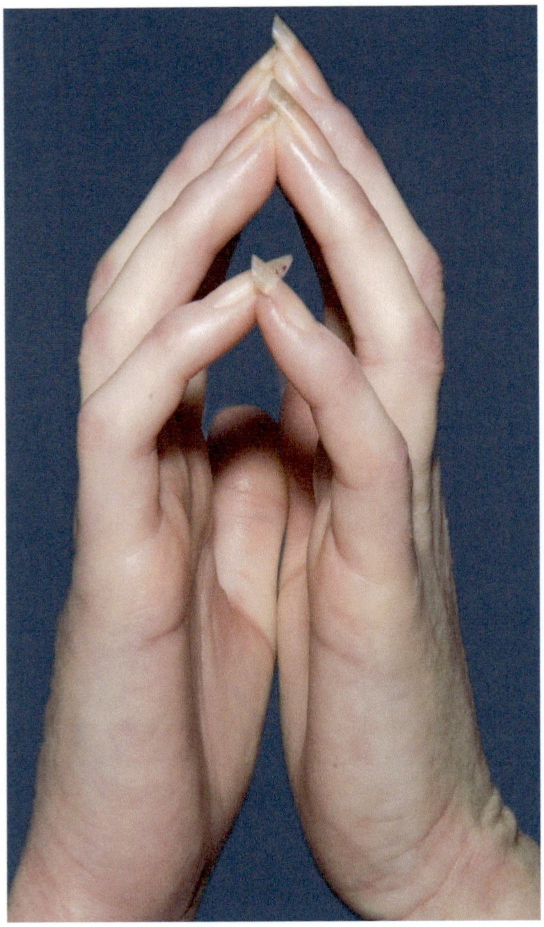

Fig. 42.1 Skin thickening of the fingers in early dcSSc, with contractures

Associated Morbidity

The pain and disability associated with skin involvement in patients with dcSSc were bench-marked by the European Scleroderma Observational Study (ESOS) of 326 patients with early dcSSc (median disease duration 11.9 months) [9]. Levels of disability including hand disability, as assessed by the Health Assessment Questionnaire-Disability Index (HAQ-DI) and the Cochin Hand Function Scale (CHFS), were high (mean HAQ-DI 1.1, SD 0.83), with fine finger movements most affected. A key point was that at baseline, both high HAQ-DI and CHFS scores were associated with high mRSS ($\rho = 0.34$, $p < 0.0001$ and $\rho = 0.35$, $p < 0.0001$ respectively). In other words, the more extensive the skin involvement, the greater the degree of disability. The extent of skin thickening was also associated with severity of pain, as assessed on a 0–100 scale ($\rho = 0.17$, $p = 0.002$) and with severity of fatigue ($\rho = -0.20$, $p = 0.0005$) as assessed by the FACIT (Functional Assessment of Chronic Illness Therapy) fatigue index. When changes over 12 months were examined, increasing overall skin thickening was strongly associated with worsening disability according to HAQ-DI ($\rho = 0.40$, $p < 0.0001$) [9]. Since then, other recent studies have confirmed the high 'skin disease burden' disease of early dcSSc. In a single centre retrospective study [10], an increase in mRSS was associated with worsening disability as measured by HAQ-DI ($\rho = 0.36$ and $p = 0.004$) in patients with early dcSSc (within 5 years of disease onset), and in a Canadian study of 154 patients with dcSSc within 5 years of onset [11], changes in mRSS correlated with changes in the HAQ-DI over 1 and 2 years ($r = 0.43$ and $r = 0.41$, respectively, $p < 0.001$).

Risk Factors for Progressive Skin Involvement

In patients with dcSSc, skin involvement progresses and then tends to plateau, usually within the first 3–5 years, and then the skin improves [12]. It is rare for skin involvement to progress after 5 years. Different trajectories have been described [3, 4]. Not all patients progress: some patients plateau early and have a relatively mild disease course. A key question for the clinician, confronted with a patient with early dsSSc, is 'How likely is this patient to have rapidly progressive disease with a poor prognosis?' And this question is important not only for the clinician who need to advise the patient, but also for the researcher, who wants to ensure that 'progressors' as opposed to 'non-progressors' are included into clinical trials aimed at identifying effective disease modifying therapy for early dcSSc. Well-recognized 'red flags' for the clinician that a patient is likely to have progressive skin disease are development of new tendon friction rubs [13, 14] and a positive anti-RNA polymerase III antibody [5].

Several recent studies have identified predictors of progressive skin disease. Maurer et al. [15] identified low mRSS, short disease duration, and joint synovitis as predictors of progression and suggested that only patients with an mRSS of 22 or lower should be included into clinical trials of early dcSSc: patients with higher scores were unlikely to progress. In the ESOS cohort [16], progressors (22.5%) compared to non-progressors (77.5%) had shorter disease duration (median 8.1 vs. 12.6 months, $p = 0.001$) and lower mRSS (median 19 vs. 21 units, $p = 0.030$). Patients who were anti-RNA polymerase III antibody positive went on to have the highest skin scores, and peaked earliest, suggesting that patients who are anti-RNA polymerase III antibody positive require especially close monitoring. Two predictive models for progressive skin thickening were derived [16]. The first included mRSS, duration of skin thickening, and their interaction, the second also included anti-RNA polymerase III positivity. The model incorporating anti-RNA polymerase III positivity was more accurate in identifying high-risk patients [16]. Both models were more accurate than a '22 mRSS' cut-off model and more flexible for a given skin score (for example, a higher baseline skin score could be compensated by a shorter disease duration) and should ensure that the most informative patients are included into clinical trials.

There has been considerable recent interest in gene expression profiling of skin biopsies to predict outcome. Higher 'fibroinflammatory' scores have been associated with higher skin scores [17]. In a phase II trial of tocilizumab, expression of several genes in forearm skin biopsies from placebo-treated patients was associated with mRSS progression [18], whereas a more recent study [19] suggested that in early dcSSc, gene expression profiles in forearm skin biopsies were associated with previous but not subsequent skin disease progression, i.e., were not predictive of future mRSS progression. The ASSET study of abatacept [20] suggested that different gene expression subsets might help to explain differences between patients in their responsiveness to immunomodulatory therapies. At present, this remains an area of active research.

In summary, we now have a much better insight than 5 years ago into the factors predicting disease progression, with progress being made towards a stratified approach to therapy.

Monitoring of Disease Progression and of Treatment Response

Monitoring of skin disease remains a challenge. The mRSS is used clinically and in research practice and is a validated outcome measure [1]. It tests 17 sites on a 0–3 scale, with a maximum score of 51. In the clinic, the mRSS is very useful to gauge whether the skin disease is progressing, plateauing, or improving. In research practice, most recent multicentre randomized controlled trials (RCTs) of early dcSSc have had the mRSS as the primary endpoint (examples include [21–23]), although a limitation of the mRSS is its substantial inter- and intra-observer variability [24], which is unsurprising due to the different ways in which clinicians perform the mRSS [25]. Standardized training is recommended to reduce this variability [26]. There is concern that the variability in mRSS reduces its ability to detect meaningful change. For example, in the recent placebo-controlled RCT of abatacept [20], active treatment was associated with significant improvement in HAQ-DI and in the American College of Rheumatology Combined Response Index in diffuse cutaneous Systemic Sclerosis (ACR CRISS: a composite measure including the mRSS [27]), but not in the mRSS itself. Despite its limitations, it is likely that the use of the mRSS will continue as it is quick to perform and very feasible. Ideally, in multicentre trials the same assessor should score the skin each time for any given patient, intra-observer variability being lower than inter-observer variability.

Other measures for assessing skin involvement include a recently developed skin patient reported outcome measure [28], which is self-administered and therefore feasible in multicentre studies. Because many patients complain of itch in early dcSSc, an itch questionnaire could also be included. There has been recent increasing interest in non-invasive measurement tools to measure skin thickness. Many cross-sectional studies have examined ultrasound [including 29–31] which reliably measures skin thickness but which requires training and is time-consuming if performed at multiple body sites: ultrasound is therefore unlikely to be feasible in later phase multicentre studies. For the same reason, optical coherence tomography (OCT) [32, 33], although a promising tool for early phase studies, is also unlikely to be a feasible option in multicentre studies. OCT can assess skin thickening and an 'extension' to the technique, polarization-sensitive OCT (PS-OCT) [34, 35] additionally assesses birefringence and can therefore measure skin fibrosis (collagen is birefringent).

'General' Treatments

Although the ultimate goal is to develop a targeted treatment to halt and ameliorate disease (as discussed below), at present a curative treatment does not exist, and 'general' measures are a very important aspect of management. Here we discuss four treatment modalities: analgesia, treatment of itch, physiotherapy and occupational therapy, and intravenous iloprost, before going on to discuss more specific therapies in the later sections.

Analgesia

The pain arising from the skin and associated contractures in patients with early dcSSc is under-recognized and under-researched. Among the 326 patients recruited into ESOS, the mean and median scores for the sHAQ pain scale (0–100, 100 most disabled) were 32.9/100 (SD 26.9) and 29.0/100 (IQR 8.7–52.7) [9]. If ulcers form over pressure points, which is often the case in early dcSSc especially over the small joints of the fingers (Fig. 42.2), then this will increase the pain. Adequate analgesia is therefore an important aspect of management. It is possible that at least in some patients there is a neurogenic component to the pain [36], and if so, gabapentin or pregabalin (for example) could be tried. Involvement of a pain management team may be helpful.

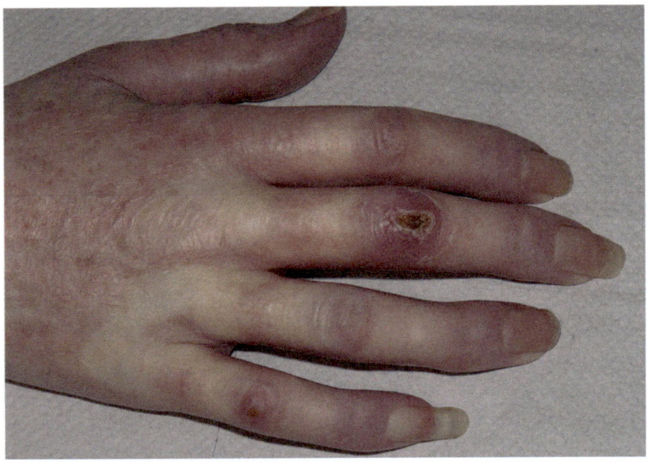

Fig. 42.2 Digital ulceration (right middle) overlying contracture in early dcSSc. Same patient as Fig. 42.1, 2 months later. The tight, shiny skin is well demonstrated

Treatment of Itch

This is very difficult. Although the itch tends to resolve as the inflammatory phase subsides, it can be troublesome for months and often for longer. In the authors' experience, antihistamines are seldom beneficial, although are worth trying. Some patients find 1% menthol in aqueous cream helpful. Low-dose prednisolone may provide relief (presumably because the itch is related to skin inflammation), but as discussed below the use of corticosteroids in early dcSSc is contentious.

Physiotherapy and Occupational Therapy

Early dcSSc has a major impact on hand function, as already discussed above, and on mobility more generally, especially if the patient has contractures. Stretching exercises are important to preserve range of movement, and anecdotal experience suggests that many patients benefit from hydrotherapy. All patients should be assessed by an occupational therapist, as it would be unusual for a patient with early dcSSc to have no functional impairment. There has been very little research examining the effects of physiotherapy (including stretching exercises), specifically in early dcSSc.

Intravenous Iloprost

The use of intravenous (IV) iloprost is well established for SS-related digital ischaemia [37]. However, it may have other beneficial effects in SSc. For example, iloprost has been shown to reduce levels of connective tissue growth factor, which is profibrotic, in the skin of patients with dcSSc [38]. In a very small minority of patients with extremely tight skin and rapidly progressive dcSSc, small superficial ulcers can occur, most commonly in the authors' experience in the upper limbs (Fig. 42.3). Our anecdotal experience is that these respond well to IV iloprost infusions, given on the assumption that these small ulcers are due to tissue ischaemia.

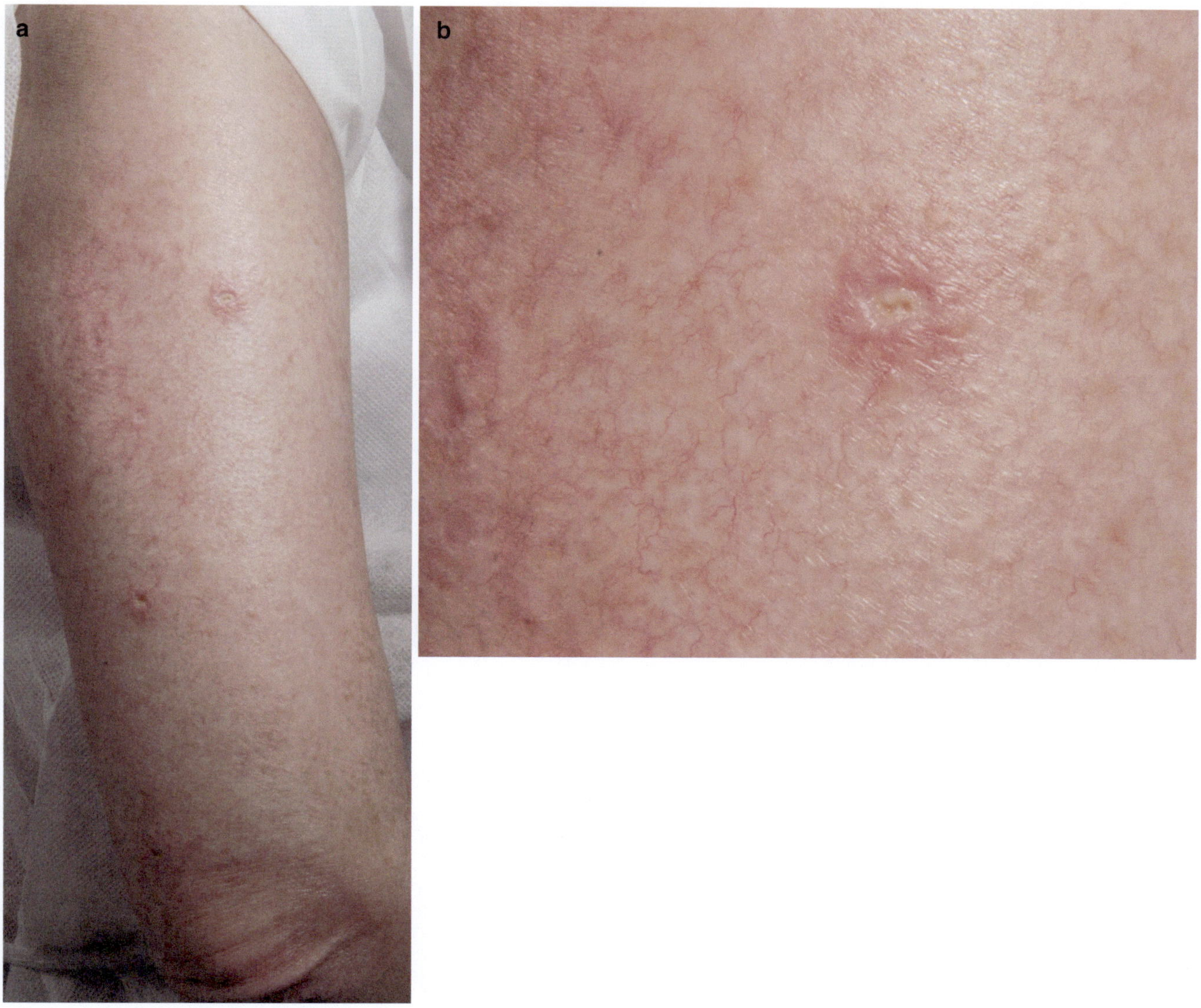

Fig. 42.3 (**a**) Superficial skin ulceration in a patient with early dcSSc with (**b**) close-up view. The skin was very itchy

Immunosuppressive Therapy

Many potential drug candidates have been tested over the last 2 decades in SSc and will be tested over the next 10 years. This is based on a better knowledge of the pathophysiology of the disease (see Fig. 42.4, Allanore et al., submitted [39]).

According to the EULAR recommendations [40], only methotrexate has an A grading of recommendation for the treatment of skin manifestations of early dcSSc. Nevertheless, an overview of the existing published data deserves to be done.

Corticosteroids

No trials have been conducted with corticosteroids in SSc. There is a controversy in using corticosteroids in early SSc due to the risk of scleroderma renal crisis, leading to many clinicians having concerns at prescribing doses above 15 mg/day of prednisone equivalent [41]. At a dose of 10 mg or less of prednisone or equivalent, corticosteroids have an anti-inflammatory effect. At a dose of 15 mg/day and above, corticosteroids have also an immunosuppressive effect. Based on the pathophysiology of skin involvement in dcSSc, their use in the early phase of the disease makes sense. In the European Scleroderma Observational Study (ESOS) in an early dcSSc population, 43% of patients were taking corticosteroids at the initial visit or previously [42]. In most RCTs conducted in recent years, corticosteroids could be used in a low-dose regimen ≤10 mg/day of prednisone or equivalent. In practice, the justification for the use of low-dose corticosteroids is based more on the presence of arthralgia or arthritis and myalgia or myositis rather than on skin involvement, with the possible exception of pruritus or recent oedematous SSc forms. Whether or not corticosteroids should be pre-

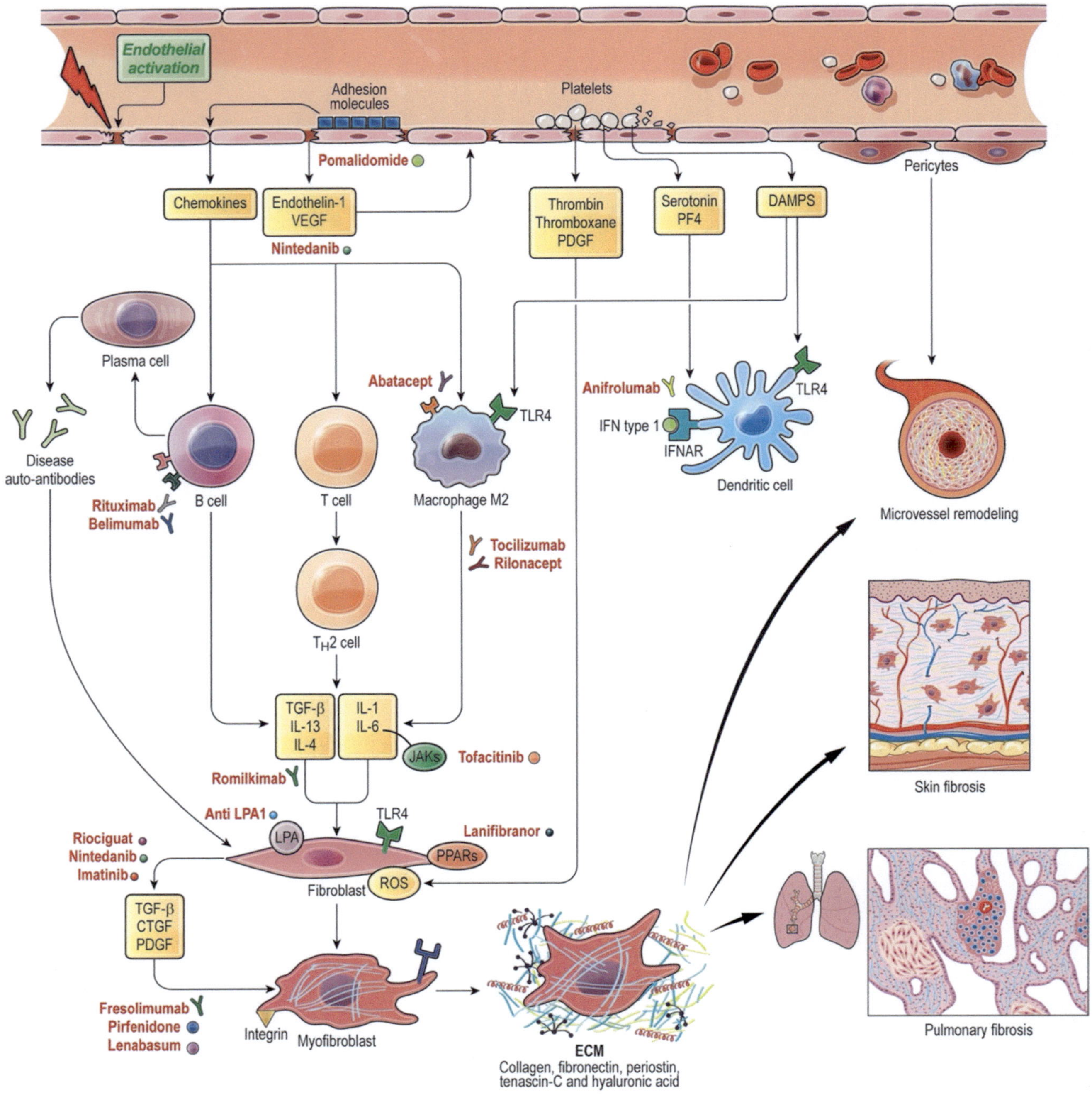

Fig. 42.4 The disease pathogenesis of SSc. The highly specific mesenchymal cell activation and related fibrosis underlying SSc are thought to be induced by vascular injury and endothelial activation leading to an uncontrolled inflammatory/ immune reaction. The main actors and players are indicated in the representation together with the targets of recently performed phase 2/phase 3 clinical trials

scribed in patients with early dcSSc is a question currently being addressed in a randomized placebo-controlled trial (ClinicalTrials.gov Identifier: NCT03708718) [43].

Methotrexate

Two small RCTs have led to the recommendation of the use of methotrexate for the skin manifestations of early dcSSc [40].

The first study published in 1996 involved 29 patients with dcSSc or lcSSc, receiving weekly injections of methotrexate 15 mg or a placebo over a 24 week-period (methotrexate = 17 patients, placebo = 12 patients). The study reached significance on a composite primary endpoint combining the Total Skin Score (TSS), DLCO, and a Visual Analogue Scale of general well-being, but did not reach significance on the TSS ($p = 0.06$ vs. placebo) [44].

The second RCT included 73 patients with dcSSc with skin involvement for less than 3 years. Thirty-five patients were randomized to receive oral methotrexate at a dose of 15 mg/week and 36 received a placebo. To improve recruitment in 2 centres, patients were allowed to take 1 tablet of 1.25 mg or 2.5 mg of active methotrexate, resulting in 11 patients in the placebo group receiving placebo +1.25–2.5 mg/week of methotrexate and the methotrexate group included 11 patients receiving 16.25–17.5 mg/week of methotrexate. After 12 months of treatment, the primary endpoint UCLA (University of California/Los Angeles) Skin Score was not significant ($p < 0.15$ versus placebo) [45]. mRSS did not reach significance at 12 months ($p < 0.17$ vs placebo). However, Bayesian reanalysis of the latter study showed that the probability that methotrexate improved overall mRSS and UCLA Skin Score was 94% and 96%, respectively [46]. This Bayesian study shows that oral methotrexate at a dose of 15 mg/week is associated with a high probability of beneficial effect on the mRSS.

In practice, if methotrexate is used, it should be prescribed with a weekly target dose of 20–25 mg as recommended in the ESOS study [42], but probably not more than 0.3 mg/kg as with rheumatoid arthritis [47] in combination with folic acid supplementation. Above 15 mg/week of methotrexate, the subcutaneous route is preferable to ensure a better bioavailability [48].

Cyclophosphamide

There are no RCTs on using cyclophosphamide for skin involvement in dcSSc as a primary endpoint. In contrast, 2 RCTs have evaluated cyclophosphamide for the treatment of SSc-interstitial lung disease (ILD).

The first RCT (Scleroderma Lung Study 1, SLS1) included 158 patients with SSc (59.5% were dcSSc) with a mean duration of 3.2 ± 0.2 years [49]. Seventy-nine patients received oral cyclophosphamide up to 2 mg/kg/day and 79 patients received placebo. At 12 months, the study was positive on the primary endpoint, which was forced vital capacity (FVC) with a treatment effect between groups of 2.53% ($p < 0.03$). In the dcSSc subgroup, there was a decrease of 5.3 ± 7.4 points in the mRSS score with a benefit of 3.6 points in the overall population, which was significant ($p < 0.05$).

The second RCT used cyclophosphamide intravenously at a dose of 600 mg/m^2 (or placebo) every 4 weeks for a total of 6 infusions followed by azathioprine at 2.5 mg/kg/day (maximum dose = 200 mg/day) as maintenance therapy. Each patient received 20 mg oral prednisolone on each other day. This study did not assess mRSS [50].

In the European observational ESOS study, [42] 326 patients with early dcSSc (within three years of onset of skin thickening) were recruited: 65 were prescribed methotrexate, 118 MMF, 87 cyclophosphamide, and 56 had no immunosuppressant. When cyclophosphamide was used, it was either IV at a dose of 500 mg/m^2 every month for 6–12 months or orally at a dose of 1–2 mg/kg/day for 12 months. There was statistically significant reduction in mRSS at 12 months in all groups: −4.0 (−5.2 to −2.7) units for methotrexate (oral or subcutaneous at a target dose of 20–25 mg/week), −4.1 (−5.3 to −2.9) for MMF (target dose 1 g twice daily), −3.3 (−4.9 to −1.7) for cyclophosphamide, and −2.2 (−4.0 to −0.3) for no immunosuppressant (p value for between-group differences = 0.346).

Based on data from the SLS1, SLS2, and EUSTAR study, Bruni et al. [51] did not find a significant difference on mRSS of the effect of cyclophosphamide used orally (n = 149) vs intravenously (n = 153), but in both groups the benefit on mRSS was modest, around −3.0 points in the oral group and − 1.9 in the IV group, but only 60% of the population had dcSSc and the mean duration of SSc was 4 ± 4 years. Therefore, no recommendation can be made on either route of administration on the basis of this analysis.

It is therefore difficult to recommend the use of cyclophosphamide for the treatment of skin progression in early dcSSc based on current published data. If cyclophosphamide is chosen as a first-line treatment, the duration of treatment should not exceed 12 months, followed by azathioprine or mycophenolate mofetil.

Mycophenolate Mofetil

There are no RCT's using mycophenolate mofetil (MMF) for skin involvement in dcSSc as a primary endpoint. The SLS-II study enrolled 126 SSc patients with an average duration of 2.6 years (range = 0.3–7.1 years), of whom 58.5% had dcSSc, and compared the 24-month FVC efficacy of MMF at the target dose of 1500 mg × 2/day administered for 24 months (n = 63) in one arm and oral cyclophosphamide (target dose: 2.0 mg/kg/day) administered for 12 months followed by placebo for 12 months in the other arm. In a post-hoc analyses, the joint model identified improvement from baseline to 24 months in each individual arm for mRSS (cyclophosphamide: −5·35 units; MMF: −4·90 units) [52].

Despite the lack of evidence, MMF is being used as a first-line treatment of progressive skin involvement in early dcSSc. Its use is of course more relevant in cases of associated ILD. The target dose should be 1500 mg twice daily. If MMF is chosen as a first-line treatment, the duration of treatment should probably not be less than 2 years [53].

Targeting Therapy

The improved knowledge of the pathophysiology of SSc (Fig. 42.4) reveals many therapeutic possibilities. So far, however, the results of the studies are rather negative or debatable, but some possible breakthroughs are emerging.

Rituximab

There are no RCT's using rituximab for skin involvement in dcSSc as a primary endpoint. In a comparative open-label observational study including 51 SSc-ILD patients (33 rituximab and 18 conventional therapy patients, mean SSc duration of 5.73 and 2.56 years, respectively, 90.9% dcSSc in the rituximab group and 77.8% dcSSc in the control group), a significant benefit was observed at 2 years on the FVC. According to the linear mixed models fitted mRSS was higher in the control group (−3.89 units, $p = 0.007$) compared to the rituximab group, therefore favouring rituximab [54].

From the EUSTAR database, it was possible to compare 254 SSc who received rituximab (63.9% dcSSc, median duration of disease progression = 4.2 years) to a control population of 9575 propensity-score matched patients (30.2% dcSSc, median duration of disease progression = 5.2 years) [55]. This study showed that patients receiving rituximab were more likely to have skin fibrosis improvement (22.7 vs. 14.03 events/100 person-years; OR = 2.79 [1.47–5.32]; $p = 0.002$). The mRSS decreased from mean ± SD 22.1 (± 9.3) to 14.1 (± 8.4) in rituximab patients ($n = 74$) vs 21.1 (±10.5) to 16.2 (±10.3) ($p < 0.0001$) in untreated patients matched according to propensity score ($n = 281$). On the other hand, no benefit was observed on FVC. It should be noted that in the rituximab group, 67.3% of patients were receiving corticosteroid at a median dose of 10 mg/d, and 53.7% of patients were receiving a DMARD in combination (methotrexate, MMF, azathioprine, or cyclophosphamide).

The safety profile of rituximab in SSc appears good with 14% of SAEs reported leading to discontinuation in 9% of cases. Of the 6 deaths observed during follow-up, 2 were possibly related to rituximab treatment (2 respiratory insufficiencies in the context of pulmonary carcinoma).

Only a RCT will make it possible to specify whether there is an indication for the use rituximab in early progressive dcSSc.

Tocilizumab

A Phase 3 RCT evaluating tocilizumab in early dcSSc was recently published [22]. This study was specifically designed to evaluate the benefit of tocilizumab on skin involvement. Two hundred and ten patients were randomized (104 in the tocilizumab group and 106 in the placebo group). Patients received weekly subcutaneous tocilizumab at a dose of 162 mg or the placebo over a 48-week period. All patients had early dcSSc for less than 60 months from the first non-Raynaud's phenomenon symptom. All patients had a mRSS between 10–35 units at screening. In the intention-to-treat population, the least square mean change from baseline to week 48 in mRSS was −6.14 for tocilizumab and − 4.41 for placebo ($p = 0.10$).

Patients had no DMARDs in combination, only corticosteroids were allowed, provided that the daily dose did not exceed 10 mg of prednisone. However, a significant benefit was observed on FVC, which may encourage a new Phase 3 trial with FVC as the primary endpoint. The overall tolerance of tocilizumab was good, with no more infection compared to the placebo group and no particular gastrointestinal complications.

Other Targeting Therapies

Romilkimab is a bispecific humanized monoclonal antibody which binds and neutralizes IL-4 and IL-13, two cytokines involved in the fibrinogenesis. A phase 2 trial was able to include 97 dcSSc patients with a mean disease course of 21.8 ± 10.7 months [23]. At study entry, the mean mRSS was 20.6 ± 6.5 in the overall population.

Patients could receive DMARDs, but at a stable dose and low doses of corticosteroids (≤10 mg/day of prednisone was allowed). Forty-eight patients received romilkimab 200 mg subcutaneously once weekly and 49 patients received placebo. Evaluation of the mRSS at 24 weeks showed a benefit in favour of romilkimab with a difference of −2.31 (−4.32 to −0.31; $p = 0.0291$). A possible additive effect of romilkimab in patients receiving an immunosuppressant has been shown by the change in mRSS at week 24 compared with patients without background medication (−5.81 vs. −3.64, respectively). There were 2 deaths in the romilkimab arm group and 1 in the placebo arm group, but unrelated to the treatment. The overall safety of romilkimab was good. These encouraging results require a Phase 3 study for confirmation.

Lenabasum is a selective type 2 cannabinoid receptor agonist. Encouraging results in animal models of SSc allowed a phase 2 RCT to be performed [56]. Patients were eligible if they had a dcSSc that had progressed for less than 3 years since the first non Raynaud's phenomenon symptom or had a disease that had progressed for more than 3 years but less than 6 years if there were biological inflammatory markers and a mRSS ≥ 16 or ≥ 12 with an increase ≥5 during the previous 6 months. Patients could be on low-dose DMARDs or prednisone at ≤10 mg/day at stable doses. This is a small trial that included 27 patients in the lenabasum arm who were taking progressive doses up to 20 mg × 2 per day and 15 patients were in the placebo group. The primary endpoint which was the CRISS score was not reached at week 16. Although there was a trend in the mRSS, significance was not achieved. The tolerance of lenabasum was good. Disappointingly, results from a recent phase 3 trial (yet to be reported in full) showed no benefit from lenabasum.

Riociguat, a guanylate cyclase agonist, did not demonstrate a benefit on mRSS in a phase 2 trial in patients with a dcSSc of <18 months duration [21].

Data are still preliminary with **tofacitinib**, which is a Januskinase inhibitor with the high degree of selectivity against JAK1 and JAK3.

There is no convincing data for **imatinib mesylate**, a tyrosine kinase inhibitor. A phase 2 pilot study that enrolled 76 patients with SSc (mean duration of progression of 3 years, extremes 1–6, 53.3% dcSSc) showed no benefit on the primary endpoint, which was FVC or mRSS. All patients had active lung disease and were non-responders to cyclophosphamide [57]. Recent data from a meta-analysis suggest some benefit on mRSS [58].

Nintedanib is a multi-tyrosine kinase inhibitor which blocks different receptors involved in fibrosis and inflammation in animal models of SSc-ILD. A recent Phase 3 trial demonstrated benefit from nintedanib in SSc-ILD [59, 60]. This large RCT which included 576 patients who received oral nintedanib at a dose of 150 mg × 2/day ($n = 288$) or placebo ($n = 288$) in patients with ILD with an extent of fibrosis ≥10% on HRCT scan showed that it significantly reduced the decline in FVC, but did not show any benefit on mRSS. It should be noted that in this study patients could receive a corticosteroid at a dose ≤ 10 mg/d of prednisone and could be on DMARDs at stable doses from ≥6 months prior to randomization. 51.9% of patients had dcSSc. A subgroup analysis of these patients (153 on nintedanib and 144 on placebo) did not show any benefit of nintedanib on mRSS.

A phase 3 trial with **pirfenidone**, another synthetic antifibrotic agent approved in idiopathic lung fibrosis, with FVC as primary endpoint in patients with SSc-ILD, and mRSS as a secondary endpoint is currently ongoing, but no benefit from pirfenidone was found in a Phase 2 trial with mRSS as a secondary endpoint [61].

Autologous Hematopoetic Stem-Cell Transplantation

Three randomized trials (ASSIST—phase 2, ASTIS—phase 3, and SCOT—phase 2) have demonstrated with a high level of evidence the efficacy of autologous hematopoietic stem-cell transplantation (HSCT) in early dcSSc with a duration of less than 4 years [62–64]. These three studies demonstrated the superiority of HSCT over standard IV cyclophosphamide treatment administered monthly for 12 months over free survival event. HSCT now has a strength of recommendation A [40] for the treatment of severe and rapidly progressive dcSSc. However, it should be noted that none of these 3 studies were designed to evaluate the benefit of HSCT on skin involvement as a primary endpoint. Only the ASSIST study considered mRSS in a composite primary endpoint at 12 months. Of the 10 patients assigned to HSCT, 8 had dcSSc versus 7 of 9 in the control group. This was a composite endpoint defined by a decrease in mRSS >25% for those who initially had mRSS >14 or an increase in FVC of more than 10%. All patients randomized to receive HSCT improved at month 12 of follow-up vs none in the CYC group ($p = 0.0001$). The benefit was also significant individually on both mRSS and DLCO.

In order to limit the initial risk of death associated with the procedure, a rigorous selection of patients prior to the procedure should be made in a multidisciplinary meeting and the international recommendations published in 2017 by the EBMT [65] must be respected. The main exclusion criteria for SSc are age > 65 years, severe cardiac disease with LVEF < 45% or pulmonary hypertension, severe pulmonary disease with FVC < 65% or DLCO < 40%, SSc renal crisis in the previous 6 months, or glomerular filtration rate < 40 ml/min/1.73 m^2.

In conclusion, although the levels of evidence are seldom good, there is a general consensus regarding the use of immunosuppressive drugs in recent dcSSc with progressive skin involvement whether or not there is associated visceral involvement. MMF is one of the best candidates for initial treatment in terms of the benefit/risk ratio. In patients with new onset, severe, and progressive dcSSc, HSCT can be discussed in a multidisciplinary meeting with a rigorous selection of patients. Targeted treatments should only be used in special cases due to their current low level of evidence and always after multidisciplinary discussion. Where at all possible, patients should be recruited into a clinical trial: only in this way will new effective and safe treatments be identified.

Overall Conclusions

Management of progressive skin involvement in early dcSSc remains a very major challenge. However, progress is being made in terms of better understanding of its associated pain and disability (highlighting the need for treatment of the skin disease itself), improved ability to identify 'progressors' (paving the way for a stratified approach to management), and a better understanding of the rationale and indications for immunosuppressant therapy and for autologous stem cell transplantation. Work is ongoing to develop better measures of outcome. Identifying safe and effective therapies for the skin disease of early dcSSc remains a major unmet need, and it is encouraging that the last five years have seen multiple collaborations between clinicians and the pharmaceutical industry to address this need, with further studies ongoing or in the planning phase.

Acknowledgement This work was supported by the NIHR Manchester Biomedical Research Centre.

References

1. Khanna D, Furst DE, Clements PJ, Allanore Y, Baron M, Czirjak L, et al. Standardization of the modified Rodnan skin score for use in clinical trials of systemic sclerosis. J Scleroderma Relat Disord. 2017;2:11–8.

2. Clements PJ, Hurwitz EL, Wong WK, Seibold JR, Mayes M, White B, et al. Skin thickness score as a predictor and correlate of outcome in systemic sclerosis. Arthritis Rheum. 2000;43:2445–54.
3. Shand L, Lunt M, Nihtyanova S, Hoseini M, Silman A, Black CM, et al. Relationship between change in skin score and disease outcome in diffuse cutaneous systemic sclerosis. Arthritis Rheum. 2007;56:2422–31.
4. Ledoult E, Launay D, Behal H, Mouthon L, Pugnet G, Lega JC, et al. Early trajectories of skin thickening are associated with severity and mortality in systemic sclerosis. Arthritis Res Ther. 2020;22:30.
5. Domsic RT, Rodriguez-Reyna T, Lucas M, Fertig N, Medsger TA. Skin thickness progression rate: a predictor of mortality and early internal organ involvement in diffuse scleroderma. Ann Rheum Dis. 2011;70:104–9.
6. Wu W, Jordan S, Graf N, de Oliveira PJ, Curram J, Allanore Y, et al. Progressive skin fibrosis is associated with a decline in lung function and worse survival in patients with diffuse cutaneous systemic sclerosis in the European Scleroderma Trials and Research (EUSTAR) cohort. Ann Rheum Dis. 2019;78:648–56.
7. Steen VD, Medsger TA. Improvement in skin thickening in systemic sclerosis associated with improved survival. Arthritis Rheum. 2001;44:2828–35.
8. Nevskaya T, Zheng B, Baxter CA, Ramey DR, Pope JE, Baron M, et al. Skin improvement is a surrogate for favourable changes in other organ systems in early diffuse cutaneous systemic sclerosis. Rheumatology. 2020;59:1715–24.
9. Peytrignet S, Denton CP, Lunt M, Hesselstrand R, Mouthon L, Silman A, et al. Disability, fatigue, pain and their associates in early diffuse cutaneous systemic sclerosis: the European Scleroderma Observational Study. Rheumatology. 2018;57:370–81.
10. Peytrignet S, Manning J, Wragg E, Moore T, Samaranayaka M, Dinsdale G, et al. Changes in disability and their relationship with skin thickening, in diffuse and limited cutaneous systemic sclerosis: a retrospective cohort study. Scand J Rheumatol. 2019;48: 230–4.
11. Zheng B, Nevskaya T, Baxter CA, Ramey DR, Pope JE, Baron M, et al. Changes in skin score in early diffuse cutaneous systemic sclerosis are associated with changes in global disease severity. Rheumatology. 2020;59:398–406.
12. Amjadi S, Maranian P, Furst DE, Wong WK, Postlethwaite AE, Khanna PP, et al. Course of the modified Rodnan skin thickness score in systemic sclerosis clinical trials. Arthritis Rheum. 2009;60:2490–8.
13. Khanna PP, Furst DE, Clements PJ, Maranian P, Indulkar L, Khanna D, et al. Tendon friction rubs in early diffuse systemic sclerosis: prevalence, characteristics and longitudinal changes in a randomized controlled trial. Rheumatology. 2010;49:955–9.
14. Avouac J, Walker UA, Hachulla E, Riemekasten G, Cuomo G, Carreira PE, et al. Joint and tendon involvement predict disease progression in systemic sclerosis: a EUSTAR prospective study. Ann Rheum Dis. 2016;75:103–9.
15. Maurer B, Graf N, Michel BA, Muller-Ladner U, Czirjak L, Denton CP, et al. Prediction of worsening of skin fibrosis in patients with diffuse cutaneous systemic sclerosis using the EUSTAR database. Ann Rheum Dis. 2015;74:1124–31.
16. Herrick AL, Peytrignet S, Lunt M, Pan X, Hesselstrand R, Mouthon L, et al. Patterns and predictors of skin score change in early diffuse systemic sclerosis from the European Scleroderma Observational Study. Ann Rheum Dis. 2018;77:563–70.
17. Assassi S, Swindell WR, Wu M, Tan FD, Khanna D, Furst DE, et al. Dissecting the heterogeneity of skin gene expression patterns in systemic sclerosis. Arthritis Rheumatol. 2015;67:3016–26.
18. Stifano G, Sornasse T, Rice LM, Na L, Chen-Harris H, Khanna D, et al. Skin gene expression is prognostic for the trajectory of skin disease in patients with diffuse cutaneous systemic sclerosis. Arthritis Rheumatol. 2018;70:912–9.
19. Skaug B, Khanna D, Swindell WR, Hinchcliff ME, Frech TM, Steen VD, et al. Global skin gene expression analysis of early diffuse cutaneous systemic sclerosis shows a prominent innate and adaptive inflammatory profile. Ann Rheum Dis. 2020;79:379–86.
20. Khanna D, Spino C, Johnson S, Chung L, Whitfield ML, Denton CP, et al. Abatacept in early diffuse cutaneous systemic sclerosis: results of a phase II investigator-initiated, multicenter, double-blind, randomized, placebo-controlled trial. Arthritis Rheumatol. 2020;72:125–36.
21. Khanna D, Allanore Y, Denton CP, Kuwana M, Matucci-Cerinic M, Pope JE, et al. Riociguat in patients with early diffuse cutaneous systemic sclerosis (RISE-SSc): randomised, double-blind, placebo-controlled multicentre trial. Ann Rheum Dis. 2020;79:618–25.
22. Khanna D, Lin CJF, Furst DE, Goldin J, Kim G, Kuwana M, et al. Tocilizumab in systemic sclerosis: a randomised, double-blind, placebo-controlled, phase 3 trial. Lancet Respir Med. 2020;8:963–74.
23. Allanore Y, Wung P, Soubrane C, Esperet C, Marrache F, Bejuit R, el. A randomised, double-blind, placebo-controlled, 24-week, phase II, proof-of-concept study of romilkimab (SAR156597) in early diffuse cutaneous systemic sclerosis. Ann Rheum Dis. 2020;79:1600–7.
24. Clements P, Lachenbruch P, Siebold J, White B, Weiner S, Martin R, et al. Inter- and intraobserver variability of total skin thickness score (modified Rodnan TSS) in systemic sclerosis. J Rheumatol. 1995;22:1281–5.
25. Showalter K, Merkel PA, Khanna D, Gordon JK. for the Scleroderma Clinical Trials Consortium. J Scleroderma Relat Disord. 2020;5:167–71.
26. Low AHL, Ng SA, Berrocal V, Brennan B, Chan G, Ng SC, et al. Evaluation of Scleroderma Clinical Trials Consortium training recommendations on modified Rodnan skin score assessment in scleroderma. Int J Rheum Dis. 2019;22:1036–40.
27. Khanna F, Berrocal VJ, Giannini EH, Seibold JR, Merkel PE, Mayes MD, et al. The American College of Rheumatology provisional composite response index for clinical trials in early diffuse cutaneous systemic sclerosis. Arthritis Care Res. 2016;68:167–78.
28. Man A, Correa JK, Ziemek J, Simms RW, Felson DT, Lafyatis R. Development and validation of a patient-reported outcome instrument for skin involvement in patients with systemic sclerosis. Ann Rheum Dis. 2017;76:1374–80.
29. Moore TL, Lunt M, McManus B, Anderson ME, Herrick AL. Seventeen-point dermal ultrasound scoring system - a reliable measure of skin thickness in patients with systemic sclerosis. Rheumatology. 2003;42:1559–63.
30. Hesselstrand R, Scheja A, Wildt M, Akesson A. High-frequency ultrasound of skin involvement in systemic sclerosis reflects oedema, extension and severity in early disease. Rheumatology. 2008;47:84–7.
31. Naredo E, Pascau J, Damjanov N, Lepri G, Gordaliza PM, Janta I, et al. Performance of ultra-high-frequency ultrasound in the evaluation of skin involvement in systemic sclerosis: a preliminary report. Rheumatology. 2020;59:1671–8.
32. Abignano G, Aydin SZ, Castillo-Gallego C, Liakouli V, Woods D, Meekings A, et al. Virtual skin biopsy by optical coherence tomography: the first quantitative imaging biomarker for scleroderma. Ann Rheum Dis. 2013;72:1845–51.
33. Liu CH, Assassi S, Theodore S, Smith C, Schill A, Singh M, et al. Translational optical coherence elastography for assessment of systemic sclerosis. J Biophotonics. 2019;12:e201900236.
34. Marjanovic E, Dinsdale G, Berks M, Moore T, Manning J, Sharma V, et al. Pilot study of polarisation sensitive optical coherence tomography as a biomarker for fibrosis in systemic sclerosis (abstract). Rheumatology. 2018;57(Suppl. 3) https://doi.org/10.1093/rheumatology/key075.382.
35. Adams DC, Szabari MV, Lagares D, McCrossan AF, Hariri LP, Tager AM, et al. Assessing the progression of systemic sclero-

sis by monitoring the tissue optic axis using PS-OCT. Sci Rep. 2020;10:2561.
36. Sousa-Neves J, Cerqueira M, Santos-Faria D, Afonso C, Teixeira F. Neuropathic pain in Systemic Sclerosis patients: A cross-sectional study. Reumatol Clin. 2019;15:e99–e101.
37. Wigley FM, Wise RA, Seibold JR, McCloskey DA, Kujala G, Medsger TA, et al. Intravenous iloprost infusion in patients with Raynaud phenomenon secondary to systemic sclerosis. A multicenter, placebo-controlled, double-blind study. Ann Intern Med. 1994;120:199–206.
38. Stratton R, Shiwen X, Martini G, Holmes A, Leask A, Haberberger T, et al. Iloprost suppresses connective tissue growth factor production in fibroblasts and in the skin of scleroderma patients. J Clin Invest. 2001;108:241–50.
39. Campochiaro C, Allanore, Y. An update on targeted therapies in systemic sclerosis based on a systematic review from the last 3 years. Arthritis Res Ther. 2021;23:155. https://doi.org/10.1186/s13075-021-02536-5.
40. Kowal-Bielecka O, Fransen J, Avouac J, Becker M, Kulak A, Allanore Y, et al. Update of EULAR recommendations for the treatment of systemic sclerosis. Ann Rheum Dis. 2017;76:1327–39.
41. Herrick AL. Controversies on the Use of Steroids in Systemic Sclerosis. J Scleroderma Relat Disord. 2017;2:84–91.
42. Herrick AL, Pan X, Peytrignet S, Lunt M, Hesselstrand R, Mouthon L, et al. Treatment outcome in early diffuse cutaneous systemic sclerosis: the European Scleroderma Observational Study (ESOS). Ann Rheum Dis. 2017;76:1207–18.
43. Herrick AL, Griffiths-Jones DJ, Ryder WD, Mason JC, Denton CP. Clinical trial protocol—PRednisolone in early diffuse cutaneous systemic sclerosis. J Scleroderma Related Disord. 2021;6(2):146–53. https://doi.org/10.1177/2397198320957552. (EPub ahead of press)
44. van den Hoogen FH, Boerbooms AM, Swaak AJ, Rasker JJ, van Lier HJ, van de Putte LB. Comparison of methotrexate with placebo in the treatment of systemic sclerosis: a 24 week randomized double-blind trial, followed by a 24 week observational trial. Br J Rheumatol. 1996;35:364–72.
45. Pope JE, Bellamy N, Seibold JR, Baron M, Ellman M, Carette S, et al. A randomized, controlled trial of methotrexate versus placebo in early diffuse scleroderma. Arthritis Rheum. 2001;44:1351–8.
46. Johnson SR, Feldman BM, Pope JE, Tomlinson GA. Shifting our thinking about uncommon disease trials: the case of methotrexate in scleroderma. J Rheumatol. 2009;36:323–9.
47. Smolen JS, Landewé RBM, Bijlsma JWJ, Burmester GR, Dougados M, Kerschbaumer A, et al. EULAR recommendations for the management of rheumatoid arthritis with synthetic and biological disease-modifying antirheumatic drugs: 2019 update. Ann Rheum Dis. 2020;79:685–99.
48. Schiff MH, Jaffe JS, Freundlich B. Head-to-head, randomised, crossover study of oral versus subcutaneous methotrexate in patients with rheumatoid arthritis: drug-exposure limitations of oral methotrexate at doses ≥15 mg may be overcome with subcutaneous administration. Ann Rheum Dis. 2014;73:1549–51.
49. Tashkin DP, Elashoff R, Clements PJ, Goldin J, Roth MD, Furst DE, et al. Cyclophosphamide versus placebo in scleroderma lung disease. N Engl J Med. 2006;354:2655–66.
50. Hoyles RK, Ellis RW, Wellsbury J, Lees B, Newlands P, Goh NS, et al. A multicenter, prospective, randomized, double-blind, placebo-controlled trial of corticosteroids and intravenous cyclophosphamide followed by oral azathioprine for the treatment of pulmonary fibrosis in scleroderma. Arthritis Rheum. 2006;54:3962–70.
51. Bruni C, Tashkin DP, Steen V, Allanore Y, Distler O, Grotts J, et al. Intravenous versus oral cyclophosphamide for lung and/or skin fibrosis in systemic sclerosis: an indirect comparison from EUSTAR and randomised controlled trials. Clin Exp Rheumatol. 2020;38(suppl. 125):161–8.
52. Tashkin DP, Roth MD, Clements PJ, Furst DE, Khanna D, Kleerup EC, et al. Mycophenolate mofetil versus oral cyclophosphamide in scleroderma-related interstitial lung disease (SLS II): a randomised controlled, double-blind, parallel group trial. Lancet Respir Med. 2016;4:708–19.
53. Mendoza FA, Lee-Ching C, Jimenez SA. Recurrence of progressive skin involvement following discontinuation or dose reduction of Mycophenolate Mofetil treatment in patients with diffuse Systemic Sclerosis. Semin Arthritis Rheum. 2020;50:135–9.
54. Daoussis D, Melissaropoulos K, Sakellaropoulos G, Antonopoulos I, Markatseli TE, Simopoulou T, et al. A multicenter, open-label, comparative study of B-cell depletion therapy with Rituximab for systemic sclerosis-associated interstitial lung disease. Semin Arthritis Rheum. 2017;46:625–31.
55. Elhai M, Boubaya M, Distler O, Smith V, Matucci-Cerinic M, Alegre Sancho JJ, et al. Outcomes of patients with systemic sclerosis treated with rituximab in contemporary practice: a prospective cohort study. Ann Rheum Dis. 2019;78:979–87.
56. Spiera R, Hummers L, Chung L, Frech TM, Domsic R, Hsu V, et al. Safety and Efficacy of Lenabasum in a Phase II, Randomized, Placebo-Controlled Trial in Adults With Systemic Sclerosis. Arthritis Rheumatol. 2020;72:1350–60.
57. Fraticelli P, Gabrielli B, Pomponio G, Valentini G, Bosello S, Riboldi P, et al. Low-dose oral imatinib in the treatment of systemic sclerosis interstitial lung disease unresponsive to cyclophosphamide: a phase II pilot study. Arthritis Res Ther. 2014;16:R144.
58. Liakouli V, Ciaffi J, Ursini F, Ruscitti P, Meliconi R, Ciccia F, et al. Efficacy and safety of imatinib mesylate in systemic sclerosis. A systematic review and meta-analysis. Expert Rev Clin Immunol. 2020;16:931–42.
59. Distler O, Highland KB, Gahlemann M, Azuma A, Fischer A, Mayes MD, et al. Nintedanib for systemic sclerosis associated interstitial lung disease. N Engl J Med. 2019;380:2518–28.
60. Seibold JR, Maher TM, Highland KB, Assassi S, Azuma A, Hummers LK, et al. Safety and tolerability of nintedanib in patients with systemic sclerosis-associated interstitial lung disease: data from the SENSCIS trial. Ann Rheum Dis. 2020;79:1478–84.
61. Khanna D, Albera C, Fischer A, Khalidi N, Raghu G, Chung L, et al. An Open-label, Phase II Study of the Safety and Tolerability of Pirfenidone in Patients with Scleroderma-associated Interstitial Lung Disease: the LOTUSS Trial. J Rheumatol. 2016;43:1672–9.
62. Burt RK, Shah SJ, Dill K, Grant T, Gheorghiade M, Schroeder J, et al. Autologous non-myeloablative haemopoietic stem-cell transplantation compared with pulse cyclophosphamide once per month for systemic sclerosis (ASSIST): an open-label, randomised phase 2 trial. Lancet. 2011;378:498–506.
63. van Laar JM, Farge D, Sont JK, Naraghi K, Marjanovic Z, Larghero J, et al. Autologous hematopoietic stem cell transplantation vs intravenous pulse cyclophosphamide in diffuse cutaneous systemic sclerosis: a randomized clinical trial. JAMA. 2014;311:2490–8.
64. Sullivan KM, Goldmuntz EA, Keyes-Elstein L, McSweeney PA, Pinckney A, Welch B, et al. Myeloablative Autologous Stem-Cell Transplantation for Severe Scleroderma. N Engl J Med. 2018;378:35.
65. Farge D, Burt RK, Oliveira MC, Mousseaux E, Rovira M, Marjanovic Z, et al. Cardiopulmonary assessment of patients with systemic sclerosis for hematopoietic stem cell transplantation: recommendations from the European Society for Blood and Marrow Transplantation Autoimmune Diseases Working Party and collaborating partners. Bone Marrow Transplant. 2017;52:1495–503.

Hematopoietic Stem Cell Transplantation

43

Jacob M. van Laar, Julia Spierings, and Oliver Distler

Clinical Effects of HSCT in Systemic Sclerosis

The concept of hematopoietic stem cell transplantation (HSCT) as a therapeutic treatment modality for autoimmune disease gained traction in the 1980s and 1990s following seminal studies in rodent models of autoimmune disease demonstrating the curative potential of allogeneic and pseudo-autologous bone marrow transplantation (BMT) and publication of case reports of positive outcomes in patients with malignancy and coexisting autoimmune disease treated with allogeneic BMT (reviewed in [1]). Advances in cell separation techniques and breakthroughs in the production of human growth factors accelerated the clinical use of peripheral blood stem cells instead of bone marrow, thus avoiding general anesthesia of the donor (Fig. 43.1). HSCT allowed dose escalation of (radio)chemotherapy to achieve immune ablation and reset the dysregulated immune system of patients with autoimmune disease. The first patient published receiving an HSCT for an autoimmune disease had systemic sclerosis (SSc) with pulmonary artery hypertension and responded satisfactorily [2] and survived in stable condition for 20 years (Alan Tyndall, personal communication). Since the start of the international collaboration in 1997, the EBMT Autoimmune Disease Working Party alone has collected data from 3855 transplants, mostly autologous, including data from 787 systemic sclerosis (SSc) patients, as treatment for severe autoimmune disease (May 2022) [3, 4]. Although many protocols were employed, they basically ranged from less aggressive, lymphoablative, e.g., CYC 200 mg/kg plus antithymocyte globulin (ATG), to more intensive, myeloablative, e.g., total body irradiation (TBI) plus CYC/ATG and CD34 selection of BU/CY plus ATG and CD34 selection. Despite its appeal as a curative treatment option, allogeneic HSCT for autoimmune disease seemed not to be more effective than autologous HSCT, while the significant risk of treatment-related mortality (TRM) and graft-versus-host disease of allogeneic HSCT precluded its wider adoption [5].

SSc was an obvious disease target for HSCT as few effective immunomodulatory conventional therapies were available for poor prognosis SSc patients at the time other than methotrexate, mycophenolate mofetil, and cyclophosphamide, and apart from the introduction of rituximab and nintedanib, little has changed in the management of SSc patients. Early case reports, case series, and registry analyses consistently showed rapid and significant improvement of skin thickening, as a surrogate measure of disease activity and severity [6, 7]. However, SSc patients also appeared particularly prone to cardiopulmonary complications attributed to fluid overload from hyperhydration, toxic effects of high-dose cyclophosphamide, and cytokine-release syndrome related to the use of ATG. TRM in SSc transplant settings was consequently high in the early days of the autoimmune transplant programme, prompting risk mitigation steps such as lung shielding in those treated with TBI-based conditioning protocols in the US and reduced intensity regimens in Europe [8, 9]. As such, important lessons were learned from the pilot studies, perhaps the main being that HSCT in SSc is a high-risk medical intervention that is best performed in tertiary referral transplant centers with expertise in managing complex SSc patients.

Three prospective randomized trials in SSc have been published, ASTIS (Autologous Stem cell Transplantation International Scleroderma), SCOT (Scleroderma Cyclophosphamide Or Transplant), and ASSIST (American Stem cell Scleroderma versus Immune Suppression Trial) . ASTIS and SCOT were similar in patient selection, control arms, and endpoints, but the transplant protocols differed. SCOT employed a more intense myeloablative regimen including TBI. The largest and longest study in this field, the ASTIS trial, involved 156 patients with a median follow-up of 5.8 years [10]. The primary endpoint of event-free sur-

J. M. van Laar (✉) · J. Spierings
Department of Rheumatology and Clinical Immunology, UMC Utrecht, Utrecht, The Netherlands
e-mail: J.M.vanLaar@umcutrecht.nl

O. Distler
Department of Rheumatology, University Hospital Zurich, Zurich, Switzerland

Y. Allanore et al. (eds.), *Scleroderma*, https://doi.org/10.1007/978-3-031-40658-4_43

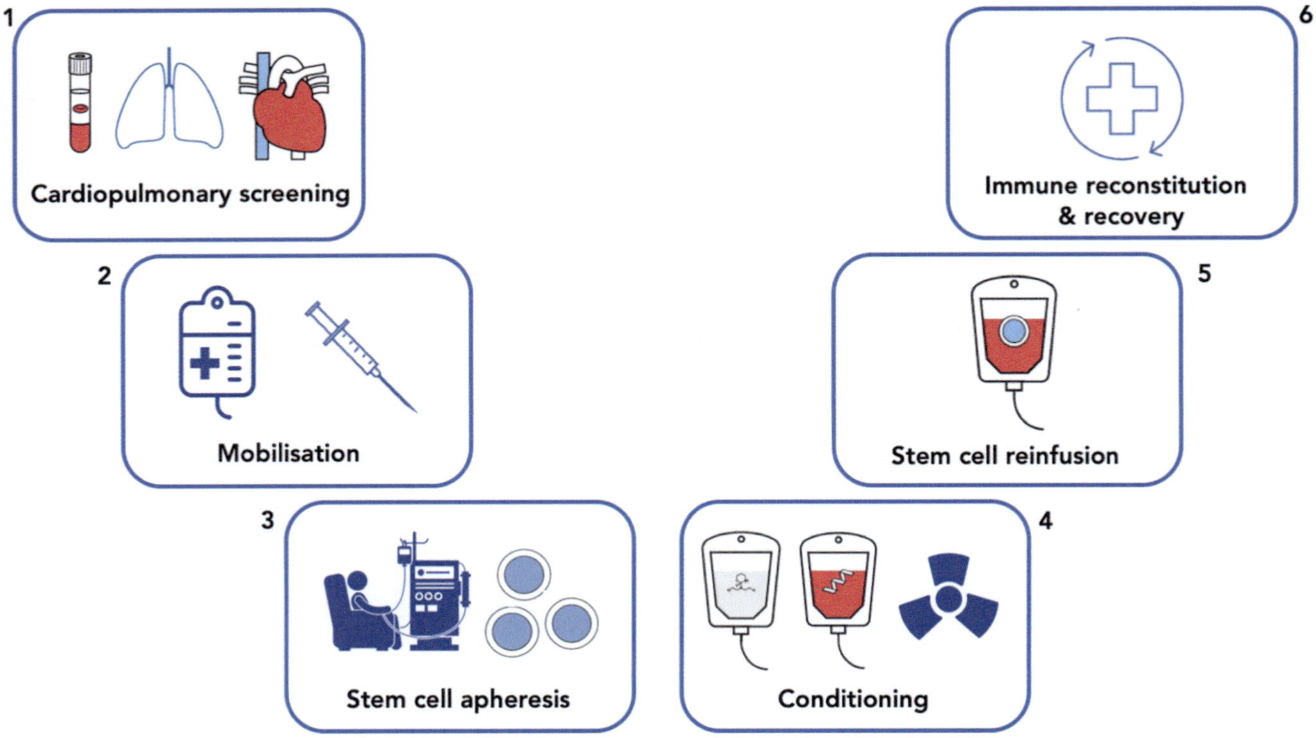

Fig. 43.1 The HSCT procedure. Step 1. To increase safety and lower the risk of severe complications, screening for (indolent) infections and heart and lung involvement are done. Step 2. The first step in HSCT is mobilization of stem cells from the bone marrow using G-CSF. Chemotherapeutic agents can be used to facilitate the release of stem cells in the peripheral circulation and prevent flaring due to G-CSF. Step 3. Stem cells are harvested using leukapheresis. Step 4. Autoreactive B- and T-cells are eliminated with the administration of myeloablative or lymphoablative regimens. Total body irradiation is used in myeloablative schemes. Chemotherapeutic agents such as cyclophosphamide and antithymocyte globulin are often included in lymphoablatic regimens. Step 5. Stem cells are (re-)infused after completion of the conditioning regimen. Step 6. Prophylactic antibiotics and symptomatic treatment are provided during the aplastic phase. Generally, neutropenia recovers in 1–3 weeks and full reconstitution of the immune system takes several months after HSCT

vival, events being defined as death or end-organ (renal, cardiac, or pulmonary) failure, was achieved long-term in the transplanted arm. Also, significantly better outcomes were seen in the HSCT group with respect to secondary outcome measures (skin score, quality of life, functional ability, vital capacity), with the exception of kidney function, which appeared worse in the first 2 years in the HSCT group. Also, more grade 3 and 4 serious adverse events were observed in the HSCT group, most related to neutropenic fever and heart-lung failure in the conditioning step. Eight patients (10%) in the HSCT group died from treatment-related complications. A post-hoc analysis revealed that the survival benefit of HSCT was only observed in those who had never smoked.

The SCOT-trial randomized 75 patients (36 to HSCT) and the primary endpoint was a global rank composite score (GRCS) at 54 months that ordered subjects based on a hierarchy of outcomes: death, event-free survival (EFS), forced vital capacity (FVC), scleroderma health assessment questionnaire, and modified Rodnan skin score (mRSS) [11]. This study demonstrated long-term superiority of myeloablative autologous HSCT over CYC on efficacy endpoints including overall survival and showed a significant reduction in use of DMARDs among HSCT recipients. Transplant-related mortality was 3% at 54 months and 6% at 72 months in the HSCT-group. Interestingly, a post-hoc analysis too showed an effect of smoking status on outcomes. A smaller phase II randomized trial in SSc, the ASSIST trial, showed a positive outcome in the 10 transplanted patients compared with 9 control patients who received CYC 1 g/m^2 for 6 months [12]. The conditioning regimen was CYC 200 mg/kg plus five doses of rabbit ATG, each one accompanied by 1 g of intravenous methylprednisolone. The primary endpoint at 12 months was based on a percentage improvement of the mRSS and/or pulmonary status. No deaths occurred in the trial. The low numbers of patients and short follow-up in the ASSIST trial precluded assessment of long-term outcomes, but it was interesting to see the effects of HSCT on lung function in the ASSIST trial corroborated by semiquantitative HRCT scores, an observation that has since been confirmed by other investigators [13, 14].

Although the randomized, controlled clinical trial remains the gold standard to determine superiority of one treatment over another, real-world data from registry analyses too have provided valuable information on practical aspects such as international trends in uptake of HSCT in SSc, potential benefit of enrichment of CD34+ stem cells from the graft, improvement of safety of HSCT of conditioning regimens, and long-term outcomes.

In a prospective non-interventional study from the European Society for Blood and Marrow Transplantation Autoimmune Disease Working Part in 80 SSc patients treated with the ASTIS-regimen, progression-free survival was 81.8%, overall survival was 90%, response was 88.7% and incidence of progression was 11.9% at two years, while the 100 day non-relapse mortality was 6.25% ($n = 5$) with four deaths from cardiac event, including three due to cyclophosphamide toxicity [15]. MRSS and FVC improved with time ($P < 0.001$). By multivariate analysis, baseline skin score > 24 and older age at transplant were associated with lower progression-free survival (Hazard ratio 3.32 and 1.77, respectively). CD34 + -selection was associated with better response (Hazard ratio: 0.46).

Better outcomes were also found in a small Japanese trial in 19 patients treated with high-dose cyclophosphamide (200 mg/kg) followed by reinfusion of either a CD34-selected autologous graft ($n = 11$) or an unmanipulated graft ($n = 8$) [16]. The 5-year progression-free survival rates of the CD34-selected and unmanipulated group were 81.8% and 50%, respectively.

Improvement of safety of conditioning has also been a priority, particularly focusing on development of potentially less cardiotoxic medication for patients with cardiac involvement [17]. A small pilot study in 6 SSc patients with cardiac involvement, a combination of a thiotepa-based regimen combined with low disease cyclophosphamide proved feasible and none of the patients died from (cardiac) complications [18]. In a larger safety study in 42 SSc patients, a regimen with fludarabine, cyclophosphamide, and ATG was relatively safe with a TRM of 2.4% and a neutropenic interval of only 5.2 days in those at risk of major cardiac toxicity according to EBMT guidelines, i.e., either a right heart catheterization PASP >40 mmHg at rest or > 45 mmHg with fluid challenge, or mPAP > 25 mmHg at rest or > 30 mmHg with fluid challenge, or diastolic interventricular septal flattening (D-sign) or septal bounce on cardiac MRI [19]. The addition of rituximab in 28/42 patients reportedly decreased 1-year relapse rate (3.6% vs. 36%), risk of late secondary autoimmune diseases (0% vs. 21%), and upper-respiratory tract infections (3.6% vs. 28%). Such exploratory studies confirm that HSCT may even be feasible in those deemed at too high risk of serious complications in the early days of HSCT in SSc. HSCT has also been successfully performed in selected SSc patients using standard conditioning, so it remains to be seen whether modifications of existing protocols are necessary [20]. Nevertheless, based on a cohort analysis of patients who received high-dose versus low-dose cyclophosphamide for mobilization showing no differences in numbers of stem cells generated nor on safety, it was deemed prudent by the UPSIDE-trial investigators (www.upsidetrial.com) to use the lower dose of cyclophosphamide for mobilization of hematopoietic stem cells [21].

Excellent long-term outcomes of transplanted SSc patients were also reported in cohorts from the Netherlands ($n = 92$) and Brazil ($n = 70$) [22, 23]. In the former study event-free survival estimates at 5, 10, and 15 years were 78%, 76%, and 66%, respectively, twenty deaths occurred, and mean FVC, DLCO, mRSS, and semiquantitative scores of lung fibrosis improved significantly. Disease progression occurred in 22 patients. TRM was lower in those transplanted after 2012 as compared to those transplanted before (7.3% vs. 13.7%), possibly due to more stringent patient selection, experience of the transplant team, and better supportive care. Overall survival was 81% at 8 years after HSCT in the Brazilian cohort, while TRM was low at 4.2%.

Nevertheless, serious toxicities from HSCT including a risk of TRM are seen by many as showstopper and unacceptable even in the face of the aforementioned positive outcome data from controlled trials and registry analyses. It is still a challenge for a rheumatologist to accept an immediate TRM of 3–10% and the risk of relapse, whether manageable or not. Furthermore, treatable complications such as viral infections and secondary autoimmune conditions, albeit rare, further tarnish the image of HSCT in some quarters. Yet the outcomes after HSCT cannot be interpreted in isolation. In a recent cohort analysis of 41 SSc patients meeting the eligibility criteria of ASTIS and SCOT but treated with conventional immunosuppressants survival rates at the time, endpoints of SCOT and ASTIS (4.5 and 7 years, respectively) were comparable to the conventionally treated SCOT/ASTIS control groups [24]. The authors concluded that if all patients with rapidly progressive SSc had undergone HSCT promptly, their overall and event-free survival rates could have increased significantly.

Apart from TRM and other serious complications, nonresponse and partial response following HSCT may pose a clinical challenge too. The factors determining this remain elusive. Whatever the underlying immune mechanisms, the occurrence of relapses bears relevance as shown in a retrospective American study of 90 SSc patients treated with the intermediate Cy/ATG regimen with an unselected graft where eight of the 13 relapses proved fatal [19]. In terms of managing relapses, most patients successfully resumed immunosuppressive medication to which they were unresponsive pre-HSCT, thus further supporting the notion that HSCT leads to a reset of an autoaggressive immune system. So far one case has been published of a SSc patient who had relapsed after HSCT who was successfully re-transplanted and put on posttransplant immunosuppression for 3 years to maintain remission which was sustained even after discontinuation of medication [25].

With the caveat that long-term follow-up beyond 25 years is not available and that loss to follow-up and underreporting may have negatively affected the quality of the data, late HSCT-related complications such as secondary autoimmunity (invariably organ-specific and treatable) and secondary malignancy have only been incidentally reported [26–28].

Mechanistic Effects of HSCT in Systemic Sclerosis

Pioneering preclinical rodent studies in arthritis and encephalitis have been instrumental in demonstrating the curative potential of BMT and elucidating its immunoablative effects, paving the way for the development of HSCT as a new treatment modality for patients with severe autoimmune disease [29]. Interestingly, no studies on the effects of BMT in animal models of SSc have ever been done, perhaps because few such models which encapsulated the complex nature of SSc with vasculopathy, autoimmunity, and fibrosis were available at the time. While clear dose-response clinical effects were shown in the aforementioned allogeneic BMT-studies in arthritis and encephalitis, very few research effort has been put into demonstrating whether tolerance to autoantigen was achieved. While immune tolerance is the holy grail of reversing autoimmunity in man, faithful biomarkers of immune tolerance do not as yet exist, hence our reliance on measuring serum autoantibodies as a surrogate measure. The ASTIS trial was the first to report the impact of HSCT, but not IV pulse cyclophosphamide, on the proportion of patients with ANA and anti-topoisomerase autoantibodies [10]. A more in-depth analysis of anti-topoisomerase antibody titers and peptide reactivities in 14 transplanted SSc patients from Germany, however, did not reveal major changes pre- and post-HSCT irrespective of clinical responses [30]. These findings are particularly important, since at the onset of the project many considered autologous HSCT to be doomed to failure, based on the preconceived and incorrect notion that HSCT from the graft automatically differentiates into 'autoaggressive' immune cells again upon transfer. Outgrowth of T- and B-cell repertoire after HSCT, however, is to a large extent determined by stochastic processes. Furthermore, the initial choice of autologous over allogeneic HSCT was mainly based on the lower toxicity of autologous HSCT, mainly due to absence of graft-vs.-host disease (GvHD). It is now appreciated that in many patients who achieved clinical remission, the autoaggressive immune system was 'debulked', rather than fully ablated, allowing reestablishment of normal immune regulation, in part due to increased Treg numbers and activity, although early data in SSc were conflicting [31–33]. A more detailed analysis of T cell reconstitution in SSc and other autoimmune conditions, however, lent further support to the importance of the regulatory T cell compartment by revealing a notable broadening of T cell repertoire after HSCT as seen in healthy individuals and immune rebound [33–35]. Of note, remission in many patients was sustained despite full immune reconstitution.

HSCT does not only induce profound changes of the T cell compartment, but also B cell lineage cells. In an analysis of peripheral blood B cell populations of 22 transplanted SSc patients, naïve B cell frequencies increased over time post-HSCT and memory B cell and plasma cell frequencies decreased during the same period [36]. IL-10-producing Bregs CD19 + CD24hiCD38hi and CD19 + CD24hiCD27+ frequencies increased. Bregs recovered their ability to suppress production of Th1 cytokines by CD4+ T cells. Finally, IL-6 and TGF-β1-producing B cells decreased following HSCT. Similar results in a smaller study in 6 patients were independently obtained by other investigators, thus lending credit to the findings [37].

A comprehensive analysis of serum cytokines and vascular biomarkers in transplanted SSc patients revealed a complex picture of changes irrespective of clinical responses [38]. Serum concentrations of IL-6, IL-10 IFN-γ, and TNF-α reportedly did not change significantly, while IL-2 levels decreased initially in all dcSSc before returning to pretransplant levels. Throughout the follow-up, IL-8 levels appeared lower than before aHSCT, with high interindividual variations. Concentrations of TGF-beta, PDGF, MCP-1, E- and P-selectin fluctuated while VEGF decreased after HSCT.

In another study in 25 transplanted SSc patients including 19 responders and 6 nonresponders, inflammatory cytokine (IL-6 and IL-1β) levels and telomere lengths decreased, whereas PD-1 expression on T-cells and the number of $CD8^+CD28^-$ cells expressing CD57 and FoxP3 increased [39]. After AHSCT, responder patients presented higher PD-1 expression on T- ($P < 0.05$) and B- ($P < 0.01$) cells and lower TGF-β, IL-6, G-CSF ($P < 0.01$), and IL-1β, IL-17A, MIP-1α, and IL-12 ($P < 0.05$) levels than nonresponders. Homeostatic proliferation after AHSCT results in transient telomere attrition and increased numbers of senescent and exhausted cells. High PD-1 expression is associated with better clinical outcomes after AHSCT.

Immunohistochemical analyses of skin and serum samples from 39 transplanted SSc patients showed increased expression of MMP-2, MMP-3, MMP-9, and TIMP-1 after HSCT, whereas expression of NF-κB p65 decreased [40]. At baseline, serum levels of COL4A1 and S100A9 were higher than in healthy controls. Serum levels of S100A9 normalized after HCST in SSc patients compared to controls. Serum levels of PDGF-AA, PDGF-BB, TIMP-1, and MMP-1 decreased, while COL1A1 increased after HSCT in SSc patients. No changes were detected in MMP-3, MMP-12, MMP-13, and FGF-1 serum levels after HSCT.

A comprehensive study of global transcripts on whole blood and a proteomic analysis on serum samples taken pre- and posttreatment from 62 SSc patients from the SCOT-trial treated with either HSCT or IV pulse therapy cyclophosphamide revealed stark changes notably in the HSCT-group, but not in patients treated with IV pulse cyclophosphamide [41]. At the baseline visit, interferon (IFN) and neutrophil transcript modules were upregulated and the cytotoxic/NK module was downregulated in SSc compared with unaffected controls. A paired comparison of the 26 months to the baseline samples revealed a significant decrease of the IFN and neutrophil modules and an increase in the cytotoxic/NK module in the HSCT arm, while there was no significant change in the CYC control arm. Also, a composite score of correlating serum proteins with IFN and neutrophil transcript modules, as well as a multilevel analysis, showed significant changes in SSc molecular signatures after HSCT while similar changes were not observed in the CYC arm. Lastly, a decline in the IFN and neutrophil modules was associated with an improvement in pulmonary FVC and an increase in the cytotoxic/NK module correlated with improvement in skin score.

Several groups have described reduced collagen deposition in skin [42, 43], although histological studies of the skin vasculature pre- and post-HSCT have shown mixed results [43, 44]. None of these observations are readily explained by either sustained immunosuppression or direct effects on fibroblasts and endothelial cells and suggest a more profound modulation of the inflammatory niche by mechanisms yet to be fully elucidated.

Early observations in small numbers of patients showed normalization of nailfold capillary abnormalities. In a recent study in 27 transplanted SSc patients who underwent nailfold capillaroscopy pre- and post-HSCT, the number of capillaries increased at 1 year, while giant capillaries decreased at 6 months and 1 year after HSCT [45]. In skin biopsies from these patients, expression of E-selectin notably decreased and Ang1 increased after HSCT. At baseline, all vascular markers evaluated in the serum were significantly higher in SSc patients when compared to healthy controls, except for ICAM-1. When compared at different time points after HSCT, thrombomodulin, pentraxin-3, vWF, and IL-18 levels remained generally stable at high levels until 36 months after HSCT.

Analyses of peripheral blood taken from 33 SSc patients treated with CYC and 30 treated with HSCT in the SCOT trial identified three subsets: a fibroproliferative subset, a normal-like subset, and an inflammatory subset [46]. Participants from the fibroproliferative subset on HSCT experienced significant improvement in EFS compared with fibroproliferative participants on CYC ($p = 0.0091$). In contrast, EFS did not significantly differ between CYC and HSCT arms for the participants from the normal-like subset ($p = 0.77$) or the inflammatory subset ($p = 0.1$). At each timepoint, we observed considerably more differentially expressed genes in the HSCT arm compared with CYC arm with HSCT arm showing significant changes in immune response pathways. This study suggests that intrinsic subset stratification of patients may be used to identify patients with a fibroproliferative subset of SSc who seem to receive the most benefit from HSCT.

Taken together, while differences were observed between results from the aforementioned studies, possibly related to timing of biosampling or technical issues, they unequivocally demonstrate that HSCT induces fundamental alterations of the immune system, microvasculature, and matrix remodeling (summarized in Fig. 43.2).

Patient and Societal Perspectives

Patients with newly diagnosed dcSSc face a mountain of challenges not just limited to their physical wellbeing and psychological stress. SSc almost universally impairs hand function and sexual activity and puts a huge strain on family relationships and ability to work and enjoy leisurely activities. None of these aspects were addressed in any of the HSCT-trials (nor other clinical trials in SSc by the way). The positive effects of HSCT on patient-reported outcomes have been hailed as very encouraging by patients and doctors alike, but it must be stressed that the superior effects on quality of life as measured by SF-36 were only found on the physical component summary scores, not on the mental component summary scores [10, 47]. In line with this, a qualitative study in the four SSc transplant centers in the Netherlands revealed that the physical and psychological impact of HSCT on dcSSc patients was greater than anticipated by the investigators with some patients needing much longer recovery and support [48]. Health care systems differ greatly in their ability to provide adequate mental support to patients and their families, let alone reimburse the necessary expenses, including those related to autologous HSCT, the costs of which vary significantly between countries, but may be prohibitively high in low- and middle-income countries [49]. Partly due to cost-issues, partly to lack of experience, access to HSCT for potentially eligible SSc patients is restricted in most countries at the moment. Unfortunately, no health economic health analyses have as yet been published to compare the costs of HSCT versus those of conventional treatment, but based on the drug-free long-term remissions seen in approximately half of transplanted SSc patients consistently seen in registry analyses and controlled trials, one would expect HSCT incurs significantly lower costs on the long-term in comparison with continued conventional immunosuppressive therapy.

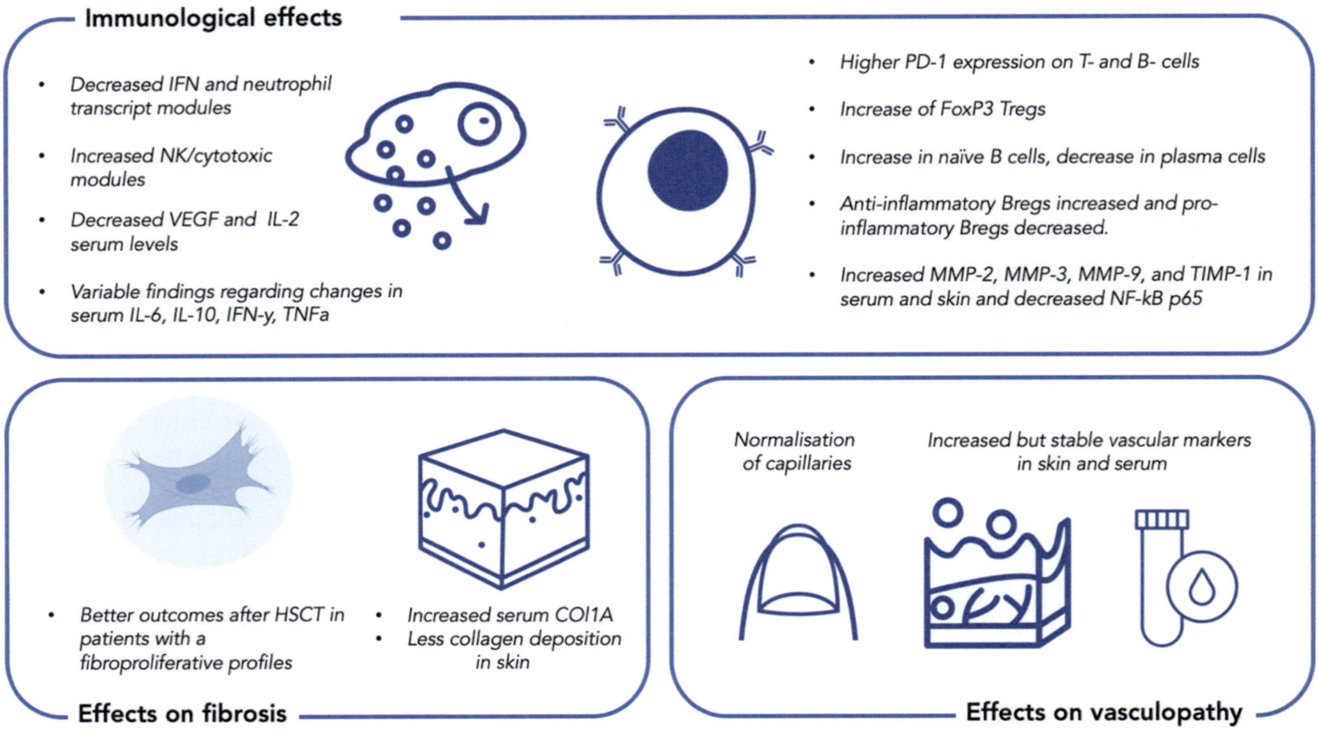

Fig. 43.2 Mechanistic effects after HSCT. Mechanistic effects on the immune system, fibrotic markers, and fibrosis in the tissues and effects on vasculopathy of HSCT. *Immunological effects.* In the SCOT trial, interferon (IFN) and neutrophil transcript modules were upregulated and the cytotoxic/NK module was downregulated in SSc compared with healthy controls at baseline. At 26 months, a significant decrease of the IFN and neutrophil modules and an increase in the cytotoxic/NK module were observed post-HSCT, but not in the CYC control arm. Cytokines and vascular biomarkers analysis in serum of transplanted SSc patients showed stable IL-6, IL-10 IFN-γ, and TNF-α levels and normalization of IL-2 levels after HSCT. In another study, IL-6 and IL-1β levels did go down and PD-1 expression on T-cells and the number of Tregs increased. After transplantation increased, expression of MMP-2, MMP-3, MMP-9, and TIMP-1 was observed in skin and serum, whereas expression of NF-κB p65 decreased. Also serum levels of S100A9 normalized. Serum levels of PDGF-AA, PDGF-BB, TIMP-1, and MMP-1 decreased, while COL1A1 increased after HSCT. B cell studies showed increased naïve B cell and IL-10-producing Bregs CD19 + CD24hiCD38hi and CD19 + CD24hiCD27+ frequencies and decreased memory B cell and plasma cell frequencies after HSCT. *Effects on fibrosis.* The SCOT trial participants with a fibroproliferative subset who were treated with HSCT had significant improvement in EFS compared to the patients on CYC. Also, studies demonstrated that collagen depositions in skin were reduced after HSCT. *Effects on vasculopathy.* Following HSCT, the number of nailfold capillaries increased, while giant capillaries decreased. In skin, serum vascular markers were increased in patients with SSc and remained stable after HSCT

Summary and Conclusions

Observational studies and (inter)national registry analyses have demonstrated the positive clinical impact of autologous HSCT in SSc patients who otherwise had few treatment options left. Two randomized controlled trials conducted in Europe and North America, respectively, have shown consistent benefits of autologous HSCT on long-term survival, skin thickening, functional ability, and quality of life when compared to pulse-therapy cyclophosphamide. The potent effects of HSCT have been mirrored by translational studies on biosamples taken from transplanted SSc patients, revealing profound effects on skin pathology, immune alterations in blood, reversal of nailfold capillary abnormalities, and alterations of cytokines and markers of matrix turnover and signalling in blood to an extent not seen in patients treated with pulse-therapy cyclophosphamide. HSCT, however, is not a routine treatment modality and given the attendant toxicities and unavoidable risk of TRM, HSCT should only be reserved as a potentially life-saving treatment option for patients with poor prognosis early diffuse cutaneous SSc following a thorough shared decision making process, as reflected by its incorporation in several guidelines [50, 51]. Patients with advanced end-stage disease are best not treated with HSCT as the benefits are unlikely to outweigh the risks. The European UPSIDE-trial has been launched to determine whether upfront HSCT is safer and more effective than HSCT as rescue treatment in those SSc patients who fail pulse therapy cyclophosphamide. The UPSIDE trial eligibility criteria are deliberately targeting patients with early dcSSc to avoid the risks of HSCT resulting from significant cumulative organ damage. Cohort studies also have merit to evaluate the added value of CD34+ selection [52], optimal conditioning regimen, posttransplantation management, timing of HSCT, selection of patients, long-term effects of HSCT, and impact of the COVID-pandemic [53].

Acknowledgments We acknowledge the Autoimmune Diseases Working Party -ADWP of the European Society for Blood and Marrow Transplantation -EBMT for its support in providing updated registry data and all EBMT member centers and their clinicians, data managers, and patients for their valuable contributions to the EBMT registry.

References

1. Alexander T, Greco R, Snowden JA. Hematopoietic stem cell transplantation for autoimmune disease. Ann Rev Med. 2021;72:215–28.
2. Tamm M, Gratwohl A, Tichelli A, Perruchoud AP, Tyndall A. Autologous haemopoietic stem cell transplantation in a patient with severe pulmonary hypertension complicating connective tissue disease. Ann Rheum Dis. 1996;55:779–80.
3. Tyndall A, Gratwohl A. Blood and marrow stem cell transplants in auto-immune disease: a consensus report written on behalf of the European league against rheumatism (EULAR) and the European Group for Blood and Marrow Transplantation (EBMT). Bone Marrow Transplant. 1997;19:643–5.
4. Alexander T, Greco R. Hematopoietic stem cell transplantation and cellular therapies for autoimmune disease: overview and future considerations from the autoimmune diseases working party (ADWP) of the European Society for Blood and Marrow Transplantation (ENMT). Bone Marrow Transpl. 2022;57:1055–62.
5. Daikeler T, Hügle T, Farge D, Andolina M, Gualandi F, Baldomero H, et al. Allogeneic hematopoietic SCT for patients with autoimmune diseases. Bone Marrow Transplant. 2009;44:27–33.
6. Binks M, Passweg JR, Furst D, McSweeney P, Sullivan K, Besenthal C, et al. Phase I/II trial of autologous stem cell transplantation in systemic sclerosis: procedure related mortality and impact on skin disease. Ann Rheum Dis. 2001;60:577–84.
7. McSweeney PA, Nash RA, Sullivan KM, Storek J, Crofford LJ, Dansey R, et al. High-dose immunosuppressive therapy for severe systemic sclerosis: initial outcomes. Blood. 2002;100:1602–10.
8. Pecher AC, Ach KR, Vogel W, Henes JC. Mobilization with reduced cyclophosphamide for autologous stem cell transplantation is feasible in patients with systemic sclerosis. Rheumatology (Oxford). 2023;62(SI):SI107–13.
9. Nash RA, McSweeney PA, Crofford LJ, Abidi M, Chen CS, Godwin JD, et al. High-dose immunosuppressive therapy and autologous hematopoietic cell transplantation for severe systemic sclerosis: long-term follow-up of the US multicenter pilot study. Blood. 2007;110:1388–96.
10. van Laar JM, Farge D, Sont JK, Naraghi K, Marjanovic Z, Larghero J, et al. Autologous hematopoietic stem cell transplantation vs intravenous pulse cyclophosphamide in diffuse cutaneous systemic sclerosis: a randomized clinical trial. JAMA. 2014;311:2490–8.
11. Sullivan KM, Goldmuntz E, Keyes-Elstein L, McSweeney PA, Pinckney A, Welch B, et al. Myeloablative autologous stem-cell transplantation for severe scleroderma. N Engl J Med. 2018;378:35–47.
12. Burt RK, Shah SJ, Dill K, Grant T, Gheorghiade M, Schroeder J, et al. Autologous non-myeloablative haemopoietic stem-cell transplantation compared with pulse cyclophosphamide once per month for systemic sclerosis (ASSIST): an open-label, randomised phase 2 trial. Lancet. 2011;378:498–506.
13. Kloth C, Thaiss WM, Preibsch H, Mark HK, Kötter I, Hetzel J, et al. Quantitative chest CT analysis in patients with systemic sclerosis before and after autologous stem cell transplantation: comparison of results with those of pulmonary function tests and clinical tests. Rheumatology (Oxford). 2016;55:1763–70.
14. Pugnet G, Petermann A, Collot S, Otal P, Lansiaux P, Abdallah NA, et al. Changes on chest HRCT in systemic sclerosis-related interstitial lung disease after autologous hematopoietic stem cell transplantation. Rheumatology (Oxford). 2023;62(SI):SI32–42.
15. Henes J, Oliveira MC, Labopin M, Badoglio M, Scherer HU, Del Papa N, et al. Autologous stem cell transplantation for progressive systemic sclerosis: a prospective non-interventional study from the European Society for Blood and Marrow Transplantation Autoimmune Disease Working Party. Haematologica. 2021;106:375–83.
16. Ayano M, Tsukamoto H, Mitoma H, Kimoto Y, Akahoshi M, Arinobu Y, et al. CD34-selected versus unmanipulated autologous haematopoietic stem cell transplantation in the treatment of severe systemic sclerosis: a post hoc analysis of a phase I/II clinical trial conducted in Japan. Arthritis Res Ther. 2019;21:30.
17. Burt RK, Oliveira MC, Shah SJ, Moraes DA, Simoes B, Gheorghiade M, et al. Cardiac involvement and treatment-related mortality after non-myeloablative haemopoietic stem-cell transplantation with unselected autologous peripheral blood for patients with systemic sclerosis: a retrospective analysis. JAMA. 2013;381:1116–24.
18. Henes JC, Koetter I, Horger M, Schmalzing M, Mueller K, Eick C, et al. Autologous stem cell transplantation with thiotepa-based conditioning in patients with systemic sclerosis and cardiac manifestations. Rheumatology (Oxford). 2014;53:919–22.
19. Burt RK, Han X, Quigley K, Arnautovic I, Shah SJ, Lee DC, et al. Cardiac safe hematopoietic stem cell transplantation for systemic sclerosis with poor cardiac function: a pilot safety study that decreases neutropenic interval to 5 days. Bone Marrow Transplant. 2021;56:50–9.
20. Shah A, Spierings J, van Laar JM, Sullivan KM. Re-evaluating inclusion criteria for autologous hematopoietic stem cell transplantation in advanced systemic sclerosis. Three successful cases and review of the literature. J Scleroderma Relat Disord. 2021;6:199–205.
21. Spierings J, van Rhenen A, Welsing PM, Marijnissen AC, De Langhe E, Del Papa N, et al. A randomised, open-label trial to assess the optimal treatment strategy in early diffuse cutaneous systemic sclerosis: the UPSIDE study protocol. BMC Open. 2021;11:e044483.
22. Van Bijnen S, de Vries-Boustra J, van den Ende CH, Boonstra M, Kroft L, Geurts B, et al. Predictive factors for treatment-related mortality and major adverse events after autologous haematopoietic stem cell transplantation for systemic sclerosis: results of a long-term follow-up multicentre study. Ann Rheum Dis. 2020;79:1084–9.
23. Henrique-Neto A, Vasconcelos MYK, Dias JBE, de Moraes DA, Gonçalves MS, Zanin-Silva DC, et al. Hematopoietic stem cell transplantation for systemic sclerosis: Brazilian experience. Adv Rheumatol. 2021;61:9.
24. Panopoulos ST, Tektonidou MG, Bournia VK, Laskari K, Sfikakis PP. Outcomes of conventionally-treated systemic sclerosis patients eligible for autologous haematopoietic stem cell transplantation. Clin Exp Rheumatol. 2021;39(Suppl. 131):S29–33.
25. van Rhijn-Brouwer FCC, Spierings J, van Rhenen A, Kuball J, van Laar JM. Second autologous haematopoietic stem cell transplantation in systemic sclerosis-a case report. Rheumatology (Oxford). 2019;58:1305–7.
26. Deligny C, Clave E, Sibon D, Daikeler T, Keshmandt H, Carmagnat M, et al. New onset of myasthenia gravis after treatment of systemic sclerosis by autologous hematopoietic stem cell transplantation: sustained autoimmunity or inadequate reset of tolerance? Hum Immunol. 2010;71:363–5.
27. Daikeler T, Labopin M, Di Gioia M, Abinun M, Alexander T, Miniati I, et al. Secondary autoimmune diseases occurring after HSCT for an autoimmune disease: a retrospective study of the EBMT autoimmune disease working party. Blood. 2011;118:1693–8.
28. De Langhe E, Lenaerts J, Dierickx D, Hendrickx P, Verleden GM, Wuyts WA, et al. Acquired haemophilia a in a patient with systemic sclerosis treated with autologous haematopoietic stem cell transplantation. Rheumatology (Oxford). 2015;54:196–7.

29. Van Bekkum DW. Stem cell transplantation for autoimmune disorders. Preclinical experiments. Best Pract Res Clin Haematol. 2004;17:201–22.
30. Glaeser L, Henes J, Kötter I, Vogel W, Kanz L, Klein R. Molecular recognition patterns of anti-topoisomerase I-antibodies in patients with systemic sclerosis before and after autologous stem cell transplantation. Clin Exp Rheumatol. 2018;36(Suppl. 113):28–35.
31. Tsukamoto H, Nagafuji K, Horicuhi T, Mitoma H, Niiro H, Arinobu Y, et al. Analysis of immune reconstitution after autologous CD34+ stem/progenitor cell transplantation for systemic sclerosis: predominant reconstitution of Th1 CD4+ T cells. Rheumatology (Oxford). 2011;50:944–52.
32. Baraut J, Grigore EI, Jean-Louis F, Khelifa SH, Durand C, Verrecchia F, et al. Peripheral blood regulatory T cells in patients with diffuse systemic sclerosis before and after autologous hematopoietic SCT: a pilot study. Bone Marrow Transpl. 2014;49:349–54.
33. Farge D, Arruda LCM, Brigant F, Clave E, Douay C, Marjanovic Z, et al. Long-term immune reconstitution and T cell repertoire analysis after autologous hematopoietic stem cell transplantation in systemic sclerosis patients. J Hematol Oncol. 2017;10:21.
34. Arruda LCM, Malmegrim KCR, Lima-Júnior JR, Clave E, Dias JBE, Moraes DA, et al. Immune rebound associates with a favorable clinical response to autologous HSCT in systemic sclerosis patients. Blood Adv. 2018;2:126–41.
35. Lutter L, Spierings J, van Rhijn-Brouwer FCC, van Laar JM, van Wijk F. Resetting the T cell compartment in autoimmune diseases with autologous hematopoietic stem cell transplantation: an update. Front Immunol. 2018;9:767.
36. Lima-Júnior JR, Arruda LCM, Gonçalves MS, Dias JBE, Moraes DA, Covas DT, et al. Autologous haematopoietic stem cell transplantation restores the suppressive capacity of regulatory B cells in systemic sclerosis patients. Rheumatology (Oxford). 2021;60:5538–48.
37. Gernert M, Tony HP, Schwaneck EC, Gadeholt O, Schmalzing M. Autologous hematopoietic stem cell transplantation in systemic sclerosis induces long-lasting changes in B cell homeostasis toward an anti-inflammatory B cell cytokine pattern. Arthritis Res Ther. 2019;21:106.
38. Michel L, Farge D, Baraut J, Marjanovic Z, Jean-Louis F, Porcher R, et al. Evolution of serum cytokine profile after hematopoietic stem cell transplantation in systemic sclerosis patients. Bone Marrow Transplant. 2016;51:1146–9.
39. Arruda LCM, Lima-Júnior JR, Clave E, Moraes DA, Douay C, Fournier I, et al. Homeostatic proliferation leads to telomere attrition and increased PD-1 expression after autologous hematopoietic SCT for systemic sclerosis. Bone Marrow Transplant. 2018;53:1319–27.
40. Zanin-Silva DC, Santana-Gonçalves M, Kawashima-Vasconcelos MY, Lima-Júnior JR, Dias JBE, Moraes DA, et al. Autologous hematopoietic stem cell transplantation promotes connective tissue remodeling in systemic sclerosis patients. Arthritis Res Ther. 2022;24:95.
41. Assassi S, Wang X, Chen G, Goldmuntz E, Keyes-Elstein L, Ying J, et al. Myeloablation followed by autologous stem cell transplantation normalises systemic sclerosis molecular signatures. Ann Rheum Dis. 2019;78:1371–8.
42. Fleming JN, Nash RA, McLeod DO, Fiorentino DF, Schulman HM, Connolly MK, et al. Capillary regeneration in scleroderma: stem cell therapy reverses phenotype? PLoS One. 2008;3:e1452.
43. Daikeler T, Kump E, Stern MM, Hügle T, Hij A, Haeuserman P, Farge D. Autologous hematopoietic stem cell transplantation reverses skin fibrosis but does not change skin vessel density in patients with systemic sclerosis. Pathol Biol (Paris). 2015;63:164–8.
44. Aschwanden M, Daikeler T, Jaeger KA, Thalkammer C, Gratwohl A, Matucci-Cerinic M, Tyndall A. Rapid improvement of nailfold capillaroscopy after intense immunosuppression for systemic sclerosis and mixed connective tissue disease. Ann Rheum Dis. 2008;67:1057–9.
45. Santana-Gonçalves M, Zanin-Silva D, Henrique-Neto Á, Moraes DA, Kawashima-Vasconcelos MY, Lima-Júnior JR, et al. Autologous hematopoietic stem cell transplantation modifies specific targets of systemic sclerosis-related microvasculopathy. Adv Musculoskelet Dis. 2022;14:1759720X221084845. https://doi.org/10.1177/1759720X221084845.
46. Franks JM, Martyanov V, Wang Y, Wood TA, Pinckney A, Crofford LJ, et al. Machine learning predicts stem cell transplant response in severe scleroderma. Ann Rheum Dis. 2020;79:1608–15.
47. Maltez N, Puyade M, Wang M, Lansiaux P, Marjanovic Z, Charles C, et al. Association of autologous hematopoietic stem cell transplantation in systemic sclerosis with marked improvement in health-related quality of life. Arthritis Rheumatol. 2021;73:305–14.
48. Spierings J, de Bresser CJ, van Rhijn-Brouwer FC, Pieterse A, Vonk MC, Voskuyl AE, et al. From "being at war" to "getting back on your feet": A qualitative study on experiences of patients with systemic sclerosis treated with hematopoietic stem cell transplantation. J Scleroderma Relat Disord. 2020;5:202–9.
49. Snowden JA, Badoglio M, Labopin M, Giebel S, McGrath E, Marjanovic Z, et al. Evolution, trends, outcomes, and economics of hematopoietic stem cell transplantation in severe autoimmune diseases. Blood Adv. 2017;1:2742–55.
50. Kowal-Bielecka O, Fransen J, Avouac J, Becker M, Kulak A, Allanore Y, et al. Update of EULAR recommendations for the treatment of systemic sclerosis. Ann Rheum Dis. 2017;76:1327–39.
51. Sullivan KM, Majhail NS, Bredeson C, Carpenter PA, Chatterjee S, Crofford LJ, et al. Systemic sclerosis as an indication for autologous hematopoietic cell transplantation: position statement from the American Society for Blood and Marrow Transplantation. Biol Blood Marrow Transplant. 2018;24:1961–4.
52. Oliveira MC, Labopin M, Henes J, Moore J, Del Papa N, Cras A, et al. Does ex vivo CD34+ positive selection influence outcome after autologous hematopoietic stem cell transplantation in systemic sclerosis patients? Bone Marrow Transplant. 2016;51:501–5.
53. Greco R, Alexander T, Burman J, Del Papa N, de Vries-Bouwstra J, Farge D, et al. Hematopoietic stem cell transplantation for autoimmune diseases in the time of COVID-19: EBMT guidelines and recommendations. Bone Marrow Transplant. 2021;56:1493–508.

Immune-Targeted Therapies in SSc

44

Voon H. Ong and Yannick Allanore

Introduction

SSc is an uncommon potentially life-threatening rheumatic disease that is considered as a prototype illness for dissecting the links between autoimmunity and fibrosis. Dysregulated innate and adaptive immune responses are key determinants to the onset and progression of SSc disease. Early infiltration of mononuclear cells including monocytes, macrophages, and CD4+ and CD8+ T cells occurs in the lesional tissues and blood. Altered expressions of key cytokines and chemokines with TGFβ, platelet-derived growth factor (PDGF), IL-4, IL-6, and IL-13 are all relevant in SSc pathology as well as altered toll-like receptors (TLR) and NOD-like receptor protein 3 (NLRP3) inflammasome.

Treatment strategies have up to now focus on skin and lung fibrosis with broad-spectrum immunosuppressive strategies. As example, mycophenolate (MMF) abrogates the molecular inflammatory signature with parallel reduction in T cell, macrophage and dendritic cell signatures, and myeloid dendritic cell and macrophage counts from active lesional skin and these signatures reappear with MMF cessation [1]. It is noteworthy that autologous stem cell transplantation and the recently FDA approved tocilizumab provide further support to the central role of immune activation in the disease pathogenesis, thus underline the potential for selective immune-mediated therapeutics while minimising the risks from non-specific immunoablation. Together with nintedanib, these new agents herald an era of exciting opportunities for translational therapeutics to halt fibrosis and prevent progression of the disease. More recently, further understanding of the immune intricacies, coupled with high-dimensional analytical tools with single cell sequencing technology, has yielded unprecedented insights into the heterogeneity of the immune responses across affected tissues in SSc. In this review, we will discuss the recent developments in the immune-mediated treatments for SSc (Table 44.1).

V. H. Ong (✉)
University College London, London, UK
e-mail: v.ong@ucl.ac.uk

Y. Allanore
Service de Rhumatologie, Hôpital Cochin,
AP-HP. Centre - Université Paris Cité, Paris, France

Innate Immunity

The innate immune system comprises a network of cellular compartments including monocytes/macrophages, neutrophils, dendritic cells embedded within a milieu of key mediators including complement network that together shape the early non-specific responses to endogenous host molecules, and danger-associated molecular patterns (DAMPs) from tissue injury. These are recognised by a variety of pattern recognition receptors (PRRs) including TLRs linked with inflammasome activation. Increased expression of inflammatory mediators by innate immune cells including type I interferon and IL-4, IL-6, and IL-13 in association with dysregulated DAMP release and PRR signalling contributes to the development and potential persistence of fibrosis.

Targeting Myeloid Cell

In this respect, myeloid cells are crucial antigen-presenting cells (APC), and increased circulating and local levels of monocytes and macrophages have been reported in SSc. Elevated CD16 + monocytes were significantly associated with the severity of skin fibrosis, pulmonary fibrosis, and restrictive pulmonary function impairment, suggesting a potential link between this subpopulation of monocytes and the pathogenesis of fibrosis in SSc [2]. In addition, increased circulating monocyte counts were reported to be significantly associated with shorter disease duration and higher mortality in SSc [3]. In parallel, elevated serum levels of M2-inducing cytokines, including IL-4, IL-13, and IL-10, are reported in patients with SSc [4, 5].

Y. Allanore et al. (eds.), *Scleroderma*, https://doi.org/10.1007/978-3-031-40658-4_44

Table 44.1 Summary of the main results from selected clinical trials investigation; the pharmacological effects of biological therapies in systemic sclerosis

Target molecule	Therapeutic agent	Mechanism (s) of action	Design	Main clinical results	Reference
B cell	Belimumab	Antagonises activity of membrane-bound BAFF, B cell survival factor leading to reduction in naïve B cells and transitional B cells	Phase II	No significant change in mRSS was observed between the belimumab and the placebo group (median reduction −10 and − 3, respectively, $p = 0.411$) at 52-week	[64]
	Rituximab	Chimeric anti-CD20 IgG1 monoclonal antibody that targets the CD20 molecule on B cells	Phase III (ClinicalTrials.gov, NCT01862926)	Results to announce	[59]
			Phase II (ClinicalTrials.gov Identifier: NCT04274257)	Significant effect on mRSS with difference − 8·44 favouring rituximab [95% CI −11·00 to −5·88]; ($p < 0{\cdot}0001$)	[60]
			Phase II (SSc- pulmonary arterial hypertension) ClinicalTrials.gov Identifier: NCT01086540	Primary outcome on mean change in 6MWD at 24-week not met (23.6 ± 11.1 m vs. 0.5 ± 9.7 m, $p = 0.12$), but was significant at 48-week (25.5 ± 8.8 m for rituximab and 0.4 ± 7.4 m for placebo, $p = 0.03$)	[61]
Immunoglobulin	Subcutaneous Ig	20% liquid formulation of human IgG with >98% IgG purity. Mechanisms specific to SSc are not well established.	Phase II—ongoing	Primary endpoint to assess safety and change in clinical assessments including lung function with weekly subcutaneous IgPro20 over 16 weeks	ClinicalTrials.gov Identifier: NCT04137224
T cells	Abatacept	Abatacept binds to CD80 and CD86, and prevents interaction with CD28 (co-stimulation signal)	Phase II	Numerically improvement on mRSS (−6.24 in the abatacept group compared to −4.49 in the placebo group, $p = 0.28$ at 12-month, $n = 88$) in early dcSSc without background immunomodulatory therapies. Significant effect on HAQ-DI was noted	[45]
Intracellular signalling pathways and cytokines/ growth factors	Nintedanib	Tyrosine kinase inhibitor that competitively binding to ATP–binding pockets of receptors, stopping intracellular signaling. It targets PDGF receptor-a/b, FGF receptor 1–3, and VEGF receptor 1–3	Phase III	Significant effect on the decline in lung function in SSc-ILD (Difference in annual rate of FVC decline of 41mls/yr., $p = 0.04$ favouring Nintedanib at 52-week, with no change in HR-QOL or skin fibrosis. Non-significant synergistic effect of mycophenolate and Nintedanib was reported	[84]
	Tofacitinib	pan-JAK inhibitor that targets JAK1, JAK2, JAK3, TYK2	Phase I/II	Achievement of 90.7% predicted FVC in tofacitinib-treated patients vs. 83.8% of the placebo group and of 82.4% predicted DLCO in tofacitinib-treated patients vs. 92.0% of the placebo group at 24 weeks	[87]
	Tocilizumab	Tocilizumab binds to both soluble and membrane-bound IL-6 receptor (trans-signaling)	Phase II and III	A statistically significant effect on preservation of FVC including those without ILD was observed	[8, 81]
	Fresolimumab	human IgG4 κ monoclonal antibody targeting all 3 TGF-β isotypes (TGF-β1–3)	OL	This small study ($n = 19$) showed dramatic skin improvement with median change in mRSS at weeks 11 and 17 (−6, $p = 0.0005$ and − 9.5, $p = 0.0024$ respectively).	[10]
	Romilkimab	Bispecific monoclonal antibody that antagonises both IL-4 and IL-13	Phase II	Statistically significant improvement in skin activity with mRSS difference − 2.31 ($p = 0.029$) at 24-week	[9]

Autotaxin and lysophosphatidic acid 1 receptor signalling pathway	*HZN-825*/ SAR100842	Selective LPA_1 receptor antagonist	Phase IIa	Numerically improvement in mRSS with active drug (treatment effect −1.2, $p = 0.46$) at week 8	[39]
	Ziritaxestat	Autotaxin inhibitor that blocks LPA activity	Phase IIa	Statistically significant improvement in mRSS: LS mean difference – 2.8 ($p = 0.041$) at week 24. No effect on FVC.	[40]
Other innate immune targets: IFNα	Anifrolumab	Human IgG1k monoclonal antibody directed against IFNAR1 and suppresses the receptor-mediated biological activity of all type I IFNs	Phase I	No measures of disease activity and patient-reported outcomes noted due to small sample size ($n = 34$) and short trial duration. Significant downregulation of T cell-associated proteins with increase type III collagen degradation marker. Whole-blood and skin microarray results also indicated the inhibition of T cell receptor and ECM-related transcripts	[15]
IL-1α	Bermekimab	Human IgG1k isotype monoclonal antibody against IL-1α	Phase II	No result available	ClinicalTrials.gov Identifier: NCT04045743
IL-1R	Rilonacept	Dimeric fusion protein consisting of the human IL-1 receptor component (IL-1R1) and IL-1 receptor accessory protein (IL-1RAcP). It neutralises IL-1β activity	Phase I/II	No effect on skin activity at 6 weeks. No change in dermal expression of the 2G SSc gene biomarkers (THBS1 and MS4A4) as surrogate for the mRSS	[21]
IL-2 receptor	Basiliximab	Chimeric monoclonal antibody directed against the α chain (CD25) of the IL-2 receptor	OL	Improvement in median mRSS from 26/51 to 11/51 at week 68, $p = 0.015$) and trend in improvement with mean FVC predicted from 82.1 to 88.4% ($p = 0.078$). However, lack of control arm negates meaningful interpretation of the results	[44]

mRSS modified Rodnan skin score, *HAQ-DI* Health assessment questionnaire-disability index, *HR-QOL* health-related quality of life, *LPA_1 receptor* lysophosphatidic acid 1 receptor, *IFNAR1* subunit 1 of the type I IFN receptor, *OL* open-label

A growing body of data has suggested that M2 macrophages play crucial roles in the activation of resident fibroblasts and the progression of fibrosis, mainly through the release of TGF-β, vascular endothelial growth factor (VEGF), connective tissue growth factor (CTGF), and PDGF [6, 7]. M2 macrophage polarisation with reduction of key markers of myeloid activation CD14, CCL2, TLR4, TLR8, and AIF1 linked to IL-6 activation has recently been proposed to underlie the therapeutic effect of Tocilizumab in early diffuse SSc [8]. Furthermore, targeting IL-4 and IL-13 with Romilkimab, a humanised bispecific immunoglobulin-G4 in a randomised placebo-controlled phase II, clinical trial with 97 patients with early diffuse SSc met its primary endpoint on skin activity with mean difference in modified Rodnan skin score (mRSS) −2.31 (90% CI −4.32 to −0.31, $p = 0.0291$) favouring Romilkimab [9]. Interestingly, fresolimumab, in addition to the direct inhibition of TGFβ-regulated gene expression, also reduces dermal expression of macrophage-associated genes (CD163 and MS4A4A), indicating an indirect effect on the differentiation of myeloid cells [10]. The tyrosine kinase inhibitor that inhibits PDGFRα and β, FGFR1–3, and VEGF1–3, Nintedanib selectively reduces M2 markers (CD11b, CD206) and CCL18 expression, but does not prevent membrane expression of M1 markers [11].

Dendritic Cell and Interferon

Dendritic cells (DCs) are potent APCs in driving activation of naive T cells and therefore maintain peripheral T cell homeostasis and shape B cell response via expression of B cell stimulatory and survival factors. DCs comprise two subsets: conventional CDs and plasmacytoid DCs (pDCs). Alterations of both DC subsets in circulation and local tissues as well as impaired DC function have been described in SSc patients. Aberrant pDCs activation manifested by IFNα signature is upregulated in early stage SSc in lesional skin, lung, and peripheral blood mononuclear cells (PBMCs) [12, 13]. While there is evidence to support IFN-inducible chemokines as biomarkers for fibrotic and vascular manifestations of SSc, its role in SSc pathogenesis remains incompletely understood but likely to involve increased activation of monocytes, increased T cell proliferation, enhanced extracellular matrix(ECM) production by fibroblasts, increased endothelial permeability, and elevated immune cells adhesion [14]. Although there is no trial on IFN antagonism, Anifrolumab a monoclonal antibody targeting IFNAR was evaluated in 34 SSc patients. Although IFN signature scores associates with skin score, this study was not powered to evaluate its effects on disease activity. Reduction of the IFN signature with downregulation of T cell receptor activation in whole blood and skin biopsy samples and reduction in IFN inducible serum proteins (CCL13, CXCL10, beta-2 microglobulin, and VCAM1) were observed [15, 16], supporting the rationale for targeting IFN activation in SSc.

Several biological agents such as abatacept affect DC-T cell interaction and T cell activation. This may support the rationale for tolerised dendritic cells as potential treatment strategy for SSc [17]. Recent study with organotypic model of human skin also showed that functional inactivation of pDC via BDCA, a type II transmembrane glycoprotein, abrogates the IFN signature and reduces the proinflammatory and profibrotic stimuli [18]. This supports the development of BDCA2-targeting as a therapeutic strategy for pDC-mediated skin inflammation and fibrosis beyond its effect on IFN and IL-6 expression.

TLR and Inflammasome

Recent years have revolutionised our understanding of TLRs and inflammasome activation as a critical part of innate immune cell response to an array of stimuli. The binding of pathogen-associated molecular patterns (PAMPs) and DAMPs to TLRs initiates downstream signalling cascades manifested by increased IL-6, IL-1β, and IL-18. TLR activation also induces NLRP3 inflammasome activation, via induction of miR-155 that in turns stimulates excessive ECM production [19, 20]. The activated NLRP3 inflammasome then cleaves procaspase-1 to caspase-1 that in turn can cleave proIL-1β and proIL-18 to produce their active forms. Once active IL-1β and IL-18 are secreted, these act in concert with IL-6 and TGF-β to promote fibrosis. A great number of inhibitors have been used to disturb the related signalling pathways, such as IL-1β blockade, IL-18 blockade, and caspase-1 inhibitors. An example is Rilonacept; the soluble decoy IL-1 receptor targeting IL-1 was evaluated in a phase I/II randomised placebo-controlled study with 19 patients [21]. Although there were no major safety concerns, there was no significant effect on mRSS with no change in gene expression (THBS1 and MS4A4) as surrogate for mRSS. Bermekimab is a novel agent which neutralises the IL-1α isoform of interleukin-1, and a trial in SSc is ongoing (ClinicalTrials.gov Identifier: NCT04045743). Most of these inhibitors appear to target the signalling pathways downstream to activation of NLRP3 inflammasome and inhibitors that directly modulate NLRP3 inflammasome may be more effective. NEK7 is a multifunctional kinase affecting centrosome duplication, mitochondrial regulation, intracellular protein transport, DNA repair, and mitotic spindle assembly [22]. Inhibitors focused on NEK7 may regulate NLRP3 to downregulate the inflammation response and NEK7 may be a potential therapeutic target for NLRP3-driven diseases including systemic lupus erythematosus [23].

Neutrophils

The role of neutrophils in SSc is largely unexplored. Transcriptomic analysis of whole blood coupled with immunophenotyping analysis revealed that neutrophils were the major determinant of the RNA abundance in two independent SSc cohorts of which 30–50% had ILD [24]. More recently, Wareing et al. showed that among the patient cohort from SLS-II indicated that higher baseline neutrophil count, independent of effects of immunosuppressives, predicted worsening of SSc-ILD, but not skin disease [25]. Beyond its potential as a biomarker, aberrant release of DNA fragments from neutrophils, NETosis, in association with oxidative stress has been reported across autoimmune diseases including SSc, but the pathogenic significance of this observation is not clear, although it may relate to the vascular and fibrotic SSc phenotypes [26, 27]. Further understanding of neutrophil biology is SSc is necessary prior to considering therapeutic targeting specifically this innate effector subset such as neutrophil elastase or NETs.

Complement Activation

Recently, altered intracellular complement signature was observed in patients with diffuse cutaneous SSc (dcSSc) with augmented C3 and C5 activation and increased autocrine C5aR1 and reduced C5aR2 activity contributing to defective Th1 contraction and hyperactive Th17 responses in early stage SSc [28]. Elevated local levels of anaphylatoxins (C3a and C5a) are reported in experimental lung fibrosis model and therapeutic blockade of receptors for C3a or C5a mitigates lung fibrosis and systemic TGF-β activity [29]. Furthermore, targeting IL-17 bioactivity reduced complement activation with further halting the progression of lung fibrosis [30]. Further support for complement activation in thrombotic microangiopathy is observed in hypertensive renal crisis with increased local and circulating levels of C5b-9 with elevated complement factor 3-d (C3d): complement factor 3 (C3) and Factor B: Factor Bb (FB:FBb) suggestive of activated alternate pathway. Anecdotal reports indicate that eculizumab, monoclonal antibody directed against C5 that disrupts formation of membrane attack complex, may be feasible in SSc hypertensive renal crisis [31, 32]. These observations provide support complement activation in disease pathogenesis and therefore present as an opportunity for complement inhibition in both vasculopathy and fibrosis in SSc [33].

Lysophosphatidic Acid Signalling

Lysophosphatidic acid (LPA) is a lysophospholipid structurally similar to sphingosine-1-phosphate (S1P), a lipid that has been well characterised to signal to immune cells and to orchestrate cell trafficking. LPA exerts various effects on parenchymal cells stimulating cell migration and ECM production, with growing evidences on a role on immune response and wound healing [34–36]. This was supported by initial pre-clinical evaluation for lung and skin fibrosis [37, 38]. A short-term exploratory biomarker study showed a good safety profile and a great target engagement, but effects on fibrotic pathways were challenging to interpret [39]. Recently, ziritaxestat, investigated in patients with early dcSSc ($n = 33$), showed some skin fibrosis interesting effects: changes in MRSS –2.8 (−5.6, −0.1), $p = 0.0411$ favouring the drug under investigation [40]. This opens the door for subsequent larger trials.

Adaptive Immune System

Aberrant activation of the adaptive immune system is well established in pathogenesis of SSc; presence of circulating autoantibodies with prominent T-lymphocytic infiltrate in lesional tissues at early stage SSc has drawn much interest in targeting these cellular immune subsets.

T-Cell-Directed Strategies

In SSc, a majority of T cell subsets including Th2 cells, Th17 cells, Th1 cells, Th22 cells, Treg cells, T follicular helper cells, mucosal-associated invariant T (MAIT), and CD8$^+$ T cells have all been implicated in the pathogenic process [41, 42]. T cells are present early on in SSc tissues and have been postulated to drive both the endothelial dysfunction and the fibrotic pathology of this disease, presumably via the production of cytokines (IL-4, IL-13, IL-6) that eventually contribute to the activation of macrophages, fibroblasts, and myofibroblasts. While most studies indicate immune polarisation skewed towards Th2/Th17 responses in SSc, perhaps indicative of an evolutionary pressure as a rapid tissue response to tissue destructive pathogens, a majority of autoimmune diseases have focussed on Th1 responses [43]. In this respect, we observed that there is less IFN-γ /IL-10 switching in activated CD4+ T cells indicative of defective Th1 contraction in early dcSSc [28]. Whether fibrosis is a consequence of parenchymal cell death and tissue remodelling or results primarily from the cytokines within an inflammatory milieu is unclear. These mechanisms are not mutually exclusive, however, and could even be sequential.

Other than recognition of the T-cell receptor of a designated antigen, activation and proliferation of naïve T cells require additional costimulatory signal. These include CD28-CD80/CD86, ICOS-B7RP1, CD70-CD27, CD40-CD154, or OX40-OX40L and also, the negative costimulatory pathways such as CTLA4-B7 or PD1-

PDL1/2 in restraining adaptive immune response. Overexpression of these co-stimulatory pathways in activated T cells induces proinflammatory (IFN-γ, IL-17) and pro-fibrotic (IL-4) cytokine synthesis, promoting fibroblast activation and ECM synthesis.

The notion that T cells are involved in SSc is exemplified by the fact that treatment with basiliximab, a chimeric monoclonal antibody that targets IL-2Rα and blocks T cell and B cell activation, showed substantial improvements in skin disease and lung function [44]. Abatacept is a soluble recombinant fusion protein that binds to CD80 and CD86 (also called B7–1 and 2, respectively), blocking T-cell co-stimulation and subsequent activation by preventing their interaction with CD28, resulting in reduced expression of proinflammatory and profibrotic cytokines such as TNF, IL-2, IL-6, and IL-10.The double blind and open extension phases of the ASSET study (mean disease duration 1.6 year) while did not met its primary endpoint on skin outcome, the exploratory outcome measures including HAQ-DI, patient- and physician-global assessment indicate potential disease-modifying effect in SSc [45]. Notably in the absence of clinical skin improvement, lesional CD4+ CTLs in affected skin were attenuated with Abatacept [46]. The mechanisms by which CD4+ CTLs may contribute to disease process are not well established, but these cells are known to express both proinflammatory and profibrotic cytokines TGFβ and IL-1β. More recently, Maehara et al. reported that these cells are located in close proximity to apoptotic endothelial cells in lesional skin, suggesting that CD4+ CTLs may have a role in endothelial cell apoptosis [47]. It is plausible that targeting the CD4+ CTLs with Elotuzumab approved for multiple myeloma is a potential therapeutic strategy.

Other agents that target inducible T cell co-stimulator (ICOS), either alone or in combination with CD28, also show promising antifibrotic activity in preclinical models of SSc [48]. However, compensatory activation of alternative pathways, such as the CD226-CD112, OX40-OX40L, CD28-B7, or 4-1BB-4-1BBL axes, which may be activated in the microenvironment, should be considered.

B Cell-Directed Therapies

Accumulating evidence suggests that B cells are involved in SSc. Failed B cell tolerance with a direct involvement of transitional B cells in autoantibody secretion has been demonstrated in autoimmune diseases including SSc [49, 50]. While it remains to be determined if autoantibodies in SSc may originate from the activation of autoreactive transitional B cells, defective autoreactive B cell selection with secretion of autoantibodies may promote fibrosis through the activation of fibroblasts via IL-6- and M-CSF-induced osteopontin secretion by macrophages [51]. Alterations to the B cell compartment maintain the hyperreactivity and chronic activation of the immune system. B cell infiltration is prominent in affected tissues including skin and lung. Increased number of naïve B cells with reduced memory B cells and plasmablasts with upregulation of the regulatory surface molecule CD19 leading to reduction in the threshold of BCR signalling is reported in SSc. More recently, altered B cell homeostasis with altered VDJ rearrangement frequencies (reduced IGHV2–5 segment usage) expanded immunoglobulin D-positive proportion with reduced mutation loads and an expanded proportion of highly antibody-secreting cells has recently been described for SSc-pulmonary arterial hypertension [52]. The imbalance of two opposing subsets of IL-6/TNF-α producing effector B cells and IL-10-producing regulatory B cells was elegantly described in an experimental model for skin and lung fibrosis, and this may be therapeutically redressed to modulate the fibrotic response [53]. Furthermore, memory B cells overexpress costimulatory CD80 and CD86 and these may be modulated by CTLA4 via internalisation and thereby impairing their capacity to co-stimulate T cells [54, 55].

Consequently, different approaches have been tested to address the hyperactivation of B cells in SSc. The specific inhibition of autoreactive, profibrotic, and chronically activated B cell subsets represents a more promising approach to achieve effective treatment of SSc.

A recent meta-analysis reported the effect of rituximab (RTX) on lung function parameters in SSc-ILD. From the 20 studies identified ($n = 575$), the authors concluded RTX was associated with a significant improvement (95% CI) from baseline in FVC and DLCO of 4.49% and 3.47% at 6 months, and with similar improvement at 12 months of 7.03% and 4.08%, respectively [56]. While it is tempting to compare the magnitude of FVC improvement with the smaller effect reported in robust RCTs such as SLS II (improvement in FVC at the end of trial was 2.19% for MMF and 2.88% for CYC), the meta-analysis is subjected to limitations including effect of concomitant steroids and lack of double-blind RCT. There is some evidence from a small retrospective study that RTX monotherapy may associate with reduction in DLCO compared to combination with MMF [57]. A trend for benefit from combination MMF with RTX was also reported in a limited number of patients in a prospective study with the European Scleroderma Trials and Research network [58]. It is therefore anticipated that results from the first randomised control trial (RECITAL) that evaluated the efficacy of RTX as first-line treatment in CTD-associated ILD will clarify its position in management of SSc lung fibrosis [59].

Specifically for skin disease, Ebata reported results from an RCT on SSc with 56 patients treated either with RTX or placebo once per week for four weeks which indicated significant benefit in change in mRSS at 24 weeks from baseline with difference in mRSS from baseline to week 24 was −6.30

for those who received RTX and 2.14 for those who received placebo, and the rate of adverse effects was similar for all participants [60]. The possible role of RTX as adjunctive therapy for SSc-PAH was evaluated in a proof-of-concept study with 57 patients. Although there was no change in 6-minute-walk distance (6MWD) at 24 weeks to rituximab from baseline, this improved at 48 weeks. Notably, haemodynamic response was not evaluated with right heart catheter [61].

Further exploration for therapeutic targets to address the imbalance of effector B cells and B-regulatory cells has been nicely illustrated with small molecule inhibitor, Bruton's TK inhibitor ibrutinib that abrogates BCR signalling by selective active-side binding. Although no specific effect on B cell subpopulation was noted, reduction of profibrotic and proinflammatory cytokines including IL-6 within the naïve B cell subset was noted [62]. Notably, downregulation of Scl-70 antibodies from stimulated B cells was observed, but it is unclear if this correlates with individuals with this specific antibody.

Two transmembrane proteins, B-cell activating factor (BAFF) with its homologous cytokine, a proliferation-inducing ligand (APRIL), are key in regulation of B cell development and homeostasis and thus impact autoreactive B cell activation and IgM- and IgG-producing populations via regulation of plasma cell survival. They are both increased in SSc albeit some inconsistency in its effect on peripheral B cell tolerance [49, 63]. BAFF antagonist attenuates skin and lung fibrosis in bleomycin-induced SSc model via reduction of IL-6-producing effector B cells [53]. Belimumab binds to soluble human BAFF and inhibits its biological activity, leading to apoptosis of B lymphocytes and decreased autoantibody production. This was evaluated in early diffuse SSc with background MMF treatment and there was greater median difference in mRSS favouring Belimumab over placebo, but this was not statistically significant [64]. Notably, there was reduction in gene expression related to B-cell signalling in addition to genes related to fibrosis among those who responded to Belimumab. Another RCT currently investigates a combination of belimumab with rituximab or background MMF over a study period of 52 weeks (NCT03844061). While consistent effects were seen on biomarkers such as lesional and circulating B cell numbers, the clinical results are, however, conflicting with some of the early studies showing a beneficial effect on skin thickening and/or lung function, but other studies reported no clinical benefit. There is a concern that anti-CD20 approach may only deplete short-lived plasmablasts sparing the long-lived plasma cells that arise from secondary immune responses and reside in survival niches with potential to express autoantibodies. Alternative approaches would include immunoproteasome inhibitors and targeting anti-CD38 antibody. The former approach may limit the toxic effects with conventional proteasome inhibitors and may have additional anti-inflammatory mechanisms. CD38++ transitional B cells have been identified in subsets of SSc and post-autologous stem cell transplantation, but further studies are required to define the pathogenic effect of targeting CD38 in SSc.

Intravenous Immunoglobulin

Immunoglobulin G (IgG) therapy has long been a treatment modality for range of autoimmune disorders [65–67]. The mechanism of action of IgG therapy in SSc is complex and not fully understood [68–70]. Potential immune-mediated mechanisms may include but not limited to neutralizing and/or increasing the catabolism of autoantibodies, blocking Fc receptors, inhibiting complement deposition and activation, inhibiting inflammatory mediators (cytokines and chemokines), and reducing immune complexes [71, 72].

Although a relatively small number of publications are available on intravenous immunoglobulin (IVIG) use in patients with SSc, IVIG even at low-dose may have a beneficial effect on multiple clinical manifestations in SSc patients [73–77] including improvement in skin thickness measured by mRSS, gastrointestinal function, muscle strength, and health-related quality of life as well as stabilisation of lung function. The safety and tolerability will be further evaluated in a prospective, randomised, open-label, crossover study of subcutaneous immunoglobulin in diffuse SSc (ClinicalTrials.gov Identifier: NCT04137224).

IL-6 Family and Janus Kinase Signalling

Feghali et al. first reported that fibroblasts from lesional skin produce from 6- to 30-fold higher levels of IL-6 than fibroblasts from unaffected skin and healthy controls [78]. However, it is clear that many innate immune cells including M2 macrophages are important in IL-6 expression, and IL-6 in turn has important roles in both T- and B-cell activation [79]. Consistent with the defective Th1 contraction reported in early dcSSc [28], IL-6-deficient mice were resistant to fibrosis in a model of acute peritoneal inflammation; transfer of polarised Th1 cells corrected this effect supporting that IL-6-dependent expansion of Th1 cells contributes to fibrosis [80].

IL-6 family of cytokines includes IL-6, IL-11, leukaemia inhibitory factor (LIF), oncostatin M (OSM), ciliary neurotrophic factor (CNTF), and cardiotrophin-1. Notably, while IL-6R is expressed mostly on cells of the immune system, IL-11 receptor subunit α (IL-11RA) is mainly expressed on non-immune cells including fibroblasts. Therefore, both receptors control distinct cellular compartments and differential biological processes.

Tocilizumab, as the IL-6 receptor inhibitor, suppresses both classical signalling and trans-signaling pathways. It recently became the first FDA-approved biologic agent for SSc-ILD based on the results of 2 clinical trials: phase II faSScinate (NCT01532896) and phase III focuSSced (NCT02453256) with patients with early dcSSc [8, 81]. Notably, for faSScinate study (n=87), the mean disease duration was 17.6 months with mean % predicted FVC 80% and %predicited DLCO 73%. In a prespecified exploratory analysis, substantially fewer participants treated with tocilizumab than placebo had decline in lung function and tocilizumab, compared to placebo, conferred significantly smaller reduction in FVC at 24 week (least square mean difference 136 mls, $p = 0.04$) and this effect was sustained numerically at 48-week (least square mean difference 120 mls, $p = 0.1$). Reassuringly, similar pattern of end point responsiveness on FVC favouring tocilizumab was observed in the larger focuSSced study ($n = 210$) with similar baseline characteristics: mean disease duration 22.2 months, mean %predicted FVC 83%, mean %predicted DLCO 76%. In this study, the %predicted FVC and FVC results were driven by the SSc-ILD cohort (representing 65% of the entire cohort). In this subgroup, tocilizumab conferred a smaller reduction in mean % predicted FVC with mean difference 6.47% compared to placebo; a smaller reduction in FVC with mean difference 241 mls was compared to placebo [81]. In this study, average % predicted FVC decline in the placebo cohort was 6.5% significantly higher than that reported in FAST (3%), SLS-I (2.6%), and SENSCIS (2.6%) [82–84].

Considering both studies did not selectively enrol patients with ILD, the robust effect of tocilizumab on lung function with preservation of FVC with mild ILD supports the immunomodulatory effect of Tocilizumab in early stage of disease in contrast to the effect of Nintedanib at later stage of disease. Notably, the mean %predicted FVC and DLCO for SENSCIS study was 72.5% and 53%, respectively, with median disease duration 3.4 years. Furthermore, post-hoc analysis of focuSSced study revealed that patients with anti-Scl70 antibody elevated baseline CRP and shorter disease duration portends a larger treatment effect with Tocilizumab [85]. This is consistent with elevated expression of IL-6 by various immune cells including $CD4^{+}$ T cells from patients with early dcSScity [86].

The promising results with tocilizumab that target the IL-6 receptor also indirectly prevent downstream activation of the JAK pathway, supporting the potential effectiveness of JAK inhibition in SSc. The potential for tofacitinib that preferentially targets JAK1 and JAK3 has been explored in two studies. A small randomised controlled trial (RCT) ($n = 15$) reported trend in improvement in mean mRSS (−5.8 Tofacitinib vs. −2.3 placebo, $p = 0.42$) with significant improvement in mean physician global assessment (−1.6 Tofacitinib vs 0.5 placebo, $p = 0.04$) at 6-month [87]. In contrast, a rapid response to Tofacitinib in mRSS was observed at 1-month in an open-label observational study in a small cohort refractory to conventional immunosuppressive therapies (MMF, cyclophosphamide) [88]. Tofacitinib was considered safe and tolerated in both studies. Further studies are warranted in light of observed cardiovascular and venous thrombotic or potential cancer risks with tofacitinib [89]. Approved for chronic graft versus host disease, Ruxolitinib as an JAK1/2 inhibitor abrogates circulating CD4+ follicular helper capacity to express the proinflammatory IL-21 and therefore reduce the proportion of plasmablasts [90]. It is also conceivable that focus on alternative upstream pathways, such as those driven by C5aR1/2, in regulating IL6 may be therapeutically relevant.

Other members of the gp130/IL6 cytokine family including IL-11 and oncostatin M (OSM) produced by variety of immune and non-immune cells including macrophages, neutrophils, activated T cells, and fibroblasts may have therapeutic potential, although their specific immune-mediated pathogenic mechanisms are less established in SSc [91–94]. An example, the presence of IL6R on macrophages without the OSM receptor, OSMRβ, indicates that the macrophage M2 phenotype may be activated by OSM in a paracrine manner by upregulating IL-6 levels [95].

Future Challenges

With the aim to restore tolerance with the dysregulated autoimmune processes in SSc that ultimately culminates in fibrosis, current approaches are limited with the lack of specificity in addition to the persistence of pathogenic immune cells and inadequate depletion of these cells in lesional tissues. Despite the complexity of the immunopathogenesis of SSc, there is growing understanding of the likely mechanisms or pathways that operate and link the different aspects of the disease. These are highlighted in Fig. 44.1 which identifies key cell types or pathways that may be targeted. The induction and maintenance of robust and specific immune tolerance remain the holy grail of immunotherapeutics in SSc. It is likely that high-dimensional characterisation of SSc blood and immune microenvironment will continue to improve our understanding of the immune-stromal cell crosstalk and to identify novel molecular factors that will enable enrichment for potential responders in clinical trials to guide treatment algorithms [41, 96].

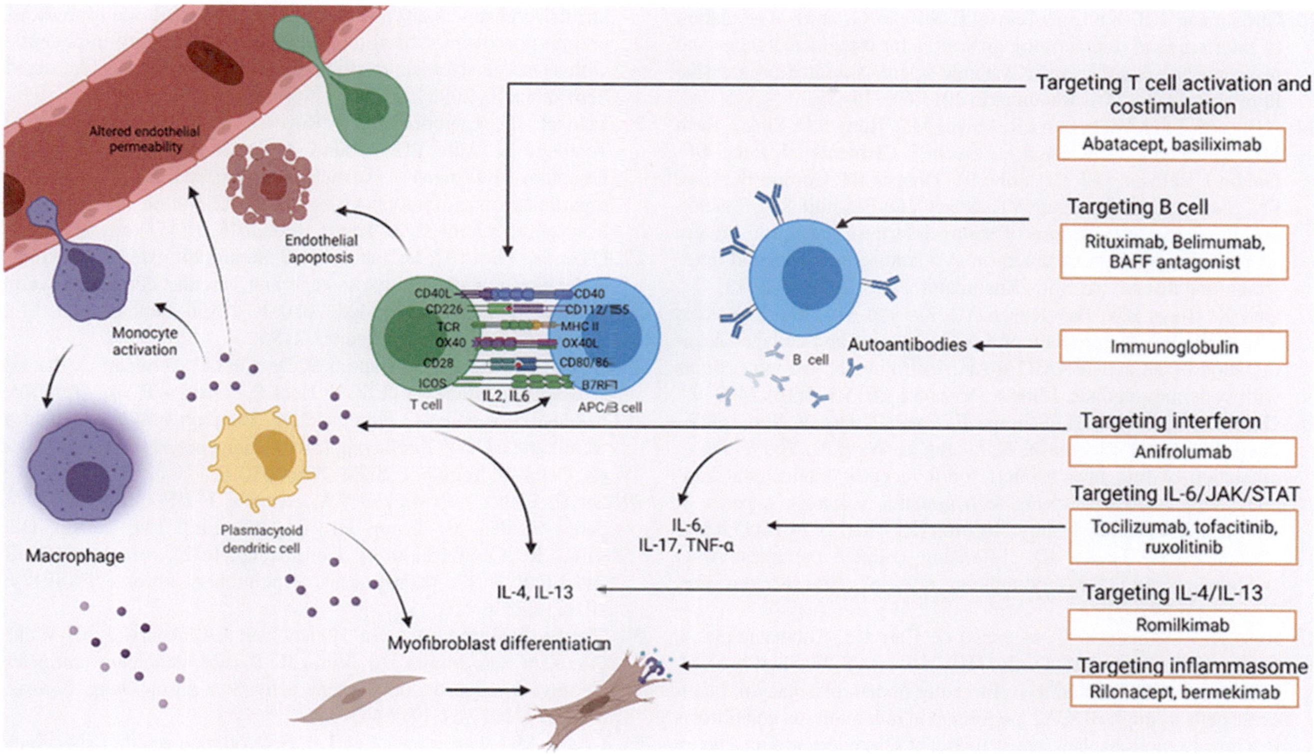

Fig. 44.1 Key SSc immunopathogenic processes that highlight potential targets for biological therapiesInitial vascular injury leads to endothelial activation with T-cell-mediated endothelial apoptosis. Inflammation and autoimmunity may be targeted by agents acting on T lymphocytes, such as abatacept, or those affecting B lymphocytes, such as rituximab and belimumab. Type I interferons play a role in autoantibody generation in SSc, and these are targeted by anifrolumab. Activated T cells, B cells, macrophages, and dendritic cells secrete profibrotic growth factors and cytokines including IL-4, IL-6, and IL-13 that in turn cause activation and differentiation of resident fibroblasts and other mesenchymal progenitor cells. Potential cytokine targets for therapy are indicated. Created with BioRender.com

References

1. Hinchcliff M, Toledo DM, Taroni JN, Wood TA, Franks JM, Ball MS, Hoffmann A, Amin SM, Tan AU, Tom K, Nesbeth Y, Lee J, Ma M, Aren K, Carns MA, Pioli PA, Whitfield ML. Mycophenolate mofetil treatment of systemic sclerosis reduces myeloid cell numbers and attenuates the inflammatory gene signature in skin. J Invest Dermatol. 2018;138(6):1301–10.
2. Lescoat A, Lecureur V, Roussel M, Sunnaram BL, Ballerie A, Coiffier G, Jouneau S, Fardel O, Fest T, Jégo P. CD16-positive circulating monocytes and fibrotic manifestations of systemic sclerosis. Clin Rheumatol. 2017;36(7):1649–54.
3. Mohan V, Khatri P, Theodore S, Charles J, Pham H, Nair D, Scott M, Reveille JD, Mayes MD, Assassi S. Higher baseline monocyte count is associated with more extensive skin involvement and higher mortality in systemic sclerosis. Arthritis Rheumatol. 2017;69(Suppl. 10) https://acrabstracts.org/abstract/higher-baseline-monocyte-count-is-associated-with-more-extensive-skin-involvement-and-higher-mortality-in-systemic-sclerosis/. Accessed September 10, 2023
4. Sato S, Hasegawa M, Takehara K. Serum levels of interleukin-6 and interleukin-10 correlate with total skin thickness score in patients with systemic sclerosis. J Dermatol Sci. 2001;27(2):140–6.
5. Huang XL, Wang YJ, Yan JW, Wan YN, Chen B, Li BZ, Yang GJ, Wang J. Role of anti-inflammatory cytokines IL-4 and IL-13 in systemic sclerosis. Inflamm Res. 2015;64(3–4):151–9.
6. Chia JJ, Lu TT. Update on macrophages and innate immunity in scleroderma. Curr Opin Rheumatol. 2015;27(6):530–6.
7. Braga TT, Agudelo JS, Camara NO. Macrophages during the fibrotic process: M2 as friend and Foe. Front Immunol. 2015;6:602.
8. Khanna D, Denton CP, Jahreis A, van Laar JM, Frech TM, Anderson ME, Baron M, Chung L, Fierlbeck G, Lakshminarayanan S, Allanore Y, Pope JE, Riemekasten G, Steen V, Müller-Ladner U, Lafyatis R, Stifano G, Spotswood H, Chen-Harris H, Dziadek S, Morimoto A, Sornasse T, Siegel J, Furst DE. Safety and efficacy of subcutaneous tocilizumab in adults with systemic sclerosis (faSScinate): a phase 2, randomised, controlled trial. Lancet. 2016;387(10038):2630–40.
9. Allanore Y, Wung P, Soubrane C, Esperet C, Marrache F, Bejuit R, Lahmar A, Khanna D, Denton CP, Investigators. A randomised, double-blind, placebo-controlled, 24-week, phase II, proof-of-concept study of romilkimab (SAR156597) in early diffuse cutaneous systemic sclerosis. Ann Rheum Dis. 2020;79(12):1600–7.
10. Rice LM, Padilla CM, McLaughlin SR, Mathes A, Ziemek J, Goummih S, Nakerakanti S, York M, Farina G, Whitfield ML, Spiera RF, Christmann RB, Gordon JK, Weinberg J, Simms RW, Lafyatis R. Fresolimumab treatment decreases biomarkers and improves clinical symptoms in systemic sclerosis patients. J Clin Invest. 2015;125(7):2795–807.
11. Bellamri N, Morzadec C, Joannes A, Lecureur V, Wollin L, Jouneau S, Vernhet L. Alteration of human macrophage phenotypes by the anti-fibrotic drug nintedanib. Int Immunopharmacol. 2019;72:112–23.
12. Vlachogiannis NI, Pappa M, Ntouros PA, Nezos A, Mavragani CP, Souliotis VL, Sfikakis PP. Association between DNA damage response, fibrosis and Type I interferon signature in systemic sclerosis. Front Immunol. 2020;11:582401.

13. Christmann RB, Sampaio-Barros P, Stifano G, et al. Association of Interferonand transforming growth factor β-regulated genes and macrophage activation with systemic sclerosis-related progressive lung fibrosis. Arthritis Rheumatol. 2014;66:714–25.
14. Assassi S, Li N, Volkmann ER, Mayes MD, Rünger D, Ying J, Roth MD, Hinchcliff M, Khanna D, Frech T, Clements PJ, Furst DE, Goldin J, Bernstein EJ, Castelino FV, Domsic RT, Gordon JK, Hant FN, Shah AA, Shanmugam VK, Steen VD, Elashoff RM, Tashkin DP. Predictive significance of serum interferon-inducible protein score for response to treatment in systemic sclerosis-related interstitial lung disease. Arthritis Rheumatol. 2021;73(6):1005–13.
15. Guo X, Higgs BW, Bay-Jensen AC, Karsdal MA, Yao Y, Roskos LK, White WI. Suppression of T cell activation and collagen accumulation by an anti-IFNAR1 mAb, Anifrolumab, in adult patients with systemic sclerosis. J Invest Dermatol. 2015;135(10):2402–9.
16. Goldberg A, Geppert T, Schiopu E, Frech T, Hsu V, Simms RW, Peng SL, Yao Y, Elgeioushi N, Chang L, Wang B, Yoo S. Dose-escalation of human anti-interferon-α receptor monoclonal antibody MEDI-546 in subjects with systemic sclerosis: a phase 1, multicenter, open label study. Arthritis Res Ther. 2014;16(1):R57.
17. Mosanya CH, Isaacs JD. Tolerising cellular therapies: what is their promise for autoimmune disease? Ann Rheum Dis. 2019;78(3):297–310.
18. Ross RL, Corinaldesi C, Migneco G, Carr IM, Antanaviciute A, Wasson CW, Carriero A, Distler JHW, Holmes S, El-Sherbiny YM, McKimmie CS, Del Galdo F. Targeting human plasmacytoid dendritic cells through BDCA2 prevents skin inflammation and fibrosis in a novel xenotransplant mouse model of scleroderma. Ann Rheum Dis. 2021;80(7):920–9.
19. Artlett CM, Sassi-Gaha S, Rieger JL, Boesteanu AC, Feghali-Bostwick CA, Katsikis PD. The inflammasome activating caspase 1 mediates fibrosis and myofibroblast differentiation in systemic sclerosis. Arthritis Rheumatol. 2011;63:3563–74. https://doi.org/10.1002/art.30568.
20. Artlett CM, Sassi-Gaha S, Hope JL, Feghali-Bostwick CA, Katsikis PD. Mir-155 is overexpressed in systemic sclerosis fibroblasts and is required for NLRP3 inflammasome-mediated collagen synthesis during fibrosis. Arthritis Res Ther. 2017;19:144. https://doi.org/10.1186/s13075-017-1331-z.
21. Mantero JC, Kishore N, Ziemek J, Stifano G, Zammitti C, Khanna D, Gordon JK, Spiera R, Zhang Y, Simms RW, Lafyatis R. Randomised, double-blind, placebo-controlled trial of IL1-trap, rilonacept, in systemic sclerosis. A phase I/II biomarker trial. Clin Exp Rheumatol. 2018;36(Suppl. 113:4):146-149.
22. Shi H, Wang Y, Li X, Zhan X, Tang M, Fina M, Su L, Pratt D, Bu CH, Hildebrand S, Lyon S, Scott L, Quan J, Sun Q, Russell J, Arnett S, Jurek P, Chen D, Kravchenko VV, Mathison JC, Moresco EM, Monson NL, Ulevitch RJ, Beutler B. NLRP3 activation and mitosis are mutually exclusive events coordinated by NEK7, a new inflammasome component. Nat Immunol. 2016;17(3):250–8.
23. Ma ZZ, Sun HS, Lv JC, Guo L, Yang QR. Expression and clinical significance of the NEK7-NLRP3 inflammasome signaling pathway in patients with systemic lupus erythematosus. J Inflamm (Lond). 2018;15:16.
24. Beretta L, Barturen G, Vigone B, Bellocchi C, Hunzelmann N, De Langhe E, Cervera R, Gerosa M, Kovács L, Ortega Castro R, Almeida I, Cornec D, Chizzolini C, Pers JO, Makowska Z, Lesche R, Kerick M, Alarcón-Riquelme ME, Martin J, PRECISESADS SSc Substudy Group; PRECISESADS Flow Cytometry Study Group. Genome-wide whole blood transcriptome profiling in a large European cohort of systemic sclerosis patients. Ann Rheum Dis. 2020;79(9):1218–26. https://doi.org/10.1136/annrheumdis-2020-217116.
25. Wareing N, Li N, Volkmann E, Lyons M, Roth M, Tashkin D, Assassi S. Serum neutrophil count predicts progression of interstitial lung disease and mortality in patients with systemic sclerosis related interstitial lung disease. Arthritis Rheumatol. 2020;72(Suppl. 10) https://acrabstracts.org/abstract/serum-neutrophil-count-predicts-progression-of-interstitial-lung-disease-and-mortality-in-patients-with-systemic-sclerosis-related-interstitial-lung-disease/. Accessed September 10, 2023
26. Maugeri N, Capobianco A, Rovere-Querini P, Ramirez GA, Tombetti E, Valle PD, Monno A, D'Alberti V, Gasparri AM, Franchini S, D'Angelo A, Bianchi ME, Manfredi AA. Platelet microparticles sustain autophagy-associated activation of neutrophils in systemic sclerosis. Sci Transl Med. 2018;10(451):eaao3089.
27. Didier K, Giusti D, Le Jan S, et al. Neutrophil extracellular traps generation relates with early stage and vascular complications in systemic sclerosis. J Clin Med. 2020;9(7):2136. Published 2020 Jul 7. https://doi.org/10.3390/jcm9072136.
28. Arbore G, Ong VH, Costantini B, Denton CP, Abraham D, Placais L, Blighe K, Mitchell L, Ellis R, Heck S, Nocerino P, Woodruff TM, Kordasti S, Kemper C, Hourcade DE. Deep phenotyping detects a pathological CD4+ T-cell complosome signature in systemic sclerosis. Cell Mol Immunol. 2020;17(9):1010–3.
29. Gu H, Fisher AJ, Mickler EA, Duerson F III, Cummings OW, Peters-Golden M, Twigg HL III, Woodruff TM, Wilkes DS, Vittal R. Contribution of the anaphylatoxin receptors, C3aR and C5aR, to the pathogenesis of pulmonary fibrosis. FASEB J. 2016;30:2336–50.
30. Cipolla E, Fisher AJ, Gu H, Mickler EA, Agarwal M, Wilke CA, Kim KK, Moore BB, Vittal R. IL-17A deficiency mitigates bleomycin-induced complement activation during lung fibrosis. FASEB J. 2017;31(12):5543–56.
31. Uriarte MH, Larrarte C, Rey LB. Scleroderma renal crisis debute with thrombotic microangiopathy: a successful case treated with Eculizumab. Case Rep Nephrol. 2018;2018:6051083.
32. Zuckerman JE, Chang A. Complement and renal thrombotic microangiopathy associated with hypertension and scleroderma. Adv Chronic Kidney Dis. 2020;27(2):149–54.
33. Clark KEN, Campochiaro C, Csomor E, Taylor A, Nevin K, Galwey N, Morse MA, Singh J, Teo YV, Ong VH, Derrett-Smith E, Wisniacki N, Flint SM, Denton CP. Molecular basis for clinical diversity between autoantibody subsets in diffuse cutaneous systemic sclerosis. Ann Rheum Dis. 2021;80(12):1584–93. annrheumdis-2021-220402
34. Rubenfeld J, Guo J, Sookrung N, Chen R, Chaicumpa W, Casolaro V, et al. Lysophosphatidic acid enhances interleukin-13 gene expression and promoter activity in T cells. Am J Physiol Lung Cell Mol Physiol. 2006;290(1):L66–74.
35. Knowlden S, Georas SN. The autotaxin-LPA axis emerges as a novel regulator of lymphocyte homing and inflammation. J Immunol. 2014;192(3):851–7.
36. Watterson KR, Lanning DA, Diegelmann RF, Spiegel S. Regulation of fibroblast functions by lysophospholipid mediators: potential roles in wound healing. Wound Repair Regen. 2007;15(5):607–16.
37. Castelino FV, et al. Amelioration of dermal fibrosis by genetic deletion or pharmacologic antagonism of lysophosphatidic acid receptor 1 in a mouse model of scleroderma. Arthritis Rheumatol. 2011;63:1405–15.
38. Swaney JS, Chapman C, Correa LD, et al. A novel, orally active LPA(1) receptor antagonist inhibits lung fibrosis in the mouse bleomycin model. Br J Pharmacol. 2010;160(7):1699–713.
39. Allanore Y, Distler O, Jagerschmidt A, Illiano S, Ledein L, Boitier E, et al. Lysophosphatidic acid receptor 1 antagonist SAR100842 for patients with diffuse cutaneous systemic sclerosis: a double-blind, randomized, eight-week placebo-controlled study followed by a sixteen-week open-label extension study. Arthritis Rheumatol. 2018;70:1634–43.
40. Khanna D, Denton C, Furst D, Mayes M, Matucci-Cerinic M, Smith V, de Vries D, Deberdt L, Stiers P, Prasad N, Ahmed S. A Phase 2a randomized, double-blind, placebo-controlled study of Ziritaxestat in early diffuse cutaneous systemic sclerosis (NOVESA). Arthritis Rheumatol. 2020;72(Suppl. 10):L09.

41. Gaydosik AM, Tabib T, Domsic R, Khanna D, Lafyatis R, Fuschiotti P. Single-cell transcriptome analysis identifies skin-specific T-cell responses in systemic sclerosis. Ann Rheum Dis. 2021;80(11):1453–60. annrheumdis-2021-220209
42. Paleja B, Low AHL, Kumar P, Saidin S, Lajam A, Nur Hazirah S, Chua C, Li Yun L, Albani S. Systemic sclerosis perturbs the architecture of the immunome. Front Immunol. 2020;11:1602.
43. Barron L, Wynn TA. Fibrosis is regulated by Th2 and Th17 responses and by dynamic interactions between fibroblasts and macrophages. Am J Physiol Gastrointest Liver Physiol. 2011;300(5):G723–8.
44. Becker MO, et al. The monoclonal anti antibody basiliximab for the treatment of progressive systemic sclerosis: an open-label study. Ann Rheum Dis. 2011;70:1340–1.
45. Khanna D, Spino C, Johnson S, Chung L, Whitfield ML, Denton CP, Berrocal V, Franks J, Mehta B, Molitor J, Steen VD, Lafyatis R, Simms RW, Gill A, Kafaja S, Frech TM, Hsu V, Domsic RT, Pope JE, Gordon JK, Mayes MD, Schiopu E, Young A, Sandorfi N, Park J, Hant FN, Bernstein EJ, Chatterjee S, Castelino FV, Ajam A, Wang Y, Wood T, Allanore Y, Matucci-Cerinic M, Distler O, Singer O, Bush E, Fox DA, Furst DE. Abatacept in early diffuse cutaneous systemic sclerosis: results of a Phase II investigator-initiated, multicenter, double-blind, randomized, placebo-controlled trial. Arthritis Rheumatol. 2020;72(1):125–36. https://doi.org/10.1002/art.41055.
46. Fox DA, Lundy SK, Whitfield ML, Berrocal V, Campbell P, Rasmussen S, Ohara R, Stinson A, Gurrea-Rubio M, Wiewiora E, Spino C, Bush E, Furst D, Pillai S, Khanna D. Lymphocyte subset abnormalities in early diffuse cutaneous systemic sclerosis. Arthritis Res Ther. 2021;23(1):10.
47. Maehara T, Kaneko N, Perugino CA, Mattoo H, Kers J, Allard-Chamard H, Mahajan VS, Liu H, Murphy SJ, Ghebremichael M, Fox D, Payne AS, Lafyatis R, Stone JH, Khanna D, Pillai S. Cytotoxic CD4+ T lymphocytes may induce endothelial cell apoptosis in systemic sclerosis. J Clin Invest. 2020;130(5):2451–64.
48. Taylor DK, et al. T follicular helper-like cells contribute to skin fibrosis. Sci Transl Med. 2018;10:eaaf5307.
49. Glauzy S, Olson B, May CK, Parisi D, Massad C, Hansen JE, Ryu C, Herzog EL, Meffre E. Defective early B cell tolerance checkpoints in patients with systemic sclerosis allow the production of self-antigen-specific clones. Arthritis Rheumatol. 2022;74(2):307–17.
50. Taher TE, Ong VH, Bystrom J, Hillion S, Simon Q, Denton CP, Pers JO, Abraham DJ, Mageed RA. Association of defective regulation of autoreactive interleukin-6-producing transitional B lymphocytes with disease in patients with systemic sclerosis. Arthritis Rheumatol. 2018;70(3):450–61.
51. Gao X, Jia G, Guttman A, DePianto DJ, Morshead KB, Sun KH, et al. Osteopontin links myeloid activation and disease progression in systemic sclerosis. Cell Rep Med. 2020;1(8):100140.
52. de Bourcy CFA, Dekker CL, Davis MM, Nicolls MR, Quake SR. Dynamics of the human antibody repertoire after B cell depletion in systemic sclerosis. Sci Immunol. 2017;2(15):eaan8289.
53. Matsushita T, Kobayashi T, Mizumaki K, Kano M, Sawada T, Tennichi M, Okamura A, Hamaguchi Y, Iwakura Y, Hasegawa M, Fujimoto M, Takehara K. BAFF inhibition attenuates fibrosis in scleroderma by modulating the regulatory and effector B cell balance. Sci Adv. 2018;4(7):eaas9944.
54. Sato S, Fujimoto M, Hasegawa M, Takehara K. Altered blood B lymphocyte homeostasis in systemic sclerosis: expanded naive B cells and diminished but activated memory B cells. Arthritis Rheumatol. 2004;50(6):1918–27.
55. Lorenzetti R, Janowska I, Smulski CR, Frede N, Henneberger N, Walter L, Schleyer MT, Hüppe JM, Staniek J, Salzer U, Venhoff A, Troilo A, Voll RE, Venhoff N, Thiel J, Rizzi M. Abatacept modulates CD80 and CD86 expression and memory formation in human B-cells. J Autoimmun. 2019;101:145–52.
56. Goswami RP, Ray A, Chatterjee M, Mukherjee A, Sircar G, Ghosh P. Rituximab in the treatment of systemic sclerosis-related interstitial lung disease: a systematic review and meta-analysis. Rheumatology (Oxford). 2021;60(2):557–67.
57. Li Y, Baig H, Rojas C, Stowell J, Lesser E, Borkar S, Abril A, Mira-Avendano I. Prospective analysis of a cohort of patients with interstitial lung disease associated with connective tissue disease and their response to immnosuppression with mycophenolate mofetil and rituximab. Arthritis Rheumatol. 2020;72(Suppl. 10) https://acrabstracts.org/abstract/prospective-analysis-of-a-cohort-of-patients-with-interstitial-lung-disease-associated-with-connective-tissue-disease-and-their-response-to-immunosuppression-with-mycophenolate-mofetil-and-rituximab/. Accessed September 1
58. Elhai M, Boubaya M, Distler O, Smith V, Matucci-Cerinic M, Alegre Sancho JJ, Truchetet ME, Braun-Moscovici Y, Iannone F, Novikov PI, Lescoat A, Siegert E, Castellví I, Airó P, Vettori S, De Langhe E, Hachulla E, Erler A, Ananieva L, Krusche M, López-Longo FJ, Distler JHW, Hunzelmann N, Hoffmann-Vold AM, Riccieri V, Hsu VM, Pozzi MR, Ancuta C, Rosato E, Mihai C, Kuwana M, Saketkoo LA, Chizzolini C, Hesselstrand R, Ullman S, Yavuz S, Rednic S, Caimmi C, Bloch-Queyrat C, Allanore Y, for EUSTAR network. Outcomes of patients with systemic sclerosis treated with rituximab in contemporary practice: a prospective cohort study. Ann Rheum Dis. 2019;78(7):979–87.
59. Saunders P, Tsipouri V, Keir GJ, et al. Rituximab versus cyclophosphamide for the treatment of connective tissue disease-associated interstitial lung disease (RECITAL): study protocol for a randomised controlled trial. Trials. 2017;18(1):275. https://doi.org/10.1186/s13063-017-2016-2.
60. Ebata S, et al. Safety and efficacy of rituximab in systemic sclerosis (DESIRES): a double-blind, investigator-initiated, randomised, placebo-controlled trial. Lancet Rheumatol. 2021;3:E489–97.
61. Zamanian RT, Badesch D, Chung L, Domsic RT, Medsger T, Pinckney A, Keyes-Elstein L, D'Aveta C, Spychala M, White RJ, Hassoun PM, Torres F, Sweatt AJ, Molitor JA, Khanna D, Maecker H, Welch B, Goldmuntz E, Nicolls MR. Safety and efficacy of B-Cell depletion with rituximab for the treatment of systemic sclerosis-associated pulmonary arterial hypertension: a multicenter, double-blind, randomized, placebo-controlled trial. Am J Respir Crit Care Med. 2021;204(2):209–21.
62. Einhaus J, Pecher AC, Asteriti E, Schmid H, Secker KA, Duerr-Stoerzer S, Keppeler H, Klein R, Schneidawind C, Henes J, Schneidawind D. Inhibition of effector B cells by ibrutinib in systemic sclerosis. Arthritis Res Ther. 2020;22(1):66.
63. Mackay F, Schneider P. Cracking the BAFF code. Nat Rev Immunol. 2009;9(7):491–502.
64. Gordon JK, Martyanov V, Franks JM, Bernstein EJ, Szymonifka J, Magro C, Wildman HF, Wood TA, Whitfield ML, Spiera RF. Belimumab for the treatment of early diffuse systemic sclerosis: results of a randomized, double-blind, placebo-controlled, pilot trial. Arthritis Rheumatol. 2018;70(2):308–16.
65. Enk AH, Hadaschik EN, Emining R, Fierlbeck G, French LE, Girolomoni G, et al. European guidelines (S1) on the use of high-dose intravenous immunoglobulin in dermatology. JEADV. 2016;30:1657–69.
66. Kerr J, Quinti I, Eibl M, Chapel H, Späth PJ, Sewell WA, et al. Is dosing of therapeutic immunoglobulins optimal? A review of a three-decade long debate in Europe. Front Immunol. 2014; 5:629.
67. Sewell WA, Kerr J, Behr-Gross ME, Peter HH; Kreuth Ig Working Group. European consensus proposal for immunoglobulin therapies. Eur J Immunol. 2014;44(8):2207–14.
68. Baleva M, Nikolov K. The role of intravenous immunoglobulin preparations in the treatment of systemic sclerosis. Int J Rheumatol. 2011;61:326–37.
69. Cantarini L, Rigante D, Vitale A, Napodano S, Sakkas LI, Bogdanos DP, et al. Intravenous immunoglobulins (IVIG) in systemic sclerosis: a challenging yet promising future. Immunol Res. 2015;61(3):326–37.
70. Gomes JP, Santos L, Shoenfeld Y. Intravenous immunoglobulin (IVIG) in the vanguard therapy of systemic sclerosis. Clin Immunol. 2019;199:25–8.

71. Galeotti C, Kaveri SV, Bayry J. IVIG-mediated effector functions in autoimmune and inflammatory diseases. Int Immunol. 2017;29(11):491–8.
72. Schwab I, Nimmerjahn F. Intravenous immunoglobulin therapy: how does IgG modulate the immune system? Nat Rev Immunol. 2013;13(3):176–89.
73. Perković D, Petrić M, Božić I, Borić K, Marasović Krstulović D, Radić M, Martinović KD. Low dose intravenous immunoglobulin in addition to cyclophosphamide in systemic sclerosis : Single centre experience. Wien Klin Wochenschr. 2021;133:1070–5.
74. Takehara K, Ihn H, Sato S. A randomized, double-blind, placebo-controlled trial: intravenous immunoglobulin treatment in patients with diffuse cutaneous systemic sclerosis. Clin Exp Rheumatol. 2013;31(2 Suppl. 76):151–6.
75. Poelman CL, Hummers LK, Wigley FM, Anderson C, Boin F, Shah AA. Intravenous immunoglobulin may be an effective therapy for refractory, active diffuse cutaneous systemic sclerosis. J Rheumatol. 2015;42(2):236–42.
76. Raja J, Nihtyanova SI, Murray CD, Denton CP, Ong VH. Sustained benefit from intravenous immunoglobulin therapy for gastrointestinal involvement in systemic sclerosis. Rheumatology (Oxford). 2016;55(1):115–9.
77. Sanges S, Riviere S, Mekinian A, Martin T, Le Quellec A, Chatelus E, et al. Intravenous immunoglobulins in systemic sclerosis: data from a French nationwide cohort of 46 patients and review of the literature. Autoimmun Rev. 2017;16(4):377–84.
78. Feghali CA, Bost KL, Boulware DW, Levy LS. Mechanisms of pathogenesis in scleroderma. I. Overproduction of interleukin 6 by fibroblasts cultured from affected skin sites of patients with scleroderma. J Rheumatol. 1992;19(8):1207–11.
79. Maier C, Ramming A, Bergmann C, Weinkam R, Kittan N, Schett G, Distler JHW, Beyer C. Inhibition of phosphodiesterase 4 (PDE4) reduces dermal fibrosis by interfering with the release of interleukin-6 from M2 macrophages. Ann Rheum Dis. 2017;76(6):1133–41.
80. Fielding CA, Jones GW, McLoughlin RM, McLeod L, Hammond VJ, Uceda J, Williams AS, Lambie M, Foster TL, Liao CT, Rice CM, Greenhill CJ, Colmont CS, Hams E, Coles B, Kift-Morgan A, Newton Z, Craig KJ, Williams JD, Williams GT, Davies SJ, Humphreys IR, O'Donnell VB, Taylor PR, Jenkins BJ, Topley N, Jones SA. Interleukin-6 signaling drives fibrosis in unresolved inflammation. Immunity. 2014;40(1):40–50.
81. Roofeh D, Lin CJF, Goldin J, Kim GH, Furst DE, Denton CP, Huang S, Khanna D, focuSSced Investigators. Tocilizumab prevents progression of early systemic sclerosis-associated interstitial lung disease. Arthritis Rheumatol. 2021;73(7):1301–10.
82. Hoyles RK, Ellis RW, Wellsbury J, Lees B, Newlands P, Goh NS, Roberts C, Desai S, Herrick AL, McHugh NJ, Foley NM, Pearson SB, Emery P, Veale DJ, Denton CP, Wells AU, Black CM, du Bois RM. A multicenter, prospective, randomized, double-blind, placebo-controlled trial of corticosteroids and intravenous cyclophosphamide followed by oral azathioprine for the treatment of pulmonary fibrosis in scleroderma. Arthritis Rheumatol. 2006;54(12):3962–70.
83. Tashkin DP, Elashoff R, Clements PJ, Goldin J, Roth MD, Furst DE, Arriola E, Silver R, Strange C, Bolster M, Seibold JR, Riley DJ, Hsu VM, Varga J, Schraufnagel DE, Theodore A, Simms R, Wise R, Wigley F, White B, Steen V, Read C, Mayes M, Parsley E, Mubarak K, Connolly MK, Golden J, Olman M, Fessler B, Rothfield N, Metersky M, Scleroderma Lung Study Research Group. Cyclophosphamide versus placebo in scleroderma lung disease. N Engl J Med. 2006;354(25):2655–66.
84. Distler O, Highland KB, Gahlemann M, Azuma A, Fischer A, Mayes MD, Raghu G, Sauter W, Girard M, Alves M, Clerisme-Beaty E, Stowasser S, Tetzlaff K, Kuwana M, Maher TM, Trial SENSCIS, Investigators. Nintedanib for systemic sclerosis-associated interstitial lung disease. N Engl J Med. 2019;380(26):2518–28.
85. Khanna D, Huang S, Ye W, Lin C, Jahreis A, Denton C. Relationship of baseline measures to the change in the forced vital capacity in a phase 3 randomised controlled trial of tocilizumab for the treatment of early systemic sclerosis. Am J Respir Crit Care Med. 2020;201(1):A2750.
86. Fava A, Cimbro R, Wigley FM, Liu QR, Rosen A, Boin F. Frequency of circulating topoisomerase-I-specific CD4 T cells predicts presence and progression of interstitial lung disease in scleroderma. Arthritis Res Ther. 2016;18(1):99.
87. Khanna D, Bush E, Nagaraja V, Koenig A, Khanna P, Young A, Moore J, Fox D, Lafyatis R. Tofacitinib in early diffuse cutaneous systemic sclerosis—results of Phase I/II investigator-initiated, double-blind randomised placebo-controlled trial. Arthritis Rheumatol. 2019;71(Suppl. 10):1493–5
88. You H, Dong X, Hou Y, Zhou J, Wang Q, Li M, Zeng X. Tofacitinib as a possible treatment for skin thickening in diffuse cutaneous systemic sclerosis. Rheumatology. 2021;60(5):2472–7.
89. Nash P, Kerschbaumer A, Dörner T, Dougados M, Fleischmann RM, Geissler K, McInnes I, Pope JE, van der Heijde D, Stoffer-Marx M, Takeuchi T, Trauner M, Winthrop KL, de Wit M, Aletaha D, Baraliakos X, Boehncke WH, Emery P, Isaacs JD, Kremer J, Lee EB, Maksymowych WP, Voshaar M, Tam LS, Tanaka Y, van den Bosch F, Westhovens R, Xavier R, Smolen JS. Points to consider for the treatment of immune-mediated inflammatory diseases with Janus kinase inhibitors: a consensus statement. Ann Rheum Dis. 2021;80(1):71–87.
90. Ricard L, Jachiet V, Malard F, Ye Y, Stocker N, Rivière S, Senet P, Monfort JB, Fain O, Mohty M, Gaugler B, Mekinian A. Circulating follicular helper T cells are increased in systemic sclerosis and promote plasmablast differentiation through the IL-21 pathway which can be inhibited by ruxolitinib. Ann Rheum Dis. 2019;78(4): 539–50.
91. Feeney M, Syed F, Khan K, Shiwen X, Sully K, Trinder S, Wilson P, Abraham D, Holmes AM, Denton CP, Oncostatin M. As a potential molecular target in systemic sclerosis. Arthritis Rheumatol. 2015;67(Suppl. 10) https://acrabstracts.org/abstract/oncostatin-m-as-a-potential-molecular-target-in-systemic-sclerosis/. Accessed September 10, 2023
92. Marden G, Wan Q, Wilks J, Nevin K, Feeney M, Wisniacki N, Trojanowski M, Bujor A, Stawski L, Trojanowska M. The role of the oncostatin M/OSM receptor β axis in activating dermal microvascular endothelial cells in systemic sclerosis. Arthritis Res Ther. 2020;22(1):179.
93. Adami E, Viswanathan S, Widjaja AA, Ng B, Chothani S, Zhihao N, Tan J, Lio PM, George BL, Altunoglu U, Ghosh K, Paleja BS, Schafer S, Reversade B, Albani S, Ling ALH, O'Reilly S, Cook SA. IL11 is elevated in systemic sclerosis and IL11-dependent ERK signaling underlies TGFβ-mediated activation of dermal fibroblasts. Rheumatology (Oxford). 2021;60(12): 5820–6.
94. Lee CG, Hartl D, Matsuura H, Dunlop FM, Scotney PD, Fabri LJ, Nash AD, Chen NY, Tang CY, Chen Q, Homer RJ, Baca M, Elias JA. Endogenous IL-11 signaling is essential in Th2- and IL-13-induced inflammation and mucus production. Am J Respir Cell Mol Biol. 2008;39(6):739–46.
95. Ayaub EA, Dubey A, Imani J, et al. Overexpression of OSM and IL-6 impacts the polarization of pro-fibrotic macrophages and the development of bleomycin-induced lung fibrosis. Sci Rep. 2017;7:13281.
96. Kobayashi S, Nagafuchi Y, Okubo M, Sugimori Y, Shirai H, Hatano H, Junko M, Yanaoka H, Takeshima Y, Ota M, Iwasaki Y, Sumitomo S, Okamura T, Yamamoto K, Shoda H, Fujio K. Integrated bulk and single-cell RNA-sequencing identified disease-relevant monocytes and a gene network module underlying systemic sclerosis. J Autoimmun. 2021; 116:102547.

Physical and Occupational Therapy

45

Luc Mouthon, Christelle Nguyen, and Janet L. Poole

Systemic sclerosis (SSc) is a connective tissue disease that causes significant disability, handicap, and worsening of quality of life [1–3]. Management of the person with SSc requires a multidisciplinary approach including rehabilitation techniques (Table 45.1) such as occupational and physical therapy. To determine the effectiveness of rehabilitation techniques, reliability and valid outcome measures are needed. This chapter will review assessments available to measure disability (Table 45.2) and participation in persons with SSc and discuss rehabilitation techniques that have been shown to be effective in improving joint motion, hand function, strength, general conditioning, and participation in daily life.

Measuring Disability and Participation Restrictions

There are a number of assessments available to measure disability and participation in persons with SSc. These assessments offer the opportunity to study joint motion, hand function, mouth disability, strength, general conditioning, and participation in daily life in order to demonstrate the effect of drugs and/or rehabilitation techniques. These measurement tools that are helpful for determining severity and outcomes following rehabilitation therapy are reviewed in the following paragraphs.

Health Assessment Questionnaire

Global disability in SSc patients is usually measured by the HAQ, a self-report questionnaire consisting of 20 items divided into eight categories [51]. Items are rated from 0 (no difficulty) to 3 (unable to do). The highest scores from each category are summed and divided by 8 to yield a disability score ranging from 0 (no disability) to 3 (maximal disability). The HAQ correlates well with the extent of skin thickening, loss of ability to close the fist, proximal muscle weakness, and tendon friction rubbing but not digital ulcers [1, 43]. In SSc patients, global disability can be measured with this scale [1, 43, 51], and an acceptable sensitivity to change has been suggested [44, 52, 53]. Steen and Medsger proposed the use of the sHAQ, a more disease-specific disability scale [44] by adding five patient-generated visual analog scales to the original HAQ, thus assessing Raynaud's phenomenon, digital-tip ulcers, gastrointestinal and lung symptoms, and overall disease severity from the patient's perspective [44].

Cochin Hand Function Scale (CHFS)

Hand disability can be evaluated with the CHFS, a functional disability questionnaire about daily activities that has been validated in rheumatoid arthritis (RA) and hand osteoarthritis [54–56]. The CHFS consists of 18 items concerning daily activities; each question is scored on a scale of 0 (performed without difficulty) to 5 (impossible to do). The total score is obtained by adding the scores of all items (range 0–90). This questionnaire has been validated in SSc [2, 47].

The CHFS has good convergent validity with global disability (HAQ and sHAQ) and global hand mobility (HFI and Kapandji indexes), a weaker correlation with patient's

L. Mouthon (✉)
Department of Internal Medicine, Centre de Référence Maladies Systémiques Autoimmunes et Autoinflammatoires Rares d'Ile de France de l'Est et de l'Ouest, Assistance Publique Hôpitaux de Paris, France (APHP-CUP), Hôpital Cochin, Paris, France

Université Paris Cité, Paris, France
e-mail: luc.mouthon@aphp.fr

C. Nguyen
Departement of Physical and Rehabilitation Medicine, Hôpital Cochin, Paris, France
e-mail: christelle.nguyen2@aphp.fr

J. L. Poole
Occupational Therapy Graduate Program, School of Medicine, University of New Mexico, Albuquerque, NM, USA
e-mail: JPoole@salud.unm.edu

Y. Allanore et al. (eds.), *Scleroderma*, https://doi.org/10.1007/978-3-031-40658-4_45

Table 45.1 Summary of studies on rehabilitation techniques for systemic sclerosis

Type of rehabilitation intervention	Authors	Description of intervention	Summary of findings
Hand exercises	Mugii et al. [4, 5]	Stretching exercises for joints of the hand	Total passive joint motion improved at 1-month post intervention which improved or was maintained at 1 year. Total hand function did not change (HAQ), but ability to perform individual items improved. At 3 years follow-up, total passive joint motion improved and was maintained or improved at 9 years after the first visit. HAQ scores did not significantly change at 9 years except in patients who also had decreased total passive finger motion. The decrease in motion was related to worse skin scores
	Piga et al. [6]	Home program consisting of mobility and strengthening exercises for the hand telemonitored as to number of repetitions, force, speed, and correctness. Control group received home program booklet and instruction on 3 strengthening and 3 mobility exercises	Both groups showed improvements in hand function and pinch and MCP ROM in the dominant hand. HAQ scores and HAMIS for the dominant hand and grip and pinch for the nondominant hand improved significantly only in the telemonitoring group. There was no difference between groups
	Stefanantoni et al. [7]	Hand exercises and information from an occupational therapist on exercises tailored to participants' goals	At 3 months, the occupational therapy group had significant improvements with perceived satisfaction and performance of daily tasks, HAQ and mental health. There were only significant differences between the OT group and the control group at 3 months was perceived performance on daily tasks
	Piga et al. [8, 9]	Home hand exercise program consisting of booklet and DVD; instructions on management of Raynaud also included	Significant improvements for pain, grip and pinch strength, RP impact, and scores on the CHFS, HAQ and SF-36 seen at 8 weeks after initial instruction. Long-term follow-up showed significant improvements from 8 to 24 weeks for CHFS, pain and pinch strength; but not for grip, HAQ, or FTP. There were significant differences in the hand exercise group for all variables compared to a control group who were evaluated at baseline and 24 weeks
Paraffin wax treatment and hand range-of-motion exercises	Askew et al. [10]	Combination of paraffin wax, friction massage, and range-of-motion for 1 session	Joint motion, skin compliance, and hand function improved more in intervention group than control group
	Pils et al. [11]	12 treatment sessions of paraffin; paraffin wax was continued for 3 months in an intervention group but discontinued in the control group	Intervention and control group received paraffin wax; joint motion increased and skin stiffness decreased. However, improvements maintained after 3 months in intervention but not control
	Sandqvist et al. [12]	Paraffin wax and hand exercises 1 time/day to one hand; other hand served as control	In the hands receiving the intervention, finger flexion and extension, thumb abduction, wrist flexion, and perceived skin thickness and elasticity significantly improved compared to baseline. Improvements from base line were greater for the intervention hands compared to the control hands for finger extension and perceived skin stiffness and elasticity
	Mancuso et al. [13]	Paraffin wax and hand exercises 5 days/week	Series of three single-case studies. Grip and pinch strength and hand function improved in all three participants, while total active joint motion increased in 2/3 of participants
	Gregory et al. [14]	Paraffin wax baths 4 times per week and 3 hand exercises for 9 weeks; control group did hand exercise only	There were no differences in HAMIS, HAQ, and CHFS scores or grip and pinch strength between groups at 9 week and 18 weeks
	Kristensen et al. [15]	Paraffin wax bath compared to lukewarm water prior to hand exercises for 6 months	HAMIS scores improved in both groups and maintained at 12-mo follow-up; however, it had no significant group differences
Hand massage and joint manipulation	Maddali Bongi et al. [16]	Combination of connective tissue massage and Mc Mennell joint manipulation and home range-of-motion exercise	Fist closure, joint motion (HAMIS), hand function, and quality of life improved significantly, while fist closure only improved significantly in the control group
	Vannajak et al. [17]	Combination of superficial heat, traditional Thai massage, and stretching. In addition, the experimental group wore nylon gloves 6 h/day for 2 weeks	Joint motion (HAMIS) significantly improved in both groups; however, thumb motion improved only in the group that wore the glove

Table 45.1 (continued)

Type of rehabilitation intervention	Authors	Description of intervention	Summary of findings
	Horvath et al. [18]	Combination of hand stretching exercises, thermal modalities (thermal and mud baths, whirlpool) and soft tissue massage for 3 weeks	At 3 weeks, both the hand exercise group and controls showed significant improvements on the DASH, pain and Raynaud's phenomenon VAS; but only the exercise group improved on the HAQ. The improvements were maintained at 6 mo of the exercise group but not the controls and there were no significant group differences at either 3 week or 6 months
	Murphy et al. [19]	Combination thermal modalities, tissue mobilization (lymphatouch) and hand and arm exercises weekly for 8 weeks plus a home exercise program	At 8 weeks, significant improvements on the QuickDASH and the PROMIS physical function
Neuromuscular/kinesio taping	Parisi et al. [20]	Neuromuscular/kinesio taping applied bilaterally on both dorsal and palmar side of the hand applied distally to proximally ending at the wrist. Tape applied 2 times weekly for 4 weeks	There were significant improvements for hand function, motion, pain and a decrease in Raynaud's phenomenon from to post intervention
Splints	Seeger et al. [21]	Dorsal splint with dynamic PIP extension outrigger worn 8 h/day for 2 months	Joint range-of-motion of the PIP joint did not improve significantly in the splinted or nonsplinted hand
Mouth and facial exercises	Naylor et al. [22]	Mouth stretching and oral augmentation exercises	At 1 month there was no significant difference in mean mouth opening between the intervention group and a control (no treatment) group
	Pizzo et al. [23]	Mouth stretching and oral augmentation exercises for 15 min twice a day	Mouth opening significantly increased; subjective improvements in eating, speaking, and ability to perform oral hygiene
	Poole et al. [24]	Mouth exercises and oral augmentation exercises in combination with education on brushing and flossing teeth and adapted dental appliances	Dental hygiene improved significantly for decreased bleeding, supragingival calculus, and increases in caries. No significant improvement in mouth opening
	Yuen et al. [25, 26]	Powered toothbrush and flosser plus mouth stretching and oral augmentation exercises if oral aperture <40 mm compared to manual toothbrush and dental floss 2 times/day for 6 months	Gingival inflammation was significantly reduced both groups. Group that used powered toothbrush showed a significantly larger reduction in inflammation than manual toothbrush group. Oral aperture significantly increased compared to controls at 3 months but not at 6 months
Massage and stretching of the face and mouth	Maddali Bongi et al. [27]	Combination of connective tissue massage, Kabat's technique, kinesitherapy, and a home exercise program	Mouth opening increased, and skin scores decreased in the intervention group compared to the home exercise only control group
Overall rehabilitation consisting of specific and global techniques	Maddali Bongi et al. [27]	Specific techniques included hand and face exercises and connective tissue massage. Those with hand edema received manual lymphatic drainage. Global techniques included respiratory exercises and land- or water-based program	Quality of life, functional ability, hand mobility and function, mouth opening, and face mobility all significantly increased at the end of the 9-week program
			At the 9 week follow-up, only improvements in mouth opening and hand mobility were maintained
			No improvements were noted in a control group who received information about scleroderma
	Schouffoer et al. [28]	Multidisciplinary intervention 1 day per week consisting of group sessions (general exercise, hand and mouth exercises, education), supervised home exercises provided by a PT 1/week, and home-based exercise program 6 days per week	Grip strength, mouth opening, distance walked in 6 min, and functional ability significantly increased at the end of the 12-week program compared to a control group who received regular outpatient care. At 24 weeks, only improvements in mouth opening was maintained

(continued)

Table 45.1 (continued)

Type of rehabilitation intervention	Authors	Description of intervention	Summary of findings
	Rannou et al. [29]	Supervised tailored multidisciplinary intervention with PT and OT consisting of aerobic, strengthening, and stretching exercises for the mouth, face, upper and lower extremities, and splints	At 12 mo, there was no significant difference in HAQ scores between the intervention and control groups. However, there were short-term effects at 1 mo for the HAQ, and other measures of functional ability, hand mobility and function and mouth opening
Generalized physical exercise	Oliveira et al. [30]	Progressive aerobic exercises 2 times/week consisting of 5-min warm-up, 40-min aerobics, and 5-min cooldown	Peak VO_2 increased significantly but no difference between an intervention group and control group of healthy individuals. No change in skin scores in the SSc group. No change in quality of life in both groups
	Pinto et al. [31]	Combination of 30 min of resistive training and 20 min of aerobic training. Resistive training consisted of bench press, leg press, lat pull down, leg extension, and seated row. The aerobic training was done on a treadmill	Dynamic strength (leg press, bench press) and isometric strength (hand and low back), and scores on the timed-stands test improved significantly after the 12-week training. There were no changes in peak VO_2, heart rate at rest was significantly reduced, time to exhaustion was increased, and workload and time of exercise at ventilatory thresholds and peak of exercise were increased. There were no changes in skin scores or muscle enzymes which stayed within normal limits
	Alexanderson et al. [32]	Combination of aerobic exercise on stationary bike and resistance training for the shoulder and hip flexor muscle groups 3 times/week for 14 weeks	Series of 4 single-case studies. Muscular endurance improved significantly in 3 participants, while aerobic capacity improved significantly in 2 participants
	Mitropoulos et al. [33]	High interval training on either a cycle leg ergometer or arm ergometer 2 times/week for 12 weeks	Peak oxygen update ↑ in both exercise groups but only significantly better in the arm ergometer group compared to control. Transcutaneous oxygen pressure increased in arm ergometer group but not significantly. Quality of life increased and pain and discomfort due to Raynaud's phenomenon decreased significantly in both exercise groups compared to controls. Endothelial-dependent vasodilation improved significantly more in the arm exercise group compared to the other groups
	Mitropoulos et al. [34]	Combination of high interval training on an arm crank and 5 upper body resistance exercises 2 times/week for 12 weeks	The exercise group had better life satisfaction, less anxiety and less pain due to Raynaud's phenomenon after 12 weeks. Compliance was 92.6% with no dropouts and participants enjoyed the program
	Filippetti et al. [35]	Combination of aerobic exercise on stationary bike, upper body resistance exercises, and hand stretching exercises plus a monthly phone call from a physiotherapist for 3 months	At 6 months, distance on the 6 min walk decreased in the exercise group and quality of life, HAQ, and grip, biceps and quadriceps strength improved compared to the control group
Occupational therapy	Zanatta et al. [36]	Occupational therapy consisted of six 90 min sessions over 3 weeks. Content included information on strategies and devices on different activities of daily living: Cooking, getting dressed, cleaning and doing personal care and leisure activities	At 24 weeks after baseline, the occupational therapy group showed improvements on the HAQ and EDAQ compared to the control group but the changes were not significant except for three items on the EDAQ (eating, indoor and outdoor mobility). The number of assistive devices used increased significantly in the occupational therapy group compared to the controls.

Table 45.1 (continued)

Type of rehabilitation intervention	Authors	Description of intervention	Summary of findings
Self-management	Samuelson and Ahlmen [37]	Self-management program consisting of seven 3-h group sessions for 5 weeks. Content included medical aspects, exercise, joint protection and energy conservation, splints, activities of daily living and assistive devices, modalities and pain control, relaxation, and diet	Participants reported improvements in self-efficacy. Course evaluations showed that participants were satisfied with the content of the program and opportunities to meet others with SSc
	Brown et al. [38]	Self-management program consisting of four 3-h group sessions. Content included medical aspects, self-management, medications, relaxation, and relationships with family and health professionals	Qualitative evaluation of the program revealed that participants felt it was valuable meeting others with SSc, the involvement of a patient educator, practical tips for daily living, fatigue and time management, and the family session
	Poole et al. [39]	Self-paced self-management program consisting of a workbook and exercise DVD. Workbook content included medical aspects and management of symptoms, coping skills, exercises, activities of daily living, and advocacy	Fatigue and pain decreased while hand function increased; however, significant improvements seen for self-efficacy for pain
	Kwakkenbos et al. [40]	Multidisciplinary intervention over 6 weeks consisting of group sessions (goal setting, education, joint protection and energy conservation, psychosocial aspects, exercise, and introduction to Tai Chi)	Participants reported less helplessness and higher acceptance of limitations post intervention and at 6 months. No changes in mood or physical function
	Poole et al. [41]	Self-paced Internet self-management program included content on medical aspects, management of symptoms, advocacy, coping, exercise and activities of daily living, an interactive discussion board, resources, learning activities, and an exercise video	Significant improvements found for ability to manage care, health efficacy, and decreases in fatigue and depression. Evaluation of the program was positive
	Khanna et al. [42]	Self-paced Internet self-management program consisting of 15 modules on medical aspects, management of symptoms, advocacy, coping, exercise and activities of daily living, caregiver tips, an interactive discussion board, resources, learning activities, and an exercise video for the face, mouth, upper and lower extremities	No significant differences between the intervention group and control conditions (book on scleroderma) for self-efficacy, depression, physical function, patient activation or quality of life. Evaluation of program positive for content, clear presentation and ease in use

CHFS Cochin Hand Function Scale, *DASH* Disabilities of the Arm Shoulder, and Hand measure, *EDAQ* Evaluation of Daily Activity Questionnaire, *HAMIS* hand mobility in scleroderma, *HAQ* health assessment questionnaire, *MCP ROM* finger metacarpophalangeal joints range of motion, *PIP* proximal interphalangeal, *PROMIS* patient-reported outcome measurement information system, SF-36 Short Form, *PT* Physical therapy, *OT* Occupational Therapy, *VAS* visual analog scale

Table 45.2 Available/validated instruments measuring disability and participation restrictions in systemic sclerosis

	Authors	Number of patients	Reliability	Validity/construct validity	Sensitivity to change
HAQ	Poole et al. [1]	211	Good	Good validity	NA
	Poole et al. [43]	80	Good	Good validity	NA
	Steen et al. [44]	1250		Good validity	Acceptable
HAMIS	Sandqvist et al. [45]	30	Good		NA
	Sandqvist et al. [46]	45	Good	Good validity	NA
CHFS	Brower et al. [47]	40	Good	Good validity	NA
	Rannou et al. [2]	50	Factor analysis extracted 2 factors that accounted for 71.63% of the total variance: activities requiring grip and pinch strength; activities requiring pinch dexterity	Good construct validity; significant correlations between CHFS, HAQ, and HFI scores. CHFS scores contribute to 75% of the HAQ variance	NA
CSF-17	Daste et al. [48]	113	Good	Good	NA
MHISS	Mouthon et al. [49]	71	Excellent three factors explore disability due to mouth opening limitation, mouth dryness, and the aesthetic concerns	Good construct validity	NA
Dash	Varju et al. [50]	128/76[a]	Good	NA	SRM: 0.64

CHFS Cochin hand function scale, *CSF-17* Cochin 17-item Scleroderma Functional scale, *DASH* disabilities of the arm, shoulder, and hand, *HAMIS* hand mobility in scleroderma, *HAQ* health assessment questionnaire, *MHISS* mouth handicap in systemic sclerosis, *NA* not assessed, *SRM* standardized response mean

[a]12-month follow-up

perceived handicap (MACTAR) and disability (SF-36 for physical function and PCS), and no correlation with anxiety (HADa), SF-36 MCS, depression (HADd), disease duration, and age [2]. Factor analysis extracted two factors that accounted for 71.6% of the total variance. The first factor represented mainly activities requiring grip and pinch strength and the second factor represented activities requiring pinch dexterity.

The CHFS has also been used as a location-specific disability scale for hand involvement in the determination of disability in SSc [2, 47]. When assessed separately, the CHFS score contributes to 75% of the HAQ variance [2]. The mean CHSF score was 16.56 ± 16.40 and 75% of the variance in the HAQ global score was explained. Significant differences were observed between patients with lcSSc and dSSc for *CHFS* (*11.07 ± 11.04* vs. *23.48 ± 19.45*) (*p = 0.01*) *and HAQ* (*0.90 ± 0.57* vs. *1.28 ± 0.75*) (*p = 0.05*) scores [2].

Cochin 17-Item Scleroderma Functional Scale (CSF-17)

SSc-specific activity limitations and participation restrictions can be evaluated with the CSF-17, a self-administered questionnaire that has been recently developed from 113 participants in the Scleroderma Patient-centered Intervention Network (SPIN) cohort [48]. The CSF-17 consists of 17 items concerning activities and participation; each question is scored on a scale of 0 (performed without limitations and/or restrictions) to 10 (impossible to perform). The total score is obtained by adding the scores of all items (range 0–170). Principal component analysis extracted two dimensions: 10 items related to mobility (CSF-17 section A, range 0–170) and seven items related to general tasks (CSF-17 section B, range 0–70). The CSF-17 has been validated in SSc [48].

The CSF-17 has a good convergent validity with global activity limitation scales (HAQ and sHAQ), hand- and mouth-specific activity limitation scales (CHFS and MHISS, respectively) patient's perceived handicap scale (MACTAR) and no correlation with anxiety (HADa), SF-12 MCS, and disease duration [48]. Factor analysis extracted two factors that accounted for *59%* and *11%* of the total variance, respectively. The first factor represented activities requiring mobility and the second factor represented general tasks.

The mean CSF-17 total score was 47.3 ± 18.5 of 170 points, the mean CSF-17 section A score was 29.8 ± 24.9 of 100 points, and the mean CSF-17 section B score was 17.9 ± 17.3 of 70 points. Significant differences were observed between patients with lcSSc and dSSc for CSF-17 total score and sections [2]. Estimates of patient acceptable symptom state thresholds calculated using the 75th percentile method were 31.0 (95% CI 18.5–37.0) for CSF-17 total score, 21.3 (95% CI 14.3–24.0) for section A and 9.3 (95% CI 5.0–12.0) for section B.

Keitel Functional Test

A German functional performance test, the Keitel Functional Test (KFT), has been developed for use in patients with RA. The KFT assesses 24 simple movement patterns for both upper and lower extremities. The 24 items are graded with a scoring system in which an index value of 100 points corresponds to normal functional ability. The test can be performed in 15–20 min and does not require any specific instrument [57]. This RA-specific measure of impairment of body functions has for several years been used by physical therapists in Denmark, for both inpatients in hospitals and outpatients in rehabilitation clinics, without prior validation. The KFT has been described as an outcome measure [58] and as a gold standard for evaluation of a new index of hand function [59]. It has been shown to have good concurrent validity [60], especially when used with the HAQ [61–63], and it has been reported to be a strong predictor of mortality [64]. To our knowledge, this score has not been used as is in patients with SSc. However, the hand functional index (HFI), which consists of the first nine questions of the KFT, might help to evaluate hand function in these patients [2].

Hand Functional Index (HFI)

The HFI consists of the first nine questions of the KFT which assesses finger and wrist flexion (four points for each hand) and extension (four points for each hand), forearm pronation and supination (three points for each forearm), and thumb abduction (three points for each thumb). The HFI score ranges from 4 (best mobility) to 42 (worst mobility). In a series of 50 patients with SSc, the HFI score was higher in patients with dSSc than in patients with lcSSc (19.35 ± 11.95 vs. 11.57 ± 8.21 ($p < 0.01$)) [2]. In this work, the correlation coefficient of the HFI with the CHFS was 0.58. This scale could be used by occupational and physical therapists for both inpatients in hospitals and outpatients in rehabilitation clinics in order to evaluate the effect of rehabilitation on hand function: finger and wrist flexion and extension, forearm pronation and supination, and thumb abduction. We have used this scale in a prospective randomized clinical trial conducted in 220 patients comparing supervised inhospital rehabilitation vs. outpatient rehabilitation. The results will be available at the end of 2011.

Kapandji Index

The Kapandji index assesses long-finger flexion (20 points for each hand) and extension (20 points for each hand) and thumb opposition (10 points for each thumb). The score ranges from 0 (worst mobility) to 100 (best mobility).

In patients with SSc, we have assessed global hand and wrist mobility by the use of the HFI and the Kapandji index [2]. In SSc patients, hand global mobility was reduced, with mean HFI and Kapandji scores of 15.08 ± 10.22 and 78.75 ± 19.94, respectively. Significant differences were observed between patients with lcSSc and dSSc for the Kapandji index which was higher in patients with dSSc than in patients with lcSSc (85.69 ± 15.50 vs. 70.00 ± 20.70 ($p < 0.01$)) [2]. In this work, the correlation coefficient of the Kapandji index with the CHFS was 0.63. Whether the HFI or the Kapandji scales will be the best scale to evaluate hand and wrist mobility in patients with SSc is not known. However, these two scales have been used in a prospective randomized clinical trial conducted in 220 patients comparing supervised inhospital rehabilitation vs. outpatient rehabilitation, the results of which will be available at the end of 2011.

Hand Mobility in Scleroderma (HAMIS)

The HAMIS is a hand function test developed for adult patients with SSc. It consists of nine items designed to measure all movements assessed in an ordinary range-of-motion-measured hand test (finger and wrist flexion and extension, thumb flexion and abduction, forearm pronation and supination). HAMIS has a demonstrated concurrent validity compared with range-of-motion and skin score. Except for the pronation and supination items, the other items on the HAMIS showed significant differences between healthy individuals and persons with SSc, attesting to the discriminating ability of the HAMIS [45]. HAMIS is a reliable instrument for evaluation of hand function on SSc patients [46]. However, in order to perform the HAMIS, a number of accessories are necessary, which is not the case for HFI or Kapandji scales. Therefore, there is a need for comparison of these three approaches for the evaluation of hand function in patients with SSc.

Disabilities of the Arm, Shoulder, and Hand (DASH)

The DASH was developed for patients with upper-extremity musculoskeletal conditions. It is a self-administered measure of symptoms and functional status, with a focus on physical function, used by clinicians in daily practice and as a research tool. The DASH consists mainly of a 30-item disability/symptom scale [65]. A short version of the DASH, the QuickDASH, has also been developed. This scale has been validated in a cohort of Hungarian patients with SSc [50]. In this study, the DASH and QuickDASH correlated strongly with the HAQ-DI and with the physical dimensions of the SF-36, providing evidence that the disability of the patient with SSc is predominantly caused by the functional impairment of the upper limb. The authors recommended the shorter and simpler QuickDASH for everyday clinical use [50]. Actually, it is difficult to get a definitive idea on the interest of the QuickDASH in patients with SSc. It would probably be of interest to use this scale as a secondary outcome measure in rehabilitation trials for the evaluation of functional impairment of the upper limb in patients with SSc.

Mouth Handicap in Systemic Sclerosis Scale (MHISS)

Mouth disability can be evaluated using the MHISS scale, a self-assessment questionnaire with 12 items concerning daily activities involving the face such as eating/drinking, speaking, oral hygiene, appearance, and condition of the mouth. Each question is scored on a scale of 0 (never) to 4 (always) [49]. The total score is obtained by adding the scores of all items (range 0–48). The mean total score obtained in a cohort of 71 SSc patients was 20.3 ± 9.7. Test–retest reliability was 0.96. Divergent validity was confirmed for global disability (Health Assessment Questionnaire [HAQ]), hand function (Cochin Hand Function Scale), interincisor distance, handicap (McMaster-Toronto Arthritis questionnaire [MACTAR]), depression (Hospital Anxiety and Depression [HAD]; HADd), and anxiety (HADa). The factor analysis extracted three factors with eigenvalues of 4.26, 1.76, and 1.47 explaining 63% of the variance. The first factor (five items) represents handicap induced by the reduction in mouth opening, the second (five items) handicap induced by sicca syndrome, and the third (three items) aesthetic concerns. In that study, the MHISS score contributed to 36% of the HAQ variance [33, 49], highlighting the need to specifically assess mouth disability in SSc patients when evaluating treatment. To our knowledge, this scale is the only available scale that allows to measure mouth disability in patients with SSc. The interest of this scale should be evaluated in rehabilitation trials.

Evaluation of Patient Priorities

Patients' priorities in disability can be assessed by use of a French version of the McMaster-Toronto Arthritis Patient Preference Disability Questionnaire (MACTAR) as described by Tugwell et al. [66]. The MACTAR questions are open ended and cover broad areas of function such as domestic care, self-care, professional activities, leisure activities, social interaction, and roles. Patients are encouraged to add activities not already listed. Patients are asked to rank these activities in order of importance by answering "Which of these activities would you most like to be able to do?" In patients with SSc, we used a "3-item priority function" and asked patients to identify and rank three situations among activities of daily living that caused them maximal trouble. In the original MACTAR, items were not scored, but patients were asked if they had noticed changes in the problem they had identified several weeks ago. In the validation study of the MACTAR, a Likert scale was added to quantify changes [67]. In order to reflect the degree of difficulty in performing a priority activity, each item was scored on an 11-point semiquantitative scale (0–10), the global score ranging from 0 (no disability) to 30 (maximal disability).

Mouthon and colleagues provided evidence that the MACTAR adds relevant information when assessing patients with SSc and has acceptable construct validity. Its weak correlation with HAQ and the large number of activities cited and ranked by patients suggests that it adds useful information about patients' perceived disability [68]. The evolution in the MACTAR global score over time for patients with SSc reflects a general feeling of deterioration over time. However, shifts in patient priorities are common and may influence the sensitivity to change of the instrument [69]. Thus, additional studies are needed to better define the usefulness of the MACTAR in prospective studies.

Rehabilitation

Rehabilitation therapies, such as occupational and physical therapy, are indicated for the person with SSc to improve joint motion, hand function, strength and general conditioning, and participation in daily activities such as self-care, home management, leisure, and work. Referral to therapy should be made early in the course of the disease especially in patients with early diffuse SSc. With disease progression, therapy referral should be made as soon as patients or physicians note decreases in joint motion and difficulty with daily tasks or work.

Hand Exercises

Because of the hand involvement and contractures observed in persons with scleroderma, range-of-motion exercises for the hand emphasize increasing flexion at the metacarpophalangeal joint, extension of the proximal interphalangeal joints, and flexion and abduction of the thumb. One study showed that total passive motion in each finger along with hand function improved after a 1-month program of stretching exercises for individual finger [4]; the changes improved or were maintained for up to 9 years [5]. Several other studies showed that hand mobility and strengthening exercises resulted in improved hand function, pinch, and metacarpophalangeal flexion [6, 8, 9] while another showed improvements in performance of specific daily tasks [7].

Heat modalities, such as paraffin wax or hot packs, may be used before commencing range-of-motion exercises to reduce pain and increase extensibility of collagen tissue. Heat is generally applied for 20 min followed by range-of-motion and stretching exercises. Each exercise is done one to two times a day and should be held in a position for stretch for 3–5 s and repeated three to five times as directed by a therapist. Several studies have evaluated the effectiveness of hand range-of-motion exercises in conjunction with paraffin wax treatments. These studies which have varied in research design, duration, and sample size generally found increased in hand motion, dexterity, and strength after treatment [11–13, 46]. However, two more recent randomized control trials did not show paraffin wax and hand exercise to have any additional benefit over hand exercise only [14] or lukewarm water and exercise [15].

Joint motion and stretching exercises (exaggerated facial movements, manual stretching of the mouth with the thumbs, and oral augmentation exercises with tongue depressors) have also been used to improve mouth opening [6, 22, 26, 70]. Two pretest-posttest design studies and two randomized controlled trials showed increases in mouth opening after stretching, augmentation exercises [22–24, 26]. In addition, one study reported subjective improvements in eating and speaking [23], while two studies showed improvements in some aspects of dental hygiene [24, 25]. In a separate study, a combination of connective tissue massage to the face, Kabat's technique (proprioceptive neuromuscular facilitation stretch and resistive techniques for the face), and face exercises (kinesitherapy) resulted in significant improvements in mouth opening and decreases in facial skin scores in the intervention group compared to a group who received a home exercise program for the mouth and face [27].

Splints are used to maintain or increase range-of-motion, particularly in the hand. Dynamic splints, which apply a constant force over a period of time to passively stretch a joint, were not shown to be effective in maintaining or improving extension of the proximal interphalangeal joint in persons with SSc [21] *and probably not recommended.* Neuromuscular taping or kinesio taping provides passive stretch through eccentric application of elastic, adhesive tape to the skin. One study applied tape on both palmar and dorsal surfaces of the hand in a distal to proximal direction. The study reported improvements for hand function, motion, pain and a decrease in frequency of Raynaud occurrences [20].

Massage has been investigated in several studies in combination with very different types of rehabilitation interventions. Connective tissue massage in conjunction with Mc Mennell joint manipulation and a home exercise program resulted in significant improvements in fist closure, hand function, and quality of life compared to a control group who received a home exercise program [27]. Thai massage along with stretching and heat improved joint motion; when combined with a nylon glove, the intervention also increased thumb motion [17]. Soft tissue mobilization in combination with thermal modalities and hand exercises resulted in improvements in grip strength, hand function and functional ability but the improvements were not significantly different from changes observed in a control group [18]. In another study, tissue mobilization delivered via a negative pressure device (LymphaTouch) in combination with thermal modalities and hand exercises resulted in improvements in hand function and physical function [19].

While studies have shown that joint motion in the lower extremities is decreased in persons with SSc, there are no studies that have focused solely on interventions to improve joint motion for the lower extremities. The few studies listed in the next section show improvements in mobility such as walking, after conditioning exercises involving the lower extremities such as treadmill walking, riding a stationary bike, and aerobic exercises.

Strengthening and General Exercise and Conditioning

Strengthening and general conditioning exercises are indicated for the person with SSc to improve cardiovascular fitness. Resistive exercises using weights, elastic bands, exercise putty, and/or exercise machines can be used to increase muscle strength. General conditioning exercises could include water exercise, swimming, walking, cycling, or other aerobic exercises. It has only been recently that the effectiveness of multidisciplinary exercise and conditioning programs was evaluated. A 9-week program combining hand- and face-specific exercises, a global water- or land-based exercise program, showed improvements in hand and face motion, hand and overall function, and quality of life compared to a control group [16]. Another study evaluated the effectiveness of a multidisciplinary program consisting primarily of physical and occupational therapy that included dexterity, stretching, strengthening and aerobic exercises and splints and adaptive devices. The 4-week program followed by home sessions resulted in short-term effects at 1 month for hand function, mobility, pain and HAQ scores but no group differences at 12 months [29]. A slightly different multidisciplinary program involving group and individually tailored exercises in combination with group education and individualized goal setting was shown to be more effective than usual care in improving grip strength, mouth opening, distance walked, and function ability [28].

Antonioli et al. [71] evaluated the effectiveness of an individualized program consisting of breathing exercises, treadmill- and land-based walking, and upper-extremity exercises including stretching. At the end of 4 months, improvements were noted in quality of life and hand mobility, and decreases seen in heart rate and dyspnea after performing the 6-min walk test. A more recent trial evaluating the effectiveness of a similar program that was home based, reported improvements for the 6-min walk test, hand, strength in select muscles, and HAQ and SF-36 scores compared to controls [35]. A series of single-case studies using a combination of aerobic exercise and proximal muscle resistance training reported improvements in muscular endurance and aerobic capacity [32]. Similar protocols involving resistive exercises for the upper and/or lower extremity musculature combined with aerobic exercises only included patients with limited SSc [33; 34]. These studies found increases in peak oxygen uptake, endothelial-dependent vasodilation, life satisfaction, enjoyment and less pain and anxiety [33; 34].

The effectiveness of an 8-week aerobic exercise program was evaluated in a group of 12 women with SSc but without lung involvement [30]. Sessions were for 40 min two times per week; each session consisted of a 5-min warm-up, aerobic exercise that was progressively increased until target heart rate was reached, followed by a 5-min cooldown. Improvements were seen in peak VO_2 and exercise intensity, but the improvements were not significantly different compared to a control group. However, a second study combining aerobic training along with a strengthening program reported improved muscle strength, function (timed-stands test),, and aerobic capacity in persons with SSc without lung involvement (pulmonary artery systolic pressure > 40 mmHg and forced vital capacity measured >75% of predicted value for age and gender). There were no significant changes in peak VO_2 or serum markers for muscle damage (CK, aldolase). Thus, these studies showed that aerobic exercise is safe in persons with SSc without lung involvement; those with lung involvement should probably get evaluated by their physicians and be monitored initially by a physical therapist or exercise physiologist.

Occupational Therapy

One study examined the effectiveness of occupational therapy only. The program consisted of six 90 min meetings over 3 weeks and consisted of strategies and devices to protect the joints and improve performance of specific activities of daily living. At the 6-mo follow-up, significant improvements on the HAQ and EDAQE were observed in the occupational therapy group compared to a control group [36].

Self-Management Programs

Management of a complex chronic disease such as SSc requires that the person with the disease become a manager of symptoms and all aspects of treatment. Because SSc is a rare disease and the symptoms are very different from other rheumatic diseases, several disease-specific self-management programs have been developed. These programs were offered in a group format in which participants met for 3 h once a week for 4–5 weeks [37, 47]. Participants reported increases in perceived self-efficacy and confidence to manage the disease and were satisfied with content. However, the sample sizes were small in these studies so statistical analyses were not preformed (12 in Brown et al. [38]; 6 in Sandqvist [72]). Kwakkenbos and colleagues [40] reported less helplessness and higher acceptance of limitations in a group of people with SSc who participated in a psychoeducation program delivered via group format. The content included disease education, goal setting, joint protection and energy conservation, and managing psychosocial aspects of SSc. Due to the challenges of participating in group sessions, a self-management program, consisting of a workbook and exercise DVD, was developed to reach persons who did not have access to support groups or education programs. Modeled after concepts used in the Arthritis Self-Management Programs, the workbook had action plans and learning activities at the end of each chapter. While improvements in fatigue, hand function, and pain were observed, the only significant improvement was for self-efficacy for managing pain [73]. A subsequent study which converted the content to an interactive Internet format (TOSS: Taking charge of systemic sclerosis) found significant improvements in the ability to manage care, health efficacy, and decreases in fatigue and depression [41]. However, a large randomized control trial compared TOSS to an educational book condition did not find significant improvements or significant differences between groups for self-efficacy, depression, physical function, patient activation, or quality of life [42]. Self-management offerings that can be accessed remotely need to be explored further using a more individualized approach as individually tailored self-management programs which incorporate goal setting have been shown to be effective.

Finally, rehabilitation professionals have expertise in non-pharmaceutical modalities to manage digital ulcers. Moran et al. [74] systematically reviewed studies using modalities including intermittent compression, topical vitamin E, hyperbaric oxygen therapy, negative pressure therapy, acoustic pressure wound therapy, exercise, and iontophoresis. However, no one modality was better than others; although vitamin E gel and iontophoresis may warrant more investigation with large sample sizes and better designed and controlled studies.

Conclusions

SSc is responsible for skin, tendon, joint, and vessel damage, which leads to disability, handicap, and worsening of quality of life [1–3]. A number of assessments are available to measure disability and participation in persons with SSc. These assessments offer the opportunity to examine and monitor joint motion, hand function, mouth disability, strength, general conditioning, and participation in daily life.

The current literature on rehabilitation techniques consists of studies evaluating the effectiveness of paraffin wax treatment, hand and face stretching exercises, connective tissue massage and joint manipulation, splints, and aerobic exercise and resistance training (for a review, see [73]). Only a small number of randomized controlled trials were identified, and the majority of studies involved small sample sizes and no control groups. However, improvement in joint motion, hand function, and cardiopulmonary endurance was clear upon analysis of the results. Hand exercises seem to offer a benefit in patients with SSc.

Based on the limited number of studies available conducted in limited numbers of patients, physical and occupational therapy might increase and maintain mobility and strength and improve functional mobility and cardiopulmonary functioning. Table 45.3 provides guidelines/recommendations for rehabilitation interventions.

Table 45.3 Guidelines/recommendations for rehabilitation interventions

Limitation	Examples of interventions
Decreased ability to fully flex and extend fingers (i.e., palm of hand does not lay flat on a table)	Modalities before exercises:
	1. Paraffin
	2. Connective tissue massage/tissue mobilization
	3. Joint manipulation
	Hand exercises:
	1. Make a fist, push down on proximal phalanx
	2. Press fingers flat against table so palmer surface of hand and fingers touch table
	3. Press fingers against each other in a prayer position
	4. Touch thumb to bottom of little finger
	5. Pads of index finger and thumb of one hand against pads of index finger and thumb of other hand; attempt to stretch web space
Difficulty reaching to wash/comb hair	Shoulder exercises:
	1. Wall fingers up a wall
	2. Lie supine and flex shoulders overhead
	3. Stretching exercises to other upper-extremity joints
	4. Strengthening exercises to upper extremities with weights, elastic bands, or machines
	Assistive devices or alternate techniques:
	1. Long-handled sponge
	2. Long-handled comb or brush
Difficulty opening mouth (difficulty to brush and floss teeth or eat)	Mouth and face exercises:
	1. Exaggerated facial movements
	2. Manual stretching of mouth with the thumbs
	3. Oral augmentation exercises
	4. Massage to facial muscles
	Assistive devices or modified oral appliances:
	1. Child toothbrushes/electric
	2. Electric flossers and water pix
Difficulty reaching to tie shoes or cut toenails	Lower extremity stretching:
	1. Hamstring stretch
	2. Cross leg with ankle of one leg above knee of other (external rotation of hip)
	3. Yoga
	Assistive devices or alternate technique:
	1. Slip on/Velcro shoes
	2. Reachers

(continued)

Table 45.3 (continued)

Limitation	Examples of interventions
Difficulty walking	Strengthening and conditioning exercises:
	1. Land based—Walking, treadmill walking, cycling, aerobics
	2. Water based—Water exercises, swimming
	3. Yoga
	Resistive exercise—Weights, elastic bands, machines:
	1. Knee extension with weights on ankles for quadriceps
	2. Sit to stand without using arms for quadriceps, hamstrings, and gluteal muscles
	3. Stand on toes for gastrocnemius muscles
	4. Exercise machines for isolated lower extremity muscles
	Assistive walking devices:
	1. Walker, cane, wheelchair
	2. Electric wheelchair, scooter
Difficulty using hands to perform daily activities	Hand exercises:
	1. See above
	2. Resistive exercises with exercise putty
	Assistive devices or alternate techniques:
	1. Built up handles on utensils
	2. Stemmed glasses
	3. Electrical appliances such as choppers
	4. Headsets/ear buds for phone, voice programs for computer and phones, touch screens
Fatigue upon doing daily activities	Education on energy conservation:
	1. Pace – Alternate activity and rest
	2. Prioritize activities
	3. Plan in advance
	4. Alternate position between sit and stand
	Strengthening and conditioning exercises and physical activity
	1. See above under walking
	Assistive devices or alternate techniques:
	1. Electrical appliances
	2. Ergonomic tools
	3. Ergonomic setups at home and work
	4. Support from family, friends, or hired help

References

1. Poole JL, Steen VD. The use of the health assessment questionnaire (HAQ) to determine physical disability in systemic sclerosis. Arthritis Care Res. 1991;4(1):27–31.
2. Rannou F, Poiraudeau S, Berezné A, Baubet T, Le-Guern V, Cabane J, et al. Assessing disability and quality of life in systemic sclerosis: construct validities of the Cochin hand function scale, health assessment questionnaire (HAQ), systemic sclerosis HAQ, and MOS SF-36. Arthritis Rheum. 2007;57(1):94–102.
3. Hudson M, Thombs BD, Steele R, Watterson R, Taillefer S, Baron M. Clinical correlates of quality of life in systemic sclerosis measured with the world health organization disability assessment schedule II. Arthritis Rheum. 2008;59(2):279–84.
4. Mugii N, Hasegawa M, Matsushita T, Kondo M, Orito H, Yanaba K, et al. The efficacy of self-administered stretching for finger joint motion in Japanese patients with systemic sclerosis. J Rheumatol. 2006;33(8):1586–92.
5. Mugii N, Matsushita T, Oohata S, Okita H, Yahata T, et al. Long-term follow-up of finger passive range of motion in Japanese systemic sclerosis patients treated with self-administered stretching. Modern Rheumatol. 2019;29(3):484–90.
6. Piga M, Tradori I, Pani D, Barabino G, Dessi A, et al. J Rheumatol. 2014;41:1324–33.
7. Stefanantoni K, Sciarra I, Iannace N, Vasile M, Caucci M, Sili Scavalli A, Massimiani MP, Passi L, Maset L, Riccieri V. Occupational therapy integrated with a self-administered stretching program on systemic sclerosis patients with hand involvement. Clin Exp Rheumatol. 2016;34(100):S157–61.
8. Landim S, Bertolo M, Marcatto de Abreu MF, del Rio A, Leme Mazon CC, Marques Neto JF, Poole JL, Magalhães E. "Hands on": a hand care guide in systemic sclerosis. J Hand Ther. 2019;32:313–21.
9. Landim S, Bértolo MR, del Rio A, Sachetto Z, Gaino J, Poole JL, Magalhães E. Sustained efficacy of a concise self-management program for hands in systemic sclerosis—a longitudinal case control observational study. Rheumatology. 2020;59: 3330–9.
10. Askew LJ, Beckett VL, An KN, Chao EY. Objective evaluation of hand function in scleroderma patients to assess effectiveness of physical therapy. Br J Rheumatol. 1983;22(4):224–32.
11. Pils K, Graninger W, Sadil F. Paraffin hand bath for scleroderma. Phys Med Rehabil. 1991;1:19–21.
12. Sandqvist G, Akesson A, Eklund M. Evaluation of paraffin bath treatment in patients with systemic sclerosis. Disabil Rehabil. 2004;26(16):981–7.
13. Mancuso T, Poole JL. The effect of paraffin and exercise on hand function in persons with scleroderma: a series of single case studies. J Hand Ther. 2009;22(1):71–7.

14. Gregory WJ, Willkinson J, Herrick AL. A randomised controlled trial of wax baths as an additive therapy to hand exercises in patients with systemic sclerosis. Physiotherapy. 2019;105:370–7.
15. Kristensen LQ, Oestergaard LG, Bovbjerg K, Rolving N, Sandergaard K. Use of paraffin instead of lukewarm water prior to hand exercises had no additional effect on hand mobility in patients with systemic sclerosis: a randomized control clinical trial. Hand Ther. 2019;24:13–21.
16. Maddali Bongi S, Del Rosso A, Galluccio F, Tai G, Sigismondi F, Passalacqua M, et al. Efficacy of a tailored rehabilitation program for systemic sclerosis. Clin Exp Rheumatol. 2009;27(3 Suppl. 54):44–50.
17. Vannajak K, Boonprakob Y, Eungpinichpong W, Ungpansattawong S, Nanagara T. The short term effect of gloving in combination with traditional Thai massage, heat, and stretching exercise to improve hand mobility in scleroderma patients. J Ayurveda Integr Med. 2014;5:505–55.
18. Horvath J, Balint Z, Szep E, Deiszinger A, Minier T, et al. Efficacy of intensive hand physical therapy in patients with systemic sclerosis. Clin Exp Rheumatol. 2017;35(Suppl. 106):S159–66.
19. Murphy SL, Barber MW, Homer K, Dodge C, Cutter CR, Khanna D. Occupational therapy treatment to improve upper extremity function in individuals with early systemic sclerosis: a pilot study. Arthritis Care Res. 2018;70:1653–60.
20. Parisi S, Celletti C, Scarati M, Prioa M, et al. Neuromuscular taking enhances hand function in patients with systemic sclerosis: a pilot study. Clin Ter. 2017;168:e371–5.
21. Seeger MW, Furst DE. Effects of splinting in the treatment of hand contractures in progressive systemic sclerosis. Am J Occup Ther. 1987;41(2):118–21.
22. Naylor WP, Douglass CW, Mix E. The nonsurgical treatment of microstomia in scleroderma: a pilot study. Oral Surg Oral Med Oral Pathol. 1984;57(5):508–11.
23. Pizzo G, Scardina GA, Messina P. Effects of a nonsurgical exercise program on the decreased mouth opening in patients with systemic scleroderma. Clin Oral Investig. 2003;7(3):175–8.
24. Poole J, Conte C, Brewer C, Good CC, Perella D, Rossie KM, et al. Oral hygiene in scleroderma: the effectiveness of a multi-disciplinary intervention program. Disabil Rehabil. 2010;32(5):379–84.
25. Yuen HK, Weng Y, Bandyopadhyay D, Reed SG, Leite RS, Silver RM. Effect of a multi-faceted intervention on gingival health among adults with systemic sclerosis. Clin Exp Rheumatol. 2011;29(Suppl. 65):S26–32.
26. Yuen HK, Marlow NM, Reed SG, Mahoney S, Summerlin LM, et al. Effect of orofacial exercises on oral aperture in adults with systemic sclerosis. Disabil Rehabil. 2012;34:84–9.
27. Maddali Bongi S, Landi G, Galluccio F, Del Rosso A, Miniati I, Conforti ML, et al. The rehabilitation of facial involvement in systemic sclerosis: efficacy of the combination of connective tissue massage, Kabat's technique and kinesitherapy: a randomized controlled trial. Rheumatol Int. 2010;31(7):895–901.
28. Schouffoer AA, Ninaber MK, Beaart-van de Voorde LJ, van der Giesen FJ, de Jong Z, Stolk J, et al. A randomised comparison of a multidisciplinary team care program with usual care in patients with systemic sclerosis. Arthritis Care Res (Hoboken). 2011;63(6):909–17.
29. Rannou F, Boutron I, Mouthon L, Sanchez K, Tiffreau V, et al. Personalized physical therapy versus usual care for patients with systemic sclerosis: a randomized controlled trial. Arthritis Care Res. 2017;69:1050–9.
30. Oliveira NC, dos Santos Sabbag LM, de Sa Pinto AL, Borges CL, Lima FR. Aerobic exercise is safe and effective in systemic sclerosis. Int J Sports Med. 2009;30(10):728–32.
31. Pinto AL, Oliveira NC, Gualano B, Christmann RB, Painelli VS, Artioli GG, et al. Efficacy and safety of concurrent training in systemic sclerosis. J Strength Cond Res. 2010;25(5):1423–8.
32. Alexanderson H, Bergegard J, Bjornadal L, Nordin A. Intensive aerobic and muscle endurance exercise in patients with systemic sclerosis; a pilot study. BMC Res Notes. 2014;7:86.
33. Mitropoulos A, Grumber A, Crank H, Akil M, Klonizakis M. The effects of upper and lower limb exercise on the microvascular reactivity in limited cutaneous systemic sclerosis. Arthritis Res Ther. 2018;20:112.
34. Mitropoulos A, Grumber A, Crank H, Akil M, Klonizakis M. Exploring the feasibility of an exercise programme including aerobic and resistance training in people with limited cutaneous systemic sclerosis. Clin Rheumatol. 2020;39:1889–98.
35. Filippetti M, Cazzoletti L, Zamboni F, Ferrari P, et al. Effect of a tailored home-based exercise program in patients with systemic sclerosis: a randomized controlled trial. Scand J Med Sci Sports. 2020;30:1675–84.
36. Zanatta E, Rodeghiero F, Pigatto E, Galozzi P, et al. Long-term improvement in activities of daily living in women with systemic sclerosis attending occupational therapy. Br J Occup Ther. 2017;80:417–22.
37. Samuelson UK, Ahlmen EM. Development and evaluation of a patient education program for persons with systemic sclerosis (scleroderma). Arthritis Care Res. 2000;13(3):141–8.
38. Brown SJ, Somerset ME, McCabe CS, McHugh NJ. The impact of group education on participants' management of their disease in lupus and scleroderma. Musculoskelet Care. 2004;2(4):207–17.
39. Poole J, Mendelson C, Skipper B. The effectiveness of a scleroderma self management program delivered via booklet and DVD. Arthritis Rheum. 2013;32:1393–8.
40. Kwakkenbos L, Bluyssen SJM, Vonk MC, van Helmond AF, van den Ende CHM, van den Hoogen FHJ, et al. Addressing patient health care demands in systemic sclerosis: pre-post assessment of a psycho-educational group programme. Clin Exp Rheumatol. 2011;29(Suppl. 65):S60–5.
41. Poole JL, Mendelson C, Skipper B, Khanna D. Taking charge of systemic sclerosis: a pilot study to assess the effectiveness of an internet self-management program. Arthritis Care Res. 2014;66(50):778–82.
42. Khanna D, Serrano J, Berrocal V, Silver RM, Cuencas P, Newbill S, Battyany J, Maxwell C, Alore M, Dyas L, Riggs R, Connolly K, Kellner S, Fisher J, Bush E, Sachdeva A, Evnin L, Raisch DW, Poole JL. A randomized controlled trial to evaluate an internet-based self-management program in systemic sclerosis. Arthritis Care Res. 2019;3:435–47.
43. Poole JL, William CA, Bloch DA, Hollak B, Spitz P. Concurrent validity of the health assessment questionnaire disability index in scleroderma. Arthritis Care Res. 1995;8(3):189–93.
44. Steen VD, Medsger TA. The value of the health assessment questionnaire and special patient-generated scales to demonstrate change in systemic sclerosis patients over time. Arthritis Rheum. 1997;40(11):1984–91.
45. Sandqvist G, Eklund M. Validity of HAMIS: a test of hand mobility in scleroderma. Arthritis Care Res. 2000;13(6):382–7.
46. Sandqvist G, Eklund M. Hand mobility in scleroderma (HAMIS) test: the reliability of a novel hand function test. Arthritis Care Res. 2000;13(6):369–74.
47. Brower LM, Poole JL. Reliability and validity of the Duruoz hand index in persons with systemic sclerosis (scleroderma). Arthritis Rheum. 2004;51(5):805–9.
48. Daste C, Abdoul H, Foissac F, Papelard A, Alami S, Kwakkenbos L, Carrier ME, Lefèvre-Colau MM, Thombs BD, Poiraudeau S, Rannou F, Mouthon L, Nguyen C. Development of a new patient-reported outcome measure to assess activities and participation in people with systemic sclerosis: the Cochin 17-item scleroderma functional scale. Br J Dermatol. 2020;183(4):710–8.
49. Mouthon L, Rannou F, Berezne A, Pagnoux C, Arene JP, Fois E, et al. Development and validation of a scale for mouth handicap in

systemic sclerosis: the mouth handicap in systemic sclerosis scale. Ann Rheum Dis. 2007;66(12):1651–5.
50. Varju C, Balint Z, Solyom AI, Farkas H, Karpati E, Berta B, et al. Cross-cultural adaptation of the disabilities of the arm, shoulder, and hand (DASH) questionnaire into Hungarian and investigation of its validity in patients with systemic sclerosis. Clin Exp Rheumatol. 2008;26(5):776–83.
51. Merkel PA, Herlyn K, Martin RW, Anderson JJ, Mayes MD, Bell P, et al. Measuring disease activity and functional status in patients with scleroderma and Raynaud's phenomenon. Arthritis Rheum. 2002;46(9):2410–20.
52. Clements PJ, Wong WK, Hurwitz EL, Furst DE, Mayes M, White B, et al. The disability index of the health assessment questionnaire is a predictor and correlate of outcome in the high-dose versus low-dose penicillamine in systemic sclerosis trial. Arthritis Rheum. 2001;44(3):653–61.
53. Khanna D, Furst DE, Clements PJ, Park GS, Hays RD, Yoon J, et al. Responsiveness of the SF-36 and the health assessment questionnaire disability index in a systemic sclerosis clinical trial. J Rheumatol. 2005;32(5):832–40.
54. Duruoz MT, Poiraudeau S, Fermanian J, Menkes CJ, Amor B, Dougados M, et al. Development and validation of a rheumatoid hand functional disability scale that assesses functional handicap. J Rheumatol. 1996;23(7):1167–72.
55. Poiraudeau S, Lefevre-Colau MM, Fermanian J, Revel M. The ability of the Cochin rheumatoid arthritis hand functional scale to detect change during the course of disease. Arthritis Care Res. 2000;13(5):296–303.
56. Poiraudeau S, Chevalier X, Conrozier T, Flippo RM, Liote F, Noel E, et al. Reliability, validity, and sensitivity to change of the Cochin hand functional disability scale in hand osteoarthritis. Osteoarthr Cartil. 2001;9(6):570–7.
57. Keitel W, Hoffman H, Weber G, Krieger U. Development of a arm functional test for rheumatologic diseases. Dtsch Gesundheitsw. 1971;26:1901–3.
58. Keysser M, Keysser C, Keitel W, Keysser G. Loss of functional capacity caused by a delayed onset of DMARD therapy in rheumatoid arthritis. Long-term follow-up results of the Keitel function test. Brief definite report. Z Rheumatol. 2001;60(2):69–73.
59. Poole JL, Cordova KJ, Brower LM. Reliability and validity of a self-report of hand function in persons with rheumatoid arthritis. J Hand Ther. 2006;19(1):12–6. quiz 17
60. Kalla AA, Kotze TJ, Meyers OL, Parkyn ND. Clinical assessment of disease activity in rheumatoid arthritis: evaluation of a functional test. Ann Rheum Dis. 1988;47(9):773–9.
61. Bombardier C, Raboud J. A comparison of health-related quality-of-life measures for rheumatoid arthritis research. The auranofin cooperating group. Control Clin Trials. 1991;12(Suppl. 4):243S–56.
62. Hakala M, Nieminen P, Manelius J. Joint impairment is strongly correlated with disability measured by self-report questionnaires. Functional status assessment of individuals with rheumatoid arthritis in a population based series. J Rheumatol. 1994;21(1):64–9.
63. Hakala M, Nieminen P. Functional status assessment of physical impairment in a community based population with rheumatoid arthritis: severely incapacitated patients are rare. J Rheumatol. 1996;23(4):617–23.
64. Soderlin MK, Nieminen P, Hakala M. Arthritis impact measurement scales in a community-based rheumatoid arthritis population. Clin Rheumatol. 2000;19(1):30–4.
65. Hudak PL, Cole DC, Haines AT. Understanding prognosis to improve rehabilitation: the example of lateral elbow pain. Arch Phys Med Rehabil. 1996;77(6):586–93.
66. Tugwell P, Bombardier C, Buchanan WW, Goldsmith CH, Grace E, Hanna B. The MACTAR patient preference disability questionnaire–an individualized functional priority approach for assessing improvement in physical disability in clinical trials in rheumatoid arthritis. J Rheumatol. 1987;14(3):446–51.
67. Verhoeven AC, Boers M, van der Liden S. Validity of the MACTAR questionnaire as a functional index in a rheumatoid arthritis clinical trial. McMaster Tor Arthritis J Rheumatol. 2000;27(12):2801–9.
68. Mouthon L, Rannou F, Berezne A, Pagnoux C, Guilpain P, Goldwasser F, et al. Patient preference disability questionnaire in systemic sclerosis: a cross-sectional survey. Arthritis Rheum. 2008;59(7):968–73.
69. Nguyen C, Mouthon L, Mestre-Stanislas C, Rannou F, Berezne A, Sanchez K, et al. Sensitivity to change in systemic sclerosis of the McMaster-Toronto arthritis patient preference disability questionnaire (MACTAR): shift in patient priorities over time. J Rheumatol. 2010;37(2):359–64.
70. Naylor WP. Oral management of the scleroderma patient. J Am Dent Assoc. 1982;105(5):814–7.
71. Antonioli CM, Bua G, Frige A, Prandini K, Radici S, Scarsi M, et al. An individualized rehabilitation program in patients with systemic sclerosis may improve quality of life and hand mobility. Clin Rheumatol. 2009;28(2):159–65.
72. Sandqvist G, Eklund M, Akesson A, Nordenskiold U. Daily activities and hand function in women with scleroderma. Scand J Rheumatol. 2004;33(2):102–7.
73. Poole JL. Musculoskeletal rehabilitation in the person with scleroderma. Curr Opin Rheumatol. 2010;22(2):205–12.
74. Moran ME. Scleroderma and evidence based non-pharmaceutical treatment modalities for digital ulcers: a systematic review. J Wound Care. 2014;23:510–6.

Psychosocial Issues and Care for Patients with Systemic Sclerosis

46

Brett D. Thombs and Linda Kwakkenbos

People living with chronic medical conditions face challenges not only with respect to their physical health, but also to their emotional and social well-being. Chronic conditions, such as systemic sclerosis (SSc, or scleroderma), often result in significant disruptions to activities of daily living, including employment and homecare, as well as social and leisure activities, and can lead to reduced health-related quality of life (HRQL). Therefore, it is important to identify factors associated with decreased HRQL and psychosocial functioning in SSc and to develop and implement strategies to help individuals with the disease manage these problems. Traditionally, there has been little research on patient-reported outcomes in SSc, and this has posed a significant clinical challenge to the field. However, recent research has highlighted important problems that have an influence on HRQL for many people living with SSc, including depression, anxiety and fear of disease progression, fatigue and sleep problems, pain, pruritus (itch), body image distress, and sexual dysfunction [1–3].

B. D. Thombs (✉)
Lady Davis Institute for Medical Research, Jewish General Hospital, Montréal, QC, Canada

Department of Psychiatry, McGill University, Montréal, QC, Canada

Department of Epidemiology, Biostatistics, and Occupational Health, McGill University, Montréal, QC, Canada

Department of Medicine, McGill University, Montréal, QC, Canada

Department of Psychology, McGill University, Montréal, QC, Canada
e-mail: brett.thombs@mcgill.ca

L. Kwakkenbos
Department of Clinical Psychology, Radboud University, Nijmegen, The Netherlands

Department of IQ Health Care, Radboud University Medical Center, Nijmegen, The Netherlands

Department of Psychiatry, Radboud University Medical Center, Nijmegen, The Netherlands
e-mail: linda.kwakkenbos@ru.nl

Depression

Depression is characterized by sadness, loss of interest or pleasure, feelings of guilt or low self-esteem, poor concentration, and disturbed sleep or appetite. The rate of major depressive disorder (MDD) among patients living with one or more chronic conditions is often reported to be as high as 15–20% [4], which is substantially greater than the approximate 5% in the general population [5] and the estimated 5–10% in primary care settings [6]. MDD and sub-threshold levels of psychological distress among patients with chronic conditions can impact physical health through biological pathways, including immune system dysfunction and inflammation, as well as through behaviors, such as poor adherence to medical treatment regimens and a reduced likelihood of adopting health-promoting lifestyles [1].

In SSc, a study from France used the Mini International Neuropsychiatric Interview (MINI) in a sample of 50 hospitalized and 50 outpatients to assess the prevalence of depression, and the authors reported rates of 19% for current and 56% for lifetime MDD [7]. SSc patients who were hospitalized had higher rates of a current major depressive episode (28%) than those who were not hospitalized (10%) [7]. In a sample of 345 SSc patients from the Canadian Scleroderma Research Group (CSRG) Registry using the Composite International Diagnostic Interview (CIDI), rates of MDD were 4% for current (30-day), 11% for 12-month, and 23% for lifetime [8]. These prevalence rates were approximately twice that of the Canadian general population, as well as higher than rates reported among patients with arthritis [8]. They were lower, however, than the rates reported from France. One possible explanation for the difference in the reported rates between the French and Canadian studies is that the MINI constitutes a brief measure, originally described by its developers as a screening interview and intended to be over-inclusive [9], rather than a comprehensive evaluation as is accomplished with the CIDI. Specifically, the MINI does not query whether symptoms of depression cause functional impairment, which

Y. Allanore et al. (eds.), *Scleroderma*, https://doi.org/10.1007/978-3-031-40658-4_46

could potentially result in higher rates than those reported from other diagnostic interviews, such as the CIDI. An independent participant data meta-analysis that included 69,405 participants (7574 [11%] with MDD) from 212 different studies found that the adjusted odds ratio of MDD diagnosis was twice as high for the MINI compared to the CIDI [10].

MDD is a serious mental health condition. Many SSc patients who meet criteria for MDD, however, may have mild to moderate MDD, and their symptoms may fluctuate with time. In the Canadian study, for instance, only three of 12 patients with MDD at baseline still met diagnostic criteria for MDD one month later [11]. These results are consistent with findings from a qualitative study where 16 women with SSc were interviewed about their emotional distress [12]. Interviewed women described their distress related to SSc as distinct from the clinical diagnosis of depression and noted that their symptoms were worse in the period directly following their SSc diagnosis [12]. Given these findings, active monitoring, or watchful waiting may be a good strategy for SSc patients with mild depression in order to avoid unnecessary treatment for those who experience transient symptoms that may resolve without a specific intervention.

Many studies have reported high rates of scores above cut-off thresholds on self-report measures of depressive symptoms [13], although the rates reported using these tools vary widely depending on the specific measure and cut-off that is used. For instance, one study of 566 CSRG Registry patients found that 34% of patients scored above a standard cut-off on the 20-item Center for Epidemiologic Studies Depression Scale (CES-D), but only 21% of the same patients exceeded the designated cut-off on the 9-item Patient Health Questionnaire (PHQ-9) [14]. Cut-offs on symptom questionnaires are designed to identify a pool of patients potentially at risk for depression, but do not assess whether any particular patient meets full diagnostic criteria for a mental health condition, such as MDD. They are also not valid proxies for clinical significance. As such, when assessing MDD, standardized clinical interviews are recommended as methods of evaluation [15].

A number of studies have examined factors associated with depressive symptoms in SSc. Cross-sectional studies have reported that both sociodemographic factors, such as being unmarried and having less education, as well as disease variables, including more tender joints and breathing and gastrointestinal problems, are associated with higher depression symptom scores [14, 16]. Other studies have documented that factors such as overall disease severity, disability, body image, pain, sexual function, disease-related cognitions, social support, and resilience are related to mental health functioning in SSc [13].

Anxiety

Few studies have assessed anxiety and the presence of anxiety disorders among persons living with SSc, and of those conducted, samples sizes were small and researchers often made use of self-report questionnaires [17–20]. One French study of 100 SSc patients reported that 49% of their sample had at least one current anxiety disorder, and that 64% of patients met criteria for one lifetime anxiety disorder based on the MINI [7]. Estimates were similar among hospitalized and outpatients and were higher than those found among a general sample of the French population; however, risk for anxiety disorders was not associated with SSc disease severity [7]. Anxiety has not been reported to relate to other common correlates of SSc, including organ involvement or functional impairment [18].

Given that the course of SSc is highly unpredictable, patients may perceive the future as uncertain. As such, for patients, worry about the future, including fear of disease progression, fear of becoming physically disabled, and fear of being dependent upon others are important sources of stress [21, 22]. Because SSc is associated with serious consequences in many patients, these concerns are realistic and in themselves do not represent anxiety disorders, for which irrational fear is typically a key component. Nonetheless, fear of progression can impact HRQL substantially. In a cross-sectional study of 215 SSc patients from the Netherlands, for instance, fear of progression was highly associated with symptoms of depression [22].

Fatigue and Sleep

Fatigue is one of the most significant factors affecting HRQL across many chronic diseases, including SSc [2, 23]. In a large cohort of Canadian patients with SSc, 89% reported fatigue at least some of the time and 72% described that fatigue had a moderate to severe impact on the ability to carry out daily activities [24]. Similarly, a survey across five European countries found that between 76% and 96% of patients in each country, fatigue is reported at least some of the time, and 63–94% reported moderate to severe impact [25]. Systematic reviews have concluded that fatigue ratings from SSc patients are similar to scores from patients with other rheumatic diseases and cancer patients currently undergoing treatment, and higher than scores from general population samples and cancer patients in remission [26, 27]. Factors that may be associated with greater fatigue in patients with SSc include diffuse disease subtype, breathing problems, severity of gastrointestinal problems, pain, functional disability, education level, and sleep quality [28–35].

While there is little research on sleep in SSc, sleep disturbances among people with the disease appear to be higher than in the general population [36–38]. Studies have reported that sleep may be associated with depression, pain, fatigue, and esophageal and gastrointestinal involvement [36–38].

Pain

Between 60–83% of SSc patients experience pain, which is comparable to rates found in other chronic pain conditions and rheumatic diseases [39]. Potential sources of pain vary widely in SSc, and include pain associated with Raynaud's phenomenon; musculoskeletal pain; pain in distal extremities due to skin tightness, calcinosis, and ulcers; and gastrointestinal problems [1]. Pain ratings are higher among patients with diffuse SSc compared to patients with limited disease, although the difference is generally small [39]. In both cross-sectional and longitudinal studies, pain in SSc has been independently associated with physical function, activity, work disability, sleep problems, fatigue, depressive symptoms, and reduced HRQL [28, 30, 33, 34, 36–43].

Pruritus

Pruritus, or itch, is described as a "poorly localized, non-adapting, usually unpleasant sensation that provokes a desire to scratch" [44]. In a recent large-scale study of 959 Canadian SSc patients, 43% of patients reported pruritus on most days within the last month. This rate was slightly higher among patients with early SSc (<5 years since onset of non-Raynaud's phenomenon symptoms; 46%) versus those with longer disease duration (≥5 years; 41%), but the difference was not statistically significant [45]. A smaller study ($N = 60$) reported that chronic itch (present for at least 6 weeks) was present in 57% of patients [46].

Pruritus in SSc has been associated with greater skin involvement, gastrointestinal symptoms, Raynaud's phenomenon, and finger ulcers, although only gastrointestinal symptoms were found to be an independent correlate of pruritus [45]. Significant pruritus may also be associated with primary biliary cirrhosis in a small percentage of people with SSc with both conditions [47]. Another study found that pruritus was associated with significantly reduced HRQL in SSc, even after controlling for disease duration, skin score, number of tender joints, gastrointestinal symptoms, breathing problems, Raynaud's phenomenon, and finger ulcers [48], although the magnitude of the relationship was small. This is consistent with a pan-Canadian patient survey, in which 69% of 400 patients reported experiencing pruritus at least sometimes in the last month, but only 27% reported that it had a moderate to severe impact on the ability to carry out daily activities [24].

Body Image Distress

People with an acquired disfigurement from an injury or medical illness often struggle with maintaining a healthy body image and many experience social anxiety and avoidance due to changes in appearance [49]. The appearance changes central to SSc (e.g., skin tightening, pigment changes, hand contractures, telangiectasias, discoloration due to Raynaud's phenomenon) commonly affect visible and socially relevant body parts (e.g., face and hands), contributing to body image distress and posing potential challenges to maintaining social interactions [50–54]. Appearance changes to the skin have been rated by patients as one of the most significant stressors associated with the disease [21]. Furthermore, low levels of self-esteem in relation to appearance and high levels of body image dissatisfaction have been reported by SSc patients, both related to the extent of physical changes and deformities to the skin [21, 50, 51]. One study specifically examined the psychosocial impact of facial changes in 171 SSc patients from England and reported that greater mouth disability, perceived noticeability of the appearance change, and worry were all associated with body image concerns [52]. In a sample of 489 Canadian SSc patients, the extent of body and face skin involvement, presence of telangiectasias and hand contractures, as well as age, were associated with body image distress and social discomfort [53]. A study of 644 patients enrolled in an international cohort reported that appearance concerns were present among 72% of patients, including 75% of 565 women and 53% of 79 men. They were present in 71% of 550 patients who identified as White and 85% of 41 who identified as Black [55]. Compared to a general population sample, the proportion of people with concerns was substantially higher for men across age groups and for younger women, but less so for older women. Differences by race/ethnicity were reduced in multivariable analysis, suggesting that they may be explained, at least partially, by more severe disease and, likely, greater pigmentation changes (e.g., perifollicular hypopigmentation, salt and pepper changes, hyperpigmentation) [55]. These findings were generally consistent with another study of 98 patients from the United States, which found that body image dissatisfaction was significantly higher among Black than White patients and that Black patients reported more concern about pigmentation changes than White patients [56].

Sexual Dysfunction

Sexual dysfunction refers to problems that may include decreased desire and enjoyment, impaired arousal, and painful sex [57]. Sexual dysfunction is a common problem among women with SSc [58–63]. Compared to women in the general population, women with SSc are significantly less likely to be sexually active, and sexually active women with SSc are significantly more likely to be sexually impaired [57, 62]. Factors that are independently associated with being sexually active include younger age, fewer gastrointestinal symptoms, and less severe Raynaud's phenomenon symptoms [63]. Among women who are sexually active, sexual impairment is associated with older age, as well as more severe skin involvement and breathing problems. Vaginal pain is eight times as common among women with impairment compared to those without impairment [63].

Among men with SSc, erectile dysfunction (ED) is common [64, 65], with onset typically occurring several years after the manifestation of the first non-Raynaud's phenomenon symptoms [65, 66]. While in the general population, ED is typically associated with atherosclerosis, in SSc, penile blood flow is impaired due to both myointimal proliferation of small arteries and corporal fibrosis [67]. Men with SSc who have ED are significantly more likely to be older than those without ED and tend to report non-SSc risk factors (e.g., alcohol consumption) at higher rates [66, 67]. SSc factors associated with ED include severe cutaneous, muscular, or renal involvement; diffuse disease; elevated pulmonary pressures; restrictive lung disease; endothelial dysfunction; and microvascular damage [66]. Most men with SSc who have ED do not receive treatment [67]. Among those who do, Sildenafil appears to be commonly used, but its efficacy has not been established in SSc [65, 66]. The reader refers Chap. 36, Overlooked Manifestations, for additional details on this topic.

Clinical Strategies for Psychosocial Care

Comprehensive, patient-centered care in chronic diseases, including SSc, involves a combination of both medical treatment of disease symptoms, as well as services and interventions to help manage the psychological, behavioral, and social aspects of living with the disease. The European League Against Rheumatism's (EULAR) recommendations for the treatment of SSc [68] have highlighted the need for these types of interventions, but no specific suggestions were made, due to the lack of high-quality evidence available.

Stepped care models of healthcare delivery involve matching interventions of differing intensities to patient needs. It entails providing services that are the least restrictive of those available, but still likely to produce significant health gain, as well as care that is self-correcting [69]. Least restrictive care typically refers to the amount of treatment intensity, but can also reflect the impact on patients in terms of cost and personal inconvenience. The self-correcting aspects of stepped care entail that the results and progress of treatments are systematically monitored and changes are made, or "stepped up," if these are not attaining gains in the specific area of treatment [69]. Thus, stepped care starts off with the simplest, least intrusive intervention available, and proceeds to more intense treatment approaches as necessary.

As part of a stepped-care approach, health care professionals should establish a relationship with a mental health practitioner, such as a psychologist, psychiatrist, or trained social worker, in order to provide more specialized treatment to patients, as needed. For instance, a skilled practitioner in cognitive behavioral therapy or a related framework would be ideal for addressing many of the psychosocial concerns common to people with SSc. This form of therapy centres on active client involvement and provides a directive and structured treatment approach to goal-setting, and emotional and behavioral change [70]. Cognitive-behavioral therapy focuses on putting into practice strategies and techniques that will improve overall functioning, and in this way, it is amenable to many conditions and settings [71]. Less-intensive sources of support may include self-help resources, self-management, and local support groups.

Psychological Interventions in SSc

Group mental health interventions in SSc, focused on practical mental health management tools, are an option that can be delivered via videoconference, which is critical during the COVID-19 pandemic, but also important, generally, in a disease like SSc, where people may live far from specialized treatment centres or have difficulty traveling [72]. In April 2020, during the initial phase of COVID-19, the Scleroderma Patient-centered Intervention Network (SPIN) tested a multifaceted group intervention delivered via videoconference to address symptoms of anxiety among people with at least mild anxiety. They randomized 172 people with SSc from 12 countries to a 4-week (3 sessions per week) intervention that was designed to provide education on mental health coping skills and foster social support to reduce isolation or to a waitlist control. The program provided educational segments on healthy information management and staying connected with others; cognitive behavioral worry management strategies; relaxation techniques; adapted home exercise; and home activity engagement. Although there were no significant differences in mental health outcomes four weeks post-randomization, both anxiety and depression symptoms were reduced significantly 6 weeks later [73].

Self-help Resources

Self-help can be a very useful first step towards addressing relatively mild problems associated with psychosocial functioning and quality of life. Providing information to both patients and those who support them regarding issues common to people living with SSc, as well as information regarding useful resources and services to address such problems, is something that can be implemented in rheumatology clinics and doctors' offices. Nurses and rheumatologists should be aware of the important psychosocial issues that affect quality of life in order to help patients access resources and facilitate conversations that address concerns of individual patients. Additionally, links to information and educational resources can be provided in clinics regarding self-help programs that are available as a first step in providing psychosocial support.

There are a number of resources that may be particularly useful for persons living with SSc. For instance, *Positive Coping with Health Conditions, A Self-Care Workbook* [74] is a general self-care manual designed for individuals living with chronic health conditions, as well as physicians, psychologists, nurses, rehabilitation professionals, and researchers who support patients. The workbook focuses on teaching skills to manage various stressors related to living with a chronic disease. It includes sections on managing anxiety, worry, anger, depressive thinking, and low mood; problem solving; relationship building; relaxation; as well as how to apply these coping skills to various aspects of having a chronic illness, such as life changes, pain, sleep, and physical activity. The workbook is based on cognitive-behavioral therapy models and framed in a manner that can be accessed by those who are not familiar with or trained in psychological interventions. Other cognitive-behavioral self-help resources available for addressing negative mood, including depressive symptoms and anxiety, are the *Mind Over Mood: Change How You Feel by Changing the Way You Think* [75] and *Thoughts & Feelings: Taking Control of Your Moods and Your Life* [76] workbooks.

A resource that may be useful in addressing physical appearance changes and body image concerns is *Changing Faces* (www.changingfaces.org.uk). *Changing Faces* is a not-for-profit organization whose mission is to provide support for individuals touched by disfigurement and to increase public awareness regarding issues related to living with a visibly different appearance. *Changing Faces* has published a range of self-help and educational resources in the form of booklets, pamphlets, and DVDs for individuals with disfigurements, their families, as well as employers and healthcare professionals. Examples of topics covered in these resources include daily challenges when living with a different appearance, intimacy, and social life. In addition, *Changing Faces* offers workshops and training on issues surrounding disfigurement, as well as more individualized services that target social anxiety, body image distress, and, generally, adjustment to living with an altered appearance.

An additional resource that may be helpful in addressing physical appearance changes and body image concerns is *About Face*, which is a Canadian-based not-for-profit organization that provides advice, education, support, and advocacy for people with facial differences (http://www.aboutface.ca). Similar to *Changing Faces, About Face* has published a range of self-help and educational resources (e.g., books, guides, and DVDs) on a variety of relevant topics for individuals with facial differences, their families, and their caregivers. Additionally, *About Face* offers further support in the form of workshops, groups, retreats, camps, teleconferences, and hotlines for individuals of all ages.

Self-Management Approaches

Self-management programs constitute another area that can be useful as a first step towards addressing relatively mild problems associated with the psychosocial aspects of living with a chronic condition. The Chronic Disease Self-Management Program (CDSMP) [77], which was developed by Kate Lorig and modeled on her Arthritis Self-Management Program [78], is designed to teach self-care techniques useful to persons with many chronic diseases. The CDSMP is delivered through face-to-face meetings or via videoconference, in small-group settings, and led by persons who have a chronic disease. The objectives of the CDSMP are to support people living with a chronic condition in taking care of the illness, carrying out normal activities, and managing emotional changes associated with living with their condition. Topics included in the CDSMP program include managing pain, fatigue, depression, and shortness of breath; exercise; relaxation techniques; healthy eating; communication skills; medication management; advanced directives; and problem-solving with specific action planning [78].

Recently, a SSc-specific self-management program was tested among 267 participants who were randomized to receive the program in a self-help internet format or to be provided with a book about SSc [79]. However, the trial did not find that the program improved self-efficacy for disease management or other outcomes. In 2021, SPIN will test a different self-management program among 440 participants who will be randomized to the intervention or usual care control. Participants in the intervention will receive access to the program and to a self-management group that will meet 8 times over 12 weeks via videoconference. The program's modules address (1) pain; (2) skin care, finger ulcers, and Raynaud's; (3) sleep problems; (4) fatigue; (5) gastrointestinal symptoms; (6) itch; (7) emotions and stress; (8) body image concerns due to disfigurement; and (9) effective communication with healthcare providers [80].

Support Groups

A large number of patients with chronic medical illnesses, including those with SSc, join support groups in order to better cope with and manage their illness [81]. Activities of support groups include giving and receiving emotional and practical support, as well as providing education and information to patients. The specific activities and focus, as well as facilitator training and competence, may vary across support groups, which are typically organized locally. Patients may differ in the acceptability of the idea of attending a support group and the degree to which they may benefit from one. Due to their grass-roots nature, support groups can be configured in a variety of ways [82]. For example, some support groups may meet face-to-face whereas others may "meet" online; some groups may be facilitated by a peer whereas others may be facilitated by a professional; and some may include structured educational activities whereas others may not. Research on the effectiveness of support groups is scant, particularly with regard to lay-led groups. However, many people who do attend support groups describe feeling more empowered, more hopeful, and less alone following their group experience [81]. In addition, some patients who attend these groups report feeling more in control of their life, as well as more knowledgeable about their illness, coping strategies, and developments in medical and self-help treatments.

Peer-led support groups have become increasingly popular in recent years [83]. Consistent with this, most SSc support groups are peer-led rather than professionally-led. Given that they may be the sole source of SSc-specific support available to many patients and that they have been effective in other conditions, attending support groups may be beneficial for some patients with SSc. It is important to keep in mind, however, that support groups are meant to complement rather than supplement standard medical care. Medical professionals may want to discuss the possible benefits of attending a support group with their patients, as well as potential pitfalls.

Recently, SPIN conducted a successful feasibility trial of the SPIN Scleroderma Support group Leader Education (SPIN-SSLED) Program [84] and has undertaken a full-scale trial, which will randomize approximately 160 participants and be completed by June 2021 [85]. The program is a 3-month group videoconference training program, designed to improve skills and self-efficacy, reduce burden, and reduce emotional distress among support group leaders. By providing key knowledge and skills, the SPIN-SSLED Program may improve the ability of SSc peer support group leaders to lead sustainable, effective support groups; reduce burden on leaders; and encourage new leaders to set up support groups where none exist, locally or via the Internet.

SSc-Specific Resources

Additional SSc-specific resources are being developed by SPIN, which is an international collaboration that was established with the aim to create an infrastructure to develop, test, and disseminate a series of psychosocial and rehabilitation interventions related to important patient-reported outcomes in SSc (https://www.spinsclero.com) [3, 72]. SPIN is comprised of SSc patient organizations, clinicians, medical professionals, and researchers from Canada, the United States, Europe, Latin America, and Australia. Building on previous research [1–3] and in consultation with patient representatives, SPIN develops online programs that address previously identified problems that are important to patients, such as those reviewed in the present chapter. Once tested, SPIN's interventions will be made widely accessible to SSc partner patient organizations around the world [70]. Recently, for instance, SPIN completed testing of its SPIN-HAND Program that offers hand exercises for people with SSc, and the program is available free-of-charge to patients in English and French on SPIN's website.

Please refer to Table 46.1 for a summary of all the self-help, self-management, support group, and scleroderma-specific resources listed in this section.

In summary, persons living with SSc face a number of challenges that affect their psychosocial well-being and quality of life. Rather than focusing only on a single issue, such as depression, approaches to psychosocial care should take into account the different levels of issues faced by patients. Self-help resources and self-management techniques can be considered as first steps towards providing patient care for a variety of psychosocial issues. Some patients may also benefit from support from other patients via support groups. Care providers should become aware of problems faced by patients and their supporters, should facilitate discussions of these problems, and should help patients access self-help material. Beyond this, rheumatology clinics should develop a relationship with a competent mental health care provider to provide more focused evaluation and intervention services for patients, as needed.

Table 46.1 Self-help, self-management, support group, and scleroderma-specific resources

Source	Purpose	Website (if applicable)
Positive coping with health conditions, a self-care workbook	A self-care workbook focusing on teaching skills to manage stressors related to living with a chronic disease (e.g., managing anxiety, anger, depressive thinking; and relationship building) and well as how to apply coping skills to various aspects of having a chronic illness (e.g., life changes, pain, sleep, and physical activity)	https://psychhealthandsafety.org/pcwhc/
Mind over mood: change how you feel by changing the way you think	Resource and workbook based on cognitive behavioral therapy to address negative mood, including depressive symptoms and anxiety	http://www.mindovermood.com
Thoughts & feelings: taking control of your moods and your life	Self-help book based on cognitive behavioral therapy and acceptance and commitment therapy to address mental health concerns (e.g., depression, anxiety, low self-esteem, anger)	
Changing faces	Not-for-profit UK-based organization created to provide support for individuals touched by disfigurement and to increase public awareness regarding issues related to living with a visibly different appearance. A range of self-help and educational resources are available online through their website	https://www.changingfaces.org.uk
About face	Non-for-profit Canadian organization created to provide advice, education, support, and advocacy for people with facial differences. A range of self-help and educational resources are available online through their website	http://www.aboutface.ca
Living a healthy life with chronic conditions: self-management of heart disease, arthritis, diabetes, asthma, bronchitis, emphysema and others	Self-management guidebook designed to help people living with chronic conditions learn the information and skills needed to manage their disease on a daily basis	
Support groups	Support groups often involve giving and receiving emotional and practical support, as well as providing education and information to patients. Patients interested in attending or joining a scleroderma support group can typically find information on local or national scleroderma organization websites (e.g., Scleroderma Society of Canada and Scleroderma Foundation in the United States)	*Scleroderma Society of Canada's website:* http://www.scleroderma.ca *Scleroderma Foundation's website:* http://www.scleroderma.org
Scleroderma Patient-centered Intervention Network (SPIN)	International research consortium aimed to create an infrastructure to develop, test, and disseminate a series of self-guided online psychosocial and rehabilitation interventions related to important patient-reported outcomes in scleroderma Access to SPIN's hand exercise program and other programs that are forthcoming, including a SSc-specific self-management program	https://www.spinsclero.com

Acknowledgements Dr. Thombs was supported by an Tier 1 Canada Research Chair.

References

1. Thombs BD, van Lankveld W, Bassel M, Baron M, Buzza R, Haslam S, et al. Psychological health and well-being in systemic sclerosis: state of the science and consensus research agenda. Arthritis Care Res. 2010;8:1181–9.
2. Kwakkenbos L, Delisle VC, Fox RS, Gholizadeh S, Jewett LR, Levis B, et al. Psychosocial aspects of systemic sclerosis. Rheum Dis Clin N Am. 2015;41:519–28.
3. Thombs BD, Jewett LR, Assassi S, Baron M, Bartlett SJ, Maia AC, et al. New directions for patient-centered care in scleroderma: The Scleroderma Patient-centered Intervention Network (SPIN). Clin Exp Rheumatol. 2012;30(2 Suppl 71):S23–9.
4. Evans DL, Charney DS, Lewis L, Golden RN, Gorman JM, Krishnan KR, et al. Mood disorders in the medically ill: scientific review and recommendations. Biol Psychiatry. 2005;58:175–89.
5. Blazer DG, Kessler RC, McGonagle KA, Swartz MS. The prevalence and distribution of major depression in a national community sample: The National Comorbidity Survey. Am J Psychiatry. 1994;151:979–86.
6. Pignone MP, Gaynes BN, Rushton JL, Burchell CM, Orleans CT, Mulrow CD, et al. Screening for depression in adults: a summary of the evidence for the U.S. Preventive Services Task Force. Ann Intern Med. 2002;136:765–76.
7. Baubet T, Ranque B, Taïeb O, Bérenzé A, Bricou O, Mehallel S, et al. Mood and anxiety disorders in systemic sclerosis patients. Presse Med. 2011;40:e111–9.
8. Jewett LR, Razykov I, Hudson M, Baron M, Thombs BD. Canadian Scleroderma Research Group. Rheumatology. 2013;52:669–75.
9. Sheehan DV, Lecrubier Y, Sheehan KH, Janavs J, Weiller E, Keskiner A, et al. The validity of the Mini International Neuropsychiatric Interview (MINI) according to the SCID-P and its reliability. Eur Psychiatry. 1997;12:232–41.
10. Wu Y, Levis B, Ioannidis JPA, Benedetti A, Thombs BD. DEPRESsion Screening Data (DEPRESSD) Collaboration. Probability of major depression classification based on the SCID, CIDI, and MINI diagnostic interviews: a synthesis of three individual participant data meta-analyses. Psychother Psychosom. 2020; https://doi.org/10.1159/000509283. Online ahead of print

11. Thombs BD, Jewett LR, Kwakkenbos L, Hudson M, Baron M, Canadian Scleroderma Research Group. Major depression diagnoses are often transient among patients with systemic sclerosis: baseline and 1-month follow-up. Arthritis Care Res. 2015;67:411–6.
12. Newton EG, Thombs BD, Groleau D. The experience of emotional distress among women with scleroderma. Qual Health Res. 2012;22:1195–206.
13. Thombs BD, Taillefer SS, Hudson M, Baron M. Depression in patients with systemic sclerosis: a systematic review of the evidence. Arthritis Rheum. 2007;57:1089–97.
14. Milette K, Hudson M, Baron M, Thombs BD, Canadian Scleroderma Research Group. Comparison of the PHQ-9 and CES-D depression scales in systemic sclerosis: internal consistency reliability, convergent validity, and clinical correlates. Rheumatology. 2010;49:789–96.
15. Thombs BD, Kwakkenbos L, Levis AW, Benedetti A. Addressing overestimation of the prevalence of depression based on self-report screening questionnaires. CMAJ. 2018;190:E44–9.
16. Thombs BD, Hudson M, Taillefer SS, Baron M, the Canadian Scleroderma Research Group. Prevalence and clinical correlates of symptoms of depression in patients with systemic sclerosis. Arthritis Rheum. 2008;59:504–9.
17. Mozzetta A, Antinone V, Alfani S, Neri P, Foglio Bonda PG, Pasquini P, et al. Mental health in patients with systemic sclerosis: a controlled investigation. J Eur Acad Dermatol Venereol. 2008;22:336–40.
18. Legendre C, Allanore Y, Ferrand I, Kahan A. Evaluation of depression and anxiety in patients with systemic sclerosis. Joint Bone Spine. 2005;72:408–11.
19. Angelopoulos NV, Drosos AA, Moutsopoulos HM. Psychiatric symptoms associated with scleroderma. Psychother Psychosom. 2001;70:145–50.
20. Faezi ST, Paragomi P, Shahali A, Akhlaghkhah M, Akbarian M, Akhlaghi M, et al. Prevalence and severity of depression and anxiety in patients with systemic sclerosis: an epidemiologic survey and investigation of clinical correlates. J Clin Rheumatol. 2017;23:80–6.
21. van Lankveld WGJM, Vonk MC, Teunissen HA, van den Hoogen FHJ. Appearance self-esteem in systemic sclerosis—subjective experience of skin deformity and its relationship with physician-assessed skin involvement, disease status and psychological variables. Rheumatology. 2007;46:972–6.
22. Kwakkenbos L, van Lankveld WGJM, Vonk MC, Becker ES, van den Hoogen FHJ, van den Ende CHM. Disease-related and psychosocial factors associated with depressive symptoms in patients with systemic sclerosis, including fear of progression and appearance self-esteem. J Psychosom Res. 2012;72:199–204.
23. Swain MG. Fatigue in chronic disease. Clin Sci. 2000;99:1–8.
24. Bassel M, Hudson M, Taillefer SS, Schieir O, Baron M, Thombs BD. Frequency and impact of symptoms experienced by patients with systemic sclerosis: results from a Canadian national survey. Rheumatology. 2011;50(4):762–7.
25. Willems LM, Kwakkenbos L, Leite CC, Thombs BD, van den Hoogen FH, Maia AC, et al. Frequency and impact of disease symptoms experienced by patients with systemic sclerosis from five European countries. Clin Exp Rheumatol. 2014;32(6 Suppl 86):S88–93. Epub 2014 Nov 3
26. Thombs BD, Bassel M, McGuire L, Smith MT, Hudson M, Haythornthwaite JA. A systematic comparison of fatigue levels in systemic sclerosis with general population, cancer and rheumatic disease samples. Rheumatology. 2008;47:1559–63.
27. Basta F, Afeltra A, Margiotta DPE. Fatigue in systemic sclerosis: a systematic review. Clin Exp Rheumatol. 2018;36(Suppl 113):150–60.
28. Thombs BD, Hudson M, Bassel M, Taillefer SS, Baron M, Canadian Scleroderma Research Group. Sociodemographic, disease, and symptom correlates of fatigue in systemic sclerosis: evidence from a sample of 659 Canadian Scleroderma Research Group Registry patients. Arthritis Rheum. 2009;61:966–73.
29. Yacoub I, Amine B, Bensabbah R, Hajjaj-Hassouni N. Assessment of fatigue and its relationship with disease-related parameters in patients with systemic sclerosis. Clin Rheumatol. 2012;31:655–60.
30. Strickland G, Pauling J, Cavill C, McHugh N. Predictors of health-related quality of life and fatigue in systemic sclerosis: evaluation of the EuroQol-5D and FACIT-F assessment tools. Clin Rheumatol. 2012;31:1215–22.
31. Harel D, Thombs BD, Hudson M, Baron M, Steele R, Canadian Scleroderma Research Group. Measuring fatigue in SSc: a comparison of the Short Form-36 vitality subscale and functional assessment of chronic illness therapy-fatigue scale. Rheumatology. 2012;51:2177–85.
32. Sandqvist G, Archenholtz B, Scheja A, Hesselstrand R. The Swedish version of the Multidimensional Assessment of Fatigue (MAF) in systemic sclerosis: reproducibility and correlations to other fatigue instruments. Scan J Rheumatol. 2011;40:493–4.
33. Sandusky SB, McGuire L, Smith MT, Wigley FM, Haythornthwaite JA. Fatigue: an overlooked determinant of physical function in scleroderma. Rheumatology. 2009;48:165–9.
34. Assassi S, Leyva AL, Mayes MD, Sharif R, Nair DK, Fischbach M, et al. Predictors of fatigue severity in early systemic sclerosis: a prospective longitudinal study of the GENISOS cohort. PLoS One. 2011;6:e26061.
35. Peytrignet S, Denton CP, Lunt M, Hesselstrand R, Mouthon L, Silman A, et al. Disability, fatigue, pain and their associates in early diffuse cutaneous systemic sclerosis: the European Scleroderma Observational Study. Rheumatology. 2018;57:370–81.
36. Frech T, Hays RD, Maranian P, Clements PJ, Furst DE, Khanna D. Prevalence and correlates of sleep disturbance in systemic sclerosis: results from the UCLA scleroderma quality of life study. Rheumatology. 2011;50:1280–7.
37. Milette K, Razykov I, Pope J, Hudson M, Motivala SJ, Baron M, et al. Clinical correlates of sleep problems in systemic sclerosis: the prominent role of pain. Rheumatology. 2011;50(5):921–5.
38. Figueiredo FP, Aires GD, Nisihara R, Skare TL. Sleep disturbance in scleroderma. J Clin Rheumatol. 2020; https://doi.org/10.1097/RHU.0000000000001437. Online ahead of print
39. Schieir O, Thombs BD, Hudson M, Boivin JF, Steele R, Bernatsky S, et al. Prevalence, severity, and clinical correlates of pain in patients with systemic sclerosis. Arthritis Care Res. 2010;62:409–17.
40. Sandqvist G, Eklund M. Daily occupations-performance, satisfaction and time use, and relations with well-being in women with limited systemic sclerosis. Disabil Rehabil. 2008;30:27–35.
41. Hudson M, Steele R, Lu Y, Thombs BD, Canadian Scleroderma Research Group, Baron M. Work disability in systemic sclerosis. J Rheumatol. 2009;36:2481–6.
42. Müller H, Rehberger P, Günther C, Schmitt J. Determinants of disability, quality of life and depression in dermatological patients with systemic scleroderma. British J Derm. 2012;166:343–53.
43. El-Baalbaki G, Lober J, Hudson M, Baron M, Thombs BD, Canadian Scleroderma Research Group. Measuring pain in systemic sclerosis: comparison of the short-form McGill Pain Questionnaire versus a single-item measure of pain. J Rheumatol. 2011;38:2581–7.
44. Weisshaar E, Kucenic MJ, Fleischer AB Jr. Pruritus: a review. Acta Derm Venereol Suppl. 2003;213:5–32.
45. Razykov I, Levis B, Hudson M, Baron M, Thombs BD, Canadian Scleroderma Research Group. Prevalence and clinical correlates of pruritus in patients with systemic sclerosis: an updated analysis of 959 patients. Rheumatology. 2011;52(11):2056–61.
46. Stull CM, Weaver LA, Valdes-Rodriguez R, Naramala S, Lavery MJ, Chan YH, et al. Characteristics of chronic itch in systemic sclerosis: a cross-sectional survey. Acta Derm Venereol. 2018;98:793–4.

47. Frech TM, Mar D. Gastrointestinal and hepatic disease in systemic sclerosis. Rheum Dis Clin N Am. 2018;44:15–28.
48. El-Baalbaki G, Razykov I, Hudson M, Bassel M, Baron M, Thombs BD, et al. Association of pruritus with quality of life and disability in systemic sclerosis. Arthritis Care Res. 2010;62:1489–95.
49. Pruzinsky T. Social and psychological effects of major craniofacial deformity. Cleft Palate Craniofac J. 1992;29:578–84.
50. Malcarne VL, Handsdottir I, Greensbergs HL, Clements PJ, Weisman MH. Appearance self-esteem in systemic sclerosis. Cognitive Ther Res. 1999;23:197–208.
51. Benrud-Larson LM, Heinberg LJ, Boiling C, Reed J, White B, Wigley FM, et al. Body image dissatisfaction among women with scleroderma: extent and relationship to psychosocial function. Health Psychol. 2003;22(2):130–9.
52. Amin K, Clarke A, Sivakumar B, Puri A, Fox Z, Brough V, et al. The psychological impact of facial changes in scleroderma. Psychol Health Med. 2011;16(3):304–12.
53. Jewett LR, Huson M, Malcarne VL, Baron M, Thombs BD, Canadian Scleroderma Research Group. Sociodemographic and disease correlates of body image distress among patients with systemic sclerosis. PLoS One. 2012;7(3):e33281.
54. Pauling JD, Domsic RT, Saketkoo LA, et al. Multinational qualitative research study exploring the patient experience of Raynaud's phenomenon in systemic sclerosis. Arthritis Care Res. 2018;70:1373–84.
55. Jewett LR, Kwakkenbos L, Carrier ME, Malcarne VL, Bartlett SJ, Furst DE, et al. Examination of the association of sex and race/ethnicity with appearance concerns: a Scleroderma Patient-centered Intervention Network (SPIN) Cohort study. Clin Exp Rheumatol. 2016;34(Suppl. 100):92–9.
56. Nusbaum JS, Gordon JK, Steen VD. African American race associated with body image dissatisfaction among patients with systemic sclerosis. Clin Exp Rheumatol. 2016;34(Suppl. 100):70–3.
57. Bancroft J. Human sexuality and its problems. 3rd ed. Edinburgh, UK: Churchill Livingstone; 2009.
58. Schouffoer AA, van der Marel J, Ter Kuile MM, Weijenborg PT, Voskuyl A, Vliet Vlieland CW, et al. Impaired sexual function in women with systemic sclerosis: a cross-sectional study. Arthritis Rheum. 2009;61:1601–8.
59. Knafo R, Thombs BD, Jewett L, Hudson M, Wigley F, Haythornthwaite JA. (Not) talking about sex: a systematic comparison of sexual impairment in women with systemic sclerosis and other chronic disease samples. Rheumatology. 2009;48:1300–3.
60. Schover LR, Jensen SR. Sexuality and chronic illness: a comprehensive approach. New York: Guilford; 1988. p. 74.
61. Saad SC, Behrend AE. Scleroderma and sexuality. J Sex Res. 1996;33:15–20.
62. Levis B, Burri A, Hudson M, Baron M, Thombs BD, Canadian Scleroderma Research Group. Sexual activity and impairment in women with systemic sclerosis compared to women from a general population sample. PLoS One. 2012;7:e52129.
63. Levis B, Hudson M, Knafo R. Rates and correlates of sexual activity and impairment among women with systemic sclerosis. Arthritis Care Res. 2012;64:640–50.
64. Jaeger VK, Walker UA. Erectile dysfunction in systemic sclerosis. Curr Rheumatol Rep. 2016;18:49.
65. Walker UA, Tyndall A, Ruszat R. Erectile dysfunction in systemic sclerosis. Ann Rheum Dis. 2009;68:1083–5.
66. Foocharoen C, Tyndall A, Hachulla E, Rosato E, Allanore Y, Farge-Bancel D, et al. Erectile dysfunction is frequent in systemic sclerosis and associated with severe disease: a study of the EULAR Scleroderma Trial and Research Group. Arthritis Res Ther. 2012;14:R37.
67. Keck AD, Foocharoen C, Rosato E, et al. Nailfold capillary abnormalities in erectile dysfunction of systemic sclerosis: a EUSTAR group analysis. Rheumatology. 2014;53:639–43.
68. Kowal-Bielecka O, Landewe R, Avouac J, Chwiesko S, Miniati I, Czirjak L, et al. EULAR recommendations for the treatment of systemic sclerosis: A report from the EULAR scleroderma trials and research group (EUSTAR). Ann Rheum Dis. 2009;68:620–8.
69. Bower P, Gilbody S. Stepped care in psychological therapies: access, effectiveness and efficiency: narrative literature review. B J Pysch. 2005;186:11–7.
70. Whitfield G, Davidson A. Cognitive behavioural therapy explained. Oxon, UK: Radcliffe Publishing Ltd; 2007.
71. Lovell K, Richards D. Multiple Access Points and Levels of Entry (MAPLE): ensuring choice, accessibility and equity for CBT services. Behav Cogn Psychoth. 2000;28:379–91.
72. Kwakkenbos L, Jewett LR, Baron M, Bartlett SJ, Furst D, Gottesman K, et al. The Scleroderma Patient-centered Intervention Network (SPIN) cohort: protocol for a cohort multiple randomised controlled trial (cmRCT) design to support trials of psychosocial and rehabilitation interventions in a rare disease context. BMJ Open. 2013;7(8):pii:e003563.
73. Thombs BD, Kwakkenbos L, Levis B, Bourgeault A, Henry RS, Levis AW, Harb S, et al. Effects of a multi-faceted education and support program on anxiety symptoms among people with systemic sclerosis with at least mild anxiety during COVID-19: a two-arm parallel partially nested randomised controlled trial. Lancet Rheumatol. 2021;3(6):e427–37.
74. Bilsker D, Samara J, Goldner E. Positive coping with health conditions: a self-care workbook. Consortium for Organizational Mental Healthcare (COMH); 2009.
75. Greenberger D, Padesky C. Mind over mood: change how you feel by changing the way you think. New York, NY: Guilford Press; 1995.
76. McKay M, Fanning P. Thoughts and feelings: taking control of your moods and your life. Oakland, CA: New Harbinger Publications, Inc; 1997.
77. Lorig KR, Sobel DS, Stewart AL, Brown BW Jr, Ritter PL, González VM, et al. Evidence suggesting that a chronic disease self-management program can improve health status while reducing utilization and costs: a randomized trial. Med Care. 1999;37:5–14.
78. Lorig K, Lubeck D, Kraines RG, Seleznick M, Holman HR. Outcomes of self-help education for patients with arthritis. Arthritis Rheum. 1985;28:680–5.
79. Khanna D, Serrano J, Berrocal VJ, Silver RM, Cuencas P, Newbill SL, et al. Randomized controlled trial to evaluate an internet-based self-management program in systemic sclerosis. Arthritis Care Res. 2019;71:435–47.
80. SPIN Self-management full-scale trial (SPIN-SELF). NCT04246528. https://clinicaltrials.gov/ct2/show/NCT04246528?term=brett+thombs&draw=2&rank=4. Accessed December 9, 2020.
81. Davison KP, Pennebaker JW, Dickerson SS. Who talks? The social psychology of illness support groups. Am Psychol. 2000;55:205–17.
82. Uccelli MM, Mohr LM, Battaglia MA, Zagami P, Mohr DC. Peer support groups in multiple sclerosis: current effectiveness and future directions. Mult Scler. 2006;10:80–4.
83. Ussher J, Kirsten L, Butow P, Sandoval M. What do cancer support groups provide which other supportive relationships do not? The experience of peer support groups for people with cancer. Soc Sci Med. 2006;62:2565–76.
84. Thombs BD, Dyas L, Pépin M, Aguila K, Carrier ME, Tao L, et al. Scleroderma Patient-centered Intervention Network-Scleroderma Support group Leader EDucation (SPIN-SSLED) program: non-randomised feasibility trial. BMJ Open. 2019;9:e029935.
85. Thombs BD, Aguila K, Dyas L, Carrier ME, Fedoruk C, Horwood L, et al. Protocol for a partially nested randomized controlled trial to evaluate the effectiveness of the Scleroderma Patient-centered Intervention Network Support Group Leader EDucation (SPIN-SSLED) Program. Trials. 2019;20:717.

Measuring Disease Activity and Outcomes in Clinical Trials

47

Dinesh Khanna and Alain Lescoat

Introduction

Systemic sclerosis (scleroderma, SSc) has seen a substantial progress in the development and validation of outcome measures [1]. This chapter will discuss the outcome measures that can be incorporated in clinical trials in SSc.

Measurement Properties of an Instrument: Feasibility, Reliability, and Validity

An outcome measure should be feasible, reliable, and valid [2]. A feasible measure is accessible, easily interpretable, and associated with low cost. Reliability is the extent to which a measure yields the same score each time it is administered if an underlying health condition has not changed. A reliability coefficient of 0.90 or higher (means that 90% of the score is accurate, while the remaining 10% denotes error) is considered satisfactory for individual comparisons and 0.70 or higher is considered satisfactory for group comparisons [3]. Validity is the extent to which a score or a health measure accurately reflects the underlying health concept. Validity includes face (measures what it purports to measure), content (comprehensive), construct (measures or correlates with a theorized health construct), and criterion validity (predicts or correlates with "gold standard"). Sensitivity to change (responsiveness) assesses the ability of an instrument to detect change when it has occurred. The ability of an instrument to detect clinically important change is crucial to its usefulness as an outcome measure in a clinical trial.

D. Khanna (✉)
Division of Rheumatology, Department of Internal Medicine, University of Michigan, Ann Arbor, MI, USA
e-mail: khannad@med.umich.edu

A. Lescoat
Department of Internal Medicine & Clinical Immunology, CHU Rennes, South Hospital, Rennes, France
e-mail: alain.lescoat@chu-rennes.fr

Measuring Disease Activity and Damage to Assess the Severity of SSc

Investigators agree that the assessment of disease activity and severity is an important goal in SSc. Based on a previous consensus reached in other rheumatic diseases [4], activity is defined as the aspect of disease that varies over time and has the potential to be reversible spontaneously or with therapy (e.g., tendon friction rubs, acute phase reactants, and inflammatory polyarthritis). Damage is a cumulative burden of a disease at a given time point and is generally irreversible (e.g., calcinosis and end-stage pulmonary fibrosis). Both activity and damage contribute to the disease severity; in early SSc, activity predominates, whereas later in the disease, damage is more likely to be the dominant part [5].

Disease Activity in SSc

The European Scleroderma Trials and Research group (EUSTAR) has recently proposed an updated composite index to assess SSc-related disease activity in routine clinical care [6–8]. This new index was published in 2016 and designed to improve a previous activity index (AI) proposed by the European Scleroderma Study Group (EScSG) in 2001. This previous index had several limitations, including a questionable face validity due to the inclusion of laboratory measures such as hypocomplementemia which is not thought to be important in SSc. The new EUSTAR-AI is feasible as it includes measures collected in routine practice (clinical parameters (such as tendon friction rubs (TFR) or mRSS), laboratory measures (such as CRP value), and altered carbon monoxide diffusing capacity or transfer factor of the lung for carbon monoxide (DL_{CO}) percent predicted. It has face and content validity. It is scored on a 0 (no activity) to 10 (severe activity) with greatest weight assigned to TFR and CRP > 1 mg/dL. The tests required to calculate index are inexpensive and easily carried out in routine clinical care. In a recent publication, EUSTAR-AI adjusted mean was the best predictor of short-term severity accrual in patients with early SSc in comparison with the EScSG-AI

Y. Allanore et al. (eds.), *Scleroderma*, https://doi.org/10.1007/978-3-031-40658-4_47

and other isolated activity parameters [9]. The revised EUSTAR-AI has a few limitations such as: (a) this index does not include extent of lung involvement, or any changes over time in laboratory, physiological or radiological parameters, preventing any consideration about the evolution of outcomes like FVC/DL_{CO}, variation of fibrosis based on lung HRCT or variation of acute-phase reactants. (b) Some included parameters such as CRP or DL_{CO} may lack of specificity, as these parameters may vary in response to events unrelated to SSc such as respiratory infection. (c) The index was not developed as an outcome measure for clinical trials, and sensitivity to change has not been published. The EUSTAR-AI is nonetheless a useful tool in observational studies to identify specific subgroups of patients with high activity and to evaluate their association with potential biomarkers and clinical features [10].

Damage Index in SSc

In 2019, the Scleroderma Clinical Trials Consortium (SCTC) developed the first damage index (DI) dedicated to SSc [11]. This DI is based on 23 items specifically associated with mortality and morbidity and selected among items rated by international experts and considered as relevant to reflect SSc-attributed damage. These items are included within the following domains: Musculoskeletal and skin, Vascular, Gastrointestinal, Respiratory, Cardiovascular and Renal. This DI is theoretically scored from 0 (no-SSc related damage) to 55 (extent damage). This DI includes a limited number of items making it easy to use in clinical trials and is the first Index capturing the concept of SSc-related cumulative, irreversible organ damage. The SCTC-DI has good internal and external validity based on the endpoints of mortality and morbidity. It also shows responsiveness to change over time in the derivation and external validation cohorts [11]. As items included in this DI were selected because of their irreversible nature, this index may not be adapted to evaluate disease modifying drugs that may reverse the disease process.

Assessment of Disease Severity

A measure of disease severity encompasses both disease activity and damage and should be associated with or predict SSc-associated morbidity and mortality [5]. The revised Medsger severity index [12] was developed by the international scleroderma experts using consensus methodology followed by prospective data collection. The authors identified nine organ systems and identified variables for each organ system that can be used to define severity. The nine organ systems are general, peripheral vascular, skin, joint/tendon, muscles, GI tract, lung, heart, and kidney. Each system is scored from 0 (uninvolved) to 4 (end-stage disease). The individual organ system severity scores have been shown to predict survival in large observational cohorts [13]. The severity index is not weighted and therefore should not be summed to have a "global" severity scale score.

Outcome Measures in SSc

This section outlines the outcome measures used in clinical trials (Table 46.1) that are feasible, reliable, valid, and sensitive to change [2, 14]. Outcome measures can be incorpo-

Table 46.1 Feasible, reliable, valid, and sensitivity to change measures that are ready for clinical trials

Instruments	Completed by patient	Completed by investigator	Laboratory or functional measurements
Composite index			
American College of Rheumatology Provisional CRISS Index for early dcSSc	X	X[b]	
Revised CRISS for early dcSSc	X	X[b]	
Global patient-reported outcome measures[a]			
SF-36	X		
UK functional score	X		
Pain visual analog scale (VAS) from health assessment questionnaire-disability index (HAQ-DI)	X		
SF-6D (scored using SF-36 data)	X		
Global assessment			
Patient global assessment using VAS or Likert scale	X		
Investigator global assessment using VAS or Likert scale		X[b]	
Skin			
Modified Rodnan skin score		X[b]	
Durometer		X[b]	

Table 46.1 (continued)

Instruments	Completed by patient	Completed by investigator	Laboratory or functional measurements
Patient assessment of skin activity	X		
Patient assessment of skin severity	X		
Scleroderma skin patient reported outcome measure	X		
Musculoskeletal			
Tendon friction rubs		X[b]	
Tender joint count		X[b]	
Serum creatinine phosphokinase			X
Cochin hand function scale	X		
Hand mobility in scleroderma scale		X[b]	
Mouth handicap in systemic sclerosis scale	X		
Health assessment questionnaire-disability index	X		
Cardiac			
Transthoracic echocardiogram with Doppler			X[c]
Right heart catheterization			X[d]
6-min walk test			X[d]
Borg dyspnea index (administered immediately after the 6-min walk test)	X[d]		
Pulmonary			
Pulmonary function test with diffusion capacity			X[c]
Forced vital capacity			X[c,e]
Total lung capacity			X[c]
High-resolution quantitative computed tomography scale			X[f]
Measures of dyspnea • Mahler dyspnea index • Saint George's respiratory questionnaire	X		
Breathing VAS from scleroderma-health assessment questionnaire (S-HAQ)	X		
Gastrointestinal			
Gastrointestinal VAS from S-HAQ	X		
UCLA Scleroderma Clinical Trials Consortium gastrointestinal instrument 2.0	X		
Body mass index		X	
NIH PROMIS® Gastrointestinal Symptoms Scale	X		
Renal			
Estimated creatinine clearance			X
Systolic and diastolic blood pressure		X	
Serum creatinine			X
Raynaud's phenomenon			
Raynaud's Condition Score	X		
Number of symptomatic Raynaud's phenomenon (RP) attacks	X		
Duration of RP attack	X		
Severity of RP attack	X		
Raynaud's VAS from S-HAQ	X		
Patient assessment of RP	X		
Physician assessment of RP		X[b]	
Digital ulcer			
Active digital tip ulcer count on the volar surface • Prevention of digital ulcers at the end of trial • New digital ulcers at the end of trial		X[b]	
Time to healing of cardinal digital ulcers or all digital ulcers at the end of trial		X[b]	
Digital ulcer VAS from S-HAQ	X		

(continued)

Table 46.1 (continued)

Instruments	Completed by patient	Completed by investigator	Laboratory or functional measurements
Hand Disability in Systemic Sclerosis-Digital Ulcers (HDISS-DU®)	X		
Biomarkers			
Acute phase reactants			X
Serum B-type natriuretic peptide (BNP/NT-proBNP)			X

Modified from [2]

[a]Measures such as Center for Epidemiologic Studies Depression Scale (CESD) and Functional Assessment of Chronic Illness Therapy (FACIT)-Fatigue have been found to be feasible, reliable, and valid, but their sensitivity to change has not been evaluated in SSc

[b]Assessed by the same investigator. Quality control strongly encouraged in multicenter RCT

[c]Standardized central reading mechanism strongly encouraged in multicenter RCT

[d]For patients with pulmonary arterial hypertension

[e]FDA approved surrogate measure for SSc-ILD

[f]Standardized performance strongly encouraged in multicenter RCT

rated to assess for early signal for go-no go decisions (such as digital perfusion for peripheral involvement in SSc) or for regulatory approval for therapeutic target. Regulatory agencies such as the Food and Drug Administration (FDA) require a primary outcome measure for regulatory approval that should reflect the way patients "feel, function or survive". Regarding psychometric and measurement properties of an instrument, we suggest that it is important to keep in mind that properties of some outcome measures may vary depending on the considered disease subset (diffuse cutaneous SSc [dcSSc] or limited cutaneous SSc [lcSSc]). For example, mRSS is considered as an acceptable endpoint in dcSSc, but its relevance (content validity and sensitivity to change) for reflecting the severity and evolution of lcSSc is not validated.

Table 46.1 provides outcome measures that can be incorporated in clinical trials in SSc. However, this does not mean that these are approvable end points for Phase III trials. Some outcome measures are direct measures of feel or function but may lack content validity in SSc such as dyspnea indices (which are largely developed for obstructive lung diseases) or may have insufficient data to support an outcome measure as surrogate end point.

Measuring Skin Disease in SSc

Modified Rodnan skin score (mRSS), a measure of skin thickness [15, 16], has been used as the primary outcome measure in numerous Phase I/II or III clinical trials of dcSSc. Measurement of skin thickness is used as a surrogate measure of disease severity and mortality in patients with dcSSc—an increase in skin thickening is associated with involvement of internal organs and increased mortality [15]. It has been well demonstrated that mRSS tends to worsen in early disease and improve in late disease [17]. "Early" dcSSc is often defined as the rapid and severe increasing induration ("thickening") of the skin, with a peak at 1–3 years after disease onset [17–19]. mRSS is feasible, reliable, valid, and sensitive to change for multicenter clinical trials [16]. Observational studies have highlighted that the probability of skin progression was higher in dcSSc patients with early disease duration (<36 months since first non-Raynaud's phenomenon symptom), a baseline mRSS ranging from 10 to 35 and progression risk factors such as recent increase of mRSS in the previous 1–6 months, involvement of new body areas or presence of TFR [20]. Nonetheless, analyses from the placebo groups of recent RCTs in early dcSSc show that mean mRSS improves over time even in patients with very early dcSSc [20–23], likely influenced by scleroderma-specific autoantibody and molecular heterogeneity. In patients with anti-RNA polymerase III antibodies, mRSS score peaks earlier and is higher than in dcSSc patients with other antibody subtypes [24]. In RCTs, the trends towards improvement in the placebo group may also be in part due to the use of background conventional immunosuppressive therapies, although it is also observed in RCTs where such background therapies were not allowed [21]. Approval agencies consider mRSS as an acceptable primary outcome for regulatory approval, but require supportive evidence for improvement in PROs and/or stabilization or prevention of internal organ involvement.

The use of mRSS in clinical trial requires training to reduce variability. For longitudinal assessment in RCTs, the same evaluator should perform the mRSS during the course of the trial, as the inter-observer variability is high. Prior clinical training for RCTs will also insure the standardization of the assessment as three approaches to rate a skin area exist: (a) considering the maximum score (0–3) for evaluated area, (b) considering the most representative score for this area, or (c) averaging the score of an area. Approaches based on the most representative score or the average score are recommended, and this should be defined prior to the beginning of the study through clinical training [25]. If mRSS is incorporated in an

RCT, the pivotal RCT should be at least 52 weeks/12 months, as post-hoc analyses of RCTs have demonstrated that time in study was an important predictor of regression of mRSS with time in study of more than 12 months being associated with higher probability of mRSS improvement. Time in study of more than 12 months may also support additional benefits of the therapy, including improvement in the functional status and internal organ involvement [26]. Nonetheless, recent phase II and III trials using mRSS as their primary outcome [20–22] have failed to reach statistical significance, whereas secondary outcomes such as FVC progression for lung involvement were able to discriminate placebo from active therapy in some of them [20]. A trend towards a numerical superior improvement in favor of the active treatment group was observed in the tocilizumab and abatacept trials (adjusted difference − 1.73 (95%CI −3.78 to 0.32); $p = 0.10$ in favor of tocilizumab after 48 weeks and treatment difference of −1.75 (95% CI −4.93 to 1.43); $p = 0.28$ in favor of abatacept after 12 months, negative score signifies an improvement). Moreover, in these trials, a composite endpoint, the American College of Rheumatology Composite Response Index for Clinical Trials in Early Diffuse Cutaneous Systemic Sclerosis (ACR-CRISS; discussed later in this chapter) also discriminated active drug from placebo. These results suggest that mRSS taken alone should not be considered as *the* primary outcome for a regulatory approvable trial but may be considered for Phase 2 trials, as recently done with Romilkimab and ziritaxestat [23, 27] for a go-no-go decision. In addition, its inclusion in combined response indices such as the ACR-CRISS may capture overall disease improvement.

Durometer for skin hardness: Durometers are handheld devices used to measure the hardness of materials using internationally standardized durometer units. Durometer was included in a multicenter study of early dcSSc and was found to be feasible, reliable, valid, and sensitive to change [28]. Durometer was found to have a higher intraobserver reproducibility compared to mRSS [29], suggesting a greater reliability. A moderate-to-high correlation was found (coefficient 0.44–0.81) between mRSS and durometer [28, 29]. Durometer was proposed as a core set measure in a recent Delphi exercise involving international scleroderma experts [30], although its use may be limited due to its cost.

The Scleroderma Skin Patient Reported Outcome (SSPRO): SSPRO has been recently developed to specifically assess the skin-related quality of life in patients with SSc [31]. This tool has been designed based on the patients' perspective and includes 18 skin-related items representing 4 health-related quality of life scales (physical, emotional, social effects and physical function). SSPRO has been prospectively validated in a phase 2 RCT (lenabasum versus placebo in dcSSc) and has shown high internal consistency, construct validity and responsiveness to change in dcSSc [32]. In this trial, as secondary efficacy outcome, SSPRO discriminated active therapy from placebo at week 12 [33]. The weak but concordant correlation of SSPRO with mRSS suggests that these two outcome measures are complementary, as SSPRO provides additional information on the patient's experience of feel that the mRSS does not.

Other methods have been proposed to measure skin disease in SSc, including skin ultrasonography, elastometry, magnetic resonance imaging, or other radiographic techniques [34], but lack data on sensitivity to change and have not been applied in a multicenter setting, which may reflect a lack of feasibility.

Measuring Musculoskeletal Involvement in SSc

TFR are a grating, "squeaking" sensation detected on passive or active motion of the affected tendon in SSc. TFR are the result of the fibrosis of tendon sheath or surrounding tissues [35]. On physical examination, TFR are most commonly present in the flexor and extensor tendons of fingers and wrists and the anterior tibial and peroneal tendons. In an RCT involving patients with early dcSSc (≤18 months from the first non-Raynaud's phenomenon symptom) [36], 14–20% of TFR were present in these three areas. This RCT also showed the dynamic nature of TFR: only 10% of patients having TFR at baseline continued to have TFR at subsequent visits, whereas 21% developed new TFR over a 2-year follow-up period. The change in TFR (decrease or increase in the number of TFR compared to baseline) over 6 and 12 months in the RCT predicted changes in skin thickening and functional disability over 12 and 24 months. In other words, an improvement/worsening of TFR at 6 and 12 months predicted an improvement/worsening in skin thickening and functional disability at 12 and 24 months. TFR should be measured by the same assessor in an RCT and incorporated as a secondary outcome measure.

Hand disability in SSc can be evaluated using the Cochin Hand Function Scale (CHFS), an 18-item instrument that relates to hand functionality or disability with various tasks in different settings (e.g., in the kitchen, dressing oneself, hygienic tasks, and in the office) [37]. Each question is scored on a scale from 0 (performed without difficulty) to 5 (impossible to do), which is administered by the physician or self-administered. The total score was obtained by adding the scores from all items (range 0–90). The instrument is feasible and has shown acceptable reliability in SSc [38]. It has three scales – dexterity, rotational movement, and flexibility of the first three fingers. CHFS was sensitive to change in an intervention study that incorporated a connective tissue hand massage and home exercises [39]. CHFS is an acceptable secondary outcome measure to assess improvement in hand function and can be incorporated with mRSS in RCTs.

Hand mobility in scleroderma (HAMIS) is a nine-item performance-based test designed to examine the effects of SSc on hand mobility and hand function, and preferably administered by an occupational therapist or research physician [40, 41]. The HAMIS consists of nine items, which assess finger flexion and extension, abduction of the thumb, pincer grip, finger abduction/swelling, dorsal extension and volar flexion of the wrist, and pronation and supination. Each task is scored from 0 (no impairment) to 3 (cannot do), yielding a total possible score of 27 for each hand and a 54 total score. HAMIS has shown acceptable reliability and validity. HAMIS was sensitive to change in an intervention study with a connective tissue hand massage and home exercises [39], and complements CHFS in studies focused on the hands.

The Mouth Handicap in Systemic Sclerosis scale has been developed to assess attributes of mouth involvement in SSc [42]. It is a 12-item scale with acceptable reliability and validity. It has three scales that represent handicap associated with reduction in mouth opening, handicap associated with sicca syndrome, and esthetic concerns. The sensitivity to change was shown in an intervention program with a connective tissue massage of the face [43].

Measuring Cardio-Pulmonary Disease in Scleroderma

Cardio-pulmonary disease is among the leading causes of death for patients with SSc [44]. Cardio-pulmonary disease in SSc falls into two major categories: interstitial lung disease (ILD) and pulmonary hypertension (PH). There have been several recent clinical trials that specifically focus on lung disease in SSc [45–47].

Pulmonary function tests (PFTs) in patients with ILD demonstrate a restrictive lung defect with decreased forced vital capacity (FVC) and DLCO [48]. PFTs are feasible in large RCTs of SSc-ILD [45–47]. FVC has been used as the main parameter of restrictive lung disease and DLCO for pulmonary vascular disease.

FVC was able to differentiate between active and placebo/background therapy group in the Scleroderma Lung Study I and II (SLS I &II), in the Nintedanib phase III trial [49] and in the Tocilizumab phase II/III and III RCTs [20, 50]. Low FVC predicts morbidity and mortality associated with SSc-ILD [44] and is sensitive to change in multicenter RCTs [45, 47]. Post-hoc analyses from SLS-II have demonstrated that the change in FVC from baseline to 12 months predicted long-term survival [51]. Therefore, FVC has been proposed by the FDA as an approvable end point (surrogate end point) for ILD trials. In addition, MCID estimates for improvement and worsening have been published in SSc-ILD [52]. MCID estimates are at a group level and a range of 3.0–5.3% for improvement in FVC% and a range of 3.0–3.3% relates to worsening in FVC% [52].

Serial measurements of lung function with PFTs are also prognostic, and a 15% decline in DLCO at 3-year follow-up corresponds to a significantly increased mortality risk in idiopathic pulmonary fibrosis [53, 54]. Nonetheless, change in DLCO from baseline to 12 months did not predict overall survival in SLS II [49]. Although DLCO provides best overall estimate of the extent of HRCT-ILD based on quantitative assessment of lung fibrosis (QLF) and ILD (QILD) [55], it is not specific for SSc-ILD or pulmonary hypertension and can decline in both diseases. In addition, it has high variability and did not differentiate between active vs. placebo groups in recent SSc-ILD phase III trials [20, 49, 56, 57]. A disproportionate decline in DLCO relative to FVC may indicate pulmonary hypertension [58].

Quality control programs are the key for studies in SSc-ILD and have been discussed in detail [57]. Briefly, such programs rely on (a) the use of equipment at each participating site that meets recommended criteria for performance characteristics [59–61], as determined and affirmed by the equipment manufacturer; (b) standardized methods of calibrating the equipment with documentation that such calibrations have been carried out; (c) certification of technicians based on local or central review of the results of tests performed on an initial sample of subjects; and (d) ongoing review by a core reading center of the graphic and numeric results of tests performed on all subjects at each site with periodic feedback to the technicians concerning the quality of the tests performed, and a plan for remedial action should test quality fall below acceptable standards. Quality control programs were implemented in SLS I with satisfactory results with respect to achievement of acceptable test quality and are feasible in RCTs.

High-resolution computed tomography (HRCT) *of lungs* was incorporated successfully in recent RCTs [45, 46]. There are three key roles of HRCT imaging in clinical trials of SSc [57]: (a) detection and staging baseline severity or patterns that can be effectively used for cohort enrichment and adjusting for baseline severity in key treatment effect analyses (as it is likely that a treatment effect may differ in cases with mild rather than extensive lung disease), (b) HRCT imaging can constitute a surrogate end point or more accurate measure of serial changes, and (c) HRCT imaging can confirm that functional changes assessed by FVC accurately reflect parenchymal involvement and are not mainly due to chest wall and/or muscle involvement. HRCT aims to diagnose and quantify the degree of fibrosis, thus supporting its face and content validity. The feasibility of HRCT for multicenter RCTs was demonstrated in many studies in SSc-ILD [20, 45, 46, 49]. The reliability of HRCT was first demonstrated in the SLS I trial [45] where there was good inter-reader agreement for determination of the absence or presence of pure ground-glass (kappa = 0.76) and fibrosis (kappa = 0.74), but fair agreement for honeycombing (kappa = 0.29). In the SLS I, a higher degree of extent of fibrosis seen on a baseline HRCT scan was predictive of the rate of decline in FVC in subjects on placebo, as well as the response to cyclophosphamide (CYC) therapy; patients with the most extensive fibrosis seen on baseline HRCT scans responded the greatest to CYC treatment. A greater extent of pulmonary fibrosis on HRCT correlated well with lower FVC and DLCO values on PFTs. The extent of pulmonary fibrosis seen on HRCT scans was significantly negatively correlated with FVC ($r = -0.22$), DLCO ($r = -0.44$), and total lung capacity ($r = -0.36$) [62]. In an analysis of 215 patients with SSc followed for 10 years [54], an increased extent of disease (as defined by the extent and coarseness of reticulation [fibrosis] and proportion of ground-glass opacity) on HRCT >20% correlated with an increase in mortality (hazard ratio [HR] 2.48, $P < 0.0005$). In the recent phase III trial evaluating tocilizumab in early dcSSc, the HRCT quantitative evaluation of interstitial lung disease on whole lung showed stabilization or improvement by active therapy in comparison with placebo, in SSc-ILD [20].

Different scoring systems have been proposed that include two visual systems and computer-based approaches and discussed in a recent review [57]. The visual quantitative assessment is based on either the division of each lung in three zones, with scoring of the extent of lung abnormalities (reticulation, honey comb cysts or/and ground glass opacities) in each zone based on a scale ranging from 0 to 4 or on the division of both lungs in five zones, with quantitative assessment of lung abnormalities based on the % of abnormal parenchyma with global extent of disease computed as the mean of the % from these five zones [54]. Several computer-based approaches have been proposed evaluating density or texture features of each pixel to define abnormal lung parenchyma and obtain quantitative evaluation of disease extent [57]. Similar to PFTs, a rigorous standardized imaging protocol needs to be implemented across multiple sites and over several time points, and reading by central radiology core is necessary. Another important aspect is the training of technologists with respect to breathing instructions given at the time of scanning to ensure the same level of inspiration at each scan examination.

The 6-min Walk Test in SSc-Related ILD

The 6-min walk test (6MWT) measures the distance a person can walk in 6 min and has been extensively used as an outcome measure in various cardiac and pulmonary diseases. The 6MWT was found to be feasible and reliable in a 1-year, multicenter, double-blind, randomized control trial, comparing bosentan to placebo in 163 patients with SSc-ILD [63], but lacked construct validity and responsiveness to change in SSc-ILD. Limitations of the 6MWT were recently highlighted by various groups, showing that pain and musculoskeletal involvement can influence the walking test and that the 6MWT is not always solely reflective of changes in the lung when used in SSc [64, 65], raising doubts about its specificity in SSc-ILD and its relevance to monitoring therapy. 6MWT is not indicated for SSc-ILD trials as a primary outcome measure.

The 6MWT and Time to Clinical Worsening: Outcome Measures for Pulmonary Arterial Hypertension

The 6MWT is presently the most widely used primary end-point for studies investigating pulmonary arterial hypertension (PAH including SSc-related PAH). The 6MWT shows good to excellent correlations with maximal cardiopulmonary exercise testing ($r \geq 0.57$) [66]. The 6MWT was able to discriminate among healthy controls, and patients with the World Health Organization class II, III, and IV disease [66]. Criterion validity was demonstrated in patients with PAH wherein the 6MWT was the only noninvasive test that correlated with survival ($p < 0.01$) [66]. The 6MWT has been successfully incorporated into trials of SSc-related PAH and was able to differentiate between active and placebo treatments in a trial of epoprostenol for SSc-related PAH [67]. Studies focusing on SSc-PAH should include hemodynamics (pulmonary vascular resistance), 6MWT, and improvement in the World Health Organization functional class as outcome measures. In this perspective, composite end-points reflecting time to clinical worsening (TTCW) have been incorporated in large RCTs on PAH [68]. Such composite definitions of disease progression or clinical worsening of PAH include, for example, the combined occurrence of ≥15% decrease in 6MWD from baseline, worsening of PAH-related symptoms (higher WHO functional class, appearance or worsening of signs of right heart failure with no response to oral diuretic therapy) and the need for additional treatment for PAH in the SERAPHIN trial (Macitentan versus placebo) [69] or ≥ 15% decrease in 6MWD from baseline combined with WHO functional class III or IV symptoms at two consecutive visits separated by at least 14 days in the AMBITION trial (Ambrisentan and tadalafil versus either alone) [70]. TTCW is thus an approved end-point for PAH therapeutic trial registration [68].

Dyspnea Indices

The *Mahler dyspnea index* [71] was used in SLS-I and II to assess dyspnea. Baseline scores depend on ratings for three different categories: functional impairment, magnitude of task, and magnitude of effort. Baseline scores were able to discriminate between moderate and severe physiological parameters of breathing (FVC and DLCO) and correlated well with the baseline breathing visual analog scale (VAS) ($r = 0.61$) [72]. The Mahler's transitional dyspnea score was able to differentiate between patients on CYC and placebo in SLS at 1 year, demonstrating its sensitivity to change [73].

Saint George's respiratory questionnaire (SGRQ) was found to be reliable, valid, and responsive to change in patients with early dcSSc, both with and without ILD in a multicenter prospective study [74]. SGRQ has four scales that assess symptoms, impairment in activity, and impact and total scale. All scales showed large correlations with breathing VAS and DLCO in overall cohort and subgroup with ILD ($r > 0.37$). Each scale is discriminated between presence/absence of ILD and restrictive lung disease ($p = <0.0001–0.03$). At follow-up, all scales were responsive to change using different anchors. Nonetheless, in two recent RCTs, SGRQ did not differentiate between active drug and placebo whereas active drugs positively impacted key pulmonary outcomes such as FVC [20, 49]. This could be explained by a lack of face and/or content validity of the SGRQ. Moreover, in these trials, active drugs (nintedanib and tocilizumab) may have lacked clinically meaningful effects on other organs that may contribute to shortness of breath, such as muscle or skin involvement [75].

Both Mahler dyspnea index and SGRQ lack in-depth cognitive debriefing or assessment of face and content validation in SSc-ILD.

The breathing VAS scale in the scleroderma health assessment questionnaire (S-HAQ) allows patients to assess their degree of difficulty in performing daily activities due to shortness of breath on a continuous 100 mm scale [76]. The VAS discriminates between moderate and severe reductions in lung function and correlates well with the Mahler dyspnea index ($r = 0.61$) and was shown to be sensitive to change in an SSc cohort [76]; it did not differentiate between CYC and placebo in the SLS I.

The University of California, San Diego, Shortness of Breath Questionnaire (UCSD SOBQ) has also been evaluated in patients with SSc-associated PAH showing strong correlation with the HAQ-DI ($r = 0.71$, $P < 0.0001$), dyspnea assessed by VAS ($r = 0.71$, $P < 0.0001$) and the SF-36 health survey component summary (PCS) score ($r = -0.77$, $P < 0.0001$). UCSD SOBQ also had moderate correlation with the 6-minute walk test distance ($r = -0.33$, $P < 0.0001$), Borg dyspnea score ($r = -0.47$, $P < 0.0001$), and DLco ($r = -0.33$, $P < 0.0001$). Change in the UCSD SOBQ at 12 months also showed significant correlation with change in HAQ-DI and SF-36 PCS in the expected direction. Multivariate analyses also suggested a trend for validity of the UCSD SOBQ to predict relative risk of death in longitudinal analyses. These results suggest that UCSD SOBQ has good construct validity and responsiveness to change in patients with SSc-related PAH [77].

Other outcome measures for cardiopulmonary disease in SSc have been proposed—exercise echocardiography and cardiac magnetic resonance imaging – but await full validation.

Measuring Gastrointestinal Disease in SSc

Disease of gastrointestinal tract (GIT) occurs in approximately 90% of patients with SSc. Although radiological tests are cornerstones for the diagnosis of specific GIT involvement, their feasibility is questionable in multicenter trials, and radiological tests may be positive in significant proportion of patients without symptoms [78]. Furthermore, many patients with SSc have multiple types of GIT disease with overlapping symptoms, making quantification of GIT involvement in SSc extremely challenging. A Delphi panel [30] and separate expert consensus [79] recommended use of patient-reported outcome measures and body mass index as core set measures. Aside from a simple GIT visual analog scale (part of the S-HAQ [76]) that assesses daily interference in daily activities, a comprehensive scleroderma gastrointestinal instrument has been recently developed using Food and Drug Administration (FDA) guidelines.

The University of California Scleroderma Clinical Trial Consortium Gastrointestinal Instrument (UCLA SCTC GIT 2.0) is a validated, patient-reported outcome measure to assess GIT symptoms and health-related quality of life (HRQOL) in SSc [80–82]. This 34-item instrument has seven scales: reflux, distention/bloating, diarrhea, fecal soilage, constipation, emotional well-being, and social functioning and a total GI score. The instrument is feasible and has shown acceptable reliability (test-retest and internal consistency) and validity [81]. All scales are scored from 0 (better HRQOL) to 3 (worse HRQOL) except diarrhea and constipation scales that range from 0–2 to 0–2.5, respectively. Participants who rated their GIT disease as mild had lower scores on all seven scales. Symptom scales were also able to discriminate subjects with corresponding clinical GIT diagnoses. The total GIT score is the average of six of the seven scales (excludes constipation), and the total GI score is scored from 0.0 (better HRQOL) to 2.8 (worse HRQOL). The instrument is sensitive to change in patient-self rated severity and is recently translated into different languages. They are available online at https://umich.qualtrics.com/jfe/form/SV_3eBP4A4umBwnSvj.

The NIH Patient-Reported Outcomes Measurement Information System (PROMIS®) Gastrointestinal Symptom Scales also offer a broad range of tools for GI evaluation of patients with SSc, some of whom were specifically involved in the instruments' development [83–85]. Eight GI symptoms scales can be used for clinical care and research. These scales assess gastroesophageal reflux, disrupted swallowing, diarrhea, bowel incontinence/soilage, nausea and vomiting, constipation, belly pain, and gas/bloat/flatulence and have been validated in SSc [86].

Other outcome measures for gastrointestinal disease in SSc have been proposed or are under development, including manometry, transit time across different regions of the gastro-intestinal tract (including gastric transit time but also whole gut transit assessment), endoscopy, and measures of malabsorption [34]. There is lack of data on the sensitivity to change in SSc.

Measuring Vascular Disease in SSc: Raynaud's Phenomenon and Digital Ulcers

Raynaud's phenomenon (RP) occurs in approximately 90% of patients with SSc. Similarly, digital ulcers (DUs) are common in SSc and traumatic ulcers, critical digital ischemia and gangrenous lesions may also develop. There have been several clinical trials examining the efficacy of various interventions for RP and DUs in SSc [83–85]. The outcome measures can be mainly divided into those assessing the digital flow with fingertip lacticemy test, laser Doppler flowmetry, laser speckle contrast imaging, thermography, power/color Doppler ultrasound, and pre-post provocative measures (cold challenge, ischemia reperfusion testing; discussed in another chapter) or clinical measures that assess feel and function directly from the patient.

For clinical measures, the symptomatic attacks of RP (also known as symptomatic digital ischemic episodes), frequency, and duration of attacks capture the face and content validity of RP. These are captured using a standardized daily RP diary for 1–2 week period (to account for variability in the attacks) using a paper or electronic diary that also includes number of times a person goes out into the cold and also includes the Raynaud's condition score (RCS) [84], calculated by averaging the daily score on the considered time period [84]. The RCS assesses the level of difficulty experienced due to RP each day (anchored from "no difficulty" to "extreme difficulty") using a 0–100 VAS or 11-point Likert scale [84]. Moreover, the clinical trials in RP are associated with marked variability in individual outcome measures [84]. This can be decreased by capturing daily RP symptoms. A preliminary composite response index in RP has been proposed, and it could improve the ability to measure efficacy of an investigational drug and facilitate the ability to compare responses across trials [87]. The index includes RCS, patient global assessment, attack symptoms (pain, numbness, and tingling), physician global assessment of RP, duration of attacks, and the average number of attacks per day. The index needs to be validated in a placebo-controlled study.

S-HAQ VAS for RP (assesses interference in daily activities due to RP) is also feasible, reliable, and valid [84].

Measuring Digital Ulcers in SSc

Methods considered for assessing digital ulcers (DUs) include standardized photographs, measuring size of ulcers, patient and physician global assessments, simple counts of ulcer frequency, and time to healing, complete healing or prevention of ulcers.

Definition of DU was initially developed using a consensus methodology [88] and recently updated in 2017 by the World Scleroderma Foundation (WSF) [89]. This updated WSF consensus-based definition of SSc-skin ulcers identifies DU as a "loss of epidermal covering with a break in the basement membrane (which separates dermis from epidermis). It appears clinically as visible blood vessels, fibrin, granulation tissue and/or underlying deeper structures (e.g. muscle, ligament, fat) or as it would appear on debridement" and did not differentiate between active (denuded area) vs. indeterminate (defined as presence of eschar over the wound). In this definition, skin ulcers overlying calcinosis were considered traumatic and excluded. This definition has acceptable validity, feasibility, and reliability. The Kappa of this new definition for inter-rater agreement ranges from 0.51 during a first round of assessment to 0.49 during a second round. The mean intra-rater reliability is 0.90. Previous studies assessing the reliability of DU definitions, as defined as active, indeterminate, and healed DUs, also found high level of intra-rater reliability (kappa = 0.81), but poor inter-rater reliability (kappa = 0.46). These results suggest that the same observer should assess DU in RCTs [90]. Some authors have more recently suggested that all types of DUs should be considered for clinical trials, including traumatic DU and calcinosis related-DU as all SSc-DUs may share an ischemic component that is potentially responsive to vascular therapy [91]. A North American working group has also proposed a consensus definition of DU, classifying DUs as "active", "healed", and "indeterminate". This classification showed robust intra-rater kappa (0.76) for classifying DU in the "not ulcer/healed ulcer" category versus "activated/indeterminate". Inter-rater kappa for the classification into the same categories was only moderate (0.53) [92]. However, the consensus now is to classify DU as present and absent and not divide it into active, indeterminate and healed due to low agreement.

DUs have a detrimental impact on quality of life and functioning of patients with SSc (both dcSSc and lcSSc) [83–85, 93]. Preventing the occurrence of new DU is thus a key aspect of DU management in SSc.

Prevention of new DUs has been assessed in the RAPIDS and DUAL studies, respectively, evaluating the impact of bosentan and macitentan on the onset of new DU [83–85]. In these trials, the primary outcome variable was the number of new DU per patients developing during the study period. Absolute and cumulative count of DU was found to be feasible, reliable, valid, and sensitive to change, and differentiated placebo from active drugs in RAPIDS-1 and 2 trials. In trials, prevention of DUs may require a beneficial effect on feel or function, such as improvement in pain or improvement in DU specific PRO.

Complete healing of DU may be a relevant endpoint. Healing of the cardinal DU (DU that is either largest in diameter and/or causing most symptoms or disability) as a dichotomous variable (*i.e.* healed or not at the end of the study) or complete healing of DUs that were present at entry have been proposed as secondary outcomes [83–85] although these outcomes did not differentiate active drugs from placebo in these trials. Healing of DU, along with beneficial effect on feel or function, may be an approvable endpoint.

Time to healing has also been proposed as a primary endpoint for RCTs. Nonetheless, the negative results of a Phase II study assessing the effect of sildenafil on the time to healing of each DU and the negative results of RAPIDS-2 concerning the second primary outcome (time to healing of the cardinal ulcer) have highlighted an unexpectedly high healing rate in the placebo group.

Considering the impact of DUs on quality of life, DU healing or number of new DU may need to be associated with assessment of functioning or feeling to have higher clinical meaning, and this may improve the ability of these outcomes to differentiate placebo from active drugs. With this regards, S-HAQ VAS for DU (assesses interference in daily activities due to DUs) is feasible, reliable, valid, and sensitive to change as was shown in a large SSc cohort [76]. A patient-reported outcome measure has recently been validated to capture the impact of SSc-DU on hand function [94]. This instrument -the Hand Disability in Systemic Sclerosis-Digital Ulcers (HDISS-DU®)-showed good content coverage as well as excellent internal consistency and test-retest reliability, with satisfactory construct validity. Based on data from two large studies of SSc-DU patients, HDISS-DU® also showed good discriminating ability and responsiveness to change. This new instrument is a promising tool for evaluating treatment outcomes in future clinical studies and clinical practice.

DU-related complications have also been proposed as candidate outcome measures for RCTs. In addition with the number of DU and the presence of new DU since last evaluation, the preliminary Digital Ulcer Clinical Assessment Score (DUCAS) includes items such as "gangrene", "need for surgical procedures beyond standard of care", "infection", "hospitalization for DU-related issues" and the use of "analgesics to control DU-induced pain" [95]. Nonetheless, this preliminary score does not include patient-reported outcomes and still need to be validated in RCTs.

Measuring Physical Function and Health-Related Quality of Life in SSc

SSc is associated with a detrimental effect on physical functioning and patients' emotional and psychological well-being, and different measures have been used.

The Short Form 36 (SF-36) and the Health Assessment Questionnaire-Disability Index (HAQ-DI)

The 36-Item Short Form Health Survey questionnaire (SF-36) is an instrument broadly used for evaluating health-related quality of Life [96]. It is a self-administrated questionnaire based on eight scales exploring physical functioning, role physical, general health, vitality, social functioning, role emotional, and mental health. Therefore, this instrument explores two main dimensions, a physical component and a mental component, with all scales contributing in different proportions to the scoring of both physical and mental dimensions.

Health assessment questionnaire-disability index (HAQ-DI) is a self-administered 20-question instrument that assesses a patient's level of functional ability and includes questions on fine movements of the upper extremities, locomotor activities of the lower extremities, and activities that involve both the upper and lower extremities [97]. The HAQ-DI score is determined by summing the highest item score in each of the eight domains and dividing the sum by 8, yielding a score ranging from 0 (no disability) to 3 (severe disability). Investigators should be aware that the scoring rules permit the scoring of two disability indices: the standard disability index, which takes into account the use of aids and devices and the alternative disability index, which does not. Investigators often do not specify which method is being used. Investigators should clearly delineate the method used to obtain the aggregate score [98]. The hand components of the HAQ-DI were able to differentiate bosentan from placebo in an RCT for digital ulcers in SSc [88].

Both the SF-36 (a measure of HRQOL) and the HAQ-DI (a measure of function) have been extensively incorporated into multicenter clinical trials of SSc [72, 99, 100]. Both instruments likely have face and content validity as they measure constructs that are important to patients with SSc but it has not been formally evaluated, and both measures are easy to administer [76]. However, some investigators have criticized the HAQ-DI for insufficiently assessing disability caused by skin tightness and muscle weakness [101, 102]. The S-HAQ has incremental content validity to the HAQ-DI, because it contains SSc-specific domains that contribute to the multifaceted conceptual framework of disability in SSc. The addition of the S-HAQ VASs enhances the ability to capture disability secondary to internal organ involvement over the HAQ-DI alone [103]. S-HAQ VASs have test–retest reliability [102] and construct validity [38]. The HAQ-DI also has good discriminant validity as SSc patients with dcSSc have a significantly worse HAQ-DI score compared with those with lcSSc (1.36 vs 0.59; $p < 0.001$) [104].

Both the SF-36 and HAQ-DI have good construct validity as the SF-36 physical component summary and HAQ-DI score in SSc patients were adversely affected by joint involvement, GI involvement, and high skin score [104]. The SF-36 has good discriminant validity as SSc patients with dcSSc had lower SF-36 scores than patients with lcSSc (40.5 vs 32.4; $p = 0.01$). Similarly, patients with dcSSc have lower SF-36 physical component summary index (32.4 vs 40.5; $p = 0.01$) and physical functioning domain scores (44.8 vs 64.1; $p < 0.01$) than patients with lcSSc [104]. Although the test-retest reliability for SF-36 has been acceptable in other rheumatologic diseases, no study has formally evaluated reliability in SSc. SF-36 and HAQ-DI were found to be responsive to change in two RCTs [99, 100]. In addition, baseline HAQ-DI scores predict mortality in early dcSSc [76, 105]. The SF-36 and HAQ-DI complement each other, and both should be incorporated as measures of HRQOL and disability in organ-specific trials in SSc [103].

UK Functional Score (UKFS) is a self-administered 11-item functional questionnaire. It includes nine items relating to upper extremity function and two items relating to muscle weakness and lower extremity function [101]. Each item is scored under four categories with both an integer and a descriptive heading, ranging from 0 (able to perform in a normal manner) to 3 (impossible to achieve) with an overall score between 0 and 33. It is feasible and has acceptable test-retest reliability (kappa ≥ 0.69). UKFS is able to differentiate between lcSSc and dcSSc ($p < 0.05$) and is highly correlated with HAQ-DI (coefficient = 0.90). UKFS was found to change during a longitudinal study with a correlation of 0.59 with HAQ-DI [106, 107].

Preference-Based Measures for HRQOL in SSc: The Short Form 6D (SF-6D)

The Short Form 6D (SF-6D) is a preference-based measure that is derived from the SF-36 by using population-based utilities of health states. Preference-based measures are used in decision and cost-effectiveness analyses. SF-6D is feasible as it only requires completion of the SF-36. The test-retest reliability assessed was acceptable. The SF-36 has face and content validity as it conforms to the guidelines by the United States Public Health Service Panel on Cost-Effectiveness in Health and Medicine [108]. Construct validity was confirmed by showing good correlation with the HAQ-DI and with patient global assessment in a recent clinical trial [109]. SF-6D was able to discriminate among the baseline severity of the HAQ-DI and patient global assessment and was sensitive to change.

Other generic and disease-specific measures have been tested in SSc, including the scleroderma assessment questionnaire, and measures of anxiety, fatigue, and depression [110]. These instruments have not yet been shown to be sensitive to change in SSc and further studies are needed to explore these dimensions [111].

Patient-Reported Outcomes Measurement Information System (PROMIS)

The NIH PROMIS® Roadmap initiative is a cooperative group program of research designed to develop, evaluate, and standardize item banks to measure patient-reported outcomes relevant across common medical conditions [112]. For adults, domains have been developed in physical, mental, and social health. There is evidence to support the feasibility and construct validity of the PROMIS® item banks in SSc [113], including a GI symptoms bank [114]. PROMIS® item banks are being incorporated in ongoing RCTs.

American College of Rheumatology Provisional Composite Response Index for Clinical Trials in Early Diffuse Cutaneous Systemic Sclerosis (CRISS) Index

Using well-accepted expert consensus and data-driven approaches, the ACR-CRISS index has been developed for dcSSc trials [30, 115]. ACR-CRISS is calculated as a two-step process. The first step evaluates clinically significant decline in renal or cardiopulmonary involvement; if present, the patient is adjudicated as non-improved. The second step assesses remaining patients and calculates the predicted probability of improvement for changes in the mRSS, FVC percent predicted, patient and physician global assessments, and HAQ-DI over 1 year on a 0.0 [no improvement] – 1.0 scale [marked improvement]. The index captures global improvement in early SSc. The index was able to differentiate the effect of tocilizumab and abatacept in a 1-year RCT ($p < 0.05$), capturing the global improvement in SSc [115].

However, ACR-CRISS has certain limitations. First, it is a probability score that was developed using expert consensus, where expert assigned the highest weight to mRSS followed by FVC. In addition, the score may be difficult to interpret and may have ceiling effect, especially in RCTs with background immunosuppressive therapy. Using the concept of the ACR 20%, 50%, and 70% response index used in rheumatoid arthritis, three RCTs were reanalyzed and a new index (revised CRISS) has been proposed - the proportion of participants who improved by a pre-defined percentage in ≥ 3 of 5 core set measures of mRSS, FVC percent predicted, patient and physician global assessments, and HAQ-DI. Each component is provided the same weight in the index. It has an advantage of easy interpretation and pre-defined cutoffs can be used to assess differences between active therapy vs. placebo [116]. This revised CRISS needs to be prospectively validated in RCT.

Biomarkers for SSc

Biomarkers in SSc can be proposed either as 1) predictive markers of progression, useful for enrichment or for patient selection/stratification or 2) responsive markers that can differentiate active therapy from placebo, highlighting the key molecular pathways influenced by active therapy and eventually associated with clinically meaningful improvement. Candidate biomarkers in SSc are comprehensively described in another chapter. Thus, we will only highlight here the role of readily available markers such as acute phase reactants Erythrocyte sedimentation rate and C-reactive protein (ESR, CRP) that are associated with disease activity [7], predict progressive ILD and mortality [76, 117] and can be used for cohort enrichment [50] as demonstrated in the tocilizumab phase III trial [20]. Scleroderma-specific autoantibodies are also valuable for predicting skin, vascular, and internal organ involvement [118]. Autoantibodies are useful for cohort enrichment [119] and could be important for patient stratification in RCTs and is discussed in another chapter.

Conclusion

This chapter outlines and discusses the outcome measures that are feasible, reliable, and valid for RCTs in SSc. Recent progress has been achieved in the assessment of patients with SSc in RCTs, including combined response indices and patients-reported outcomes, as well as validated functional or radiological outcome measures such as FVC and HRCT findings.

Acknowledgments The previous edition of this chapter was co-authored with Sindhu R. Johnson MD, PhD, FRCPC from Toronto Scleroderma Program, Mount Sinai Hospital, Toronto Western Hospital, Toronto, ON, Canada.

References

1. Khanna D, et al. Measures of response in clinical trials of systemic sclerosis: the Combined Response Index for Systemic Sclerosis (CRISS) and outcome measures in pulmonary arterial hypertension related to systemic sclerosis (EPOSS). J Rheumatol. 2009;36:2356–61.
2. Khanna D. In: Hochberg M, Silman A, Smolen J, Weinblatt M, Weisman M, editors. Rheumatology. St. Louis: Mosby; 2010. p. 1367–71.
3. Khanna D, Tsevat J. Health-related quality of life—an introduction. Am J Manag Care. 2007;13(Suppl. 9):S218–23.
4. Symmons DP. Disease assessment indices: activity, damage and severity. Baillieres Clin Rheumatol. 1995;9:267–85.
5. Medsger TA Jr. Natural history of systemic sclerosis and the assessment of disease activity, severity, functional status, and psychologic well-being. Rheum Dis Clin N Am. 2003;29:255–73.
6. Valentini G, et al. The European Scleroderma Trials and Research group (EUSTAR) task force for the development of revised activity criteria for systemic sclerosis: derivation and validation of a preliminarily revised EUSTAR activity index. Ann Rheum Dis. 2017;76:270–6.
7. Valentini G, et al. European multicentre study to define disease activity criteria for systemic sclerosis. II. Identification of disease activity variables and development of preliminary activity indexes. Ann Rheum Dis. 2001;60:592–8.
8. Valentini G, D'Angelo S, Della Rossa A, Bencivelli W, Bombardieri S. European Scleroderma Study Group to define disease activity criteria for systemic sclerosis. IV. Assessment of skin thickening by modified Rodnan skin score. Ann Rheum Dis. 2003;62:904–5.
9. Fasano S, et al. Revised European Scleroderma Trials and Research Group Activity Index is the best predictor of short-term severity accrual. Ann Rheum Dis. 2019;78:1681–5.
10. García-Martín A, et al. EHP-101, an oral formulation of the cannabidiol aminoquinone VCE-004.8, alleviates bleomycin-induced skin and lung fibrosis. Biochem Pharmacol. 2018;157:304–13.
11. Ferdowsi N, et al. Development and validation of the Scleroderma Clinical Trials Consortium Damage Index (SCTC-DI): a novel instrument to quantify organ damage in systemic sclerosis. Ann Rheum Dis. 2019;78:807–16.
12. Medsger TA Jr, et al. A disease severity scale for systemic sclerosis: development and testing. J Rheumatol. 1999;26:2159–67.
13. Geirsson AJ, Wollheim FA, Akesson A. Disease severity of 100 patients with systemic sclerosis over a period of 14 years: using a modified Medsger scale. Ann Rheum Dis. 2001;60:1117–22.
14. Sumpton D, et al. Scope and consistency of outcomes reported in trials of patients with systemic sclerosis. Arthritis Care Res (Hoboken). 2020;72:1449–58.
15. Clements PJ, et al. Skin thickness score as a predictor and correlate of outcome in systemic sclerosis: high-dose versus low-dose penicillamine trial. Arthritis Rheum. 2000;43:2445–54.
16. Clements P, et al. Inter and intraobserver variability of total skin thickness score (modified Rodnan TSS) in systemic sclerosis. J Rheumatol. 1995;22:1281–5.
17. Dobrota R, et al. Prediction of improvement in skin fibrosis in diffuse cutaneous systemic sclerosis: a EUSTAR analysis. Ann Rheum Dis. 2016;75:1743–8.
18. Ledoult E, et al. Early trajectories of skin thickening are associated with severity and mortality in systemic sclerosis. Arthritis Res Ther. 2020;22:30.
19. Clements P, Medsger TA, Feghali C. Cutaneous involvement in systemic sclerosis. In: Clements P, Furst DE, editors. Systemic sclerosis. Philadelphia: Lippincott Williams & Wilkins; 2004. p. 129–50.
20. Khanna D, et al. Tocilizumab in systemic sclerosis: a randomised, double-blind, placebo-controlled, phase 3 trial. Lancet Respir Med. 2020;8:963–74.
21. Khanna D, et al. Abatacept in early diffuse cutaneous systemic sclerosis: results of a phase II investigator-initiated, multicenter, double-blind, randomized, placebo-controlled trial. Arthritis Rheumatol (Hoboken, N.J.). 2020;72:125–36.
22. Khanna D, et al. Riociguat in patients with early diffuse cutaneous systemic sclerosis (RISE-SSc): randomised, double-

blind, placebo-controlled multicentre trial. Ann Rheum Dis. 2020;79:618–25.
23. Allanore Y, et al. A randomised, double-blind, placebo-controlled, 24-week, phase II, proof-of-concept study of romilkimab (SAR156597) in early diffuse cutaneous systemic sclerosis. Ann Rheum Dis. 2020;79:1600–7.
24. Herrick AL, et al. Patterns and predictors of skin score change in early diffuse systemic sclerosis from the European Scleroderma Observational Study. Ann Rheumatic Dis. 2018;77:563–70.
25. Khanna D, et al. Standardization of the modified Rodnan skin score for use in clinical trials of systemic sclerosis. J Scleroderma Rel Disord. 2017;2(1):11–8.
26. Amjadi S, et al. Course of the modified Rodnan skin thickness score in systemic sclerosis clinical trials: analysis of three large multicenter, double-blind, randomized controlled trials. Arthritis Rheum. 2009;60:2490–8.
27. Khanna D, et al. A phase 2a randomized, double-blind, placebo-controlled study of ziritaxestat in early diffuse cutaneous systemic sclerosis (NOVESA). Arthritis Rheumatol (Hoboken, NJ). 2020;72(Suppl. 10):L09.
28. Merkel PA, et al. Validity, reliability, and feasibility of durometer measurements of scleroderma skin disease in a multicenter treatment trial. Arthritis Rheum. 2008;59:699–705.
29. Kissin EY, et al. Durometry for the assessment of skin disease in systemic sclerosis. Arthritis Rheum. 2006;55:603–9.
30. Khanna D, et al. Development of a provisional core set of response measures for clinical trials of systemic sclerosis. Ann Rheum Dis. 2008;67:703–9.
31. Man A, et al. Development and validation of a patient-reported outcome instrument for skin involvement in patients with systemic sclerosis. Ann Rheum Dis. 2017;76:1374–80.
32. Man A, Dgetluck N, White B. Prospective validation of the systemic sclerosis skin symptoms patient-reported outcome (SSPRO) in a Phase 2 trial of anabasum (JBT-101) in diffuse cutaneous systemic sclerosis (dcSSc). Arthritis Rheumatol (Hoboken, N.J.). 2017;69(11) https://acrabstracts.org/abstract/prospective-validation-of-the-systemic-sclerosis-skin-symptoms-patient-reported-outcome-sspro-in-a-phase-2-trial-of-anabasum-jbt-101-in-diffuse-cutaneous-systemic-sclerosis-dcssc/. Accessed September 11, 2023
33. Spiera R, et al. Safety and efficacof Lenabasum in a Phase II, randomized, placebo-controlled trial in adults with systemic sclerosis. Arthritis Rheumatol (Hoboken, N.J.). 2020;72:1350–60.
34. Merkel PA, et al. Current status of outcome measure development for clinical trials in systemic sclerosis. Report from OMERACT 6. J Rheumatol. 2003;30:1630–47.
35. Lescoat A, et al. Synovial involvement assessed by power Doppler ultra-sonography in systemic sclerosis: results of a cross-sectional study. Rheumatology (Oxford). 2018;57:2012–21.
36. Khanna PP, et al. Tendon friction rubs in early diffuse systemic sclerosis: prevalence, characteristics and longitudinal changes in a randomized controlled trial. Rheumatology (Oxford). 2010;49:955–9.
37. Rannou F, et al. Assessing disability and quality of life in systemic sclerosis: construct validities of the Cochin Hand Function Scale, Health Assessment Questionnaire (HAQ), Systemic Sclerosis HAQ, and Medical Outcomes Study 36-Item Short Form Health Survey. Arthritis Rheum. 2007;57:94–102.
38. Brower LM, Poole JL. Reliability and validity of the Duruoz Hand Index in persons with systemic sclerosis (scleroderma). Arthritis Rheum. 2004;51:805–9.
39. Bongi SM, et al. Efficacy of connective tissue massage and Mc Mennell joint manipulation in the rehabilitative treatment of the hands in systemic sclerosis. Clin Rheumatol. 2009;28:1167–73.
40. Sandqvist G, Eklund M. Validity of HAMIS: a test of hand mobility in scleroderma. Arthritis Care Res. 2000;13:382–7.
41. Sandqvist G, Eklund M. Hand Mobility in Scleroderma (HAMIS) test: the reliability of a novel hand function test. Arthritis Care Res. 2000;13:369–74.
42. Mouthon L, et al. Development and validation of a scale for mouth handicap in systemic sclerosis: the Mouth Handicap in Systemic Sclerosis scale. Ann Rheum Dis. 2007;66:1651–5.
43. Maddali-Bongi S, et al. The rehabilitation of facial involvement in systemic sclerosis: efficacy of the combination of connective tissue massage, Kabat's technique and kinesitherapy: a randomized controlled trial. Rheumatol Int. 2011;31:895–901.
44. Steen VD, Conte C, Owens GR, Medsger TA Jr. Severe restrictive lung disease in systemic sclerosis. Arthritis Rheum. 1994;37:1283–9.
45. Tashkin DP, et al. Cyclophosphamide versus placebo in scleroderma lung disease. N Engl J Med. 2006;354:2655–66.
46. Seibold JR, et al. Randomized, prospective, placebo-controlled trial of bosentan in interstitial lung disease secondary to systemic sclerosis. Arthritis Rheum. 2010;62:2101–8.
47. Hoyles RK, et al. A multicenter, prospective, randomized, double-blind, placebo-controlled trial of corticosteroids and intravenous cyclophosphamide followed by oral azathioprine for the treatment of pulmonary fibrosis in scleroderma. Arthritis Rheum. 2006;54:3962–70.
48. Berry CE, Wise RA. Interpretation of pulmonary function test: issues and controversies. Clin Rev Allergy Immunol. 2009;37:173–80.
49. Distler O, et al. Nintedanib for systemic sclerosis-associated interstitial lung disease. N Engl J Med. 2019;380:2518–28.
50. Khanna D, et al. Safety and efficacy of subcutaneous tocilizumab in adults with systemic sclerosis (faSScinate): a phase 2, randomised, controlled trial. Lancet. 2016;387:2630–40.
51. Volkmann ER, et al. Short-term progression of interstitial lung disease in systemic sclerosis predicts long-term survival in two independent clinical trial cohorts. Ann Rheum Dis. 2019;78:122–30.
52. Kafaja S, et al. Reliability and minimal clinically important differences of forced vital capacity: results from the Scleroderma Lung Studies (SLS-I and SLS-II). Am J Respir Crit Care Med. 2018;197:644–52.
53. Latsi PI, et al. Fibrotic idiopathic interstitial pneumonia: the prognostic value of longitudinal functional trends. Am J Respir Crit Care Med. 2003;168:531–7.
54. Goh NS, et al. Interstitial lung disease in systemic sclerosis: a simple staging system. Am J Respir Crit Care Med. 2008;177:1248–54.
55. Tashkin DP, et al. Relationship between quantitative radiographic assessments of interstitial lung disease and physiological and clinical features of systemic sclerosis. Ann Rheum Dis. 2016;75:374–81.
56. Khanna D, et al. Systemic sclerosis-associated interstitial lung disease: lessons from clinical trials, outcome measures, and future study design. Curr Rheumatol Rev. 2010;6:138–44.
57. Khanna D, et al. Systemic sclerosis-associated interstitial lung disease-proposed recommendations for future randomized clinical trials. Clin Exp Rheumatol. 2010;28:S55–62.
58. Khanna D, et al. Recommendations for screening and detection of connective tissue disease-associated pulmonary arterial hypertension. Arthritis Rheum. 2013;65:3194–201.
59. Wanger J, et al. Standardisation of the measurement of lung volumes. Eur Respir J. 2005;26:511–22.
60. Miller MR, et al. Standardisation of spirometry. Eur Respir J. 2005;26:319–38.
61. Macintyre N, et al. Standardisation of the single-breath determination of carbon monoxide uptake in the lung. Eur Respir J. 2005;26:720–35.
62. Goldin J, et al. Treatment of scleroderma-interstitial lung disease with cyclophosphamide is associated with less progressive fibro-

sis on serial thoracic high-resolution CT scan than placebo: findings from the scleroderma lung study. Chest. 2009;136:1333–40.
63. Buch MH, et al. Submaximal exercise testing in the assessment of interstitial lung disease secondary to systemic sclerosis: reproducibility and correlations of the 6-min walk test. Ann Rheum Dis. 2007;66:169–73.
64. Schoindre Y, et al. Lack of specificity of the 6-minute walk test as an outcome measure for patients with systemic sclerosis. J Rheumatol. 2009;36:1481–5.
65. Garin MC, Highland KB, Silver RM, Strange C. Limitations to the 6-minute walk test in interstitial lung disease and pulmonary hypertension in scleroderma. J Rheumatol. 2009;36:330–6.
66. Miyamoto S, et al. Clinical correlates and prognostic significance of six-minute walk test in patients with primary pulmonary hypertension. Comparison with cardiopulmonary exercise testing. Am J Respir Crit Care Med. 2000;161:487–92.
67. Badesch DB, et al. Continuous intravenous epoprostenol for pulmonary hypertension due to the scleroderma spectrum of disease. A randomized, controlled trial. Ann Intern Med. 2000;132:425–34.
68. Sitbon O, et al. Clinical trial design and new therapies for pulmonary arterial hypertension. Eur Respir J. 2019;53(1):1801908.
69. Pulido T, et al. Macitentan and morbidity and mortality in pulmonary arterial hypertension. N Engl J Med. 2013;369:809–18.
70. Galie N, et al. Initial use of Ambrisentan plus Tadalafil in pulmonary arterial hypertension. N Engl J Med. 2015;373:834–44.
71. Mahler DA, Weinberg DH, Wells CK, Feinstein AR. The measurement of dyspnea. Contents, interobserver agreement, and physiologic correlates of two new clinical indexes. Chest. 1984;85:751–8.
72. Khanna D, et al. Correlation of the degree of dyspnea with health-related quality of life, functional abilities, and diffusing capacity for carbon monoxide in patients with systemic sclerosis and active alveolitis: results from the Scleroderma Lung Study. Arthritis Rheum. 2005;52:592–600.
73. Khanna D, et al. Minimally important differences in the Mahler's Transition Dyspnoea Index in a large randomized controlled trial—results from the Scleroderma Lung Study. Rheumatology (Oxford). 2009;48:1537–40.
74. Wallace B, et al. Reliability, validity and responsiveness to change of the Saint George's Respiratory Questionnaire in early diffuse cutaneous systemic sclerosis. Rheumatology (Oxford). 2015;54:1369–79.
75. Volkmann ER, et al. Treatment with mycophenolate and cyclophosphamide leads to clinically meaningful improvements in patient-reported outcomes in scleroderma lung disease: results of Scleroderma Lung Study II. ACR Open Rheumatol. 2020;2:362–70.
76. Steen VD, Medsger TA Jr. The value of the Health Assessment Questionnaire and special patient-generated scales to demonstrate change in systemic sclerosis patients over time. Arthritis Rheum. 1997;40:1984–91.
77. Chung L, Chen H, Khanna D, Steen VD. Dyspnea assessment and pulmonary hypertension in patients with systemic sclerosis: utility of the University of California, San Diego, Shortness of Breath Questionnaire. Arthritis Care Res. 2013;65:454–63.
78. Clements PJ, Becvar R, Drosos AA, Ghattas L, Gabrielli A. Assessment of gastrointestinal involvement. Clin Exp Rheumatol. 2003;21:S15–8.
79. Baron M, et al. Screening and therapy for malnutrition and related gastro-intestinal disorders in systemic sclerosis: recommendations of a North American expert panel. Clin Exp Rheumatol. 2010;28:S42–6.
80. Khanna D, et al. Development of a preliminary scleroderma gastrointestinal tract 1.0 quality of life instrument. Arthritis Rheum. 2007;57:1280–6.
81. Khanna D, et al. Reliability and validity of the University of California, Los Angeles Scleroderma Clinical Trial Consortium Gastrointestinal Tract Instrument. Arthritis Rheum. 2009;61:1257–63.
82. Bodukam V, et al. Association of gastrointestinal involvement and depressive symptoms in patients with systemic sclerosis. Rheumatology (Oxford). 2011;50:330–4.
83. Wigley FM, et al. Intravenous iloprost infusion in patients with Raynaud phenomenon secondary to systemic sclerosis. A multicenter, placebo-controlled, double-blind study. Ann Intern Med. 1994;120:199–206.
84. Merkel PA, et al. Measuring disease activity and functional status in patients with scleroderma and Raynaud's phenomenon. Arthritis Rheum. 2002;46:2410–20.
85. Fries R, Shariat K, von Wilmowsky H, Bohm M. Sildenafil in the treatment of Raynaud's phenomenon resistant to vasodilatory therapy. Circulation. 2005;112:2980–5.
86. Nagaraja V, et al. Construct validity of the Patient-Reported Outcomes Measurement Information System gastrointestinal symptom scales in systemic sclerosis. Arthritis Care Res (Hoboken). 2014;66:1725–30.
87. Gladue H, Maranian P, Paulus HE, Khanna D. Evaluation of test characteristics for outcome measures used in Raynaud's phenomenon clinical trials. Arthritis Care Res (Hoboken). 2013;65:630–6.
88. Korn JH, et al. Digital ulcers in systemic sclerosis: prevention by treatment with bosentan, an oral endothelin receptor antagonist. Arthritis Rheum. 2004;50:3985–93.
89. Suliman YA, et al. Defining skin ulcers in systemic sclerosis: systematic literature review and proposed World Scleroderma Foundation (WSF) definition. J Scleroderma Relat Disord. 2017;2:115–20.
90. Matucci-Cerinic M, et al. Bosentan treatment of digital ulcers related to systemic sclerosis: results from the RAPIDS-2 randomised, double-blind, placebo-controlled trial. Ann Rheum Dis. 2011;70:32–8.
91. Hughes M, Murray A, Denton CP, Herrick AL. Should all digital ulcers be included in future clinical trials of systemic sclerosis-related digital vasculopathy? Med Hypotheses. 2018;116:101–4.
92. Baron M, et al. Consensus opinion of a North American Working Group regarding the classification of digital ulcers in systemic sclerosis. Clin Rheumatol. 2014;33:207–14.
93. Mouthon L, et al. Ischemic digital ulcers affect hand disability and pain in systemic sclerosis. J Rheumatol. 2014;41:1317–23.
94. Mouthon L, et al. Psychometric validation of the Hand Disability in Systemic Sclerosis-Digital Ulcers (HDISS-DU(R)) patient-reported outcome instrument. Arthritis Res Ther. 2020;22:3.
95. Bruni C, et al. Preliminary Validation of the Digital Ulcer Clinical Assessment Score in Systemic Sclerosis. J Rheumatol. 2019;46:603–8.
96. Lins L, Carvalho FM. SF-36 total score as a single measure of health-related quality of life: Scoping review. SAGE Open Med. 2016;4:2050312116671725.
97. Fries JF, Spitz P, Kraines RG, Holman HR. Measurement of patient outcome in arthritis. Arthritis Rheum. 1980;23:137–45.
98. Johnson SR, Lee P. The HAQ disability index in scleroderma trials. Rheumatology (Oxford). 2004;43:1200–1.
99. Khanna D, et al. Impact of oral cyclophosphamide on health-related quality of life in patients with active scleroderma lung disease: results from the scleroderma lung study. Arthritis Rheum. 2007;56:1676–84.

100. Khanna D, et al. Responsiveness of the SF-36 and the Health Assessment Questionnaire Disability Index in a systemic sclerosis clinical trial. J Rheumatol. 2005;32:832–40.
101. Silman A, et al. Assessment of functional ability in patients with scleroderma: a proposed new disability assessment instrument. J Rheumatol. 1998;25:79–83.
102. Poole JL, Williams CA, Bloch DA, Hollak B, Spitz P. Concurrent validity of the Health Assessment Questionnaire disability index in scleroderma. Arthritis Care Res. 1995;8:189–93.
103. Johnson SR, Hawker GA, Davis AM. The health assessment questionnaire disability index and scleroderma health assessment questionnaire in scleroderma trials: an evaluation of their measurement properties. Arthritis Rheum. 2005;53:256–62.
104. Johnson SR, Glaman DD, Schentag CT, Lee P. Quality of life and functional status in systemic sclerosis compared to other rheumatic diseases. J Rheumatol. 2006;33:1117–22.
105. Clements PJ, et al. The Disability Index of the Health Assessment Questionnaire is a predictor and correlate of outcome in the high-dose versus low-dose penicillamine in systemic sclerosis trial. Arthritis Rheum. 2001;44:653–61.
106. Smyth AE, et al. A cross-sectional comparison of three self-reported functional indices in scleroderma. Rheumatology (Oxford). 2003;42:732–8.
107. Serednicka K, Smyth AE, Black CM, Denton CP. Using a self-reported functional score to assess disease progression in systemic sclerosis. Rheumatology (Oxford). 2007;46:1107–10.
108. Weinstein MC, Siegel JE, Gold MR, Kamlet MS, Russell LB. Recommendations of the Panel on Cost-effectiveness in Health and Medicine. JAMA. 1996;276:1253–8.
109. Khanna D, et al. Reliability, validity, and minimally important differences of the SF-6D in systemic sclerosis. Qual Life Res. 2007;16:1083–92.
110. Thombs BD, Hudson M, Taillefer SS, Baron M, G. Canadian scleroderma research, prevalence and clinical correlates of symptoms of depression in patients with systemic sclerosis. Arthritis Rheum. 2008;59:504–9.
111. Stamm T, Mosor E, Omara M, Ritschl V, Murphy SL. How can fatigue be addressed in individuals with systemic sclerosis? Lancet Rheumatol. 2020;2:e128–9.
112. Khanna D, et al. The future of measuring patient-reported outcomes in rheumatology: Patient-Reported Outcomes Measurement Information System (PROMIS). Arthritis Care Res (Hoboken). 2011;63(Suppl. 11):S486–90.
113. Khanna D, et al. Feasibility and construct validity of PROMIS and "legacy" instruments in an academic scleroderma clinic. Value Health. 2012;15:128–34.
114. Spiegel BM, et al. Development of the NIH Patient-Reported Outcomes Measurement Information System (PROMIS) gastrointestinal symptom scales. Am J Gastroenterol. 2014;109:1804–14.
115. Khanna D, et al. The American College of Rheumatology Provisional composite response index for clinical trials in early diffuse cutaneous systemic sclerosis. Arthritis Rheumatol (Hoboken, NJ). 2016;68:299–311.
116. Khanna D, Huang S, Lin CJF, Spino C. New composite endpoint in early diffuse cutaneous systemic sclerosis: revisiting the provisional American College of Rheumatology Composite Response Index in Systemic Sclerosis. Ann Rheum Dis. 2021;80(5):641–50.
117. Scussel-Lonzetti L, et al. Predicting mortality in systemic sclerosis: analysis of a cohort of 309 French Canadian patients with emphasis on features at diagnosis as predictive factors for survival. Medicine (Baltimore). 2002;81:154–67.
118. Nihtyanova SI, et al. Using Autoantibodies and cutaneous subset to develop outcome-based disease classification in systemic sclerosis. Arthritis Rheumatol (Hoboken, N.J.). 2020;72:465–76.
119. Steen VD. Autoantibodies in systemic sclerosis. Semin Arthritis Rheum. 2005;35:35–42.

Recommended Reading

Allanore Y, et al. A randomised, double-blind, placebo-controlled, 24-week, phase II, proof-of-concept study of romilkimab (SAR156597) in early diffuse cutaneous systemic sclerosis. Ann Rheum Dis. 2020;79:1600–7.

Distler O, et al. Nintedanib for systemic sclerosis-associated interstitial lung disease. N Engl J Med. 2019;380:2518–28.

Gladue H, Maranian P, Paulus HE, Khanna D. Evaluation of test characteristics for outcome measures used in Raynaud's phenomenon clinical trials. Arthritis Care Res (Hoboken). 2013;65:630–6.

Johnson SR, Glaman DD, Schentag CT, Lee P. Quality of life and functional status in systemic sclerosis compared to other rheumatic diseases. J Rheumatol. 2006;33:1117–22.

Johnson SR, Hawker GA, Davis AM. The health assessment questionnaire disability index and scleroderma health assessment questionnaire in scleroderma trials: an evaluation of their measurement properties. Arthritis Rheum. 2005;53:256–62.

Kafaja S, et al. Reliability and minimal clinically important differences of forced vital capacity: results from the Scleroderma Lung Studies (SLS-I and SLS-II). Am J Respir Crit Care Med. 2018;197:644–52.

Khanna D, et al. Responsiveness of the SF-36 and the Health Assessment Questionnaire Disability Index in a systemic sclerosis clinical trial. J Rheumatol. 2005;32:832–40.

Khanna D, et al. Development of a provisional core set of response measures for clinical trials of systemic sclerosis. Ann Rheum Dis. 2008;67:703–9.

Khanna D, et al. Measures of response in clinical trials of systemic sclerosis: the Combined Response Index for Systemic Sclerosis (CRISS) and outcome measures in pulmonary arterial hypertension related to systemic sclerosis (EPOSS). J Rheumatol. 2009;36:2356–61.

Khanna D, et al. The future of measuring patient-reported outcomes in rheumatology: Patient-Reported Outcomes Measurement Information System (PROMIS). Arthritis Care Res (Hoboken). 2011;63(Suppl. 11):S486–90.

Khanna D, et al. Feasibility and construct validity of PROMIS and "legacy" instruments in an academic scleroderma clinic. Value Health. 2012;15:128–34.

Khanna D, et al. Recommendations for screening and detection of connective tissue disease-associated pulmonary arterial hypertension. Arthritis Rheum. 2013;65:3194–201.

Khanna D, et al. Safety and efficacy of subcutaneous tocilizumab in adults with systemic sclerosis (faSScinate): a phase 2, randomised, controlled trial. Lancet. 2016;387:2630–40.

Khanna D, et al. The American College of Rheumatology Provisional composite response index for clinical trials in early diffuse cutaneous systemic sclerosis. Arthritis Rheumatol (Hoboken, N.J.). 2016;68:299–311.

Khanna D, et al. Tocilizumab in systemic sclerosis: a randomised, double-blind, placebo-controlled, phase 3 trial. Lancet Respir Med. 2020;8:963–74.

Khanna D, et al. Abatacept in early diffuse cutaneous systemic sclerosis: results of a phase II investigator-initiated, multicenter, double-blind, randomized, placebo-controlled trial. Arthritis Rheumatol (Hoboken, N.J.). 2020;72:125–36.

Khanna D, et al. Riociguat in patients with early diffuse cutaneous systemic sclerosis (RISE-SSc): randomised, double-blind, placebo-controlled multicentre trial. Ann Rheum Dis. 2020;79:618–25.

Khanna PP, et al. Tendon friction rubs in early diffuse systemic sclerosis: prevalence, characteristics and longitudinal changes in a randomized controlled trial. Rheumatology (Oxford). 2010;49:955–9.

Matucci-Cerinic M, et al. Bosentan treatment of digital ulcers related to systemic sclerosis: results from the RAPIDS-2 randomised, double-blind, placebo-controlled trial. Ann Rheum Dis. 2011;70:32–8.

Medsger TA Jr, et al. A disease severity scale for systemic sclerosis: development and testing. J Rheumatol. 1999;26:2159–67.
Mouthon L, et al. Development and validation of a scale for mouth handicap in systemic sclerosis: the Mouth Handicap in Systemic Sclerosis scale. Ann Rheum Dis. 2007;66:1651–5.
Mouthon L, et al. Psychometric validation of the Hand Disability in Systemic Sclerosis-Digital Ulcers (HDISS-DU(R)) patient-reported outcome instrument. Arthritis Res Ther. 2020;22:3.
Nihtyanova SI, et al. Using autoantibodies and cutaneous subset to develop outcome-based disease classification in systemic sclerosis. Arthritis & rheumatology (Hoboken, N.J.). 2020;72:465–76.
Poole JL, Williams CA, Bloch DA, Hollak B, Spitz P. Concurrent validity of the health assessment questionnaire disability index in scleroderma. Arthritis Care Res. 1995;8:189–93.
Rannou F, et al. Assessing disability and quality of life in systemic sclerosis: construct validities of the Cochin Hand Function Scale, Health Assessment Questionnaire (HAQ), Systemic Sclerosis HAQ, and Medical Outcomes Study 36-Item Short Form Health Survey. Arthritis Rheum. 2007;57:94–102.
Silman A, et al. Assessment of functional ability in patients with scleroderma: a proposed new disability assessment instrument. J Rheumatol. 1998;25:79–83.
Spiegel BM, et al. Development of the NIH Patient-Reported Outcomes Measurement Information System (PROMIS) gastrointestinal symptom scales. Am J Gastroenterol. 2014;109:1804–14.
Steen VD, Medsger TA Jr. The value of the Health Assessment Questionnaire and special patient-generated scales to demonstrate change in systemic sclerosis patients over time. Arthritis Rheum. 1997;40:1984–91.
Sumpton D, et al. Scope and consistency of outcomes reported in trials of patients with systemic sclerosis. Arthritis Care Res (Hoboken). 2020;72:1449–58.
Tashkin DP, et al. Cyclophosphamide versus placebo in scleroderma lung disease. N Engl J Med. 2006;354:2655–66.
Tashkin DP, et al. Relationship between quantitative radiographic assessments of interstitial lung disease and physiological and clinical features of systemic sclerosis. Ann Rheum Dis. 2016;75:374–81.
Volkmann ER, et al. Short-term progression of interstitial lung disease in systemic sclerosis predicts long-term survival in two independent clinical trial cohorts. Ann Rheum Dis. 2019;78:122–30.
Wallace B, et al. Reliability, validity and responsiveness to change of the Saint George's Respiratory Questionnaire in early diffuse cutaneous systemic sclerosis. Rheumatology (Oxford). 2015;54:1369–79.
Wigley FM, et al. Intravenous iloprost infusion in patients with Raynaud phenomenon secondary to systemic sclerosis. A multicenter, placebo-controlled, double-blind study. Ann Intern Med. 1994;120:199–206.

Evolving Clinical Trial Design and Innovative Approaches

48

Christopher P. Denton, Daniel E. Furst, Ulf Muller-Ladner, and Dinesh Khanna

Introduction

An area of substantial progress in systemic sclerosis (SSc) therapeutics over the past two decades has been the completion of successful clinical trials that have supported successful application for marketing authorisation from Health Authorities for drugs to treat complications of systemic sclerosis including pulmonary arterial hypertension, digital ulceration, Raynaud's phenomenon, and lung fibrosis [1–3]. This has depended upon positive pivotal phase 3 clinical trials. However, this success is tempered by the disappointing results from several trials of therapeutics that had promised. This reflects the challenge of phase 3 trials in SSc and the difficulty in moving from a promising phase 2 study to a successful pivotal trial [4]. It is important to consider that some of these negative trials showed promising trends of benefit that may suggest that a different trial design could have been positive, and this possibility of a type 2 error is especially disappointing in a disease with high unmet medical need.

C. P. Denton (✉)
UCL Division of Medicine, University College London, London, UK

Centre for Rheumatology, University College London, Royal Free Hospital, London, UK
e-mail: c.denton@ucl.ac.uk

D. E. Furst
University of California, Los Angeles, Los Angeles, CA, USA
e-mail: dan@furst.us.com

U. Muller-Ladner
Justus-Liebig Universität Giessen, Kerckhoff-Klinik GmbH, Bad Nauheim, Germany
e-mail: u.mueller-ladner@kerckhoff-klinik.de

D. Khanna
University of Michigan, Ann Arbor, MI, USA
e-mail: khannad@med.umich.edu

Historical Perspective

Much can be learnt from the long history of clinical trial design in SSc. Historically, trials illustrate the progress that has been made in understanding the classification, natural history, and pathobiology of SSc. In addition, clinical trials and successful therapeutic advances in other areas of rheumatology and medicine have informed trial design and development.

Early attempts to test drugs in systemic sclerosis were hampered by a lack of understanding of the basic clinical diversity of SSc. The appreciation that this condition could be dichotomised into limited and diffuse subsets based upon the extent and pattern of skin involvement was a major step forward. This led to a better appreciation of disease natural history and of the timing and risk of certain key complications. However, there was still incomplete understanding of heterogeneity within subset that has become clearer in recent studies and is especially informed by autoantibody profile.

Once the basic disease classification was established, it became possible to consider clinical trial design [5]. First, there needed to be definition of endpoints and the development of a semi-quantitative tool for the assessment of skin severity, the skin score, that offered the potential for development of trials to assess impact on skin disease. This was most applicable to cases of dcSSc and has led to the major focus on this subset for studies exploring treatment in SSc [6].

The skin score was first developed by Rodnan and later revised and modified into the current 17 site MRSS. This has been studied and validated [7]. One of the key strengths of this measure was demonstration that it associated with outcome including survival and function and that changes in MRSS predicted worsening. Nevertheless, it was appreciated that measurement was potentially subjective, prone to variability, and shows heterogeneity at a group level and there has been a major focus on standardisation of MRSS assessment for clinical trial purposes.

The application of MRSS as a primary endpoint for SSc trials was based upon the contemporary view that skin fibrosis would not improve spontaneously and that treatments

Y. Allanore et al. (eds.), *Scleroderma*, https://doi.org/10.1007/978-3-031-40658-4_48

may prevent worsening or possibly improve the status of established disease. This led to several early comparative studies that explored MRSS change on treatments.

The first trial performed examined N-acetyl –cysteine [8]. This was not positive and paved the way for later studies such as chlorambucil [9], D-penicillamine and others [10–13]. The challenge was that differentiating placebo from active treatment was not possible. The D-penicillamine study was well conducted and was among the first studies that used the modified Rodnan skin score as a primary endpoint [13]. This is important as it represents progress from the chlorambucil and earlier studies that assessed skin tethering as the predominant outcome using a 10-site score. The move from assessor rating of skin tethering to skin thickness is an important step in the development of skin assessment tools in clinical trials and practice. There has now been a careful expert consensus publication that standardises the procedure for training skin score assessors in clinical trials and this is supported by major international research groups including the Scleroderma Clinical Trials Consortium (SCTC) and World Scleroderma Foundation (WSF) [7]. Later studies with MTX and other agents proved similarly challenging, and there was an overall nihilism to the treatment for SSc and to the likelihood of demonstrating treatment benefit in a trial [14].

Following these early disappointing studies, there was a phase of open label trials, or studies with only small placebo cohorts [15–18]. These proved similarly challenging because, although generally MRSS improved over time, it was not possible to separate treatment effect from natural history [19]. The concept of placebo response emerged, although later this was appreciated to be the natural history of group level skin score change in dcSSc. It was also appreciated that patients were able to discern when their disease was particularly active, so they tended to enter studies at their worst. This meant that majority of patients tended to improve, even when in the control group, making differentiation of treatment effects even more difficult [20, 21].

In more recent years, it became apparent that placebo comparators were critical to trial interpretations and that modern studies should be of sufficient duration and recruit enough cases to be interpretable. Even with this, diversity of outcomes in early dcSSc related to disease or subgroup heterogeneity was a confounder. Studies defined subgroups better and allowed the most informative cases to be identified. This led to greater success but still the problem remained that group level changes were hard to assess and likely depended on the population structure in the trial.

The variability of mRSS assessment has been a challenge but with standardised training it has been shown that the inter-observer variability can be reduced to between 3 and 5 skin score units and the intra-observer variability to between 2 and 3 skin score units. Among other improvements, this information led to a strict need to have the same evaluator examining a given patient throughout a study. This information has been informative in determining likely sample size requirements for clinical trials in dcSSc that evaluate mRSS [21].

The variable natural history of mRSS has been a challenge to clinical trials design and interpretation in SSc. This was highlighted from the assessment of mRSS in the CAT-192 trial of an anti-TGFbeta1 monoclonal antibody [17]. Diversity in mRSS over 6 months was observed in all treatment groups but was especially variable in placebo treated patients. This led to a pooled data meta-analysis that better defined the group level and individual patient changes in skin score over time that are seen in SSc trials [19]. In addition, there was a detailed analysis of skin score trajectories in an observational cohort of early stage dcSSc that identified clinically relevant subgroups. It is important to understand this subgrouping as it suggests that if informative patients are not included in sufficient numbers in a clinical trial or are diluted by non-informative subjects, these non-informative, unchanging patients may confound treatment effects, leading to negative trials.

Detailed analysis of observational trial cohorts has also identified the characteristics that are more likely to be associated with progression of mRSS. Thus, early-stage disease with a low mRSS seems important to avoid a ceiling effect for mRSS and to reflect the fact that, often, skin score peaks in the first 12–18 months and then stabilises or even improves [21, 22]. These cohorts are generally on active treatment, and this may result in a ceiling effect which precludes finding a response [23]. The ESOS trial provides excellent data about the current natural history of dcSSc cases including those on active background treatment [24]. The data also corroborate the EUSTAR analysis in predicting disease progression but suggest that some cases, notably those with anti-RNA polymerase III (ARA+) serology, can still progress even with higher baseline skin scores. Disease duration overall seems to be the most important determinant of skin score progression, and the optimal disease duration may vary by autoantibody subset [24, 25]. In another RCT, skin molecular gene expression, based on bulk RNA-seq, is associated with heterogeneity in mRSS trajectory in the placebo group [26].

It should be noted however that at a group level, all recent trials have shown improvement in mRSS over 6–12 months that likely reflects natural history of skin disease in placebo controlled trials. Thus, treatment benefit might be possible through seeing greater improvement, as in some recent trials, and this appears to be more feasible than demonstrating a lack of progression at a group level so that there is no clear reason to focus only on worsening disease in skin-based SSc trials. Indeed, since all recent studies, including placebo controlled and early disease, show group level improvement and that we see trends or significant treatment effect on active drug, the goal of preventing worsening probably is not feasible in future trials, especially if background treatment is permitted [27, 28]. This may of course depend in part on the mechanisms of action of a candidate therapeutic [29, 30].

Thus, despite the clear evidence of association of mRSS with outcome in dcSSc and the value of skin extent in subset classification, there remains concern that just showing that a drug improves or benefits mRSS may not be sufficient to convince health authorities and clinicians that the intervention is truly meaningful for patients. This has led to greater interest in patient reported outcomes and composite response indices that are discussed further below. It also led to the development of the SSPRO which is a patient reported outcome assessing skin impact [31]. Once validated, this is attractive as a measure that could be applied to clinical trials, especially in later phases when impact on how patients feel and function have high priority for efficacy assessment from both the patient's and regulatory perspectives. Recent cohort studies have assessed the correlation between the SSPRO and mRSS [32]. In addition, a recent study has explored patient self-assessment of skin using a novel PASTUL (patient assessment of skin thickness in the upper limb) tool and shown good construct validity by comparing it with physician assessed mRSS and the SSPRO domains [32]. It is likely that SSPRO and other self-assessment methods may become more widely used in forthcoming clinical trials although they await full validation, especially to define minimally clinically important difference and sensitivity to change over time, but such measures may be useful in future trials and also might reduce need for face to face assessment that can be limited, for example due to coronavirus necessitated changes in practice.

Considerations in Trial Design

There have been several exercises that focus on developing or harmonising the methods used for clinical trials in systemic sclerosis. The first of these was an expert group that focused on diffuse cutaneous SSc and developed a suggested template for trials over 12 months. This was published and provided useful guidance [22]. However, as outlined above, there are many challenges and limitations in study design and the conduct of trials was further considered in much more detail in a collaborative international exercise. This followed an agreed methodology to assess the overall conduct of trials as well as specific study design for trials that might be focused on one aspect or manifestation of SSc. This exercise produced a general guidance document and a detailed roadmap for trials that might be considered in SSc [22]. The general principles of SSc trial design are included in the schematic in Fig. 48.1.

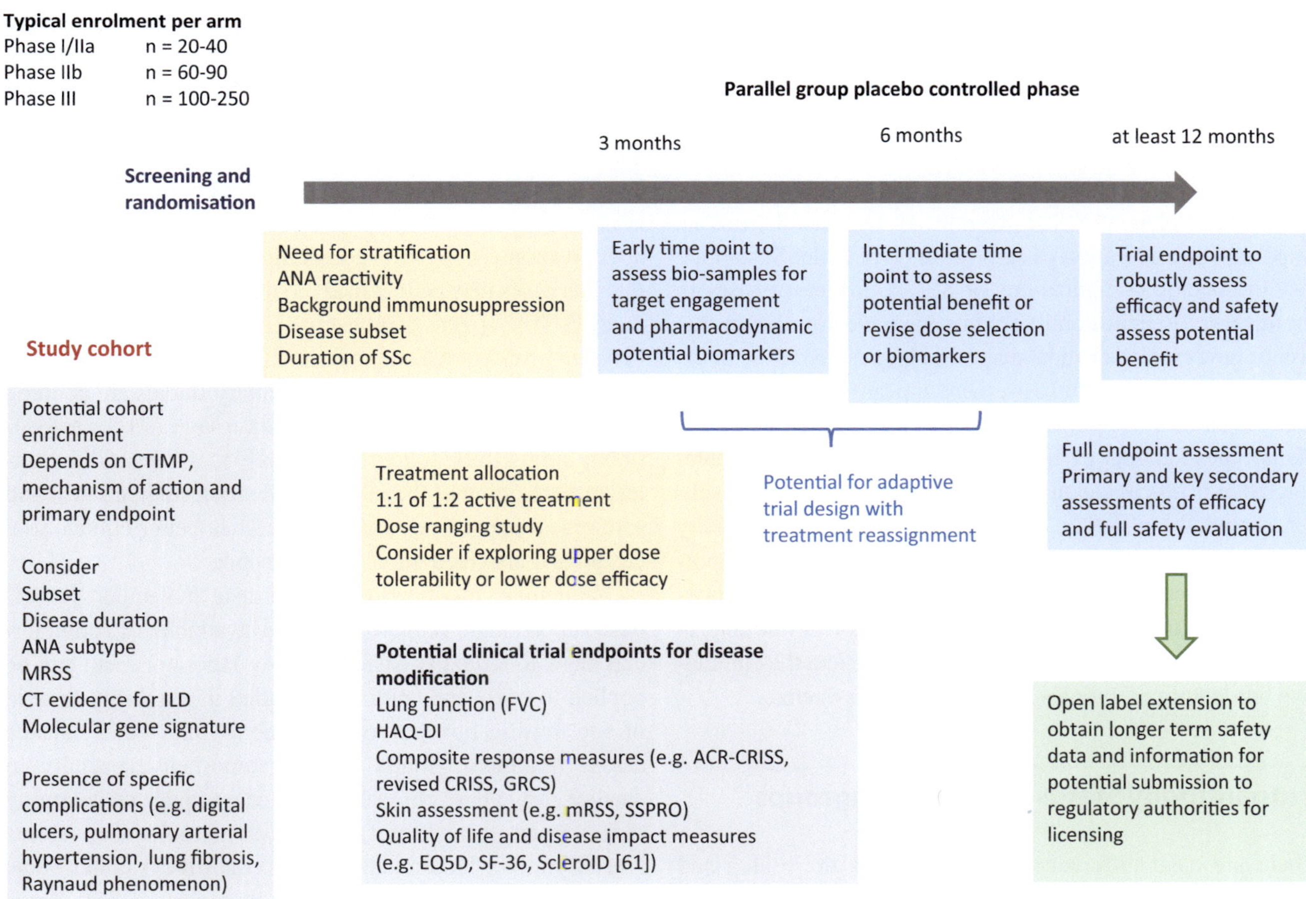

Fig. 48.1 Trial design template for evaluating potential disease modifying therapy in systemic sclerosis. Potential approaches to trials in systemic sclerosis are summarised depending upon the stage of development and target being examined. There is potential for adaptive design and also bio-sampling with associated studies of target engagement or mechanism of action that may be especially valuable in early phase trials. Novel endpoints such as the ScleroID may assess patient reported outcome and disease impact (see text for more details and Ref. [57])

The clinical heterogeneity of SSc is an important factor to consider in clinical trial design. This is important because different patient groups may respond differently to a trial therapeutic or to background standard of care treatment. In this way, the population architecture and structure are very important in considering trial design. It is also important because a change in population structure in moving from an early-stage trial to a pivotal study may have major implications. This could impact power calculations and recruitment ability as well as treatment effect.

Scleroderma Subset

In general, most studies have focused on dcSSc. This is logical when skin is considered as an endpoint because the lower burden of skin involvement in lcSSc, lack of validation of the skin score in lcSSc and the relative stability of mRSS over time in lcSSc can be problematic. In addition, other complications may occur more often in dcSSc than lcSSc and so event rates are likely to be higher in dcSSc. Recent trials have given additional information and highlighted the differences between these subsets. For some complications of SSc such as lung fibrosis, PAH or digital ulcer disease, subset stratification approaches may be considered to balance subsets between treatment arms [33, 34].

Stage

The distinct phases of SSc are relevant because there is an important consideration of skin score peak in dcSSc and the risk of specific complications of SSc at different phases in the disease. Recent cohort studies have clearly shown that risk of new cardiac or renal disease is highest in dcSSc in the first 3 years. For lung fibrosis, there appear to be two distinct phases: an early stage in the first 3 years that links to risk phenotypes such as particular ANA reactivities and a later stage that is less associated with ANA but linked to skin subset, especially in dcSSc. Other factors such as comorbidity and severity of gastro-oesophageal reflux may also be important. Some complications such as PH appear to be time-dependent variables and have greater risk of developing in later stage disease. These differences may reflect the cumulative burden of pathologies in various organ systems.

Autoantibody Status and ANA Subgroups

There are clear differences with respect to the timing and frequency of major complications of SSc for the mutually exclusive serological subgroups including antinuclear antibodies. This may reflect that some ANA patterns such as anti-topoisomerase (Scl-70, ATA) are associated with lung fibrosis or anti-fibrillarin (U3-RNP, AFA) with pulmonary hypertension and ARA with scleroderma renal crisis [35]. These differences may be an opportunity to enrich cohorts for increased risk of a specific complication of for progression of established disease. In turn, this may lead to more uniform patient groups and an opportunity to improve the likelihood of showing differences in treatments (e.g. placebo versus test medication).This is important and means that trials could be stratified by ANA. This is feasible because most ANA are mutually exclusive and present from diagnosis [36, 37]. Therefore, stratification is possible, and this should be considered in forthcoming trials. It should be noted, on the other hand, that such careful stratification may limit the ultimate approval of therapeutics to specific subgroups, so the application of such groupings may best be applied in phase 2 studies during registration.

Molecular Stratification

There has been a growing interest in the potential for molecular stratification in SSc. This has been fuelled by studies from skin biopsies that show molecular subgroups. It has further been shown that as well as providing insight into pathogenesis the intrinsic subgroups of SSc might have different response to treatment [38, 39]. This has been reported for cohort studies as well as interventional trials. Although first described in skin biopsies, the molecular subgroups have also been derived from other biopsies such as gut tissue obtained at endoscopy or from peripheral blood sampling. Recent data about response in trials is compelling. For example, the normal like cases may be less likely to respond to HSCT [40] and the ASSET [27] trials demonstrated clear differential response between proliferative and inflammatory subsets derived from baseline biopsy profiles. Complementary studies are defining molecular subgroups that link to disease stage [41] or autoantibody subset [42]. Together, it is likely that there will be better understanding of the inks between molecular, clinical and serological phenotypes that will facilitate better clinical trial design and also feed into clinical practice.

Molecular classification to "intrinsic molecular subset" based upon single skin biopsy is now available on a commercial basis in a quality assured testing laboratory and can be applied to trials and could be included in eligibility criteria of for stratification purposes. It seems likely that balance across treatment groups will be important especially in smaller early phase clinical trials. Recent trials and emerging data support the concept that different molecular subsets ("proliferative; inflammatory or normal-like") could show differential response to candidate therapies in SSc. Once again, this stratification has both positive and negative aspects, as noted above.

Biomarkers for Stratification and Pharmacodynamic Evaluation

In SSc, although several recent trials have used biomarkers or unvalidated molecular markers, these have been of limited value. Markers that link to target engagement are helpful in early stage and proof of concept trials because they increase confidence in data and facilitate interpretation of directional change and trends of benefit in clinical or other endpoints [43, 44]. Pharmacodynamic markers have proved more challenging and, at least for skin, the changes in markers of fibrosis seem to occur after clinical benefit rather than anticipating skin changes [29, 30]. This may be limiting but more sophisticated approaches are being pursued to develop novel markers that may more closely align with relevant disease biology or composite approaches. A molecular skin score marker has been developed and already shown to be useful in some clinical trials. This was originally developed to include four gene transcripts [45] but later developed into a two gene composite that has been shown to reflect clinical change in skin score in two trials and may anticipate the clinical assessment [30, 45, 46]. Stratification markers have been more successful and may be used alongside clinical or ANA features to enrich for response or better understand subgroup response in clinical trials.

Cohort Enrichment in Clinical Trials

Based upon the stage, subset, and ANA type together with molecular profile, it might be possible to enrich effectively in trials, especially when a medication's mechanism of action suggests likely differential treatment response. This is an important trial consideration, but other aspects need to be considered such as the generalisability of the results. In practice, stratification can be used and pre-specified in an analysis plan, but it is always likely to be useful to know if a subset of cases has increased or decreased response and this is likely to be the most robust way for testing a hypothesis. It also offers the possibility of seeing directional trends that will support generalisability beyond a specific subgroup of cases in the trial. As noted above, this may have important implications in pivotal trials that link to marketing authorisation and labelling of drugs for specific indication or in a certain disease. Enrichment for progressive or improving cases has been used for mRSS as outlined above. It is however important to consider whether derivation cohorts reflect trial populations or clinical practice [25]. This has been a limitation.

Composite Endpoints

Composite endpoints are methodologically and conceptually challenging in clinical trials because there are difficulties in comparing outcomes across domains and determining the extent to which components of composite outcome measures are equivalent or may individually drive apparent treatment effect in the endpoint. ACR CRISS was developed and has performed well in some studies but has ceiling effect in those that have background treatment [47]. This may reflect the population that the CRISS was developed in and the cohorts used for validation. These development cohorts included lower levels of background immunosuppression. Very recently, a simpler modified CRISS has been proposed, which assesses the proportion of patients who improve by a certain percentage (e.g. 20%) in at least 3 or 4 of 5 core set items (similar to ACR 20% responder index for rheumatoid arthritis). This may be a more feasible or relevant endpoint but performance in trials has not yet been explored prospectively [48].

Other composite endpoints such as time to clinical worsening have been proposed but this too has not yet been validated. In fact, time to clinical worsening is analogous to step 1 of ACR CRISS. It has the potential to operate across disease subsets and give extremely robust data for long-term clinical benefit [47]. Analogy with PAH would suggest this could overcome some of the limitations of biomarker or short-term clinical surrogates (e.g. SMWT) [49]. Its limitation is that time to clinical worsening is a relatively infrequent event, thus requiring larger and may be longer trials.

Stem cell transplant trials ASTIS and SCOT have proven the validity of composite clinical endpoints. This composite endpoint looks at event free survival and it has been partially validated against overall survival [50]. In SCOT a much smaller number of cases achieved statistical significance by using a novel ranked composite score (GRCS) endpoint [51] but required 54 months to show a statistical difference, and the utility of this endpoint beyond trials of less intensive treatments is unclear.

Recent Experience in Systemic Sclerosis Trials

Table 48.1 summarise the outcome data for recent trials focused on skin and lung disease and highlights the most informative endpoints.

These studies demonstrate the progress that has been made in developing clinical trial templates that are capable of distinguishing active drug from placebo. This is a step forward and allows both positive and negative trials to be interpreted clearly. However, reflecting that there is much to be done to improve study design, it has been difficult to reliably demonstrate the feasibility of trial endpoints in the context of background treatment with immunosuppression. Further, it has been challenging to determine the best or most informative endpoint for primary analysis in a pivotal trial. In addition, there are several examples of recent trials that show trends of benefit that would potentially have been positive if

Table 48.1 Summary of recent phase II and phase III clinical trial results for systemic sclerosis

Trial	Total (n)	Duration (weeks)	Drug	MRSS	Change MRSS	FVC	CRISS	HAQ-DI	Global-patient	Global-physician
faSScinate	86	48	Tocilizumab	0.06	−3.5	**0.03**	**0.002**	0.53	0.51	0.03
focuSSced	212	48	Tocilizumab	0.1	−1.73	**0.002**	**0.02**	NS	NS	NS
ASSET	88	52	Abatacept	0.28	−1.75	0.11	**0.03**	**0.005**	0.73	**0.03**
RISE-SSc [62]	121	52	Riociguat	0.08	−2.34	NS	NS	NS	NS	NS
JBT-101-SSc [63]	38	4	Lenabasum	0.085	−2.6	NS	**0.04**	**0.03**	0.1	**0.02**
FASST	145	48	Lanifibranor	NS	+0.9	NS	NA	NA	0.08	NA
SENSCIS	580	52	Nintedanib	0.58	−0.2	**0.035**	NS	NA	NA	NA
Sanofi IL4/13	97	24	Romilkimab	**0.03**	−2.31	0.10	NS	0.4	0.1	NA
NOVESA	33	24	Ziritaxestat	**0.04**	−2.60	NA	NA	NA	NA	NA

Primary and key secondary endpoint data (*p*-values shown) are summarised for recent clinical trials in systemic sclerosis targeting skin or lung disease. Based upon the phase 3 trial data for forced vital capacity (FVC), both nintedanib and tocilizumab are now approved by FDA for prevention of decline in lung function tests in systemic sclerosis. Some of analyses included are pre-specified whilst others are post hoc. The magnitude of treatment effect is below the minimal clinically meaningful threshold for MRSS, even where differences are statistically significant. Where available, papers that describe the primary trial outcomes are cited in parentheses

the study were larger. In this way it has been important to discriminate studies that show no suggestion of efficacy from those that may warrant further analysis. The absence of clear MCID for most potential endpoints is also a critical problem in moving forward [4].

Trials Examining a Single Disease Manifestation

There are now approved therapies for three complications of SSc including lung fibrosis, pulmonary arterial hypertension and digital ulcers. This has been due to the development of trial templates and acceptance of the results of statistically positive studies by regulators. For lung complications of fibrosis and PAH, the trial templates have been adopted from other forms of the conditions. This has been useful because larger studies have been possible and it has allowed group level treatment effect to benefit multiple forms of disease with overlapping pathobiology. For digital ulcers, there was development of an SSc specific trial template.

Pulmonary Arterial Hypertension (PAH)

Pulmonary arterial hypertension is an important complication of SSc that represents a time-dependent risk for patients. Thus, overall 1–2% of SSc cases develop pulmonary hypertension per year beginning after approximately 3 years of disease. Thus, SSc appears to represent a susceptibility phenotype. The pathobiology of PAH is shared across the different forms of the condition included in the group I PH subgroup of the current classification system. This made it logical to include SSc-PAH in pivotal clinical trials and this has allowed therapies to be approved for PAH-SSc. The first trials used gain in exercise capacity measured by six-minute walk test (SMWT) to gain approval. In idiopathic PAH, this endpoint correlated with survival [1, 49, 52]. However, multiple factors in SSc determine exercise capacity including musculoskeletal deconditioning and this has resulted in less impact on SMWT in SSc-PAH in most trials. The adoption of a clinical endpoint of time to clinical worsening as a composite morbidity-mortality endpoint has been better able to demonstrate treatment benefit in SSc-PAH as shown in recent trials and subgroup analyses [53–55]. This provides a robust template for studies but is challenged by the need for background treatment and need for large trials, as time to clinical worsening is a relatively uncommon event, requiring many patients to accrue sufficient patients with this endpoint for statistical analysis as addressed above.

Digital Ulcers (DU)

One drug, bosentan, has received regulatory approval for treatment of digital ulcers in SSc. This was based on two clinical trials showing reduced new ulcer formation in a subset of patients on bosentan compared with placebo over 16–24 weeks [2, 56]. The drug did not increase ulcer healing and so is licensed as a preventive treatment. This has been challenging to use but a large evidence base now supports efficacy. In addition, it seems likely that, as for PAH combination treatment, better response is possible when using drugs working by distinct or overlapping mechanisms of action. DU trials have been less successful once effective treatments were available because less informative cases are recruited and additional benefit above background can be hard to demonstrate [57]. Therefore, more refinement and improvement of DU trials such as using ultra-sound to define ulcers is likely to be essential for clinical progress and a number of efforts are underway to improve assessment, classification and study design.

Lung Fibrosis (SSc-ILD)

As for PAH, lung fibrosis in SSc is now treated with agents that are approved for use in other forms of interstitial lung fibrosis. Nintedanib is currently the only approved treatment for SSc-ILD although trials have previously shown benefit for cyclophosphamide and mycophenolate mofetil (MMF) in academic studies [58, 59]. As for PAH, it has been shown that adding an additional treatment is beneficial on top of MMF. Group level impact on FVC is now accepted as the best measure in SSc-ILD trials although the magnitude of treatment effect has been less that seen in other progressive forms of ILD. In recent trials of Tocilizumab in early active dcSSc, FVC has robustly outperformed MRSS as a trial endpoint discriminating active treatment from placebo [29, 60]. Additional measures that reflect symptoms or burden of SSc-ILD are important and may be incorporated into future trials. Some of these showed positive effect in cyclophosphamide trials. Lung fibrosis can be assessed by well-controlled lung function with robust central quality assurance, as has become standard for IPF trials, and the place of imaging has also been considered as this can now be quantified using several computerised systems. This provides an additional potential biomarker or surrogate in ILD trials. It should be noted that FVC decline is accepted as an endpoint in SSc-ILD because it has even validated against mortality in IPF. Thus, for both SSc-PAH and SSc-ILD, the approvable endpoint in trials has depended on data from the same clinical entity outside SSc.

Assessing Quality of Life in Clinical Trials

Quality of life (QoL) is important in rationed healthcare and cost effectiveness models. This is important for payers as well as for regulators and is increasingly important to include in clinical trials. It has been challenging to improve QoL due to the use of generic measures rather than disease specific tools and also because, in a multifaceted disease, the impact on QoL may depend on aspects of the disease that are not reversible or do not respond to a candidate therapeutic. Nevertheless, encouraging data are available for SCT treatment in registry cohorts and trials, with strong indications that HSCT improves QoL. It is notable that a much less invasive treatment abatacept showed a strong positive benefit for the HAQ-DI measure when given over 48 weeks [27]. There are promising new assessment tools being developed such as the EULAR Scleroderma Impact of Disease tool (ScleroID) that may be validated in the future and be useful additional outcomes for trials that assess how patients feel and function [61].

Future Strategies

As discussed above, trial templates now exist and successful trials have been performed in SSc. This represents major progress over the past three decades. However, clinical development remains difficult. In part, this reflects the multisystem disease represented by SSc. This means that improvement in one domain may not be sufficient to impact generic measures such as PROs or QoL tools. Thus, SSc has been harder to benchmark, especially in health economic driven markets where generic tools allow benefits across diseases to be compared and validated. HSCT is associated with such major benefits that it exemplifies the potential for major treatment effect and has been positive in trials with active comparators. This provides a standard of treatment effect that can be potentially replicated but that seems likely to require combination treatments. The fundamental goal is achieving HSCT level benefit with a simpler and less toxic treatment, thus allowing treatment for more patients.

Other approaches that may be considered are trial designs using molecular or biomarkers to enrich cohorts for treatment response. Emerging data from experimental medicine and cohort studies is unravelling the link between molecular profiles in skin or blood and clinical phenotype, disease stage and outcome, and hallmark autoantibody reactivity and this may underpin trial design in the future. For example, in early phase studies, this may include markers that enrich for activation of a target pathway, as has been applied for Tocilizumab and IL-6 or use of gene expression profiles in skin or blood as look promising in other recent studies. In addition it may be possible to develop more innovative or adaptive study designs that group SSc cases with other relevant immune mediated or fibrotic diseases. Although attractive in concept this may be challenging due to differences in outcome between SSc and other diseases such as idiopathic lung fibrosis. Randomised cohort designs are attractive as better standard treatments emerge or therapies become approved because it allows incremental progress by randomly adding new candidate treatments but providing contemporaneous comparator patients that receive standard of care management. Overall, there is reason for cautious optimism related to future trial design in SSc but potential treatments will need to be carefully selected as for any rare disease because the number of patients available and willing to participate in clinical trials is challenging.

References

1. Rubin LJ, Badesch DB, Barst RJ, Galie N, Black CM, Keogh A, Pulido T, Frost A, Roux S, Leconte I, Landzberg M, Simonneau G. Bosentan therapy for pulmonary arterial hypertension. N Engl J Med. 2002;346:896–903. https://doi.org/10.1056/NEJMoa012212.

2. Matucci-Cerinic M, Denton CP, Furst DE, Mayes MD, Hsu VM, Carpentier P, Wigley FM, Black CM, Fessler BJ, Merkel PA, Pope JE, Sweiss NJ, Doyle MK, Hellmich B, Medsger TAJ, Morganti A, Kramer F, Korn JH, Seibold JR. Bosentan treatment of digital ulcers related to systemic sclerosis: results from the. Ann Rheum Dis. 2011;70:32–8. https://doi.org/10.1136/ard.2010.130658.
3. Distler O, Highland KB, Gahlemann M, Azuma A, Fischer A, Mayes MD, Raghu G, Sauter W, Girard M, Alves M, Clerisme-Beaty E, Stowasser S, Tetzlaff K, Kuwana M, Maher TM. Nintedanib for systemic sclerosis-associated interstitial lung disease. N Engl J Med. 2019;380:2518–28. https://doi.org/10.1056/NEJMoa1903076.
4. Denton CP. Challenges in systemic sclerosis trial design. Semin Arthritis Rheum. 2019;49:S3–7. https://doi.org/10.1016/j.semarthrit.2019.09.019.
5. LeRoy EC, Black C, Fleischmajer R, Jablonska S, Krieg T, Medsger TAJ, Rowell N, Wollheim F. Scleroderma (systemic sclerosis): classification, subsets and pathogenesis. J Rheumatol. 1988;15:202–5.
6. White B, Bauer EA, Goldsmith LA, Hochberg MC, Katz LM, Korn JH, Lachenbruch PA, LeRoy EC, Mitrane MP, Paulus HE. Guidelines for clinical trials in systemic sclerosis (scleroderma). I. Disease-modifying interventions. The American College of Rheumatology Committee on design and outcomes in clinical trials in systemic sclerosis. Arthritis Rheum. 1995;38:351–60. https://doi.org/10.1002/art.1780380309.
7. Khanna D, Furst DE, Clements PJ, Allanore Y, Baron M, Czirjak L, Distler O, Foeldvari I, Kuwana M, Matucci-Cerinic M, Mayes M, Medsger TJ, Merkel PA, Pope JE, Seibold JR, Steen V, Stevens W, Denton CP. Standardization of the modified Rodnan skin score for use in clinical trials of systemic sclerosis. J Scleroderma Relat Disord. 2017;2:11–8. https://doi.org/10.5301/jsrd.5000231.
8. Furst DE, Clements PJ, Harris R, Ross M, Levy J, Paulus HE. Measurement of clinical change in progressive systemic sclerosis (PSS): a one year double-blind placebo controlled trial of N-acetylcysteine. Annals of Rheumatic Disease. 1979;38:356–61. PMID: 386962
9. Furst DE, Clements PJ, Hillis S, Lachenbruch PA, Miller BL, Sterz MG, Paulus HE. Immunosuppression with chlorambucil, versus placebo, for scleroderma. Results of a three-year, parallel, randomized, double-blind study. Arthritis Rheum. 1989;32:584–93. https://doi.org/10.1002/anr.1780320512.
10. Seibold JR, Korn JH, Simms R, Clements PJ, Moreland LW, Mayes MD, Furst DE, Rothfield N, Steen V, Weisman M, Collier D, Wigley FM, Merkel PA, Csuka ME, Hsu V, Rocco S, Erikson M, Hannigan J, Harkonen WS, Sanders ME. Recombinant human relaxin in the treatment of scleroderma. A randomized, double-blind, placebo-controlled trial. Ann Intern Med. 2000;132(11):871–9. https://doi.org/10.7326/0003-4819-132-11-200006060-00004.
11. Amjadi S, Maranian P, Furst DE, Clements PJ, Wong WK, Postlethwaite AE, Khanna PP, Khanna D. Investigators of the D-penicillamine, human recombinant Relaxin, and Oral bovine type I collagen clinical trials. Course of the modified Rodnan skin thickness score in systemic sclerosis clinical trials: analysis of three large multicenter, double-blind, randomized controlled trials. Arthritis Rheum. 2009;60(8):2490–8. https://doi.org/10.1002/art.24681. PMID: 19644851; PMCID: PMC2725229
12. Khanna D, Furst DE, Hays RD, Park GS, Wong WK, Seibold JR, Mayes MD, White B, Wigley FF, Weisman M, Barr W, Moreland L, Medsger TA Jr, Steen VD, Martin RW, Collier D, Weinstein A, Lally EV, Varga J, Weiner SR, Andrews B, Abeles M, Clements PJ. Minimally important difference in diffuse systemic sclerosis: results from the D-penicillamine study. Ann Rheum Dis. 2006;65(10):1325–9. https://doi.org/10.1136/ard.2005.050187. Epub 2006 Mar 15. PMID: 16540546; PMCID: PMC1798331
13. Clements PJ, Furst DE, Wong WK, Mayes M, White B, Wigley F, Weisman MH, Barr W, Moreland LW, Medsger TAJ, Steen V, Martin RW, Collier D, Weinstein A, Lally E, Varga J, Weiner S, Andrews B, Abeles M, Seibold JR. High-dose versus low-dose D-penicillamine in early diffuse systemic sclerosis: analysis of a two-year, double-blind, randomized, controlled clinical trial. Arthritis Rheum. 1999;42:1194–203. https://doi.org/10.1002/1529-0131(199906)42:6<1194::AID-ANR16>3.0.CO;2-7.
14. Pope JE, Bellamy N, Seibold JR, Baron M, Ellman M, Carette S, Smith CD, Chalmers IM, Hong P, O'Hanlon D, Kaminska E, Markland J, Sibley J, Catoggio L, Furst DE. A randomized, controlled trial of methotrexate versus placebo in early diffuse scleroderma. Arthritis Rheum. 2001;44:1351–8. https://doi.org/10.1002/1529-0131(200106)44:6<1351::AID-ART227>3.0.CO;2-I.
15. Denton CP, Engelhart M, Tvede N, Wilson H, Khan K, Shiwen X, Carreira PE, Diaz Gonzalez F, Black CM, van den Hoogen FH. An open-label pilot study of infliximab therapy in diffuse cutaneous systemic sclerosis. Ann Rheum Dis. 2009;68:1433–9. https://doi.org/10.1136/ard.2008.096123.
16. Khanna D, Saggar R, Mayes MD, Abtin F, Clements PJ, Maranian P, Assassi S, Saggar R, Singh RR, Furst DE. A one-year, phase I/IIa, open-label pilot trial of imatinib mesylate in the treatment of systemic sclerosis-associated active interstitial lung disease. Arthritis Rheum. 2011;63:3540–6. https://doi.org/10.1002/art.30548.
17. Denton CP, Merkel PA, Furst DE, Khanna D, Emery P, Hsu VM, Silliman N, Streisand J, Powell J, Akesson A, Coppock J, van den Hoogen F, Herrick A, Mayes MD, Veale D, Haas J, Ledbetter S, Korn JH, Black CM, Seibold JR. Recombinant human anti-transforming growth factor beta1 antibody therapy in systemic sclerosis: a multicenter, randomized, placebo-controlled phase I/II trial of CAT-192. Arthritis Rheum. 2007;56:323–33. https://doi.org/10.1002/art.22289.
18. Gordon J, Udeh U, Doobay K, Magro C, Wildman H, Davids M, Mersten JN, Huang W-T, Lyman S, Crow MK, Spiera RF. Imatinib mesylate (Gleevec™) in the treatment of diffuse cutaneous systemic sclerosis: results of a 24-month open label, extension phase, single-centre trial. Clin Exp Rheumatol. 2014;32:S-189-193.
19. Merkel PA, Silliman NP, Clements PJ, Denton CP, Furst DE, Mayes MD, Pope JE, Polisson RP, Streisand JB, Seibold JR. Patterns and predictors of change in outcome measures in clinical trials in scleroderma: an individual patient meta-analysis of 629 subjects with diffuse cutaneous systemic sclerosis. Arthritis Rheum. 2012;64:3420–9. https://doi.org/10.1002/art.34427.
20. Khanna D, Clements PJ, Furst DE, Korn JH, Ellman M, Rothfield N, Wigley FM, Moreland LW, Silver R, Kim YH, Steen VD, Firestein GS, Kavanaugh AF, Weisman M, Mayes MD, Collier D, Csuka ME, Simms R, Merkel PA, Medsger TA Jr, Sanders ME, Maranian P, Seibold JR, Relaxin Investigators and the Scleroderma Clinical Trials Consortium. Recombinant human relaxin in the treatment of systemic sclerosis with diffuse cutaneous involvement: a randomized, double-blind, placebo-controlled trial. Arthritis Rheum. 2009;60(4):1102–11. https://doi.org/10.1002/art.24380. PMID: 19333948; PMCID: PMC3711466
21. Kaldas M, Khanna PP, Furst DE, Clements PJ, Kee Wong W, Seibold JR, Postlethwaite AE, Khanna D, Investigators of the human recombinant relaxin and oral bovine collagen clinical trials. Sensitivity to change of the modified Rodnan skin score in diffuse systemic sclerosis--assessment of individual body sites in two large randomized controlled trials. Rheumatology (Oxford). 2009;48(9):1143–6. https://doi.org/10.1093/rheumatology/kep202. Epub 2009 Jul 14. PMID: 19605370; PMCID: PMC2734267
22. Nihtyanova SI, Brough GM, Black CM, Denton CP. Mycophenolate mofetil in diffuse cutaneous systemic sclerosis—a retrospective analysis. Rheumatology (Oxford). 2007;46(3):442–5. https://doi.org/10.1093/rheumatology/kel244. Epub 2006 Aug 9. PMID: 16899504
23. Khanna D, Furst DE, Allanore Y, Bae S, Bodukam V, Clements PJ, Cutolo M, Czirjak L, Denton CP, Distler O, Walker UA, Matucci-Cerinic M, Müller-Ladner U, Seibold JR, Singh M, Tyndall

A. Twenty-two points to consider for clinical trials in systemic sclerosis, based on EULAR standards. Rheumatology (Oxford). 2015;54:144–51. https://doi.org/10.1093/rheumatology/keu288.

24. Herrick AL, Peytrignet S, Lunt M, Pan X, Hesselstrand R, Mouthon L, Silman AJ, Dinsdale G, Brown E, Czirják L, Distler JHW, Distler O, Fligelstone K, Gregory WJ, Ochiel R, Vonk MC, Ancuța C, Ong VH, Farge D, Hudson M, Matucci-Cerinic M, Balbir-Gurman A, Midtvedt Ø, Jobanputra P, Jordan AC, Stevens W, Moinzadeh P, Hall FC, Agard C, Anderson ME, Diot E, Madhok R, Akil M, Buch MH, Chung L, Damjanov NS, Gunawardena H, Lanyon P, Ahmad Y, Chakravarty K, Jacobsen S, MacGregor AJ, McHugh N, Müller-Ladner U, Riemekasten G, Becker M, Roddy J, Carreira PE, Fauchais AL, Hachulla E, Hamilton J, İnanç M, McLaren JS, van Laar JM, Pathare S, Proudman SM, Rudin A, Sahhar J, Coppere B, Serratrice C, Sheeran T, Veale DJ, Grange C, Trad G-S, Denton CP. Patterns and predictors of skin score change in early diffuse systemic sclerosis from the European scleroderma observational study. Ann Rheum Dis. 2018;77:563–70. https://doi.org/10.1136/annrheumdis-2017-211912.
25. Maurer B, Graf N, Michel BA, Müller-Ladner U, Czirják L, Denton CP, Tyndall A, Metzig C, Lanius V, Khanna D, Distler O. Prediction of worsening of skin fibrosis in patients with diffuse cutaneous systemic sclerosis using the EUSTAR database. Ann Rheum Dis. 2015;74:1124–31. https://doi.org/10.1136/annrheumdis-2014-205226.
26. Stifano G, Sornasse T, Rice LM, Na L, Chen-Harris H, Khanna D, Jahreis A, Zhang Y, Siegel J, Lafyatis R. Skin gene expression is prognostic for the trajectory of skin disease in patients with diffuse cutaneous systemic sclerosis. Arthritis Rheumatol. 2018;70(6):912–9. https://doi.org/10.1002/art.40455. PMID: 29858547; PMCID: PMC6731768. 674
27. Khanna D, Spino C, Johnson S, Chung L, Whitfield ML, Denton CP, Berrocal V, Franks J, Mehta B, Molitor J, Steen VD, Lafyatis R, Simms RW, Gill A, Kafaja S, Frech TM, Hsu V, Domsic RT, Pope JE, Gordon JK, Mayes MD, Schiopu E, Young A, Sandorfi N, Park J, Hant FN, Bernstein EJ, Chatterjee S, Castelino FV, Ajam A, Wang Y, Wood T, Allanore Y, Matucci-Cerinic M, Distler O, Singer O, Bush E, Fox DA, Furst DE. Abatacept in early diffuse cutaneous systemic sclerosis: results of a phase II investigator-initiated, multicenter, double-blind, randomized, placebo-controlled trial. Arthritis Rheumatol. 2020d;72:125–36. https://doi.org/10.1002/art.41055.
28. Khanna D, Allanore Y, Denton CP, Kuwana M, Matucci-Cerinic M, Pope JE, Atsumi T, Bečvář R, Czirják L, Hachulla E, Ishii T, Ishikawa O, Johnson SR, De Langhe E, Stagnaro C, Riccieri V, Schiopu E, Silver RM, Smith V, Steen V, Stevens W, Szücs G, Truchetet M-E, Wosnitza M, Laapas K, de Oliveira Pena J, Yao Z, Kramer F, Distler O. Riociguat in patients with early diffuse cutaneous systemic sclerosis (RISE-SSc): randomised, double-blind, placebo-controlled multicentre trial. Ann Rheum Dis. 2020a;79:618–25. https://doi.org/10.1136/annrheumdis-2019-216823.
29. Khanna D, Denton CP, Jahreis A, van Laar JM, Frech TM, Anderson ME, Baron M, Chung L, Fierlbeck G, Lakshminarayanan S, Allanore Y, Pope JE, Riemekasten G, Steen V, Müller-Ladner U, Lafyatis R, Stifano G, Spotswood H, Chen-Harris H, Dziadek S, Morimoto A, Sornasse T, Siegel J, Furst DE. Safety and efficacy of subcutaneous tocilizumab in adults with systemic sclerosis (faSScinate): a phase 2, randomised, controlled trial. Lancet. 2016b;387:2630–40. https://doi.org/10.1016/S0140-6736(16)00232-4.
30. Rice LM, Padilla CM, McLaughlin SR, Mathes A, Ziemek J, Goummih S, Nakerakanti S, York M, Farina G, Whitfield ML, Spiera RF, Christmann RB, Gordon JK, Weinberg J, Simms RW, Lafyatis R. Fresolimumab treatment decreases biomarkers and improves clinical symptoms in systemic sclerosis patients. J Clin Invest. 2015;125:2795–807. https://doi.org/10.1172/JCI77958.
31. Man A, Correa JK, Ziemek J, Simms RW, Felson DT, Lafyatis R. Development and validation of a patient-reported outcome instrument for skin involvement in patients with systemic sclerosis. Ann Rheum Dis. 2017;76(8):1374–80. https://doi.org/10.1136/annrheumdis-2016-210534. Epub 2017 Feb 17
32. Spierings J, Ong V, Denton CP. PASTUL questionnaire: a tool for self-assessment of scleroderma skin during the COVID-19 pandemic. Ann Rheum Dis. 2021; https://doi.org/10.1136/annrheumdis-2020-219775. annrheumdis-2020-219775; Epub ahead of print
33. Johnson SR, Soowamber ML, Fransen J, Khanna D, Van Den Hoogen F, Baron M, Matucci-Cerinic M, Denton CP, Medsger TAJ, Carreira PE, Riemekasten G, Distler J, Gabrielli A, Steen V, Chung L, Silver R, Varga J, Müller-Ladner U, Vonk MC, Walker UA, Wollheim FA, Herrick A, Furst DE, Czirjak L, Kowal-Bielecka O, Del Galdo F, Cutolo M, Hunzelmann N, Murray CD, Foeldvari I, Mouthon L, Damjanov N, Kahaleh B, Frech T, Assassi S, Saketkoo LA, Pope JE. There is a need for new systemic sclerosis subset criteria. A content analytic approach. Scand J Rheumatol. 2018;47:62–70. https://doi.org/10.1080/03009742.2017.1299793.
34. Johnson SR, van den Hoogen F, Devakandan K, Matucci-Cerinic M, Pope JE. Systemic sclerosis: to subset or not to subset, that is the question. Eur J Rheumatol. 2020;7:S222–7. https://doi.org/10.5152/eurjrheum.2020.19116.
35. Nihtyanova SI, Sari A, Harvey JC, Leslie A, Derrett-Smith EC, Fonseca C, Ong VH, Denton CP. Using autoantibodies and cutaneous subset to develop outcome-based disease classification in systemic sclerosis. Arthritis Rheumatol. 2020;72:465–76. https://doi.org/10.1002/art.41153.
36. Bunn CC, Denton CP, Shi-Wen X, Knight C, Black CM. Anti-RNA polymerases and other autoantibody specificities in systemic sclerosis. Br J Rheumatol. 1998;37:15–20. https://doi.org/10.1093/rheumatology/37.1.15.
37. Caetano J, Nihtyanova SI, Harvey J, Denton CP, Ong VH. Distinctive clinical phenotype of anti-centromere antibody-positive diffuse systemic sclerosis. Rheumatol Adv Pract. 2018;2:rky002. https://doi.org/10.1093/rap/rky002.
38. Milano A, Pendergrass SA, Sargent JL, George LK, McCalmont TH, Connolly MK, Whitfield ML. Molecular subsets in the gene expression signatures of scleroderma skin. PLoS One. 2008;3:e2696. https://doi.org/10.1371/journal.pone.0002696.
39. Assassi S, Swindell WR, Wu M, Tan FD, Khanna D, Furst DE, Tashkin DP, Jahan-Tigh RR, Mayes MD, Gudjonsson JE, Chang JT. Dissecting the heterogeneity of skin gene expression patterns in systemic sclerosis. Arthritis Rheumatol. 2015;67:3016–26. https://doi.org/10.1002/art.39289.
40. Franks JM, Martyanov V, Wang Y, Wood TA, Pinckney A, Crofford LJ, Keyes-Elstein L, Furst DE, Goldmuntz E, Mayes MD, McSweeney P, Nash RA, Sullivan KM, Whitfield ML. Machine learning predicts stem cell transplant response in severe scleroderma. Ann Rheum Dis. 2020;79:1608–15. https://doi.org/10.1136/annrheumdis-2020-217033.
41. Skaug B, Khanna D, Swindell WR, Hinchcliff ME, Frech TM, Steen VD, Hant FN, Gordon JK, Shah AA, Zhu L, Zheng WJ, Browning JL, Barron AMS, Wu M, Visvanathan S, Baum P, Franks JM, Whitfield ML, Shanmugam VK, Domsic RT, Castelino FV, Bernstein EJ, Wareing N, Lyons MA, Ying J, Charles J, Mayes MD, Assassi S. Global skin gene expression analysis of early diffuse cutaneous systemic sclerosis shows a prominent innate and adaptive inflammatory profile. Ann Rheum Dis. 2020;79(3):379–86. https://doi.org/10.1136/annrheumdis-2019-215894. Epub 2019 Nov 25. PMID: 31767698; PMCID: PMC7386329
42. Clark KEN, Campochiaro C, Csomor E, Taylor A, Nevin K, Galwey N, Morse MA, Singh J, Teo YV, Ong VH, Derrett-Smith E, Wisniacki N, Flint SM, Denton CP. Molecular basis for clinical diversity between autoantibody subsets in diffuse cutaneous systemic sclerosis. Ann Rheum Dis. 2021; https://doi.org/10.1136/annrheumdis-2021-220402. Epub ahead of print

43. Allanore Y, Distler O, Jagerschmidt A, Illiano S, Ledein L, Boitier E, Agueusop I, Denton CP, Khanna D. Lysophosphatidic acid receptor 1 antagonist SAR100842 for patients with diffuse cutaneous systemic sclerosis: a double-blind, randomized, eight-week placebo-controlled study followed by a sixteen-week open-label extension study. Arthritis Rheumatol. 2018;70:1634–43. https://doi.org/10.1002/art.40547.
44. Allanore Y, Wung P, Soubrane C, Esperet C, Marrache F, Bejuit R, Lahmar A, Khanna D, Denton CP. A randomised, double-blind, placebo-controlled, 24-week, phase II, proof-of-concept study of romilkimab (SAR156597) in early diffuse cutaneous systemic sclerosis. Ann Rheum Dis. 2020;79:1600–7. https://doi.org/10.1136/annrheumdis-2020-218447.
45. Farina G, Lafyatis D, Lemaire R, Lafyatis R. A four-gene biomarker predicts skin disease in patients with diffuse cutaneous systemic sclerosis. Arthritis Rheum. 2010;62(2):580–8. https://doi.org/10.1002/art.27220. PMID: 20112379; PMCID: PMC3018285
46. Rice LM, Ziemek J, Stratton EA, McLaughlin SR, Padilla CM, Mathes AL, Christmann RB, Stifano G, Browning JL, Whitfield ML, Spiera RF, Gordon JK, Simms RW, Zhang Y, Lafyatis R. A longitudinal biomarker for the extent of skin disease in patients with diffuse cutaneous systemic sclerosis. Arthritis Rheumatol. 2015;67(11):3004–15. https://doi.org/10.1002/art.39287. PMID: 26240058; PMCID: PMC5522178
47. Khanna D, Berrocal VJ, Giannini EH, Seibold JR, Merkel PA, Mayes MD, Baron M, Clements PJ, Steen V, Assassi S, Schiopu E, Phillips K, Simms RW, Allanore Y, Denton CP, Distler O, Johnson SR, Matucci-Cerinic M, Pope JE, Proudman SM, Siegel J, Wong WK, Wells AU, Furst DE. The American College of Rheumatology Provisional Composite Response Index for clinical trials in early diffuse cutaneous systemic sclerosis. Arthritis Rheumatol. 2016a;68:299–311. https://doi.org/10.1002/art.39501.
48. Khanna D, Huang S, Lin CJF, Spino C. New composite endpoint in early diffuse cutaneous systemic sclerosis: revisiting the provisional American College of Rheumatology Composite Response Index in systemic sclerosis. Ann Rheum Dis. 2020b; https://doi.org/10.1136/annrheumdis-2020-219100.
49. Denton CP, Humbert M, Rubin L, Black CM. Bosentan treatment for pulmonary arterial hypertension related to connective tissue disease: a subgroup analysis of the pivotal clinical trials and their open-label extensions. Ann Rheum Dis. 2006;65:1336–40. https://doi.org/10.1136/ard.2005.048967.
50. van Laar JM, Farge D, Sont JK, Naraghi K, Marjanovic Z, Larghero J, Schuerwegh AJ, Marijt EWA, Vonk MC, Schattenberg AV, Matucci-Cerinic M, Voskuyl AE, van de Loosdrecht AA, Daikeler T, Kötter I, Schmalzing M, Martin T, Lioure B, Weiner SM, Kreuter A, Deligny C, Durand J-M, Emery P, Machold KP, Sarrot-Reynauld F, Warnatz K, Adoue DFP, Constans J, Tony H-P, Del Papa N, Fassas A, Himsel A, Launay D, Lo Monaco A, Philippe P, Quéré I, Rich É, Westhovens R, Griffiths B, Saccardi R, van den Hoogen FH, Fibbe WE, Socié G, Gratwohl A, Tyndall A. Autologous hematopoietic stem cell transplantation vs intravenous pulse cyclophosphamide in diffuse cutaneous systemic sclerosis: a randomized clinical trial. JAMA. 2014;311:2490–8. https://doi.org/10.1001/jama.2014.6368.
51. Sullivan KM, Goldmuntz EA, Keyes-Elstein L, McSweeney PA, Pinckney A, Welch B, Mayes MD, Nash RA, Crofford LJ, Eggleston B, Castina S, Griffith LM, Goldstein JS, Wallace D, Craciunescu O, Khanna D, Folz RJ, Goldin J, St Clair EW, Seibold JR, Phillips K, Mineishi S, Simms RW, Ballen K, Wener MH, Georges GE, Heimfeld S, Hosing C, Forman S, Kafaja S, Silver RM, Griffing L, Storek J, LeClercq S, Brasington R, Csuka ME, Bredeson C, Keever-Taylor C, Domsic RT, Kahaleh MB, Medsger T, Furst DE. Myeloablative autologous stem-cell transplantation for severe scleroderma. N Engl J Med. 2018;378:35–47. https://doi.org/10.1056/nejmoa1703327.
52. Sitbon O, Gomberg-Maitland M, Granton J, Lewis MI, Mathai SC, Rainisio M, Stockbridge NL, Wilkins MR, Zamanian RT, Rubin LJ. Clinical trial design and new therapies for pulmonary arterial hypertension. Eur Respir J. 2019;53 https://doi.org/10.1183/13993003.01908-2018.
53. Pulido T, Adzerikho I, Channick RN, Delcroix M, Galiè N, Ghofrani H-A, Jansa P, Jing Z-C, Le Brun F-O, Mehta S, Mittelholzer CM, Perchenet L, Sastry BKS, Sitbon O, Souza R, Torbicki A, Zeng X, Rubin LJ, Simonneau G. Macitentan and morbidity and mortality in pulmonary arterial hypertension. N Engl J Med. 2013;369:809–18. https://doi.org/10.1056/NEJMoa1213917.
54. Galiè N, Barberà JA, Frost AE, Ghofrani H-A, Hoeper MM, McLaughlin VV, Peacock AJ, Simonneau G, Vachiery J-L, Grünig E, Oudiz RJ, Vonk-Noordegraaf A, White RJ, Blair C, Gillies H, Miller KL, Harris JHN, Langley J, Rubin LJ. Initial use of Ambrisentan plus tadalafil in pulmonary arterial hypertension. N Engl J Med. 2015;373:834–44. https://doi.org/10.1056/NEJMoa1413687.
55. Gaine S, Chin K, Coghlan G, Channick R, Di Scala L, Galiè N, Ghofrani H-A, Lang IM, McLaughlin V, Preiss R, Rubin LJ, Simonneau G, Sitbon O, Tapson VF, Hoeper MM. Selexipag for the treatment of connective tissue disease-associated pulmonary arterial hypertension. Eur Respir J. 2017;50 https://doi.org/10.1183/13993003.02493-2016.
56. Korn JH, Mayes M, Matucci Cerinic M, Rainisio M, Pope J, Hachulla E, Rich E, Carpentier P, Molitor J, Seibold JR, Hsu V, Guillevin L, Chatterjee S, Peter HH, Coppock J, Herrick A, Merkel PA, Simms R, Denton CP, Furst D, Nguyen N, Gaitonde M, Black C. Digital ulcers in systemic sclerosis: prevention by treatment with bosentan, an oral endothelin receptor antagonist. Arthritis Rheum. 2004;50:3985–93. https://doi.org/10.1002/art.20676.
57. Khanna D, Denton CP, Merkel PA, Krieg T, Le Brun F-O, Marr A, Papadakis K, Pope J, Matucci-Cerinic M, Furst DE. Effect of Macitentan on the development of new ischemic digital ulcers in patients with systemic sclerosis: DUAL-1 and DUAL-2 randomized clinical trials. JAMA. 2016c;315:1975–88. https://doi.org/10.1001/jama.2016.5258.
58. Tashkin DP, Elashoff R, Clements PJ, Goldin J, Roth MD, Furst DE, Arriola E, Silver R, Strange C, Bolster M, Seibold JR, Riley DJ, Hsu VM, Varga J, Schraufnagel DE, Theodore A, Simms R, Wise R, Wigley F, White B, Steen V, Read C, Mayes M, Parsley E, Mubarak K, Connolly MK, Golden J, Olman M, Fessler B, Rothfield N, Metersky M, Scleroderma Lung Study Research Group. Cyclophosphamide versus placebo in scleroderma lung disease. N Engl J Med. 2006;354(25):2655–66. https://doi.org/10.1056/NEJMoa055120.
59. Tashkin DP, Roth MD, Clements PJ, Furst DE, Khanna D, Kleerup EC, Goldin J, Arriola E, Volkmann ER, Kafaja S, Silver R, Steen V, Strange C, Wise R, Wigley F, Mayes M, Riley DJ, Hussain S, Assassi S, Hsu VM, Patel B, Phillips K, Martinez F, Golden J, Connolly MK, Varga J, Dematte J, Hinchcliff ME, Fischer A, Swigris J, Meehan R, Theodore A, Simms R, Volkov S, Schraufnagel DE, Scholand MB, Frech T, Molitor JA, Highland K, Read CA, Fritzler MJ, GHJ K, Tseng CH, Elashoff RM, Sclerodema Lung Study II Investigators. Mycophenolate mofetil versus oral cyclophosphamide in scleroderma-related interstitial lung disease (SLS II): a randomised controlled, double-blind, parallel group trial. Lancet Respir Med. 2016;4(9):708–19. https://doi.org/10.1016/S2213-2600(16)30152-7. Epub 2016 Jul 25. PMID: 27469583; PMCID: PMC5014629
60. Khanna D, Lin CJF, Furst DE, Goldin J, Kim G, Kuwana M, Allanore Y, Matucci-Cerinic M, Distler O, Shima Y, van Laar JM, Spotswood H, Wagner B, Siegel J, Jahreis A, Denton CP. Tocilizumab in systemic sclerosis: a randomised, double-blind, placebo-controlled, phase 3 trial. Lancet Respir Med. 2020c;8:963–74.

61. Becker MO, Dobrota R, Fligelstone K, et al. The EULAR systemic sclerosis impact of disease (ScleroID)—a new patient reported outcome measure for patients with systemic sclerosis. Ann Rheum Dis. 2020;79:158–9.
62. Spiera R, Hummers L, Chung L, Frech TM, Domsic R, Hsu V, Furst DE, Gordon J, Mayes M, Simms R, Lafyatis R, Martyanov V, Wood T, Whitfield ML, Constantine S, Lee E, Dgetluck N, White B. Safety and efficacy of lenabasum in a phase II, randomized, placebo-controlled trial in adults with systemic sclerosis. Arthritis Rheumatol. 2020;72(8):1350–60. https://doi.org/10.1002/art.41294. Epub 2020 Jul 17. PMID: 32336038; PMCID: PMC7497006

49 Drug Development and Regulatory Considerations for Systemic Sclerosis Therapies

Peter K. Wung and Jean-Marc Guettier

Drug discovery and development is an expensive and risky endeavor. It is estimated that only 10–15% of therapeutic compounds that enter clinical development ever reach the market. The challenge of developing an effective and safe drug for a rare disease such as systemic sclerosis (SSc) is arguably even greater, given the number of challenges including but not limited to relatively rare occurrence of this complex disease, the multiple proposed pathogenic mechanisms, the heterogeneity in its phenotypic manifestation, the absence of a proven "gold standard" effective therapy against which to benchmark, the lack of validated, widely accepted instruments to measure disease activity from the clinician's and the patient's perspective, and the scarcity of clinical research infrastructure with deep experience in the disease to efficiently conduct relatively large studies (Table 49.1). As such and to no surprise, there are no drugs approved for the broad indication of SSc. However, with our ever expanding knowledge of biological disease pathways and increasing number of therapeutic modalities to target these pathways, there is a real reason for optimism and enthusiam. With the right therapeutic candidate(s), there is now, more than ever, an opportunity to bring safe and effective drugs to the market for a patient population that desperately needs it. This chapter will highlight the drug development process as well as the regulatory considerations when developing potential therapies for SSc.

Table 49.1 Challenges for developing SSc therapies

Complex pathogenesis: vasculopathy, autoimmunity, fibrosis
Disease heterogeneity—limited vs. diffuse subtype, kinetics of disease progression, autoantibodies, organ system involvement
Lack of predictive animal models
Natural improvement of the skin over time (most patients)
Lack of validated biomarkers for disease activity, progression, and remission
Limitations of available clinical (e.g., mRSS, CRISS) and patient-centric (e.g., SHAQ) endpoints
Long duration (more than a year) required to achieve clinically meaningful endpoints (e.g., time to death or end-organ damage)
Insufficient high-quality global sites with thorough understanding of the disease to conduct the clinical trials in a short period of time

Drug Development Overview

From Molecule to Market: Time and Risk

The process to discover and develop a new drug (*new molecular entity* or NME) from initial concept to a marketed product is lengthy and complex, typically extending over a period of 10–15 years [1, 2]. A prototypical timeline for drug discovery and development is illustrated in Fig. 49.1. Timelines will vary depending on the amount of time spent in the pre-clinical phase optimizing the molecule and the complexity of the development phase (e.g., treatment duration, background therapy, sample size, and selected endpoints). In general, biologics and some of the newer drug platform modalities (i.e., gene silencing) require less optimization time and undergo the pre-clinical phase more rapidly than chemically synthesized small molecules. Development programs for drugs to treat rare, serious or life-threatening, orphan diseases will generally be smaller and require a shorter duration of exposure to the novel drug to support an initial approval.

Analyses of the success of drug development programs indicate that approximately 11% of NMEs entering human testing will make it to the market [3–5]. The reported success rates for biologics are approximately twice the rates for small molecules, and the highest rates for success from Phase 1 (33%) are for molecules with orphan drug designation [4, 5].

P. K. Wung (✉)
Immunology Clinical Development, AbbVie, North Chicago, IL, USA
e-mail: peter.wung@abbvie.com

J.-M. Guettier
Precision Medicine, Sanofi, Boston, MA, USA
e-mail: Jean-Marc.Guettier@sanofi.com

Y. Allanore et al. (eds.), *Scleroderma*, https://doi.org/10.1007/978-3-031-40658-4_49

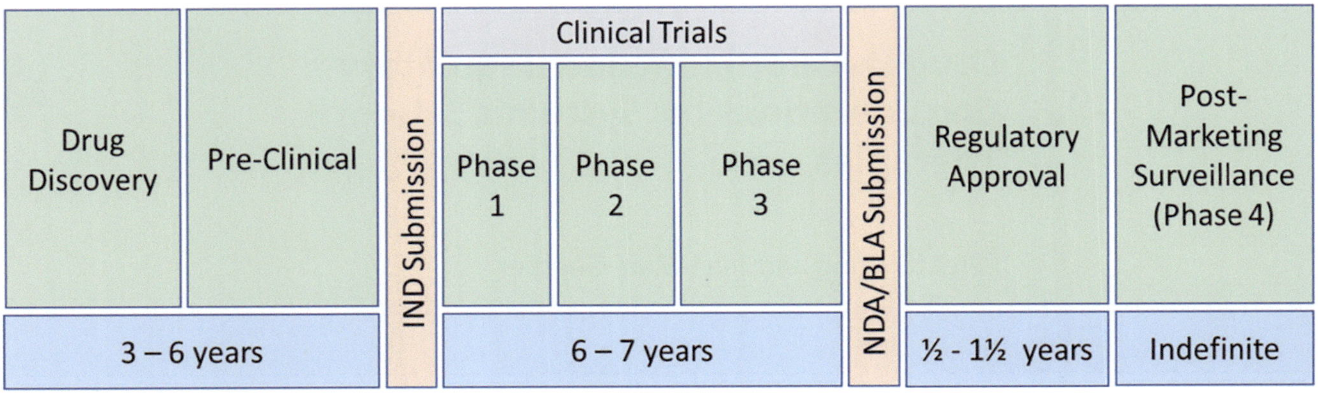

Fig. 49.1 Timeline of drug development

Cost of Drug Development

Considerable investments are required to develop NMEs and bring them to market, with the cost having doubled in the last decade [3]. The average cost needed to develop a single approvable drug is estimated to be in the range of $1.8–2.9B over the entire product and development lifecycle, depending on whether the cost of capital and failures are included [3, 6]. Also, it is more often the case than not that NMEs, once marketed, will not generate the commercial return needed to cover the fully loaded R&D costs.

At the time of a new product launch, the systems of patents and exclusivities protect, for a limited time, the innovator from competitors who may seek to market the same or a highly similar version of the innovative NME. The innovator company will generally use this time to attempt to recoup R&D costs. It is worth noting that the time elapsed between when a molecule is patented to the time it is marketed may leave little patent life remaining to recoup R&D investments. With regards to exclusivities in the US, the Hatch-Waxman Act, passed in 1984, provides an innovator company that develop a new chemical entity 5 years' worth of marketing exclusivity at the time of approval. Drugs which are approved to treat orphan diseases however, defined as diseases that affect fewer than 200,000 individuals in the United States, qualify for 7 years of marketing exclusivity. In the EU, the time frame of minimum exclusivity for orphan drugs is 10 years after approval.

There are other financial incentives besides patents and exclusivities granted to innovators of orphan disease drugs, including a 25% US federal tax credit for qualified clinical trial costs, a waiver of the US Federal Drug Administration (FDA) Prescription Drug User Fee Act (PDUFA) filing fee (~$3 million) and eligibility for research grants designated to support orphan product research. Similar financial incentives are in effect for EU orphan drug approvals [7]. Based on the prevalence of SSc, new drugs for this indication are regarded as "orphan disease" therapeutics by regulators in major markets [8]. Since 2016, orphan drug status was granted to 13 compounds in the development for the treatment of SSc [9]. The above-mentioned exclusivity and regulatory incentives should continue to promote drug development innovation in SSc.

Drug Discovery Phases

Initiation of New Programs

Drug discovery programs can originate from many parts of the scientific ecosystem. Initial concepts often arise from published research findings derived from academic laboratories. These can range from basic observations in genetics, genomics, cellular, or pathway biology that point to a potentially relevant target for disease control or to observations made in a different therapeutic area (e.g., pulmonary, oncology) that suggest a benefit on a key component of the disease. Others may be more translational in nature and describe phenotypes in animal models or humans and their association with certain gene signatures or specific T-cell mediated pathways, for instance. What follows from these fundamental observations can vary but usually involves an independent replication of the promising findings by private, public, or public/private entities interested in embarking on a drug discovery program. Depending on the availability of resources, expertise to confirm the findings and timing considerations, an early drug discovery program may be initiated in parallel to the confirmatory work. The strength of the data, biologic plausibility, and ultimately independent confirmation will drive the investment for a full drug discovery effort.

Many considerations go into the decision to embark on a new therapeutic program including but not limited to (1) the degree of target validation, (2) the ability to generate modulators (agonists or antagonists, as appropriate) of the target using available therapeutic modalities and technology, (3) the likelihood that the therapeutic approach will deliver an overall benefit for the patient that is on par with, if not better than the current standard of care, (4) whether the profile of the drug will be acceptable for the intended use, and (5) the potential to be either first-in-class or best-in-class. Some companies will also initiate a commercial assessment relatively early in the drug discovery process to determine the potential future commercial value of the product, although it is clear that such value forecasts are highly inaccurate especially for early programs [10–12]. Together these considerations shape what is often referred to as a "target product profile" or "TPP" that serves as a guide for the drug discovery team. It is important at this stage of developing novel therapeutics to remain flexible in the TPP so as not to restrict the exploration of novel therapeutics and their applications, since drug discovery involves a great deal of empiricism as well as serendipity.

New programs may originate in academic labs with the transfer of assays to central screening facilities in the private sector (e.g., NIH, NCI, some universities, and institutes), biotechs, or pharmaceutical companies. Alternatively, the screening assays may be created in the industry labs, themselves. These assays and appropriate counter-screens for selectivity, off-target effects, and cellular toxicity are used to generate the initial molecules (referred to as "compounds" until regulatory approval) for pre-clinical testing. The use of high-throughput robotic screening now enables the evaluation of millions of small molecules and natural products rapidly in enzyme-based or cellular assays [13]. Alternatively, monoclonal antibodies can be generated from millions of potential candidates using in vivo selection of hyperimmunized humanized mice or in vitro screening of recombinant human antibody libraries (e.g., phage or yeast display). Therapeutic peptides can be designed based on native sequences and modified to improve duration of action and potency and to alter their specificity (including dual specificity in some cases). Novel nucleic acid and cell therapeutic candidates can be generated in a matter of a few months using recombinant methods, an array of gene transduction approaches (viral and nonviral), and gene-editing techniques. Lastly, with the combination of available large data sets and improved algorithms to enhance machine learning, artificial intelligence is beginning to be employed in the search for new compounds. While traditional approaches are still important and vital, the use of AI will become increasingly commonplace and undoubtedly change the landscape of drug discovery [14].

Validation and Optimization Phase

The next phase of drug discovery is a highly iterative one in which the compounds identified from initial screens are profiled extensively in vitro using enzyme and cellular assays, as appropriate. Often significant structural modifications are made to improve compound qualities (cell permeability, plasma stability, target selectivity, etc.), and this process can continue for months to years, depending on the desired profile. Subsequently, compounds are selected for testing in animals to examine pharmacokinetics (PK), pharmacodynamics (PD), and preliminary toxicology. These tool compounds are also used to confirm that modulating the target originally identified as linked to a human disease process or phenotype has the desired efficacy in vitro and in vivo (ideally in a relevant animal model of human disease). The other major goal of the profiling at this stage is to understand the preliminary safety and tolerability of the compound in animals (in short-term tolerability studies). Together, these data are compared to the TPP described above and begin to inform the benefit-risk profile of the drug.

Years may elapse validating the new therapeutic target based on the generation of genetically modified animals, in vitro testing in cellular systems reflective of human disease processes (cellular knockdown or overexpression, in vitro) or through the evaluation of tool compounds in vitro and in vivo. Indeed, many programs never make it out of this early phase of drug discovery due to the failure of target validation or the inability to generate suitable molecules with "drug-like" properties that satisfy the TPP.

Candidate Selection and Profiling

Once advanced compounds have passed the initial battery of evaluations, a few of these are taken into the next round of more intensive pre-clinical profiling to determine whether they will be suitable for clinical testing. This phase includes extensive evaluation of the pharmaceutical properties of the compounds including manufacturing scalability, formulation, stability, metabolism, and more formal toxicology studies in vitro and in vivo. It is during this period using the most advanced compounds that estimates, based on pre-clinical data, are made of the human dose and exposure needed for a desired level of efficacy (often using PK-PD modeling). This work is greatly facilitated by the availability of biomarkers that can serve as reliable surrogates for human disease activity, monitor early beneficial response to treatment, and/or predict potential unwanted toxicity [15]. In the absence of such biomarkers and animal models that accurately reproduce disease mechanisms important in human diseases, the drug program advances with great uncertainty with respect to the ultimate translatability to human efficacy and safety.

In nearly all cases, a single most promising compound is selected as the clinical candidate for manufacturing scale up under "current good manufacturing practices" or cGMP and further pre-clinical testing of the compound under "good laboratory practices" or GLP. This phase of late pre-clinical development requires rigorous documentation and monitoring for quality, reproducibility, and reliability to meet regulatory standards to support human testing. Failure of compounds at this stage is not uncommon due to the inability to achieve consistent blood or tissue exposure (across pre-clinical species) at the levels projected for human efficacy or due to unacceptable toxicity in GLP pre-clinical safety studies performed to support human studies. Termination of a late pre-clinical program due to an unexpected finding can mean going back to earlier-stage compounds with a different chemical scaffold that may have improved pharmaceutical properties or lack a specific toxicity. Alternatively, it can lead to abandonment of the entire program due to uncertainty that a backup will address the shortcomings of the initial candidate or because the timeline of the program is no longer competitive with that of other companies.

Initiating SSc Targeted Drug Discovery Programs

Considering the current state of knowledge and the complex pathogenesis of SSc, it may be challenging to embark on a focused de novo drug discovery program in SSc. A more common scenario is a program that targets one or more of the fundamental mechanisms underpinning SSc biology (e.g., vasculopathy, autoimmunity, or fibrosis) with the goal to slow down or even reverse disease course. Once early compounds are identified from screens, it would be essential to have access to primary cells from SSc patients (endothelial cells, PBMCs, and fibroblasts from the skin and lung) to interrogate their utility in secondary assays. This is particularly important since the next phase of pre-clinical validation, evaluation in SSc animal models, is not a straightforward (or clinically relevant) process.

Moving from in vitro cell culture assays to examining the effects of compounds in vivo in animal models is a valuable step to select compounds for advancement to the clinic. As described above, testing in animal models provides data that can enable PK-PD modeling and establish whether the degree of target modulation by the compound is likely to elicit the sought after clinical effect. The big challenge with SSc in this regard is selecting among the many animal models that best reflects the human disease mechanism. Although there is no specific model that recapitulates all of the pathogenic mechanisms, existing models can be used to probe specific pathogenic components of SSc and establish a PK-PD-efficacy relationship that can serve as a guide for human testing.

In the absence of availability of suitable models to interrogate a novel disease target and mechanism of action, it may be adequate to establish that exposures in vivo sufficiently modulate the target to achieve the desired cellular or tissue effect in normal animals. The gap created by this approach can reduce confidence (and support) for pursuing the SSc indication. One way to supplement the disease-relevant pre-clinical information and potentially bridge to the clinic is with the use of biomarkers that reflect disease activity. Further work to better define disease activity (e.g., vascular damage, immune, fibrosis) biomarkers and profiling them in pre-clinical models can help close the gap between in vitro cellular assays and human studies.

Clinical Development Phases

Exploratory Clinical Development: Phases 1 and 2a

After compiling the package of pre-clinical data satisfying the requirements for safeguarding human testing and providing reasonable confidence that the compound will achieve adequate human exposure in the dosage form and route chosen, an application to perform the first in human (FIH) Phase 1 clinical trial is made to the regulatory authority and independent ethics committee (e.g., Institutional Review Board or IRB) with oversight responsibilities of studies conducted in humans. In the USA, this is in the form of an Investigational New Drug (IND) application submitted to the Food and Drug Administration (FDA), and elsewhere this has other regulatory formats, such as the Clinical Trial Application (CTA) in Europe. Clinical trials for worldwide drug development are conducted according to "Good Clinical Practice" (GCP) guidelines, a standard critical to the ethical conduct of research involving human subjects.

Before a novel drug can be tested in humans, animal toxicity studies from two species (rodent and a higher non-rodent species) that involve dosing the drug at multiple times higher than the highest anticipated human exposure to achieve a benefit are required. These studies ideally identify organ system(s) sensitive to drug toxicity and allow for first in human dose setting and prospective planning for the monitoring for early signs of toxicity in future first in human tests. Exceptions can be made to the two species toxicology testing depending on species cross-reactivity of the compound. The initial GLP toxicology studies are usually of 2–4 weeks in duration and support human testing up to the duration of animal dosing. Since in most chronic conditions, the duration of human dosing will be in the order of months to years, longer-term non-clinical toxicology studies (i.e. 6–9 months depending on the species) will be required to support longer-term clinical trials. If the compound moves forward in development, several other toxicology studies (i.e., carcinogenicity, reproductive toxicology, etc.) will also generally be required before a compound can be approved. Toxicology studies are expensive to conduct and are the most demanding of the

GMP compound supply in the early stage of development. Therefore, toxicology studies are usually conducted in a staggered fashion with increasing duration of dosing after promising Phase 1 human data have been generated.

The goal of early human testing is to establish human safety, tolerability, and pharmacokinetics of the investigational compounds. In parallel, an important secondary objective of Phase 1 studies, whenever possible, is to determine the drug concentration that corresponds to the desired level of biologic target engagement so that a preliminary human PK-PD relationship can be established. The FIH trial is generally a single ascending dose (SAD) study. In this phase, small groups of subjects (e.g., 8) are exposed to increasing single doses of the new drug (e.g., 6) or placebo (e.g., 2) with careful clinical monitoring and frequent sampling for PK, PD and common clinical laboratories. Once a single dose has been shown to be bioavailable, safe, and well-tolerated, a multiple ascending dose (MAD) study can be initiated to examine the effect of repeat dosing on the same or similar parameters over a period of 1–2 weeks. Safety, tolerability, PK, and PD across dose groups are carefully reviewed to assess the potential of the compound to deliver its intended effect when evaluated in longer-term studies in patients. Compounds that are unsafe or do not achieve the desired human PK exposure profile may require reformulation or may be discontinued.

To limit the influence of external factors (i.e., disease or concomitant drugs) on experimental results in Phase 1 studies, the FIH trials are usually conducted on healthy volunteer subjects (with appropriate safeguards and informed consent) in a domiciled setting in order to closely monitor them for safety and tolerability. In the case of compounds projected to have a narrow therapeutic index (e.g., most oncology compounds) or novel therapeutics (i.e., cell and gene therapies) for the treatment of rare, serious, life-threatening diseases, it may be preferrable and justifiable to initiate testing in the patient population.

If the Phase 1 objectives are met, the compound enters Phase 2 to establish "Proof of Concept" (PoC) that the drug will have its intended effect in diseased individuals (i.e., Phase 2a). The result of this study will provide the critical evidence needed to justify the large investments required for Phase 2b/3. The PoC study is typically a randomized, placebo-controlled, double-blind trial performed in a well-defined and often relatively homogeneous patient population (generally less than 100–200 subjects) whose objective is to generate sufficient evidence that the highest tolerated dose from the Phase 1 trial has the desired effect in individuals with the disease. A lower dose may be included to get a preliminary assessment of the therapeutic range, part of a dose-ranging trial often seen in Phase 2b to guide future development.

In designing and analyzing PoC trials, which are considered exploratory in nature, considerable flexibility is possible including planned interim analyses, exploratory analyses across dose groups, reduced statistical power, and level of statistical significance for declaring a positive study (commonly a $p < 0.1$). The determination of PoC may be made on one or more endpoints (clinical, imaging, or laboratory) that gives confidence that subsequent longer duration trials will deliver the evidence needed to establish clinical efficacy. Whenever feasible, PoC trials include "registration endpoints," i.e., those established by regulatory authorities as the basis for approval in a specific condition, although the trial design and duration may not support rigorous statistical analysis of these endpoints. While there is no universal method to determine PoC in this early phase of drug development, the three-outcome decision model can be employed as an effective tool utilizing a systematic approach [16]. The three-outcome decision model allows quantitative decision-making (Go or No-Go for next phase) in a controlled and efficient manner, based upon pre-determined parameters of the Target Value (TV) and Lower Reference Value (LRV) associated with the TPP.

Each of the exploratory aspects of PoC trial design and data analysis comes with some risk when extrapolating results to larger studies. The tolerance for risk of replicating PoC results in subsequent Phase 2b or of accepting a false-positive POC study is established on a case-by-case basis. On average, one-third of compounds that reached Phase 1 (FIH) will pass PoC and enter the confirmatory phase of clinical development.

Confirmatory Clinical Development: Phases 2b and 3

Having achieved PoC, the next phase of clinical development can be considered. This is a major inflection point in the investment for a development program and represents a period of intense analysis of available clinical and preclinical data in the context of the TPP and commercial assessment, which is more mature at this stage, factoring in the available data and the competitive landscape. In Phase 2b and 3 trials, the rigor of statistical design and analyses comes into play since these are considered trials that are core to the regulatory review and approval process. Although regulatory advice can be sought throughout the research and development process, it is a key component for the confirmatory phase of clinical development since the stakes (cost for designing an inadequate set of trials) are highest at this stage. Complicating matters is the fact that there is no global harmonization of regulatory requirements, endpoints, inclusion of comparators, and duration of follow-up for approval. Thus, discussions with the regulatory bodies from the different regions are needed to fine tune the key elements of the study design, including primary and key secondary endpoints which will serve as the basis for establishing evidence of efficacy and safety and will inform labeling. These major regulatory bodies generally include the FDA (USA), European Medicines Agency (EMA in Europe), Pharmaceuticals and Medical Devices Agency (PMDA in Japan), and National Medical Products Administration (NMPA in China), formerly known as the Chinese Food and Drug Administration (CFDA), if authorization in these major markets is sought. Each region may have a specific set of requirements that needs to be met, necessitating a carefully designed study that can encompass and address as many of the key essential regulatory elements required to obtain an authorization in these markets. Specific elements of study design may need to be carefully negotiated with the authorities themselves or handled disparately across regions in the protocol. For example, in China, the exportation of biological and genetic samples collected during the study and analyzed abroad is controlled by the Human Genetic Resources Administration of China (HGRAC) and the use of samples for exploratory analyses is not permitted. This poses logistic challenges if genetic testing is required and can only be performed outside of China or if exploratory analyses are key to support the application. Thus, global trials should take such points into consideration while assessing the evolving regulatory landscape.

For the majority of compounds (exceptions in oncology and some orphan indications), the Phase 2b trial is a randomized placebo-controlled dose ranging study in patients designed to establish the effective dose(s) of the compound using the intended registrational endpoint(s). It also serves to expand the safety database in the target population and ideally to identify a minimally effective (or ineffective) dose to guide dose selection for Phase 3. Because these studies typically extend beyond 6 months and also since continued treatment via open-label extension of dosing for patients who respond to the therapy, chronic toxicology studies need to be completed before initiating Phase 2b (6 months in rodents, 9 months in non-rodents). For most clinical indications, the sample size needed to define the dose response with a high degree of confidence ($p < 0.05$) is on the order of a hundred subjects per arm, depending on many variables including the effect size, variance, the shape of the dose-response curve, and where on the curve the chosen doses fall. It is common for Phase 2b studies to require 1.5–2 years for completion. At the end of Phase 2b, if the data are promising, they are presented to regulatory authorities to get input and agreement on the design of the Phase 3 program.

The final investigational leg of the clinical development journey is Phase 3 in which one or two studies (i.e., depends on the indication and whether the Phase 2b results are robust enough to act as supportive evidence for an approval) are performed in the target patient population to confirm the efficacy and characterize the safety of the compound at the proposed dose(s) for registration. The phase 3 program often involves 500–1000+ subjects (though this is highly dependent on disease prevalence and can be much smaller [200–400] for rare conditions such as SSc) in global multicenter trials and last 2–3 years when the time for recruitment and duration of follow-up necessary for efficacy and safety assessments are factored in. Overall success rate for compounds entering Phase 3 is roughly 70%, and assuming no surprises, the data will support regulatory approval [4].

Regulatory Submission and Review

After the completion of a successful Phase 3 program, the sponsor assembles an application with all the evidence generated from manufacturing, pre-clinical and clinical studies to support the regulatory review and approval processes. Due to the volume of data, the complexity of integrating the evidence and the time required to assemble all supporting data, documents, and cross-references in a functioning application, the preparation of a dossier for a New Drug Application (NDA) or Biologic License Application (BLA) can take several months to complete. Once filed and accepted by the regulatory authorities, the review clock begins. For the USA, the review timeline is 10 months for standard applications [17] and 6 months for priority review applications [18] from the time the application is filed. Priority review is granted to applications for drugs that treat serious or life-threatening diseases and where the preliminary clinical evidence suggest they offer a benefit over available therapies. The EMA review is usually completed over a period of 12–14 months, and faster review is possible based on the unmet medical need and data. The PMDA is similar to FDA in its review timelines. Through a series of reforms over the last 5 years, the NMPA has significantly decreased its review and approval timelines from the previous average of nearly 2 years to the current duration of 8 and 6 months for standard and priority reviews, respectively. With such an improvement in the review and approval timelines and streamlining of its regulatory procedures for market access, China is commonly included in the global development program within the last 5 years.

Post-approval Studies: Phase 4 and Beyond

After approval, clinical research on the new drug continues and includes a variety of studies that further characterize the safety and efficacy of the new product. There may be commitments or requirements placed on the sponsor to perform additional studies or post marketing surveillance by health authorities as a condition of approval. This is standard in certain countries and is more often the case when the approval has been accelerated, the primary indication is a small patient population (limited number of exposure years of safety follow-up), or if the new drug is first in a new class with a novel mechanism for which long-term safety is unknown [19–21]. Phase 4 studies build on the data generated in highly monitored and controlled trials during the earlier phases of clinical development and add to this important information generated in the "real-world" setting [21].

Once a drug has reached the market, the sponsor is more likely to entertain exploratory studies in additional patient populations. Some companies include indication expansion strategies earlier in development (e.g., Phase 2a), and this can lead to parallel Phase 2b and Phase 3 programs in more than one indication [22]. The more likely scenario is the willingness of the company to consider the evaluation of their drug following initial regulatory approval in novel indications based on pre-clinical (in vitro or in vivo) data, case reports, or compelling disease mechanism related rationale. These new studies may originate within the company as the result of internal scientific work or indication expansion strategy, or they may originate externally—typically from the academic community. Investigator-initiated trials (IITs, also referred to as investigator-sponsored trials) represent important mechanisms for exploratory clinical research for new drugs. These studies, if positive, can form the basis for pivotal studies that result in supplemental regulatory approvals in expanded patient populations or new indications [23].

Strategies for SSc Drug Development

As described above, the path to clinical testing of new compounds requires careful coordination of pre-clinical and clinical research activities and is enabled by a clear understanding of anticipated clinical and laboratory outcomes that define as "success". It is appropriate to include patients in Phase 1 studies if there is the potential to observe a measurable response of clinical benefit to the test compound being evaluated during the short period of treatment and observation (typically up to 2–4 weeks). Currently we lack evidence that SSc would exhibit a significant clinical or biomarker (laboratory or imaging) response in this time frame, making it likely that new compounds designed for SSc would be evaluated first in healthy volunteers (if safety profile was favorable) or in patients with another disease for which an earlier clinical or PD (e.g., biomarker) response may be observed.

In the absence of predictive biomarkers or disease outcome measures useful in Phase 1, the earliest studies of novel compounds to generate preliminary evidence of efficacy in SSc patients will take place in Phase 2 when PK and safety for the compounds has been established and toxicology studies have been performed to support human dosing of 6 months or longer. The identification of reliable short-term predictive biomarkers of disease activity and/or response to therapy would be an important enabler for SSc drug discovery and would encourage earlier and rapid exploration of novel compounds for use in SSc patients.

The complication of disease heterogeneity is another challenge in the design of SSc clinical trials. As noted above, most PoC trials are conducted in relatively small and homogeneous disease populations for which the mechanism of action of the compound is hypothesized to be of benefit. The desire to ensure strict homogeneity (SSc subtype, disease duration, organ system involvement) in order to achieve key objectives and endpoints must be acknowledged and balanced with the feasibility of recruitment, along with operational execution. It is worth noting and learning from the recent success of efforts made in trials of homogeneous patient populations with idiopathic pulmonary fibrosis and SSc-interstitial lung disease (ILD) leading to the approval of two NMEs [24–27].

Another key strategy is to identify the primary and key secondary endpoints that will be acceptable to regulatory bodies. In the early part of the last decade, the modified Rodnan Skin Score (mRSS) was commonly accepted and used as the primary endpoint to establish benefit in SSc pivotal trials. However, as the number of failed studies that employed this endpoint continued to mount, regulatory bodies such as the FDA have questioned the appropriateness of this surrogate endpoint and recommended coming up with additional relevant endpoint(s) that better assesses the impact of the drug on a how a SSc patient functions, feels, or survives. A good example of a patient-centric endpoint is the Scleroderma Health Assessment Questionnaire (SHAQ) which is composed of the standard Health Assessment Questionnaire (HAQ) and additional visual analog scales to measure symptoms specific to SSc and overall disease severity, but it has its limitations. The Composite Response Index in Systemic Sclerosis (CRISS) [28] is a relatively newer endpoint that summarizes the changes in clinical and patient-reported outcomes in a single composite score which conveys the probability of improvement from disease but its effectiveness remains to be determined and may have an associated ceiling effect; as a result, a revised CRISS is in development. When considering the various SSc endpoints, it is good to identify the appropriateness for the target population of interest, ability to cover the clinical spectrum of limited and diffuse subtypes, and the duration required to assess a beneficial effect. For example, endpoints such as the mRSS and CRISS are more suited for a study involving diffuse SSc, whereas an endpoint focused on mortality will require a much longer study.

Other key elements of the study design that are important to consider in SSc trials are the allowance of background therapy during the trial and instituting some type of post-trial access to the compound after a patient has completed the trial. In the absence of therapies with clearly established efficacy, most regulatory bodies assess SSc trials relying on a strict placebo comparator arm, but this could pose an ethical dilemma to SSc patients who have potentially serious and life threatening disease. As such, most regulatory bodies require that standard of care treatment be allowed as background therapy during the trial; stratification can be used to ensure equal distribution of patients on background therapy between the different trial arms, if needed. Recent trials in SSc have employed this strategy and are able to still demonstrate a significant effect of the compound vs. placebo [29]. Additionally, the ability to provide post-trial access to the compound, especially in the post-PoC phase, is another essential element to consider in the study design as it increases both site and patient participation as well as fulfilling a regulatory requirement for certain countries, given that this is a life-threatening disease largely without approved therapies. Post-trial access may come in different forms including bridging the primary study(ies) to a long-term safety study or open label extension study where long-term safety (and efficacy) of the patients can be closely monitored in a clinical trial setting. Provided the benefit continues to outweigh the risks in the individual receiving the experimental therapy, treatment can continue under a post-trial access mechanism until regulatory approvals in the respective countries have been achieved.

Another approach for developing novel therapeutics for SSc is to pursue organ system specific or symptomatic therapeutics, rather than overall disease modifying drugs. There are many examples of clinical trials evaluating marketed products targeting mechanisms of relevance for the vasculopathy (Raynaud's, digital ulcer), gastroesophageal reflux, ILD, and pulmonary arterial hypertension in SSc patients. Working with companies that have novel compounds in their pipeline to conduct trials for organ-specific benefit may lead to important therapeutic step wise advances for SSc patients.

Lastly, the operational execution of the trial must be diligently planned in order to optimize its success, particularly for a rare and complicated disease such as SSc. First, experienced and well-qualified sites with appropriate access to ancillary services (e.g., pulmonary function test (PFT), echocardiogram, high resolution computed tomography (HRCT)) must be properly identified. This can be done with a well-planned and thorough feasibility assessment and/or by collaborating with different organizations (e.g., Scleroderma Clinical Trials Consortium (SCTC) [30] and/or Scleroderma Research Foundation (SRF) [31]), which are often connected to the top SSc centers or experts around the world. Second, for a commonly used primary or key secondary endpoint such as the mRSS which can be associated with a great degree of intra-rater and inter-rater variability, it is imperative to make sure that the identified investigators are qualified to perform this assessment and have prior experience with it, as there is an associated learning curve for novice users. This assessment should be performed on a regular basis in their respective clinical practice and they should be re-trained on it at the beginning and possibly during the course of the study to ensure uniformity of the assessment across all sites. For the other commonly used endpoint, forced vital capacity, it is a necessity that the PFT is captured by the same skilled pulmonary technician using the same machine for each timepoint in order to ensure consistency of data.

Conclusion

There is continued interest on the part of industry and academia to pursue the development of new drugs for SSc. It is essential that basic and clinical research continue to address gaps in our knowledge related to the disease pathogenesis and markers of disease activity, while quantitative outcome measures, especially ones that are patient-centric in nature, need to be further developed or improved in order to enhance the feasibility and success of future SSc drug discovery programs.

Acknowledgments The authors would like to acknowledge Dr. Timothy Wright, the previous author of this chapter. The current chapter is built upon his previous work with additional updates and insights.

References

1. Corr P, Williams D. The pathway from idea to regulatory approval: examples for drug development. In: Lo B, Field MJ, editors. Institute of medicine committee on conflict of interest in medical research, education, and practice. Washington, DC: National Academies Press; 2009. p. 375–83.
2. Woosley RL, Cossman J. Drug development and the FDA's critical path initiative. Clin Pharmacol Ther. 2007;81:129–33.
3. DiMasi JA, Grabowski HG, Hansen RW. Innovation in the pharmaceutical industry: New estimates of R&D costs. J Health Econ. 2016;47:20–33.
4. Hay M, Thomas DW, Craighead JL, Economides C, Rosenthal J. Clinical development success rates for investigational drugs. Nat Biotechnol. 2014;32(1):40–51.
5. Kola I, Landis J. Can the pharmaceutical industry reduce attrition rates? Nat Rev Drug Discov. 2004;3:711–5.
6. Munos B. Lessons from 60 years of pharmaceutical innovation. Nat Rev Drug Discov. 2009;8:959–68.
7. EMA Website: Orphan Incentives https://www.ema.europa.eu/en/human-regulatory/research-development/orphan-designation/orphan-incentives. Access 22 Dec 2020.
8. Field MJ, Boat TF, editors. Rare diseases and orphan products: accelerating research and development. Washington, DC: National Academies Press; 2010. p. 29–33.
9. US Food and Drug Administration. Search for orphan drug designations and approvals: https://www.accessdata.fda.gov/scripts/

opdlisting/oopd/listResult.cfm?StartRow=1&EndRow=25. Accessed 22 Dec 2020.
10. Nigro GL, Morreale A, Enea G. Open innovation: a real option to restore value to the biopharmaceutical R&D. Int J Prod Econ. 2014;149:183–93.
11. Walker A, Turner S, Johnson R. Pharma and biotech valuations: divergent perspectives. Bus Dev Lic J. 2015;22:10–3.
12. Cha M, Rifai B, Sarraf P. Pharmaceutical forecasting: throwing darts? Nat Rev Drug Disc. 2013;12:737–8.
13. Hughes JP, Rees S, Kalindjian SB, Philpott KL. Principles of early drug discovery. Br J Pharm. 2011;162:1239–49.
14. Fleming N. How artificial intelligence is changing drug discovery. Nature. 2018;557(7707):S55–7.
15. Mina-Osorio P. Basics of drug development in rheumatology. Arth Rheum. 2015;67:2581–90.
16. Frewer P, Mitchell P, Watkins C, Matcham J. Decision-making in early clinical drug development. Pharm Stat. 2016;15(3):255–63.
17. US Food and Drug Administration. The Drug Development Process website: https://www.fda.gov/patients/learn-about-drug-and-device-approvals/drug-development-process. Access 22 Dec 2020.
18. US Food and Drug Administration. Fast track, breakthrough therapy, accelerated approval, Priority Review. https://www.fda.gov/patients/learn-about-drug-and-device-approvals/fast-track-breakthrough-therapy-accelerated-approval-priority-review. Accessed 22 Dec 2020.
19. Curtin F, Schultz P. Assessing the benefit:risk ratio of a drug—randomized and naturalistic evidence. Dialogues Clin Neurosci. 2011;13:183–90.
20. Glasser SP, Salas M, Delzell E. Importance and challenges of studying marketed drugs: what is a phase IV study? Common clinical research designs, registries, and self-reporting systems. J Clin Pharmacol. 2007;47:1074–86.
21. Suvarna V. Phase IV of drug development. Perspect Clin Res. 2010;1:57–60.
22. Miossec P, Kolls JK. Targeting IL-17 and T_H17 cells in chronic inflammation. Nat Rev Drug Disc. 2012;11:763–76.
23. Wang B, Kesselheim AS. Characteristics of efficacy evidence supporting approval of supplemental indications for prescription drugs in United States, 2005–14: systematic review. BMJ. 2015;351:h4679.
24. Richeldi L, Costabel U, Selman M, Kim DS, Hansell DM, Nicholson AG, et al. Efficacy of a tyrosine kinase inhibitor in idiopathic pulmonary fibrosis. N Engl J Med. 2011;365:1079–87.
25. Richeldi L, du Bois RM, Raghu G, Azuma A, Brown KK, Costabel U, et al. Efficacy and safety of nintedanib in idiopathic pulmonary fibrosis. N Engl J Med. 2014;370:2071–82.
26. Aravena C, Labarca G, Venegas C, Arenas A, Rada G. Pirfenidone for idiopathic pulmonary fibrosis: a systematic review and meta-analysis. PLoS One. 2015;10(8):0136160.
27. Distler O, Highland KB, Gahlemann M, Azuma A, Fischer A, Mayes MD, Raghu G, Sauter W, Girard M, Alves M, Clerisme-Beaty E, Stowasser S, Tetzlaff K, Kuwana M, Maher TM, Senscis Trial Investigators. Nintedanib for systemic sclerosis-associated interstitial lung disease. N Engl J Med. 2019;380(26):2518–28.
28. Khanna D, Berrocal VJ, Giannini EH, Seibold JR, Merkel PA, Mayes MD, Baron M, Clements PJ, Steen V, Assassi S, Schiopu E, Phillips K, Simms RW, Allanore Y, Denton CP, Distler O, Johnson SR, Matucci-Cerinic M, Pope JE, Proudman SM, Siegel J, Wong WK, Wells AU, Furst DE. The American College of Rheumatology provisional composite response index for clinical trials in early diffuse cutaneous systemic sclerosis. Arthritis Rheumatol. 2016;68(2):299–311.
29. Allanore Y, Wung P, Soubrane C, Esperet C, Marrache F, Bejuit R, Lahmar A, Khanna D, Denton CP, Investigators. A randomised, double-blind, placebo-controlled, 24-week, phase II, proof-of-concept study of romilkimab (SAR156597) in early diffuse cutaneous systemic sclerosis. Ann Rheum Dis. 2020;79(12):1600–7.
30. Scleroderma Clinical Trial Consortium website: https://sclerodermaclinicaltrialsconsortium.org/. Accessed 22 Dec 2020.
31. Scleroderma Research Foundation website: https://srfcure.org/. Accessed 22 Dec 2020.

Part IX

Case Studies: Approach to Complex Clinical Problems

John Varga and Christopher P. Denton

Managing the Ischemic Finger in Scleroderma

50

Fredrick M. Wigley and Thomas Reifsnyder

The case to be presented is not an actual case but was created from experience to represent an uncommon situation confounding the specialist caring for patients with scleroderma vascular disease.

Case Presentation

The patient is a 48-year-old Caucasian woman with limited scleroderma. The features of her disease include stiff puffy fingers, gastrointestinal reflux disease (GERD), severe Raynaud's phenomenon (RP), and a sicca syndrome. On her initial examination, the blood pressure was 120/69, weight 130 lb., pulse 79, temperature 98°, and normal respiratory rate. Sclerodactyly, numerous cutaneous telangiectasia on the palms and face and definite abnormal nailfold capillaries with dilatation and areas of void of capillaries. The remainder of her examination was completely normal. The general laboratory testing was unremarkable but serology demonstrated high-titer anti-centromere antibodies. Both lung function testing and echocardiograph were normal. She was managed with a proton pump inhibitor for her GERD and artificial tears for her dry eyes.

Initial Therapy

When deciding the treatment of the RP, one must consider measures to both improve quality of life and prevent ischemic injury to the digits and tissues. The foundation of the initial therapy for every patient with Raynaud's is nondrug management. Several types of daily activities, the effects of various drugs, and environmental factors greatly influence the severity of RP. Educating the patient about what to expect, the cause and potential complications of RP in the patient with scleroderma and the various "triggers" that aggravate RP not only reduces anxiety but also provides the framework for the patient to actively participate in management. Patients have an improved quality of life after they understand why RP is happening and what they can do to avoid aggravating factors that precipitate Raynaud's events. A major factor in triggering events in scleroderma is the ambient temperature. In fact, managing the environmental exposures is still the most effective method to reduce the severity of RP. For example, shifting temperatures (moving into the cold of air conditioning or sitting in a cool breeze) is a major trigger for RP. In cold environments wearing layered clothing, gloves, and covering the head will help keep the core body temperature normal (the central body process of temperature regulation) and protect the surface skin (the local response to regulation of body temperature) from cold exposure. Emotional stress is another factor that can trigger RP even if the patient is warm. Clinical observations show that provocation of anxiety (e.g. sudden noise; a visit to the doctor) will provoke RP even if the patient is in a warm environment. Our patient is not a smoker, but smoking cessation is essential to reduce the risk of a severe digital ischemic event. Certain drugs and agents that may cause peripheral vasoconstriction need to be avoided (Table 50.1). Interestingly, there are few formal studies to define the exact impact of managing anxiety and stress. Interventions such as acupuncture, biofeedback, and techniques to help relaxation are not proven to be helpful, but sensible advice and good communication are clearly important [1].

Raynaud's phenomenon associated with scleroderma is a manifestation of peripheral vascular disease that is complicated by both abnormal vasoreactivity and underlying structural vascular disease [2]. This vasculopathy increases the risk of ischemic tissue injury due to severe repeated episodes of vasoconstriction, vascular occlusion, loss of cutaneous ves-

F. M. Wigley (✉)
Division of Rheumatology, Department of Medicine, The Johns Hopkins University School of Medicine,, Baltimore, MD, USA
e-mail: fwig@jhmi.edu

T. Reifsnyder
Department of Surgery/Vascular Surgery and Endovascular Therapy, The Johns Hopkins University School of Medicine, Baltimore, MD, USA
e-mail: treifsn1@jhmi.edu

Y. Allanore et al. (eds.), *Scleroderma*, https://doi.org/10.1007/978-3-031-40658-4_50

sels, and defective vascular repair. While all patients with scleroderma should be considered at risk for complications from RP and peripheral vascular disease, certain subsets of patients are at greater risk for severe ischemic events which can lead to digital amputation (Fig. 50.1). The patients at greatest risk of digital amputation from macrovascular disease are those like our case with limited scleroderma and anti-centromere antibodies [3]. However, recurrent ischemic digital ulcers are more likely to occur in patients with diffuse skin disease [4]. Patients do appear to follow a consistent pattern of either no ischemic ulcers or one of recurring lesions. To best guide management, it is important to recognize various types of lesions that mimic ischemic digital ulcers (Fig. 50.2) that occur on the fingers of patients with scleroderma. Dry thickened skin can fissure mimicking an ischemic ulcer; painless digital pits occur after ulcer healing; paronychia can occur at the nailfold; the skin over joint contractures can thin and ulcerate from local trauma; avascular thicken skin can ulcerate on the shaft of the finger; underlying cutaneous calcinosis is common on the fingertips and can rupture to the surface and ulcerate; and any open wound can get secondarily infected. A digital ischemic ulcer (Fig. 50.3) is generally at the tip secondary to both vasospasm and occlusion in small arterioles and arteries with loss of blood flow and tissue hypoxia. Disease in more proximal digital vessels, palmar arch, or distal forearm arteries may also occur. This vascular disease may be occult with repeat RP alone or lead to repeated small ischemic ulcers or it may cause prolonged deep tissue ischemia necessitating digital amputation (Fig. 50.1).

Table 50.1 Drugs that may aggravate Raynaud's phenomenon

Migraine headache drugs (serotonin agonist; blocking calcitonin gene-related peptide)
Cold preparations (sympathetic agonist)
Beta-blockers (controversial)
Caffeine (controversial)
ADHD: Methylphenidate, dextroamphetamine-amphetamine, and atomoxetine
Weight-reducing drugs: Ephedra
Estrogens (undefined)
Interferons, opiates, cocaine, polyvinyl chloride exposure, and chemotherapeutic drugs including cisplatin, bleomycin, or gemcitabine

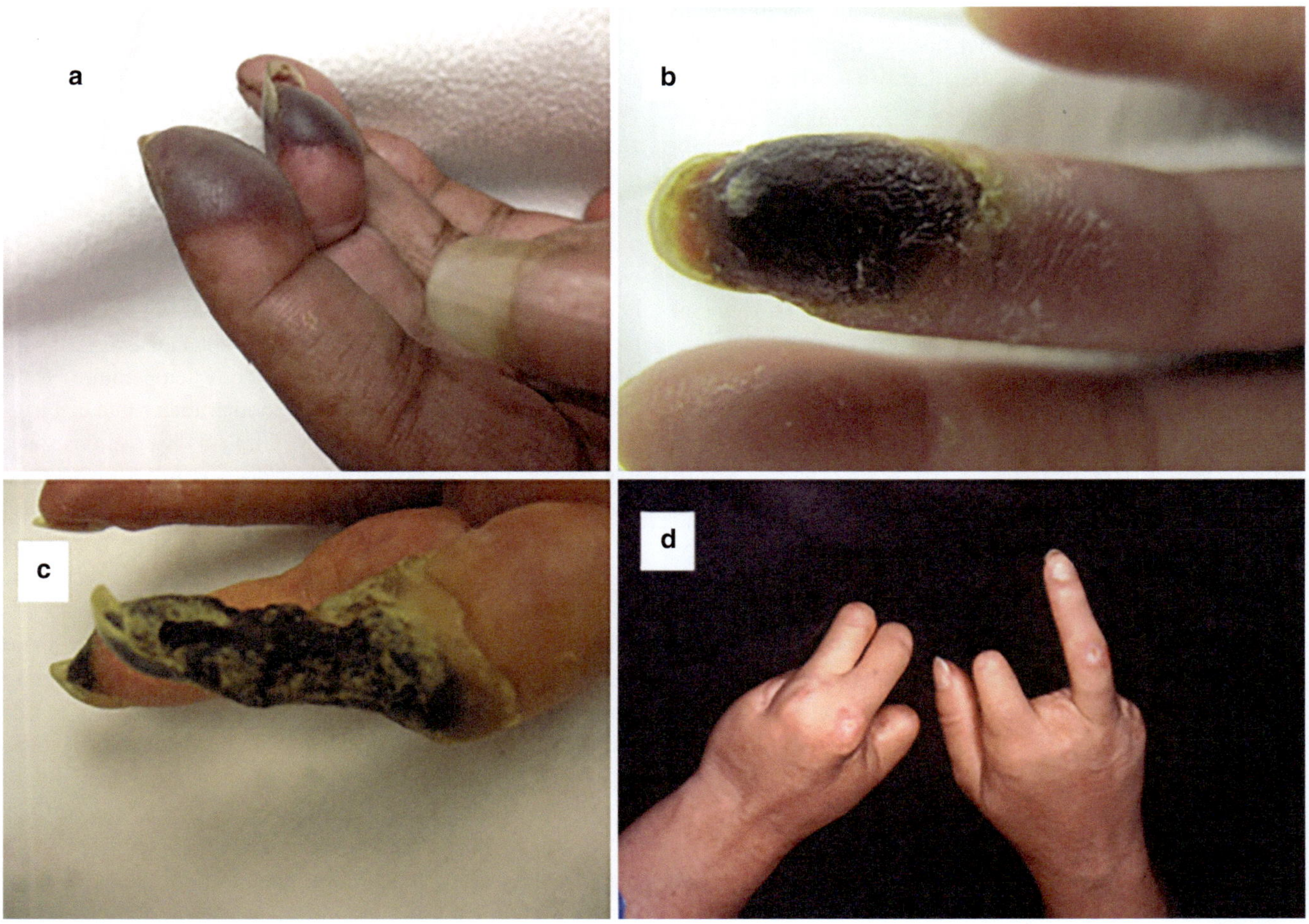

Fig. 50.1 (**a**) Cyanosis of the index finger due to digital ischemia in a patient with limited scleroderma. (**b**) Note the hyperemia of an acute ischemic finger demarcated to the distal finger. (**c**) Advancing ischemia with cyanotic fingertip (**d**) Loss of multiple fingers from scleroderma vascular disease

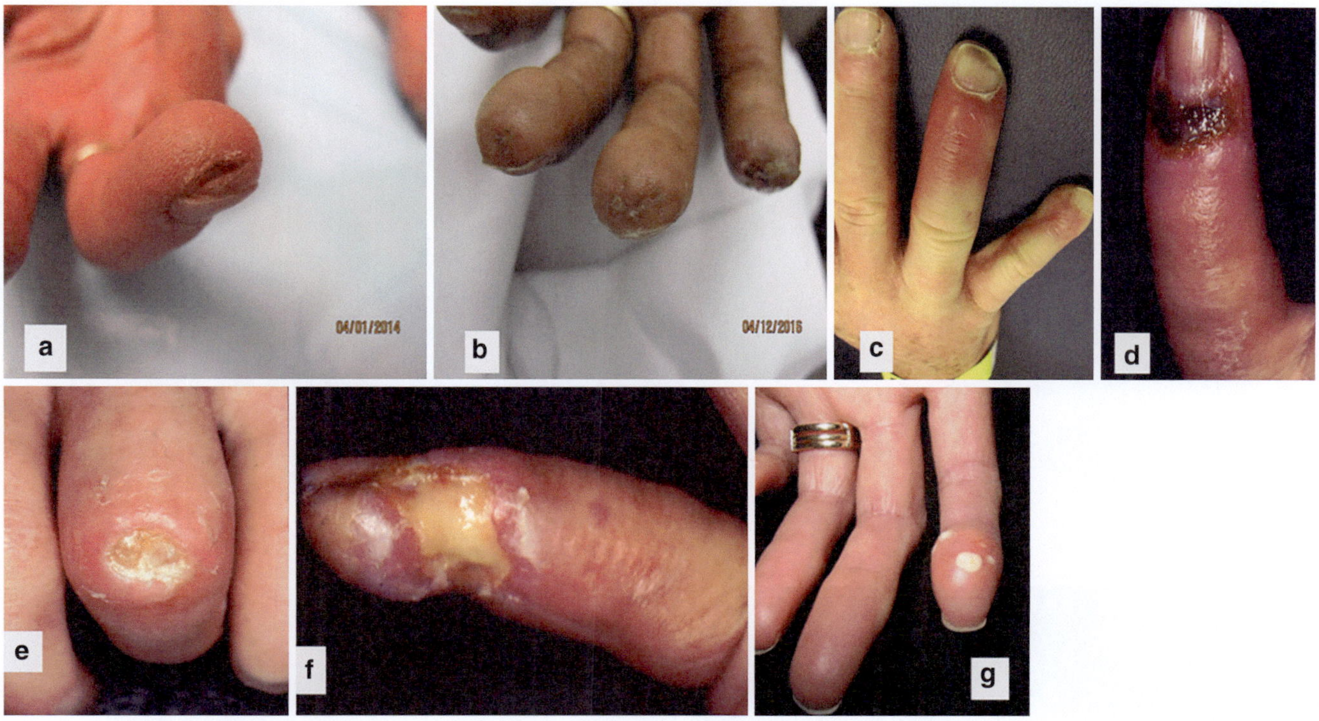

Fig. 50.2 (**a**) Fissure. (**b**) Digital pit form previous ischemic ulcer. (**c**) Perinychia. (**d**) Erosion secondary to perinychia. (**e**) Traumatic ulcer over PIP joint. (**f**) Ulceration on shaft of finger. (**g**) Calcinosis on fingertip

When first seen, our patient had no signs of an ischemic event and was started on a calcium channel blocker (amlodipine 5 mg daily). Amlodipine was selected because it is a dihydropyridine-type calcium channel blocker, a class that is shown to have benefit for RP secondary to scleroderma [5]. The use of vasoactive agents is used to target the vasospasm component of the vascular disease and improve regional blood flow. Given the risk of occlusive vascular disease, she was also started on low-dose aspirin (81 mg daily). Studies to specifically define the role of antiplatelet therapy do not exist, but there is good rationale to use aspirin or similar agents because of the evidence of platelet activation in scleroderma [6, 7]. While the insult to the vessels is thought to be mediated by an immune insult, there is no clear evidence that standard immunosuppression prevents progression of the vascular disease. Other strategies to treat the vascular disease and prevent progression such as prostaglandin therapy, a endothelin-1 inhibitor, or a statin are usually not used in the subtype of patients who do not have clinically defined ischemic events with tissue injury. Anti-antioxidants (e.g. N-acetylcysteine) may be helpful, but there is limited evidence of benefit [8]. She required a titration to 15 mg of amlodipine to have a notable reduction in the severity of her RP. Our patient tolerated this dose, but at this higher dose side effects such as lower systemic blood pressure and peripheral edema are more common.

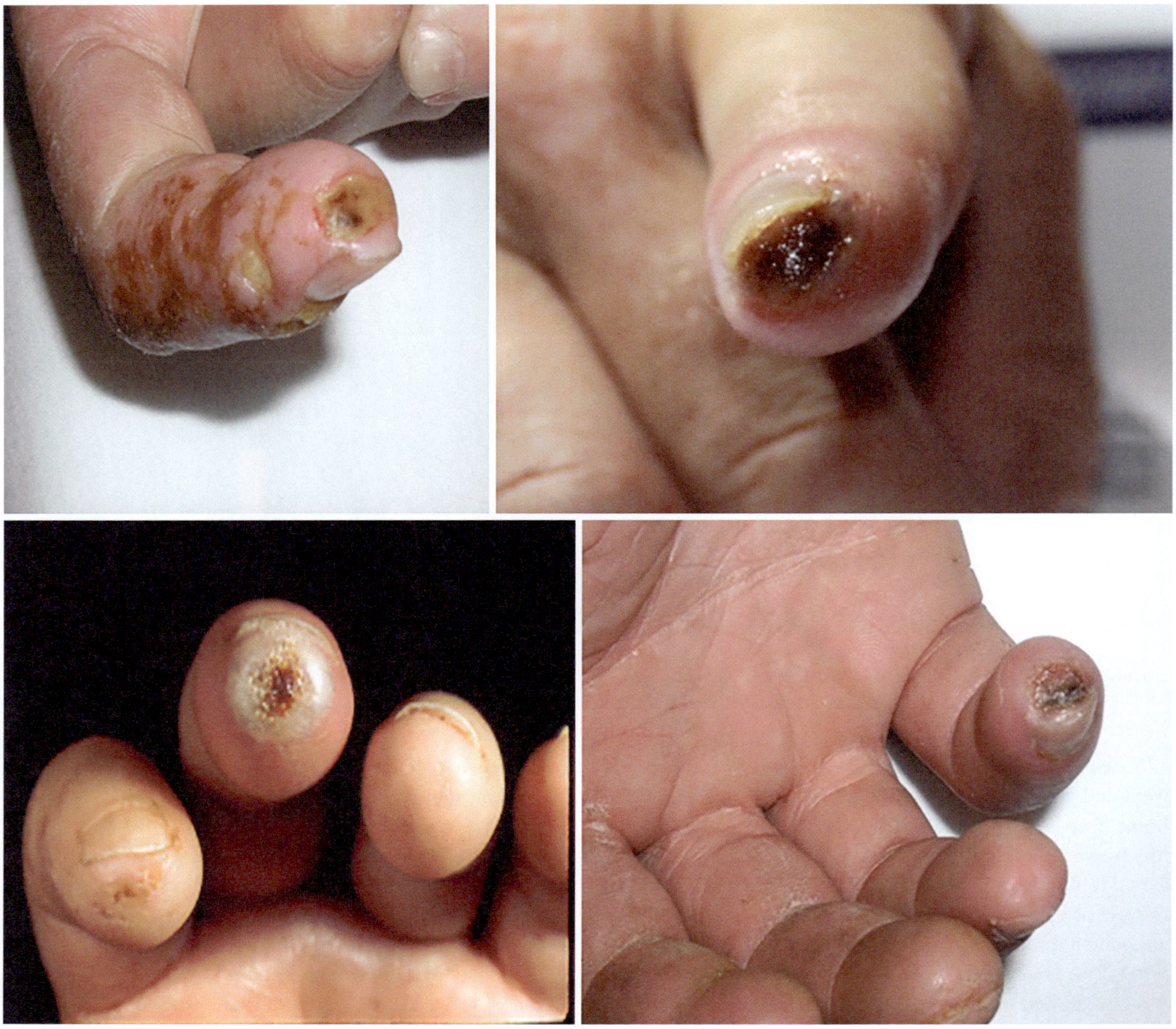

Fig. 50.3 Typical ischemic digital ulcers in patients with scleroderma

The Ischemic Digital Crisis

While the patient was improved on this treatment, she suddenly developed a painful right index finger with persistent discoloration. The pain was intense and radiated from the fingertip to the palm of the hand. Despite resting and keeping very warm, the finger did not improve after several hours. On examination, the finger appeared ischemic with a discolored swollen fingertip typical of impending tissue necrosis and was exquisitely tender to palpation (Fig. 50.1). There was no capillary refill following release of gentle pressure on the fingertip. The other fingers were cool but not ischemic. There were no lower extremity lesions and the examination of large vessels was normal. This included strong pulses in the upper and lower extremities. An Allen's test disclosed bilateral attenuation of the ulnar flow but with good reflow through the radial and palmar arteries (Fig. 50.4).

This patient presents with a medical urgency which in all likelihood will ultimately lead to a digital amputation from critical ischemia secondary to underlying micro- and macrovascular disease. It is important to remember that while there is clearly significant vaso-occlusive disease in scleroderma, vasospasm plays a major role in acute ischemic events and quick action has the potential of reversing critical ischemia and tissue damage or digital loss. In this case, her amlodipine and low-dose aspirin alone failed to prevent the ischemic crisis. In order to manage the crisis, pain control is critical. This was rapidly accomplished with a digital block. Local anesthetic such as lidocaine or bupivacaine is injected at the base of the finger on both the medial and lateral sides. This simple procedure not only provides immediate pain relief, but also induces a sympathetic nerve block which may help to

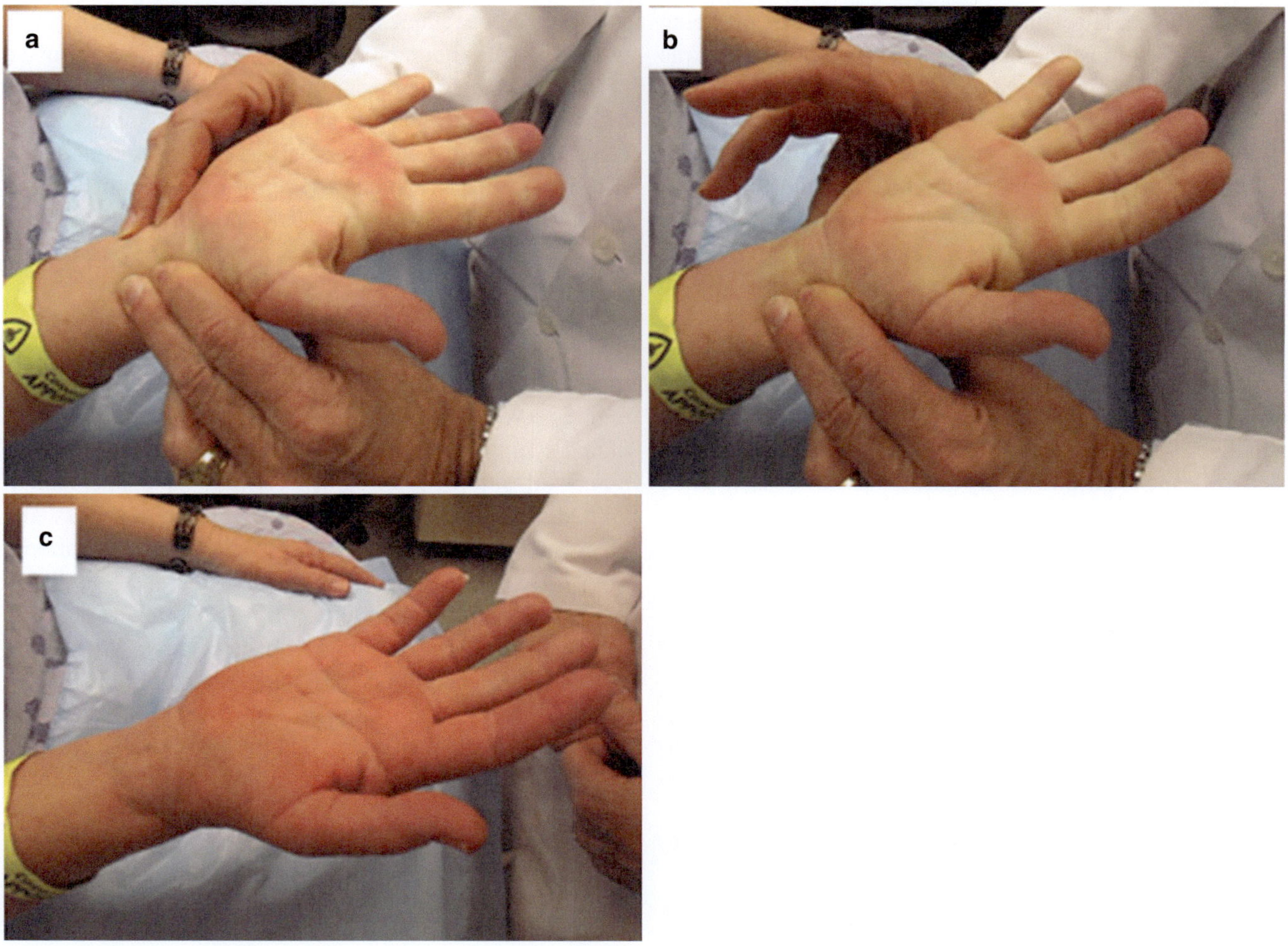

Fig. 50.4 Allen's test demonstrating compromise to ulnar flow to the hand. (**a**) Both arteries are occluded by pressure and the hand is pale. (**b**) The ulnar artery is released but the hand remains pale due to reduced blood flow. (**c**) The radial artery is released and blood flow returns and the hand flushes

improve blood flow to the distal portion of the finger.. Once the block dissipates, longer-term pain control can be accomplished with a nonsteroidal anti-inflammatory drug and/or an opiate such as low-dose oxycodone (5–10 mg q6h).

In our case, with the local finger block, we obtained rapid but transient pain control, and we did not see immediate improvement in digital blood flow. Evaluation for a correctable lesion was done because the examination suggested ulnar artery compromise, a situation known to occur in patients with scleroderma [9]. Most of the time, both medium-sized arterial and diffuse small vessel disease occurs together in scleroderma, and therefore, it is uncommon to find an isolated correctable large proximal lesion alone. The first study recommended is a Doppler ultrasound and then angiography only if the initial evaluation suggests a high suspicion of larger vessel occlusion or thrombus. A CT angiogram is not likely to have the resolution to accurately see digital and palmer arteries, so usually a digital subtraction angiogram will be needed. If the imaging studies demonstrate a thrombus or correctable large vessel lesion, then open surgical or endovascular correction of the lesion should be the next step. Thrombolytic therapy for an acute thrombosis can be done, but there is no good evidence to give specific guidance for this approach in scleroderma. In our case, the non-invasive testing confirmed that there was not a large vessel problem.

She had no contraindication to anticoagulation, and because the prolonged vasospasm with endothelial dysfunction is associated with thrombosis, she was acutely anticoagulated using intravenous heparin. This was continued for the next 48 h. Chronic anticoagulation in patients with scleroderma for digital ischemic events is not recommended unless a hypercoagulable state or defined large thrombus is discovered.

Indication for Intravenous Therapy

Despite this therapy, the finger continued to appear ischemic and was not improving. In this situation, intravenous prostacyclin (either epoprostenol or iloprost) is begun [10, 11]. It is best not to delay, and therefore, the infusion via a peripheral vein can be started while other diagnostic tests are being done. The rapid institution of the prostacyclin can stop the progression of the lesion and relieve acute vasoconstriction if occlusion or structural disease is not advanced. In non-acute situations, we administer epoprostenol (available in the USA) via a peripheral vein in an outpatient infusion center. Hospitalizing the patient provides the opportunity to deliver continuous therapy of prostacyclin (0.5–2 ng/kg/min for 3–5 days), and also controls the patient's environment to reduce provocation of vasospasm by limiting physical activity, avoiding temperature fluctuations, and controlling pain. Each institution will have their own requirements and guidelines for the administration of intravenous prostacyclin which is approved for the treatment of pulmonary hypertension by experts in pulmonary medicine. An observational study demonstrated that 12% of patients in a scleroderma cohort required at least one hospitalization for administration of IV prostacyclin in an 18-month period [12]. If prostacyclin therapy is not available, then rapidly maximizing other vasodilating therapy in a controlled warm setting is an alternative. One option is to move to a rapid acting calcium channel blocker and titrating rapidly to maximum tolerated dose; for example, nifedipine 10 mg po tid increased to 20–30 mg po tid in a 24 h period. Another option is to combine the current extended release calcium channel blocker with another vasodilator. The most popular drugs to use in combination are a phosphodiesterase (PDE-5) inhibitor such as sildenafil 20–40 mg po tid or topical nitroglycerin (1/2 in. every 6 h of 2% ointment with 12 h nitrate-free interval daily). In our case, acute administration of botulinum toxin (Botox) injected locally by a hand surgeon into the base of the involved finger was done, while prostaglandin infusion was underway. Uncontrolled experience in this setting has suggested that botulinum toxin is helpful, usually seeing benefit in 48 h, but this recommendation is not evidence based [13]. The potential delayed benefit of botulinum toxin warrants the use of more acutely vasoactive agents when confronted with an acutely ischemic finger. A controlled clinical trial of botulinum toxin in patients with scleroderma who had RP but no signs of critical ischemia or an active digital ulcer found no improvement in digital blood flow compared to placebo [14]. If vasoconstriction/vasospasm is not quickly reversed in patients with scleroderma, then vascular occlusion and digital tissue injury will occur. The consequences can be loss of the involved digit (Fig. 50.1).

Indications for Digital Sympathectomy

If rest, pain control, and vasodilation therapy are not rapidly working, then surgical sympathectomy is an option. Improvement is measured by clinical signs and level of deep tissue pain; if pain disappears, then tissue ischemia is improved. For example, if there is persistent digital ischemia with pain that is not rapidly responding to a 3-5 day infusion of prostacyclin or if prostacyclin therapy is not available, then it is recommended to move to digital sympathectomy [15, 16]. Delay in doing a sympathectomy may result in loss of the digit if the ischemic phase of vasospasm is not reversed quickly and irreversible thrombosis or occlusion occurs. It is no longer recommended to use a proximal sympathectomy because of the increased morbidity of the procedure and the effectiveness of an approach right at the level of the digit. Sympathectomy provides both a decrease in sympathetic tone but also release of peri-vascular fibrosis that may entrap digital vessels. If vasodilator therapy is not effective, then a digital sympathectomy can be done with or without botulinum toxin injection. In our experience, rapid intervention with digital sympathectomy can prevent digital loss and quickly reverse a critical ischemic event. Digital peri-arterial sympathectomy can be done using a regional anesthesia which reduces the risk of airway manipulation and also acts as a temporary chemical limb sympathectomy. Whether the procedure is done on the palm to do common digital artery sympathectomy or distally on the finger, infection and delayed healing are risks. In the long term, a digit or digits that have undergone a sympathectomy procedure will continue to have episodes of RP, but the severity is less and new ischemic events are less common. A skilled hand surgeon should be able to do the procedure with low morbidity.

Prevention of Recurrent Digital Ischemic Events

In our case, the prostacyclin therapy and acute anticoagulation were successful and the finger ischemia rapidly improved. The first indication of success was the resolution of pain with reduction in the need for pain medications. Tissue ischemia is painful and when blood flow returns, pain rapidly improves. The other signs followed with improved tissue color and decreased soft tissue swelling. The next issue then was the prevention of a relapse or new episodes. Maximizing the oral vasodilator therapy to maintain control of vasospasm is critical. In this case, she was on a full dose of a calcium blocker, but was tolerating it with normal blood pressure and no peripheral edema. We elected to add the PDE-5 inhibitor, sildenafil at 20 mg daily with slow titration to 20 mg tid [17, 18]. Often sildenafil or another PDE-5 inhibitor is not available. In such cases, topical nitrates (2% nitroglycerin cream/ointment) can be applied starting with 1/2 in. and titrating to 2 in. at 6 h intervals twice a day with 12 h nitrate-free interval daily [19]. Oral prostacyclin (treprostinil) is an option with evidence of reducing ulcer burden in scleroderma [20]. Riociguat, a soluble guanylate cyclase stimulator, increases nitric oxide and can improve RP [21].

In cases that cannot tolerate intense oral or topical vasodilator due to intolerance or low blood pressure, then we recommend preventive therapy with intermittent intravenous prostacyclin, for example, every 1–3 months depending on the severity of the RP. However, prostacyclin may be difficult to have readily available and alternatives need to be considered. There is some evidence that a selective serotonin reuptake inhibitor (SSRI) like fluoxetine 20–40 mg daily may be helpful [22], although controversial. Another prevention strategy is the institution of a statin, a class of drugs that may protect vessels and in theory reduce the risk of ischemic digital lesions [23, 24]. Anti-platelet agents such as aspirin (81 mg po daily) should be continued if there is no contraindication such as a confirmed allergy or previous episodes of gastrointestinal bleeding while on aspirin. The endothelin receptor inhibitor Bosentan is reported to prevent new digital ulcers from occurring in patients with scleroderma, but there is no solid evidence that this class of agents will prevent acute digital ischemia as in our case or reverse the acute vasospasm of RP [25].

In our case, the finger improved after the prostacyclin infusion and continues to do well on the combination therapy of amlodipine and sildenafil with both improvement in the severity of her RP and no new severe ischemic events. In cases that do not respond to this aggressive approach and who go on to develop advanced digital injury with dry gangrene (Fig. 50.1), then surgical amputation is the only option. This procedure should be done only after the digit has completely demarcated. Indications for earlier surgery would be intractable pain or conversion from dry gangrene to wet gangrene.

Key Principle Lessons of the Case

1. A subset of patients with scleroderma is at risk for major vascular events presenting with digital ischemia.
2. Rapid and aggressive intervention in cases of digital ischemia is essential to prevent tissue damage or loss of digit.
3. Rest, warm temperature, pain control, antiplatelet therapy, and vasodilation therapy are all important components of care. This may require hospitalization.
4. Intravenous prostacyclin can rapidly reverse acute vasospasm in the setting of digital ischemia.
5. Acute anticoagulation may also be helpful but full evidence for this approach is still needed. Chronic anticoagulation is not recommended in the absence of a hypercoagulable state.
6. If medical therapy is not rapidly working, then digital sympathectomy should be done if vasoconstriction is still present.
7. Once the acute episode is resolved, then preventive therapy needs to be in place including either oral vasodilator therapy or intermittent intravenous prostacyclin.
8. Preventive therapy with antiplatelet therapy or statins may have a role but more evidence is needed to define their role.

References

1. Daniels J, Pauling JD, Eccleston C. Behaviour change interventions for the management of Raynaud's phenomenon: a systematic literature review. BMJ Open. 2018;8(12):e024528.
2. Matucci-Cerinic M, Kahaleh B, Wigley FM. Evidence that systemic sclerosis is a vascular disease. Arthritis Rheumatol. 2013;65:1953–62.
3. Wigley FM, Wise RA, Miller R, et al. Anticentromere antibody as a predictor of digital ischemic loss in patients with systemic sclerosis. Arthritis Rheum. 1992;35:688–93.
4. Denton CP, Krieg T, Guillevin L, DUO Registry Investigators, et al. Demographic, clinical and antibody characteristics of patients with digital ulcers in systemic sclerosis: data from the DUO Registry. Ann Rheum Dis. 2012;71:718–21.
5. Rirash F, Tingey PC, Harding SE, et al. Calcium channel blockers for primary and secondary Raynaud's phenomenon. Cochrane Database Syst Rev. 2017;12:CD000467.
6. Pauling JD, O'Donnell VB, McHugh NJ. The contribution of platelets to the pathogenesis of Raynaud's phenomenon and systemic sclerosis. Platelets. 2013;24:503–15.
7. Ntelis K, Solomou EE, Sakkas L, Liossis SN, Daoussis D. The role of platelets in autoimmunity, vasculopathy, and fibrosis: implications for systemic sclerosis. Semin Arthritis Rheum. 2017;47:409–17.
8. Rosato E, Borghese F, Pisarri S, et al. The treatment with N-acetylcysteine of Raynaud's phenomenon and ischemic ulcers therapy in sclerodermic patients: a prospective observational study of 50 patients. Clin Rheumatol. 2009;28:137984.
9. Lescoat A, Yelnik CM, Coiffier G, et al. Ulnar artery occlusion and severity markers of vasculopathy in systemic sclerosis: a multicenter cross-sectional study. Arthritis Rheumatol. 2019;71:983–90.
10. Wigley FM, Wise RA, Seibold JR, et al. Intravenous iloprost infusion in patients with Raynaud phenomenon secondary to systemic sclerosis. A multicenter, placebo-controlled, double-blind study. Ann Intern Med. 1994;120(3):199–206.
11. Ingegnols F, Schioppo T, Allanore Y, et al. Practical suggestions on intravenous iloprost in Raynaud's phenomenon and digital ulcer secondary to systemic sclerosis: systematic literature review and expert consensus. Semin Arthritis Rheum. 2019;48:686–93.
12. Nihtyanova SI, Brough GM, Black CM, et al. Clinical burden of digital vasculopathy in limited and diffuse cutaneous systemic sclerosis. Ann Rheum Dis. 2008;67:120–3.
13. Zebryk P, Puszczewicz MJ. Botulinum toxin a in the treatment of Raynaud's phenomenon: a systematic review. Arch Med Sci. 2016;12:864–70.
14. Bello RJ, Cooney CM, Melamed E, et al. The therapeutic efficacy of botulinum toxin in treating scleroderma-associated Raynaud's phenomenon: a randomized, double-blind, placebo-controlled clinical trial. Arthritis Rheumatol. 2017;69:1661–9.
15. Merritt WH. Role and rationale for extended periarterial sympathectomy in the management of severe Raynaud syndrome: techniques and results. Hand Clin. 2015;31:101–20.

16. Momeni A, Sorice SC, Valenzuela A, et al. Surgical treatment of systemic sclerosis-is it justified to offer peripheral sympathectomy earlier in the disease process? Microsurgery. 2015;35:441–6.
17. Roustit M, Blaise S, Allanore Y, et al. Phosphodiesterase-5 inhibitors for the treatment of secondary Raynaud's phenomenon: systematic review and meta-analysis of randomized trials. Ann Rheum Dis. 2013;72:1696–9.
18. Hachulla E, Hatron P-Y, Carpenter P, et al. Efficacy of sildenafil on ischaemic digital ulcer healing in systemic sclerosis: the placebo-controlled SEDUCE study. Ann Rheum Dis. 2016;75:1009–2015.
19. Anderson ME, Moore TL, Hollis S, et al. Digital vascular response to topical glyceryl trinitrate, as measured by laser doppler imaging, in primary Raynaud's phenomenon and systemic sclerosis. Rheumatology (Oxford). 2002;41:324–8.
20. Shah AA, Schiopu E, Chatterjee S, et al. The recurrence of digital ulcers in patients with systemic sclerosis after discontinuation of oral treprostinil. J Rheumatol. 2016;43:1665–71.
21. Huntgeburth M, Kiesling J, Weimann G, et al. Riociguat for the treatment of Raynaud's phenomenon: a single-dose, double-blind, randomized, placebo-controlled cross-over pilot study (DIGIT). Clin Drug Invest. 2018;38:1061–9.
22. Coleiro B, Marshall SE, Denton CP, et al. Treatment of Raynaud's phenomenon with the selective serotonin reuptake inhibitor fluoxetine. Rheumatology (Oxford). 2001;40:1038–43.
23. Kuwana M. Potential benefit of statins for vascular disease in systemic sclerosis. Curr Opin Rheumatol. 2006;18:594–600.
24. Abou-Raya A, Abou-Raya S, Helmii M. Statins: potentially useful in therapy of systemic sclerosis-related Raynaud's phenomenon and digital ulcers. J Rheumatol. 2008;35:1801–8.
25. Matucci-Cerinic M, Denton CP, Furst DE, et al. Bosentan treatment of digital ulcers related to systemic sclerosis: results from the RAPIDS-2 randomised, double-blind, placebo-controlled trial. Ann Rheum Dis. 2011;70:32–8.

Scleroderma Renal Crisis: A Case Study

51

Edward P. Stern and Christopher P. Denton

Case

Mrs. M is a 53-year-old nurse who was previously fit and well. Her only prior medical history is of essential hypertension, for which she has been taking ramipril 5 mg daily for 2 years. She was referred to a rheumatologist with a 3-month history of puffy fingers and Raynaud's phenomenon. Physical examination demonstrated skin thickening bilaterally on the upper limbs, extending proximal to the elbows—modified Rodnan skin score (MRSS) of 21/51—and palpable tendon friction rubs anteriorly at both ankles and in the right wrist. Examination of the cardiovascular, respiratory, and abdominal systems was unremarkable. Her blood pressure (BP) was 130/70 mmHg, and her urine dipstick analysis was normal.

Full blood count and routine biochemistry tests were normal. Serum creatinine was 61 μmol/L (0.69 mg/dL), with an eGFR of >90 mL/min. Antinuclear antibodies (ANA) were strongly positive (>1:1000) with a fine speckled/nucleolar staining pattern. Abnormal nailfold capillaroscopy with dilated capillary loops and reduced vessel density confirmed the diagnosis of diffuse cutaneous systemic sclerosis (dcSSc).

She was started on therapy with mycophenolate mofetil (MMF) primarily for active skin disease at a dose of 500 mg twice daily, which was titrated up to 1 g twice daily the following month. At this stage, she was also started on prednisolone 15 mg daily, for joint pain and pruritis, and omeprazole 20 mg twice daily was added for gastroesophageal reflux. Given the risk of scleroderma renal crisis (SRC) in patients with dcSSc, she was advised to buy a home BP monitor and to check her BP at least 3 times a week.

Three weeks after this, she presented to the emergency department complaining of shortness of breath and headache. Her blood pressure had been at its baseline level 24 h previously, but that afternoon, she had measured it as 180/110 mmHg. Oxygen saturations were 88% on room air. On auscultation of the chest, she had coarse crepitations to the midzones bilaterally. Fundoscopy demonstrated cotton-wool spots, consistent with Grade 3 hypertensive retinopathy. Skin thickening had worsened since her last clinic visit and her fingers were poorly perfused distally.

Urinalysis was positive for both blood and protein, and serum creatinine was 195 umol/L (2.2 mg/dL). As this was >3 times her stable baseline creatinine, she was classified as having Stage 3 acute kidney injury (AKI). Haemoglobin concentration was 102 g/L, platelet count was 73 and red cell fragments were seen on her blood film.

A chest radiograph confirmed moderate pulmonary oedema and she went on to have an echocardiogram. This showed left ventricular systolic dysfunction (estimated ejection fraction 25%) and a high estimated pulmonary artery systolic pressure of 45 mmHg.

Ramipril was titrated-up over the following 48 h to 10 mg daily. She was also started on continuous low-dose iloprost infusion to treat her severe Raynaud's phenomenon. Despite this, her blood pressure remained significantly above her baseline clinic values at 160/100. In addition, her renal function continued to deteriorate with a creatinine of 455 μmol/L (5.2 mg/dL) and declining urine output on day 3 after admission. The angiotensin receptor blocker losartan was added-in, resulting in a modest decline in systolic blood pressure and some improvement in her respiratory symptoms. On day 5, she was started on intermittent haemodialysis (IHD), initially to treat refractory hyperkalaemia.

Her BP subsequently stabilized with the addition of a third vasodilator (the alpha-blocker doxazosin); thrombocytopenia and haemolysis resolved. She continued to be oliguric and dependent on IHD. Percutaneous renal biopsy was performed on day 20. This demonstrated fibrinoid necrosis and adventitial fibrosis in the medium-sized and small intrarenal arteries, occasional collapsed glomeruli and a relatively preserved tubulointerstitium.

She was discharged home on day 30 but continued to attend for three times weekly IHD as an outpatient. Once she was established on long-term dialysis, her antihypertensive

E. P. Stern (✉) · C. P. Denton
Centre for Rheumatology, UCL Royal Free Campus, London, UK
e-mail: e.stern@ucl.ac.uk; c.denton@ucl.ac.uk

Y. Allanore et al. (eds.), *Scleroderma*, https://doi.org/10.1007/978-3-031-40658-4_51

requirements reduced, and losartan and doxazosin were eventually stopped. A follow-up echocardiogram demonstrated that her estimated left ventricular systolic function and pulmonary artery pressure had normalized. Pulmonary function tests were normal.

However, 12 months after initial presentation with SRC, Mrs. M was still on dialysis. Her sister approached the nephrology team to be considered as a donor for live-related renal transplantation and was found to be a suitable donor. However, over the following months, Mrs. M's urine output increased somewhat and her pre-dialysis creatinine levels were noted to be falling each week. She had a trial off dialysis after 18 months and her creatinine stabilized around 225 umol/L (2.5 mg/dL) giving her an eGFR of 21 mL/min. Renal function continued to improve over the subsequent year and eGFR was stable at 35 mL/min 3 years after diagnosis of SRC with no significant haematuria or proteinuria.

Discussion

Mrs. M is an archetypal patient at high risk of SRC. At presentation, she had early diffuse SSc, rapidly progressive skin score and a nucleolar staining pattern on ANA (anti-RNA polymerase III antibodies were later confirmed). Her rheumatologist appreciated this risk, choosing to minimize the dose of corticosteroid, she was prescribed and arranged for her to do home BP monitoring [1–3].

She was on angiotensin converting enzyme (ACE) inhibitor therapy prior to the diagnosis of systemic sclerosis, for essential hypertension. There is no evidence that "prophylactic" ACE-inhibitor therapy reduces the risk of SRC and in fact, it is associated with a higher mortality (although there are many reasons that this finding may be confounded) [4].

A rise in systolic BP > 20 mmHg above her baseline and an increase of >10% from her baseline creatinine mean that she fulfilled the consensus criteria for a diagnosis of SRC when she presented to the emergency department. Pulmonary oedema, hypertensive retinopathy and microangiopathic haemolytic anaemia are all supportive of this diagnosis [5, 6].

A renal biopsy was not performed at this stage because uncontrolled hypertension confers a high risk of bleeding complications. Biopsy may be considered once blood pressure and coagulation have normalized. The most important indication for this is to exclude an alternative cause for renal impairment. Differential diagnoses for AKI in this context would include allergic tubule-interstitial nephritis (TIN) caused by one of her recently introduced medications (proton pump inhibitors are among the most common causes of TIN in developed countries) or a co-existing glomerular disease, e.g., ANCA-associated vasculitis or lupus nephritis. ANCA positivity or overlap serology would be clues in such cases and they are less likely to be associated with severe hypertension [7, 8]. Biopsy may also give prognostic information regarding the chance of renal recovery [2].

The team caring for this patient continued to titrate up her ACE inhibitor despite worsening renal function, which is appropriate. However, her BP was not sufficiently well-controlled on maximal dose of ramipril. In this setting, there is no consensus regarding the best add-in agents but there are some general considerations. Beta-blockers are contraindicated in SRC as they can cause catastrophic circulatory collapse in the context of very high peripheral resistance.

Angiotensin receptor blockers (ARBs) may be beneficial given the survival benefit conferred by antagonizing another part of the same renin-angiotensin system (RAS), but they have not been demonstrated to be of equivalent benefit to ACE-inhibitors when used alone [9]. Furthermore, dual RAS inhibition (ARB + ACE inhibitor) is associated with a significantly increased risk of hyperkalaemia, as was seen in this case [10]. Iloprost has been demonstrated to be an effective renal vasodilator in patients with SSc and our practice is to give 10 days of low-dose continuous iloprost in SRC; however, the specific benefits in this setting are unproven [11].

Finally, this case illustrates that the uncertain long-term prognosis for patients with renal crisis has a specific impact on their renal replacement therapy planning: unlike in other causes of end-stage renal failure, early transplantation may not be appropriate. Recovery of independent renal function more than 2 years after being established on dialysis is not uncommon. In such patients, the GFR may continue to improve for several years, and they appear to be relatively protected from the gradual decline in renal function that is typical in other forms of chronic kidney disease [2, 12, 13].

References

1. Trang G, Steele R, Baron M, Hudson M. Corticosteroids and the risk of scleroderma renal crisis: a systematic review. Rheumatol Int. 2012;32:645–53.
2. Penn H, et al. Scleroderma renal crisis: patient characteristics and long-term outcomes. QJM: Monthly J Assoc Phys. 2007;100:485–94.
3. Stern EP, et al. Analysis of anti-RNA Polymerase III antibody-positive systemic sclerosis and altered GPATCH2L and CTNND2 expression in scleroderma renal crisis. J Rheumatol. 2020;47(11):1668–77.
4. Hudson M, Baron M, Tatibouet S, Furst DE, Khanna D. Exposure to ACE inhibitors prior to the onset of scleroderma renal crisis-results from the International Scleroderma Renal Crisis Survey. Semin Arthritis Rheumatism. 2014;43:666–72.
5. Butler E-A, et al. Generation of a core set of items to develop classification criteria for scleroderma renal crisis using consensus methodology. Arthritis Rheumatol. 2019;71(6):964–71.
6. Hoa S, et al. Towards developing criteria for scleroderma renal crisis: a scoping review. Autoimmunity Rev. 2017;16:407–15.

7. Torpey N, Barker T, Ross C. Drug-induced tubulo-interstitial nephritis secondary to proton pump inhibitors: experience from a single UK renal unit. Nephrol Dial Transplant. 2004;19:1441–6.
8. Derrett-Smith EC, Nihtyanova SI, Harvey J, Salama AD, Denton CP. Revisiting ANCA-associated vasculitis in systemic sclerosis: clinical, serological and immunogenetic factors. Rheumatology (Oxford). 2013;52:1824–31.
9. Caskey FJ, Thacker EJ, Johnston PA, Barnes JN. Failure of losartan to control blood pressure in scleroderma renal crisis. Lancet. 1997;349:620.
10. Makani H, Bangalore S, Desouza KA, Shah A, Messerli FH. Efficacy and safety of dual blockade of the renin-angiotensin system: meta-analysis of randomised trials. BMJ (Clin Res Ed). 2013;346:f360.
11. Scorza R, et al. Effect of iloprost infusion on the resistance index of renal vessels of patients with systemic sclerosis. J Rheumatol. 1997;24:1944–8.
12. Steen VD. Long-term outcomes of scleroderma renal crisis. Ann Intern Med. 2000;133:600.
13. Guillevin L, et al. Scleroderma renal crisis: a retrospective multicentre study on 91 patients and 427 controls. Rheumatology (Oxford). 2012;51:460–7.

Rapid Diffuse Skin Disease with Progressive Joint Contractures

52

Faye N. Hant and Richard M. Silver

Case Presentation

The patient is a 64-year-old Caucasian female diagnosed with diffuse cutaneous systemic sclerosis (dcSSc). She developed tight swelling in her hands, feet, wrists, and arms with subsequent involvement of the face and trunk over the ensuing 2 months. She reported difficulty with hand grip and could not make a fist. She could not fully extend her elbows or knees. She denied joint swelling or pain but did note pain in both arms and legs along with a severe "rubbing" sensation while moving her extremities. She had Raynaud phenomenon (RP), nonproductive cough, gastroesophageal reflux, and sicca symptoms. Physical examination was notable for facial telangiectasias and sclerodactyly with flexion contractures at the proximal interphalangeal (PIP) and metacarpophalangeal (MCP) joints of hands (Fig. 52.1) and elbows; skin was diffusely taut and the modified Rodnan skin score (mRSS) was 25 (maximum 51); tendon friction rubs (TFRs) were palpable at her elbows, knees, and ankles; no joint tenderness or swelling was noted. Laboratory evaluation revealed a positive ANA (1:160 titer, speckled pattern) and the presence of RNA polymerase III auto-antibodies. Comprehensive metabolic panel, complete blood count, CK, aldolase, thyroid testing, and urinalysis were all within normal limits. On pulmonary assessment, the 6 min walk distance was limited to 316 m, forced vital capacity (FVC) was 83% predicted, total lung capacity (TLC) was 89% predicted, and diffusion lung capacity for carbon monoxide (DLCO) was 58% predicted. High-resolution CT scan (HRCT) of the chest showed mild bibasilar interstitial lung changes with septal thickening and scattered ground glass opacities, and the esophagus was dilated and gas-filled. Echocardiogram was normal except for stage 1 (mild) left ventricular diastolic dysfunction. She was started on a proton pump inhibitor for gastroesophageal reflux and a calcium channel blocker and low-dose aspirin for RP. She was placed on low-dose prednisone (10 mg daily) for her tendon friction rubs. We emphasized to the patient that she was at an increased risk for scleroderma renal crisis, given her positive RNA-polymerase III antibody, and that she should not take prednisone in doses ≥15 mg daily. She was prescribed a blood pressure (BP) cuff and counseled on the importance of close monitoring of her BP and to report to us any new onset BP > 150/85 mmHg or ≥ 20 mmHg from usual systolic BP, obtained at least twice over 24 h. We also discussed initiation of mycophenolate mofetil (MMF) for her lung and skin disease.

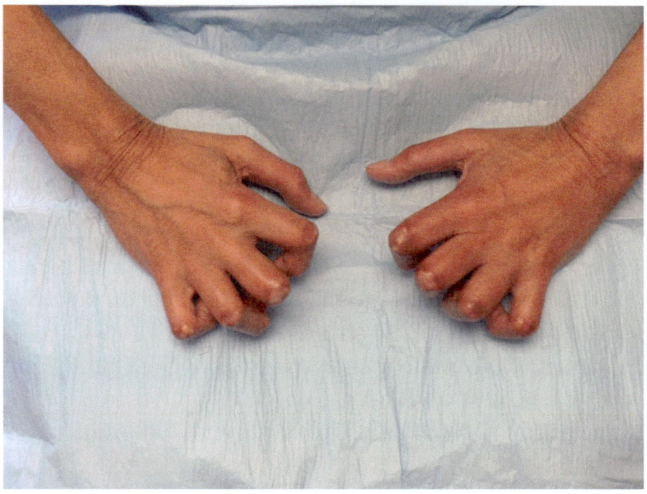

Fig. 52.1 Typical hand changes of diffuse cutaneous systemic sclerosis with contractures and skin sclerosis

Introduction and Background

This case presents one of the most challenging situations in caring for a patient with scleroderma: how to manage the early rapidly progressive phase of skin disease. While there are no proven disease-modifying drugs that are approved for the

F. N. Hant (✉) · R. M. Silver
Division of Rheumatology and Immunology, Medical University of South Carolina, Charleston, SC, USA
e-mail: hant@musc.edu; silverr@musc.edu

Y. Allanore et al. (eds.), *Scleroderma*, https://doi.org/10.1007/978-3-031-40658-4_52

management of skin disease, most believe early intervention with an immunosuppressive/anti-inflammatory agent can alter the course of the skin disease. Recognizing the limitations of proven options, the fact that there are no FDA-approved therapies or established standard of care, treatment is often designed by one's own experience or it is based on the current bias of the community of experts caring for patients with scleroderma. Whenever possible, the authors recommend that patients in the early phase of skin disease be referred to a scleroderma specialty center to participate in organized research including clinical trials. The ideal therapy be discovered only by a community effort. In the absence of a research option, we recommend the following principles: (1) establish the current phase of the skin disease (i.e., is the disease active and progressive or late, fibrotic and inactive?), (2) document the extent of the disease using a modified Rodnan skin score to allow a measure of outcome, (3) consider the association with internal organ involvement and disease-related consequences, (4) take measures to prevent further morbidity and improve quality of life (e.g., control pain, physical, and occupational therapy), and (5) initiate intervention.

SSc patients with diffuse cutaneous disease have a higher risk of death compared to patients with limited cutaneous involvement. Diffuse SSc patients typically develop significant internal organ involvement with the highest proportion of new organ systems affected (pulmonary, cardiac, and renal complications) within the first 3 years [1]. An association of scleroderma-specific auto-antibodies with certain prognostic, clinical, and laboratory characteristics is well known [2]. Joint involvement and tendon friction rubs (TFRs) are most often seen in dcSSc patients with anti-topoisomerase (Scl-70), anti-RNA polymerase III (Pol-3), or anti-U3-RNP auto-antibodies [2]. Patients with anti-Pol-3 antibodies have the highest frequency of scleroderma renal crisis and rapidly develop the most severe skin disease with the highest mRSS [2]. This particular scleroderma auto-antibody is frequently associated with the presence of a speckled ANA (can also have a nucleolar ANA), extensive skin and tendon involvement early in the disease course, negative anti-topoisomerase (Scl-70) auto-antibodies, and sometimes an associated cancer; severe interstitial lung disease is rare [2]. There is also concern about an increased risk of gastrointestinal bleeding for GAVE. Our case presentation illustrates some of these associations.

The natural course of skin thickening in patients with dcSSc is variable. Skin thickness typically progresses over the first 2–5 years of disease, and then gradually improves [3]. The prospective Pittsburgh Scleroderma Databank revealed that patients in the "improved group" (skin thickening improved by >25% of peak skin score and a rate of change of at least 5 units/year) had an average improvement of 50% of their peak skin score at 2 years after initial visit and, importantly, survival was significantly better in the "improved group" at 5 and 10 years (90% and 80%, respectively) compared to the "unimproved group" (increased skin thickening or no improvement) (77% and 60%, respectively, at 5 and 10 years; $p < 0.0001$) [4]. A skin thickness progression rate (STPR), defined as the mRSS at the first patient visit divided by duration of skin thickening (in years) by patient report, may be a useful measure to perform at initial evaluation to identify patients who may be at increased risk of death and more likely to develop scleroderma renal crisis within the next 2 years [5]. A "rapid" STPR of ≥45 has been reported to be an independent predictor of both scleroderma renal crisis within 2 years from first evaluation (OR 2.05, 95% CI 1.10–3.85) as well as of mortality (OR 1.72, 95% CI 1.13–2.62) [5]. STPR is an easy measure that can be obtained at the initial visit that allows the identification of those at increased risk of scleroderma renal crisis and death [5].

Our case has findings of loss of joint mobility, an early sign that joint contractures will develop if the disease is not controlled. Joint contracture is an abnormal typically permanent shortening of scar tissue or muscle, especially within a joint, resulting in deformity [6]. Joint contractures are common in dcSSc patients, affecting large and small hand joints, and they can be a major source of morbidity and disability [7]. As the disease progresses, there may be tethering of the skin and contracture of the underlying joints, leading to a decrease in function and motor abilities [6]. The EULAR Scleroderma Trials and Research (EUSTAR) registry found in a cross-sectional examination that 31% of patients had joint contractures, more prevalent in dcSSc patients with severe renal, muscular, vascular, and interstitial lung involvement [8]. A recent study of 131 patients with three-year follow-up found a high frequency of baseline joint contractures in the shoulders (50%), wrists (75%), and small joints of hands (82%) and noted a significant decrease in ROM of the dominant hand (suggesting impaired function) compared to the non-dominant hand [9].

Our case has active TFRs suggesting to us that aggressive therapy is warranted. The presence of palpable TFRs is associated with diffuse skin involvement, reduced survival, shorter disease duration, and both cardiac and renal involvement [10–12]. One study comparing early dcSSc patients having TFRs to early dcSSc patients without TFRs found that that the presence of one or more TFRs was associated with an increased risk of cardiac (OR 3.26, 95% CI 1.35–7.84), gastrointestinal (OR 5.14, 95% CI 1.74–15.17), and renal involvement (OR 2.66, 95% CI 1.23–5.75), as well as with an increased rate of mortality after age and sex adjustments, TFR cases had a 5-year mortality 1.8 times greater than those without TFRs (95% CI 1.21–2.58, $p = 0.003$) [12]. SSc patients with TFRs are not more likely to have joint contractures than those SSc patients without TFRs [12].

Treatment Considerations

A number of different therapeutic agents have been assessed in the treatment of scleroderma skin disease, most with limited evidence for efficacy [13]. Limitations of the reported studies in SSc include small numbers, lack of placebo-controlled design, the heterogeneity of the stage of the skin disease under study, and the lack of appropriate timing of a therapeutic intervention [13]. We will approach our case using agents that are available as if there is no research trial option available. First, we noted that on the low-dose steroids, there was an improvement in joint pain and motion, but the nature of the skin disease was unchanged. For the pruritis, we started both an antihistamine (hydroxyzine 25 mg oral every 6 h) and gabapentin (100 mg oral at bedtime). We instituted a physical therapy program to improve ADL and relieve pain. A nonsteroidal anti-inflammatory (ibuprofen 600 mg oral every 8 h) was given to use only as needed due to concerns about gastrointestinal side effects including gastrointestinal bleeding.

Methotrexate

We started our patient on methotrexate (MTX) by subcutaneous injection of 1 ml at 25 mg/ml once weekly. We elected to use methotrexate because of our experience that it can help both active skin disease and the inflammatory joints/tendon process; it is our first option for early, mild skin disease. MTX has been reported to be efficacious in the treatment of skin progression in two randomized, placebo-controlled, double-blind, multi-center trials [14, 15]. In a 24-week trial followed by an observational period of 24 weeks, van den Hoogen et al. randomized 29 patients (11 dcSSc and 18 lcSSc with <3 years of skin thickening) to receive MTX 15 mg intramuscular weekly ($n = 17$) or placebo ($n = 12$) [15]. Patients who had a favorable response defined as an improvement of total skin score (TSS) by ≥30%, of DLCO by ≥15%, or of the score on a visual analogue scale of general well-being (VAS) by ≥30%) after 24 weeks continued with the same regimen for another 24 weeks. Participants who showed a poor response on placebo were crossed over to MTX, and those who responded poorly to treatment with MTX 15 mg weekly had an increase in dose to 25 mg weekly [15]. After 24 weeks, a significantly greater number of patients receiving MTX ($n = 8$, 53%) who completed the first 24 weeks of the study had responded favorably compared to patients receiving placebo ($n = 1$, 10%, $p = 0.03$). In an intention-to-treat analysis, TSS decreased in the MTX group and increased in the placebo group ($p = 0.06$); however, this difference was not stratified by subset of SSc [15]. Another study of 71 patients with dcSSc <3 years duration randomized 35 patients to MTX and 36 to placebo for 12 months, with the primary outcome being skin score and physician global assessment (PGA) [16]. At 12 months, results slightly favored the MTX group (mean ± SEM mRSS 21.4 ± 2.8 in the MTX group vs. 26.3 ± 2.1 in the placebo group [$p < 0.17$], and PGA results also favored MTX ($p < 0.035$) [14]. The authors concluded that the results of their trial demonstrated a trend in favor of MTX vs. placebo but did not provide evidence that MTX is significantly effective in the treatment of patients with early dcSSc [14]. MTX is now considered a treatment option for skin manifestations of early dcSSc (strength of recommendation = A), based on a report from the European League Against Rheumatism (EULAR) and the EULAR Scleroderma Trials and Research group (EUSTAR) [17].

Mycophenolate Mofetil (MMF)

After 2 months of therapy, the patient clearly has progressed with advancing skin changes now on the proximal arms and legs with intense pruritis and decreased flexibility of major joints. Truncal skin on the chest and abdomen worsened with sparing of the back. At this point, our options were to continue MTX and low-dose prednisone or to move to or add another agent. Given the intensity of our patient's skin disease, we elected to add mycophenolate mofetil (MMF) beginning at a dose of 500 mg oral twice daily and slowly titrated to a full dose of 1500 mg oral twice daily over several months. We check safety laboratory data (complete blood count (CBC) and liver profile) every 2 weeks during this titration phase of therapy. A retrospective study looked at a single center experience using MMF comparing the change in mRSS in a MMF cohort at baseline with scores at 3, 6, 9, and 12 months to those of historical controls from a pooled analysis of three negative large, randomized controlled clinical trials of other medications (recombinant human relaxin, oral bovine type I collagen, and d-penicillamine [16]). The mean mRSS of the patients treated with MMF decreased progressively over time from baseline, 3, 6, 9, and 12 months (mean mRSS: 24.4 ± 9.5, 23.4 ± 10.1, 21.4 ± 10.6, 17.5 ± 10.3, and 17.5 ± 10.4, respectively). Compared to baseline, there was no statistically significant change in mRSS at 3 months ($p = 0.255$); however, statistical significance was reached at 6, 9, and 12 months when compared to baseline mRSS (all $p < 0.001$) [16]. The mRSS of the MMF cohort did not differ from the historical controls at 6 months but was significantly lower at 12 months (MMF −7.59 ± 10.1 vs d-penicillamine −2.47 ± 8.6, $p < 0.001$; collagen −3.4 ± 7.12, $p = 0.002$) [16]. In an open-label study to evaluate the efficacy and safety of using MMF (titrated to 3000 mg daily) to treat dcSSc over 12 months, 15 patients were recruited with the primary outcome being mRSS; a statistically significant improvement in mRSS was noted in those patients who tolerated the medication for >3 months ($p < 0.0001$) [18]. In a pilot study of 16 patients with early SSc with either active ILD or extensive skin disease, a protocol-based treatment strategy combined the use of MMF, intravenous (IV) methylprednisolone (MP) pulses, and low-dose glucocorticoids [19]. Here, patients received three consecutive daily IV MP pulses, followed by five additional monthly IV MP pulses; MMF (titrated to 1000 mg twice daily) and low-dose (5–10 mg daily) oral prednisolone were prescribed for 1 year; such treatment resulted in a statistically significant improvement in mRSS [19]. A 2007 retrospective analysis examined the duration, indications, and tolerability of MMF to treat dcSSc ($n = 109$) compared with a control cohort ($n = 63$) treated with other immunosuppressive medications [20]. MMF was well tolerated with a lower frequency of clinically significant pulmonary fibrosis in the MMF-treated cohort ($p = 0.037$) and significantly better 5-yr survival from disease onset and from commencement of treatment ($p = 0.027$ and $p = 0.012$, respectively); no significant difference in mRSS was noted between the two groups [20].

The Scleroderma Lung Study II ((SLS-II) was a double-blind, parallel group, randomized controlled trial comparing MMF vs. oral cyclophosphamide (CYC) in the treatment of early SSc and SSc-related ILD [21]. Secondary outcome variables included change in mRSS. Applying the primary analysis approach (i.e., the longitudinal joint model), no significant between-treatment differences were identified for the course of the mRSS (diffuse and limited cutaneous patients combined) over the 24 months of the study [21]. However, similar to the primary outcome, in post-hoc analyses, the joint model identified improvements from baseline to 24 months in each individual arm for the mRSS (CYC: −5.35; MMF: −4.9). The mRSS decreased (i.e., improved) in 73.6% of subjects on CYC and 71.7% of subjects on MMF and in the majority (78% and 64%, respectively) the improvements were ≥5 units [21]. Thus, both immunosuppressive treatments resulted in improvements from baseline to 24 months in skin thickness, even though no between-treatment differences were found for this outcome. This trial emphasized the better tolerability and toxicity profile of MMF compared to CYC, making this the preferred agent [21].

Cyclophosphamide

We considered the use of cyclophosphamide (CYC) but decided to use MMF, given its preferred toxicity profile and similar efficacy. The Scleroderma Lung Study (SLS-I) was a multicenter randomized, double-blind, placebo-controlled trial that looked at the safety and efficacy of daily oral cyclophosphamide (CYC) versus placebo for 1 year in SSc patients with ILD, followed by 1 year off therapy [22]. In the trial, 145 of 158 patients completed at least 6 months of treatment and were included in the analysis. Following a year of treatment with CYC, dyspnea, skin thickening, functional ability and some health-related measures of the quality of life also improved [22]. In an effort to assess whether these effects were sustained at 24 months, a longitudinal assessment was performed and found that the beneficial effects of CYC on pulmonary function and health status continued to increase through 18 months, after which they ceased, and skin improvements also ceased after 12 months [23]. The effect of CYC on musculoskeletal involvement was also evaluated in the SLS, and the proportion of patients with large joint contractures did not change [24]. Small hand joint contractures did seem to improve (as measured by ability to make a fist) over 24 months but this was independent of treatment, either CYC or placebo [24]. Given these data and our desire to avoid side effects from CYC, we chose to use MMF instead. We expected if the MMF were to be effective, the patient would sense stabilization in 1–3 months and a decrease in mRSS in 6–12 months. In other words, the first sign of dampening of the skin disease activity would be reduced pruritis, pain, and the lack of new areas of skin involvement. Following this, the patent should note improved flexibility, new hair growth, and a sense of well-being that precedes any change in measurable skin texture or skin score.

Intravenous Immunoglobulin (IVIg)

In the next 8 weeks, the patient did not improve on this combination therapy with worsening joint flexibility and early contractures, progressive skin changes, and continued fatigue with discomfort in the muscles and soft tissues. The mRSS worsened. There was no evidence of any additional internal organ involvement. The options at this point were to continue on the same therapy hoping that with time, there would be a response, to stop MMF and move to a new approach or to add yet a third agent to the current regimen. Consideration of novel therapy was considered including immunoablative therapy, rituximab, other biologics, or IVIg. We elected to continue MMF and to institute intravenous immunoglobulin (IVIg). The IVIg was given monthly at 400 mg/kg daily over 5 days. IVIg is used to treat a variety of different autoimmune conditions as well as scleromyxedema, another fibrosing skin condition [25]. IVIg is also used when patients with SSc have an overlap syndrome with an inflammatory myopathy. It has also been reported as adjunctive therapy for refractory skin disease. In a "tight-skin" mouse model, IVIg administration led to a significant decrease in type I collagen gene expression and collagen deposition and inhibition of TGFβ1 [26]. IVIg may also decrease fibrosis through the presence of anti-Fas and anti-fibroblast antibodies in the

IVIg preparation itself [27]. In a randomized, double-blind placebo-controlled trial of a single cycle infusion dose of IVIg (400 mg/kg/day for five consecutive days: a single course) vs. placebo in 63 patients with dcSSc, there was no difference in mRSS between the groups at 12 weeks [28]. Trial participants whose mRSS did not improve by 5 points at 12 weeks were dosed an additional cycle of IVIg, and it was noted that those who received two IVIg treatments had a greater improvement in mRSS over time than those who received placebo followed by a later IVIg infusion. The authors concluded that although their primary outcome was not attained, repeated administration of IVIG for two courses may be effective for diffuse skin disease [28]. A retrospective study of IVIg (2 g/kg/month) to treat refractory, active dcSSc patients ($n = 30$) unresponsive to current traditional therapies compared the mRSS at baseline to the mRSS at 6, 12, 18, and 24 months after starting IVIg, and also compared the changes in mRSS at 6 and 12 months to historical controls data from three negative large, randomized controlled clinical trials of other medications (relaxin, collagen, and D-penicillamine), as well as to patients on MMF alone [29]. The authors noted significant changes in mRSS over time in patients treated with IVIg and also in comparison to historical controls in their cohort. In those treated with IVIg, the mean baseline mRSS was 29.6 ± 7.2, and this decreased to 24.1 ± 9.6 ($n = 29$, $p = 0.0011$) at 6 months, 22.5 ± 10.0 ($n = 25$, $p = 0.0001$) at 12 months, 20.6 ± 11.8 ($n = 23$, $p = 0.0001$) at 18 months, and 15.3 ± 6.4 ($n = 15$, $p < 0.0001$) at 24 months [29]. Compared to historical controls, the mean change in mRSS at 6 months was not significantly different in the IVIg group (−5.3 ± 7.9), compared to the relaxin trial (−4.8 ± 6.99, $p = 0.74$) or MMF group (−3.4 ± 7.4, $p = 0.26$); however, at 12 months, the mean change in mRSS was significantly better in the IVIG group (−8 ± 8.3) than in the D-pen (−2.47 ± 8.6, $p = 0.005$) and collagen (−3.4 ± 7.12, $p = 0.005$) groups, and was comparable to the group of primary MMF responders (−7.1 ± 9, $p = 0.67$) [29].

Tyrosine Kinase Inhibitors

We considered starting Imatinib mesylate, a tyrosine kinase (TK) inhibitor with activity against c-abl, platelet-derived growth factor receptor (PDGFR), or another TK inhibitor, but we decided against using a TK inhibitor because of the lack of evidence of benefit in early skin disease and the high frequency of side effects. However, due to its ability to interfere with PDGF and TGF-β signaling, there has been interest in imatinib as a therapeutic agent in SSc [30–32]. In a phase IIa, single arm, open-label clinical trial, dcSSc patients were treated with imatinib mesylate 400 mg daily [32]. Of 30 participants, 24 completed 12 months of therapy. Many (171) adverse events (AE) with possible relation to imatinib were identified, 97.6% being classified as mild to moderate. In addition, 24 serious AE (SAE) were identified, two of which were attributed to imatinib mesylate. The mRSS decreased by 6.6 points (22.4%) at 12 months ($p = 0.001$), and this change was noted beginning at the 6-month time point ($\Delta = -4.5$; $p < 0.001$) and was seen in patients with both early and late-stage disease. A 6-month, randomized, double-blind, placebo-controlled, proof-of-concept pilot study aimed to further investigate the role of imatinib mesylate for patients with dcSSc [33]. These investigators found imatinib mesylate to be poorly tolerated due to AE which included edema, fluid retention, nausea, cramps/myalgia, diarrhea among others, and furthermore, no significant difference was observed in the mean mRSS in all patients who took imatinib mesylate (31.1 at baseline vs. 29.4 at 6 months) or in those that completed 6 months of the drug (31 at baseline vs. 30.3 at 6 months) [33]. In a recent 24-month open label, extension phase, single-center trial to assess the long-term tolerability and safety of imatinib mesylate in dcSSc, 17 patients were enrolled. Forty of the 92 AE and none of six serious SAEs were possibly related to medication, and overall the mRSS decreased from a median of 21–16 ($p = 0.002$) [34].

Rituximab

We also considered treating our patient with rituximab (RTX) given that several small studies have investigated the efficacy of RTX for the treatment of dcSSc, including three open-label studies, one multi-center nested case control trial and three randomized controlled trial [35–41]. The rationale for use of this agent stems from evidence that B cells and auto-antibodies contribute to fibrosis in the lungs and skin of patients with SSc [39, 42]. Daoussis et al. performed a study to assess the efficacy of RTX in SSc and randomized eight patients with dcSSc and ILD to receive two cycles (each cycle was four weekly infusions of RTX 375 mg/m^2) at baseline and at 24 weeks in addition to standard of care treatment, and six control subjects received standard of care treatment alone [36]. Skin scores improved significantly in the RTX group compared with the baseline score (mean ± SD = 13.5 ± 6.84 vs. 8.37 ± 6.45 at baseline vs. 1-year, respectively, $p < 0.001$), contrasted to the control group, where no significant change in mRSS was noted (mean ± SD = 11.50 ± 2.16 vs. 9.66 ± 3.38 at baseline vs. 1 year, respectively, $p = 0.16$) [36]. Analysis of skin tissue showed a significant reduction in dermal collagen at 24 weeks compared with baseline in the RTX-treated group (mean ± SD: 51.75 ± 19.78 vs. 31.68 ± 14.02 at baseline vs. week 24, respectively, $p = 0.030$) [36]. The control group showed no change in collagen deposition at 24 weeks compared with baseline values (mean ± SD = 46.53 ± 22.43 vs. 46.27 ± 10.49 at baseline vs. week 24, respectively,

$p = 0.980$). In an open-label study of RTX (2 doses of 1000 mg IV, 2 weeks apart) in 15 patients with recent onset dcSSc (mean 14.5 months (range 9–18 months), there was no improvement in skin score at baseline compared to 6 months, despite noting both circulating and dermal B cell depletion [39]. In another open-label pilot study, after a two-treatment course of RTX (2 doses of 1000 mg IV, 2 weeks apart, at months 0 and 6) in patients with early dcSSc, there was a clinically significant change in skin score (decrease in mRSS of 11.2 at 24 months vs. baseline, mRSS 13.6 and 24.8, respectively; $p < 0.0001$), equating to a 45% mean improvement in mRSS at month 24 vs. baseline [41] with no significant progression in internal organ involvement [41]. A small, 24-month, randomized, double-blind, placebo-controlled, single-center trial in patients with SSc diagnosed <2 years was conducted in the Netherlands with patients receiving RTX or placebo infusions, (2 doses of 1000 mg IV, 2 weeks apart, at months 0 and 6) [43]. In total, 16 patients (rituximab ($n = 8$), placebo ($n = 8$)) were included with 12 patients having dcSSc. Baseline mRSS (mean ± SE) was 16.4 ± 4.4 in the rituximab group vs. 14.0 ± 3.8 in the placebo group ($p = 0.88$), and in this trial, the mean skin score over time did not differ between the groups [43]. A recent double-blind, randomized placebo-controlled trial evaluating RTX was performed at four hospitals in Japan with the primary endpoint of the absolute change in mRSS 24 weeks after initiation of study treatment, measured in all patients who received at least one dose of study treatment and who had at least one endpoint assessment [42]. In this study, 80 individuals were screened and 56 (70%) were enrolled and randomly assigned. Twenty-seven (96%) of 28 patients in the rituximab group and 22 (79%) of 28 patients in the placebo group received at least one dose of their allocated treatment and completed 24 weeks of follow-up [42]. The absolute change in mRSS 24 weeks after initiation of study treatment was greater in the rituximab group than in the placebo group (−6.30 vs. 2.14, respectively); difference − 8.44 ([95% CI −11.0 to −5.88]; $p < 0.0001$) and adverse events were similar in both groups, most commonly upper respiratory infection occurring in 11 (39%) patients in the rituximab group and 10 (38%) patients in the placebo group [42]. Although promising, further evaluation of RTX is necessary in the form of large, multi-center, international randomized, placebo-controlled trials.

Abatacept

We also considered giving our patient abatacept, based on a 12 month, randomized, double-blind, placebo-controlled Phase II trial to assess the safety and efficacy of abatacept in patients with diffuse cutaneous systemic sclerosis (dcSSc), where patients were randomized 1:1 to receive either subcutaneous abatacept 125 mg or matching placebo, stratified by duration of dcSSc [44]. Of interest, skin biopsies obtained from participants at baseline were classified into intrinsic gene expression subsets. Among the 88 participants, the adjusted mean change in the MRSS at 12 months was −6.24 units for those on abatacept and −4.49 units for those on placebo, with an adjusted mean treatment difference of −1.75 units ($p = 0.28$). In the inflammatory and normal-like skin gene expression subsets, decline in the MRSS over 12 months was clinically and significantly greater in the abatacept group versus the placebo group ($p < 0.001$ and $p = 0.03$, respectively) [44]. In the normal-like skin gene expression and inflammatory subsets, the decline in mRSS over 12 months was clinically and significantly greater in the abatacept versus the placebo group ($p < 0.001$ and $p = 0.03$, respectively) [44]. The authors concluded that abatacept was well-tolerated, but change in the mRSS was not statistically significant, but that secondary outcome measures, including gene expression subsets, showed evidence in support of abatacept [44]. Although promising, further study in a phase III clinical trial is warranted to evaluate the effectiveness of abatacept for skin disease in SSc.

Tocilizumab

We also considered the use of tocilizumab for our patient, based on a multicentre, randomised, double-blind, placebo-controlled, phase 3 trial, where participants were recruited from 75 sites in 20 countries around the world [45]. In this trial, adults with dcSSc for 60 months or less and a modified Rodnan skin score (mRSS) of 10–35 at screening were randomly assigned (1:1) with a voice-web-response system to receive subcutaneous tocilizumab 162 mg or placebo weekly for 48 weeks, stratified by IL-6 levels; participants and investigators were masked to the treatment group [45]. Primary endpoint was the difference in change from baseline to week 48 in mRSS. Secondary endpoints included FVC% predicted at week 48, time to treatment failure, and patient-reported and physician-reported outcomes [45]. In the trial, 210 individuals were randomly assigned to receive tocilizumab ($n = 104$) or placebo ($n = 106$). In the intention-to-treat population, least squares mean (LSM) change from baseline to week 48 in mRSS was −6.14 for tocilizumab and −4.41 for placebo (adjusted difference −1.73 [95% CI −3.78 to 0.32]; $p = 0.10$) [45]. The shift in the distribution of change from baseline in FVC% predicted at week 48 favoured tocilizumab (van Elteren nominal $p = 0.002$ vs placebo), with a difference in LSM of 4.2 (95% CI 2.0–6.4; nominal $p = 0.0002$), as did time to treatment failure (hazard ratio 0.63 [95% CI 0.37–1.06]; nominal $p = 0.08$) [45]. The primary skin fibrosis endpoint was not met. Findings for the secondary endpoint of FVC% predicted indicated that tocilizumab might preserve lung function in people with early SSc-ILD and elevated acute-phase reactants [45]. The latter finding led to the FDA approval of tocilizumab for the treatment of Scleroderma associated interstitial lung disease.

Immunoablation with Stem Cell Rescue

Given the aggressive nature of the skin disease in our patient and her failure to respond to MTX and MMF, we also considered immunoablation therapy but decided not to use it due to the absence of life-threatening internal organ disease and the reported treatment-related mortality risk. High-dose immunosuppressive therapy and hematopoietic autologous stem cell transplantation (HSCT) are established treatments for various hematologic and oncologic conditions, and the potential role of this as a treatment in SSc has been studied. The European Group for Blood and Marrow Transplantation and EULAR published results from the Autologous Stem Cell Transplantation International Scleroderma (ASTIS) trial, which was the first international, randomized controlled trial of autologous HSCT vs. pulse monthly cyclophosphamide in early dcSSc [46]. A total of 156 patients were randomly assigned to receive HSCT ($n = 79$) or cyclophosphamide ($n = 77$), with the primary end point of event-free survival, defined as time from randomization until the occurrence of death or persistent major organ failure [44]. During a median follow-up of 5.8 years, 53 events occurred: 22 in the HSCT group (19 deaths, 3 irreversible organ failures) and 31 in the control group (23 deaths, 8 irreversible organ failures). Time-varying hazard ratios for event-free survival were 0.35 (95% CI, 0.16–0.74) at 2 years and 0.34 (95% CI, 0.16–0.74) at 4 years. The investigators concluded that among patients with early dcSSc HSCT was associated with increased treatment-related mortality in the first year after treatment but provided a significant long-term, event-free survival benefit [44]. The results of the multicenter National Institutes of Health–funded clinical trial Myeloablative Autologous Stem-Cell Transplantation for Severe Scleroderma [SCOT] randomly assigned adults with severe scleroderma to undergo myeloablative autologous stem-cell transplantation (36 participants) or to receive cyclophosphamide (39 participants) with a primary endpoint of a global rank composite score comparing participants with each other on the basis of hierarchy of disease features assessed at 54 months: death, event-free survival (survival without respiratory, renal, or cardiac failure), forced vital capacity, the score on the Disability Index of the Health Assessment Questionnaire, and the mRSS [47]. Baseline characteristics reflected severe scleroderma with a mean mRSS of 30. Results revealed that both among participants who had survived event-free (at least 54 months) and among those who had died or had had organ failure (at last assessment), the transplantation group was more likely than the cyclophosphamide group to show improvements on prespecified secondary clinical end points, including the mRSS, 100% vs. 82% among those who survived event-free and 71% vs. 29% among those who had died or had had organ failure [47]. Conclusions of the SCOT trial were that myeloablative autologous stem-cell transplantation achieved long-term benefits in patients with scleroderma, including improved event-free and overall survival, at a cost of increased expected toxicity. Post-transplantation use of DMARDs and rates of treatment-related death were lower than in previous reports of nonmyeloablative transplantation [47]. In a previous editorial, several issues had been raised as to whether HSCT is ready for clinical practice [48]. The authors emphasize that the optimal conditioning regimen for autologous HSCT in SSc is unknown, and there may be a specific "window of therapeutic opportunity" in which a patient with progressive SSc and internal organ involvement might be considered for HSCT [48, 49]. Potential candidates to be considered for HSCT might include: (a) patients with dcSSc within the first 4–5 years of onset with mild-moderate internal organ involvement or (b) lcSSc patients with progressive internal organ involvement, and this should be limited to patients who have failed standard immunosuppressive therapies [48].

After IVIg was started, our patient had definite improvement and the skin texture improved gradually over the next 6 months. We discontinued IVIg after 6 monthly infusions and continued the MMF. The low-dose prednisone was slowly tapered off. After 12 months, the patient continued in remission with only residual hand and finger involvement and mild skin texture changes on the forearm and dorsum of the feet (mRSS of 6); more importantly, the skin did not have an inflammatory quality, new hair growth was noted on the forearms and the patient had a marked improvement in well-being. The patient was maintained on MMF but the dose was reduced to 1000 mg twice daily for the next 6 months. The duration of MMF therapy needed is unknown, but we elect to continue therapy for a minimum of 2–3 years in severe cases due to an experience of skin and disease flares following discontinuation of MMF in the early recovery phase of the disease.

Rehabilitation Therapy

Despite the lack of robust studies, we routinely engage our patients in physical and occupational therapy. Also, we try to have family members play a role in helping and understanding the needs of the patient by educating them as to what is needed. As noted above, deformities and contractures of the hand are major factors in reduced quality of life and disability in patients with SSc. Physical (PT) and occupational therapy (OT) are often utilized to address impairment of hand function. A Canadian study sought to determine the proportion of patients with SSc who had hand involvement and who were referred to and used OT and PT services. Of 317 patients with hand involvement, only 90 (28%) reported a referral to PT or OT, and only 39 (12%) reported actually utilizing these services [50]. Much of the recent literature on rehabilitation techniques in SSc have small sample sizes with no control groups and consist of studies evaluating the effectiveness of face and hand stretching exercises, paraffin wax treatment, connective tissue joint massage and manipulation, splints, and resistance training and aerobic exercise [49]. Several studies show improvement in joint motion, hand function, and cardiopulmonary endurance, except for dynamic splinting which failed to maintain PIP extension in patients with PIP flexion contractures [51, 52]. A recent study looking at the role of PT in SSc from a patient perspective using questionnaires revealed significant variation in the use and content of PT for patients in a primary care setting, suggesting the potential under-use of PT care, in particular for hand and oral dysfunction, and expressed the need for initiatives to improve the quality and accessibility of PT care for SSc patients [53]. More robust studies are required in the area of rehabilitative therapy as an adjunctive modality in the overall comprehensive care of the patient with SSc.

Key Principle Lessons of the Case

1. Skin disease is best treated in the early phase before irreversible fibrosis, skin damage, and contractures occur.
2. We strongly recommend that patients with early skin disease have a comprehensive evaluation for internal organ involvement.
3. In the absence of proven disease-modifying therapy, it is recommended that patients with early skin disease be referred to specialty centers for the opportunity to participate in organized clinical trials.
4. Evidence suggests that immunosuppression/anti-inflammatory agents can dampen the progression of scleroderma skin disease.
5. Novel approaches to controlling skin disease are under study and more evidence is needed to define their role.
6. Managing a patient with early skin disease requires a comprehensive approach that includes managing pain, providing physical and occupational therapy, as well as emotional support for the patient and family.

References

1. Steen VD, Medsger TA Jr. Severe organ involvement in systemic sclerosis with diffuse scleroderma. Arthritis Rheum. 2000;43:2437–44.
2. Steen VD. Autoantibodies in Systemic sclerosis. Semin Arthritis Rheum. 2005;35:35–42.
3. Medsger TA Jr, Steen VD, Ziegler G, Rodnan GP. The natural history of skin involvement in progressive systemic sclerosis. Arthritis Rheum. 1980;23:720–1.
4. Steen VD, Medsger TA Jr. Improvement in skin thickening in systemic sclerosis associated with improved survival. Arthritis Rheum. 2001;44(12):2828–35.
5. Domsic RT, Rodriguez-Reyna T, Lucas M, Fertig N, Medsger TA Jr. Skin Thickness progression rate: a predictor of mortality and early internal organ involvement in diffuse scleroderma. Ann Rheum Dis. 2011;70:104–9.
6. Avouac J, Clements PJ, Khanna D, Furst DE, Allanore Y. Articular involvement in systemic sclerosis. Rheumatology. 2012;51:1347–56.
7. Malcarne VL, Hansdottir I, McKinney A, Upchurch R, Greenbergs HL, Henstorf GH, et al. Medical Signs and Symptoms associated with disability, pain, and psychosocial adjustment in systemic sclerosis. J Rheumatol. 2007;34:359–67.
8. Avouac J, Walker U, Tyndall A, et al. Characteristics of joint involvement and relationships with systemic inflammation in systemic sclerosis: results from the EULAR Scleroderma Trial and Research Group (EUSTAR) database. J Rheumatol. 2010;37(7):1488–501.
9. Balint Z, Farkas H, Farkas N, Minier T, Kumanovics G, Horvath K, Solyom AI, Czirjak L, Varju C. A three-year follow-up study of the development of joint contractures in 131 patients with systemic sclerosis. Clin Exp Rheumatol. 2014;32(6 Suppl. 86):68–74.
10. Steen VD, Powell DL, Medsger TA Jr. Clinical Correlations and prognosis based on serum autoantibodies in patients with systemic sclerosis. Arthritis Rheum. 1988;31:196–203.
11. Steen VD, Medsger TA Jr. The palpable tendon friction rub: an important physical examination finding in patients with systemic sclerosis. Arthritis Rheum. 1997;40:1146–51.
12. Dore A, Lucas M, Ivanco D, Medsger TA Jr, Domsic RT. Significance of palpable tendon friction rubs in early diffuse cutaneous systemic sclerosis. Arthritis Care Res. 2013 Aug;65(8):1385–9.
13. Frech TF, Shanmugam VK, Shah AA, Assassi S, Gordon JK, Hant FN, Hinchcliff ME, Steen V, Khanna D, Kayser C, Domsic RT. Treatment of early diffuse systemic sclerosis skin disease. Clin Exp Rheumatol. 2013;31:166–71.
14. Pope JE, Bellamy N, Seibold JR, Baron M, Ellman M, Carette S, Smith CD, Chalmers IM, Hong P, O'Hanlon D, Kaminska E, Markland J, Sibley J, Catoggio L, Furst DE. A randomized, controlled trial of methotrexate versus placebo in early diffuse scleroderma. Arthritis Rheum. 2001;44(6):1351–8.
15. van den Hoogen FH, Boerbooms AM, Swaak AJ, Rasker JJ, van Lier HJ, van de Putte LB. Comparison of methotrexate with placebo in the treatment of systemic sclerosis: a 24 week randomized double-blind trial, followed by a 24 week observational trial. Br J Rheumatol. 1996;35(4):364–72.
16. Le EN, Wigley FM, Shah AA, Boin F, Hummers LK. Long-term experience of mycophenolate mofetil for treatment of diffuse cutaneous systemic sclerosis. Ann Rheum Dis. 2011;70(6):1104–7.
17. Kowal-Bielecka O, Landewé R, Avouac J, Chwiesko S, Miniati I, Czirjak L, Clements P, Denton C, Farge D, Fligelstone K, Földvari I, Furst DE, Müller-Ladner U, Seibold J, Silver RM, Takehara K, Toth BG, Tyndall A, Valentini G, van den Hoogen F, Wigley F, Zulian F, Matucci-Cerinic M, EUSTAR Co-Authors. EULAR recommendations for the treatment of systemic sclerosis: a report from the EULAR Scleroderma Trials and Research group (EUSTAR). Ann Rheum Dis. 2009;68(5):620–8.
18. Derk CT, Grace E, Shenin M, Naik M, Schulz S, Xiong W. A prospective open-label study of mycophenolate mofetil for the treatment of diffuse systemic sclerosis. Rheumatology (Oxford). 2009;48(12):1595–9.
19. Vanthuyne M, Blockmans D, Westhovens R, Roufosse F, Cogan E, Coche E, Nzeusseu Toukap A, Depresseux G, Houssiau FA. A pilot study of mycophenolate mofetil combined to intravenous methyl-

prednisolone pulses and oral low-dose glucocorticoids in severe early systemic sclerosis. Clin Exp Rheumatol. 2007;25(2):287–92.
20. Nihtyanova SI, Brough GM, Black CM, Denton CP. Mycophenolate mofetil in diffuse cutaneous systemic sclerosis—a retrospective analysis. Rheumatology (Oxford). 2007;46(3):442–5.
21. Tashkin DP, Roth MD, Clements PJ, Furst DE, Khanna D, Kleerup EC, for the Scleroderma Lung Study II Investigators, et al. Mycophenolate mofetil versus oral cyclophosphamide in scleroderma-related interstitial lung disease: Scleroderma Lung Study II (SLS-II), a double-blind, parallel group, randomized controlled trial. Lancet Respir Med. 2016;4(9):708–19.
22. Tashkin DP, Elashoff R, Clements PJ, Goldin J, Roth MD, Furst DE, for the Scleroderma Lung Study Research Group, et al. Cyclophosphamide versus placebo in scleorderma lung disease. N Engl J Med. 2006;354:2655–66.
23. Tashkin DP, Elashoff R, Clements PJ, Goldin J, Roth MD, Furst DE, for the Scleroderma Lung Study Research Group, et al. Effects of 1-year treatment with cyclophosphamide on outcomes at 2 years in scleroderma lung disease. Am J Respir Crit Care Med. 2007;176(10):1026–34.
24. Au K, Mayes MD, Maranian P, Clements PJ, Khanna D, Steen VD, Tashkin D, Roth MD, Elashoff R, Furst DE. Course of dermal ulcers and musculoskeletal involvement in systemic sclerosis patients in the scleroderma lung study. Arthritis Care Res. 2010;62(12):1772–8.
25. Baleva M, Nikolov K. The role of intravenous immunoglobulin preparations in the treatment of systemic sclerosis. Int J Rheumatol. 2011;2011:829751. Article ID 829751:PubMed: 22121376
26. Blank M, Levy Y, Amital H, Shoenfeld Y, Pines M, Genina O. The role of intravenous immunoglobulin therapy in mediating skin fibrosis in tight skin mice. Arthritis Rheum. 2002;46(6):1689–90.
27. Molina V, Blank M, Shoenfeld Y. Intravenous immunoglobulin and fibrosis. Clin Rev Allergy Immunol. 2005;29(3):321–6.
28. Takehara K, Ihn H, Sato S. A randomized, double-blind, placebo-controlled trial: intravenous immunoglobulin treatment in patients with diffuse cutaneous systemic sclerosis. Clin Exp Rheumatol. 2013;31(2 Suppl 76):151–6.
29. Poelman CL, Hummers LK, Wigley FM, Anderson C, Boin F, Shah AA. Intravenous immunoglobulin may be an effective therapy for refractory, active diffuse cutaneous systemic sclerosis. J Rheumatol. 2015;42:236–42.
30. Distler JH, Distler O. Intracellular tyrosine kinases as novel targets for anti-fibrotic therapy in systemic sclerosis. Rheumatology (Oxford). 2008;47(Suppl. 5):v10–1.
31. Rosenbloom J, Castro SV, Jiminez SA. Narrative review: fibrotic diseases: cellular and molecular mechanisms and novel therapies. Ann Intern Med. 2010;152:159–66.
32. Spiera RF, Gordon JK, Mersten JN, Magro CM, Mehta M, Wildman HF, Kloiber S, Kirou KA, Lyman S, Crow MK. Imatinib mesylate (Gleevec) in the treatment of diffuse cutaneous systemic sclerosis: results of a 1-year, phase IIa, single-arm, open-label clinical trial. Ann Rheum Dis. 2011;70(6):1003–9. https://doi.org/10.1136/ard.2010.143974.
33. Pope J, McBain D, Petrlich L, Watson S, Vanderhoek L, de Leon F, Seney S, Summers K. Imatinib in active diffuse cutaneous systemic sclerosis: results of a six-month, randomized, double-blind, placebo-controlled, proof-of-concept pilot study at a single center. Arthritis Rheum. 2011;63(11):3547–51.
34. Gordon J, Udeh U, Doobay K, Magro C, Wildman H, Davids M, Mersten JN, Huang WT, Lyman S, Crow MK, Spiera RF. Imatinib mesylate (Gleevec) in the treatment of diffuse cutaneous systemic sclerosis: results of a 24-month open label, extension phase, single-centre trial. Clin Exp Rheumatol. 2014;32(6 Suppl. 86):S189–93.
35. Jordan S, Distler JHW, Maurer B, et al. Effects and safety of rituximab in systemic sclerosis: an analysis from the European Scleroderma Trial and Research (EUSTAR) group. Ann Rheum Dis. 2014; https://doi.org/10.1136/annrheumdis-2013-204522.
36. Daoussis D, Liossis S-NC, Tsamandas AC, et al. Experience with rituximab in sclerodrema: results from a 1-year, proof-of-principle study. Rheumatology. 2010;49:271–80.
37. Daoussis D, Liossis S-NC, Tsamandas AC, et al. Effect of long-term treatment of rituximab on pulmonary function and skin fibrosis in patients with diffuse systemic sclerosis. Clin Exp Rheumatol. 2012;30(2 Suppl 71):S17–22.
38. Bosello S, De Santis M, Lama G, et al. B cell depletion in diffuse progressive systemic sclerosis: safety, skin score modification and IL-6 modulation in an up to thirty-six months follow-up open-label trial. Arthritis Res Ther. 2010;12:R54.
39. Lafaytis R, Kissin E, York M, et al. B cell depletion with rituximab in patients with diffuse cutaneous systemic sclerosis. Arthritis Rheum. 2009;60:578–83.
40. Smith V, Van Praet JT, Vandooren B, et al. Rituximab in diffuse cutaneous systemic sclerosis: an open-label clinical and histopathological study. Ann Rheum Dis. 2010;69:193–7.
41. Smith V, Piette Y, van Praet JT, et al. Two-year results of an open label pilot study of a 2-treatment course with rituximab in patients with early systemic sclerosis with diffuse skin involvement. J Rheumatol. 2013;40:52–7.
42. Ebata S, Yoshizaki A, Oba K, Kashiwabara K, et al. Safety and efficacy of rituximab in systemic sclerosis (DESIRES): a double-blind, investigator-initiated, randomized, placebo-controlled trial. Lancet Rheumatol. 2021;3:e489–97.
43. Boonstra M, Meijs J, Dorjée AL, et al. Rituximab in early systemic sclerosis. RMD Open. 2017;3:000384.
44. Khanna D, Spino C, Johnson S, Chung L, et al. Abatacept in early diffuse cutaneous systemic sclerosis: results of a phase II investigator initiated, multicenter, double-blind, randomized, placebo-controlled trial. Arthritis Rheumatol. 2020;72:125–36.
45. Khanna D, Lin CJF, Furst DE, Goldin J, et al. Tocilizumab in systemic sclerosis: a randomised, double-blind, placebo-controlled, phase 3 trial. Lancet Resp Med. 2020;8:963–74.
46. van Laar JM, Farge D, Sont JK, EBMT/EULAR Scleroderma Study Group, et al. Autologous hematopoietic stem cell transplantation vs intravenous pulse cyclophosphamide in diffuse cutaneous systemic sclerosis: a randomized clinical trial. JAMA. 2014;311(24):2490–8.
47. Sullivan KM, Goldmuntz EA, Keyes-Elstein L, McSweeney PA, et al. Myeloablative autologous stem-cell transplantation for severe scleroderma. N Engl J Med. 2018;378:35–47.
48. Khanna D, Georges GE, Couriel DR. Autologous hematopoietic stem cell therapy in severe systemic sclerosis ready for clinical practice? JAMA. 2014;311(24):2485–7.
49. Khanna D, Denton CP. Evidence-based management of rapidly progressing systemic sclerosis. Best Pract Res Clin Rheumatol. 2010;24(3):387–400.
50. Bassel M, Hudson M, Baron M, Taillefer SS, Mouthon L, Poiraudeau S, Poole JL, Thombs BD. Physical and occupational therapy referral and use among systemic sclerosis patients with impaired hand function: results from a Canadian national survey. Clin Exp Rheumatol. 2012;30(4):574–7.
51. Poole JL. Musculoskeletal rehabilitation in the person with scleroderma. Curr Opin Rheumatol. 2010;22(2):205–12.
52. Seeger MW, Furst DE. Effects of splinting in the treatment of hand contractures in progressive systemic sclerosis. Am J Occup Ther. 1987;41(2):118–21.
53. Liem SI, van Leeuwen NM, Vliet Vlieland TP, Boerrigter GM, et al. Physical therapy in systemic sclerosis: the patient perspective. Arthritis Care Res. 2022. Accepted Author Manuscript; https://doi.org/10.1002/acr.24741.

53 Management of the Scleroderma Patient with Pulmonary Arterial Hypertension Failing Initial Therapy

Christopher J. Mullin and Stephen C. Mathai

Case

Our patient is a 53-year-old Caucasian woman with limited cutaneous systemic sclerosis (SSc) who is referred to the pulmonary hypertension clinic for evaluation of continued shortness of breath. She first developed Raynaud's phenomena around the age of 25, and she was diagnosed with limited cutaneous systemic sclerosis at the age of 41 in the setting of symptoms of gastroesophageal reflux, sclerodactyly, and telangiectasias. She was found to have positive antinuclear antibody with a 1:160 titer, a positive anticentromere antibody, and negative anti Scl-70 antibody; other antibodies were all negative. She was managed with a low-dose calcium channel blocker and a proton pump inhibitor for her Raynaud's and esophageal reflux symptoms, respectively.

She initially presented to our clinic with six months of gradually increasing exertional dyspnea to the point where she noticed that she was becoming short of breath after walking up two flights of stairs; in retrospect noted that she had become increasingly sedentary over the past two years despite previously enjoying a more active lifestyle. Her physical exam was notable for an elevated jugular venous pulsation at 7 cm H_2O, a loud second heart sound, a systolic murmur at the left sternal border, fourth intercostal space, clear lungs, trace peripheral edema, sclerodactyly without digital ulcers or evidence of active synovitis, and telangiectasias on her face and chest.

Her initial evaluation included pulmonary function testing showed no evidence of obstructive or restrictive lung disease, though her diffusing capacity was moderately reduced at 60% of predicted; her forced vital capacity-to-diffusing capacity ratio was elevated at 1.7. A chest CT showed no parenchymal abnormalities or pulmonary fibrosis, and a ventilation-perfusion (VQ) scan was low probability for pulmonary embolism. An N-terminal pro-brain natriuretic peptide (NT-proBNP) was 2165 pg/ml. A transthoracic echocardiogram showed normal left ventricular size and function, normal diastolic function, a normal left atrium, but a mildly dilated right atrium (RA), a mildly dilated right ventricle (RV) with preserved RV function including a tricuspid annular plane systolic excursion (TAPSE) of 2.2 cm, and a RV systolic pressure estimated at 50 mmHg.

Given the concern for pulmonary hypertension, she underwent a right heart catheterization (RHC), which showed a RA pressure of 6, pulmonary artery (PA) pressure of 58/31 (mean PA pressure of 39), and a pulmonary arterial wedge pressure (PAWP) of 10 mmHg. Cardiac output (CO) was 3.78 ml/min, cardiac index (CI) was 2.25 ml/min/m^2, and pulmonary vascular resistance (PVR) was 7.67 Wood units. Based upon these findings, she was felt to have pulmonary arterial hypertension in the setting of SSc (SSc-PAH), World Health Organization Group 1 disease, with World Health Organization functional class (WHO FC) II symptoms. With a six-minute walk distance (6MWD) of 390 m, she was classified as intermediate risk by both the REVEAL (Registry to Evaluate Early and Long-Term PAH Disease Management) risk score and 2015 European Society of Cardiology/European Respiratory Society (ESC/ERS) guidelines. She was subsequently started on combination therapy with oral tadalafil therapy 40 mg daily and ambrisentan 10 mg daily, with furosemide 20 mg daily and now returns for follow-up 3 months after starting PAH specific therapies.

Discussion

Our patient has a diagnosis of pulmonary arterial hypertension (PAH), with borderline cardiac function as indicated by her cardiac index of 2.25 ml/min/m^2, and intermediate risk as

C. J. Mullin
Division of Pulmonary, Critical Care, and Sleep Medicine, Alpert Medical School of Brown University, Providence, RI, USA
e-mail: christopher_mullin@brown.edu

S. C. Mathai (✉)
Division of Pulmonary and Critical Care Medicine, Department of Medicine, Johns Hopkins University School of Medicine, Baltimore, MD, USA
e-mail: smathai4@jhmi.edu

Y. Allanore et al. (eds.), *Scleroderma*, https://doi.org/10.1007/978-3-031-40658-4_53

assessed by several PAH risk scores. Based on her symptoms, functional class, and risk assessment, initiation of PAH specific therapies is clearly indicated. Initiating therapy requires first, determining which therapies to initiate and second, assessing the response to the initiated treatment. The choice of initial PAH therapy is based on a clinical risk assessment in conjunction with patient and provider preference. Over the past decade, there has been development and validation of several risk assessment tools in PAH that provide an estimate of risk and/or predict mortality at any time during the disease. These tools can provide both an initial risk stratification and an assessment of response to therapy to assist with therapeutic decision making. The two most commonly used risk assessment tools in PAH are the ESC/ERS risk table and the REVEAL risk score (Fig. 53.1).

The REVEAL risk score was derived from a multivariable regression analysis that predicted one-year survival in a large North American PAH registry which contained over 13% SSc-PAH [1, 2]. The initial REVEAL risk score was examined in a cohort of incident SSc-PAH patients, and found to have a good discrimination, but poor calibration, particularly in regards to the risk assigned to high natriuretic peptide levels and reduced 6MWD, suggesting the REVEAL score and attendant risk of death at 1 year may be overestimated in these patients [3]. The REVEAL risk score has been updated to improve predictive performance [4]; however, the REVEAL 2.0 risk score has yet to be validated specifically in SSc-PAH. The ESC/ERS risk table from the 2015 guidelines [5] is purposed to guide PAH treatments to achieve a low-risk status, using parameters that have been accepted as treatment goals in PAH [6]. Methods for calculating a risk score from this table were proposed and validated in a several diverse cohorts of PAH patients [7, 8]. An analysis of this ESC/ERS risk stratification specifically in incident SSc-PAH patients found this to be accurate in predicting survival [9]. In our practice, these multimodal risk assessment tools are used to complement our clinical assessment and may be challenging to interpret when there are discrepancies between the severity of some of the individual parameters- as in our case where our patient has a markedly elevated NT-proBNP but WHO FC II symptoms. As stated, our patient is intermediate risk by both REVEAL 2.0 and ESC/ERS risk assessment, which is congruent with our clinical impression of her PAH and helps guide our initial treatment decisions.

There are many approved PAH specific therapies that are available by either oral, inhaled, subcutaneous, or intravenous deliveries; however, for our patient, upfront combination therapy with a phosphodiesterase type 5 (PDE-5) inhibitor and endothelin receptor antagonist (ERA) is recommended based on her functional class, risk assessment, and lack of high-risk features [5, 10]. The recommendation is based on the AMBITION study, a blinded, randomized trial of WHO FC II and III incident PAH patients where upfront combination therapy with tadalafil and ambrisentan reduced time to clinical worsening (defined as the first occurrence of death, hospitalization for worsening PAH, disease progression, or unsatisfactory long-term clinical response) compared to pooled monotherapy of each agent [11]. A post-hoc analysis of the 118 SSc-PAH patients in the trial demonstrated a 57% risk reduction for time to clinical worsening with combination therapy compared to the monotherapy groups, along with significant reduction in NT-proBNP and improvement in 6MWD [12]. Further supporting upfront combination therapy in SSc-PAH was a multicenter study of 24 treatment-naïve SSc-PAH patients, where initial combination therapy with tadalafil and ambrisentan for 36 weeks improved hemodynamics, RV structure and function assessed by cardiac magnetic resonance imaging (CMR), NT-proBNP, and 6MWD [13].

The assessment of response to treatment is as equally important as deciding on initial PAH therapy. This is typically done with a multimodal evaluation that includes patient symptoms and functional class, along with objective measures such as NT-proBNP, exercise capacity as measured by distance on the six-minute walk test (6MWT) or cardiopulmonary exercise testing (CPET), imaging assessment of RV structure and function, and reassessment of cardiopulmonary hemodynamics. Most of these parameters are included in the ESC/ERS risk table, and guidelines recommend goals of PAH treatment are to achieve a low-risk status [10].

There are caveats for the application of these treatment goals and achieving a low-risk status specifically in SSc-PAH. The 6MWT is a simple way to measure submaximal exercise tolerance [14], and has been used as an endpoint in many of the clinical trials for treatment of PAH. However, the 6MWT is influenced not only by cardiopulmonary status, but also by the statuses of the peripheral vasculature, nerves, and musculature, and thus there are concerns with the use of this test in assessing response to therapies in SSc-PAH. In a study assessing limitations of 6MWT in SSc, over one-third of small number of SSc-PAH patients reported limitations on 6MWT for reasons other than dyspnea, the majority of which were from lower extremity pain [15]. Therefore, interpretation of 6MWT in SSc should include considerations of pulmonary, vascular, and musculoskeletal involvement, as the distance walked may not be a direct assessment of cardiopulmonary limitations. Similarly, it is important to consider what degree of change in distance on 6MWT is clinically relevant. Using data from a large clinical trial of tadalafil in PAH, the minimal important difference for the 6MWT was determined to be around 33 m; interestingly, the estimate for connective tissue disease-related PAH (CTD-PAH) was smaller, around 24 m, highlighting the differences in response to therapy between these groups of PAH patients [16]. It is our practice to obtain 6MWT at three months after initiation of PAH specific therapy, and then subsequently at 3 or

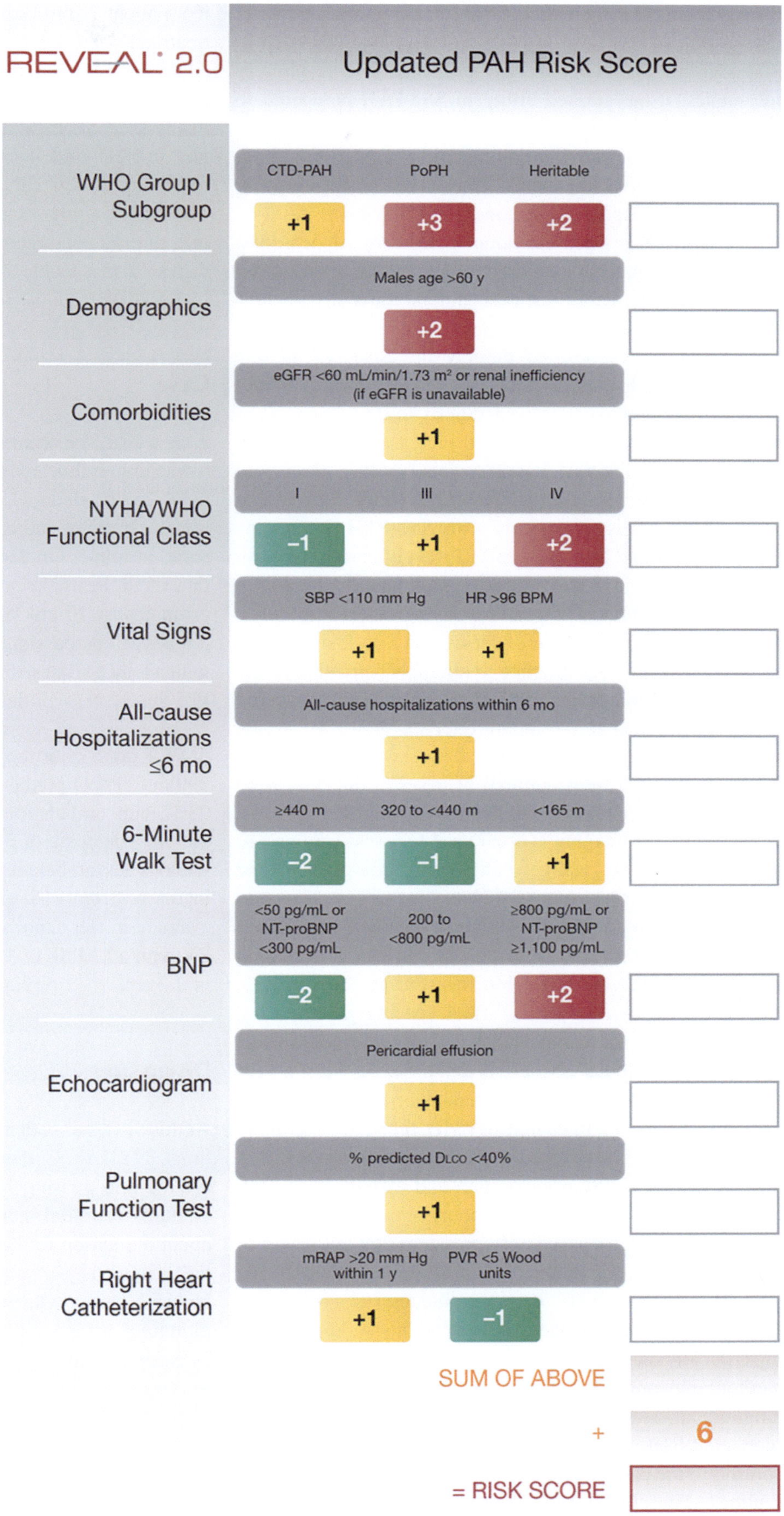

Fig. 53.1 REVEAL 2.0 Risk ScoreFrom Benza et al. [4]. Low risk = 0–6, Intermediate Risk = 7–8, High risk ≥9. *REVEAL* Registry to Evaluate Early and Long-Term Pulmonary Arterial Hypertension Disease Management. *PAH* Pulmonary arterial Hypertension. *WHO* World Health Organization. *CTD-PAH* PAH associated with connective tissue disease. *PoPH* portopulmonary hypertension. *eGFR* estimated glomerular filtration rate. *NYHA* New York Heart Association, *SBP* systolic blood pressure. *HR* heart rate. *BNP* brain natriuretic peptide, *NT-proBNP* N-terminal prohormone of brain natriuretic peptide, D_{LCO} diffusing capacity of the lungs for carbon monoxide. *mRAP* mean right atrial pressure. *PVR* pulmonary vascular resistance

6 month intervals thereafter. While cardiopulmonary exercise testing (CPET) can provide an integrative approach to assessing cardiac function, gas exchange and respiratory mechanics, it has limited utility in SSc-PAH compared to IPAH and other forms of pulmonary hypertension largely due to the risk of vascular complications related to arterial line placement in SSc patients. Thus, CPET is not routinely used to assess response to treatment in SSc-PAH.

NT-proBNP is a pro-hormone secreted by myocardium in response to mechanical stretch, hypoxia, and stimuli by neurohormonal factors such as endothelin and catecholamines. It has a role in diagnosis, prognostication, and assessment of response to therapy in SSc-PAH. In one cohort of 109 SSc patients, an NT-proBNP level of >395 pg/ml was found to have a 95% specificity for the diagnosis of PAH [17]. In that study, a 10-fold increase in NT-proBNP while on PAH therapy was associated with a three-fold increased risk of death. Another study comparing NT-proBNP levels in patients with SSc-PAH to patients with IPAH found that NT-proBNP levels correlated with hemodynamics in SSc-PAH were significantly higher in SSc-PAH despite less severe hemodynamic abnormalities, and were a strong predictor of survival in SSc-PAH, but not in IPAH [18]. It is our practice to obtain NT-proBNP levels on SSc-PAH patients 3 months after initiating PAH specific therapies and then at 3–6 month intervals thereafter. While no specific threshold for clinically-relevant changes in NT-proBNP have been defined, in general, our goal is to attain normal or near-normal levels with therapy.

Non-invasive imaging is often used to assess response to therapy in PAH, using both echocardiography and CMR. Multiple measures of RV size, structure, and function have been shown to predict outcome in PAH. Specific to SSc-PAH, the tricuspid annular plane systolic excursion (TAPSE), an echocardiographic measure of RV function, assessed prior to initiation of PAH specific therapy, is a strong predictor of survival [19]. In a cohort of a PAH patients that included SSc-PAH, a TAPSE >2.0 cm a year after initiation of PAH therapy predicted improved survival [20]. The ventricular mass index (VMI), the ratio of the mass of the RV to the LV assessed by CMR, predicted survival in a small cohort of SSc patients with and without PAH [21]. However, estimates of more commonly obtained parameters, such as RV or pulmonary artery pressures, are not useful in the longitudinal evaluation of SSc-PAH, regardless of the modality with which these estimates are obtained. Importantly, to our knowledge, there are no studies describing clinically relevant responses to therapy using either echocardiography or CMR in SSc-PAH, emphasizing the need for longitudinal studies employing these modalities. While sequential RHC can be performed, the invasive nature, discomfort to the patient, and associated risks often preclude its routine use in follow-up. In our practice, we may repeat RHC if a patient is failing therapy and requires additional PAH treatment.

Serial risk assessment can aide in evaluating a patient's response to PAH therapy. The achievement of a low-risk status by the ESC/ERS risk table is a recommended treatment goal in PAH guidelines [10], based on data that risk score in follow-up is associated with improved survival in PAH [8]. There are no prospective trials examining a treatment regimen or protocol targeting a low risk status in PAH, but nonetheless is reasonable strategy to pair with clinical judgment in assessing response to therapies in SSc-PAH.

Case

At her visit, she reports tolerating the medications but notes worsening reflux symptoms. She has no exertional chest pain, lightheadedness, or palpitations, but has noticed new lower extremity and a 3 kg weight gain on her scale measured at home. On exam, she is normotensive with a heart rate of 96 beats per minute and a jugular venous pressure estimated at 10 cm H_2O. Her lungs are clear without any dullness to percussion at the bases, and her heart is regular with a loud s2, but without any parasternal heave or palpable P2. She has 1+ pitting edema to the midshins bilaterally, without any calf tenderness, warmth, or erythema. On a 6MWT done prior to the initiation of therapies, she walked 390 m (69% of predicted) with a nadir oxygen saturation of 93% with ambulation. Her distance on 6MWT today is 335 m, a decrease of 55 m since the time of her RHC, again without any ambulatory desaturations. Her NT-proBNP has increased from 2165 pg/ml to 3415 pg/ml since her initial evaluation. Her echocardiogram shows a moderately dilated RV with a TAPSE of 1.8 cm; prior studies showed a TAPSE of 2.2 cm.

Discussion

At this visit, our patient has worsened, in terms of her symptoms, NYHA FC (from II to III), declining distance on 6MWT and a rising NT-proBNP. Before labeling her as a "failure" of initial therapy, it is important to think broadly about the reason for her clinical deterioration. The differential diagnosis for worsening symptoms for our patient includes issues with volume overload, hypoxemia, deconditioning, or the possibility of another disease process, such as cardiac arrhythmias, pulmonary embolism (PE), or pulmonary veno-occlusive disease (PVOD).

In addition to specific pharmacotherapies, treatment of PAH includes several general, or supportive measures, such as diuretics, supplemental oxygen therapy, and rehabilitation and exercise training. Other general measures that may be appropriate for IPAH are not recommended for SSc-PAH, namely, routine anticoagulation [22]. Diuretics are not necessarily required for patients who are compensated and lack elevated filling pressures or RV failure, but they are routinely required as patients develop peripheral edema, systemic venous congestion, severe tricuspid regurgitation, and/or RV failure [5]. Loop diuretics are the first line of treatment, and require adequate dosing and appropriate monitoring of renal function and serum electrolytes. Spironolactone, a potassium-sparing aldosterone antagonist, is useful in patients with hypokalemia and/or ascites, and post-hoc analysis of the ARIES trial showed trends towards improved exercise capacity, functional class, and clinical outcomes when spironolactone was used in conjunction with ambrisentan [23].

Supplemental oxygen therapy is used based on the assumption of that hypoxia stimulates vasoconstriction in the pulmonary vasculature [24]. The role of oxygen therapy has not been specifically studied in PAH, but several published guidelines recommend supplemental oxygen be used to maintain oxygen saturations greater that 88%–92%, or a partial pressure of oxygen in arterial blood of >55-60 mmHg at rest, during sleep, or with exertion [5, 25]. Hypoxemia intermittently with exercise or with sleep is common in patients with PAH, and clinicians must also be aware that nocturnal hypoxemia may be seen in up to 60% of patients with PAH who do not have exertional hypoxemia [26].

Pulmonary rehabilitation and exercise training are another forms of supportive therapy in PAH. The most recent treatment guidelines for PAH [5, 10] strongly recommend exercise training and rehabilitation based on the evidence of multiple controlled and uncontrolled trials that have shown improvements in exercise capacity, fatigue, cardiorespiratory function, and quality of life using varying models of exercise training [27–30]. One study looked at exercise training in only patients with CTD-PAH, 43% of whom had SSc-PAH, and found improvements in distance on 6MWT, quality of life, resting heart rate, and peak oxygen consumption [30]. Thus, despite the systemic and musculoskeletal manifestations of SSc, patients with SSc-PAH appear to benefit from rehabilitation and exercise training. There is no consensus as to the specific method of exercise training; however, patients should be referred to rehabilitation centers that have experience with care and rehabilitation of PAH patients.

In addition to optimizing these supportive therapies, clinicians must consider other diagnostic possibilities when a patient with SSc-PAH has a clinical deterioration. The risk of pulmonary embolism (PE) is increased in systemic sclerosis; a population-based cohort study showed a seven-fold increased risk of PE in patients with systemic sclerosis compared to healthy controls, after adjusting for age, sex, and comorbidities [31]. A more recent cohort study found that PAH was a risk factor for venous thromboembolism with a large SSc cohort [32]. Not only should the initial work-up for pulmonary hypertension include an evaluation for thromboembolic disease, but also the possibility of PE should be considered in the setting of clinical deterioration and appropriately evaluated and treated.

Cardiac arrhythmias are an important cause of morbidity and mortality in PAH, and thought to be caused by modulation in autonomic activity, delayed cardiac repolarization, and RV myocardial ischemia related to remodeling of the RV and the right atrium (RA) in response to longstanding pressure and volume overload [33]. Supraventricular arrhythmias, such as atrial fibrillation, atrial flutter and atrioventricular re-entry tachycardia (AVNRT) are typically seen in the setting of longstanding PAH, and onset of atrial tachyarrhythmias is often related to clinical deterioration [34]. Restoration of normal sinus rhythm is imperative in patients with PAH and is associated with a dramatic improvement in mortality [34, 35]. However, in one study, over 40% of patients with a first episode of supraventricular tachycardia (SVT) required an increase in their specific PAH therapy after conversion to sinus rhythm [36], suggesting that SVT is potentially a harbinger for deteriorating RV function. In addition to PAH, patients with SSc can have other mechanisms of arrhythmias such as myocardial fibrosis and autoantibody-mediated processes [37], and ventricular ectopy is associated with increased mortality [38]. The management of cardiac arrhythmias in PAH can be challenging as beta-blocker and calcium channel blocker therapies are relatively contraindicated because of their negative inotropic effects. Many antiarrhythmic agents, such as amiodarone, must be used judiciously because of their side effect profiles and negative inotropy, but are often administered at the lowest possible effective dose given that arrhythmias are so poorly tolerated [33, 35]. Digoxin is often used in our experience to manage atrial tachyarrhythmias. There is minimal data for its use in PAH, although one study showed an acute improvement in cardiac output and the neurohormonal axis when administered in the setting of RV failure [39]. Its use requires close monitoring of renal function and electrolytes, as it can cause hypomagnesemia and hypokalemia that can be arrhythmogenic [40].

Finally, pulmonary veno-occlusive disease (PVOD) is a rare cause of pulmonary hypertension in systemic sclerosis, and is likely under recognized because it is often difficult to distinguish from PAH [41]. It is pathologically characterized by patchy intense capillary congestion in the alveolar parenchyma, and obliterative intimal fibrosis of small veins and venules [41], histopathology that is frequently discovered on SSc patients undergoing lung transplantation [42]. Patients typically present with severe hypoxia, pulmonary edema and pleural effusions [43], often after initiation of PAH specific therapies, particularly during infusions of prostacyclin [44]. Diagnosis can be obtained by lung biopsy, although this is typically not done as patients are quite ill, and diagnosis can be suspected based on clinical scenario in conjunction with chest imaging that shows centrilobular ground glass nodules, septal lines, and adenopathy [45]. There is debate as to whether intravenous prostacyclin should be used as treatment [43, 46], but this is an indication for referral for lung transplantation evaluation.

Thus, when a patient with PAH deteriorates, or has worsening symptoms, the clinician must consider other diagnostics possibilities, as well as optimize volume status, correct hypoxemia, and ensure adequate exercise training and rehabilitation prior to labeling that patient as a failure of PAH specific therapy.

Case

Our patient has a chest radiograph that does not show pleural effusions, interstitial edema, or adenopathy. Her furosemide dose is increased to 40 mg daily and then to 40 mg twice daily, ultimately with improvement in her lower extremity edema, and a decrease in her weight back to her previous baseline. She is continued on tadalafil 40 mg daily and ambrisentan 10 mg daily, and begins a program of pulmonary rehabilitation.

She returns to clinic after another three months, where she reports being improved since her previous visit; however, she has not noticed much, if any improvement from the time of her initial diagnosis. She can walk up about one-and-a-half flights of stairs before stopping because of shortness of breath, and on occasion will has some lightheadedness when doing so. She has no chest pain, and her peripheral edema is resolved. Her physical exam is notable for trace pedal edema, a jugular venous pulse estimated at 6 cm H_2O, and a cardiac exam with regular rate and rhythm, but now with a II/VI systolic murmur heart best at the left lower sternal border, a fixed split second heart sound and a palpable P2. During a 6MWT, she ambulates 364 m, with a nadir in her ambulatory saturations to 86% on room air. Her NT-proBNP is 2433 pg/ml, and a repeat echocardiogram shows moderate RA dilation, a moderately dilated RV with a TAPSE of 1.7 cm, and trace tricuspid regurgitation. She asks what the next steps are for treating her pulmonary hypertension and improving her symptoms.

Discussion

Our patient unfortunately has not had the desired response to 6 months of tadalafil and ambrisentan. Her exercise tolerance has decreased since her diagnosis, her NT-proBNP remains elevated, and her distance on 6MWT is reduced. She now has evidence of hypoxemia with exertion, but this is a reflection of the progression of her disease. It will be important to address this with an appropriate dose of supplemental oxygen, but this may not improve her symptoms. Additionally, she has evidence of worsening RV function both on exam and on her repeat echocardiogram. When considering the treatment goals for PAH and achieving a low-risk status, it is quite evident that she has failed initial therapy. It is a common practice, and in accordance with treatment guidelines [10], to add additional therapies when patients fail to improve or worsen. Her options would be to consider a switch from a PDE5 inhibitor to the soluble guanylate cyclase (sGC) stimulator, riociguat, or to add a prostacyclin analogue.

Riociguat, is an oral s-CG stimulator approved for use in PAH. The subgroup analysis of the 111 CTD-PAH patients (66 with SSc-PAH) in the Pulmonary Arterial Hypertension sGC stimulator Trial (PATENT)-1 and PATENT-2 studies showed riociguat improved functional capacity, 6MWD, and hemodynamics, with improvement persisting for 2 years [47]. In our practice, riociguat is not typically a first-line therapy in SSc-PAH, given the less favorable cost and side effect profile compared to PDE5 inhibitors, as well as the data supporting the combination of PDE5 inhibitors and ERA in the initial treatment of SSc-PAH. The recently published REPLACE study randomized intermediate risk PAH patients on PDE5 inhibitors to replace PDE5 inhibitor with riociguat [48]. The group switched to riociguat was more likely to have clinical improvement compared to the group continued on PDE5 inhibitors. Over 70% of the enrolled patients were concurrently on ERA with PDE5I, and 19% of enrolled patients had CTD-PAH; subgroup analyses of CTD-PAH in this study have not been reported. Thus, in cases like our patient, we typically will add a prostacyclin analogue rather than switching PDE5 inhibitor to riociguat.

Several forms of prostacyclin analogues are available for delivery intravenously, subcutaneously, inhaled, and orally, and include epoprostenol, treprostinil, iloprost, and selexipag. In SSc-PAH, continuous infusion of epoprostenol improves exercise capacity and hemodynamics [49] although in contrast to the IPAH population, a mortality benefit has yet to be demonstrated [50]. Treprostinil is an epoprostenol analogue that can be delivered intravenously or subcutaneously via continuous infusion, inhaled, or orally. Subcutaneous treprostinil was shown to improve symptoms, exercise capacity, and hemodynamics in 90 patients who had CTD-PAH, 50% of whom has SSc-PAH [51]. Less is known about the effects of either the intravenous, inhaled, or oral forms of treprostinil in CTD-PAH as disaggregated data specific to this population from the pivotal clinical trials have not been reported [52, 53]. Intravenous and subcutaneous deliveries of prostaglandins can be burdensome, and come with the risks of catheter-associated infections for intravenous delivery, and infusion site pain, bleeding, and infection for subcutaneous delivery. Manipulation of the medications and delivery devices can be challenging in SSc patients with digital ulcers and limited manual dexterity, and can increase the patients' burden of their disease. As such, intravenous prostaglandins may be less commonly used in SSc-PAH compared to other forms of PAH due to these limitations [54]. Currently, intravenous prostaglandins are recommended for patients with high-risk disease, and survival remains poor in SSc-PAH patients requiring intravenous prostanoids [55].

Selexipag is an oral, selective prostacyclin receptor agonist approved for use in PAH in 2015. A subgroup analysis of the 334 CTD-PAH patients in the GRIPHON study showed that compared to placebo, selexipag reduced the risk of a composite outcomes (of death, disease progression defined by worsening 6MWD and FC, hospitalization, initiation of parenteral prostanoid therapy or long-term oxygen therapy, or the need for lung transplantation or balloon atrial septostomy) by 41% [56]. Importantly, the treatment effect was similar between SSc-PAH and other CTD-PAH subgroups, and between PAH therapy at baseline. Given these data, along with the established benefit of initial oral combination therapy of ERA and PDE5 inhibitors, upfront triple combination therapy was recently examined in TRITON (The Efficacy and Safety of Initial Triple Versus Initial Dual Oral Combination Therapy in Patients With Newly Diagnosed Pulmonary Arterial Hypertension) [57]. In this randomized, placebo controlled study which included 34% CTD-PAH patients, initial triple therapy with macitentan, tadalafil, and selexipag showed no difference in hemodynamics at 26 weeks compared to initial double therapy with macitentan and tadalafil. In exploratory secondary analyses, there was a decreased risk of disease progression in the triple therapy group, despite no difference in 6MWD. These data do not support the routine use of upfront triple combination therapy for PAH, but additional studies assessing long-term outcomes in triple vs double therapy are warranted.

Given her decline despite appropriate combination therapy, referral for lung transplantation evaluation should be considered at this time as well, as per the 6th World Symposium guidelines (see below) [11].

Case

Our patient is started on oral selexipag, uptitrated to a maximally tolerated dose of 1200mcg twice daily, while continued on oral tadalafil 40 mg daily and ambrisentan 10 mg daily. She is prescribed supplemental oxygen, and with 2 L NC maintains her oxygen saturation > 92% when checked with exertion and with nocturnal oximetry. She tolerates the selexipag, albeit with some headache, nausea, and mild jaw pain.

Six months after initiation of selexipag, she reports her exercise tolerance has slightly improved and she is able to walk up two flights of stairs again, and she has not had any chest pain, lightheadedness, or palpitations. Her exam remains generally unchanged from her previous visit, and her distance on 6MWT is 376 m. A pro-BNP is 1785 pg/ml. Her improvement with the addition of selexipag is marginal at best, and she certainly has not met treatment goals to suggest that she has had an adequate response. Given this, the possibility of initiation of a parenteral prostaglandin therapy is discussed with her, and the specifics of subcutaneous and intravenous options are reviewed. She says that she is not quite ready for a therapy requiring infusion and pump management and asks to take some time to think about this and see if she has an additional improvement on her triple oral agent therapy. Additionally, referral for lung transplant evaluation is also suggested, but the patient declines and asks to consider this at a later date.

Unfortunately, at her next appointment three months later, she reports continued decline, with an exercise tolerance that gradual decreased to less than a full flight of stairs. She has had episodes of lightheadedness with exertion, and despite feeling presyncopal has not had any episodes of syncope. She remains adherent to her medications, never missing any doses, and has not observed any changes with daily weights. Her exam is notable for a fixed split second heart sound, an increase in her systolic murmur to III/IV, and a palpable RV heave. Her lungs remain clear to auscultation and she has no peripheral edema. On a repeat 6MWT, she walks 310 m without any desaturations. A repeat transthoracic echocardiogram shows a severe RA dilation, severe RV dilation with reduced RV systolic function (TAPSE 1.4 cm), septal hypertrophy with septal bowing, and moderate tricuspid regurgitation with preserved left ventricular systolic function.

She undergoes a repeat RHC, which shows a RA pressure of 10, pulmonary artery (PA) pressure of 54/23 (mean PA pressure of 34), and a pulmonary arterial wedge pressure (PAWP) of 12 mmHg. Cardiac output (CO) was 2.64 ml/min, cardiac index (CI) was 1.57 ml/min/m^2, and pulmonary vascular resistance (PVR) was 8.33 Wood units. She is admitted to the hospital where intravenous epoprostenol is initiated and cross-titrated with her selexipag as this agent is weaned off. During this admission, she asks about the possibility of lung transplantation.

Discussion

Our patient has had a continuous deterioration of her cardiopulmonary status, and in the setting of relatively rapid clinical worsening and severely reduced right ventricular function, the decision was made to transition her to intravenous prostanoid therapy. In patients who are naïve to prostacyclin, initiation requires a gradual uptitration of dose, limited by side effects, to achieve a symptomatic benefit. In a patient like ours already on a prostacyclin analogue, cross-titration is performed by simultaneously increasing epoprostenol dose while decreasing selexipag dose under close monitoring for symptoms of prostacyclin excess or worsening pulmonary hypertension with dose changes. After the transition of therapy is performed, and her dose of epoprostenol is uptitrated, she will be receiving maximal medical therapy, at which point, the clinician needs to consider what other therapies or interventions are available to her.

Given the immune dysregulation implicated in the pathogenesis of both PAH and systemic sclerosis, the use of immunomodulatory therapies for the treatment of PAH and specifically SSc-PAH remains of interest. In a recent study, 57 SSc-PAH patients with predominantly NYHA FC II and III disease were randomized to two infusions of rituximab or placebo 2 weeks apart [58]. There was a trend towards improvement in the primary outcome of 6MWD at 24 weeks, although there was a statistically and clinically significant improvement of 6MWD at 48 weeks, and rituximab was safe and well-tolerated. This study does not support the use of rituximab currently for the treatment of SSc-PAH.

Lung transplantation is considered to be the only definitive and curative treatment for PAH. PAH accounts for less than 4% of all lung transplants, and the majority of these cases are patients with IPAH [59, 60]. There is a reluctance to perform lung transplantation in SSc patients because of the systemic nature of the disease and the risk of peri- and postoperative complications such as renal dysfunction, impaired wound healing, and an increased risk of microaspiration due to esophageal disease that can lead to organ rejection [61, 62]. However, several cohort studies have demonstrated that for appropriately screened and approved SSc patients, outcomes for lung transplantation in patients with SSc and SSc-PAH in particular are similar to other PAH populations [61–65].

Current guidelines for referral for lung transplantation evaluation and timing of transplant listing in all pulmonary vascular diseases [66] are included in Table 53.1. There are no standardized guidelines for SSc specific contraindications to lung transplantation; however, several centers have proposed and implemented criteria based on skin, musculoskeletal, renal, and gastrointestinal manifestations of the disease [61, 63, 67]. The number of lung transplant centers with significant experience in transplanting patients with SSc is small [65], and this can be a consideration when referring SSc-PAH patients for lung transplant evaluation.

Balloon atrial septostomy (BAS) is considered a last resort therapy, and it typically only used as a palliative procedure or as a bridging to transplantation [68]. The procedure involves creation of a right-to-left interatrial shunt which unloads the right heart, increases cardiac output, and improves systemic oxygen transport despite decreased arterial oxygen saturation [68, 69]. The procedure is contraindicated for patients with a RA pressure > 20 mmHg and resting oxygen saturation < 85% on room air. Studies have shown improvement in hemodynamics and exercise capacity with BAS in IPAH patients who were NYHA FC IV with right heart failure refractory to medical therapy [69–71]. There are case reports of the use of a BAS in SSc-PAH [72], but the impact on overall survival remains uncertain.

Table 53.1 Guidelines for referral and listing for lung transplant in pulmonary vascular diseases (Adapted from Weill D et al. JHLT 2015 [66])

Timing of referral	Timing of transplant listing
NYHA FC III or IV symptoms during escalating therapy	NYHA Functional Class III or IV despite a trial of at least 3 months of combination therapy including prostanoids
Rapidly progressive disease (assuming weight and rehabilitation concerns not present)	Cardiac index of <2 L/min/m^2
Use of parenteral targeted (PAH) therapy regardless of symptoms or NYHA Functional Class	Mean right atrial pressure of >15 mmHg
Known or suspected pulmonary veno-occlusive disease (PVOD) or pulmonary capillary hemangiomatosis	6-minute walk test of <350 m
	Development of significant hemoptysis, pericardial effusion, or signs of progressive right heart failure (renal insufficiency, increasing bilirubin, brain natriuretic peptide, or recurrent ascites)

Finally, referral and involvement of palliative care is a valuable resource that is underused in PAH. Palliative care is defined as "patient and family-centered care that optimizes quality of life by anticipating, preventing, and treating suffering," and "involves addressing physical, intellectual, emotional, social, and spiritual needs and to facilitate patient autonomy, access to information, and choice" [73]. Despite PAH and SSc-PAH portending a poor prognosis, a high degree of symptom burden, and poor or sub-optimal health related quality of life [74, 75], there is very limited formal investigation of the incorporation of palliative care into a PAH treatment plan. Several surveys have shown that palliative care awareness and use by both providers and patients is low [76–78], and that patients who die from PAH have a high degree of symptom burden, particularly dyspnea, at the time of their deaths [79]. A referral to palliative care should be considered for patients with rapidly progressing disease, NYHA FC III or IV symptoms, or who express interest, regardless of the stage of their disease. A referral to palliative care should not indicate to the clinician or the patient that either is "giving up," but instead providing an additional resource to ensure that all patient needs and symptoms are being adequately addressed.

Case

Our patient was referred both for a lung transplant evaluation and a palliative care consultation. She has now developed a good rapport with her palliative care physician, who has helped manage her dyspnea and provided her with many coping mechanisms for dealing with the burdens of the symptoms and treatments of her diseases. With the uptitration of epoprostenol to its effective dose, her symptoms have stabilized; however, she remains NHYA FC III. She underwent a comprehensive transplant evaluation, and ultimately, the decision was made to list her for double lung transplantation. She is continuing her current therapies-tadalafil, ambrisentan, and intravenous epoprostenol-and is anxiously awaiting the possibility of receiving a lung transplant.

Key Principle Lessons of the Case

1. Choice of initial therapy in SSc-PAH requires knowledge of the treatment guidelines in PAH, understanding risk assessment in PAH and the data behind the use of initial upfront combination therapy with ERA and PDE5 inhibitor in SSc-PAH.
2. Assessment of response to therapy in SSc-PAH is typically done with a combination of evaluation of a patient functional class, NT-proBNP, distance on 6MWT, echocardiographic and/or CMR assessments of RV structure and function, reassessment of cardiopulmonary hemodynamics, and use of multimodal risk scores that include many of these parameters.
3. When a SSc-PAH patient is worsening, the clinician must consider possibilities of other diagnoses such as PE, cardiac arrhythmias, PVOD, and ensure that volume status, oxygenation, and exercise training and rehabilitation have been optimized prior to labeling the patient as failing PAH therapy.
4. While it is common practice and recommendation of current guidelines to change or add therapies to a SSc-PAH patient who is failing therapy, there is no consensus as to which combination of agents is preferred, and typically is guided by physician and patient preferences.
5. Prostaglandin therapies are available by intravenous, subcutaneous, inhaled, or oral deliveries and are typically reserved for patients failing dual therapies, who are NYHA FC IV, or have other high risk features. Continuous intravenous epoprostenol has the most robust evidence in SSc-PAH, and data exists for the use of selexipag in SSc-PAH. The use of other prostaglandins in combination therapies are extrapolated from PAH population in general.
6. Referral for lung transplantation in SSc-PAH should be done accordance with current guidelines. Despite concerns for SSc specific-related complications, for appropriately screened SSc-PAH patients, outcomes for lung transplantation appear to be similar to other PAH populations.
7. Palliative care is an underused resource in SSc-PAH and a referral should be considered for patients with progressive or advanced disease, or a high burden of symptoms and treatments from their diseases.

References

1. Benza RL, Gomberg-Maitland M, Miller DP, Frost A, Frantz RP, Foreman AJ, et al. The REVEAL Registry risk score calculator in patients newly diagnosed with pulmonary arterial hypertension. Chest. 2012;141(2):354–62.
2. Benza RL, Miller DP, Gomberg-Maitland M, Frantz RP, Foreman AJ, Coffey CS, et al. Predicting survival in pulmonary arterial hypertension: insights from the Registry to Evaluate Early and Long-Term Pulmonary Arterial Hypertension Disease Management (REVEAL). Circulation. 2010;122(2):164–72.
3. Mullin CJ, Khair RM, Damico RL, Kolb TM, Hummers LK, Hassoun PM, et al. Validation of the REVEAL prognostic equation and risk score calculator in incident systemic sclerosis-associated pulmonary arterial hypertension. Arthritis Rheumatol. 2019;71(10):1691–700.
4. Benza RL, Gomberg-Maitland M, Elliott CG, Farber HW, Foreman AJ, Frost AE, et al. Predicting survival in patients with pulmonary arterial hypertension: The REVEAL risk score calculator 2.0 and comparison with ESC/ERS-based risk assessment strategies. Chest. 2019;156(2):323–37.
5. Galie N, Humbert M, Vachiery JL, Gibbs S, Lang I, Torbicki A, et al. 2015 ESC/ERS Guidelines for the diagnosis and treatment of pulmonary hypertension: The Joint Task Force for the Diagnosis and Treatment of Pulmonary Hypertension of the European Society of Cardiology (ESC) and the European Respiratory Society (ERS): Endorsed by: Association for European Paediatric and Congenital Cardiology (AEPC), International Society for Heart and Lung Transplantation (ISHLT). Eur Heart J. 2016;37(1):67–119.
6. McLaughlin VV, Gaine SP, Howard LS, Leuchte HH, Mathier MA, Mehta S, et al. Treatment goals of pulmonary hypertension. J Am Coll Cardiol. 2013;62(Suppl. 25):D73–81.
7. Kylhammar D, Kjellstrom B, Hjalmarsson C, Jansson K, Nisell M, Soderberg S, et al. A comprehensive risk stratification at early follow-up determines prognosis in pulmonary arterial hypertension. Eur Heart J. 2018;39(47):4175–81.
8. Hoeper MM, Kramer T, Pan Z, Eichstaedt CA, Spiesshoefer J, Benjamin N, et al. Mortality in pulmonary arterial hypertension: prediction by the 2015 European pulmonary hypertension guidelines risk stratification model. Eur Respir J. 2017;50(2):1–10.
9. Mercurio V, Diab N, Peloquin G, Housten-Harris T, Damico R, Kolb TM, et al. Risk assessment in scleroderma patients with newly diagnosed pulmonary arterial hypertension: application of the ESC/ERS risk prediction model. Eur Respir J. 2018;52(4):1800497.
10. Galie N, Channick RN, Frantz RP, Grunig E, Jing ZC, Moiseeva O, et al. Risk stratification and medical therapy of pulmonary arterial hypertension. Eur Respir J. 2019;53(1):1801889.
11. Galie N, Barbera JA, Frost AE, Ghofrani HA, Hoeper MM, McLaughlin VV, et al. Initial use of Ambrisentan plus tadalafil in pulmonary arterial hypertension. N Engl J Med. 2015;373(9):834–44.
12. Coghlan JG, Galie N, Barbera JA, Frost AE, Ghofrani HA, Hoeper MM, et al. Initial combination therapy with ambrisentan and tadalafil in connective tissue disease-associated pulmonary arterial hypertension (CTD-PAH): subgroup analysis from the AMBITION trial. Ann Rheum Dis. 2017;76(7):1219–27.
13. Hassoun PM, Zamanian RT, Damico R, Lechtzin N, Khair R, Kolb TM, et al. Ambrisentan and tadalafil up-front combination therapy

in scleroderma-associated pulmonary arterial hypertension. Am J Respir Crit Care Med. 2015;192(9):1102–10.
14. Guyatt GH, Sullivan MJ, Thompson PJ, Fallen EL, Pugsley SO, Taylor DW, et al. The 6-minute walk: a new measure of exercise capacity in patients with chronic heart failure. Can Med Assoc J. 1985;132(8):919–23.
15. Garin MC, Highland KB, Silver RM, Strange C. Limitations to the 6-minute walk test in interstitial lung disease and pulmonary hypertension in scleroderma. J Rheumatol. 2009;36(2):330–6.
16. Mathai SC, Puhan MA, Lam D, Wise RA. The minimal important difference in the 6-minute walk test for patients with pulmonary arterial hypertension. Am J Respir Crit Care Med. 2012;186(5):428–33.
17. Williams MH, Handler CE, Akram R, Smith CJ, Das C, Smee J, et al. Role of N-terminal brain natriuretic peptide (N-TproBNP) in scleroderma-associated pulmonary arterial hypertension. Eur Heart J. 2006;27(12):1485–94.
18. Mathai SC, Bueso M, Hummers LK, Boyce D, Lechtzin N, Le Pavec J, et al. Disproportionate elevation of N-terminal pro-brain natriuretic peptide in scleroderma-related pulmonary hypertension. Eur Respir J. 2010;35(1):95–104.
19. Mathai SC, Sibley CT, Forfia PR, Mudd JO, Fisher MR, Tedford RJ, et al. Tricuspid annular plane systolic excursion is a robust outcome measure in systemic sclerosis-associated pulmonary arterial hypertension. J Rheumatol. 2011;38(11):2410–8.
20. Mazurek JA, Vaidya A, Mathai SC, Roberts JD, Forfia PR. Follow-up tricuspid annular plane systolic excursion predicts survival in pulmonary arterial hypertension. Pulm Circ. 2017;7(2):361–71.
21. Hagger D, Condliffe R, Woodhouse N, Elliot CA, Armstrong IJ, Davies C, et al. Ventricular mass index correlates with pulmonary artery pressure and predicts survival in suspected systemic sclerosis-associated pulmonary arterial hypertension. Rheumatology (Oxford). 2009;48(9):1137–42.
22. Olsson KM, Delcroix M, Ghofrani HA, Tiede H, Huscher D, Speich R, et al. Anticoagulation and survival in pulmonary arterial hypertension: results from the Comparative, Prospective Registry of Newly Initiated Therapies for Pulmonary Hypertension (COMPERA). Circulation. 2014;129(1):57–65.
23. Maron BA, Waxman AB, Opotowsky AR, Gillies H, Blair C, Aghamohammadzadeh R, et al. Effectiveness of spironolactone plus ambrisentan for treatment of pulmonary arterial hypertension (from the [ARIES] study 1 and 2 trials). Am J Cardiol. 2013;112(5):720–5.
24. Sylvester JT, Shimoda LA, Aaronson PI, Ward JP. Hypoxic pulmonary vasoconstriction. Physiol Rev. 2012;92(1):367–520.
25. Sauler M, Fares WH, Trow TK. Standard nonspecific therapies in the management of pulmonary arterial hypertension. Clin Chest Med. 2013;34(4):799–810.
26. Minai OA, Pandya CM, Golish JA, Avecillas JF, McCarthy K, Marlow S, et al. Predictors of nocturnal oxygen desaturation in pulmonary arterial hypertension. Chest. 2007;131(1):109–17.
27. Mereles D, Ehlken N, Kreuscher S, Ghofrani S, Hoeper MM, Halank M, et al. Exercise and respiratory training improve exercise capacity and quality of life in patients with severe chronic pulmonary hypertension. Circulation. 2006;114(14):1482–9.
28. Ehlken N, Lichtblau M, Klose H, Weidenhammer J, Fischer C, Nechwatal R, et al. Exercise training improves peak oxygen consumption and haemodynamics in patients with severe pulmonary arterial hypertension and inoperable chronic thrombo-embolic pulmonary hypertension: a prospective, randomized, controlled trial. Eur Heart J. 2016;37(1):35–44.
29. Grunig E, Ehlken N, Ghofrani A, Staehler G, Meyer FJ, Juenger J, et al. Effect of exercise and respiratory training on clinical progression and survival in patients with severe chronic pulmonary hypertension. Respiration. 2011;81(5):394–401.
30. Grunig E, Maier F, Ehlken N, Fischer C, Lichtblau M, Blank N, et al. Exercise training in pulmonary arterial hypertension associated with connective tissue diseases. Arthritis Res Ther. 2012;14(3):R148.
31. Chung WS, Lin CL, Sung FC, Hsu WH, Yang WT, Lu CC, et al. Systemic sclerosis increases the risks of deep vein thrombosis and pulmonary thromboembolism: a nationwide cohort study. Rheumatology (Oxford). 2014;53(9):1639–45.
32. Johnson SR, Hakami N, Ahmad Z, Wijeysundera DN. Venous thromboembolism in systemic sclerosis: prevalence, risk factors, and effect on survival. J Rheumatol. 2018;45(7):942–6.
33. Rajdev A, Garan H, Biviano A. Arrhythmias in pulmonary arterial hypertension. Prog Cardiovasc Dis. 2012;55(2):180–6.
34. Tongers J, Schwerdtfeger B, Klein G, Kempf T, Schaefer A, Knapp JM, et al. Incidence and clinical relevance of supraventricular tachyarrhythmias in pulmonary hypertension. Am Heart J. 2007;153(1):127–32.
35. Reddy SA, Nethercott SL, Khialani BV, Grace AA, Martin CA. Management of arrhythmias in pulmonary hypertension. J Interv Card Electrophysiol. 2021;62(2):219–29.
36. Ruiz-Cano MJ, Gonzalez-Mansilla A, Escribano P, Delgado J, Arribas F, Torres J, et al. Clinical implications of supraventricular arrhythmias in patients with severe pulmonary arterial hypertension. Int J Cardiol. 2011;146(1):105–6.
37. Patane S, Marte F, Sturiale M, Dattilo G, Luzza F. Atrial flutter, ventricular tachycardia and changing axis deviation associated with scleroderma. Int J Cardiol. 2011;153(2):e25–8.
38. Kostis JB, Seibold JR, Turkevich D, Masi AT, Grau RG, Medsger TA Jr, et al. Prognostic importance of cardiac arrhythmias in systemic sclerosis. Am J Med. 1988;84(6):1007–15.
39. Rich S, Seidlitz M, Dodin E, Osimani D, Judd D, Genthner D, et al. The short-term effects of digoxin in patients with right ventricular dysfunction from pulmonary hypertension. Chest. 1998;114(3):787–92.
40. Smith TW, Antman EM, Friedman PL, Blatt CM, Marsh JD. Digitalis glycosides: mechanisms and manifestations of toxicity. Part I. Prog Cardiovasc Dis. 1984;26(5):413–58.
41. Overbeek MJ, Vonk MC, Boonstra A, Voskuyl AE, Vonk-Noordegraaf A, Smit EF, et al. Pulmonary arterial hypertension in limited cutaneous systemic sclerosis: a distinctive vasculopathy. Eur Respir J. 2009;34(2):371–9.
42. Gupta S, Gupta A, Rehman S, Ocak I, Domsic RT, Schneider F, et al. Pulmonary veno-occlusive disease is highly prevalent in scleroderma patients undergoing lung transplantation. ERJ Open Res. 2019;5(1):00168-2018. https://doi.org/10.1183/23120541.00168-2018.
43. Johnson SR, Patsios D, Hwang DM, Granton JT. Pulmonary veno-occlusive disease and scleroderma associated pulmonary hypertension. J Rheumatol. 2006;33(11):2347–50.
44. Farber HW, Graven KK, Kokolski G, Korn JH. Pulmonary edema during acute infusion of epoprostenol in a patient with pulmonary hypertension and limited scleroderma. J Rheumatol. 1999;26(5):1195–6.
45. Resten A, Maitre S, Humbert M, Rabiller A, Sitbon O, Capron F, et al. Pulmonary hypertension: CT of the chest in pulmonary veno-occlusive disease. AJR Am J Roentgenol. 2004;183(1):65–70.
46. Okumura H, Nagaya N, Kyotani S, Sakamaki F, Nakanishi N, Fukuhara S, et al. Effects of continuous IV prostacyclin in a patient with pulmonary veno-occlusive disease. Chest. 2002;122(3):1096–8.
47. Humbert M, Coghlan JG, Ghofrani HA, Grimminger F, He JG, Riemekasten G, et al. Riociguat for the treatment of pulmonary arterial hypertension associated with connective tissue disease: results from PATENT-1 and PATENT-2. Ann Rheum Dis. 2017;76(2):422–6.

48. Hoeper MM, Al-Hiti H, Benza RL, Chang SA, Corris PA, Gibbs JSR, et al. Switching to riociguat versus maintenance therapy with phosphodiesterase-5 inhibitors in patients with pulmonary arterial hypertension (REPLACE): a multicentre, open-label, randomised controlled trial. Lancet Respir Med. 2021;9(6):573–84.
49. Badesch DB, Tapson VF, McGoon MD, Brundage BH, Rubin LJ, Wigley FM, et al. Continuous intravenous epoprostenol for pulmonary hypertension due to the scleroderma spectrum of disease. A randomized, controlled trial. Ann Intern Med. 2000;132(6):425–34.
50. Badesch DB, McGoon MD, Barst RJ, Tapson VF, Rubin LJ, Wigley FM, et al. Longterm survival among patients with scleroderma-associated pulmonary arterial hypertension treated with intravenous epoprostenol. J Rheumatol. 2009;36(10):2244–9.
51. Oudiz RJ, Schilz RJ, Barst RJ, Galie N, Rich S, Rubin LJ, et al. Treprostinil, a prostacyclin analogue, in pulmonary arterial hypertension associated with connective tissue disease. Chest. 2004;126(2):420–7.
52. McLaughlin VV, Benza RL, Rubin LJ, Channick RN, Voswinckel R, Tapson VF, et al. Addition of inhaled treprostinil to oral therapy for pulmonary arterial hypertension: a randomized controlled clinical trial. J Am Coll Cardiol. 2010;55(18):1915–22.
53. White RJ, Jerjes-Sanchez C, Bohns Meyer GM, Pulido T, Sepulveda P, Wang KY, et al. Combination therapy with oral treprostinil for pulmonary arterial hypertension. A double-blind placebo-controlled clinical trial. Am J Respir Crit Care Med. 2020;201(6):707–17.
54. Rubenfire M, Huffman MD, Krishnan S, Seibold JR, Schiopu E, McLaughlin VV. Survival in systemic sclerosis with pulmonary arterial hypertension has not improved in the modern era. Chest. 2013;144(4):1282–90.
55. Vlachou M, Fayed H, Dawson A, Reddecliffe S, Stevenson A, Thomson RJ, et al. Intravenous prostanoids in systemic sclerosis-associated pulmonary arterial hypertension: a single centre experience. Rheumatology (Oxford). 2022;61(3):1106–14.
56. Gaine S, Chin K, Coghlan G, Channick R, Di Scala L, Galie N, et al. Selexipag for the treatment of connective tissue disease-associated pulmonary arterial hypertension. Eur Respir J. 2017;50(2):1602493.
57. Chin KM, Sitbon O, Doelberg M, Feldman J, Gibbs JSR, Grunig E, et al. Three- versus two-drug therapy for patients with newly diagnosed pulmonary arterial hypertension. J Am Coll Cardiol. 2021;78(14):1393–403.
58. Zamanian RT, Badesch D, Chung L, Domsic RT, Medsger T, Pinckney A, et al. Safety and efficacy of B-cell depletion with rituximab for the treatment of systemic sclerosis-associated pulmonary arterial hypertension: a multicenter, double-blind, randomized, placebo-controlled trial. Am J Respir Crit Care Med. 2021;204(2):209–21.
59. Yusen RD, Edwards LB, Kucheryavaya AY, Benden C, Dipchand AI, Dobbels F, et al. The registry of the International Society for Heart and Lung Transplantation: thirty-first adult lung and heart-lung transplant report--2014; focus theme: retransplantation. J Heart Lung Transplant. 2014;33(10):1009–24.
60. Chambers DC, Perch M, Zuckermann A, Cherikh WS, Harhay MO, Hayes D Jr, et al. The International Thoracic Organ Transplant Registry of the International Society for Heart and Lung Transplantation: Thirty-eighth adult lung transplantation report—2021; focus on recipient characteristics. J Heart Lung Transplant. 2021;40(10):1060–72.
61. Saggar R, Khanna D, Furst DE, Belperio JA, Park GS, Weigt SS, et al. Systemic sclerosis and bilateral lung transplantation: a single centre experience. Eur Respir J. 2010;36(4):893–900.
62. Schachna L, Medsger TA Jr, Dauber JH, Wigley FM, Braunstein NA, White B, et al. Lung transplantation in scleroderma compared with idiopathic pulmonary fibrosis and idiopathic pulmonary arterial hypertension. Arthritis Rheum. 2006;54(12):3954–61.
63. Miele CH, Schwab K, Saggar R, Duffy E, Elashoff D, Tseng CH, et al. Lung transplant outcomes in systemic sclerosis with significant esophageal dysfunction. A comprehensive single-center experience. Ann Am Thorac Soc. 2016;13(6):793–802.
64. Bernstein EJ, Peterson ER, Sell JL, D'Ovidio F, Arcasoy SM, Bathon JM, et al. Survival of adults with systemic sclerosis following lung transplantation: a nationwide cohort study. Arthritis Rheumatol. 2015;67(5):1314–22.
65. Khan IY, Singer LG, de Perrot M, Granton JT, Keshavjee S, Chau C, et al. Survival after lung transplantation in systemic sclerosis. A systematic review. Respir Med. 2013;107(12):2081–7.
66. Weill D, Benden C, Corris PA, Dark JH, Davis RD, Keshavjee S, et al. A consensus document for the selection of lung transplant candidates: 2014—an update from the Pulmonary Transplantation Council of the International Society for Heart and Lung Transplantation. J Heart Lung Transplant. 2015;34(1):1–15.
67. Launay D, Savale L, Berezne A, Le Pavec J, Hachulla E, Mouthon L, et al. Lung and heart-lung transplantation for systemic sclerosis patients. A monocentric experience of 13 patients, review of the literature and position paper of a multidisciplinary Working Group. Presse Med. 2014;43(10 Pt 2):e345–63.
68. Keogh AM, Mayer E, Benza RL, Corris P, Dartevelle PG, Frost AE, et al. Interventional and surgical modalities of treatment in pulmonary hypertension. J Am Coll Cardiol. 2009;54(1 Suppl):S67–77.
69. Sandoval J, Gaspar J, Pulido T, Bautista E, Martinez-Guerra ML, Zeballos M, et al. Graded balloon dilation atrial septostomy in severe primary pulmonary hypertension. A therapeutic alternative for patients nonresponsive to vasodilator treatment. J Am Coll Cardiol. 1998;32(2):297–304.
70. Khan MS, Memon MM, Amin E, Yamani N, Khan SU, Figueredo VM, et al. Use of balloon atrial septostomy in patients with advanced pulmonary arterial hypertension: a systematic review and meta-analysis. Chest. 2019;156(1):53–63.
71. Kurzyna M, Dabrowski M, Bielecki D, Fijalkowska A, Pruszczyk P, Opolski G, et al. Atrial septostomy in treatment of end-stage right heart failure in patients with pulmonary hypertension. Chest. 2007;131(4):977–83.
72. Allcock RJ, O'Sullivan JJ, Corris PA. Palliation of systemic sclerosis-associated pulmonary hypertension by atrial septostomy. Arthritis Rheum. 2001;44(7):1660–2.
73. Centers for M, Medicaid Services HHS. Medicare and Medicaid programs: hospice conditions of participation. Final rule. Fed Regist. 2008;73(109):32087–220.
74. Campo A, Mathai SC, Le Pavec J, Zaiman AL, Hummers LK, Boyce D, et al. Hemodynamic predictors of survival in scleroderma-related pulmonary arterial hypertension. Am J Respir Crit Care Med. 2010;182(2):252–60.
75. Chung L, Farber HW, Benza R, Miller DP, Parsons L, Hassoun PM, et al. Unique predictors of mortality in patients with pulmonary arterial hypertension associated with systemic sclerosis in the REVEAL registry. Chest. 2014;146(6):1494–504.
76. Fenstad ER, Shanafelt TD, Sloan JA, Novotny PJ, Durst LA, Frantz RP, et al. Physician attitudes toward palliative care for patients with pulmonary arterial hypertension: results of a cross-sectional survey. Pulm Circ. 2014;4(3):504–10.
77. Swetz KM, Shanafelt TD, Drozdowicz LB, Sloan JA, Novotny PJ, Durst LA, et al. Symptom burden, quality of life, and attitudes toward palliative care in patients with pulmonary arterial hypertension: results from a cross-sectional patient survey. J Heart Lung Transplant. 2012;31(10):1102–8.
78. Anand V, Vallabhajosyula S, Cheungpasitporn W, Frantz RP, Cajigas HR, Strand JJ, et al. Inpatient palliative care use in patients with pulmonary arterial hypertension: temporal trends, predictors, and outcomes. Chest. 2020;158(6):2568–78.
79. Grinnan DC, Swetz KM, Pinson J, Fairman P, Lyckholm LJ, Smith T. The end-of-life experience for a cohort of patients with pulmonary arterial hypertension. J Palliat Med. 2012;15(10):1065–70.

Pseudo-obstruction with Malabsorption and Malnutrition

54

Tracy M. Frech

Case Study

The patient is a 73-year male with past medical history of prostate cancer and a 12-year history of limited cutaneous systemic sclerosis who underwent robot-assisted laparoscopic right hemicolectomy for a high-grade dysplastic polyp found on screening colonoscopy. He was discharged to home 2 days after this procedure. He was re-admitted to the hospital 1 week later for presumed ileus, when he presented to the emergency department with nausea, vomiting, abdominal pain, and distention where abdominal imaging was consistent with pseudo-obstruction (Fig. 54.1a). At admission, a nasogastric tube was placed for decompression and gastrografin confirmed full movement of contrast throughout the bowel consistent with pseudo-obstruction (Fig. 54.1b).

Rheumatology was consulted to evaluate whether SSc is the cause of ileus, which was treated with bowel rest and intravenous hydration. Two months after hospital discharge, the patient reports persistent nausea, alternating obstipation with loose stools, and an additional 10.6 kg weight loss at his rheumatology visit.

T. M. Frech (✉)
Vanderbilt University Medical Center and Tennessee Valley Healthcare System Veterans Affairs, Nashville, TN, USA
e-mail: tracy.frech@vumc.org

Y. Allanore et al. (eds.), *Scleroderma*, https://doi.org/10.1007/978-3-031-40658-4_54

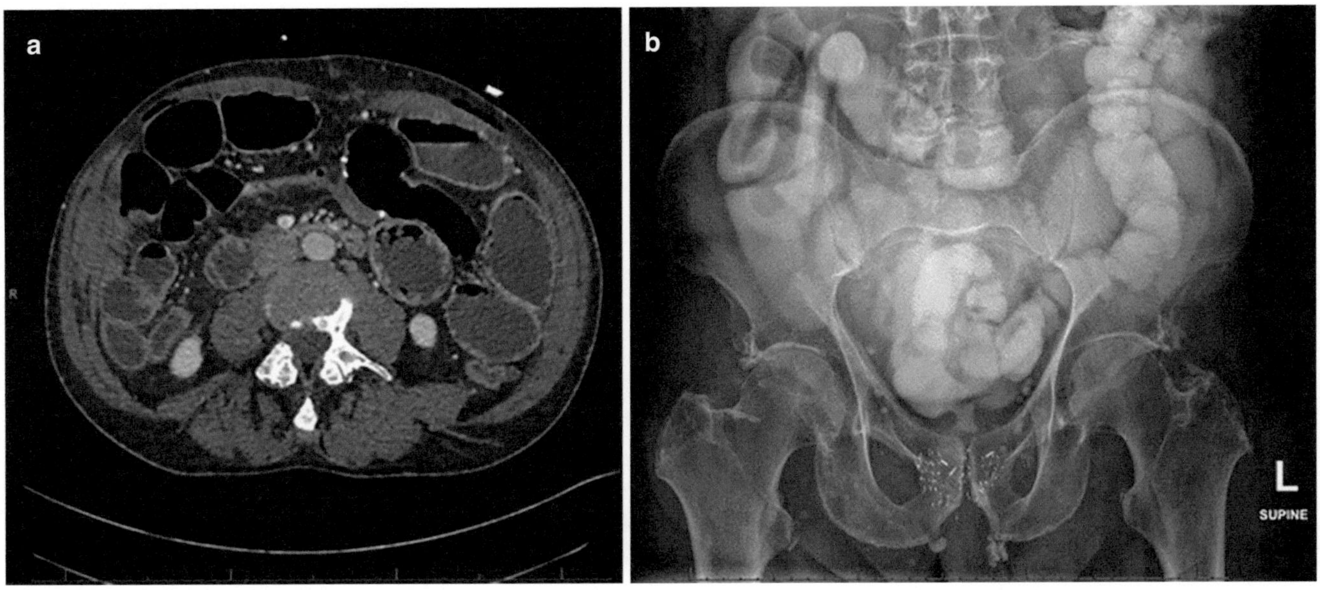

Fig. 54.1 (**a**) Computed tomography of abdomen. (**b**) Gastrografin study

Introduction

Intestinal pseudo-obstruction is defined by the presence of ineffective propulsion with symptoms of altered bowel movements, pain, and distention with radiographic appearance of intestinal obstruction in the absence of occluding lesions of the intestinal lumen [1]. Intestinal pseudo-obstruction is due to enteric nervous system dysfunction and can be either acute or chronic. In systemic sclerosis (SSc), the pathogenesis may be due to autoantibodies, smooth muscle cell inflammation and atrophy, and the characteristic fibrosis of the enteric connective tissue [2]. Acute intestinal pseudo-obstruction cares a mortality rate of approximately 15% and can be seen in the postoperative setting of systemic sclerosis (SSc) patients [3, 4]. Chronic intestinal pseudo-obstruction represents an important cause of persistent functional intestinal failure leading to malnutrition in SSc patients. Detection of intestinal pseudo-obstruction requires the evaluating physician to have a high index of suspicion and an understanding of diagnostic and management strategies.

Diagnosis

Medical history is the first step in making a diagnosis of pseudo-obstruction. The classical clinical symptoms for pseudo-obstruction are abdominal pain, nausea and emesis, abdominal distention, and (if lower tract involvement) constipation-to-obstipation [5–7]. If intermittent diarrhea or steatorrhea is reported, the presence of small intestinal bacterial overgrowth (SIBO) due to intestinal stasis should be considered [8]. The Scleroderma Clinical Trials Consortium Gastrointestinal Tract Questionnaire (GIT 2.0) is a validated instrument for evaluation of patient-reported outcomes involving the gastrointestinal tract and is useful for evaluating the presence of gastrointestinal tract symptoms in the clinical setting [9]. However, GIT 2.0 does not assess for weight loss or malnutrition. The Malnutrition Universal Screening Tool (MUST), a validated nutrition-screening tool assesses weight loss to help identify adults at risk of undernutrition and the need for intervention, has successfully been used in SSc [10, 11]. It is important to highlight that while a low serum albumin may not be useful for identifying patients that are malnourished, it is associated with a higher mortality in patients with pseudo-obstruction [4, 11].

The physical exam in pseudo-obstruction often reveals signs of dehydration, such as tachycardia, hypotension, orthostasis, dry mucous membranes, and an abdominal assessment notable for distention and hypoactive bowel sounds. However, severe direct tenderness, involuntary guarding, abdominal rigidity, and rebound tenderness with leukocytosis, neutrophilia, bandemia, and lactic acidosis should raise suspicion of perforation [5]. A comorbidity assessment should include an assessment of diabetes, hypothyroidism, hypoparathyroidism, celiac disease, radiation therapy for malignancy, and the use of narcotics for pain management [6]. Additionally, if malabsorption is suspected, serum methylmalonic acid (elevated in malabsorption), zinc (decreased in malabsorption), 25-OH vitamin D levels, vitamin K level or prothrombin time, and a C14 xylose breath test or a hydrogen breath test can be considered [12].

In current clinical practice, computerized tomography (CT) scan of the abdomen is more accurate than conventional radiology to demonstrate air-fluid levels, while ruling out mechanical causes as well as provides more information to exclude an extra luminal, gut wall or intraluminal mechanically obstructive lesion [8]. Manometry may provide pathophysiologically relevant information on neuropathic versus myopathic mechanisms underlying dysmotility but is best completed at highly specialized centers that care for SSc patients [6]. Histological analysis of intestinal tract tissue is generally not helpful in SSc patients [6].

Management

For acute pseudo-obstruction, medical resuscitation includes intravenous hydration, correcting electrolyte abnormalities, nil per os, and nasoenteral suction [5]. Most pro-kinetic drugs have not proven efficacy in restoring intestinal propulsion; however, cyclic course of selective antibiotics for malabsorption due to concurrent SIBO are sometimes effective [2]. Octreotide is sometimes prescribed in refractory small intestinal pseudo-obstruction and bacterial overgrowth [13]. For chronic pseudo-obstruction, enteral nutrition (EN) or long-term parenteral nutrition (PN) should be considered to prevent deterioration in nutritional status [2]. The main indication for prescribing PN is antibiotic-refractory and prokinetic-refractory chronic intestinal pseudo-obstruction and SIBO [14]. It is, however, notable that long-term PN carries risk of complications in SSc [15].

The ability of the gastrointestinal tract to receive and process nutrients is impaired in pseudo-obstruction. Malnutrition may follow from malabsorption as well as food avoidance because of severe postprandial symptoms. Dietary measures include the recommendation of small, frequent meals that are low in fat and fiber, and avoiding carbonated drinks or lactose (in intolerant individuals) that can alter gastrointestinal motility [16]. An elemental diet and vitamin/mineral supplementation may be necessary, thus cases of suspected malnutrition should be referred to a dietitian with expertise in assessing and managing nutrient malabsorption and other issues specific to SSc is essential [12]. The nutrition intervention is largely dependent on the segment of the GI tract affected and the severity and progressive nature of the specific disease process, thus similarly a gastroenterologist with expertise in SSc is important for including in the management of patients with pseudo-obstruction [12, 16].

Conclusions

The case study highlights the importance of considering both acute and chronic pseudo-obstruction when assessing SSc patients complaining of nausea, vomiting, abdominal pain, and distention. A higher tract lesion may not result in obstipation. As highlighted in this patient's presentation, acute pseudo-obstruction should be considered in an SSc patient that has recently been hospitalized or had surgery. Hydration and bowel rest requires hospitalization, but prior to discharge a nutrition plan and follow-up are imperative. In the outpatient setting, the routine use of the GIT 2.0 and MUST can help identify patients with chronic pseudo-obstruction (Fig. 54.2).

Chronic or recurrent pseudo-obstruction may result in malabsorption and malnutrition. Thus, it is particularly important, in addition to asking about gastrointestinal tract

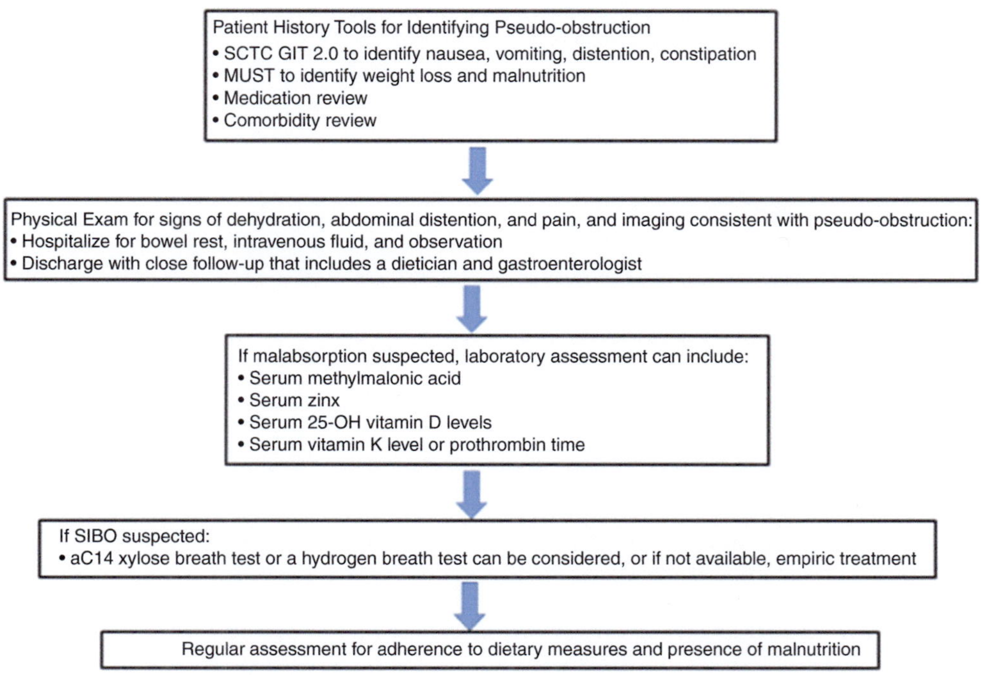

Fig. 54.2 Approach to identifying pseudo-obstruction, malabsorption, and malnutrition in SSc

symptoms, to query SSc patients at every visit about weight loss and dietary intake. Laboratory assessment can help identify malabsorption is present. If a patient has intermittent diarrhea or soilage, concurrent SIBO may be present. The management of SSc patients with pseudo-obstruction requires a comprehensive care plan that should include a dietician and gastroenterologist to ensure nutrition and procedural diagnostics/therapeutics are appropriate. In summary, as highlighted by this case presentation, the rheumatologist plays a critical role in identification and management of pseudo-obstruction and malnutrition.

Acknowledgment Dr. Tracy Frech gratefully acknowledges the contribution of Dr. John O. Clark to a related chapter included in a previous edition of this textbook.

References

1. Coulie B, Camilleri M. Intestinal pseudo-obstruction. Annu Rev Med. 1999;50:37–55.
2. Bharadwaj S, Tandon P, Gohel T, Corrigan ML, Coughlin KL, Shatnawei A, et al. Gastrointestinal manifestations, malnutrition, and role of enteral and parenteral nutrition in patients with scleroderma. J Clin Gastroenterol. 2015;49(7):559–64.
3. Fazel A, Verne GN. New solutions to an old problem: acute colonic pseudo-obstruction. J Clin Gastroenterol. 2005;39(1):17–20.
4. Mecoli C, Purohit S, Sandorfi N, Derk CT. Mortality, recurrence, and hospital course of patients with systemic sclerosis-related acute intestinal pseudo-obstruction. J Rheumatol. 2014;41(10):2049–54.
5. Rami Reddy SR, Cappell MS. A systematic review of the clinical presentation, diagnosis, and treatment of small bowel obstruction. Curr Gastroenterol Rep. 2017;19(6):28.
6. Downes TJ, Cheruvu MS, Karunaratne TB, De Giorgio R, Farmer AD. Pathophysiology, diagnosis, and management of chronic intestinal pseudo-obstruction. J Clin Gastroenterol. 2018;52(6):477–89.
7. Antonucci A, Fronzoni L, Cogliandro L, Cogliandro RF, Caputo C, De Giorgio R, et al. Chronic intestinal pseudo-obstruction. World J Gastroenterol. 2008;14(19):2953–61.
8. Di Nardo G, Karunaratne TB, Frediani S, De Giorgio R. Chronic intestinal pseudo-obstruction: Progress in management? Neurogastroenterol Motil. 2017;29(12)
9. Khanna D, Hays RD, Maranian P, Seibold JR, Impens A, Mayes MD, et al. Reliability and validity of the University of California, Los Angeles scleroderma clinical trial consortium gastrointestinal tract instrument. Arthritis Rheum. 2009;61(9):1257–63.
10. Murtaugh MA, Frech TM. Nutritional status and gastrointestinal symptoms in systemic sclerosis patients. Clin Nutr. 2013;32(1):130–5.
11. Baron M, Hudson M, Steele R, Canadian Scleroderma Research G. Is serum albumin a marker of malnutrition in chronic disease? The scleroderma paradigm. J Am Coll Nutr. 2010;29(2):144–51.
12. Baron M, Bernier P, Cote LF, Delegge MH, Falovitch G, Friedman G, et al. Screening and therapy for malnutrition and related gastro-intestinal disorders in systemic sclerosis: recommendations of a North American expert panel. Clin Exp Rheumatol. 2010;28(2 Suppl 58):S42–6.
13. Kirby DF, Chatterjee S. Evaluation and management of gastro-intestinal manifestations in scleroderma. Curr Opin Rheumatol. 2014;26(6):621–9.
14. Brown M, Teubner A, Shaffer J, Herrick AL. Home parenteral nutrition—an effective and safe long-term therapy for systemic sclerosis-related intestinal failure. Rheumatology (Oxford). 2008;47(2):176–9.
15. Ishikawa M, Okada J, Kondo H. Five cases of systemic sclerosis with associated with intestinal pseudo-obstruction. Ryumachi. 1999;39(5):768–73.
16. Krasaelap A, Kovacic K, Goday PS. Nutrition management in pediatric gastrointestinal motility disorders. Nutr Clin Pract. 2020;35(2):265–72.

Progressive Interstitial Lung Disease Non-Responsive to Immunosuppressive Therapy

55

Katherine C. Silver, Kristin B. Highland, and Richard M. Silver

Case Presentation

A 27-year-old Caucasian woman presented at 23 6/7 weeks gestational age with seizures and hypoxic respiratory failure. She had no relevant past medical history, but family history was significant for a mother and sister with lupus. On initial examination, her blood pressure was 200/130 mmHg and on chest exam she had bibasilar inspiratory crackles. Laboratory workup revealed acute kidney injury, thrombocytopenia, and microangiopathic hemolytic anemia. She was originally thought to have eclampsia; however, she did not improve following delivery. Upon further investigation, she was found to have a positive ANA (1:320, homogeneous pattern), a positive anti-Scl-70 antibody, and abnormal capillary morphology. In the absence of initial skin changes, she was diagnosed with systemic sclerosis *sine* scleroderma presenting as scleroderma renal crisis (SRC). An angiotensin-converting enzyme (ACE) inhibitor was prescribed, and she had complete recovery from SRC. Within several months of initial presentation, she developed skin changes consistent with diffuse cutaneous SSc. She was noted to have a decrease in forced vital capacity (FVC) and diffusing capacity for carbon monoxide (DL_{CO}), so she underwent high-resolution computed tomography (HRCT) chest scan that showed mild interstitial lung disease (ILD) (Fig. 55.1a). Bronchoalveolar lavage fluid contained 12.5% neutrophils consistent with active alveolitis.

K. C. Silver · R. M. Silver (✉)
Department of Medicine, Medical University of South Carolina, Charleston, SC, USA
e-mail: silverk@musc.edu; silverr@musc.edu

K. B. Highland
Department of Pulmonary Medicine, Cleveland Clinic, Cleveland, OH, USA
e-mail: highlak@ccf.org

Y. Allanore et al. (eds.), *Scleroderma*, https://doi.org/10.1007/978-3-031-40658-4_55

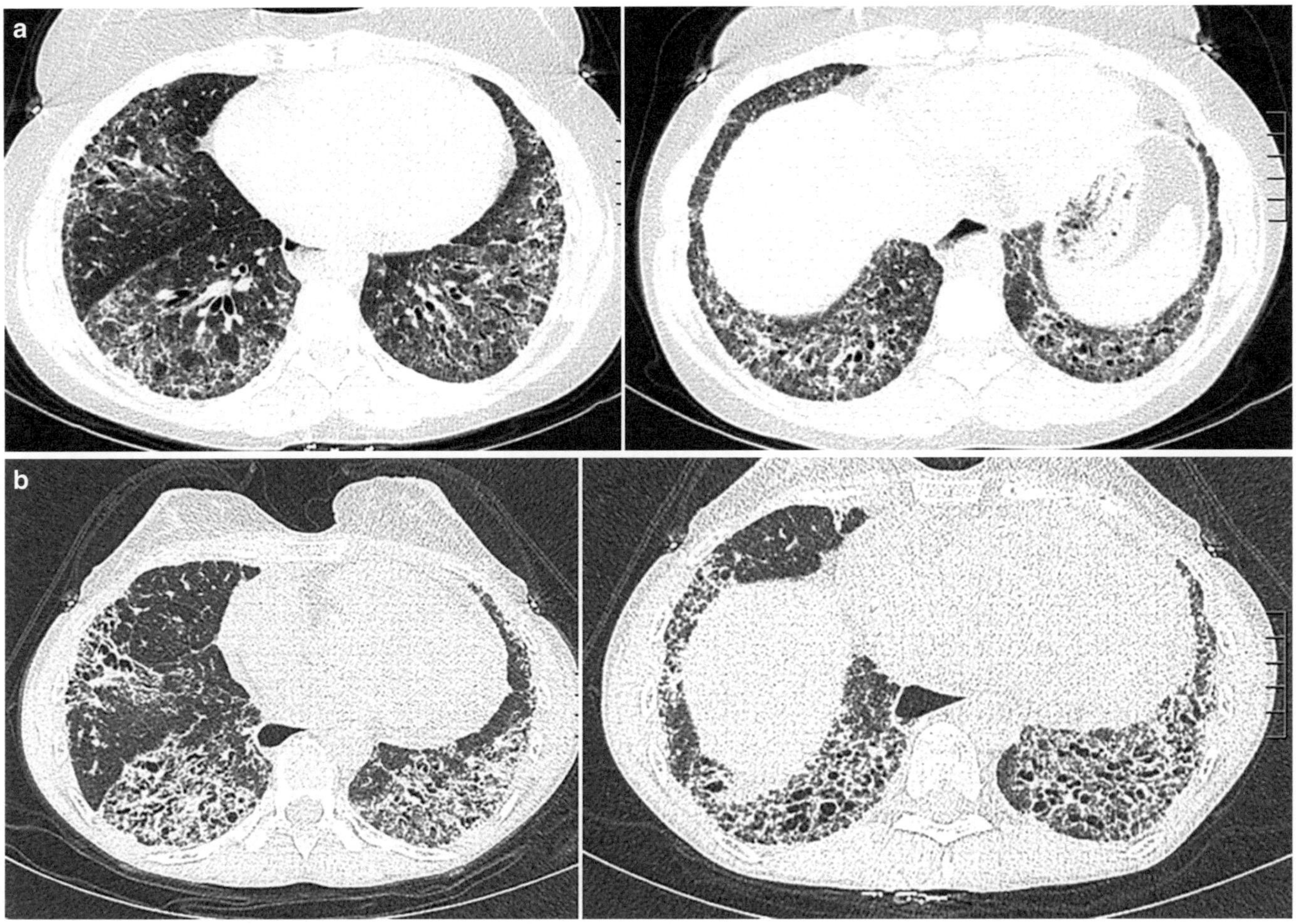

Fig. 55.1 (**a**) HRCT chest scan showing mild systemic sclerosis-associated interstitial lung disease (SSc-ILD) with ground glass opacification at both lung bases. (**b**) HRCT chest scan 8 years later and despite treatment showing honeycomb changes, traction bronchiectasis, and severe SSc-ILD. Compliments of Dr. Dhiraj Baruah, Department of Radiology, Medical University of South Carolina

Treatment Course

Eight months after her initial presentation, the patient was started on oral cyclophosphamide for SSc-ILD. She had improvement in her pulmonary function tests (PFTs) (Fig. 55.2), dyspnea, and modified Rodnan skin score on daily oral cyclophosphamide (2 mg/kg), but this treatment was discontinued after 18 months out of concern for long-term toxicity. Within several months of discontinuing cyclophosphamide, her PFTs worsened so she then received a course of intravenous cyclophosphamide (750 mg/m^2 body surface area monthly) for a total of 6 months. Dyspnea remained stable following treatment with intravenous cyclophosphamide; however, PFTs continued to decline and so she was started on mycophenolate mofetil (MMF) titrated up to a dose of 1.5 g twice daily. PFTs and HRCT chest scan continued to worsen (Fig. 55.1b) and she developed anemia. MMF was stopped after just a few months and intravenous cyclophosphamide was resumed. Over the next several months, the patient had a decrease in her exercise capacity and increasing oxygen requirement. FVC decreased to 41% predicted and DL_{CO} decreased to just 23% predicted. Thus, experimental therapy with a tyrosine-kinase inhibitor, imatinib, was begun (prior to the availability of nintedanib [vide infra], in addition to oral cyclophosphamide. After 1 year, she developed pancytopenia so both cyclophosphamide and imatinib were discontinued. Her oxygen requirement had increased to 6 L/min, so she was referred for lung transplant evaluation. She was initially rejected due to severe esophageal dysmotility and gastroesophageal reflux disease (GERD). A second lung transplant center recommended surgical management of GERD prior to proceeding with lung transplant, so she underwent a Roux-en-Y gastric bypass to manage her GERD. During this time, her ILD appeared to remain stable. The patient continued pulmonary rehabilitation and was able to be weaned off supplemental oxygen. PFTs improved as well, with FVC increasing to 51% predicted and DL_{CO} increasing to 52% predicted (Fig. 55.2).

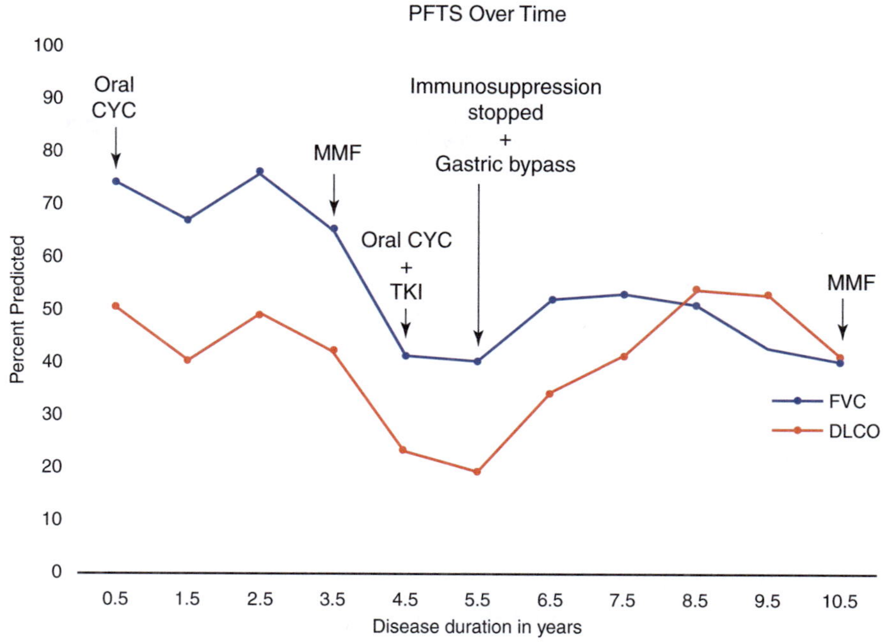

Fig. 55.2 Pulmonary function tests (PFT) over time. *FVC* Forced Vital Capacity, *DLCO* Diffusing Capacity for Carbon Monoxide, *MMF* Mycophenolate mofetil, *CYC* Cyclophosphamide, *TKI* Tyrosine kinase inhibitor

After doing well for several years, her FVC and DL_{CO} began to trend downward, and she once again required supplemental oxygen. Right heart catheterization revealed mild pulmonary hypertension with a mean PA pressure of 32 mmHg. MMF was resumed and tadalafil was added to her medical regimen. She is once again undergoing evaluation for lung transplant.

Discussion

Since the introduction of angiotensin-converting enzyme (ACE) inhibitor therapy as the first effective treatment for scleroderma renal crisis (SRC), ILD has become a leading cause of morbidity and mortality in scleroderma (SSc) [1, 2]. Our patient had a number of risk factors for the presence and progression of SSc-ILD (Table 55.1). Interstitial lung disease may occur in all subtypes of SSc, but the prevalence of SSc-ILD is higher in patients with diffuse cutaneous SSc [3]. Although our patient originally presented as systemic sclerosis *sine* scleroderma, she quickly went on to develop dcSSc with a high modified Rodnan skin score. She also was found to have anti-topoisomerase I (anti-Scl-70) auto-antibodies, the presence of which is strongly linked to SSc-ILD with over 85% of Scl-70+ patients going on to develop pulmonary fibrosis [4]. Soon after her diagnosis of SSc, our patient was found to have ILD as evident by a decline in her FVC and abnormalities on both chest CT and bronchoalveolar lavage studies. Studies show that the greatest risk of progression of SSc occurs within the first 5 years of disease, with an abnormal FVC during this time-frame being an important predictor for eventual end-stage lung disease [5]. Patients with more extensive fibrosis (>20%) on CT are also at significantly higher risk to experience rapid decline in pulmonary function and death [6]. Likewise, patients with increased granulocytes on BAL have greater dyspnea and reduction in lung volumes and diffusion capacity that persists over time [7]. Although our patient did not have the classical symptoms of gastroesophageal reflux disease (GERD), she eventually was found to have severely abnormal esophageal function on testing during evaluation for lung transplantation. Aggressive treatment with proton pump inhibitors (PPIs), histamine (H2) blockers and eventually a Roux-en-Y gastric bypass significantly improved her pulmonary function and reduced her supplemental oxygen requirement. An association between GERD and several different ILDs including SSc-ILD exists, and the extent of SSc-ILD as assessed by pulmonary function and CT has been correlated to the degree of esophageal reflux. The sum of these risk factors may explain in part why our patient did not respond to conventional immunosuppressive treatment.

Table 55.1 Risk factors for presence and progression of interstitial lung disease

- Male gender
- African ancestry
- Diffuse skin involvement
- Auto-antibodies
  - Topoisomerase (Scl-70)
  - U1-RNP
  - U3-RNP
  - Th/To
  - PM/Scl
- Early SSc (<5 years from initial non-Raynaud phenomenon symptom)
- Abnormal forced vital capacity
- Extensive fibrosis on HRCT (>20%)
- GERD

The decision to begin cyclophosphamide in our patient was based on data from the Scleroderma Lung Study I [8], which was designed as a randomized multicenter, double-blind, placebo-controlled trial to evaluate the efficacy and safety of oral cyclophosphamide for 1 year in patients with symptomatic SSc-ILD and evidence of disease activity by BAL and/or CT chest scan. This was the first positive study in SSc-ILD and showed a modest improvement in FVC, the primary endpoint (2.53% adjusted FVC % predicted, $p < 0.03$) and improvement in a number of secondary endpoints including total lung capacity, modified Rodnan skin score, Transition Dyspnea Index, extent of fibrosis on chest HRCT, and several quality-of-life measures [8, 9]. Unfortunately, like in our patient, the treatment effect was lost by 24 months [10]. In an attempt to mitigate some of the long-term side-effects of oral cyclophosphamide, we then treated our patient with intravenous cyclophosphamide, in part based on data from the Fibrosing Alveolitis in Scleroderma Trial (FAST) [11]. This small study randomized patients to receive either intravenous cyclophosphamide for 6 months followed by daily oral azathioprine, or placebo infusions followed by oral placebo. At 12 months, a modest but non-statistically significant improvement in FVC was seen in the actively treated group ($p = 0.08$).

Cyclophosphamide has been quoted as "arguably the most toxic immunosuppressive agent currently used to treat autoimmune diseases" [12], which prompted investigation into safer, less toxic alternatives. In a number of uncontrolled, prospective or retrospective case series, mycophenolate mofetil (MMF) was shown to stabilize or improve lung function in patients with SSc-ILD [13–24]. Scleroderma Lung Study II was designed to evaluate the efficacy and safety of MMF for 2 years in comparison with oral cyclophosphamide for 1 year followed by placebo for an additional year [25]. Subjects in each treatment arm demonstrated an improvement in FVC % predicted at month 24 (2.2% with MMF and 2.9% with cyclophosphamide) together with improvement in dyspnea and a reduction of the extent of ILD on chest CT scan. MMF had better tolerability than cyclophosphamide with fewer withdrawals due to adverse events and fewer treatment-related serious adverse events. More than twice as many deaths occurred in the cyclophosphamide group with most attributed to progression of ILD [25]. Unfortunately, MMF is also not without side-effects, and our patient developed anemia while on this drug.

There has been interest in the use of tyrosine kinase inhibitors for SSc-ILD because of downstream effects to inhibit transforming growth factor-beta and platelet-derived growth factor, key signaling molecules in the pathogenesis of SSc-ILD. In a study of 30 consecutive SSc-ILD patients non-responsive to cyclophosphamide, treatment with low-dose imatinib for 6 months resulted in stabilization or improvement in 22 patients (73%) [26]. Other studies, as in our patient, showed poor tolerability of imatinib [27–32]. Nintedanib, a different tyrosine kinase inhibitor, along with another anti-fibrotic agent, pirfenidone, have been approved by the FDA to slow the decline in pulmonary function in idiopathic pulmonary fibrosis (IPF) patients [33, 34]. Subsequently, nintedanib was approved by the FDA and the European Commission to slow the rate of decline in pulmonary function for adults with SSc-ILD. Approval was based on the results of the pivotal phase III clinical trial SENSCIS (Safety and Efficacy of Nintedanib in Systemic SClerosIS) [35]. In this placebo-controlled trial comprised of 576 patients with SSc-ILD, nintedanib significantly reduced the annual rate of decline of FVC compared to placebo (−52.4 mL/year versus −93.3 mL/year, difference 41.0 mL/year [95% CI 2.9, 41.0, $p = 0.04$]) [35]. Nintedanib was effective in reducing the rate of decline of FVC in patients who were or were not receiving MMF, with a greater treatment effect in those who were receiving background therapy with MMF [35]. Gastrointestinal side-effects were common and similar to those observed in patients receiving nintedanib for IPF. In our patient, nintedanib was not available until later in the course of her disease, and an earlier trial with imatinib was inefficacious. Pirfenidone, another anti-fibrotic agent approved for IPF had been under study for SSc-ILD in the Scleroderma Lung Study III (ClinicalTrials.gov Identifier: NCT03221257), however, that clinical trial was halted due to recruitment issues centered around the COVID-19 pandemic. Additional studies are needed to determine a role for combination (immunosuppressive and antifibrotic) therapies for SSc-ILD.

A number of other immunosuppressive agents which were not tried in our patient have recently become of interest in treating SSc-ILD. Several small studies [36, 37] suggest that rituximab may improve or stabilize PFTs and CT chest scan changes. A prospective study from the EUSTAR cohort looked at rituximab in SSc patients, 58% of whom were treated for SSc-ILD, found no effects on FVC or DL_{CO} [38]. Compared to more than 9500 matched control patients, rituximab-treated patients were more likely to have improvement in skin score but did not demonstrate different rates of decline in FVC or DL_{CO} [38]. Several ongoing clinical trials of rituximab and other biologic agents in patients with CTD-ILD are currently underway [39].

IL-6 has been implicated in the pathogenesis of SSc as well as with declines in FVC and DL_{CO} in SSc-ILD, so there has been interest in using the monoclonal anti-IL-6R antibody tocilizumab to treat SSc. FaSScinate was a phase II trial of tocilizumab in early dcSSc patients [40]. While the trial failed to meet its primary endpoint of decrease in skin score over 48 weeks, there was a suggestion of preservation of FVC in the tocilizumab group compared to the placebo group. FocuSSced, a phase III trial clinical in a similar patient population, demonstrated in a key secondary analysis an effect of tocilizumab on lung function preservation [41]. A post-hoc analysis of the 136 FocuSSced subjects with ILD found that the patients in the tocilizumab group demonstrated preserved

FVC over 48 weeks compared to the patients in the placebo group. For mild, moderate, and severe QILD (chest CT quantitative ILD), the mean decline in the FVC % predicted with tocilizumab was −4.1, 0.7, and 2.1, respectively, compared to placebo where the mean decline in the FVC % predicted was −10.0, −5.7, and −6.7, respectively [42]. In these early disease patients, tocilizumab appeared to be effective in preserving lung function irrespective of the degree of quantitative ILD or fibrosis at baseline [42].

Because both conventional and nonconventional treatments for SSc-ILD failed, our patient chose to pursue lung transplantation. Many centers, as our patient encountered, are reluctant to perform lung transplantation in scleroderma patients because of the high prevalence of esophageal dysfunction that is believed to contribute to allograft dysfunction. Nevertheless, transplant outcomes have been shown to be similar in carefully selected SSc patients compared to patients with IPF and patients with pulmonary arterial hypertension (PAH). For SSc patients undergoing lung transplantation, the 2-year and 5-year survival was reported to be 72% and 55%, respectively [43, 44], although the severity of GERD was shown to impact the 1-year survival rate [45]. There have been no reports of recurrence of SSc-ILD in the lung allograft [46].

Autologous hematopoietic stem cell transplantation (aHSCT) is another potential therapy for selected patients with scleroderma. The Autologous Stem Cell Transplantation International Scleroderma Trial (ASTIS) [47] included a high percentage of patients with mild to moderate restrictive lung disease (86.5% of 156 subjects). At 5.8 years of follow-up, a statistically significant difference favoring aHSCT was found in lung function (mean change in FVC 6.3% vs −2.8% predicted and TLC 5.1% vs −1.3% predicted). Treatment-related mortality was high in the first year (10.1% with aHSCT versus 0% with cyclophosphamide) [47]. In contrast, the Scleroderma: Cyclophosphamide Or Transplantation Study (SCOT) had a treatment-related mortality in the first year that was much lower than in the ASTIS study (0% versus 10.1%), and aHSCT was associated with improved event-free and overall survival [48]. At 72 months, the rate of event-free survival was 74% in the aHSCT group and only 47% in the cyclophosphamide group ($p = 0.03$), and the rate of overall survival was 86% and 51%, respectively ($p = 0.02$), Whole lung quantitative ILD scores decreased significantly in the transplantation group, while there was no change in the cyclophosphamide group ($p = 0.02$), and there was a significant difference in whole lung quantitative lung fibrosis, increasing in the cyclophosphamide arm versus stability in the aHSCT arm ($p = 0.047$) [48, 49].

In the smaller non-myeloablative Autologous Stem Cell Systemic Sclerosis Immune Suppression Trial (ASSIST) trial [50], 10 patients demonstrated improvement in lung function as well as reduction in the extent of lung disease on chest HRCT. Eight of 9 control patients (cyclophosphamide-treated) showed disease progression, and 7 of these patients then crossed over to aHSCT therapy. After 2 years, 11/18 patients showed persistent improvement in HRCT and FVC (but not TLC or DLCO).

Our patient later presented with increased dyspnea and worsened exercise tolerance without substantial change in PFTs or chest CT. This prompted investigation for pulmonary hypertension (PH), a co-morbid condition seen in approximately 45% of patients with SSc-ILD [51], and one that carries a significant increase in morbidity and mortality. Our patient had a number of clinical risk factors for the development of SSc-ILD-PH: female, Caucasian, dcSSc, disease duration more than 10 years, presence of telangiectasia and severe Raynaud phenomenon. DL_{CO} <40% predicted or FVC % predicted/DL_{CO} % predicted >1.6 may be predictive of the presence of pulmonary hypertension in the background of interstitial lung disease (Table 55.2) [52–55]. Echocardiogram is often inaccurate in patients with advanced lung disease [56], so the clinician should have a low clinical threshold to obtain right heart catheterization, the gold standard to establish the diagnosis of pulmonary arterial hypertension, whenever pulmonary hypertension is suspected. Identification of pulmonary hypertension in our patient increased her lung allocation score moving her higher up on the transplantation list.

The safety and efficacy of pulmonary arterial hypertension (PAH)-specific vasodilator therapy in patients with SSc-ILD-PH has been questioned owing to concern that these drugs might be associated with worsening hypoxemia due to a V/Q mismatch. In a retrospective analysis of 70 patients with SSc-ILD-PH, no benefit was observed in WHO functional class, 6-min walk distance and hemodynamics with prostanoids, phosphodiesterase-5 inhibitors, or endothelin receptor antagonists [53]. Nevertheless, in small case series some patients have received benefit from reducing pulmonary vascular resistance without significantly reducing oxygen tension [51]. A larger, single-center cohort found that a large proportion of patients with >20% extent of ILD on HRCT may have features of both PAH and WHO Group III PH. When such patients were treated with

Table 55.2 Clinical risk factors for development of SSc-ILD-PH

- Female gender
- European ancestry
- Diffuse skin involvement
- Late age of onset of systemic sclerosis
- Disease duration greater than 10 years
- Presence of telangiectasias
- Severe Raynaud phenomenon
- Auto-antibodies
  - Anti-nucleolar antibody
  - U3RNP
  - Cardiolipin

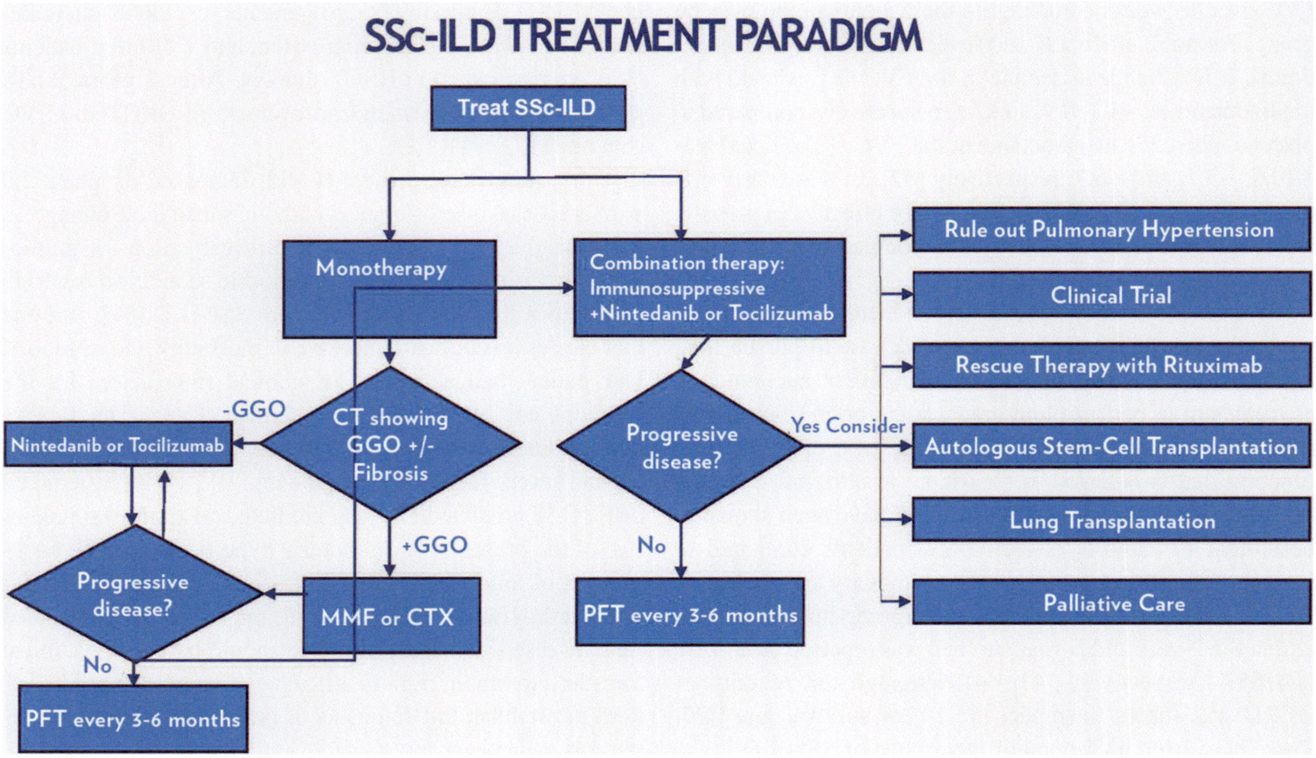

Fig. 55.3 SSc-ILD Treatment Paradigm. A schema of treatment for patients with scleroderma-associated interstitial lung disease (SSc-ILD). Abbreviations: *CT* Computed tomography, *GGG* Ground glass opacification, *PFT* Pulmonary function tests, *MMF* Mycophenolate mofetil, *CTX* Cyclophosphamide

PAH-specific therapies along with immunosuppressive agents for ILD, the majority were found to tolerate PAH-specific therapy regardless of simultaneous or prior ILD treatment, with stability in WHO functional class and/or 6-min walk test [57]. INCREASE was a recently completed placebo-controlled trial of inhaled trepostinil that enrolled more than 325 ILD patients with PH, some of whom had SSc-ILD with WHO group III PH [58]. Inhaled trepostinil therapy was found to improve exercise capacity as assessed by the 6-min walk test (at week 16, the least-squares mean difference between the trepostinil group and the placebo group in the change from baseline was 31.1 m [95% confidence interval 16.85–45.39, $p < 0.001$). In addition to the improvement noted in exercise capacity, inhaled trepostinil treatment was associated with a reduction in NT-proBNP levels from baseline, as well as with a reduction in time to clinical worsening [58]. Sotatercept, a fusion protein that binds to and sequesters select TGF-beta superfamily ligands, is a promising new therapy for PAH, including CTD-related PAH [59].

Lastly, patients with SSc-ILD should receive supportive care including supplemental oxygen, pneumococcal vaccinations, and viral vaccinations (shingles, influenza, RSV and COVID-19), referral for pulmonary rehabilitation, psychosocial counseling, pregnancy prevention and, in some cases, palliative care. Patients treated with cyclophosphamide should also receive prophylaxis antibiotic therapy to prevent *Pneumocystis jirovecii* infection. Palliative care aimed at improving and maintaining quality of life should be discussed and initiated early in the disease course depending on the individual patient's needs, preferences, culture, and religion [60].

One example of a treatment decision paradigm is presented in Fig. 55.3, with the following caveats: (1) formal treatment guidelines have yet to be established; (2) treatment decisions should be based on multidisciplinary discussions among pulmonologists, rheumatologists, radiologists, etc., and (3) it is critically important to include input from the patient and family in all treatment decisions.

References

1. Steen VD, Medsger TA Jr. Changes in causes of death in systemic sclerosis. Ann Rheum Dis. 2007;66:940–4.
2. Ferri C, Valentini G, Cozzi F, et al. Systemic sclerosis: demographic, clinical, and serologic features and survival in 1,012 Italian patients. Medicine (Baltimore). 2002;81:139–53.
3. Walker UA, Tyndall A, Czirják L, et al. Clinical risk assessment of organ manifestations in systemic sclerosis: a report from the EULAR scleroderma trials and research group database. Ann Rheum Dis. 2007;66:754–63.

4. Briggs DC, Vaughan RW, Welsh KI, Myers A, duBois RM, Black CM. Immunogenetic prediction of pulmonary fibrosis in systemic sclerosis. Lancet. 1991;338:661–2.
5. Morgan C, Knight C, Lunt M, Black CM, Silman AJ. Predictors of end stage lung disease in a cohort of patients with scleroderma. Ann Rheum Dis. 2003;62:146–50.
6. Goh NS, Desai SR, Veeraraghavan S, et al. Interstitial lung disease in systemic sclerosis: a simple staging system. Am J Respir Crit Care Med. 2008;177:1238–54.
7. Silver RM, Miller KS, Kinsella MB, Smith EA, Schabel SI. Evaluation and management of scleroderma lung disease using bronchoalveolar lavage. Am J Med. 1990;88:47–76.
8. Tashkin D, Elashoff R, Clements P, et al. Cyclophosphamide versus placebo in scleroderma lung disease. N Engl J Med. 2006;25(354):2655–66.
9. Goldin JG, Lynch DA, Strollo DC, et al. Follow-up HRCT after treatment of scleroderma-interstitial lung disease with cyclophosphamide demonstrates evidence for treatment effect. Am J Respir Crit Care Med. 2008;177(A768):91.
10. Tashkin DP, Elashoff R, Clements PJ, et al. Effects of 1-year treatment with cyclophosphamide on outcomes at 2 years in scleroderma lung disease. Am J Respir Crit Care Med. 2007;176:1026–34.
11. Hoyles RK, Ellis RW, Wellsbury J, et al. A multicenter, prospective, randomized, double-blind, placebo-controlled trial of corticosteroids and intravenous cyclophosphamide followed by oral azathioprine for the treatment of pulmonary fibrosis in scleroderma. Arthritis Rheum. 2006;54:3962–70.
12. Martinez FJ, McCune WJ. Cyclophosphamide for scleroderma lung disease. N Engl J Med. 2006;345:2707–9.
13. Swigris JJ, Olson AL, Fischer A, et al. Mycophenolate mofetil is safe, well tolerated, and preserves lung function in patients with connective tissue disease-related interstitial lung disease. Chest. 2006;130:30–6.
14. Liossis SN, Bounas A, Andonopoulos AP. Mycophenolate mofetil as first-line treatment improves clinically evident early scleroderma lung disease. Rheumatology (Oxford). 2006;45:1005–8.
15. Nihtyanova SI, Brough GM, Black CM, Denton CP. Mycophenolate mofetil in diffuse cutaneous systemic sclerosis—a retrospective analysis. Rheumatology (Oxford). 2007;46:442–5.
16. Zamora AC, Wolters PJ, Collard HR, et al. Use of mycophenolate mofetil to treat scleroderma-associated interstitial lung disease. Respir Med. 2008;102:150–5.
17. Gerbino AJ, Goss CH, Molitor JA. Effect of mycophenolate mofetil on pulmonary function in scleroderma-associated interstitial lung disease. Chest. 2008;133:455–60.
18. Derk CT, Grace E, Shenin M, Naik M, Schulz S, Xiong W. A prospective open-label study of mycophenolate mofetil for the treatment of diffuse systemic sclerosis. Rheumatology. 2009;48:1595–9.
19. Koutroumpas A, Ziogas A, Alexiou I, Barouta G, Sakkas LI. Mycophenolate mofetil in systemic sclerosis-associated interstitial lung disease. Clin Rheumatol. 2010;29:1167–8.
20. Le EN, Wigley FM, Shah AA, Boin F, Hummers LK. Long-term experience of mycophenolate mofetil for treatment of diffuse cutaneous systemic sclerosis. Ann Rheum Dis. 2011;70:1104–7.
21. Simeon-Aznar CP, Fonollosa-Pia V, Tolosa-Vilella C, Selva-O'Callaghan A, Solans-Laque R, Vilardeli-Tarres M. Effect of mycophenolate sodium in scleroderma-related interstitial lung disease. Clin Rheumatol. 2011;30:1393–8.
22. Mendoza FA, Nagle SJ, Lee JB, Jimenez SA. A prospective observational study of mycophenolate mofetil treatment in progressive diffuse cutaneous systemic sclerosis of recent onset. J Rheumatol. 2012;39:1241–7.
23. Henes JC, Horger M, Amberger C, et al. Enteric-coated mycophenolate sodium for progressive systemic sclerosis—a prospective open-label study with CT histography for monitoring pulmonary fibrosis. Clin Rheumatol. 2013;32:673–8.
24. Panopoulos ST, Bournia VK, Trakada G, Giavri I, Kostopoulos C, Sfikakis PP. Mycophenolate versus cyclophosphamide for progressive interstitial lung disease associated with systemic sclerosis: a 2-year case control study. Lung 2013;191:483–489.
25. Tashkin DP, Roth MD, Clements PJ, et al. Mycophenolate mofetil versus oral cyclophosphamide in scleroderma-related interstitial lung disease (SLS II): a randomized controlled, double-blind, parallel group trial. Lancet Respir Med. 2016;4:708–19.
26. Fraticelli P, Gabrielli B, Pomponio G, et al. Low-dose oral imatinib in the treatment of systemic sclerosis interstitial lung disease unresponsive to cyclophosphamide: a phase II pilot study. Arthritis Res Ther. 2014;16:R144.
27. Pope J, McBain D, Petrlich L, Watson S, Vanderhoek L, de Leon F, Seney S, Summers K. Imatinib in active diffuse cutaneous systemic sclerosis: results of a six-month, randomized, double-blind, placebo-controlled, proof-of-concept pilot study at a single center. Arthritis Rheum. 2011;63:3547–51.
28. Spiera RF, Gordon JK, Mersten JN, Magro CM, Mehta M, Wildman HF, Kloiber S, Kirou KA, Lyman S, Crow MK. Imatinib mesylate (Gleevec) in the treatment of diffuse cutaneous systemic sclerosis: results of a 1-year, phase IIa, single-arm, open-label clinical trial. Ann Rheum Dis. 2011;70:1003–9.
29. Khanna D, Saggar R, Mayes MD, Abtin F, Clements PJ, Maranian P, Assassi S, Saggar R, Singh RR, Furst DE. A one-year, phase I/IIa, open-label pilot trial of imatinib mesylate in the treatment of systemic sclerosis-associated active interstitial lung disease. Arthritis Rheum. 2011;63:3540–6.
30. Distler O, Distler JHW, Varga J, Denton CP, Lafyatis RA, Wigley FM, Schett G. A multi-center, open-label, proof of concept study of imatinib mesylate demonstrate no benefit for the treatment of fibrosis in patients with early, diffuse systemic sclerosis. [abstract]. Arthritis Rheum. 2010;62:560.
31. Guo L, Chen XX, Gu YY, Zou HJ, Ye S. Low-dose imatinib in the treatment of severe systemic sclerosis: a case series of six Chinese patients and literature review. Clin Rheumatol. 2012;31: 1395–400.
32. Prey S, Ezzedine K, Doussau A, Grandoulier AS, Barcat D, Chatelus E, Diot E, Durant C, Havchulla E, de Korwin-Krokowski JD, Kostrzewa E, Quemeneur T, Paul C, Schaeverbeke T, Seneschal J, Solanilla A, Sparsa A, Bouchet S, Lepreux S, Mahon FX, Chene G, Taïeb A. Imatinib mesylate in scleroderma-associated diffuse skin fibrosis: a phase II multicentre randomized double-blinded controlled trial. Br J Dermatol. 2012;167:1138–44.
33. King TE, Bradford WZ, Castro-Bernardini S, et al. A phase 3 trial of pirfenidone in patients with idiopathic pulmonary fibrosis. N Engl J Med. 2014;370:2083–92.
34. Richeldi L, du Bois RM, Raghu G, et al. Efficacy and safety of nintedanib in idiopathic pulmonary fibrosis. N Engl J Med. 2014;370:2071–82.
35. Distler O, Highland KB, Gahlemann M, et al. Nintedanib for scleroderma-associated interstitial lung disease. N Engl J Med. 2019;380:2518–28.
36. Daoussis D, Liossis SN, Tsamandas AC, et al. Experience with rituximab in scleroderma: results from a 1-year, proof-of-principle study. Rheumatology (Oxford). 2010;49:271–80.
37. Jordan S, Distler JHW, Maurer B, Huscher D, van Laar JM, Allanore Y, Distler O, on behalf of the EUSTAR rituximab study group. doi: https://doi.org/10.1136/annrheumdis-2013-204522.
38. Elhai M, Boubaya M, Distler O, et al. Outcomes of patients with systemic sclerosis treated with rituximab in contemporary practice: a prospective cohort study. Ann Rheum Dis. 2019;78: 979–87.
39. Distler O, Volkmann ER, Hoffmann-Vold AM, Maher TM. Current and future perspectives on management of systemic sclerosis-associated interstitial lung disease. Exp Rev Clin Immunol. 2019;15(10):1009–17.

40. Khanna D, Denton CP, Jahreis A, et al. Safety and efficacy of subcutaneous tocilizumab in adults with systemic sclerosis (fascinate): a phase 2 randomised, controlled trial. Lancet. 2016;387:2630–40.
41. Khanna D, Lin CJF, Furst DE, et al. A randomized, double-blind, placebo-controlled phase 3 trial of tocilizumab in systemic sclerosis. Lancet Respir Med. 2020;8:P963–74.
42. Roofeh D, Lin CJF, Goldin J, et al. Tocilizumab prevents progression of early systemic sclerosis associated interstitial lung disease. Arthritis Rheumatol. 2021;73:1301. https://doi.org/10.1002/art.41668.
43. Shitrit D, Amitai A, Peled N, et al. Lung transplantation in patients with scleroderma: case series, review of the literature, and criteria for transplantation. Clin Transpl. 2009;23:178–83.
44. Schachna L, Medsger TA Jr, Dauber JH, et al. Lung transplantation in scleroderma compared with idiopathic pulmonary fibrosis and idiopathic pulmonary arterial hypertension. Arthritis Rheum. 2006;54:3954–61.
45. Fisichella PM, Reder NP, Gagermeier J, Kovacs EJ. Usefulness of pH monitoring in predicting the survival status of patients with scleroderma awaiting lung transplantation. J Surg Res. 2014;189:232–7.
46. Khan IY, Singer LG, de Perrot M, et al. Survival after lung transplantation in systemic sclerosis. A systematic review. Respir Med. 2013;107:2081–7.
47. Van Laar JM, Farge D, Sont JK, et al. For the EBMT/EULAR Scleroderma Study Group. Autologous hematopoietic stem cell transplantation vs intravenous pulse cyclophosphamide in diffuse cutaneous systemic sclerosis. A randomized clinical trial. JAMA. 2014;311:2490–8.
48. Sullivan KM, Goldmuntz EA, Keyes-Elstein L, et al. Myeloablative stem-cell transplantation for severe scleroderma. N Engl J Med. 2018;378:35–47.
49. Goldin J, Keyes-Elstein L, Crofford L, et al. Changes in quantitative scleroderma lung CT measures in patients treated with cyclophosphamide or transplantation. Abstract 901, American College of Rheumatology Annual Meeting; 2018.
50. Burt RK, Shah SJ, Dill K, et al. Autologous non-myeloablative haemopoietic stem-cell transplantation compared with pulse cyclophosphamide once per month for systemic sclerosis (ASSIST): an open-label, randomized phase 2 trial. Lancet. 2011;378:498–506.
51. Ryu JH, Krowka MJ, Pellikka PA, Swanson KL, McGoon MD. Pulmonary hypertension in patients with interstitial lung diseases. Mayo Clin Proc. 2007;82:342–50.
52. Chang B, Wigley FM, White B, Wise RA. Scleroderma patients with combined pulmonary hypertension and interstitial lung disease. J Rheumatol. 2003;30:2398–405.
53. Le Pavec J, Girgis RE, Lechtzin N, et al. Systemic sclerosis-related pulmonary hypertension associated with interstitial lung disease: impact of pulmonary arterial hypertension therapies. Arthritis Rheum. 2011;63:2456–64.
54. Shlobin OA, Nathan. Pulmonary hypertension secondary to interstitial lung disease. Expert Rev Respir Med. 2011;5:179–89.
55. Hinchcliff M, Fisher A, Schiopu E, Steen VD, PHAROS Investigators. Pulmonary hypertension assessment and recognition of outcomes in scleroderma (PHAROS): baseline characteristics and description of study population. J Rheumatol. 2011;38:2172–9.
56. Arcasoy SM, Christie JD, Ferrari VA, Sutton MS, et al. Echocardiographic assessment of pulmonary hypertension in patients with advanced lung disease. Am J Respir Crit Care Med. 2003;167:735–40.
57. Young A, Vummidi D, Visovatti S, et al. Prevalence, treatment, and outcomes of coexistent pulmonary hypertension and interstitial lung disease in systemic sclerosis. Arthritis Rheumatol. 2019;8:1339–49.
58. Waxman A, Restrepo-Jaramillo R, Thenappan T, et al. Inhaled treprostinil in pulmonary hypertension due to interstitial lung disease. N Engl J Med. 2021;384:325–34.
59. Humbert M, McLaughlin V, Gibbs JSR, et al. Sotatercept for the treatment of pulmonary arterial hypertension: PULSAR open-label extension. Eur Resp J. 2023;61:2201347. https://doi.org/10.1183/13993003.01347-2022.
60. Kreuter M, Bendstrup E, Russell AM, et al. Palliative care in interstitial lung disease: living well. Lancet Resp Med. 2017;5:968–80.

Body Image Distress in Scleroderma

56

Shadi Gholizadeh, Rina S. Fox, Sarah D. Mills,
Lisa R. Jewett, Brett D. Thombs, and Vanessa L. Malcarne

Case Study

A 41-year-old woman with scleroderma presented to her rheumatologist for her 12-month follow-up. At the time of her first symptoms, a little more than a year prior, she had presented to her primary care physician with fatigue, gastrointestinal complaints, and numbness in her fingertips and hands. She had also reported cold sensitivity with dramatic color changes of pallor and cyanosis of her fingers with recent onset. Due to the fact that her job as a case manager in a small law firm required many hours of typing each day, she had attributed the growing numbness and tingling in her hands to carpal tunnel syndrome. She had not been overly concerned about most of her symptoms and had a theory that her fatigue and gastrointestinal issues resulted from an undiagnosed thyroid disorder because her symptoms mirrored those of a friend with Hashimoto's Disease. However, her cold fingers were worrisome, and she consequently had sought help from her doctor.

The patient's physician had noted puffy fingers and requested a full blood panel. General laboratory tests were normal, but serological tests were remarkable for a positive antinuclear antibody (ANA). Because the woman had been experiencing new onset Raynaud's and had a positive ANA, the potential for an autoimmune disease, like scleroderma, was immediately recognized, and a rheumatologist was consulted. The rheumatologist had made the diagnosis of scleroderma based on abnormal skin thickening of the fingers (sclerodactyly), abnormal nailfold capillaries, and a confirmation of her positive ANA with a positive anti-SCL70. The patient reported having been shocked, as she had no family history of autoimmune or rheumatic diseases, and she had believed that her generally healthy lifestyle would have protected her from these kinds of diseases. At the time of diagnosis, the patient had described frustration with the uncertainty around living with scleroderma, particularly in terms of its unpredictable course. Furthermore, as she was the mother of two young daughters, she had expressed anxi-

S. Gholizadeh (✉)
Clinical PsyD Program, California School of Professional Psychology/Alliant International University-Los Angeles, Alhambra, CA, USA
e-mail: shadi@thekey.com

R. S. Fox
Department of Medical Social Sciences, Northwestern University Feinberg School of Medicine, Chicago, IL, USA
e-mail: rsfox@arizona.edu

S. D. Mills
Department of Health Behavior, University of North Carolina at Chapel Hill, Chapel Hill, NC, USA

Lineberger Comprehensive Cancer Center, University of North Carolina at Chapel Hill, Chapel Hill, NC, USA
e-mail: sarahmills@unc.edu

L. R. Jewett
Department of Psychiatry, Institute of Community and Family Psychiatry, Jewish General Hospital, Montreal, QC, Canada
e-mail: lisa.jewett@mcgill.ca

B. D. Thombs
Lady Davis Institute for Medical Research, Jewish General Hospital, Montreal, QC, Canada

Departments of Psychiatry; Epidemiology, Biostatistics, and Occupational Health; Medicine; Psychology; Educational and Counselling Psychology; and Biomedical Ethics Unit, McGill University, Montreal, QC, Canada
e-mail: brett.thombs@mcgill.ca

V. L. Malcarne
SDSU/UC San Diego Joint Doctoral Program in Clinical Psychology, San Diego, CA, USA

Department of Psychology, San Diego State University, San Diego, CA, USA
e-mail: VMALCARNE@sdsu.edu

Y. Allanore et al. (eds.), *Scleroderma*, https://doi.org/10.1007/978-3-031-40658-4_56

ety about not knowing the etiology of the illness and whether it was possible that her daughters might also develop the disease. The rheumatologist had told her that scleroderma had no curative treatment and that it could shorten her life expectancy. He had ordered special testing of her lung and heart function and started her on medication to help reduce her gastrointestinal reflux and the frequency of her Raynaud's episodes.

The patient spent the next few months pursuing second opinions and consulting alternative medicine practitioners with the hope that she could discover an approach that would reverse the illness. She had returned to the rheumatologist after 3 months due to exacerbation of her symptoms, including noticeably advancing skin tightening in her fingers, hands, arms, face, and lower legs, thinning lips, and telangiectasias. At that appointment, she was highly distressed about the skin changes, specifically the skin thickening on her face and hands. She explained to her rheumatologist that she had searched for images associated with the disease on the Internet and had been quite shaken up by the prospect of further changes to her appearance. She also reported the onset of pruritus as well as worsening heartburn and fatigue although she wondered if the fatigue was psychogenic and related to depression secondary to her diagnosis. The patient reported feeling "down" most days and described being unsure as to whether this was normal and expected, given her diagnosis. The rheumatologist found signs of disease progression that explained the worsening symptoms. He ordered new testing that showed progression of lung disease with fibrosis on a high-resolution CT scan. He suggested starting immunosuppression therapy and provided an explanation of the potential benefits, as well as the possible adverse effects, of this approach. The patient had read about various treatments on patient blogs, and she asked her rheumatologist if he would refer her to a scleroderma specialty center at a nearby large university to see if she would qualify for any experimental treatments in addition to immunosuppression therapy.

Over the course of the next several months, the patient's capacity for exercise decreased due to shortness of breath. At her 12-month follow-up appointment, although her rheumatologist reported that the patient's lung function and skin thickening had stabilized, her depression and anxiety had worsened. Now, the patient described feeling "a little guilty" that she was not taking advantage of resources offered to her. She described having access to a support group, but she reported that, whereas she regularly attended her medical appointments and adhered to prescribed medication, dietary, and lifestyle regimens, she had avoided patient support groups and patient networks. She described walking into a support meeting towards the beginning of the first year after her diagnosis and feeling "absolutely terrified" after seeing several women who appeared to be close to her age who had severe manifestations of the disease in the face and hands. The patient also reported feeling guilty that she had not been able to fully perform in her roles as a professional, mother, and wife, as fatigue and discomfort were limiting her physical capacity.

The patient reported finding the progression of facial changes and disfigurement of her hands to be the most alarming aspects of her disease. She described avoiding mirrors and feeling a deep sense of grief around her changing appearance, as well as concerns about the potential that her appearance changes would become even more dramatic. She was interested in potentially exploring cosmetic options for her thinning lips but admitted feeling uncomfortable discussing this with her rheumatologist. She explained, "it seems petty…you know, in light of the other health problems, like my lungs."

When asked about daily activities, the patient reported avoiding social situations, especially in recent months, and spending more time alone. While she remained an active mother in the home, she had stopped going to her children's school events and was concerned about her limited involvement with her children outside of the home. Her withdrawal had impacted her level of physical activity as well, as she no longer went on the long walks that used to be her primary form of exercise. The patient described an upsetting situation in which she had been out walking and had run into someone from her neighborhood who she had not seen for several months. When she greeted this person, the person did not initially recognize her, which the patient attributed to her changed facial features. She also was avoiding sexual encounters with her husband due to discomfort about her appearance. She reported being unable to openly discuss her distress with him for fear of rejection.

In addition, the patient reported that her appearance changes had caused her discomfort at work. She did not like discussing the disease with her co-workers but realized that it was not possible to fully conceal the visible changes in her appearance from them. She felt that people were beginning to treat her differently, and also that some people seemed less comfortable interacting with her. Also, her hand contractures had become quite problematic, not only aesthetically but also practically in that she was no longer able to type. Although her supervisors had been supportive, she had had to reduce her work status to part-time and relinquish many of her job duties. She described that, while her doctor had not explicitly warned her about what the progression of her contractures could mean, she had seen special devices on patient blogs for patients with severe contractures and other hand changes, and feared the day when, "…I won't even be able to open a bottle of water without help."

Discussion

Living with a serious, chronic illness can have numerous implications for a patient's self-concept, and often necessitates role redefinition as the patient experiences the physical manifestations of the disease and adapts to the associated limitations (e.g., social, occupational) [1]. In the case presented above, the patient is clearly distressed by the present and anticipated changes to her appearance, and this distress is contributing to lowered mood, increased anxiety, and social withdrawal. Despite the prevalence of illnesses that cause changes in appearance, the role of disease-related changes to appearance in body image and other quality of life domains in these conditions remains relatively under-investigated [2]. This is true in scleroderma, where research into body image dissatisfaction and distress remains in the early stages [3, 4]. However, greater attention to psychosocial outcomes in scleroderma, including the development of scleroderma-specific measurement tools to evaluate appearance dissatisfaction, has contributed to a growing research base in this area in recent years. Generally, research has demonstrated that body image dissatisfaction is common in scleroderma [2, 5–9], and that changes in appearance can negatively impact psychosocial well-being and increase psychological distress [1–9], underscoring the importance of clinician awareness of the potential for significant body image concerns in scleroderma.

The word scleroderma is derived from the Greek words skleros (hard) and dermos (skin) [10]. Effects of excessive collagen production associated with the disease and skin thickening and hardening are hallmarks of the disease. Other appearance changes in scleroderma can include [1]:

1. Loss of skin folds
2. Shiny appearance to the skin
3. Hypo- or hyperpigmentation of the skin
4. Loss of flexibility of the lips and decreased ability to fully open the mouth
5. Pinched appearance to the nose and eyes
6. Telangiectasias
7. Subcutaneous calcinosis, often in the fingers, elbows, and knees
8. Sclerodactyly
9. Deformity of the digits
10. Limited range of motion in the hands caused by contractures and/or non-healing ulcers, or surgical amputation to manage digital ischemia

Many scleroderma patients experience similar changes to the appearance of their face, contributing to a facial appearance unique to the disease. In a study of scleroderma facial involvement, standardized digital photographs of 117 patients with scleroderma were rated for degree of disfigurement by three independent health professionals, and these ratings were highly concordant with ratings by the patients themselves [6]. The authors suggested that this agreement may reflect the presence of a characteristic facial "look" in scleroderma, including common features, such as a pinched nose, thinning lips, shiny and taut skin, and shrunken mouth opening. This characteristic pattern of appearance may also contribute to the fears of future appearance changes and disease progression because patients may recognize that other patients with more advanced disease have the same types of involvement (e.g., thinning lips) with greater severity.

Although less common in scleroderma than in some other diseases (e.g., cancer), treatment may also lead to changes in appearance, as well. For example, long-term steroid use can contribute to moon facies, or a rounded appearance of the face, and some of the immunosuppressant drugs (e.g., Cyclophosphamide) can cause hair loss. While appearance changes are common in both limited and diffuse scleroderma, patients with limited scleroderma tend to experience skin thickening only in the face and extremities, whereas patients with the diffuse subtype experience more widespread thickening, including trunk involvement [2, 11].

The numerous appearance changes that can occur and the variable and unpredictable nature of disfigurement in scleroderma contribute to the complexity of managing body image distress in this disease. However, advances in assessment methods and greater awareness of the role of body image distress in scleroderma have contributed to a slowly growing research base that can inform clinical practice.

Body Image in Scleroderma

It is important to distinguish among a number of key terms used in the body image literature, namely body image dissatisfaction and body image distress. The construct of body image includes both an evaluative (i.e., perceptions and attitudes) and investment (i.e., salience) component. Body image dissatisfaction is a product of the evaluative process whereas body image distress also incorporates investment and can include stronger negative body image emotions [12]. Thus, it is possible for a patient to be dissatisfied with their appearance but not distressed if the patient is not highly invested in their appearance. Severity of visible disfigurement does not always predict dissatisfaction or distress [13, 14]. Moreover, while the modified Rodnan skin score [15] is sometimes used as a proxy for severity of disease or degree of skin involvement in research settings, in clinical settings there is no single score from which clinicians can draw inferences about body image dissatisfaction or distress. Thus, body image distress may be a concern for patients with any level of disease-related changes in appearance. For example, in a study of 93 patients with scleroderma, which investigated appearance self-esteem and treatment for disease-related changes in scleroderma, skin thickening in the right hand and fingers was the strongest predictor of appearance self-esteem [1]. In another study of 127 women with scleroderma, correlates of body image dissatisfaction were identified as younger age, skin tightening above the elbows, and functional disability [2]. Another study of 171 patients with scleroderma found facial changes to be the most worrisome aspect of scleroderma [6]. In a mailed survey study of 303 patients with scleroderma who were asked more specifically about their level of concern relating to various changes in appearance, the following percentages of respondents noted concern for a specific body area: mouth furrows (80%), thin lips (73%), smaller mouth (77%), telangiectasias (76%), loss of facial lines (68%), skin darkening (50%), and finger ulcers (33%) [16]. Another study with 141 patients with scleroderma that included qualitative interviews in addition to quantitative assessment found that poor body image was higher among patients with diffuse scleroderma versus limited disease, and that patients with telangiectasias reported higher levels of appearance dissatisfaction [17]. Thus, it is important to consider the role of both disease-related factors (e.g., facial involvement) and social context (e.g., younger age) in body image dissatisfaction and distress [18]. In our case study, the patient displays specific concerns about changes in her appearance, such as her telangiectasias and thinning lips, but also reports social concerns around having to explain her appearance to others, evidencing the social impacts of the disease and multidimensional nature of body image concerns. There can also be profound feelings of loss and sadness associated with the changes in appearance. That the patient in the case study avoided looking in mirrors speaks to the sense of loss that many patients have around their previous appearance and difficulty adjusting to the disease and its physical changes.

An underexplored area is the role of cultural/sociodemographic context in body image outcomes related to changes in appearance caused by scleroderma. There has been research showing that Black scleroderma populations have more severe disease [19] and higher rates of body image dissatisfaction [20] compared to White scleroderma populations. A study examining the association of appearance concerns in scleroderma with sex and race/ethnicity found that women were more likely than men to endorse appearance concerns compared with men [21]. There have been no studies on the role of gender identity on body image outcomes. Black patients were also more likely to endorse appearance concerns than White patients; however, Black patients also can have more severe appearance impacts (e.g., greater hyperpigmentation) [21, 22].

Social Impacts of Poor Body Image

Generally, problems (or perceptions of problems) with social interactions are among the most frequently endorsed challenges reported by individuals living with visible differences (i.e., disfigurement) [23]. Disfigurement in scleroderma often occurs in areas of the body that are both visible and socially relevant (e.g., face, hands), which can contribute to increased social anxiety and avoidance [1–3, 5, 7]. Thus, understanding and anticipating the social impacts of the disease are important, especially because dissatisfaction with appearance and social discomfort are separate, although often related, problems [8, 14]. Changes in appearance can lead to numerous challenges in social interactions to which the individual had not been exposed prior to diagnosis (e.g., staring, avoidance, negative comments, unsolicited advice or questions, unwanted attention), and these can leave patients feeling a sense of loss of control [23]. Many patients may not realize that they are engaging in social avoidance or isolation due to body image distress, and it can be difficult to disentangle these behaviors from underlying depressive symptomatology, underscoring the importance of referrals to mental health services when patients describe withdrawal or avoidance behaviors. This is especially important because the withdrawal behaviors themselves can contribute to depression.

Examples of avoidance behaviors are present throughout our clinical case study. The patient reported limiting interactions outside of the home and in professional contexts in an effort to avoid having to explain her condition or potentially awkward encounters with others. For individuals who are partnered or who have children, avoidance can contribute to dyadic or family problems. The patient in the case described being a less involved parent as a result of her body image distress in that she stopped attending school events for her children. Acquired changes in appearance can also contribute to questions about one's identity and roles. There can be feelings of loss related both to one's previous physical appearance and the ability to engage in social interactions more readily [19, 24].

Self-Esteem and Mood Impacts of Body Image Distress

Self-esteem, or the appraisal of one's worth or significance as compared to others [25], is an important construct in that self-concept has been shown to be associated with various outcomes in chronic illness, most notably depression [1]. Appearance self-esteem is a subtype of self-esteem that is important to consider in the context of physical illnesses that cause changes in appearance [1, 26]. Appearance self-esteem has the potential to influence treatment decision-making; one study in rheumatoid arthritis demonstrated that negative self-perceptions of one's hands predicted reparative surgery desires, controlling for disease duration and objective measures of hand attractiveness [27]. There are no studies of how common cosmetic procedures are for patients with scleroderma; however, many patients do express a desire for cosmetic reconstructive options [16, 28]. The patient in the case study reported interest in cosmetic options for her thinning lips. Understanding the role of self-esteem in treatment seeking and decision-making is an important area for further exploration.

The first study exploring appearance self-esteem in scleroderma found that women with scleroderma had lower scores on self-report measures of appearance self-esteem than healthy controls, although men with scleroderma had scores similar to the healthy control group [1]. Further, appearance self-esteem was found to mediate the relationship between skin thickening and distress. Appearance self-esteem relating to acquired conditions has been most often studied in the context of acute changes (e.g., mastectomy, burns) [1], and thus there may be longitudinal processes of self-esteem changes unique to scleroderma given that the physical changes can be quite variable in severity and duration, and may develop over an extended period of time. In one study, individuals with scleroderma reported lower self-esteem than hospitalized burn patients, which may be attributed to the progressive, rather than stable nature of scleroderma, although another possible explanation is the relatively small scale of the burn injuries among many patients studied [6].

Body image dissatisfaction has been shown to relate directly to depressive symptomatology, which has, in turn, been associated with poorer psychosocial functioning [2]; thus, depression may mediate the relationship between body image dissatisfaction and psychosocial function. Further, the unpredictable and uncontrollable nature of the physical changes may cause individuals to feel helpless over their condition, which has also been associated with higher levels of depression in scleroderma [29]. In addition, there is little control over how others will react to one's changed appearance. Fear of negative evaluation by others was identified as an important contributor to the presence of anxiety symptomatology in scleroderma [30]. The patient in the case study reported depressive symptomatology associated with her body image distress, withdrawal from social situations, feeling "down on most days," and feelings of guilt.

Sexual Impacts of Body Image Dissatisfaction

Sexual dysfunction is common in scleroderma, with over 50% of women reporting impairment in sexual functioning [31] and over 80% of men reporting erectile dysfunction [32]. Despite the prevalence of sexual dysfunction, the lack of validated measures in this area precludes a research base elucidating correlates and predictors of sexual dysfunction [3, 4]. Various physical manifestations of scleroderma, such as shrinking of the mouth, skin tightening and discomfort, and vaginal tightening and dryness, can contribute to diminished sexual function [31, 33, 34]. While one study did not find a significant association between body image dissatisfaction and increased sexual impairment (dissatisfaction with appearance was associated with reduced sexual function in bivariate analysis, but became nonsignificant in multivariate analysis after including pain, disease duration, and unmarried status as correlates of sexual function) [35], the strong link between body image and sexual functioning, generally, and in other chronic illnesses, warrants further attention [36]. In the case study, the patient reports decreased sexual activity with her husband and associated feelings of guilt. Given the likely interface between physical contributors (e.g., vaginal tightening) and psychological contributors (e.g., body image distress, depressive symptomatology) to her sexual problems, it would be important to address each area of potential concern. As with body image distress in general, this may be an area that patients will not discuss unless directly assessed (i.e., "Are you experiencing sexual problems as a result of your disease?"), given the sensitive nature of the topic.

Fear of Physical Progression

The unpredictable course of the disease coupled with the availability of online images depicting severe changes in appearance in scleroderma can contribute to elevated worries and fears of progression of the physical manifestations of the disease. The patient in the case study described feelings of helplessness around the unclear progression of her symptoms and fears around increasing severity of her facial and hand changes. Patients may avoid potentially helpful resources, such as patient support groups, because seeing patients in more advanced stages of disease can be worry-inducing. Patients may engage in comparative pursuits, assessing how their own physical changes relate to those of other patients. This type of comparison is not limited to in-person support groups, and it can also occur in the context of Internet searches. Thus, asking patients about their perceptions of physical progression in scleroderma and what changes they may be expecting can be important in highlighting potential misconceptions or areas for education. This is especially important because, as described in the present case study, some patients may not feel that it is appropriate to raise concerns around body image or sexual dysfunction with their medical providers. However, given the aforementioned significant impacts of body image distress on various psychosocial domains, the importance of addressing these concerns should be evident.

Assessments of Body Image

Clinicians can foster a more open environment by simply asking all patients specifically about appearance-related concerns. Clinicians should inquire about appearance-related concerns among all patients who experience changes in their appearance due to scleroderma, not just patients with the most severe disfigurement. Simply asking the patient rather than using a "screening tool" is recommended because there are no established clinical cut-offs to detect clinically significant body image distress or evidence that screening in this way would improve outcomes for patients. Being proactive in asking about body image and appearance concerns is especially important because, as described in the case study, body image may not always be an area that the patient feels comfortable broaching with the clinician. Although there is no standard protocol for how to talk to patients about appearance concerns and what to do if such concerns are voiced, it is recommended that health professionals ask patients if they have concerns about changes in appearance that have occurred or might occur, perhaps by first normalizing that such concerns are common among individuals with scleroderma. Health professionals can then engage in a dialogue around this topic more openly with patients who have this concern or provide a referral to a mental health specialist as appropriate.

A consensus statement on research in scleroderma called for the development and validation of disease-specific measures that assess multiple dimensions of body image, such as social avoidance, appearance investment, and evaluation of appearance [3]. While such measures are important to researchers so that psychometrically robust instruments can be utilized to identify predictors and correlates of body image dissatisfaction and distress, there are also clinical uses for these measures. For example, in clinical care, assessments of body image can be used to track progress in treatment. However, such measures are not required, or necessarily appropriate, in all clinical settings. It is not recommended that a measure be administered unless there is a clear purpose for doing so. For many clinical encounters, simply asking the patient about concerns related to changes in their appearance or fears of changes that might occur is sufficient. However, because of the role of these measures in the growing research on body image in scleroderma and their potential for use by qualified professionals treating body image concerns, having an awareness of what measures exist and what constructs they assess can be important for providers to understand.

Existing general body image measures described for other populations may not be appropriate for use with scleroderma patients, as they may include items relating to weight concerns, and often do not measure disfigurement-related avoidance or social anxiety that would be important to explore in scleroderma [3]. Since the publication of the aforementioned consensus statement, the 14-item Satisfaction with Appearance Scale (SWAP) [12] and the abbreviated 6-item Brief-SWAP [7] have been validated in patients with scleroderma [7–9]. These measures require respondents to rate the extent to which they agree with items about their appearance on a seven-point scale ranging from 1 = strongly disagree to 7 = strongly agree. Higher scores indicate greater personal and social body image dissatisfaction. Originally developed for body image dissatisfaction relating to burn injuries, the SWAP and its abbreviated form the Brief-SWAP have been shown to yield the following two subscales: Dissatisfaction with Appearance and Social Discomfort [7, 9]. A recent study compared the two measures and concluded that both versions can be used with patients although the Brief-SWAP is the more parsimonious option [9]. On the Brief-SWAP, the Dissatisfaction with Appearance subscale measures patient self-reported dissatisfaction with specific areas of the body (e.g., "I am satisfied with the appearance of my face"), while the Social Discomfort subscale measures the social impacts of concerns around body image (e.g., "Because of changes in my appearance caused by my scleroderma, I am uncomfortable in the presence of strangers."). The two subscales of the Brief-SWAP have been psychometrically supported for use in both limited and diffuse scleroderma [37].

Research using the SWAP and Brief-SWAP to explore outcomes associated with specific disease-related changes in appearance has demonstrated that there are differential impacts not only for severity of disfigurement but also for specific body areas and patient characteristics. For example, in a study examining sociodemographic correlates of body image distress in 489 patients with scleroderma using the Brief-SWAP, upper-body telangiectasias and younger age were associated with greater social discomfort, finger-to-palm distance and hand contractures were associated with dissatisfaction with appearance, and extent of skin involvement and facial involvement were associated with both of these aspects of body image distress [8].

Three studies have been published using data from the Scleroderma Patient-centered Intervention Network (SPIN) Cohort to validate a number of existing measures that can contribute to our understanding of the social impacts of body image dissatisfaction. The Brief Fear of Negative Evaluation (BFNE; [38]), Social Appearance Anxiety Scale (SAAS; [39]), and Social Interaction Anxiety Scale-6 (SIAS-6; [40]) have all been validated for use with people with scleroderma. A measure called the Body Concealment Scale for Scleroderma (BCSS; [41]) has also been developed to assess body concealment behaviors related to avoidance for individuals with visible differences due to scleroderma. A recent review exploring the measurement and management of appearance anxiety in scleroderma noted that a validated measures to assess appearance investment is needed, given that those patients for whom appearance is especially salient and valued may be at elevated risk for negative psychosocial outcomes [42].

Clinical Strategies for Body Image Distress

Increasing awareness of body image distress among providers so that there can be open discourse and greater facilitation of referrals to appropriate healthcare providers and interventions is essential if patients are to receive appropriate and needed services. Psychosocial treatments for body image distress, as well as cosmetic and surgical approaches, provide important options for patients.

Psychosocial Treatments

While the need for psychosocial interventions in the treatment of scleroderma has been highlighted, there are currently no specific guidelines regarding referral for such interventions [43]. An important first strategy, as described above, is simply to evaluate the presence and degree of body image dissatisfaction and distress. In cases where distress is present, referral to a mental health professional may be indicated. The stepped care model has been recommended as a framework for psychosocial treatments in scleroderma ([18], see also Chap. x in this volume). Per the stepped care model, treatment may range on a spectrum from self-guided intervention through online programs or books (i.e., no therapist involvement) to long-term individual face-to-face therapy with a clinical team with expertise in body image distress. Chapter 46 in this volume lists a range of self-help resources for general psychosocial distress and one online resource specific to body image distress resulting from visible differences, Changing Faces (www.changingfaces.org.uk).

There are currently no evidence-based, disease-specific body image interventions available for scleroderma. Three systematic reviews have examined the effectiveness of psychological interventions developed for individuals with visible differences due to various conditions (e.g., vitiligo, psoriasis) [28, 44, 45]. A 2007 review on psychosocial interventions for individuals with visible differences [28] identified only one randomized controlled trial (RCT) [37] examining the effectiveness of a psychosocial intervention for body image distress although this trial was too small to draw conclusions with any degree of confidence [28]. A 2015 update to the review [45] identified only four additional studies, two of which were RCTs, but similarly had methodological limitations that precluded conclusions as to the optimal type and duration of psychosocial treatment for individuals with visible differences [46]. A third systematic review [44] broadly examined the use of self-help interventions (i.e., interventions requiring no or minimal therapist contact) for individuals with visible differences. Eight RCTs were identified and the authors qualitatively synthesized the findings and concluded that there was some support for the use of self-help tools for the reduction of anxiety but noted that efficacy across other outcomes was less clear. There is currently a review underway to specifically examine the effectiveness of psychological interventions to improve appearance-related and psychological outcomes in individuals living with visible differences that will focus on RCTs [47].

There are components of therapeutic modalities that may be useful to target body image distress, especially relating to social concerns. For example, cognitive-behavioral therapy (CBT) for social anxiety, social skills training programs, and psycho-educational support around body image distress have been suggested as useful interventions in scleroderma although none have been empirically tested [7]. CBT focuses on the interplay among cognitions, emotions, and behaviors. In a review of studies of both acquired and congenital disfigurement, negative emotions (e.g., social anxiety), maladaptive cognitions (e.g., fear of negative judgments from others), and negative behaviors (e.g., social isolation) were frequently reported [23], underscoring the relevance of this approach. A 2013 text titled "CBT for Appearance Anxiety: Psychosocial Interventions for Anxiety due to Visible Difference" is an excellent resource for mental health professionals that can be used as a clinical manual to guide CBT-based treatment for individuals with visible differences [46]. The book is grounded in a stepped care model that is useful for health professionals hoping to deliver more intensive psychosocial interventions and those who want to deliver more basic psychological treatments. Another therapeutic approach that is increasing in popularity, particularly for chronic illnesses, is Acceptance and Commitment Therapy (ACT). Unlike CBT, which provides tools to challenge and change unhelpful thoughts, ACT focuses on accepting these thoughts without judgment and learning how to live a valued life despite them. ACT may be useful in scleroderma, as CBT may feel invalidating for some patients because many underlying "negative" thoughts are not irrational thoughts to be challenged (e.g., "My appearance has changed quite a bit in the past five years"), but rather rational thoughts for which acceptance can be practiced.

Social skills training may also be appropriate. It is important to emphasize that this is not because individuals with scleroderma have a social deficit, but rather because (1) they are now living with added social challenges that they did not have prior to their diagnosis that may necessitate new skills (e.g., how to react to rude comments or stares) and (2) these skills can be helpful in managing the negative or hurtful social reactions of others. An issue that has not received scholarly attention but may contribute to difficulties in social interactions is that of restrictions in expressing facial non-verbal emotions given limited mouth function in scleroderma. The facial changes in scleroderma can sometimes contribute to an "expressionless face," and research on facial disfigurement has suggested that this may contribute to "difficulty in 'reading' the faces of disfigured people, which in turn results in hesitancy, awkwardness, and an abbreviated interchange" ([23], p. 86; [20]). For patients experiencing difficulties with social interactions, it is important that interventions expand their repertoire of social skills, so that they have more available resources to respond to the myriad challenges posed by social situations, rather than assuming that their social coping strategies are somehow deficient [23].

Cosmetic Camouflage and Surgical Options

As previously stated, models that assume a general, positive correlation between the severity of disfigurement and body image distress can be misleading because of individual differences that promote differential levels of distress [23]. In scleroderma, patients with the most severe changes in appearance are not necessarily the most distressed. Further, while cosmetic camouflage and surgical options (described briefly below) may sometimes be an option for some scleroderma-related appearance concerns, clinicians should offer psychosocial interventions in addition to any cosmetic camouflage or surgical options that may be available to address body image concerns.

The role of cosmetic camouflage (also referred to as makeup) has not been studied in scleroderma although many patient support groups offer cosmetic education days with tips and guidance around downplaying or highlighting certain features (e.g., lining the lips to make them appear thicker). Experts in body image acknowledge that some conditions "…are amenable to camouflage using make-up, prosthetics, clothes or hair. However, for some, camouflage can bring its own problems in relation to issues of identity." (p. 86) [23]. Clinicians hoping to educate themselves about the role of cosmetic camouflage can look to the burn literature, which includes numerous case studies and examples of how cosmetic camouflage can improve aesthetic balance and help to restore symmetry to facial and bodily areas of concern [48]. A systematic review exploring the effectiveness of non-surgical cosmetic interventions to improve appearance-related and psychological outcomes in adults with visible differences identified six RCT trials, but all had high risk of bias across several key domains, precluding a meaningful synthesis of the findings. The authors concluded that until evidence from methodologically rigorous trials is available, clinicians can engage with patients interested in cosmetic interventions in shared decision-making, noting the pros and the cons and emphasizing the lack of evidence [49].

Another area that has received relatively little attention in scleroderma-related body image distress is the role of surgical options to address body image concerns. There are procedures that may be of interest to patients with specific concerns. For example, lip thinning can be a very distressing change for many patients, who may explore surgery as a means to recreate their previous lip thickness [50]. There has been a call for a more systematic approach to the surgical management of facial disfigurement in scleroderma. For example, some clinicians do not advise that patients with scleroderma undergo surgical procedures given concerns such as poor wound healing, while other experts argue that such concerns are unfounded [16]. Various laser and surgical options exist for patients, such as carbon dioxide laser (Coherent 5000-C Ultra Pulse laser at 300 mJ/60 W) for peri-oral rhytidosis [51], pulsed dye laser for treatment of telangiectasias [51, 52], and autologous fat transfer for isolated skin areas [16, 53]. There has been a call for collaboration among various clinical specialties, including plastic surgery, rheumatology, dermatology, and internal medicine, to develop guidelines for best practices for the management of patients with scleroderma who desire surgical treatments to address changes in appearance [16].

At present, there are no guidelines for discussing such interventions with patients who desire them. Some argue that when clinicians offer cosmetic or surgical options to patients exhibiting body image distress, or assume that patients with more severe physical manifestations of the disease must be experiencing body image distress, this can be a means by which, "care providers are colluding with the myth that quality of life necessarily improves when physical appearance is enhanced" (p. 91) [23]. This is an area that deserves further attention so that clinicians can know how to respond to patient requests for surgical or cosmetic options. It is also important for health professionals to know when and how to present patients with surgical or less invasive cosmetic options when patients present with body image distress but do not know what options are available to them. Finally, clinicians who do present such options should be ready to address the clinical and psychosocial impacts of such treatments.

Conclusion

In summary, changes in appearance and associated concerns are common for many people with scleroderma. It is important for all those providing clinical care in scleroderma to be aware of body image impacts and to be mindful that dissatisfaction and distress do not necessarily correlate with severity of appearance changes. As such, open communication around changes in appearance is important to ensure that patients with body image concerns who are not being asked about body image do not fall between the cracks. The recent development of scleroderma-specific body image assessments has contributed to a growing literature base that demonstrates the multidimensional nature of body image dissatisfaction and distress, and the personal and social impacts that can be associated with changes in appearance. Referrals to mental health professionals may be indicated when patients have concerns related to body image distress. Furthermore, there are resources for patients wanting to take a self-managed approach to understanding and coping with body image distress. Future efforts should focus on identification of evidence-based scleroderma-specific interventions to aid patients struggling with body image due to disease-related changes in appearance.

Acknowledgments Dr. Thombs was supported by a Tier 1 Canada Research Chair.

References

1. Malcarne VL, Handsdottir I, Greensbergs HL, Clements PJ, Weisman MH. Appearance self-esteem in systemic sclerosis. Cognitive Ther Res. 1999;23(2):197–208.
2. Benrud-Larson LM, Heinberg LJ, Boiling C, Reed J, White B, Wigley FM, et al. Body image dissatisfaction among women with scleroderma: extent and relationship to psychosocial function. Health Psychol. 2003;22(2):130–9.
3. Thombs BD, van Lankveld W, Bassel M, Baron M, Buzza R, Haslam S, et al. Psychological health and Well-being in systemic sclerosis: state of the science and consensus research agenda. Arthritis Care Res. 2010;8:1181–9.
4. Malcarne VM, Fox RS, Mills SD, Gholizadeh S. Psychosocial aspects of systemic sclerosis. Curr Opin Rheumatol. 2013;25(6):707–13.
5. Heinberg LJ, Kudel I, White B, Kwan A, Medley K, Wigley F, Haythornthwaite J. Assessing body image in patients with systemic sclerosis (scleroderma): validation of the adapted satisfaction with appearance scale. Body Image. 2007;4(1):79–86.
6. Amin K, Clarke A, Sivakumar B, Puri A, Fox Z, Brough V, et al. The psychological impact of facial changes in scleroderma. Psychol Health Med. 2011;16(3):304–12.
7. Jewett LR, Hudson M, Haythornthwaite JA, Heinberg L, Wigley FM, Baron M, Thombs BD, Canadian Scleroderma Research Group. Development and validation of the Brief-Satisfaction with Appearance Scale (Brief-SWAP) for systemic sclerosis (SSc). Arthritis Care Res. 2010;62(12):1779–86.
8. Jewett LR, Huson M, Malcarne VL, Baron M, Thombs BD, Canadian Scleroderma Research Group. Sociodemographic and disease correlates of body image distress among patients with systemic sclerosis. PLoS One. 2012;7(3):e33281.
9. Mills SD, Fox RS, Merz EL, Clements PJ, Kafaja S, Malcarne VL, Furst DE, Khanna D. Evaluation of the satisfaction with appearance scale and its short form in systemic sclerosis: analysis from the UCLA scleroderma quality of life study. 2015;42:1624–30.
10. Seibold J, Harris ED, Budd RC, Genovese MC, Sergent JS. Kelley's textbook of rheumatology. Philadelphia: Elsevier; 2007.
11. Poole JL, Steen VD. The use of the Health Assessment Questionnaire (HAQ) to determine physical disability in systemic sclerosis. Arthritis Care Res. 1991;4(1):27–31.
12. Cash TF, Melnyk SE, Hrabosky JI. The assessment of body image investment: an extensive revision of the Appearance Schemas Inventory. Int J Eat Disord. 2004;35(3):305–16.
13. Robinson E. Psychological research on visible differences in adults. In: Lansdown R, Rumsey N, Bradbury E, Carr T, Partridge J, editors. Visibly different: coping with disfigurement. London: Butterworth; 1997. p. 102–11.
14. Rumsey N, Clarke A, Musa M. Altered body image: the psychosocial needs of patients. Br J Community Nurs. 2002;7(11):563–6.
15. Clements PJ, Hurwitz EL, Wong WK, Seibold JR, Mayes M, et al. Skin thickness scores as a predictor and correlate of outcome in systemic sclerosis: high-dose versus low-dose penicillamine trial. Arthritis Rheum. 2000;43(11):2445–54.
16. Paquette DL, Falanga V. Cutaneous concerns of scleroderma patients. J Dermatol. 2003;30(6):438–43.
17. Ennis H, Herrick AL, Cassidy C, Griffiths CE, Richards HL. A pilot study of body image dissatisfaction and the psychological impact of systemic sclerosis-related telangiectases. Clin Exp Rheumatol. 2013;31(2 Suppl 76):12–7.
18. Jewett LR, Haythornthwaite JA, Thombs BD. Psychosocial issues and care for patients with systemic sclerosis. In: Varga J, Denton CP, Wigley FM, editors. Scleroderma: From pathogenesis to comprehensive management. New York: Springer; 2012. p. 641–8.
19. Morgan ND, Shah AA, Mayes MD, et al. Clinical and serological features of systemic sclerosis in a multicenter African American cohort: analysis of the genome research in African American scleroderma patients clinical database. Medicine (Baltimore). 2017;96(51):e8980.
20. Nusbaum JS, Gordon JK, Steen VD. African American race associated with body image dissatisfaction among patients with systemic sclerosis. Clin Exp Rheumatol. 2016;34(8):70–3.
21. Jewett LR, Kwakkenbos L, Carrier ME, Malcarne VL, Bartlett SJ, Furst DE, Gottesman K, Mayes MD, Assassi S, Harcourt D, Williamson H. Examination of the association of sex and race/ethnicity with appearance concerns: a Scleroderma Patient-centered Intervention Network (SPIN) Cohort study. Clin Exp Rheum. 2016;34(5):PI-0092.
22. Shapiro L, Saketkoo LA, Steen VD. Scleroderma in pigmented skin populations. In: Orfanos C, Zouboulis C, Assaf C, editors. Pigmented ethnic skin and imported dermatoses. Cham: Springer; 2018.
23. Rumsey N, Harcourt D. Body image and disfigurement: issues and interventions. Body Image. 2004;1(1):83–97.
24. Bradbury E. Understanding the problems. In: Lansdown R, Rumsey N, Bradbury E, Carr A, Partridge J, editors. Visibly different: coping with disfigurement. Oxford: Butterworth-Heinemann; 1997. p. 180–93.
25. Coopersmith S. Studies in self-esteem. Sci Am. 1968;218(2):96–106.
26. Vamos M. Body image in chronic illness: a re-conceptualization. Int J Psychiat Med. 1993;23(2):163–78.
27. Vamos M. Body image in rheumatoid arthritis: the relevance of hand appearance to desire for surgery. Br J Med Psychol. 1990;6(3):267–77.
28. Bessell A, Moss TP. Psychosocial interventions for visible differences: a 453 systematic review. Body Image. 2007;4(3):227–38.
29. Nicassio PM, Wallston KA, Callahan LF, Herbert M, Pincus T. The measurement of helplessness in rheumatoid arthritis: the development of the arthritis helplessness index. J Rheumatol. 1985;12(3):462–7.

30. Richards HL, Herrick AL, Griffin K, Gilliam PDH, Fortune DG. Psychological adjustment to systemic sclerosis—exploring the association of disease factors, functional ability, body related attitudes and fear of negative evaluation. Psychol Health Med. 2004;9(1):29–39.
31. Saad SC, Pietrzykowski JE, Lewis SS, Stepien AM, Latham VA, Messick S, et al. Vaginal lubrication in women with scleroderma and Sjögren's syndrome. Sex Disabil. 1999;17(2):103–13.
32. Walker UA, Tyndall A, Ruszat R. Erectile dysfunction in systemic sclerosis. Ann Rheum Dis. 2009;68(7):1083–5.
33. Schover LR, Jensen SR. Sexuality and chronic illness: a comprehensive approach. New York: Guilford; 1988.
34. Saad SC, Behrend AE. Scleroderma and sexuality. J Sex Res. 1996;33(3):15–20.
35. Knafo R, Haythornthwaite JA, Heinberg L, Wigley F, Thombs BD. The association of body image dissatisfaction and pain with reduced sexual function in women with systemic sclerosis. Rheumatol. 2011;50(6):1125–30.
36. Passik SD, Newman ML, Brennan M, Tunkel R. Predictors of psychological distress, sexual dysfunction and physical functioning among women with upper extremity lymphedema related to breast cancer. Psychooncology. 1995;4(4):255–63.
37. Fox RS, Mills SD, Gholizadeh S, Merz EL, Roesch SC, Clements PJ, Kafaja S, Khanna D, Furst DE, Malcarne VL. Validity and correlates of the brief satisfaction with appearance scale for patients with limited and diffuse systemic sclerosis: analysis from the University of California, Los Angeles Scleroderma Quality of Life Study. J Scleroderma Relat Disord. 2020;5(2):143–51.
38. Fox RS, Kwakkenbos L, Carrier ME, Mills SD, Gholizadeh S, Jewett LR, Roesch SC, Merz EL, Assassi S, Furst DE, Gottesman K. Reliability and validity of three versions of the brief fear of negative evaluation scale in patients with systemic sclerosis: a Scleroderma Patient-Centered Intervention Network cohort study. Arthritis Car Res. 2018;70(11):1646–52.
39. Mills SD, Kwakkenbos L, Carrier ME, Gholizadeh S, Fox RS, Jewett LR, Gottesman K, Roesch SC, Thombs BD, Malcarne VL. Scleroderma patient-centered intervention network investigators. Validation of the social appearance anxiety scale in patients with systemic sclerosis: a scleroderma patient-centered intervention network cohort study. Arthritis Care Res. 2018;70(10):1557–62.
40. Gholizadeh S, Kwakkenbos L, Carrier ME, et al. Validation of the 520 social interaction anxiety scale in scleroderma: a scleroderma patient-centered intervention network cohort study. J Scleroderma Related Dis. 2018;3(1):98–105.
41. Jewett LR, Malcarne VL, Kwakkenbos L, et al. Development and validation of the body concealment scale for scleroderma. Arthritis Care Res. 2016;68(8):1158–65.
42. Gholizadeh S, Meier A, Malcarne VL. Measuring and managing appearance anxiety in patients with systemic sclerosis. Expert Rev Clin Immun. 2019;15(4):341–6.
43. Kowal-Bielecka O, Landewe R, Avouac J, Chwiesko S, Miniati I, Czirjak L, et al. EULAR recommendations for the treatment of systemic sclerosis: a report from the EULAR scleroderma trials and research group (EUSTAR). Ann Rheum Dis. 2009;68(5):620–8.
44. Muftin Z, Thompson AR. A systematic review of self-help for disfigurement: effectiveness, usability, and acceptability. Body Image. 2013;10:442–50.
45. Norman A, Moss TP. Psychosocial interventions for adults with visible differences: a systematic review. Peer J. 2015;3:e870.
46. Clarke A, Thompson AR, Jenkinson E, Rumsey N, Newell R. CBT for appearance anxiety: psychosocial interventions for anxiety due to visible difference. Oxford: John Wiley & Sons; 2013.
47. Gholizadeh S, Rice D, Carboni Jiménez A, Kwakkenbos L, Boruff J, Malcarne V, Thombs, and Scleroderma Patient-centered Intervention Network (SPIN) Body Image Patient Advisory Team. Examining the effectiveness of psychological interventions to improve appearance-related and psychological outcomes among adults with visible differences: a systematic review. PROSPERO 2018 CRD42018100632. https://www.crd.york.ac.uk/prospero/display_record.php?ID=CRD42018100632
48. Rose EH. Aesthetic restoration of the severely disfigured face in burn victims: a comprehensive strategy. Plast Reconstr Surg. 1994;96(7):1573–85.
49. Gholizadeh S, Rice DB, Carboni-Jiménez A, Kwakkenbos L, Boruff J, Krishnan A, Malcarne VL, Thombs BD. Effects of cosmetic and other camouflage interventions on appearance-related and psychological outcomes among adults with visible differences in appearance: A systematic review. BMJ Open. 2021;11:e046634.
50. Spackman GK. Scleroderma: what the general dentist should know. Gen Dent. 1999;47(6):576–9.
51. Apfelberg DB, Varga J, Greenbaum SS. Carbon dioxide laser resurfacing of peri-oral rhytids in scleroderma patients. Dermatol Surg. 1998;24:517–9.
52. Murray AK, Moore TL, Richards H, Ennis H, Griffiths CEM, Herrick AL. Pilot study of intense pulsed light for the treatment of systemic sclerosis-related telangiectases. Br J Dermatol. 2012;167(3):563–9.
53. Glogau RG. Microlipoinjection: autologous fat grafting. Arch Dermatol. 1988;124(9):1340–3.

57 Managing Complicated Digital Ulcers

John D. Pauling and Marco Matucci-Cerinic

The Spectrum of DU in Systemic Sclerosis

Digital ulcers (DU) are a major cause of disease-related morbidity in SSc, leading to pain, emotional distress and impaired hand function [1–3]. DU, that occur in over half of SSc patients during their disease course with a point prevalence of around 10% [4–6], are a poor prognostic indicator associated with a more severe disease course and increased mortality [7]. The pattern of DU occurrence differs between patients, with approximately half of patients experiencing solitary/episodic DU with the remainder experiencing recurrent or even chronic DU disease [8]. The clinical features, pathogenesis and management of SSc-DU are covered in detail in Chap. 20. In this chapter, we shall consider some of the challenges facing clinicians in the management of SSc-DU under the three proposed distinct types of SSc-DU [6]. Our cases highlight the potential contribution of different aetiopathogenic drivers of SSc-DU and how clinical, laboratory and imaging modalities can be used to identify factors implicated in SSc-DU occurrence and targeted therapeutic intervention.

Ischaemic (Fingertip) DU

Fingertip DUs (typically distal to the distal interphalangeal joint of the fingers and toes) are considered the archetypal complication of persistent digital ischaemia [6]. They are the most common form of SSc-DU, occurring approximately three-fold more commonly that extensor DU [9]. They are also considered the most responsive to vasodilator therapy and successful clinical trial programmes for secondary SSc-DU prevention have typically applied definitions for sentinel DU that indicate a likely ischaemic origin [10, 11]. Nonetheless, ischaemic ulcers can be refractory to treatment, sometimes necessitating treatment escalation with combination therapy and consideration of potential additional modifiable aggravating factors.

Case 1: Refractory Ischaemic Digital Ulceration

A 50-year-old female had features of paronychia at the time of her presentation with limited cutaneous SSc (anticentromere antibody, ACA). She had already developed sclerodactyly and proximal scleroderma of dorsal hands at presentation. Within 1 year of diagnosis, she had experienced recurrent DUs affecting multiple digits despite trials of nifedipine, amlodipine, fluoxetine, three hospital admissions for intravenous iloprost, surgical debridement, and digital sympathectomies. She continued to experience new DU (Fig. 57.1a) and microvascular imaging confirmed impaired digital perfusion (Fig. 57.1b). She experienced significant pain, impaired hand function and work absenteeism. She described her experience as follows:

> 'my life became intolerable with regard to all daily living activities. I was in excruciating pain for which I was prescribed morphine, which only dulled the pain. I could not sleep. I became depressed'

She was commenced on bosentan therapy which resulted in an immediate 50% improvement in pain levels and improved quality of life, allowing her to stop her to return to work and stop her opiate analgesia and neuromodulatory drugs. There was healing of her existing DU (Fig. 57.1c) and objective evidence of improved digital perfusion (Fig. 57.1d). She continued on bosentan, amlodipine and fluoxetine; only experiencing a single DU in the ensuing 8 years of follow-up.

J. D. Pauling (✉)
Department of Rheumatology, North Bristol NHS Trust, Bristol, UK

Musculoskeletal Research Unit, Bristol Medical School Translational Health Sciences, University of Bristol, Bristol, UK
e-mail: JohnPauling@nhs.net

M. Matucci-Cerinic
Unit of Immunology, Rheumatology, Allergy and Rare diseases (UnIRAR), IRCCS San Raffaele Hospital, Milan, Italy
e-mail: marco.matuccicerinic@unifi.it

Y. Allanore et al. (eds.), *Scleroderma*, https://doi.org/10.1007/978-3-031-40658-4_57

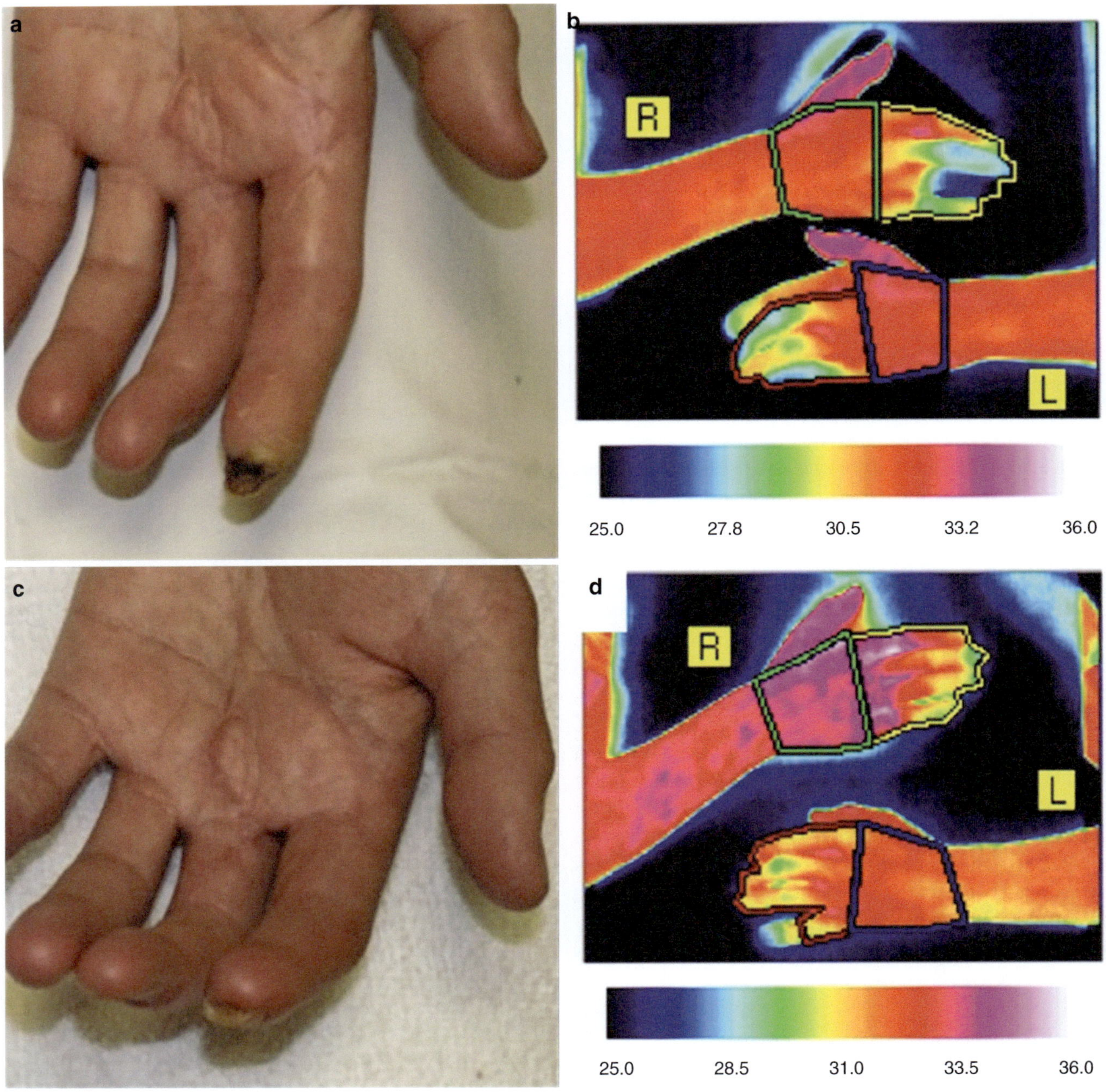

Fig. 57.1 (**a**) Refractory ischaemic digital ulceration of left index finger in patient with limited cutaneous SSc (anti-centromere antibody); (**b**) Corresponding thermal image revealing significantly impaired basal perfusion of multiple digits (including site of active ulceration); (**c**) Appearance of hands after 6 months treatment with bosentan revealing healing of prior ulceration; (**d**) Corresponding improvement in digital perfusion on thermal imaging

This case highlights the severe pain and broader impact on health-related quality of life caused by ischaemic SSc-DU, as well as the need to escalate pharmacological management with combination vasodilator therapies. Her SSc-DU were eventually controlled with endothelin receptor antagonist therapy which has been shown to reduce the mean number of new DU by 30–48% in controlled trials of SSc patients with ischaemic DU (particularly in patients with a high burden of active DU at study entry) [10, 11]. Important, these trials adopted a definition for 'cardinal' DU that enriched the trial for patients with DU considered to have a predominantly ischaemic aetiology [10, 11]. The case also highlights the issue of delayed diagnosis of SSc, with patients continuing to only achieve a diagnosis of SSc once features of disease damage such as DU occur (akin to joint erosions previously being identified at diagnosis in rheumatoid arthritis). SSc-DU are associated with nailfold capillary drop out and indicative of advanced progression of the microangiopathy of SSc [12]. Unfortunately, diagnostic delay remains an unmet need in SSc, precluding intervention with vasodilator therapies which may modify the evolution of microangiopathy in SSc [13, 14] and help prevent the future development of organ-specific complications [15, 16]. Delay to initiating vasoactive therapy in SSc is associated with an increased burden of SSc-DU [6, 17]. Many patients are 'diagnosed' with Raynaud's in primary care prior to the identification of SSc, with the interval prior to formal SSc diagnosis exceeding 10 years in around 20% of such patients [18].

Case 2: Associated Macrovascular Disease

A 57-year-old smoker with established diffuse cutaneous SSc (dcSSc) with anti-Scl-70 antibodies, complicated by recurrent DU and interstitial lung disease (ILD), presented with refractory DU of her right great toe (Fig. 57.2), despite current treatment with intravenous prostacyclin, sildenafil, bosentan, fluoxetine and aspirin therapy. Her feet were cool and pedal pulses were absent. Her ankle brachial pressure index (ABPI) was reduced at 0.75. Vascular studies revealed proximal popliteal artery occlusion which was managed with balloon angioplasty. This resulted in prompt healing of the DU, enhanced clinical perfusion of the foot with an improved capillary refill time and an increased ABPI of 0.88.

The microangiopathy of SSc has been closely studies but clinicians must also be alert to the possibility of modifiable macrovascular involvement. Indeed, macrovascular and microvascular co-exist in patients with SSc-DU [19, 20]. A worsening ABPI in SSc has been associated with advancing age, lcSSc, ACA and smoking [21]. Smoking cessation advice is an essential component of management of all patients with SSc, but particularly those with DU. Other cardiovascular risk factors should be modified and vascular imaging undertaken to identify large vessel abnormalities that may be amenable to angioplasty.

Case 3: Pro-coagulant Tendency

A 63-year-old non-smoking male with lcSSc (ACA) presented with ischaemic subungal ulceration of the right ring finger (Fig. 57.3a). There was reduced capillary density on nailfold capillaroscopy with dilated capillaries and micro-haemorrhages (Fig. 57.3b) and evidence of delayed digital reperfusion following local cold challenge on thermal imaging (Fig. 57.3d). Magnetic resonance imaging (MRI) of the hand revealed moderate marrow oedema with expansion of the distal phalanx of ring finger (Fig. 57.3d) which healed with subsequent acro-osteolysis (Fig. 57.3e). Investigation

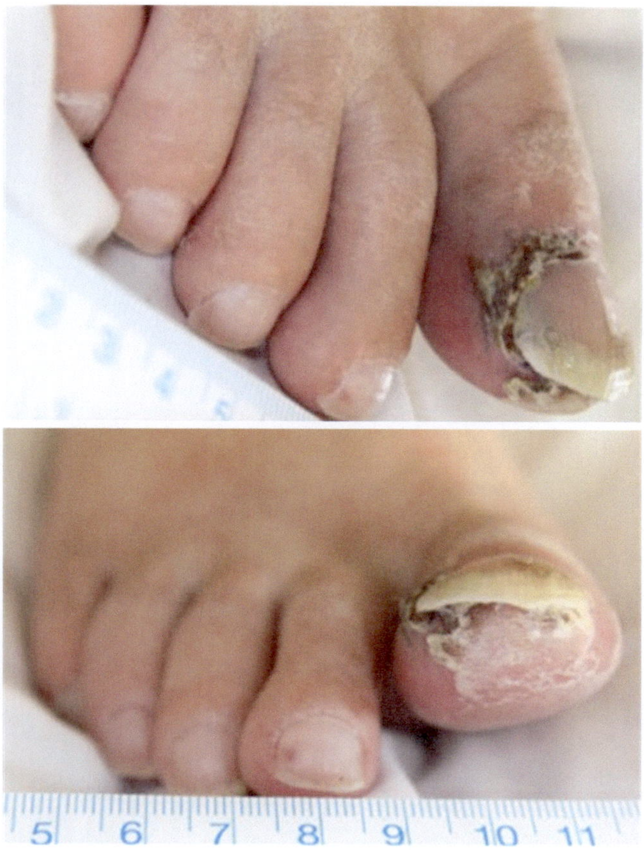

Fig. 57.2 Ischaemic digital ulceration of great toe in a 57-year-old smoker with longstanding diffuse cutaneous systemic sclerosis (Scl-70 antibody) despite treatment with intravenous prostacyclin, sildenafil, bosentan, fluoxetine and aspirin therapy. Vascular studies revealed proximal popliteal short occlusion treated with popliteal balloon angioplasty. This resulted in prompt healing of ulceration and an increase in ankle brachial pressure index from 0.75 to 0.88

revealed a strongly positive anticardiolipin IgG (64.6 GPL/mL and 99.1 GPL/mL, 12 weeks apart), and a weakly positive anti-β2-GP1 IgG (15 MPL/mL). Vasodilator therapies were optimised and warfarin commenced to prevent further ischaemic events.

Anti-phospholipid syndrome (APS) antibodies should be routinely assessed in all SSc patients at diagnosis and repeated in those with active DU or necrosis (or other potential thrombotic events) [22]. In this case, digital ischaemia was sufficient to cause osteonecrosis and acro-osteolysis. The prevalence of APS antibodies in SSc is ~13%; with ~1–2% for lupus anti-coagulant, ~9% for anticardiolipin (with an IgM and IgG isotype prevalence of 7.8 percent and 12.8 percent, respectively) and ~9% prevalence of anti-B2-GP1 [23, 24]. SSc-associated APS (particularly anti-B2-GP1 antibodies) has been associated with worse Raynaud's phenomenon and SSc-DU disease [25]. Digital ischaemic events are generally uncommon features of established APS, except in the context of 'catastrophic' disease [26–28]. Nonetheless, APS has been implicated in ~5% of

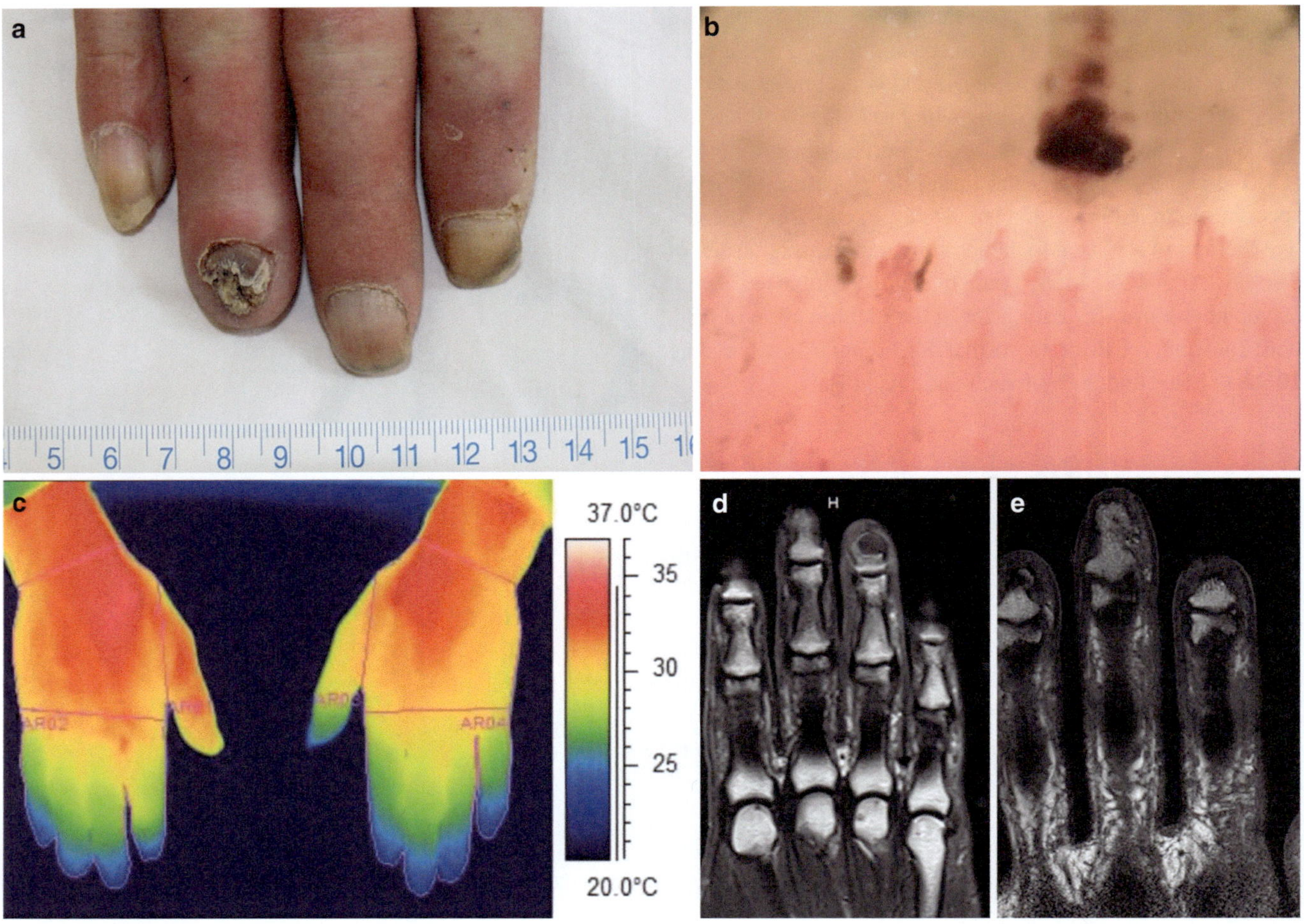

Fig. 57.3 (**a**) Ulceration of ring finger in a 63-year-old non-smoking male with limited cutaneous systemic sclerosis (anti-centromere) and anti-phospholipid syndrome; (**b**) Dilated capillary loops with micro-haemorrhage and some reduced capillary density on nailfold capillaroscopy; (**c**) Delayed digital reperfusion following local cold challenge on thermal imaging; (**d**) Moderate marrow oedema with expansion of the distal phalanx of ring finger on MRI; (**e**) Subsequent acro-osteolysis of the distal phalanx

patients presenting with unexplained digital ischaemia [29, 30]. Other intravascular factors are thought to be relevant to the pathogenesis of digital vasculopathy in SSc, including platelet activation and anti-platelet/anti-coagulant therapy have been proposed in recommendations on the management of patients with refractory SSc-DU disease [31, 32].

Calcinosis-associated DU

Another distinct type of SSc-DU proposed is that associated with calcinosis cutis, that relate to ischaemic, mechanical and inflammatory phenomena [6]. A detailed analysis of calcinosis cutis is provided in Chap. 34. There is increasing evidence to indicate calcinosis cutis form at ischaemic foci within the skin, hence their propensity to form at the distal extremities. The presence of calcinosis is strongly associated with the severity of digital vasculopathy, extent of capillary loss and, unsurprisingly, DU occurrence [33–36]. The mechanical and local inflammatory effects of calcinotic deposits can further promote spontaneous extrusion and emergence of ulceration. These calcinosis-associated digital ischaemic lesions are very painful and take longer to heal than 'pure' ischaemic DUs (93.6 vs. 76.2 days) and can be more refractory to intervention [29].

Case 4: Refractory Calcinosis-associated DU

A 70-year-old female with lcSSc (anti-centromere) diagnosed 1990s, presented with a 2-year history of persistent ulceration on radial and ulnar border of left index finger at level of DIP (Fig. 57.4a,b). The lesions were refractory to intervention with sildenafil and intravenous iloprost (neither of which were tolerated). There were intermittent episodes of local inflammation, treated with antibiotics to eradicate potential local infection. These episodes would typically lead to small flecks of hard calcinotic material spontaneously exuding from the surface of the skin. There were calcinotic deposits at the elbows. Plain films confirmed the presence of calcinotic deposits below the surface of the cutaneous ulcers (Fig. 57.4c).

This case highlights the multi-faceted nature of calcinosis-associated DU. The site of the DU differs from ischaemic DU and the fingertips themselves were reasonably well perfused without digital pitting. The efficacy of pharmacological intervention such as endothelin receptor antagonists is unknown as patients with such as DU would usually be ineligible for clinical trial programmes in this field. Nonetheless, management should include optimisation of vasodilatory therapy and aggressive modification of existing cardiovascular risk factors (including smoking cessation advice where required). Clinicians should have a low threshold for treating any suspected local infection but should also consider treatments targeting local inflammation when present. Surgical debridement can be effective but wound healing can be slow and recurrence frequently occurs.

Case 5: Inflammatory Calcinosis-associated DU

A 42-year-old female with a 7-year history of dcSSc (RNA Pol III antibody), complicated by scleroderma renal crisis (requiring renal replacement therapy) and lower gastrointestinal pseudo-obstruction, presented with severe cutaneous ulceration of the hands and digits (Fig. 57.5a). The combination of sildenafil and bosentan did not impact on symptoms and was discontinued. Plain films revealed widespread calcinotic deposits, particularly at the sites of cutaneous ulceration (Fig. 57.5b). A trial of minocycline resulted in rapid and sustained healing and secondary prevention of further cutaneous ulcers (Fig. 57.5c), with marked improvement in pain, functional capacity and body image satisfaction.

This case highlights the inflammatory and pro-infectious potential of calcinotic deposits and the potential role of treatments such as minocycline [37]. Other treatments targeting local inflammation have been trialled in CTD-associated cal-

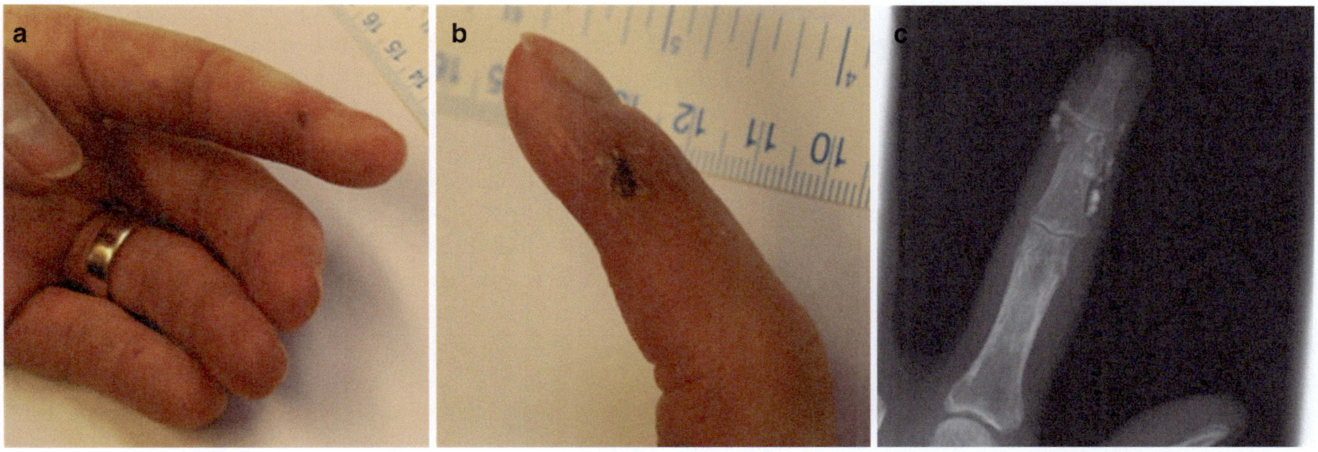

Fig. 57.4 (**a**, **b**) Ulceration of index finger in a 70-year-old female with limited cutaneous systemic sclerosis (anti-centromere) with recurrent spontaneous exudation of calcinotic material; (**c**) Plain films revealed calcinosis cutis at the site of the refractory ulceration

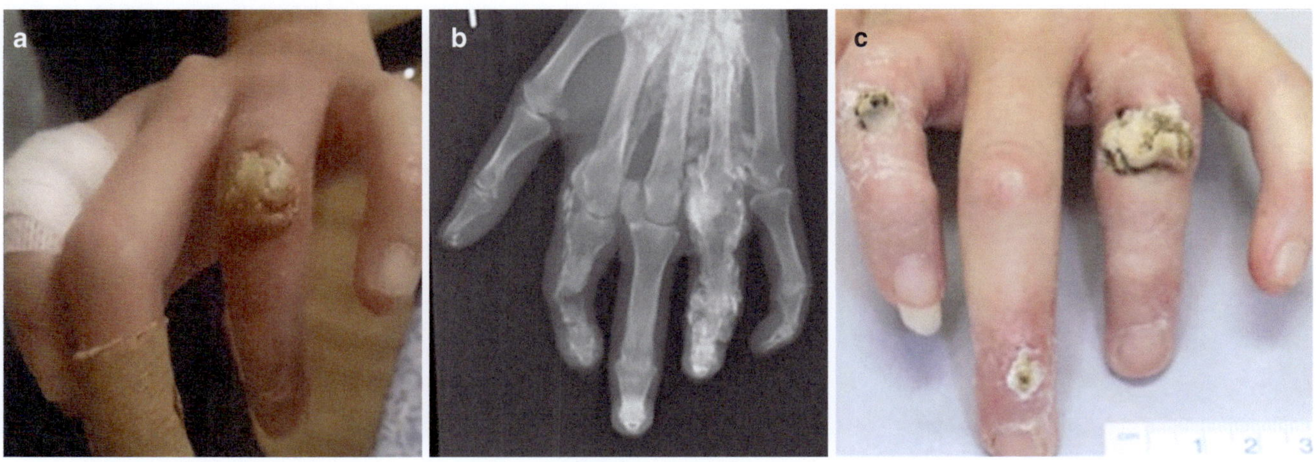

Fig. 57.5 (**a**) Multiple refractory digital ulcers despite treatment with conventional vasodilator therapy including trials of sildenafil and bosentan; (**b**) Plain films confirmed widespread calcinosis cutis; (**c**) Marked improvement within 2 months of commencing minocycline. Adapted and reproduced with permission from previously reported case [44].

cinosis including infliximab [38] and intravenous immunoglobulin [39–41].

Extensor Digital Ulcers in SSc

The third subtype of DU proposed by Hachulla et al. was the 'extensor' DU which are thought to occur secondary to recurrent microtrauma/increased tension from skin sclerosis. This type of DU is less common the 'ischaemic' DU and typically associated with the presence of joint contractures in patients with diffuse cutaneous SSc (particularly in the context of RNA Pol III) [2, 13, 14, 24]. Both types can be found simultaneously and the prevalence of both fingertip and extensor DUs was 6% in one observation study [5]. Increased tension of the skin across fixed-flexion deformities leads to vascular compromise and assessment of cutaneous perfusion using laser Doppler suggests both fingertip and extensor DUs are characterised by an ischaemic core [17, 18]. In a 4-year prospective study of 1614 digital lesions, approximately half were DUs, and over half of the DUs were ischaemic fingertip DUs (with round 30% of all DUs being extensor DUs) [15].

Case 6: Extensor-aspect SSc-DU in dcSSc

A 37-year-old female presented with early dcSSc (RNA Pol III) with a skin score of 21/51 at diagnosis, rising within 6 months to 45/51. Treatment of her skin disease was commenced with pulsed intravenous cyclophosphamide (6 infusions of 750 mg) followed by mycophenolate mofetil (1.5 g bd). Her skin disease resulted in fixed flexion deformities of the fingers (finger-to-palm distance 2 cm on the left and 0.5 cm on the right side) and a positive prayer sign. She developed ulceration over the extensor aspect of her left fifth digit proximal interphalangeal joint (PIP) that was complicated by soft tissue infection (Fig. 57.6a). She was treated with intravenous iloprost, intravenous antibiotics and commenced on sildenafil 50 mg tds. The ulcer took 4 months to completely heal but her fixed flexion deformity in this finger persisted (Fig. 57.6b). She did not experience any ulcer recurrence at this site over the ensuing 12 months but has fixed flexion deformities at several digits resulting in blanching of the skin overlying several PIPs that remain vulnerable to potential ulceration (Fig. 57.6c,d).

Skin disease in SSc and its relationship with fixed flexion deformities is described in detail in Chap. 32. As with calcinosis-related DU, treatment with vasodilatory therapies should be used but interventions targeting skin involvement and hand therapy to maintain joint function is also imperative in the primary and secondary prevention of these lesions.

Conclusions

The cases described highlight the major morbidity associated with SSc-DU. SSc is a vascular disease, but whilst all DU have a potentially reversible ischaemic component, clinicians must remain alert to the possibility of other factors contributing to DU development such as infection, thrombosis, proximal vascular stenosis, calcinosis and mechanical forces around joints compromising cutaneous perfusion. Appreciating the multi-faceted nature of cutaneous ulceration in SSc can help identify targeted interventions tailored to the aetiopathogenic factors leading to ulceration within individual patients [13, 14]. Optimising vasodilator therapies is vital in the management of SSc-DU and may modify the progression of SSc-related microangiopathy [13, 14]. Indeed, failure to fully exploit the range of treatment options now available for the management of SSc-associated vasculopathy results in an increased burden of SSc-DU [6, 17]. Careful assessment and aggressive management of SSc-DU is vital as 'chronic DU' disease (DU present at every follow-up visit) is associated with higher rates of work absenteeism, disability, need for assistance (paid and unpaid), analgesic requirements and rates of hospitalisation [8, 42, 43].

Acknowledgements We are grateful to each of the patients described in this chapter who each provided written informed consent for their clinical histories and medical images to be used.

Disclosures: Dr. John Pauling has undertaken consultancy work, received speaker's honoraria, educational support and unrestricted research grant support (totalling £25,000) from Janssen (formerly Actelion Pharmaceuticals). Dr John D Pauling has undertaken consultancy work for Astra Zeneca, Boehringer Ingelheim, IsoMab, Permeatus Inc., and Sojournix Pharma.

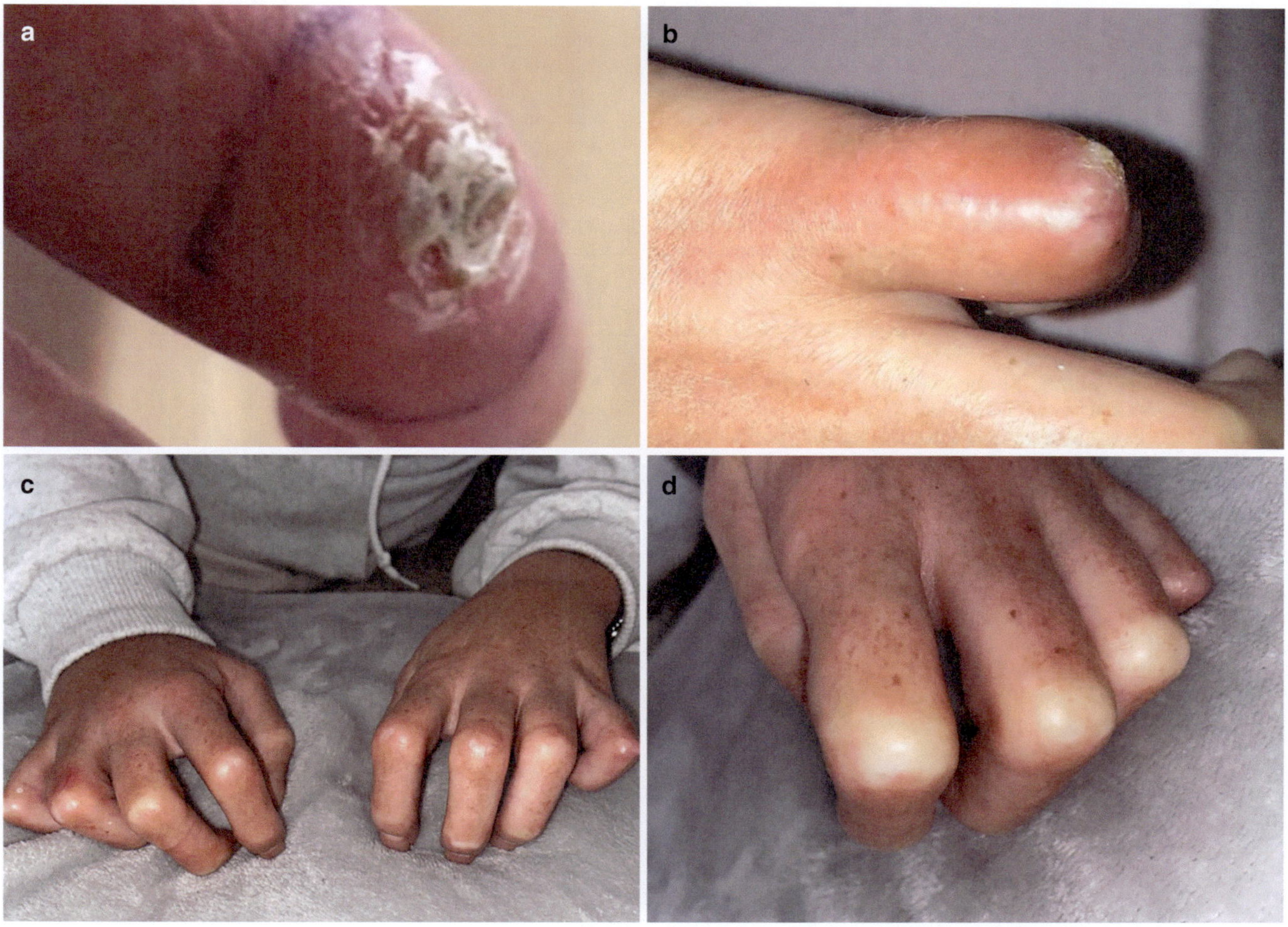

Fig. 57.6 (**a**) Ulceration of dorsal aspect of left fourth finger proximal interphalangeal joint in a 38-year-old female with diffuse cutaneous systemic sclerosis (RNA Pol III with mRSS of 45/51), complicated by local infection; (**b**) Improvement following intravenous antibiotics, iloprost and commencement of sildenafil 50 mg tds, despite ongoing fixed flexion of the finger; (**c**, **d**) Sustained improvement at 1 year but sclerous skin overlying fixed flexion deformities of digits resulting in blanching of skin on dorsal aspect of PIPs which remain vulnerable sites for future ulceration

References

1. Hughes M, Allanore Y, Chung L, Pauling JD, Denton CP, Matucci-Cerinic M. Raynaud phenomenon and digital ulcers in systemic sclerosis. Nat Rev Rheumatol. 2020;16(4):208–21. https://doi.org/10.1038/s41584-020-0386-4.
2. Hughes M, Pauling JD, Jones J, Denton CP, Domsic RT, Frech TM, et al. Multicenter qualitative study exploring the patient experience of digital ulcers in systemic sclerosis. Arthritis Care Res (Hoboken). 2020;72(5):723–33. https://doi.org/10.1002/acr.24127.
3. Hughes M, Pauling JD. Exploring the patient experience of digital ulcers in systemic sclerosis. Semin Arthritis Rheum. 2019;48(5):888–94. https://doi.org/10.1016/j.semarthrit.2018.08.001.
4. Steen V, Denton CP, Pope JE, Matucci-Cerinic M. Digital ulcers: overt vascular disease in systemic sclerosis. Rheumatology (Oxford). 2009;48(Suppl 3):iii19–24. https://doi.org/10.1093/rheumatology/kep105.
5. Ennis H, Vail A, Wragg E, Taylor A, Moore T, Murray A, et al. A prospective study of systemic sclerosis-related digital ulcers: prevalence, location, and functional impact. Scand J Rheumatol. 2013;42(6):483–6. https://doi.org/10.3109/03009742.2013.780095.
6. Hachulla E, Clerson P, Launay D, Lambert M, Morell-Dubois S, Queyrel V, et al. Natural history of ischemic digital ulcers in systemic sclerosis: single-center retrospective longitudinal study. J Rheumatol. 2007;34(12):2423–30.
7. Mihai C, Landewe R, van der Heijde D, Walker UA, Constantin PI, Gherghe AM, et al. Digital ulcers predict a worse disease course in patients with systemic sclerosis. Ann Rheum Dis. 2016;75(4):681–6. https://doi.org/10.1136/annrheumdis-2014-205897.
8. Matucci-Cerinic M, Krieg T, Guillevin L, Schwierin B, Rosenberg D, Cornelisse P, et al. Elucidating the burden of recurrent and chronic digital ulcers in systemic sclerosis: long-term results from the DUO Registry. Ann Rheum Dis. 2016;75(10):1770–6. https://doi.org/10.1136/annrheumdis-2015-208121.
9. Lambova S, Batalov A, Sapundzhiev L, Muller-Ladner U. Digital ulcers in systemic sclerosis—frequency, subtype distribution and

clinical outcome. Curr Rheumatol Rev. 2013;9(4):268–73. https://doi.org/10.2174/157339710904140417125627.
10. Matucci-Cerinic M, Denton CP, Furst DE, Mayes MD, Hsu VM, Carpentier P, et al. Bosentan treatment of digital ulcers related to systemic sclerosis: results from the RAPIDS-2 randomised, double-blind, placebo-controlled trial. Ann Rheum Dis. 2011;70(1):32–8. https://doi.org/10.1136/ard.2010.130658.
11. Korn JH, Mayes M, Matucci Cerinic M, Rainisio M, Pope J, Hachulla E, et al. Digital ulcers in systemic sclerosis: prevention by treatment with bosentan, an oral endothelin receptor antagonist. Arthritis Rheum. 2004;50(12):3985–93. https://doi.org/10.1002/art.20676.
12. Paxton D, Pauling JD. Does nailfold capillaroscopy help predict future outcomes in systemic sclerosis? A systematic literature review. Semin Arthritis Rheum. 2018;48(3):482–94. https://doi.org/10.1016/j.semarthrit.2018.02.005.
13. Cutolo M, Ruaro B, Pizzorni C, Ravera F, Smith V, Zampogna G, et al. Long-term treatment with endothelin receptor antagonist bosentan and iloprost improves fingertip blood perfusion in systemic sclerosis. J Rheumatol. 2014;41(5):881–6. https://doi.org/10.3899/jrheum.131284.
14. Trombetta AC, Pizzorni C, Ruaro B, Paolino S, Sulli A, Smith V, et al. Effects of Long-term treatment with bosentan and iloprost on nailfold absolute capillary number, fingertip blood perfusion, and clinical status in systemic sclerosis. J Rheumatol. 2016;43(11):2033–41. https://doi.org/10.3899/jrheum.160592.
15. Steen V, Medsger TA Jr. Predictors of isolated pulmonary hypertension in patients with systemic sclerosis and limited cutaneous involvement. Arthritis Rheum. 2003;48(2):516–22. https://doi.org/10.1002/art.10775.
16. Allanore Y, Meune C, Vonk MC, Airo P, Hachulla E, Caramaschi P, et al. Prevalence and factors associated with left ventricular dysfunction in the EULAR Scleroderma Trial and Research group (EUSTAR) database of patients with systemic sclerosis. Ann Rheum Dis. 2010;69(1):218–21. https://doi.org/10.1136/ard.2008.103382.
17. Caramaschi P, Martinelli N, Volpe A, Pieropan S, Tinazzi I, Patuzzo G, et al. A score of risk factors associated with ischemic digital ulcers in patients affected by systemic sclerosis treated with iloprost. Clin Rheumatol. 2009;28(7):807–13. https://doi.org/10.1007/s10067-009-1155-6.
18. Pauling JD, McGrogan A, Snowball J, McHugh NJ. Epidemiology of systemic sclerosis in the UK: an analysis of the clinical practice research datalink. Rheumatology (Oxford). 2020;60:2688. https://doi.org/10.1093/rheumatology/keaa680.
19. Silva I, Loureiro T, Teixeira A, Almeida I, Mansilha A, Vasconcelos C, et al. Digital ulcers in systemic sclerosis: role of flow-mediated dilatation and capillaroscopy as risk assessment tools. Eur J Dermatol. 2015;25(5):444–51. https://doi.org/10.1684/ejd.2015.2605.
20. Gigante A, Bruni C, Lepri G, Tesei G, Maestripieri V, Guiducci S, et al. The renal resistive index: a new biomarker for the follow-up of vascular modifications in systemic sclerosis. J Rheumatol. 2020;48:241. https://doi.org/10.3899/jrheum.191101.
21. Wig S, Wilkinson J, Moore T, Manning J, Chevance A, Vail A, et al. A longitudinal study of ankle brachial pressure indices in a cohort of patients with systemic sclerosis. Rheumatology (Oxford). 2014;53(11):2009–13. https://doi.org/10.1093/rheumatology/keu227.
22. Chatterjee S, Pauling JD. Anti-phospholipid syndrome leading to digital ischaemia and rare organ complications in systemic sclerosis and related disorders. Clin Rheumatol. 2020;40:2457. https://doi.org/10.1007/s10067-020-05399-4.
23. Sobanski V, Lemaire-Olivier A, Giovannelli J, Dauchet L, Simon M, Lopez B, et al. Prevalence and clinical associations of antiphospholipid antibodies in systemic sclerosis: new data from a French cross-sectional study, systematic review, and meta-analysis. Front Immunol. 2018;9:2457. https://doi.org/10.3389/fimmu.2018.02457.
24. Merashli M, Alves J, Ames PRJ. Clinical relevance of antiphospholipid antibodies in systemic sclerosis: a systematic review and meta-analysis. Semin Arthritis Rheum. 2017;46(5):615–24. https://doi.org/10.1016/j.semarthrit.2016.10.004.
25. Martin M, Martinez C, Arnaud L, Weber JC, Poindron V, Blaison G, et al. Association of antiphospholipid antibodies with active digital ulceration in systemic sclerosis. RMD Open. 2019;5(2):e001012. https://doi.org/10.1136/rmdopen-2019-001012.
26. Cervera R, Piette JC, Font J, Khamashta MA, Shoenfeld Y, Camps MT, et al. Antiphospholipid syndrome: clinical and immunologic manifestations and patterns of disease expression in a cohort of 1,000 patients. Arthritis Rheum. 2002;46(4):1019–27. https://doi.org/10.1002/art.10187.
27. Cervera R, Boffa MC, Khamashta MA, Hughes GR. The euro-phospholipid project: epidemiology of the antiphospholipid syndrome in Europe. Lupus. 2009;18(10):889–93. https://doi.org/10.1177/0961203309106832.
28. Stojanovich L, Marisavljevic D, Rovensky J, Djokovich A, Kozakova D, Milinic N. Clinical and laboratory features of the catastrophic antiphospholipid syndrome. Clin Rev Allergy Immunol. 2009;36(2–3):74–9. https://doi.org/10.1007/s12016-008-8108-8.
29. Keo HH, Umer M, Baumgartner I, Willenberg T, Gretener SB. Long-term clinical outcomes in patients diagnosed with severe digital ischemia. Swiss Med Wkly. 2011;141:w13159. https://doi.org/10.4414/smw.2011.13159.
30. Marchal A, Mahe E, Sin C, Bagan P, Bilan P, Linder JF, et al. Acute finger ischemia: a retrospective study of 13 patients. Annales de dermatologie et de venereologie. 2015;142(5):332–9. https://doi.org/10.1016/j.annder.2015.02.018.
31. Pauling JD, O'Donnell VB, McHugh NJ. The contribution of platelets to the pathogenesis of Raynaud's phenomenon and systemic sclerosis. Platelets. 2013;24(7):503–15. https://doi.org/10.3109/09537104.2012.719090.
32. Hughes M, Ong VH, Anderson ME, Hall F, Moinzadeh P, Griffiths B, et al. Consensus best practice pathway of the UK Scleroderma Study Group: digital vasculopathy in systemic sclerosis. Rheumatology (Oxford). 2015;54(11):2015–24. https://doi.org/10.1093/rheumatology/kev201.
33. Valenzuela A, Baron M, Rodriguez-Reyna TS, Proudman S, Khanna D, Young A, et al. Calcinosis is associated with ischemic manifestations and increased disability in patients with systemic sclerosis. Semin Arthritis Rheum. 2020;50(5):891–6. https://doi.org/10.1016/j.semarthrit.2020.06.007.
34. Baron M, Pope J, Robinson D, Jones N, Khalidi N, Docherty P, et al. Calcinosis is associated with digital ischaemia in systemic sclerosis-a longitudinal study. Rheumatology (Oxford). 2016;55(12):2148–55. https://doi.org/10.1093/rheumatology/kew313.
35. Valenzuela A, Baron M, Canadian Scleroderma Research G, et al. Calcinosis is associated with digital ulcers and osteoporosis in patients with systemic sclerosis: a Scleroderma Clinical Trials Consortium study. Semin Arthritis Rheum. 2016;46(3):344–9. https://doi.org/10.1016/j.semarthrit.2016.05.008.
36. Morardet L, Avouac J, Sammour M, Baron M, Kahan A, Feydy A, et al. Late nailfold videocapillaroscopy pattern associated with hand calcinosis and acro-osteolysis in systemic sclerosis. Arthritis Care Res (Hoboken). 2016;68(3):366–73. https://doi.org/10.1002/acr.22672.
37. Robertson LP, Marshall RW, Hickling P. Treatment of cutaneous calcinosis in limited systemic sclerosis with minocycline. Ann Rheum Dis. 2003;62(3):267–9. https://doi.org/10.1136/ard.62.3.267.
38. Tosounidou S, MacDonald H, Situnayake D. Successful treatment of calcinosis with infliximab in a patient with systemic sclerosis/myositis overlap syndrome. Rheumatology (Oxford). 2014;53(5):960–1. https://doi.org/10.1093/rheumatology/ket365.

39. Galimberti F, Li Y, Fernandez AP. Intravenous immunoglobulin for treatment of dermatomyositis-associated dystrophic calcinosis. J Am Acad Dermatol. 2015;73(1):174–6. https://doi.org/10.1016/j.jaad.2015.03.047.
40. Touimy M, Janani S, Rachidi W, Etaouil N, Mkinsi O. Calcinosis universalis complicating juvenile dermatomyositis: improvement after intravenous immunoglobulin therapy. Joint Bone Spine. 2013;80(1):108–9. https://doi.org/10.1016/j.jbspin.2012.07.001.
41. Penate Y, Guillermo N, Melwani P, Martel R, Hernandez-Machin B, Borrego L. Calcinosis cutis associated with amyopathic dermatomyositis: response to intravenous immunoglobulin. J Am Acad Dermatol. 2009;60(6):1076–7. https://doi.org/10.1016/j.jaad.2008.09.051.
42. Matucci-Cerinic M, Seibold JR. Digital ulcers and outcomes assessment in scleroderma. Rheumatology (Oxford). 2008;47(Suppl 5):v46–7. https://doi.org/10.1093/rheumatology/ken310.
43. Guillevin L, Hunsche E, Denton CP, Krieg T, Schwierin B, Rosenberg D, et al. Functional impairment of systemic scleroderma patients with digital ulcerations: results from the DUO Registry. Clin Exp Rheumatol. 2013;31(2 Suppl 76):71–80.
44. Pauling JD. Vasodilation is not the only approach to the management of cutaneous ulceration in systemic sclerosis. Rheumatology (Oxford). 2017;56(9):1559. https://doi.org/10.1093/rheumatology/kex175.

Lower Limb Ulceration

58

Muditha Samaranayaka, Ariane L. Herrick, and Nuala O'Donoghue

Introduction

Lower limb ulcers are uncommon in patients with systemic sclerosis (SSc) [1–3]. However, when they do occur, they can be very difficult to heal due to a combination of poor blood supply and (in some patients) the tightness of the surrounding skin. They have been relatively little researched. A multicentre retrospective study of 45 patients with SSc and lower limb ulcers [3] reported that in 22 patients (49%) these were predominantly venous and in 21 (47%) ischaemic (macrovascular in 7 [16%]). An earlier study of 60 patients with SSc and 'lower limb cutaneous lesions' (41 of whom had ulcers) similarly showed that while some patients had venous and others arterial insufficiency, SSc-related microangiopathy (leading to ischaemia) was often the major contributory factor [2].

The purpose of this chapter is not to review the pathogenesis and epidemiology of SSc-related lower limb ulcers but rather to present four short cases, each describing a type of lower limb ulcer which can occur in patients with SSc and which can present challenges in both assessment and management. In addition, we provide some practical tips for the clinician. These four types of ulcers are: ischaemic toe ulcers, ulcers overlying areas of calcinosis, 'mechanical' ulcers over the malleoli in patients with diffuse cutaneous SSc, and small superficial ulcers/erosions in patients with early diffuse cutaneous SSc and rapidly progressive scleroderma. After each case, we include a general discussion about the type of ulcer in question, including investigation and management. Other types of lower limb ulcer can of course occur in patients with SSc, for example (as mentioned earlier), venous ulcers, and (rarely) vasculitic ulcers. Lower limb ulcers in patients with SSc pose particular management challenges irrespective of aetiology. We have therefore included a section entitled 'general approach to the management of lower limb ulceration in the patient with SSc'.

M. Samaranayaka · N. O'Donoghue
Northern Care Alliance NHS Foundation Trust, Salford, UK
e-mail: muditha.samaranayaka@nca.nhs.uk; Nuala.O'Donoghue@nca.nhs.uk

A. L. Herrick (✉)
Division of Musculoskeletal and Dermatological Sciences, The University of Manchester, Northern Care Alliance NHS Foundation Trust, Manchester Academic Health Science Centre, Manchester, UK
e-mail: ariane.herrick@manchester.ac.uk

Case 1: Ischaemic Toe Ulceration

A 32-year-old woman was reviewed urgently in view of deterioration of a left great toe ulcer. This ulcer, present for more than 6 months despite regular dressings by nursing staff and short courses of oral antibiotics, had become more symptomatic, and she described throbbing pain at night requiring opiates. The patient had a 6-year history of diffuse cutaneous SSc (anti Scl70 positive) with inflammatory arthritis/myositis overlap and a probable lupus component evidenced by elevated double stranded DNA (dsDNA) antibodies. She had a complicated disease course including severe digital vasculopathy with recurrent digital ulcers. She was a non-smoker.

Current treatment included nifedipine (sustained release), sildenafil, clopidogrel, mycophenolate mofetil, and moderate dose prednisolone. Bosentan was not considered as she was planning conception. Previous treatments included intravenous (IV) iloprost infusions and rituximab.

On examination, she had an infected necrotic ulcer mainly over the medial border of the left great toe (Fig. 58.1). She was systemically well with good peripheral pulses.

Investigations: Arterial Doppler scan showed normal Doppler waveforms and pressures. The wound swab grew *Staphylococcus aureus* and mixed coliforms sensitive to flucloxacillin and co-trimoxazole. Plain radiography of the left foot (Fig. 58.2) showed no findings such as bone destruction or demineralisation which might be related to osteomyelitis. Magnetic resonance (MR) imaging of the left foot (Fig. 58.3) showed oedema of the distal aspect of the proximal phalanx;

Y. Allanore et al. (eds.), *Scleroderma*, https://doi.org/10.1007/978-3-031-40658-4_58

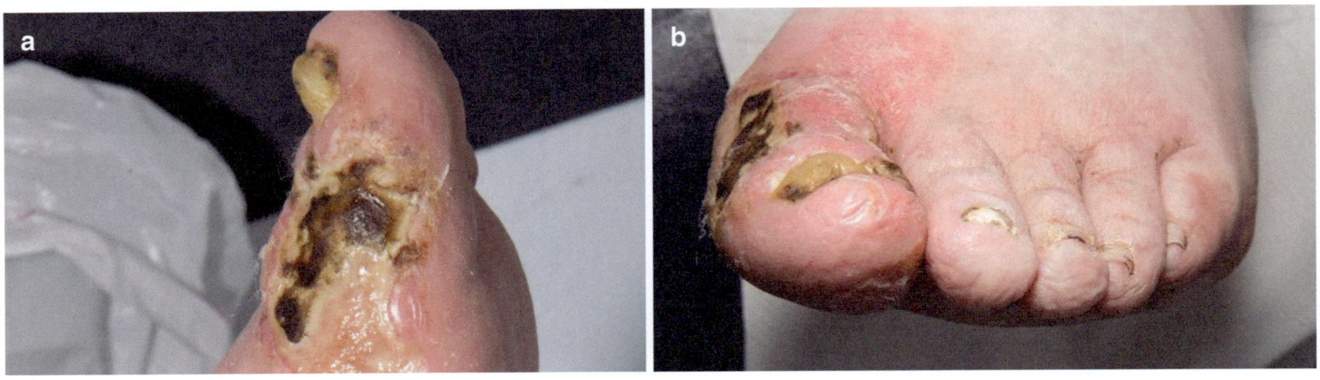

Fig. 58.1 (**a**) Lateral view of the angulated necrotic ischaemic ulcer with overlying eschar on medial great toe. Note the thickened dystrophic great toenail. (**b**) Frontal view of the same ischaemic ulcer with surrounding ill-defined erythema and oedema compared to normal looking skin on the rest of the foot. Images copyright of Northern Care Alliance NHS Foundation Trust

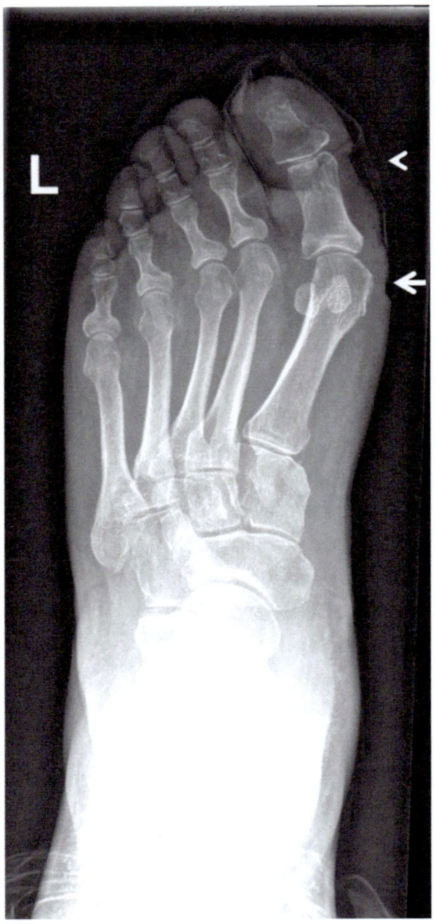

Fig. 58.2 Dorsoplantar X-ray of the left foot with soft tissue ulceration (arrow) and dressing (arrow head) but no bone destruction or demineralisation

early osteomyelitis could not be excluded. C-reactive protein (CRP) was 12 mg/l (reference 0–7). Antineutrophil cytoplasmic antibodies (ANCA), lupus anticoagulant, anticardiolipin IgG and IgM antibodies, and anti-beta 2 glycoprotein IgG and IgM antibodies were negative, C3 and C4 normal, dsDNA 11 iu/mL (reference <8).

Management and outcome: Over the previous 8 weeks, she had already received three courses of oral antibiotics: firstly, flucloxacillin 500 mg four times daily for 2 weeks followed by a 1-week course of cephalexin and a 1-week course of co-amoxiclav. Mycophenolate mofetil was temporarily discontinued.

As advised by microbiology, oral flucloxacillin 1 g four times daily was prescribed for 6 weeks, given the clinical concern (together with the MR appearances) of underlying osteomyelitis. She declined hospital admission for IV iloprost and IV antibiotic therapy due to the Covid 19 pandemic.

Remote monitoring via patient feedback and digital photographs, in view of the ongoing pandemic (Fig. 58.4) confirmed slow and steady improvement of this ulcer following the prolonged course of flucloxacillin, with frequent careful nursing care and dressing changes.

Discussion

Ischaemic toe ulcers in patients with SSc are always a major concern. They may reflect severe vascular compromise, and often become infected, sometimes progressing to osteomyelitis which can be very refractory to treatment.

Therefore, the first step in assessment, especially in patients with associated critical ischaemia as in this patient, is to exclude large (proximal) vessel disease (e.g. femoral or tibial artery [4] stenosis or occlusion) requiring immediate intervention [5]. And so the key point on examination is to assess the peripheral arterial circulation by feeling for the peripheral pulses. This patient had good peripheral pulses, confirmed on lower limb arterial Doppler examination, and so did not require urgent referral to the vascular surgical

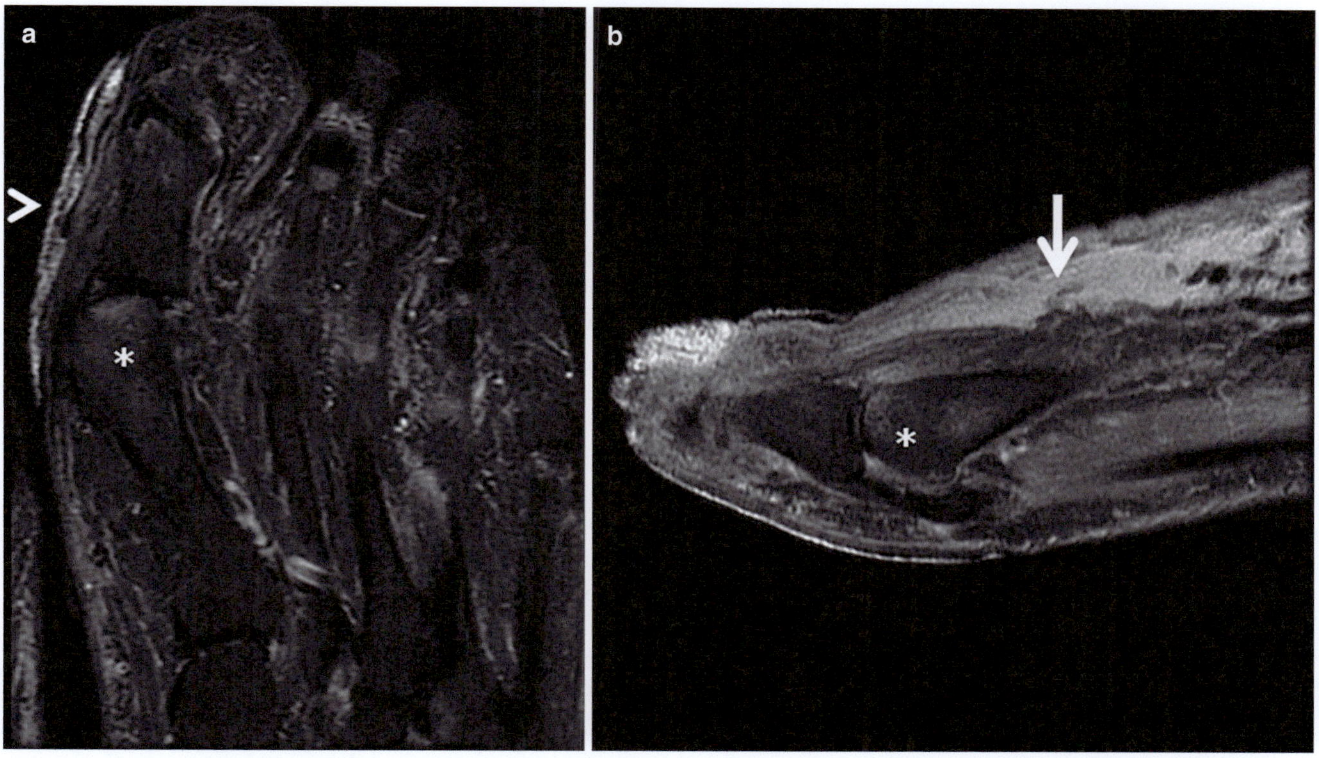

Fig. 58.3 Sagittal (**a**) and axial (**b**) STIR images showing mild oedema in the head of the great toe metatarsal (*), marked subcutaneous oedema (arrow), and dressing (arrow head). Courtesy of Professor Jonathan Harris, Northern Care Alliance NHS Foundation Trust

team. Patients most likely to have proximal large vessel disease are those with cardiovascular risk factors, for example, smoking. A combination of large vessel atherosclerosis and SSc-related microangiopathy puts patients at high risk of severe digital ischaemia which, if left untreated, may progress rapidly and necessitate below knee amputation. The patients with large vessel disease described by Boheley et al. [3] had a particularly poor prognosis with amputation (toe or transmetatarsal) required in 4 out of 7 (57%).

Another important step is to determine whether the ulcer is secondarily infected and if so whether the infection has spread to bone. Assessment of soft tissue infection is on the basis of the history and examination (increasing pain, purulent discharge, erythema, swelling). The ulcer should be swabbed for bacterial culture and sensitivity to direct antibiotic therapy. Ongoing/increasing severe pain and tenderness (as in this patient) should raise suspicion of development of osteomyelitis. Plain radiography is an insensitive tool for detection of early osteomyelitis, which is often well demonstrated on MR scanning. Whether or not bone infection has developed, an exquisitely tender toe often indicates the need for surgical debridement to remove necrotic tissue.

Management of SSc-related ischaemic toe ulcers is similar to that recommended for finger ulcers [6] and includes local wound care, analgesia, antibiotics if any clinical suspicion of infection, optimising vasodilator treatment and (when appropriate) surgery. In the case described, surgery proved not to be necessary, but would have been indicated had the ulcer not improved on optimal antibiotic therapy. This case demonstrates that with optimal medical and nursing care even large, necrotic toe ulcers can heal in patients with SSc [7].

Practical Tips—Ischaemic Toe Ulcers

1. Feel for the peripheral pulses—if absent, and a toe ulcer is associated with critical ischaemia, then this is a vascular surgical emergency.
2. Maintain a high index of suspicion of underlying bone infection, especially if the ulcer is very painful and tender (remember that plain radiographs are insensitive to early osteomyelitis).

Case 2: Ulceration Overlying Calcinosis

A 58-year-old woman was seen urgently because of an infected ulcer overlying calcinosis related to the left knee. She described local swelling, erythema, and night pain for 2 days preceded by a discharge of white material from the ulcer.

She had first presented 15 years earlier with classic features of dermatomyositis and new onset Raynaud's phenomenon and was found to be anti-PM-Scl 100 positive. Two years later, she developed puffy fingers, distal skin tightness,

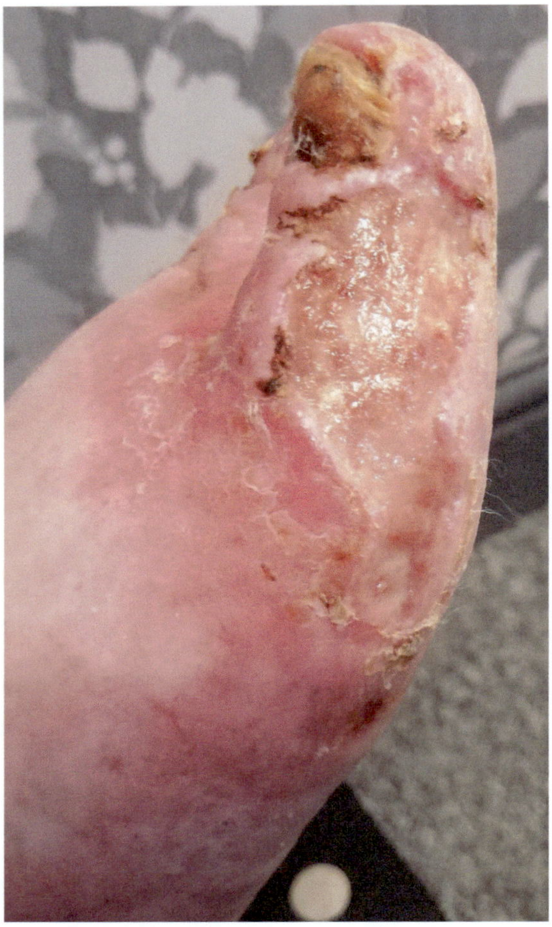

Fig. 58.4 Mobile phone photograph demonstrating gradual healing by secondary intention with the erosion now visibly more superficial 4 months after starting higher dose flucloxacillin. Images copyright of Northern Care Alliance NHS Foundation Trust

and telangiectases and a diagnosis of SSc was made. Rapidly progressive calcinosis later became a major issue requiring surgical debulking of fingertip and right elbow calcinosis to reduce infections and pain. Treatment comprised azathioprine, prednisolone (low dose), nifedipine (sustained release), sildenafil, and latterly minocycline. She had intermittently required courses of oral antibiotics for infection related to calcinosis and IV iloprost infusions.

On examination, the left knee demonstrated a hard irregular swelling typical of calcinosis anterior to the left knee, the overlying skin was erythematous and extremely tender with a bead of calcium about to extrude just beneath the skin (Fig. 58.5a). Her temperature was 37.4 °C.

Management and outcome: She was admitted for IV antibiotics and urgent orthopaedic review. The orthopaedic surgeons were satisfied that no immediate surgical intervention was indicated. She was treated with intravenous flucloxacillin, to which the *Staphylococcus aureus* grown on a bacterial swab from her knee was fully sensitive.

The CRP which was 17 (reference <10 mg/L) on admission fell to <4. Plain radiographs showed very extensive calcinosis (Fig. 58.5b). The skin overlying the calcinosis subsequently ulcerated. After 12 days in hospital, she was well enough to go home with resolving ulceration (Fig. 58.5c) to complete a further 1-week course of oral flucloxacillin.

Discussion

SSc-related calcinosis (subcutaneous or intracutaneous deposition of calcium salts) often ulcerates through skin, and in the lower limb most commonly occurs anterior to the

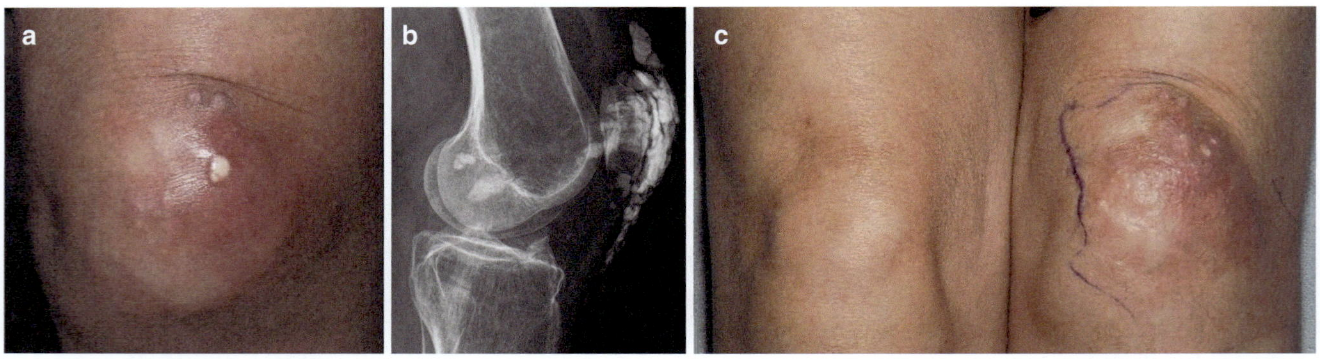

Fig. 58.5 (**a**) Incipient superficial erosion overlying chalky white intradermal papule of calcinosis, lying within a tight, shiny erythematous and swollen plaque of calcinosis on the knee. Note the multiple, much smaller white perforating papules with surrounding hyperkeratosis and hyperpigmentation at the borders of the plaque. (**b**) Lateral X-ray of knee showing extensive calcinosis. (**c**) Healing punctate tiny ulcers and resolving surrounding soft tissue infection following treatment with IV antibiotics; see marker pen marks delineating previous cellulitic changes, now resolved. Images copyright of Northern Care Alliance NHS Foundation Trust

knee. At sites of calcinosis, the skin and subcutaneous tissue can feel very hard and related ulcers are therefore often under tension. Finger ulcers have been studied more than lower limb ulcers, and in the fingers calcinosis-related ulcers take longer to heal than those not associated with calcinosis [8]. Perhaps not surprising given the additional gravitational factors at play, lower limb calcinosis-related ulceration can be very difficult to heal.

Calcinosis is well demonstrated on plain radiographs, and so if there is any doubt as to whether there is underlying calcinosis then this can be easily resolved by a radiograph. At present, there are no effective medical treatments for SSc-related calcinosis [9]. Therefore, the mainstay of current management is expert wound care. Surgery is only rarely required. Prevention of ulceration is important, by protecting vulnerable areas and optimising vasodilator therapy, as ischaemia may contribute to calcinosis [10–12].

Practical Tips—Ulcers Associated with Underlying Calcinosis

1. Have a low threshold for prescribing an antibiotic for calcinosis-related ulcers because these are often secondarily infected. Topical antiseptics can be helpful.
2. Surgery debulks but does not remove calcinosis, and so the patient should be told that the calcinosis can 'regrow'.

Case 3: Ulcers Overlying the Malleoli

A 56-year-old man was admitted with rapidly progressive diffuse cutaneous SSc and myositis, with the onset of skin thickening and Raynaud's phenomenon around 2 months earlier. Shortly after admission, he developed ulcers over both lateral malleoli (Fig. 58.6). They resembled arterial ulcers but arterial Doppler findings were normal reflecting normal large arteries (despite his chronic smoking habit). The ulcers became secondarily infected with methicillin-resistant *Staphylococcus aureus*, requiring treatment with systemic and topical antibiotics.

His hospital stay was complicated by asymptomatic Covid-19 infection. He was discharged on moderate-dose prednisolone (for myositis) with the intention of commencing mycophenolate mofetil (delayed due to Covid-19). However, he was re-admitted shortly after with renal crisis and developed cardiac problems. Two months later, the lower limb ulcerations continued to heal slowly with tissue viability nurse input; however, he required opiates for pain management.

Discussion

In our experience, ulcers over pressure points are far less common in the lower than in the upper limb, where they are commonly found over the extensor aspects of the fingers [8, 13]

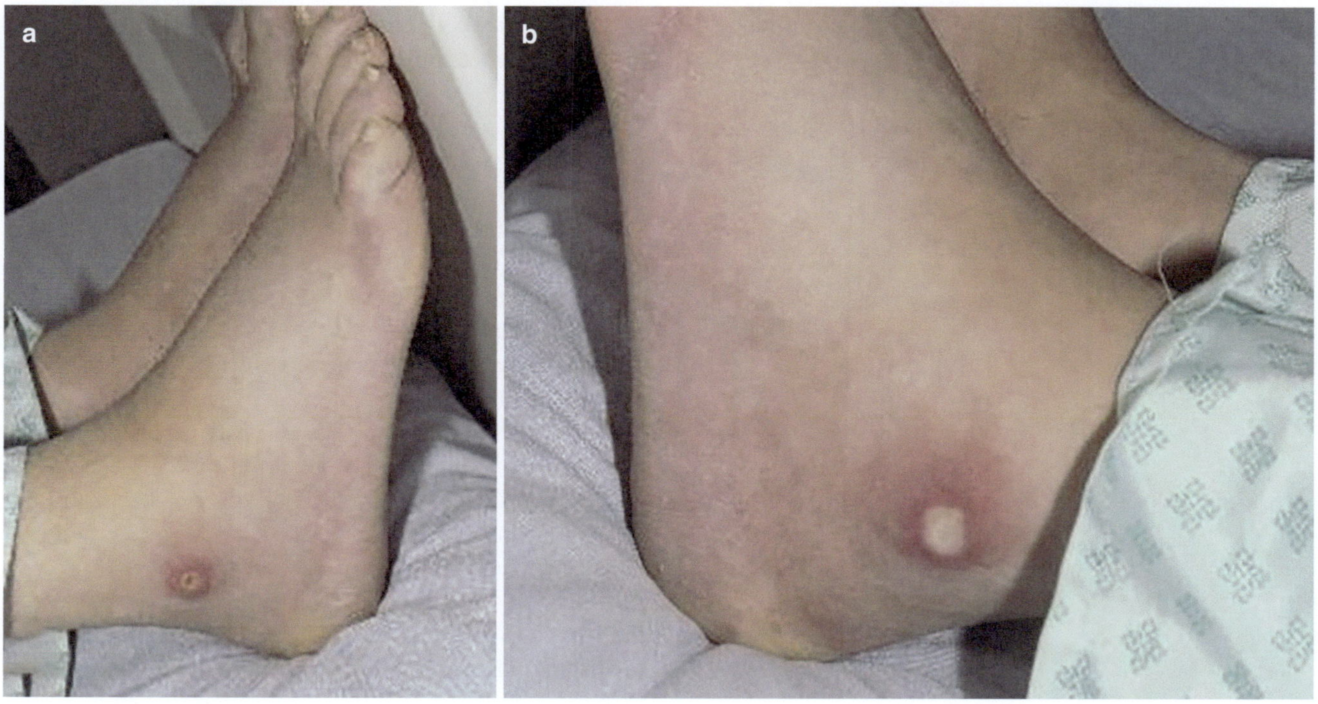

Fig. 58.6 (**a, b**). Punched-out ulcers with surrounding erythema on both lateral malleoli, with surrounding oedema causing loss of normal bony prominences. Note the skin pallor and reduced hair growth. Images copyright of Northern Care Alliance NHS Foundation Trust

and have an ischaemic component [14]. However, ulcers can (rarely) occur over the malleoli as described in this case, especially in the context of early diffuse cutaneous disease: the likely cause is the underlying microvascular disease, with the skin being stretched over the bony prominence causing biomechanical stresses contributing to the ulceration. Several series and case reports specifically mention and/or illustrate malleolar ulcers [1, 15–17], possibly reflecting their refractoriness to treatment. The mainstays of management are excluding significant arterial disease, local wound care, analgesia, the use of antiseptics, prompt treatment of secondary cutaneous infection, and consideration of immunosuppression if there is progressive skin disease, if the patient is not already on this.

Case 4: Superficial Ulceration/Erosion in Early Diffuse Cutaneous SSc

A 63-year-old woman with diffuse cutaneous SSc (anti-RNA polymerase III positive) and inflammatory myositis diagnosed 6 months previously was noted to have a worsening modified Rodnan skin score (which had progressed from 24 to 34) and severe pruritus. She had also developed recurrent superficial skin ulcerations where the skin was very tight (Fig. 58.7).

She was admitted for IV iloprost infusions on the assumption that these ulcers were partly due to microangiopathy. The dermatology team prescribed clobetasol-propionate cream, soft white paraffin as an emollient, and oral antihistamines for the itching. After iloprost, the ulcers and itch were less troublesome.

After autologous stem cell transplantation, skin tightness and itching gradually improved but the superficial ulcers recurred and were again treated with IV iloprost 5-month post-transplantation (Fig. 58.8) to good clinical effect. She has since been free of ulcers and is no longer requiring systemic immunosuppression.

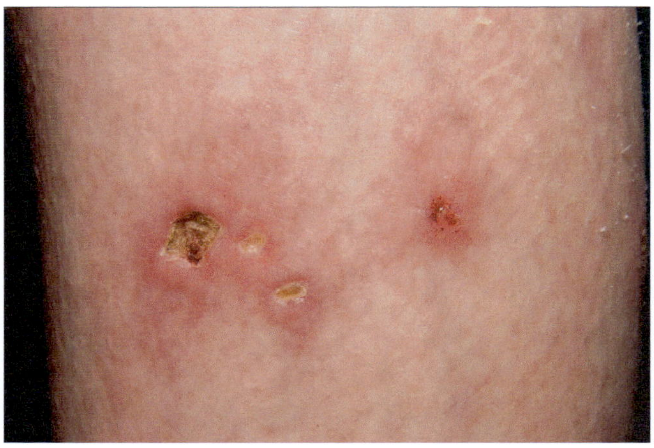

Fig. 58.7 Superficial ulceration of the lower leg with marked surrounding erythema in early diffuse cutaneous SSc. Image copyright of Northern Care Alliance NHS Foundation Trust'

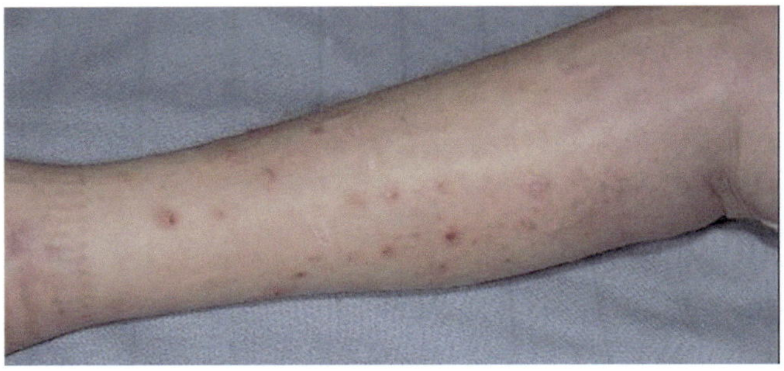

Fig. 58.8 Diffuse superficial erosions, shiny-surfaced papules and small atrophic scars overlying tight, pale skin on the calves. Note the contrasting erythema distally and proximally. Oedema is demonstrated by the pitted clothing marks on the ankle. Images copyright of Northern Care Alliance NHS Foundation Trust

Discussion

In our experience, small superficial ulcers/erosions can occur in very rapidly progressive early diffuse cutaneous disease, more commonly in the upper than in the lower limbs. On the assumption that there is an ischaemic component to these ulcers, we have tried IV infusions of iloprost, usually with good effect as in the case described. It is important to assess the patient for pruritus to determine if these lesions represent primarily excoriations associated with SSc, as 43–62% patients with SSc [18–20] describe itch which is associated with the degree of skin involvement [19].

General Approach to the Management of Lower Limb Ulceration in the Patient with Systemic Sclerosis

The first step in management is to diagnose the type of ulcer. In addition to considering ulceration associated with SSc, other causes of ulceration must be considered (see Table 58.1), and also the possibility of contribution of comorbidities as a multifactorial pathogenesis is not uncommon [2]. For instance, venous stasis may be partially responsible for an ulcer and may be associated with lipodermatosclerosis changes to the ankle and gaiter areas which may complicate the clinical picture. A careful history should include assessing for comorbidities such as diabetes, hypertension, thyroid disease, deep vein thrombosis (and pro-thrombotic states), arterial disease, inflammatory conditions which can be associated with ulcerating conditions such as pyoderma gangrenosum, and underlying causes of itch, if present. Examination should include a full skin check, assessment of the ulcer to look for diagnostic clues, examination of the peripheral pulses, and the legs whilst the patient is standing to look for evidence of varicose veins. Patients with SSc are often treated with immunosuppressants, which may predispose to primary or secondary infection, or an ulcerating skin

Table 58.1 Causes of lower limb ulceration (to be considered when assessing an ulcer in systemic sclerosis)

• Trauma/pressure
• Infection including atypical organisms/leprosy/tuberculosis/fungae/leishmaniasis
• Chronic venous insufficiency
• Chronic arterial insufficiency
• Neuropathic ulcer (including secondary to diabetes)
• Hypertension
• Skin malignancy
• Inflammatory causes of ulceration including pyoderma gangrenosum; vasculitis; rheumatoid ulceration; necrobiosis lipoidica diabeticorum; livedoid vasculopathy associated with coagulation disorders; warfarin and heparin induced necrosis; cholesterol or septic embolism; calciphylaxis; dysglobulinaemias and primary blistering conditions of the skin such as epidermolysis bullosa acquisita

malignancy such as squamous cell carcinoma. Systemic steroid therapy (which may be prescribed in patients with SSc overlap syndromes, and all four cases described here had a myositis overlap, one with inflammatory arthritis) may be associated with hypertension and diabetes, which in turn may be associated with ulceration.

Investigations to consider include those tailored towards the possible differential cause of ulceration, and a dermatology opinion and skin biopsy may be required. The authors would recommend assessment of the peripheral vasculature by Doppler ultrasound in most cases: arterial disease may require specific treatment and may preclude compression bandaging (discussed below).

The authors also recommend skin swabs for bacterial culture as secondary infection is not infrequent, as well as serological markers of inflammation such as erythrocyte sedimentation rate/CRP. Investigations for underlying bony involvement should be requested if there is any concern about osteomyelitis. Itch, where present, should be investigated to exclude and manage other causes for itch such as anaemia, renal impairment, and hypothyroidism. We would also recommend checking for lupus anticoagulant and anticardiolipin antibodies: Shamugan et al. [1] reported that of 10 patients with non-digital lower limb ulcers, 5 had antiphospholipid antibodies, and 7 a positive genetic prothombotic screen.

Treatment of ulceration needs to be tailored to the cause of the ulceration and any concomitant large vessel disease should be treated [21]. Expert wound care is probably the most important aspect of management, this includes skilled nursing support to provide topical treatments and dressings. Compression, given the frequency of co-existence of venous disease in particular [3], is often advised to support wound healing in the absence of arterial disease.

The patient's smoking status, diet, and exercise should be reviewed and where appropriate, addressed, as well as general medical problems such as anaemia and heart failure which would delay healing. These general measures should be combined with optimising blood flow with vasodilator therapies, analgesia, and antiseptics. Where appropriate, following swabs, antibiotic therapy may be required: it is the authors' experience that bacterial infection is not uncommon in this immunosuppressed cohort of patients. Analgesia is another important aspect of management. Low-dose naltrexone has been found to be efficacious in patients with chronic pruritus related to numerous dermatological conditions, and one small series of three patients taking this for pruritus in the context of SSc reported substantial response [22]: this is relevant because scratching itchy areas will exacerbate ulceration.

Case reports and small series have reported benefit from a number of other treatment modalities, both local and systemic, including platelet gel [15], the endothelin receptor antagonist bosentan [16], hyperbaric oxygen therapy [17], spinal cord stimulation [23], and skin grafting [21, 24].

Practical Tips—General Assessment and Management of Lower Limb Ulcers in Patients with SSc

1. Always consider the possibility of comorbidities (e.g. arterial or venous disease) which may be contributory or causative.
2. Look for (and treat) secondary infection.
3. Before applying compression bandaging, exclude concomitant large vessel disease which poses additional risk in patients with SSc who already have a compromised vasculature.

Conclusions

Lower limb ulcers are unusual in patients with SSc, but when they do occur, it can be a major source of morbidity because they are often very painful and slow/difficult to heal. At worst, they can necessitate amputation. The main 'disease-specific' issues which can be contributory are microangiopathy (leading to ischaemia), mechanical factors (stretching of taught skin over pressure points), and underlying calcinosis. However, other factors/comorbidities should also be considered including large vessel arterial disease and venous disease, and secondary infection. Expert nursing care is a key aspect of management.

Acknowledgement This work was supported by the NIHR Manchester Biomedical Research Centre.

References

1. Shanmugam VK, Price P, Attinger CE, Steen VD. Lower extremity ulcers in systemic sclerosis: features and response to therapy. Int J Rheumatol. 2010;2010:747946.
2. Blagojevic J, Piemonte G, Benelli L, Braschi F, Fiori G, Bartoli F, et al. Assessment, definition, and classification of lower limb ulcers in systemic sclerosis: a challenge for the rheumatologist. J Rheumatol. 2016;43(3):592–8.
3. Bohelay G, Blaise S, Levy P, Claeys A, Baudot N, Cuny JF, et al. Lower-limb ulcers in systemic sclerosis: a multicentre retrospective case-control study. Acta Derm Venereol. 2018;98(7):677–82.
4. Deguchi J, Shigematsu K, Ota S, Kimura H, Fukayama M, Miyata T. Surgical result of critical limb ischemia due to tibial arterial occlusion in patients with systemic scleroderma. J Vasc Surg. 2009;49(4):918–23.
5. Sharp C, Akram Q, Hughes M, Muir L, Herrick AL. Differential diagnosis of critical digital ischemia in systemic sclerosis: report of five cases and review of the literature. Sem Arthritis Rheum. 2016;46:209–16.
6. Hughes M, Ong VH, Anderson ME, Hall F, Moinzadeh P, Griffiths B, et al. Consensus best practice pathway of the UK Systemic Sclerosis Study Group: digital vasculopathy in systemic sclerosis. Rheumatology. 2015;54:2015–24.
7. Abignano G, Mennillo G, Letteri G. Foot ulcers in systemic sclerosis escape surgical amputation. Lancet. 2020;396:E29.
8. Amanzi L, Braschi F, Fiori G, Galluccio F, Miniati I, Guiducci S, et al. Digital ulcers in scleroderma: staging, characteristics and subsetting through observation of 1614 digital lesions. Rheumatology. 2010;49:1374–82.
9. Valenzuela A, Song P, Chung L. Calcinosis in scleroderma. Curr Opin Rheumatol. 2018;30:554–61.
10. Baron M, Pope J, Robinson D, Jones N, Khalidi N, Docherty P, et al. Calcinosis is associated with digital ischaemia in systemic sclerosis - a longitudinal study. Rheumatology. 2016;55:2148–55.
11. Valenzuela A, Baron M, Rodriguez-Reyna TS, Proudman S, Khanna D, Young A, et al. Calcinosis is associated with ischemic manifestations and increased disability in patients with systemic sclerosis. Sem Arthritis Rheum. 2020;50:891–6.
12. Manning JB, Marjanovic E, Moore TL, Dinsdale G, Wilkinson S, Dickinson MR, et al. A pilot study of cutaneous oxygenation and perfusion in systemic sclerosis-related digital calcinosis (letter). Rheumatology. 2020;59:3109–11.
13. Ennis H, Vail A, Wragg E, Taylor A, Moore T, Murray A, et al. A prospective study of systemic sclerosis-related digital ulcers: prevalence, location, and functional impact. Scand J Rheumatol. 2013;42(6):483–6.
14. Murray A, Moore T, Wragg E, Ennis H, Vail A, Dinsdale G, et al. Pilot study assessing pathophysiology and healing of digital ulcers in patients with systemic sclerosis using laser Doppler imaging and thermography. Clin Exp Rheumatol. 2016;34(Suppl 100):S100–5.
15. Giuggioli D, Colaci M, Manfredi A, Mariano M, Ferri C. Platelet gel in the treatment of severe scleroderma skin ulcers. Rheumatol Int. 2012;32(9):2929–32.
16. Naert A, De Haes P. Successful treatment with bosentan of lower extremity ulcers in a scleroderma patient. Case Reports Med 2013:690591.
17. Mirasoglu B, Bagli BS, Aktas S. Hyperbaric oxygen therapy for chronic ulcers in systemic sclerosis - case series. Int J Dermatol. 2017;56:636–40.
18. El-Baalbaki G, Razykov I, Hudson M, Bassel M, Baron M, Thombs B, et al. Association of pruritus with quality of life and disability in systemic sclerosis. Arthritis Care Res. 2010;62:1489–95.
19. Razykov I, Levis B, Hudson M, Baron M, Thombs B, On Behalf of the Canadian Scleroderma Research Group. Prevalence and clinical correlates of pruritus in patients with systemic sclerosis: an updated analysis of 959 patients. Rheumatology. 2013;52:2056–61.
20. Thérèné C, Brenaut E, Sonbol H, Pasquier E, Saraux A, Devauchelle V, et al. Itch and systemic sclerosis: frequency, clinical characteristics and consequences. Br J Dermatol. 2017;176:1392–3.
21. Hafner J, Schneider E, Burg G, Cassina PC. Management of leg ulcers in patients with rheumatoid arthritis or systemic sclerosis: the importance of concomitant arterial and venous disease. J Vasc Surg. 2000;32:322–9.
22. Frech T, Novak K, Revelo MP, Murtaugh M, Markewitz B, Hatton N, et al. Low-dose naltrexone for pruritus in systemic sclerosis. Int J Rheumatol. 2011;2011:804296.
23. Provenzano DA, Nicholson L, Jarzabek G, Lutton E, Catalane DB, Mackin E. Spinal cord stimulation utilization to treat the microcirculatory vascular insufficiency and ulcers associated with scleroderma: a case report and review of the literature. Pain Med. 2011;12:1331–5.
24. Grossman JA, Barrall DT, Dennison A, Lally EV. Successful combined medical and surgical treatment of a lower extremity sclerodermal ulcer. Ann Plastic Surg. 1988;20(6):582–5.

Index

Y. Allanore et al. (eds.), *Scleroderma*, https://doi.org/10.1007/978-3-031-40658-4

B

C

D

E

F

G

J

K

L

M

N

Q

R

X

Y

Z

MIX
Papier aus verantwortungsvollen Quellen
Paper from responsible sources
FSC® C105338

If you have any concerns about our products,
you can contact us on
ProductSafety@springernature.com

In case Publisher is established outside the EU,
the EU authorized representative is:
Springer Nature Customer Service Center GmbH
Europaplatz 3, 69115 Heidelberg, Germany

Printed by Libri Plureos GmbH
in Hamburg, Germany